VOLUME I

# DISEASES OF THE CAT

## MEDICINE & SURGERY

JEAN HOLZWORTH, D.V.M.

ANGELL MEMORIAL ANIMAL HOSPITAL
MASSACHUSETTS SOCIETY FOR THE
PREVENTION OF CRUELTY TO ANIMALS

1987
W. B. Saunders Company
Philadelphia • London • Toronto • Mexico City • Rio de Janeiro • Sydney • Tokyo • Hong Kong

W. B. Saunders Company: West Washington Square
Philadelphia, PA 19105

**Library of Congress Cataloging-in-Publication Data**

Holzworth, Jean.

Diseases of the cat.

1. Cats—Diseases. I. Title. [DNLM: 1. Cat Diseases.
SF 985 H762d]

SF985.H66 1986 636.8′089 85–14606

ISBN 0–7216–4763–4

*Editor:* John Dyson
*Designer:* Terri Siegel
*Production Manager:* Bob Butler
*Manuscript Editor:* Constance Burton
*Illustration Coordinator:* Walt Verbitski

Diseases of the Cat: Medicine and Surgery (Volume I) ISBN 0–7216–4763–4



Last digit is the print number: 9 8 7 6 5 4 3 2 1

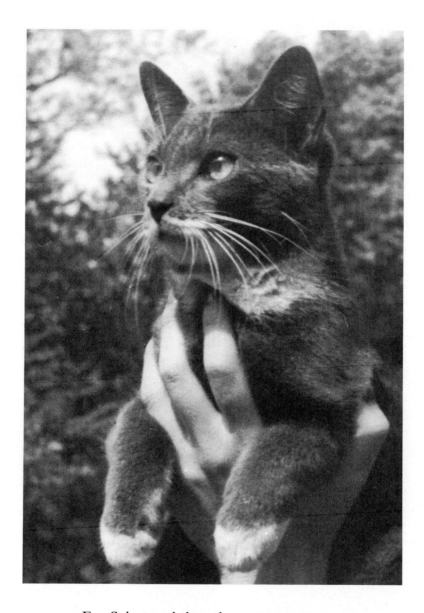

For Sabot and the other cats
that have gladdened my life
And for the multitude of Angell patients
from whom I have learned

# CONTRIBUTORS

## MELVIN K. ABELSETH, D.V.M., Ph.D.

Director, Laboratories for Veterinary Science, Division of Laboratories and Research, State of New York Department of Health, Albany, New York

*Rabies*

## LAURA K. ANDREWS, D.V.M.

Diplomate, American College of Veterinary Pathologists. Pathologist, Department of Pathology and Experimental Toxicology, Warner Lambert/Parke Davis, Ann Arbor, Michigan

*Tumors and Tumor-like Lesions*

## DAMON R. AVERILL, JR., D.V.M.

Diplomate, American College of Veterinary Internal Medicine; Diplomate, American College of Veterinary Pathologists. Associate Professor of Comparative Pathology and Laboratory Animal Medicine, University of Michigan Medical School, Ann Arbor, Michigan

*Tumors and Tumor-like Lesions*

## ERNST L. BIBERSTEIN, D.V.M., Ph.D.

Professor of Microbiology, School of Veterinary Medicine; Microbiology Service, Veterinary Medical Teaching Hospital, University of California, Davis, California

*Bacterial Diseases*

## PAULE BLOUIN, D.M.V., Ph.D.

Diplomate, American College of Veterinary Ophthalmologists. Hôpital Vétérinaire Rive Sud, Brossard, Quebec

*Mycotic Diseases: Cryptococcosis*

## NANCY O. BROWN, V.M.D.

Diplomate, American College of Veterinary Surgeons. Consultant in Surgery, The Animal Medical Center, New York, New York; Owner, Hickory Veterinary Hospital, Plymouth Meeting, Pennsylvania

*Management of Feline Neoplasms*

## JAMES L. CARPENTER, D.V.M.

Diplomate, American College of Veterinary Pathologists. Assistant Professor of Comparative Pathology, Harvard Medical School; Director of Pathology, Angell Memorial Animal Hospital, Boston, Massachusetts

*Tumors and Tumor-like Lesions*

## MICHAEL W. CONNER, D.V.M.

Assistant Professor of Pathology, Boston University School of Medicine; Adjunct Assistant Professor of Pathology, Tufts University School of Veterinary Medicine; Consultant in Pathology, Angell Memorial Animal Hospital, Boston, Massachusetts

*Mycotic Diseases: Cryptococcosis*

## SUSAN M. COTTER, D.V.M.

Diplomate, American College of Veterinary Internal Medicine. Associate Professor of Medicine, Tufts University School of Veterinary Medicine; Visiting Lecturer in Cancer Biology, Harvard University, School of Public Health, Boston, Massachusetts

*The Hematopoietic System*

## CATHERINE G. FABRICANT, M.S.

Senior Research Associate, Department of Microbiology, New York State College of Veterinary Medicine, Cornell University, Ithaca, New York

*Feline Urolithiasis*

## J. K. FRENKEL, M.D., Ph.D.

Professor of Pathology, University of Kansas School of Medicine; University of Kansas Medical Center, Kansas City, Kansas

*Protozoan Diseases: The Coccidia*

## DONALD P. GUSTAFSON, D.V.M., Ph.D.

Leo P. Doyle Professor of Virology, Purdue University School of Veterinary Medicine, West Lafayette, Indiana

*Pseudorabies*

## MARGARET L. HARBISON, V.M.D.

Research Associate and Director of Diagnostics, Laboratory Animal Research Center, Rockefeller University, New York, New York

*Tumors and Tumor-like Lesions*

## WILLIAM D. HARDY, JR., V.M.D.

Head, Laboratory of Veterinary Oncology, Memorial Sloan-Kettering Cancer Center, Cornell University, New York, New York

*Oncogenic Viruses*

## NEIL K. HARPSTER, V.M.D.

Diplomate, American College of Veterinary Internal Medicine. Director of Cardiology, Angell Memorial Animal Hospital, Boston, Massachusetts

*The Cardiovascular System*

MARK E. HASKINS, V.M.D., Ph.D.

Associate Professor of Pathology and Medical Genetics, School of Veterinary Medicine, University of Pennsylvania, Philadelphia, Pennsylvania

*Inherited Metabolic Diseases*

AUDREY A. HAYES, V.M.D.

Diplomate, American College of Veterinary Internal Medicine. Staff, Department of Medicine, The Donaldson-Atwood Cancer Clinic of The Animal Medical Center, New York, New York

*Management of Feline Neoplasms*

K. C. HAYES, D.V.M., Ph.D.

Professor of Biology (Nutrition); Director, Foster Biomedical Research Laboratory, Brandeis University, Waltham, Massachusetts

*Nutrition and Nutritional Disorders*

MATTIE J. HENDRICK, V.M.D.

Diplomate, American College of Veterinary Pathologists. Assistant Professor, Department of Pathobiology, School of Veterinary Medicine, University of Pennsylvania, Philadelphia, Pennsylvania

*The Hematopoietic System*

JEAN HOLZWORTH, D.V.M.

Diplomate, American College of Veterinary Internal Medicine. Clinical Staff, Angell Memorial Animal Hospital, Boston, Massachusetts

*The Sick Cat; Viral Diseases; Bacterial Diseases; Mycotic Diseases; Protozoan Diseases; Tumors and Tumor-like Lesions; The Ear; The Hematopoietic System*

EDWARD A. HOOVER, D.V.M., Ph.D.

Professor and Chairman, Department of Pathology, Colorado State University, Fort Collins, Colorado

*Viral Respiratory Diseases and Chlamydiosis*

ANN B. KIER, D.V.M., Ph.D.

Associate Professor, Departments of Veterinary Pathology and Veterinary Microbiology; Veterinary Medical Diagnostic Laboratory, College of Veterinary Medicine, University of Missouri, Columbia, Missouri

*Protozoan Diseases: Cytauxzoonosis*

ROBERT L. LEIGHTON, V.M.D.

Diplomate, American College of Veterinary Surgeons. Emeritus Professor of Surgery, School of Veterinary Medicine, University of California, Davis, California

*Orthopedic Surgery*

E. GREGORY MacEWEN, V.M.D.

Diplomate, American College of Veterinary Internal Medicine. Associate Professor of Oncology, Department of Medical Sciences, School of Veterinary Medicine, University of Wisconsin, Madison, Wisconsin

*Management of Feline Neoplasms*

EDWARD A. MAHAFFEY, D.V.M., Ph.D.

Diplomate, American College of Veterinary Pathologists. Associate Professor, Department of Veterinary Pathology, College of Veterinary Medicine, University of Georgia, Athens, Georgia

*The Hematopoietic System*

SAMANTHA C. MOONEY, M.A.

Research Associate, The Donaldson-Atwood Cancer Clinic of The Animal Medical Center, New York, New York

*Management of Feline Neoplasms*

FRANCES M. MOORE, D.V.M.

Diplomate, American College of Veterinary Pathologists. Staff Pathologist, Angell Memorial Animal Hospital, Boston, Massachusetts

*Tumors and Tumor-like Lesions*

JOSEPH A. O'DONNELL III, Ph.D

Vice President, Basic Product Research, United Dairy Industry Association, Rosemont, Illinois

*Nutrition and Nutritional Disorders*

DONALD F. PATTERSON, D.V.M., D.Sc.

Diplomate, American College of Veterinary Internal Medicine. Charlotte Newton Sheppard Professor of Veterinary Medicine, School of Veterinary Medicine; Professor of Human Genetics, School of Medicine, University of Pennsylvania, Philadelphia, Pennsylvania

*Inherited Metabolic Diseases*

MICHAEL M. PAVLETIC, D.V.M.

Diplomate, American College of Veterinary Surgeons. Associate Professor of Small Animal Surgery and Section Head, Small Animal Surgery, Tufts University School of Veterinary Medicine, North Grafton, Massachusetts

*Soft Tissue Surgery*

NIELS C. PEDERSEN, D.V.M., Ph.D.

Professor, Department of Clinical Sciences; Clinician, Veterinary Medical Teaching Hospital, School of Veterinary Medicine, University of California, Davis, California

*Basic and Clinical Immunology; Coronavirus Diseases; Feline Syncytium-Forming Virus Infection; Mycoplasmal Infections*

KEITH W. PRASSE, D.V.M., Ph.D.

Diplomate, American College of Veterinary Pathologists. Professor of Veterinary Pathology, College of

Veterinary Medicine, University of Georgia, Athens, Georgia
*The Hematopoietic System*

MIODRAG RISTIC, D.V.M., Ph.D.
Professor, Department of Veterinary Pathobiology, College of Veterinary Medicine, University of Illinois, Urbana, Illinois
*Bacterial Diseases: Hemobartonellosis*

GORDON W. ROBINSON, V.M.D.
Head, Department of Surgery, Bergh Memorial Animal Hospital, New York, New York
*Orthopedic Surgery*

DANNY W. SCOTT, D.V.M.
Diplomate, American College of Veterinary Dermatology. Associate Professor of Medicine, Department of Clinical Sciences, New York State College of Veterinary Medicine, Cornell University, Ithaca, New York
*The Skin*

FREDRIC W. SCOTT, D.V.M., Ph.D.
Diplomate, American College of Veterinary Microbiologists. Professor of Virology; Director, Cornell Feline Health Center, Department of Microbiology, New York State College of Veterinary Medicine, Cornell University, Ithaca, New York
*Panleukopenia*

ERWIN SMALL, D.V.M., M.S.
Diplomate, American College of Veterinary Internal Medicine; Diplomate, American College of Veterinary Dermatology. Associate Dean and Professor, College of Veterinary Medicine, University of Illinois, Urbana, Illinois
*Bacterial Diseases: Hemobartonellosis*

BARBARA SYDNEY STEIN, D.V.M.
Director, Chicago Cat Clinic, Chicago, Illinois
*The Sick Cat*

CAROL SZYMANSKI, D.V.M.
Diplomate, American College of Veterinary Ophthalmologists. Associate Professor, Department of Veterinary Clinical Sciences, The Ohio State University College of Veterinary Medicine, Columbus, Ohio
*The Eyes*

RICHARD J. TODOROFF, D.V.M., Ph.D.
Diplomate, American College of Veterinary Surgeons. Surgeon, Contra Costa Veterinary Surgical Service, Concord, California
*Soft Tissue Surgery*

CYNTHIA M. TRIM, B.V.Sc.
Diplomate in Veterinary Anaesthesia (U.K.); Diplomate, American College of Veterinary Anesthesiologists. Professor, College of Veterinary Medicine; Anesthesiologist, Veterinary Teaching Hospital, College of Veterinary Medicine, University of Georgia, Athens, Georgia
*Sedation and Anesthesia*

JANE M. TURREL, D.V.M., M.S.
Diplomate, American College of Veterinary Radiology. Assistant Professor, Department of Radiological Sciences, School of Veterinary Medicine; Radiation Oncologist, Veterinary Medical Teaching Hospital, University of California, Davis, California
*Management of Feline Neoplasms*

JOSEPH E. WAGNER, D.V.M., Ph.D.
Professor of Veterinary Pathology, College of Veterinary Medicine, University of Missouri, Columbia, Missouri
*Protozoan Diseases: Cytauxzoonosis*

BERNARD C. ZOOK, D.V.M.
Diplomate, American College of Veterinary Pathologists. Department of Pathology, The George Washington University Medical Center, Washington, D.C.
*The Cardiovascular System*

# FOREWORD

In 1954, when I came as an intern to the Angell Memorial Animal Hospital in Boston, the editor and chief author of this book, though herself only a few years out of veterinary school, was already an authority on diseases of the cat. Many of us whose interest in the medicine and surgery of the cat has been stimulated by Dr. Jean Holzworth's knowledge and enthusiasm have anticipated that she would produce the definitive book on the subject. It has also been clear to the interns and close colleagues who have admired and, perhaps, squirmed at times under Dr. Holzworth's insistence on the scholarly, clear, and economical use of words that it would be a readable book. And, we expected that it would be as comprehensive and well-documented a book as can be written on the subject, for Jean Holzworth is an incurable perfectionist.

Over the years, it gradually became clear to Dr. Holzworth and to her expectant colleagues and editors at Saunders that two strong forces were conspiring to delay completion of *Diseases of the Cat.* The first was her desire for thoroughness, the second was the rising tide of new knowledge. By the early 1960s, clinical specialization in small animal medicine was well under way, and the growth in basic scientific knowledge had vastly increased the useful information available to the clinician. For example, special knowledge of electrocardiography, cardiac catheterization, angiocardiography, and, recently, echocardiography has become essential for the accurate diagnosis of cardiovascular disease in the cat. A detailed understanding of virology and immunology is now necessary for the recognition and treatment of a large number of infectious diseases, including feline leukemia, a disorder whose etiology and complex nature have only recently become clear through basic and clinical research. New developments in genetics and biochemistry have led to the detection and characterization of an increasing variety of inherited metabolic diseases in cats.

Veterinarians and others interested in the cat will not be disappointed at having waited so long. To solve the problem of the proliferation and specialization of knowledge, Dr. Holzworth has enlisted recognized experts in special fields bearing on feline medicine and surgery. While welcoming individuality of style from chapter to chapter, the editor has suggested, cajoled, and where necessary, enforced a standard of clarity that is unusual in multi-authored volumes in the medical sciences.

The idea for this work can be traced to a farm in Connecticut where a young girl organized a hospital to treat the cats in her parents' barn. Reflecting her training as a PhD in Latin at Bryn Mawr College, developed through a veterinary education and long experience in one of the world's leading small animal hospitals, and brought to completion with the cooperation of many specialists, this work will long stand as the definitive written word on medicine and surgery of the cat.

DONALD F. PATTERSON, DVM, DSC
*Charlotte Newton Sheppard Professor of Veterinary Medicine*
*University of Pennsylvania*

# PREFACE

Passionate cat lovers are legion, but very few are lucky enough to make cats their life work. I am one of these, and this book is, above all, for cat lovers.

Pictures of my forebears, and of me at various ages, show us cuddling cats. The farm cats of my childhood were prone to fatal fits in bedroom closets (a propensity I am still at a loss to explain), and at 10 years I composed a Cat's Funeral March, of which, unhappily, there were many performances. At 15 I had to be excused from the painful experience of dissecting a cat in biology class; at that time I could not have believed that one day I would feel as much anticipation when starting the autopsy of an ill-fated cat patient as one does when the curtain goes up in the theater.

I owe my admission to veterinary school to two timely coincidences. I applied in the last year of World War II, when most would-be veterinarians were still overseas and admissions committees were "scraping the bottom of the barrel." The other favorable circumstance was that the agents of feline panleukopenia and pneumonitis had recently been identified, and the humble cat, my reason for wanting to be a veterinarian, was at last launched on its way into the realm of serious research.

Coming, after graduation, to the Angell Memorial Animal Hospital in Boston, I found myself in a city of multitudes of devoted cat owners and at the best possible institution for developing my interest in cats. Many, many years later, I can still say that hardly a day passes there when one does not encounter some feline curiosity that one has never seen before. I soon decided that cats deserved a serious book to themselves, and I have ever since had support and encouragement from many quarters in this long-time project.

As fast as I completed a draft, however, it was outstripped by the torrent of research and clinical reports of which my favorite species increasingly became the subject. Ultimately I realized that only a band of specialists could handle the project, and I became, as well as author, the editor of a collaborative text, and I have numerous co-authors to thank for their interest and help.

Many others have had important roles in this undertaking. Heading the list are colleagues at Angell, both clinicians and pathologists, and most especially Dr. Gerry B. Schnelle and Dr. Gus W. Thornton, who as chiefs-of-staff permitted me to concentrate exclusively on cats and encouraged my special interest with patience, indulgence, and much time off for researching, writing, and editing.

Veterinarians all over the world have contributed valuable bits and pieces never published elsewhere or have given helpful leads to work in progress. Dr. Robert Habel, former chairman of the Department of Anatomy at the New York State College of Veterinary Medicine, has advised on up-to-date terminology in gross and microscopic anatomy.

As well as being a practical text for veterinary practitioners, this book is also intended, by virtue of its extensive bibliographies, to serve as a resource for researchers. Since the 1960s, "searching the literature" has been greatly facilitated by computerization of bibliographies. However, much important work with diseases of cats was done before this time, particularly by Europeans, and the contributions of these earlier workers are well represented.

Librarians to whom I can never sufficiently express thanks have been those of the National Libraries of Agriculture and of Medicine, the Flower Veterinary Library at Cornell University, and the libraries of the Harvard Medical School, the New England Regional Primate Research Center, the University of Massachusetts Medical School, and the Tufts University School of Veterinary Medicine.

The late Leo Goodman, photographer extraordinary at the Mallory Institute of Boston City Hospital, was responsible for many fine photographs; thanks go also to Martin Snyder of the same laboratory and to Kathleen Driscoll, formerly of the Angell Memorial Animal Hospital.

The loyalty and confidence of three very special friends gave crucial support to my labors. Dr. James Carpenter, as well as organizing a review of Angell's feline tumors that deserves a book to itself, responded instantaneously and enthusiastically to my every appeal for help or consultation, and his painstaking contributions are represented in several chapters other than his own. Second, Mr. Thomas Mancuso, a long-time neighbor and a seasoned editor of books on all manner of subjects, introduced me to the nuts and bolts of publishing, alerted me to many pitfalls, and by sheer proximity and stern discipline kept my nose to the grindstone. An artist as well, he created the cat that adorns the book's cover. Finally, Mr. John Dyson, my editor at Saunders, remained ever hopeful, indulgent, and unflappable, no matter what the problem; our mutual purpose was implemented by the other patient and conscientious members of the Saunders team—Constance Burton, Walter Verbitski, Terri Siegel, Bob Butler, and Cass Stamato.

Financial support toward this project was provided by grants from the American Philosophical Society, the US Public Health Service (E1157), and the National Institutes of Health (2R01GM11941-02).

This preface, like so many, concludes with the rueful reflection that no matter how hard we all have tried, some errors and omissions are inevitable. *Please* let me hear about them.

JEAN HOLZWORTH

# CONTENTS

CHAPTER **1**

## THE SICK CAT

Jean Holzworth and Barbara S. Stein



CHAPTER **2**

## NUTRITION AND NUTRITIONAL DISORDERS

Joseph A. O'Donnell III, and K. C. Hayes



CHAPTER **3**

## SEDATION AND ANESTHESIA

Cynthia M. Trim

CHAPTER **4**

## SOFT TISSUE SURGERY

Richard J. Todoroff

Contributing Author: Michael M. Pavletic



CHAPTER **5**

## ORTHOPEDIC SURGERY

Robert L. Leighton and Gordon W. Robinson

CHAPTER 6
## BASIC AND CLINICAL IMMUNOLOGY
Niels C. Pedersen



CHAPTER 7
## VIRAL DISEASES



CHAPTER 8
## BACTERIAL DISEASES
Ernst L. Biberstein and Jean Holzworth

Contributing Authors: Erwin Small, Miodrag Ristic, and Niels C. Pedersen

CHAPTER **11**

## TUMORS AND TUMOR-LIKE LESIONS

James L. Carpenter, Laura K. Andrews, and Jean Holzworth
Contributing Authors: Damon R. Averill, Jr., Margaret L. Harbison, and Frances M. Moore



CHAPTER **12**

## MANAGEMENT OF FELINE NEOPLASMS



CHAPTER **13**

## THE SKIN

Danny W. Scott

CHAPTER **14**

## THE EYE

Carol Szymanski



CHAPTER **15**

## THE EAR

Jean Holzworth



CHAPTER **16**

## THE HEMATOPOIETIC SYSTEM

CHAPTER **17**

## INHERITED METABOLIC DISEASES

Mark E. Haskins and Donald F. Patterson



CHAPTER **18**

## THE CARDIOVASCULAR SYSTEM

Neil K. Harpster
Contributing Author: Bernard C. Zook

# 1
# CHAPTER
# THE SICK CAT

JEAN HOLZWORTH and BARBARA S. STEIN

As the human population has exploded so also has the pet population, and both humans and animals have less and less living space. It is not surprising then that the cat is gaining on the dog as man's favored housemate. Cats are less apt than dogs to disturb the peace or damage property. They cost less to feed than most dogs, do not have to be exercised, can often live happily all their lives indoors, and can be left alone at home for a day or two, or for longer periods with only a daily visit from a trusted person who waters and feeds the cat and attends to the litter box.

Another significant trend is reflected in the naming of pets. Fluffy, Tippy, Mittens, and Whiskers are now George, Otis, Mildred, and Dorothy—a clear sign that, however psychiatrists interpret anthropomorphism, pets are considered people. Their families, not surprisingly, expect medical care comparable to that available for humans.

If a veterinarian has not been lucky enough to grow up with cats, he should acquire one or two and become familiar with feline behavior in health and disease. An understanding of cats' ways and assurance in handling them are quickly sensed by both animal and owner and go far to win the confidence of both.

## AN OUNCE OF PREVENTION

Life itself, we are told, is a fatal illness, but good stock and a healthy start can smooth and lengthen the course. Veterinarians are often asked by would-be cat owners how they can acquire a healthy pet. Cats from shelters, pet shops, and catteries are at risk of exposure to a variety of parasitic and infectious diseases and should be acquired with a written understanding that they may be returned if they are found to have some serious infection or illness. Knowledgeable buyers of purebreds today ask the seller for a veterinarian's certification that a cat has tested negative for feline leukemia (FeLV) and feline infectious peritonitis (FIP-coronavirus) within a month before purchase. Some veterinarians advise similar testing of any new cat, especially a stray, for many an appealing waif has introduced illness into a previously healthy household of cats.

Private homes and small "closed" catteries in which breeding is strictly limited to their own stock are the most likely to have healthy kittens. Both breeders and cat owners should be aware that the larger a "herd," the greater the risk of infectious disease and behavioral conflicts. A cat that is to be alone much of the time, especially if it is young, may well enjoy the companionship of another cat, but an established cat may jealously resent sharing the affection and attention of its owners and may live more happily as an "only" cat.

The sex of a cat is also a factor to be considered in disease prevention. Because castration is less costly than spaying, males have traditionally been preferred to females; however, the risk of urinary obstruction in males and the expense, bother, and uncertain outcome of treatment lead many veterinarians to recommend females in order to avert this problem.

Kittens are best left with their mother and littermates until they are seven or eight weeks of age. Younger or orphaned kittens require special care and may retain infantile habits, such as suckling on their own or another animal's toes or tail or on an owner's clothing.

There can even be advantages in getting a mature cat. All kittens appear charming, but with time many lose their playfulness and some actually develop into self-centered dullards. A person adopting a grown pet can be more sure of what he is getting. An adult cat with spirit, intelligence, and responsiveness is likely always to stay that way.

However a cat is acquired, it should be examined at once by a veterinarian for evidence of parasitism or illness. At this time any necessary vaccinations may be given, with advice that the check-up and vaccinations be repeated yearly.

"Complete" commercial cat foods, such as those manufactured by large national companies, should be recommended as the principal component of the diet, but a cat's individual taste and whims may be indulged by limited supplementation with "gourmet" canned foods or "human" delicacies or food scraps, provided that the cat does not become overweight or addicted to any one food that would lead to a dietary imbalance, excess, or deficiency. Vitamin-mineral supplements should not be needed by a healthy cat receiving such a diet, and owners should be warned that certain vitamins and minerals can actually be dangerous if given in excess. They should be warned too that milk or liver may cause diarrhea in many cats.*

Owners should be advised to give short-haired cats a brief daily brushing. Longhairs should be carefully combed with a coarse comb before brushing. If, despite regular grooming, a cat tends to vomit hairballs, the safest lubricant is plain or malt-flavored petroleum jelly, which can be squeezed onto a cat's nose or paw for the cat to lick down itself. Mineral oil should be given only when mixed with food, as this (or any oil) may cause fatal pneumonia if inhaled because of an owner's unskilled method of administration.

A first-time cat owner should also be given information about the special indoor and outdoor hazards to which cats are exposed by their excessive curiosity and penchant for living dangerously. Identification tags and bells attached to collars that are at least partly elastic should be a requirement for all outdoor cats. A rabies vaccination tag bearing a veterinary hospital's name may also be lifesaving identification for a lost or injured pet.

Owners should be emphatically cautioned that cats may be poisoned by drugs or other preparations that are harmless to other species and that *nothing* should ever be applied to a cat's skin or given internally except on the advice of a veterinarian.

Much valuable and practical advice of this sort may be given in handout form by veterinarians and is also available in books written for laymen on the care of cats, two of which are *The Well Cat Book* by Dr. Terri McGinnis (1975) and *Pet Medicine* by Roger Caras and a number of veterinary specialists (1977).

Routine examinations and procedures give the perceptive owner a chance to satisfy himself as to the concern and skill of a veterinarian and his personnel, the character of the hospital, and the services and coverage available, so that in case of emergency or illness there will be no question as to where to get help.

Also in the realm of preventive medicine is caution about boarding, which may expose a cat to the risk of infectious disease, most often upper respiratory infection against which vaccination does not always confer solid immunity. A far better solution is to leave the cat at home and arrange for a "cat sitter" or have a trustworthy person visit daily to provide food and fresh water and attend to the litter pan.

## RECORD KEEPING

A cat's record, started at the first visit, should contain accurate identifying data as to breed, length and color of hair coat, sex, and age, as well as information about origin and any medical history. Weighing at each visit provides useful data as to growth and also baseline information in case of illness. The record, written in ink, should be updated in adequate detail at each subsequent visit or hospitalization, both as good medical practice and as a precaution in the event of medicolegal problems, which arise occasionally even in the most efficient and conscientiously maintained practices. Radiographs and reports on diagnostic work are an essential part of this record.

Detailed suggestions for record keeping have been provided by Ettinger (1983). A variety of systems are possible, depending on the veterinarian's preference and practice.

## HOSPITAL VISITS

For all but a few extroverted cats, visits to a veterinarian are disturbing. The cat will be less frightened by sights and sounds if confined in a carrier. Carriers also afford protection against possible transmission of infection in the waiting room and discourage owners from handling one another's pets.

A few "bad actors" require special arrangements. If a cat is known to be difficult, a tranquilizer tablet (2 mg/kg acepromazine) may be dispensed to the owner to be given an hour before the visit, and the cat may wait in the owner's car or in the seclusion of an examination room rather than in the reception room.

If a cat is found to be impossible to examine when presented, it may be given a low intramuscular dose of ketamine (total, 10 to 25 mg). Or, provided that the cat has not eaten for several hours, it may be placed in an anesthesia chamber and briefly anesthetized with halothane. It is a wise precaution to trim the cat's claws while it is under sedation or anesthesia.

A blanket or a large, thick bath towel is the best aid in handling an uncooperative cat, and owners should be encouraged to bring their own. Heavy protective gloves are clumsy and in any case can be penetrated by a cat's teeth. Poles with snares are barbarous and may injure a cat. Instead, a fishnet is used by some veterinarians to capture and immobilize a belligerent escapee, which can then be grasped with a blanket.

## SIGNS OF ILLNESS

Cats are creatures of routine, and most owners are quick to notice any departure from the usual. Sudden and alarming signs, such as convulsions or choking, leave no doubt that a veterinarian should be consulted, but owners should be aware that less dramatic manifestations such as inactivity, "hiding," and lack of appetite may also be clues to illness. Other unmistakable abnormalities include swellings, disturbances in gait, respiratory difficulties, vomiting, diarrhea, straining to defecate or urinate, and excessive drinking.

Owners should understand that such developments are a signal to take the cat's temperature and then telephone their veterinarian with a well-organized description of the cat's trouble. In most cases the doctor will recommend an office visit or possibly a house call, for it is far better to examine a hundred cats and find nothing wrong than to miss one case of serious illness.

*It is the experience of both authors that dry foods are sometimes implicated in cases of cystitis or urethral obstruction. One of us (Stein) advises that dry food should not constitute more than 25 per cent of the diet for any cat. The other (Holzworth) advises feeding no dry food to a male cat over a year old. Both advise against dry food for any cat subject to cystitis or urolithiasis.

## HISTORY TAKING

Except in life-threatening situations that require immediate emergency measures, history taking should precede the examination. Meanwhile, if the cat stays quietly in its carrier or on the owner's lap, it will have a chance to adjust to the strange surroundings and become accustomed to the examiner's voice.

An orderly, chronologic history should be elicited. In a complicated case, a written history prepared by the owner in advance may provide valuable information that might otherwise be overlooked. If a cat has been treated elsewhere, it is important to learn what the diagnosis was and exactly what treatment was given. If the case is a referral, a letter of information with relevant diagnostic data and radiographs should be sent with the owner from the referring veterinarian.

A good history alone sometimes establishes or suggests a diagnosis. In any case, it is a guide for the examination and possible diagnostic procedures.

Although certain preliminary data can be obtained by a receptionist or assistant, a complete history in a case of illness can be taken only by the veterinarian. He should begin by verifying that the cat's breed, color, hair length, age, and sex have been correctly recorded. Owners of domestic cats (the term "alley" is frowned upon) are sometimes unable to describe their cat correctly and also occasionally are mistaken about its sex. Owners of purebreds, on the other hand, expect a veterinarian to recognize the pure breeds and variants and to describe them correctly. The veterinarian will also be aware of certain breed predispositions—for example, that Persians may be tardy breeders and that their shortened faces may mean impatent tear ducts, that taillessness in the Manx is often associated with other anatomic abnormalities, and that certain strains of Siamese are cloth-eaters.

Information as to whether the cat came from a breeder, pet shop, or shelter; where it originated or traveled; and whether it has recently been boarded may raise the possibility of infectious disease or parasitism. Information about the cat's life style—what it is fed, whether it goes out of doors, and whether it is an "only" cat or lives with related or unrelated housemates—is also essential, as are dates of vaccinations and spaying or castration and medical history.

The owner should then relate the history of the present problem from the time it was first noticed, with questions as necessary from the veterinarian to amplify or clarify the information. It is not enough to know, for instance, that a cat has been vomiting. One must know for how long, how often, the character of the vomitus, and what, if any, relationship there is to time of eating and type of food. Diarrhea and urinary frequency are other common complaints about which the veterinarian must elicit qualifying details.

Never should the veterinarian underestimate what may seem to be fanciful or irrelevant observations on the part of an owner. A cat that "makes a noise like a duck honking" may have a cryptococcal granuloma of the nose, and a cat that "doesn't know his way around his own house," a meningioma of the cerebrum.

## EXAMINATION

Examination should begin by simple observation of the cat in its carrier, on its owner's lap, on the examination table, or moving about. The cat's general appearance and behavior, the character of its respirations, and its carriage and gait may provide important information. Having the owner set the cat on the floor and coax it to walk about may raise the possibility of blindness or aid in distinguishing between simple weakness, lameness, and incoordination. To give an example, a cat that has suffered an aortic embolism is likely to walk feebly, if at all, to breathe with difficulty, and to trail its hind legs in a characteristic manner.

Many cats can be handled by one person. Otherwise the owner, if not too timid or awkward, makes the best assistant, because his presence is reassuring to the cat. If an attendant is needed for help, it should be someone who likes cats and is experienced in their ways. A cat that is grasped too firmly, held by the legs, or restrained in an unnatural position reacts by struggling. A towel or blanket is an invaluable aid in capturing, grasping, or controlling an unruly cat. Temporarily covering the head or cupping it in the hands so that the cat cannot see may have a favorably inhibiting effect.

The temperature should, if possible, be taken at the beginning of the examination before the cat has been disturbed by handling. Except when a cat is excited or overheated, its temperature should not normally exceed 39 C (102.2 F). The temperature of elderly cats may normally be lower than that of young, active animals. If the significance of an elevated temperature is in doubt, the temperature should be checked later at several intervals. Fevers occasionally exceed the scale on the thermometer but do not appear to inflict the lasting brain damage that may occur in the human and do not call for heroic measures such as icy baths (except in heat stroke) or dangerous antipyretic drugs.

While taking the temperature, the veterinarian may verify the owner's information as to the cat's sex and note the condition of the perineum and anal sacs. If no stool sample has been brought by the owner, enough material may often be obtained on the thermometer for direct microscopic examination and for information on the character of the stool.

While talking soothingly to the cat, scratching it hypnotically under the chin, or stroking it, the veterinarian may also be examining the coat and skin; estimating body condition; noting dehydration, edema, or emphysema, if present; and feeling for wounds, swellings, enlarged superficial lymph nodes, or skin tumors.

At this point in the examination most cats are sufficiently reassured so that the veterinarian may cup the head between his hands and inspect it face to face for asymmetry or abnormalities. It is important to note the character of a nasal discharge and whether it is unilateral or bilateral. Incipient lesions of eosinophilic granuloma on the upper lips should not be overlooked.

It is usually apparent on rapid inspection whether the outer structures of the eye are normal, and the reaction of the pupils to light may be checked by placing a hand over first one eye and then the other. Owners commonly complain of a film or "cataract" over the eye, referring to the puzzling phenomenon of prolapsed third eyelids. In some cases this is associated with parasitism or other disorders of the gastrointestinal tract. The owner may be assured, however, that in time the eyelids will return to normal without treatment. A squint, discharge, or inflammation may require a local anesthetic so that a foreign body, wound, or ulcer can be looked for. Growths involving the visible parts of the eye, as well as bulging or enlargement of the globe, are usually apparent. Ocular signs that may accompany systemic disease are pallor or jaundiced discoloration of the sclera, exudates or hemorrhage in the anterior chamber, and dullness or abnormal coloration of the iris. Ophthalmoscopic examination is then required so that the vitreous and retina can be inspected for abnormalities that might be caused by localized or systemic infection or malignancy. Impaired vision with pupillary dilatation and retinal changes may also be associated with nutritional deficiencies.

The ears should be examined next, the pinna being drawn laterally to permit a good look into the canal. The most common and most often neglected aural disorder is parasitism of the ear canal with ear mites, signs of which are head-shaking, scratching, a dry brown exudate, and occasionally a hematoma. A diagnosis of ear mite infestation should not be made, however, unless mites are demonstrable. A crepitant sound when the external ear canal is massaged suggests the presence of a liquid exudate. A unilateral aural discharge is a signal to look into the external canal for a foreign body or growth. Infection or neoplasm of the inner ear usually causes a head tilt or circling. Small, dark "blisters" at the orifice of the ear canal in older cats suggest the presence of cysts or neoplasms of ceruminous glands. Many ear disturbances call for otoscopic examination of the meatus and tympanum, often under sedation or anesthesia and with preliminary cleansing.

It is amazing how rarely it occurs to an owner to look into a pet's mouth, although foul odor, drooling, pawing at the mouth, and difficulty in eating are clues to trouble. To open a cat's mouth, it is usually sufficient to place one hand over the head and force the jaws apart by pressing inward on the commissures of the lips with thumb and middle finger, and pulling the mandible down with the thumbnail of the other hand. If the cat resists opening its mouth, the lower jaw may often be pulled down by hooking a piece of gauze over the lower canines (Fig. 1–1). Sedation or anesthesia may be required for thorough examination of difficult cats.

Common localized problems are dental tartar, alveolar disease, and chronic gingivitis. Thin sheets of inflamed gingiva proliferating over the molars usually hide erosions in the enamel. Foreign bodies are frequent but may not be readily apparent if they have penetrated the soft tissue. A good look under the tongue is essential, for string or thread looped about the frenum and extending into the gastrointestinal tract may lead to fatal complications. The frenum is also the site of cancer in elderly cats, but in the early stage this may escape notice unless the tongue is pushed aside or lifted for examination. Fusospirochetal infection may be suspected by its foul odor, even before lesions appear.

Signs of systemic illness recognizable in the mouth are odors of acetone and uremia and abnormal mucosal color such as cyanosis, pallor, and jaundice. Tongue ulcers may be associated with upper respiratory infection, and bleeding may suggest a clotting disorder. Characteristic eosinophilic granulomas involving the lips, tongue, palate, or pharynx, and even the larynx may be associated with lesions already noted in the skin.

If there is a history of abnormal nasal sounds or gagging, one should try to apply upward pressure to the soft palate to determine whether a mass, such as a polyp, granuloma, or tumor, is present in the posterior nasal passages.

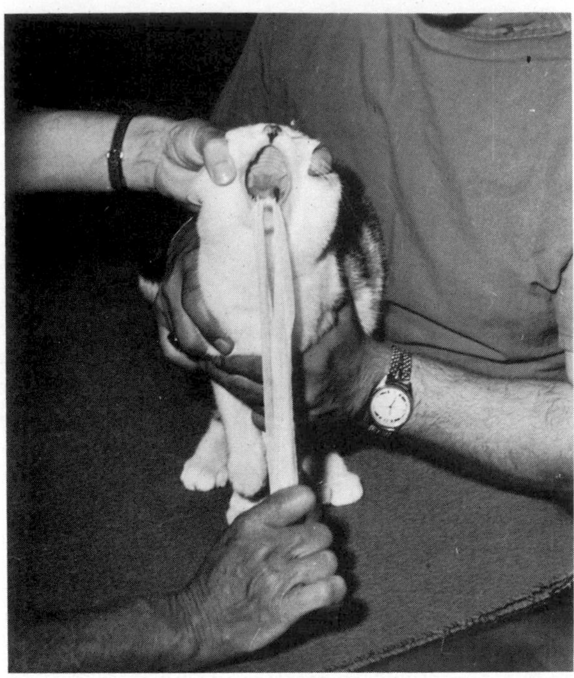

**Figure 1–1.** A length of gauze looped over the lower canines helps to open the mouth wide for examination of the throat.

A cooperative cat may permit the examiner to get a good glimpse of the tonsils and larynx. Examination of the larynx for inflammation or a growth is especially important if there has been a change in quality of a cat's purr.

External palpation of the throat should include salivary glands, cervical nodes, larynx, and trachea. Elderly cats with signs suggestive of hyperthyroidism should be carefully examined for enlarged thyroid lobes, which may slide elusively behind the trachea or down into the thoracic inlet. Occasionally a lymphoma of the anterior mediastinum can be palpated where it has bulged forward through the thoracic inlet.

Before examining the thorax, the veterinarian should already have observed the cat's respirations and listened for any abnormal sounds suggesting the site of a respiratory difficulty. A cat breathes more deeply when purring. The respiratory rate in a cat peacefully at rest may be as slow as 25 per minute but is accelerated if the cat is handled or nervous. Examination of the chest may be complicated by a cat's persistent purring. This can sometimes be stopped by covering the nostrils briefly with a hand or pressing upward on the larynx. By laying the palms flat on either side of the cat's thorax or grasping the thorax from below between thumb and fingers, the examiner may detect pronounced cardiac enlargement, an abnormally forceful cardiac impulse, and loud murmurs as well as loud pulmonary râles or the unyielding density of a mediastinal tumor. Because of the cat's thick fur and the relatively small size of its chest, percussion is rarely informative unless sizable areas of density are present.

The heart should be auscultated on both sides of the chest. There is great variability in the heart rate of normal cats and considerable variation from moment to moment in the same cat, sometimes with slight irregularities. A consistently slow heart rate is usually a sign of disease. Careful auscultation will also identify murmurs and a variety of arrhythmias. If embolic disease is suspected, the femoral pulses and temperature of the feet should be checked.

Auscultation of the lungs in a normal cat at rest may detect no sound at all or only the faintest vesicular murmur. Therefore when abnormal sounds are heard, they must be carefully assessed as to origin and significance. Especially notable, for example, are the labored abdominal breathing and harsh lung sounds characteristic of toxoplasmal pneumonia. Because of the high incidence of disorders of the chest cavity in cats, dullness on percussion and auscultation is frequent owing to the presence of fluids of various etiologies or of lymphomas that occupy the lower part of the chest, muffling heart and lung sounds. Injuries resulting in the presence of air, blood, chyle, or herniated abdominal organs may produce a similar effect. All such signs that are accompanied by severe dyspnea call for prompt diagnostic measures, such as radiography or even immediate thoracocentesis.

The small size of the cat makes it an ideal subject for abdominal palpation unless it is very fat or the abdomen is tense. Palpation should be gentle; otherwise the cat will show sensitivity that may be misinterpreted as actual tenderness. Excessively heavy-handed palpation or successive examinations by a number of interested persons may even inflict serious injury.

With one hand steadying the cat in a standing position, the other hand may palpate from below. Beginning with the cranial abdomen, one should ascertain position, size, and shape of the kidneys. The right is usually firmly attached cranially partly under the rib cage so that only the posterior pole may be palpable. The left is caudal to the right and is usually freely movable. If the kidneys cannot be located by palpation from below, one may palpate from above with a hand on either side of the back. If a cat's forepart is lifted, the kidneys usually drop back far enough so that they can be identified. A tiny hypoplastic kidney may elude palpation. Polycystic or lymphomatous kidneys are sometimes so large that they bulge visibly on either side of the spinal column.

A normal liver should not extend caudal to the rib cage unless forced back by some disorder in the thorax. Its edges should be sharp. Irregularity or a significant decrease or increase in size is abnormal. In the standing cat, the stomach is dorsal to the liver within the rib cage and is usually palpable only if distended (for example, with food or a hairball) or if its wall is greatly thickened.

Behind the stomach and liver is the freely movable spleen, which is most easily palpated if it is enlarged, as in hemobartonellosis or hematopoietic malignancy. With massive enlargement, it moves from a transverse position to lie on the floor of the abdomen, stretching from the liver to the pubis. In mastocytosis, the spleen is especially friable and may be ruptured by even gentle palpation or by carrying the cat without care to avoid pressure on the abdomen. Massive homogeneous enlargement of both liver and spleen is almost invariably a sign of hematopoietic neoplasm.

Much of the abdomen is occupied by the freely movable small intestine and colon. In enteritis, abnormal amounts of gas or fluid may be present. The walls may be spastically thickened and tender in panleukopenia. Thickening may also be present in chronic bowel disease as a result of inflammation or diffuse neoplastic change, e.g., eosinophilic enteritis or diffuse lymphomatous infiltration. Localized disorders such as foreign bodies, intussusception, and tumors are usually readily detected, although further diagnostic study may be needed for differentiation. Distinguishing between a foreign body and a fecal mass is not always easy, and in a wasted cat the ileocolic junction and its associated lymph nodes may sometimes be mistaken for a foreign body or tumor. The mesenteric nodes may be prominently enlarged with a variety of infections and tumors. A strong suspicion of intussusception or of pleating of the intestine by string or thread is an indication for prompt surgical exploration. The pancreas, if abnormally firm and thickened, may sometimes be palpated along the initial segment of the duodenum.

Prominent in the posterior part of the abdomen are the terminal portion of the large intestine, which often contains masses of hard stool, and the urinary bladder. Thickening, flaccidity, and contraction of the bladder are easily recognized. Urinary "sand" is not ordinarily palpable, but occasionally small stones are detected. After an injury to the hind parts, it is most important to ascertain whether the urinary bladder is intact. A persistently distended bladder and paralyzed tail are evidence of neural damage for which the outlook is uncertain.

A normal uterus is not ordinarily palpable. Pregnancy is first detectable at three weeks. Endometrial hyperplasia, neoplastic changes, and distention with fluid are pathologic changes easily detected by palpation. A uterus tensely distended with pus is at risk of rupture. This occasionally occurs during examination or may already have occurred when a cat is presented.

Accumulation of fluid in the abdominal cavity is a common finding in cats. Small amounts are difficult to distinguish from fat, but larger amounts are usually easily recognized by palpation and ballottement. If a cat is febrile, peritonitis is a strong probability; one should remember, however, that the feline infectious peritonitis (FIP) virus is not the only possible cause and that confirmatory laboratory study of fluid is required and perhaps other procedures as well. Other important causes of abdominal effusion are heart and liver disease (ascites) and abdominal tumors (modified transudates). Fluid associated with a tumor is frequently bloody, and a diagnosis may often be made by identification of neoplastic cells. Milky-looking fluids are rarely the result of injury but are most often associated with inflammation or tumor; only laboratory examination can determine whether they are truly chylous. In some cases of extremely tense distention of the abdomen with fluid, the fluid is not actually in the abdomen but within an enormous cyst such as occasionally arises from bile ducts. Hygroma renis, a rare complication involving injured or chronically diseased kidneys, also gives an initial impression of tense abdominal distention.

Straining to defecate, passage of stool coated with bright red blood, and pelvic injury are indications for digital rectal examination. This is so resented by a cat that it should be postponed until the end of the examination.

Examination of the spinal column and limbs for painful conditions should also be postponed until the end of the examination. Owners often interpret lameness as a sign of a fracture or sprain, but if fever is present, a careful search, often requiring clipping of the fur, usually discloses bite marks and incipient or advanced infection.

Only when the examination is completed should one

arouse a cat's displeasure by collecting samples for diagnostic studies or by carrying out minor procedures, such as cleaning ears, scaling teeth, and emptying anal sacs.

## FEVER OF UNKNOWN CAUSE

Cats are notorious for developing fevers of unknown cause. Fever is often the sole abnormality detected during physical examination of a cat that is apathetic and has stopped eating. If the elevation of temperature is so slight that its significance is uncertain, the temperature should be taken again a few hours later before any medication is given. A complete blood count (CBC) or rapid inspection of a blood film is indicated. Leukopenia, leukocytosis, or an abnormal differential count suggests that the fever may indeed reflect illness.

In the majority of cases, if a broad-spectrum antibiotic is given, the cat and the temperature return rapidly to normal—whether because of the treatment one can never be sure. In some cases it is possible that the cat has had a very mild form of one of the infections that we are accustomed to recognizing only when severe or fatal, for instance, panleukopenia, toxoplasmosis, or feline infectious peritonitis (FIP).

Persistent or recurrent fever calls for monitoring of the CBC, analysis and possible culture of urine, and even blood cultures. Tests for FeLV, FIP, and toxoplasmosis may be considered. Antipyretics should not be given. At best their only effect is to mask signs of illness; at worst they are so poorly tolerated by cats that they may well prove fatal if given to an animal that is already ill.

## OUTPATIENT VERSUS HOSPITAL TREATMENT

Except when an owner is unable to give adequate care or when serious injury or severe illness requires constant veterinary supervision and skilled nursing, a sick cat is usually better off at home. Treatment may be started at the time of the office visit and the cat returned as necessary for follow-up outpatient treatment. This may often be given by a technician, who keeps the veterinarian informed of the progress of the case. Large hospitals may set aside a specially equipped room where outpatient treatment can be given independently of other clinic and hospital activities.

Hospitalization should be kept to a minimum. Many procedures lend themselves to management of the patient as a day case, and the owner should be informed if preliminary vaccination or overnight fasting is needed. In this category are routine castration and spaying, Caesarean section, dentistry, grooming under sedation or anesthesia, abscess drainage, biopsy or removal of superficial growths, radiographic examination requiring anesthesia, and certain laboratory tests. Mastectomies and surgery for pyometra can usually be done with an overnight stay. Because of the possibility of hemorrhage, cats being declawed should usually stay for two days, the dressing being removed after the first night.

The hospital stay is longer if a seriously ill animal needs tests, radiographs, and follow-up treatment until the diagnostic possibilities have been narrowed down. In this group are cases of persistent vomiting or diarrhea and dyspnea of almost any sort. A cat with urethral blockage must be carefully monitored until it is again urinating freely, and a diabetic cat until a suitable regimen for insulin has been established.

Every cat admitted to the hospital should wear an identification collar, and its cage should be similarly identified.

## SUGGESTIONS FOR DIAGNOSTIC PROCEDURES

Cats from which samples must be obtained are often in a precarious state, especially if anemic or dyspneic, and many have died during heavy-handed struggles to obtain samples. Compassionate handling, quiet surroundings, and skill are essential. A guard should be posted against noisy persons and banging doors, and barking, bouncing dogs should not be led by, terrorizing the cat just as a blood sample is being drawn!

Samples of several milliliters or more, such as are needed for some blood studies and for surveys of chemical values, must be obtained from a jugular vein (Fig. 1–2); samples of a few drops to 1 or 2 ml may be drawn from a cephalic (Fig. 1–3) or saphenous vein. It is better to clip the fur over a vein than to try to demonstrate one's virtuosity by aiming for a vein that cannot be seen. A gentle, deliberate technique that first penetrates the skin and then the vein is most successful with cats. If the skin is dehydrated or the vein small and collapsed, a 25-gauge needle may serve better than a 20-gauge. Suction should be moderate or the vein will collapse.

For small or for very ill cats undergoing tests requiring only a few drops of blood, a marginal ear vein or toe pad may be pricked. The area should not be disinfected with an aqueous material but should simply be smoothed with mineral oil or petrolatum so that the drops of blood will

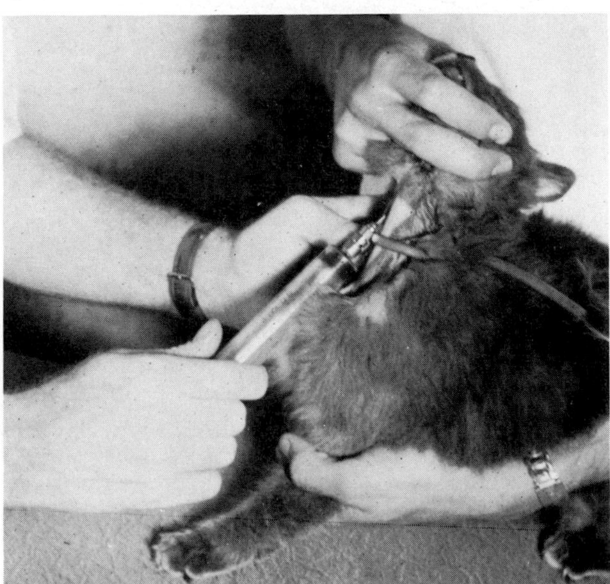

**Figure 1–2.** Substantial samples of blood for testing must be obtained from a jugular vein. The vein may be compressed either by a tourniquet or by the operator's thumb. (Courtesy of Dr. Eugene Jones.)

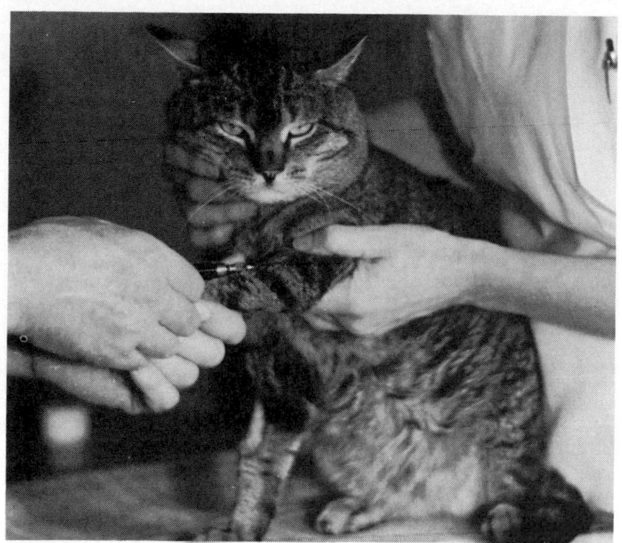

**Figure 1–3.** A cat lightly restrained in a normal sitting position while several milliliters of blood are drawn from the cephalic vein.

well up over the pricked area and not spread into the surrounding fur. This technique is the least stressful and most practical for obtaining small samples for blood films; for total solids, hematocrit, or hemoglobin determinations; for total WBC by pipette method; and for dipstick screening tests (e.g., Ames Azostix) that require only a drop or two of blood. If a microlancet does not elicit sufficient blood, the tip of a curved scalpel blade is more effective. The collector's index finger under the ear is protected from the stab of the lancet or blade by a small gauze pad, which is also used to pinch off the flow of blood when the sample has been collected (Fig. 1–4). Ear pricks should be used as much as possible if veins are in poor condition and must be preserved for intravenous therapy. An uncooperative cat should be lightly sedated; otherwise the excitement of a struggle distorts the results obtained.

Sampling of blood and marrow is discussed in detail in the chapter on blood disorders.

Urine samples that are not to be cultured may be obtained from a clean, empty sanitary pan or from a sheet of plastic spread over the litter. Samples for culture are best collected by needle aspiration from the bladder. The skin at the site of puncture should be clipped and thor-

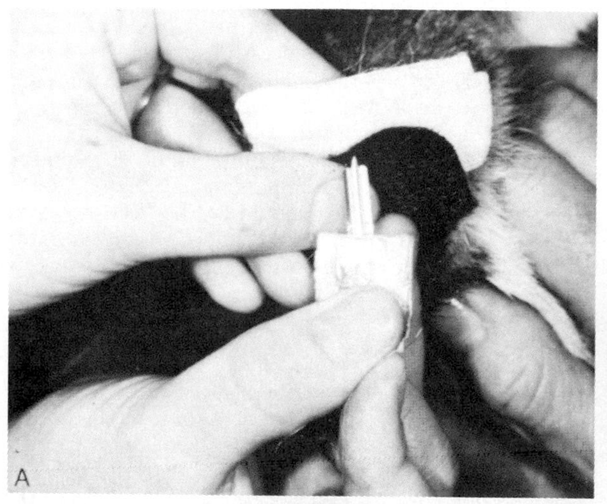

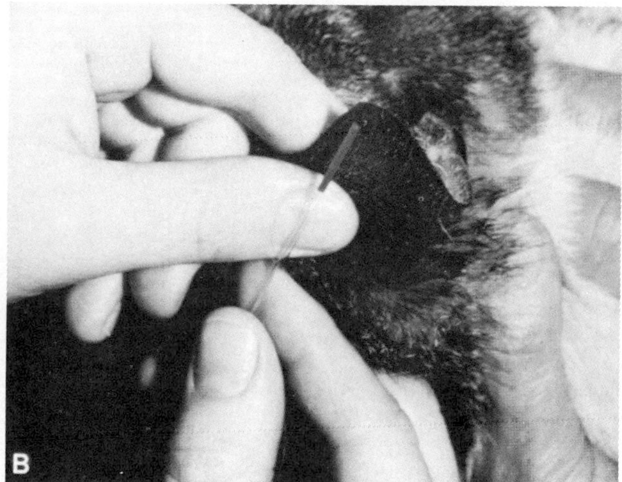

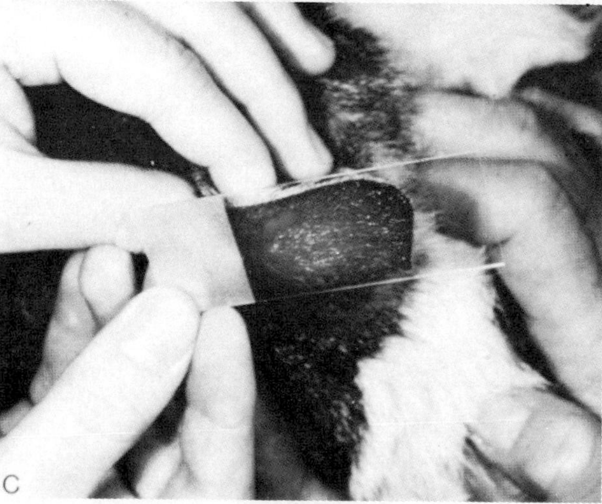

**Figure 1–4.** *A*, After the fur has been smoothed with petroleum jelly to prevent the blood from spreading, a marginal ear vein is pricked with a disposable lancet (or curved scalpel blade). The gauze pad under the ear protects the operator's finger. *B* and *C*, As drops of blood well up from the vein, a microhematocrit tube and vials for WBC and platelet counts (Unopette, Becton-Dickinson) are filled and blood films are made.

oughly disinfected. Although it is most desirable to obtain a sample by needle aspiration, experience with many samples indicates that a "clean catch" obtained by expressing the bladder manually and collecting the latter part of the flow is unlikely to be contaminated, since most samples so obtained prove to be bacteriologically sterile. The chance of contamination can be further reduced if the entire vulvar or preputial area is clipped and thoroughly cleansed with a Betadine wash. Only when an irritating cystitis causes a cat to urinate frequently should catheterization be resorted to on the chance of aspirating a few drops of urine from a bladder that is almost constantly contracted and empty.

Whenever physical examination or a radiograph suggests that fluid is present in a swelling or body cavity, a suitable area should be clipped and thoroughly disinfected and a sample obtained for study (and, in the case of excessive thoracic fluid, as a lifesaving measure). Many a cat on the verge of suffocation with a chestful of fluid has died because of unskilled attempts at aspiration. The cat, sedated if necessary, is steadied, with a minimum of restraint, in the crouching or sternal position that it naturally prefers (Fig. 1–5). A 14- or 15-gauge, ¾-inch needle is introduced gently through an intercostal space caudal to the heart on either side or on the fluid-filled side if a radiograph indicates that the effusion is unilateral. The large-gauge needle is advisable in case the fluid is thick or flocculent, and it should be just long enough to penetrate the chest wall so that there will be no puncture or injury of the heart or lung. Samples of fluid must always be saved for laboratory study. Because some fluids clot rapidly (notably in feline infectious peritonitis), several films should be made at once. Some of the fluid should be put into a heparinized tube, and more in thioglycolate liquid medium for culture and sensitivity testing.

Although an abdomen may be full of fluid, abdominal structures, such as loops of intestine, mesentery, and especially omentum, are apt to block the opening of a needle, trocar, or catheter when suction is applied, so that repeated attempts may produce only a few drops. One fairly successful method is to allow the cat to lie on its sternum or side in the position it prefers and to introduce a large-gauge needle without a syringe into the most dependent portion of the abdomen in the hope that without suction the fluid will simply drip from the hub of the needle, where it should be collected for diagnostic purposes. If there is little or no flow, it can usually be stimulated by gentle, moving pressure on the abdomen. If no fluid can be obtained from one side, an attempt should be made on the other side. Restraining a cat on its back for this purpose apparently causes extreme discomfort. Any struggle should be avoided.

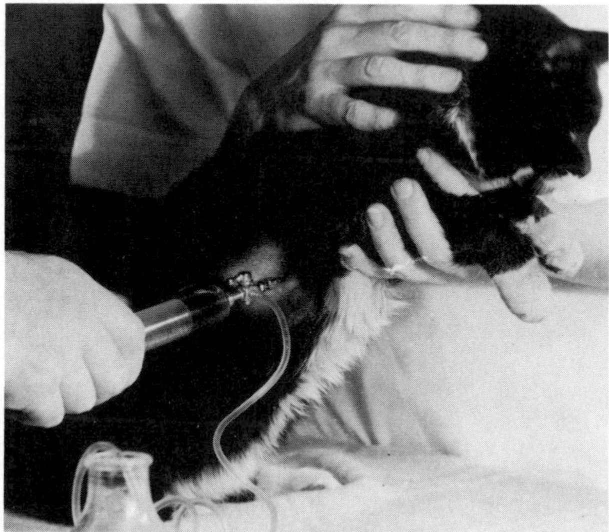

**Figure 1–5.** For thoracocentesis the cat is lightly restrained in a natural upright position, and fluid is aspirated from the lower part of the chest, where it tends to accumulate by gravity.

If fluid cannot be obtained with a needle, one can sometimes succeed by passing an intravenous catheter through a large-gauge needle and moving the catheter around gently in the thoracic or abdominal cavity.

Whether obtained from the chest or abdomen, a milky-looking fluid must not automatically be presumed to be chyle or necessarily of traumatic origin, and it should be submitted for multiple diagnostic tests. Even autopsy in some cases may fail to disclose the pathogenesis of the condition.

Radiographs, in the majority of cases, may be taken without anesthesia or sedation if technicians are expert and gentle. When absolutely accurate positioning is essential, as for views of the middle and inner ear or nasal passages and sinuses, general anesthesia is required for good relaxation and immobilization. Food must be withheld for at least 12 hours before the procedure.

For contrast studies of the digestive, urinary, and biliary tracts, it is necessary that food be withheld for 12 to 24 hours; in addition, the intestine must be emptied of stool. The owner may administer a milk of magnesia tablet the night before bringing the cat to the hospital, where small soap-and-water enemas must be given until a scout film indicates that all stool has been removed. Several small enemas are preferable to one employing so much fluid that the cat vomits. Enemas of high-concentration sodium phosphate solutions (e.g., Fleet) are occasionally followed shortly by severe, even fatal, reactions due to hypovolemia, hypernatremia, and hyperphosphatemia, the last binding and precipitating calcium so that hypocalcemia results. Prompt intravenous injection of 10 per cent calcium gluconate is required (Schaer et al., 1977).

Many cats will lap a mixture of barium and strained baby food meat or will accept it if given by dropper or syringe (e.g., Sherwood Medical Curved Tip Syringe). An uncooperative cat may have to be given a small dose of ketamine or a tranquilizer so that the barium can be given by stomach tube. One must be absolutely certain that the stomach tube is in the digestive tract before administering the barium. Too great an amount may cause the cat to vomit, and if any barium is inhaled, the outcome is usually fatal pneumonia.

If perforation of the digestive tract is a possibility, a nonirritating form of barium (e.g., Gastrografin, Squibb) should be used. This is also indicated if a rapid gastrointestinal scan is desired, as it moves through the tract much more quickly than barium. It should not be used in a dehydrated animal, however, as it aggravates that condition. If a cat is vomiting only after eating food, it is advisable to mix some of the food with the barium.

## MEDICATING CATS

Injection is the easiest method for giving medication both for the cat and for the veterinarian or technician. An injection is practical, however, only when a cat is hospitalized or is returned as an outpatient as often as the medication is required. Many veterinarians* never use the intramuscular route in cats for any injection except rabies vaccination. They are apprehensive of injury to the sciatic nerve and of phlebitis, which occasionally results from injections into the caudal thigh muscles. They have found that most drugs recommended for intramuscular injection in other species can be administered effectively to cats by the subcutaneous route.

If the intramuscular route is chosen, a more substantial mass in young or thin cats is that of the cranial thigh muscle (quadriceps femoris). A needle inserted obliquely into this muscle encounters no large nerve or vessel, and injections at this site are more likely to be truly intramuscular than those into the caudal thigh muscle (biceps femoris), where the medication has been shown to be deposited, in many cases, between fascial planes (Baxter and Evans, 1973). Rabies vaccine can usually be injected into the cranial thigh muscle with little or no sign of discomfort from the cat.

Satisfactory for most injections in cats is a 3/4-inch, 22-gauge, disposable needle and syringe, the needle being inserted to only half its length.

Most owners do best in medicating cats with pills, and less well with capsules. Some capsules contain an irritant material that may be hazardous if a cat bites into them and inhales the contents. Occasionally, clients find it easier to give liquids by dropper than to administer pills. Such liquids must be reasonably palatable to the cat. Medicines with sweet or aromatic flavors, such as Pepto-Bismol or Kaopectate, will be promptly spewed into the environment. Liquids should be given into the side of the mouth behind a canine tooth with the cat's head steadied in a natural position (Fig. 1–6). The head should never be forced back, and no more liquid should be given at one time than the cat can easily swallow. Jelly-like preparations that come in tubes may be squeezed onto a cat's nose or forepaw, from which the cat will often lick it.

The veterinarian or assistant should take time to teach an owner how to give medication.

For uncooperative cats it is sometimes possible to mix liquid medication, powder, or crushed tablets with the food. Cats are less likely than dogs to be fooled into swallowing little balls of food that contain pills or capsules but may do so if first given a small piece of favorite food with no medication in it.

A struggle over medication is counterproductive and even dangerous, for inhaled material, especially if oily, can lead to pneumonia.

There are some cats—luckily few—to which it is impossible to administer oral medication of any kind, and both owner and veterinarian must accept that there are limitations to what can be done for such an animal.

## HANDLING CATS

Most cats are easily handled if they are allowed to assume natural positions and are subjected to a minimum of restraint. They should be carried firmly but gently in an upright position with paws under control and the body weight supported by an arm (Fig. 1–7). If a cat's spleen is greatly enlarged, there should be no pressure on the abdomen, lest the organ be ruptured. Severely anemic and dyspneic cats must be handled with special consideration, since any struggling may end fatally.

Wire carriers that can be disinfected should be available for in-hospital purposes and should be used for carrying uncooperative or aggressive cats.

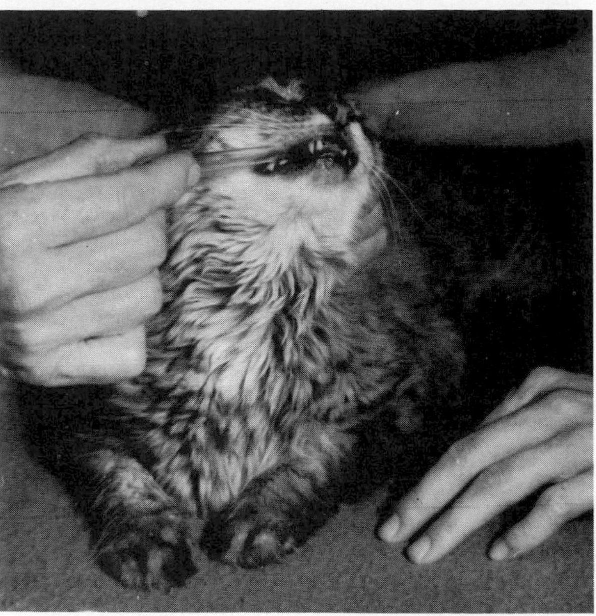

**Figure 1–6.** Liquid medication is given by plastic dropper in the space behind a canine tooth. The head should be kept almost level, not forced up and back.

## HOSPITAL ACCOMMODATIONS FOR CATS

In a well-planned hospital for both dogs and cats, or for cats exclusively, a ward should accommodate no more than 10 animals, so that if upper respiratory infection breaks out, it can more easily be contained. Under no circumstances should there be any circulation of air from ward to ward. Each ward should have a dozen changes of fresh air per hour, with separate intakes and exhausts for each ward. An even temperature of 22 to 24 C (72 to 75 F) and a humidity of 30 to 40 per cent should be maintained. If it is the practice to hospitalize cats with panleukopenia and upper respiratory tract infections, there must be two isolation wards. Of the two infections, the latter is more apt to spread among cats because vaccination against panleukopenia gives the better immunity. Practitioners who have around-the-clock ultraviolet lighting in their wards believe that it materially reduces the chance of outbreak of respiratory infection for both dogs and cats. To be both safe and effective, the lights must be adequate for the area to be protected, professionally installed, kept free of dust, and replaced at regular intervals.

Fiberglass cages are preferable to stainless steel because of the difference in heat loss from the occupant. Advo-

*Including one of the authors (Holzworth).

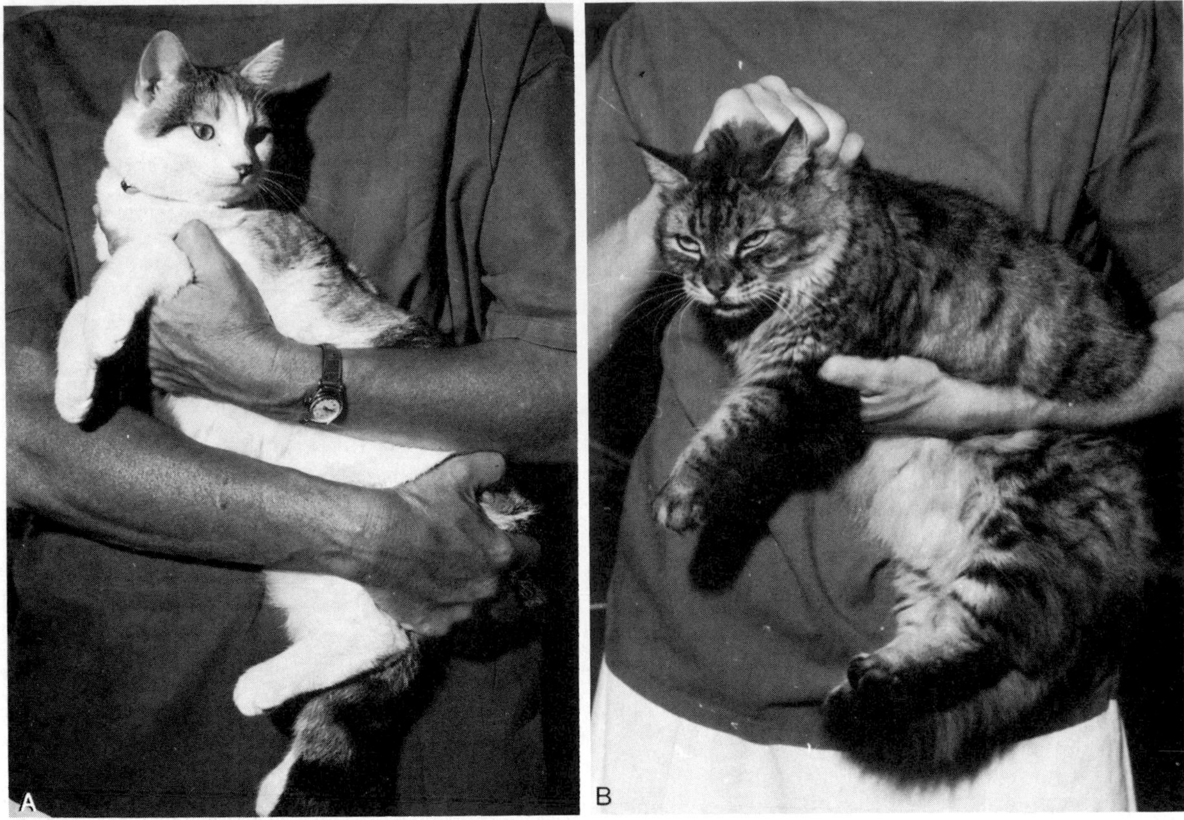


**Figure 1–7.** *A*, Carrying a gentle cat, an attendant holds the paws between the fingers of one hand and supports the cat's body securely with the other hand and arm. *B*, A cat that may be inclined to leap away or bite is grasped firmly by the nape of the neck.

cates of fiberglass maintain that cold, sick cats get colder and sicker in steel cages. Moreover, owners (if not the cats) find the pleasant color of the fiberglass more cheerful. Regardless of the type of cage, the rods of the cage doors should be close enough so that small kittens cannot get their heads wedged between. Cages should measure at least 2 × 2 × 2 feet, but some should be larger for the comfort of big cats and those staying for longer periods.

The cages should not face other cages, and upper cages should not be open at the top. If they are constructed to slope slightly to the back, fluids will not drip out.

Newspapers are more economical for lining cages than are special corrugated sheets of lining paper. A timid cat is reassured by having a "house" to hide in. This can be made by turning a lidless cardboard carton upside down and cutting an opening in one side or end. When it is necessary to handle the cat, the box is simply lifted off the occupant. If a cat is difficult to handle, such a box is also useful in pulling the cat forward out of the cage into an open-topped carrier. Heavy paper bags also provide reassuring retreats and may also be used for removing a difficult cat from a cage.

Although it may be a nuisance to keep track of and launder "personal possessions," some cats are reassured by having a familiar blanket, towel, or woolen sweater to sleep on.

Disposable dishes are the most practical. If stainless steel bowls are used, they must be autoclaved after each use.

A sanitary pan or box should be provided lest a cat accustomed to this amenity or to going outdoors be inhibited from defecating and urinating. A lining of newspaper or white paper towels absorbs moisture and makes it possible to detect blood in the urine. Cat litter is put into the box on top of the paper if that is what a cat is accustomed to. Cardboard packing boxes may be of suitable dimensions or can be cut down and taped at the corners. It is also possible to buy heavy paper trays of the type used in markets to package fruits and vegetables. Metal or plastic pans must be disinfected when used for another cat because of the hazards of urine-transmitted infectious agents.

For collecting urine samples, a plastic bag or sheet of plastic wrap may be spread over the litter, or a clean empty pan may be placed in the cage.

Cleanliness is the best weapon for combating the odor of cat urine. A solution of vinegar may be used to neutralize the powerful scent of a tomcat's urine.

The disinfectant most effective against the pathogens of cats (of which the panleukopenia virus is the most resistant) is Clorox diluted 1:32 with water. It is more easily used for cleaning if combined with a detergent-disinfectant. For this purpose A33 (Airkem, Airwick

Industries, Carlstadt, New Jersey 07072) may be added to make a final concentration of Clorox 1:32 and A33 1:64 (4 oz/gal and 2 oz/gal, respectively).

## HOSPITALIZATION OF CATS

Information should always be obtained about the food a cat is most likely to eat, and if it is not stocked, the owner should be asked to provide it. In general, ill cats do not take to changes in diet but are more likely to eat if tempted with their favorite treats. Sometimes a cat will eat only from its own dishes. Because most cats are nibblers, food as well as water should be kept in the cage. Frightened cats may sometimes be coax-fed in the quiet of the evening. Visits from the owner can boost the morale of both, and the owner should be encouraged to coax-feed and hold the cat, preferably in a quiet examination room or some other comfortable and secluded corner of the hospital.

With exceptions only for critical cases, visits should take place during office hours and by advance arrangement. An owner is greatly reassured by being able to see his animal and its quarters, and extreme manifestations of concern should receive sympathetic understanding if a pet's survival is in doubt. Denying an owner the right to visit an animal may arouse ill feeling or even suspicions that could have serious consequences. It is even possible that refusal to let an owner visit could be interpreted as a denial of his legal rights.

Successful communication with owners is essential. In some hospitals, progress reports are available at a certain hour for owners who telephone. Any unexpected findings or unfavorable development should be reported promptly to the owner, preferably by the veterinarian. Except in emergencies, the need and cost for additional tests or special treatment should be explained to the owner and his agreement obtained.

Instructions for aftercare should be carefully explained by an experienced assistant or by the veterinarian. Often they should be clearly and simply written out and may be supplemented by handouts that describe the illness and its cause, treatment, and prevention. If medication is dispensed, it should be identified and directions for use clearly written.

Instructions should be given, drugs dispensed, the bill paid, and any follow-up appointment made before the cat is brought from the ward. Otherwise the owner will pay attention only to the cat.

## INTENSIVE CARE

An area where severely injured or ill cats can receive special care and monitoring is desirable. An oxygen cage or a cage with an "oxygen door" is essential.

Hot water bottles are unsatisfactory providers of warmth. Several baby incubators (for instance, the Armstrong type) should be available for seriously ill or injured cats and may also be used for short periods for the administration of oxygen. An electrocardiograph machine and resuscitative equipment should be within easy access.

In many hospitals the special care area adjoins or is combined with the surgical recovery area.

## SUPPLEMENTARY FEEDING

Caloric requirements can be met most easily if nutrients are taken orally. Food can be supplied in several ways to cats that have stopped eating voluntarily. Concentrated nutrients are available in jelly or pastelike form, e.g., Nutri-Cal (Evsco) and Pet Kalorie (Haver-Lockhart), and may be squeezed into the mouth or onto a paw for the cat to lick. A single tablespoonful may supply the daily maintenance requirements for a 5 kg (10 lb) cat. (Some cats develop a real liking for these preparations, which may also be given in small quantities as a treat or when a vitamin-mineral source is needed to supplement an inadequate diet.)

Strained baby food meats or other puréed foods may be supplemented with vitamins and minerals and fed by dropper or syringe into the side of the mouth.

If a cat does not cooperate with forced feeding, a stomach tube may be used if only a few such feedings are anticipated. Suitable for this purpose is a rubber feeding-tube-and-urethral-catheter (Sherwood Medical) or a rectal tube (size 12 to 14 French for the average cat, and size 9 for a kitten). Used with a suitable mouth gag (modeled after one formerly available from Jen-Sal), the tube will be tolerated by most cats (Fig. 1–8). When the feeding is concluded, the tube must be pinched off as it is withdrawn, lest food be inhaled.

Tube feeding is also occasionally done with a fine human male catheter (number 8 Bard) passed through the nose (Clark, 1975). A drop or two of a topical anesthetic (no more, or serious side effects may result) is introduced into a nostril; alternatively, the cat may be given ketamine to facilitate passage of the catheter, which is inserted with the tip bent slightly down so that it will pass along the floor of the nasal passage and into the esophagus. If the cat swallows and does not gag or cough, one may assume that the catheter has not by mischance entered the respiratory tract but is safely in the esophagus. Liquid alimentation is then given by means of a 12-gauge needle and a 10- to 30-ml syringe, depending on the cat's size. Many cats tolerate having the tube left in place so that feeding may be done at frequent intervals. This method should not be used, however, for cats with nasal disorders; another disadvantage is that only a thin liquid will pass through the catheter.

More widely used in recent years is feeding by a pharyngostomy tube, which can remain in place for days and through which foods of puréed consistency are easily passed. The technique for pharyngostomy was described by Böhning et al. (1970) and Stein (1980). With ketamine anesthesia (1 to 4 mg/kg IV) and a speculum to hold the mouth open, the examiner's gloved index finger is inserted into the pouchlike cavity behind the base of the tongue and lateral to the hyoid apparatus. The tip of the finger pressing outward indicates the site on the side of the neck that should be prepared for surgery (Fig. 1–9*A*). A large, curved artery forceps substituting for the finger is directed outward at that spot, and a small skin incision is made over the forceps, which is then jabbed out through the pharyngeal mucosa. The tip of the feeding tube is grasped by the forceps and directed down the esophagus to just within the stomach, the length from stoma to last rib having been previously marked on the tube. The skin is tightened around the tube by a pursestring suture, and

The deficit figure indicates how many milliliters should be administered in a 24-hour period to restore the water deficit. Once a cat's hydration is restored to normal, 40 to 50 ml/kg/day (20 to 25 ml/lb/day) divided into amounts given intravenously, subcutaneously, or intraperitoneally will meet the requirements for maintenance of fluids and electrolytes. With fever the requirement is moderately increased.

Cats that are not eating should receive regular supplementation with B-complex vitamins. When undiluted, these solutions sting acutely and therefore, in order to be diluted, should be injected by way of the same tube as the fluid. With prolonged lack of food intake, intramuscular administration of fat-soluble vitamins may be indicated as well.

As already noted, caloric requirements are best met by the oral route or by a pharyngostomy tube.

## EUTHANASIA

If a cat is injured beyond hope of salvage, or incurably ill to the point at which it can no longer be maintained in reasonable comfort, euthanasia should be suggested. Often an owner knows that this is the right course but is unwilling to take the initiative, and the veterinarian may have to assume the responsibility for suggesting it.

If the owner desires, he should be encouraged to be with his pet at the end, for it can be an enormous comfort to know with certainty that a beloved animal died quickly and peacefully.

Injection of a barbiturate solution is the only humane method. Whether euthanasia is performed at the hospital or at the owner's home in order to avoid a final stressful trip for the cat, a skilled assistant should be present to help with the intravenous injection. If a cat is likely to be nervous, distressed, or difficult to handle, the owner may give a preliminary dose of phenobarbital or a tranquilizer. If the cat struggles or a vein cannot be entered easily, attempts should not be prolonged, for a less stressful alternative is injection of the barbiturate into the thorax or peritoneal cavity—an alternative that should be explained in advance to the owner. The needle should be no longer than 3/4 inch and should be introduced gently just through the body wall while the cat's attention is distracted by stroking of the head. If the thoracic route is chosen, a needle this short is unlikely to puncture the lung and cause pain. There should be no probing in an attempt to enter the heart, which may also cause distress. The cat should be stroked soothingly as it becomes drowsy; and it will be dead in two or three minutes. Whatever the owner's wishes about disposal of the body, the veterinarian should cooperate in carrying them out.

In some cases the veterinarian will be anxious to have an autopsy performed. Few owners object to this if it is explained that something helpful to other animals may be learned; in fact, they are often grateful for the suggestion, as long as they are assured that the body can still be returned to them for burial if they wish. In this event, it is important that the body be neatly sutured, cleaned, wrapped in a towel or blanket, and returned to the owner in a suitable box. This final act of consideration is important because of the very real possibility that the owner will wish to have one final look at the pet and be certain that it is indeed his.

### REFERENCES

Baxter JS, Evans JM: Intramuscular injection in the cat. J Small Anim Pract 14 (1973) 297–302.

Böhning RH Jr, DeHoff WD, McElhinney A, Hofstra, PC: Pharyngostomy for maintenance of the anorectic animal. J Am Vet Med Assoc 156 (1970) 611–615.

Caras R, Cavanagh PG, Fisher LE, Fox MW, Frye FL, Holzworth J, Hyman JD, Mathey WJ, Schuchman SM: Pet Medicine. New York, McGraw-Hill Book Company, 1977.

Clark CH: Fluid therapy. *In* Catcott EJ (ed): Feline Medicine and Surgery, 2nd ed. Santa Barbara, American Veterinary Publications, 1975.

Ettinger SJ (ed): Textbook of Veterinary Internal Medicine. Philadelphia, WB Saunders Company, 1983.

McGinnis T: The Well Cat Book. New York, Random House–Bookworks, 1975.

Muir WW, Di Bartola SP: Fluid therapy. *In* Kirk RW (ed): Current Veterinary Therapy VIII. Philadelphia, WB Saunders Company, 1983.

Schaer M, Cavanagh P, Hause W, Wilkins R: Iatrogenic hyperphosphatemia, hypocalcemia and hypernatremia in a cat. J Am Anim Hosp Assoc 13 (1977) 39–41.

Scott FW: Virucidal disinfectants and feline viruses. Am J Vet Res 41 (1980) 410–424.

Stein BS: A method for continuous intravenous fluid therapy in a cat. Feline Pract 4(4) (1974) 12–15.

Stein BS: Feline respiratory disease complex. *In* Kirk RW (ed): Current Veterinary Therapy VII. Philadelphia, WB Saunders Company, 1980.

#### ADDITIONAL REFERENCES

Burrows CF: Techniques and complications of intravenous and intraarterial catheterization in dogs and cats. J Am Vet Med Assoc 163 (1973) 1357–1363.

Collette WL, Meriwether WF: Oral alimentation of cats. *In* Kirk RW (ed): Current Veterinary Therapy III. Philadelphia, WB Saunders Company 1968.

Edney ATB: The management of euthanasia in small animal practice. J Am Anim Hosp Assoc 15 (1979) 645–649.

# 2
# CHAPTER
# NUTRITION AND NUTRITIONAL DISORDERS

JOSEPH A. O'DONNELL, III, and K.C. HAYES

The cat secured its position within the ecosystem, in part, by adapting its metabolism to efficient utilization of a strictly carnivorous diet. As a consequence, it long ago lost the capacity to obtain all essential nutrients solely from plants and relies instead on animal tissues to meet certain nutritional requirements. In its natural habitat the cat usually secures its most appropriate diet as prey; however, in a domestic environment it is not always so fortunate. To provide food for domesticated animals in the least costly manner, man has formulated diets consisting largely of plant-derived nutrients. Although the cat has adapted to most manmade diets, the limitations of total substitution of nutrients of vegetable origin for those of animal origin are now being realized.

The following discussion identifies currently appreciated aspects of these limitations while describing known specific nutrient requirements in the cat. Emphasis is placed on the nutritional consequences of the peculiarities of metabolism that distinguish the cat from most other mammals.

## ENERGY

In energy requirements, cats adhere to general norms according to their size and metabolic activity. As in other species, energy needs on a body weight basis are greatest during growth of the kitten, when maintenance, new tissue formation, and vigorous physical activity contribute to a caloric demand of about 300 kcal/kg. The adult cat has a basal need of about 75 kcal/kg, but pregnancy and lactation raise the requirement to 100 to 200 kcal/kg, the level depending on litter size and condition of the queen. A typical queen may lose as much as a quarter of her body weight before her kittens are weaned as she attempts to meet their growth requirements through lactation. The actual energy needs of kittens and adult cats are detailed in Table 2–1, along with a translation of these requirements into feeding portions of dry ration or canned food and extra water.

Since longevity is increased and obesity is usually averted by slightly underfeeding caloric requirements, it is safer to err on the low side, especially when feeding relatively expensive canned cat foods that become unpalatable if not eaten when fresh.

Because of the high water content of canned products, the caloric density is low (about 1.1 kcal/gm) compared with that of soft-moist (3 kcal/gm) and dry products (3.5 kcal/gm) (see Table 2–1). Most cats regulate their food intake to match energy needs. Otherwise, cats maintained on dry products would be fatter than those eating an equal amount of canned products. The high palatability of canned products, however, occasionally causes cats to overeat.

If caloric density is diminished by an ingredient other than water, a different result may occur. Whereas the feeding behavior of cats is sensitive to dietary compositional changes, especially in protein, they do not appear to be responsive to changes in caloric density of their food (Hirsch et al., 1978). When non-nutritive kaolin was added to the diet, reducing caloric density, food consumption was similar to that for diets without kaolin. As a result, the cats lost weight. Kanarek (1975) reported similar results. Conversely, Skultety (1969) found that increasing the caloric density of the diet did not lower the food intake. These observations need further corroboration by studies using other diluents. If valid, they suggest a means of treating obese cats by increasing non-nutritive vegetable fiber in dietary formulations.

**Table 2–1 Energy and Water Requirements of Cats Fed Dry or Canned Food**

| AGE | APPROXIMATE BODY WEIGHT | | DAILY ENERGY REQUIREMENT | | APPROXIMATE FEED AND WATER REQUIRED | | | | | |
|---|---|---|---|---|---|---|---|---|---|---|
| | | | | | Dry Diet (10% water) 3.5 kcal/gm | | | Canned Diet (74% water) 1.1 kcal/gm | | |
| wk | kg | lb | kcal/kg | kcal | gm | cup | ml $H_2O$ | gm | 6½ oz can | ml $H_2O$ |
| 5 | 0.5 | 1.1 | 300 | 150 | 44 | 1/2 | 175 | 121 | 2/3 | 10 |
| 6 | 0.75 | 1.6 | 275 | 206 | 60 | 2/3 | 100 | 166 | 9/10 | 10 |
| 10 | 1.0 | 2.2 | 250 | 250 | 73 | 3/4 | 100 | 202 | 1 1/10 | 10 |
| 14 | 1.5 | 3.3 | 200 | 300 | 88 | 1 | 120 | 242 | 1 1/3 | 20 |
| 18 | 2.0 | 4.4 | 140 | 280 | 82 | 9/10 | 150 | 226 | 1 1/4 | 30 |
| 24* | 3.0 | 6.6 | 100 | 300 | 88 | 1 | 200 | 242 | 1 1/3 | 30 |
| 32 | 4.0 | 8.8 | 85 | 340 | 100 | 1 1/10 | 250 | 274 | 1 1/2 | 50 |
| 48 | 5.0 | 10.0 | 75 | 375 | 110 | 1 1/4 | 275 | 302 | 1 2/3 | 50 |

*Weight gain is reduced sharply between 36 and 48 weeks. Final weights are somewhat breed-dependent. As in other species, weights also vary according to an individual cat's skeletal size and constitution. Substantial weight gain beyond one year of age is probably undesirable, because it generally reflects adiposity.

The cat differs from most species in that much of its energy is normally derived from fat and protein, with a small component contributed by carbohydrate as the glycogen found in meat. Commercial diets alter this relationship without apparent detriment to the cat by including a significant portion of calories as carbohydrate, usually from cereals and grains, with a reduced portion as fat. This acceptable variation in energy source assumes that certain other nutrient requirements are met.

Kittens can begin weaning at four to five weeks and are often totally weaned by eight weeks. Weaning is facilitated by provision of moistened food (canned or dry with water added) from four weeks and by gradually shortening the kittens' time with the queen. Most kittens need moistened food (1 oz of water per 1½ cups) until 10 to 12 weeks of age and should be fed at least three or four times daily. As they mature, constantly available dry food will allow them to satisfy their hunger ad libitum. Fresh water should be available at all times, particularly when dry food is used. Canned food generally provides most of a cat's water requirement (Table 2–1), which is minimal in comparison with that of most mammalian species. The cat normally consumes two to three times as much water as dry matter (Burger et al., 1980; Seefeldt and Chapman, 1979).

## PROTEINS AND AMINO ACIDS

### Dietary Protein Requirement

**BASIC PRINCIPLES.** Protein requirement is usually defined as the requirement for essential amino acids and nonspecific α-amino nitrogen, the latter being necessary for synthesis of dispensable amino acids. Since protein synthesis is primarily responsible for consumption of both dispensable and indispensable amino acids in most animals, whether carnivore, herbivore, or omnivore, this definition appears to be valid. The cat, however, requires far more protein (as a percentage of its daily food intake) than is presumably needed for protein synthesis (Miller, 1957), so that its protein requirement appears more complex than that defined for other animals.

A dietary protein level below 16 to 18 per cent of total calories in either the growing kitten (Anderson et al., 1980a; Smalley et al., 1981) or the adult cat (Greaves and Scott, 1960) leads to classic signs of protein deficiency. These figures, if correct, are extraordinary, since the young of most other animals require diets of 8 to 12 per cent protein, whereas most adult animals have a minimal protein requirement for maintenance of about 4 per cent of calories (Table 2–2). Thus the minimal protein requirement of the adult cat is at least four times that of other adult animals, while the kitten requires at least 50 per cent more protein than the young of other species.

Even though the dietary protein requirement of cats was estimated as early as 1960, experimental determination of specific amino acid requirements was not feasible until some years later, when purified crystalline amino acids became available. Hardy et al. (1977) were the first to describe a purified experimental diet acceptable to cats that provided only crystalline amino acids as the nitrogen source. Later studies identified the essential amino acids and estimated their requirement.

Eleven amino acids are considered essential in the diet of cats (Rogers and Morris, 1979) (Table 2–3). Experimental evidence indicates that three more—cystine, glycine, and serine—are inadequately synthesized by the kitten (Rogers and Morris, 1980), but their essentiality for kittens and adult cats remains to be established. In examining the values listed in Table 2–3, it is important to note that although the protein requirement of cats greatly exceeds that of other animals, with four exceptions the requirements for specific essential amino acids are not significantly greater than those of other animals (e.g., rats and pigs). The cat is unique with its high total protein

**Table 2–2 Comparison of the Minimal Protein Requirement of Cats and Other Mammals***

| | WEANLING | ADULT |
|---|---|---|
| | (percentage of kcal) | |
| Cat | 18† | 19 |
| Dog | 12 | 4 |
| Rat | 12 | 4 |
| Human | 8 | 4 |

*Data from National Research Council publications on dietary requirements (1974, 1978).

†Anderson et al. (1980a).

**Table 2–3 Comparison of Essential Amino Acid Requirements and Recommended Allowances for Growing Kittens, Rats, and Pigs (gm per 100 gm diet)**

| AMINO ACID | KITTEN* | PIG† | RAT† |
|---|---|---|---|
| Arginine | 0.80 (1.10) | 0.28 | 0.60 |
| Asparagine | ? | — | 0.40 |
| Histidine | 0.30 (0.40) | 0.25 | 0.30 |
| Isoleucine | 0.30 (0.60) | 0.69 | 0.50 |
| Leucine | 1.20 (1.20) | 0.83 | 0.75 |
| Lysine | 0.80 (0.90) | 0.96 | 0.70 |
| Methionine plus cystine | 0.75 (0.90) | 0.69 | 0.60 |
| Phenylalanine plus tyrosine | 1.00 (1.10) | 0.69 | 0.80 |
| Proline | — | — | 0.40 |
| Taurine | 0.05 (0.07) | — | — |
| Threonine | 0.70 (0.85) | 0.62 | 0.50 |
| Tryptophan | 0.15 (0.18) | 0.18 | 0.15 |
| Valine | 0.60 (0.70) | 0.69 | 0.60 |
| Total essential amino acids | 6.65 | 5.88 | 5.50‡ |

*Based on data in text and a diet containing 25 per cent animal fat on a calculated metabolizable energy of 4.7 kcal per gm. Values in parentheses represent a recommended allowance, per data of Rogers and Morris (personal communication).

†Based on data from the National Research Council: Nutrient Requirements of Domestic Animals (1973, 1978).

‡Excluding asparagine and proline.

requirement and special need for arginine, leucine, threonine, methionine, and taurine.

Studies by Rogers et al. (1977) reconciled these peculiarities by revealing that the cat, unlike the rat, does not adjust its metabolism in response to the level of dietary protein. With few exceptions, key amino acid–metabolizing enzymes and urea-cycle enzymes in the cat maintain a constant level of activity comparable to that found in rats fed high-protein diets. That is, the cat constantly metabolizes large amounts of protein regardless of dietary protein availability. As might be expected, in addition to basic requirements for essential amino acids, this carnivore requires a considerable level of nonspecific α-amino nitrogen to satisfy these nitrogen-catabolizing enzymes. Hence the extraordinary protein requirement of the cat apparently results from a metabolic system obliged to catabolize protein. For most animals, survival advantage is gained by efficiently down-regulating metabolic pathways to compensate for reduced consumption of protein. The cat, however, has lost this adaptive trait characteristic of omnivores and has assumed the metabolic burden of an obligate carnivore.

A question that follows from the foregoing discussion is: How does the cat metabolize this abundance of dietary amino acids? Since the amount of amino acids required for protein synthesis in the cat does not appear to differ from that for most other animals, the excess amino acids might simply be utilized for energy (Greaves, 1965). Enzyme activity values in cat liver suggest that glucogenic amino acids are deaminated and converted to glucose rather than being oxidized directly for energy (Beliveau et al., 1981). Most of the energy needs, however, appear to be met by catabolism of the high fat content in the diet. Hence the cat forgoes nitrogen efficiency for energy efficiency, amino acids being oxidized directly or converted to glucose that is then oxidized, while fats provide the primary source of energy for the body as a whole.

**PRACTICAL ASPECTS OF THE PROTEIN REQUIREMENT.** Whereas an amino acid requirement is established by feeding highly digestible purified diets containing known quantities of crystalline amino acids, this experimental approach represents an obviously artificial situation. Natural foodstuffs contain complex proteins rather than purified amino acids and may in fact be less than ideal with respect to digestibility or composition. Furthermore, a source of protein that contains an ideal mixture of essential amino acids may not ensure optimal availability of those amino acids for metabolism, especially after the product has been commercially processed and heat-treated. To circumvent this problem, dietary allowances have been recommended that provide a margin of safety to accommodate reasonable individual variation in digestibility, absorption, processing, or other factors that interfere with optimal assimilation of nutrients. One should be aware that these allowances are established for growing kittens, whose demands for protein synthesis exceed those of nonpregnant, nonlactating adults.

It is also apparent that the higher quality meat and fish proteins, which cats tend to prefer, are better suited to the metabolic pathways that have evolved in this carnivorous species. With continued research, it is probable that protein considered of lesser quality (i.e., not containing optimal proportions of the essential amino acids) will be found useful, inexpensive sources of supplemental protein for the adult cat. This speculation is based on the knowledge that the cat (with its high protein intake and high capacity for nitrogen catabolism) readily metabolizes excess amino acids while retaining the essential components needed for protein synthesis.

It is noteworthy that until recently, before the actual essential amino acid and total protein requirements of cats were appreciated, maximal growth and reproductive performance were assured by diets that typically contained 25 to 30 per cent of calories as protein, i.e., about 10 per cent more protein calories than are required when all essential amino acids are present in balanced fashion. Ultimately it may be possible to feed less total dietary protein (16 to 18 per cent of calories), with far-reaching implications for overall nitrogen metabolism in cats, especially in reducing urea formation by a diseased liver and the nitrogen load on damaged kidneys.

Nonetheless, for practical purposes, diet formulation from crude protein sources (meat, fish, poultry, cereals) must still include substantial protein to ensure adequate essential amino acid intake by this species, with its "wasteful" amino acid–catabolizing system. An allowance of 28 per cent protein on a dry basis is currently recommended (Table 2–4).

## Basic Amino Acids

**ARGININE.** As indicated in Table 2–3, the cat's requirement for arginine far exceeds that of other animals, being as much as 1.1 per cent of the dry diet. This value reflects the relationship between dietary arginine levels and the processes of growth, nitrogen retention (Anderson et al., 1979a), food intake, and orotic acid excretion (Costello et al., 1980; Morris and Rogers, 1978a, b). This high level of arginine is required in part because the cat,

**Table 2–4 Recommended Nutrient Allowances for Cats (Percentage or Amount per Kilogram of Diet, Dry Basis,* and Daily Amount for an Adult Cat Eating 100 gm of Dry Food or Semi-moist or Canned Equivalent)**

| NUTRIENT | UNIT | AMOUNT | DAILY PER CAT |
|---|---|---|---|
| Protein† | % | 28 | 28 gm |
| Fat‡ | % | 9 | 9 gm |
| Linoleic Acid§ | % | 1 | 1 gm |
| Minerals | | | |
| Calcium | % | 1 | 1 gm |
| Phosphorus | % | 0.8 | 800 mg |
| Potassium | % | 0.3 | 300 mg |
| Sodium chloride‖ | % | 0.5 | 500 mg |
| Magnesium | % | 0.05 | 50 mg |
| Iron | mg | 100 | 10 mg |
| Copper | mg | 5 | 500 μg |
| Manganese | mg | 10 | 1 mg |
| Zinc | mg | 30 | 3 mg |
| Iodine | mg | 1 | 100 μg |
| Selenium | mg | 0.1 | 10 μg |
| Vitamins | | | |
| Vitamin A | IU | 10000 | 1000 IU (333 μg) |
| Vitamin D | IU | 1000 | 100 IU (2.5 μg) |
| Vitamin E¶ | IU | 80 | 8 IU (7.2 mg) |
| Thiamin | mg | 5 | 500 μg |
| Riboflavin | mg | 5 | 500 μg |
| Pantothenic acid | mg | 10 | 1 mg |
| Niacin | mg | 45 | 4.5 mg |
| Pyridoxine | mg | 4 | 400 μg |
| Folic acid | mg | 1 | 100 μg |
| Biotin | mg | 0.05 | 5 μg |
| Vitamin $B_{12}$ | mg | 0.02 | 2 μg |
| Choline | mg | 2000 | 200 mg |

*From National Research Council: Nutrient Requirements of the Cat (1978). Based on a diet with an ME concentration of 4 kcal/gm of dry matter. If dietary energy density exceeds this value, it may be necessary to increase nutrient concentrations proportionately (e.g., the recommended protein allowance for a diet with an ME concentration of 5 kcal/gm of dry matter would be 35 per cent). Nutrient levels selected have satisfactorily maintained adult cats and have supported the growth of kittens. It is probable that they would be adequate for gestation and lactation, but few such studies have been conducted. Since diet processing (such as extruding or retorting) may destroy or impair the availability of some nutrients, sufficient amounts of such nutrients should be included to ensure the presence of recommended allowances at the time the diet is eaten.

†Quality equivalent to that derived from unprocessed mammalian, avian, or fish muscle. Processing may lower protein quality and necessitate higher concentrations. See text for discussion of amino acid requirements.

‡No requirement for fat, apart from the need for essential fatty acids and as a carrier of fat-soluble vitamins, has been demonstrated. The figure of 9 per cent fat is listed because approximately this amount is necessary to develop a diet with a caloric density of 4 kcal ME/gm of dry matter. Fat favorably influences diet palatability.

§It may also be important to include 0.1 per cent arachidonic acid (see text).

‖Since reliable individual estimates of the need for sodium and chloride are not available, the need for both elements has been expressed as a recommended allowance for sodium chloride.

¶Higher levels may be necessary when large concentrations of unsaturated lipids, such as in tuna oil, are included in the diet (see text).

unlike most species (Featherston et al., 1973; Rogers et al., 1972), can neither synthesize ornithine de novo nor readily regenerate arginine from ornithine (Fig. 2–1). The latter observation is puzzling because feeding citrulline seems to supply adequate substrate for arginine biosynthesis. Apparently the citrulline synthesized from ornithine during removal of ammonia by the cat liver can neither leave the hepatocyte to be converted to arginine by the kidney nor be converted to arginine in sufficient quantity by the liver to supply extrahepatic needs for growth (Rogers and Morris, 1980). In most animals, glutamate and proline act as precursors to ornithine. With an adequate supply of these precursors and appropriate enzyme activity to convert them to ornithine, arginine becomes a dispensable amino acid for most adult mammals. The cat, however, apparently does not synthesize ornithine from either glutamate or proline (Morris and Rogers, 1978a, b) so that net synthesis of arginine does not occur. Thus arginine is essential for the cat.

Of all the essential amino acids, an acute deficiency of arginine in the cat has the most dramatic repercussions (Morris and Rogers, 1978a, b). Cats fed a balanced amino acid diet lacking arginine develop severe ammonia toxicity with vomiting, hyperesthesia, tetanic spasms, ataxia, apnea with cyanosis, convulsions, and coma within three hours. The reasons for this become clear when one considers the involvement of arginine in the urea cycle, which utilizes ornithine to convert toxic ammonia (an end product of amino acid catabolism) to relatively nontoxic urea. For the cycle to function effectively, each intermediate (including arginine) must be present (Fig. 2–1). As emphasized, the cat, unlike the rat, is unable to synthesize arginine or its precursor, ornithine, from glutamate or proline. Therefore a diet limiting in arginine causes malfunction of the urea cycle. Amino acids ingested in the absence of any one essential amino acid, including arginine, are unable to enter protein anabolic pathways, yet are rapidly deaminated by the high catabolic enzyme activity for amino acids maintained by the cat. Accordingly, a large load of dietary amino acids (in the absence of arginine) generates a level of ammonia that surpasses the capability of the suppressed urea cycle to detoxify it, producing ammonia intoxication. Thus, in addition to the requirement for protein synthesis, the unusual demand for arginine arising from the disposal of excess dietary nitrogen via the urea cycle explains the relatively high requirement of the cat for dietary arginine—a requirement met by consumption of extra animal protein.

**LYSINE AND HISTIDINE.** In addition to arginine, two other basic amino acids, lysine and histidine, are essential for the cat. Fox et al. (1973) and Jansen et al. (1975) demonstrated that growth of kittens depends on the addition of lysine to a wheat-gluten, lysine-poor diet, thus establishing the essentiality of this amino acid. Anderson et al. (1979a), using weight gain and nitrogen retention, estimated the lysine requirement of growing kittens to be about 0.80 per cent of the diet, a level that has been corroborated and more clearly defined by Morris and Rogers (1980).

A histidine requirement for normal growth in kittens has been reported to be about 0.3 per cent of the dry diet (Anderson et al., 1980b). Additional data are necessary, however, before the requirement can be firmly established. At present, an allowance of 0.4 per cent dietary histidine is recommended (Morris and Rogers, 1980).

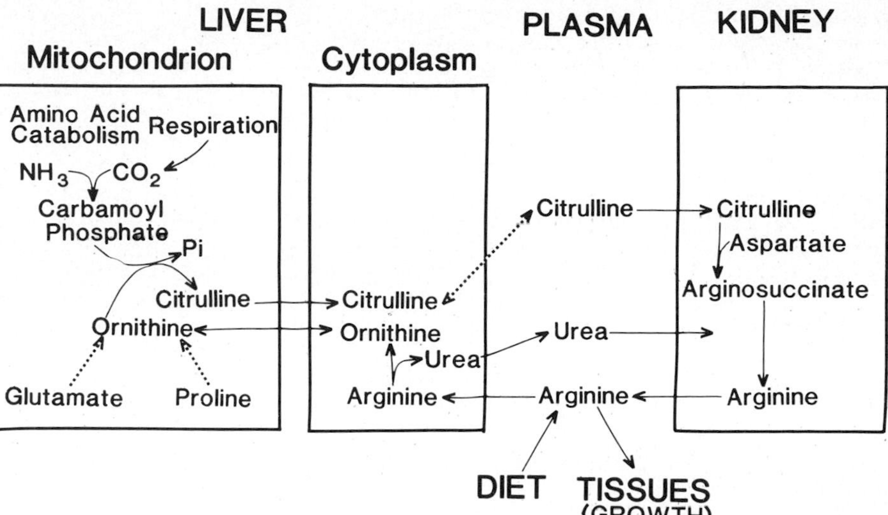


**Figure 2–1.** Metabolic pathway for arginine in the cat. Unlike the metabolism in most species, hepatic synthesis of ornithine and subsequent synthesis and secretion of citrulline (dotted lines) by the cat are apparently inadequate to satisfy renal arginine synthesis needed for growth of all tissues and resupply of the liver for nitrogen disposal. Ammonia accumulation and toxicity may result.

## Sulfur Amino Acids

**METHIONINE AND CYSTINE.** In addition to appreciating the requirement for sulfur amino acids (SAA) in protein synthesis, integrating the interactions within SAA metabolism is particularly challenging to the nutritionist. In most animals, methionine is the only essential SAA since it can be converted to the other sulfur-containing amino acids, including cysteine and taurine (Fig. 2–2). Methionine also provides sulfate for macromolecules such as mucopolysaccharides and is the primary donor of methyl groups for synthesis of hundreds of compounds, an example of which is choline. Thus the degree to which these numerous interactions depend on a source of methionine is directly reflected in the methionine requirement. For example, in a diet containing appreciable choline, inorganic sulfate, and cystine, the requirement for methionine is low by comparison with one in which one or more of these methionine-derived compounds is limiting.

The establishment of the methionine requirement in cats has had a rather confusing history. Early studies suggested that adult cats did not need this sulfur amino acid (Miller, 1957; Rambaut and Miller, 1965, 1966) or that the requirement was possibly less than 0.12 per cent of the dry diet (Dymsza and Miller, 1964). Further studies in kittens found maximal growth when methionine supplied approximately 0.9 per cent of the dry diet fed in conjunction with 0.06 per cent cystine (Ritter and Owens, 1974). Teeter et al. (1978a, b) indicated that growing kittens need 0.9 per cent sulfur amino acids, either as methionine alone or in combination with 0.45 per cent cystine, thus establishing the latter amino acid as dispensable. They also demonstrated that the cat utilizes D-methionine nearly as well as the more commonly occurring L-methionine. A study by Smalley et al. (1980) measured growth and nitrogen retention in cats to demonstrate that in a diet containing 0.6 per cent cystine and adequate choline (0.3 per cent), methionine in the amount of 0.33 per cent provides for maximal body weight gain and in the amount of 0.39 per cent for maximal nitrogen retention. The rate of weight gain was found to be much greater in males than in females, but no sex difference existed when the methionine requirement was expressed as percentage of dietary dry weight. Schaeffer et al. (1980, 1982) provided data consistent with the observations of Teeter et al. (1978a) that cystine is a dispensable amino acid, which nonetheless can supply as much as half the total sulfur amino acid requirement. In the absence of

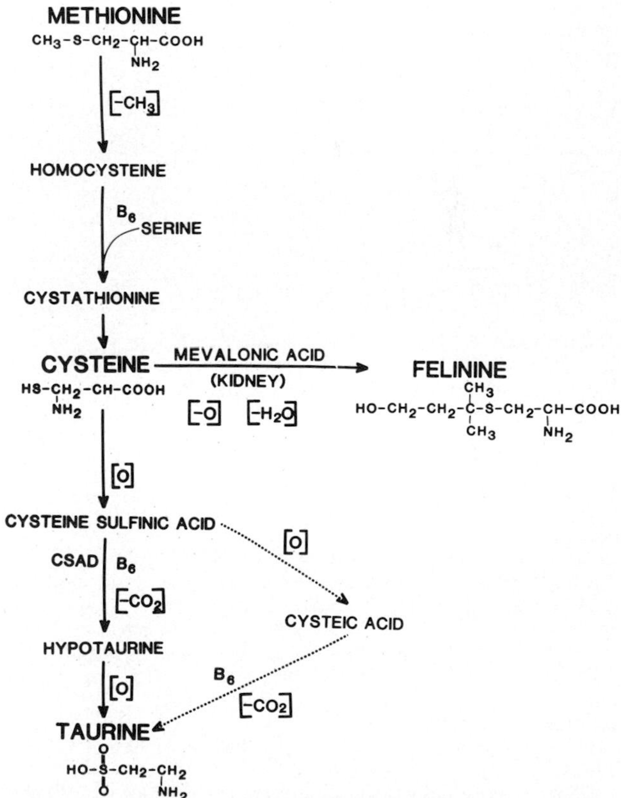


**Figure 2–2.** The cat's unique transulfuration pathway includes methionine, cysteine, felinine, and taurine. Conversion of cysteine to taurine is limited in cats owing to the low activity of the vitamin $B_6$-dependent enzyme, cysteine sulfinic acid decarboxylase (CSAD).

cystine, the methionine requirement was 0.7 per cent (Schaeffer et al., 1980, 1982). This value is considerably less than the 0.9 per cent value reported by Teeter et al. (1978b) and Ritter and Owens (1974), which was determined with diets of lower caloric density that induce greater food intake. These discrepancies have yet to be reconciled.

**TAURINE.** In keeping with its other metabolic peculiarities, the cat further complicates its sulfur metabolism by being incapable of adequate taurine biosynthesis. As a result, this β-amino sulfonic acid is a dietary essential, without which cats become blind (Hayes et al., 1975a). This deficiency may occur because taurine biosynthesis must compete with felinine biosynthesis for available cysteine. The cat is unique in its substantial excretion of felinine (Westall, 1953), synthesized from cysteine and mevalonic acid (a cholesterol precursor) (Fig. 2–2). Felinine, which is formed in the kidney (Tallan et al., 1954), may function as a territorial marker, since male cats excrete more than females. The amount excreted varies, but it often exceeds the daily taurine requirement (20 to 30 mg). Cat urine has small amounts of other sulfur-containing organic compounds (Mizuhara and Oomori, 1961) that add to the drain of sulfur from metabolic pools and consequently contribute to the dietary sulfur requirement (including methionine) of the cat.

Taurine deficiency in cats has gained attention because of the retinal degeneration (feline central retinal degeneration, FCRD) that results from its absence from the diet (Fig. 2–3). Originally thought to be an hereditary defect (Rubin and Lipton, 1973) or an expression of vitamin A deficiency (Scott et al., 1964; Scott, 1975), the retinopathy represents disruption and loss of photoreceptor outer segments (Hayes et al., 1975b) coupled with disintegration of the highly structured rods of the tapetum lucidum (Sturman and Hayes, 1980). Growth in newborn kittens is markedly depressed by taurine depletion (Hayes, unpublished data), a circumstance that does not seem to pertain in weanling or young adult cats (Hayes et al., 1975b; Rogers and Morris, 1980). The latter presumably have a greater capacity for synthesizing taurine, a slower growth velocity, and larger tissue reserves at the onset of depletion.

The cellular role of taurine is unknown, but it appears to function in the stabilization of cell membranes and in the excitatory process as a free amino acid that is not incorporated into peptides in the manner of the carboxylic α-amino acids. The cat appears uniquely susceptible to deficiency of taurine because of its poor synthetic capacity and because feline bile acids are obligatory taurine conjugators (Hayes and Sturman, 1982; Rabin et al., 1976). Essentially unexplored is the relationship of taurine to the sense of smell and the effect of taurine depletion on atrophy of the olfactory lobe (Anderson et al., 1979c).

The actual dietary requirement for taurine in cats depends somewhat on the level of total SAAs present in

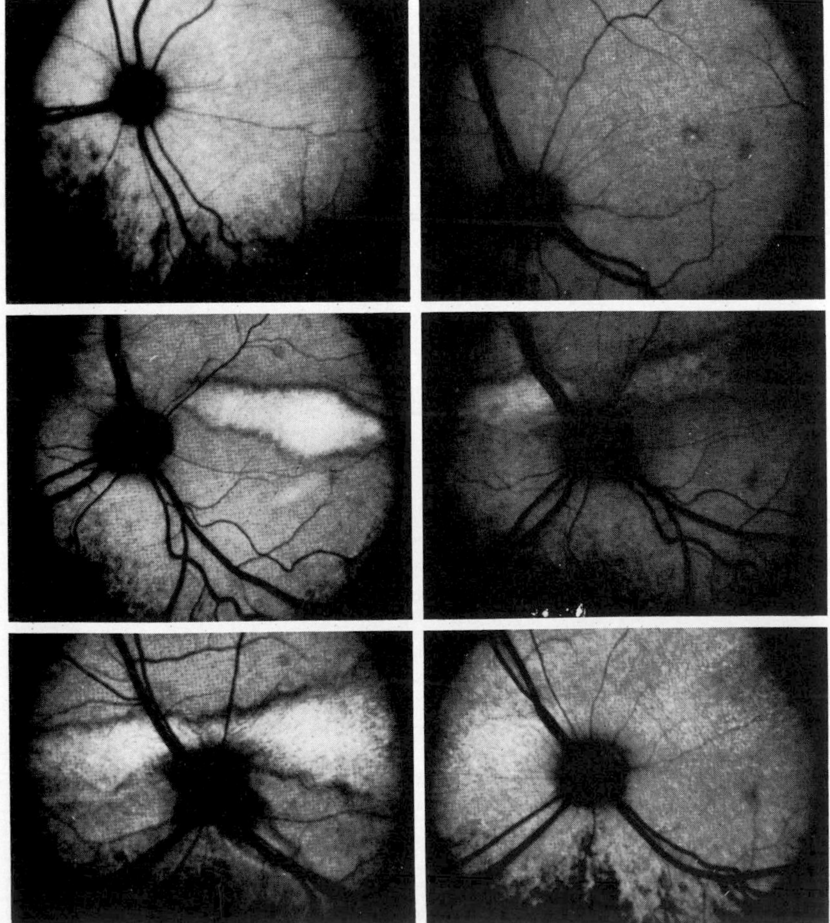

**Figure 2–3.** Progressive feline central retinal degeneration develops in cats fed diets that lack taurine. Normal tapetum (top left) develops focal hyperreflective spot (top right) and subsequent zonal degeneration in the dorsolateral and dorsomedial quadrants. This condition is sometimes observed clinically in cats eating vegetable-based dog food or, in extreme cases, those forced to eat vegetarian diets by their owners.

the diet. The dietary requirement increases when the total SAA content drops below 1.55 per cent of the diet in young adult cats (O'Donnell et al., 1981). Younger, growing kittens apparently need significantly more taurine than they can synthesize, even when supplemental methionine or cystine is fed (Berson et al., 1976). The best estimates suggest that growing kittens require a dietary level of taurine between 500 and 750 ppm (NRC, 1981) or about 20 to 30 mg per day. These estimates are based on the response of the plasma taurine to changes in dietary levels.

Since taurine is practically absent from the plant kingdom, it is not surprising that a number of clinical cases of FCRD have resulted from feeding cereal-based dog foods to cats (Aguirre, 1978). High concentrations of taurine (200 to 400 mg/kg wet weight) are normally present in meat (including poultry) and fish, with extraordinary levels (up to 2500 mg/kg) reported for shellfish. Clams and clam juice are excellent sources of taurine. Ironically, the normal carnivorous diet of cats would preclude their developing taurine deficiency. It is also interesting that taurine is the most concentrated free amino acid in milk of early lactation in cats and several other species (Hayes and Sturman, 1981), assuring the newborn of a ready supply of this sulfur amino acid for growth and development.

### AROMATIC AMINO ACIDS

**PHENYLALANINE AND TYROSINE.** Although tryptophan is an essential aromatic amino acid, the phenylalanine and tyrosine requirements have traditionally been referred to as the total aromatic amino acid (TAAA) requirement because tryptophan is needed in relatively small amounts. In fact, the cat is normally capable of deriving tyrosine from phenylalanine, so that only the latter is actually essential. Anderson et al. (1980b) reported that the TAAA requirement is about 1 per cent of the dry diet, which is considerably greater than that reported for other species. This value, however, is at best an approximation, since the increments tested were large (i.e., the nearest experimentally tested levels of dietary tyrosine differed from the suggested optimal value by 40 per cent) and the sample size was rather small (four or five kittens per group). Thus the TAAA requirement may be the same for cats as for other animals.

**TRYPTOPHAN.** The essentiality of tryptophan for cats has been shown by Anderson et al. (1980b), who estimated the requirement as 0.15 per cent of the dry diet, a value comparable to that for the rat. Adding a 20 per cent margin of safety, a tryptophan allowance of 0.18 per cent has been recommended (Morris and Rogers, 1980). It is noteworthy that the cat, unlike most other animals, cannot utilize tryptophan as a precursor for niacin synthesis. Experimental evidence indicates that kynurenic acid, an intermediate in the synthesis of niacin from tryptophan, is neither metabolized (Gordon et al., 1936) nor synthesized (Jackson, 1939) by cats. Accordingly, tryptophan failed to substitute for niacin in experimental cat diets (Braham et al., 1962; Carvalho da Silva et al., 1952; Leklem et al., 1969). Ikeda et al. (1965) reported that the cat possesses a pathway for niacin synthesis, but that a second tryptophan catabolic pathway (the picolinic acid decarboxylase pathway) exhibits far greater activity. Thus niacin synthesis from tryptophan catabolism is functionally absent in cats.

### BRANCHED-CHAIN AMINO ACIDS

**VALINE.** On the basis of weight gain, nitrogen balance, and plasma amino acid values, Hardy et al. (1977) suggested that the valine requirement of kittens is about 0.6 per cent of the diet. Later, Anderson et al. (1980c) supported this observation by recommending an allowance of 0.7 per cent of the dry diet.

**LEUCINE.** The kitten's requirement for leucine has also been estimated by Anderson et al. (1980c) as 1.2 per cent of the dry diet, a value considerably greater than the 0.83 per cent required by the pig or 0.75 per cent needed by the rat. As with TAAA requirement, the data are inconclusive owing to the large increments fed during experimental balance studies.

**ISOLEUCINE.** The requirement for the third essential branched-chain amino acid, isoleucine, has been estimated as 0.3 per cent of the dry diet (Anderson et al., 1980c). This value is lower than that reported for other species (Table 2–3), but as for valine and leucine, the data are inconclusive. A dietary isoleucine allowance for the cat of 0.6 per cent has been recommended (Baker, 1980; Morris and Rogers, 1980).

### HYDROXY AMINO ACIDS

**THREONINE.** Three separate studies estimated the threonine requirement for growing kittens as 0.7 per cent of the diet (Anderson et al., 1980c; Rogers and Morris, 1979, 1980; Titchenal et al., 1980). Titchenal et al. (1980) also described neurologic malfunction presenting as marked lameness of the limbs that responded to threonine supplementation. Since threonine is often the second or third limiting amino acid in both animal and vegetable protein, an awareness of the threonine requirement will increase its importance in commercially formulated diets. The recommended allowance for threonine is 0.85 per cent of the dry diet (Morris and Rogers, 1980).

## CARBOHYDRATE

An appropriate level of carbohydrate in the diet of the cat is dictated more by palatability than by nutritional requirement. In fact, a requirement for dietary carbohydrate in the cat has not been demonstrated and is assumed to be nonexistent as long as glucogenic precursors (glycerol and amino acids) are available. Newborn kittens require considerable lactose in their diet if they are to consume an osmotically balanced formula and a digestible form of carbohydrate. More complex polysaccharides have been used for many years in commercial and experimental rations for weanling and adult cats without deleterious effect.

A comparison of the apparent digestibility of starch, dextrin, glucose, sucrose, lactose, and cellulose fed as 20 per cent of the dry diet revealed that all except cellulose are readily digested by the mature cat (more than 96 per cent) (Trudell and Morris, 1975). Pencovic and Morris (1975) examined the effect of milling and cooking on the digestibility of corn and wheat starch at 35 per cent dry weight and found that both substances are well digested by the cat, especially when finely ground. These values reflect only apparent digestibility and do not account for losses such as that from colonic fermentation; however, since no gastrointestinal disorders were reported, one can assume that digestibility was maximal.

With the advent of semimoist cat foods there has been renewed interest in the taste response of cats and their tolerance for mono- and disaccharides, since these sugars are important in the formulation of such diets. Sucrose is less palatable for cats than for other species (Carpenter, 1956; Pfaffmann, 1955; Zotterman, 1956) because there are few sucrose-sensitive nerve endings in feline taste buds. Nevertheless, interactions between sucrose and other dietary components can affect taste preference (Bartoshuk et al., 1971, 1975; Frings, 1951), and diets containing dextrin are more readily eaten by cats than diets containing sucrose, although the reason remains unclear (Greaves and Scott, 1963).

Studies of intestinal disaccharidase activity indicate that the cat possesses a high potential for digesting sugars (Hore and Messer, 1968). As the cat approaches maturity, the activity of intestinal β-fructofuronidase (sucrose-hydrolyzing enzyme) decreases from the level in the kitten (Morris et al., 1977). In addition, neither this enzyme nor β-galactosidase (lactose-hydrolyzing enzyme) activity was affected by addition of sucrose or lactose to the diet, an indication that activities of these disaccharidases are not responsive to dietary levels of their substrate sugars. Sucrose and glucose are accepted and tolerated by kittens at 15 per cent of the diet (Drochner and Muller-Schlosser, 1980). Significantly, the gastrointestinal tract became intolerant when these sugars constituted 25 per cent of the diet. Although causing no trouble in the newborn kitten, lactose was poorly tolerated at both levels and promoted severe diarrhea in these weanling kittens. Similar results were obtained with solutions of sugars (Passe and Lee, 1982). The discrepancy between the results of these researchers and those of Trudell and Morris (1975) mentioned previously may be due to the method of administration. Trudell and Morris (1975) included lactose in the dry diet, whereas Passe and Lee (1982) added lactose to the water. In veterinary practice, milk is recognized as an important cause of diarrhea in many kittens and cats.

## FAT

### Dietary Level and Source

Meat (on a dry weight basis) is essentially devoid of carbohydrate, its two major components being protein and fat. Not surprisingly, fat normally provides most of the energy in the feline diet, and the level of dietary fat plays a major role in diet palatability and acceptance (Greaves, 1965; Schneck and Cumberland, 1968; Scott, 1966). For this reason a dietary allowance of 9 to 10 per cent is recommended (Table 2–4). Digestibility of fat in the cat is high, varying between 85 and 99 per cent (Kane et al., 1981a; NRC, 1978), and high levels of dietary fat (64 per cent dry weight) have not resulted in adverse clinical signs (Scott and Humphreys, 1962).

Both the amount and the source of dietary fat influence food acceptance and growth in kittens (Kane et al., 1981a; MacDonald et al., 1981a). Diets containing 25 per cent hydrogenated coconut oil were found unpalatable and failed to support growth. Even when acceptance was improved by adding small amounts of essential fatty acids as safflower oil or chicken fat, normal growth was not restored. By contrast, hydrogenated beef tallow did support growth in kittens, although tested for only seven weeks. Again, growth was not improved by addition of safflower oil or tuna oil. This difference between fats was attributed to palatability, since the hydrogenated beef tallow diet was consumed at almost five times the level of the hydrogenated coconut oil diet. Similarly, kittens chose beef tallow (nonhydrogenated) over chicken fat (3:1), although no significant difference in palatability was noted between diets containing 35 per cent fat as hydrogenated tallow and those containing regular beef tallow (MacDonald et al., 1981a).

### Essential Fatty Acids

Certain polyunsaturated fatty acids are key components of phospholipids and, as such, represent an important component of membranes and precursors for a group of metabolic regulators, the prostaglandins and leukotrienes. Since the basic configuration (i.e., the location of certain double bonds) for most of these fatty acids cannot be formed by the cat, they must be provided in the diet and are referred to as essential fatty acids (EFA).

Essential fatty acids are categorized as belonging to the γ-linoleic acid (18:2ω6) series or the α-linolenic acid (18:3ω3) series. In most animals, all other EFAs are derived from these two parent molecules by 2-carbon elongation and specific desaturase enzymes (Fig. 2–4). Since significant metabolic effort is required to maintain an enzyme system, the cat has taken advantage of the circumstance that the phospholipids in its meat diet contain the required EFAs, thus eliminating the need for the synthetic machinery. As a consequence, the cat (Hassam et al., 1977; Rivers et al., 1975) and the lion (Rivers et al., 1976b) no longer readily convert α-linolenic or γ-linoleic acid to other EFAs. Thus, as with its peculiar requirement for amino acids, the cat relies on a high meat content in the diet to supply most of its EFAs.

Fatty acid requirements of the cat were first reported by Rivers et al. (1975, 1976a, c), who compared several diets containing different amounts of linoleic acid, linolenic acid, and their derivative fatty acids. On the basis of the fatty acid composition of plasma phospholipids, these investigators determined that the cat could elongate essential fatty acids, but lacked sufficient Δ6- or Δ8-desaturase activity to desaturate them into needed derivative fatty acids. Thus, linoleic and α-linolenic were elongated to dihomo-γ-linoleic (20:2ω6) or dihomo-α-linolenic (20:3ω3), but were not desaturated to form arachidonic (20:4ω6) or eicosopentaenoic (20:5ω3) acid.

MacDonald et al. (1981b) detected only minimal activity of Δ6- and Δ5-desaturases in the cat (about 1/40 of that in the rat) and proposed that this low activity may have nutritional implications. Sinclair (1979) and Sinclair et al. (1981) also reported minimal Δ5- and Δ8-desaturase activity, and Frankel and Rivers (1978) made a similar finding concerning Δ4-desaturase activity. As in other species, Δ9-desaturase activity is found in cats, and although the resulting fatty acid (oleic, 18:1ω9) is not a dietary essen-

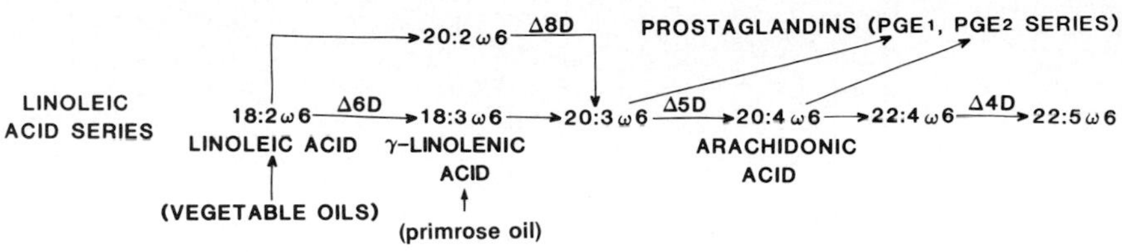


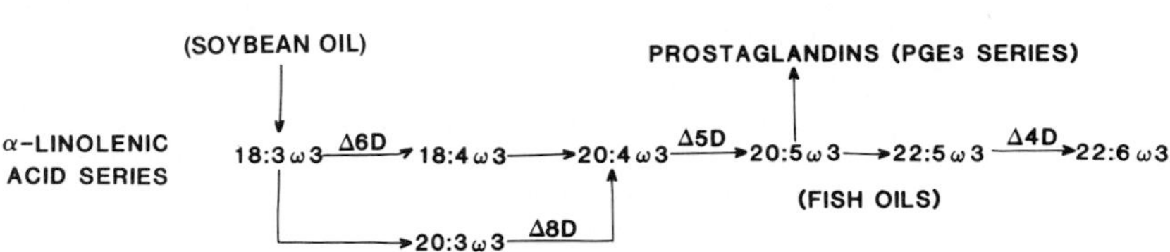


**Figure 2–4.** Pathway for essential fatty acid metabolism in cats. Unlike most species, the cat lacks adequate desaturase enzymes to generate arachidonic acid and other required long-chain polyunsaturated fatty acids.

tial, it is thought to be necessary for the phospholipids incorporated into nervous tissue (Rivers and Frankel, 1980).

MacDonald et al. (1983) have further demonstrated that dietary linoleate is essential for regulating water permeability of cat skin, independent of any conversion to other fatty acids. They also found that dietary arachidonic acid was needed by cats for reproductive function in females but not males (MacDonald et al., 1984c). Queens lacking dietary arachidonic acid failed to deliver viable kittens, whereas 18:2ω6 alone maintained seminiferous tubule architecture and spermatogenesis in males because the testes were able to form 20:4ω6 from linoleic acid. Thus, unlike the liver hepatocyte, the testes appeared to have Δ5-desaturase activity.

The foregoing data indicate major qualitative differences in the types of fatty acids required by the cat as compared with other species, but exact quantitative estimates of a requirement are difficult to make because several months of feeding an EFA–free diet are needed to induce clinical signs of deficiency. Clinical manifestations of EFA deficiency are reported to be a greasy and scruffy hair coat with dandruff, slow wound healing, flaccid testes, retarded growth and weight loss, anestrus, fatty liver, mineralization of kidneys, impaired platelet aggregation, and an elevated white blood cell count (MacDonald et al., 1981b, 1984a,b; Rivers and Frankel, 1980; Sinclair et al., 1981). The implication is that cats require a source of animal fat.

Extremely painful steatitis, advanced hyperkeratosis of the footpads, and mild alopecia with scaly dermatosis developed in kittens made deficient in EFA and vitamin E by feeding of safflower oil stripped of vitamin E (Fig. 2–5). Although tocopherol supplementation prevented the clinical signs of deficiency, the EFA level in RBC fatty acids from the experimental cats fed the presumably adequate semi-purified diet was only one-sixth the level found in RBC from kittens fed a commercial diet. Growth in tocopherol-supplemented kittens was essentially normal, a finding that suggests that growth may not be a sensitive index of depressed EFA availability in this species. More detailed histologic and biochemical characterizations are needed before firm conclusions are drawn regarding the EFA requirement in cats. Accordingly, an attempt to establish specific requirements for each EFA is unrealistic at this time. A rather generous level (2.5 per cent of calories) fed as linoleic acid has been suggested as safe (Rivers and Frankel, 1980). From the data of Rivers et al. (1975) and the content of EFA in commercial products, the National Research Council (1978) calculated the arachidonic acid requirement as 0.10 per cent of the dry weight, whereas the data of MacDonald et al. (1984c) suggest that 0.04 per cent of the energy supplied as 20:4ω6 would assure pregnancy and lactation except when fish oil was added. Fish oil contains ω3 fatty acids (20:5ω3, 22:6ω3), which can displace 20:4ω6 and inhibit Δ6 and Δ5 desaturase enzymes. In most species 1 per cent of calories are recommended as linoleate to supply the entire EFA requirement. Collectively the data suggest that most of the EFA requirement in the cat can be satisfied by linoleic acid with a probable dietary requirement for fatty acids of the α-linolenic acid series (18:3ω3, 20:5ω3), arachidonic acid, and eicosotrienoic acid under certain dietary circumstances. The peculiar EFA requirement of the cat may be increased by the tendency of mono- and polyunsaturated fatty acids to inhibit desaturase enzyme activity. Feeding polyunsaturated vegetable oils or fish oils that do not contain all the necessary EFAs may slow biosynthesis of those that are needed and lead to peroxidative damage of those already present if sufficient vitamin E is not supplied.

## VITAMINS

### Fat-Soluble Vitamins

Deficiencies of the fat-soluble vitamins should be considered whenever exocrine pancreatic insufficiency is diagnosed and when chronic diarrhea or other evidence of fat malabsorption is present, since adequate absorption of fat is required for the absorption of these vitamins. Vitamin E deficiency is probably the most commonly encountered of these deficiencies in cats owing to inclusion of polyunsaturated fish oils in certain diets. Ironically, hypervitaminosis A and, potentially, vitamin D excess are more likely complications than their deficiencies because these vitamins can be stored in the body to reach dangerous concentrations. Clients should be informed that the use of cod liver oil, rather than mineral oil, for prevention

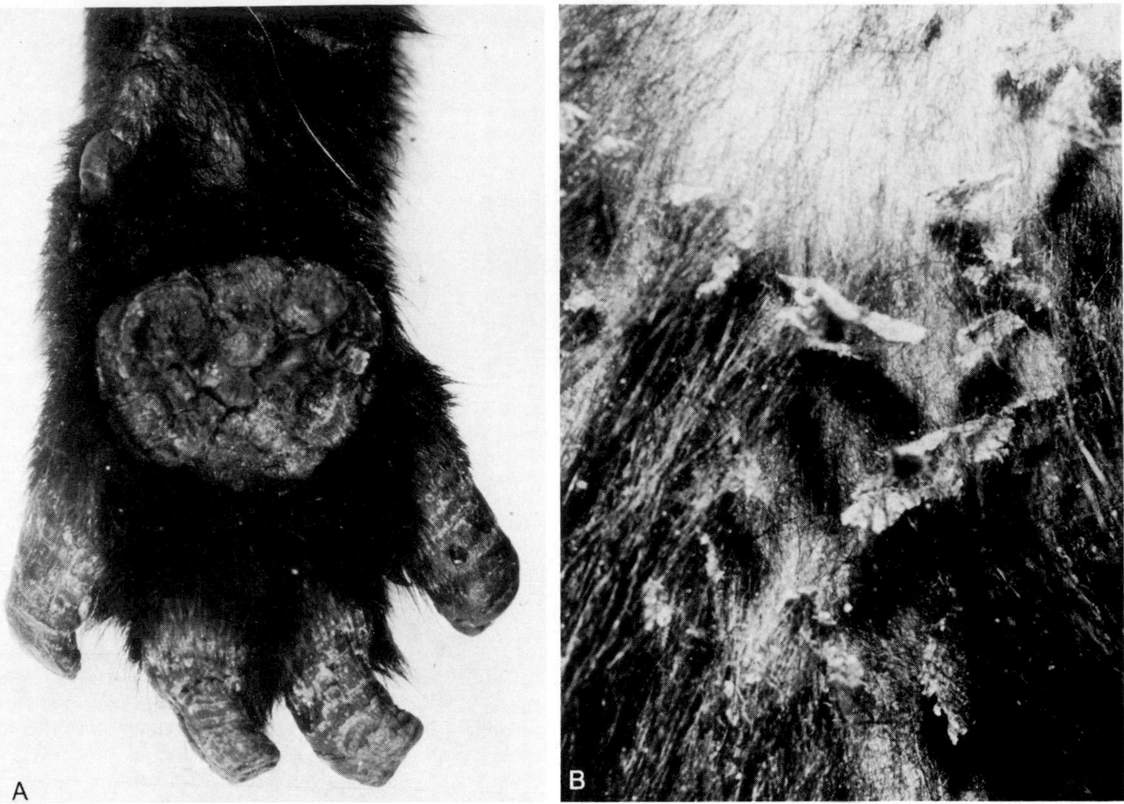


**Figure 2–5.** Advanced hyperkeratosis of the claws and footpads (*A*) and scaly dermatosis with alopecia (*B*) were observed in kittens made deficient in vitamin E and essential fatty acids.

of hairball formation is contraindicated because of the high level of vitamins A and D in the former. Excessive use of mineral oil, however, can interfere with absorption of the fat-soluble vitamins.

**VITAMIN A.** Vitamin A has marked effects on cell growth and differentiation, especially on the epithelial tissues of the body. The cat lacks the enzyme required to convert the vitamin A precursor β-carotene to the active compound **retinol** (Gershoff et al., 1957a). Thus it ordinarily relies on preformed retinyl palmitate stored in the liver of mammals or fish it consumes to meet its vitamin A needs. This form of vitamin A is stable to heat exposure during cooking but may be oxidized by extended exposure to sunlight and air.

Spontaneous vitamin A deficiency is seldom diagnosed in the domestic cat, probably because cats do not ordinarily eat a low-fat, low–vitamin A diet, and signs of debilitating inanition and lethargy would most likely precede those of overt deficiency.

Experimental deficiency has been induced in kittens fed high-fat, high-protein purified diets (Gershoff et al., 1957a). The younger the kittens, the more rapidly the deficiency developed. The first signs were loss of weight, serosanguineous exudates about the eyelids, and weakness and incoordination, especially in the hindquarters. The muscular weakness was sometimes associated with a well-defined increase in muscle tonus. Most of the kittens had some degree of bronchopneumonia. Bizarre subpleural cysts lined with squamous epithelium bulged above the surface of the lungs. Corneal ulceration was present in advanced deficiency. Microscopic studies disclosed squamous metaplasia of the conjunctiva, salivary glands, uterus, and respiratory tract. It is of interest that no pathologic changes were present in the urinary tract, for vitamin A deficiency is often listed among possible causes of urinary tract infection and the formation of calculi.

Previous descriptions of night blindness in vitamin A–deficient cats (Morris, 1965; Scott et al., 1964) are complicated by the fact that these diets were based on casein, so that taurine deficiency was presumably concurrent and unrecognized. Vitamin A depletion in most species often leads to epithelial infections, since this vitamin is required for mitosis and differentiation of mucous cells that secrete surface antibody in the form of IgA. Deficiency is clinically accompanied by anorexia and emaciation with ataxia, and the diagnosis is best confirmed by a low plasma vitamin A concentration (less than 40 μg/dl is suspect; less than 15 μg/dl, deficient) (Knox, 1982).

**Hypervitaminosis A.** More often the cat develops hypervitaminosis A, also referred to as deforming cervical spondylosis because of its most prominent feature. A bone disease caused by a diet exclusively or mostly of beef or sheep liver, it is a striking and easily recognized clinical entity of domestic cats. Experimental studies have reproduced the condition by feeding of liver with both normal and high levels of vitamin A and by feeding of excessive doses of vitamin A itself.

The condition appears to have been first recognized in Uruguay (Christi, 1957), but it received serious veterinary attention only after publication of a group of studies from Australia, where beef and sheep liver is an abundant, inexpensive food for cats. Subsequently, numerous clinical and experimental reports of the disease appeared in New Zealand, the United States, Great Britain, and Western Europe.

Cats with naturally occurring hypervitaminosis A have ranged in age from two to nine years (English and Seawright, 1964; Riser et al., 1968). No breed or sex predilection has been recognized. Months or years of liver diet precede signs of toxicity. When first affected, cats are lethargic, seek isolation, lie down almost constantly, and resent handling. After several months, stiffness of the neck or lameness in one or both forelegs is the first specific sign of skeletal abnormality. It has been suggested that the neck may be affected first because of the cat's constant licking activity, but in time ankylosis of the cervical diarthrodial joints prevents grooming, and the cat's coat becomes unkempt and matted. Because the cat cannot turn its head, it must, to change its line of vision, move its entire body. Lameness in the forelegs is due to ankylosis of the elbow and occasionally shoulder joints and probably also to pinching of spinal nerves. If the elbow joints become fixed in flexion, the cat may assume a kangaroo-like sitting position with forelegs elevated. Inactivity and the restricted character of the diet frequently cause constipation, and fusion of the cervical vertebrae makes eating difficult so that the cat loses weight. Bone changes involving the hip and stifle joints occasionally cause an abnormal crouching gait of the hind legs.

On physical examination, cutaneous hyperesthesia is sometimes apparent along the back of the neck and thorax and occasionally on the dorsum of the forelegs. The neck cannot be flexed, and exostoses immobilizing vertebral joints may be palpated from as far forward as the atlanto-occipital articulation to the midthoracic region. After cervical fusion, ankylosis of the elbow is next in frequency, then ankylosis of other limb joints. The sternebrae and ribs are often involved by osseocartilaginous proliferations, and occasionally also the surface of the long bones, scapulae, and pelvis, so that they are abnormally enlarged (e.g., Riser et al., 1968).

Although it was early recognized that a diet consisting wholly or largely of liver would also be deficient in calcium (e.g., Riser et al., 1968), experimental studies with diets high in liver or vitamin A as well as deficient or adequate in calcium clearly established the essentially different characteristics of hypervitaminosis A and calcium deficiency (e.g., Seawright and Hrdlicka, 1974).

Lesions can be produced in as little as 15 weeks of experimental vitamin A supplementation. In trials with very young kittens it was also discovered that hypervitaminosis A, whether from feeding of a liver diet or excessive supplementation with the vitamin, caused edema and inflammation of the gums, faulty alveolar development, and loosening of incisor teeth—features not typical of the naturally occurring disease in older cats (Seawright and Hrdlicka, 1974). Damage to the epiphyseal plates of the long bones and consequent shortening also occur in young kittens given massive doses of vitamin A (Clark and Seawright, 1968).

Radiographs are diagnostic in cases of naturally occurring toxicity, demonstrating the striking cervical ankylosis (Fig. 2–6*A*) and subperiosteal new bone deposition (Fig. 2–6*B*).

Data on serologic values are limited. In a naturally occurring case the calcium level was 8.8 mg/dl, phosphorus 3.6 mg/dl, and alkaline phosphatase significantly elevated (Riser et al., 1968). The normal plasma level of vitamin A is given as about 70 μg/dl (Riser et al., 1968; Scott, 1975) or 100 μg/dl (Scott, 1964), but in cats receiving liver diets, plasma levels ranged from 451 to 1281 μg/dl (Seawright et al., 1967).

The pathologic changes have been described in detail (e.g., English and Seawright, 1964; Lucke et al., 1968; Riser et al., 1968; Seawright et al., 1967). Proliferating cartilaginous and subperiosteal tissue invades joints, causing enlargement and ankylosis. A similar proliferation may occur on the surfaces of sternebrae, scapulae, pelvis, and long bones. The subperiosteal osseous hyperplasia suggests that the periosteum is especially sensitive to high concentrations of vitamin A and can be stimulated by trauma and exertion of attached ligaments and muscles. There is concurrent absorption of cortical bone and replacement by new cancellous bone, resulting in remodeling of the original bone. The proliferation may also extend to involve the origins of muscles, producing localized myositis ossificans. Extensive involvement of vertebrae impinges on nerve roots and may cause atrophy of the spinal cord. Normal marrow adjacent to affected bone is replaced by relatively acellular fibrous and vascular tissue.

The liver is enlarged and pale. Hepatocytes and reticuloendothelial cells of the liver, hepatic node, lungs, and spleen, as well as renal epithelial cells, are infiltrated with lipid that contains fluorescent particles of vitamin A.

Change to a balanced diet when cervical stiffness and lameness first develop gives clinical relief, prevents further progression of the disorder, and in time promotes regression of appositional bone. Established ankyloses, however, are irreversible, but discomfort has been alleviated without ill effect by administration of phenylbutazone 12 to 16 mg/kg body weight twice a day (English and Seawright, 1964). Food dishes should be elevated to make eating and drinking easier. Owners should be warned of the dangers of feeding excessive amounts of liver. To judge from the amounts of vitamin A itself required to induce toxicity in kittens, it is unlikely that harmful overdosing of the vitamin would occur under natural conditions.

The minimal amount of vitamin A needed to prevent deficiency is 15 μg (or 45 IU)/kg body weight/day in essentially all species, and a practical allowance would be 100 μg (or 300 IU)/kg (about 10,000 IU/kg diet). Toxicity occurs only when intake exceeds 20,000 μg (or 60,000 IU)/kg body weight/day for a prolonged period. Serum and liver vitamin A levels become greatly elevated and provide the most direct means of making a diagnosis.

In experimental studies, plasma levels of vitamin A ranged from 180 μg/dl in control cats (vitamin A intake from beef and milk apparently not known) to more than 1200 μg/dl in toxic cats (Seawright et al., 1967). Liver levels ranged respectively from about 800 μg/gm to more than 35,000 μg/gm. Additional experiments with kittens given doses of about 40,000 μg/kg/day for four weeks induced acute toxicity with depression of appetite and reluctance to walk (Clark et al., 1970). The latter resulted from arrested growth of epiphyseal cartilage and a distorted tibial crest dorsally, causing abnormal restriction of stifle joint extension. Such changes are not typical of spontaneous toxicity.

The role of a high-liver diet in spontaneous disease is

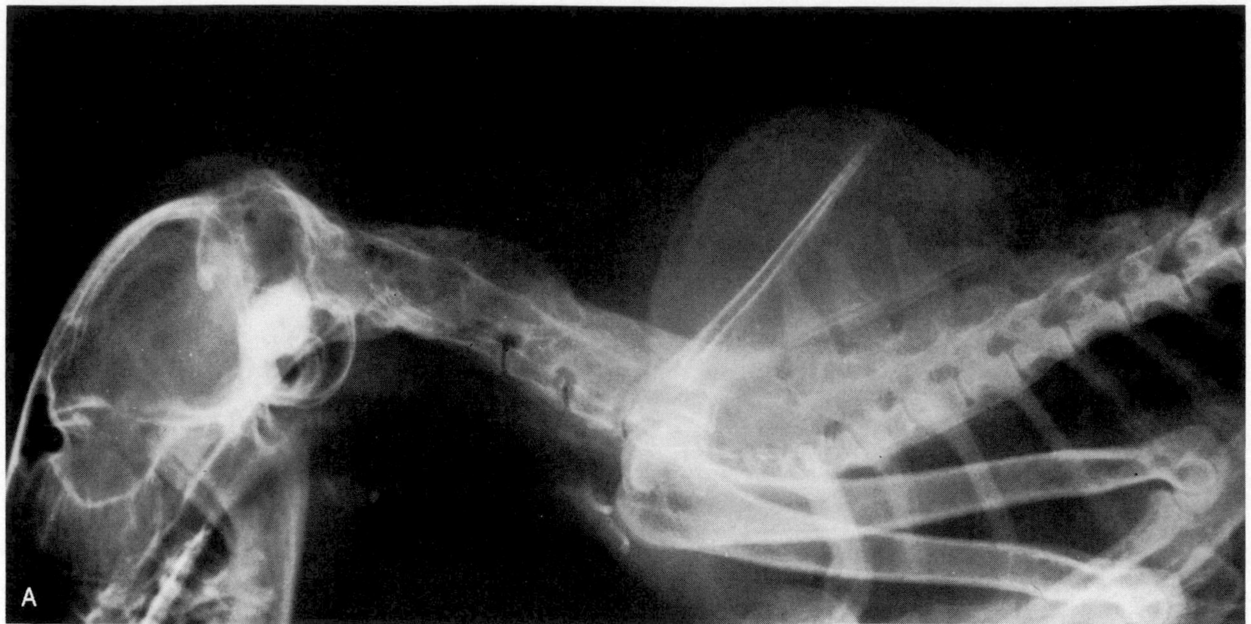


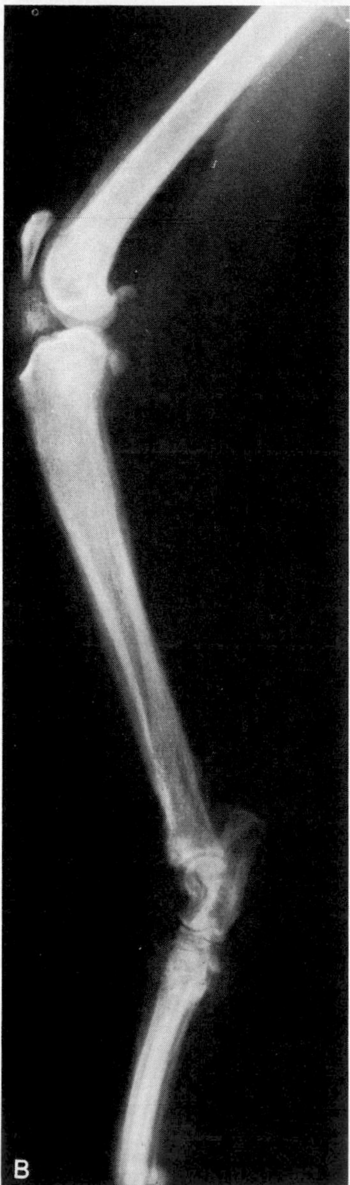


**Figure 2–6.** *A*, Dorsal exostoses and fusion of the cervical vertebrae (spondylosis) in a three-year-old female cat with chronic vitamin A toxicity. (Courtesy Dr. Frederick Busch.) *B*, Subperiosteal bony proliferation is present along the femur, tibia, tarsus, and metatarsus and on the patella in a cat fed beef liver and suffering from chronic vitamin A toxicity. (Courtesy Dr. Robert S. Brodey.)

not fully understood, since under controlled conditions, a greater amount of vitamin A than is usual in liver is required to induce comparable toxicity.

**VITAMIN D.** Vitamin D plays a major role in the mobilization of calcium and in the mineralization of bones in both young and adult. A deficiency of vitamin D or an imbalance in the calcium:phosphorus (Ca:P) ratio results in deficient calcification, which takes the form of rickets in the young and osteomalacia in older animals. Vitamin D occurs abundantly in fish-liver oils and is synthesized by the action of sunlight on 7-dehydrocholesterol in the skin. Vitamin D is added to pasteurized milk and is also present in small amounts in the fat fraction of milk.

Naturally occurring rickets and osteomalacia are rare in cats. Experimentally produced rickets has been studied by Gershoff et al. (1957b), and certain peculiarities of its pathogenesis in kittens have been noted. Although it is generally accepted that the rachitogenicity of a diet increases as the Ca:P ratio deviates from 1 to 1.5:1, and that such deviations are essential for producing rickets in rats, severe rickets was produced in kittens given vitamin D–deficient diets with Ca:P ratios of 1:1 and 2.0:0.65. Surprisingly, the more severe rickets was associated with the 1:1 ratio. A possible explanation for this was that the cats fed the 2.0:0.65 ratio diet ate less well and therefore grew more slowly. In the cats receiving the 1:1 ration, rickets generally became progressively severe, whereas a curious cycle of spontaneous exacerbations and remissions occurred in cats given the 2.0:0.65 ratio diet.

The most severe changes involved the costochondral junctions of the ribs and were the same as in man—a markedly irregular costochondral line; a thick, irregular layer of mature cartilage; disorganization in the region of new bone formation; excessive osteoid; an increased number of osteoblasts; and a swollen costochondral junction.

Radiographic changes are likewise the same as in man. There is an initial rarefaction and irregular fraying of the epiphyseal plate, which fades into the soft tissue density of the adjacent epiphyseal cartilage. Later, more pronounced changes include enlargement of the ends of the long bones, haziness and cupping of the diaphyses, and a wide, radiolucent shadow between the epiphyseal ossification center and the end of the shaft. These changes were associated with increased activity of alkaline phosphatase.

Ultimately, in both vitamin D–deficient groups, the rickets of the kittens that survived was healed, even though vitamin D was never supplied—a circumstance suggesting that the requirement of grown cats for vitamin D is low. Although the exact quantitative requirement of cats for vitamin D was not determined, 250 IU of vitamin $D_3$ given orally twice a week was adequate for the control cats. Carvalho da Silva et al. (1952) met the requirement experimentally by giving 2 ml of cod liver oil three times a week. Addition of 1 per cent cod liver oil to the ration appears to accomplish the same purpose (Gershoff, 1959).

Effects of overdosage of vitamin D were observed at autopsy in a cat that over a six-month period had been given 5 million IU of vitamin $D_3$ and 2.5 million IU of vitamin A by mouth. The cat was given these vitamins as treatment for a skin ailment, but gradually lost weight and suddenly died. The most outstanding changes occurred in the circulatory system. The great vessels, including aorta and the carotid arteries, had calcified, the adrenals were almost completely calcified, and calcium was deposited in the stomach wall and parathyroids. There was no increased fragility of the bones (Suter, 1957).

**VITAMIN E.** Vitamin E, known chemically as **α-tocopherol,** is a biologic antioxidant that is synthesized by plants and found in vegetable oils. It is stored in egg yolk and liver. The deficiency of this vitamin, referred to as steatitis, pansteatitis, or "yellow fat disease," was first reported in young cats fed commercially canned cat food, presumably fish (Cordy and Stillinger, 1953) or known to be fish-based (Coffin and Holzworth, 1954). In these cases the conspicuous findings were firmness and an orange or brownish yellow discoloration of the fat of the subcutis and body cavities. Histologically the fat was heavily infiltrated with neutrophils and some macrophages, and an acid-fast pigment was demonstrated (Fig. 2–7). Subsequently Cordy produced the disease experimentally by feeding a commercial canned cat food and demonstrated that it could be prevented by supplementation with vitamin E (Cordy, 1954).

Vitamin E deficiency did not become a significant clinical problem until 1957, when the red (dark) meat of tuna was introduced into canned cat foods. These became the most palatable foods on the market, many cats preferring them to any other. Cases of steatitis were soon encountered on the west coast of the United States where the food was first marketed, but red tuna had become widely distributed and very popular by the time its association with naturally occurring steatitis was first brought to the attention of the veterinary profession in 1958 by Munson et al. and later by Griffiths et al. (1960). The

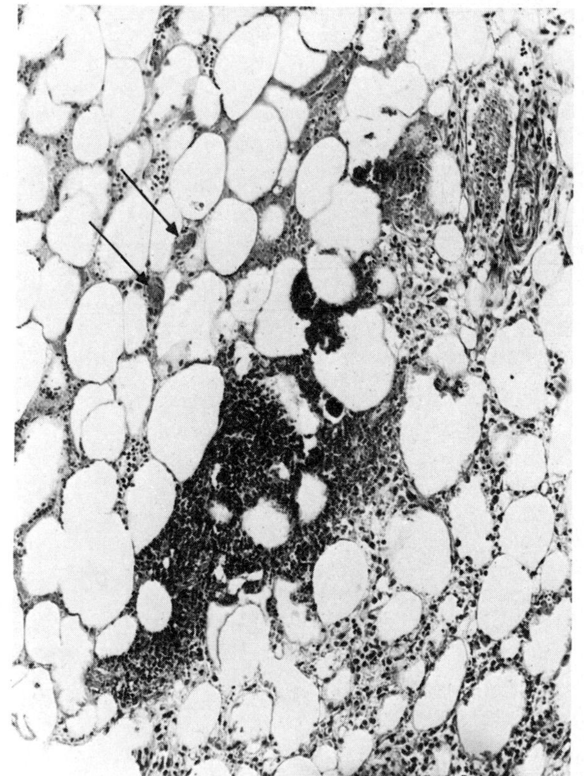

**Figure 2–7.** Steatitis due to chronic vitamin E deficiency. Section of adipose tissue demonstrating interstitial inflammatory cells, necrosis, and aggregates of peroxidized lipid-ceroid (arrows).

association with red tuna is presumably linked to the higher content of polyunsaturated fish oils in the dark meat of tuna, and although supplements of vitamin E are added to these diets, steatitis still occurs occasionally in cats (Gaskell et al., 1975).

During a 10-year period (1958 to 1968), 63 cases were observed at the Angell Memorial Animal Hospital (P.T. Theran, unpublished data). Most of the cats affected were young adults (average age, 2.5 years), the majority females (41 of 63), that received red-meat tuna as all or part of their diet for weeks or months. Rather infrequently older animals were affected, and the food was occasionally a mixture of red- and white-meat tuna, or other fish or fish-base food. In rare instances the diet was primarily liver.

Typically the owner first notices that the cat is eating poorly and is unwilling to move about and jump onto its favorite place. It is then discovered that the cat is sore to the point of hypersensitivity over almost its entire body. It will not tolerate even the lightest stroking over its backbone, and abdominal palpation is so painful that it cannot be performed. When the condition is far advanced, the lumpiness of the subcutaneous fat is easily detectable, particularly in the groin, where it may even be mistaken for an inguinal hernia. Frequently the cat has a rather high fever that persists in spite of antibiotic treatment. In untreated cases the white-cell count tends to climb progressively and may reach 70,000 to 100,000/μl just before death. The increase is mostly in neutrophils, but the eosinophils are sometimes moderately elevated.

Biopsy specimens should be taken from the area of greatest tenderness, usually the groin or back. A tractable cat may require only a local anesthetic. In the early stages the fat, although lumpy or "lobulated," is not discolored; later it becomes dirty yellowish or grayish white and ultimately assumes the characteristic mustard-yellow color imparted by ceroid, the inert peroxidation product of the polyunsaturated fatty acids deposited in adipose tissue.

Treatment consists most importantly of a change in diet. The cat must be coaxed by all possible inducements to eat, for the painful and inflamed condition of the subcutis does not permit administration of fluids by that route. The inflammation in the subcutis, which is essentially a foreign-body reaction, may be reduced by oral administration of cortisone. The vitamin E deficiency is treated by daily oral administration of one or two capsules of α-tocopheryl acetate (100 IU vitamin E).

The response to treatment is gradual, recovery requiring weeks or even months, owing to the difficulty in getting cats to accept a change in diet. Occasionally there is little or no response, and the cat slowly wastes away until it dies or is destroyed by the discouraged owner. Sudden and unexpected death may occur.

In cats that die or are destroyed in advanced stages of the disease, the subcutaneous fat, except that of the head and neck, is a dirty orange or mustard-yellow and is lumpy. The fat within the body cavities has a similar character. Occasionally there is an inflammatory effusion in the abdomen.

The characteristic microscopic lesion consists of infiltration of the fat with neutrophils and numerous mononuclear cells (lymphocytes, plasma cells, and macrophages). The ceroid pigment, an end-product of lipid peroxidation, is found in macrophages, in fat cells, in Langhans-type giant cells, and extracellularly (Fig. 2–7). Macrophages in liver, spleen, and mesenteric lymph nodes may also contain the pigment (Cordy and Stillinger, 1953). It is best demonstrated with acid-fast stains. In some cases, microscopic studies have disclosed degenerative changes of the myocardium.

Gershoff and Norkin (1962) tested the effects of tuna oil in the diet on the vitamin E requirement. Cats fed a diet containing 20 per cent lard (vitamin E–free) as the sole lipid source did not develop steatitis after 13½ months, although mild degenerative myopathy was noted in skeletal and cardiac muscles. They concluded that the cat fails to exhibit clinical signs of vitamin E deficiency seen in other animals and suggested that 34 IU of vitamin E/kg dry diet prevented all lesions of deficiency under their conditions (i.e., 20 per cent lard). However, when 5 per cent of the lard was replaced with tuna oil, severe steatitis developed precipitously in the tenth month. Under these circumstances, vitamin E added at 136 IU/kg dry diet prevented all lesions. Thus it was concluded that the steatitis associated with fish oils is a function of the increased need for dietary vitamin E to prevent lipid peroxidation caused by diets high in polyunsaturated fats. Scott and Humphreys (1962) also provided experimental evidence consistent with this concept. In the study by Stephan and Hayes (1978), tocopherol fed at 100 IU/kg diet prevented signs of deficiency when a diet containing 15 per cent stripped safflower oil was fed.

Since vitamin E availability and utilization depend on the diet and the sensitivity of an individual animal to peroxidation, more data, including the effect of various polyunsaturated:saturated fat ratios and levels of dietary fat on vitamin E status, must be accumulated before an accurate (practical) vitamin E requirement can be established. In addition, the sparing effect provided by artificial antioxidants should prove to be a nutritionally significant aspect of the vitamin E requirement. Pending further experimental evidence, the current NRC recommendation of 80 IU/kg diet appears rather generous, particularly since some commercial cat foods presumably meet performance standards with as little as 10 or 33 IU/kg in dry and canned foods, respectively. The losses due to processing of cat food have not been tested.

**VITAMIN K.** It appears that cats do not require a dietary source of vitamin K, as evidenced by their maintenance of normal prothrombin times in the absence of dietary vitamin K (Reber and Malhotra, 1961). It is reasonable to assume that the needs for this vitamin are met through synthesis by the intestinal microflora of the cat (Scott, 1966). Accordingly, caution should be exercised during long-term oral therapy with antibiotics that effectively sterilize the gut.

## WATER-SOLUBLE VITAMINS

**THIAMINE (Vitamin $B_1$).** Thiamine in the form of thiamine pyrophosphate is a coenzyme involved in the oxidative decarboxylation of pyruvate and α-ketoglutarate and in the transketolation of glucose, processes concerned with the utilization of carbohydrates. Good sources are yeast, lean pork, fowl, beef, kidney, liver, egg yolk, legumes (especially peas), potatoes, milk, and whole-grain cereals. The vitamin may sometimes be destroyed in heat-processing of foods or by thiaminase, an enzyme present in a wide variety of fish (Jubb et al., 1956). Storage in the body is limited.

Thiamine deficiency predominantly affects the nervous system, the gastrointestinal tract, and the cardiovascular system. It was first produced experimentally in cats fed a diet of canned dog food and brewers' yeast, autoclaved to destroy the thiamine. The condition produced was prevented and cured by administration of thiamine (Everett, 1944; Odom and MacEachern, 1942).

Three stages are distinguishable in acute thiamine deficiency (Everett, 1944). In the first, which may last for several days, the cat, although acting interested in food, stops eating and salivates. It also loses weight, vomits, and develops slight ataxia or "weaving" of the hindquarters. The second, critical stage develops suddenly with the appearance of neurologic disturbances—impaired righting and vestibulo-ocular reflexes, spasticity, dilatation of the pupils with a slow response to light, circling, dysmetria, and spinal hypersensitivity. Early in the critical stage there is a rapid succession of short tonic convulsions in which the cat is curled rigidly with ventriflexion of the head and neck (Fig. 2–8). Even when the cat is held suspended by the hindlegs it maintains the ventriflexion of the head. This phase is succeeded by spasticity of the limbs, so that the cat seems to walk on its toes, and by a spinal hypersensitivity so acute that a tap on the back may elicit a sudden extensor thrust. The retinal veins are dilated, and sometimes there are retinal hemorrhages.

Toman et al. (1945) reported that cardiac disorders in thiamine deficiency in cats include abnormal slowing and acceleration of the heart rate, sinus irregularity, excitement syndrome, and ectopic rhythm.

All signs of thiamine deficiency disappear within a day if thiamine is administered (1 mg IM or 5 mg orally). Otherwise the cat passes into a third stage of semicoma, continuous crying, opisthotonos, and maintained extensor tone and dies within a day or two. If thiamine deficiency is suspected, the diagnosis is easily confirmed clinically by the rapid response to injection of B-complex vitamins if thiamine alone is unavailable.

In cats destroyed in extremis, there were nonspecific changes of dehydration and malnutrition (Jubb et al., 1956). A lesion ordinarily rare in cats was observed—ulceration of the mucosa of the pylorus. The brain lesions in acute cases were typically focal, bilaterally symmetric hemorrhages in the periventricular gray matter. The only consistent and most severe involvement occurred in the inferior colliculi where the hemorrhages were visible. Lesions also occurred in the medial vestibular, lateral geniculate, habenular, and oculomotor nuclei; in the accessory vestibular, cuneate, and red nuclei; and irregularly in the mamillary bodies, accessory cuneate nucleus, superior colliculi, and commissures of the nucleus reuniens and ciliary nucleus. Occasionally there were hemorrhages in the medial and small pyramidal cell layers of the occipital cortex.

Microscopically the lesions exhibited varicose dilatation of the blood vessels, especially the veins, with focal extravasations, hemorrhages, and edema. Reparative changes were represented by vascular hypertrophy, gliosis, and "gitter" cell formation. The vascular dilatation was a general phenomenon within the brain and spinal cord and, as already noted, appeared in the retina too. Acute neuronal necrosis was observed in the olivary nuclei only in the naturally occurring cases and was thought perhaps to be due to niacin deficiency.

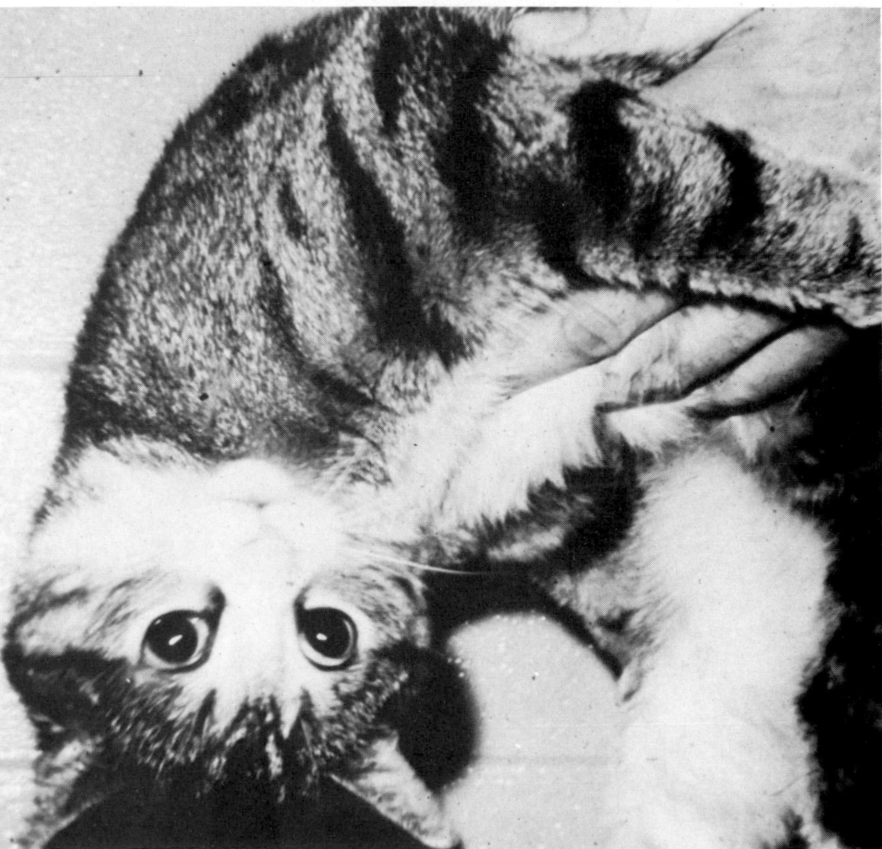

**Figure 2–8.** Ventriflexion of the head and neck in a cat suffering from thiamine deficiency. (From Loew F et al.: Can Vet J 11 [1970] 109.)

Many kinds of fish, from both salt and fresh water, contain thiaminase (Deutsch and Hasler, 1943; Jubb et al., 1956) (Table 2–5). Since as many as 60 species of fish from the Atlantic and Pacific coasts may be used in commercial cat foods at various times of the year, a real possibility exists that certain lots will be deficient in thiamine (Jubb et al., 1956).

Thiamine may also be destroyed in processing or during prolonged storage of canned cat food (Baggs et al., 1978). It is fairly resistant to high temperature and oxygen in a weakly acid medium, but if the pH is allowed to rise above 6.0, there may be considerable loss of the vitamin in the presence of heat and sulfite (Loew et al., 1970). It would thus appear that processing must be regulated with great care or that supplements of thiamine should be added after cooking.

**Table 2–5 Fish Reported to Contain Thiaminase***

| STUDIES | FRESHWATER FISH | SALTWATER FISH |
|---|---|---|
| America | Buckeye shiner<br>Bullhead<br>Burbot<br>Carp<br>Catfish<br>Chub<br>Goldfish<br>Minnow spp<br>Sauger pike<br>Smelt<br>Sucker<br>White bass<br>Whitefish | Herring |
| Scandinavia | "Bjorkna"<br>Carp<br>Crucian<br>Perch†<br>Pike<br>Roach<br>Rudd<br>Tench<br>"Vimma" | Bream<br>Cod‡<br>Garfish<br>Herring<br>Sprat |
| Japan | Carp<br>Catfish<br>Eel<br>Gray mullet<br>Goby | A variety of shellfish, including:<br>Clams<br>Crab<br>Lobster |
| Russia | Carp | Flounder, Herring, Smelt, Skate } White Sea<br>Black Sea shark, Some sturgeon spp } Black Sea |

*Compiled from Deutsch and Hasler (1943) and Jubb et al. (1956). The whole fish of some species contains thiaminase (in some the viscera only [Deutsch and Hasler]). Smelt and herring would be important among saltwater fish. Feeding any of the fish listed, whole or raw, to cats would be dangerous. In processed food the danger is that the thiaminase acts to destroy the thiamine before processing.

†Thiaminase was not found in *Perca flavescens* by Deutsch and Hasler but was found in *Perca fluviatilis* by Suomalainen and Philgren (1955; cited by Jubb et al.).

‡Thiaminase was not found in *Gadus morrhua* by Deutsch and Hasler but was found in *Gadus callarias* by Suomalainen and Philgren.

Owing to intestinal synthesis and biologic variability, the requirement for thiamine is difficult to establish. Nevertheless Loew et al. (1970) estimated a requirement of 0.36 mg/day for a 3 kg cat. The NRC (1978) set an allowance of 5 mg thiamine/kg diet, which would provide about 0.44 mg per day.

An interaction exists between thiamine and glutamate intake (Deady et al., 1981a, b) such that glutamate fed at a level greater than 9 per cent of the diet can induce thiamine deficiency in kittens supplemented at a level of 4.4 mg/kg of diet (the NRC recommended allowance available at that time was published in 1972). The mechanism is unknown. Observed signs included vomiting, anorexia, depressed growth, and opisthotonos. The potential hazard implied by this observation is that cat foods formulated with high vegetable protein, which contains more glutamate than most animal proteins, may increase the risk of thiamine deficiency. In a product subjected to retorting (i.e., high-heat sterilization), the loss of thiamine is appreciable, so that the risk of deficiency is even greater with canned cat foods.

A preferred treatment for otherwise normal anorexic and lethargic cats is to provide supportive fluid therapy and an injection of B-complex vitamins. The positive response of many such cats may reflect their marginal thiamine status.

**RIBOFLAVIN (Vitamin $B_2$).** Riboflavin is a necessary component of the physiologically active coenzymes involved in essential oxidation-reduction reactions during energy metabolism. It occurs in muscle, liver, kidney, milk, eggs, and leafy vegetables. Gershoff et al. (1959a) described marginal riboflavin deficiency (1 to 2 mg/kg diet) in the cat, with signs that included rather acute cataract formation, testicular hypoplasia, and limited periauricular alopecia with histologic evidence of epidermal atrophy, as well as fatty infiltration of the liver. In contrast, acute deficiency resulted in nonspecific emaciation. Cats were maintained satisfactorily on high carbohydrate diets for 34 months with 3 mg riboflavin/kg diet, or on high-fat diets for two years with 4 mg riboflavin/kg diet, the different requirement being attributed to greater intestinal synthesis of riboflavin during high-carbohydrate feeding. Leahy et al. (1967) proposed that cats fed a low-fat diet require no more than 100 μg/day. The NRC (1978) recommended 5 mg riboflavin/kg dry diet.

**NIACIN (Nicotinic Acid, Nicotinamide, Niacinamide).** Niacin enters into the formation of coenzymes I and II, involved in carbohydrate metabolism. It is present in yeast, raw meat, milk, eggs, leafy vegetables, and cereals (except corn). It seems reasonable that because the cat cannot synthesize niacin from tryptophan it would be particularly sensitive to niacin deficiency, but this relationship has not been explored fully. Heath et al. (1940) first described pellagra in cats. Signs include inappetence, erosions of the tongue and palate, drooling of thick foul saliva, diarrhea, emaciation, and death within 20 days. Carvalho da Silva et al. (1952) suggested 10 mg of niacin per day as an adequate dietary intake. Braham et al. (1962) estimated a requirement of 5 mg per day. NRC (1978) recommended an allowance of 45 mg niacin/kg diet or about 2 to 3 mg/day. It is probable that niacin, thiamin, and riboflavin deficiencies often occur in combination (Scott, 1964), since these vitamins are derived from similar food sources and are sensitive to similar destructive processes during diet processing. Since raw meat is an excellent source of B vitamins, cats that hunt are probably in little danger of developing these deficiencies; however, the feeding of raw meat is not recommended because of possible transmission of toxoplasmosis.

Niacin in massive doses may cause a distressing degree of transient vasodilation. A 50 mg tablet of niacin administered to an anorexic cat by its physician-owner evoked, within five minutes, signs of intense agitation and discomfort. The cat ran around, jumped, and rolled, with skin twitching. Its pupils were dilated, and it appeared frightened and licked frantically at itself. Within 15 minutes all signs had resolved. The veterinarian to whom the cat was taken for consultation found that the disturbance was consistently reproduced when he gave 50 mg niacin tablets to his own cats (Sheffield, 1983).

**PYRIDOXINE (Vitamin $B_6$).** Pyridoxine, which is primarily a cofactor for enzymes concerned with the intermediary metabolism of protein, is found in muscle and glandular meats, legumes, potatoes, and wheat germ but in only moderate amounts in milk and eggs. Carvalho da Silva et al. (1959a) and Gershoff et al. (1959b) described pyridoxine deficiency in cats. Because pyridoxal phosphate plays such a key role in transamination and decarboxylation of amino acids, its shortage results in signs that include growth depression and depressed red blood cell formation expressed as a microcytic, hypochromic anemia with an elevated serum iron and hemosiderosis of the liver. Convulsive seizures have been reported. Advanced renal disease may also develop, characterized histologically by renal tubular atrophy and dilatation with fibrosis surrounding intratubular deposits of calcium oxalate crystals. These crystals are readily observed in the urine as well. Since consumption of ethylene glycol or oxalate-containing plants can result in similar crystals, a veterinary clinician should inquire as to possible exposure or access to ethylene glycol–containing chemicals (e.g., antifreeze) or oxalate-containing plants.

Available data suggest that the requirement for vitamin $B_6$ is low (less than 2 mg/kg diet) (Gershoff et al., 1959b). NRC (1978) recommended 4 mg/kg diet.

**PANTOTHENIC ACID.** Gershoff and Gottlieb (1964) induced pantothenate deficiency in cats and reported weight loss, fatty liver, and blunting of villi in the small intestine. They estimated the requirement to be no more than 5 mg/kg dry diet. NRC (1978) recommended an allowance of 10 mg pantothenic acid/kg dry diet; but since the cat's requirement is so low and the vitamin so prevalent, there is little concern that a clinical deficiency will ever be observed.

**FOLIC ACID.** The lack of sensitive methods for analysis of highly purified diets may explain the inability of Carvalho da Silva et al. (1955) to demonstrate a folate requirement in the cat unless they also included sulfonamide drugs to block synthesis of folate by the intestinal microflora. Schalm (1974) described severe anemia and a megaloblastic bone marrow in a cat that responded to folate and vitamin $B_{12}$ administration. Thenen and Rasmussen (1978) induced folate deficiency in kittens by feeding a casein-based diet containing lard, sucrose, and dextrin as the source of energy. They followed plasma, red blood cell, and liver folate depletion in these kittens and observed megaloblastic erythropoiesis and increased urinary formiminoglutamic acid excretion (after injection of the precursor, histidine) without overt anemia. Their control diet contained 2 mg/kg folic acid and maintained normal tissue stores. NRC (1978) recommended an allowance of 1 mg folate/kg dry diet.

**CYANOCOBALAMIN (Vitamin $B_{12}$).** This vitamin, abundant in liver and kidney and in lesser amounts in milk, muscle, and fish, combines with intrinsic factor from the stomach to ensure its absorption across the ileum. Once absorbed, it is involved in DNA synthesis, including that needed for red cell production. Long-term deficiency in humans is associated with peripheral neuropathy, but this aspect of the deficiency has not been demonstrated in domestic animals. Keesling and Morris (1975) produced vitamin $B_{12}$ deficiency in cats by feeding a soy protein diet, since vegetable protein does not contain this vitamin. The onset of deficiency was evidenced by progressive weight loss and inappetence, a wet appearance to the hair coat, and occasional pica. Hematologic values and bone marrow morphology remained normal. Injection of 10 μg/day induced immediate and dramatic weight gain. These investigators did not estimate a requirement, but NRC (1978) recommended an allowance of 20 μg vitamin $B_{12}$/kg dry diet.

Many veterinary practitioners believe that vitamin $B_{12}$ is helpful (or at least they employ it) for a variety of clinical conditions; however, an inappetent and cachectic cat is likely to be suffering from multiple deficiencies and would be more apt to benefit from a multivitamin preparation than from vitamin $B_{12}$ alone.

**BIOTIN.** Carey and Morris (1977) were unable to produce a biotin deficiency in cats fed a diet containing all nutrients except biotin. However, by feeding dried egg white (presumably containing avidin, which binds biotin) and succinylsulfathiazole, they successfully induced biotin deficiency associated with depressed hepatic activity of propionyl-CoA carboxylase, a biotin-dependent enzyme needed in the conversion of propionic acid to succinic acid. Daily subcutaneous injection of 0.25 mg D-biotin prevented all signs of deficiency, which included dried discharges about the eyes, nose, and mouth; alopecia with generalized xerosis and dandruff; and anorexia resulting in weight loss. Miliary dermatitis in cats has been reported to respond to biotin treatment at a level of 50 to 200 mg IM weekly (Joshua, 1965). In the healthy cat most of the biotin requirement is presumably met by intestinal synthesis.

**CHOLINE.** Choline is present in animals and vegetables as a base component of lecithin, which is required in the mobilization of fat from the liver and contributes methyl groups to the synthesis of methionine. Choline is also a part of acetylcholine, involved in neuroexcitation.

Carvalho da Silva et al. (1959b) described fatty liver and poor growth due to choline deficiency in the cat. They found that 30 mg of choline/day could prevent hepatic lipid accumulation and restore normal growth. Hypoalbuminemia was also described (Mansur Guérios and Hoxter, 1962). As mentioned earlier, methionine contributes methyl groups for the synthesis of choline. Anderson et al. (1979b) have shown that in the cat a level of dietary methionine (0.37 per cent), providing methyl groups equivalent to 0.1 per cent choline, completely replaced the dietary need for choline by donating the methyl groups needed for choline biosynthesis. The diet contained 25 per cent turkey fat, whereas that of Carvalho da Silva et al. (1959b) contained 24 per cent hydrogenated coconut oil and a low level of methionine. Thus the difference in the two observations is explained. Furthermore, it is clear from the previous discussion of lipids that hydrogenated coconut oil is EFA–deficient and is poorly tolerated by the cat, factors that may have further complicated the experimental results. Until it is known to what extent methionine can replace or spare choline under varying dietary conditions, especially those related to the level and type of fat, an allowance of 2 gm choline/kg dry diet is recommended (NRC, 1978).

**INOSITOL.** Inositol is synthesized by most species, especially by the accessory reproductive organs in males, and is incorporated into phosphatidyl inositol, which is important to cellular secretory processes, such as lipoprotein secretion.

Scott (1964) reported an inositol deficiency manifested as a fatty liver in the cat regardless of the choline status. Approximately 10 mg inositol per day (0.02 per cent of diet) offered adequate protection.

**OTHER VITAMINS.** No other chemicals have been reported to have vitamin activity in the cat. Ascorbic acid (vitamin C), which cannot be synthesized by primates and guinea pigs, is synthesized by the cat from glucose, but according to Scott (1975), depressed production during severe infection may result in a deficiency. Ascorbic acid is recommended by some clinicians as a urinary acidifier, but its efficacy is extremely limited (see discussion of the feline urolithiasis syndrome).

As mentioned earlier, the mechanism of taurine function remains obscure. Its requirement in the cat is somewhat greater than that for the vitamins, but considerably less than that for other essential amino acids. Furthermore, cats are capable of synthesizing a variable amount of taurine depending on the available sulfur amino acid pool, a fact that removes it from vitamin status.

## MINERALS

Of the many minerals known to be essential nutrients in most species, only a few have been studied in the cat. Undoubtedly the concepts being generated by continuing research in trace mineral metabolism with humans and laboratory animals will increase our understanding of mineral requirements in the cat. The current estimated allowances for several minerals are included in Table 2–4.

### Major Minerals

Several minerals are required in the diet in rather large quantities and are important determinants of fluid pH and osmotic balance in tissues. They are accordingly referred to as electrolytes and include sodium, potassium, chloride, calcium, phosphorus, and magnesium.

**SODIUM, POTASSIUM, AND CHLORIDE.** These three electrolytes are best appreciated for their role in fluid and ionic balance in individual cells and the whole body. Weight loss, dry skin, and alopecia have been associated with a deficiency of sodium chloride. Following the suggestions of Scott (1960, 1964) and Morris (1968) and incorporating a margin of safety, NRC (1978) recommended an allowance of 0.5 per cent sodium chloride in the dry diet. Most commercial diets contain three to four times that amount.

The feline requirement for potassium is linked to the protein level in the diet (Hills et al., 1982). Whereas 0.3 per cent potassium was required in diets containing 33 per cent protein, the requirement increased to 0.47 per cent potassium in diets containing 68 per cent protein. The mechanism for this interaction with protein remains to be determined. Without benefit of these data NRC (1978) recommended an allowance of 0.3 per cent.

The signs of potassium deficiency in the cat resemble those in other species: anorexia, depressed growth, emaciation, lethargy, unkempt fur, and locomotive disorders (ventriflexion of the head, ataxia of the hind limbs, reduced flexion of the joints, and eventual inability to stand or walk) (Hills et al., 1982). Since animal tissues generally contain considerable potassium, deficiency is unlikely with a carnivorous diet. However, because plant-derived ingredients constitute a larger percentage of the diet, potassium supplementation may become an increasingly important consideration.

**CALCIUM AND PHOSPHORUS.** Calcium is one of the most ubiquitous and versatile minerals found in higher organisms. Together with phosphorus, magnesium, and fluoride it contributes to bone and tooth structure. As a part of the cell membrane and cytoskeleton it contributes actively to the control of cell metabolism. It also plays an essential role in blood clotting. In addition, neuromuscular transmission requires calcium, as do countless other metabolic reactions. With so many critical functions at stake, calcium homeostasis is tightly controlled and provides one of the more complex examples of intermediary metabolism.

Little work has been done regarding the control of calcium metabolism in the cat, but it is assumed that the mechanisms are the same as in other species. Any differences in calcium metabolism between the cat and dog, for example, appear to be in magnitude. The kitten is born with about 750 mg of calcium in storage (Jackson, 1968). Considering that the weanling kitten is one of the fastest growing mammals, requiring 200 to 400 mg of calcium per day (Scott, 1965), this reserve would be depleted quickly if the diet were limiting in calcium. The burden of providing calcium (and all other nutrients) to the kitten rests with the lactating queen, whose calcium requirement under this stress is over 600 mg daily (Scott, 1975). If the lactating cat does not ingest adequate calcium, her bone reserves are mobilized, with ultimate depletion of the bone mass (Humphreys and Scott, 1964). It is noteworthy that the lactating queen and growing kitten demonstrate an exemplary efficiency of calcium absorption, exceeding 80 per cent (compared with the usual 30 per cent in the nonlactating adult) (Scott, 1964, 1975). Urinary excretion of calcium is also decreased during lactation (Roberts and Scott, 1961).

It is inappropriate to discuss calcium homeostasis without including phosphorus, which usually takes the form of phosphate in biologic systems. Phosphate combines with calcium and other inorganic compounds to form bones and teeth. It is an integral part of many molecules, including genetic material (DNA, RNA), phospholipids, and phosphoproteins, and is central to energy transfer as a component of ATP and creatine phosphate. In the unbound form, phosphate plays a major role in the buffering capacity of the body and acts as an effector for certain enzyme activities.

Because of the close association between phosphorus

and calcium, both in the food supply and in metabolism, it is not surprising that those factors controlling calcium homeostasis also affect that of phosphorus. This interdependence between calcium and phosphorus is reflected in their requirements, particularly in the dietary calcium to phosphorus ratio. As in other species, metabolism in cats is most efficient when the ratio approximates 1.1:1 (Scott and Scott, 1967).

Since meat contains much more phosphorus than calcium and is a relatively rich source of protein, a **calcium deficiency** may be induced or aggravated by an all-meat diet. High protein consumption increases urinary excretion of calcium in man (Allen et al., 1979). Further, when a large amount of dietary phosphorus is absorbed, a relative hyperphosphatemia is induced, and a depression in the serum calcium concentration results according to the law of constant ion product. The parathyroid responds to the low serum calcium level by secreting parathyroid hormone (PTH), which increases phosphate excretion by the kidney. The high phosphate concentration in the kidney tubule depresses conversion of 25-hydroxycholecalciferol (25-OH $D_3$) to the active 1,25-OH $D_3$. The reduced level of the latter is significant because 1,25-OH $D_3$ would normally evoke an increase in the blood calcium level by absorption from the gut in addition to promoting calcium removal from bone. Because bone is the only source of calcium under these dietary conditions, continued PTH action on bone releases calcium while the excess phosphorus continues to be excreted in urine. Unfortunately, relative hyperphosphatemia persists unless the dietary Ca:P ratio is corrected to a level greater than 1.0. Bones eventually become brittle and then fibrous as they demineralize, becoming susceptible to multiple fractures.

Early descriptions of calcium deficiency in cats (e.g., Coop, 1958) wrongly assumed that it was analogous to osteogenesis imperfecta of humans and that it was hereditary. Scott was the first to suggest (1957) that the condition actually resulted from a low calcium intake, and subsequent reports by Riser (1961) and Scott et al. (1963) provided definitive evidence that inadequate calcium consumption or a Ca:P imbalance could cause the syndrome. Other reports contributed to the description of this metabolic derangement (e.g., Jowsey and Gershon-Cohen, 1964; Palmer, 1968; Rowland et al., 1968). Because parathyroid hypertrophy is secondary to the dietary Ca:P imbalance (a high-meat diet typically has a Ca:P ratio of 1:20), the condition was also called nutritional secondary hyperparathyroidism and fits the classic pathologic description of osteitis fibrosa (Krook et al., 1963).

Since the deficiency is most dramatic in the growing kitten, labels of juvenile osteoporosis, osteodystrophy, and osteomalacia have been used somewhat inaccurately. In essence, a dietary calcium insufficiency forces removal of bone calcium to meet essential metabolic needs. A high incidence has been reported in Siamese and Burmese kittens—probably the result of the misguided practices of breeders who fed a diet of lean beef and no milk, rather than of any genetic predisposition.

Under natural conditions, signs of the deficiency are seen most often in kittens aged 16 to 20 weeks, after they have been fed diets deficient to varying degrees in calcium for periods of one to three months. Nursing kittens as young as eight weeks of age may be affected if the queen's own diet is deficient. Typically kittens are well and in good body condition with sleek coats, but they become inactive and evince tenderness when handled. In some the first sign of trouble is a limp in a limb or weakness or unsteadiness in the hind parts, developing suddenly after playing, a jump from a step or chair, or a trivial injury resulting in fractures (Fig. 2–9). As the condition advances, lordosis may develop in the lumbar region, so that the kitten is recognizably deformed and may suffer from posterior incoordination or paralysis due to compression fractures of the vertebrae and pressure on the spinal cord. Lordosis of the thoracic spine may compress the lungs, causing severe dyspnea (Fig. 2–10). Palpable deformation or "winging" of the scapulae may result from muscles pulling on the softened bone. Pelvic collapse may cause severe constipation with distention of the intestinal tract and eventual death from inappetence, wasting, and dehydration. A paralyzed and distended bladder occasionally results from impaired innervation.

Adult cats fed a calcium-deficient diet, especially lactating females, undergo a more prolonged skeletal depletion and are less apt to develop the severe lesions seen in kittens.

Together with a history of a calcium-deficient diet, radiographs of kittens are diagnostic. An abnormal lack of density is evident in the entire skeleton, with marked thinning of cortical bone. There are bowing and folding fractures of the long bones, especially at the proximal and distal ends of the metaphyses. In more advanced deficiency, compression fractures of the vertebrae are evident as well as narrowing of the pelvic canal.

Values for serum calcium, phosphorus, and alkaline phosphatase do not seem to be diagnostically significant. They were followed consistently in only one experimental study (Rowland et al., 1968). A mild hypocalcemia was present by the time the deficiency was advanced. Alkaline phosphatase activity was higher in deficient kittens than in controls in weeks two through five, and was then lower until the thirteenth week of the 14-week study. Single determinations performed at the twelfth week of another experiment indicated mild hypocalcemia and hyperphosphatemia in two kittens and elevation of alkaline phosphatase in one (Krook et al., 1963). In severe cases the calcium level may fall below 8 mg/dl (Scott, 1969), a level that may precede the development of convulsions.

At autopsy the bones appear grossly hyperemic. They are soft and easily bent or cut. Microscopic changes have been most thoroughly studied by Rowland et al. (1968). In kittens fed only ground beef heart, providing a Ca:P ratio of about 1:20, alterations appeared first in the maxillae and last in the cervical and thoracic vertebrae. The lesion is generalized osteitis fibrosa (fibrous osteodystrophy), characterized by excessive osteocytic and osteoclastic resorption, increased osteoblastic proliferation, demineralization of bone, and replacement by fibrous connective tissue. In adult cats the bone lesion is osteoporosis.

The parathyroid glands are hyperplastic. There is also hyperplasia of the thyroid due to the low iodine content of meat.

Although kittens with severe skeletal deformities or neurologic damage must usually be destroyed, many others can be rehabilitated. In acute cases, intravenous injection of 10 ml of 10 per cent calcium borogluconate is remarkably effective, giving relief from pain and restoring activity within 48 hours (Riser, 1961). The kitten must be converted as quickly as possible to a balanced diet.

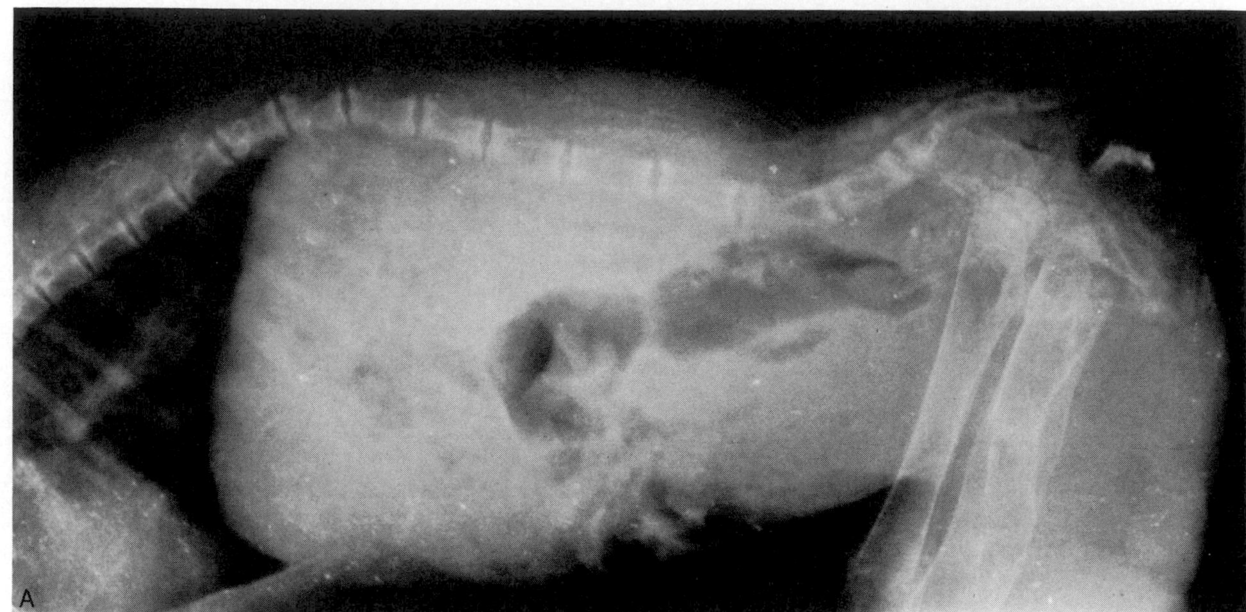


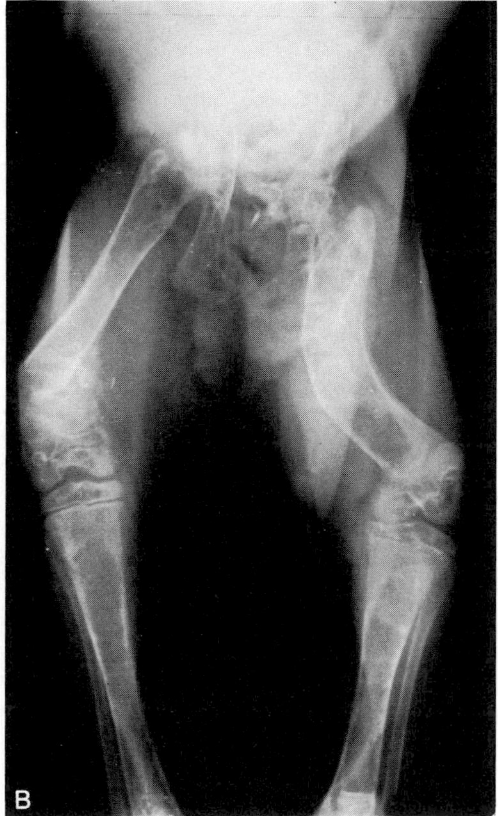


**Figure 2–9.** Calcium deficiency (nutritional secondary hyperparathyroidism). *A*, Extreme calcium depletion in a kitten manifested by radiolucent vertebrae, pelvis, and femurs. *B*, Note the thin cortices, decreased calcification, and folding fractures of the femur, as well as abdominal distention due to collapse and narrowing of the pelvic canal.

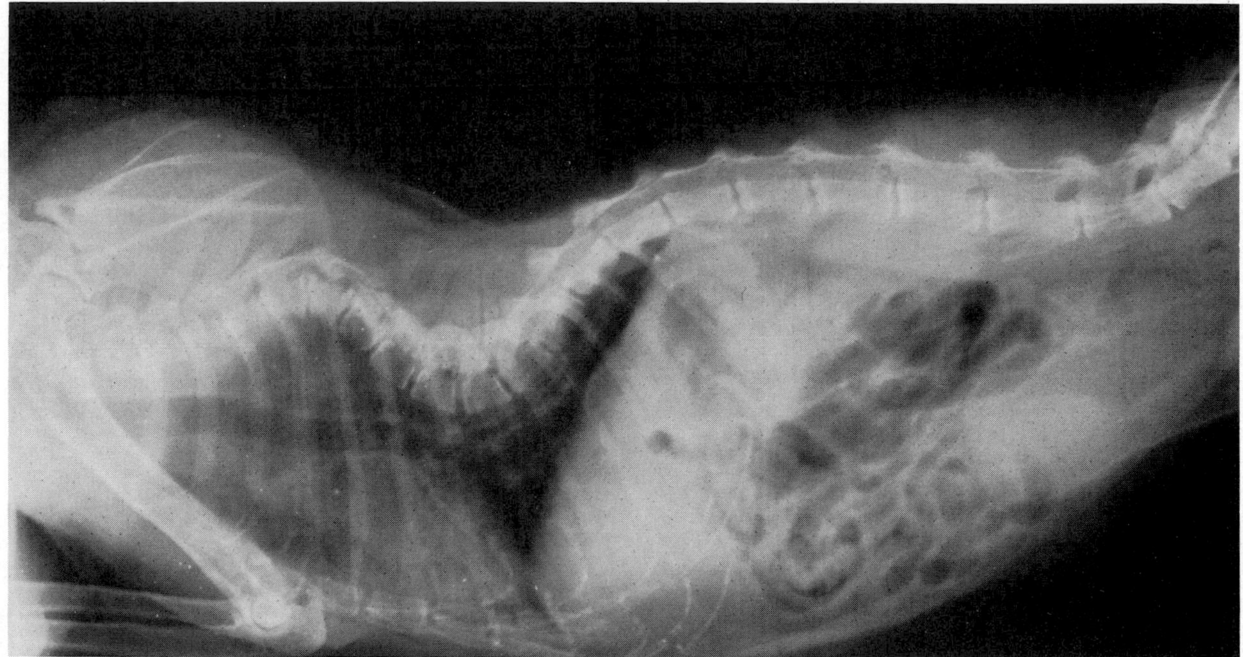

**Figure 2–10.** A 13-year-old spayed female Siamese cat suffered extreme calcium deficiency as a kitten and developed a deformed thoracic spine that resulted in severe dyspnea.

Calcium carbonate, calcium gluconate, or calcium lactate (1 to 2 gm/day) is also given orally in tablet form or crushed in food for two or three weeks (Scott, 1975). Small bones from fish or fowl, cooked until soft, are a source of calcium that many cats relish.

Splinting or pinning of fractures is contraindicated because of the softness of the bones. Instead, the kitten should be confined for two or three weeks in a cage or limited area where it cannot injure itself. Females in which the pelvic canal has undergone constriction should be neutered to prevent dystocia. Resourceful surgeons have occasionally salvaged cats suffering from chronic obstipation due to a collapsed pelvis by removing the floor of the pelvis, or splitting it and widening the outlet by spreading the ischial bones with a horizontal steel bar (see Chapter 5).

Not surprisingly, a frequent cause of nutritionally induced bone disease is an exclusive meat diet with a Ca:P ratio as high as 1:20 or 1:30 in some tissues such as beef heart, which may be fed by uninformed owners or keepers. In the feral state, cats and other predators eat their prey whole, including bones and intestinal contents, thereby obtaining the necessary calcium while maintaining an adequate Ca:P ratio. Calcium deficiency in domestic or captured cats is prevented and treated by a well-balanced diet.

To achieve a Ca:P ratio near unity, a calcium allowance of 1 per cent and a phosphorus allowance of 0.8 per cent of the dry diet are recommended (NRC, 1978).

**MAGNESIUM.** Like calcium and phosphorus, magnesium contributes to bone structure as well as to several metabolic reactions, some of which also involve phosphate. This relationship is understandable, since magnesium and calcium belong to the same elemental period and thus share similar chemical properties. Neither magnesium deficiency nor an estimate of its requirement has been reported for the cat. On the basis of successful experimental diets, NRC (1978) recommended an allowance of 0.05 per cent magnesium in the dry diet. An elevated magnesium intake (>0.5 per cent, often associated with a diet high in by-products from meat- and fishbone) can be a factor in precipitating urolithiasis (see further on); especially when the dietary calcium level is low.

## Trace Elements

Other minerals are needed in the diet in small quantities (less than 100 ppm) and serve a variety of metabolic functions, often as cofactors in enzymes. The requirement for many of these so-called trace elements has not been studied in cats, but they can be assumed to be needed in this species.

**IRON AND COPPER.** These two elements are closely associated in several physiologic functions usually involving electron transfer, cellular oxidation, and overall metabolism of oxygen. Animal tissues of a reddish color (blood, red muscle, liver) are a good source of both iron and copper (Moore, 1962) and often represent the initial site of pathologic change during nutritional deficiency of these trace minerals. If red meat is replaced in the diet by plant-derived ingredients, inorganic salts of iron and copper are often added to the diet. Data concerning the utilization of these salts by cats are lacking, but in other species the efficiency of absorption of inorganic iron is far less than that of iron bound in an organic matrix, such as hemoglobin. Therefore, when diets for cats are formulated, the source of iron, and probably copper, should be a matter for concern. The classic hallmark of iron deficiency is a microcytic, hypochromic anemia, which if severe can lead to retarded growth. NRC (1978) recommended allowances of 100 mg iron and 5 mg copper/kg dry diet.

**ZINC.** A preliminary report indicated that kittens fed vegetable protein–based diets require supplemental zinc (Aiken et al., 1978); however, Kane et al. (1981b) were unable to induce gross zinc deficiency in weanling cats. Therefore a naturally occurring zinc deficiency would be a rare occurrence in adult cats, but may be a problem during pregnancy and lactation. The question of how increased amounts of dietary fiber affect zinc status remains unanswered. Slow and thin hair growth, scaly skin, ulcers of the buccal margins, weight loss, testicular degeneration, depressed food intake, and histologic evidence of parakeratosis have been correlated with low plasma and liver zinc levels (Kane et al., 1981b). Interestingly, no changes in the activity of the zinc-containing enzyme glutamate dehydrogenase were found. The authors estimated the zinc requirement to be between 15 and 50 ppm, which is reasonably consistent with the older NRC (1978) recommended allowance of 30 mg/kg dry diet (30 ppm) that was based on preliminary evidence.

**IODINE.** Iodine combines with tyrosine to form thyroid hormone. It also appears to be necessary for optimal utilization of calcium by the cat (Roberts and Scott, 1961). Occasionally, cats maintained on high-meat diets develop a deficiency manifested by goiter, alopecia, abnormal calcium metabolism, fetal resorption, and death (Greaves et al., 1959; Scott, 1965; Scott et al., 1961). The inclusion of seafood in the diet precludes the development of deficiency (Scott and Scott, 1967), but the influence of iodine on calcium metabolism is unexplained. The danger of iodine toxicity is very slight in normal cats, levels of up to 5 mg/day of iodine having been tolerated. Cats rendered experimentally hypothyroid are sensitive to iodine toxicity and react to such large doses with anorexia, weight loss, fever, and rapid pulse and respiration (Scott, 1964). The allowance recommended by NRC (1978) is 1 mg/kg dry diet.

**OTHER MINERALS.** Manganese has been measured in nutritionally adequate diets at 2 mg/kg dry diet (Morris, 1968) and 4 mg/kg dry diet (Scott, 1960). No thorough studies have been reported. NRC (1978) recommended an allowance of 10 mg/kg dry diet.

In the absence of data concerning selenium requirements of cats, NRC (1978) considered the high polyunsaturated fatty acid content of many cat foods and the potential for peroxidation and steatitis in cats and recommended an allowance of 0.1 mg selenium per kg of dry diet.

As research continues, the various trace minerals known to be essential in other species can be expected to be essential in the cat. Perhaps those minerals that function as antioxidants (e.g., selenium) or in glucose homeostasis (e.g., chromium) will be found to have surprising nutritional implications and technically useful applications. Similarly, the interactions and availability of minerals present in diets containing increased levels of vegetable fiber should be studied.

## Feline Urolithiasis Syndrome

Feline urolithiasis has long been an urgent problem. Its etiology has been considered to be multifactorial, with diet and mineral metabolism, especially that of magnesium, playing a pre-eminent role (e.g., Jackson, 1971; Kallfelz et al., 1980; Lewis et al., 1978; Lewis and Morris, 1984). The characteristic features and possible contributing factors have been reviewed, with extensive reference to the literature, by Finco et al. (1975), Greene and Scott (1983), and Osborne and Lees (1980).

Urolithiasis is manifested, most often between one and six years as dysuria, hematuria, and cystitis, often leading in males to urethral obstruction and fatal uremia. Males are predisposed to obstruction because of their long, narrow urethra and its constriction at the ischium and penis, but cats of both sexes may develop severe cystitis due to concretions of sand or stones in the bladder.

It has been estimated that about 1 per cent of the total feline population is affected, and possibly up to 10 per cent of males among hospital admissions. One study reported a recurrence rate of obstruction between 35 and 50 per cent (Foster, 1967). Mortality rates in the feline urolithiasis syndrome from 22 to 50 per cent have been recorded, but in 250 cases in which the standard treatment was a lifelong regimen of canned low-ash diet and acidification, the mortality was less than 1 per cent (Engle, 1977).

A strong predisposing factor is the cat's well-known tendency to drink relatively little fluid and produce urine of a high specific gravity. Urination is usually infrequent, and a cat's reluctance to use an unclean litter pan or to go out of doors in cold weather contributes further to concentration and stasis of urine.

Evidence exists that crystals of microscopic size may actually form in the renal tubules (Osbaldiston and Taussig, 1970) and become enmeshed in a colloid matrix in the lower urinary tract. Since struvite, the common calculus in the cat, becomes progressively less soluble with increasing urine alkalinity, the urinary pH is an important variable in stone formation and is often elevated (above pH 6.8) in afflicted cats owing to dietary factors, urinary stasis, or inflammation. Inflammation, possibly related to alkaline urine, can also contribute dead cells and other matter that can form the nucleation center and colloid matrix for calculus formation.

Bacterial infection has not been shown to be a primary factor but may develop as a result of instrumentation or in chronic cases. Certain viruses, acting synergistically, have been directly implicated in the etiology of the feline urolithiasis syndrome (e.g., Fabricant, 1977; see also Chapter 7), but these studies have not been uniformly reproducible.

Because the most prevalent component of the stones is struvite (magnesium ammonium phosphate hexahydrate, $Mg(NH_4)PO_4 \cdot 6H_2O$) (Fig. 2–11), many investigators have focused attention on the total ash content and mineral composition of the diet (e.g., Kallfelz et al., 1980; Lewis et al., 1978). The data indicate that a high ash content per se cannot be incriminated, but that a high magnesium content ($>$0.75 per cent) in a diet otherwise favoring subclinical alkalosis readily induces stone formation in most cats, particularly when the dietary Ca:P ratio is less than 1.0. On the other hand, calculi seldom form (even with alkaline diets) if the magnesium concentration is less than 0.1 per cent on a dry weight basis (Rich et al., 1974).

Dry rations appear more calculogenic than canned foods. Because the dry foods contain somewhat less acid-producing animal protein, the cat must eat more of the food to meet its caloric protein needs and thus also

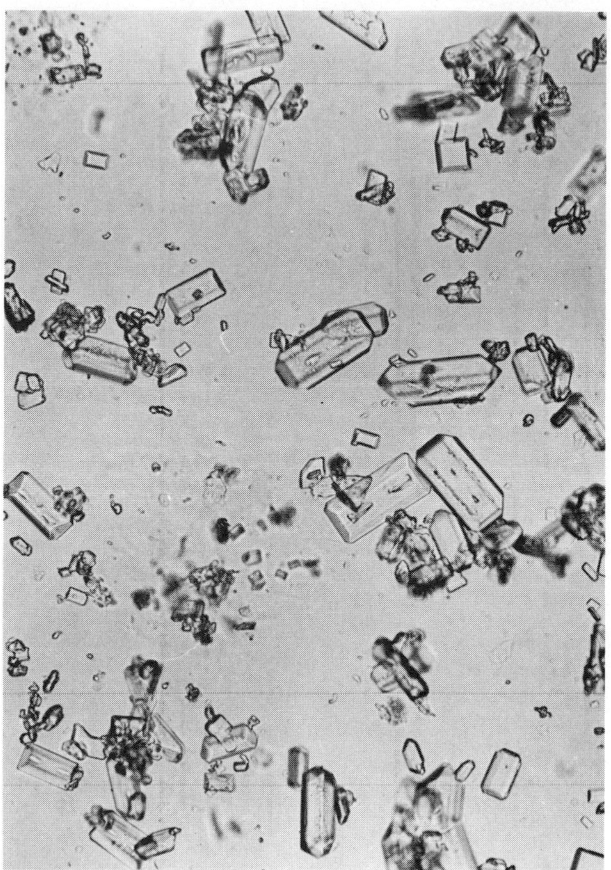

**Figure 2–11.** Struvite crystals are readily seen in the urinary sediment of cats. Increased concentration of these crystals causes urethral plugs that result in life-threatening obstruction in male cats.

consumes more of the alkaline-producing major minerals (Ca, Mg, Na, K). The result is a urine of higher pH (>6.8) with a high concentration of urinary protein and mineral and increased urine osmolality (Cook et al., 1985; Lewis, 1981; Palmore et al., 1978; Seefeldt and Chapman, 1979). The percentage of protein calories in the diet may be an important variable.

On the one hand, a high amount of animal protein contains substantial sulfur amino acids (methionine, cystine), which are oxidized to sulfate and contribute significantly to urine acidification, whereas vegetable protein and low-protein diets tend to be low in SAA and high in $K^+$ and $Mg^{++}$, resulting in more alkaline urine and struvite precipitation. Both urinary ammonium and phosphate are positively correlated with the amount of protein metabolized, and magnesium intake and excretion generally would be higher during consumption of vegetable protein. As indicated earlier (see discussion of protein), since the typical cat diet contains an exceptional amount of protein (more than 30 per cent dry weight), a high contribution from vegetable protein without proper consideration of mineral balance would have deleterious effects.

Decreased water excretion by the kidney leading to increased "sludging" of urine has been incriminated, particularly since cats, as already noted, are notorious for their capacity to conserve fluid and decrease urine output by forming hyperosmolar urine (Palmore et al., 1978; Scott, 1980). Although most cats do not drink much water, they will do so when given an adequate supply and when thirst is induced, as by salting the food.

Whether the lower moisture content of dry cat foods (9 to 12 per cent) represents a potential problem is a matter of some disagreement. Burger et al. (1980) suggested that cats may not completely compensate for water intake when the diet changes from about 75 per cent water (typical animal carcass or canned food) to less than 10 per cent; i.e., cats tended to consume only half as much total water (food and drinking) when fed a dry diet as when fed a high-moisture diet. On the contrary, other investigators failed to find an appreciable decrease in the water intake as the diet moisture content decreased (Jackson and Tovey, 1977; Seefeldt and Chapman, 1979; Thrall and Miller, 1976). Also, most of the experimental diets referred to elsewhere in this chapter were fed as a dry ration without harmful consequences when water was provided ad libitum.

Corrective measures for urolithiasis include attempts to decrease struvite formation, to reduce mineral concentration by increasing urine volume, and to acidify the urine to enhance struvite solubility. Struvite excretion has been reduced empirically by lowering the dietary intake of base-producing magnesium (Kallfelz et al., 1980; Lewis, 1981) in a diet tending toward alkalosis. Attempts to increase urine volume by adding salt (NaCl) to the diet to induce thirst and enhance water consumption have met with partial success, for although volume can be increased and the incidence of stone formation may decline, the problem is not corrected if excessive magnesium intake and a Ca:P imbalance (i.e., acid-base imbalance) are allowed to persist (Hamar et al., 1976). Feeding semimoist cat food has proved beneficial in that the concentration of urinary solutes declines to one-tenth while daily water intake increases as much as 50 per cent and urine volume increases 100 per cent (Bressett et al., 1979; Kallfelz, 1981). It is noteworthy that hunting cats normally consume a high–animal protein (more than 50 per cent kcal), high-fat (more than 34 per cent kcal) and low-ash (about 2 per cent) diet containing approximately 75 per cent water in the form of an animal carcass. The ash content of such a diet implies that a balanced, low-ash intake is an important deterrent to struvite formation. Feeding up to 1 gm (¼ teaspoon) of ammonium chloride per day has proved to be the most effective means of clinically acidifying the urine of an affected cat, maintaining an acid pH more consistently than ascorbic acid, DL-methionine, or acid phosphate (Chow et al., 1978; Taton et al., 1984a,b).

In summary, the feline urolithiasis syndrome seems to be associated with a low volume of hyperosmolar (high specific gravity) alkaline urine coupled with an increased urinary excretion of certain metabolites, especially magnesium ion in the form of struvite crystals. The most successful clinical approach attempts (1) to lessen the formation of struvite by correcting the acid-base components of the diet, (2) to enhance the solubility of the struvite formed by acidifying the urine clinically with ammonium chloride (or, less effectively, with methionine), and (3) to increase water consumption and urine output. The first two objectives are met by selecting a cat food with a high animal protein and low magnesium (<0.1 per cent dry matter) content and supplementing the ration with 0.75 to 1 gm of ammonium chloride daily. Adequate water intake may be achieved by adding water to a dry diet (3 oz per cup) or feeding a canned diet with a normally high (74 to 78 per cent) water content. Water intake may be increased by adding salt to the diet (2 per cent dry weight, or ½ teaspoon per day) (Hamar et al., 1976), or by feeding a semimoist product having a moderate (35 per cent) water content and osmotically active binders that promote greatly increased water consumption. Fresh water in a clean bowl must be available at all times.

## FORMULATION AND PRODUCTION OF COMMERCIAL CAT FOODS

To make recommendations for feeding cats, it is important to have some understanding of cat food production. Product quality depends most importantly on whether the food is nutritionally complete. In order to be marketed in the United States as nutritionally complete, it must either contain the recommended allowances for all nutrients as listed by the National Research Council (1978) or satisfy the performance protocol of the American Association of Feed Control Operators (1980). Whichever the standard, there is apt to be variability in digestibility, caloric density, and crude estimates of dietary nutrients as well as breed, age, and sex variabilities in the cats consuming the food.

The energy requirements of cats for growth, pregnancy, lactation, and adult maintenance have been discussed already and have been summarized by the National Research Council (1978). Products claiming to be nutritionally complete should satisfy the nutritional demands of cats during the various stages of life.

Commercial pet foods are also categorized into three basic types—dry, semimoist (soft-moist), and canned. The dry foods of "kibble" type contain about 8 to 12 per cent moisture, about 32 to 36 per cent protein (dry-weight basis), and 8 to 12 per cent fat (dry-weight basis). The major brands are usually nutritionally complete. To judge from the order in which ingredients are listed for most dry foods, plant nutrients predominate over those of animal origin, thus making these foods the least expensive for providing cats with balanced diets. Since dry cat foods rely heavily on vegetable-derived ingredients, they must therefore be carefully formulated to provide all the nutrients required by the cat (e.g., amino acids and possibly EFA) as described in other sections. Special foods with small-sized kibbles and increased levels of protein and calcium are marketed for kittens, and for palatability are preferred by many adult cats.

Semimoist (soft-moist) foods are marketed in sealed, foil-lined containers or in individual, meal-sized, sealed foil packets, the latter best preserving moisture and freshness. The moisture content (30 to 35 per cent) is higher than in dry foods, and the food would spoil if unrefrigerated, except for the inclusion of certain osmotically active sugars as well as other natural and synthetic stabilizers. The use of sugars in cat food has been discussed in the section on carbohydrate. The consequences of using stabilizers such as sorbate and propylene glycol are uncertain, although they have been in use without apparent harm for many years. On a dry basis the protein content is usually 34 to 40 per cent, and fat, 10 to 15 per cent. Animal products appear to predominate over those of vegetable origin. The major brands are nutritionally complete. Whatever the reason, there is a conspicuous increase in water drinking and output by cats eating semimoist foods.

Canned cat foods may or may not be nutritionally complete. Owners should be advised to look carefully for a label stating whether this is the case. Some labels list the total ash content, which is of limited value; rather, the amounts and ratios of individual minerals are the critical consideration. Canned foods contain 72 to 78 per cent moisture, 35 to 41 per cent protein (dry-weight basis), and 9 to 18 per cent fat (dry-weight basis). Animal-derived ingredients usually predominate over those of vegetable origin in order to maintain a high protein and low carbohydrate content.

Specialty ("gourmet") canned foods may have crude protein levels from 40 to 65 per cent and crude fat levels from 15 to 40 per cent on a dry-weight basis. They consist largely of animal or marine products such as beef, liver, kidney, chicken, or fish, sometimes with some soy protein. Mineral or vitamin supplements are sometimes added. Occasionally such a product is designated as nutritionally complete, but the labels of many make clear that the food should be used only as a "treat" or as a supplement to a complete diet. Because of the high quality of the protein content, and sometimes the packaging in 3 oz tins suitable for a single meal, the specialty foods are the costliest of all the cat foods and understandably appeal to the most finicky eaters.

The major nutritional disadvantage of canned food is that the retort (heating under pressure) process significantly reduces the nutritional quality of the protein and impairs the integrity of the heat-sensitive vitamins. The decrease in protein quality is usually offset by the high quantity of protein, while the vitamin loss is offset by vitamin supplementation during the formulation.

## PRACTICAL RECOMMENDATIONS FOR FEEDING CATS

A cat diet should consist of nutritionally complete commercial foods, with only limited "gourmet" treats and table scraps. Commercial diets highly touted to cat owners, but not labeled as either meeting NRC requirements or being "nutritionally complete," should be regarded with caution and fed only occasionally as "snack food."

Recommendations for approximate amounts of food for normal cats are suggested in Table 2–1 and also on the containers of commercial foods. Adjustments should be made "to effect," in accordance with the age, activity, and genetic constitution of the individual cat, some being, like humans, naturally lean or pleasantly plump. Obese cats, as a general rule, should have their daily intake reduced by one-third until the desired weight is attained.

Cat owners should be discouraged from supplementing a balanced (complete) food with vitamins, minerals, meat, or other ingredients, unless their veterinarian has identified some special indication to do so. Home-prepared diets may appeal to the taste buds of a cat or owner, but such preparations often contain harmful excesses or deficiencies of certain nutrients that can have devastating results if fed for a prolonged period.

Cats, like people, sometimes have strong individual predilections for certain foods, e.g., olives, melon, lettuce, cucumber, corn, asparagus, cheese, pizza, or bacon. Contrary to what owners believe, these cravings do not represent an instinctive effort to satisfy a nutritional need, but there is no harm in indulging them occasionally. Indeed, encouraging a cat's taste for a variety of foods may foster an adaptability that could be helpful if gastrointestinal, liver, heart, or kidney disease, for example, should some day require dietary modifications that are refused by many a cat that has become unalterably accustomed to a fixed dietary regimen.

Modifications desirable for such conditions are discussed in the chapters dealing with these disorders.

## ORPHAN KITTENS

Commercial formulas for rearing orphan kittens or supplementing unthrifty members of a litter are available from veterinarians and pet supply stores, together with suitable "kitten bottles" and schedules for feeding. Formulas for human infants and puppies do not supply the high levels of protein and fat required by kittens. A homemade formula that may be used in an emergency is composed of nonfat dried milk (1/3 cup), cottage cheese (1/4 cup), and corn oil (1/8) cup). Add water to make up to 2 cups, blend, and refrigerate, making the mixture fresh every two days. Before feeding, heat to body temperature. Two teaspoonsful of formula per ounce of kitten will meet its daily needs. Vitamins may be supplied by one fifth of the daily dose of infant vitamin drops added to the formula or placed on the back of the tongue. At first the kittens should be fed five or six times a day, but after two weeks, three or four times daily should suffice.

## REFERENCES


Aguirre GD: Retinal degeneration associated with the feeding of dog foods to cats. J Am Vet Med Assoc 172 (1978) 791–796.

Aiken TD, Schnepper LE, Forbes RM, Corbin JE: The effect of a low-zinc diet on growth and skin condition in cats. Proc 11th Ann Meet Am Soc Anim Sci, Midwest Section (1978) 27.

Allen LH, Oddoye EA, Margen S: Protein-induced hypercalciuria: A longer term study. Am J Clin Nutr 32 (1979) 741–749.

American Association of Feed Control Operators, Inc.: Official Publication, College Station, TX, 1980.

Anderson PA, Baker DH, Corbin JE: Lysine and arginine requirements of the domestic cat. J Nutr 109 (1979a) 1368–1372.

Anderson PA, Baker DH, Sherry PA, Corbin JE: Choline-methionine interrelationship in feline nutrition. J Anim Sci 49 (1979b) 522–527.

Anderson PA, Baker DH, Corbin JE, Helper LC: Biochemical lesions associated with taurine deficiency in the cat. J Anim Sci 49 (1979c) 1227–1234.

Anderson PA, Baker DH, Sherry PA, Corbin JE: Nitrogen requirement of the kitten. Am J Vet Res 41 (1980a) 1646–1649.

Anderson PA, Baker DH, Sherry PA, Corbin JE: Histidine, phenylalanine-tyrosine, and tryptophan requirements for growth of the young kitten. J Anim Sci 50 (1980b) 479–483.

Anderson PA, Baker DH, Sherry PA, Teeter RG, Corbin JE: Threonine, isoleucine, valine and leucine requirements of the young kitten. J Anim Sci 50 (1980c) 266–271.

Baggs RB, de Lahunta A, Averill DR: Thiamine deficiency encephalopathy in a specific-pathogen–free cat colony. Lab Anim Sci 28 (1978) 323–326.

Baker DH: Some essentials of the kitten diet. Petfood Industry 22 (2) (1980) 20–32.

Bartoshuk LM, Harned MA, Parks LH: Taste of water in the cat: Effects on sucrose preference. Science 171 (1971) 699–701.

Bartoshuk LM, Jacobs HL, Nichols TL, Hoff LA, Ryckman JJ: Taste rejection of nonnutritive sweeteners in cats. J Comp Physiol Psychol 89 (1975) 971-975.

Beliveau GP, Morris JG, Rogers QR, Freedland RA: Metabolism of serine, threonine, and glycine in isolated cat hepatocytes. Fed Proc 40 (1981) 847 (abstr).

Berson EL, Hayes KC, Rabin AR, Schmidt SY, Watson G: Retinal degeneration in cats fed casein. II. Supplementation with methionine, cysteine, or taurine. Invest Ophthalmol 15 (1976) 52–58.

Braham JE, Villarreal A, Bressani R: Effect of lime treatment of corn on the availability of niacin for cats. J Nutr 76 (1962) 183–186.

Bressett JD, Kallfelz FA, Lubar J, Wallace RL: Relation of ration type and mineral content to the incidence of feline urologic syndrome. Proc Cornell Nutr Conf (1979) 108–112.

Burger IH, Anderson RS, Holme DW: Nutritional factors affecting water balance in the dog and cat. *In* Anderson RS (ed): Nutrition of the Dog and Cat. New York, Pergamon Press, 1980.

Carey CJ, Morris JG: Biotin deficiency in the cat and the effect on hepatic propionyl CoA carboxylase. J Nutr 107 (1977) 330–334.

Carpenter JA: Species differences in taste preferences. J Comp Physiol Psychol 49 (1956) 139–144.

Carvalho da Silva A, Fried R, de Angelis RC: The domestic cat as a laboratory animal for experimental nutrition studies. III. Niacin requirements and tryptophan metabolism. J Nutr 46 (1952) 399–409.

Carvalho da Silva A, de Angelis RC, Pontes MA, Mansur Guérios MF: The domestic cat as a laboratory animal for experimental nutrition studies. IV. Folic acid deficiency. J Nutr 56 (1955) 199–213.

Carvalho da Silva A, Fajer AB, de Angelis RC, Pontes MA, Giesbrecht AM, Fried R: The domestic cat as a laboratory animal for experimental nutrition studies. VII. Pyridoxine deficiency. J Nutr 68 (1959a) 213–229.

Carvalho da Silva A, Mansur Guérios MF, Monsao SR: The domestic cat as a laboratory animal for experimental nutrition studies. VI. Choline deficiency. J Nutr 67 (1959b) 537–547.

Chow FHC, Taton GF, Lewis LD, Hamar DW: Effect of dietary ammonium chloride, DL-methionine, sodium phosphate and ascorbic acid on urinary pH and electrolyte concentrations of male cats. Feline Pract 8 (4) (1978) 29–34.

Christi GA: Ann Fac Vet Med Montevideo 6 (1957) 95. Cited by Seawright AA, et al., 1967.

Clark L, Seawright AA: Skeletal abnormalities in the hindlimbs of young cats as a result of hypervitaminosis A. Nature (Lond) 217 (1968) 1174–1176.

Clark L, Seawright AA, Gartner RJW: Longbone abnormalities in kittens following vitamin A administration. J Comp Pathol 80 (1970) 113–121.

Coffin DL, Holzworth J: "Yellow fat" in two laboratory cats: Acid-fast pigmentation associated with a fish-base ration. Cornell Vet 44 (1954) 63–71.

Cook N, Kane E, Rogers QR, Morris JG: Selfselection of dietary casein and soy-protein by the cat. Physiol Behav 34 (1985) 583–588.

Coop MC: A treatment for osteogenesis imperfecta in kittens. J Am Vet Med Assoc 132 (1958) 299–300.

Cordy DR: Experimental production of steatitis (yellow fat disease) in kittens fed a commercial canned cat food and prevention of the condition by vitamin E. Cornell Vet 44 (1954) 310–318.

Cordy DR, Stillinger CJ: Steatitis ("yellow fat disease") in kittens. North Am Vet 34 (1953) 714–716.

Costello MJ, Morris JG, Rogers QR: Effect of dietary arginine level on urinary orotate and citrate excretion in growing kittens. J Nutr 110 (1980) 1204–1208.

Deady JE, Anderson B, O'Donnell JA III, Morris JG, Rogers QR: Effects of level of dietary glutamic acid and thiamin on food intake, weight gain, plasma amino acids and thiamin status of growing kittens. J Nutr 111 (1981a) 1568–1579.

Deady JE, Rogers QR, Morris JG: Effect of high dietary glutamic acid on the excretion of 35S-thiamin in kittens. J Nutr 111 (1981b) 1580–1585.

Deutsch HF, Hasler AD: Distribution of a vitamin $B_1$ destructive enzyme in fish. Proc Soc Exp Biol Med 53 (1943) 63–65.

Drochner W, Muller-Schlosser S: Digestibility and tolerance of various sugars in cats. *In* Anderson RS (ed): Nutrition of the Dog and Cat. New York, Pergamon Press, 1980.

Dymsza HA, Miller SA: Dietary methionine requirement of the cat. Fed Proc 23 (1964) 186(abstr).

Engle GC: A clinical report on 250 cases of feline urological syndrome. Feline Pract 7 (4) (1977) 24–27.

English PB, Seawright AA: Deforming cervical spondylosis of the cat. Aust Vet J 40 (1964) 376–381.

Everett GM: Observations on the behavior and neurophysiology of acute thiamin deficient cats. Am J Physiol 141 (1944) 439–448.

Fabricant CG: Herpesvirus-induced urolithiasis in specific-pathogen–free male cats. Am J Vet Res 38 (1977) 1837–1842.

Featherston WR, Rogers QR, Freedland RA: Relative importance of kidney and liver in synthesis of arginine by the rat. Am J Physiol 224 (1973) 127–129.

Finco DR, Kneller SK, Crowell WA: Diseases of the urinary system. *In* Catcott EJ (ed): Feline Medicine and Surgery, 2nd ed. Santa Barbara, American Veterinary Publications, 1975.

Foster SJ: The "urolithiasis" syndrome in male cats: A statistical analysis of the problems, with clinical observations. J Small Anim Pract 8 (1967) 207–214.

Fox LAD, Jansen GR, Knox KL: Effect of variations in protein quality on growth, PER, NPR and NPU in growing kittens, Nutr Rep Int 7 (1973) 621–631.

Frankel TL, Rivers JPW: The nutritional and metabolic impact of γ-linolenic acid (18:3ω6) on cats deprived of animal lipid. Br J Nutr 39 (1978) 227–231.

Frings H: Sweet taste in the cat and the taste-spectrum. Experientia 7 (1951) 424–426.

Gaskell CJ, Leedale AH, Douglas SW: Pansteatitis in the cat: a report of four cases. J Small Anim Pract 16 (1975) 117–121.

Gershoff SN: The nutritional requirements of cats. J Am Vet Med Assoc 134 (1959) 139–141.

Gershoff SN, Andrus SB, Hegsted DM, Lentini EA: Vitamin A deficiency in cats. Lab Invest 6 (1957a) 227–240.

Gershoff SN, Andrus SB, Hegsted DM: The effect of the carbohydrate and fat content of the diet upon the riboflavin requirement of the cat. J Nutr 68 (1959a) 75–88.

Gershoff SN, Faragalla FF, Nelson DA, Andrus SB: Vitamin $B_6$ deficiency and oxalate nephrocalcinosis in the cat. Am J Med 27 (1959b) 72–80.

Gershoff SN, Gottlieb LS: Pantothenic acid deficiency in cats. J Nutr 82 (1964) 135–138.

Gershoff SN, Legg MA, O'Connor FJ, Hegsted DM: The effect of vitamin D–deficient diets containing various Ca:P ratios on cats. J Nutr 63 (1957b) 79–93.

Gershoff SN, Norkin SA: Vitamin E deficiency in cats. J Nutr 77 (1962) 303–308.

Gordon WG, Kaufman RE, Jackson RW: The excretion of kynurenic acid by the mammalian organism. A method for the identification of small amounts of kynurenic acid. J Biol Chem 113 (1936) 125–134.

Greaves JP: Protein and calorie requirements of the feline. *In* Graham-Jones O (ed): Canine and Feline Nutritional Requirements. London, Pergamon Press, 1965.

Greaves JP, Scott MG, Scott PP: Thyroid changes in cats on a high protein diet, raw heart. J Physiol 148 (1959) 73P–74P.

Greaves JP, Scott PP: Nutrition of the cat. 3. Protein requirements for nitrogen equilibrium in adult cats maintained on a mixed diet. Br J Nutr 14 (1960) 361–369.

Greaves JP, Scott PP: The influence of dietary carbohydrate on food intake of adult cats. Proc Nutr Soc 22 (1963) iv (abstr).

Greene RW, Scott RC: Diseases of the bladder and urethra. *In* Ettinger SJ (ed): Textbook of Veterinary Internal Medicine, 2nd ed. Philadelphia, W.B. Saunders Company, 1983.

Griffiths RC, Thornton GW, Willson JE: Pansteatitis ("yellow fat") in cats fed canned red tuna. J Am Vet Med Assoc 137 (1960) 126–128.

Hamar D, Chow FHC, Dysart MI, Rich LJ: Effect of sodium chloride in prevention of experimentally produced phosphate uroliths in male cats. J Am Anim Hosp Assoc 12 (1976) 514–517.

Hardy AJ, Morris JG, Rogers QR: Valine requirement of the growing kitten. J Nutr 107 (1977) 1308–1312.

Hassam AG, Rivers JPW, Crawford MA: Metabolism of gamma-linolenic acid in essential fatty acid–deficient rats. J Nutr 107 (1977) 519–524.

Hayes KC, Carey RE, Schmidt SY: Retinal degeneration associated with taurine deficiency in the cat. Science 188 (1975a) 949–951.

Hayes KC, Rabin AR, Berson EL: An ultrastructural study of nutritionally induced and reversed retinal degeneration in cats. Am J Pathol 78 (1975b) 505–524.

Hayes KC, Sturman JA: Taurine in metabolism: Ann Rev Nutr 1 (1981) 401–425.

Hayes KC, Sturman JA: Taurine deficiency: A rationale for taurine depletion. *In* Huxtable RJ, Pasantes-Morales H (eds): Taurine in Nutrition and Neurology. New York, Plenum Publishing Corporation, 1982, 79–87.

Heath MK, MacQueen JW, Spies TD: Feline pellagra. Science 92 (1940) 514.

Herron MR: The musculoskeletal system. *In* Catcott EJ (ed): Feline Medicine and Surgery, 2nd ed. Santa Barbara, American Veterinary Publications, 1975.

Hills DL, Morris JG, Rogers QR: Potassium requirement of kittens as affected by dietary protein. J Nutr 112 (1982) 216–222.

Hirsch E, Dubose C, Jacobs HL: Dietary control of food intake in cats. Physiol Behav 20 (1978) 287–295.

Hore P, Messer M: Studies on disaccharidase activities of the small intestine of the domestic cat and other carnivorous mammals. Comp Biochem Physiol 24 (1968) 717–725.

Humphreys ER, Scott PP: Variations in the distribution of calcium in the femurs of growing and adult cats on high and low calcium intakes. Proc Nutr Soc 23 (1964) xxxv–xxxvi (abstr).

Ikeda M, Tsuji H, Nakamura S, Ichiyama A, Nishizuka Y, Hayaishi O: Studies on the biosynthesis of nicotinamide adenine dinucleotide. II. A role of picolinic carboxylase in the biosynthesis of nicotinamide adenine dinucleotide from tryptophan in mammals. J Biol Chem 240 (1965) 1395–1401.

Jackson OF: Nutritional requirements of cats with special reference to the skeleton. J S Afr Vet Med Assoc 39 (4) (1968) 18–24.

Jackson OF: An experimental study of factors promoting the formation of uroliths in the cat. PhD thesis, University of London, 1971.

Jackson OF, Tovey JD: Water balance studies in domestic cats. Feline Pract 7 (4) (1977) 30–33.

Jackson RW: The excretion of kynurenic acid by members of various families of the order carnivora. J Biol Chem 131 (1939) 469–478.

Jansen GR, Deuth MA, Ward GM, Johnson DE: Protein quality studies in growing kittens. Nutr Rep Internat 11 (1975) 525–536.

Joshua JO: The Clinical Aspects of Some Diseases of Cats. London, William Heinemann, 1965.

Jowsey J, Gershon-Cohen J: Effect of dietary calcium levels on production and reversal of experimental osteoporosis in cats. Proc Soc Exp Biol Med 116 (1964) 437–441.

Jubb KV, Saunders LZ, Coates HV: Thiamine deficiency encephalopathy in cats. J Comp Pathol 66 (1956) 217–227.

Kallfelz FA: Personal communication, 1981.

Kallfelz FA, Bressett JD, Wallace RJ: Urethral obstruction in random source and SPF male cats induced by high levels of dietary magnesium or magnesium and phosphorus. Feline Pract 10(4) (1980) 25–35.

Kanarek RB: Availability and caloric density of the diet as determinants of meal patterns in cats. Physiol Behav 15 (1975) 611–618.

Kane E, Morris JG, Rogers QR: Acceptability and digestibility by adult cats of diets made with various sources and levels of fats. J Anim Sci 53 (1981a) 1516–1523.

Kane E, Morris JG, Rogers QR, Ihrke PJ, Cupps PT: Zinc deficiency in the cat. J Nutr 111 (1981b) 488–495.

Keesling PT, Morris JG: Vitamin $B_{12}$ deficiency in the cat. J Anim Sci 41 (1975) 317(abstr).

Knox K: Personal communication, 1982.

Krook L, Barrett RB, Usui K, Wolke RE: Nutritional secondary hyperparathyroidism in the cat. Cornell Vet 53 (1963) 224–240.

Leahy JS, Shillam KWG, Waterhouse CE, Partington H: Studies of the riboflavin requirements of the kitten. J Small Anim Pract 8 (1967) 351–363.

Leklem JE, Woodford J, Brown RR: Comparative tryptophan metabolism in cats and rats: Differences in adaptation of tryptophan oxygenase and in vivo metabolism of tryptophan, kynurenine and hydroxykynurenine. Comp Biochem Physiol 31 (1969) 95–109.

Lewis LD: Nutritional causes and management of feline urolithiasis. Proc Am Anim Hosp Assoc 48 (1981) 273–284.

Lewis LD, Chow FHC, Taton GF, Hamar DW: Effect of various dietary mineral concentrations on the occurrence of feline urolithiasis. J Am Vet Med Assoc 172 (1978) 559–563.

Lewis LD, Morris ML, Jr: Feline urologic syndrome. *In* Small Animal Clinical Nutrition, 2nd ed. Topeka, Mark Morris Associates, 1984.

Loew FM, Martin CL, Dunlop RH, Mapletoft RJ, Smith SI: Naturally occurring and experimental thiamin deficiency in cats receiving commercial cat food. Can Vet J 11 (1970) 109–113.

Lucke VM, Baskerville A, Bardgett PL, Mann PGH, Thompson SY: Deforming cervical spondylosis in the cat associated with hypervitaminosis A. Vet Rec 82 (1968) 141–142.

MacDonald ML, Rogers QR, Morris JG: Influence of dietary fat and essential fatty acids on growth in kittens. Fed Proc 40 (1981a) 882 (abstr).

MacDonald ML, Rogers QR, Morris JG: Clinical signs of essential fatty acid deficiency in the cat. Twelfth Int Cong Nutr, San Diego (1981b) 90 (abstr).

MacDonald ML, Rogers QR, Morris JG: Role of linoleate as an essential fatty acid for the cat independent of arachidonate synthesis. J Nutr 113 (1983) 1422–1433.

MacDonald ML, Anderson BC, Rogers QR, Buffington CA, Morris JG: Essential fatty acid requirements of cats: Pathology of essential fatty acid deficiency. Am J Vet Res 45 (1984a) 1310–1317.

MacDonald ML, Rogers QR, Morris JG: Effects of dietary arachidonate deficiency on the aggregation of cat platelets. Comp Biochem Physiol 78C (1984b) 123–126.

MacDonald ML, Rogers QR, Morris JG, Cupps PT: Effects of linoleate and arachidonate deficiencies on reproduction and spermatogenesis in the cat. J Nutr 115 (1984c) 719–726.

Manitius A, Pigeon G, Epstein FH: Mechanism by which dietary protein enhances renal concentrating ability. Am J Physiol 205 (1963) 101–106.

Mansur Guérios MF, Hoxter G: Hypoalbuminemia in choline deficient cats. Protides Biol Fluids Proc Colloq 10 (1962) 199–201.

Miller SA: The development of a semi-synthetic diet and its use in a study of protein metabolism in the cat. PhD thesis, Rutgers University, 1957.

Mizuhara S, Oomori S: A new sulfur-containing amino acid. Arch Biochem Biophys 92 (1961) 53–57.

Moore T: Copper deficiency in rats fed upon meat. Br Med J 5279 (1962) 689–691.

Morris JG, Rogers QR: Ammonia intoxication in the near-adult cat as a result of a dietary deficiency of arginine. Science 199 (1978a) 431–432.

Morris JG, Rogers QR: Arginine: An essential amino acid for the cat. J Nutr 108 (1978b) 1944–1953.

Morris JG, Rogers QR: Amino acid requirements of the kitten. Royal Netherlands Vet Assoc, Voorjaaredagen, Amsterdam, 1980.

Morris JG, Trudell J, Pencovic T: Carbohydrate digestion by the domestic cat *(Felis catus)*. Br J Nutr 37 (1977) 365–373.

Morris ML Jr: Feline degenerative retinopathy. Cornell Vet 55 (1965) 295–308.

Morris ML Jr: Feline Dietetics: Nutritional management in health and disease. Topeka, Mark Morris Associates, 1968.

Munson TO, Holzworth J, Small E, Witzel S, Jones TC, Luginbühl H: Steatitis ("yellow fat") in cats fed canned red tuna. J Am Vet Med Assoc 133 (1958) 563–568.

National Research Council: Nutrient Requirements of Cats. Washington, DC, National Academy of Sciences, 1972.

National Research Council: Nutrient Requirements of Swine. Washington, DC, National Academy of Sciences, 1973.

National Research Council: Nutrient Requirements of Cats. Washington, DC, National Academy of Sciences, 1978.

National Research Council: Nutrient Requirements of Laboratory Animals. Washington, DC, National Academy of Sciences, 1978.

National Research Council: Taurine Requirement of Cats. Washington, DC, National Academy of Sciences, 1981.

Odom G, MacEachern D: Subarachnoid injection of thiamine in cats; unmasking of brain lesions by induced thiamine deficiency. Proc Soc Exp Biol Med 50 (1942) 28–31.

O'Donnell JA III, Rogers QR, Morris JG: Effect of diet on plasma taurine in the cat. J Nutr 111 (1981) 1111–1116.

Osbaldiston GW, Taussig RA: Clinical report on 46 cases of feline urological syndrome. Vet Med Small Anim Clin 65 (1970) 461–468.

Osborne CA, Lees GE: Feline urologic syndrome: medical aspects of prophylaxis. *In* Kirk RW (ed): Current Veterinary Therapy VII. Philadelphia, WB Saunders Company, 1980.

Palmer NC: Osteodystrophia fibrosa in cats. Aust Vet J 44 (1968) 151–155.

Palmore WP, Gaskin JM, Nielson JT: Effects of diet on feline urine. Lab Anim Sci 28 (1978) 551–555.

Passe D, Lee HS: Personal communication, 1982.

Pencovic TA, Morris JG: Corn and wheat starch utilization by the cat. J Anim Sci 41 (1975) 325 (abstr).

Pfaffmann C: Gustatory nerve impulses in the rat, cat and rabbit. J Neurophysiol 18 (1955) 429–440.

Rabin B, Nicolosi RJ, Hayes KC: Dietary influence on bile acid conjugation in the cat. J Nutr 106 (1976) 1241–1246.

Rambaut PC, Miller SA: Studies of sulfur amino acid nutrition in the adult cat. Fed Proc 24 (1965) 373 (abstr).

Rambaut PC, Miller SA: Studies in feline sulfur amino acid metabolism. Proc Seventh Int Cong Nutr (Hamburg) 5 (1966) 164. (Braunschweig, Pergamon Press, 1967).

Reber EF, Malhotra OP: Effect of feeding a vitamin K–deficient ration containing irradiated beef to rats, dogs and cats. J Nutr 74 (1961) 191–193.

Rich LJ, Dysart I, Chow FHC, Hamar D: Urethral obstruction in male cats: Experimental production by addition of magnesium and phosphate to diet. Feline Pract 4 (5) (1974) 44–47.

Riser WH: Juvenile osteoporosis (osteogenesis imperfecta)—a calcium deficiency. J Am Vet Med Assoc 139 (1961) 117–119.

Riser WH, Brodey RS, Shirer JF: Osteodystrophy in mature cats: A nutritional disease. J Am Vet Radiol Soc 9 (1968) 37–46.

Ritter SM, Owens FN: Methionine requirements of the growing cat. J Anim Sci 39 (1974) 981 (abstr).

Rivers JPW, Frankel TL: Fat in the diet of cats and dogs. *In* Anderson RS (ed): Nutrition of the Dog and Cat. New York, Pergamon Press, 1980.

Rivers JPW, Hassam AG, Alderson C: The absence of Δ6-desaturase activity in the cat. Proc Nutr Soc 35 (1976a) 67A–68A.

Rivers JPW, Hassam AG, Crawford MA, Brambell MR: The inability of the lion, *Panthera leo* L., to desaturate linoleic acid. FEBS Lett 67 (1976b) 269–270.

Rivers JPW, Sinclair AJ, Crawford MA: Inability of the cat to desaturate essential fatty acids. Nature (Lond) 258 (1975) 171–173.

Rivers JPW, Sinclair AJ, Moore DP, Crawford MA: The abnormal metabolism of essential fatty acids in the cat. Proc Nutr Soc 35 (1976c) 66A–67A.

Roberts AH, Scott PP: Nutrition of the cat. 5. The influence of calcium and iodine supplements to a meat diet on the retention of nitrogen, calcium and phosphorus. Br J Nutr 15 (1961) 73–82.

Rogers QR, Freedland RA, Symmons RA: In vivo synthesis and utilization of arginine in the rat. Am J Physiol 223 (1972) 236–240.

Rogers QR, Morris JG: Essentiality of amino acids for the growing kitten. J Nutr 109 (1979) 718–723.

Rogers QR, Morris JG, Freedland RA: Lack of hepatic enzymatic adaptation to low and high levels of dietary protein in the adult cat. Enzyme 22 (1977) 348–356.

Rogers QR, Morris JG: Why does the cat require a high protein diet? *In* Anderson RS (ed): Nutrition of the Dog and Cat. New York, Pergamon Press, 1980.

Rowland GN, Capen CC, Nagode LA: Experimental hyperparathyroidism in young cats. Pathol Vet 5 (1968) 504–519.

Rubin LF, Lipton DE: Retinal degeneration in kittens. J Am Vet Med Assoc 162 (1973) 467–469.

Schaeffer MC, Rogers QR, Morris JG: Methionine requirement of weanling kittens in the absence of dietary cystine. Fed Proc 39 (1980) 794 (abstr).

Schaeffer MC, Rogers QR, Morris JG: The choline requirement of the growing kitten in the presence of just adequate dietary methionine. Nutr Res 2 (1982) 289–299.

Schalm OW: Megaloblastic marrow cytology in the cat: Vitamin $B_{12}$ and folic acid deficiencies [and] erythroleukemia. Feline Pract 4 (5) (1974) 16–19.

Schneck GW, Cumberland V: The effect of 10 per cent dietary fat addition on the growth rate of cats. Vet Rec 83 (1968) 486–488.

Scott PP: Problems encountered in studying the nutrition of the cat. Proc Nutr Soc 16 (1957) 77–83.

Scott PP: Some aspects of the nutrition of the dog and cat. II. The cat. Vet Rec 72 (1960) 6–9.

Scott PP: Nutritional requirements and deficiencies. *In* Catcott EJ (ed): Feline Medicine and Surgery. Santa Barbara, American Veterinary Publications, 1964.

Scott PP: Minerals and vitamins in feline nutrition. *In* Graham-Jones O (ed): Canine and Feline Nutritional Requirements. London, Pergamon Press, 1965.

Scott PP: Nutrition. *In* Wilkinson GT (ed): Diseases of the Cat. London, Pergamon Press, 1966.

Scott PP: Osteodystrophies. Vet Rec 84 (1969) 333–335.

Scott PP: Nutrition and disease. *In* Catcott EJ (ed): Feline Medicine and Surgery, 2nd ed. Santa Barbara, American Veterinary Publications, 1975.

Scott PP: The influence of feeding on the incidence of urolithiasis in the cat. *In* Anderson RS (ed): Nutrition of the Dog and Cat. New York, Pergamon Press, 1980.

Scott PP, Greaves JP, Scott MG: Nutrition of the cat. 4. Calcium and iodine deficiency on a meat diet. Br J Nutr 15 (1961) 35–51.

Scott PP, Greaves JP, Scott MG: Nutritional blindness in the cat. Exp Eye Res 3 (1964) 357–364.

Scott PP, Humphreys ER: The addition of herring and vegetable oils to the diet of cats. Proc Nutr Soc 21 (1962) xiii.

Scott PP, McKusick VA, McKusick AB: The nature of osteogenesis imperfecta in cats. Evidence that the disorder is primarily nutritional, not genetic, and therefore not analogous to the disease in man. J Bone Joint Surg 45A (1963) 125–134.

Scott PP, Scott MG: Nutritive requirements for carnivora. *In* Conalty ML (ed): Husbandry of Laboratory Animals. London, Academic Press, 1967.

Seawright AA, English PB, Gartner RJW: Hypervitaminosis A and deforming cervical spondylosis of the cat. J Comp Pathol 77 (1967) 29–39.

Seawright AA, Hrdlicka J: Pathogenetic factors in tooth loss in young cats on a high daily oral intake of vitamin A. Aust Vet J 50 (1974) 133–141.

Seefeldt SL, Chapman TE: Body water content and turnover in cats fed dry and canned rations. Am J Vet Res 40 (1979) 183–185.

Sheffield MG: Personal communication, 1983.

Sinclair AJ: Metabolism of linoleic acid in the cat. Lipids 14 (1979) 932–936.

Sinclair AJ, Slattery W, McLean JG, Monger EA: Essential fatty acid deficiency and evidence for arachidonate synthesis in the cat. Br J Nutr 46 (1981) 93–96.

Skultety FM: Alterations of caloric intake in cats following lesions of the hypothalamus and midbrain. Ann NY Acad Sci 157 (1969) 861–874.

Smalley KA, Rogers QR, Morris JG: Methionine requirement of weanling kittens fed adequate cystine. Fed Proc 39 (1980) 435 (abstr).

Smalley K, Rogers QR, Morris JG, Buria L, Eslinger L: The nitrogen requirement of the kitten using crystalline amino acid diets or casein diets. Twelfth Int Cong Nutr, San Diego (1981) 117 (abstr).

Smith DC, Proutt LM: Development of thiamine deficiency in the cat on a diet of raw fish. Proc Soc Exp Biol Med 56 (1944) 1–3.

Stephan ZF, Hayes KC: Vitamin E deficiency and essential fatty acid (EFA) status of cats. Fed Proc 37 (1978) 706 (abstr).

Sturman JA, Hayes KC: The biology of taurine in nutrition and development. Adv Nutr Res 3 (1980) 231–299.

Suter P: Zur Gefähr der Überdosierung von Vitamin-D-Präparaten. Schweiz Arch Tierheilkd 99 (1957) 421–433.

Tallan HH, Moore S, Stein WH: Studies on the free amino acids and related compounds in the tissues of the cat. J Biol Chem 211 (1954) 927–939.

Taton GF, Hamar DW, Lewis LD: Evaluation of ammonium chloride as a urinary acidifier in the cat. J Am Vet Med Assoc 184 (1984a) 433–436.

Taton GF, Hamar DW, Lewis LD: Urinary acidification in the prevention and treatment of feline struvite urolithiasis. J Am Vet Med Assoc 184 (1984b) 437–443.

Teeter RG, Baker DH, Corbin JE: Methionine and cystine requirements of the cat. J Nutr 108 (1978a) 291–295.

Teeter RG, Baker DH, Corbin JE: Methionine essentiality for the cat. J Anim Sci 46 (1978b) 1287–1292.

Thenen SW, Rasmussen KM: Megaloblastic erythropoiesis and tissue depletion of folic acid in the cat. Am J Vet Res 39 (1978) 1205–1207.

Thrall BE, Miller LG: Water turnover in cats fed dry rations. Feline Pract 6 (1) (1976) 10–17.

Titchenal C, Rogers QR, Indrieri RJ, Morris JG: Threonine imbalance in the kitten. Fed Proc 39 (1980) 794 (abstr).

Toman JEP, Everett GM, Oster RH, Smith DC: Origin of cardiac disorders in thiamine-deficient cats. Proc Soc Exp Biol Med 58 (1945) 65–67.

Trudell JE, Morris JG: Carbohydrate digestion in the cat. J Anim Sci 41 (1975) 329 (abstr).

Westall RG: The amino acids and other ampholytes of urine. 2. The isolation of a new sulphur-containing amino acid from cat urine. Biochem J 55 (1953) 244–248.

Zotterman Y: Species differences in the water taste. Acta Physiol Scand 37 (1956) 60–70.

# 3
CHAPTER
# SEDATION AND ANESTHESIA

CYNTHIA M. TRIM

## PREPARATION

Success in anesthesia is not measured merely by survival rate. Good anesthesia provides conditions that allow a procedure to be performed efficiently and safely with minimal stress or pain for the cat. Equally important, anesthesia must not cause residual organ depression, which would result in a slow return to health, prolonged hospitalization time, greater cost in drugs, and labor and worry for the veterinarian and the client.

Adequate preparation increases the chance of meeting these goals. It includes examination of the cat and its medical history, correct interpretation of information from relevant laboratory tests, and consideration of the procedure to discover anything that would preclude the use of specific drugs or influence the course of anesthesia and recovery. A history of an unsatisfactory anesthetic experience or an unusual drug reaction warrants careful choice of drugs. Use of agents with easily reversible actions, such as narcotic or inhalant drugs, may be indicated. Kittens are less able to metabolize anesthetic drugs owing to immaturity of their liver enzyme systems, and the use of barbiturates in particular should be avoided in the first three months of life.

Certain physical characteristics of the cat may forewarn of potential problems. The thin or emaciated cat is likely to have a prolonged recovery from barbiturate anesthesia, the obese cat will probably hypoventilate during general anesthesia, and the Persian cat may experience airway obstruction when anesthetized. Auscultation of the heart and lungs in every cat requiring anesthesia is advisable to identify cardiac abnormalities or early changes of respiratory disease. It is important to perform the examination in a room where the cat will relax and the heart rate will slow, enabling a more accurate evaluation of these systems. For every cat that requires major surgery, has a history of organ malfunction, or is middle-aged or older, blood should be submitted for a complete blood count (CBC) and determination of blood urea nitrogen (BUN), creatinine, and liver enzymes. Further tests before anesthesia may be warranted, depending on other laboratory results or the particular patient's problem. It is essential that the blood be collected from the unsedated cat in a quiet, nonstressful environment, since both stress and sedation alter many blood values (Frankel and Hawkey, 1980).

The course of anesthesia and the postoperative recovery can be greatly improved if abnormalities of fluid, electrolyte, and acid-base status are corrected as much as possible before induction of anesthesia. Restoration of circulating blood volume is essential before further cardiovascular depression from anesthetic drugs is imposed. In many cases it is better to administer intensive care for several days before surgery. For example, before a perineal urethrostomy is created in a cat with urethral obstruction, the bladder should be catheterized under sedation or light anesthesia and the cat hospitalized for two or three days for fluid therapy to correct dehydration and to lower the serum potassium level.

Any complications that might arise directly from the medical or surgical procedure should be considered. Will the duration of anesthesia be prolonged? Will positioning of the cat interfere with breathing? How much muscle relaxation is needed? What degree of pain or blood loss is associated with this operation? At the same time one should consider whether there are any drugs that should be avoided in this cat or for this procedure. One must bear in mind that ketamine increases intracranial pressure and must not be used in animals with cranial or spinal cord trauma; that methoxyflurane decreases hepatic blood flow by 50 per cent and should be avoided with liver disease; that xylazine causes bradycardia and pulmonary hypertension and must be used cautiously in the presence of cardiac disease. It cannot be overemphasized that the few minutes spent in planning for the use of each anesthetic will greatly reduce the incidence of complications.

Before induction of anesthesia, in all but emergencies, food must be withheld for 8 to 12 hours and water for 2 hours to reduce the likelihood of vomiting or regurgitation and pulmonary aspiration. Whenever possible, the surgical site should be clipped well in advance to decrease anesthesia time. All equipment needed to carry out anesthesia and surgery should be collected and, when used, the anesthetic machine and circuit checked. Antibiotics and drugs other than anesthetics must be administered before anesthesia. Adverse reactions or drug interactions are difficult to identify and diagnose while the cat is anesthetized.

Finally, it must be stressed that greater cooperation is obtained from most cats through gentle, quiet handling than through a show of dominance or force.

## INJECTABLE DRUGS

The majority of cats can be quietly removed from their cages and comfortably and securely held for transport or for injections as shown in Figure 3–1. Excited or aggressive cats can be restrained with the use of gloves, blankets, and towels. Only rarely should a snare be necessary. Subcutaneous and intramuscular injections, even intravenous injections, can usually be given by one person (Figs. 3–2 and 3–3) but can be accomplished more rapidly if a second person holds the cat. For intramuscular injection involving two people, a method of restraint is illustrated in Figure 3–4. Stretching the cat diminishes the effectiveness of its muscular movements and minimizes the range of the forepaws.

The most common site for intramuscular injection is the biceps femoris muscle caudal to the shaft of the femur; however, a study of intramuscular injections has shown that drug injected at that site lies more often in the fascial tissue than in the muscle (Baxter and Evans, 1973). A more reliable site has been found to be the quadriceps muscle mass cranial to the femur (Fig. 3–5). Beside providing more reliable drug absorption, use of this site avoids damage to the sciatic nerve.

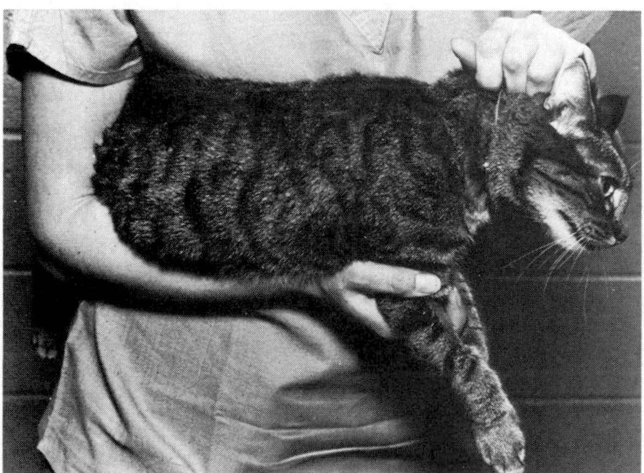

**Figure 3–1.** This method of holding the cat provides maximal restraint. The hand holds the forelimbs while the forearm supports the body. The hindlimbs are immobilized because the elbow maintains the stifles in extension. The head cannot move because of the secure hold on the scruff of the neck.

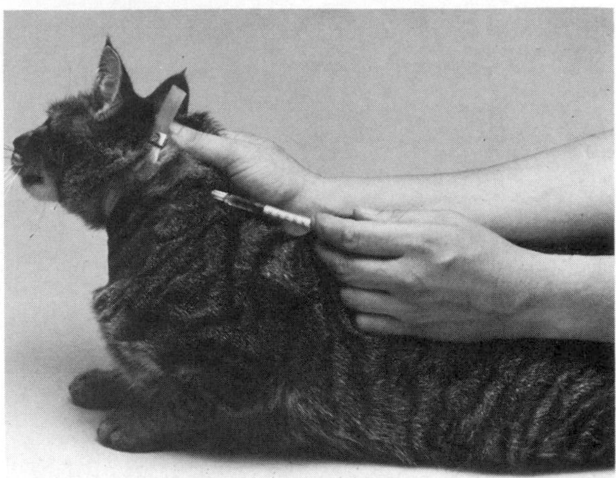

**Figure 3–2.** For subcutaneous injection, the cat is faced away from the operator. The skin over the neck is tented for injection while the forearm presses the cat to the table.

Anesthetic drugs to be administered intravenously to the cat are usually injected into the cephalic or saphenous vein (Figs. 3–6 and 3–7). Use of the cephalic vein causes minimal disturbance by allowing the cat to sit in a normal position, but a greater length of saphenous vein is available for venepuncture. A 25-gauge needle is adequate for most intramuscular or intravenous injections; however, a 25- or 21-gauge butterfly infusion set or a 20-gauge indwelling catheter is more likely to ensure a patent vein for the duration of the procedure (Fig. 3–8).

The person responsible for administering drugs should be familiar with the properties of each drug and the recommended route of administration, because the onset and duration of action may be affected by alternative use. The rest of this section therefore deals with the pharmacology of injectable anesthetic drugs.

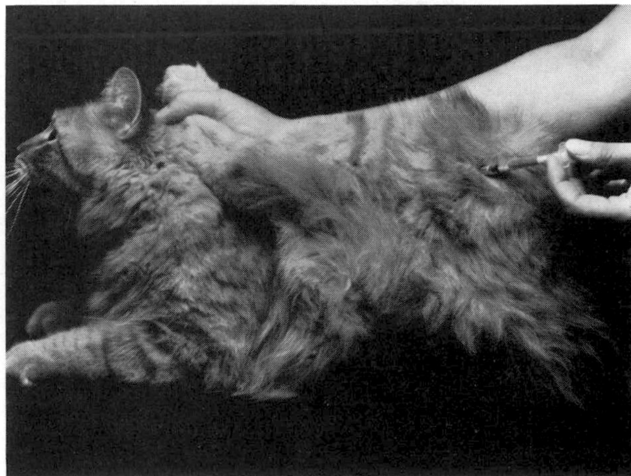

**Figure 3–3.** For intramuscular injection, the hand restraining the cat by the scruff of the neck also holds one hindlimb. The intramuscular injection is made into the restrained limb.

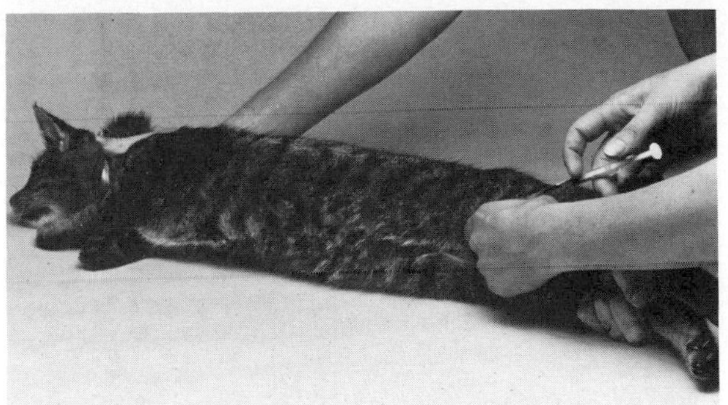

**Figure 3–4.** One person restrains the cat fully stretched by holding the scruff in one hand and the hocks in the other hand. Intramuscular injection is performed by a second person.

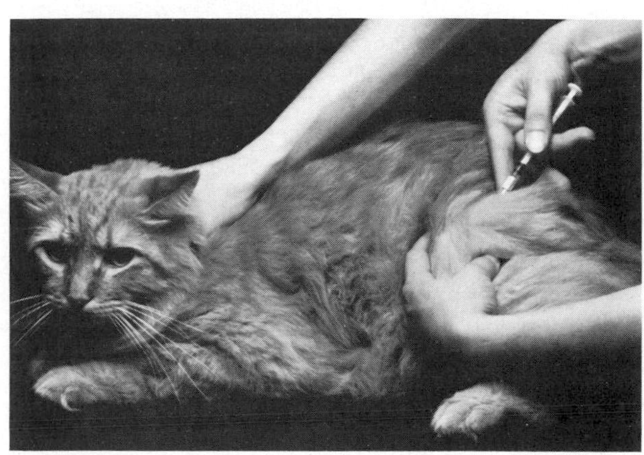

**Figure 3–5.** Quiet cats require little restraint. Intramuscular injection is into the muscle mass cranial to the shaft of the femur.

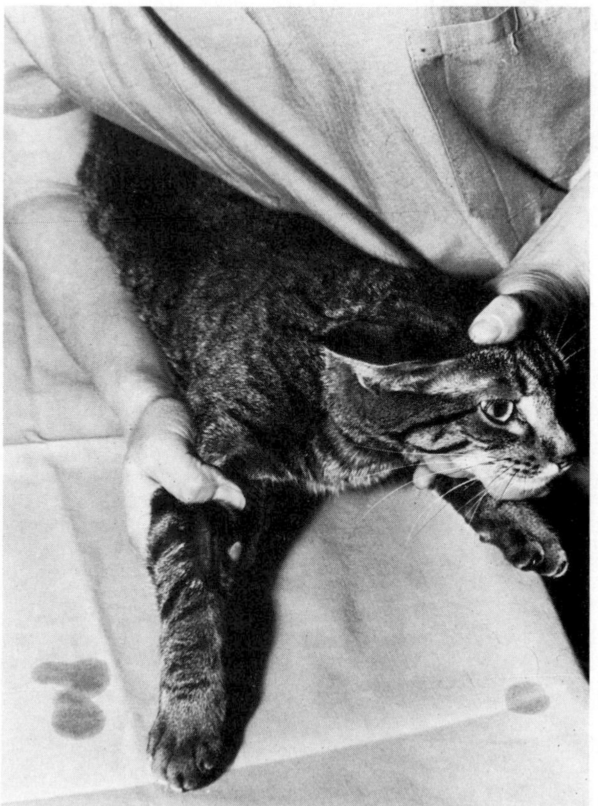

**Figure 3–6.** Restraint for intravenous injection into the cephalic vein. The cat is enclosed by the handler's body, right arm, and left hand. The right hand cups the cat's elbow to immobilize the limb, and thumb pressure occludes the vein.

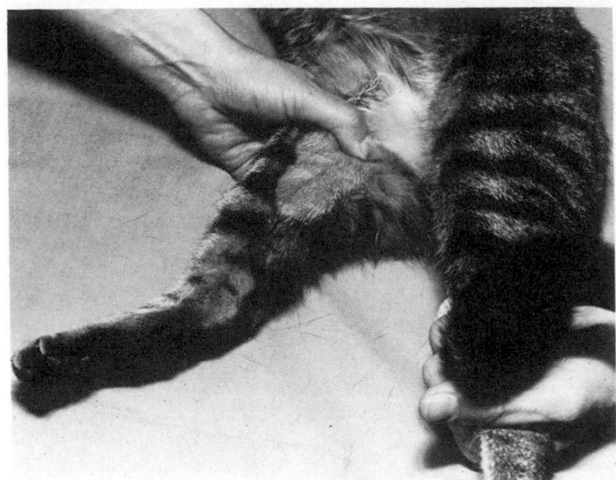

**Figure 3–7.** The saphenous vein lying on the medial surface of the hindlimb is very prominent. Finger and thumb pressure above the stifle prevents flexion of the limb and occludes the vein.

## ANTICHOLINERGIC DRUGS

Atropine and glycopyrrolate are the two anticholinergic drugs most commonly used in veterinary anesthesia. Glycopyrrolate's activity in the cat is similar to that in dogs (Miller, 1981). These drugs are used for three main reasons: to prevent reflex bradycardia arising from surgical manipulation of organs, particularly during oophorohysterectomy, intestinal repair, thoracotomy, and eye enucleation; to slow gastrointestinal motility and thus reduce the incidence of vomiting; and to diminish salivary and bronchial secretions, which may cause airway obstruction during anesthesia. These drugs are best given before induction of anesthesia to allow sufficient time for full effect. Atropine injected at the usual dose (0.04 mg/kg IM, SC) becomes effective 20 minutes after intramuscular administration, and its action continues for about one hour. An intramuscular injection of glycopyrrolate (0.01 mg/kg) is adequately absorbed in about 45 minutes, but subcutaneous injection often does not provide levels adequate to prevent drug-induced bradycardia.

The advantages of glycopyrrolate over atropine are its longer duration of action, the absence of tachycardia, and the alteration in gastric secretion. In the event of pulmonary aspiration, the severity of tissue reaction may be less when the pH of gastric fluid is higher. Glycopyrrolate, however, is considerably more expensive than atropine. Unlike atropine, it is incompatible in the same syringe with acetylpromazine and barbiturates.

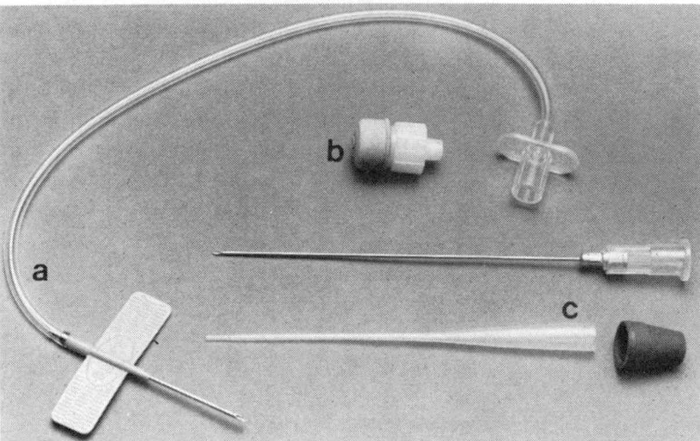


**Figure 3–8.** a, Butterfly infusion set. b, Catheter plug. c, Indwelling catheter.

## TRANQUILIZERS, SEDATIVES, AND HYPNOTICS

This group of drugs includes the phenothiazine derivatives acetylpromazine (acepromazine), promazine (Sparine), piperacetazine (Psymod), and triflupromazine (Vetame), and also diazepam (Valium) and xylazine (Rompun). Most of these drugs are used both for sedation alone and before general anesthesia, with a lower dose for the latter purpose. Combined with gentle handling, use of the phenothiazine tranquilizers for preanesthetic medication produces an unconcerned cat likely to have a smooth anesthetic induction. In addition, the tranquilizers have an antiarrhythmic effect on the heart. Their effect usually persists into the recovery period to ease disorientation and prevent nausea and vomiting. Acetylpromazine is at present the most widely used phenothiazine tranquilizer because it has a predictable action and is relatively safe within the dose range now recommended for premedication (0.1 to 0.22 mg/kg IM). Piperacetazine is useful in producing greater sedation than acetylpromazine at the same dose, but this is reflected in greater somnolence during recovery from general anesthesia. In the healthy cat these drugs have a minimal depressant effect on the cardiovascular and respiratory systems, but they should be used cautiously in depressed or hypovolemic cats, which cannot compensate for the decreased myocardial contractility and peripheral vasodilation. The phenothiazine tranquilizers alter the threshold for convulsions and should not be used in cats with elevated intracranial pressure or toxic reactions characterized by seizures.

Diazepam is a long-acting drug and is methylated into active metabolites. In cats given an oral or slow intravenous dose of 0.2 to 0.5 mg/kg, offensive behavior is decreased, some muscle relaxation is produced, and appetite is stimulated. Diazepam has been documented as producing a mixture of central nervous system depressant and facilitatory effects, which seem to vary with the state of consciousness of the cat. Sometimes excitement occurs in the awake cat. Smaller quantities of other drugs used for induction must be given when diazepam is used for premedication, and ketamine-induced sleep time is prolonged. Diazepam, 0.1 mg/kg, has been shown to decrease myocardial contractile force in cats by 25 per cent, as well as mildly reducing heart rate and arterial blood pressure (Chai and Wang, 1966). Respiratory depression is common, but the degree is partly determined by the combination of drugs used. Cats anesthetized with pentobarbital show a pronounced decrease in ventilation after intravenous injection of diazepam (0.5 mg/kg), whereas those anesthetized with ketamine do not.

Xylazine produces more profound sedation and muscle relaxation than either the phenothiazine tranquilizers or diazepam and is therefore particularly useful for manipulative procedures such as radiography or casting (0.5 to 2 mg/kg IM). Xylazine premedication (0.5 mg/kg IM) greatly reduces the dosage of anesthetic drugs. Many cats vomit soon after administration, but this vomiting must not be relied on to empty the stomach. The onset of maximal action occurs within five minutes after intravenous injection and within 15 minutes after intramuscular injection. Intravenous injection results in an immediate significant reduction in heart rate and cardiac output, which remain depressed for 25 minutes and gradually return to preinjection values (McLeish and Steffey, 1977). Xylazine must therefore be used very cautiously in depressed cats. When given alone it has little effect on arterial carbon dioxide values, but when combined with general anesthetic drugs may cause considerable respiratory depression. Xylazine sedation is accompanied by up to a 500 per cent increase in the plasma glucose level (Feldberg and Symonds, 1980) and should be avoided in diabetic cats. Urine production is increased six fold within two hours after intramuscular injection of xylazine, 1.1 mg/kg (Hartsfield, 1980), an effect that might preclude its use in the dehydrated cat or the cat with urethral obstruction.

## Narcotics and Narcotic Antagonists

Narcotic analgesics are valuable to alleviate pain during and after surgery. Excitement and restlessness may be produced in any animal receiving a narcotic in the absence of pain, but excitement in the cat may be due to incorrect extrapolation of dosage information from another species. For example, administration of morphine at one-tenth the dose used for dogs (0.1 mg/kg) produces analgesia for about four hours without excitement (Davis and Donnelly, 1968). Meperidine (Demerol) has a wider safety margin and is the narcotic most commonly used in cats. Intramuscular injection of meperidine (2 to 4 mg/kg IM, SC) provides analgesia for about two hours. When used for premedication, meperidine produces little sedation but reduces the subsequent requirement for inhalation anesthetics. The rapid biotransformation means that additional drug is usually needed to control pain after surgery. Acetylpromazine and meperidine injected together form a neuroleptanalgesic mixture with synergistic actions and provide excellent preanesthetic control of the cat. Oxymorphone is also used in the cat (0.2 mg/kg IM) both alone and combined with a tranquilizer (Palminteri, 1965).

A major advantage of the use of narcotics in the sick cat is the ability at any time to reverse their effects. Several narcotic antagonists are available, but naloxone, a derivative of oxymorphone, reverses the effects of all opiates or opioids. In addition, unlike nalorphine or levallorphan, naloxone does not have sedative properties. It is short-acting (about 15 minutes), and more than one injection may be needed (0.01 to 0.02 mg/kg IM IV).

## Barbiturates

The ultra-short-acting barbiturates—thiopental, thiamylal, and methohexital—are useful and reliable anesthetics for the cat. They may be used alone for short procedures or as induction drugs with inhalation anesthesia, preferably with a preanesthetic sedative or tranquilizer to reduce the dose needed and to ensure a smooth recovery. Dilute solutions of 2.5, 2, or 1 per cent provide a sufficient volume of drug to allow accurate titration to effect. Dilution also reduces the severity of tissue damage following accidental perivascular injection. The dosage for each drug depends on the degree of preanesthetic sedation and existing central nervous system depression. Acidosis and hypoproteinemia alter the ionization and protein-binding of the drugs and also reduce the amount of barbiturate required to produce anesthesia. Approximate dosages of the thiobarbiturates and methohexital for the unpremedicated healthy cat are 20 mg/kg and 12 mg/kg, respectively. Moderate preanesthetic sedation (e.g., acetylpromazine, 0.2 mg/kg IM) reduces the requirement by half. The speed of injection of barbiturate significantly influences the total dose needed to achieve anesthesia. Rapid injection of only a small amount results in a high blood level and causes apnea. One third to one half of the calculated dose should be injected steadily. Then, after a pause of 20 seconds, additional amounts should be injected to achieve the desired effect. Injection of barbiturate into an infusion line containing lactated Ringer's solution reduces the potency of the barbiturate and renders induction of anesthesia less precise. The change is due to mixing of acidic solution with alkaline barbiturate, which causes precipitation of the free acid. Interaction with calcium in the solution may also occur.

Recovery to consciousness occurs when redistribution into major organs and muscle lowers blood level. Full recovery is due to further distribution into fat, followed by metabolism. Consequently the thin cat is slow to recover and barbiturates are best avoided. Methohexital is more rapidly metabolized than are the thiobarbiturates. Its half-life is one-tenth that of thiopental or thiamylal, and complete recovery is more rapid. Methohexital is therefore preferable for very young or old cats or animals in which airway obstruction or aspiration might be a problem, e.g., those undergoing oral surgery.

Pentobarbital differs from the previously mentioned barbiturates in two respects. First, because it is slow to cross the blood-brain barrier, it must be injected more slowly over several minutes to avoid overdosing. Second, the duration of action is about 40 minutes after a single anesthetic dose, and recovery depends on metabolism by the liver rather than redistribution. Pentobarbital depresses hypothalamic thermoregulation, and hypothermia is a common effect. A reduction in circulating blood volume accompanies major surgery owing to fluid loss and evaporation from exposed viscera. Prevention of hypothermia and hypovolemia minimizes the effects of anesthesia on liver function and avoids prolonged sleep time.

The extent of cardiovascular and ventilatory depression induced by barbiturates depends on the total dose of the drug used and the rapidity and duration of administration. Thiopental, for example, possesses negative inotropic properties but also induces reflex tachycardia. The result is only a small depression in cardiac function. Venous dilation occurs, reducing venous return to the heart and depressing systemic blood pressure. Ventilation may be nearly normal, but arterial oxygenation is usually lowered in response to the decrease in cardiac output. Barbiturate anesthesia has a minimal effect on hepatic function, but the presence of severe hepatic disease greatly prolongs sleeping time even with thiobarbiturates. Renal disease also prolongs the action of barbiturates. The effect is multiple through changes in blood pH, plasma protein levels, and hepatic function. Concurrent administration of chloramphenicol has been shown to extend anesthesia time from barbiturates (Adams and Dixit, 1970).

Tissue damage resulting from extravascular injection of a barbiturate may be prevented by subcutaneous infiltration of the area with an equal amount of a solution of 1 ml of 2 per cent lidocaine in 4 ml physiologic saline solution.

## KETAMINE

Ketamine, a dissociative drug, differs from traditional anesthetics in that failure to react to painful stimuli is not associated with general central nervous system depression. It has been shown to be analgesic in subanesthetic doses in man, but neither in humans nor in cats does it prevent the hemodynamic response to abdominal pain. Although muscle relaxation is incomplete (Fig. 3–9), most surgical procedures can be accomplished with ketamine alone. However, the quality of anesthesia is improved by addition of a sedative or tranquilizer. Several drugs have been recommended in order to reduce the ketamine dose or to prolong the duration of anesthesia, provide muscle relaxation, and promote a smooth recovery (Reid and Frank, 1972). Useful drugs are acetylpromazine (0.1 mg/kg), piperacetazine (0.1 mg/kg), promazine (1 mg/kg), and xylazine (0.5 mg/kg), all of which are given intramuscularly. Diazepam (0.2 to 0.5 mg/kg, IM or IV) is useful with ketamine for compromised cats. The onset of action of the phenothiazines is much slower than that of ketamine, and they should therefore be administered at least 20 minutes before ketamine for best effect. Since xylazine induces vomiting in most cats, a delay before the administration of ketamine is advisable to avoid aspiration. Because ketamine usually causes profuse salivation, pretreatment with atropine is recommended.

In the healthy cat an intramuscular injection of ketamine (25 to 30 mg/kg), after sedation with one of the drugs recommended, takes effect within several minutes and provides 40 minutes of anesthesia. Recovery of coordinated movement takes several hours. When the ketamine is injected intravenously (10 mg/kg), anesthesia time is shortened to 20 minutes, and complete recovery is considerably more rapid. In either case, anesthesia can be prolonged by giving additional ketamine. Ketamine (2 mg/kg) injected intravenously prolongs anesthesia by about 10 minutes. Dosages should be lowered for sick cats. If a cat is extremely difficult to handle, ketamine may be administered by squirting the drug into the cat's open mouth. Initially one uses the same dose as for intramuscular injection, allowing 20 minutes for effect. Accidental introduction into the eyes does not cause corneal damage despite the low pH of ketamine (Macy and Siwe, 1977). Ketamine is, however, absorbed through the conjunctiva, contributing to the anesthetic effect.

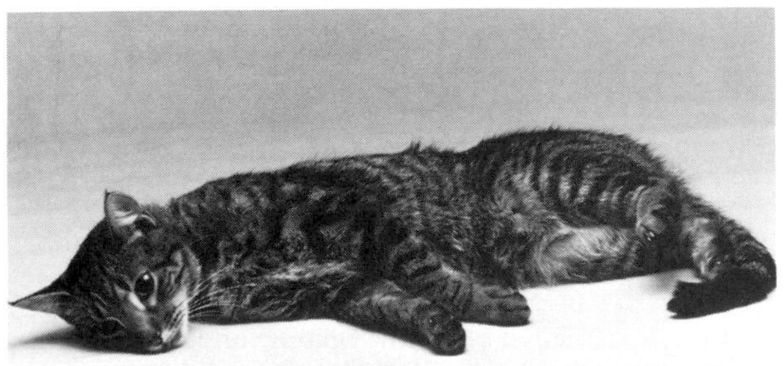

**Figure 3–9.** Ketamine anesthesia. Incomplete muscle relaxation and dilated pupils are characteristic.

Application of ophthalmic ointment is necessary during ketamine anesthesia to prevent corneal drying and ulceration because the eyes remain wide open (Fig. 3–9). The effect of ketamine on pharyngeal and laryngeal reflexes is unpredictable and varies from complete suppression with potential for aspiration to retention of ability to both cough and swallow. Ketamine alone causes central sympathetic stimulation, which increases heart rate and blood pressure. Concurrent use of sedatives or hypnotics blocks this effect, so that the ketamine anesthesia depresses the cardiovascular system.

An apneustic pattern of breathing (inspiratory breath-holding) is characteristic of ketamine anesthesia. Complete cessation of breathing occurs sometimes, particularly with the xylazine-ketamine combination. Provided the apnea is recognized early and artificial ventilation is instituted, recovery is uneventful. Respiratory depression is less if the dose of xylazine does not exceed 0.5 mg/kg. I also recommend that any cat receiving ketamine be kept under observation from the time of injection.

The Ontario Veterinary Association has recorded its concern about the increasing number of reports of unexplained deaths in cats and dogs associated with xylazine-ketamine anesthesia (Gillick, 1981). The article emphasized the cardiovascular effects of the drug combination and recommended a thorough preanesthetic examination as a step toward identifying animals likely to have difficulty with anesthesia. Personal communications from practitioners indicate that cats have died both during anesthesia with xylazine-ketamine and later, after returning home. In most cases no obvious reason for death was given, but signs of severe pulmonary edema and cardiac failure have been described.

Initial recovery from ketamine is due to lowering of brain and blood levels as a result of redistribution into tissues. At least part of the elimination in cats is by metabolism in the liver, and most of the ketamine and metabolites are excreted in the urine (Heavner and Bloedow, 1979). One metabolite of ketamine possesses similar central depressant effects, but the degree of contribution to anesthesia in the cat is yet unknown. Hyperreflexia and "hallucinations" often occur during recovery. If the cat claws at its mouth, additional tranquilizer may be indicated. Self-damage may be prevented by bandaging the paws or applying an Elizabethan collar until full awareness returns. Seizures induced by ketamine are uncommon in the cat but occasionally develop irrespective of the type of premedication. If cyanosis is produced, oxygen must be supplied by face mask or, rarely, by endotracheal tube. The seizure can be controlled by diazepam (0.2 to 0.5 mg/kg) given slowly intravenously or by the inhalation of small quantities of halothane or methoxyflurane. Elimination of ketamine can be speeded by infusing lactated Ringer's solution (10 ml/kg) intravenously over 10 to 15 minutes.

### Alphadione

A steroid anesthetic, alphadione (CT 1341) is licensed for use in cats, primates, and man in Great Britain (Saffan, Althesin) and in man in Canada (Alfathesin) but is not yet commercially available in the United States. It has no progestational or mineralocorticoid activity. Alphadione consists of two pregnanedione derivatives, alphaxalone and alphadalone, which are solubilized in saline by polyoxyethylated castor oil. Alphaxalone is principally responsible for the anesthetic activity; alphadalone, which is slower acting and less potent, is necessary to improve solubility. The mixture is a clear, slightly viscous solution of approximately neutral pH. Each milliliter of solution contains 12 mg of total steroids, composed of 9 mg alphaxalone and 3 mg alphadalone.

The drug can be used both for heavy sedation and for general anesthesia and compares favorably with xylazine or ketamine (Haskins et al., 1975). Alphadione can be administered intramuscularly or intravenously. Surgical anesthesia begins within 30 seconds after intravenous injection. The duration of anesthesia is proportional to the dose; 9 mg/kg given intravenously provides about 20 minutes of surgical anesthesia, with good mobility regained after one and one-half hours. Generally no more than 2 ml (24 mg) is needed for an initial intravenous dose. Anesthesia can be prolonged with minimal cumulative effect by additional injections, in contrast to the situation with barbiturates or ketamine, and recovery time is almost the same as from a single injection (Dodds and Twissell, 1973). The drug is not irritating to tissues and does not cause necrosis if accidentally injected perivascularly. Intramuscular injection may cause discomfort owing to the large volume of drug needed to produce general anesthesia. It may be easier to inject a smaller volume to induce sedation and then follow with an intravenous injection to provide general anesthesia.

General anesthesia with alphadione is accompanied by excellent muscle relaxation and minimal cardiovascular or respiratory depression. The margin of safety is high, as shown by the therapeutic index (anesthetic dose: lethal dose) for alphadione, which is 30.6 compared with 4.6 for thiopental and 8.5 for ketamine. Good conditions for surgery are produced; however, like ketamine, alphadione does not block the sympathetic nervous system response to pain from major abdominal procedures. Elimination is entirely through metabolism, mainly in the liver, with excretion of metabolites in bile and urine.

The castor oil solubilizing agent of alphadione may cause histamine release. In some cats this is manifested by hyperemia and swelling of the nose, ears, and paws and is of little significance. Premedication with acetylpromazine usually prevents these effects. There are, however, a few reports of complications, mainly pulmonary edema and pharyngeal and laryngeal swelling causing airway obstruction (Dodman, 1980; Stogdale, 1978).

The use of alphadione with barbiturates is absolutely contraindicated.

## INHALATION ANESTHESIA

Anesthesia maintained with an inhaled anesthetic allows good control of the cat while providing analgesia and muscle relaxation. The technique also offers some advantages over the use of injectable drugs alone. In the event of surgical complications, and at the termination of surgery or a treatment procedure, the level of anesthesia can be altered readily by adjusting the delivered concentration of anesthetic drug. The use of a high concentration of oxygen as a carrier gas produces good arterial oxygenation throughout anesthesia even when ventilation is below normal. The lungs can be intermittently hyperinflated to reverse the inevitable lung collapse associated with general anesthesia. If the trachea is intubated, the risk of pulmonary aspiration of blood, saliva, or gastric fluid is reduced. Finally, the cost of most inhalation methods is less than that of some ketamine combinations.

### Nitrous Oxide

Nitrous oxide, one of the earliest inhalation anesthetics to be discovered, was first used in the cat in 1779 (Smithcors, 1971). It cannot provide adequate anesthesia for surgery when used alone, except perhaps in the very sick cat, and thus is used as an adjunct to injectable or other inhalation anesthetics. The maximal concentration of nitrous oxide that should be used in a nitrous oxide–oxygen mixture is 66 per cent. The reason is that in all types of general anesthesia, 10 to 15 per cent of the cardiac output is shunted through the lungs, primarily as a result of perfusion of completely collapsed alveoli, and an inspired oxygen concentration of about 33 per cent is necessary to maintain full hemoglobin saturation. This is also the reason for continuing oxygen administration after discontinuing the anesthetic (irrespective of whether nitrous oxide is used) until the cat is able to maintain good ventilation.

The addition of nitrous oxide to halothane or methoxyflurane at the beginning of anesthesia creates a phenomenon known as the second gas effect. The effective blood concentration of halothane or methoxyflurane (the second gas) is reached more rapidly than when nitrous oxide is not used. The phenomenon is a consequence of passage of large volumes of nitrous oxide into the blood, transiently causing a relative increase in second gas concentration in the alveolar gas and rapid passage of molecules down the greater concentration gradient. The effect ceases in about five minutes when equilibrium between nitrous oxide in the alveoli and blood is approached. Clinically, this property of nitrous oxide is utilized effectively for face mask or chamber induction of anesthesia in the cat. When administration of nitrous oxide is discontinued, a large volume of nitrous oxide is available to leave the blood, and oxygen administration must be continued for about five minutes to prevent hypoxia. The release of nitrous oxide from the blood causes a pronounced reduction in oxygen in the alveoli, known as diffusion hypoxia.

Although nitrous oxide is not as potent in the cat as in man or the dog, it reduces the concentration needed of another inhalant anesthetic. This effect is desirable because nitrous oxide causes less respiratory or cardiovascular depression than the other agents. In light anesthesia, nitrous oxide has slight sympathomimetic effects, and mild cardiovascular stimulation occurs.

Use of nitrous oxide is contraindicated in cats with pneumothorax (except at the time of a thoracotomy), pneumoperitoneum, or intestinal obstruction with gaseous distention. Any air bubble within the body will be greatly expanded as a result of diffusion of nitrous oxide into it, because nitrous oxide is 20 to 30 times more soluble in blood or tissues than nitrogen. Use of nitrous oxide should therefore also be avoided during air ventriculography or cystography.

## Diethyl Ether

Ether is a volatile anesthetic agent that has enjoyed great popularity for anesthesia in the cat. Its great solubility in blood and tissues results in a slow change in depth of anesthesia and therefore a wide safety margin. Administration of ether is accompanied by increased activity of the sympathetic nervous system and an increase in blood concentration of catecholamines, both of which help to stabilize the cardiovascular system during anesthesia. In addition, ventilation is increased during light planes of anesthesia with ether, whereas almost all other inhalation anesthetics decrease ventilation.

The risk of explosion with the use of electrical diathermy and the introduction of agents such as halothane or enflurane that result in rapid induction and recovery have rendered the use of ether almost obsolete. In cat practice, the major use for ether anesthesia is for Caesarean section, in the absence of facilities for halothane anesthesia.

## Halothane and Methoxyflurane

Halothane was introduced for the induction of anesthesia in 1956 and methoxyflurane in 1960. The potencies of inhalation anesthetics may be compared by measurement of the minimal alveolar concentration (MAC) of an anesthetic that prevents response to a standard painful stimulus in 50 per cent of a population. The MAC value is different for each anesthetic and remains constant from animal to animal within a species but may vary between species. Thus, because a higher concentration of halothane is needed to produce anesthesia (MAC 1.14 per cent), it is less potent than methoxyflurane (MAC 0.23 per cent). Halothane, however, has a lower solubility in blood and tissues and rapidly reaches equilibrium. Face mask or chamber induction of anesthesia is consequently a rapid and easy technique with halothane. By contrast, methoxyflurane has a very high solubility in tissues, which prolongs induction of anesthesia. An injection of barbiturate or ketamine is usually used to facilitate anesthesia with methoxyflurane.

Halothane causes a dose-dependent reduction in cardiac output and blood pressure by depression of the myocardium and peripheral vasodilation. A cat lightly anesthetized with halothane has minimal respiratory depression, but an increased concentration of halothane characteristically causes rapid, shallow breathing. The effect of methoxyflurane on the cardiovascular system is also dose-dependent, but unfortunately the signs and stages of anesthesia are not as well defined as with halothane. Thus a common fault is to maintain the level of anesthesia deeper than necessary. In deep anesthesia with methoxyflurane, the cardiovascular system is severely depressed, and the arterial carbon dioxide level is invariably increased. The capacity of these two agents to "sensitize" the myocardium to epinephrine and cause ventricular dysrhythmias varies among species. In dogs the myocardium is less sensitive with methoxyflurane than with halothane, whereas in humans there is little difference between their effects (Wong, 1981).

Both halothane and methoxyflurane are excreted from the lungs. Much more methoxyflurane (up to 50 per cent of the inhaled dose) than halothane undergoes hepatic biotransformation. The high uptake of methoxyflurane into tissues during anesthesia results in elevated blood levels long after administration of the anesthetic is discontinued—an advantage after painful surgery because methoxyflurane is analgesic at subanesthetic blood levels.

## Enflurane and Isoflurane

Enflurane and isoflurane are new inhalation anesthetics currently used in humans but not yet licensed for veterinary medicine. Enflurane is more potent in the cat (MAC 1.2 per cent) than in the dog or man (MAC 2.2 and 1.68 per cent, respectively). The anesthetic requirement for isoflurane in the cat is slightly greater than that for the dog (MAC 1.61 per cent compared with 1.2 per cent). Both agents are less soluble in blood than halothane; however, induction may be slower because their mild pungency tends to provoke breath-holding or coughing. Studies using isolated cat papillary muscles have demonstrated that enflurane depresses myocardial contraction more than halothane, whereas isoflurane causes less depression (Eger, 1981). Excretion of both agents occurs almost entirely by the lungs.

One aspect of enflurane anesthesia in the cat that needs further investigation is the appearance of high-voltage spikes on the electroencephalogram. These changes have not been correlated with motor activity during anesthesia. Cats are alert and apparently normal four hours after anesthesia; however, behavioral changes have been reported to develop in cats for 2 to 16 days after enflurane anesthesia (Julien and Kavan, 1972).

## Anesthetic Machines and Circuits

A thorough understanding of the function of the components of an anesthesia machine is essential in order to avoid complications. The outward appearance of anesthesia machines varies with the manufacturer, but the basic components are always the same—oxygen source, pressure regulator, gas flowmeter, and vaporizer (Figure 3–10). The pressure of oxygen in a full cylinder is about 2000 pounds per square inch (p.s.i.) and declines linearly with use. The small E cylinder attached to the anesthetic machine contains 625 liters of oxygen when full, and a simple calculation determines the volume of gas available at the beginning of a procedure. A large H cylinder contains about 6000 liters of oxygen and is less expensive per liter. (Note, however, that nitrous oxide compresses into a liquid, and therefore the pressure cannot be used to calculate the volume of the contents.) The regulator maintains the pressure of gas leaving the cylinder to between 50 and 60 p.s.i. irrespective of the contents or the flowmeter setting.

Many different vaporizers are available that can be used to induce anesthesia in the cat. The draw-over type of vaporizer, such as the number 8 type for methoxyflurane

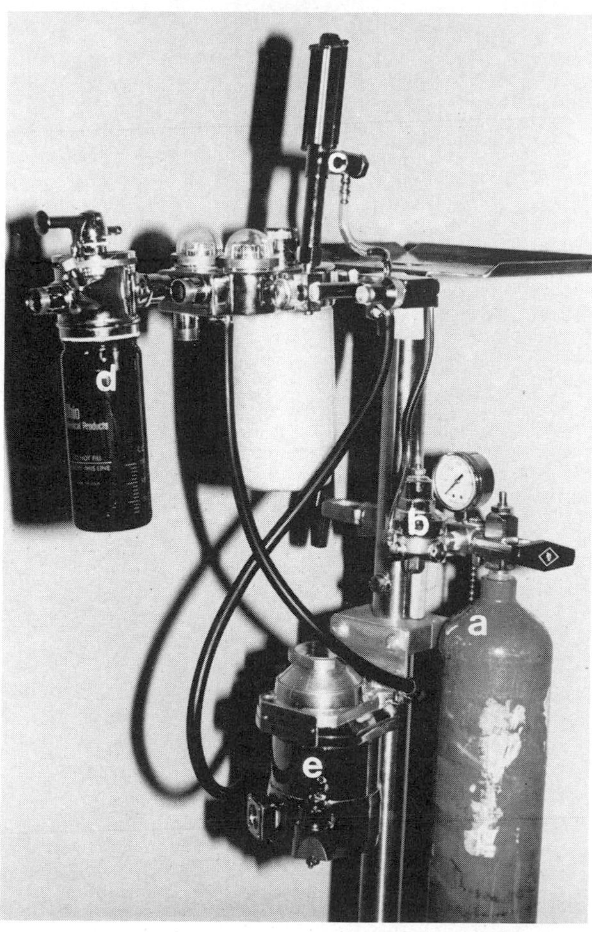


**Figure 3–10.** Ohio anesthesia machine. a, E size oxygen cylinder. b, Reducing valve/regulator. c, Oxygen flowmeter. d, Methoxyflurane vaporizer. e, Halothane vaporizer. (Courtesy Ohio Medical Products, Madison, WI.)

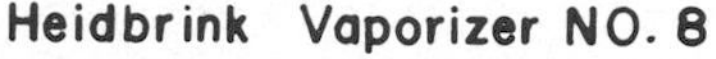


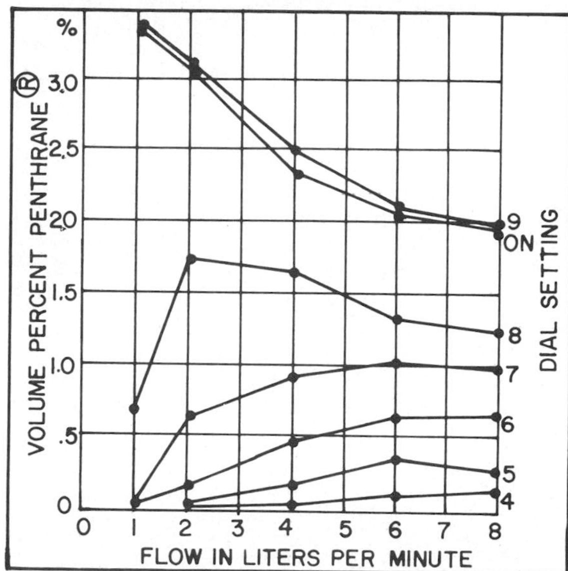


**Figure 3–11.** Methoxyflurane (Penthrane) vapor concentrations leaving an Ohio No. 8 vaporizer at a temperature of 20 C (68 F) and a constant gas flow through the vaporizer (nonrebreathing system only). (Courtesy Abbott Laboratories.)

on Ohio 960 and 970 machines, can be difficult to use, because the flow rate through the vaporizer generated by the cat's breathing will not carry sufficient methoxyflurane to maintain a satisfactory level of anesthesia. The graph in Figure 3–11 shows the vaporizer output in percentage of methoxyflurane for different gas flow rates. At flows less than 6 l/minute, a change in flow rate alters the vaporizer output independently of the dial setting. An oxygen flow of 2 to 3 l/minute has proven to be the most useful for cats.

The anesthetic gases are usually delivered through a nonrebreathing system. The basic T-piece design is common to the Ayre, Norman Elbow, Kuhn, and Jackson-Rees circuits (Fig. 3–12). In this design, the volume of gas remaining in the endotracheal tube connector (apparatus dead space) is small, and there are no valves or soda lime to impede gas flow. The addition of a reservoir bag to the expiratory tube does not alter circuit function but facilitates artificial ventilation. The circuit is connected to the machine on the outlet side of the vaporizer. However, the Ohio 980, 970, and 960 anesthetic machines must be adjusted to allow use of a nonrebreathing system (Fig. 3–13).

A flowmeter setting of two and one-half to three times the cat's minute ventilation volume is needed to ensure elimination of carbon dioxide from the circuit and to provide fresh gas for inhalation. The flow required is calculated as a minimum of 450 ml/kg body weight/minute, and oxygen may be used alone or nitrous oxide and oxygen together.

An adult circle circuit demands greater respiratory effort to maintain adequate ventilation than does the

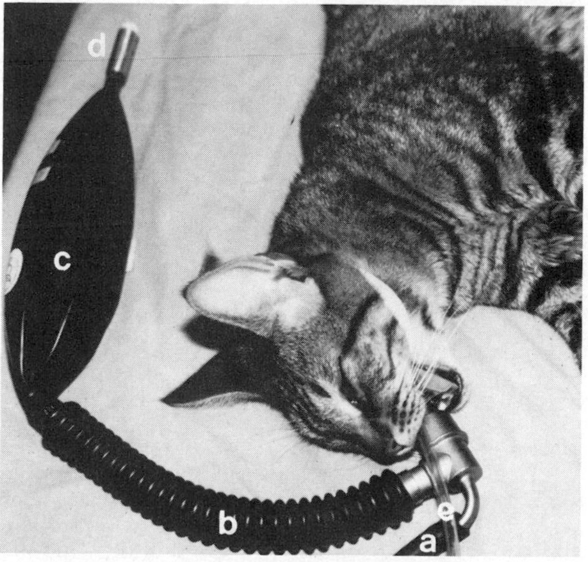


**Figure 3–12.** Nonrebreathing circuit (Norman Elbow). a, Gas inflow. b, Expiratory tube. c, Reservoir bag. d, Outlet. e, Esophageal stethoscope.

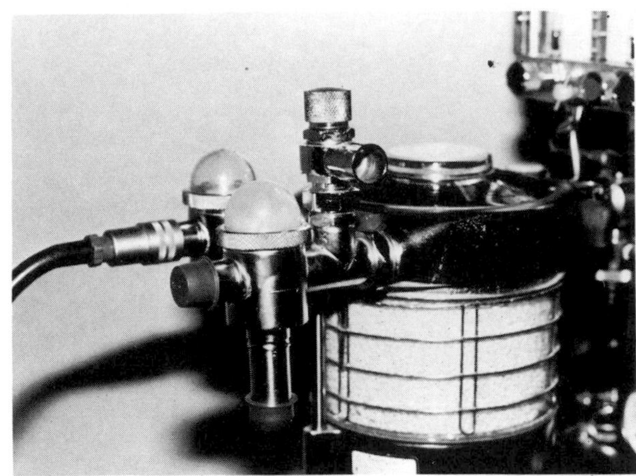

**Figure 3–13.** Ohio 980 anesthesia machine adapted for a nonrebreathing circuit. The pop-off valve is closed, the expiratory and rebreathing bag outlets are plugged, and the circuit is attached to the inspiratory outlet. (Courtesy Ohio Medical Products, Madison, WI.)

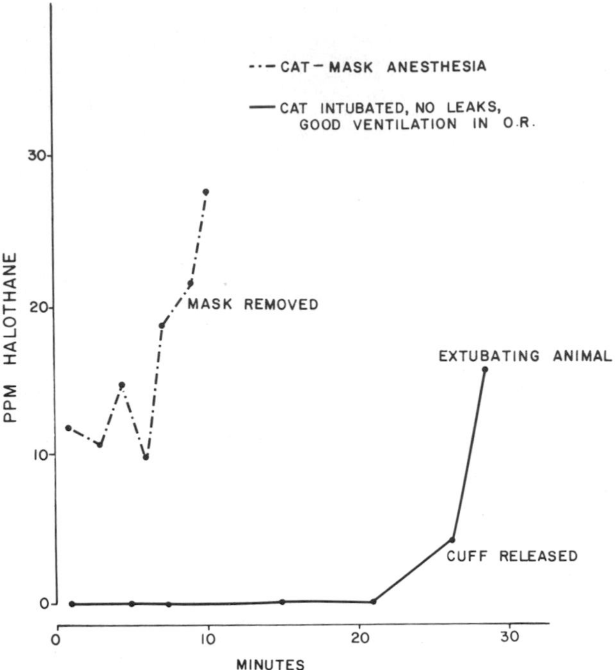


**Figure 3–14.** Measurement of halothane (ppm) in air close to anesthetized cats. Administration of halothane by face mask without scavenging results in high levels in ambient air. Tracheal intubation, connection to a circuit without leaks, and scavenging of waste gases minimize operating room pollution. (Courtesy Dr. S. V. Manley, University of California, Davis.)

nonrebreathing system. This can be achieved by healthy adult cats anesthetized with halothane with no adverse effect on cardiopulmonary function (Hartsfield and Sawyer, 1976). For cats that are depressed preoperatively or have respiratory disease, use of the adult circle may result in inadequate spontaneous ventilation. The pediatric circle offers less resistance and is more suitable for the cat.

Gas flow into a circle need only provide adequate oxygen for metabolism. This volume, however, is very small (11 ml/kg/minute), and therefore the gas flow is usually determined by the flow required for accurate vaporizer output (a minimum of 500 ml/minute through a Fluotec 3 or Fluomatic, 300 ml/minute through the Vapor vaporizers, and 250 ml/minute through the Pentec 2). A gas flow of 1 to 2 l/minute is needed to vaporize sufficient methoxyflurane from an Ohio 8 vaporizer (Figure 3–11).

Irrespective of the system used, some effort must be made to reduce anesthetic gas pollution of the operating room. Considerable evidence suggests that chronic exposure of personnel to these gases is a potential health hazard. The results of several surveys confirm that without scavenging of waste anesthetic gas, the concentrations in veterinary operating rooms are well above the minimal standards recommended by the National Institute of Safety and Health of 25 ppm of nitrous oxide and 0.5 ppm of halothane (when used with nitrous oxide), or less than 2 ppm for halogenated agents used alone (Manley, 1981; Manley and McDonell, 1980; Milligan and Sablan, 1979; Wingfield et al., 1981). For example, measurements of halothane in the air close to a cat anesthetized with halothane delivered through a face mask, and especially when the mask is removed, show how the anesthetic gases in the room can quickly climb to concentrations far in excess of those believed "safe" (Fig. 3–14). In contrast, with a cat intubated and connected to a leak-free circuit, with a simple scavenging system and good operating room ventilation, the atmosphere was not polluted with halothane. However, room halothane concentrations rapidly rose when the endotracheal cuff was deflated and when the intubated cat exhaled anesthetic into the room. To reduce pollution, waste gases must be captured from the expiratory tube of the nonrebreathing circuit or the pop-off valve of the circle and disposed of outside the room. The methods employed vary from commercially available systems to personal inventions; some of these were reviewed by Manley and McDonell (1980).

## Induction of Anesthesia

Both halothane and methoxyflurane can be used to induce anesthesia with either a chamber or a face mask. Excess anesthetic gas is more easily scavenged from a chamber, an important advantage because the greatest pollution occurs at this time. Chamber inductions are also often better tolerated by the cat. Since anesthetic concentration increases more rapidly in a smaller chamber, the chamber should be of a size to accommodate the cat comfortably but with little excess space. Anesthetic chambers can be homemade or bought commercially (Fig. 3–15). Chambers are available in plexiglass (Fraser-Harlake) and in soft plastic (Snyder). Pediatric or small-animal incubators can also be adapted as anesthetic chambers (Kim and Clifford, 1980).

A gas flow of 3 to 5 l/minute with 4 per cent halothane or 3 per cent methoxyflurane should be introduced into the chamber. When nitrous oxide is used, good results are obtained with 3 l/minute nitrous oxide and 2 l/minute oxygen. The cat should be removed from the chamber when lightly anesthetized and anesthesia main-

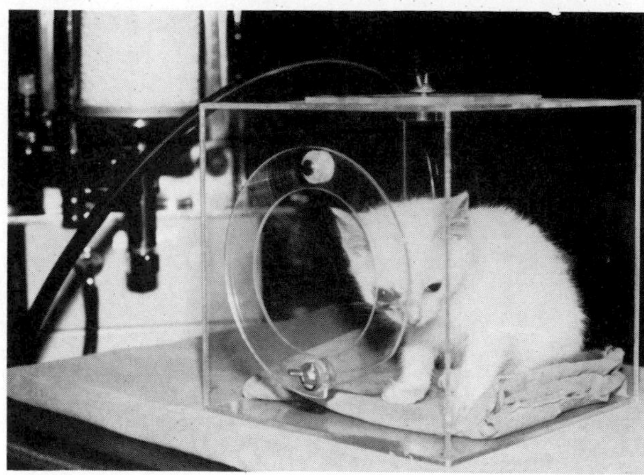

**Figure 3–15.** Anesthesia chamber (home construction) for induction of anesthesia with halothane or methoxyflurane.

tained with a face mask or endotracheal tube. The vaporizer setting must be reduced at this time to avoid overdosing (down to 1 to 2 per cent halothane or 0.3 to 0.7 per cent methoxyflurane). The nitrous oxide may be conditioned throughout anesthesia or shut off once anesthesia has been achieved.

Several different sizes and shapes of face masks are marketed for cats (Fig. 3–16). The face mask should be chosen to fit snugly over the nose and mouth (to be airtight and minimize rebreathing) but must not occlude the nostrils. Lower gas flows than those used for the whole-body chamber suffice for induction by mask because the anesthetic concentration is delivered directly to the cat. Additionally, to avoid breath-holding, the concentration of halothane administered should be increased stepwise over one minute, allowing the cat to breathe several times at each concentration. Use of a head chamber (e.g., Connell, Pitman Moore) is not recommended because the large apparatus dead space results in excessive rebreathing of carbon dioxide.

On some occasions halothane may be used for induction and methoxyflurane for maintenance of anesthesia to provide a rapid induction and good analgesia intraoperatively. As the halothane is discontinued, the vaporizer setting for methoxyflurane can be placed at the level customarily used for maintenance of anesthesia, since halothane is eliminated rapidly and methoxyflurane accumulates slowly. If the reverse (transfer from methoxyflurane to halothane) is desired, when methoxyflurane is discontinued the halothane concentration must be increased slowly. Otherwise overdosage will occur.

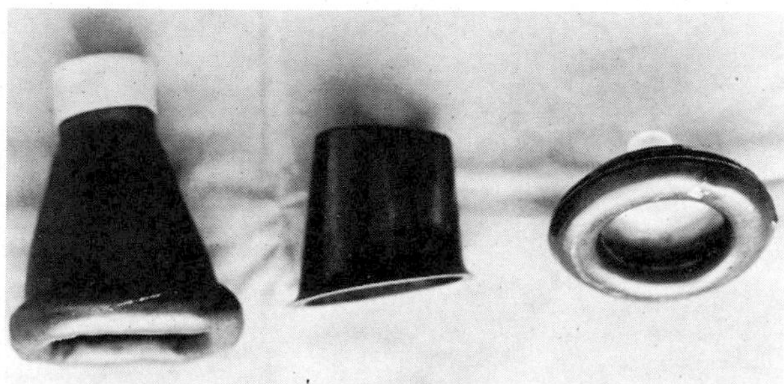

**Figure 3–16.** Anesthesia face masks for cats. Hall's mask of malleable rubber (*left*). Hard rubber mask (*center*). Clear plastic mask with foam rubber rim (*right*).

Induction of anesthesia with a barbiturate, ketamine, or alphadione and maintenance with an inhalant agent constitute a popular and reliable technique. In each case the amount of halothane or methoxyflurane needed to maintain anesthesia is less than when the inhalation agent is used alone. Generally a prolonged effect is obtained from the intravenously administered drug because the inhalant delays plasma clearance and metabolism. In addition, the signs of anesthesia will be modified according to the agent used.

## Endotracheal Intubation

The objectives of endotracheal intubation are to ensure a patent airway and to prevent aspiration of regurgitated material, secretions, or blood. Intubation also allows greater control of anesthetic depth and favors economy by preventing dilution of inspired gases with room air.

A Cole endotracheal tube, which has no cuff to occupy valuable tracheal space, is preferred for small cats (Fig. 3–17). The tube is available from most suppliers of anesthetic equipment, including North American Dräger, Fraser-Harlake, and Foregger. A 4.0 or 4.5 mm (internal diameter) tube is satisfactory for a 3 kg cat. Larger cats can accommodate cuffed endotracheal tubes (5.0 mm for a 5 kg cat) with a proportionately smaller reduction in airway diameter. To avoid endobronchial intubation, most tubes must be cut so that the tip will not extend beyond the thoracic inlet when the endotracheal tube connector is level with the incisors. Tubes that are soft and flexible are more easily controlled if a plastic or metal stylet is used.

Endotracheal intubation can be accomplished with the cat in any position. Laying the cat on its abdomen is often preferred when an assistant is available. Placing the cat on its side is preferable when the procedure is performed by one person. Rapid and easy intubation requires optimal positioning and good lighting. The oropharynx and tra-

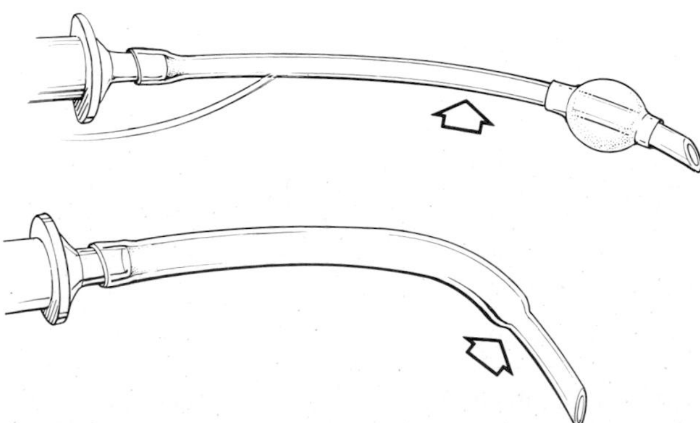

**Figure 3–17.** Endotracheal tubes. *Top*, Cuffed tube. *Bottom*, Cole tube. The arrows indicate the level of the laryngeal entrance when the tubes are in place. The tubes shown here are the same size (the internal diameter is identical).

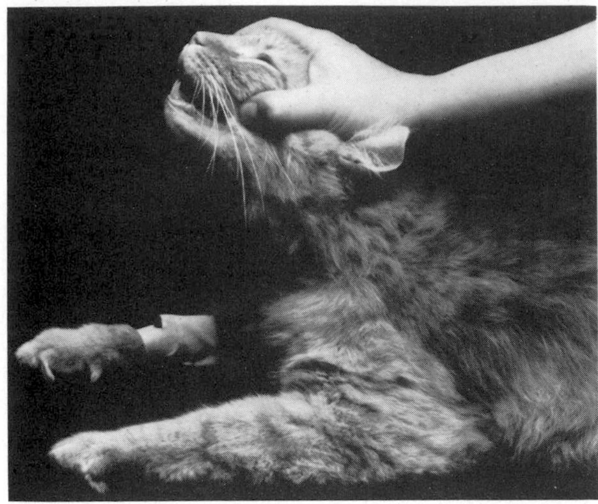

**Figure 3–18.** Restraint for endotracheal intubation must provide easy access by positioning the pharynx, larynx, and trachea in a straight line. The fingers and thumb grasping the zygomatic arches stabilize the head.

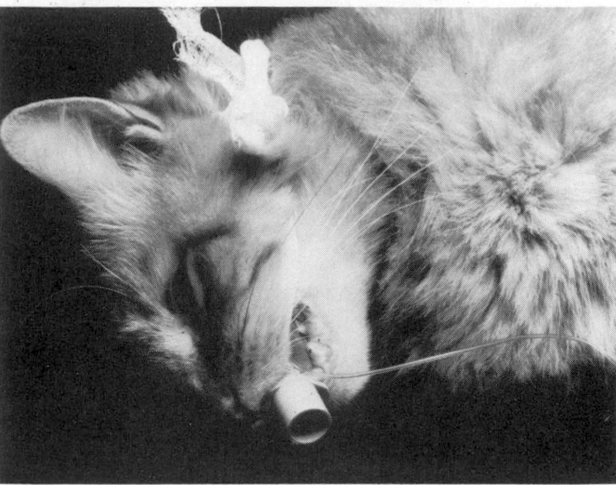

**Figure 3–20.** The endotracheal tube is secured by gauze bandage tied behind the head. The tube is inserted so that the connector is level with the incisors. Any tube projecting beyond this point increases apparatus dead space.

chea are positioned in a straight line (Fig. 3–18), and the tongue is pulled out (excessive traction will damage lingual nerves) to move the larynx forward. The laryngeal opening can then be seen with the help of an overhead light or a laryngoscope. When a laryngoscope is used, the blade tip is placed between the root of the tongue and the epiglottis. Laryngeal activity is more pronounced in the cat than in the dog, and laryngospasm occurs commonly during induction of anesthesia with volatile anesthetic agents, especially ether and halothane. The suggestion that barbiturates may increase the sensitivity of the laryngeal reflex has not been confirmed (Rex, 1973). The laryngospasm obstructs early passage of the tracheal tube, which may bruise the epiglottis and laryngeal mucosa. Preliminary densensitization of the larynx by topical application of lidocaine by spray or cotton-tip swab will

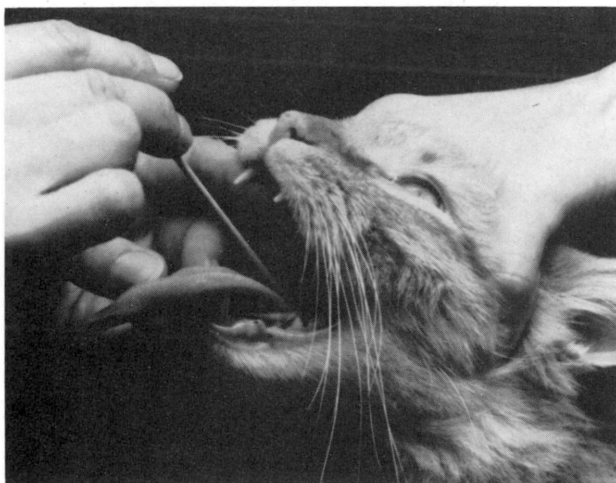

**Figure 3–19.** Endotracheal intubation. The jaws are opened by hand or with a speculum. The tongue is gently pulled forward. The larynx can be desensitized by the topical application of lidocaine with a cotton-tipped swab.

prevent this (Fig. 3–19). The endotracheal tube is moistened with sterile lubricant or water, and the tip is used to depress the epiglottis and expose the larynx. At the entrance to the larynx, the tube is rotated 90 degrees so that the bevel spreads the arytenoids. The tube is returned to its original position upon entering the trachea and is advanced to its depth. The endotracheal tube is loosely secured to the head with gauze bandage or a rubber band (Fig. 3–20). The cuff, if present, is inflated with just enough air to prevent leakage of air around the tube when the lungs are artificially inflated.

An alternative technique preferred by some incorporates the administration of a muscle relaxant (succinylcholine) to paralyze the larynx and facilitate tracheal intubation. An intravenous injection of succinylcholine (2 to 5 mg total dose) given to the anesthetized cat results in complete paralysis and eliminates laryngospasm. Because spontaneous breathing is abolished for about five minutes, artificial ventilation must be quickly instituted after intubation.

The systemic effects of intubation common to all species are tachycardia and hypertension. These are likely to be of significance in cats with cardiac disease. In such cases, lidocaine (2 mg/kg) should be applied topically to the larynx before intubation to decrease the blood pressure response.

## Care of Equipment

Prevention of infection following anesthesia and operation is the responsibility of surgeons, anesthetists, and nurses alike. Infection is transmitted by direct contact, and the use of aseptic equipment without frequent handwashing is futile. Equipment for anesthesia, inhalation therapy, and intensive care carries a high potential for transmission of respiratory disease. Care should be taken to identify cats with active respiratory infection or a recent history of respiratory disease, and equipment used for these animals should be sterilized. Unfortunately, it is now known that at least 69 per cent of cats that recover from feline rhinotracheitis retain the virus in a latent form and that the stress of an environmental change results in shedding of the virus into ocular, nasal, and oral secretions (Povey, 1977). Cleaning endotracheal tubes inside and out with a brush to remove mucus and thoroughly washing the anesthetic equipment with soap, such as povidone-iodine (Betadine), after each use help to prevent the inadvertent transmission of disease. The practice of not using the endotracheal tubes for 72 hours between cases improves protection. Endotracheal tubes and circuits can be effectively sterilized with ethylene oxide. Adequate airing of tubes is important because gas residue causes tissue irritation or damage (Trim and Simpson, 1982). The speed of diffusion of ethylene oxide from different materials varies, and some equipment must be aired for 12 days. Manufacturers' instructions should be followed to avoid injury to patients.

## CARE OF THE ANESTHETIZED CAT

In this section monitoring, supportive treatment, and recovery of the anesthetized cat will be discussed.

### MONITORING

The value of consistent monitoring of the anesthetized cat cannot be overemphasized; it is the basis of safe clinical anesthesia. Not one but several functions should be monitored and frequent comparisons of serial recordings made to evaluate a patient's status or to arrive at a decision to increase or decrease anesthetic administration. Four major systems should be regularly monitored: central nervous, respiratory, cardiovascular, and urinary.

The signs of anesthesia produced by barbiturates and inhalation agents differ from those produced by ketamine. Barbiturates and the inhalants produce predictable CNS depression with progressive, dose-dependent reductions in palpebral and pedal reflexes and skeletal muscle tone. Reflex twitching of the ear in response to touch should be ignored. Jaw mobility is not a reliable measure of muscle relaxation, and pupil size and eyeball position are less predictable signs in the cat than in the dog.

The anesthetic state produced by an injection of ketamine bears no resemblance to the CNS signs during barbiturate or inhalation anesthesia. Monitoring in the cat must be directed at the respiratory and cardiovascular systems. Redosing with ketamine is based on obvious responses (usually movement) to surgical stimulation.

Several functions of the cardiovascular system can be monitored with a minimum of expense. The oxygen-carrying capacity of the blood can be assessed by preoperative measurement of the packed cell volume (PCV), red cell count, and hemoglobin level. During anesthesia, monitoring of pulse rate, blood pressure, capillary refill time, and mucous membrane color provides information about tissue perfusion. An esophageal stethoscope simplifies auscultation of heart rate (Fig. 3–21). It can be connected to a battery-powered monitor that produces an audible "beep." To some extent, a reduction in sound intensity indicates reduced cardiac contractility. Heart rates that are considered normal are strongly influenced

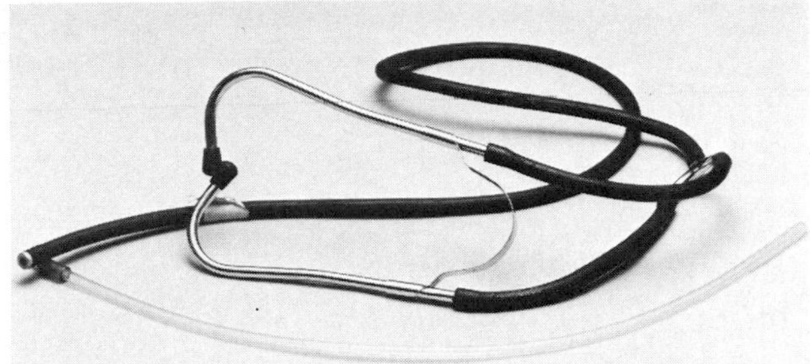

**Figure 3–21.** Esophageal stethoscope with headpiece. The tip of the probe is passed down the esophagus until it is level with the heart.

by the drug or drug combination in use. With barbiturate anesthesia about 140 beats/minute is usual, whereas with halothane the heart rate is often 160 to 180. Ketamine further increases the rate to 180 to 200 beats/minute.

Arterial blood pressure is easily measured indirectly by the Doppler technique. The probe can be placed at any of several sites—over the median caudal (coccygeal), cranial tibial, saphenous, or ulnar artery (Figs. 3–22 and 3–23). Determinations are easier when the hair over the artery is first clipped. The blood pressure values obtained are determined by the anesthetic agent used, halothane and methoxyflurane producing more hypotension than barbiturates or ketamine, but all efforts should be made to maintain a systolic pressure at or above 70 mm Hg. The cost of blood pressure equipment varies enormously. The units most frequently used are made by Parks Electronics; others are available from Kontron (Arteriosonde), Medsonics (Versatone), and Applied Medical Research (Dinamap).

If the anesthetist were to maintain a finger on a peripheral pulse, almost all dysrhythmias would be detected. This procedure is not always possible in veterinary practice, but the audible sound from the blood pressure probe

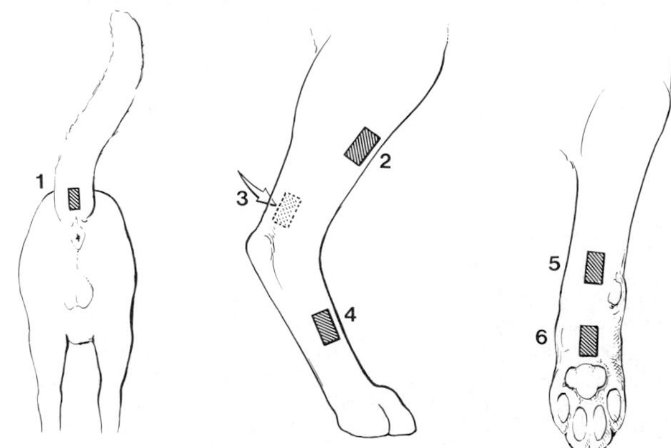


**Figure 3–22.** Sites for application of the Doppler probe for indirect measurement of arterial blood pressure. *1*, Median caudal (coccygeal) artery on the ventral surface of the tail. *2*, Cranial tibial artery on the craniolateral surface of the hindlimb. *3*, Saphenous artery on the medial surface of the flexor tendons. *4*, Metatarsal artery. *5* and *6*, Ulnar artery on the caudal surface of the forelimb, above and below the carpal pad.

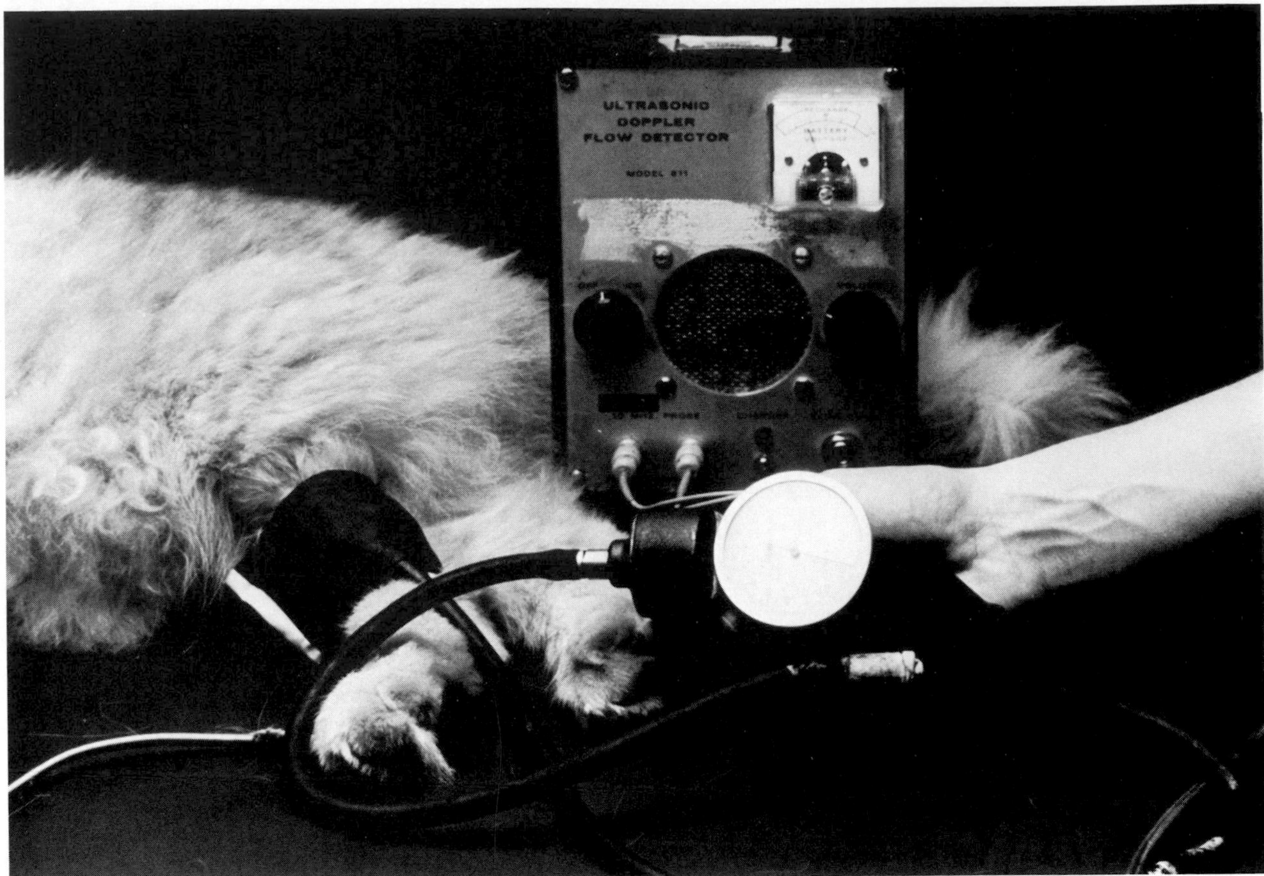


**Figure 3–23.** Indirect measurement of blood pressure using the saphenous artery. (Courtesy Parks Electronics, Aloha, OR.)

is almost as effective. Heart sounds detected by an esophageal stethoscope or an electrocardiograph (ECG) are not as useful but indicate a change in rhythm. The ECG also provides early warning of myocardial difficulty through S-T segment depression or elevation of the T wave. Prompt treatment may avert cardiac arrest. Furthermore, surveys of human anesthesia records have shown that a surprisingly high proportion of instances of cardiac arrest occurs in healthy people. For all these reasons, when an ECG is available, its use should not be limited to the high-risk case.

Evaluation of ventilation can be difficult without sophisticated equipment, especially since the respiratory rate of the cat is usually rapid. Observation of the mucous membranes may confirm good oxygenation but tells nothing about the carbon dioxide levels. Therefore conditions that depress or obstruct breathing (namely, deep anesthesia or pressure on the thorax or abdomen) must be avoided, and cats with disorders that interfere with ventilation should be artificially ventilated. General anesthesia abolishes the physiologic "sigh" and thus invariably is accompanied by progressive lung collapse. An artificial sigh (hyperinflation of the lungs) effectively reopens collapsed alveoli. This can be done at approximately 10-minute intervals if the cat is connected to an anesthetic machine.

## Supportive Treatment

Some positions that facilitate surgery produce undesirable effects in the anesthetized cat. A head-up or head-down position has hemodynamic consequences that may be tolerated by the healthy cat, but the cat with cardiac disease, low circulating blood volume, obesity, or lung disease can be expected to react adversely. If anesthesia is deep, cardiovascular depression occurs even in the healthy cat, because the reflex response of the cardiovascular system through the baroreceptors and peripheral vasculature is blunted. In the head-up position the heart is elevated and caudal vena cava flow decreased. In the head-down position pooling of blood in the head and forelimbs results in decreased cranial vena cava flow. In either position, the reduction in venous return to the heart leads directly to changes in myocardial contractility and heart rate. Additionally, in the head-down position the abdominal organs press on the diaphragm, limiting ventilation. The increase in the arterial carbon dioxide level also depresses myocardial contractility.

An example of the effect of position on the cardiovascular system is provided by a cat anesthetized for a perineal urethrostomy, as demonstrated in Figure 3–24). This four-year-old, 8.2 kg cat, premedicated intramuscularly with atropine (0.3 mg) and acetylpromazine (0.8 mg)

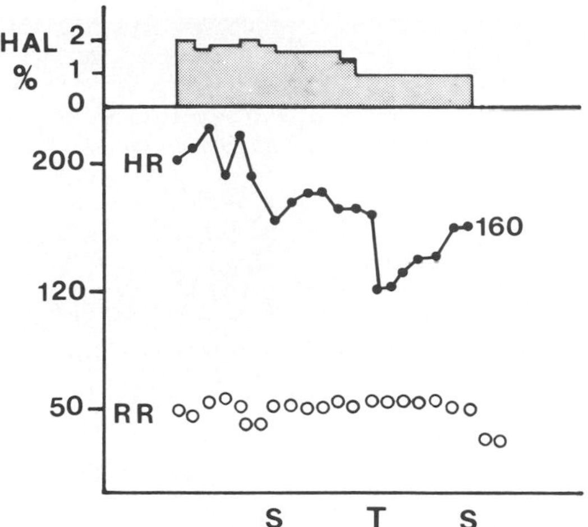


**Figure 3–24.** Anesthesia record of a cat anesthetized with atropine, acetylpromazine, halothane, and nitrous oxide for perineal urethrostomy. S–S was the surgery time. Tilting the table at point T resulted in a marked drop in the heart rate (HR). The table was returned almost to its original position and the heart rate was restored.

and anesthetized with halothane and nitrous oxide, was placed in the prone position and during the surgery was tilted (at point T on the anesthetic record) into a head-down position. Almost immediately the heart rate dropped from 165 to 120 beats/minute, indicating a compromised cardiovascular system. Within a few minutes after the tilt of the table was reduced, the heart rate gradually increased. To limit the adverse effects on the cardiovascular system, it is recommended that the cat not be tilted more than 30 degrees from the horizontal. Mechanical interference with breathing can be minimized by placing a pad under the pelvis to support the cat's weight.

Heat loss is a major problem in the anesthetized cat. Hypothermia decreases anesthetic requirements, depresses ventilation, and prolongs recovery. The major decrease in body temperature occurs early, mainly during clipping and preparing of the surgical area. Once hypothermia develops, it is difficult to reverse during the intraoperative period. It is better to try to prevent hypothermia by keeping preparation time as short as possible, by placing the cat on a circulating warm-water blanket from the beginning of anesthesia, and by using warmed intravenous fluids. Several methods of preventing and treating hypothermia in the cat during anesthesia have been studied (Haskins, 1981). During recovery, wrapping the cat in a warm-water blanket was found to be the most effective. Laying the cat on the warm-water blanket under a 250 watt infrared heat lamp or under a hot-water bottle heat tent prevented heat loss, but simply cocooning the cat in cotton hand towels or a space blanket* did not. A hot air dryer attached to the cage door and run on medium setting has been found to rapidly warm a cat. An incubator with controlled temperature and humidity also serves well.

*King-Seeley Thermos Co., Norwich, CT.

During anesthesia all aspects of renal function (renal blood flow, glomerular filtration rate, electrolyte secretion, and urine production) are altered to varying degrees. These effects are not entirely the result of anesthetic drugs, because different types of surgery have a variable influence on the sympathetic nervous system, endocrine function, and "third-space" water loss. The major depression of renal function is reversed when the cat recovers from anesthesia; however, after anesthesia and surgery, in all cases, the capacity of the kidney to regulate urine volume and content is impaired for several days (Trim, 1979). Administration of a balanced electrolyte solution (e.g., lactated Ringer's solution), is recommended for all surgery over an hour long, all major surgery, and all surgery on old cats and cats with a history of urinary or hepatic malfunction. A useful guide to the volume of fluid is 10 ml/kg/hour for the first two hours, then 5 ml/kg/hour. Blood loss is estimated and replaced with a balanced electrolyte solution at two to three times the lost volume. The anesthetized healthy cat, if given fluid, can usually adjust to a loss of 20 per cent of the circulating blood volume (11 ml/kg), but some cats may need a blood transfusion at an earlier time.

When ventilation is inadequate, artificial ventilation (intermittent positive pressure ventilation) is necessary. This, however, causes hemodynamic changes, because the negative pressure that normally occurs during inspiration is abolished and the positive pressure needed to inflate the lungs impedes blood flow back to the heart. Figure 3–25 presents a comparison of correctly (a) and incorrectly (b,c) applied artificial ventilation. In (b) the lungs were held inflated at a greater pressure for two seconds, which is too long. In (c) both inflation time and pressure were

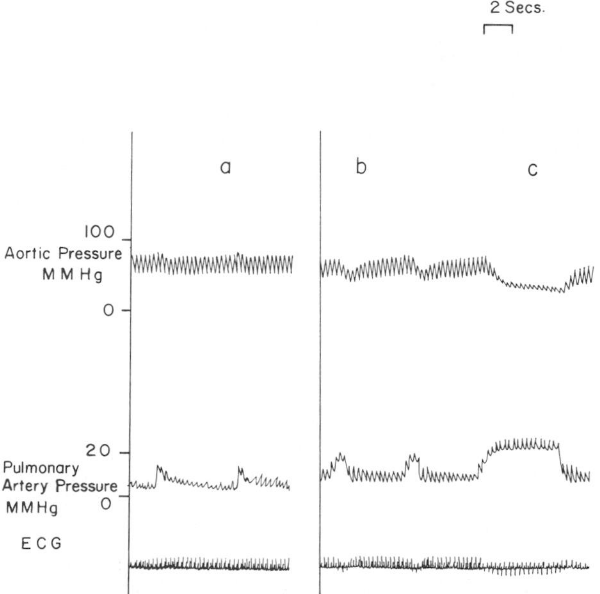


**Figure 3–25.** Aortic blood pressure, pulmonary artery pressure, and ECG measured in a cat anesthetized with halothane. a, Artificial ventilation correctly applied. b, Inspiratory time prolonged to 2 seconds. c, Lungs held hyperinflated for 6 seconds. (Redrawn from a recording.)

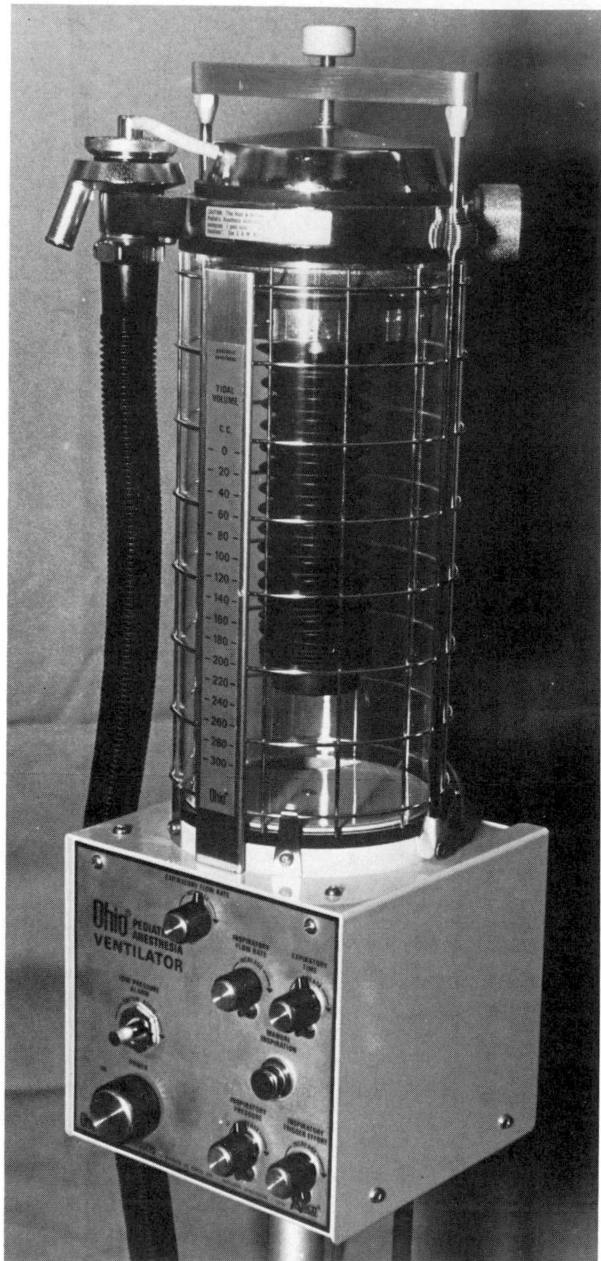


**Figure 3–26.** Ohio pediatric anesthesia ventilator. Note the small-sized bellows, capacity 200 ml, with 20 ml graduations. (Courtesy Ohio Medical Products, Madison, WI.)

excessive, severely depressing arterial pressure and causing electrocardiographic changes.

Whether artificial ventilation is accomplished by manual compression of the rebreathing bag or by a mechanical ventilator, adequate ventilation with minimal effect on the cardiovascular system is most often provided by a rate of 12 to 15 breaths per minute at a tidal volume of 15 to 20 ml/kg. The time ratio for inspiration to expiration should be 1:2 or 1:3. An adequate tidal volume is usually achieved with an inspiratory pressure of 20 cm $H_2O$ (15 mm Hg), but a higher inspiratory pressure is needed by obese cats and by those in which positioning for surgery compromises ventilation. It is rarely necessary to exceed 30 cm $H_2O$ for the cat. If artificial ventilation is needed because of hypoventilation, the vaporizer setting should be reduced to prevent deepening of anesthesia.

Many types of mechanical ventilators marketed for human use have been adapted for animal anesthesia. Not all are suitable for the cat because of its small size, but the pressure-limited ventilator manufactured by Bird can be used. Tidal volume is regulated indirectly by controlling the inspiratory pressure. Set at 15 mm Hg, this produces an adequate tidal volume in most cats. The inspiratory time is regulated by controlling the inspiratory flow rate, which is adjusted until inspiration occupies about one third of the total respiratory cycle. Mechanical ventilators on which the tidal volume is directly set should have a small bellows of the size produced for pediatric anesthesia (Fig. 3–26).

When the cat is weaned from the ventilator, anesthesia is lightened to reduce central respiratory depression. Then, with the tidal volume remaining the same, the respiratory rate is decreased to four to six per minute to allow accumulation of carbon dioxide to the normal level. Hypoventilation at this time may be due to anesthetic depression, hypocarbia, or hypothermia.

### RECOVERY

A quiet, pain-free recovery is desirable. If necessary, small doses of a tranquilizer or narcotic (e.g., meperidine 2.5 mg/kg IM) may be given before consciousness is regained.

As a precaution against aspiration, extubation should be delayed until the cat can swallow, but not until the cat is awake, when the risk of laryngospasm is higher.

Bandages applied around the head and neck or thorax and abdomen are easily applied too tightly when the cat is anesthetized. They should be checked periodically to make sure that they are not obstructing the airway or impeding breathing.

A pharyngostomy tube is easily kinked in the pharynx and may obstruct breathing. After the tube has been inserted, it must be viewed from the mouth, not just palpated, to ensure correct placement. A tube inserted from the left side of the neck is less likely to obstruct breathing than one entering from the right.

Cats recover best from anesthesia in a quiet environment and do not need stimulating, a common practice with the dog. The animal recovering from major surgery is more comfortable with a blanket or synthetic sheepskin (available from hospital suppliers). Efforts may be needed at this time to restore body temperature. There should be no food, water, or litter pan in the cage, and the cat should be kept under continuous observation until it is effectively mobile.

## RECOGNITION, TREATMENT, AND PREVENTION OF COMPLICATIONS

Vigilant monitoring of the anesthetized cat ensures early recognition of a complication. Usually several possible causes must be considered to arrive at an accurate diagnosis and appropriate treatment. In every case, a change in anesthetic management to prevent the complication is desirable.

## Complications During Induction of Anesthesia

Vomiting or regurgitation when laryngeal reflexes are abolished can result in death from asphyxia or pulmonary aspiration of food. In the event of regurgitation, the pharynx must be cleared immediately by lowering the cat's head to drain fluid and extracting solid material with a forceps or suction. An endotracheal tube may have to be inserted into the esophagus to divert fluid sufficiently to permit unobstructed tracheal intubation. When aspiration has occurred, surgery should be postponed, if at all possible, and the cat allowed to recover from anesthesia to make possible immediate treatment and assessment of the severity of the complication.

The risk of vomiting or regurgitation is slight if the cat has not been fed for 6 to 12 hours before anesthesia but should always be anticipated in the cat with a ruptured diaphragm, intestinal foreign body, or dilated esophagus. In these animals, rapid induction of anesthesia is essential. The cat should be held in a head-up position and the trachea intubated before the head is lowered. Occluding the esophagus by pressure against the cricoid cartilage of the larynx is an added precaution.

Apnea must first be distinguished from cardiopulmonary arrest by palpation of a femoral pulse. Transient apnea may not require treatment, but when cyanosis is present or when apnea exceeds 45 seconds, artificial ventilation must be instituted. A face mask and resuscitator (Ambu bag) using room air (Fraser-Harlake, North American Dräger) are adequate if an endotracheal tube and anesthetic machine are not immediately available. Apnea and hypoventilation caused by anesthetic overdose or a xylazine-ketamine combination require artificial ventilation for a variable time until drug redistribution occurs and adequate spontaneous breathing resumes. Apnea following endotracheal intubation often results from tracheal irritation by the tube or sometimes from bronchial irritation by methoxyflurane or halothane, and is self-limiting. Gentle movement of the endotracheal tube elicits a modified cough in the form of thoracic and abdominal muscle contraction, differentiating this apnea from drug-induced apnea, in which there is no response to movement of the tube.

## Complications During Anesthesia

Inadequate depth of anesthesia may complicate surgery when movement results in contamination of the operative site or inadvertent injury to tissues. Sympathetic stimulation and catecholamine released in response to pain produce cardiac dysrhythmias. Insufficient administration of drugs is often responsible. Poor absorption from intramuscular injection and hypoventilation or endobronchial intubation (limiting uptake of inhalation anesthetics) must be considered.

Deep general anesthesia from excessive drug administration is invariably accompanied by cardiovascular and respiratory depression. Cerebral or other organic damage, particularly to liver or kidney, may occur. Furthermore, the prolonged recovery following deep anesthesia is accompanied by slow return of protective reflexes and increased incidence of pulmonary complications and renal malfunction. Fluid therapy and artificial ventilation during anesthesia minimize the immediate effects and, when continued at the end of anesthesia, promote detoxification of barbiturates or ketamine and elimination of halothane or methoxyflurane.

Analeptic drugs have been advocated as treatment for deep or prolonged anesthesia. They have CNS-stimulant properties through action on the medullary centers and carotid body chemoreceptors. They are primarily respiratory stimulants but produce a moderate rise in blood pressure and arousal from anesthesia. They should never be used as substitutes for artificial ventilation, if that is needed, and cannot be relied on to treat cerebral hypoxia because cerebral blood flow is decreased by hypocapnia.

Doxapram has a greater margin of safety than other analeptic drugs and is considered the most effective, although, unfortunately, the response is not as marked in the cat as in the dog or horse (Jensen and Klemm, 1967). Doxapram (7.5 mg/kg IV) has been reported to increase both rate and depth of breathing in cats anesthetized with thiopental or alphadione (Curtis and Evans, 1981). The study demonstrated a more rapid return of ability to raise the head and of righting reflex, but in the cats anesthetized with thiopental, the time to standing was not shortened by doxapram. Doxapram also speeds recovery from the effects of inhalation agents by causing hyperventilation; however, the elevated blood catecholamine levels it produces increase the probability of dysrhythmias. Hence a lower dose is used (1 mg/kg). CNS stimulation from doxapram lasts from 5 to 12 minutes. In some situations a second injection as indicated.

The anticholinergic drug physostigmine has been used as a nonspecific analeptic to treat CNS depression from drugs such as diazepam, narcotic analgesics, and ketamine. Further investigation is needed to determine the appropriate dosage for the cat.

### Cardiovascular Complications

The immediate nonspecific treatment of circulatory depression includes a reduction in anesthetic administration, an initial challenge of lactated Ringer's solution (10 ml/kg) and sodium bicarbonate (1.5 mEq/kg) given separately intravenously, and artificial ventilation. Atropine (0.02 mg/kg IV) reverses bradycardia. When circulatory collapse is associated with hemorrhagic or septic-endotoxic shock, corticosteroids, such as methylprednisolone (30 mg/kg) or dexamethasone (5 mg/kg), are indicated to stabilize endothelial membranes and to prevent initiation of arachidonic acid metabolism and prostaglandin release. These steroids produce vasodilation, aggravating hypotension, and are therefore administered after fluid therapy has begun.

Stimulation of the cardiovascular system is sometimes necessary. Dopamine is at present considered to be the most useful vasoactive agent, because it increases cardiac output and arterial blood pressure while selectively improving the coronary, mesenteric, and renal circulations. The drug is extremely potent. Dilution (1 or 2 ml in 500 ml physiologic saline solution) aids accurate administration. An infusion rate of 5 μg/kg/minute is usually sufficient, but more can be used. The infusion rate must be decreased if tachycardia develops.

Blood loss during surgery can be an insidious cause of hypotension, culminating in unexpected circulatory collapse and death. Initially blood loss can be effectively replaced with two to three times that volume of lactated Ringer's solution, but eventually a blood transfusion becomes necessary. Crossmatching is not routinely practiced before blood transfusion in the cat. Personal experience with many single transfusions during anesthesia has not included adverse reactions; however, one case report of a fatal reaction to blood transfusion indicates that incompatible transfusion is a possibility. (Auer et al., 1982). (See also the chapter on the hematopoietic system.) When severe hemorrhage is anticipated, a reasonable alternative in some cases is a form of autotransfusion, for which blood is drawn from the cat several hours or a day before surgery. A fluid infusion after the blood is collected restores the circulating blood volume before anesthesia. Heparin is often used as an anticoagulant for cat blood, but it is easy to use too much and heparinize the patient. Acid citrate dextrose and citrate phosphate dextrose are safer anticoagulants. Blood can be injected directly if it is done within two hours after collection, but stored blood must be filtered. Regular blood transfusion recipient sets can be used, but a smaller filter marketed by Fenwal for cryoprecipitate and platelet infusion has proved more convenient. To avoid aggregation of red cells as the calcium antagonizes the anticoagulant, the flow of lactated Ringer's solution must be temporarily discontinued if the transfusion is to be made through the same catheter. The volume of blood required to restore cardiovascular stability is determined by a variety of factors but rarely equals the volume lost. A PCV of at least 20 per cent should be achieved.

Fortunately, cardiac dysrhythmias are less common in the anesthetized cat than in the dog. Premature ventricular contraction (PVC) is the most frequent. Thiamylal and, to a lesser extent, thiopental produce PVCs which, although cause for concern, generally have little effect on the blood pressure. Their appearance is short-lived, and they disappear as drug redistribution occurs. Endotracheal intubation evokes tachycardia and hypertension, occasionally with PVCs, but these effects are prevented when the larynx is desensitized with lidocaine. Deep anesthesia (resulting in poor coronary perfusion) and hypoventilation (resulting in elevated carbon dioxide levels) are probably the most common causes of PVCs occurring during anesthesia. Treatment in this situation should include supplying oxygen and artificial ventilation. The blood volume should be expanded with fluids, and sodium bicarbonate should be administered if metabolic acidosis is suspected. Premature ventricular contractions occurring two in succession or more than five in one minute require additional treatment with lidocaine (1 to 2 mg/kg) injected intravenously over at least one minute. Diluting the lidocaine with physiologic saline solution or using a 1 ml syringe ensures accurate administration and avoids overdosage. The antiarrhythmic activity of lidocaine lasts about 10 minutes. Repeated injections may be necessary if the cause of the PVCs has not been eliminated.

## Respiratory Complications

Paradoxical breathing, movement of the thoracic wall inward during inspiration, is characteristic of upper airway obstruction. An abnormal position of the head and neck, laryngospasm, a kinked endotracheal tube, a mucus plug in the endotracheal tube, or an endotracheal tube misplaced in the esophagus may be responsible.

Hypoventilation is easily treated with artificial ventilation if it is recognized. The shape of the oxyhemoglobin dissociation curve is such that a severe decrease in ventilation must occur before the arterial $PO_2$ is low enough for cyanosis to develop. Before this extreme, the $PCO_2$ will have risen sufficiently to produce adverse effects.

## Cardiopulmonary Arrest and Resuscitation

Asystole, ventricular fibrillation, and electrical mechanical dissociation are indications for immediate institution of artificial ventilation and cardiac massage. The ABC sequence, in which A stands for patent airway, B for breathing, and C for cardiac massage and circulation, is a helpful memory aid that is generally applicable. Drugs are used later if ventilation and massage are ineffective or require augmentation; however, modification of this regimen may be desirable on certain occasions, depending on the cause of the arrest.

For example, when arrest immediately follows injection of an intravenous anesthetic such as thiamylal, the most effective treatment is cardiac massage to stimulate circulation and redistribution of the drug. If the heart does not start beating within one minute, the trachea should be intubated and positive-pressure ventilation begun. When circulatory collapse and cardiac arrest result from release of vasoactive substances during manipulation of an intussusception, an infected uterus, or a pancreatic abscess, ventilation and cardiac massage must be followed as soon as possible by administration of sodium bicarbonate and dopamine or isoproterenol (1 ml, 0.2 mg, in 500 ml lactated Ringer's solution) to counteract the effects of these substances. Treatment of cardiac arrest due to tension pneumothorax from accidental rupture of a lung must first include insertion of a catheter into the pleural space to reduce the intrathoracic pressure and permit blood to return to the heart.

Cardiac massage is performed by external lateral compression of the thorax between the fourth and sixth ribs. A rate of 60 compressions per minute is combined with 12 breaths per minute. This procedure often suffices to restore cardiac activity, especially when asystole is due to anesthetic overdose. Many recommendations for sodium bicarbonate dosage are excessive, and overdosage should be avoided, since alkalosis may predispose the cat to arrhythmia, constrict coronary arteries, and shift the oxygen dissociation curve to the left. An initial dose of 1.5 mEq/kg sodium bicarbonate is sufficient, to be followed by 1 mEq/kg for every 10 minutes of inadequate circulation, unless measurements of blood pH and $PCO_2$ are available.

Epinephrine (0.25 to 0.5 ml of 1:10,000 solution), the drug of choice for asystole refractory to external massage, is injected into the left ventricle. It should be given every five minutes during an episode of arrest, since the circulating life of catecholamines is two and one-half to three minutes. The risk that epinephrine will convert asystole to fibrillation is quite high in a cat anesthetized with halothane or methoxyflurane. It is wiser to withhold the epinephrine longer in these animals or to substitute dopamine. An injection of lidocaine before the epinephrine may reduce the incidence of fibrillation.

The motions of intubation and massage produce unduly high vagal tone, which interferes with resuscitation. For this reason atropine (0.02 mg/kg IV) is indicated during asystole.

Ventricular fibrillation can be diagnosed only from an ECG or by visual observation of the heart. The ability to restore stable activity appears to be directly related to the duration of the fibrillation. Therefore, if a defibrillator is available, it should be applied immediately (25 to 50 watts/second). One electrode is placed over the left sixth intercostal space near the sternum and the other over the right fourth intercostal space, but more dorsally. If electrical defibrillation is unsuccessful, artificial ventilation and external cardiac massage should be resumed. Epinephrine to coarsen the fibrillation and sodium bicarbonate to reverse acidosis should be given before a second attempt. If sinus rhythm is restored but then relapses into fibrillation, injections of atropine and lidocaine before the next electrical shock may preserve the rhythm.

In the absence of electrical defibrillation, external massage alone may be effective in the cat. Some success has been obtained in chemical defibrillation in dogs with acetylcholine bromide or an acetylcholine chloride–potassium chloride mixture (Breznock et al., 1978). Further evaluation of this treatment is needed.

Electrical mechanical dissociation occurs when electrical activity of the heart continues without producing an effective cardiac output. Calcium chloride or calcium gluconate increases the availability of calcium ion and enhances myocardial contractility. Sodium bicarbonate must be given to maintain the blood pH between 7.3 and 7.4. A vasoactive drug such as isoproterenol or dopamine must be infused until improvement is obtained. Dexamethasone (5 mg/kg) has also been recommended for this condition.

In all types of cardiac arrest, intravenous fluid administration is needed to maintain blood volume and venous return while providing a route for drug administration. However, when an intravenous catheter is not already in place or when venepuncture is difficult, epinephrine, lidocaine, and atropine can be instilled into the endotracheal tube and forced into the lungs by positive-pressure ventilation. Absorption is more efficient when the drug is diluted in 2 ml of distilled water, thereby spreading the medication over a larger absorptive area.

## Complications During Recovery

The time for recovery from anesthesia varies with the anesthetic used and the total dose administered. Recovery from halothane and methoxyflurane anesthesia is more predictable than it is from injectable drugs. Usually up to 15 or 20 minutes elapse after halothane or methoxyflurane is discontinued until a return to consciousness, and a maximum of one hour to ambulation. A slow return to

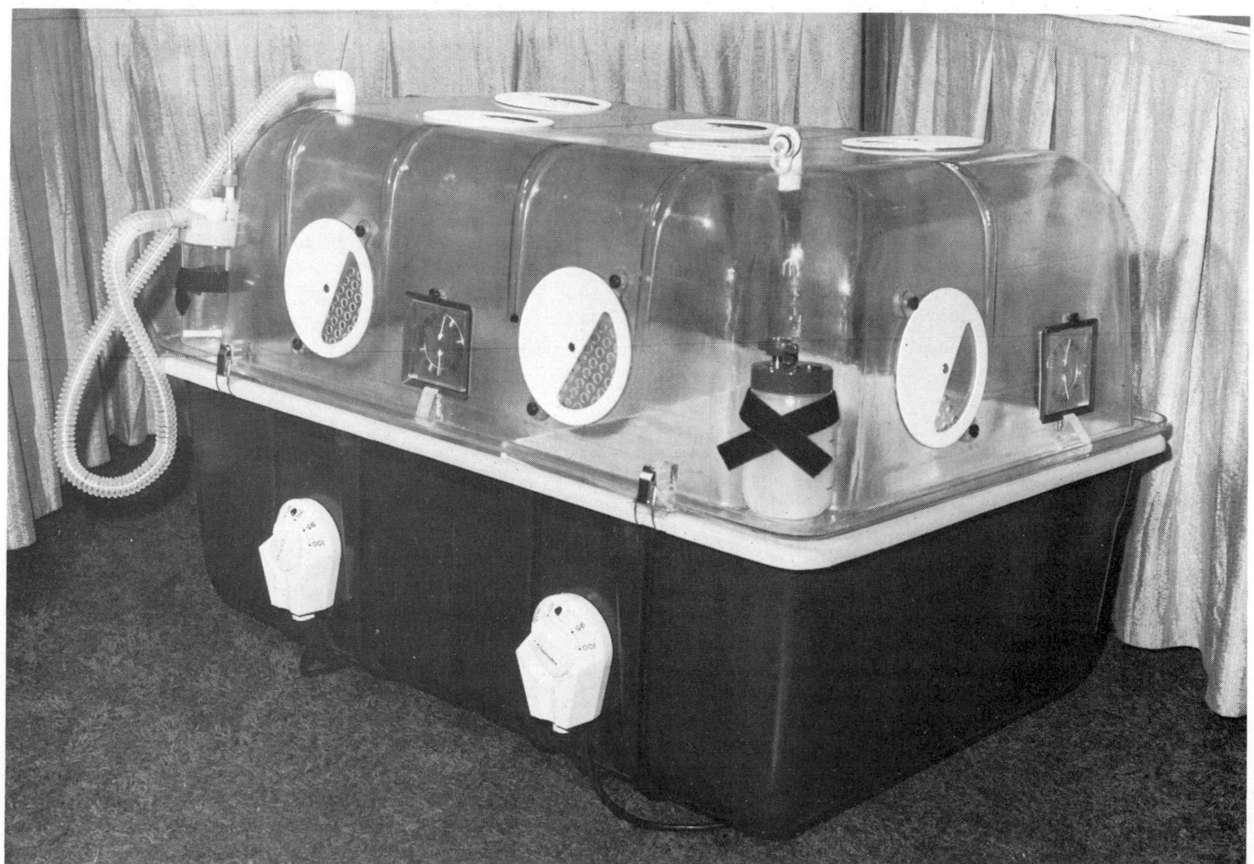

**Figure 3–27.** Incubator for intensive care and recovery from anesthesia. Smaller units are available. (Courtesy Thermocare, Inc, Incline Village NV.)

consciousness is usually the result of excessive anesthetic. Lingering effects can also be due to heavy premedication, inadequate intraoperative fluid therapy, or slow detoxification of drugs in a cat with impaired hepatic or renal function. Physiologic support is necessary to prevent long-term adverse effects. Oxygen (with artificial ventilation, if needed), fluids, and warmth form the basis of treatment. An incubator, like that marketed by Thermocare, Inc., is ideal for cats (Fig. 3–27). The floor contains a warm-water bath with an adjustable thermostat; the top is clear plastic for good visibility and incorporates an inlet for oxygen. Immobile cats should be turned hourly to reverse lung congestion and collapse. Corneal ulceration can be prevented by periodic application of a lubricant or ointment. Urine production must be closely monitored to allow early recognition and treatment of renal malfunction.

Seizures occasionally develop after ketamine anesthesia or myelography. Their danger lies in hypoxia from changes in cerebral perfusion or from restricted breathing during the muscle spasms. Oxygen is supplied by a face mask while diazepam (0.2 to 0.5 mg/kg) is given slowly intravenously to control the seizure. Fluids are started to speed elimination of the ketamine or contrast material. Persistent seizures may have to be controlled with barbiturates and the cat managed as for anesthesia. Monitoring body temperature is especially important at this time, because the exaggerated muscle activity may cause hyperthermia.

Laryngospasm occurs more often in the cat than in any other domestic species. Usually it causes partial airway obstruction, recognized as a "crowing" sound on inspiration. Breathing can be assisted by extending the cat's head and neck and pulling the tongue forward. Usually the laryngospasm resolves spontaneously. Topical application of lidocaine to the larynx may abolish persistent laryngospasm, but tracheal intubation is necessary when complete airway obstruction occurs.

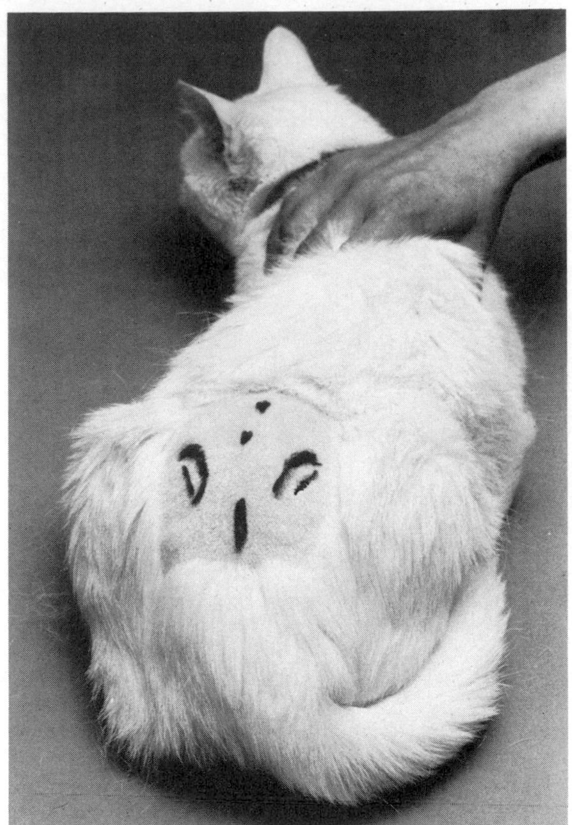

**Figure 3–28.** The cat is restrained in the sternal position. The lumbosacral space is located by palpating the right and left cranial dorsal iliac spine, then (cranial to them) the spinous process of the seventh lumbar vertebra, and finally the prominent spinous process of the first sacral vertebra (more easily palpable than in the dog).

## LOCAL ANALGESIA TECHNIQUES

Local or regional anesthesia is useful for some operations. Lidocaine is the drug most often used for the cat, despite the many analgesics available, and is satisfactory for our purposes. It is infiltrated at the surgical site for excision of small tumors, suturing of lacerations, and, in some cases, for laparotomy. However, it is easy to overdose the cat and produce toxic symptoms. Thus, the quantity of drug injected must be kept small. Dilution of the lidocaine with physiologic saline solution to 1 or 0.5 per cent helps to reduce the dose.

### Epidural Nerve Block

Sedation may or may not be necessary with epidural nerve block. Local anesthetic can be easily injected into the epidural space at the lumbosacral junction. After the hair is clipped from the lumbosacral area, the cat is restrained squarely in a normal crouching position. One locates the point for injection by palpating the cranial dorsal iliac spines and the spinous processes of the seventh lumbar vertebra and sacrum (Fig. 3–28). The lumbosacral space in a cat is immediately cranial to the sacrum (Figs. 3–28 and 3–29), in contrast to its position in the dog, in which it is halfway between L7 and S1.

The skin is cleaned and a small bleb of lidocaine is injected subcutaneously with a 25-gauge needle. For the epidural injection one uses a needle specifically designed for spinal anesthesia with a stylet that prevents injection of a tissue plug into the epidural space. From the notch on the hub one can determine the direction of the bevel. Aseptic technique is essential to avoid meningitis, and this includes not touching the needle except at the hub. The needle (22-gauge, 1½ inch) is inserted perpendicular to the skin to a depth of about 1 cm. The resistance to penetration followed by loss of resistance (a "pop") as the needle passes through the ligamentum flavum is characteristic of the procedure in the dog but is not obvious in the cat.

The spinal cord ends in most cats at a level varying from the seventh lumbar to the third sacral vertebra, and the dural sac continues through the sacrum (Habel, 1978). Therefore, when the stylet is removed from the needle, it should be carefully inspected, as well as the needle hub, for signs of cerebrospinal fluid (CSF) or blood; then an empty 3 ml syringe is attached and aspiration carried out. If either CSF or blood is seen, the needle is slightly withdrawn. Then the syringe is detached and filled with

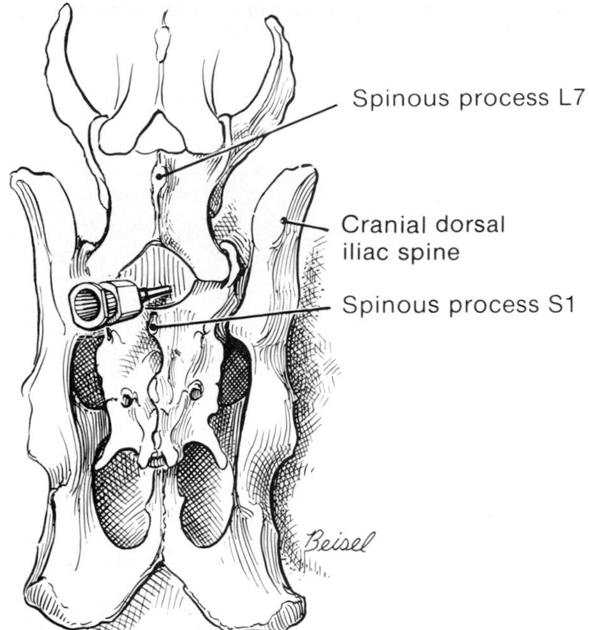


**Figure 3–29.** Drawing of the seventh lumbar vertebra, sacrum, and ilia of the cat, showing the site for injection of local anesthetic through the lumbosacral intervertebral space. To avoid the cranially sloping spinous process of the seventh lumbar vertebra, the needle is introduced perpendicularly to the skin just cranial to the sacrum. The pointed spinous process of the first sacral vertebra is used as a landmark.

0.5 ml air for a test injection. Correct placement of the needle in the epidural space is reasonably certain when the air can be injected with no resistance, provided the needle point is deep enough. The bevel of the needle is directed cranially and lidocaine (2 per cent, 0.2 ml/kg) is injected slowly but steadily. Both the amount of drug and the rate of injection may be varied, depending on the site and nature of the surgical procedure (Klide, 1971). Lack of muscle tone in the anus and tail should be apparent within two minutes, but full analgesia does not develop for 10 to 12 minutes. The duration of surgical anesthesia is about 45 minutes with lidocaine alone, but it can be extended by addition of epinephrine (1:200,000). This dilution is approximated by flushing the syringe with a small amount of epinephrine (1:1000) before drawing the lidocine into the syringe (Klide, 1971).

Possible difficulties in administration and complications of epidural anesthesia are discussed by Klide (1971).

The cat is confined during recovery. Excessive activity is prevented to avoid spinal injury.

## ANESTHESIA FOR CAESAREAN SECTION

A discussion on anesthetic management for Caesarean section is difficult because there have been few detailed reports published on placental drug transfer in the cat. This section is therefore a composite of personal experience and information extrapolated from other species.

### Basic Considerations

Certain physiologic changes occur in the pregnant cat that alter anesthetic management in Caesarean section from that for routine laparotomy. The increase in blood volume and cardiac output caused by pregnancy is offset by a lower than normal arterial blood pressure. When the cat is placed on its back for surgery, venous return to the heart is decreased as the uterus compresses the caudal vena cava and aorta (supine hypotensive syndrome). The hypotension is reflected in the fetuses and causes hypoxia and bradycardia. To prevent these effects, the weight of the uterus may be redirected by tilting the cat 30 degrees to the left about the long axis of the body, or the operation may be performed by a flank incision. Premedication with atropine and intraoperative use of fluids help to maintain adequate blood pressure.

As the uterus increases in size, the diaphragm is displaced and lung volume is reduced. With the increased oxygen demand from the fetuses, only a slight decrease in ventilation results in a large decrease in arterial oxygenation. Oxygen supplied to the anesthetized cat through a face mask or endotracheal tube is not only a sensible precaution but essential for success in some cases.

Investigations in several other species have shown that pregnant animals require less drug for anesthesia than when nonpregnant. In sheep, for example, the magnitude of the reduction is 25 per cent for halothane and 32 per cent for methoxyflurane (Palahniuk et al., 1974). The anesthetic requirement also appears to be reduced for the cat. The increase in ventilation produced by pregnancy and the decreased anesthetic requirement facilitate rapid induction of anesthesia with inhalation anesthetics, but also introduce the risk of excessive depth or overdose of anesthesia.

Intestinal motility diminishes with the onset of labor, slowing emptying of the stomach, and predisposes the cat to vomiting before or, more often, during recovery from anesthesia.

### Drugs and Techniques

All anesthetic drugs cross the placenta. The degree of transfer depends on the ionization, lipid solubility, and protein-binding properties of the drug. It depends also to a great extent on the magnitude of the dose. The route of administration has some influence on the fetal concentration, in that intramuscular injections usually produce lower concentrations than do intravenous injections. Consequently calculation of dosages must allow for the decreased requirements of the pregnant cat and the necessity for maintaining sedation and anesthesia as light as possible to decrease placental transfer. Dosages are usually based on 75 per cent of the cat's weight. The longer the cat is anesthetized before the kittens are removed, the greater the amount of drug transferred to them. Therefore it is advisable to clip the hair and prepare the skin for incision before administering anesthesia.

Premedication with atropine or glycopyrrolate followed by chamber induction and maintenance of anesthesia with halothane, with or without nitrous oxide, is my preference. Halothane anesthetizes the kittens, but is soon eliminated because of its low solubility. Because it causes vasodilation, it may potentiate uterine bleeding, but if uterine involution is rapid, the bleeding is minimal. If necessary, involution can be promoted with an intravenous or intrauterine injection of oxytocin (0.5 to 3 units slowly IV). Diffusion hypoxia occurs in the newborns as a result of excretion of nitrous oxide and should be prevented by giving them oxygen for a few minutes. Meperidine can be used as premedication for halothane anesthesia, but because its metabolites also depress the fetus, surgery should be performed within an hour of administration.

Methoxyflurane should not be used for Caesarean section because it is eliminated too slowly from the kittens. An alternative method of analgesia is recommended until the kittens are removed from the uterus.

Oxymorphone sedation, with or without a phenothiazine tranquilizer, has been used successfully with local anesthetic infiltration. When narcotics have been used, naloxone can be injected into the kittens to reverse depression. Epidural nerve block also provides satisfactory analgesia for Caesarean section with little effect on kittens.

Thiobarbiturates readily cross the placenta, producing a high fetal blood level within one minute. The resulting fetal depression may not be significant in elective surgery but predisposes to kitten deaths when surgery has been delayed and placental separation has begun. Methohexital is a more useful barbiturate because of its much shorter half-life.

Xylazine-ketamine anesthesia has been found in general to be too depressant, even when very low doses of ketamine are used. An alternative is to use xylazine sedation with local analgesic infiltration initially, and then to inject the ketamine for completion of surgery after the kittens have been removed.

The usefulness of diazepam is in question. In human infants it has several severe adverse effects, including reduced suckling reflex and impairment of thermoregulation for 24 hours.

A technique used by some veterinarians incorporates succinylcholine (Goodger and Levy, 1973). Premedication with atropine is followed by induction of anesthesia with a barbiturate, intubation of the trachea, and institution of artificial ventilation with 60 per cent nitrous oxide and 40 per cent oxygen. Succinylcholine is injected (3 to 5 mg total dose) and surgery performed immediately. By the time the kittens are removed, the effect of the barbiturate is waning, and methoxyflurane or halothane must be administered for analgesia. Succinylcholine provides complete muscle relaxation, which facilitates surgery. Disadvantages are the necessity for artificial ventilation and the speed required for surgery. The kittens must be removed before the effect of the barbiturate wears off and the cat feels pain.

## THE INJURED OR SICK CAT

The prospects for anesthetic and surgical success are enhanced if abnormalities of fluid, electrolyte, and acid-base balance are corrected before induction of anesthesia. The time required for this varies from a few hours for rehydration of the cat with an intestinal foreign body to several days for intensive care of the cat with a fractured femur and cardiac dysrhythmias from thoracic trauma.

Restoration of the circulating blood volume before anesthesia is of primary importance to enable the cardiovascular system to withstand subsequent depression from anesthetic drugs. Response to intravenous fluid administration may be gauged by changes in the cat's behavior, arterial blood pressure, and urine production, as well as by serial measurements of PCV and total protein (TP). Both the cephalic and the saphenous veins are easily accessible for catheterization, but flexion of the limb must be prevented to allow continuous infusion. A wooden tongue depressor taped to the limb immobilizes the carpus (Fig. 3–30) or the hock. A half-circle metal splint can be applied to the forelimb to restrict movement at the elbow. A Thomas splint attached to the hindlimb effectively immobilizes hock and stifle and is well tolerated by cats. An Elizabethan collar can be used if the cat chews at the catheter.

Metabolic acidosis should be corrected with sodium bicarbonate, 1 mEq/kg given intravenously over five minutes and repeated 30 minutes later. More sodium bicarbonate is needed for severe acidosis, but, if facilities are available, should be given only after confirmation of acidosis by laboratory tests. The cat differs from other domestic species in that it is normally in metabolic acidosis. A naturally occurring respiratory alkalosis offsets the metabolic acidosis so that normal arterial blood pH of the cat is $7.34 \pm 0.1$ (Middleton et al., 1981). Measurement of pH and $P_{CO_2}$ permits exact calculation of the base deficit. In the absence of facilities for blood gas analysis, measurement of the total carbon dioxide ($T_{CO_2}$) content of the blood can be used as an approximate estimation of the metabolic status. This value is approximate because it is increased when $CO_2$ accumulates because of ventilatory depression from disease or drugs. The $T_{CO_2}$ can be measured easily and cheaply with the $CO_2$ apparatus set manufactured by Harleco (Division of American Hospital Supply). This test has been compared with a recognized standard method of $CO_2$ measurement (Van Slyke) using bovine and canine blood and has been found to be accurate (Gentry and Black, 1975).

The normal $T_{CO_2}$ of cat arterial blood is $18.4 \pm 3.9$

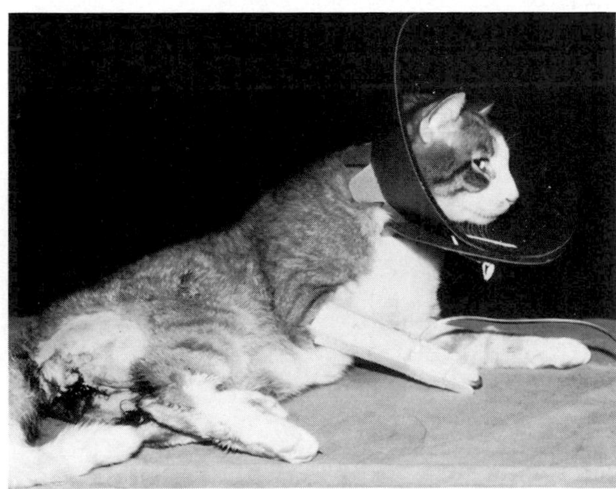

**Figure 3–30.** Intravenous administration of fluids through the cephalic vein. A tongue depressor is taped to the leg above and below the carpus to prevent flexion and to secure the catheter. The Elizabethan collar protects both the catheter and the surgical site from the cat.

mMol/l (mEq/l) and of venous blood, 20.1 ± 2.4 mMol/l. Subtraction of the measured value from the normal value gives the base deficit. A deficit of 5 mMol/l indicates mild metabolic acidosis, a deficit of 10 mMol/l moderate acidosis, and 15 mMol/l severe acidosis. The total mEq of bicarbonate needed to correct the acidosis is calculated from the formula: deficit × kg body weight × 0.3. This amount is given in two infusions 30 minutes apart for the correction of mild or moderate acidosis, but over several hours for severe acidosis, to avoid paradoxical cerebral acidosis.

## Trauma

With a few urgent exceptions, a severely traumatized cat should not be anesthetized for at least 24 hours. The reason is twofold—so that fluid distribution and cardiovascular and endocrine functions altered by stress and injury may return toward normal, and so that the extent of injury can be more adequately assessed. Signs of myocardial contusion do not develop for 24 hours. The appearance of premature ventricular contractions confirms myocardial damage, and anesthesia may have to be delayed pending return of normal cardiac function. Inadequate urine production may indicate kidney damage, for which treatment will be necessary before anesthesia.

Anesthetic management depends on the damage incurred. Pulmonary contusion impairs oxygenation, so that oxygen must be supplied before, during, and after anesthesia. Heavy sedation from premedication must be avoided because it will cause ventilatory depression. Fluids infused during surgery are limited to half the amount used in a healthy cat to reduce the risk of pulmonary edema.

Every cat, but especially those with fractures of limb bones or pelvis, should be checked for pneumothorax. Unless ventilation is severely compromised, artificial ventilation is not recommended when pneumothorax or pulmonary blebs are present, owing to the risk of lung rupture. Nitrous oxide must not be used in cases of pneumothorax.

The cat that has sustained head trauma requires special management. The intracranial pressure can be lowered by supporting the cat's head slightly above the level of the body and by maintaining arterial $P_{CO_2}$ at or below normal. Diazepam and thiopental both lower intracranial pressure; however, ketamine not only raises the pressure but also increases cerebral metabolic oxygen demands. Phenothiazine tranquilizers should be avoided in cases of severe head damage because they lower the convulsive threshold.

## Ruptured Diaphragm

The cat undergoing surgery for repair of a ruptured diaphragm is most at risk during induction of anesthesia and during removal of the abdominal organs from the thoracic cavity. Induction of anesthesia sometimes precipitates complete collapse of the lungs and inability to ventilate. To shorten the time from induction to removal of organs from the thorax, anesthesia should be preceded by preparation of the surgical site, the cat being held upright. The cat is then given oxygen to breathe for three to five minutes (preoxygenation) to ensure adequate oxygenation during intubation. Anesthesia is induced rapidly with a small dose of thiobarbiturate or ketamine to reduce the delay between awake, spontaneous breathing and artificial ventilation. The cat must be held head up until the trachea is intubated, to avoid regurgitation and aspiration.

The second danger period is during removal of abdominal organs from the chest, when cardiovascular collapse is a common complication. Atropine or glycopyrrolate prevents vagal effects of surgical manipulation; however, the hypotension apparently more often results from blood loss from the systemic circulation as a result of pooling in the involved organs. Temporary discontinuance of anesthetic and increased fluid administration usually suffice to restore blood pressure. In some instances dopamine stimulation is necessary, and if hypotension persists, corticosteroids and sodium bicarbonate must be administered.

The cat should be placed in an oxygen cage for the first hour of recovery until it is able to regulate its breathing. Administration of analgesic drugs must strike a balance, avoiding respiratory depression, yet preventing excitement, which might cause sutures to tear loose.

For the small percentage of cats in which repair cannot be delayed because of a life-threatening displacement of abdominal viscera, the anesthetist has the difficult tasks of assessing the decreased requirement for anesthetic and of working with an unstable cardiovascular system.

## Oral Surgery

To prevent airway obstruction and aspiration of blood, endotracheal intubation is advisable during oral surgery. The tube may interfere with surgical exposure and assessment of jaw alignment during repair of mandibular fractures. This difficulty may be circumvented by passing the endotracheal tube through the site commonly used for pharyngostomy (Fig. 3–31). The tube can be inserted through the opening in either direction. A forceps may be needed to direct the tip of the tube into the larynx.

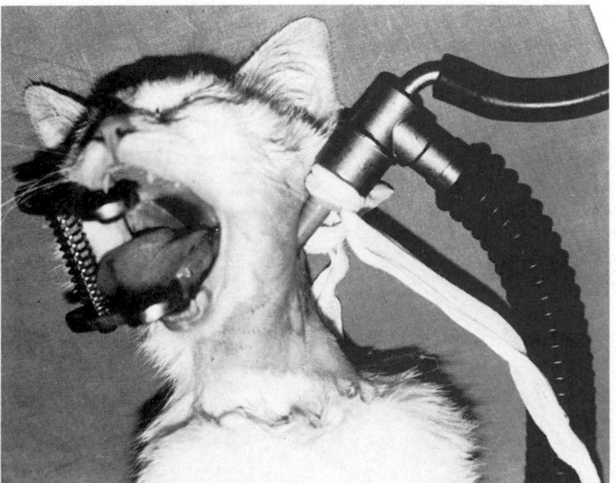

**Figure 3–31.** Cat anesthetized with halothane for repair of a laceration of the hard palate. The endotracheal tube is inserted through the pharyngostomy site to provide greater exposure for surgery.

## Urolithiasis With Obstruction

Fluid and electrolyte balances are invariably disturbed in urinary obstruction. Hypovolemia with elevation of PCV and TP is common. Notable increases in serum potassium occur early and are of great significance to anesthesia. In 15 uremic cats with urethral obstruction, the serum potassium exceeded 6 mEq/l within 48 hours after the reported onset of obstruction; in seven of these, the potassium exceeded 9 mEq/l (Parks, 1975). Electrocardiographic abnormalities appear when the serum potassium concentration reaches 7 mEq/l, and cardiac arrest is likely to occur at a concentration of 9 to 10 mEq/l. Metabolic acidosis develops secondary to retention of metabolic products and contributes to the hyperkalemia by shifting potassium from cells to the intravascular space. Other undesirable effects of acidosis are depression of the myocardium and a shift in the oxygen dissociation curve. The serum potassium levels can be lowered by treatment of the acidosis and infusion of glucose-containing solutions. A specific regimen using glucose and insulin has been described (Schaer, 1975).

The CNS depression caused by azotemia reduces the anesthetic requirement. Also the actions of many drugs are altered by changes in pH and plasma protein level, and their effects are lengthened by reduced renal excretion. In addition, renal function is not immediately restored when the urethral obstruction is relieved. Both barbiturates and ketamine can be expected to produce deeper and longer anesthesia, and greatly reduced quantities of drug must be used to avoid complications. A popular drug combination for analgesia in the cat for catheterization of the urethra is atropine (0.1 ml), ketamine (0.1 ml), and promazine (0.1 ml) or acepromazine (0.05 ml). They are mixed in the same syringe and injected slowly intravenously until sufficient immobilization is achieved. A combination of oxymorphone, triflupromazine, and ketamine has also been recommended (Reid and Frank, 1972). Epidural analgesia is preferred by others. Several days should elapse between catheterization and anesthesia for perineal urethrostomy, to allow correction of fluid, electrolyte, and acid-base abnormalities.

## Hepatic Disease

Identification of cats with hepatic malfunction is of twofold importance. First, anesthesia and surgery may increase the severity of the disease. Second, changes in protein synthesis and metabolism may alter the action and duration of action of drugs used for anesthesia. Coagulation may also be impaired, causing excessive blood loss during surgery.

Most techniques of regional, local, and general anesthesia cause some alteration in liver function attributable to reduced hepatic blood flow; ether and methoxyflurane cause the greatest reductions in splanchnic flow. The closer the surgical procedure is to the liver, the greater is its influence on liver function.

Anesthesia in the cat with liver disease must be planned to maintain good arterial oxygenation and normal $Pco_2$ and to avoid hypotension. Even when local analgesia is used, a large-bore catheter should be installed as a precaution. Decreased glycogen stores may occur with liver disease and result in intraoperative hypoglycemia. Dextrose (5 per cent in water, 5 ml/kg/hour) can be used as the primary fluid for intraoperative replacement, unless blood loss is significant, in which case a balanced electrolyte solution is indicated. In patients with obstructive jaundice, there is an increased incidence of renal failure following surgery. This may be prevented if diuresis is induced before anesthesia and continued postoperatively. An infusion of fresh blood or plasma before surgery reduces the risk of hemorrhage even when prothrombin time is prolonged. Parenteral administration of vitamin K restores prothrombin production impaired by biliary obstruction but may not be effective if hepatocellular disease is severe.

The optimal anesthetic regimen for cats with hepatic disease is not known. Local analgesia, narcotics, halothane, and nitrous oxide are safer than barbiturates, ketamine, or methoxyflurane. Balanced anesthesia using narcotics, nitrous oxide, and muscle relaxants may be the best form of anesthesia for cats with severe liver disease. Succinylcholine is contraindicated in liver disease. Pancuronium, probably the drug of choice, is partially metabolized in the liver, so that a half dose (0.03 mg/kg) will suffice.

## REFERENCES


Adams HR, Dixit BM: Prolongation of pentobarbital anesthesia by chloramphenicol in dogs and cats. J Am Vet Med Assoc 156 (1970) 902–905.

Auer L, Bell K, Coates S: Blood transfusion reactions in the cat. J Am Vet Med Assoc 180 (1982) 729–730.

Baxter JS, Evans JM: Intramuscular injection in the cat. J Small Anim Pract 14 (1973) 297–302.

Breznock EM, Kagan KG, Attix ES: Effects of ionic salts or acetylcholine, or both, on electrically induced ventricular fibrillation in dogs. Am J Vet Res 39 (1978) 977–980.

Chai CY, Wang SC: Cardiovascular actions of diazepam in the cat. J Pharmacol Exp Ther 154 (1966) 271–280.

Curtis R, Evans JM: The effect of doxapram hydrochloride on cats anaesthetised with either Saffan or thiopentone sodium. J Small Anim Pract 22 (1981) 77–83.

Davis LE, Donnelly EJ: Analgesic drugs in the cat. J Am Vet Med Assoc 153 (1968) 1161–1167.

Dodds MG, Twissell DJ: CT 1341 and thiopentone compared in feline anaesthesia by an intermittent injection technique. J Small Anim Pract 14 (1973) 487–492.

Dodman N: Complications of Saffan anesthesia in cats. Vet Rec 107 (1980) 481.

Eger EI: Isoflurane: A review. Anesthesiology 55 (1981) 559–576.

Feldberg W, Symonds HW: Hyperglycaemic effect of xylazine. J Vet Pharmacol Ther 3 (1980) 197–202.

Frankel T, Hawkey CM: Haematological changes during sedation in cats. Vet Rec 107 (1980) 512–513.

Gentry PA, Black WD: Evaluation of Harleco $CO_2$ apparatus: comparison with the Van Slyke method. J Am Vet Med Assoc 167 (1975) 156–157.

Gillick A: High frequency complaints. Ontario Vet Assoc Newsletter 5 (1)(1981) 12.

Goodger WJ, Levy W: Anesthetic management of the cesarean section. Vet Clin North Am 3 (1)(1973) 85–99.

Habel RE: Applied Veterinary Anatomy, 2nd ed. Ithaca, NY, RE Habel, 1978.

Hartsfield SM: The effects of acetylpromazine, xylazine, and ketamine on urine production in cats. Proceedings, American College of Veterinary Anesthesiologists Meeting, St Louis, October 1980.

Hartsfield SM, Sawyer DC: Cardiopulmonary effects of rebreathing and non-rebreathing systems during halothane anesthesia in the cat. Am J Vet Res 37 (1976) 1461–1466.

Haskins SC: Hypothermia and its prevention during general anesthesia in cats. Am J Vet Res 42 (1981) 856–861.

Haskins SC, Peiffer RL, Stowe CM: A clinical comparison of CT 1341, ketamine, and xylazine in cats. Am J Vet Res 36 (1975) 1537–1542.

Heavner JE, Bloedow DC: Ketamine pharmacokinetics in domestic cats. Vet Anesth 6(2) (1979) 16–19.

Jensen EC, Klemm WR: Clinical evaluation of the analeptic, doxapram, in dogs and cats. J Am Vet Med Assoc 150 (1967) 516–525.

Julien RM, Kavan EM: Electrographic studies of a new volatile anesthetic agent: Enflurane. J Pharmacol Exp Ther 183 (1972) 393–403.

Kim DH, Clifford DH: Use of a small animal incubator as an anesthetic chamber for cats. Vet Med Small Anim Clin 75 (1980) 1274–1277.

Klide AM: Epidural analgesia. *In* Soma LR (ed): Textbook of Veterinary Anesthesia. Baltimore, The Williams & Wilkins Company, 1971.

Macy DW, Siwe ST: The use of ketamine as an oral anesthetic in cats. Feline Pract 7(1) (1977) 44–66.

Manley SV: Anesthetic pollution in veterinary practice in northern California. Presented at American College of Veterinary Anesthesiologists Meeting, New Orleans, 1981.

Manley SV, McDonell WN: Recommendations for reduction of anesthetic gas pollution. J Am Vet Med Assoc 176 (1980) 519–524.

McLeish I, Steffey EP: Recent developments and expectations in feline anesthesia. Vet Anesth 4(2) (1977) 28–34.

Middleton DJ, Ilkin JE, Watson ADJ: Arterial and venous blood gas tensions in clinically healthy cats. Am J Vet Res 42 (1981) 1609–1611.

Miller RL: Personal communication, 1981.

Milligan JE, Sablan JL: A survey of waste anesthetic gas levels in selected USAF veterinary surgeries. Report OEHL 79-33, USAF Occupational and Environmental Health Laboratory, Aerospace Medical Division, 1979.

Palahniuk RJ, Shnider SM, Eger EI II: Pregnancy decreases the requirement for inhaled anesthetic agents. Anesthesiology 41 (1974) 82–83.

Palminteri A: Oxymorphone, an effective analgesic in dogs and cats. J Am Vet Med Assoc 143 (1963) 160–163.

Parks J: Electrocardiographic abnormalities from serum electrolyte imbalance due to feline urethral obstruction. J Am Anim Hosp Assoc 11 (1975) 102–106.

Povey RC: Differential diagnosis and control of infectious respiratory disease in cats. Bi-weekly Small Animal Veterinary Medicine Update Series. 1. Princeton, Veterinary Publications, Inc, 1977.

Reid JS, Frank RJ: Prevention of undesirable side reactions of ketamine anesthesia in cats. J Am Anim Hosp Assoc 8 (1972) 115–119.

Rex MAE: Laryngeal activity during the induction of anaesthesia in the cat. Aust Vet J 49 (1973) 365–368.

Schaer M: The use of regular insulin in the treatment of hypokalemia in cats with urethral obstruction. J Am Anim Hosp Assoc 11 (1975) 106–109.

Smithcors JF: History of veterinary anesthesia. *In* Soma LR (ed): Textbook of Veterinary Anesthesia. Baltimore, The Williams & Wilkins Company, 1971.

Stogdale L: Laryngeal edema due to Saffan in a cat. Vet Rec 102 (1978) 283–284.

Trim CM: Anesthesia and the kidney. Compend Contin Ed 1 (1979) 843–848.

Trim CM, Simpson ST: Complications following ethylene oxide sterilization: a case report. J Am Anim Hosp Assoc 18 (1982) 507–510.

Wingfield WE, Ruby DL, Buchan RM, Gunther BJ: Waste anesthetic gas exposure to veterinarians and animal technicians. J Am Vet Med Assoc 178 (1981) 399–402.

Wong KC: Sympathomimetic drugs. *In* Smith NT, Miller RD, Corbascio AN (eds): Drug Interactions in Anesthesia. Philadelphia, Lea & Febiger, 1981.

**Additional Reading**

Sawyer DC, Rech RH: Analgesia, sedation, and behavioral changes in the cat produced by butorphanol or nalbuphine injection. Proc. 2nd Int Congress Veterinary Anesthesia, Sacramento, October 1985.

Trim CM: Anesthesia and the endocrine system. *In* Slatter DH (ed): Textbook of Small Animal Surgery. Philadelphia, WB Saunders Company, 1985.

# 4
CHAPTER
# SOFT TISSUE SURGERY

RICHARD J. TODOROFF

CONTRIBUTING AUTHOR:
MICHAEL M. PAVLETIC

Cats are gratifying surgical patients. They are small, light, and nimble and adapt well to the adversity imposed by surgical disease and surgery. Their anatomy is discrete, with easily identified tissue planes that simplify surgical dissection.

Sound surgical principles must be followed as carefully in the cat as in any other species. Aseptic technique is used in every instance. Adequate exposure and meticulous hemostasis are critical, for blood in the surgical field can obscure important anatomic details and provides a substrate for bacteria in establishing wound infections. Gentle tissue handling with appropriate instruments (Table 4–1) and frequent moistening of exposed tissues minimize hemorrhage, swelling, and wound dehiscence. Sutures should be swaged onto needles and kept to the necessary minimum in numbers, tightness, and size.

Anesthesia must be closely monitored and must provide adequate analgesia and relaxation. An indwelling intravenous catheter is used for all major surgery. The cat's small size and relatively large surface area render it susceptible to hypothermia, which is best countered with a circulating warm-water heating pad.

Many surgical procedures are identical in dogs and cats and are well described in standard texts on canine surgery. This chapter concentrates on procedures that are unique to, or deserve emphasis in, the cat.

## THE INTEGUMENT*

Skin wounds are the most common injuries seen by veterinarians. Most skin injuries are treated by primary closure, by delayed closure, or by contraction and epithelialization. The choice of closure depends on the size and condition of the wound and the area of the body involved. Considerations of cost may play a role in choice of closure but do not give the veterinarian license to choose a method contrary to good surgical judgment. The common cat abscess, for example, is best treated by establishing adequate ventral drainage and allowing the open infected wound to heal by second intention. Suture closure is both unnecessary and inadvisable.

Skin grafting is necessary when direct or second-intention closure techniques cannot be used. Few discussions deal specifically with skin grafting in the cat. Although there are microscopic differences between cat and dog skin, the anatomic structure and blood supply are similar and most grafting techniques can be successfully extrapolated. The cat's loose, elastic skin, mobile limbs, and capacity to accept full-thickness grafts make it an excellent candidate for skin grafting procedures.

### Basic Wound Management

Wounds can be assigned to one of four categories according to their cause and condition (Hunt and Dunphy, 1979).

1. A clean wound is an uninfected operative wound made aseptically and without entrance into the respiratory, alimentary, or genitourinary tract or the oropharyngeal cavity. It is usually closed without drains.

**Table 4–1 Instruments Useful in Feline Surgery**

| |
|---|
| Adson tissue forceps, 1 × 2 teeth, 4¾ inches |
| Brown-Adson tissue forceps, 4¾ inches |
| Metzenbaum scissors, curved, 5½ inches |
| Stevens tenotomy scissors, straight, blunt, 4½ inches |
| Ryder needle holders, 6 inches |
| Frazier suction tip, 7F |
| Poole suction tip, pediatric, 18F outer cannula |
| Weitlaner retractor, blunt, 5½ inches |
| Baby Gossett abdominal retractor, ¾ by 1½ inch blades, 4 inch spread |

*By Michael M. Pavletic.

2. A clean-contaminated wound is an operative wound in which the respiratory, alimentary, or genitourinary tract is entered without unusual contamination.

3. Contaminated wounds include open, fresh traumatic wounds and operative wounds with a break in aseptic technique or contact with acute, nonpurulent inflammation.

4. Dirty and infected wounds include old traumatic wounds and those involving abscesses or perforated viscera, pus, or the preoperative presence of organisms that may cause postoperative infection.

The type of wound determines the proper method of closure. There are four basic methods of closure exclusive of grafting procedures:

1. Primary closure (healing by first intention) is reserved for wounds created under aseptic conditions. Contaminated wounds less than four to six hours old can often be converted to clean wounds with judicious débridement and copious lavage with sterile isotonic solutions. Wounds less than four to six hours old, even if contaminated, are considered acceptable candidates for primary closure.

2. Wounds with borderline contamination may be left unsutured and covered with a sterile dressing to allow time for adequate drainage and improved tissue resistance to infection (delayed primary closure). If no devitalized tissue or infection is evident on the fourth or fifth day, primary closure may be attempted.

3. Secondary closure is generally reserved for infected wounds and can be attempted between the fifth and tenth days with direct suture apposition of the two granulation surfaces (healing by third intention) or granulation tissue excision and primary closure. The latter technique is preferred by many surgeons because of the relative ease in mobilization of the wound edges for closure, better cosmetic results, and lower incidence of infection.

4. Healing by second intention or contraction and epithelialization is a technique common in veterinary surgery for grossly contaminated and infected wounds. Large skin defects may be left to contract and epithelialize—a practical and economical course if the wound is adequately cared for. Excessive scarring and a fragile epithelial surface are possible complications. Healing by second intention is not advisable for large areas subject to constant motion or abuse but is best suited for the feline trunk, where loose skin will not impede wound contraction. The distal extremities may lack sufficient skin for adequate healing by second intention (Hunt and Dunphy, 1979; Johnston, 1977, 1979; Schilling, 1976; Spreull, 1968).

It should be kept in mind that partial-thickness skin losses resulting from scrapes or burns (e.g., with automobile fan belt injuries) may re-epithelialize from remnants of the germinal layer of the epidermis or by migration of epithelial cells lining hair follicles and other adnexa in the surviving dermal layer. Such a wound must be protected from added insult that could convert it into a full-thickness skin loss.

## Wound Care

Healthy tissue can withstand a considerable bacterial inoculum, but poorly perfused and devitalized tissue is fertile ground for infection. The presence of foreign debris also impairs resistance to bacterial invasion (Hunt and Dunphy, 1979; Schilling, 1976). Detergents and strong antiseptic agents further injure compromised tissues (Hunt and Dunphy, 1979; Swaim, 1980). Heroic attempts to destroy bacteria at the expense of damaged tissues are a common error of veterinarians. The old adage, "Above all, do no harm," favors débridement, gentle tissue handling, copious lavage with isotonic solutions (lactated Ringer's), adequate drainage, treatment with appropriate topical and systemic antibiotics, and adequate postsurgical "tissue rest."

Dressings, bandages, or splints may be needed to protect the wound from added injury and movement. Bandages, however, can collect bacteria and excessive moisture, promoting tissue maceration and infection, and can also abrade the wound in areas subject to motion. These problems can be minimized by frequent bandage changes and application of massive bandages or splints to prevent motion of the area involved (Schilling, 1976).

Adequate wound drainage is important in the management of soft tissue injuries. As a general rule, drains are used whenever an abnormal accumulation of fluid is present or anticipated (Warren, 1963)—soft latex Penrose drains for drainage of soft tissue "cavities" or noncollapsible rigid drains for areas requiring suction or infusion. Most are removed in two to five days (Hunt and Dunphy, 1979; Schilling, 1976). Drains are not to be used arbitrarily and cannot substitute for sound surgical judgment and technique. With prolonged use, they elicit a foreign body, fibroplastic response and may provide entrance for infection. Their routine use in the treatment of cat abscesses is unnecessary.

## Abscesses

Foreign bodies and irritants can stimulate abscess formation without the presence of microorganisms, but most feline abscesses are due to bacterial infection secondary to bite wounds from other cats. Many of these infections are caused by *Pasteurella multocida*, the dominant feline oral pathogen, but mixed bacterial infections are common. (See chapter on bacterial diseases.)

Most cat abscesses are simple unilocular swellings, but occasionally the infection spreads along fascial planes and causes extensive soft tissue injury. The management of an uncomplicated abscess calls for thorough history taking and complete physical examination. Sedation or light anesthesia is given unless contraindicated by the history or signs of serious illness. The hair is clipped liberally from the abscess and adjacent skin, and the area is gently prepared for surgery. The ventral wall of the abscess is lanced with a sterile scalpel blade and emptied of pus, a sample being taken for culture if desired. With a sterile forceps the abscess cavity is gently probed to ensure that the entire cavity is confluent with the drainage opening. Necrotic tissue is excised and the opening enlarged by trimming its edges to ensure adequate postoperative drainage. The abscess cavity is then flushed with isotonic saline solution. A systemic, broad-spectrum antibiotic (or the antibiotic indicated by Gram stain or by culture and sensitivity testing) is given for 7 to 10 days.

Gram stains and culture and sensitivity tests are not routinely performed. Cauterization of the cavity with concentrated iodine solutions or packing with gauze impregnated with an antimicrobial drug has been used successfully, but from the author's experience, these measures seem to offer no advantage over the foregoing procedure for uncomplicated abscesses. Adequate drainage is the single most important measure.

The cat is returned to the owner with instructions to apply moist, warm compresses to the area for 10 minutes two or three times daily for a week. These help to keep the area clean, prevent premature closure of the drainage opening, and improve local circulation to the wound.

History or signs of other illness, severe depression, anemia, and very high fever are contraindications to anesthesia. The abscess should simply be opened by a stab wound and emptied, and an antibiotic and supportive treatment given until the necessary diagnostic tests have been done and the cat is in better condition for more thorough surgical treatment.

Foreign bodies, bone sequestra, immunologic defects or suppression (as with feline leukemia virus infection), associated neoplasia, inaccessibility of the microorganisms to antibiotics, or resistant fungal or bacterial organisms may be involved in unresponsive abscesses, causing recurrence of infection or persistent drainage at the site. These complicated infections require thorough laboratory evaluation, Gram stains, culture and sensitivity testing of the organisms, and radiographic examination. Aggressive treatment of the wound, including extensive exploration, débridement, and ingress-egress drains, may be necessary in such cases. Additional therapy may be required if neoplasia is evident on biopsy.

## Reconstructive Surgery

### Anatomy

The skin is composed of the epidermis and dermis. The cat's epidermis varies in thickness from 12 to 45 μ, (with an average of 25 μ) (Crouch, 1969; Strickland and Calhoun, 1963). The dermis contains collagenous, elastic, and reticular fibers, as well as nerve components, blood vessels, and skin adnexa (Creed, 1958; Crouch, 1969; Strickland and Calhoun, 1963).

Skin differs in thickness in various areas of the cat's body, being thickest along the dorsal cervical, lumbar, and sacral regions and thinnest along the lateral sides of the lower hindlimb, thigh, and lower forelimb. In general, skin thickness decreases in a dorsal to ventral direction on the trunk and a proximal to distal direction on the limbs. Skin thickness varies from 1900 μ on the dorsal neck to 375 μ on the lower lateral hindlimb (Strickland and Calhoun, 1963).

The cat has two major cutaneous muscles of surgical importance, the large cutaneus trunci (cutaneus maximus) and the platysma muscle of the neck and head (Crouch, 1969; Field and Taylor, 1974; Gilbert, 1977; McClure et al., 1973). The cutaneous musculature is intimately attached to the skin and functions in twitching the skin, erecting the fur, moving the vibrissae, and giving expression to the face (Crouch, 1969).

### Cutaneous Circulation

Adequate circulation to tissue is essential for optimal healing and resistance to infection. Most graft failures result from poor vascular perfusion during flap development or transfer. A basic understanding of the cutaneous circulation will enable the veterinary surgeon to manipulate skin with less risk of necrosis.

The cutaneous circulation is composed of three plexuses, the deep or subdermal, the middle or cutaneous, and the superficial or subpapillary. They are interconnected to supply nourishment to the skin. The deep plexus is the major conduit to the cutaneous circulation and is intimately associated with the cutaneous muscle. In areas where this muscle is present, the surgeon should undermine it. Preservation of the muscle and overlying skin as a unit will help to ensure the integrity of the deep plexus (Pavletic, 1980a).

### Simple Direct Closure Techniques

Many cutaneous defects can be closed by undermining and direct suturing. An irregular defect can be converted into a conventional geometric design to facilitate closure (Fig. 4–1) (Spreull, 1968). Direct closure of elliptical and circular defects occasionally forms skin elevations ("dog ears") at the ends of the incision. These are rarely a problem in the cat, because its elastic and pliable skin adapts to irregular closures. Offensive "dog ears" are easily excised if necessary; small "dog ears" may disappear in time. Areas not amenable to undermining and direct closure may require pedicle grafts (skin flaps) or free skin grafts.

### Pedicle Grafts

A pedicle graft (skin flap) is a portion of skin and underlying subcutaneous tissue attached to the body by a vascular pedicle (base). Survival of the graft depends on maintenance of adequate vascular perfusion pressure from the pedicle until new vessels establish a secondary blood supply from the recipient bed (Converse, 1977; Grabb and Myers, 1975; Grabb and Smith, 1973).

In selected cases, a pedicle graft can rapidly restore anatomic function and tissue continuity to an area, so that

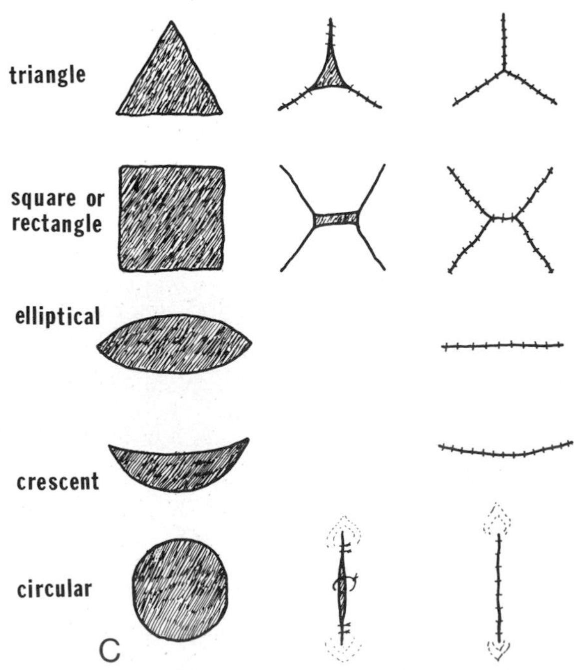


**Figure 4–1.** Closure of simple geometric skin defects.

the prolonged time and potential complications associated with second intention healing can be avoided.

Pedicle grafts can be classified according to blood supply, location, method of transfer, method of development, and configuration. Flaps in the cat and dog are commonly developed without consideration of the cutaneous blood supply. Flaps that include a direct cutaneous artery and vein are termed axial pattern flaps or direct cutaneous arterial pedicle grafts. Direct cutaneous arteries are capable of nourishing sizable axial pattern flaps. Flaps lacking a direct cutaneous artery and vein are termed subdermal plexus flaps. These are less robust, for survival depends primarily on preservation of the pedicle's subdermal plexus. A delay procedure is required to develop long subdermal plexus flaps safely (Pavletic, 1980a, b; 1981).

Local pedicle grafts can be advanced (advancement flaps) into a defect with a single (Fig. 4–2) or bipedicle attachment (Fig. 4–3). Bipedicle flaps have the advantage of two sources of circulation. Necrosis, however, can occur at the vascular interface in a long bipedicle flap when the circulation from the pedicles is insufficient to supply the entire flap. The necrotic area may not be at the center of the flap. Other flaps are best transplanted to the adjacent defect in a lateral or rotational fashion (rotation type flaps) (Bistner et al., 1977; Converse, 1977; Grabb and Myers, 1975; Grabb and Smith, 1973; Keefe, 1946; Krahwinkel, 1976; Quigley and Voight, 1976; Ross, 1968).

To avoid technical errors, all flaps should be carefully planned before surgery with cloth or foam rubber models. The simplest method that safely covers the defect should be chosen, the prime consideration being to establish an adequate blood supply (Converse, 1977; Grabb and Smith, 1973; Pavletic, 1980a).

## Distant Flaps

Distant flaps are those created a distance from the recipient bed (Converse, 1977; Grabb and Myers, 1975; Grabb and Smith, 1973). These are less desirable in veterinary surgery than local flaps. The major problem is the method of graft transfer. A common technique is to raise the affected limb to the donor site (direct transfer). Single pedicle flaps or bipedicle distant flaps can be developed from the lateral thoracic or abdominal skin (see Fig. 4–3). Two incisions are made as far apart as the width of the skin defect, and the flap is undermined beneath the cutaneous muscle. The prepared recipient bed on the limb is placed under the graft, and the edges of graft and bed are sutured. After the graft "takes" (in about two weeks), the two pedicles are severed in four stages (half every two days) to avoid vascular compromise of the established graft (Alexander et al., 1976; Converse, 1977; Grabb and Myers, 1975; Grabb and Smith, 1973; Johnston, 1976; Krahwinkel, 1976; Ross, 1968, Yturraspe et al., 1976). The major difficulty of direct transfer is adequate limb immobilization to ensure a proper "take."

The tube graft is another form of distant graft (Arnall, 1960; Cawley and Francis, 1958; Converse, 1977; Grabb and Myers, 1975; Grabb and Smith, 1973; Jensen, 1959; Keefe, 1946; Ross, 1968; Spreull, 1968; Swaim and Bushby, 1976). The tube is gradually developed for two to three weeks to enhance its blood supply before severing and "opening" one end of the tube and applying it to the defect (indirect transfer). The remaining tube pedicle is severed when the graft has completely healed to the defect. Tube grafts are costly and time-consuming to perform and may fail. Kinking or twisting of the transfer pedicle can result in graft necrosis. Proper planning of tube grafts is critical to their success. Fortunately, they are rarely necessary in the cat.

## Free Skin Grafts

Free skin grafts are skin transplants lacking a vascular attachment to the recipient bed. They survive by absorbing tissue fluid from the recipient bed for the first 48 hours. A thin fibrin film serves as "glue" between the graft and the bed, until capillaries from the bed unite with those in the graft to re-establish circulation. The vascular channels later remodel, and fibrous connective tissue forms to hold the graft securely in place. Accumulation of pus, serum, blood, or foreign matter between the graft and the bed can prevent revascularization of the graft, with resulting necrosis. Motion between the graft and bed has similar effects. Improper graft contact from stretching or folding also prevents adequate revascularization.

All grafts require a vascular recipient bed for survival. Healthy, fresh, pink granulation tissue makes an excellent bed for skin grafts. Chronic granulation tissue, however, has a poor vascular supply and should be excised to promote formation of fresh granulation tissue. Infection should be controlled, and the granulation surface must be free of any epithelial cover before graft application.

Free grafts can be classified according to source, thickness, and shape. Autogenous grafts are used for permanent free grafts in the cat and dog. Allografts (homografts) and xenografts (heterografts) can serve as temporary biologic dressing but are rarely used in the cat.

Free grafts can be harvested as full- or split-thickness grafts and vary according to the amount of dermis included with the overlying epidermis. Split-thickness grafts "take" more readily than full-thickness grafts but lack durability and proper hair growth and are more susceptible to secondary graft contraction than full-thickness grafts. For these reasons, full-thickness grafts are preferred by many veterinary surgeons (Jensen, 1959; Ross, 1968; Spreull, 1968; Wallace et al., 1962). Free grafts "take" better in the cat than in other species (Howard et al., 1976).

A free graft can be applied as a sheet over the entire recipient bed or divided into various shapes or patterns. Multiple small grafts or mesh grafts are useful for a recipient bed with low-grade infection; these permit drainage until the bed is covered by advancing epithelial cells originating from the graft. They also conform to irregular recipient beds, which are normally difficult to graft over. Unfortunately, the resulting epithelialized areas may lack the durability and cosmetic appearance achieved with full-thickness grafts (Alexander and Hoffer, 1976; Converse, 1977, Grabb and Smith, 1973; Hanselka and Boyd, 1976; Hoffer and Alexander, 1976; Jensen, 1957; Keefe, 1946; Ross, 1968; Self, 1934).

Coverage of the entire defect with a full-thickness graft is usually preferred by the author for cats and is carried out in five steps: (1) The recipient bed is prepared for

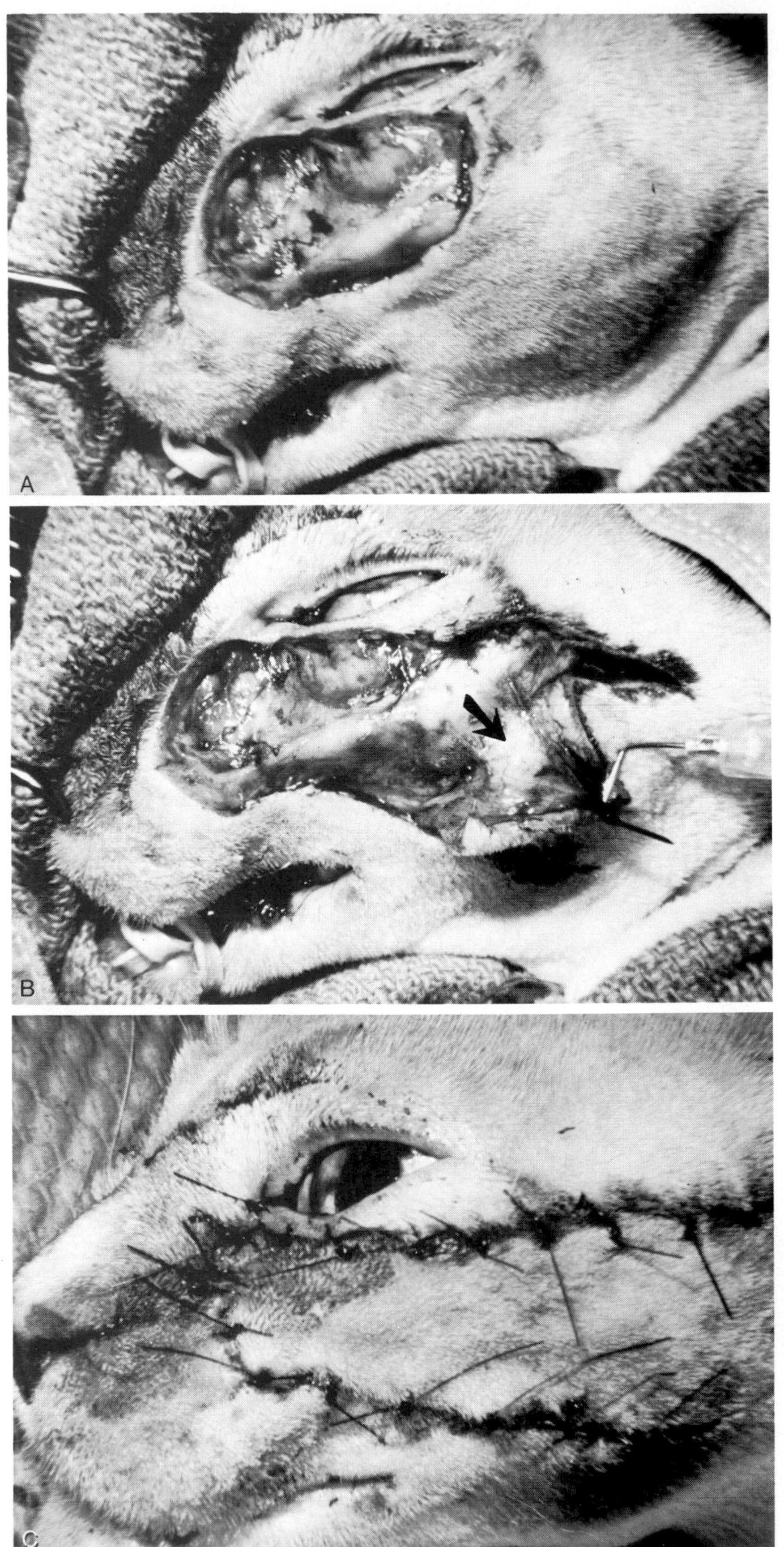


**Figure 4–2.** *A*, A large basal cell carcinoma was excised from the lower eyelid and cheek. *B*, Development of a single-pedicle advancement flap from adjacent loose skin of the cheek and neck (arrow). Notice the skin hook made from a hypodermic needle held in a hemostat, an atraumatic means of graft manipulation. *C*, Closure of the large defect was accomplished with excellent functional and cosmetic results.

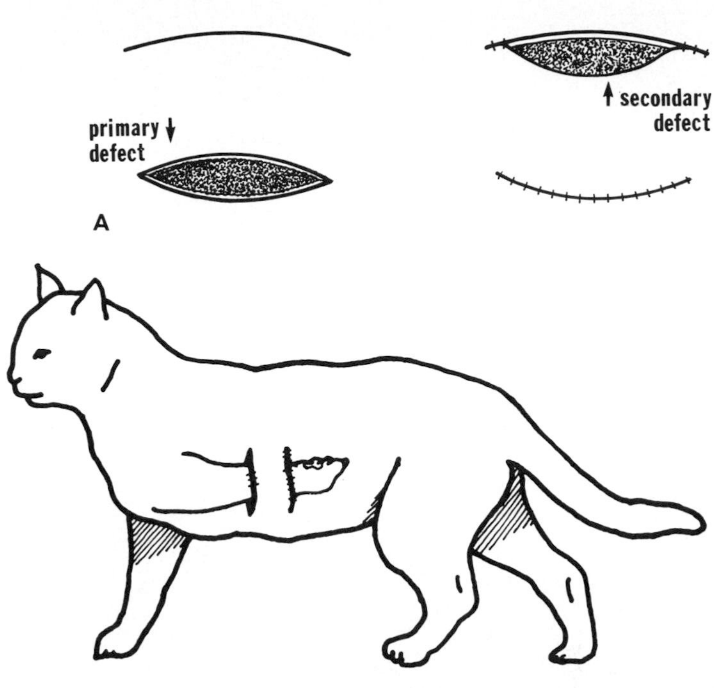


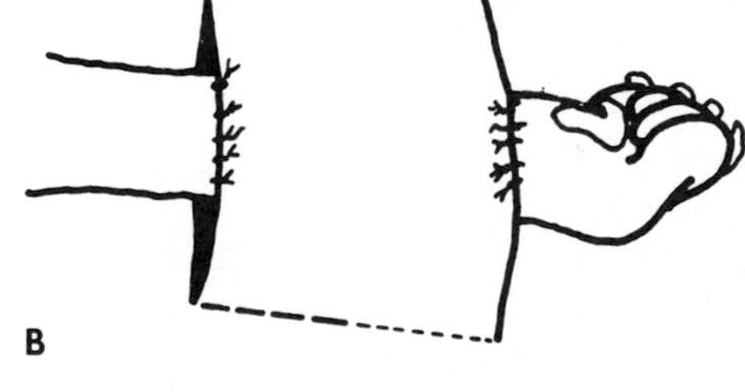


**Figure 4–3.** *A*, Bipedicle advancement flap to close an elliptical (primary) defect. The secondary defect is closed by undermining the adjacent skin margin and suturing it to the opposing flap margin. *B*, Distant bipedicle (tunnel) graft.

grafting. (2) With a paper or gauze template of the defect, the skin to be harvested is outlined. (The author includes an additional 1-cm border on the template to ensure an adequate harvest.) (3) All subcutaneous tissue is removed from the underlying surface of the graft to promote rapid graft revascularization. (4) The graft is applied to the recipient bed, overlapping the wound edges, and is secured to the adjacent skin with a simple interrupted or continuous suture pattern. A few small drainage holes are made to prevent postoperative fluid accumulation under the graft. (5) A nonadherent dressing impregnated with petrolatum or antimicrobial ointment is covered by a soft, bulky, layered bandage of cotton, supported if necessary by a splint, to secure the graft from motion.

Proper postoperative graft protection is essential. The cat should be confined to a cage, and sedatives administered if it is excitable. The bandage is changed four or five days after surgery, with the cat under light anesthesia. Earlier changes risk moving the graft during the critical 48-hour period of revascularization. Bandages are changed in similar fashion every two to four days, depending on the condition of the graft. After about two weeks, a lighter bandage is used for another 10 to 14 days.

## HEAD AND NECK

Maintenance of form and function is especially important in surgery of the head and neck. Anticipated alteration in appearance must be discussed with the cat's owner before surgery, as this is an emotion-laden topic. Failure to anticipate alterations in function may lead to disaster. The airway must be protected and maintained with a cuffed endotracheal tube. Hemorrhage from major vessels can usually be avoided with proper exposure. Complications of both functional and cosmetic significance may arise if the facial, vestibulocochlear, glossopharyngeal, vagosympathetic, or hypoglossal nerve is damaged; again, such problems can be avoided by proper exposure and a knowledge of regional anatomy. Because monitoring of anesthesia depth can be difficult when the head is draped, some form of electronic monitoring is strongly recommended.

## Nose and Sinuses

Chronic discharge, deformity, sneezing, and obstruction are the major signs of nasal or sinus disease. Thorough evaluation with radiographs, cultures, cytologic examination, rhinoscopy, and biopsy usually establishes the etiology and directs treatment. Chronic infections, foreign bodies, oronasal fistulae, and neoplasms may be encountered (Cook, 1964), and surgery may play a diagnostic or therapeutic role in their management.

### Rhinoscopy

The vestibule and rostral nasal fossa may be examined directly with an otoscope and small cone. The nasopharynx and choanae should be examined by pulling the soft palate forward or with a small, angled dental mirror.

### Nasal Flushing

Cytologic examination of discharge or tissue fragments can give valuable information. Samples may be obtained by direct aspiration through a 3½F urinary catheter. Alternatively a 5F feeding tube may be inserted through the nostril to the pharynx, where it is grasped and tied to the tip of an 8F feeding tube, which is pulled over the soft palate to the choanae. Pressure is applied over the soft palate to occlude the nasopharynx, and the larger tube is flushed with saline to irrigate the nasal passage. Fragments of tissue or exudate may be collected in a sponge at the nostril.

### Biopsy

Samples for microscopic examination can be obtained by several methods. If abnormal tissue is seen at rhinoscopy, it may be grasped with an alligator forceps or retrieved with a 2-0 Buck ear curette. Another method may be used when a lesion deep within the nasal fossa is seen radiographically. The distance from the nostril to the lesion is measured on the radiograph and marked on a 2 mm laryngeal cup forceps or an ear curette, and a piece of tissue harvested blindly from that area. Brisk bleeding usually ensues but rapidly abates. A simple incisional biopsy may be performed when the bone over the nose or sinus has been eroded.

### Sinus Trephination

Bacterial sinusitis is usually secondary to occlusion of the nasofrontal opening by a nasal foreign body, tumor, or viral infection (Carpenter, 1974). Sinus trephination has been used to obtain culture or biopsy specimens, remove exudate, irrigate the sinus and nasal passages, and relieve any partial vacuum that may interfere with drainage. A ⅛-inch Steinmann pin is used to perforate the involved sinus just off the midline at the level of the supraorbital process (Leighton, 1958; Startup, 1963). Pus is removed and cultured and irrigation performed. The sinuses and nasal passages may be irrigated for several days if the openings are maintained.

A more extensive skull opening (Fig. 4–4) may be created with a pneumatic drill in order to see and enlarge the nasofrontal opening, which is often occluded with inflamed mucosa or discharge. This opening, a small slit,

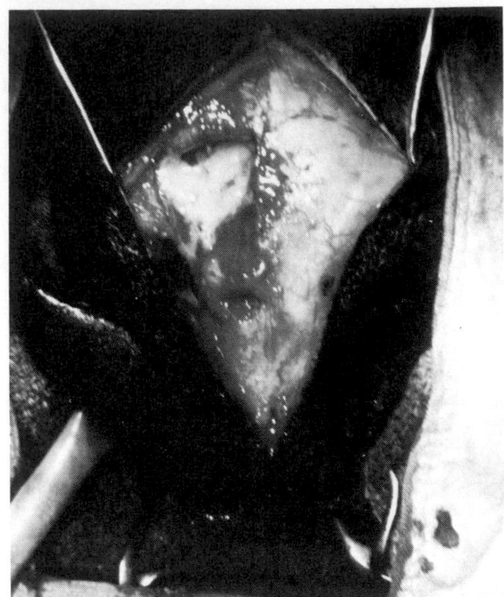

**Figure 4–4.** Empyema of the right frontal sinus exposed by removal of the bone over the sinus and caudal nasal fossa. The pus accumulated because of obstruction of the right nasal passage by an adenocarcinoma.

is located rostrally on a shelf of bone and is not in the lowest part of the sinus (Proud, 1974); it should be enlarged to permit drainage (Carpenter, 1974). Removal of the sinus mucosa and packing of the sinus with autogenous fat (Tomlinson and Schenck, 1975) may be helpful in the rare case of primary sinusitis.

The results of trephination have not been objectively assessed but are poor in many instances of chronic discharge (Bajer, 1973; Winstanley, 1974), and the procedure is gradually being supplanted by nasal exploration and curettage (Baker, 1973; Delmage, 1973; Ford and Walshaw, 1980; Spreull, 1963).

### Nasal Exploration and Curettage

A midline incision is made from the nasal pad to the confluence of the frontal crests, and bleeding is controlled by electrocautery. A Freer elevator is used to lift the periosteum laterally. A bone flap, which may uncover both nasal fossae and frontal sinuses, is created with a pneumatic drill and should be as wide as possible for optimal exposure. The usual caudal limit is just behind the supraorbital processes; laterally the orbital margin should be preserved. The flap is lifted and left attached to its rostral soft tissues, exposing the frontal sinus and turbinates. The ventral conchae (maxilloturbinates) are removed first. Brisk, thorough curettage and packing of the cavity will control the profuse hemorrhage that ensues. Next the ethmoid conchae (ethmoturbinates) are removed with a curette and rongeur, care being taken to avoid the underlying cribriform plate. Suction and irrigation are invaluable for clearing debris and estimating blood loss. If more than 75 ml of blood is lost, it is replaced with whole blood—a measure necessary in about one third of cases. Turbinate remnants and shreds of mucosa should be thoroughly removed (Fig. 4–5*A*), and any bleeding points touched with the electrocautery. In most cases,

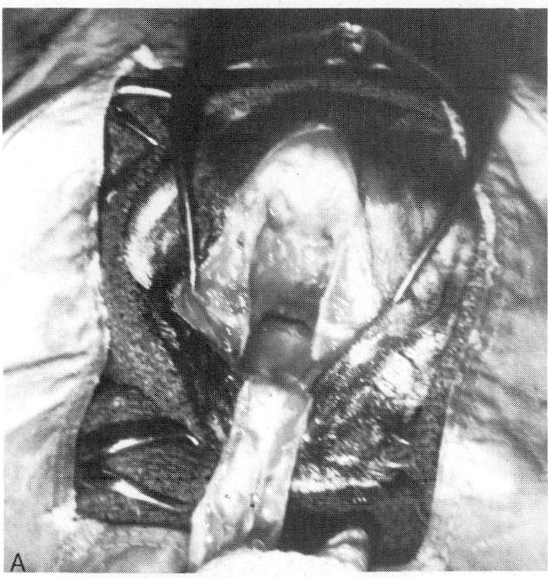


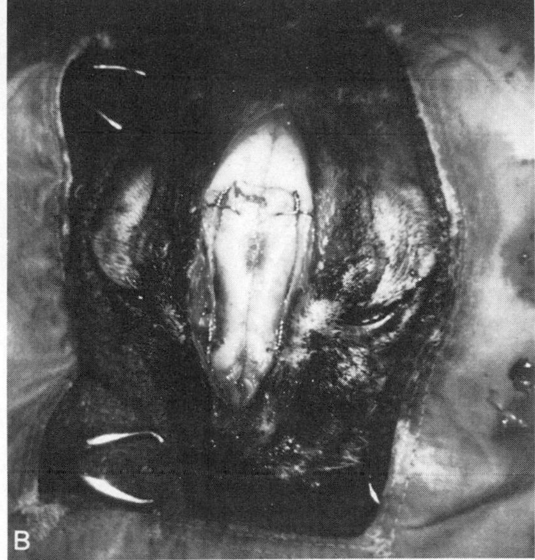


**Figure 4–5.** *A*, Completed bilateral curettage of turbinates in a cat with chronic rhinitis. The bone flap is reflected rostrally, disclosing the frontal sinuses, remnants of the ethmoid conchae, and the hard palate. *B*, The bone flap is wired back in place.

careful hemostasis eliminates the need for nasal packing. The nostrils must be cleared of any obstructing turbinate fragments, and a curved hemostat should pass easily into the nasopharynx. The bone flap may be wired into place (Fig. 4–5*B*) or discarded. The overlying periosteum and subcutis are closed with a continuous suture of 4-0 gut. The skin is closed routinely.

Before the tracheal tube is removed, the pharynx should be cleared of any debris that could be aspirated. After surgery, most cats are able to breathe comfortably. Serosanguineous nasal discharge should decrease in 10 days. Subcutaneous emphysema may develop if there is a gap in the bone flap and the nostrils are partly obstructed; this is a harmless complication that resolves spontaneously.

## Oral Cavity and Pharynx

### Lip Avulsion

Repair of separation of the lower lip from the mandible has been described (Farrow, 1973). After the torn lip and exposed mandible are debrided and cleaned, the subcutaneous tissue at the center of the lip is attached to the fascia under the mandibular symphysis by a single 3-0 gut suture. A braided wire suture is passed through a section of polyethylene tubing (cut from a fluid administration set), up through the mucocutaneous junction of the lip at the level of the canine tooth, behind both canines, down through the other lip, and tied. The tubing is slipped over the knot and acts as a stent. This suture is removed when healing is complete, usually in about 10 days. Another method is to secure the lip against the mandible by a mattress suture tied around each lower canine tooth.

Other lip lesions, such as tumors or eosinophilic granulomas that fail to respond to medical treatment, are occasionally encountered. Some may be treated with electrocautery or cryosurgery. Excision of such lesions may require reconstructive surgery to minimize distortion; surgical techniques designed for the eyelid (Bistner et al., 1977) are easily adapted to such uses.

### Tumors

Oral tumors in cats are most often squamous cell carcinomas, which are invasive and may spread to regional lymph nodes and the lungs. Surgical management may range from simple incisional biopsy to wide local excision, including curettage, fulguration, or cryosurgery of the tumor bed, and must be approached with palliation as the major goal. Extensive en bloc resection of the tumor with underlying invaded bone is a more radical possibility that has come into use. (See chapter on neoplasms.)

### Cleft Palate

The majority of palatal clefts in cats result from trauma. Those less than 2 mm wide usually heal spontaneously. Larger clefts may be narrowed by wiring the canine teeth (occasionally the carnassial teeth) together across the hard palate (see Fig. 5–45), care being taken to maintain dental occlusion. If a symptomatic cleft persists, closure by suturing is sometimes successful. The epithelial edges of the cleft must be trimmed. Narrow clefts may be closed in two layers, with a relaxing incision along one alveolar margin and with undermining of the tissue overlying the palate to effect a tension-free closure. The deep (mucoperiosteal) layer is closed with absorbable sutures. The palatal epithelium is best closed with everting mattress sutures of nonabsorbable material swaged onto a cutting needle (Sinibaldi, 1979). Larger clefts are best managed with a mucoperiosteal flap technique (Howard et al., 1974). Aftercare consists of a soft diet for two weeks; pharyngostomy tube feeding may be necessary to protect more difficult repairs.

## Pharyngostomy

Cats that cannot, will not, or should not eat may be fed by a pharyngostomy tube (Bohning et al., 1970). A 12F rubber feeding tube is used, with the distance from the angle of the jaw to the thirteenth rib marked on the tube with a tag of adhesive tap. The skin caudal to the angle of the jaw is clipped and scrubbed, and a gloved finger is inserted into the piriform recess (fossa) of the pharynx, the area lateral to the base of the tongue. The epihyoid bone is palpated, and the finger is replaced with a curved forceps that is pushed through the pharyngeal wall just rostral to the epihyoid. A small stab wound is made through the skin to allow the forceps to protrude and grasp the tip of the feeding tube, which is pulled into the pharynx and pushed down the esophagus. The tape marker is sutured to the skin, a light dressing applied, and the tube clamped.

## Pharyngeal Examination

Pharyngeal disorders manifested by coughing, gagging, dysphagia, and nasal discharge are often unrecognized. Thorough evaluation of the pharynx requires deep general anesthesia, because the gag reflex interferes with the examination. The oropharynx is examined first with a laryngoscope. The piriform recesses, including the areas just lateral to the glossoepiglottic folds, and the tonsillar crypts are common sites of lodgment of foreign bodies and must not be overlooked. The nasopharynx is examined by pulling the soft palate rostrally with a Snook hook or Allis forceps (Fig. 4–6).

## Pharyngeal Polypectomy

Pharyngeal polyps are benign inflammatory growths that usually arise within the middle ear or auditive (Eustachian) tube (e.g., Lane et al., 1981). The mass is grasped and pulled away from its attachment by gently increasing traction with a curved hemostat or Allis forceps; if this fails, the soft palate may be slit and the stalk of the polyp twisted free. Recurrence is common because the pedicle is not always totally removed (Sumner-Smith and Eger, 1975). Associated ear polyps that have pushed through the tympanum into the external ear canal must be searched for and removed by twisting and traction. Sometimes bulla osteotomy and a lateral resection of the external ear canal must be performed to gain access to the polyp.

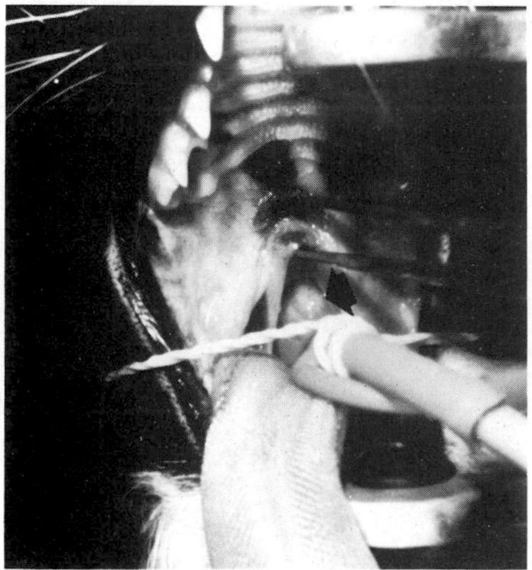

**Figure 4–6.** Pharyngeal extension of an ear polyp (arrow) exposed by retraction of the soft palate with an Allis forceps.

## Salivary Glands

Ranulae, mucoceles, and salivary fistulae are far less common in cats than in dogs but are treated similarly. Ranulae are marsupialized (Leighton, 1975). Mucoceles, which result from damaged ducts, are treated by removal of the mandibular and caudal sublingual salivary glands and drainage of the mucocele sac. An attempt at removal of the sac is contraindicated, for it would require major dissection among vital structures. Parotid duct injury may cause a salivary fistula, characterized by persistent serous discharge through a sinus on the side of the face. This is best controlled by ligation of the parotid duct proximal to the fistula (Harvey, 1977).

# The Ear

Injury, infections, and tumors may affect the pinna, ear canal, or middle ear and are common causes of discomfort or disfigurement.

## Trauma

Lacerations of the pinna are repaired after it has been prepared for aseptic surgery and any dead tissue débrided. The cartilage is apposed with 4-0 gut sutures starting at the margin of the pinna. The skin of the convexity is sutured with fine monofilament nylon; that on the inner surface need not be sutured.

## Hematoma

An ear hematoma, a collection of blood between the cartilage and inner surface of the pinna, occasionally results from a fight injury but more often from self-trauma secondary to parasitic irritation of the external ear canal. A variety of surgical treatments are used, but it is virtually impossible to restore the ear to its pristine appearance or to prevent some fibrosis and shriveling. Any successful method must treat the underlying cause and provide drainage of any accumulated fluid while coapting the skin and cartilage to allow healing. The classic method is to incise the length of the hematoma and obliterate dead space with mattress sutures (Leighton, 1975). Some veterinarians claim good results with suturing or stapling through conformers of x-ray film or balsa wood. A better cosmetic appearance may be achieved by passing a small Penrose drain through stab wounds at the top and bottom of the hematoma and coapting the surfaces of the hematoma with a dressing that conforms to the shape of the ear, e.g., by taping a partly used roll of gauze bandage upright within the pinna. The drain should be removed in 10 days and the dressing replaced for another 10 days. An Elizabethan collar is usually necessary to prevent the cat from disrupting the dressing.

## Tumors

Squamous cell carcinoma of the pinna occurs most often in white-eared cats in sunny climates and represents the end stage of actinic dermatitis (e.g., Muller, 1967). It is an invasive tumor and often recurs unless widely excised; if it is extensive, amputation of the entire pinna is recommended (Scott, 1980). An incision is made around the base of the pinna to a point opposite the horizontal ear canal. The muscles of the ear and the scutiform cartilage are severed at their insertions on the vertical canal, until the pinna is attached only by the ear canal. The ear canal is severed at the junction of its vertical and horizontal parts, and the ventral edge of the horizontal canal is sutured to the skin. Dorsally the auricular muscles and subcutis are closed with fine surgical gut, and the suturing of the skin to the horizontal canal is completed (Fig. 4–7).

## Lateral Ear Canal Resection

This procedure is indicated to provide access to tumors or polyps deep within the ear canal or drainage and aeration for recurrent or refractory otitis externa. The shape of the vertical canal differs from that of the dog; the cat's external meatus flares, and the vertical canal tapers ventrally instead of forming a cylinder, but the operation is essentially the same in both species. A rectangle of skin is removed over the lateral surface of the vertical canal, starting at the pretragic (tragohelicine) and intertragic incisures and extending rostroventrally to a point 5 mm ventral to the floor of the horizontal canal. Subcutaneous tissue is incised and bluntly separated from the vertical canal; ventrally the parotid gland is simply pushed away. The lateral auricular vein, which courses across the tragus, must be ligated (Habel, 1978). Exposure of the vertical canal permits the use of accurate rostral and caudal cartilage incisions to develop the lateral flap. The incisions should continue into the horizontal canal for 3 mm to ensure adequate drainage. The lateral flap is reflected ventrally, excess length trimmed to leave a 5 mm "drainboard," and the edges of the skin defect are sutured to the ear cartilage and integument, care being taken that no cartilage is left exposed. After surgery the site should be left open, but an Elizabethan collar may be used to prevent self-trauma. Sutures are removed in two weeks.

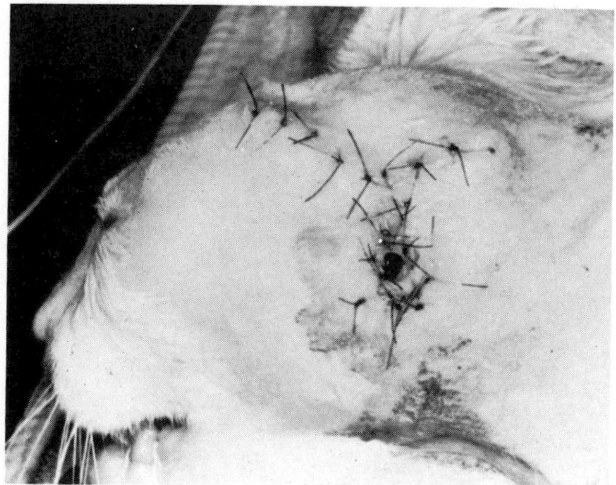

**Figure 4–7.** Amputation of the pinna for advanced squamous cell carcinoma. The horizontal ear canal was anastomosed to the skin.

## Ear Canal Ablation

This procedure is preferred when the horizontal ear canal is stenotic or deeply invaded by tumor. Perforation of the tympanum and otitis media are common when the horizontal ear canal is occluded, and the tympanic bulla should be evaluated radiographically before ablation. Density within the bulla may represent infection or extension of tumor and indicates the need for middle ear drainage at the time of ablation.

An incision is made through the inner skin and cartilage around the opening of the vertical ear canal and extended over its lateral wall. The cartilage of the vertical canal is grasped and freed from surrounding tissues with Metzenbaum scissors. As the horizontal canal is exposed, the dissection plane is confined to the perichondrium to avoid the parotid salivary gland and the trunk of the facial nerve, which courses just ventral to the canal. Blunt dissection with a Freer periosteal elevator helps to expose the deep part of the horizontal canal (Fig. 4–8*A*) and separates the cartilage of the horizontal canal from the bony external acoustic meatus by breaking the annular ligament. If middle ear disease is present (Fig. 4–8*B*), a lateral bulla osteotomy is performed at this point by deflecting the soft tissues ventrally and using a fine rongeur to remove the lateral wall of the bulla, starting at the external acoustic meatus. An ear curette or Frazier suction tip is used to remove the contents of the bulla. After thorough irrigation of the cavity with physiologic saline solution, a Penrose drain is placed to emerge ventral to the primary incision, which is closed routinely. The drain is removed in about five days, and specific antibiotic treatment, based on culture and sensitivity testing of the middle ear contents, is continued for at least three weeks.

## Bulla Osteotomy

Ventral bulla osteotomy is performed when clinical and radiographic evidence indicates the need for drainage or exploration of the tympanic bulla. The surgical approach is similar to that for the dog but is technically easier in the cat (Ader and Boothe, 1979). With the cat on its back and the hair clipped on the affected side, the ventral wall of the bulla can usually be palpated caudomedial to the angular process of the mandible. The skin incision over the bulla parallels the midventral line, and the underlying muscles are separated by blunt dissection to expose the bulla, the hypoglossal nerve and hyoglossal muscle being retracted medially. The bulla is penetrated with a Steinmann pin and the opening enlarged with a small rongeur. The transverse septum should be opened to facilitate aspiration, curettage, or exploration of the entire middle ear. A drainage tube from the bulla is sutured to the skin. The muscles and skin incision are closed separately.

# THYROIDECTOMY

Thyroidectomy is performed with increasing frequency as more clinicians recognize hyperthyroidism in older cats

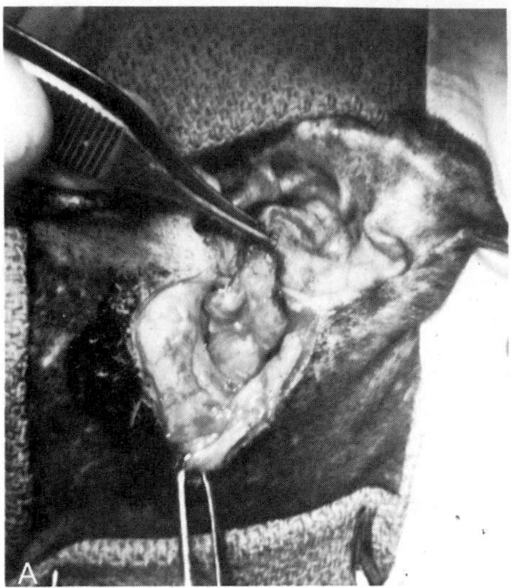

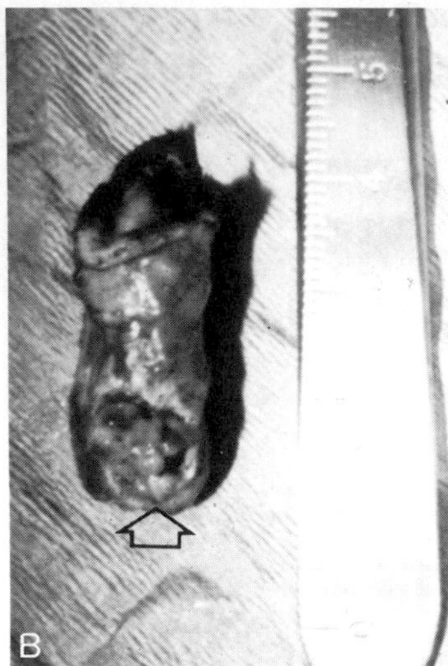

**Figure 4–8.** *A*, Ablation of the ear canal for recurrent ceruminous gland adenocarcinoma in a cat that previously had undergone a lateral resection. The overlying skin and subcutaneous tissue are reflected ventrally by an Allis forceps. The horizontal canal, held by the thumb forceps, has been dissected from the surrounding tissue. *B*, The ablated ear canal with the tumor (arrow), which pushed through the tympanum into the tympanic bulla. The bulla was thoroughly curetted, and when the cat died two years later of an unrelated cause, there had been no recurrence of the tumor.

(Holzworth et al., 1980). The same surgical approach is used for removal of other neck masses and for access to the cervical parts of the trachea and esophagus.

The cat is placed on its back with forelegs drawn caudally, the neck extended over a rolled towel, and the chin immobilized with a piece of adhesive tape. A midline incision is made from the larynx to the manubrium. The sternocephalicus and sternohyoideus muscles are separated along the midline. Lateral retraction of the sternothyroideus muscles exposes the lobes of the thyroid gland. Enlarged thyroid lobes often descend toward or even into the thoracic inlet or may slip dorsal to the trachea; they are easily retrieved and lifted from either location. The enlarged lobe is separated from the surrounding loose areolar tissue after isolation and severing of the caudal thyroid vessels. The recurrent laryngeal nerves, which are less than 1 mm in diameter and course dorsomedial to the thyroid lobes, should be identified and avoided during this dissection. If both thyroid lobes are abnormal and must be removed (Fig. 4–9*A*), at least one cranial parathyroid gland and its blood supply must be spared (Fig. 4–9*B*). For this purpose the surgeon may use small eye instruments to incise the delicate thyroid capsule and dissect or tease out the thyroid lobe (Birchard et al., 1984). Closure is done by apposing the sternohydoideus muscles, then the sternocephalicus muscles, and the subcutis with 4-0 surgical gut sutures; the skin is then sutured. After surgery, cats from which only one lobe was removed usually recover uneventfully. After bilateral lobectomy, cats must be watched closely for hypocalcemic tetany, even when a parathyroid gland has been spared. Acute hypoparathyroidism usually develops 12 to 24 hours after surgery and responds well to the intravenous administration of calcium followed by oral calcium and vitamin D therapy, which may have to be continued for long periods in some cats. Trauma to the recurrent laryngeal nerves may cause temporary or permanent voice changes, impaired purring, or coughing.

## UPPER AIRWAY

### Devocalization (Removal of Vocal Fold, "Ventriculocordectomy")

Occasionally devocalization is requested, usually for a raucous, apartment-dwelling Siamese. This may be done by an oral approach or through a laryngotomy incision. In the oral approach, the cat is anesthetized with a thiobarbiturate and the vocal folds ("cords") medial to the vestibular folds are identified with a laryngoscope. A 2-mm offset laryngeal cup forceps is used to remove all

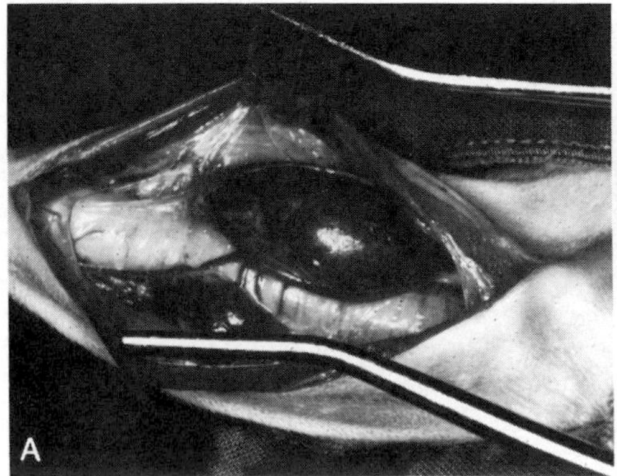

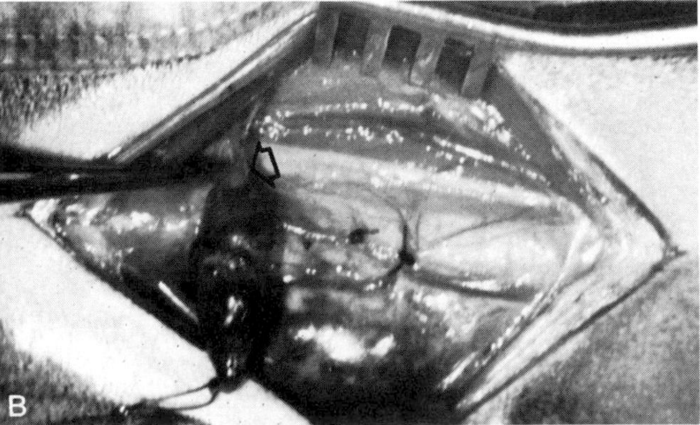

**Figure 4–9.** Adenomatous hyperplasia of both thyroid lobes in a hyperthyroid cat. *B*, A cranial parathyroid gland (arrow) has been isolated and spared.

of one vocal fold and the dorsal half of the other, biting deeply into the vocalis muscle. An endotracheal tube is then placed, its cuff inflated, and the cat allowed to recover normally. In the ventral approach (Chabot and Weaver, 1966), a midline incision is made over the larynx. The laminae of the thyroid cartilage are separated, the endotracheal tube retracted, and one vocal fold excised from its arytenoid attachment. The endotracheal tube is replaced, the halves of the thyroid cartilage are reunited with 3-0 surgical gut sutures, and the skin is closed routinely. Complete removal of both vocal folds by either approach should be avoided, lest laryngeal webbing or stenosis ensue.

### Tracheostomy

Tracheostomy may be done as an emergency procedure for laryngeal obstruction or as an elective procedure in surgery of the larynx, pharynx, or oral cavity, or when the mouth cannot be opened for tracheal intubation. Whenever possible, general anesthesia should be induced and an endotracheal tube placed before tracheostomy. The skin is incised for 2 cm caudal to the larynx, and the neck muscles are separated along the midline to expose the trachea. The endotracheal tube is retracted and an incision is made between two tracheal rings. A stay suture may be placed through the skin and around the proximal ring for stabilization of the trachea in case the tracheostomy tube has to be changed during convalescence; it is not tied. A 2-0 or 3-0 tracheostomy tube is then inserted and held in place with umbilical tape (Harvey and O'Brien, 1972). Cats with tracheostomy tubes in place must be continuously monitored, because the tiny tubes are likely to become obstructed with respiratory secretions and need frequent cleaning, especially if left in place for more than one or two days. The tube is removed when the upper airway is patent, and the skin incision is left to close by contraction. For elective tracheostomy, a sterile 3.5 mm endotracheal tube may be substituted for the tracheostomy tube and removed at the end of surgery. Again the tracheostomy site is left to heal by second intention to avoid subcutaneous emphysema.

### Tracheal Foreign Bodies

Occasionally a foreign body, such as a tooth, bead, or small bone, may be aspirated and lodged deep within the trachea or at the carina, causing intermittent obstruction and paroxysmal coughing. These are best retrieved through a ventilating bronchoscope with a long-handled forceps; the only alternative is thoracotomy (Eyster et al., 1976). A repeat chest radiograph must be obtained immediately before surgery in case the cat has already coughed up the foreign body.

## THORACIC AND CARDIOVASCULAR SURGERY

Thoracic surgery is subject to the same conditions in the cat as in any other species. Positive-pressure anesthesia and controlled ventilation by a mechanical respirator or manual compression of a rebreathing bag must be used whenever the pleural space is opened. Pressure should not exceed 15 cm of water, and a rate of 8 to 12 breaths per minute is appropriate. Anesthesia depth must be monitored closely when ventilation is controlled, for the tendency is to overanesthetize the cat. A chest tube should usually be placed after thoracic surgery and removed only when the operator is sure that there will be no accumulation of air or fluid to restrict ventilation. Careful postoperative observation is mandatory.

### THORACOCENTESIS

The frequent occurrence of pleural effusions in cats makes thoracocentesis a common diagnostic and therapeutic procedure. Except in cases of life-threatening dyspnea, preliminary lateral and dorsoventral radiographs should be obtained. If possible, the lateral view should be taken with a horizontal beam with the cat in a standing or sternal position. In addition to indicating the level of the fluid line, radiography in this position is less stressful to the cat. A cat with a chest full of fluid may struggle and die if forcibly restrained on its side.

Restraint for thoracocentesis must be gentle, as cats with limited lung expansion do not tolerate stress. An unanesthetized cat should never be forcibly restrained on its side but should be allowed to assume the sitting or sternal position that it prefers. Fluid will obviously gravitate to the ventral part of the chest cavity while air rises to the upper portion of the cavity. An area over the appropriate intercostal space, usually the seventh, should be clipped and prepared aseptically. A 19-gauge butterfly catheter, attached to a three-way stopcock and large syringe, is inserted into the pleural space and as much fluid or air as possible is removed. (Editor's note. Some veterinarians prefer a ¾-inch, 15-gauge needle as being less apt to puncture heart or lung, and the large gauge permits aspiration of thick exudates. Occasionally, inspissated material requires use of a trocar for incision and aspiration with a chest tube.)

Samples of fluid are reserved for laboratory examination.

### CHEST TUBE INSERTION

An indwelling chest tube is used when continued accumulation of air or fluid restricts ventilation and also for lavage. General anesthesia is preferred for the placement of such tubes (Sherding, 1979; Withrow et al., 1975), but local anesthesia may be used if necessary. Whenever possible, thoracocentesis, with the removal of as much air or fluid as possible, should be followed by an interval for the cat to recover and relax before the chest tube is placed. The thorax is clipped widely and prepared aseptically. A 10- or 12F rubber feeding tube is prepared by cutting extra side holes near its tip; this is done by kinking the tube and trimming off a corner. A catheter adapter and three-way stopcock are inserted into the large end, and a serrefine clamp or hemostat is used to occlude the tube (Fig. 4–10*A*). A subcutaneous tunnel with a purse-string suture surrounding a stab wound at either end is created between the seventh and eleventh intercostal spaces, and the catheter is brought through it (Fig. 4–10*B*).

The pleural space is entered by inserting a closed hemostat through the stab wound and spreading its jaws;

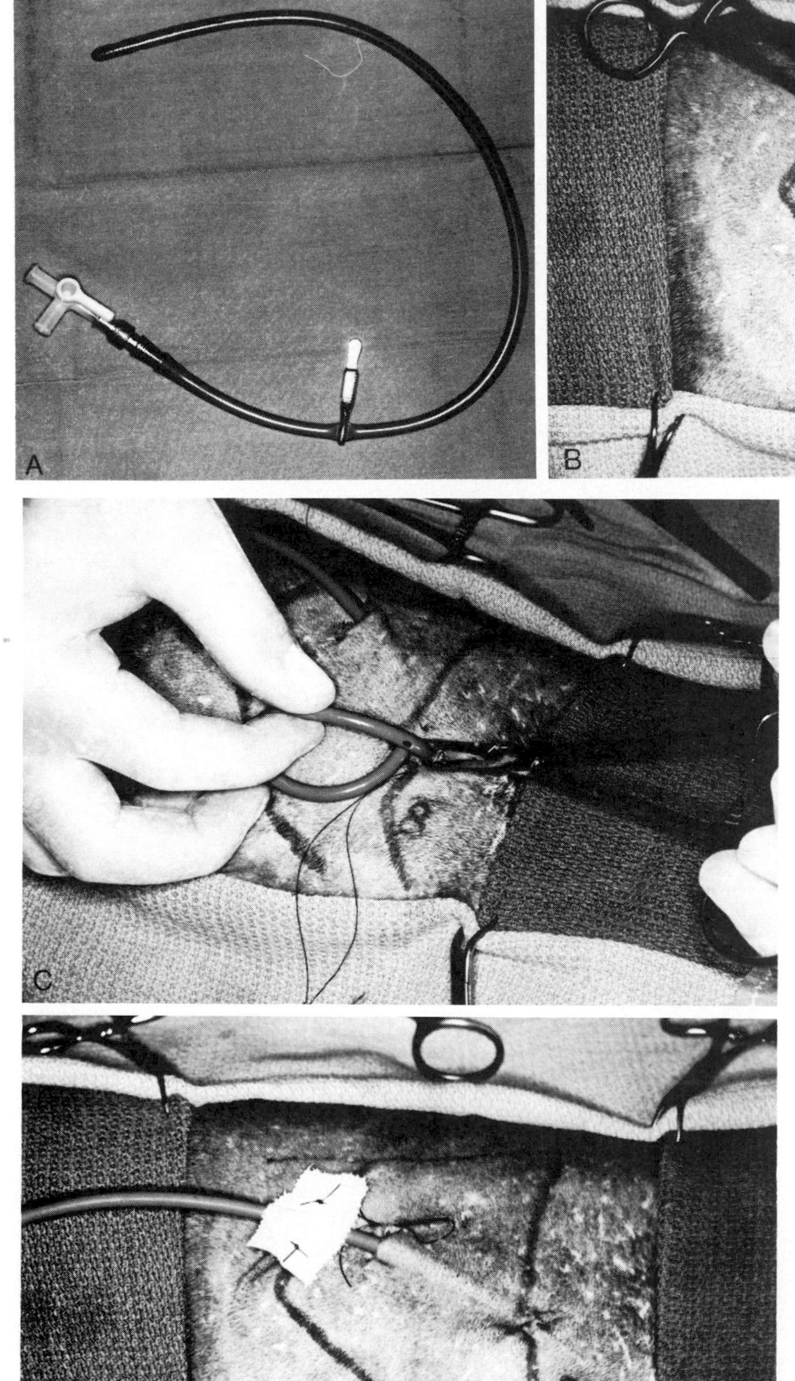


**Figure 4–10.** *A*, A 10F perforated feeding tube, catheter adapter, three-way stopcock, and serrefine clamp assembled for use as an indwelling chest tube. *B*, Incisions are made and pursestring sutures placed at both ends of the subcutaneous tunnel (ribs are marked and numbered). *C*, The chest tube is drawn through the subcutaneous tunnel and introduced into the pleural space between the jaws of a hemostat. *D*, The pursestring suture over the seventh intercostal space is tied. The chest tube is anchored to the skin with a tape butterfly before a dressing is applied.

the tip of the chest tube is rapidly inserted and advanced as the hemostat is withdrawn (Fig. 4–10*C*). The purse-string suture over the seventh space is tied, but the suture around the eleventh space is left untied. The chest tube is anchored with sutures through an adhesive tape tag (Fig. 4–10*D*), and a light dressing is applied (Harvey and O'Brien, 1972). A trocar catheter may be used in a similar manner, without the need for a stab wound over the site of entry into the pleural space (Sherding, 1979). The clamp is removed for aspiration of the chest tube and then replaced.

A cat with a chest tube in place must never be left unattended lest it dislodge or chew through the tube, perhaps causing fatal pneumothorax. The preplaced suture around the chest tube is tied when the chest tube is removed, to avoid pneumothorax from the ingress of air through the subcutaneous tunnel.

## THORACOTOMY

The indications and techniques for thoracotomy in the cat parallel those for the dog. A Weitlaner retractor is preferable to the heavier Finochietto retractor for spreading the ribs or sternum.

### Pyothorax

In cases of pyothorax that do not respond to conservative treatment with indwelling chest tubes and lavage (Withrow et al., 1975), thoracotomy is used to assess the extent of disease, débride necrotic mediastinal and pleural debris, release adhesions, and perform lung lobectomy if a lung abscess is found. Stripping the visceral pleura of fibrinous material that restricts lung expansion usually results in massive tearing of the lung and intractable tension pneumothorax and cannot be recommended. After thoracotomy, new chest tubes should be placed and postoperative care directed at maintaining nutrition and fluid and electrolyte balance as well as pleural lavage (Crane, 1976).

### Chylothorax

Chylous effusions arise from a variety of causes, including direct trauma to large intrathoracic lymphatic vessels, their erosion or obstruction by tumors, and thrombosis of the cranial vena cava. Chylothorax must be differentiated from the pseudochylous effusions of chronic inflammation, cardiomyopathy, or lymphoma by examination of both the cytologic and the physical properties of the fluid (Creighton and Wilkins, 1975). Cats with true chylous effusions that fail to resolve with conservative treatment consisting of chest tube drainage, fasting for four to seven days, and dietary management for another one to three weeks are candidates for thoracotomy. The goal of thoracotomy is to discover, if possible, the source of the effusion and, if indicated, to ligate the thoracic duct (Creighton and Wilkins, 1980; Graber, 1965; Patterson and Munson, 1968). The cat's duct, usually single and located to the left and dorsal to the aorta in the caudal mediastinum, is best approached through a left tenth intercostal thoracotomy (Lindsay, 1974). The lymph within the duct may be made visible by feeding a light meal of cream or butter three hours before surgery, injection of 1 ml of 1 per cent Evans blue dye into the dorsum of a hindpaw (Lindsay, 1974), or injection of 2.5 ml of patent blue dye with 0.1 ml of hyaluronidase subserosally into the esophagus during surgery (Leighton, 1975). The duct is doubly ligated with 4-0 silk; adequate ligation is usually evidenced by dilation of the duct distal to the ligatures. Recurrence of chylous effusions after surgery is common, and the prognosis must be guarded or poor (Creighton and Wilkins, 1980: Leighton, 1975).

### Patent Ductus Arteriosus

The signs of patent ductus arteriosus in the cat are similar to those in the dog. Successful surgical correction has been described, with the approach usually through the left fifth or sixth intercostal space (Cohen et al., 1975; Jeraj et al., 1978; Jones and Buchanan, 1981). In a group of five cases the outcome was successful in only one of three cats undergoing surgery (Cohen et al., 1975); thus the prognosis must be guarded.

### Persistent Right Aortic Arch

Vascular ring anomalies have been diagnosed and treated surgically in cats and must be differentiated from esophageal achalasia (Clifford et al., 1971) by radiographic studies before surgery. A left fourth or fifth intercostal thoracotomy gives access to the ligamentum arteriosum, which is ligated and severed (Burke et al., 1978; Knecht, 1967). Mediastinal adhesions are carefully broken down and a 16F feeding tube passed through the site of the stricture to demonstrate patency. Some esophageal dilatation may persist after surgery (Reed and Bonasch, 1962), but clinical improvement is gratifying if the condition is diagnosed early and treated promptly.

## PERIPHERAL ARTERIOVENOUS FISTULA

Peripheral arteriovenous fistulae have been described in the forelegs of cats, two involving communication between the cranial superficial antebrachial artery (formerly termed the proximal collateral radial artery) and the cephalic vein (Slocum et al., 1973) and one between the same artery (also once termed the accessory radial artery) and ulnar vein (Furneaux et al., 1974). Each was secondary to trauma and caused swelling of the paw and a palpable thrill in the distended cephalic vein. Angiography was necessary to define the exact area of the fistula; removal of the communicating vascular shunts was curative in all three cases.

## AORTIC EMBOLECTOMY

The surgical removal of emboli occluding the distal aorta remains a controversial procedure. These emboli originate in the left atrium in cats with cardiomyopathy or bacterial endocarditis. Occlusion of the aortic trifurcation results in loss of femoral pulses, firmness and pain in the gastrocnemius muscles, paralysis of the hindlegs, and coolness and pallor of the hindfeet. Such cats have an unstable cardiovascular system owing to their primary cardiac disease and are extremely poor anesthesia risks. Surgery is reserved for those lacking spinal reflexes or with emboli extending proximal to the renal arteries that do not respond to a brief trial of medical therapy.

Cardiac arrhythmias and pulmonary edema must be controlled before anesthesia (Harpster, 1977). (See also the chapter on the cardiovascular system.) The surgical technique is straightforward (Leighton, 1975; McCurnin and Seeli, 1972). A midline incision is made from the umbilicus to the pubis; viscera are displaced with the mesocolon and laparotomy pads. The peritoneum over the distal aorta and its trifurcation is incised, care being taken to avoid the left ureter. Rumel tourniquets of ¼-inch umbilical tape threaded through sterile intravenous tubing or delicate serrefine clamps are used to occlude the aorta proximal to the embolus and the external and common iliac arteries distal to it. The distal aorta is incised longitudinally and the embolus removed with a smooth forceps or suction. The tourniquets are briefly released from each iliac artery and finally from the aorta to demonstrate patency and flush out any clot fragments or air. The aortic incision is closed with 6-0 vascular silk in a simple interrupted pattern with minimal handling of the incision edges. The iliac tourniquets are slowly released and the incision line inspected for leakage; additional sutures are placed if necessary. Finally, the aortic tourniquet is released. Fluids with bicarbonate added must be given intravenously throughout surgery to minimize the vasomotor effects of accumulated lactic acid and vasoactive amines that are flushed into the general circulation as blood flow is restored to the ischemic extremities (declamping acidosis). A rapid, layered closure of the abdomen is then done with continuous suture patterns. Postoperative care is directed at controlling the cardiomyopathy and preventing further thrombus formation.

## Diaphragmatic Hernia

The majority of diaphragmatic hernias result from trauma and may cause variable degrees of respiratory distress. Such hernias may be immediately obvious or may not become evident for months, as cats limit their activity to compensate for the loss of tidal volume. Long-standing hernias may not be recognized clinically until an incarcerated organ becomes strangulated or obstructed. Plain radiographs of the chest usually confirm the diagnosis by disclosing the presence of abdominal organs. Occasionally drainage of any pleural fluid followed by a barium study or a positive contrast peritoneogram is needed.

Time may usually be taken to treat associated injuries and shock before surgical repair of the hernia is undertaken, but continuous observation is important. Aspiration of pleural fluid often aids in stabilizing a cat's condition by decreasing the ventilation-perfusion imbalance and increasing cardiac output. Incarceration of the stomach through a left-sided tear may cause rapidly progressive respiratory failure as it fills with swallowed air, and this constitutes the major indication for immediate surgery. The stomach should be emptied of air by stomach tube or by percutaneous aspiration before induction of anesthesia.

Anesthesia management is similar to that for any thoracic procedure. Controlled ventilation is necessary from the onset of anesthesia, which obtunds the cat's conscious mechanisms for respiratory compensation. Overinflation of the lungs must be avoided; in acute herniation, inspiratory pressure should not exceed 20 cm of water (Leighton and Steffey, 1972). In long-standing hernias, pressures in excess of 15 cm of water may tear adhesions between lung lobes and cause severe pneumothorax after surgery.

The surgical field extends from the manubrium to the pubis. An abdominal approach, with the initial incision from the xiphoid through the umbilicus, is satisfactory for most repairs and may be extended with a midline sternotomy if further thoracic exposure is needed. Herniated portions of the gastrointestinal tract are easily reduced with gentle traction and are isolated from the diaphragm with moistened laparotomy pads. Reduction of herniated liver lobes is more difficult and is best done by enlarging the hernial opening in an easily sutured area, inserting a finger, and gently pushing the liver back into the abdomen. Once the viscera are reduced, the edges of the tear are grasped with a Babcock forceps or stay sutures and lifted to facilitate closure. The rent is closed with simple interrupted sutures of 2-0 gut or polypropylene, starting at its dorsal extremity. The posterior vena cava, aorta, esophagus, and liver must be avoided. Tears along the costal margin are repaired by sutures passed around the rib. Before the diaphragm is completely closed, a chest tube should be inserted for removal of air and fluid. Once the abdominal wall is closed, air and fluid are aspirated to re-establish negative intrathoracic pressure and spontaneous respiration.

Long-standing traumatic hernias and congenital diaphragmatic and peritoneopericardial hernias (Fig. 4–11) are managed similarly. If there is too little diaphragm to close the defect, a flap of internal oblique muscle may be developed along the lateral edge and rotated to supplement the costal margin of the diaphragm (Furneaux and Hudson, 1976), or the affected hemidiaphragm may be anchored several ribs cranial to its usual attachment. Depending on the nature of a peritoneopericardial hernia, the surgeon may or may not close the pericardium.

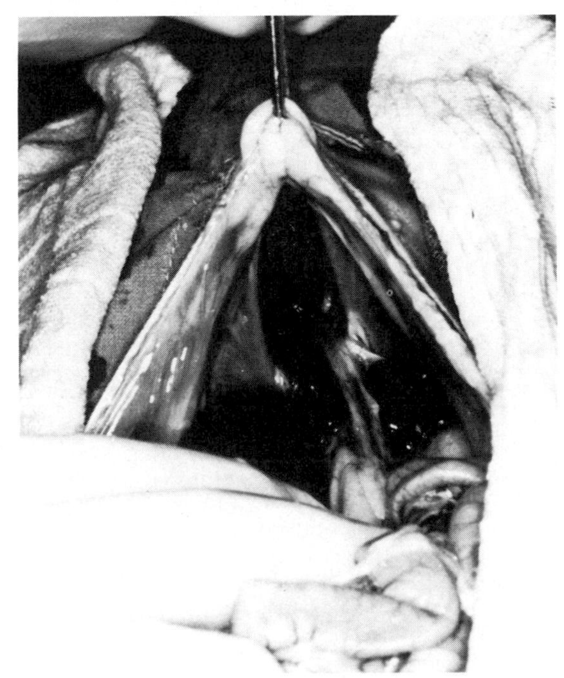

**Figure 4–11.** Peritoneopericardial diaphragmatic hernia. One liver lobe is still incarcerated.

After surgery, the chest tube is aspirated frequently and removed when less than 10 ml of air or fluid is recovered over a two-hour period. The mortality rate in treated cases in one survey was 17.2 percent (Wilson et al., 1971). About one-third of the deaths were related to anesthesia, the rest occurring within a day after surgery for reasons including recurrence of herniation and shock.

# THE ABDOMEN

## EXPLORATORY LAPAROTOMY

Abdominal exploration is a valuable diagnostic and therapeutic technique. The decision to explore the abdomen may be based on clinical, radiographic, or laboratory abnormalities; the likelihood of positive findings is enhanced when all three types of abnormalities are present (Piedrahita and Butterfield, 1976). A well-conducted exploratory laparotomy embraces techniques useful in all abdominal surgery.

A ventral midline approach is preferred and is easily extended to give the necessary exposure. A flank approach is useful for exposing the kidney or adrenal, and combined ventral midline and paracostal incisions are occasionally needed to remove liver masses or approach the esophagogastric junction (Lipowitz and Schenck, 1979). Once the abdomen has been opened, the incision edges are protected with moist laparotomy pads. A self-retaining retractor may be used to spread the incision and enhance exposure. Systematic exploration of all the abdominal contents is important. All surfaces of the liver are palpated and inspected. The duodenum is then lifted and its mesentery used to retract the viscera to the left, exposing the right upper urogenital tract, adrenal, pancreas, and bile duct.

Next the descending colon is lifted and its mesentery used to retract the viscera to the right to expose the left upper urogenital tract and adrenal. The greater omentum and spleen are then exteriorized and inspected. The stomach is examined both visually and by palpation and then the rest of the alimentary canal, its mesentery, and lymph nodes. As this is done, the tract is lifted from the abdomen and protected with moist laparotomy pads. After evaluation of the distal urogenital tract and descending colon, the viscera are gently returned to the abdomen. Biopsies, resections, or repairs are then performed.

The use of intraoperative biopsy and microscopy, when available, is a potent adjunct to exploratory laparotomy. In a series of 23 cases, the operative plan was altered in 13 on the basis of examination of frozen sections (Stone et al., 1978). If suction is needed to remove irrigating solutions or pathologic fluid accumulations, a fenestrated metal (Poole) suction tip is helpful. Midline incisions may be closed by a variety of techniques, depending on the surgeon's preference. The classic method is to use 2-0 chromic gut in a simple interrupted pattern, but continuous 2-0 polypropylene has been used successfully in many cats (Crowe, 1978). Subcutis and skin are sutured separately.

If available, laparoscopy may often substitute for exploratory laparotomy (Wildt et al., 1977). It must be done with careful aseptic technique.

## GASTROINTESTINAL TRACT

Whenever the alimentary canal is opened, contamination of the abdomen with bacteria or irritants is likely, but is minimized by isolating the segment to be opened from the general peritoneal cavity with several layers of moist laparotomy sponges, irrigating the isolated segment after surgery, and removing soiled laparotomy sponges and changing gloves and instruments before closure. Gross contamination requires irrigation of the abdominal cavity with 1 or 2 liters of warm isotonic fluid, to which an antibiotic may be added.

### Gastrotomy

The most common indication for gastric surgery in the cat is removal of foreign bodies and hairballs. Once the stomach has been isolated, the ends of the proposed incision site are elevated with stay sutures or Babcock forcepses. The initial incision is made with a pointed scalpel blade and extended with scissors. Liquid gastric content is aspirated by suction and any foreign material is removed. The stomach is best closed in two layers with 3-0 absorbable suture material with a swaged-on, curved tapered needle with a cutting tip. A deep, continuous Connell suture line provides hemostasis and a watertight closure; this is reinforced with a superficial row of seromuscular Lembert sutures.

Gruel-like food may be given in small amounts after 24 hours, softened canned food after 48 hours, and a regular diet after a week.

### Gastroesophageal Intussusception

Gastroesophageal intussusception occurs occasionally in young cats with persistent vomiting and represents a surgical emergency, because strangulation of the incarcerated stomach or respiratory compromise may rapidly ensue. The intussusception is reduced by traction. A large stomach tube is passed through the cardia, and the diameter of the esophageal hiatus is reduced with several interrupted sutures of 2-0 gut. Finally, a gastropexy between the greater curvature of the stomach and the left abdominal wall is performed.

### Intestinal Surgery

The basic techniques of enterotomy and resection with anastomosis are used for intestinal foreign bodies, intussusceptions, and tumor. The affected segment should be exteriorized and isolated from the peritoneal cavity; with mid-duodenal lesions, the duodenocolic fold (ligament) must be cut. The intestine proximal and distal to the proposed incision should be gently occluded by an assistant's fingers, by hair clips, or by Allis forcepses with the bars closed over gauze sponges to avoid the reflux of chyme during surgery; Doyen forcepses are unwieldy and tend to crush or bruise the bowel. A broad-spectrum antibiotic should be administered parenterally whenever the intestine is opened.

**ENTEROTOMY.** Incisions are made on the antimesenteric aspect and must be handled minimally and gently to avoid crushing of tissue that could lead to failure of the suture line. They are closed in a single layer with 4-0 medium chromic gut or polyglycolic acid swaged onto a tapered needle with a cutting tip. Standard curved taper needles require such force to penetrate the tough submucosa that the intestinal edge is often crushed with a thumb forceps; the thumb forceps should support rather than grasp the edge. The suture pattern should appose or minimally invert the edges to avoid stenosis; a single layer closure of simple interrupted (DeHoff et al., 1973) or Gambee suture pattern is preferred.

**LINEAR FOREIGN BODIES.** Pieces of string, tinsel, or thread are common foreign bodies in cats and may have devastating consequences. They can cause chronic partial obstruction that is difficult to diagnose even with contrast studies or may perforate the intestine and cause peritonitis. String or thread may often be seen looped tautly under the tongue or it may form a mass lodged at the pylorus or in the proximal small intestine with one or more strands passing distally. With peristalsis, the intestine "climbs" up the strand, which often becomes imbedded in its mesenteric border. As time passes, the strand may perforate the intestine in multiple sites, with an ensuing chemical and bacterial peritonitis and septicemia. Simple and compound intussusceptions are common along the strand.

It is risky simply to cut string or thread looped under the tongue in the hope that the foreign material will be eliminated uneventfully; prompt surgical removal is the safest course.

If possible, the affected segment of intestine should be isolated with laparotomy pads. The proximal anchoring mass of foreign material is removed through a gastrotomy or enterotomy. The intestine is gently pulled free as far as possible off the remaining strand; vigorous pulling must be avoided, for perforation may ensue. Multiple enterotomies (Fig. 4–12), often needed to remove the strand piecemeal, are done on the antimesenteric border if the strand is within the lumen. If the strand is buried along the mesenteric border, small enterotomies may be effected over it, at right angles to the long axis of the intestine. In cases of long-standing linear foreign bodies, a ridge of scar tissue develops along the mesenteric border and may be mistaken for another buried strand. The enterotomies are closed as described previously. If peritonitis is present, a suture material that resists enzymatic digestion, such as polyglycolic acid, is preferred. Resection of severely affected segments is often necessary. The abdomen should be irrigated with large volumes of isotonic fluid; "sump" drains for postoperative irrigation may be placed in cats with severe, generalized peritonitis. The abdominal wall is closed with a monofilament nonabsorbable suture material (Withrow and Black, 1979).

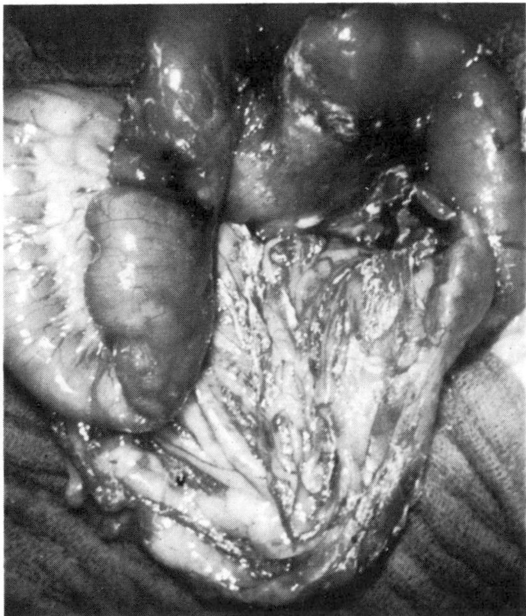

**Figure 4–12.** Linear foreign body. Multiple perforations that caused local peritonitis were sutured after the foreign body was removed.

**RESECTION AND ANASTOMOSIS.** This procedure is done whenever there is severe damage or a tumor involving the intestine. Special skill is required with the cat because of the small diameter of the organ and the risk of postoperative stenosis. The blood supply to the anastomosis site must be carefully preserved. The incisions, made well into healthy tissue, are angled at about 60 degrees from the mesenteric surface, which has the richest blood supply. This maneuver, by increasing the diameter of the bowel at the anastomosis site, helps to avoid stenosis (DeHoff et al., 1973). If segments of unequal caliber are to be anastomosed, the smaller segment is incised along its antimesenteric border to create a larger circumference. For suture material, 3-0 or 4-0 medium chromic surgical gut or polyglycolic acid is commonly used, although some surgeons prefer monofilament nylon. The first suture is placed through the mesenteric border; a suture is then placed, but not tied, on the antimesenteric border, to ensure accurate approximation of the entire circumference of the bowel. The edges of the segments are apposed with simple interrupted sutures. After the anastomosis has been completed, the mesenteric incision should be closed to avoid the risk of an internal hernia.

An end-to-end anastomosis of ileum to colon is occasionally followed by intussusception. To avoid this, some surgeons tack the ileum to the abdominal wall or to the proximal colon in the manner of a U.

Side-to-side or end-to-side anastomosis is also a possibility although generally reserved for gastroenterostomy or cholecystoenterostomy after resection of tumors in the proximal duodenum or pylorus, or when the common bile duct is damaged or occluded by a benign process such as chronic fibrosing pancreatitis.

**MEGACOLON.** Surgical treatment of megacolon is occasionally undertaken in cats with obstipation that is refractory to medical treatment. For cases in which the colon is not constricted by distortion of the pelvic canal or a colonic tumor, several surgical options have been reported.

After the colon is emptied of impacted feces, an ellipse of seromuscular tissue may be removed sufficient to restore the normal diameter of the colon; the excess mucosa is not excised but is folded into the lumen, and the margins of the ellipse are closed with 3-0 gut sutures (Leighton, 1975).

If the fecal mass cannot be removed through the anus, the colon may be exposed and thoroughly isolated with laparotomy pads. An antimesenteric colotomy is done along the entire distended segment, the impacted feces are removed, and the redundant colon is resected to restore the normal diameter. The colon is closed with two layers of 3-0 gut in a Cushing pattern. Good results have been claimed (Leighton, 1975.)

Resection and anastomosis of the descending colon were successful in a cat in which a 12-cm stricture developed after removal of a full-thickness strip of colon (Leighton and Grain, 1978). In another case 70 per cent of the colon was resected, with good results for at least 10 months (Yoder et al., 1968).

If obstipation results from constriction of the bony pelvic canal, osteoplastic reconstructive procedures such as removal of the ventral pubis and ischium, partial transection of the ilium, and mechanical spreading of the ischia may be resorted to (Leighton, 1969).

**RECTAL PROLAPSE.** Straining from parturition, irritation of the rectal lining, or urinary tract obstruction may cause rectal prolapse. This must be differentiated from prolapse of an intussception; in the latter case a lubricated probe or thermometer will pass easily lateral to the intussusceptum. Fresh prolapses may be reduced and the anus partially closed with a pursestring suture tied with a rectal thermometer in place. Any underlying cause must be treated as well. The suture is removed in three to five days. In about half the cases the prolapse recurs. Recurrent prolapses or those with necrotic mucosa should be resected. The rectum may be prolapsed intentionally for the removal of polyps or tumors (Fig. 4–13), or for repair of rectal lacerations.

**COLOPEXY.** Colopexy may be necessary if rectal prolapse occurs repeatedly and no underlying cause can be treated. The colon is approached through a caudal midline incision and its wall anchored to the peritoneum by several 2-0 gut sutures passed from the seromuscular layer of the colon to the incision edge (Leighton, 1975). The lumen of the colon is avoided.

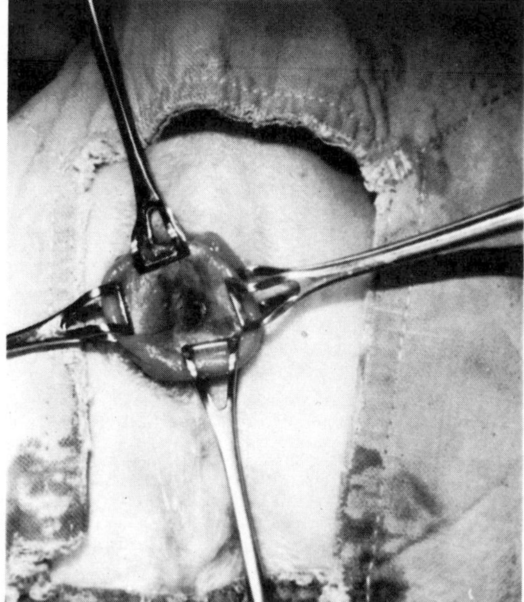

**Figure 4–13.** Prolapse of the rectum and distal descending colon with four Babcock forcepses to expose a constricting carcinoma for resection.

## Liver

### Lobectomy

Biliary retention cysts, solitary tumors, and severe trauma may necessitate the removal of part or all of a liver lobe. The liver lobes are easily approached in the cat; if necessary, the hepatorenal or coronary ligament may be severed, or the midline incision may be extended paracostally to enhance exposure. The affected tissue is easily removed after preplacing, and then tying, a row of overlapping 2-0 gut mattress sutures proximal to the lesion.

### Biliary Tract Obstruction

Obstructive jaundice is frequent in the cat. Sometimes the cause is within the biliary tree, e.g., congenital anomalies, cholangitis, parasites, inspissated bile (Holzworth and Gilmore, 1969), tumors (Barsanti et al., 1976), gallstones (O'Brien and Mitchum, 1970; Wigderson, 1955), or blood clots (Furneaux, 1974a). Obstruction may also result from external pressure, as with acute or chronic pancreatitis or pancreatic tumors (Holzworth and Gilmore, 1969). Exploratory laparotomy often provides the answer, but occasionally the bile duct must be explored.

### Bile Duct Exploration

The biliary tree is approached through a cranial midline incision. Retraction with the mesoduodenum exposes the gallbladder, cystic duct, and common bile duct. Palpation of the common duct may reveal masses, stones, or inspissated bile. The duodenal opening of the common bile duct may be exposed through a duodenotomy opposite the major duodenal papilla, which is on the dorsal wall of the duodenum 3 cm distal to the pylorus (Crouch, 1969). The bile duct may be cannulated and irrigated, or obstructions at the papilla removed. Patency may be confirmed by pressing on the gallbladder and watching bile flow through the papilla. An incision may be made into the gallbladder to remove inspissated bile or stones and for irrigation. The cholecystotomy incision is closed with two layers of 4-0 gut in a continuous pattern (Leighton, 1975).

Obstruction of the common bile duct by fibrosis is managed by anastomosing the gallbladder to the duodenum (cholecystoduodenostomy), to create an alternate path for the drainage of bile.

### Cholecystectomy

Removal of the gallbladder is occasionally required in the cat for acute or chronic inflammation or tumor.

## Splenectomy

The major indications for splenectomy in the cat are tumors and trauma. Mast cell tumors may cause massive splenomegaly, and splenectomy has been of benefit in some cases, even in the presence of circulating mast cells (Confer and Langloss, 1978; Guerre et al., 1979; Liska et al., 1979.) The technique of splenectomy in the cat is similar to that in the dog, but extra care must be taken to avoid damaging the left limb of the pancreas, which is much nearer the splenic hilus.

### Adrenalectomy

A case of Cushing's syndrome due to a functional adrenal cortical adenoma has been reported (Meijer et al., 1978). Bilateral paracostal laparotomies were used to expose and examine the adrenals; the right adrenal, measuring 7 × 9 × 13 mm, was removed. Postoperative care included maintenance with Hartmann's solution and injectable hydrocortisone for 48 hours and oral doses of cortisone for three weeks. The paracostal approach is easier and gives better exposure in the cat than in the dog.

A midline approach is preferred by some surgeons, since a single incision permits inspection of both glands.

### Hernias

Some hernias may be congenital, but most that come to surgery result from trauma.

#### Umbilical Hernia

This common congenital hernia may range in extent from a small, inconsequential defect to the absence of a large part of the ventral abdominal wall (omphalocele). Small umbilical hernias are common in the cat and are easily repaired by bluntly exposing the hernia sac and its contents at the umbilical ring, inverting the sac into the abdomen, and suturing the ring closed. Monofilament, nonabsorbable suture material is preferred. In females an umbilical hernia is often repaired at the time of spaying.

#### Ventral Hernia

This term refers to any hernia through the abdominal wall. The most common sites of traumatic disruption are along the costal margins, at the inguinal rings and brim of the pelvis, and along the dorsal attachments of the abdominal muscles to the wing of the ilium and the lumbodorsal fascia. Such hernias are often multiple and associated with damage to underlying viscera. They are repaired by widely exposing the torn edges and débriding necrotic tissue. Underlying viscera should be inspected and the abdominal wall palpated to detect associated hernias. Whenever possible, the layers of the abdominal muscles should be reconstituted. Because paracostal hernias may be accompanied by diaphragmatic hernias, positive pressure anesthesia must be available (Peiffer and Stickle, 1975). The torn muscles are anchored to the costal margin cranially and to the lumbodorsal fascia dorsally if corresponding muscle edges cannot be identified.

Another common ventral hernia results when the abdominal muscles are torn from their pelvic attachments. In most cases the rectus sheath can be reattached to the obturator foramina by vertical mattress sutures of monofilament nonabsorbable suture material. Sutures may also be anchored to holes drilled in the pubis and the wing of the ilium. Care must be taken to avoid perforating the femoral vessels or occluding the caudal superficial epigastric vessels when suturing in the inguinal region. Rarely synthetic mesh is needed to help close such defects (Furneaux, 1974b).

#### Perineal Hernia

Perineal hernias, rare in the cat, should be repaired if they are symptomatic (Ashton, 1976; Leighton, 1979). They may be unilateral or bilateral and are repaired by the same technique used for dogs.

## UROGENITAL TRACT

### Kidney

Renal surgery in cats includes needle biopsy to aid in the diagnosis and management of renal disease, and nephrectomy for severe trauma, abscesses, solitary tumors, hydronephrosis, and refractory unilateral pyelonephritis.

#### Needle Biopsy

Percutaneous kidney biopsy is of diagnostic value in diffuse renal disease and is easily performed in most cats by use of a Franklin-modified Vim-Silverman needle. The flank is prepared aseptically, and the kidney is grasped and immobilized with the fingers against the abdominal wall. The biopsy needle is inserted through a stab wound in the skin and directed under the greater curvature of the kidney to avoid the hilus. An assistant is needed to harvest the sample. In two thirds of the samples thus procured in one series, transitional epithelium was present, indicating penetration of the renal pelvis (Osborne, 1971). In one cat a blood clot obstructed the ureter and caused mild hydronephrosis; the others recovered uneventfully.

#### Nephrectomy

If removal of a kidney is anticipated, normal function of the other kidney should be demonstrated by excretory urography. Nephrectomy is usually performed through a ventral midline incision; the renal vessels are isolated, ligated, and severed and the ureter is ligated and severed as far distally as possible (Leighton, 1975). A flank approach is useful to gain early exposure of the renal vessels in the dissection of large, vascular renal masses, especially when adhesions to the dorsal body wall are present.

#### Perirenal Cysts (Perirenal Hygroma)

Bilateral fluid-filled perirenal cysts are a rare finding of uncertain pathogenesis. In some cases they are associated with polycystic kidneys (Bloom, 1954) or with advanced chronic kidney disease. The fluid, which appears from analysis to be urine, is thought to leak from cysts or cystic collecting tubules on the kidney surface, loosening and distending the kidney capsule. If renal decompensation is present, treatment is fruitless. In some cases, especially if unilateral, the accumulation of fluid appears to be associated with previous injury to the kidney. In a cat with a history of urethral obstruction and automobile injury, kidney function was apparently unimpaired, and the cysts were drained and most of the walls removed (Chastain and Grier, 1975). Although the kidneys did not appear entirely normal in photographs taken at laparotomy, the cat recovered, with no sign of trouble later.

### Ectopic Ureter

Bilateral ureteral ectopia, manifested by dribbling of urine, has been reported in three kittens, two males and one female (Bebko et al. 1977; Biewinga et al., 1978). Contrast radiography indicated that the ureters emptied into the urethra. Urinary continence was restored in two of the kittens by reimplantation of the distal ureters into the bladder wall (Biewinga et al., 1978).

## Bladder

Congenital anomalies, calculi, tumors, and trauma are the principal indications for bladder surgery.

The most common congenital anomaly, some form of urachal remnant, has been reported to occur in 24 per cent of cats undergoing autopsy (Hansen, 1977). Few have related clinical signs, but if recurrent infection or hematuria is present, excision of the urachal diverticulum is often curative. Persistent urachus with dribbling of urine at the umbilicus has also been reported (Bachrach and Kleine, 1974; Greene and Bohning, 1971).

Cystic calculi are not uncommon in adult cats of either sex and may be detected by plain or contrast radiography; the majority are radiopaque (Bohonowych et al., 1978). Clinical signs include persistent or recurrent hematuria and pyuria.

Primary bladder tumors are rare in cats. Malignant tumors, including transitional cell carcinoma (Dill et al., 1972), leiomyosarcoma (Burk et al., 1975), and squamous cell carcinoma (Dorn et al., 1978), are generally advanced at the time of diagnosis and often inoperable. Benign tumors have been successfully resected (Patnaik and Greene, 1979). (See also the chapter on tumors.)

Rupture of the urinary bladder may be associated with blunt trauma or may be iatrogenic. Intraperitoneal extravasation of urine results in severe shock, probably associated with the marked hypertonicity of cat urine and the presence of postrenal uremia in obstructed cats. The prognosis is guarded, but early detection, intensive fluid replacement, and repair of the rent, together with intraoperative peritoneal lavage with large volumes of warm isotonic solution, saves most cats.

### Cystotomy

The bladder is approached through a caudal midline incision. To aid in mobilizing the bladder, the median ligament should be severed, beginning cranially with its cordlike edge (the urachal remnant) and continuing caudally along the ventral surface of the bladder. (This procedure is also a precaution against the occasional catastrophe of postoperative torsion of the bladder if the median ligament is accidentally torn while the tougher urachal remnant remains intact.)

The bladder is then exteriorized and isolated with moist laparotomy pads to avoid spillage of urine. Urine may be aspirated with a hypodermic needle or by a suction tube introduced through a small nick in the bladder wall.

The site of the fundic incision varies with the purpose of the surgery, but as a rule the incision is made in the least vascular area. If the cystotomy is performed to remove or explore for stones, it is important to search the neck of the bladder and also to ensure patency of the urethra by flushing.

The cystotomy incision or the débrided margin of a rupture is closed with 3-0 chromic gut on a curved tapered needle. A two-layer closure of interrupted Lembert sutures over a continuous Cushing pattern is preferred, although a thickened, tightly contracted bladder may sometimes be closed by a single continuous suture line.

After cystotomy the cat should be carefully observed to be sure that it is voiding urine without difficulty and in an appropriate volume.

## Urethra

### Urethral Rupture

The urethra may be perforated or severed by catheters or by pelvic trauma. Positive-contrast urethrography is necessary to define the extent and location of the tear. Perforations or linear tears heal over an indwelling catheter within 10 days; continuity may be confirmed by urethrography before removal of the catheter.

The treatment of a severed urethra depends on the site of the tear and the amount of urethral tissue lost. Ruptures distal to the ischium are repaired with a perineal urethrostomy. More proximal ruptures are approached through a caudal abdominal midline incision. If necessary, the pelvic floor can be lifted by cutting the acetabular rami of the pubis and the pubic symphysis at the caudal extremity of the obturator foramina. The bone flap thus formed is reflected caudally to expose the intrapelvic urethra. A preplaced urethral catheter helps to identify the distal segment. Devitalized urethral tissue is débrided, the catheter is passed into the proximal segment, and the urethra is anastomosed around it with six to eight simple interrupted sutures of 4-0 chromic gut. The pelvic bone flap is then wired back in place and the abdomen closed routinely. The urinary catheter is removed after 10 days, when healing of the anastomosis has been confirmed with urethrography.

If too much urethral tissue has been lost to permit a tension-free anastomosis, or if the distal segment of the urethra cannot be identified, antepubic urethrostomy is the treatment of choice.

### Antepubic Urethrostomy

The bladder and urethra are approached through a caudal midline incision. The abdominal urethra is exposed by dissecting away the periurethral fat, vessels, and nerves and is transected as far caudally as possible after ligation of the distal remnant. The caudal end of the abdominal urethra is brought out through the abdominal incision or through a separate stab incision, care being taken to avoid twisting, kinking, or tension. The abdominal wall is then closed routinely. The urethra is next passed through a separate opening from which a 1-cm ellipse of skin has been removed. A 1-cm incision is made along the ventral midline of the urethra, which is anastomosed to the skin with simple interrupted sutures of 5-0 braided nonabsorbable suture material (McCully, 1955). In a series of 32 cats undergoing antepubic urethrostomy for urethral obstruction, complications arose in 12 (Mendham, 1970). Recurrent bacterial cystitis, urine scalding, and subcutaneous urine infiltration were the most common. Other sequelae included incontinence, stricture, kinking of the urethra, and dysuria.

(Editor's note. If such sequelae of antepubic urethrostomy are serious or persistent, a modification developed by Whitehead [1961] might be considered as a measure of last resort. A sterile 8F polyethylene tube is introduced into the urethra to pass just through the abdominal wall but not into the bladder. It is anchored by a simple interrupted suture of 3-0 braided stainless steel placed directly through the center of the urethra and its enclosed tubing and tied snugly to the outer urethral wall. Another suture is placed just outside the abdominal wall and another just below the skin. The subcutis is closed with 2-0 chromic gut and the skin with the stainless steel. The tube is allowed to protrude for about 4 cm in obese cats and can be shortened after convalescence according to individual requirements. Tubes have functioned for six months to three years and are easily replaced.)

## Urethral Obstruction

The surgical management of urethral obstruction in male cats has been the topic of more debate in the literature than any other feline surgical problem. Every conceivable form of anatomic manipulation has been tried, including ureterocolostomy (Beamer, 1959), cystocolostomy (Nayar and Wilson, 1974), urethrocolostomy (Barnes and Bone, 1963; Beamer, 1959; Nayar, 1974), trigone translocation (Beamer, 1959). antepubic urethrostomy (McCully, 1955; Mendham, 1970; Whitehead, 1961), prostheses for drainage of urine from the bladder (Manziano and Manziano, 1967) or urethra (Richards, 1976; Robinette, 1973), preputial urethrostomy (Biewinga, 1975; Christensen, 1964), and perineal urethrostomy. Translocation of the urinary tract into the colon often causes liquid, frequent stools and ascending infection; antepubic urethrostomy may be plagued by recurrent cystitis, urine scalding, and incontinence; preputial urethrostomy is technically difficult and predisposes to the formation of fistulae and strictures (Johnston, 1974). The use of prostheses when sound conventional techniques exist is unjustifiable.

Perineal urethrostomy is currently the favored technique and is likely to remain so. Many modifications have been applied to the earliest reported procedure, in which the penis and crura were left intact and the pelvic urethra was sutured to the skin (Carbone, 1963). These include amputation of the entire penis to avoid recanalization and stricture (Carbone, 1965), the use of separate incisions for dissection and formation of the urethral opening (Carbone, 1967), longitudinal bisection of the penis with lateral anchorage of the flaps thus formed and healing by second intention (Blake, 1968), meticulous dissection and suturing to achieve primary healing and avoid stenosis (Johnston, 1974; Wilson and Harrison, 1971), and the use of "smilers," "wrinkles," and elaborate suture techniques (Rickards et al., 1972; Rickards and Hinko, 1974). The most significant contributions were those that stressed the application of the science of wound healing to perineal urethrostomy, in the recognition that gentle tissue handling, thorough dissection to avoid tension, hemostasis, and meticulous suturing to achieve primary healing between the urethra and the skin are necessary to ensure consistently good results (Johnston, 1974; Wilson and Harrison, 1971). The most recent technique (Long, 1977; 1979) and the technique presented here represent this philosophy.

## Perineal Urethrostomy

Perineal urethrostomy should not be performed as an emergency measure for an obstructed cat that is azotemic and in shock. Fluid and electrolyte imbalances should first be corrected. If it is impossible to relieve the obstruction by catheterization, urine can be aspirated from the bladder by a 22-gauge needle (a larger needle permits leakage); however, a safer and more satisfactory emergency measure is implantation of an 8F Foley catheter into the bladder by way of abdominal and cystotomy incisions. In a severely depressed cat this may be done with local anesthesia, sometimes with no anesthesia at all. The catheter is firmly secured in the bladder with a pursestring suture. When the perineal urethrostomy is done, the catheter is removed and the openings in the bladder and abdominal wall are sutured.

For perineal urethrostomy the anesthetized cat, with perineum clipped and scrubbed, is placed on its sternum with hindquarters elevated and tail pulled forward. Positioning is important; the cat must lie straight, with the perineum tilted slightly upward. A pursestring suture is tied about the anus and anal sac orifices, and final surgical preparation completed. An elliptical skin incision is made about the scrotum and prepuce (Fig. 4–14*A*) and deepened through the subcutaneous tissue. If the cat is an intact male, it is castrated at this point. The skin is removed along with the preputial reflection and a hemostat is placed on the penis for ease of manipulation. The distal penis and attached skin are amputated and discarded. Blunt and sharp dissection through subcutaneous fat exposes the ischiocavernosus muscles covering the crura (Fig. 4–14*B*). The penis is lifted with the hemostat, superficial ventral midline attachments are severed, and the penis is reflected to the right to expose the left crus of the penis, which is cut with Metzenbaum scissors at its insertion on the ischium (Fig. 4–14*C*). This procedure is repeated for the right crus. A finger may then be inserted ventral to the urethra and into the pelvic canal to break down the ventral ligaments that run between the pelvic urethra and the pelvic symphysis. Gentle traction and blunt dissection further expose the superficial longitudinal muscle of the perineum (levator scroti), the fascial extension of the external anal sphincter, and fibers of the retractor penis. These are lifted (Fig. 4–14*D*) and transected so that the bulbourethral glands and dorsal urethra are completely exposed. The soft tissues running to the bulbourethral glands are severed next (Fig. 4–14*E*); a small branch of the urogenital artery is usually severed and should be ligated or cauterized.

The completed dissection exposes at least 2 cm of the pelvic urethra proximal to the bulbourethral glands (Fig. 4–14*F*), which easily reach the level of the skin without traction. Next the urethra is partly transected just distal to the crura, and a tomcat catheter is introduced. The

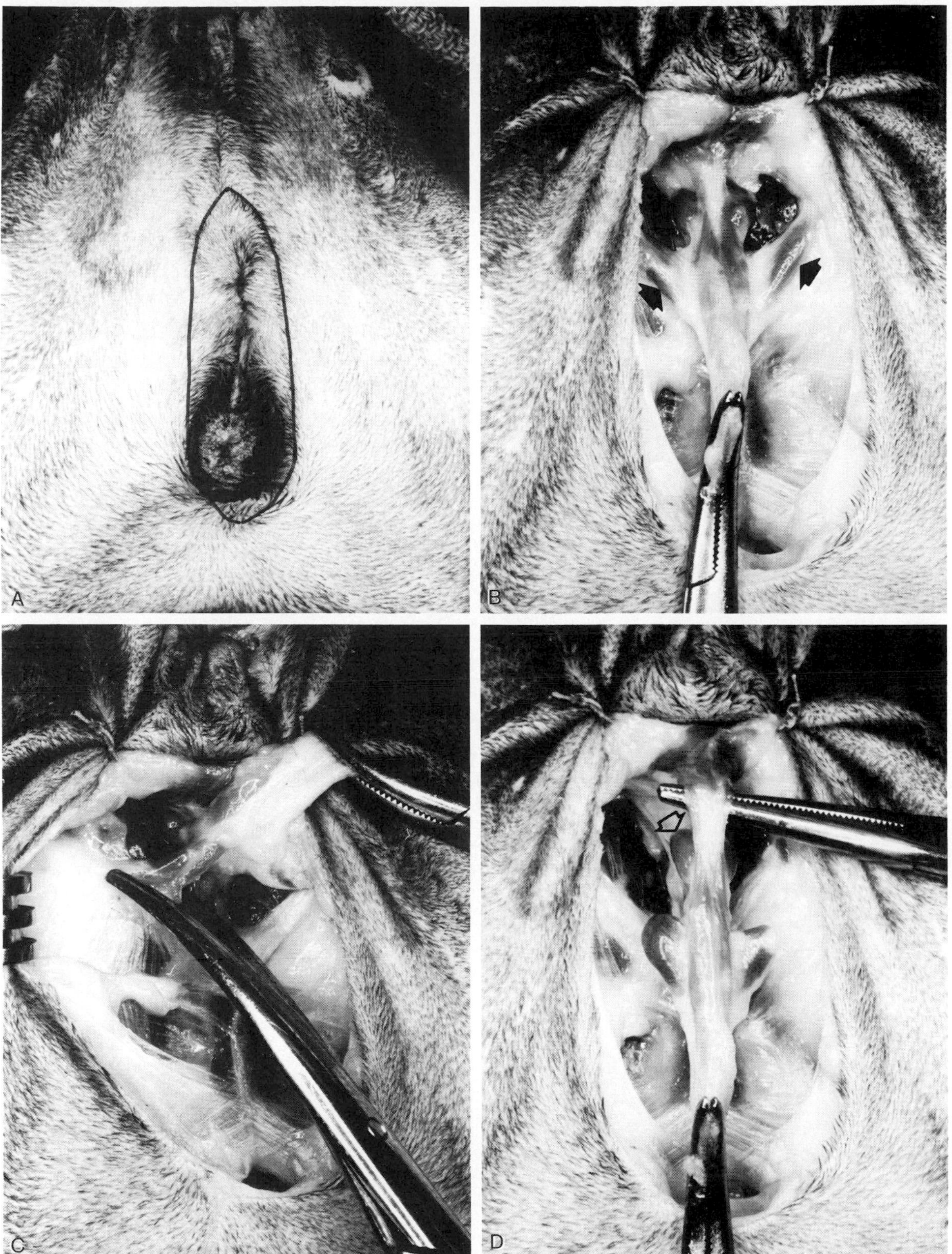


**Figure 4–14.** *A*, Perineal urethrostomy: operative field and location of skin incision. *B*, A hemostat is placed across the penis for manipulation after the preputial skin is removed. Stay sutures were placed and perineal fat around the crura (arrows) removed for these illustrations. *C*, The left crus of the penis is transected with Metzenbaum scissors at its ischial insertion. *D*, The retractor penis and superficial longitudinal muscle of the perineum (levator scroti) are elevated with a hemostat before their transection. This will completely expose the bulbourethral glands (arrow).

*Illustration continued on following page*

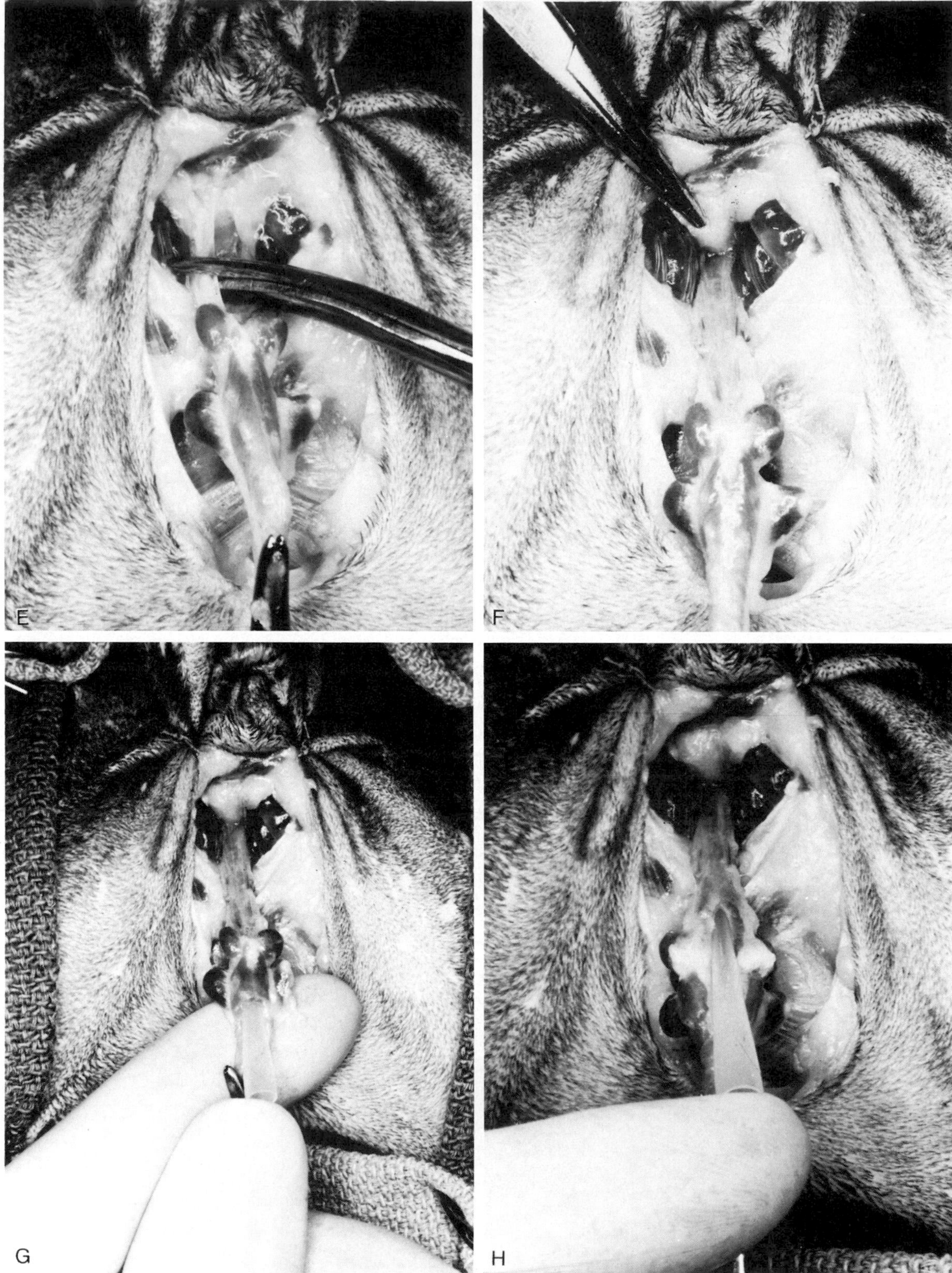


**Figure 4–14** *Continued. E*, Attachments to the bulbourethral glands are severed to further expose and mobilize the pelvic urethra. *F*, Completed dissection. Two cm of pelvic urethra is exposed and mobilized. The hemostat points to the rectum. *G*, The penis is partially transected distal to the crura to allow insertion of a tomcat catheter in the urethra. The catheter is impacted into the urethra and cut down upon. *H*, The urethral incision extends 5 mm cranial to the bulbourethral glands.

*Illustration continued on opposite page*

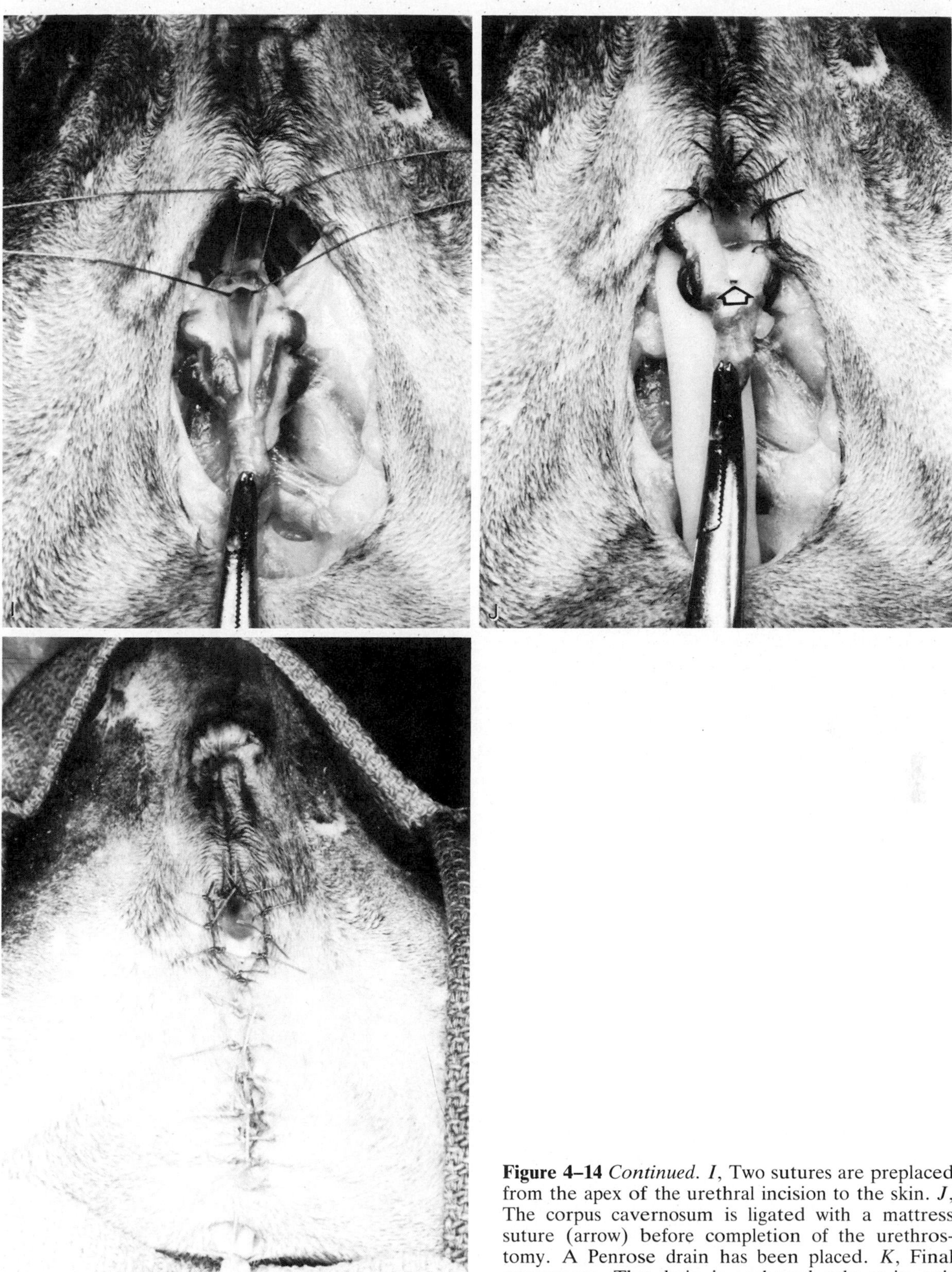


**Figure 4–14** *Continued. I*, Two sutures are preplaced from the apex of the urethral incision to the skin. *J*, The corpus cavernosum is ligated with a mattress suture (arrow) before completion of the urethrostomy. A Penrose drain has been placed. *K*, Final appearance. The drain is anchored only at its exit site.

flared end is impacted against the urethra (Fig. 4–14*G*); by cutting down on the impacted catheter, the surgeon makes a smooth incision through the urethra to a point 5 mm cranial to the bulbourethral glands (Fig. 4–14*H*). The catheter is withdrawn and suturing begun by preplacing two sutures of 4-0 braided nonabsorbable material next to the apex of the urethral incision (Fig. 4–14*I*). Suturing is then continued distally. The placement of the sutures is critical: They must incorporate a small bite (less than 1 mm) of urethral mucosa, a large bite of cavernous tissue, and minimal periurethral muscle. They are brought through the skin 3 mm from the cut edge and tied snugly to compress the cavernous tissue, bringing the skin and mucosal edges into apposition. The urethral mucosa is too weak to support sutures; incorporating the cavernous tissue adds strength and provides hemostasis. Before suturing is completed, a mattress suture of 3-0 gut is tied around the corpus cavernosum just distal to the crura, and a ¼-inch Penrose drain is placed ventral to the urethra (Fig. 4–14*J*), to emerge through a separate stab incision ventral to the primary incision. The penis is amputated distal to the mattress suture, and the urethrostomy completed (Fig. 4–14*K*). The pursestring suture is then removed.

After surgery, antibiotics are continued to combat any urinary tract infection. Catheterization is avoided. A bland antibiotic ointment is applied to the urethrostomy site several times a day, and an Elizabethan collar should be used if the cat licks at the sutures. Urethral patency should be checked frequently for the first two days; it is not unusual for a blood clot to adhere to the sutures and obstruct the urethra, but such a clot is easily removed. The drain is removed after 48 hours and sutures after 8 to 10 days.

Complications may develop immediately after surgery or may be delayed. Persistent bleeding, which has resulted in exsanguination, may occur if the cavernous tissue along the edges of the incision has not been adequately compressed. Proper suture placement avoids this, but any bleeding should be controlled with additional sutures. Leakage of urine under the skin may occur if the urethral mucosa or the apex of the urethral incision is not included in the sutures. Leakage becomes obvious when urine drips out around the drain and is managed by diverting the flow of urine with an 8F Foley catheter for five days. By then, any urethral defect will have healed. Undetected urine leakage in the absence of a drain can result in huge areas of skin loss from the medial thighs and perineum, thus some surgeons take the precaution of routine use of a Penrose drain.

Later complications include bacterial cystitis and stricture of the urethral opening. Postoperative bacterial cystitis was reported in 26 per cent of the cases in one series and was managed medically (Smith and Schiller, 1978). Stricture of the urethrostomy occurred in over half the cases in which urethral catheters were used after surgery. The incidence of stricture with the Wilson-Harrison technique was 11.5 per cent; this figure fell to 2 per cent if cats with postoperative urethral catheters were excluded. Most strictures were recognized between four and six weeks after surgery and were managed by dilatation or reoperation, the latter being preferred.

Stricture of the urethrostomy site may cause straining but more often dribbling of urine secondary to chronic partial obstruction (paradoxic incontinence). The bladder is distended, and inspection of the urethrostomy site reveals a flat, epithelialized scar, with a barely perceptible urethral orifice that is often impossible to catheterize (Fig. 4–15*A*). A secondary urethrocutaneous fistula may be present. Surgical reconstruction is easily done in most cases.

## Repair of a Stenotic Urethrostomy

Positioning and preparation are the same as for perineal urethrostomy. A 1-cm, round incision is made about the stenotic orifice and deepened through the scar tissue; then 2 to 3 cm of healthy urethra is exposed by blunt dissection (Fig. 4–15*B*). The scarred distal urethra is resected, a dorsal incision made in the healthy urethra (Fig. 4–15*C*), and the urethrostomy reformed. The resultant urethral orifice is usually much larger than in the initial surgery, because the urethra is dilated from the chronic obstruction (Fig. 4–15*D*).

It cannot be overemphasized, both for the initial urethrostomy and for any subsequent repairs, that the surgeon must carefully appose the urethral mucosa to the skin edges (because exposed connective tissue predisposes to granulation and stricture); that handling of tissue must be gentle and efficient; and that only nonreactive suture material must be used.

## Castration

Male cats are castrated to prevent objectional behavioral patterns such as fighting, roaming, and urine spraying, as well as for population control. The age at which castration should be done is controversial because of concern that early castration may retard development of the penile urethra and predispose to urinary tract obstruction.

This possibility has been the subject of only limited study (Herron, 1971, 1972). Although the penile urethral circumference of cats castrated at five months did not appear to be less at 10 months than in uncastrated cats of the same age, sections were not measured at the level of the os penis, nor did the study concern itself with the possible effect on urethral distensibility or differences in the size of the penis itself. Finally, both groups of cats were destroyed before maturity rather than being followed into the adult age range, when urethral obstruction most often develops. One incidental disadvantage of castration at five months was identified: In some of these cats adhesions persisted between the prepuce and the penis, giving rise to "pockets" in which debris and urine could collect and cause irritation or infection (Herron, 1971).

Castration has proven effective in decreasing fighting, roaming, and urine spraying in males over one year of age (Hart and Barrett, 1973). The usual recommendation is to castrate cats between 8 and 10 months of age (e.g., Stein, 1975) but to do so earlier at the first sign of objectionable behavior.

Many techniques are available for castration. Whatever the procedure, it should be aseptic and provide for the control of hemorrhage from the spermatic vessels. The scrotum and adjacent area are plucked or closely clipped, scrubbed, and draped. The scrotal skin is tensed by pinching it over a testis, and an incision is made just to one side of the median raphe through skin, subcutis, and tunics. The tunics are separated from the testis by break-

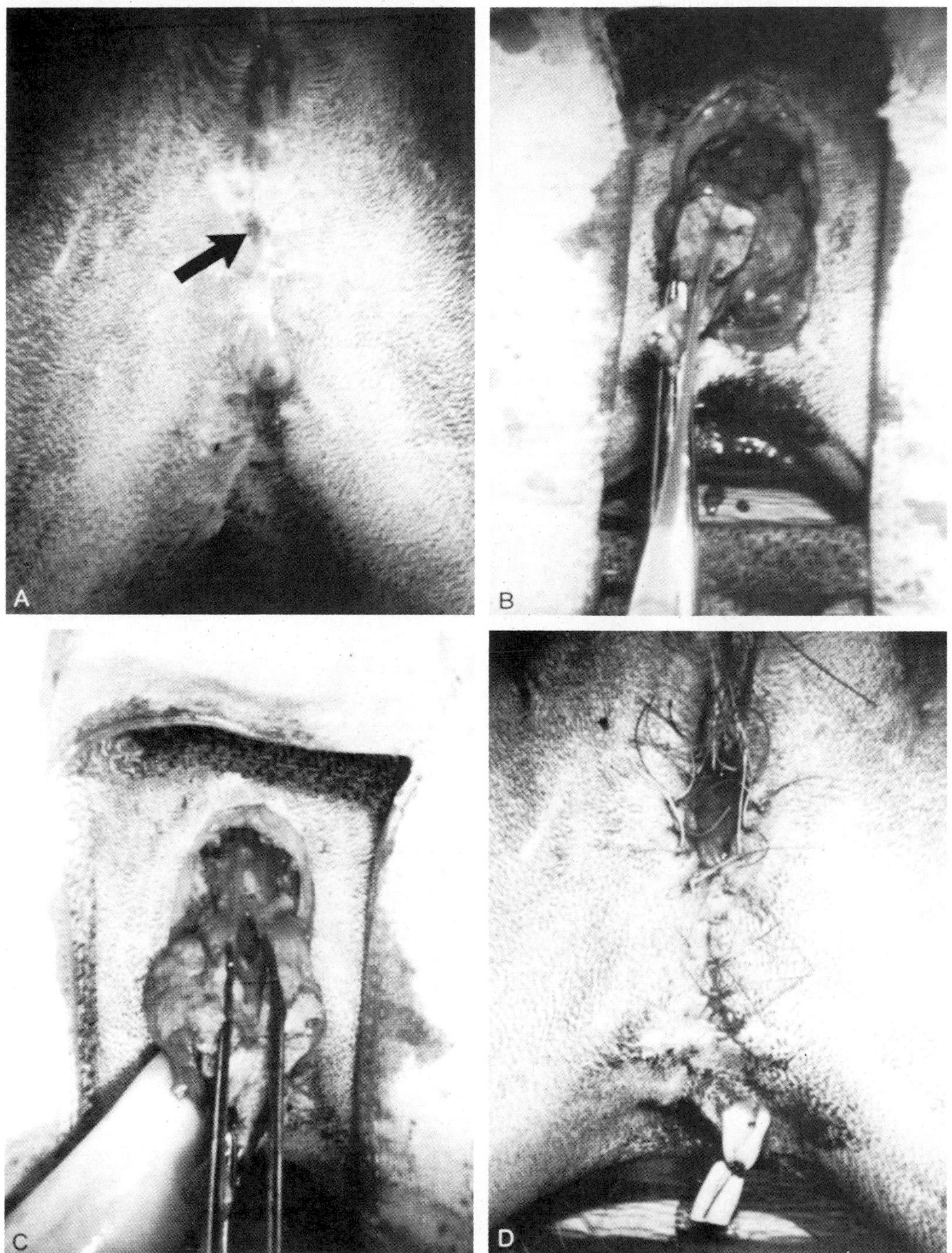


**Figure 4–15.** *A*, Strictured perineal urethrostomy (arrow). The urethrostomy is nearly obliterated by scar tissue. *B*, An incision is made about the stenotic orifice and deepened through the scar tissue; the urethra is mobilized by blunt and sharp dissection. *C*, A 1-cm incision is made into the dilated urethra proximal to the stricture. Scarred skin and urethral tissue are then amputated and discarded. *D*, Repair of the stenotic urethrostomy is completed in a manner similar to that in a routine urethrostomy.

ing the scrotal ligament and are amputated or replaced in the scrotum. The ductus deferens is separated from the spermatic vessels by running the point of a hemostat between them; the hemostat is placed across the spermatic vessels near the testis, and the spermatic vessels are cut distal to the hemostat, leaving the testis attached to the ductus deferens. The two pedicles thus formed are securely knotted together; the testis, ductus, and vessels distal to the knot are amputated. The other testis is exposed through the same skin incision by cutting through the scrotal septum and is removed in a similar fashion (Mandelker, 1978). The scrotum is not sutured.

Many veterinarians prefer simply to free the spermatic cord and ligate it with 2-0 or 3-0 chromic gut, although this method is less economical in that suture material and instruments in addition to a simple scalpel blade are required. A simpler variant of this method has been described—knotting the spermatic cord on itself (Blake, 1969).

Postoperative infection is uncommon, but since the ideal of aseptic technique is not always assured, many veterinarians give a prophylactic injection of long-acting penicillin.

## Vasectomy

The only indication for vasectomy is to prepare teaser toms for catteries, to terminate estrus in female cats in which it is desired to postpone conception. The surgical approach is identical to that for the removal of cryptorchid testes. The spermatic cords are exposed and the vaginal tunics incised to expose the ductus deferens. A 1-cm segment of each duct is isolated from its accompanying artery and spermatic vessels, ligated, and removed. Closure is routine (Herron and Herron, 1972). Clients requesting this procedure must understand that it in no way alters the objectionable aspects of male cat behavior.

## Cryptorchidism

Cryptorchidism is common in cats. The majority of undescended testes lie in the inguinal area, where they may or may not be palpable, or just inside the inguinal ring.

The presence of masculine external genitalia is always confirmed before surgery. After routine preparation, a 6-cm incision is made on the midline, centered over the pubis. Inguinal fat is lifted to expose the inguinal ring, 1 cm lateral to the midline and 2 cm cranial to the pubis. If the spermatic cord is seen, it may be followed to the inguinal testis, which is then removed. If only the gubernaculum is seen, it is pulled caudally, as the inguinal ring is gently dilated with a hemostat, to withdraw the testis from the abdominal cavity. If neither structure is seen, the incision is extended cranially and the abdomen is entered on the midline. The bladder is exteriorized and reflected caudally, and the ductus deferens is traced from the ampulla of the prostate cranially to the testis (Noffsinger and Carbone, 1978). If this procedure fails to reveal the retained testis, the caudal abdomen should be thoroughly explored to the level of the kidneys. In a search for cryptorchid testes, a case of intersexuality with normal male external genitalia but an apparently female internal genital tract was discovered (Diegmann et al., 1978).

Fatal torsion of the bladder has been known to follow exploration for a cryptorchid testis—the median ligament having been torn and the bladder subsequently filling and rotating on the axis formed by the surviving urachal remnant. This disaster can be prevented by severing both the urachal remnant and the median ligament as already described for cystotomy.

## Phimosis

Kittens with phimosis are usually presented with a history of straining to urinate and dribbling urine. The prepuce is distended (Fig. 4–16*A*), and a tiny stream or bead of urine may be seen at the stenotic orifice. The perineum is prepared for aseptic surgery and the prepuce incised, care being taken to avoid the penis (Fig. 4–16*B*). The preputial mucosa is sutured to the skin with 5-0 surgical gut to achieve primary healing without scarring, and antibiotic ointment is instilled daily for a week. If the prepuce scars repeatedly or the mucosa is destroyed by infection, perineal urethrostomy may be necessary.

## Oophorohysterectomy (Spaying)

This is the most commonly performed abdominal surgery in the cat and warrants respect, for there is no greater disaster than when routine surgery performed in a young, healthy cat goes awry.

Most surgeons favor a midline approach. The entire abdomen is clipped and prepared for aseptic surgery. An

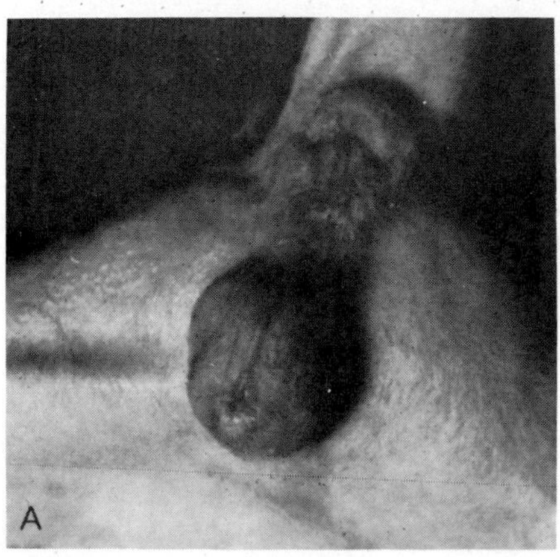


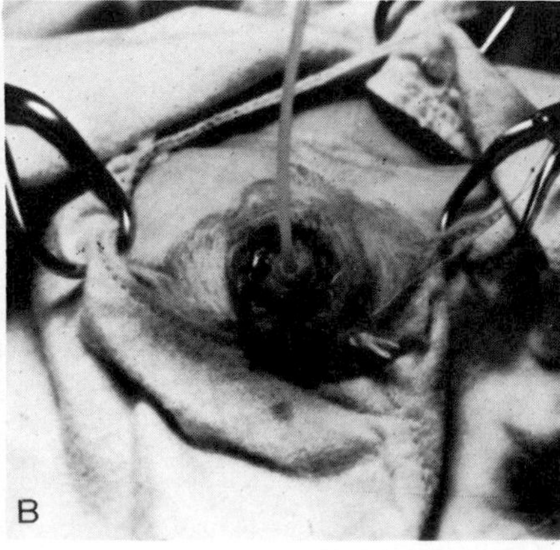


**Figure 4–16.** *A*, Phimosis in a kitten. The prepuce is distended with urine. *B*, The prepuce is incised on the midline, to expose a normal penis (catheterized). The preputial mucosa is then sutured to the skin.

incision of 2 or 3 cm is made on the midline, starting 2 cm caudal to the umbilicus, and deepened through the linea alba. A Snook hook is then introduced along the body wall opposite the surgeon, swept dorsally and medially along it, and gently lifted. The hook usually engages the broad ligament, and gentle traction on the ligament exposes the uterine horn. This is lifted and pulled caudally to expose the ovary, its vessels, and suspensory ligament. Gentle traction exposes 2 or 3 cm of mesovarium; it is rarely necessary to break the suspensory ligament. The mesometrium is perforated alongside the ovarian vessels, which are occluded with two mosquito forcepses. A third forceps is passed through the rent in the mesometrium and clamped across the proper ovarian ligament to control retrograde bleeding from the uterine vessels. The ovarian vessels are severed between the ovary and the first clamp, 1 mm of tissue being left above the clamp to avoid slippage. A ligature of 2-0 monofilament nylon or surgical gut is tied around the ovarian pedicle below the second clamp, and a second ligature is placed in the crushed area under the second clamp as it is removed. Some surgeons prefer to ligate the ovarian vessels before they are severed. The pedicle is slowly released and observed for hemorrhage.

The uterine horn is then reflected caudally to expose the uterine body and the other horn; if this is not possible without undue force, thé abdominal incision is extended caudad. The other horn is lifted and its ovarian pedicle managed like the first.

Next the uterine horns and their attached forcepses are reflected caudally to expose the uterine body, which is clamped and doubly ligated with 2-0 monofilament nylon and severed. If the uterine body is enlarged and turgid, as during estrus, or thinned, as in older cats that have had many litters, it should not be clamped, because the myometrium is friable and could break and slip out of the clamp. In such cases the uterine vessels are ligated separately before the uterine body is ligated. After the uterine pedicle is returned to the abdomen, the area is again inspected for hemorrhage before routine closure.

Pyometra and mucometra are managed similarly, but more generous exposure is required.

The flank approach for oophorohysterectomy, used by many with good results (e.g., Dorn, 1975; Krzaczynski, 1974), has the disadvantage of limited exposure but may be valuable when the surgeon desires to avoid the midline site, as in cats with massive mammary hyperplasia or extensive malignant tumor, and for some Caesarean sections (e.g., Stein, 1975).

In the technique of Schwartz (1982), the cat is placed on its left side with the forelimbs extended cranially and the hindlimbs caudally. The entire right side of the abdomen is prepared for aseptic surgery. After routine draping of the abdomen, a 2-cm dorsoventral skin incision is made at a point halfway between the dorsal and ventral midlines and between the last rib and the fold of the flank. Subcutaneous tissues are dissected bluntly to the level of the external abdominal oblique muscle. The surgeon bluntly separates the fibers on their long axes (first the external abdominal oblique muscle, running craniodorsad, and then the internal abdominal oblique muscle, running cranioventrad). A retractor is inserted to maintain this opening, while the transversus abdominis muscle and peritoneum are incised for a distance of about 1.5 cm in a dorsoventral direction. An Allis tissue forceps may be placed on the cranial edge of the transversus-peritoneum layer for retraction. Subsequently a spay hook is inserted carefully and moved dorsally to reach the right uterine horn. The latter and the right ovary are withdrawn through the incision and the ovarian pedicle clamped, ligated, and severed as for the ventral abdominal approach.

To expose the body of the uterus, the caudal aspect of the transversus-peritoneum layer is drawn caudad with a Senn retractor or spay hook while tension is applied first cranially and then laterally on the exposed right uterine horn. This usually allows exposure of the uterine body and the most caudal portion of the left uterine horn. The latter is then grasped and drawn from the body cavity, and the left ovarian pedicle is clamped, ligated, and severed. The body of the uterus and the associated uterine blood vessels are then clamped and ligated as described for the ventral approach. Some surgeons prefer to ligate the body of the uterus after the right ovarian pedicle, in order to exteriorize the left uterine horn properly (Dorn, 1975).

The abdomen is closed by suturing of the transversus abdominis–peritoneum layer with one or two 3-0 catgut sutures in a simple interrupted pattern. The external abdominal oblique muscle is then sutured similarly, and the skin is closed with nonabsorbable sutures.

The flank approach has both advantages and disadvantages (Dorn, 1975; Krzaczynski, 1974). By separating rather than severing the muscles of the abdominal wall, both hemorrhage and tissue trauma are minimized. The right side is preferred to the left because of the more cranial location of the right ovary, which may be difficult to reach from a left-sided incision. The presence of the omentum over the viscera on the left side and the left-sided location of the spleen (which may be enlarged if barbiturates are administered) also make the right side a more practical approach. Flank incisions are fast and carry a very low incidence of wound dehiscence.

Disadvantages include limited exposure of the abdomen, more difficulty in controlling hemorrhage arising from the left ovarian pedicle if the ligature slips from the latter, and inadequate exposure in the case of ovarian or uterine disease, such as pyometra or neoplasia. It must be noted, however, that by incising the external and internal abdominal oblique muscles, rather than separating the fibers, a rather substantial incision may be made in the flank allowing adequate exposure in such cases. Should there be hemorrhage secondary to slippage of a left ovarian pedicle ligature, it may be necessary to do a left flank incision to retrieve it (Dorn, 1975). Rarely hair at the surgical site may grow back in a different color (Dorn, 1975).

Under no circumstances should a veterinarian accede to an owner's request to "tie the tubes" in lieu of oophorohysterectomy. Although the procedure prevents pregnancy, it does not prevent recurrent or constant heat and predisposes to ovarian and uterine disease.

Congenital anomalies are occasionally encountered during routine oophorohysterectomy (Todoroff, 1979), most often aplasia or hypoplasia of a uterine horn, which may be associated with aplasia of the kidney on the same side (e.g., Robinson, 1965). The ovary is usually present in such cases and must be removed.

Complications of spaying are common, but most are minor. A survey of 476 cats undergoing elective abdominal oophorohystererctomy at a teaching institution yielded the following incidences: delayed healing or incisional swelling, 45 per cent; self-trauma or licking at sutures, 43 per cent; seroma, 6 per cent; intraoperative hemorrhage, 4 per cent; nonfatal anesthetic complications, 3 per cent; incisional hernia, postoperative hematuria, vaginal hemorrhage, recurrent estrus, uterine stump infection, and endocrinopathy, 1 per cent or less (Berzon, 1979). Most of these were minor problems related to rough tissue handling by inexperienced surgeons, but intraoperative hemorrhage is life-threatening. If such bleeding occurs, the incision is immediately lengthened. The ovarian pedicles are exposed for inspection by retraction of the viscera with the mesoduodenum and then the mesocolon. The uterine pedicle is exposed by exteriorizing the bladder and reflecting it caudally. The offending vessel is ligated and all other pedicles re-examined.

Recurrent estrus is invariably caused by a remnant of ovarian tissue. Exploratory laparotomy with exposure of both pedicles as already described is necessary to identify and remove the offending remnant.

A case of primary abdominal pregnancy, probably the result of dislodged fertile ova, was encountered in a cat 18 months after oophorohysterectomy (Carrig et al., 1972).

Although many cats are spayed when in heat or even when pregnant, it is preferable to spay in anestrus, when the tissues are less turgid. Since heat periods are of unpredictable occurrence once they start, a good case can be made for spaying before the first heat. It is also a safety precaution, for a sheltered indoor cat that escapes from home during one of its first heats runs a high risk of injury or of getting lost.

Spaying should be strongly urged for all but breeders' females. Unspayed cats not mated and cycling repeatedly till old age may be predisposed to endometritis, pyometra, and tumors of the ovaries, uterus, and mammary glands.

## Caesarean Section

This operation is performed as in the dog. When a cat with dystocia is presented, the owner should be offered the option of spaying, unless a breeding queen is involved. Provided that milk is already present in the mammary glands, spaying does not usually interfere with lactation.

## Uterine Prolapse

This rare but dramatic sequel to parturition is easily recognized. The prolapse should be reduced with gentle application of cold or hypertonic solutions and lubrication, and oophorohysterectomy done when the cat's condition permits. Simple amputation of the prolapsed organ does not remove the ovaries, which are excised by an abdominal approach (Egger, 1978; Leighton, 1975).

## Mastectomy

Several conditions affecting the mammary glands may require surgery. Feline mammary fibroepithelial hyperplasia (hypertrophy, "fibroadenoma") occasionally involves one, several, or all glands and may reach tremendous proportions. (e.g., Allen, 1973; Bloom, 1954). The affected glands are usually large, often painless, and rubbery in consistency owing to ductal proliferation and edema. Most cats are less than a year old and in or just past estrus. The masses slowly regress spontaneously or within eight weeks of oophorohysterectomy. An identical or very similar lesion occasionally follows oral administration of progestogens such as megestrol acetate to older cats of either sex (Hinton and Gaskell, 1977). (See also the chapter on tumors.)

The condition in young unbred females is so characteristic in appearance and sudden onset that it should not be mistaken for tumor. Approaches to treatment vary. Mastectomy should be limited to cases with ulceration or abscesses. In some cats immediate spaying has been performed to terminate the hormonal stimulation. Sudden death from pulmonary embolism has occurred in severely affected cats, both untreated and shortly after spaying (e.g., at the Angell Memorial Hospital). Since fibrin thrombi may be a prominent feature in the hyperplastic and edematous tissue and overlying skin, it has been suggested that the manipulation of the tissue during surgery may predispose to embolization. Since the condition tends to recur with successive heats, oophorectomy is the ultimate solution, but unless performed by the flank approach should be delayed until the mammary hyperplasia is reduced (Stein, 1975). Measures suggested for the purpose are repeated cold applications, reduced food and water intake, and a diuretic or corticosteroid (Harvey, 1981; Stein, 1975). Repositol testosterone gives variable results (Stein, 1975).

Because the hyperplasia induced in neutered cats by administration of progestogens occasionally progresses to cancer, some surgeons prefer to perform a biopsy or remove involved glands without awaiting regression.

Mammary tumors are the third most common neoplasm in the female cat, and 86 per cent are malignant. In two-thirds of the cats in one series multiple glands were involved, with both chains affected in a third (Hayes, 1977). In the absence of metastasis this surgeon's preferred treatment is wide excision of the entire affected chain with its draining axillary and inguinal lymph nodes. Some surgeons (e.g., Harvey, 1981) remove the axillary nodes only if they are firm or fixed to surrounding tissue. If both chains of glands are involved, the second is removed four weeks later; simultaneous bilateral mastectomy does not, in my opinion, permit a wide enough excision. The entire chest and abdomen well up the side of the cat are clipped and prepared for surgery. The skin incision, an ellipse, extends from the axilla to the groin, from the midline medially to at least 1 cm lateral to any recognizable mammary tissue. Subcutaneous tissue is removed down to the pectoral muscles cranially and fascia caudally, and cranial and caudal superficial epigastric vessels are isolated and ligated before they are severed. Any fascia or muscle attached to the tumor is included in the resection. Some surgeons (e.g., Harvey, 1981) flush the wound copiously with sterile saline solution in the belief that an important cause of recurrence of otherwise adequately excised tumors is viable exfoliated malignant cells that grow in the wound bed. Subcutaneous tissue is closed with 3-0 gut in a simple interrupted pattern, and the skin is closed in a routine manner. Drains are rarely needed except in very obese cats.

The prognosis is guarded to poor; over half the cats thus treated suffer recurrence at a median of five and a half months after surgery; monthly re-evaluation is recommended (Hayes, 1977).

Because glands that appear grossly normal sometimes prove on microscopic examination to have foci of cancer cells, some surgeons prefer to remove both chains together with the inguinal nodes and to do so in a single-stage procedure to lessen anesthetic and surgical immunosuppression. With bilateral excision, inguinal drains are routinely used.

If a cat is to be spayed at the same time mastectomy is done, the spay should be performed first and the skin incision then extended to form the ellipse around the breasts (Harvey, 1981). If the midline incision site is involved with tumor, the spay should be performed by the flank approach.

## REFERENCES


Ader PL, Boothe HW: Ventral bulla osteotomy in the cat. J Am Anim Hosp Assoc 15 (1979) 757–762.

Alexander JW, Hoffer RE: Pinch grafting in the dog. Canine Pract 3(1) (1976) 27–30.

Alexander JW, Hoffer RE, MacDonald JM: The use of tubular flap grafts in the treatment of traumatic wounds on the extremity of the cat. Feline Pract 6(3) (1976) 29–32.

Allen HL: Feline mammary hypertrophy. Vet Pathol 10 (1973) 501–508.

Arnall L: Repair of an extensive brachial skin slough by a cervical pedicle flap graft. J Small Anim Pract 1 (1960) 286–290.

Ashton DG: Perineal hernia in the cat—a description of two cases. J Small Anim Pract 17 (1976) 473–477.

Bachrach A, Kleine LJ: "What is your diagnosis?" [patent persistent urachus]. J Am Vet Med Assoc 165 (1974) 1099–1100.

Baker GJ: Nasal surgery in the dog and cat. Vet Annu 14 (1973) 129–133.

Barnes JW, Bone JK: Urethrocolostomy of the cat. Small Anim Clin 3 (1963) 31–32.

Barsanti JA, Higgins RJ, Spano JS, Jones BD: Adenocarcinoma of the extrahepatic bile duct in a cat. J Small Anim Pract 17 (1976) 599–605.

Beamer RJ: Ureterocolostomy for relief of urinary stenosis in the domestic cat. J Am Vet Med Assoc 134 (1959) 201–204.

Bebko RL, Prier JE, Biery DN: Ectopic ureters in a male cat. J Am Vet Med Assoc 171 (1977) 738–740.

Berzon JL: Complications of elective ovariohysterectomies in the dog and cat at a teaching institution: Clinical review of 853 cases. Vet Surg 8 (1979) 89–91.

Biewinga WJ: Preputial urethroplasty for relief of urethral obstruction in the male cat. J Am Vet Med Assoc 166 (1975) 460–462.

Biewinga WJ, Rothuizen J, Voorhout G: Ectopic ureters in the cat—a report of two cases. J Small Anim Pract 19 (1978) 531–537.

Birchard SJ, Peterson ME, Jacobson A: Surgical treatment of feline hyperthyroidism: results of 85 cases. J Am Anim Hosp Assoc 20 (1984) 705–709.

Bistner SI, Aguirre G, Batik G: Atlas of Veterinary Ophthalmic Surgery. Philadelphia, WB Saunders Company, 1977.

Blake JA: Perineal urethrostomy in cats. J Am Vet Med Assoc 152 (1968) 1499–1506.

Blake JA: A technique for castrating cats. J Am Vet Med Assoc 154 (1969) 25.

Bloom F: Pathology of the Dog and Cat: The Genitourinary System, with Clinical Considerations. Evanston, Illinois, American Veterinary Publications, 1954.

Bohning RH, DeHoff WD, McElhinney A, Hofstra PC: Pharyngostomy for maintenance of the anorectic animal. J Am Vet Med Assoc 156 (1970) 611–615.

Bohonowych RO, Parks JL, Greene RW: Features of cystic calculi in cats in a hospital population. J Am Vet Med Assoc 173 (1978) 301–303.

Bojrab MJ (ed): Current Techniques in Small Animal Surgery. Philadelphia, Lea & Febiger, 1975.

Burk RL, Meierhenry EF, Schaubhut CW: Leiomyosarcoma of the urinary bladder in a cat. J Am Vet Med Assoc 167 (1975) 749–751.

Burke TJ, Froehlich PS, Chambers JN: Congenital esophageal disease in two kittens. Feline Pract 8(6) (1978) 18–27.

Carbone MG: Perineal urethrostomy to relieve urethral obstruction in the male cat. J Am Vet Med Assoc 143 (1963) 34–39

Carbone MG: Perineal urethrostomy in the male cat. A report on 20 cases. J Am Vet Med Assoc 146 (1965) 843–853.

Carbone MG: A modified technique for perineal urethrostomy in the male cat. J Am Vet Med Assoc 151 (1967) 301–305.

Carpenter JL: Sinusitis. *In* Kirk RW (ed): Current Veterinary Therapy V. Philadelphia, WB Saunders Company, 1974.

Carrig CB, Gourley IM, Philbrick AL: Primary abdominal pregnancy in a cat subsequent to ovariohysterectomy. J Am Vet Med Assoc 160 (1972) 308–310.

Cawley AJ, Francis SM: Pedicle graft in a dog. A case report. Cornell Vet 48 (1958) 12–16.

Chabot JF, Weaver RA: Unilateral ventriculochordectomy in the cat. Anim Hosp 2 (1966) 120–121.

Chastain CB, Grier RL: Bilateral retroperitoneal perirenal cysts in a cat. Feline Pract 5(4) (1975) 51–53.

Christensen NR: Preputial urethrostomy in the male cat. J Am Vet Med Assoc 145 (1964) 903–908.

Clifford DH, Soifer FK, Wilson CF, Waddell ED, Guilloud GL: Congenital achalasia of the esophagus in four cats of common ancestry. J Am Vet Med Assoc 158 (1971) 1554–1560.

Cohen JS, Tilley LP, Liu SK, DeHoff WD: Patent ductus arteriosus in five cats. J Am Anim Hosp Assoc 11 (1975) 95–101.

Confer AW, Langloss JM: Long-term survival of two cats with mastocytosis. J Am Vet Med Assoc 172 (1978) 160–161.

Converse JM: Reconstructive Plastic Surgery. Philadelphia, WB Saunders Company, 1977, Vol I.

Cook WR: Observations on the upper respiratory tract of the dog and cat. J Small Anim Pract 5 (1964) 309–329.

Crane SW: Surgical management of feline pyothorax. Feline Pract 6(2) (1976) 13–19.

Creed RFS: The histology of mammalian skin, with special reference to the dog and cat. Vet Rec 70 (1958) 171–175.

Creighton SR, Wilkins RJ: Thoracic effusions in the cat. J Am Anim Hosp Assoc 11 (1975) 66–76.

Creighton SR, Wilkins RJ: Pleural effusions. *In* Kirk RW (ed): Current Veterinary Therapy VII. Philadelphia, WB Saunders Company, 1980.

Crouch JE: Text-Atlas of Cat Anatomy. Philadelphia, Lea & Febiger, 1969.

Crowe DT: Closure of abdominal incisions using a continuous polypropylene suture: Clinical experience in 550 dogs and cats. Vet Surg 7 (1978) 74–77.

DeHoff WD, Nelson AW, Lumb WN: Simple interrupted approximating technique for intestinal anastomosis. J Am Anim Hosp Assoc 9 (1973) 483–489.

Delmage DA: Some conditions of the nasal chambers of the dog and cat. Vet Rec 92 (1973) 437–442.

Diegmann FG, Loo BJ, Grom PA: Female pseudohermaphroditism in a cat. Feline Pract 8(5) (1978) 45.

Dill GS, McElyea U, Stookey JL: Transitional cell carcinoma of the urinary bladder in a cat. J Am Vet Med Assoc 160 (1972) 743–745.

Dorn AS: Ovariohystererctomy by the flank approach. Vet Small Anim Clin 70 (1975) 569–573.

Dorn AS, Harris SG, Olmstead ML: Squamous cell carcinoma of the urinary bladder in a cat. Feline Pract 8(5) (1978) 14–17.

Egger EL: Uterine prolapse in a cat. Feline Pract 8(1) (1978) 34–37.

Eyster GE, Evans AT, O'Handley P, Steffes J: Surgical removal of a foreign body from the tracheal bifurcation of a cat. J Am Anim Hosp Assoc 12 (1976) 481–483.
Farrow CS: Surgical treatment of lower-lip avulsion in the cat. Vet Med Small Anim Clin 68 (1973) 1418–1419.
Field HE, Taylor ME: An Atlas of Cat Anatomy. Chicago, University of Chicago Press, 1974.
Ford RB, Walshaw R: Feline upper respiratory disease. *In* Kirk RW (ed): Current Veterinary Therapy VII. Philadelphia, WB Saunders Company, 1980.
Furneaux RW: Obstructive jaundice in a cat. Feline Pract 4(1) (1974a) 9–14.
Furneaux RW: Abdominal wall reconstruction in a cat. Feline Pract 4(4) (1974b) 28–32.
Furneaux RW, Hudson MD: Autogenous muscle flap repair of a diaphragmatic hernia. Feline Pract 6(1) (1976) 20–24.
Furneaux RW, Pharr JW, McManus JL: Arteriovenous fistulation following declaw removal in a cat. J Am Anim Hosp Assoc 10 (1974) 569–573.
Gilbert SG: Pictorial Anatomy of the Cat. Seattle, University of Washington Press, 1977.
Grabb WC, Myers MB: Skin Flaps. Boston, Little, Brown and Company, 1975.
Grabb WC, Smith JW: Plastic Surgery. Boston, Little, Brown and Company, 1973.
Graber ER: Diagnosis and treatment of a ruptured thoracic duct in the cat. J Am Vet Med Assoc 146 (1965) 242–245.
Greene RW, Bohning RH: Patent persistent urachus associated with urolithiasis in a cat. J Am Vet Med Assoc 158 (1971) 489–491.
Guerre R, Millet R, Groulade P: Systemic mastocytosis in a cat: remission after splenectomy. J Small Anim Pract 20 (1979) 769–772.
Habel RE: Applied Veterinary Anatomy, ed 2. Ithaca, New York, RE Habel, 1978.
Hanselka DV, Boyd CL: Use of mesh grafts in dogs and horses. J Am Anim Hosp Assoc 12 (1976) 650–653.
Hansen JS: Urachal remnant in the cat: occurrence and relationship to the feline urological syndrome. Vet Med Small Anim Clin 72 (1977) 1735–1746.
Harpster NK: Feline cardiomyopathy. Vet Clin North Am 7 (1977) 355–371.
Hart BL, Barrett RE: Effects of castration on fighting, roaming, and urine spraying in adult male cats. J Am Vet Med Assoc 163 (1973) 290–292.
Harvey CE: Parotid salivary duct rupture and fistula in the dog and cat. J Small Anim Pract 18 (1977) 163–168.
Harvey CE, Goldschmidt MH: Inflammatory polypoid growths in the ear canal of cats. J Small Anim Pract 19 (1978) 669–677.
Harvey CE, O'Brien JA: Management of respiratory emergencies in small animals. Vet Clin North Am 2 (1972) 252–254.
Harvey HJ: Personal communication to J Holzworth, 1981.
Hayes A: Feline mammary gland tumors. Vet Clin North Am 7 (1977) 205–212.
Herron MA: A potential consequence of prepuberal feline castration. Feline Pract 1 (1) (1971) 17–19.
Herron MA: The effect of prepubertal castration on the penile urethra of the cat. J Am Vet Med Assoc 160 (1972) 208–211.
Herron MA, Herron MR: Vasectomy in the cat. Mod Vet Pract 53 (6) (1972) 41–43.
Hinton M, Gaskell CJ: Non-neoplastic mammary hypertrophy in the cat associated either with pregnancy or with oral progestagen therapy. Vet Rec 100 (1977) 277–280.
Hoffer RE, Alexander JW: Pinch grafting. J Am Anim Hosp Assoc 12 (1976) 644–647.
Holzworth J: Personal communication, 1980.
Holzworth J, Gilmore CE: Jaundice in cats. Proc Am Anim Hosp Assoc (1969) 109–110.
Holzworth J, Theran P, Carpenter JL, Harpster NK, Todoroff RJ: Hyperthyroidism in the cat: ten cases. J Am Vet Med Assoc 176 (1980) 345–353
Howard DR, Davis DG, Merkley DF, Krahwinkel DJ, Schirmer RG, Brinker WO: Mucoperiosteal flap technique for cleft palate repair in dogs. J Am Vet Med Assoc 165 (1974) 352–354.
Howard DR, Lammerding JL, Bloomberg MS: Principles of pedicle flaps and grafting techniques. J Am Anim Hosp Assoc 12 (1976) 573–575.
Hunt TK, Dunphy JE: Fundamentals of Wound Management. New York, Appleton-Century-Crofts, 1979.
Jensen EC: Skin grafting in the dog. Iowa State Coll Vet 3 (1957) 163–169.
Jensen EC: Canine autogenous skin grafting. Am J Vet Res 20 (1959) 898–908.
Jeraj K, Ogburn P, Lord PF, Wilson JW: Patent ductus with pulmonary hypertension in a cat. J Am Vet Med Assoc 172 (1978) 1432–1436.
Johnston DE: Feline urethrostomy—a critique and new method. J Small Anim Pract 15 (1974) 1–15.
Johnston DE: The repair of skin loss on the foot by means of a double-pedicle abdominal flap. J Am Anim Hosp Assoc 12 (1976) 593–596.
Johnston DE: The processes in wound healing. J Am Anim Hosp Assoc 13 (1977) 186–196.
Johnston DE: The healing processes in open skin wounds. Compend Contin Ed 1 (1979) 789–795.
Jones CL, Buchanan JW: Patent ductus arteriosus: Anatomy and surgery in a cat: J Am Vet Med Assoc 179 (1981) 364–369.
Keefe F: Skin grafting in a cat. J Am Vet Med Assoc 108 (1946) 43–48.
Knecht CD: Persistent right aortic arch with rotation of the vena cava. Anim Hosp 3 (1967) 243–247.
Krahwinkel DJ: Reconstruction of skin defects by the use of pedicle grafts. J Am Anim Hosp Assoc 12 (1976) 844–846.
Krzaczynski J: The flank approach to feline ovariohysterectomy. Vet Med Small Anim Clin 69 (1974) 572–574.
Lane JG, Orr CM, Lucke VM, Gruffyd-Jones TJ: Nasopharyngeal polyps arising in the middle ear of the cat. J Small Anim Pract 22 (1981) 511–522.
Leighton RL: Trephining the frontal sinus in the cat. Mod Vet Pract 39(8) (1958) 44–45.
Leighton RL: Symphysectomy in the cat and use of a steel insert to increase pelvic diameter. J Small Anim Pract 10 (1969) 355–356.
Leighton RL: Surgical procedures. *In* Catcott EJ (ed): Feline Medicine and Surgery, 2nd ed. Santa Barbara, American Veterinary Publications Inc, 1975.
Leighton RL: Perineal hernia in a cat. Feline Pract 9 (1) (1979) 44.
Leighton RL, Grain E: Partial colectomy for the treatment of feline megacolon. Feline Pract 8(3) (1978) 31–33.
Leighton RL, Steffey EP: Successful management and repair of a diaphragmatic hernia in a cat. Feline Pract 2 (2) (1972) 40–43.
Lindsay FEF: Chylothorax in the domestic cat—a review. J Small Anim Pract 15 (1974) 241–258.
Lipowitz AJ, Schenck MP: Surgical approaches to the abdominal and thoracic viscera. Vet Clin North Am 9 (1979) 169–194.
Liska WD, MacEwen EG, Zaki FA, Garvey M: Feline systemic mastocytosis: a review and results of splenectomy in seven cases. J Am Anim Hosp Assoc 15 (1979) 589–597.
Long RD: A technique for perineal urethrostomy in the cat. J Small Anim Pract 18 (1977) 407–413.
Long RD: A technique for perineal urethrostomy in the cat. Feline Pract 9(1) (1979) 27–31.
Mandelker L: A sterile surgical procedure for feline castration. Vet Med Small Anim Clin 73 (1978) 904–906.
Manziano CF, Manziano JR: A bladder prosthesis to relieve urethral blockage in the male cat. J Am Vet Med Assoc 151 (1967) 218–222.

McClure RC, Dallman MJ, Garrett PD: Cat Anatomy. Philadelphia, Lea & Febiger, 1973.

McCully RM: Antepubic urethrostomy for the relief of recurrent urethral obstruction in the male cat. J Am Vet Med Assoc 126 (1955) 173–179.

McCurnin DM, Seeli DE: Surgical treatment of aortic embolism in a cat. Vet Med Small Anim Clin 67 (1972) 387–390.

Meijer JC, Lubberink AAME, Gruys E: Cushing's syndrome due to adrenocortical adenoma in a cat. Tijdschr Diergeneeskd 103 (1978) 1048–1051.

Mendham JH: A description and evaluation of antepubic urethrostomy in the male cat. J Small Anim Pract 11 (1970) 709–721.

Muller GH: Basal cell epithelioma and squamous cell carcinoma in animals. Arch Dermatol 96 (1967) 386–390.

Nayar SR, Wilson FD: Experimental studies on urinary diversions in canines and felines. Indian Vet J 51 (1974) 545–553.

Noffsinger GR, Carbone MG: Nonabdominal approach to castration of the cryptorchid cat. J Am Vet Med Assoc 173 (1978) 303–304.

O'Brien TR, Mitchum GD: Cholelithiasis in a cat. J Am Vet Med Assoc 156 (1970) 1015–1017.

Osborne CA: Clinical evaluation of needle biopsy of the kidney and its complications in the dog and cat. J Am Vet Med Assoc 158 (1971) 1213–1228.

Patnaik AK, Greene RW: Intravenous leiomyoma of the bladder in a cat. J Am Vet Med Assoc 175 (1979) 381–383.

Patterson DF, Munson TO: Traumatic chylothorax treated by ligation of the thoracic duct. J Am Vet Med Assoc 133 (1958) 452–458.

Pavletic MM: The vascular supply to the skin of the dog. Vet Surg 9 (1980a) 77–80.

Pavletic MM: Caudal superficial epigastric arterial pedicle grafts in the dog. Vet Surg 9 (1980b) 103–107.

Pavletic MM: Canine axial pattern flaps utilizing the omocervical, thoracodorsal, and deep circumflex iliac direct cutaneous arteries. Am J Vet Res 42 (1981) 391–406.

Peiffer RL, Stickle JE: Traumatic lateral hernia and diaphragmatic tear in a kitten. Feline Pract 5 (3)(1975) 27–29.

Piedrahita P, Butterfield WC: Abdominal exploration as a diagnostic procedure. Am Surg 131 (1976) 181–184.

Proud AJ: Frontal sinuses and rhinitis in the cat [corresp]. Vet Rec 95 (1974) 426.

Quigley PT, Voight RP: Skin transplantation in two cats. Vet Rec 98 (1976) 52–53.

Reed JH, Bonasch H: Surgical correction of a persistent right aortic arch in a cat. J Am Med Assoc 40 (1962) 142–144.

Rickards DA: The feline urethral shunt technique. Feline Pract 6 (4)(1976) 48–53.

Rickards DA, Hinko PJ, Morse EM: Feline perineal urethrostomy—a new techinque for an old problem. J Am Anim Hosp Assoc 8 (1972) 66–73.

Rickards DA, Hinko PJ: Feline perineal urethrostomy: "The Cleveland technique." Feline Pract 4 (2) (1974) 41–48.

Robinette JD: A silicone rubber prosthesis for replacement of the urethra in male cats. J Am Vet Med Assoc 163 (1973) 285–289.

Robinson GW: Uterus unicornis and unilateral renal agenesis in a cat. J Am Vet Med Assoc 147 (1965) 516–518.

Ross GE: Clinical canine skin grafting. J Am Vet Med Assoc 153 (1968) 1759–1765.

Schilling JA: Wound healing. Surg Clin North Am 56 (1976) 859–874.

Schwartz A: Personal communication to J Holzworth, 1982.

Scott DW: Feline dermatology 1900–1978: a monograph. J Am Anim Hosp Assoc 16 (1980) 331–459.

Self RA: Skin grafting in canine practice. J Am Vet Med Assoc 84 (1934) 163–167.

Sherding RG: Pyothorax in the cat. Compend Contin Ed 1 (1979) 247–252.

Sinibaldi KR: Cleft palate. Vet Clin North Am 9 (1979) 245–257.

Slocum B, Colgrove DJ, Carrig CB, Suter PF: Acquired arteriovenous fistula in two cats. J Am Vet Med Assoc 162 (1973) 271–276.

Smith CW, Schiller AG: Perineal urethrostomy in the cat: a retrospective study of complications. J Am Anim Hosp Assoc 14 (1978) 225–228.

Spreull JSA: Surgery of the nasal cavity of the dog and cat. Vet Rec 75 (1963) 105–113.

Spreull JSA: The principles of transplanted skin in the dog. J Am Anim Hosp Assoc 4 (1968) 71–84.

Startup CM: Trephining the frontal sinus in the cat. Vet Rec 75 (1963) 752–754.

Stein BS: The genital system. *In* Catcott EJ (ed): Feline Medicine and Surgery, 2nd ed. Santa Barbara, American Veterinary Publications Inc, 1975.

Stone EA, Rawlings CA, Prasse KW, Duncan JR: Intraoperative biopsy and microscopy during exploratory laparotomies. Vet Surg 7 (1978) 93–96.

Strickland JH, Calhoun LM: The integumentary system of the cat. Am J Vet Res 24 (1963) 1018–1029.

Sumner-Smith G, Eger C: The respiratory system. *In* Catcott EJ (ed): Feline Medicine and Surgery, 2nd ed. Santa Barbara, American Veterinary Publications Inc, 1975.

Swaim SF: Surgery of Traumatized Skin: Management and Reconstruction in the Dog and Cat. Philadelphia, WB Saunders Company, 1980.

Swaim SF, Bushby PA: Principles of bipedicle tube grafting in the dog. J Am Anim Hosp Assoc 12(1976) 600–603.

Swaim SF, Henderson RA, Sutton HH: Correction of triangular and wedge shaped skin defects in dogs and cats. J Am Anim Hosp Assoc 16 (1980) 225–232.

Todoroff RJ: Congenital urogenital anomalies. Compend Contin Ed 1 (1979) 780–787.

Tomlinson MJ, Schenck NL: Autogenous fat implantation as a treatment for chronic frontal sinusitis in a cat. J Am Vet Med Assoc 167 (1975) 927–930.

Wallace AB, Spreull JSA, Hamilton HA: The use of autogenous free full thickness skin graft in the treatment of a chronic inflammatory lesion in a dog. Vet Rec 74 (1962) 286–289.

Warren R: Surgery. Philadelphia, WB Saunders Company, 1963.

Whitehead JE: Urolithiasis in the feline. Small Anim Clin 1 (1961) 307–319.

Wigderson FJ: Cholelithiasis in a cat. J Am Vet Med Assoc 126 (1955) 287.

Wildt DE, Kinney GM, Seager SWJ: Laparoscopy for direct observation of internal organs of the domestic cat and dog. Am J Vet Res 38 (1977) 1429–1432.

Wilson GP, Harrison JW: Perineal urethrostomy in cats. J Am Vet Med Assoc 159 (1971) 1789–1793.

Wilson GP, Newton CD, Burt JK: A review of 116 diaphragmatic hernias in dogs and cats. J Am Vet Med Assoc 159 (1971) 1142–1145.

Winstanley EW: Trephining frontal sinuses in the treatment of rhinitis and sinusitis in the cat. Vet Rec 95 (1974) 289–292.

Withrow SJ, Black AP: Generalized peritonitis in small animals. Vet Clin North Am 9 (1979) 363–379.

Withrow SJ, Fenner WR, Wilkins RJ: Closed chest drainage and lavage for treatment of pyothorax in the cat. J Am Anim Hosp Assoc 11 (1975) 90–94.

Yoder JT, Dragstedt LR, Starch CJ: Partial colectomy for correction of megacolon in a cat. Vet Med Small Anim Clin 63 (1968) 1049–1052.

Yturraspe DJ, Creed JE, Schwoch RP: Thoracic pedicle skin flap for repair of lower limb wounds in dogs and cats. J Am Anim Hosp Assoc 12 (1976) 581–587.

# 5
CHAPTER

# ORTHOPEDIC SURGERY

ROBERT L. LEIGHTON and GORDON W. ROBINSON

## GENERAL PRINCIPLES OF FELINE ORTHOPEDICS

The cat is a wonderful orthopedic patient. It responds to injury by retiring to a safe place and remaining inactive until well. This trait, together with a remarkable innate ability to heal, encourages solid union among even widely separated bone fragments.

The cat has no consistently well-defined gait, moving with graceful ease from a slow crouching walk, to a trot, to bursts of high-speed running, all commensurate with its role as a patient hunter, stealthy stalker, and sudden attacker. It is capable of adapting to and concealing considerable joint and bone deformities that would be instantly observable in the dog. Joints that have been surgically invaded or rigidly pinned for weeks or months usually return to function in three weeks or so with minimal evidence of arthritic changes.

In general:

1. The simplest effective method of repair is best.
2. Many simple fractures, such as those of the digits, metacarpals, and metatarsals, as well as uncomplicated pelvic fractures respond well to cage confinement for two to four weeks.
3. Plaster casts and Schroeder-Thomas splints should be avoided, as they are heavy and unwieldy for the cat, frequently soiled, and difficult to maintain.
4. Bone plating may present difficulties because the thin cortices of the long bones offer very little purchase for the screw threads.
5. Cerclage wiring is very effective. The wire must be single-strand orthopedic wire, usually 20- to 22-gauge, and effectively tightened and secured. Several wires should be used to ensure stability.
6. With a round intramedullary pin, the largest possible diameter should be used to ensure fixation and control rotation, and the pin should be seated as deeply and securely as possible.
7. Indications for surgical repair increase with the degree of fragment displacement, but very severely comminuted fractures often do better with conservative care.
8. Contaminated and infected fractures can be managed by thorough débridement and use of local and systemic antibiotics. Immobilization is the prime concern, since healing can take place in the face of infection but not where there is motion.

Cats appear to have more fractures of the pelvis and mandible and relatively fewer of the radius and ulna than dogs. An English survey of 298 fractures in 285 cats showed femur 28.2 per cent, pelvis 24 per cent, mandible 11.4 per cent, tibia 5.8 per cent, and all others 29.8 per cent (Phillips, 1979). Other surveys report similar percentages (Hill, 1977).

## SPECIAL INSTRUMENTATION

In addition to the standard orthopedic instruments, such as an intramedullary pin drill with Jacob's chuck, Steinmann (intramedullary) pins, Kirschner wires, orthopedic wire, wire scissors, wire tightener, small wire guide, and a pin cutter, some special instruments may be very useful:

- Small bone reduction forceps with points*
- Small pin guide†
- Kirschner (K) wire vise for inserting K wire
- Small intramedullary pins (1/16 inch) used as drills for orthopedic wiring
- Lever-action K-wire cutter†
- Rush pins of 1/16-inch diameter in 1/2-inch increments in lengths from two to four inches†

In the cat the Rush pin is inserted in an introduction hole made with a 1/16-inch intramedullary pin and is driven in with a wire-holding forceps or Smillie pin extractor.‡ The latter two instruments may also be used to remove Rush pins and K wires (Fig. 5–1).

*Synthes Ltd. (USA), Wayne, PA 19087.
†Kirschner, Aberdeen, MD 21601.
‡Richards Manufacturing Company, Memphis, TN 38116.

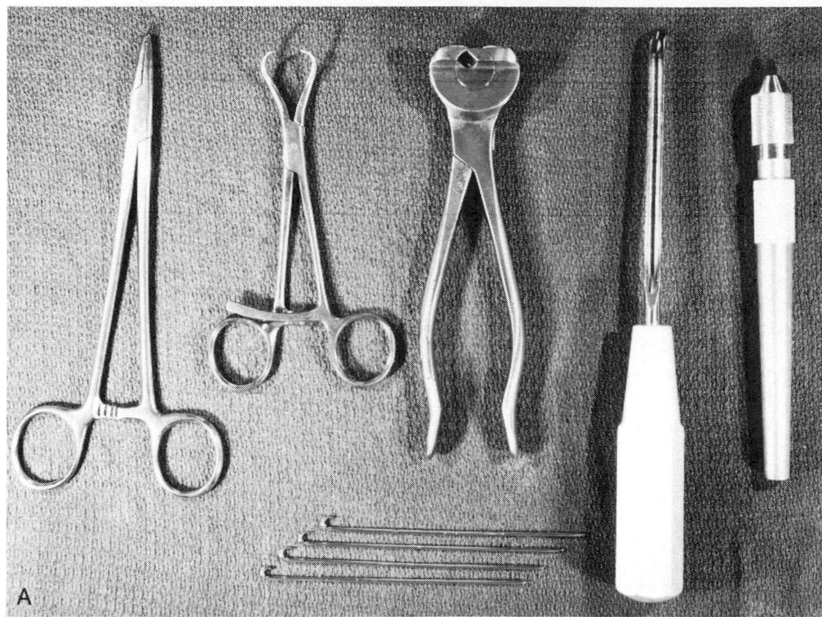


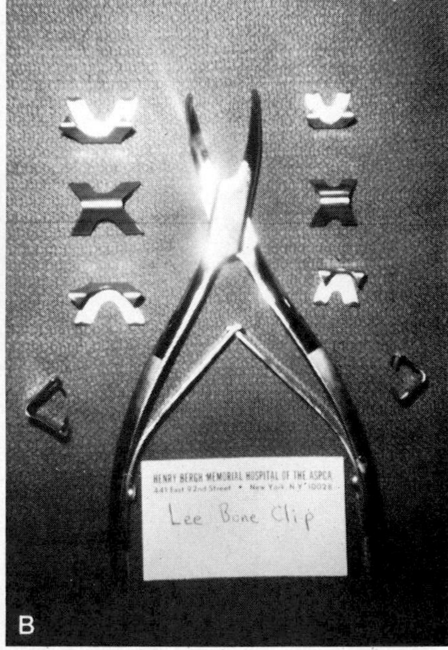


**Figure 5–1** Special orthopedic instruments: *A* (left to right), Wire twister, small bone-reduction forceps with points, K wire cutter, pin guide, K wire vise, and Rush pins. *B,* Lee bone clip.

## CAUTIONS IN THE MANAGEMENT OF ACUTE TRAUMA IN THE CAT

Cats with fractures have usually been involved in a severe traumatic episode. Unlike small dogs, they rarely sustain fractures from minor events, such as falling from the owner's arms or jumping from furniture. In urban areas many fractures result from falls from the windows of high-rise apartment buildings (Robinson, 1976). In suburban and rural areas they most often occur when the cat is struck by a car (Phillips, 1979).

It is essential to look for concomitant injuries, particularly pneumothorax (Fig. 5–2), and rupture of abdominal viscera, especially of the bladder. Observation of the cat for one to two days will allow physiologic stabilization

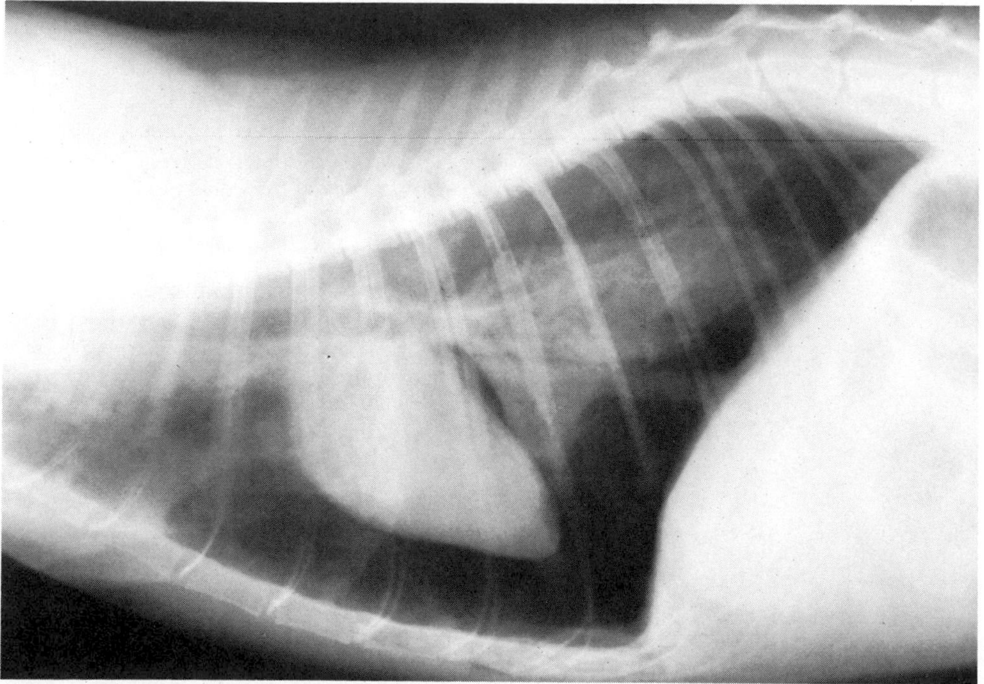

**Figure 5–2** Pneumothorax, with significant features of cardiac elevation and atelectasis of the lung lobes.

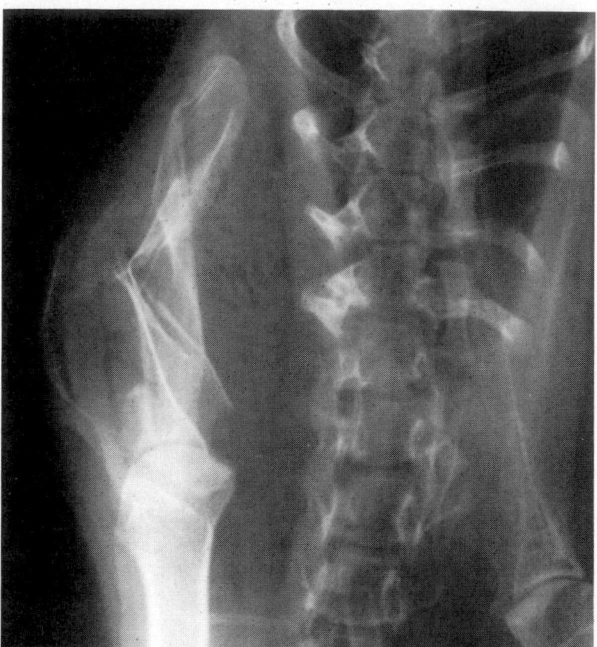

**Figure 5–3** Comminuted fracture of the scapula. Treatment with a Velpeau shoulder bandage resulted in good functional recovery. (Courtesy Dr. M. H. Engen.)

and determination of the extent of other more potentially life-threatening injuries by a thorough examination including radiographs and clinicopathologic tests. Sedation or anesthesia may be interdicted or require extreme caution. This course of action may appear as an objectionable delay to the owner, who will need to be informed and shown that it is for the animal's benefit.

# MANAGEMENT OF SPECIFIC FRACTURES

## FORELIMB

### Scapula

Fractures of the scapula are rare in the cat. The normal remnant of the clavicle should not be confused with a bone fragment. Usually only conservative care by means of a shoulder bandage or simple cage rest is required (Fig. 5–3).

### Humerus

**PROXIMAL EPIPHYSEAL FRACTURE.** This uncommon condition is very disabling. Closed reduction should be attempted in recent cases and is often successful. The leg is held flexed in a Velpeau bandage for two to three weeks (Fig. 5–4).

If open reduction is required, the approach is made craniolaterally over the proximal end of the humerus. Retraction of the brachiocephalic muscle and entry through the underlying fascia expose the fracture. After reduction, one or two small pins or Kirschner (K) wires are inserted parallel to the shaft of the humerus to secure the epiphyseal fragment. The physeal plate will tolerate a small round pin without fusing (Fig. 5–5). The pins are cut close to the bone. They may be left in for considerable time but are usually removed some time between three

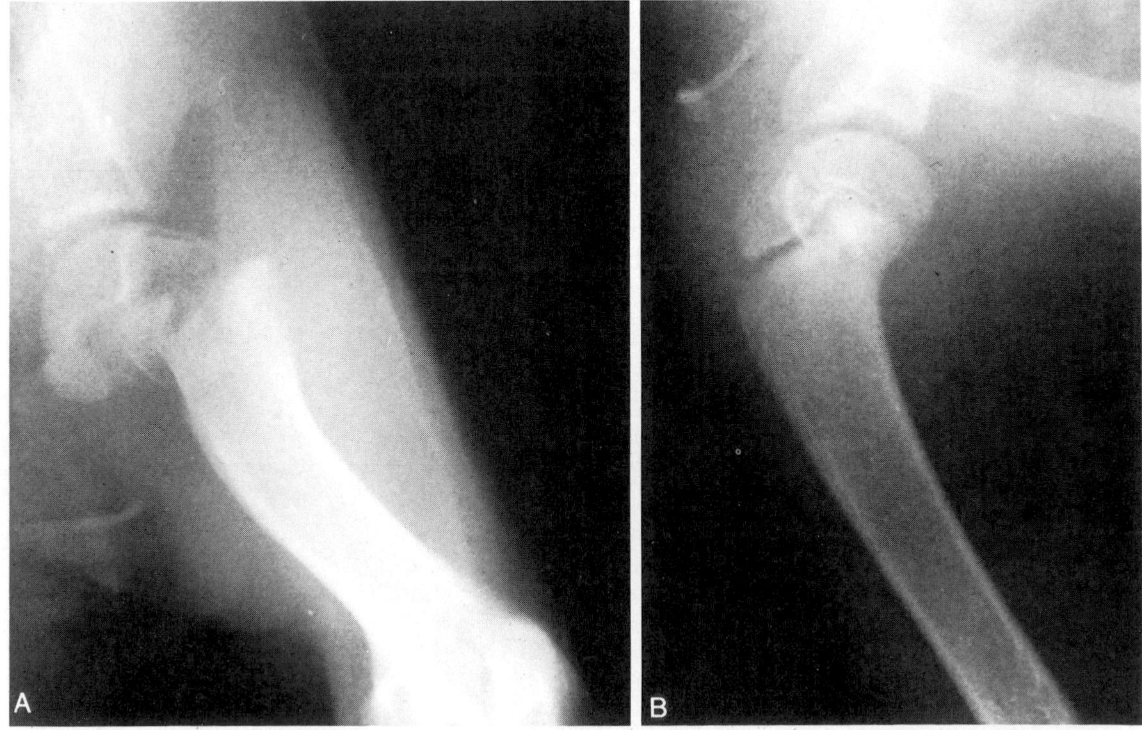


**Figure 5–4** *A,* Proximal epiphyseal fracture of the humerus. *B,* After manual closed reduction the leg was placed in a Velpeau shoulder bandage for two weeks with an excellent result. (Courtesy Dr. P. C. Gambardella.)

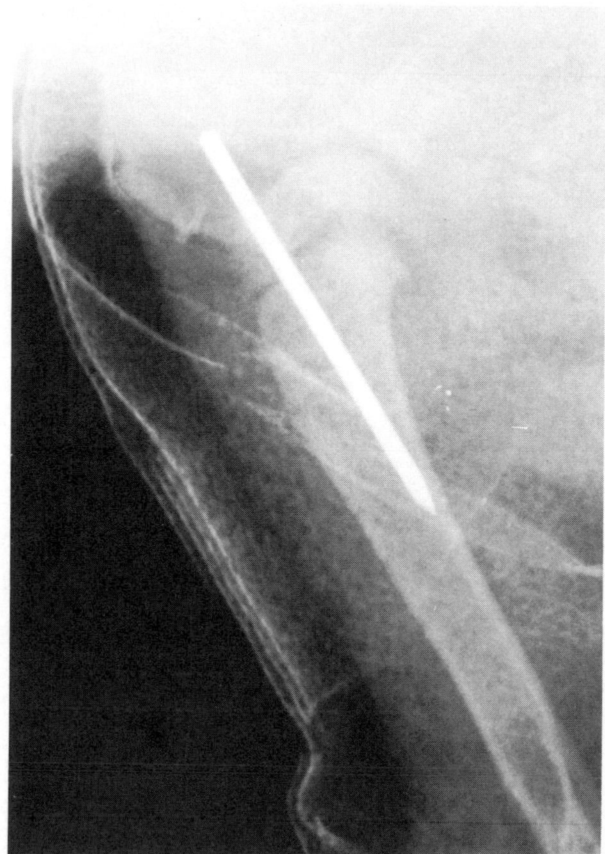

**Figure 5–5** Proximal epiphyseal fracture of the humerus treated by open reduction and fixation with a single intramedullary pin. Complete functional recovery was reported. (Courtesy Dr. S. G. Brown.)

and six months. The leg is supported in a full forelimb coaptation splint. Healing is usually excellent with return of full function.

**SIMPLE TRANSVERSE OR SHORT OBLIQUE FRACTURES.** These are fairly frequent. They are exposed through a ventrolateral approach to the humerus. An intramedullary pin of a diameter to fill the medullary cavity of the distal fragment is driven retrograde up the proximal fragment and directed to exit somewhat to the lateral side of the greater tubercle. This ensures that the pin, when seated into the distal fragment, will be in the area of the medial aspect of the condyle and less likely to penetrate into the olecranon fossa. The pin is cut off close enough to the bone to allow subcutaneous tissue and skin coverage. No rotation should be possible (Fig. 5–6).

The placement of a half Kirschner-Ehmer (K/E) device may be required to provide rigid fixation (Fig. 5–7). The proximal short pin is inserted dorsal to the intramedullary pin, and the distal short pin is inserted across the distal condyle. This device is removed a week before removal of the intramedullary pin, which is usually kept in place for a month to six weeks. It may be allowed to remain longer until radiographic proof of healing is present. It should ultimately be removed.

**LONG OBLIQUE FRACTURES.** These are common. A ventrolateral approach to the shaft of the humerus is made. Care must be taken to avoid injury to the radial nerve, which could be damaged by manipulation of the long, sharp, pointed ends of the fragments. Introduction of a suitably sized intramedullary pin down the proximal fragment from its cranial aspect avoids excessive manipulation of the fragments. The reduction can often be more easily obtained with a pin guide. After the tip of the instrument is placed in the medullary cavity of the distal fragment, the tip of the intramedullary pin extending from the proximal fragment is placed in the groove of the pin guide. Slow gentle leverage will fatigue the surrounding muscles and permit introduction of the intramedullary pin into the distal fragment. The guide is slowly removed and the pin is seated.

The fragments are held reduced by a small bone reduction forceps. Two or more cerclage wires are placed to provide additional stability. With removal of the reduction forceps the fixation should be checked for any vestige of motion. The fracture site should be thoroughly flushed with physiologic saline or Ringer's solution. With a long completely reduced oblique fracture, fixation with several cerclage wires may suffice, but dependence upon cerclage wires alone is usually risky.

**COMMINUTED FRACTURES.** These are the most common humeral fractures. A ventrolateral approach to the shaft is made. The fragments and their muscle and tissue attachments should be preserved. Larger butterfly fragments are fitted in place to the appropriate proximal or distal fragment and secured with cerclage wires. With the fragments replaced, the resulting two-piece fracture is fixed with an intramedullary pin driven down from the proximal fragment or up the proximal fragment and then seated in the distal fragment. The pin guide may be required. Additional cerclage wires may be needed to ensure complete stability (Fig. 5–8).

**SEVERELY COMMINUTED FRACTURES.** These are relatively common. Where there are multiple small fragments, as in gunshot fractures, attempts to achieve anatomic replacement may be self-defeating. These fractures are usually best treated conservatively with a full forelimb coaptation splint to immobilize the entire limb. The leg is wrapped in cotton and covered with bandage continuing dorsally into a similar chest bandage, which passes just caudal to the opposite forelimb. A thin piece of aluminum rod is bent to conform to the lateral surface of the forelimb and then bent to extend over the withers. The rod is secured to the limb and chest bandage with adhesive tape. In some cases simple cage confinement has brought good results. If possible an external fixation splint (K/E apparatus) should be applied to give good fragment control until healing occurs.

**T OR Y FRACTURES.** These fractures are not common. The choice of treatment depends on the degree of separation of the fragments. Good results have been reported in less severe cases with a full forelimb coaptation splint. The cat tolerates a limited degree of flexion and extension of the elbow surprisingly well.

For the severely displaced fracture in a small cat, an open reduction is done through a caudolateral incision of the elbow joint followed by either tenotomy of the insertion of the triceps muscle or osteotomy of the olecranon. With the triceps retracted the medial and lateral condylar fragments are exposed. Two K wires are drilled from the fracture surface of the lateral fragment through to its lateral surface. The condylar fracture is reduced and both

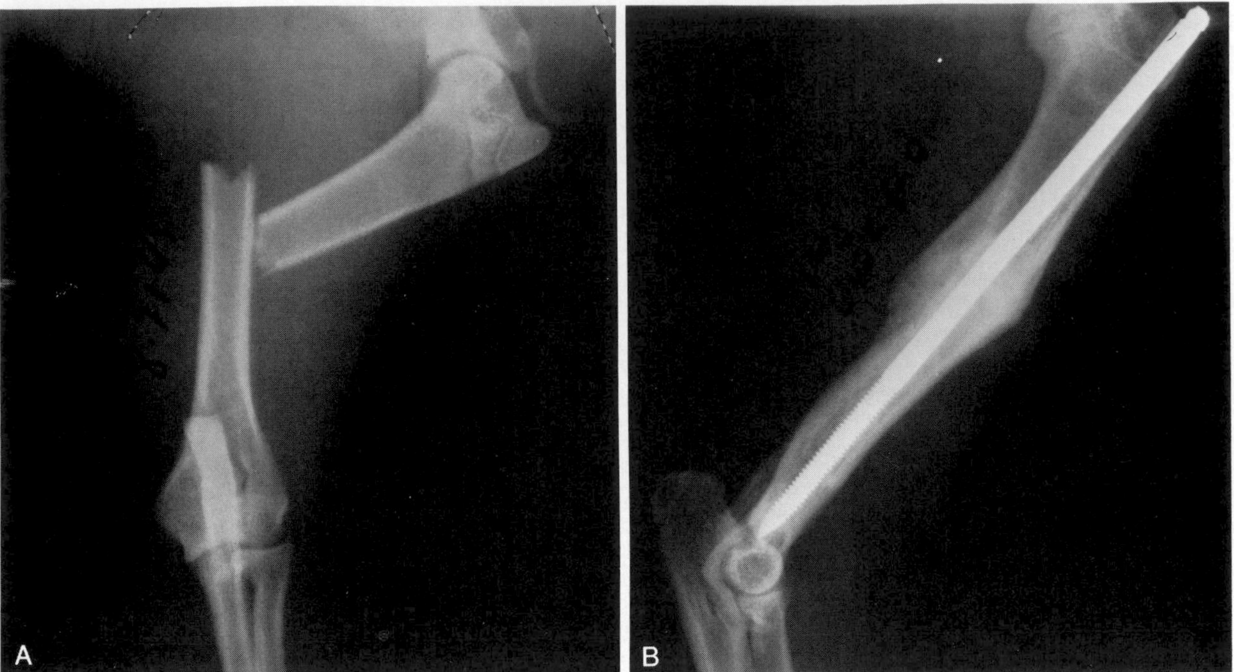


**Figure 5–6** *A,* Transverse midshaft fracture of the humerus. *B,* The fracture was treated with a single large intramedullary pin. Excellent healing six weeks after surgery. (Courtesy Dr. P. B. Vasseur.)

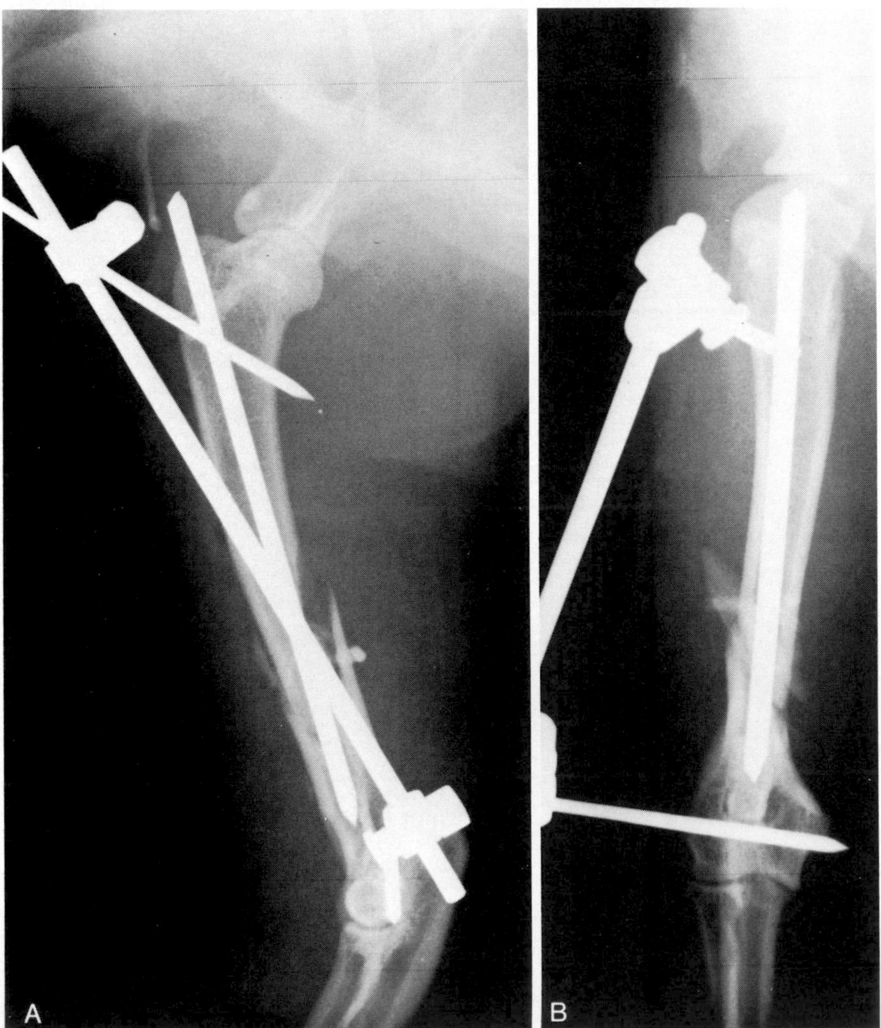


**Figure 5–7** *A,* Midshaft oblique fragmented fracture of the humerus treated with an intramedullary pin and ½ K/E apparatus. Proximal locations of the intramedullary and ½ K/E pins are shown. *B,* Placement of the distal portions of the intramedullary and ½ K/E pins is shown. Rigid stability and excellent control of rotation and collapse are provided. (Courtesy Dr. S. G. Brown.)

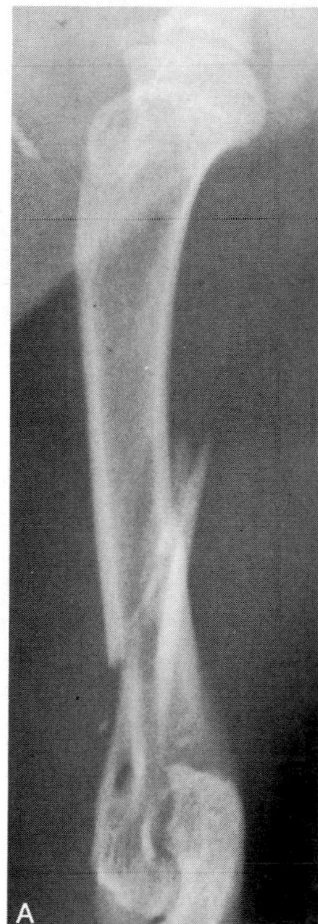


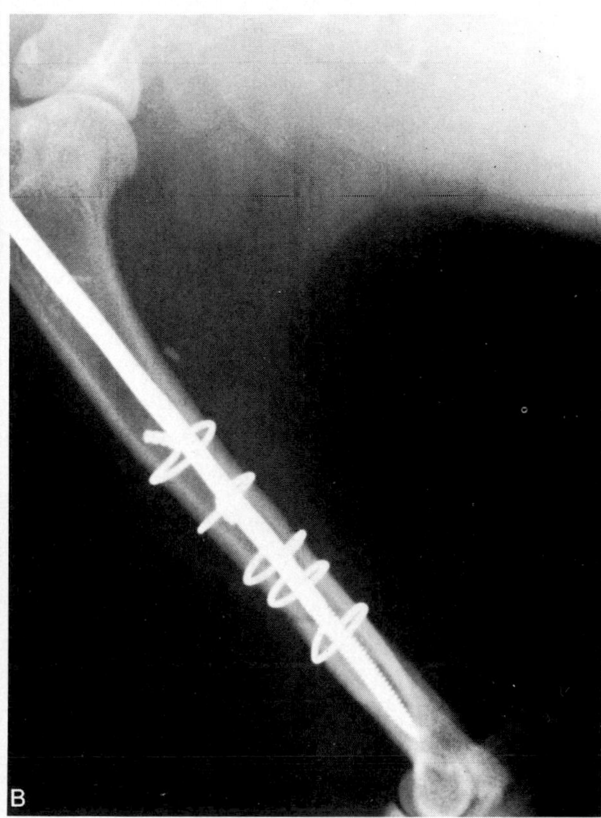


**Figure 5–8** *A,* Comminuted oblique humeral fracture. *B,* Intramedullary pinning and multiple cerclage wires have achieved a complete anatomic reduction with subsequent excellent healing and function. The pin was removed in six weeks. The wires remain permanently. (Courtesy Dr. P. C. Gambardella.)

K wires are driven into the medial condylar fragment until the ends can be palpated under the skin over the medial surface of the condyle. The proximal and distal fragments are aligned, and a K wire is inserted from the caudomedial aspect of the medial condylar fragment into the medullary cavity of the proximal fragment. Further stability is achieved with a short K wire from the caudolateral aspect of the humeral condyle penetrating into the distal end of the proximal fragment. The severed tendon of the triceps is replaced and sutured with nonabsorbable material, or the osteotomized portion of the olecranon is anchored with pins and a tension band wire. The leg is placed in a full forelimb coaptation splint.

For the severely displaced fracture in a larger cat, the olecranon is osteotomized and the triceps muscles are elevated to permit clearing of damaged tissues and reflection of the surrounding muscles to expose the condylar separation. The fragments are carefully aligned to provide the joint congruency essential to the repair and are held with a small bone-holding forceps. A transverse lag screw is inserted to stabilize the condylar fragments. Further exposure must be done carefully to avoid injury to the radial, median, and ulnar nerves. The proximal fragment is aligned with the combined condylar fragments, and two cerclage wires are placed to prevent misalignment while placing the prebent intramedullary pins, which are inserted from the caudolateral surfaces of the lateral and medial condylar fragments and through them into the medullary cavity of the proximal fragment. The pins are cut off close to the bone. The olecranon osteotomy is repaired with an intramedullary pin and a figure-eight wire tension band. The leg is placed in a full forelimb splint for three weeks (Fig. 5–9).

**HUMERAL CONDYLE FRACTURE.** Lateral fractures are uncommon. A caudolateral approach is used. The small size of the lateral condylar fragment often precludes a standard lag screw technique. Repair is done with a K wire driven from the center of the cranial fracture site of the condylar fragment to exit distolaterally. The end of the pin to be reinserted into the proximal fragment is bent with a slight lateral bowing so that when the fracture is reduced the wire will travel up the medullary canal. To ensure proper entry of the pin, the medullary canal is predrilled with an intramedullary pin of somewhat larger diameter. The fragment may be secured to the medial condylar fragment with a transverse K wire. The wire or wires are cut off close to the bone. The leg is placed in a full forelimb coaptation splint.

**MEDIAL FRACTURE.** Medial fractures are somewhat more frequent. A caudomedial approach is used. Repair can be done with K wires, but a lag screw is better. The incision extends through the underlying medial head of the triceps into the joint. A fragment is replaced and immobilized with a small bone-holding forceps. A transverse hole is drilled through the fragment into the lateral portion of the condylar fragment. The hole in the loose fragment is overdrilled. A small bone screw is inserted and tightened. This lags the fragment tightly into position. Additional stability is gained by inserting a short transverse K wire proximally. After routine closure, the limb is placed in a full forelimb coaptation splint (Fig. 5–10).

## Radius and Ulna

**PROXIMAL ULNA/OLECRANON FRACTURES.** These fractures are not common. Exposure is obtained by a caudal incision directly over the fracture site. If the fracture is distal to the elbow joint, fixation can be obtained by introducing an intramedullary pin up the

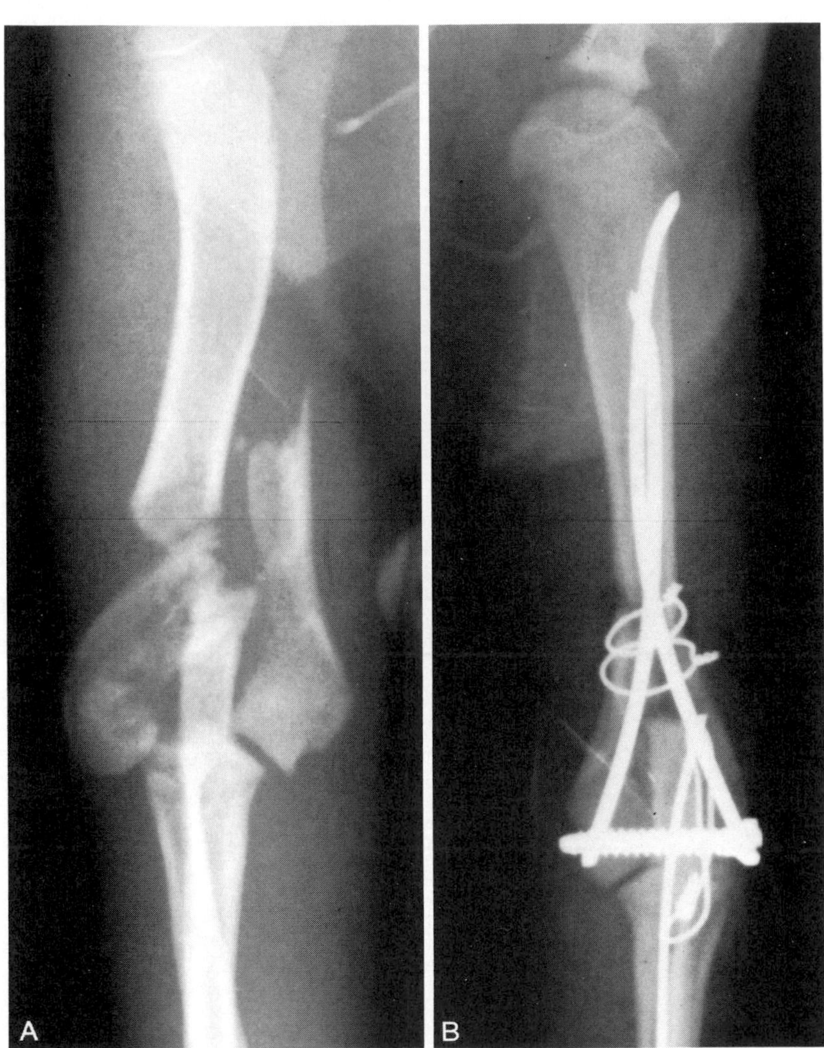

**Figure 5–9** *A,* Y fracture of the humerus. *B,* Stabilization of the condylar fragments with a lag screw and fixation with cerclage wires and prebent intramedullary pins directed from the lateral surfaces of the condylar fragments. (Courtesy Dr. P. C. Gambardella.)

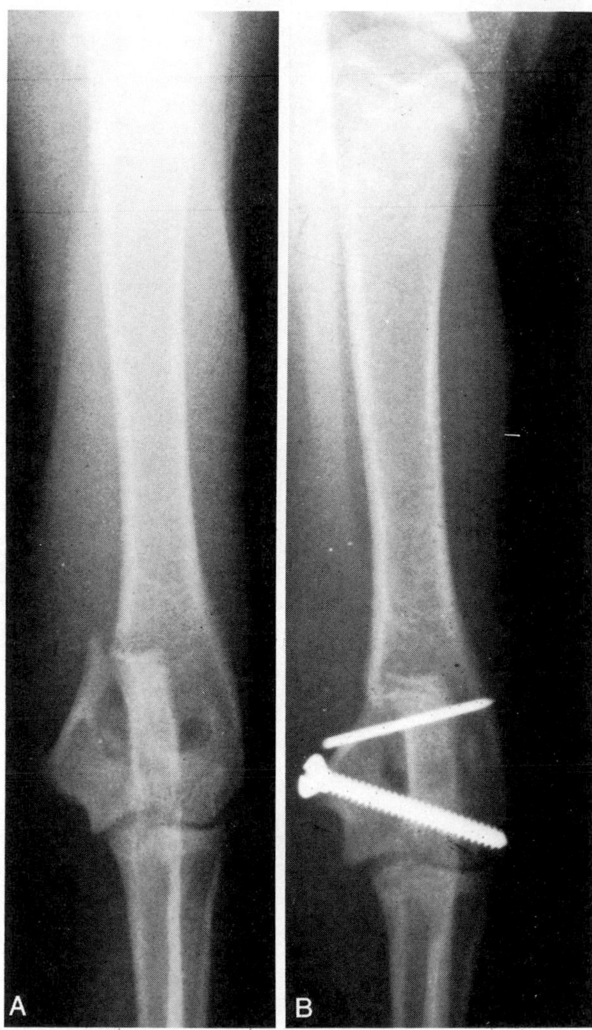


**Figure 5–10** *A*, Medial condylar fracture of the humerus. *B*, The fracture is treated with a lag screw and stabilized with a proximal transverse K wire. (Courtesy Dr. P. C. Gambardella.)

proximal fragment to exit at the top of the olecranon. The fracture is reduced and the pin is driven into the distal fragment. A full forelimb coaptation splint is applied. The pin is removed in a month to six weeks. If the fracture is above the head of the radius, repair will include a tension band (Fig. 5–11).

In the small cat two parallel K wires are driven about 2 to 3 mm apart from the fracture site out the olecranon and then with reduction of the fracture are driven into the shaft of the ulna. A figure-eight tension band of 22-gauge orthopedic wire is placed from cranial to the K wires (going cranial to the insertion of the triceps tendon) to cross over the caudal aspect of the olecranon and pass lateral to medial through a transversely drilled hole in the caudal aspect of the ulna 1 cm below the fracture site and is returned to bring the two wire ends together. They are then drawn tightly together and twisted with a wire twister. It is suggested that a loop be formed on the opposite limb of the figure-eight so that it and the ends of the wire can be twisted to bring about an equal degree of tension (Birchard and Bright, 1981).

In the very small cat it may be possible to place only one K wire with a smaller tension band. Although not quite so stable, it will function satisfactorily. The K wires are removed in three months. The tension band does not need to be removed.

**PROXIMAL RADIUS AND ULNA FRACTURES.** These infrequent fractures are treated by pinning the ulna, which is approached caudally. An intramedullary pin of the largest size that will fit into the distal ulna fragment is driven up the proximal fragment out the olecranon. Predrilling the medullary cavity of the distal ulnar fragment ensures proper direction of the pin when it is seated after the two fragments are aligned. The pin is cut off at the olecranon. A fracture of the proximal ulna with luxation of the radial head (Monteggia fracture) is treated in the same way. The radial head is replaced as the fracture is reduced. A coaptation splint that immobilizes the forelimb gives further support (Fig. 5–12).

**MIDSHAFT RADIUS AND ULNA FRACTURES.** These are rather common. Greenstick fractures and those that can be reduced manually and remain reduced can often be well managed by a coaptation splint. Such treatment should not be too greatly relied upon if there appears to be a chance of excess motion. Fractures with significant overriding should be treated by open reduction and fixation. The approach is made medially over the radius between the flexor and extensor muscles. The radius is pinned by inserting a suitably sized intramedullary pin down the canal of the distal fragment to exit just above the radial carpal bone as the carpus is held completely flexed. Both fractures are reduced and the pin is introduced into the proximal radial fragment to be seated deeply and securely. A pin must have a diameter of at least 3/32 inch to give adequate support. The pin is cut off so that it lies under the skin at the carpus. The limb is placed in a coaptation splint with the carpus flexed just enough to prevent the pin from damaging the radial carpal bone. In larger animals, pinning only the radius may result in nonunion because of rotational movement. A small bone plate or an external fixation (K/E) splint consisting of a single rod with four pins will provide adequate stability. No external splinting will be required with the K/E apparatus (Fig. 5–13).

**DISTAL RADIUS AND ULNA FRACTURES.** These are quite common. If there is little displacement, closed reduction can be obtained and a coaptation splint may suffice. Usually there is considerable displacement and open reduction is required. The approach is over the craniomedial aspect of the distal radius at the fracture site. An intramedullary pin is driven out the distal fragment to exit above the radial carpal bone while the carpus is held in acute flexion. Care should be taken to make sure that the pin is parallel to the long axis of the fragment and exits centrally. The fracture is reduced with care not to damage the distal fragment. The pin is driven up the radius as far as possible and is cut off so as to lie under the skin of the carpus. If the ulna interferes with reduction, a small portion of the distal ulnar fragment may be removed to allow good contact at the site of the radial fracture. A coaptation splint is applied with the carpus held in some degree of flexion. The pin is removed in about a month.

## Metacarpals

With these common fractures a closed reduction can usually be obtained. The leg is placed in a coaptation

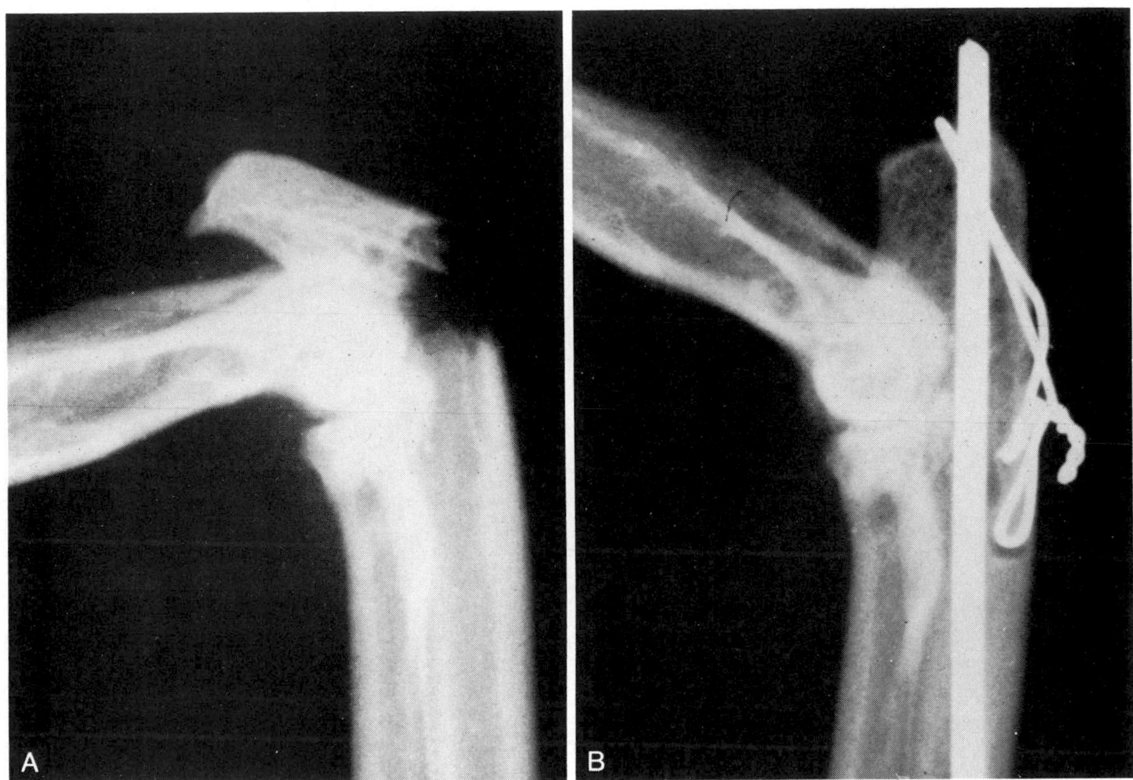


**Figure 5–11** *A,* Fracture of the olecranon showing marked distraction from the pull of the triceps muscles. *B,* Fixation with an intramedullary pin and tension band wire.

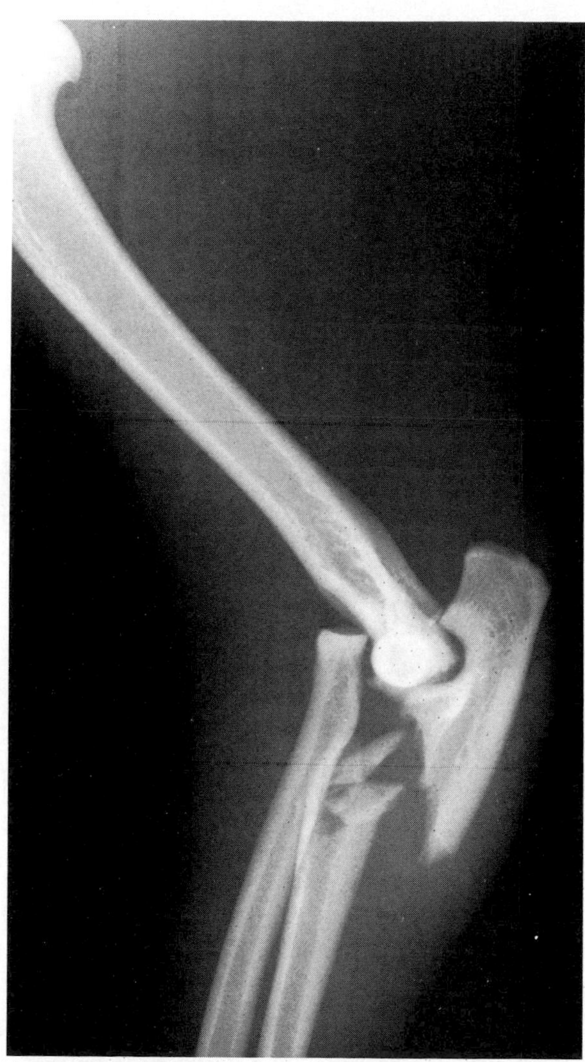

**Figure 5–12** Monteggia fracture. Treatment is with an intramedullary pin in the ulna. The luxated head of the radius is replaced as the fracture is reduced. (Courtesy Dr. P. C. Gambardella.)

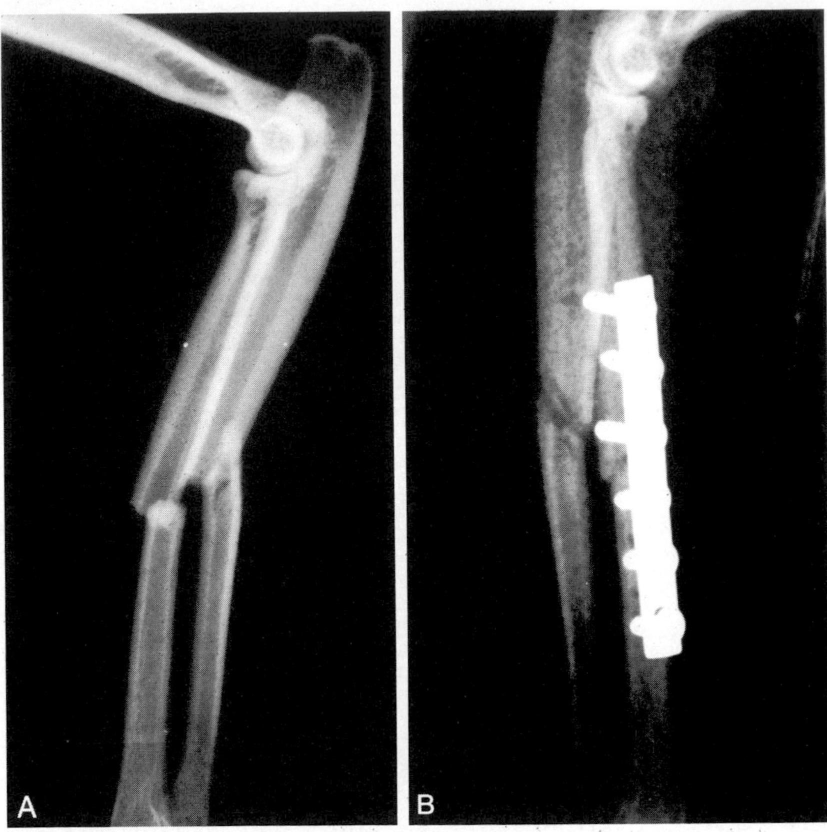


**Figure 5–13** *A,* Transverse midshaft fracture of the radius and ulna. *B,* Fixation with a small bone plate. Excellent stability is obtained. Additional protection is provided by a coaptation splint. The plate is removed after healing. (Courtesy Dr. S. G. Brown.)

splint. Even if some of the metacarpals are intact, the leg is splinted to provide support, reduce pain, and control motion at the fracture site. In some cases it is advisable to provide immobilization by introducing small intramedullary pins at the distal articular surface of each injured metacarpal. This procedure may not provide enough stability even with a suitable splint, and bone plating will need to be done. The small plates are introduced on the lateral and medial sides of the metacarpal area.

## Digits

Fractures or dislocations of the digits are not uncommon and can be quite painful. The usual treatment is the application of a firm padded bandage and cage confinement. Dislocations often recur, causing pain and a limp. Chronic luxations are best treated by amputation of the digit. The digital pads should be preserved. If there is not sufficient tissue coverage with a simple disarticulation, the distal end of the second metacarpal may have to be removed. The surgery should be carried out as an aseptic procedure with good surgical closure.

## Nails

Neglected and ingrown dewclaws are frequently infected and a source of annoyance. They are best amputated. These appendages, especially the supernumerary ones, often have a significant blood supply requiring ligation.

Broken claws are removed. The exposed nail bed will be painful and open to infection, so an antibiotic dressing is applied under a soft bandage. Deformed claws that cause lameness should also be amputated.

**DECLAWING (ONYCHECTOMY).** Requests for declawing have increased with the increase in apartment and condominium living. Cats deprived of an outdoor opportunity to sharpen their claws on trees or wear them down to the ground may develop the bad habit of clawing furniture, draperies, and rugs. Declawing should be performed only on indoor cats, since it deprives them of one of their principal defences and impairs their ability to climb trees.

If owners are loath to have the surgery, fearing that it may be cruel, they should be reminded that other surgeries such as castration and spaying are commonly accepted to adapt the pet to household living. Under the circumstances of city dwelling this surgery is often justifiable in order to keep an otherwise desirable pet.

There is some difference of opinion as to whether all the third phalanx should be amputated (Herron, 1975b). It is imperative that the base of the claw with the germinal epithelium be removed. Some veterinarians believe that removal of the entire third phalanx most reliably prevents regrowth, and they disarticulate the third phalanx with a scalpel (see chapter on soft tissue surgery). The majority prefer a White or Resco nail clipper.

The cat is anesthetized and a tourniquet is applied to the forelimb after the quantity of venous blood in the limb has been reduced by encircling the leg with the thumb and index finger and stripping toward the elbow. Except in longhaired cats, it is not necessary to trim the hair around the foot. The foot is prepared with surgical soap and rinsed in disinfectant solution.

The digit is pressed between a thumb and forefinger to extend it fully, or traction may be applied to the claw with a small hemostat. If a clipper is used the claw is amputated by seating the instrument in the small notch 2

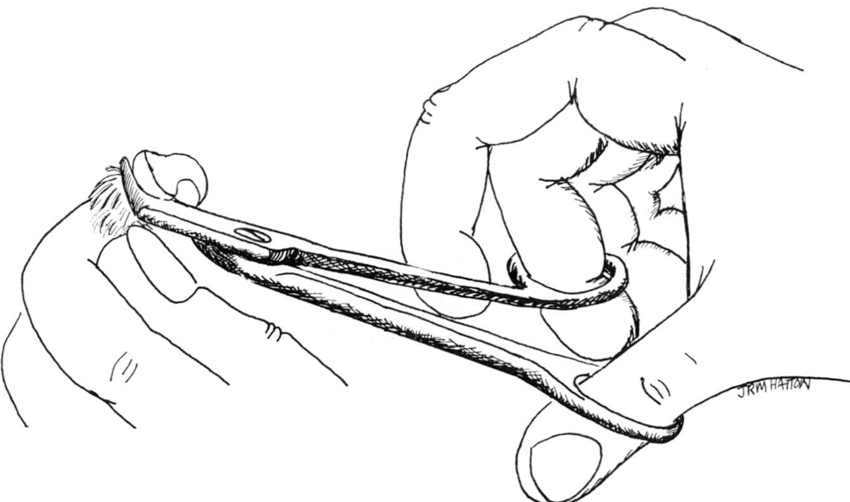

**Figure 5–14** Declawing with a nail clipper. The cutting edge of the instrument is placed in the small notch proximal to the unguicular crest.

to 3 mm proximal to the unguicular crest, removing all the base of the claw and part of the third phalanx. It is important that none of the digital pad be removed, as healing will be painful and prolonged (Fig. 5–14).

The amputated claws should be counted to be certain that all are removed. Antibiotic powder is applied to each cut surface. A single catgut suture engaging the digital flexor helps to control hemorrhage and ensures good coverage of the exposed joint. The foot is wrapped in a pressure bandage for 24 hours. The cat is released the day after bandage removal. Shredded paper in the litter box for a week is recommended to prevent clay particles from entering the wound. Recently the use of a cyanoacrylate (Nexaband*) has shown great promise in controlling hemorrhage and eliminating the need to bandage the feet.

## Hindlimb

### Femur

**FEMORAL HEAD FRACTURES AND SLIPPED EPIPHYSES.** Fractures of the femoral head and slipped capital epiphyses (physeal separation) are relatively rare. Ostectomy of the femoral head is recommended, with a craniolateral approach. The damaged femoral head is removed and the femoral neck is trimmed away with a small rongeur to leave a smooth surface to prevent bone contact with the acetabulum. Aftercare consists of a short period of confinement. Functional use of the limb usually returns quickly (Fig. 5–15).

**FEMORAL NECK FRACTURES.** These are common in cats, particularly those under two years of age. If displacement is significant a femoral head osteotomy is indicated. Fractures with minimal displacement often heal spontaneously. Treatment is cage rest and home confinement. If a fracture does not heal a femoral head osteotomy can still be done. Femoral neck fracture in cats less than a year old may also result in an avulsion of the greater trochanter. With removal of the femoral head the trochanteric fragment is replaced with a small Steinmann pin (Fig. 5–16).

Femoral neck fractures are also successfully treated by fixation with two K wires. At open reduction the neighboring tissues are cleared from the fracture site to provide direct visualization. The fracture is held reduced, and two K wires are inserted at an angle from the lateral surface of the proximal femoral shaft through the femoral neck and into the femoral head. The pins should not penetrate

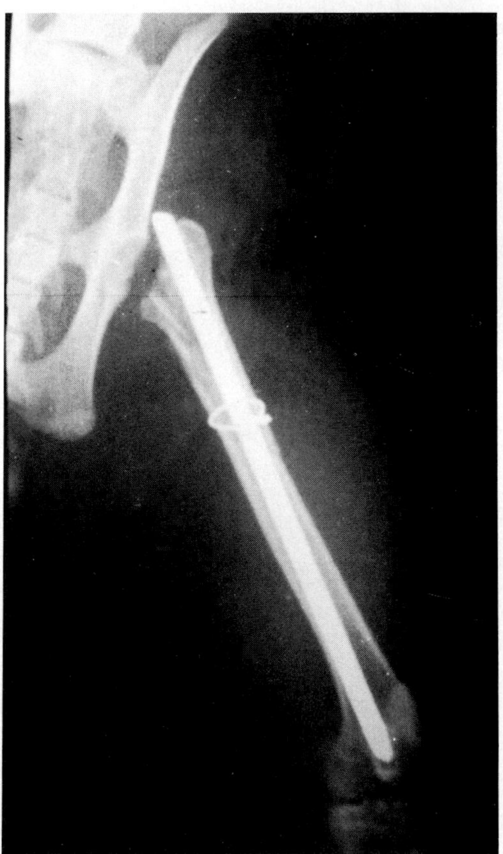

**Figure 5–15** A proximal femoral fracture has been pinned and reinforced with a cerclage wire. The fractured femoral head has been excised.

*Bionexus, Inc., Vet. Products Div., 5257 North Boulevard, P.O. Drawer 58517, Raleigh, NC 27658–8517.

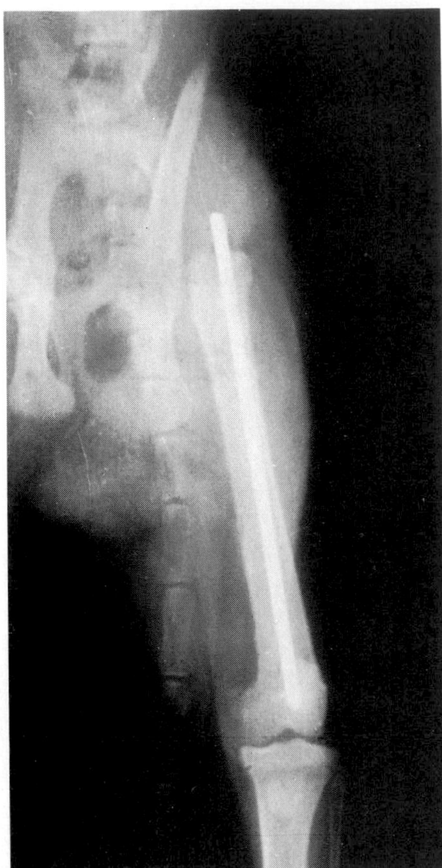

**Figure 5–16** A femoral head ostectomy was done for treatment of a femoral neck fracture. The avulsed greater trochanter was replaced and secured with an intramedullary pin.

the joint. They are cut off close to the bone and remain permanently. Aftercare consists of cage confinement for two weeks (Fig. 5–17).

**TRANSVERSE OR SHORT OBLIQUE FEMORAL FRACTURES.** These injuries are frequent. They are managed with a lateral approach and insertion of a large intramedullary pin. If the fracture is very proximal, the proximal segment should be predrilled with progressively larger pins to prevent splitting the fragment. The pin should be of sufficient diameter to fill the medullary canal and should be deeply and securely seated to prevent rotation. External splinting is not necessary. A single Rush pin inserted through the proximal fragment and seated well down the shaft of the distal fragment works equally well. The intramedullary pin may be left in for several months if it is cut off close to the femur. The Rush pin is removed after healing has occurred (Fig. 5–18).

**LONG OBLIQUE FEMORAL FRACTURES.** For these very common fractures, intramedullary pinning is recommended with a standard lateral approach. To prevent possible tissue damage during exposure of a long sharp femoral fragment, the intramedullary pin is introduced proximally at the trochanteric fossa. The fracture is reduced and the pin is driven down the medullary canal of the distal fragment. A small pin guide is often very helpful. The pin is seated deeply in the distal fragment. Cerclage wires are placed to maintain the reduction and prevent collapse of one fragment along the other. The pin is removed after healing (Fig. 5–19).

**COMMINUTED FEMORAL FRACTURES.** These are probably the most common long-bone fractures. A standard lateral approach is used. Large fragments are added to the proximal or distal fragment by use of cerclage wires so as to build up a two-fragment fracture. A large intramedullary pin is carefully introduced up the medullary canal of the proximal fragment and then down into the distal fragment. Patience and the use of a small pin guide permit a deep secure seating in the distal fragment (Fig. 5–20). Bone plating is an excellent alternative method of repair (Fig. 5–21).

**SEVERELY COMMINUTED FEMORAL FRACTURES.** These fractures are unfortunately very common. A lateral approach is used. The fragments are reconstructed with multiple cerclage wiring as long as anatomic reduction can be obtained. Cancellous bone graft material from the humerus is used to stimulate healing. The number of cerclage wires is not important, but stability

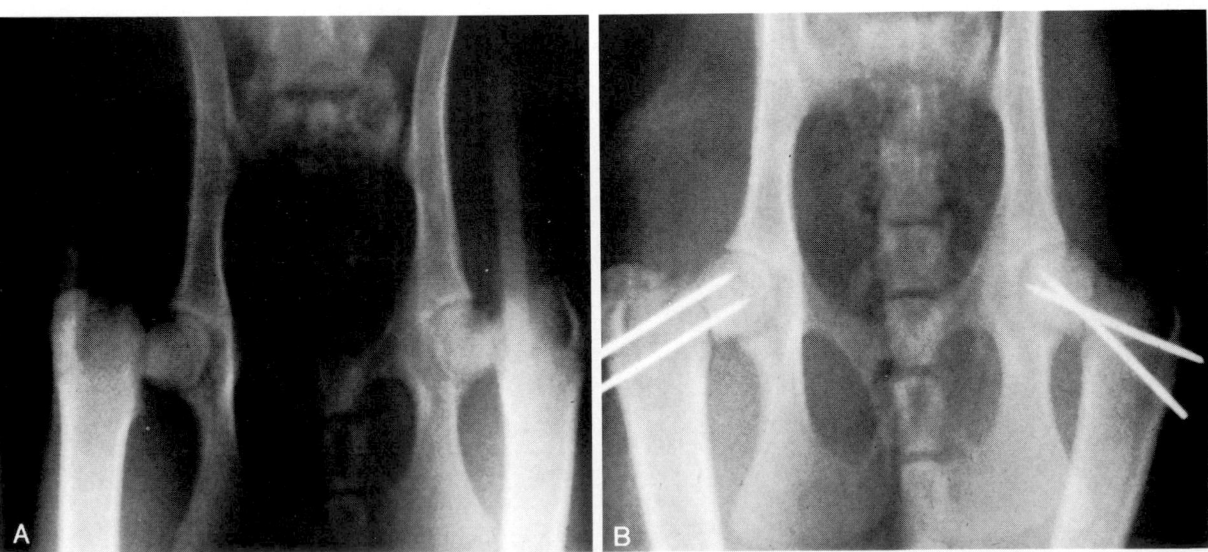


**Figure 5–17** *A,* Bilateral femoral neck fractures. *B,* Reduction and fixation with two angled K wires. (Courtesy Dr. P. C. Gambardella.)

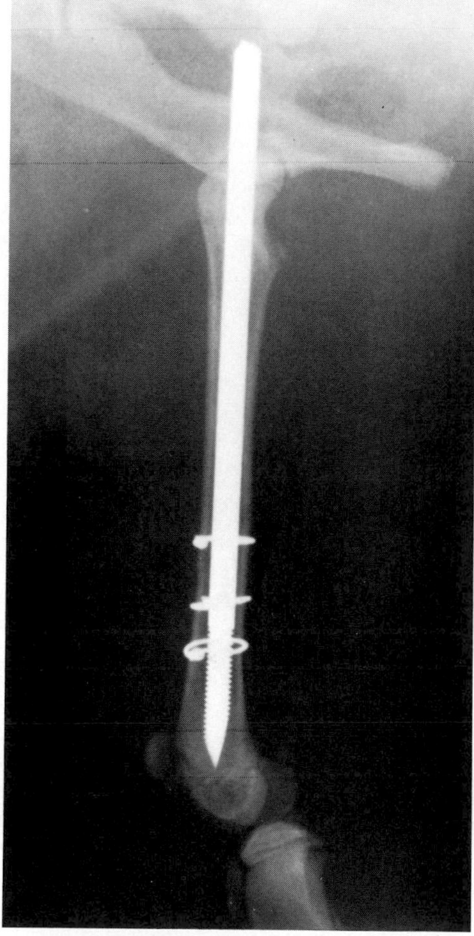

**Figure 5–18** A short oblique femoral fracture anatomically reduced and stabilized with an intramedullary pin. The distal two cerclage wires are reinforcing a slight crack in the distal fragment. (Courtesy Dr. P. C. Gambardella.)

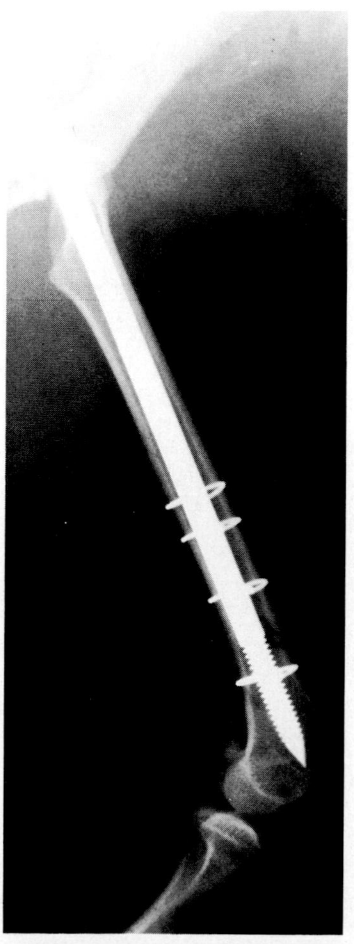

**Figure 5–19** A long oblique femoral fracture has been anatomically reduced and stabilized with an intramedullary pin and cerclage wires.

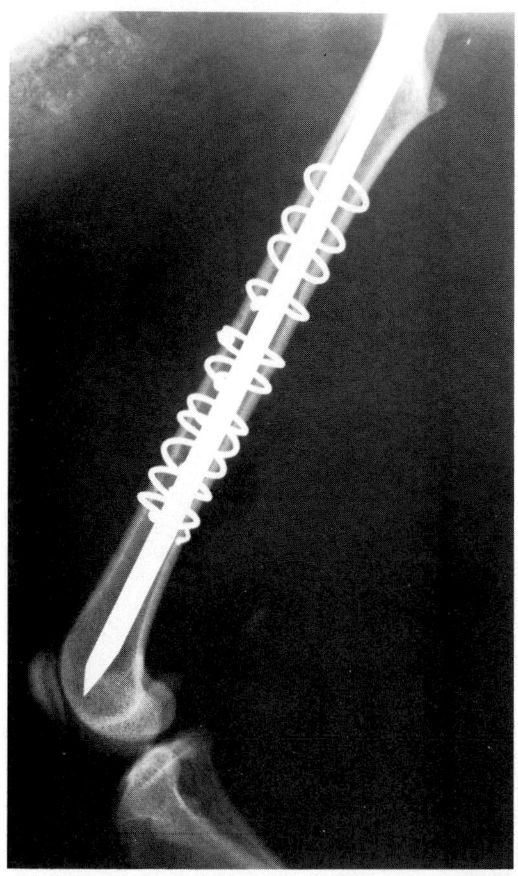

**Figure 5–20** A comminuted femoral fracture has been anatomically reduced and stabilized with an intramedullary pin and 11 cerclage wires. Healing was excellent. (Courtesy Dr. P. C. Gambardella.)

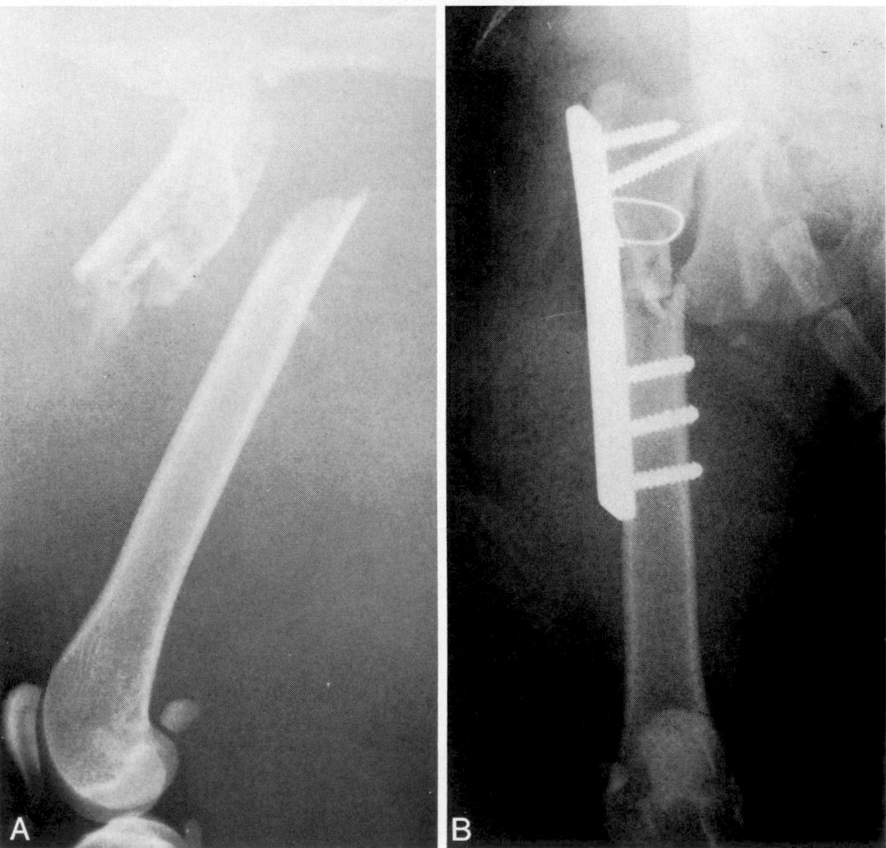


**Figure 5–21** *A,* Proximal comminuted femoral fracture. *B,* Fixation with a bone plate. The extra-long screw extending into the femoral neck and head is essential to provide support for the short proximal fragment. (Courtesy Dr. S. G. Brown.)

is. Nonstable reductions cannot be compensated for by a coaptation or Schroeder-Thomas splint.

If an anatomic reduction cannot be obtained, multiple cerclage wiring and an intramedullary pin should not be used alone. Instead, a full or one-half K/E apparatus is applied as well to prevent rotation and collapse. The selected pin should be small enough in diameter to allow the proximal external pin to pass through the femur caudal to the intramedullary pin just distal to the trochanter major. The other external pin is placed transversely through the distal condyles (Fig. 5–22). The use of a full K/E alone or bone plates is also successful in these fractures (Fig. 5–23).

In some cases severely comminuted fractures are best managed with a coaptation splint fastened to a padded abdominal bandage. A piece of aluminum rod is bent to conform to the lateral surface of the leg and then bent to go over the back. The rod is taped to the leg and abdominal bandage. This immobilizes the entire limb and may have to be kept in place as long as six weeks. Some shortening and nonanatomic healing will have to be accepted. Functional use will usually return, sometimes with a limp (Fig. 5–24).

A relatively new technique uses entire-segment cortical bone transplants (diaphyseal tubular allografts) to repair severely comminuted fractures of the femur and, occasionally, other long bones (Wadsworth and Henry, 1976). The femoral shafts of young mature cats are harvested in a sterile manner, stripped of all attachments, double-bagged in plastic sterilized bags, and frozen in an ordinary food freezer or the freezing compartment of a regular refrigerator. They are thawed for use at the time of surgery by immersion in a bowl of room-temperature physiologic saline solution. The comminuted fragments of the recipient's femur are removed and discarded. The proximal and distal ends of the femur are cut transversely. The donor bone is cut to fill the gap exactly. To reduce the antigen load and immune response to the graft, the medullary canal of the donor bone is flushed clean of marrow with Ringer's solution. The graft is anchored by a bone plate with three screws above the graft, at least two in the graft, and three below the graft. No external support is required. Aftercare consists of systemic antibiotic administration and cage confinement.

The allograft functions as a structural template and will eventually be totally replaced by bone from the recipient by the process of creeping substitution. The bone plate is left in place for a year or more to allow the replacement process to progress to completion. Failures have occurred because of inadequate fixation, infection, and placement of allograft bone on fragmentary reconstructed bone.

**SUPRACONDYLAR FEMORAL FRACTURES.** These common fractures usually require open reduction and fixation. A poor reduction with a large callus inter-

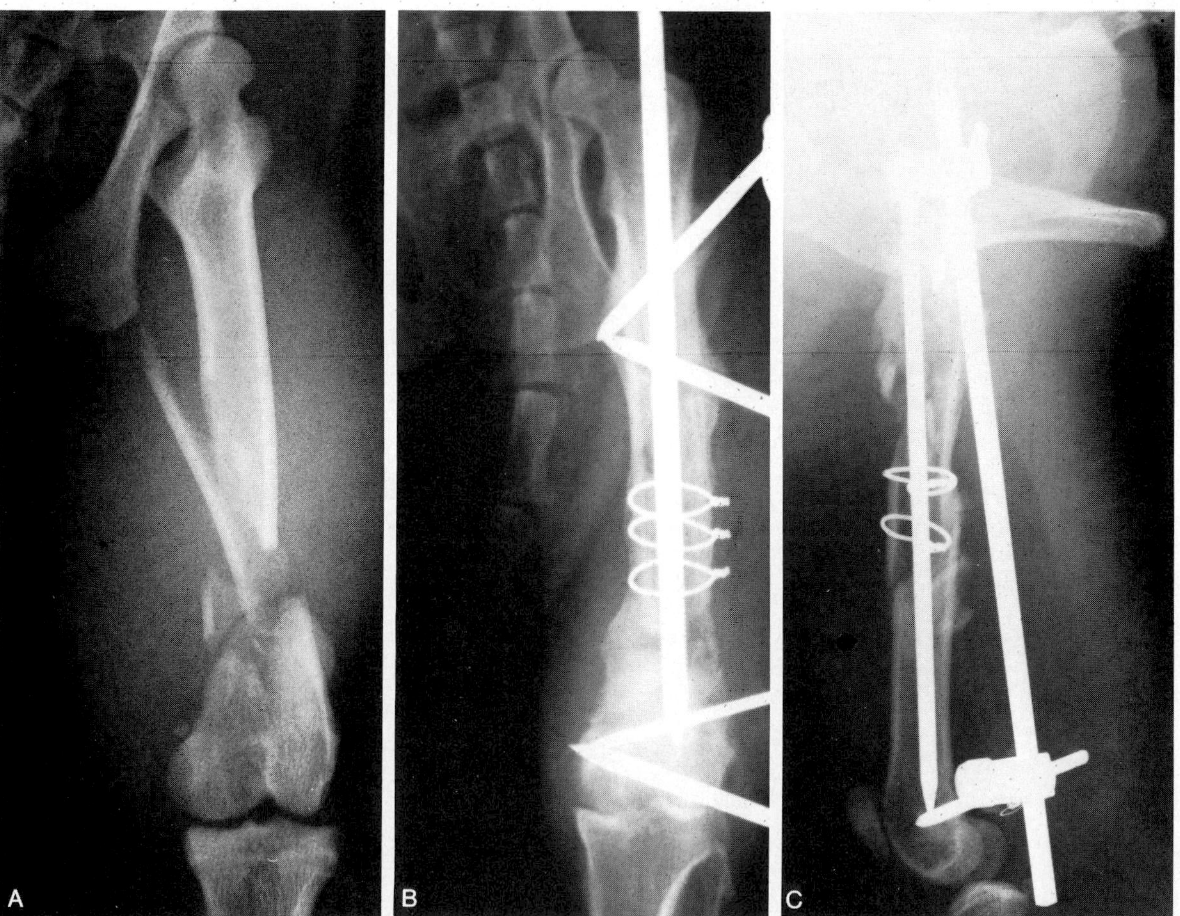


**Figure 5–22** *A,* Severely comminuted femoral fracture. *B,* Fixation with an intramedullary pin, cerclage wires, and a full K/E splint. The radiograph was taken about 10 weeks later, when the splint was removed. *C,* Another severely comminuted femoral fracture treated with an intramedullary pin, cerclage wires, and a half K/E splint. (Courtesy Dr. P. C. Gambardella.)

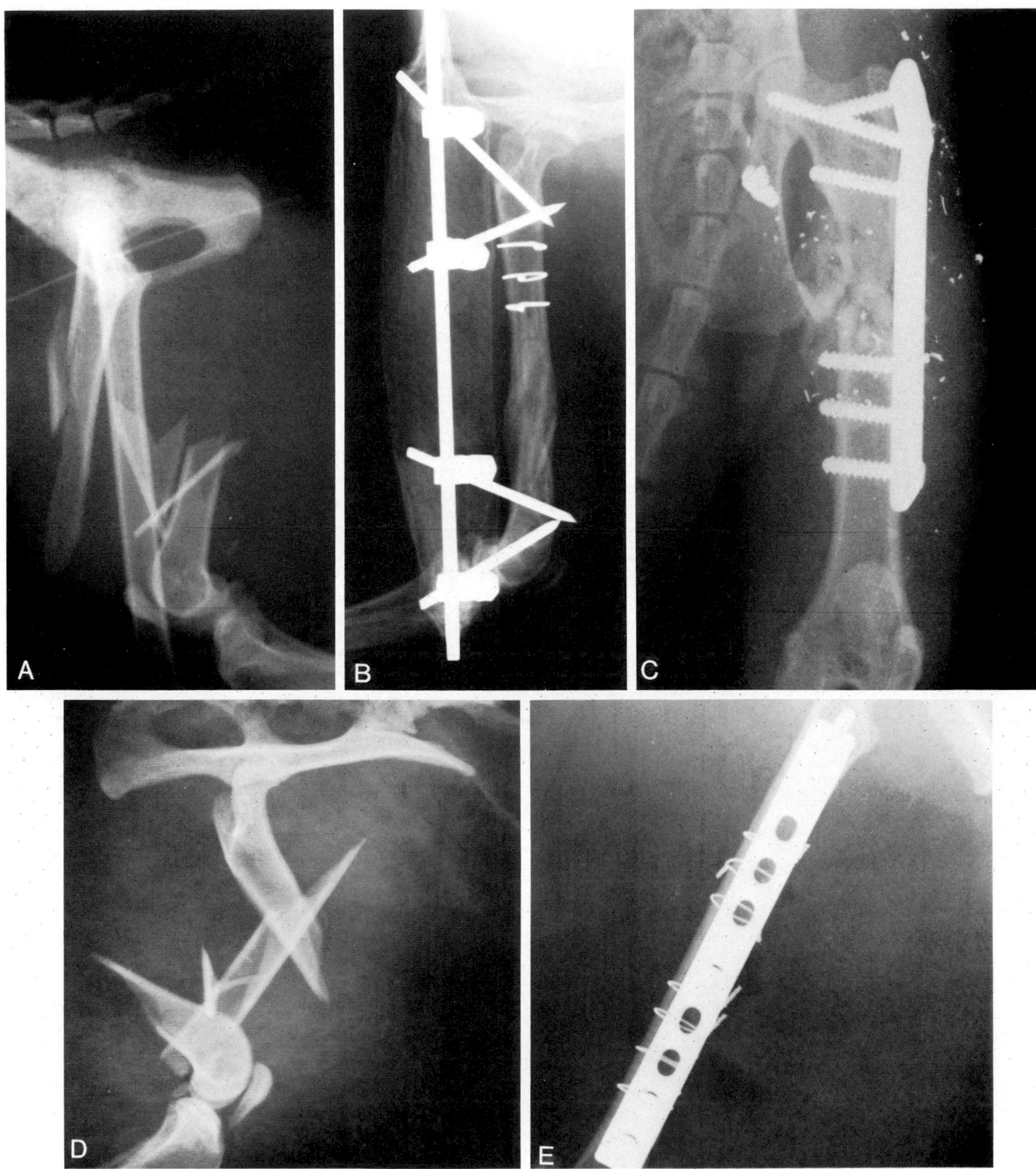


**Figure 5–23** *A*, Severely comminuted femoral fracture. *B*, Fixation by cerclage and a full K/E splint. *C*, Severely comminuted gunshot femoral fracture treated with a bone plate and cancellous bone grafting. *D*, Severely comminuted femoral fracture. *E*, Fixation with cerclage wires and a neutralization bone plate. (*A* and *B*, Courtesy Dr. P. C. Gambardella; *C*, Courtesy Dr. R. J. Todoroff; *D* and *E*, Courtesy Dr. S. G. Brown.)

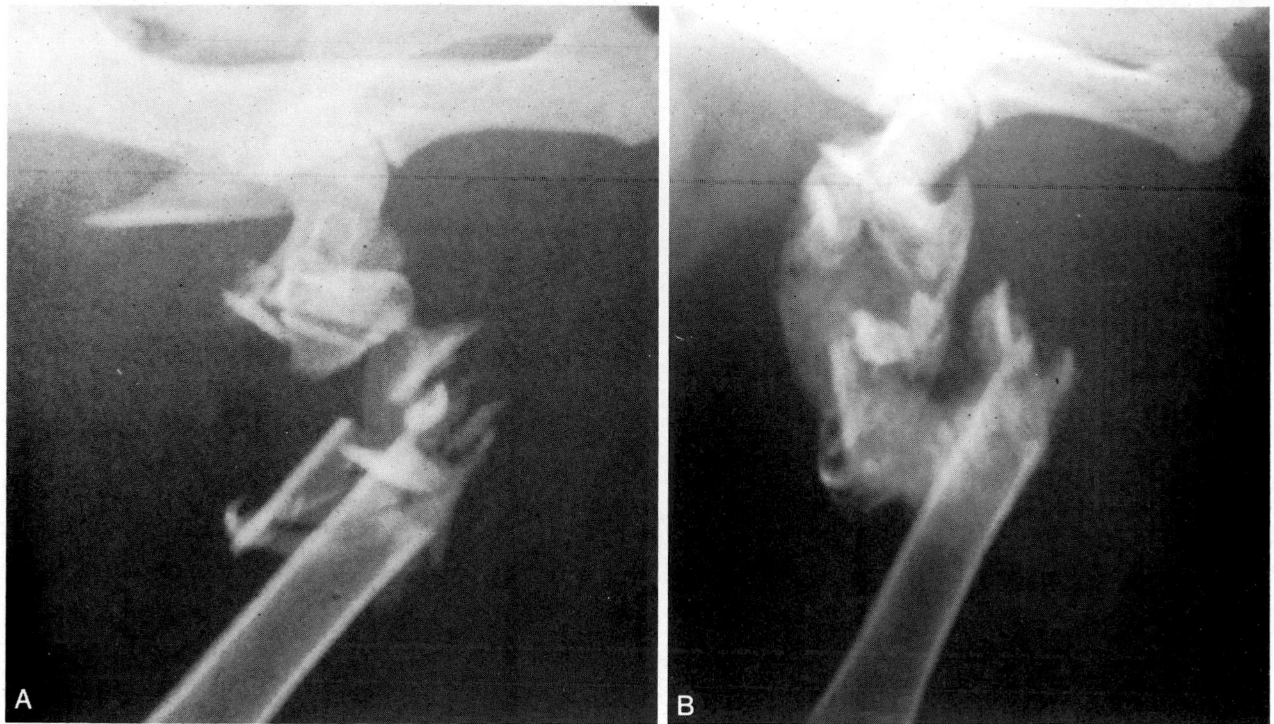


**Figure 5–24** *A,* Severely comminuted proximal femoral fracture. *B,* Without treatment a bony union resulted that was quite functional despite the bizarre radiographic appearance. (Courtesy Dr. P. C. Gambardella.)

feres with patellar function, causing a marked limp. The approach is by a medial arthrotomy of the stifle joint. The distal fragment is small and can be easily damaged, so care must be taken not to crush the bone while maneuvering it into position with a large towel clamp or small bone-holding forceps. An intramedullary pin with one blunt end is prepared. The pin is introduced centrally into the distal fragment just above the intercondylar fossa and is driven through the distal fragment across the fracture site and up the shaft of the proximal femoral fragment to exit at the trochanteric fossa. The pin is withdrawn until the blunt end is flush with the bone surface. A bone-reduction forceps is kept in place on the lower fragment to prevent it from splitting while the intramedullary pin is driven. The pin in the distal fragment should not be used to lever the fracture into reduction, as this may split the distal fragment. The proximal end of the pin is cut off before closure, since the pin may move in the process and may need to be readjusted. Closure of the joint capsule is not necessary, but the retinacular structure and the fascia of the knee should be securely sutured. No coaptation splinting is needed (Fig. 5–25).

Paired 1/16-inch Rush pins can be used to repair these fractures (Alcantara and Stead, 1975; Larsen, 1958). The pins are prebent and introduced from the condyles through predrilled holes and driven up the medullary canal of the proximal fragment, producing a very stable fixation. They are difficult and somewhat traumatic to remove but can be left in permanently (Fig. 5–26). If the fragment is comminuted, K wires are used. In placing the K wires, one prebent wire is introduced into each condyle just lateral to the apex and driven through the distal fragment to the fracture site. The fracture is reduced and the pins are driven up the shaft of the femur to exit at the trochanteric fossa. The wires are now pulled dorsally until only 1 to 3 mm protrudes from the condyle. The proximal ends are cut off under the skin. The pins must be driven alternately 1 cm at a time to avoid affecting the line-up of the distal fragment. The pins are removed from the proximal end to avoid reinvading the joint (Fig. 5–27).

**T OR Y FRACTURES.** These difficult fractures are not uncommon. The condyle may be split into several fragments. Repair is directed toward reconstruction of the condyles to preserve the trochlear groove and the articular surfaces. The distal fragment is then secured to the proximal shaft. The two condyles are held in reduction by a bone-reduction forceps or large towel clamp. A small K wire is inserted from medial to lateral to fix the two fragments in position. The combined condylar fragments are then fatigued into position. This maneuver can be difficult, and several millimeters of the distal end of the proximal fragment may be trimmed off to achieve reduction. Precurved K wires are used in the fashion of Rush pins, being inserted from the lateral surfaces of the condyles up the shaft of the femur. The pins are cut off 2 to 3 mm from each condylar surface (Shires and Hulse, 1980). Loose smaller fragments involving the trochlear surface may be pressed into place to be held down by the patella. These pins are removed when healing takes place. No external splinting is required. The animal is confined to a cage for two weeks (Fig. 5–28).

**SLIPPED DISTAL FEMORAL EPIPHYSIS.** This condition is fairly common in young cats between four and eight months of age. Manual reduction can be obtained if the condition is not over two days old. With the cat under deep anesthesia the joint is grasped as for obtaining the drawer sign when checking the anterior

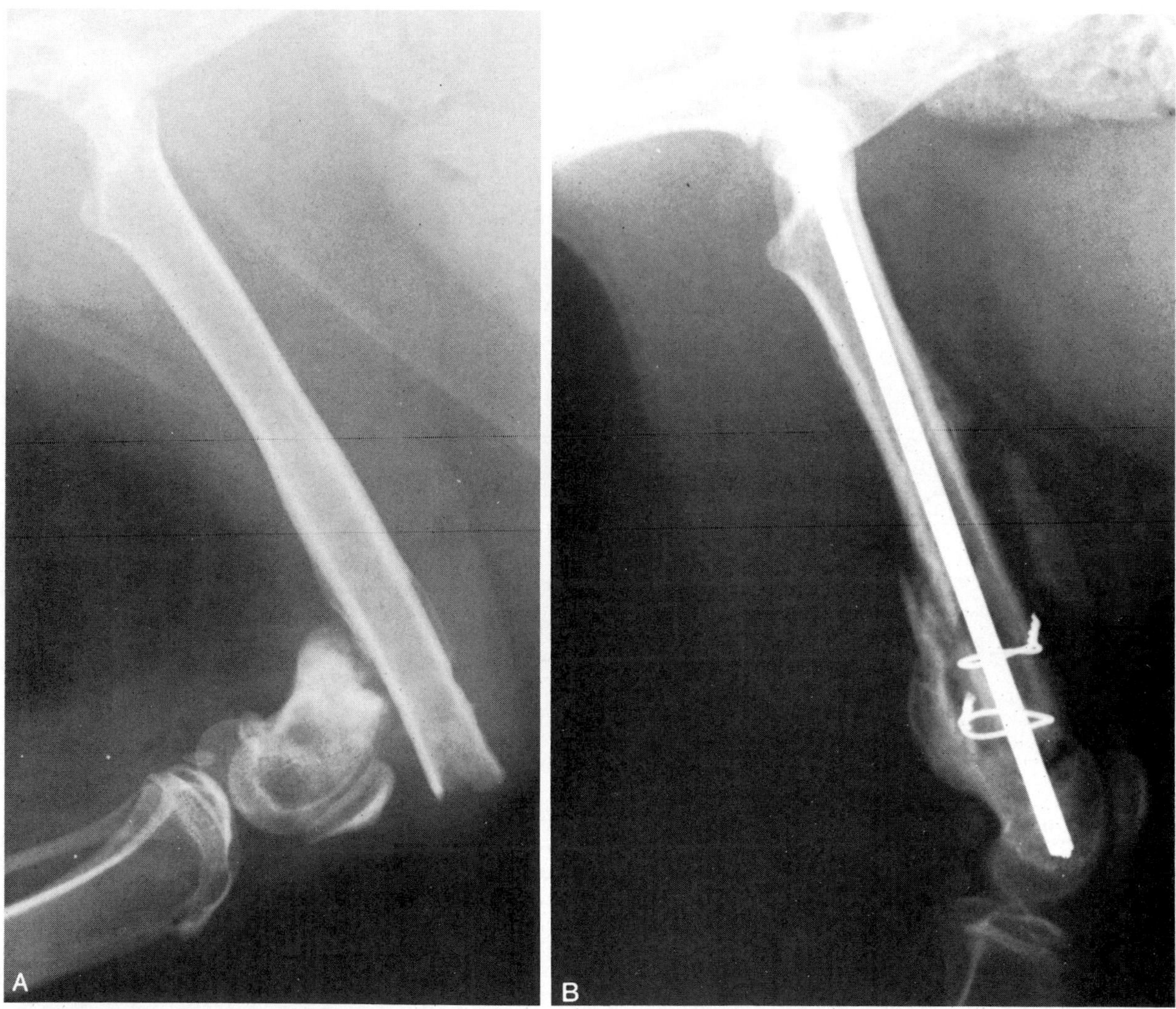


**Figure 5–25** *A*, An old supracondylar femoral fracture. Patellar function is compromised. *B*, Fixation with an intramedullary pin and two cerclage wires. Function of the patella and use of the leg improved greatly. (Courtesy Dr. S. G. Brown.)

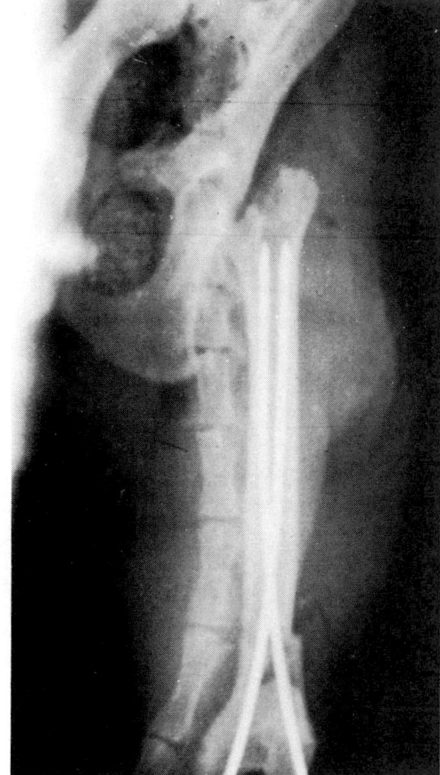
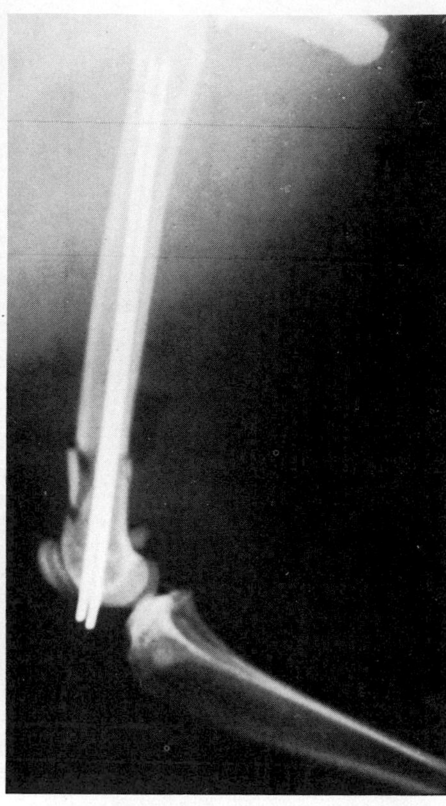

**Figure 5–26** A pair of small intramedullary pins have been introduced in the manner of Rush pins to stabilize a distal supracondylar femoral fracture.

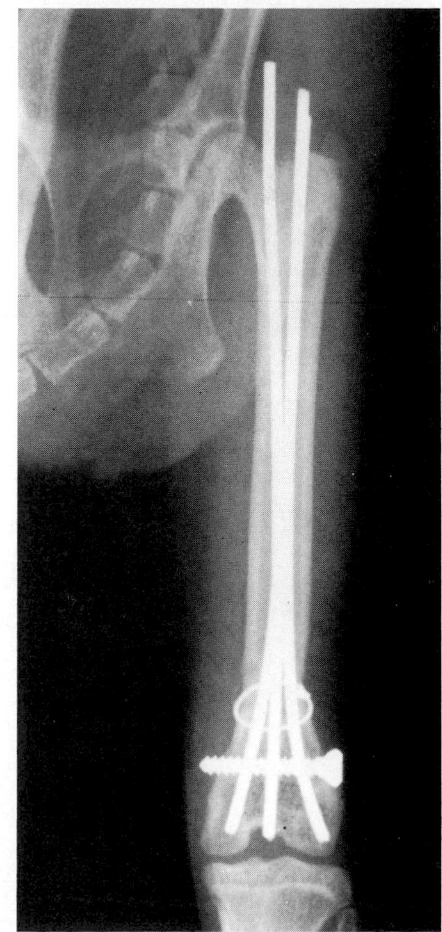

**Figure 5–27** A distal supracondylar femoral fracture was treated with small intramedullary pins introduced from the condyles and centrally. The distal fragment has been reinforced with a lag screw and cerclage wire. (Courtesy Dr. P. C. Gambardella.)

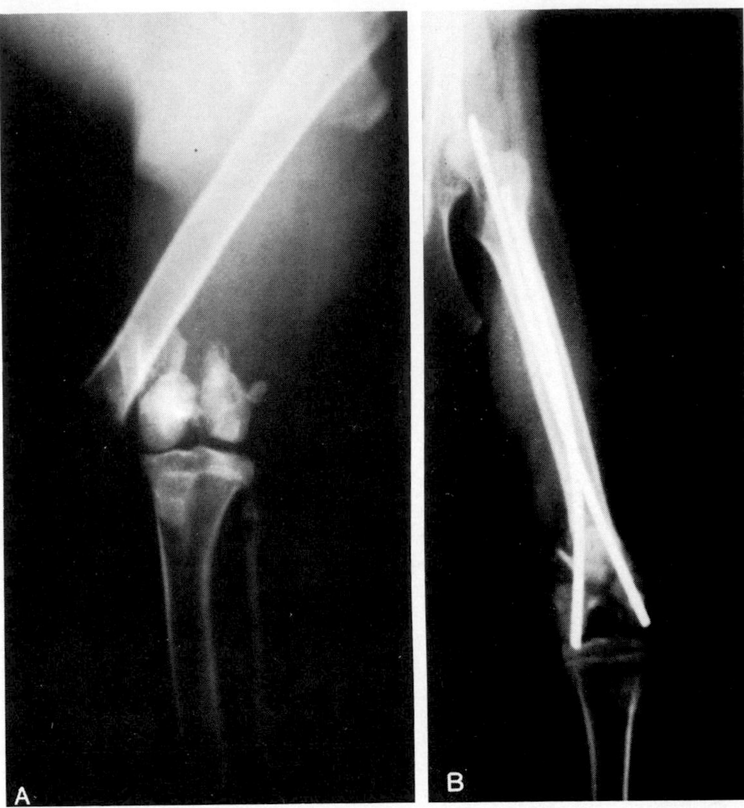


**Figure 5–28** *A,* T fracture of the distal femur. *B,* Fixation with prebent K wires inserted in the manner of Rush pins.

cruciate ligament. With proper manipulation the reduction can be felt as it goes into place. A radiograph should be taken. An Ehmer sling is applied to maintain the reduction. Healing occurs rapidly and the sling is removed in two weeks (Fig. 5–29). If reduction cannot be obtained, open reduction and fixation with a single intramedullary pin as with a supracondylar fracture are done (Fig. 5–30).

## Patella

Fracture of the patella is rare. To avoid severe lameness, surgical repair is necessary because of the distraction of the fragments by the quadriceps muscles. The fracture is treated by open reduction and fixation with a K wire and tension band. A parapatellar incision is made and the underlying tissues are reflected to expose the fragments. With the leg extended to permit apposition of the fragments, a K wire is inserted longitudinally and centrally. The wire ends are cut off to leave small proximal and distal projections. A figure-eight tension band is placed around the projecting wire ends. The K wire maintains the alignment, and the tension band compacts the fragments, counteracting the pull of the quadriceps muscles. Aftercare consists of cage confinement for two weeks. The pin and wire remain permanently (Fig. 5–31).

## Tibia

**PROXIMAL TIBIAL FRACTURES.** These are not common. If the displacement is minimal, especially if the fibula is intact, a fresh fracture can be reduced manually and immobilized with a coaptation splint. When displacement is significant, the fracture is treated by open reduction and fixation. The approach is by a craniomedial incision. After reduction, fixation is obtained by introducing a small Rush pin or intramedullary pin medial to the straight patellar ligament, through the proximal fragment, and down the shaft of the tibia. If needed, a second pin may be inserted to provide additional stability. These pins are cut off under the tissues, fairly close to the bone. They may be difficult to remove but can be left in permanently as long as the ends do not interfere with joint function (Fig. 5–32). A buttress bone plate provides excellent support (Fig. 5–33).

**TRANSVERSE AND SHORT OBLIQUE TIBIAL FRACTURES.** These are common, usually with significant overriding. The surgical approach is medial over the fracture site. Fixation is done with the largest possible pin to fit into the distal fragment. With the stifle held in acute flexion the pin is driven up the proximal fragment to exit just medial to the straight patellar ligament. The fragments are aligned and the pin is driven down and seated securely in the distal fragment. The pin is cut off as close as possible to the head of the tibia to prevent interference with motion of the stifle. However, a coaptation splint may be applied to protect the leg from stress. The repair must be stable.

A full K/E splint, a half K/E consisting of a rod with four pins, or a bone plate also provides excellent fixation (Fig. 5–34). Distal fractures may be pinned with an intramedullary pin introduced through the hock joint into the distal fragment and seated in the proximal fragment. The pin is removed after healing. The joint is not permanently affected (Fig. 5–35).

**COMMINUTED OR LONG OBLIQUE TIBIAL FRACTURES.** These common fractures are managed by intramedullary pinning combined with placement of several cerclage wires. Large fragments may be built up on

*Text continued on page 127*

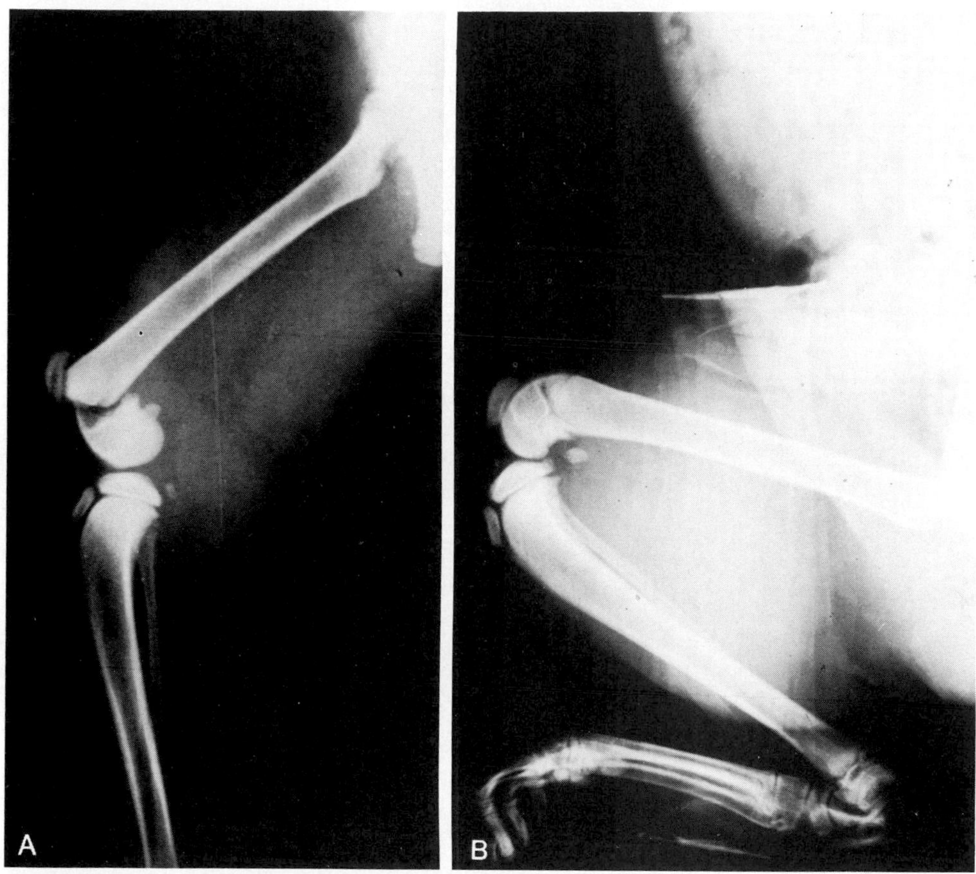


**Figure 5–29** *A,* Slipped distal femoral epiphysis with typical fragment location. *B,* After closed manual reduction the leg is placed in an Ehmer sling.

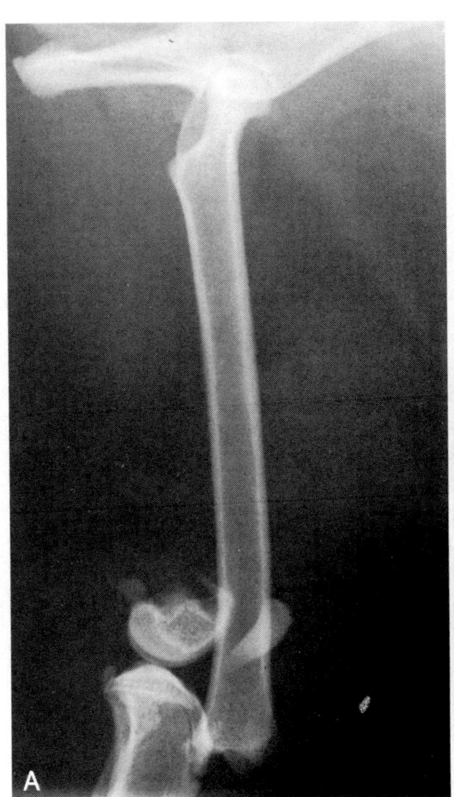


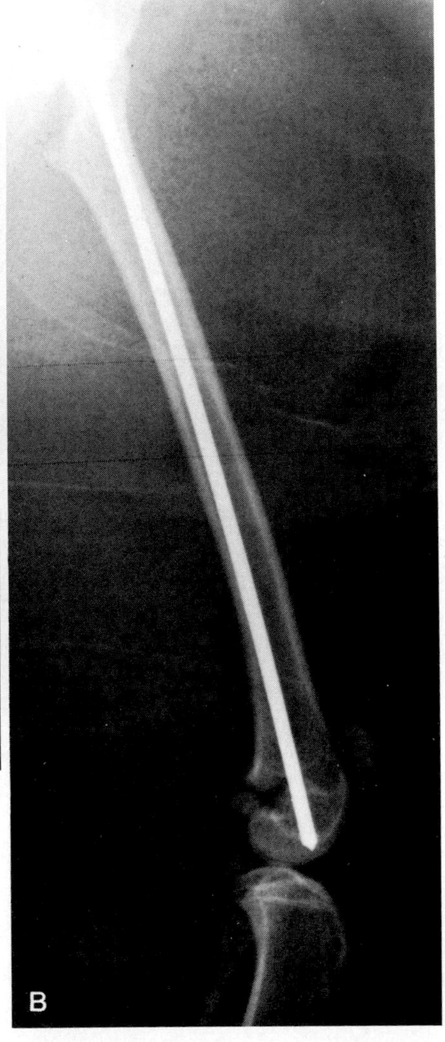


**Figure 5–30** *A,* Slipped distal femoral epiphysis. *B,* Open reduction and fixation with a single intramedullary pin. (Courtesy Dr. R. J. Todoroff.)

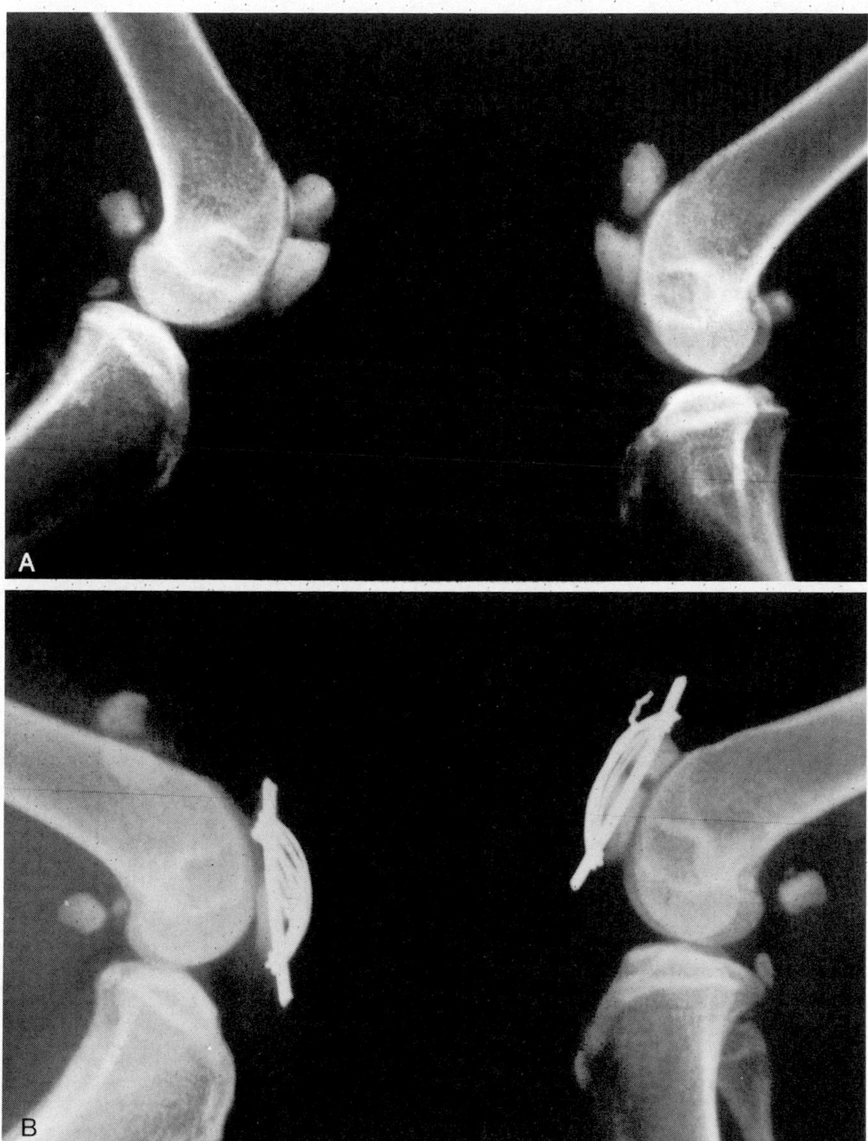


**Figure 5–31** *A,* Transverse fracture of the patella. *B,* Fixation with a longitudinally placed K wire and a wire tension band. (Courtesy Dr. R. C. Griffiths.)

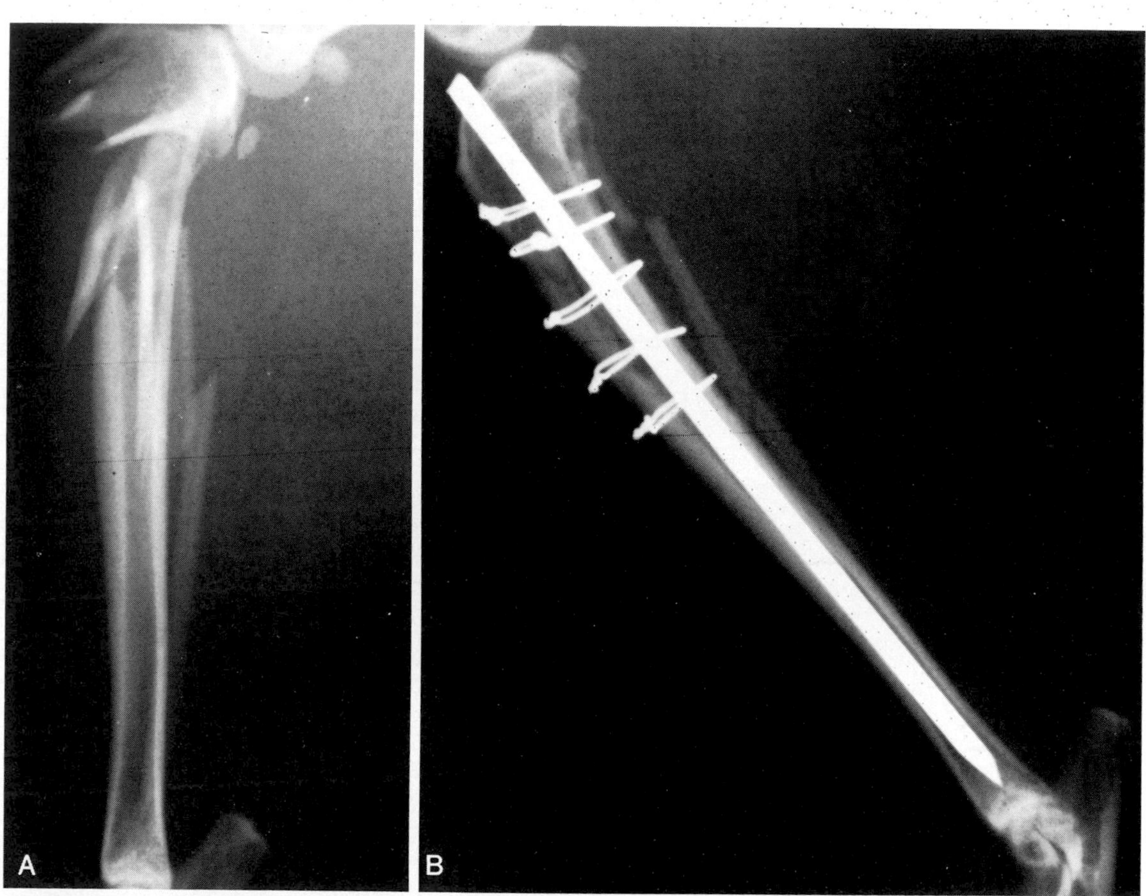


**Figure 5–32** *A,* Severely comminuted fracture of the proximal tibia. *B,* Fixation with an intramedullary pin and cerclage wires. Excellent reduction has been achieved. (Courtesy Dr. P. C. Gambardella.)

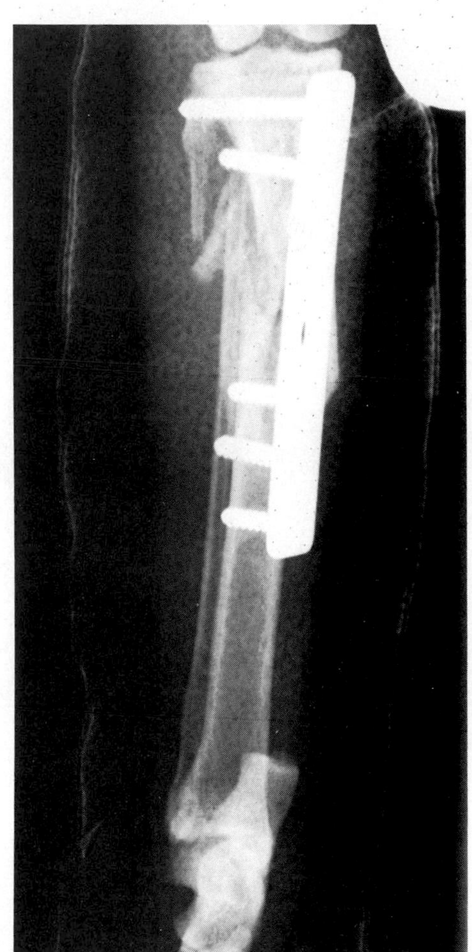

**Figure 5–33** Comminuted proximal fracture of the tibia treated with a buttress bone plate. Further protection of the leg has been provided with a coaptation splint. (Courtesy Dr. S. G. Brown.)

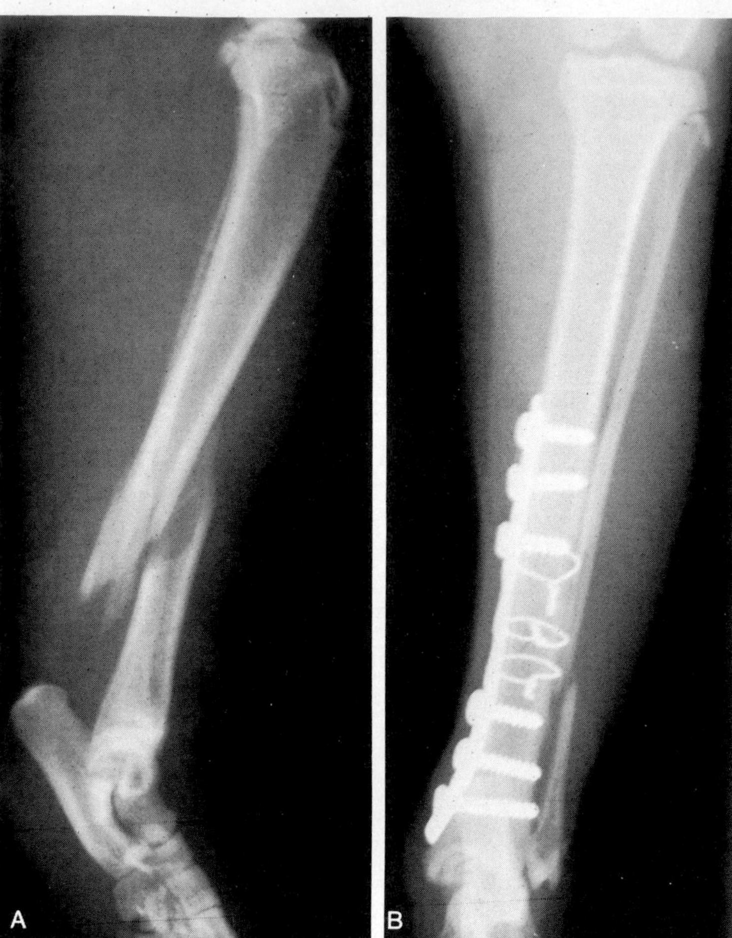


**Figure 5–34** *A*, Oblique midshaft fracture of the tibia. *B*, Fixation with a bone plate. The fragments have been anatomically replaced and held with cerclage wires. Adequate support of the bone plate is provided by three screws above and below the fracture. (Courtesy Dr. S. G. Brown.)

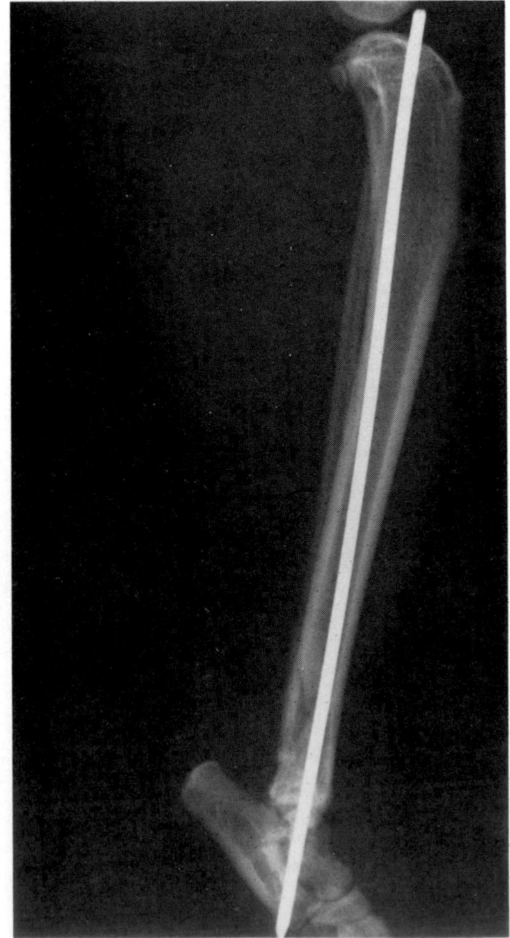

**Figure 5–35** Distal tibial fracture treated with a transtalar pin. Excellent fracture fixation is achieved. The pin is removed after the fracture has healed. The tibiotarsal joint will not be permanently affected. (Courtesy Dr. P. B. Vasseur.)

the proximal or distal fragment until a two-piece fracture is formed, which is then reduced and the intramedullary pin inserted. External fixation with the K/E apparatus is often effective. Transfixing pins allowing placement of a supporting rod both medially and laterally provide excellent rigidity. This method is effective when the fragments are contaminated or infected or when tissue coverage is inadequate. Wound dressings, drain adjustments, and débridement can be easily done as required (Fig. 5–36).

**SLIPPED DISTAL TIBIAL EPIPHYSIS.** This is fairly common in cats from four to nine months of age. Displacement is usually medial, and the condition should not be confused with luxation of the hock. Manual reduction may be possible within the first 48 hours with application of a coaptation splint.

Open reduction is usually required. The approach is over the site of the fracture. Intramedullary pins may split a small epiphysis, so care must be exercised in introducing them. The pin is inserted across the joint from the ventral surface of the hock into the medullary canal of the tibia, and a coaptation splint is applied. The pin is withdrawn in two to three weeks.

### Tarsus

A fractured calcaneus (fibular tarsal bone) is rare. The surgical approach is ventrolateral over the site of the fracture. A small intramedullary pin is inserted up the proximal fragment to exit at the point of the hock (tuber calcanei). The fracture is reduced and the pin is seated in the distal fragment as far as the heads of the metatarsals. A figure-eight wire tension band is looped over the pin at the point of the hock and through a hole drilled through the distal fragment (Fig. 5–37).

Fractures of the talus (tibial tarsal) bone are extremely rare. Ideally they are stabilized with a lag screw. If the bone is too small to be so treated, one or two small K wires are placed to maintain fracture alignment. The hock is placed in a coaptation splint (Fig. 5–38).

Fractures and luxations of other tarsal bones occasionally occur and are treated by open reduction and fixation with K wires or lag screws (Fig. 5–39).

### Metatarsals

Metatarsal fractures are fairly common and are treated in the same fashion as metacarpal fractures (Fig. 5–40).

## Pelvis

Pelvic fractures are very common in the cat. Most do not need to be repaired surgically, as they respond well to cage rest or confinement indoors. Surgical repair should be done if narrowing of the pelvic canal is significant and there are medially displaced sharp fragments that may damage the pelvic viscera. Involvement of the acetabulum is not so troublesome as in the dog, since the cat responds well to femoral head ostectomy. Pelvic fractures often damage the urinary tract and nearby nerves. If the cat is an intact female, spaying to prevent dystocia should be recommended.

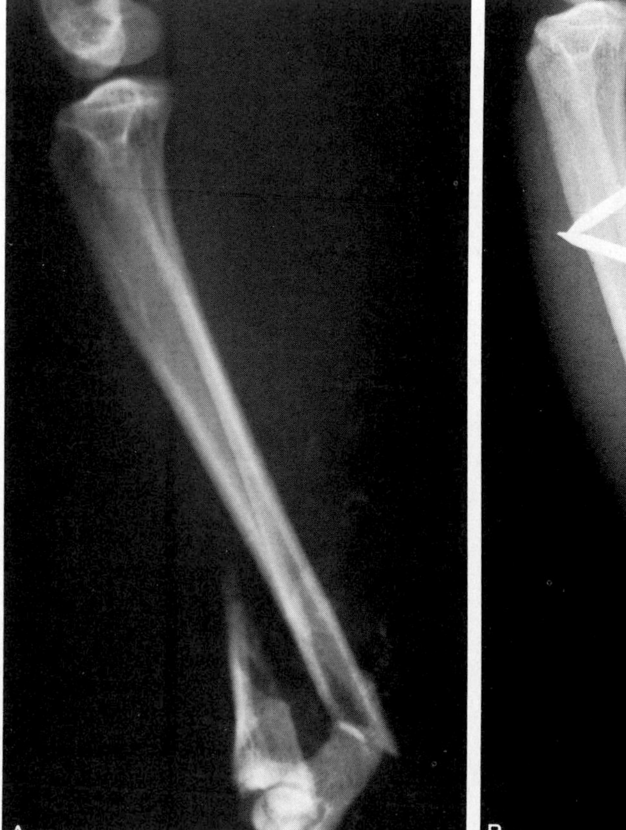


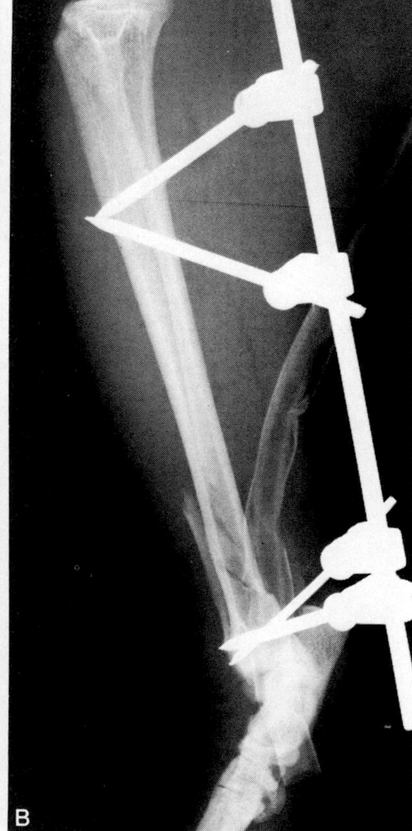


**Figure 5–36** *A,* Oblique distal fracture of the tibia. *B,* Fixation with a full K/E splint. A drain is present for treatment of infection in the surrounding soft tissues. (Courtesy Dr. P. C. Gambardella.)

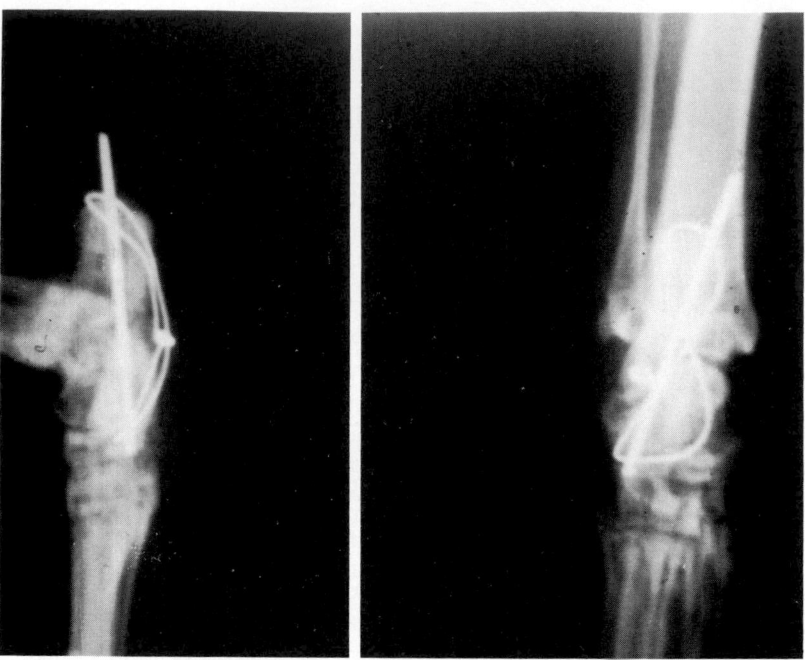

**Figure 5–37** A small intramedullary pin has been inserted to maintain reduction of a fracture of the calcaneus (fibular tarsal bone). A wire tension band counteracts the pull of the muscles attached to the tuber calcanei (tuber calcis).

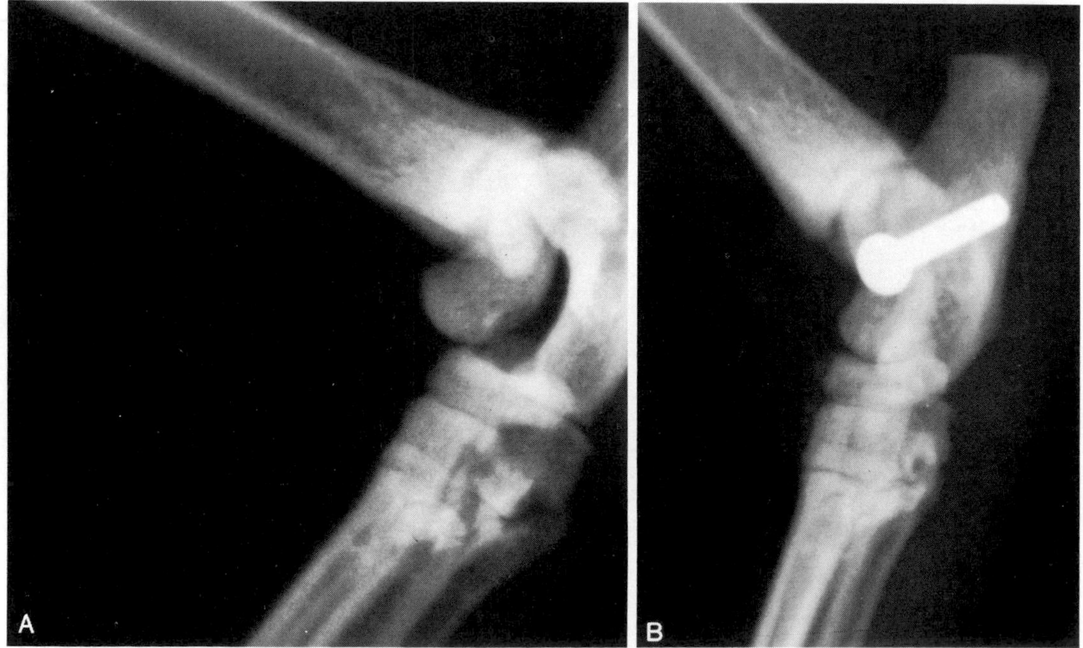


**Figure 5–38** *A*, Fracture luxation of the tibial tarsal bone. *B*, Reduction with a single lag screw. (Courtesy Dr. R. J. Todoroff.)

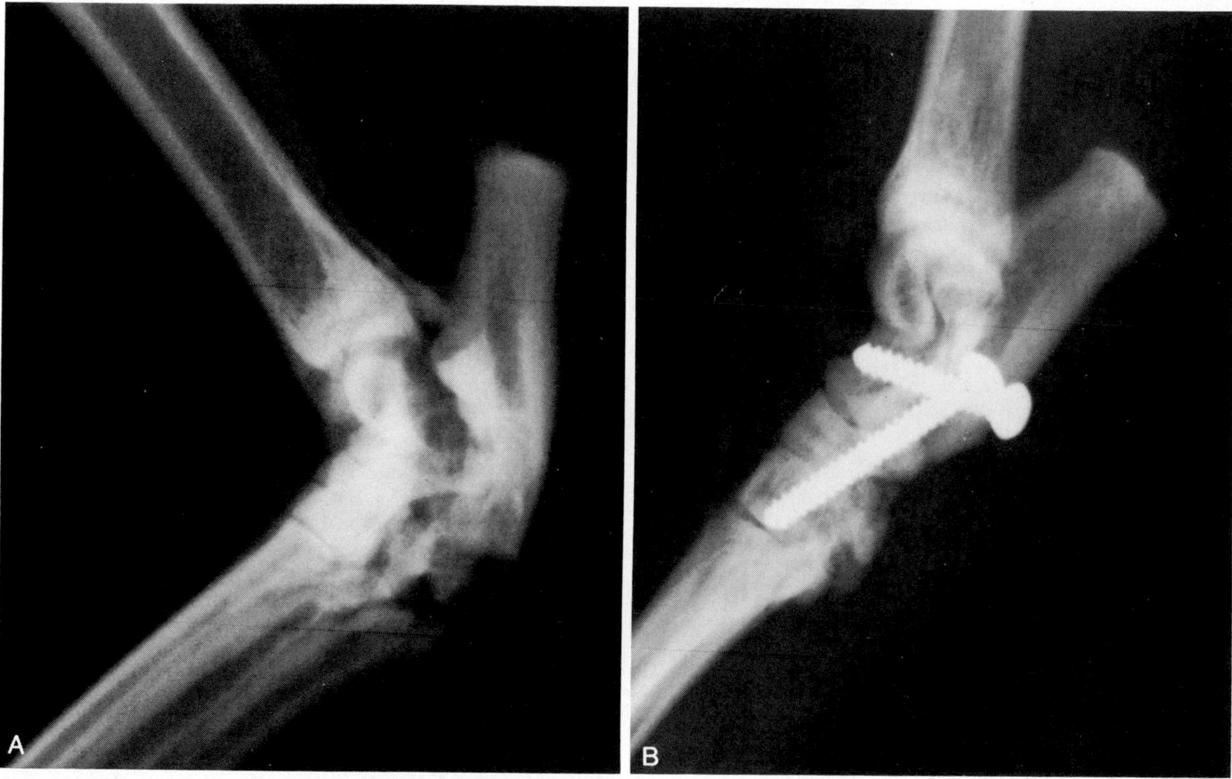


**Figure 5–39** *A,* Fracture and luxation of the calcaneus (fibular tarsal) and adjacent small tarsal bones. *B,* The luxation of the calcaneus has been reduced and stabilized with the proximal bone screw. The distal tarsal bones have been immobilized with the distal bone screw. Solid union and good joint function were obtained. (Courtesy Dr. R. J. Todoroff.)

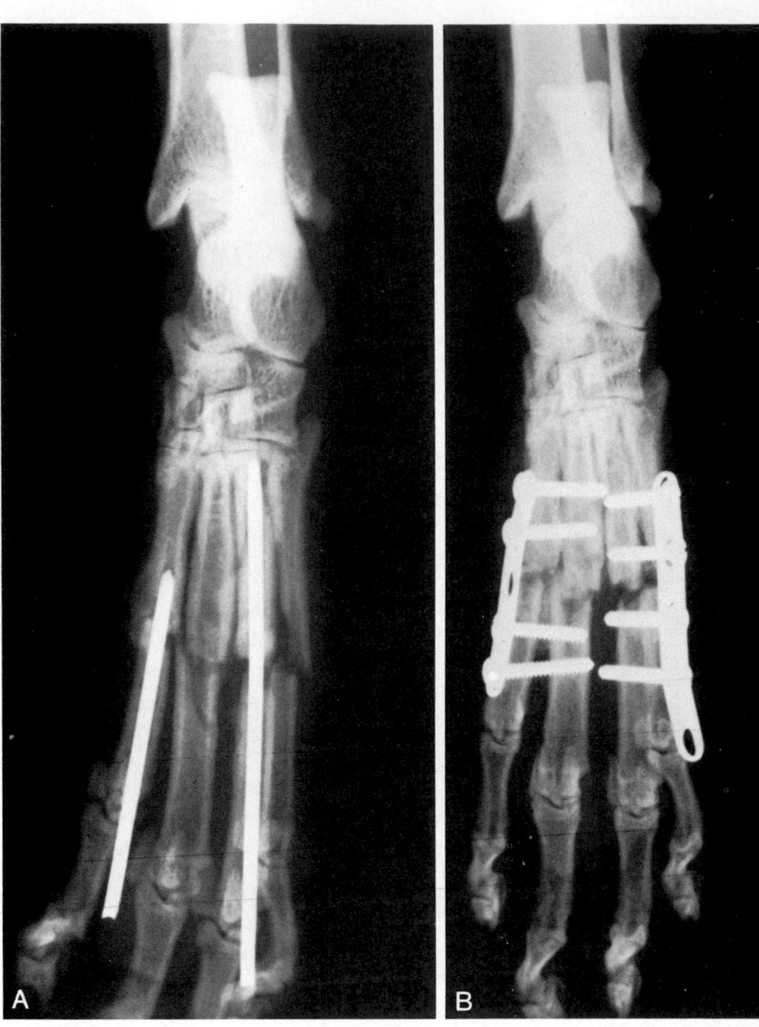


**Figure 5–40** *A,* Fractured metatarsals treated with small intramedullary pins. The foot is placed in a coaptation splint. (Courtesy Dr. S. G. Brown.) *B,* Fractured metatarsals treated with two small bone plates. Previous attempts to achieve healing had failed. Successful union was obtained.

## Oblique Iliac Shaft Fractures

The ilium is a common site for pelvic fractures. Treatment is by introduction of an intramedullary pin. The approach is dorsal between the superficial and middle gluteal muscles. An intramedullary pin is introduced from the fracture site into the proximal iliac fragment to exit at the medial aspect of the tuber coxae. To do this more readily, a closed straight hemostat is carefully passed caudally over the femoral neck along the body of the ischium and out through a small incision made in the skin over the tuber ischii. The pin is grasped and guided to the fracture site, parallel to the body of the ischium and in line with the ilium to avoid injury to the sciatic nerve. It is quite difficult to enter the craniomedial aspect of the tuber coxae and have the pin exit at the fracture site. After the pin is driven retrograde from the fracture site, the fracture is reduced and the pin is driven across the fracture and seated in the caudal iliac fragment. It should not enter the acetabulum. The pin is cut off close to the bone under the skin. The cat is confined to a cage for three or four weeks. Excellent results can also be obtained with bone plates (Fig. 5–41).

## Ipsilateral Fractures of the Ilium and Ischium

These fractures allow the acetabular fragment to be displaced inwardly. The iliac fracture is repaired with an intramedullary pin or bone plate. The ischium rarely needs fixation (Fig. 5–42).

The acetabular fragment or fragments can be maintained in position by a rolled bandage splint. A padded roll of bandage is placed longitudinally between the thighs against the pelvic symphysis. The roll should be large enough so that when the stifles are adducted the acetabular fragment is forced laterally by the lever action of the femur. The adduction is maintained by a loop of adhesive tape placed from one hindlimb to the other just above the stifles. The padded roll is further secured by strips of tape passed between the legs to cross over the back. Cage confinement is maintained for three weeks.

## Fractures of the Pubis or Ischium

Surgical repair of these common fractures is not often needed. Damage to the bladder or urethra should be ruled out. In those cases where the displacement is severe

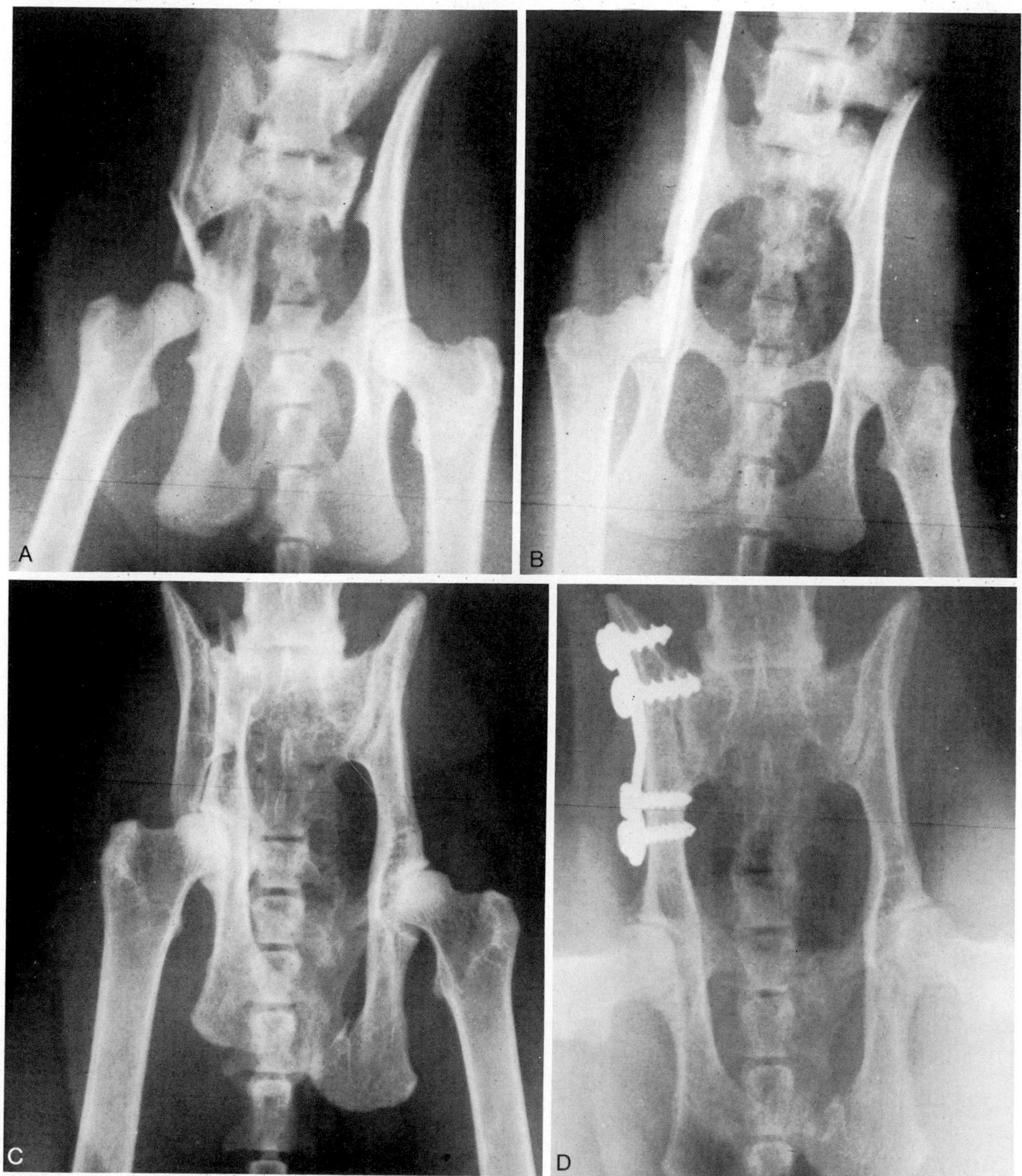


**Figure 5–41** *A,* Fracture of the ilium, ischium, and pubis. *B,* Fixation with an intramedullary pin. *C,* Fracture of the ilium, ischium, and pubis. *D,* Fixation by plating of the body of the ilium gave excellent results. (*C* and *D,* Courtesy Dr. S. G. Brown.)

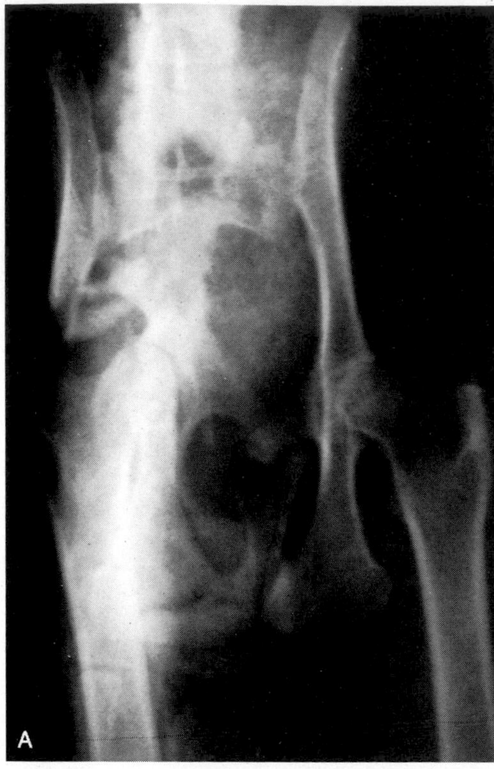


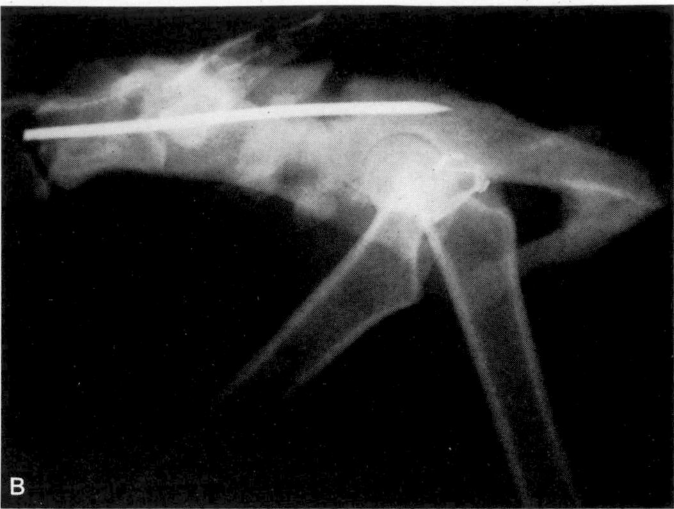


**Figure 5–42** *A,* Multiple fractures of the pelvis with the acetabular fragment forced medially require repair to avoid narrowing of the pelvic canal and hindlimb lameness. *B,* The fracture of the ilium has been treated with an intramedullary pin, and ischial fragments have been wired together. The pelvic canal is not obstructed, and the hindlimb has complete function. (Courtesy Dr. R. C. Griffiths.)

enough to result in obstipation or the symphysis pubis is so widely separated that the animal is unable to stand, the pubis may be wired together with 22-gauge orthopedic wire. Small holes are drilled in the opposing fragments. The wire is introduced and tightened, drawing the symphysis or fragments together. Improvement in walking and speed of healing are soon observed. Ischial fractures rarely cause damage to the sciatic nerve. Ordinarily, conservative treatment will suffice, but large, loose, painful fragments are immobilized with a pin and wire (Fig. 5–43).

## Multiple Fractures of the Pelvis

These are very common, and urinary tract and neurologic injury are of utmost concern. Orthopedic repair is

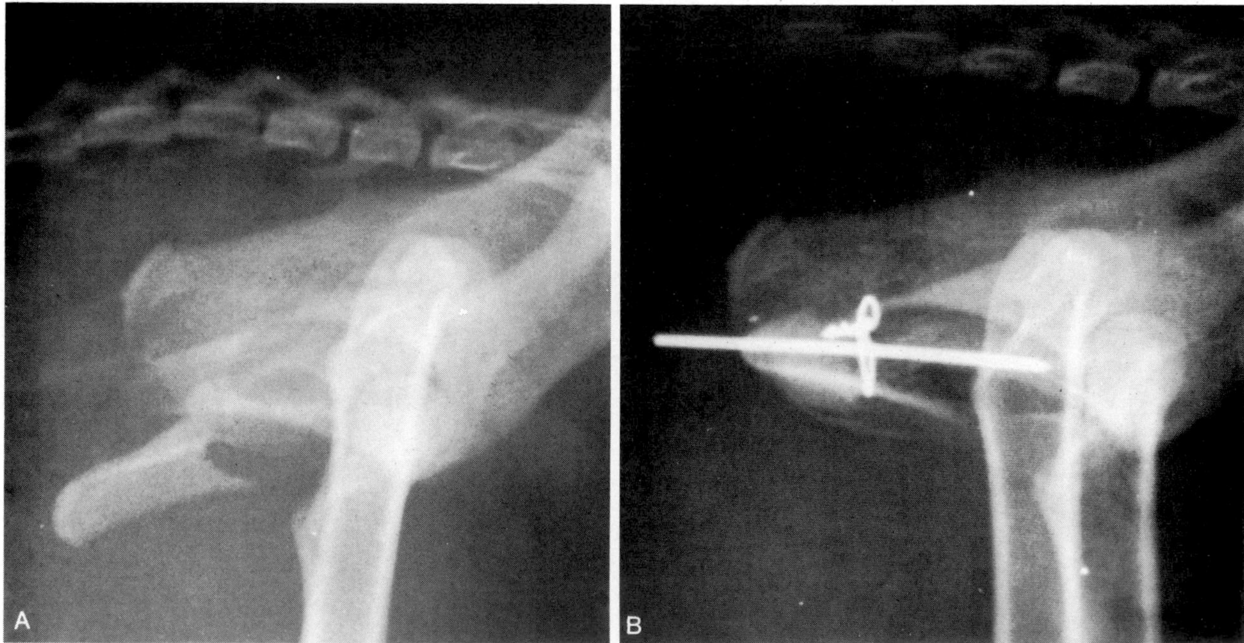


**Figure 5–43** *A,* Displaced fracture of the ischium. *B,* Fixation with a K wire and a loop of orthopedic wire. Pain from movement of the fragment was relieved. (Courtesy Dr. R. J. Todoroff.)

oriented toward maintaining the diameter of the pelvic canal. Control of constipation during the healing period requires a lubricant or stool softener. Combinations of pins, wires, and plates are used.

## Sacrococcygeal Separations

These are fairly frequent and may occur with other pelvic injuries. Cats crouch with tail paralysis and can have urinary stasis from damage to the sacral nerve plexus. Paralysis of the anal sphincter may result in fecal incontinence (Bennett, 1975). The sacrococcygeal separation may be 2 to 3 cm long. Initial treatment is conservative with physical and medical aid to control the bladder and bowel functions. The likelihood of recovery is slight after four weeks. If the tail develops dry gangrene or remains totally paralyzed it should be amputated (Fig. 5–44).

## Pelvic Symphysiotomy

Occasionally cats suffer chronic obstipation when the pelvic inlet diameter is decreased as a result of collapse from nutritional calcium deficiency or old malaligned fractures. Relief is obtained by splitting or excising the pubic symphysis and placing a notched metal spreader (Ward, 1967; Leighton, 1969) or by the use of an iliac bone graft (Herron, 1975a) or an iliac allograft (Evans, 1980).

For symphysiotomy with a bone graft the symphysis is exposed through a ventral incision. It is split with a small bone chisel or osteotome and spread apart. If it cannot be forced apart sufficiently it is excised with a rongeur. Two holes are drilled in the ischium on each side and each is threaded with 20-gauge orthopedic wire. Matching holes are drilled in the bone graft, and the corresponding wires are inserted in them. The graft is forced into place and the wires twisted tightly. Specially prepared self-retaining metal spreaders may be inserted instead. Vascular adhesions to bone in malaligned pelvic fractures should be removed with great care because of the danger of hemorrhage. The interference with passage of stool is removed and normal defecation restored.

# MAXILLA AND MANDIBLE

## Split Hard Palate

This condition is particularly common in urban areas where cats fall from high buildings (Robinson, 1976). The hard palate splits longitudinally, often with extensive separation. A minor separation often heals without treatment. Complications of hemorrhage and pneumothorax are common and must be dealt with before anesthesia or surgery can be considered.

A mattress suture of orthopedic wire is placed across the roof of the mouth from one second or third premolar to the other at the location of widest separation. Small holes are drilled through the gums, one rostral and one caudal to the second or third premolar on each side. The wire is passed through these holes with a blunt hypodermic needle as a guide and is twisted tightly to draw the maxillary separation together. The twisted portion of the wire ends is cut off and bent back parallel to the buccal gum line. The wire is removed in two weeks (Fig. 5–45).

## Other Fractures of the Maxilla

Most maxillary fractures are treated conservatively. Occasionally a depressed fracture of the zygomatic arch must be retracted laterally to relieve pressure on the eye or permit movement of the mandible. A small incision is made over the fracture site, and the depressed fragments are drawn into position with a towel clamp or Snook spay hook.

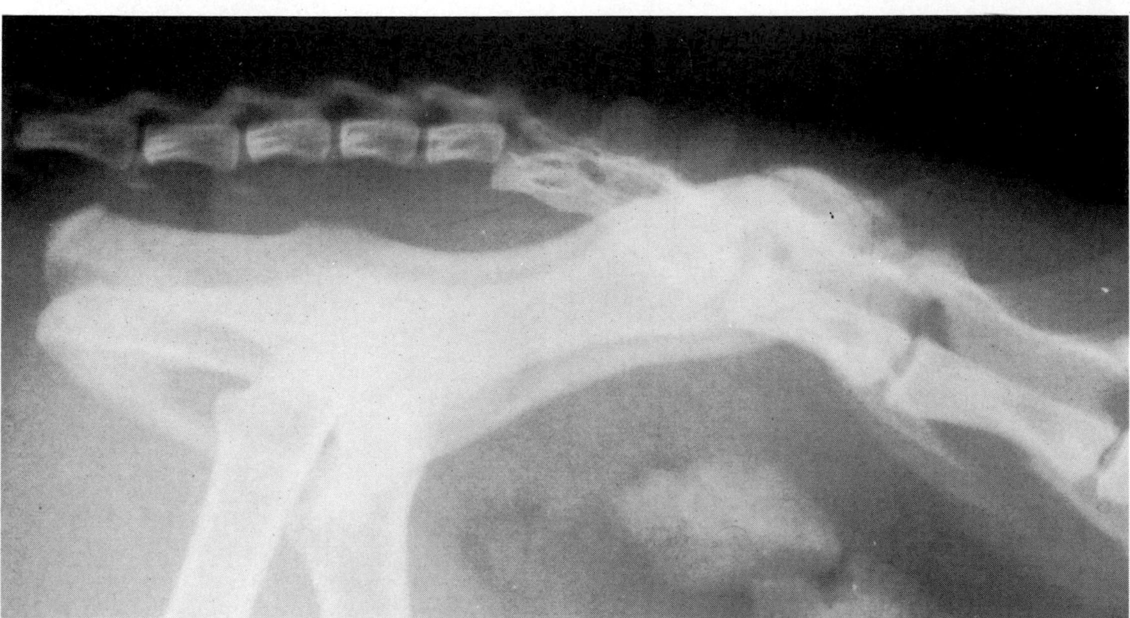

**Figure 5–44** A minor sacrococcygeal separation. Major separations will usually have the more severe neurologic complications.

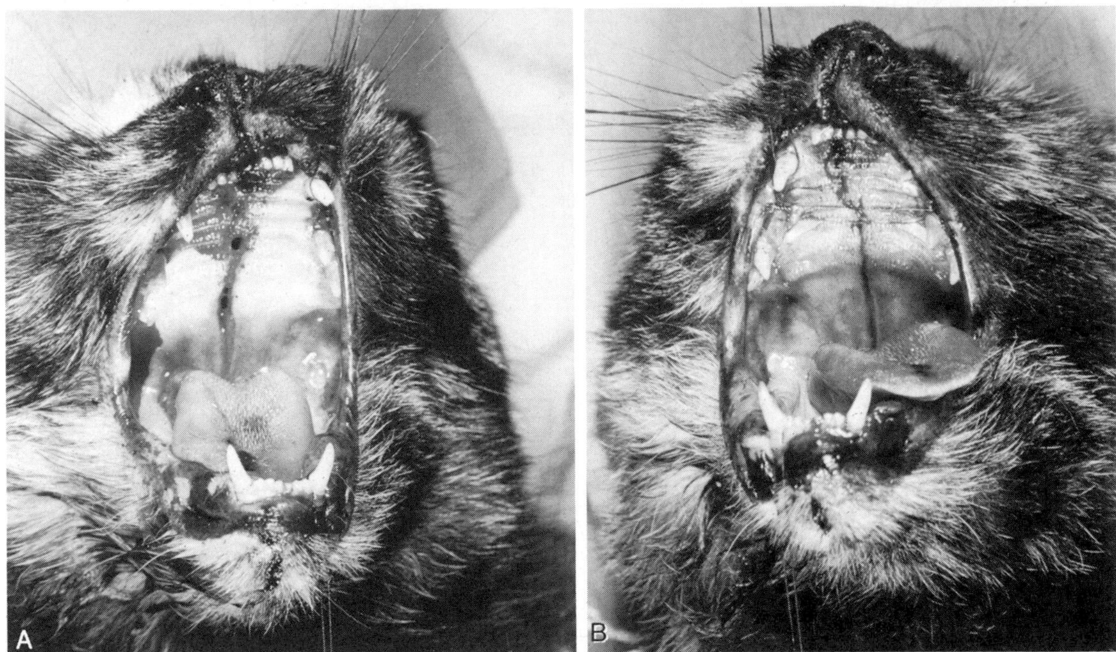


**Figure 5–45** *A,* Fracture of the maxilla (split hard palate). *B,* Immobilization with a mattress suture of orthopedic wire across the roof of the mouth. (Courtesy Dr. T. O. Munson.)

## Split Mandibular Symphysis

This very common injury is best treated by wiring the two fragments together. A simple figure-eight around the lower canines is seldom satisfactory because the wire works loose and when tightened tends to distract the fracture. Several other wiring techniques work satisfactorily.

A 20-gauge needle is passed subgingivally caudal to each lower canine from buccal to lingual side. From the lingual side the free ends of a piece of 24-gauge orthopedic wire are passed through the needles, which are then withdrawn. The ends of the wire are brought together in front of the mandible as far down on the gingiva as possible and tightened to fix the fracture. The twisted wire is cut and bent to lie close to the gum line. The wire will cut into the gingiva, but this is of no consequence. Placing the wire subgingivally keeps it from coming off and being swallowed by the cat, with possible harmful complications in the digestive tract (Fig. 5–46).

Another method of wiring approaches the fractured symphysis from the ventral aspect. The tissues are separated from the underlying bone enough to allow a wire stitch to be placed in holes drilled in the end of each half of the mandible centering on the exposed split surfaces. When the wire is tightened the fragments are drawn together. The twisted ends are cut and bent flat to the bone. The wire remains permanently.

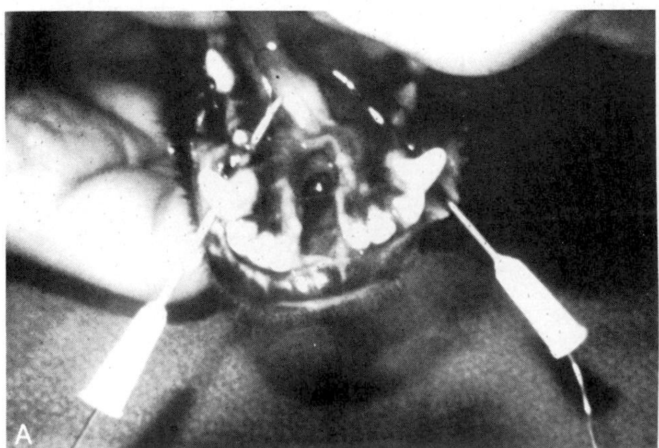


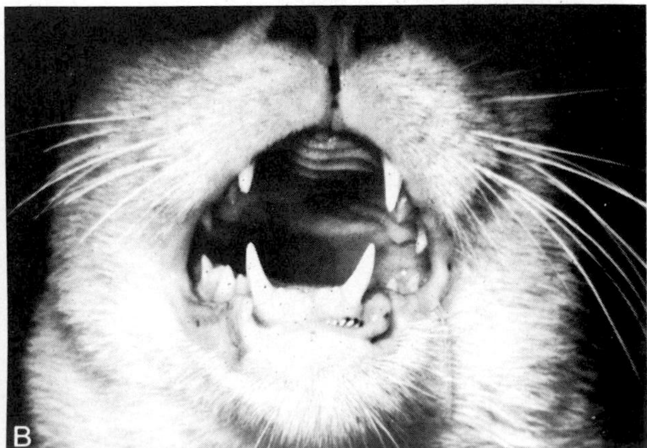


**Figure 5–46** *A,* Split mandibular symphysis, dog. Two 22-gauge needles are used to guide the wire subgingivally caudal to the lower canines. *B,* Same procedure in a cat. The orthopedic wire passed subgingivally caudal to the lower canines is brought rostrally and twisted together to draw the separated symphysis together. Excellent healing has occurred.

Transfixion of the two sides of the mandible through the fracture site with a small K wire improves stability and is combined with a figure-eight wire. The pin and wire are removed after healing.

## Fractures of the Mandible

These relatively common fractures are often best managed by placing the teeth in proper occlusion and applying a muzzle. The cat is able to eat foods of fairly liquid consistency. The canines remain in contact, but the tongue can be extended between the incisors. A pharyngostomy tube can be placed but is rarely needed.

A tape muzzle is made from a strip of adhesive tape 1-inch wide with an equal length of 24-gauge wire placed longitudinally in the center. The tape is folded longitudinally on itself over the wire, providing a fairly stiff 1/2-inch double thickness piece, from which a tight form-fitting muzzle may be made (Fig. 5–47).

Multiple or unstable fractures may require that the jaw be wired shut. A small hole is drilled transversely through the maxilla just rostral to the roots of the upper canines. A piece of 22-gauge wire is introduced with an 18-gauge needle as a guide. The wire is similarly passed through a hole drilled transversely through the mandible just rostral to the roots of the lower incisors. The mouth is closed to get normal occlusion with the lower canines rostral and medial to the upper ones. The wire is tightened and twisted closed. A pharyngostomy tube could be used but is rarely needed if the cat is allowed just enough space to extend the tongue over the incisors. A semiliquid diet is provided. Normal function of the jaw will return in two to three weeks (Hobart, 1979) (Fig. 5–48).

Fracture of the body of the mandible may require some form of external fixation, especially if bilateral and complicated by loss of, or damage to, teeth. A small-diameter pin is placed transversely across the rostral fragment, avoiding the roots of the canines. A similar pin is placed across the most caudal portion of the mandible just under the skin of the intermandibular space. Other small pins are placed at an angle in a location to obtain the best additional fragment control. These pins are cut off about 1 cm from the skin.

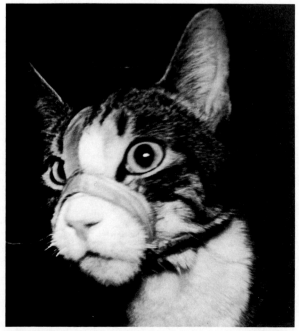

**Figure 5–47** A wire-reinforced tape muzzle will help to hold a mandibular fracture in position and still allow ingestion of liquid.

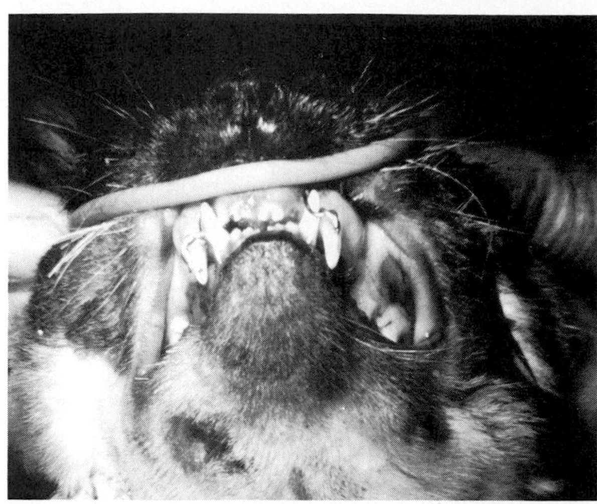

**Figure 5–48** Fracture of the mandible. The upper lip is retracted to show that the upper and lower jaws have been wired together. Space enough is provided so that the cat can extend the tongue over the incisors and ingest liquid.

A soft mixture of methyl methacrylate is prepared and injected by syringe into a piece of plastic tubing. The filled tubing is impaled on the projecting pins. The fragments are aligned first by finger pressure in the mouth and then by holding the mouth shut with the canine teeth in proper occlusion. The plastic will quickly harden, holding the pins solidly. To remove the splint, the pins are cut between the skin and the plastic and then carefully withdrawn (Fig. 5–49).

# SPINE

Spinal fractures are uncommon and require a good neurologic workup to determine whether surgical repair is indicated. Great care should be taken in handling spinal fractures, especially when radiographing the anesthetized patient.

External splinting and bandaging are poorly tolerated and rarely effective. Internal fixation is done with a spinal rod made from an intramedullary pin, with plastic spinal plates, or with methyl methacrylate applied to the ends of K wires inserted into the vertebral bodies near the fracture site.

The patient is firmly positioned on its sternum. A dorsal midline incision is made and the dorsal vertebral spinous processes exposed by sharp and blunt dissection. A dorsal laminectomy is done only if immediate decompression or inspection of the cord is needed. A 5/64-inch diameter intramedullary pin is cut to a length to extend over three vertebrae cranial and caudal to the fracture. A rounded

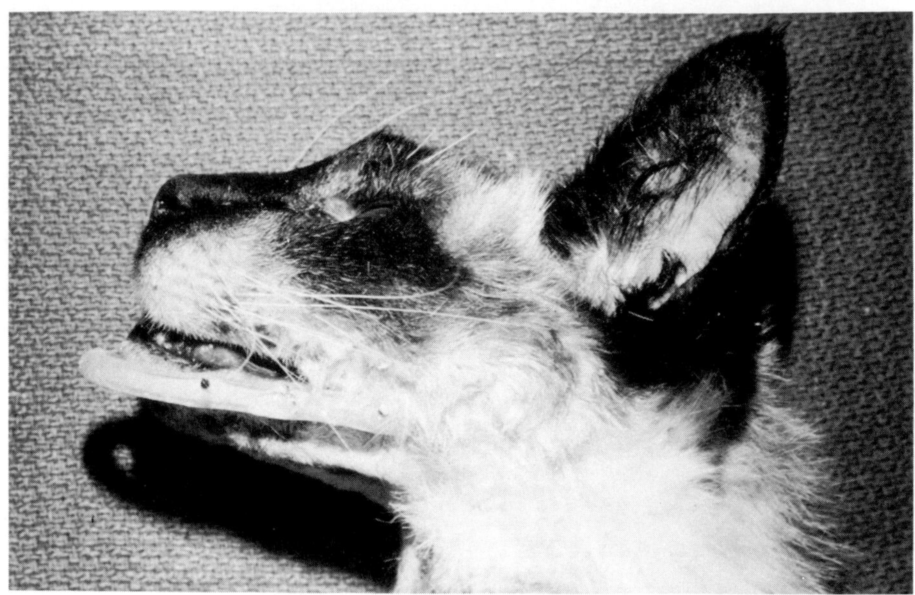

**Figure 5–49** A bilateral fracture of the mandible treated by inserting small intramedullary pins into the fragments. The pins are secured externally with methyl methacrylate. The plastic has been inserted into tubing that has been impaled on the pin ends.

hook is formed at one end. As an assistant holds the fracture in alignment with bone-holding forceps, the curved end of the wire rod is hooked in front of the dorsal spine two vertebrae cranial to the fracture. The wire rod is placed along the dorsal spinal processes as close to the lamina as possible. The caudal end of the wire is bent to hook caudally around the dorsal spinal process two vertebral bodies caudal to the fracture. Small wires are placed through holes drilled in the dorsal processes and then twisted tightly around the rod to hold it securely. The device is left in place permanently. Muscle spasm and the natural arching of the back tend to increase the tension on the rod. After closure the cat is confined in a well-padded cage with intensive nursing care for three weeks. The prognosis is guarded (Fig. 5–50).

An alternative procedure provides stability with paired plastic spinal plates, Lubraplates,* which are compressed onto the exposed dorsal spinous processes by interspaced nuts and bolts. The device is left in place permanently (Fig. 5–51).

A new procedure involves inserting bilaterally paired K wires into the vertebral body cranial and caudal to the fracture. These must be firmly seated in the entire body and must avoid the vertebral canal. The dorsally projecting pin ends are cut off a bit shorter than the dorsal spines. A soft mass of methyl methacrylate is molded over the projecting pin ends. The hardening process is exothermic. Chilled physiologic saline or Ringer's solution is flushed over the area. None of the methyl methacrylate is allowed to contact the cord at a laminectomy site. After the plastic has set, a regular closure is done. The material remains permanently. No different aftercare is needed.

## MANAGEMENT OF LUXATIONS

### Mandibular Luxation

This condition is fairly common, especially in urban areas where cats fall from high buildings. The displacement is caudal, permitting the lower canines to strike the hard palate. With the cat well relaxed under anesthesia, a pencil or a piece of 1/4-inch wooden dowel is placed across the mouth in the area of the molar teeth. With the dowel serving as a fulcrum, the nose and tip of the mandible are squeezed together and the dowel is rotated so that the mandible is distracted and drawn forward. When the luxation is of less than 48 hours duration, reduction to normal occlusion is usually easy. A muzzle is applied for a week (Fig. 5–52).

### Scapular Luxation

This condition, infrequent in the cat, produces a significant although painless lameness. The supporting structures of the scapula are torn away, so that it is loosened from the body and moves freely under the skin, especially in an upward direction. Treatment consists of anchoring the scapula to the fifth rib (Leighton, 1975) (Fig. 5–53).

With the cat on its side, the scapula is placed in its normal position. An incision is made along the dorsal half of the caudal edge of the scapula, and a 2-cm section of the caudodorsal edge of the scapula is freed of muscle. A rib directly beneath, usually the fifth or sixth, is exposed by blunt dissection. A piece of 22-gauge wire is passed around it with care not to invade the pleural cavity. Two holes are drilled in the exposed edge of the scapula. The ends of the wire are passed through them and tightened and twisted together, anchoring the scapula to the thoracic cage in correct anatomic position. No bandaging is needed. The functional result is usually good.

### Elbow Luxation

This condition is rare in the cat (Mainster, 1980). A much more common injury is subluxation secondary to a fracture of the lateral or occasionally the medial aspect of the humeral condyle. In a true luxation the anconeal process is displaced caudolaterally over the lateral aspect of the humeral condyle. Manual reduction requires deep

*The Lubra Company, 1905 Mohawk, Fort Collins, CO 80525.

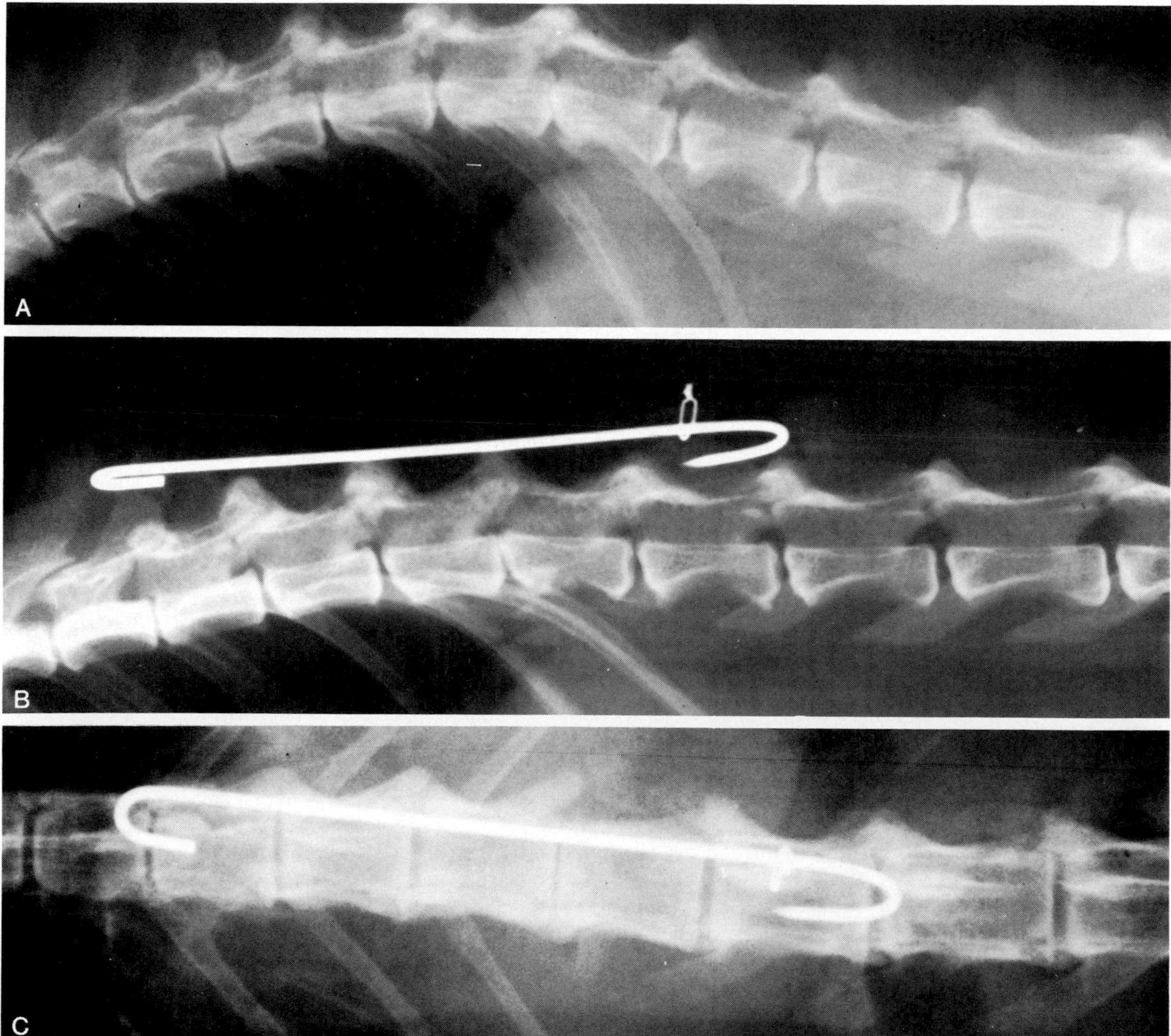


**Figure 5–50** *A,* A collapsed disk space is present at T13–L1, the result of an injury of unknown origin. *B,* A steel pin has been inserted along the side of the base of the dorsal spinous processes to stabilize T13–L1. *C,* The dorsal view shows the steel pin at the base of the spinous processes hooked around the dorsal spines above and below the unstable space at T13–L1. (Courtesy Dr. P. C. Gambardella.)

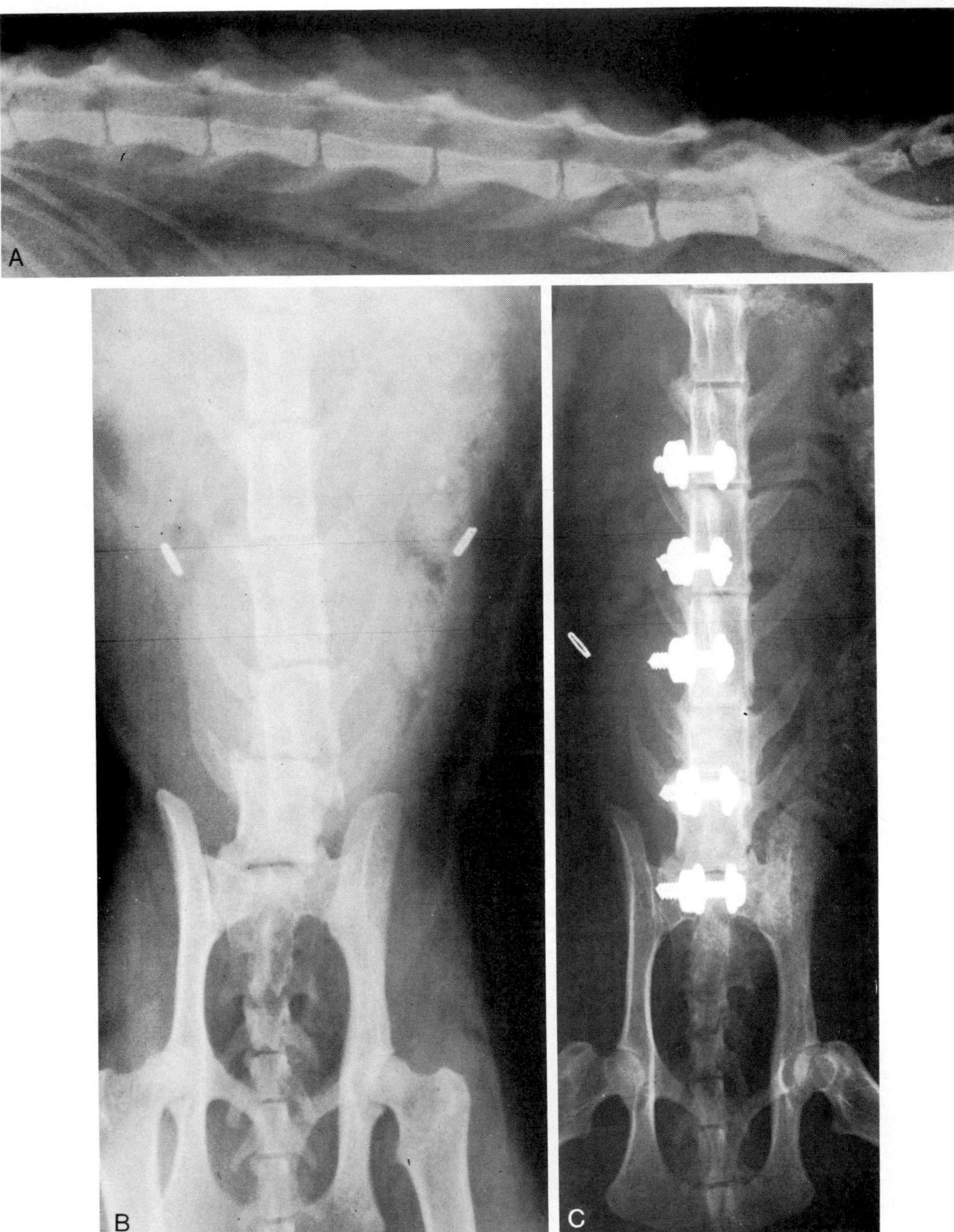

**Figure 5–51** *A*, Lateral view of an oblique fracture of L6 with cranioventral displacement. *B*, Dorsoventral view showing lateral displacement. *C*, Dorsoventral view of repair of the fracture of L6 with Lubraplates. The nuts and bolts are placed between the dorsal spines, compressing the paired plates against them. The device remains permanently. Good healing and recovery were reported. (Courtesy Angell Memorial Animal Hospital.)

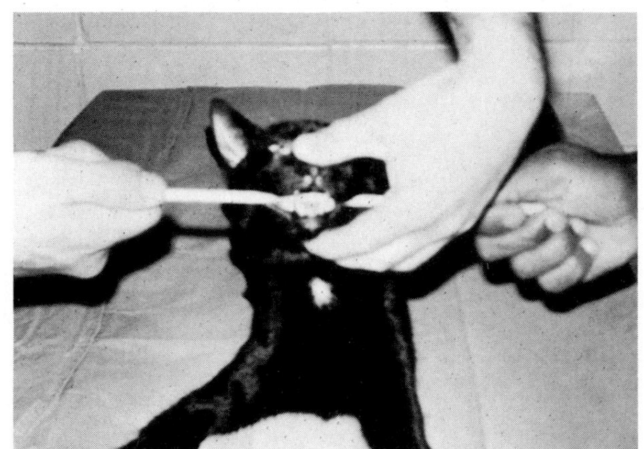

**Figure 5–52** A small dowel or pencil is placed across the back of the mouth in treatment of luxation of the jaw. As the mouth is forced shut, the dowel is rotated to bring the lower jaw forward.

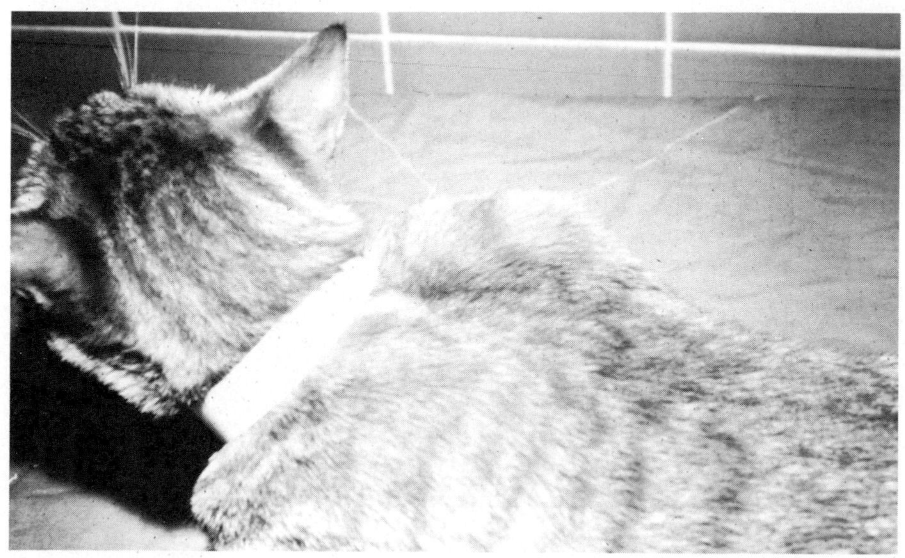

**Figure 5–53** The luxated right scapula moves freely under the skin and projects above the withers as the cat walks on the limb.

anesthesia. The elbow is flexed while the ulna is pushed medially until the anconeal process engages the caudal aspect of the lateral aspect of the humeral condyle. The elbow is slightly extended, and the radial head is pushed medially and distally. As the anconeal process is guided into the olecranon fossa the radial head is reduced. A full range of motion indicates successful replacement. The elbow is bandaged in extension for 10 days.

Elbow luxations over a few days old require surgical reduction by a caudolateral approach with a tenotomy of the triceps tendon. Considerable scar tissue must be removed. With the pull of the triceps relieved, the anconeal process is more readily replaced into normal position. The radial head follows into position at the same time. The tenotomy is closed with nonabsorbable suture material, and the elbow is immobilized in a splint for 10 to 14 days (Fig. 5–54).

## Carpal Luxations

These are rare in the cat. Caudal luxations are usually stable when reduced and are treated by splinting for about four weeks. Cranial luxations usually involve injuries to the supportive ligaments of the carpus and show varying degrees of hyperextension sometimes associated with small fractures of the carpal bones. Reduction and splinting in a moderately flexed position may bring some improvement, but in general results may be unfavorable (Fig. 5–55).

## Sacroiliac Luxation

This is a fairly common condition in the cat and, when minor, frequently does not require surgical replacement.

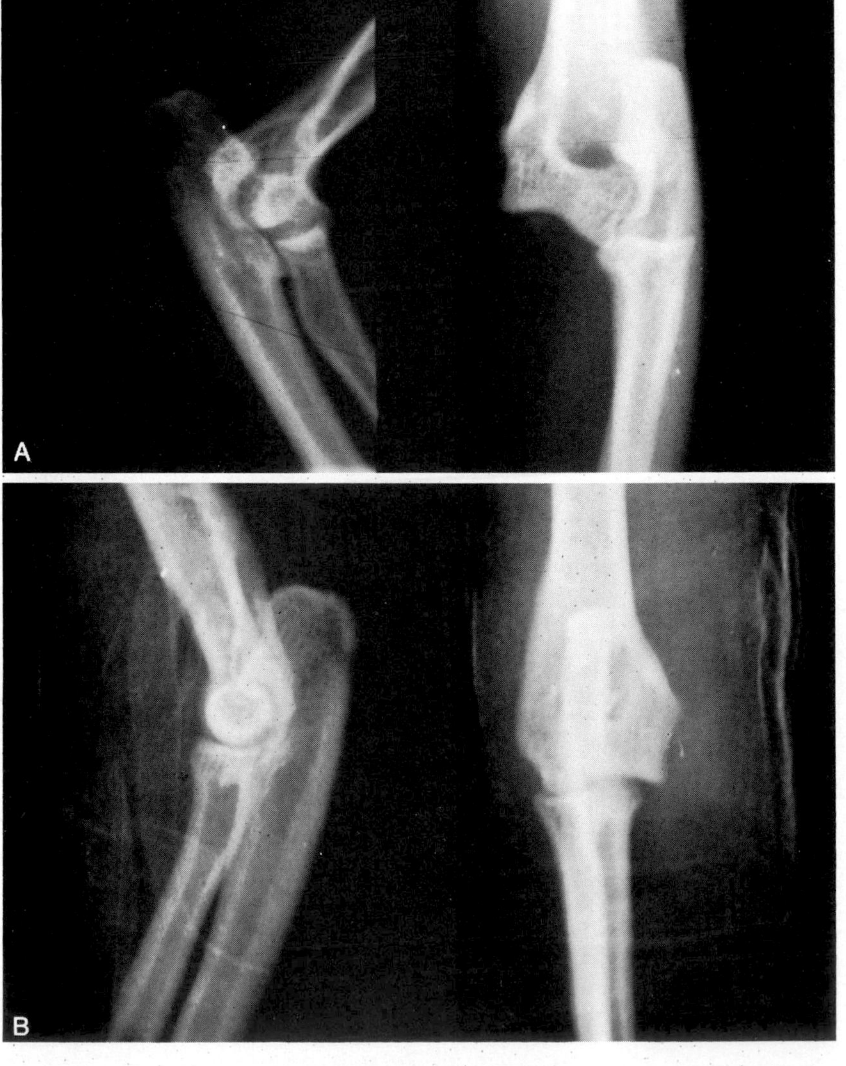


**Figure 5–54** *A,* Complete elbow luxation. The diagnostic value of the A-P view is well demonstrated. *B,* The luxation has been reduced manually and the leg placed in a coaptation splint. (Courtesy Dr. R. C. Griffiths.)

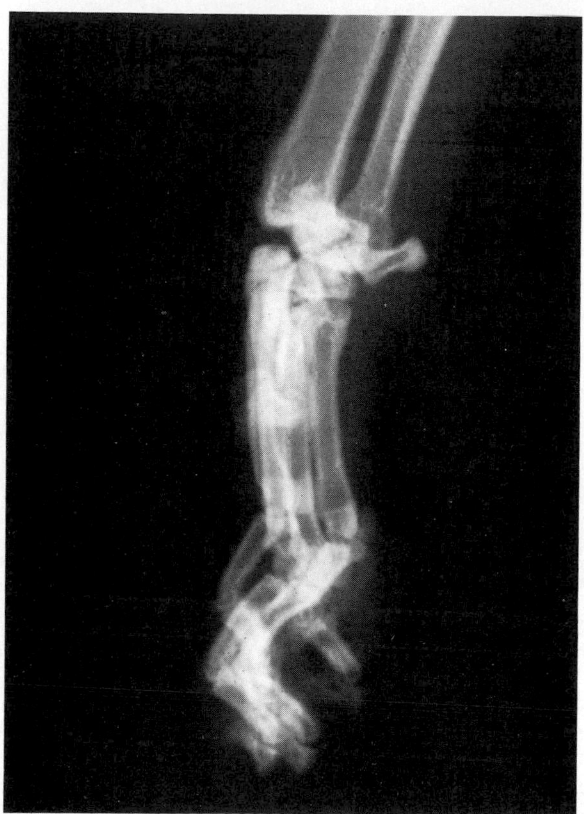

**Figure 5–55** Carpal luxations in a cat. Most may be managed by closed reduction and splinting. (Courtesy Dr. R. C. Griffiths.)

Of greater concern is the possibility of neural injury impairing the autonomic control of the rectum, anus, and bladder and resulting variously in urinary and fecal incontinence or urinary retention. Concomitant fractures of the pelvis allow the hemipelvis to move forward. Fresh luxations can sometimes be treated by closed reduction (Herron, 1976). Surgical repair is indicated in more severe cases.

Fixation can be obtained by inserting a 3/32-inch diameter intramedullary pin transversely from the lateral side of the wing of the ilium, which serves as a handle to shift the hemipelvis caudally. The pin is placed in the middle to ventral portion of the wing of the ilium so that it may be driven medially to anchor into the sacrum when the luxation is reduced. A towel clamp secured to the tuber ischii or the greater trochanter provides a grip to assist in moving the hemipelvis into position. The body of the cat must be immobilized by an assistant. The index finger placed in the rectum by an assistant aids in guiding the fragment and stabilizing the cat's body. The pin is removed in three weeks. Perfect reduction is rare. If the pelvic canal is narrowed, spaying of intact females should be recommended.

## Coxofemoral Luxations

Hip luxations are common in mature cats, but fractures of the femoral neck are more frequent than luxations in younger cats. Craniodorsal luxation is usual. Closed reduction is possible when the injury is not over two to three days old and there is no obstructing material in the acetabulum. Reduction is obtained by rotating the femur outward and pulling it caudoventrally until the femoral head is seated in the acetabulum. Then the leg is rotated inward and flexed. It is important for the surgeon to push upward (laterally) on the lesser trochanter with the thumb of the opposite hand while the leg is pulled caudoventrally. The fingers of this hand then press downward on the trochanter after the femoral head is over the acetabulum. An Ehmer sling is applied for 7 to 10 days. It is difficult to keep such a device on a fat cat unless it is integrated into an abdominal bandage. Reduction is often unstable, usually because torn joint capsule or remnants of the ligament of the femoral head remain in the acetabulum.

Recurrent or unstable luxation requires one of several possible surgical procedures:

### Open Reduction with Suturing

An open reduction is done by a craniolateral approach. The acetabulum is exposed so that it may be cleared of blood clots, tissue debris, and remnants of the ligament of the femoral head. The luxation is reduced. The surrounding tissues are sutured to keep the hip in place. There may not be enough capsule or deep gluteal muscle remnants for a secure reduction. An Ehmer sling is applied for 10 to 14 days.

### Open Reduction with Transarticular Pinning

An open reduction is performed by a craniolateral approach, and the acetabulum is cleared of obstructing material. A 1/16-inch intramedullary pin is driven from the lateral base of the greater trochanter through the femoral neck to exit centrally at the fovea capitis; for more accurate placement it is inserted retrograde from the fovea capitis to exit laterally at the base of the greater trochanter. After the luxation is reduced, the leg is held in an anatomically correct position, and the pin is driven across the joint through the acetabulum for approximately 1 cm. The pin is retracted slightly and held in a strong forceps while a right-angled bend is produced. The pin is cut off to leave a small L-shaped tip and is seated firmly. The bent tip will prevent migration of the pin into the pelvic cavity. If the pin is placed correctly, flexion of the hip is allowed, but medial and lateral rotation and luxation are prevented. The cat is kept in a cage for two weeks, after which time the pin should be removed.

### Femoral Head Ostectomy

If damage to the acetabulum or femoral head precludes a good chance of maintaining a reduction, the femoral head is removed. Cats respond very well to such surgery, usually walking without a limp if the neck is removed flush with the femoral shaft (Berzon, 1980).

## Tibiotarsal Joint Luxation

This luxation is fairly common and is usually medial, with a fracture of the lateral malleolus. Transtalar pinning is effective in maintaining a reduction. The pin may be inserted through the tarsus, across the tibiotarsal joint, and into the medullary canal of the tibia. A more precise way of accurately placing the pin is to drive it up the medullary canal of the tibia from the distal joint surface to exit just medial to the straight patellar ligament. With the knee held flexed, the luxation is reduced and the pin is driven into the hock until its tip can be palpated on the ventral surface of the hock. The pin is cut off under the tissues of the knee close to the bone. After healing, the pin is withdrawn from either the knee or the hock. A coaptation splint may be applied for a month to reduce stress on the joint. Function will return in one to two weeks after pin removal.

For the fractured malleolus excellent results can be obtained by reduction and fixation with a K wire and tension band wire. Damaged collateral ligaments are replaced with a figure-eight of nonabsorbable suture material placed between the malleolus and a small bone screw in the talus (tibial/tarsal) bone. (Fig. 5–56).

## TENDON AND LIGAMENT SURGERY

### Repair of the Triceps Tendon

Injury to the triceps tendon is uncommon and must be differentiated from damage to the brachial plexus or radial nerve. The cat carries the affected limb. For surgical repair an approach is made over the injury site. The torn or lacerated ends of the tendon are apposed and sutured with nonabsorbable suture material. Sutures may have to be passed through a small hole drilled in the olecranon. If more immobilization than can be obtained from a forelimb splint is needed, an intramedullary pin is introduced proximally into the humeral medullary canal and is driven across the olecranon fossa just through the olecranon. The joint is held so as to be fixed in extension. Proximally the pin is cut off just under the skin. The pin is removed in six to eight weeks. Normal function returns in about three weeks.

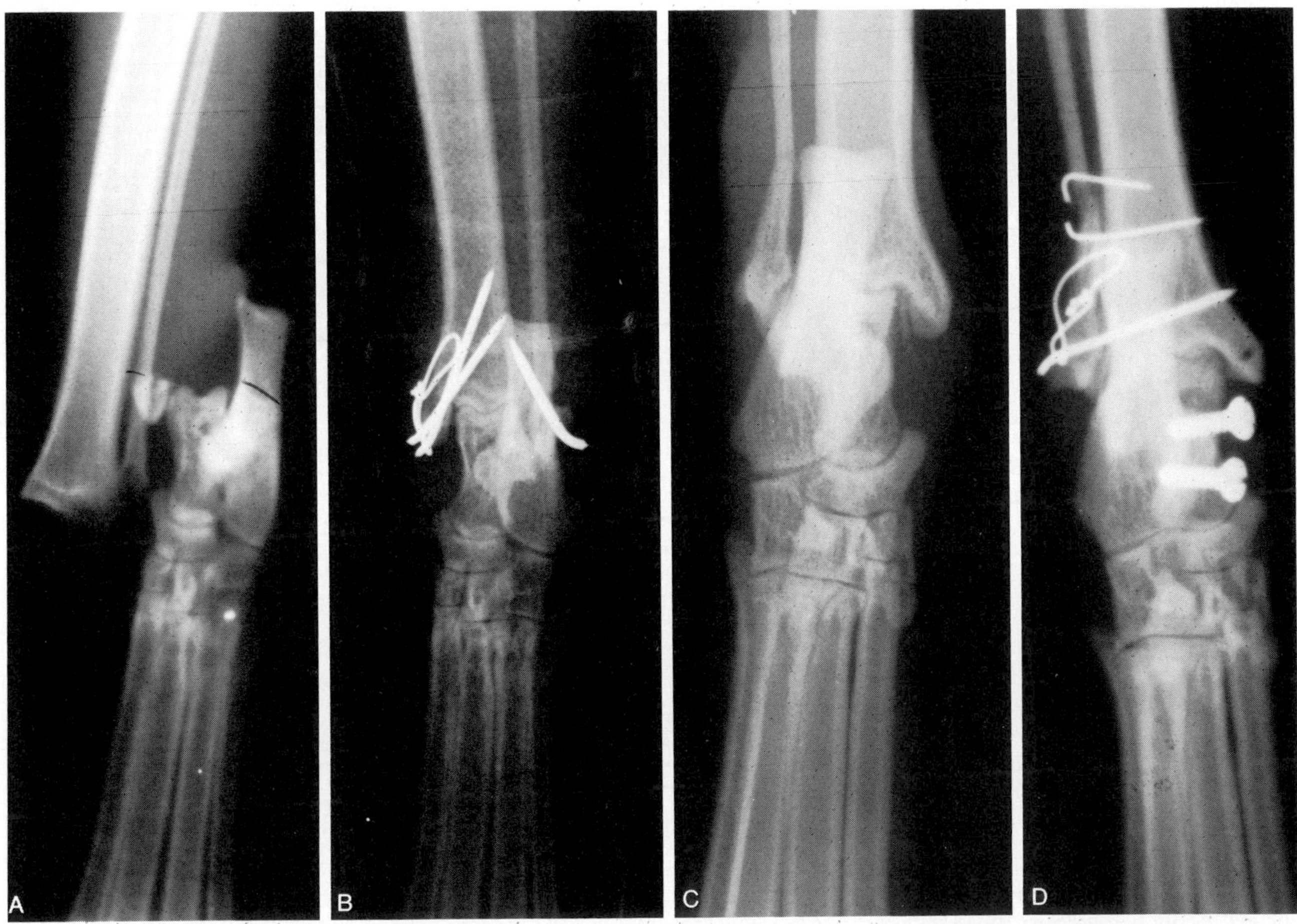


**Figure 5–56** *A,* Luxation of the tibiotarsal joint with fractures of both malleoli. *B,* The luxation has been reduced and the malleoli pinned in place with K wires. A tension band wire has been applied to the lateral malleolus. *C,* The lateral malleolus has been fractured, and the medial collateral ligament has been damaged in this tibiotarsal subluxation. *D,* The lateral malleolus and fibula fractures have been stabilized with K wires and a figure-eight tension band. The medial collateral supporting ligaments have been replaced by nonabsorbable sutures. These have been placed through a hole drilled in the medial malleolus and secured to the bone screws. (*C, D,* Courtesy Dr. S. G. Brown.)

### REPAIR OF THE COMMON CALCANEAL (ACHILLES) TENDON

With this relatively common injury part of the tendon complex may be torn from the calcaneus, or the tendon may be entirely severed or torn from the muscle groups at its origin. The injury must be differentiated from sciatic nerve paralysis or the results of iliac embolism.

The hock is held in extension and immobilized by introducing an intramedullary pin across the tibiotarsal joint. This transtalar pinning reduces stress on the surgical repair of the tendons. The pin may be introduced proximally at the knee just medial to the straight patellar ligament and driven down the medullary canal of the tibia across the tibiotarsal joint to exit through the talus (tibial tarsal) bone, until the point of the pin can be just palpated beneath the skin. The pin is cut off short at the knee.

Each of the tendons making up the common calcaneal tendon (Achilles tendon) is repaired separately by an appropriate technique. Nonabsorbable suture of small diameter is used. Considerable proximal dissection may be necessary to obtain the retracted tendon ends. A small hole is drilled transversely through the end of the calcaneus to receive a suture if the tendon is torn directly from its insertion on the bone. Severe cuts in this area may also necessitate repair of the digital flexor. The pin is removed in two months. Normal flexion usually returns in about three weeks.

### REPAIR OF RUPUTURED ANTERIOR CRUCIATE LIGAMENT

This is a fairly common injury in cats. The diagnostic feature is the "drawer" sign—an excessive cranial motion of the tibial plateau in relation to the femoral condyles. Unless the rupture is treated, osteoarthritis will result from joint instability. "Repair" is a misnomer. All the surgical procedures replace the ligament or its function, because it is usually so damaged that true repair is not feasible.

Some techniques provide anatomic replacement of the ligament with fascia, skin, tendon, ligament, or artificial material. Others provide functional replacement with fascia, suture pattern, or artificial material placed in a nonanatomic position (extra-articular location). All techniques are designed to produce joint stability and most are suitable for the cat.

A relatively simple method of stabilization is done with an extra-articular nonabsorbable suture placed laterally from the tibial crest to the lateral fabella. This permits complete joint function but prevents cranial motion of the tibial plateau. The joint is approached by a parapatellar incision 2 to 3 mm lateral to the patella. The joint is entered and the patella luxated medially. The remnants of the ruptured cruciate ligament are removed, the menisci are examined for damage, and the joint is flushed clear of any debris. A hole is drilled transversely through the proximal tip of the tibial crest, and a 0 to 1 size nonabsorbable suture such as Supramid (Vetafil) is passed through a hole from the lateral side and then returned under the straight patellar ligament. Another hole is drilled through the caudolateral portion of the lateral femoral condyle to exit just under the lateral fabella. The suture is threaded through this hole and is tied so that it does not restrict movement of the stifle but does stop the "drawer" sign. Medial rotation of the tibia is also controlled. The joint capsule and fascia are closed with a nonabsorbable suture material in an overlapping vertical mattress pattern. Imbricating the capsule and retinaculum in an oblique plane aids in stabilizing the joint (DeAngelis and Lau, 1970). No bandaging or splinting is needed. The cat is confined at home for about four weeks.

### MULTIPLE STIFLE DAMAGE (DERANGED STIFLE)

Occasionally cats are presented with multiple ligamentous injuries to the stifle—ruptures of both cruciate ligaments, collateral ligaments, and other supporting structures. Abnormal motion of the stifle can be obtained in all directions with an especially exaggerated "drawer" sign. After repair of the cruciate and collateral ligaments, the joint is stabilized by placing an intramedullary pin across the stifle joint.

The distal cranial femoral shaft is exposed for 2 to 3 cm above the trochlear surface. A 3/32-inch intramedullary pin is guided through the distal quadriceps to this location with a closed hemostat that has been pushed bluntly through the muscle from the cranial surface of the distal femur to the skin surface. The patella is replaced and the pin is driven obliquely into the cranial surface of the femoral shaft 2 to 3 cm above the trochlear surface. The patella is replaced and the pin is driven obliquely into the cranial surface of the femoral shaft 2 to 3 cm above the trochlear surface. The pin should exit into the intercondylar fossa. The stifle is aligned in a physiologic position with the tibia at an angle to allow functional use of the leg without bending of the stifle. The pin is driven across the joint into the tibial plateau to exit on the tibial crest. The pin is cut off, leaving about 1 cm extending from the femoral shaft. The joint is closed. No bandage or splint is necessary. The pin is removed in two months. Results are usually good, with weight bearing, although there is sometimes a persistent limp.

## FELINE BANDAGING AND SPLINTING

Cats are difficult to bandage or splint because of their thick haircoat, loose skin, and active nature. Bandaging a limb involves bandaging the apex of an inverted triangle. A "Bergh bandage" has been developed to overcome some of the difficulties. The leg must be dry, loose hair must be removed, and very long hair trimmed. Longitudinal strips of anchoring tape are placed cranially and caudally extending several inches below the foot. The wound is dressed and the leg is wrapped over the tapes with cotton and then with gauze, leaving the toes exposed (Fig. 5–57 *A*). The bandage is wrapped with tape from top to bottom (Fig. 5–57 *B*). The exposed ends of the anchor strips are reflected back onto the bandage (Fig. 5–57 *C*). The bandage is not tight and therefore does not irritate the limb. It is almost impossible for the cat to remove it. Interdigital irritation does not occur, and any swelling of the foot can be observed immediately. No constriction of the limb occurs. If the foot must be covered, an additional bandage may be applied and is

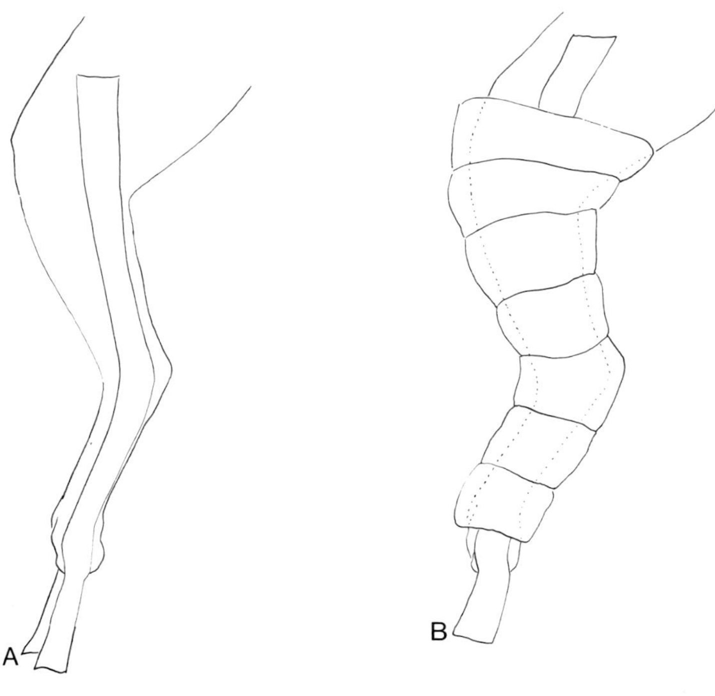


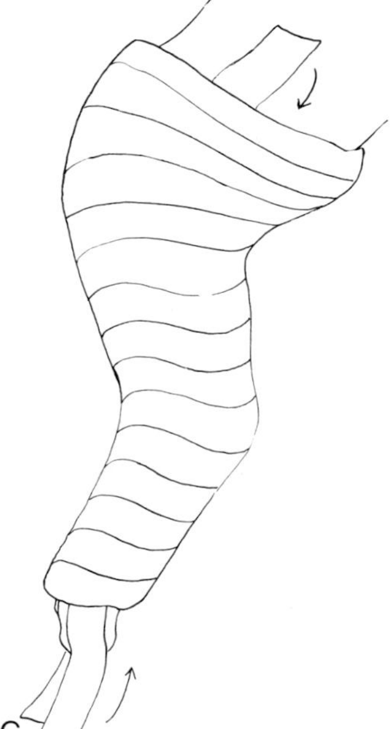


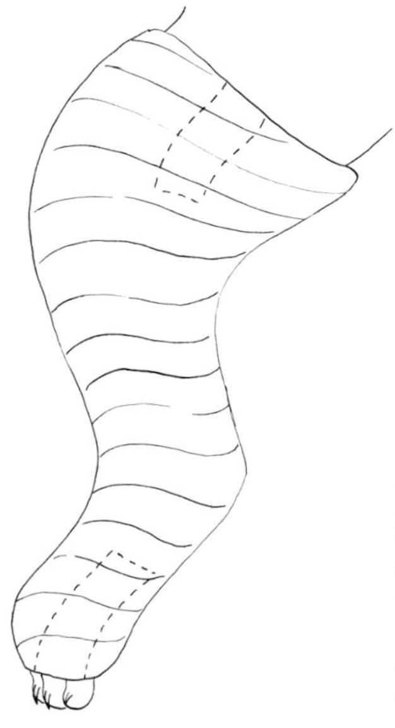

**Figure 5–57** "Bergh bandage." *A*, Two anchoring tapes are placed, and the limb is wrapped with cotton covered with bandage in the first stage of a specialized leg bandage for the cat. *B*, The bandage is wrapped with tape. *C*, The anchor strips are reflected onto the bandage and covered with a second layer of tape.

*Illustration continued on opposite page*

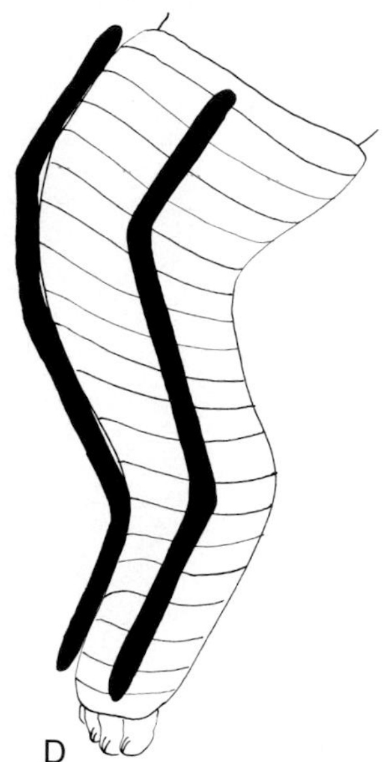

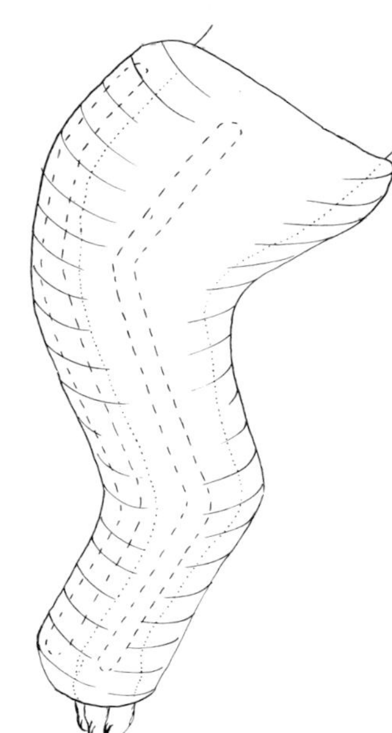

**Figure 5–57** *Continued. D,* The specialized bandage is reinforced, when needed, with a piece of aluminum rod placed laterally over the bandage and secured with additional circling pieces of adhesive tape.

secured to the leg bandage. This bandage may be removed to inspect the foot without disturbing the rest of the bandage. A similar technique works well for keeping a bandage on the tail.

If necessary, this type of bandage can be reinforced with a piece of aluminum splint rod bent to conform to the lateral aspect of the limb. The rod is secured to the bandage by encircling pieces of adhesive tape (Fig. 5–57 *D*). The two cental toes are not covered by bandage. This type of light splint is very well tolerated by cats and, being open-toed, is easily checked. If the cotton padding becomes compacted, allowing the splint to loosen, additional tape is applied.

## REFERENCES

Alcantara PJ, Stead AC: Fractures of the distal femur in the dog and cat. J Small Anim Pract 16 (1975) 649–659.

Bennett D: Orthopaedic disease affecting the pelvic region of the cat. J Small Anim Pract 16 (1975) 723–738.

Berzon JL: A retrospective study of the efficacy of femoral head and neck excision in 94 dogs and cats. Vet Surg 9 (1980) 88–92.

Birchard SJ, Bright RM: The tension band wire for fracture repair in the dog. Compend Contin Ed 3 (1981) 37–41.

DeAngelis M, Lau RE: A lateral retinacular imbrication technique for the surgical correction of anterior cruciate ligament rupture in the dog. J Am Vet Med Assoc 157 (1970) 79–84.

Evans I: Use of an allogenic bone graft to enlarge the pelvic outlet in a cat. Vet Med Small Anim Clin 75 (1980) 218–220.

Herron MR: Orthopedic surgery. *In* Catcott EJ (ed): Feline Medicine and Surgery, 2nd ed. Santa Barbara, American Veterinary Publications, Inc, 1975a, 592.

Herron MR: Feline onychectomy. *In* Bojrab MJ (ed): Current Techniques in Small Animal Surgery, 1st ed. Philadelphia, WB Saunders Company, 1975b, 274.

Herron MR: Sacroiliac luxations: Methods of closed repair. Feline Pract 6 (5) (1976) 46–49.

Hill FWG: A survey of bone fractures in the cat. J Small Anim Pract 18 (1977) 457–463.

Hobart JC: The repair of comminuted fractures of the vertical ramus of the mandible in the dog and cat. Aust Vet Pract 9 (1979) 147–149.

Larsen DD: The use of Rush pins in the management of fractures of the dog and cat. Vet Rec 70 (1958) 760–763.

Leighton RL: Symphysectomy in the cat and use of a steel insert to increase pelvic diameter. J Small Anim Pract 10 (1969) 355–356.

Leighton RL: Luxation of the scapula. *In* Bojrab MJ (ed): Current Techniques in Small Animal Surgery, 1st ed. Philadelphia, Lea & Febiger, 1975, 497–499.

Mainster ME: An unusual orthopedic problem in the feline. Texas Vet Med J 42 (5) (1980) 18.

Phillips IR: A survey of bone fractures in the dog and cat. J Small Anim Pract 20 (1979) 661–674.

Robinson GW: The high rise trauma syndrome in cats. Feline Pract 6 (5) (1976) 40–43.

Shires PK, Hulse DA: Internal fixation of physeal fractures using the distal femur as an example. Compend Contin Ed 2 (1980) 858.

Wadsworth PL, Henry WB: Entire segment cortical bone transplant. J Am Anim Hosp Assoc 12 (1976) 741–745.

Ward GW: Pelvic symphysiotomy in the cat—a steel insert to increase pelvic diameter. Can Vet J 8 (1967) 81–84.

**Additional References**

Leighton RL: Repair of skeletal lesions. *In* Catcott EJ (ed): Feline Medicine and Surgery. Santa Barbara, American Veterinary Publications, Inc, 1964, 462–483.

Robinson GW: The Bergh bandaging technique—feline bandaging and splinting. Feline Pract 7 (6) (1977) 41–43.

Roush J C II: Orthopedic problems of the cat—a review. Feline Pract 10 (3) (1980) 10–12, 16–26.

# 6
CHAPTER

# BASIC AND CLINICAL IMMUNOLOGY

NIELS C. PEDERSEN

## NORMAL IMMUNE SYSTEM

### Anatomy

#### Lymph Nodes

The lymph nodes of cats resemble those of other species in form and function. Their location has been described by Crouch (1969). A network of coalescing afferent lymphatic vessels transports to the nodes lymph derived from capillary filtrate (interstitial fluid) and containing a small number of lymphocytes and macrophages. These cells traversing the tissues are believed to function in peripheral immunosurveillance.

Entering the periphery of the node from afferent lymphatics, the lymph flows into the cortical and perifollicular sinuses, percolates through and around the cortex and across the paracortical areas, then enters the medullary sinus in the hilus. Lymph drains through one or two major lymphatic ducts that leave the node at its hilus. Efferent lymph from unstimulated nodes resembles afferent lymph except that it contains no macrophages and has about 10 times more lymphocytes.

Efferent ducts ultimately coalesce to form two major lymphatic trunks (Crouch, 1969). The right lymphatic duct, which receives lymphatic drainage from the right foreleg and the right side of the head and neck, enters the right jugulosubclavian venous trunk. The thoracic duct carries lymph from the rest of the body to the left jugulosubclavian venous trunk.

The resting lymph node consists of cortical, paracortical, and medullary regions (Fig. 6–1). The cortex is characterized by follicles made up of lymphocytes and phagocytes that encircle small accumulations of large pyroninophilic lymphoid cells (germinal centers). The paracortical region is made up of dense accumulations of small lymphocytes. The medulla is composed of cords of tissue lined with phagocytes and plasma cells.

Antigenic material, in the form of particulate matter or soluble substances, triggers major changes in the structure of the node. It enters the node by afferent lymphatics, either free in the lymph or carried by macrophages. Particulate antigens are processed to smaller, more antigenic molecules by phagocytes. Antigen-lymphocyte-macrophage interactions stimulate a vast influx of lymphocytes from the blood. This cell recruitment brings more specific antigen-responsive cells into the site of antigen localization, greatly increasing the size of the perifollicular and paracortical regions of the node. This enlargement, noticeable within 24 hours after stimulation, peaks in four to seven days.

Within 48 hours after stimulation the germinal centers begin to enlarge because of increased mitosis of lymphoblasts, and additional (secondary) germinal centers appear in the cortex. These reach their greatest size by 7 to 10 days and then, like the paracortical lymphoid accumulations, slowly regress over the next several weeks. As the germinal centers enlarge, increased numbers of plasma cells appear along the medullary cords. Fluorescent antibody staining shows that immunoglobulin is being synthesized by lymphoblasts in the germinal centers and by plasma cells in the medullary cords (Fig. 6–1).

Products of antigen stimulation include immunoglobulin and cells active in cell-mediated immune phenomena, i.e., lymphoblasts, plasma cells, neutrophils, macrophages, and small lymphocytes that can respond at a later time to the original eliciting stimulus. Plasma cells remain within the node, while lymphoblasts migrate through the paracortical area, enter the medullary sinuses, and leave the node in efferent lymph. The lymphoblasts, along with the smaller specific-antigen-responsive cells, are disseminated throughout the body, where some of the lymphoblasts may change into plasma cells, participate in cell-mediated immunity, or revert into stem cells awaiting future antigenic stimulation. Cells leaving the node are responsible

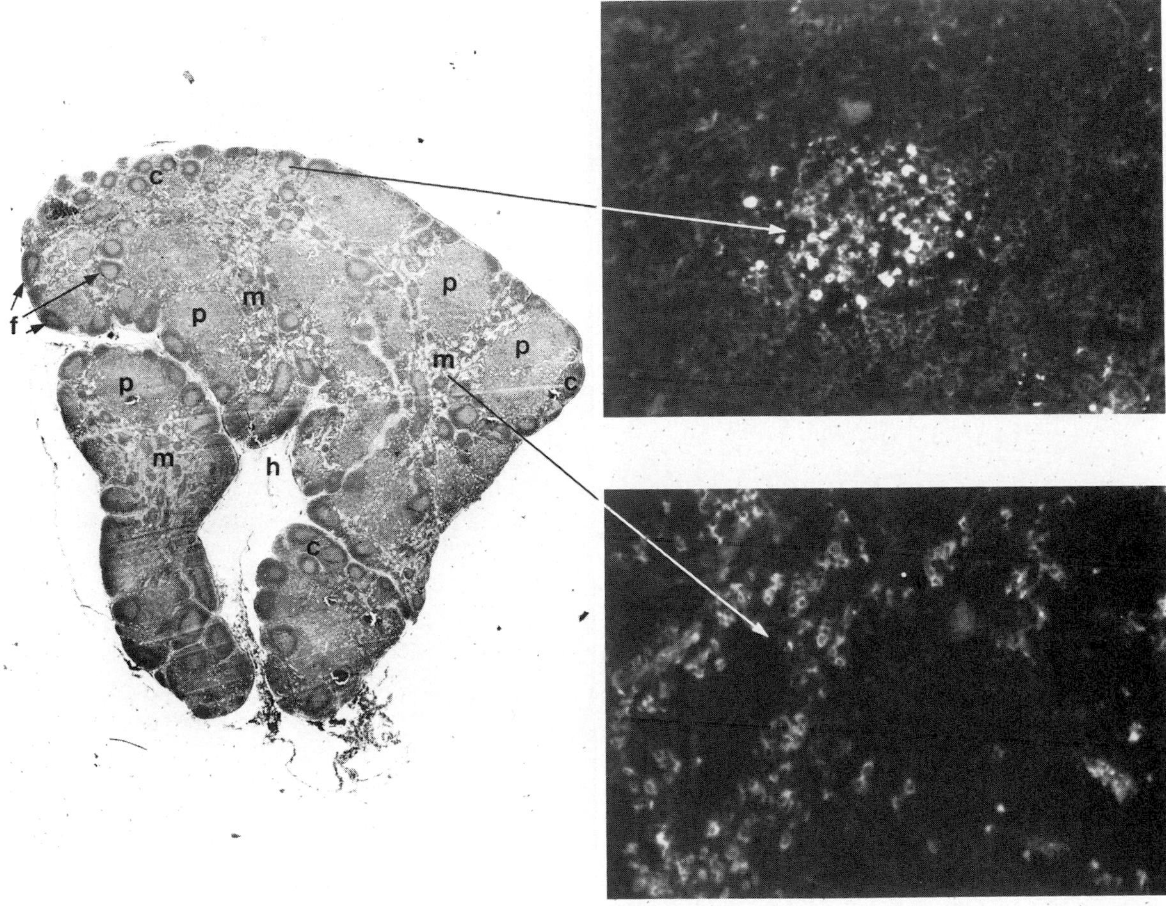


**Figure 6–1** *Left*, Normal mesenteric lymph node of a cat. The cortex (c) is made up of a thin rim of tissue containing numerous primary lymphoid follicles (f). The paracortical region (p) consists of dense accumulations of small lymphocytes. The medullary area (m) is made up of cords of tissue extending to the hilus (h). H&E, × 8.5. *Upper right*, Primary lymphoid follicle in the cortex. Fluorescence is seen in large lymphoblasts in the center of the follicle. Rabbit anti-cat IgM globulin–fluorescein isothiocyanate (FITC) stain, × 250. *Lower right*, Medullary area of a lymph node. Fluorescent antibody staining is seen mainly in plasma cells. Rabbit anti-cat IgM globulin–FITC stain, × 250.

for amplifying the immune response and for conferring immunologic memory on other lymphoid tissues (Smith et al., 1970b).

## Spleen

Beside acting as a reservoir for red cells, the spleen functions similarly to the lymph node, but it filters blood, whereas lymph nodes filter lymph. The cat's spleen resembles that of other mammals. The splenic artery ramifies into smaller arterioles, which with surrounding accumulations of lymphoid cells form the white pulp. Primary germinal centers are found in the lymphoid cuffs (Fig. 6–2). The splenic arterioles give rise to a swamplike meshwork of vascular sinuses (red pulp) containing sequestered red cells, phagocytes, and plasma cells. This area is analogous to the medullary cords of the lymph nodes. Antigenic stimulation causes changes in the lymphoid cuffs, germinal centers, and sinuses similar to those in the stimulated lymph node.

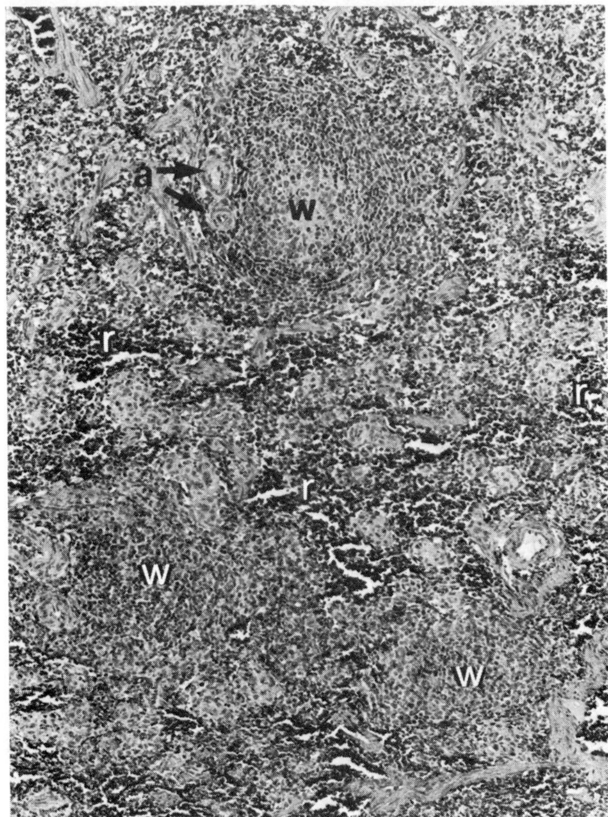


**Figure 6–2** Normal cat's spleen. The white pulp (w) is made up of lymphoid cell accumulations around splenic arterioles (a). The red pulp (r) is composed of tortuous endothelium-lined venous sinuses. The cords of tissue constituting these sinuses contain phagocytes as well as plasma cells. This area is analogous to the medullary area of lymph nodes. H & E, × 100.

## Diffuse Lymphoid Aggregates

Just as lymph nodes receive antigenic stimuli from the skin, muscles, and parenchyma of organs, the diffuse lymphoid aggregates are situated so as to survey the mucous membranes of the body.

**TONSILS.** The tonsils (palatine, lingual, and para-epiglottic) are well-developed lymphoid aggregates covered by the oropharyngeal mucosa and can be stimulated by ingested antigenic material and infectious agents. The tonsils resemble lymph nodes in structure and respond similarly to stimulation.

**PEYER'S PATCHES.** Peyer's patches, most numerous in the middle and lower parts of the small bowel, are composed of numerous lymphoid follicles similar to those in the lymph nodes (Fig. 6–3) and respond like lymph nodes to antigenic stimulation. They lie just below the muscularis mucosae but in certain areas break through to lie adjacent to the intestinal epithelium (Fig. 6–3). The epithelium overlying such areas is flatter than the surrounding villous epithelium, a characteristic indicating that it has a different biologic function. Here the closeness of the bowel lumen to the lymphoid tissue and the altered epithelium probably facilitate contact between the immune apparatus of the Peyer's patch and antigenic substances in the bowel lumen as well as movement of immunoglobulin from the Peyer's patch to the bowel lumen. The chief protein produced by lymphoid cells in the Peyer's patch is IgA (Fig. 6–3), although IgG- and IgM-producing cells are also abundant (Klotz et al., 1985).

Peyer's patches are also the site of origin of precursor cells that ultimately become IgA-secreting plasma cells. After antigenic stimulation small precursor lymphocytes and lymphoblasts leave the germinal centers in efferent lymphatics and pass through the blood to the mucous membranes and mammary glands (Lamm, 1976). Part of this migration has been documented by studies of intestinal lymph of cats showing that lymph draining areas near Peyer's patches contains many more lymphocytes than lymph draining other areas of the intestine (Baker, 1932–1933). The plasma cell progeny of these cells, found mainly between the epithelium and the underlying lamina propria (Fig. 6–3), are responsible for the continuous secretion of immunoglobulins by the mucosa.

**CECUM.** The shortness and structure of the cat's cecum preclude any digestive function, and it is probably primarily concerned with immune reactions. Its entire wall is infiltrated with lymphoid cells and in structure resembles Peyer's patches. It is noteworthy that the cecum is situated at the entrance of the large intestine, which contains most of the bacterial flora of the bowel. Products of viral infection, which usually involves the small bowel, are also likely to come into contact with the cecum.

**BRONCHIAL LYMPHOID TISSUE.** There are also small aggregates of lymphoid cells around the bronchi and bronchioles, but they are less numerous and less well organized than those in the intestine. In normal lungs they are not conspicuous, but in infections they become more prominent. In addition to these diffuse lymphoid aggregates, plasma cells are often seen under the mucosa of the bronchi and bronchioles (Fig. 6–4).

**OTHER LYMPHOID AGGREGATES.** Diffuse and poorly organized lymphoid aggregates are present under the urogenital epithelium and in the dermis. They are not normally noticeable but can become conspicuous in conditions of local antigenic stimulation. In the central nervous system they are capable of considerable local production of immunoglobulin. For example, in some cases of feline infectious peritonitis (FIP), the cerebrospinal

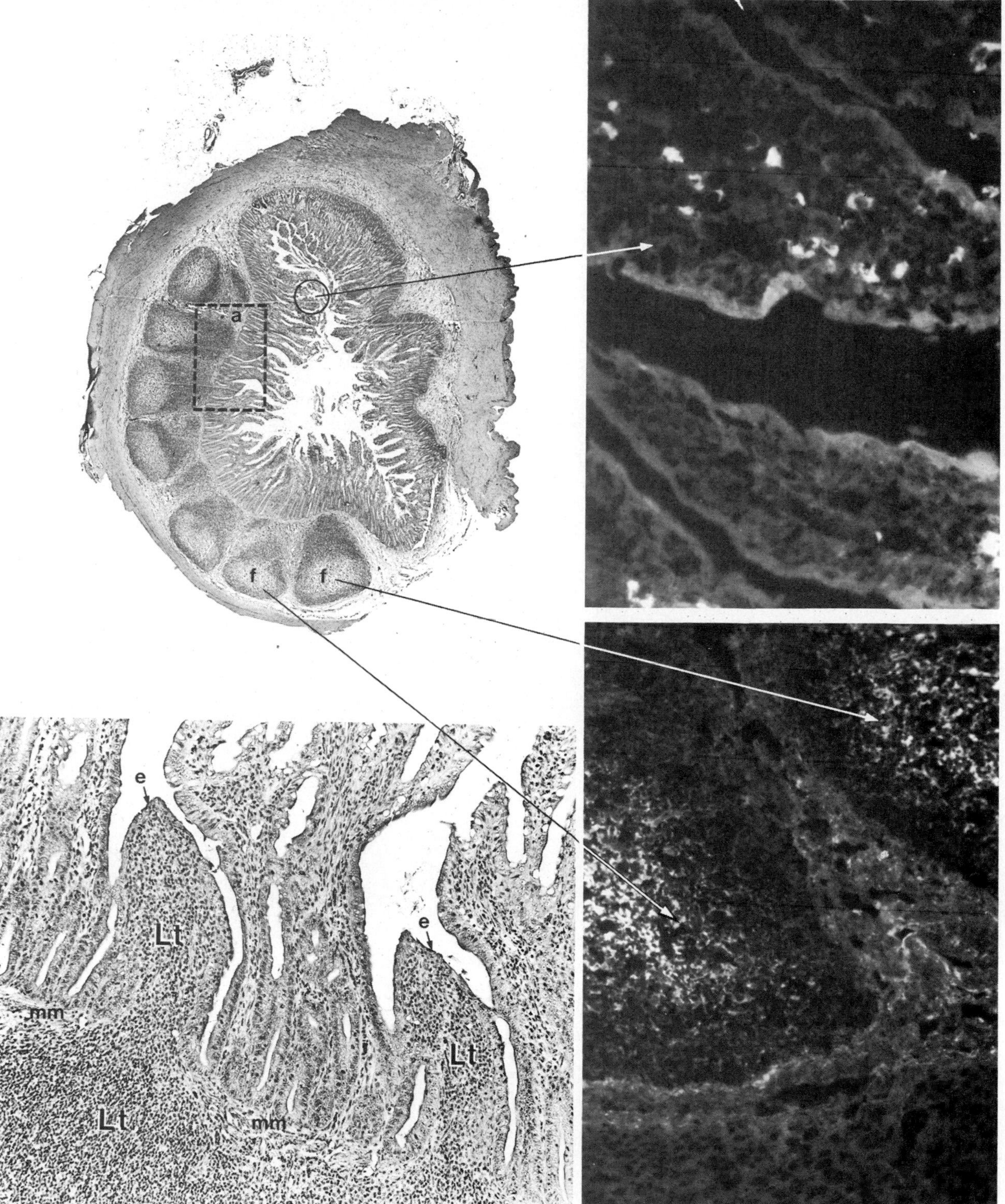


**Figure 6–3** *Upper left*, Section of the ileum of a cat through an area containing a Peyer's patch. Peyer's patches are made up of lymphoid follicles (f). The central pale-staining area in each follicle is made up of lymphoblasts, and the darker-staining peripheral area consists of dense accumulations of small lymphocytes. These lymphoid follicles lie below the muscularis mucosae (mm), except for certain areas (a) where lymphoid tissue penetrates the muscularis mucosae and becomes congruent with the mucosa. H & E, × 13.5. *Lower left*, Higher power view of area designated (a) in the photomicrograph above. Lymphoid tissue (Lt) projects through the muscularis mucosae (mm) and comes into contact with the epithelium. The epithelium (e) overlying this area is more cuboidal and less vacuolated than that overlying the surrounding absorptive villi. H & E, × 100.

*Upper right*, Villus in the ileum of a cat. Fluorescing, antibody-containing plasma cells can be found under the epithelium. Rabbit anti-cat IgA globulin–FITC stain, × 250.

*Lower right*, Peyer's patch in the ileum of a cat. The central region of each of the two lymphoid follicles contains numerous fluorescing, antibody-producing lymphoblasts. Rabbit anti-cat IgA globulin–FITC stain, × 250.

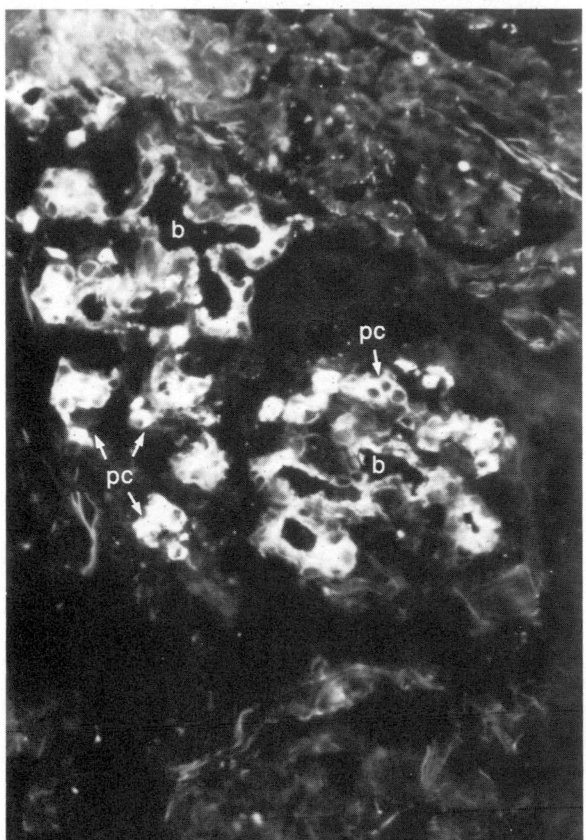


**Figure 6–4** Two bronchioles (b) in the lung of a cat. Fluorescent antibody staining is seen in the mucosal cells of the bronchioles and in plasma cells (pc) adjacent to the epithelium. The fluorescent staining of bronchiolar mucosal cells is associated with the uptake, transport, and secretion of IgA by these cells. Rabbit anti-cat IgA globulin–FITC stain, × 250.

fluid titers to the virus may be as high as the blood titers. Although some of this antibody may result from transudation or exudation of serum, much of it is apparently locally produced.

## Bone Marrow

Many of the circulating lymphocytes destined to produce antibody originate in bone marrow (B-lymphocytes, B cells). Although the marrow contains a few plasma cells (Klotz et al., 1985), antibody production, except in some diseases, is not significant.

## Thymus Gland

The thymus gland of the cat appears at about the twenty-eighth day of gestation and continues to grow until sexual maturity, after which it slowly involutes. The feline thymus is morphologically similar to that of other mammalian species (Fig. 6–5). During embryogenesis the thymic epithelium becomes infiltrated with lymphoid cells that migrate from the marrow.The thymic epithelium influences the differentiation of certain lymphocytes for specialized functions. These cells (T-lymphocytes, T cells) are important in cell-mediated immunity and in regulation of the immune response, e.g., suppression or facilitation of imunoglobulin production.

# Cells Involved in the Immune Response

## Lymphocytes

The small lymphocyte is the main cell involved in immune phenomena. Lymphocytes are in continuous migration in the body (Yoffey and Courtice, 1970). About 10 per cent are traversing nonlymphoid tissues at any given time and the rest are in transit through lymphoid tissue. Lymphocytes ultimately return to the blood by the right and thoracic lymphatic ducts. In a typical 4-kg cat about $1.6 \times 10^8$ lymphocytes enter the blood by way of the thoracic duct every hour (Reinhardt, 1964). Lymphocytes within this vast recirculating pool originate from lymphoid tissue and bone marrow. They can be recruited into any area of antigenic stimulation, their numbers increasing in lymphoid structures 10 to 60 times over resting levels (Smith et al., 1970a).

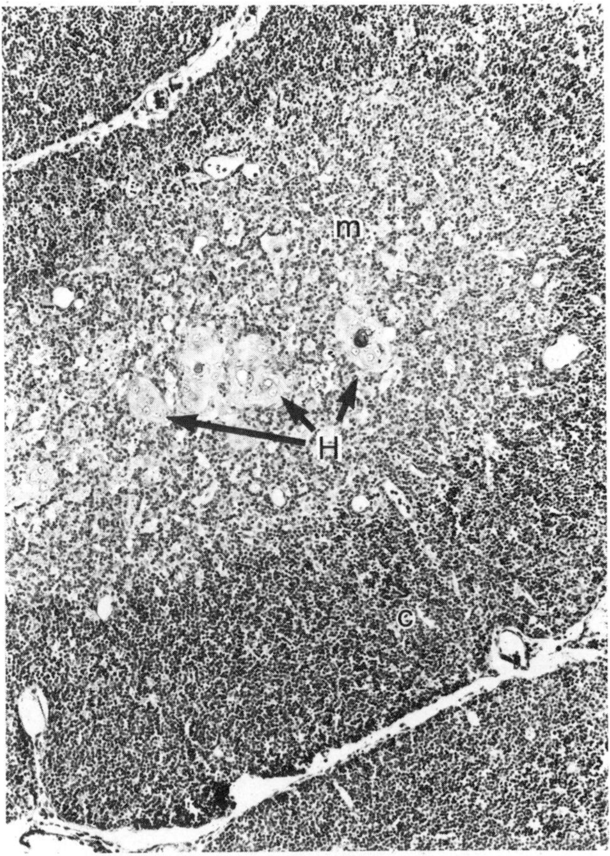


**Figure 6–5** Thymus of a 10-week-old kitten. The thymus consists of lobules made up of darker-staining cortex (c) and lighter-staining medulla (m). The cortex is composed of small lymphocytes and the medulla of large and small lymphoid cells. Hassall's corpuscles (H) are present in the medulla. H & E, × 40.

Several subpopulations of lymphocytes can be distinguished on the basis of surface antigens and immunoglobulin or complement receptors. Each has a specific role in the immune response. B-lymphocytes possess membrane-bound immunoglobulin detectable by fluorescent antibody staining (Klotz et al., 1985). Feline B-lymphocyes also have membrane receptors that recognize complement, and they can be detected, therefore, by their capacity to bind heterologous erythrocytes (E) coated with antibody (A) and complement (C) to form EAC rosettes. With membrane-fluorescence tests and EAC binding it has been determined that 40 to 45 per cent of the cat's peripheral blood lymphocytes are B-lymphocytes (Holmberg et al., 1976; Taylor et al., 1975; Taylor and Siddiqui, 1977). Methods for the separation and characterization of peripheral blood mononuclear cells have been described by Tham and Studdert (1985).

The development of B-lineage cells in the domestic cat has been studied by Klotz and coworkers (1985). They concluded that the pattern of development from embryonic through adult life is the same as in other species. Pre–B-lymphocytes were first seen in 42-day fetal liver and later in spleen and bone marrow, where they remained throughout life. Adult levels of B-lymphocytes were attained in the spleen by 12 weeks of age. The only major difference between B cells of cats and other species was in the much greater expression of lambda- compared with kappa-type light chains on secreted immunoglobulins.

The immunoglobulin receptors on any given B-lymphocyte will bind only one specific antigen, and in the entire pool of recirculating B-lymphocytes, every possible antigenic determinant is represented. Only B-lymphocytes bearing the correct antibody receptor will bind the specific antigen and will be triggered to differentiate into antibody-forming cells. After this differentiation, some cells revert into small lymphocytes with the same antigenic responsiveness as their parent cells. B-lymphocytes in lymphoid tissues are found primarily in the follicular regions.

Lymphocytes influenced in differentiation by thymic factors (T-lymphocytes) possess specific antigens on their surfaces (theta-antigen and lymphocyte-differentiation antigens). T-lymphocytes also have surface receptors that will recognize and bind foreign red cells; guinea pig and rat red cells bind particularly well to feline T-lymphocyte membranes (Cockerell et al., 1976b). The receptors for rat red cells appear to be present on more differentiated feline T cells, whereas the receptors for guinea pig red cells react with both differentiated and undifferentiated feline T cells. With fluoresceinated anti-cat thymocyte globulin of rabbit origin or guinea pig erythrocyte-binding (E-rosette) tests, it has been shown that 32 to 41 per cent of the peripheral blood lymphocytes of cats are T cells (Schultz and Adams, 1978; Taylor and Siddiqui, 1977; Taylor et al., 1975). T-lymphocytes are further subclassified into T-effector cells, T-suppressor cells that depress the function of B-lymphocytes in antibody formation, and T-helper cells that collaborate with B-lymphocytes to facilitate antibody production. T-effector lymphocytes function in antibody-independent and antibody-dependent cell-mediated immune reactions. T-effector lymphocyte activity has been demonstrated in the blood of cats with regressing virus-induced fibrosarcomas (Johnson et al., 1985). Feline T-suppressor lymphocytes have been induced with concanavalin A treatment of blood leukocytes (Langweiler and Cockerell, 1982). T-lymphocytes tend to congregate in the paracortical regions of lymph nodes.

T-lymphocytes are stimulated to grow by a 30,000 to 35,000 dalton protein, interleukin 2 (IL2, T-cell growth factor, TCGF). Interleukin 2 is produced by cellular interactions between T-lymphocytes and macrophages. This protein has been recognized in cats (Yamamoto, et al., 1986).

A third class of lymphocytes ("null cells") also exists in mammals (Betton, 1980). They lack identifiable surface markers such as are found on T- and B-lymphocytes. About 20 per cent or more of feline lymphocytes are probably null cells. It has been noted that some can destroy tumor cells and virus-infected cells in a cell-mediated reaction. Because such cells are present in both nonimmune and immune animals, they have been called "natural killer cells." They thus differ from T-lymphocytes, which also act as killer cells but are found in detectable levels only after a specific antigenic stimulus. Hu and coworkers (1982) failed to demonstrate natural killer-cell activity in domestic cats against homologous and heterologous tumor cells and antigen-coated red cells. Tompkins and associates (1983), however, demonstrated natural killer-cell activity in cats against herpes simplex virus–infected cells.

Lymphocyte function has been measured by so-called mitogen-stimulation tests. Certain substances such as phytohemagglutinin (PHA), pokeweed mitogen, concanavalin A (con-A), and *E. coli* lipopolysaccharide stimulate lymphocytes to undergo blastogenesis in culture. Con-A and PHA are reportedly T-lymphocyte mitogens; pokeweed mitogen stimulates both T- and B-lymphocytes, and *E. coli* lipopolysaccharide stimulates mainly B-lymphocytes. Feline lymphocytes, however, respond poorly to PHA and to *E. coli* lipopolysaccharide in comparison with those of other animals (Schultz, 1977; Schultz and Adams, 1978). The poor response to PHA is uniform over a wide range of mitogen concentration (Cockerell et al., 1975).

In theory, it should be possible to estimate T- and B-lymphoctyte function in cats by measuring the responsiveness of peripheral lymphocytes to con-A and pokeweed mitogen. A good blastogenic response would indicate intact function and a poor response, impaired function. Actually, however, lymphocyte function of cats as measured by such tests is often nonspecifically impaired in many chronic debilitating illnesses, malignancies, and infectious diseases. These conditions are not due to impaired lymphocyte function, and impaired lymphocyte function in vitro does not necessarily mean that normal immune responses will also be impaired in vivo. Immune function tests of this type should therefore be interpreted with caution in ill cats.

## Plasma Cells

Plasma cells, end-stage cells in the antigen-induced differentiation of B-lymphocytes, are found in the medullary cords of lymph nodes, in the red pulp of the spleen, and under the epithelium of mucous membranes. They appear in nonlymphoid tissue in cases in which there is a chronic localized antigenic stimulus, e.g., chronic stomatitis, hepatitis, dermatitis, and synovitis. Plasma cells do not migrate from the tissues into the blood except in certain diseases such as myeloma. During their relatively short life span they are very efficient secretors of immunoglobulin. A myeloma is a plasma cell tumor that arises

**Table 6–1 Immunoglobulin Levels in Serum and Bile of Cats**

| SPECIMEN | NUMBER | SOURCE | IMMUNOGLOBULIN MG/ML ($\bar{X}$ AND RANGE) IgG | IgA | IgM |
|---|---|---|---|---|---|
| Serum | 36 | Household cats (1/2 to 1-1/2 years) | 9.48 (3.88–20.0) | 0.71 (0.25–1.88) | 0.81 (0.2–1.95) |
| Serum | 12 | Cattery cats (specific pathogen-free adults) | 9.94 (8.83–11.40) | 2.77 (0.42–6.0) | 1.93 (0.8–3.6) |
| Serum | 15 | Cattery cats (specific pathogen–free 12-week-olds) | 7.26 (5.8–9.0) | 1.23 (0.3–2.54) | 1.11 (0.69–1.35) |
| Serum | 36 | Cattery cats (conventionally reared purebred adults) | 19.72 (5.67–38.33) | 1.75 (0.35–5.0) | 1.16 (0.15–3.0) |
| Bile | 12 | Cattery cats (conventionally reared domestics, 3 to 10 months old) | 0.35 (0.005–2.85) | 1.65 (0.37–3.35) | .68 (0–1.66) |

as a clone of a single malignant cell and can therefore produce a single type of immunoglobulin.

## Lymphoblasts

Lymphoblasts are large, pyroninophilic, primitive-appearing cells found in active germinal centers in lymphoid tissues. Like the plasma cell, they are progeny of small lymphocytes. Some produce immunoglobulin, while others function in cell-mediated immunity. Unlike plasma cells, they migrate in large numbers into the lymph draining antigen-stimulated lymph nodes and lymphoid aggregates (Hay et al., 1972; Murphy et al., 1972). They circulate only briefly and, except in cases of intense antigenic stimulation, do not appear in significant numbers in the blood. They migrate to lymphoid tissues throughout the body, some differentiating into plasma cells, others reverting into small, antigen-responsive lymphocytes (T- or B-lymphocytes). Lymphomas arise from lymphoblasts, and some B-cell lymphomas can produce monoclonal immunoglobulin.

## Macrophages

Macrophages, beside serving as phagocytes, are important in antigen processing. They also facilitate antigen presentation to B-lymphocytes (Unanue, 1980) and function in the same way as T-effector lymphocytes in some antigen-dependent and independent cell-mediated immune reactions (Nathan et al., 1980). Macrophages also participate in the production of interleukins 1 and 2 (Aarden et al., 1979).

# PHYSIOLOGY

## Humoral Antibody Production

Immunoglobulin responses of cats resemble those of other animals. Antibodies of the IgG, IgM, and IgA classes have been identified in cat serum and secretions. Reaginic antibodies, presumably IgE or IgE-like, have also been described in cats. Immunoglobulin G, A, and M Levels in serum, bile, colostrum, and milk of cats are given in Tables 6–1 and 6–2.

Cats are not immunocompetent to all antigens at birth. The newborn kitten produces antibodies when injected with bovine and human fibrinogen, rat collagen, and *Salmonella typhi* flagella (Miller–Ben Shaul, 1965). It does not respond, however, to egg albumin, human gamma globulin (HGG), or bovine serum albumin (BSA). Kittens do not make antibodies to injected BSA and HGG until 25 to 28 days of age (Miller–Ben Shaul, 1965). Oral administration of these antigens to one-day-old kittens either produces no response (bovine or human fibrinogen) or induces tolerance (BSA, HGG). This tolerogenic effect can be induced only during the first 20 to 38 days of life (Miller–Ben Shaul, 1965).

Normal immunoglobulin levels of cats vary considerably, depending on the environment in which they are reared. Specific-pathogen-free (SPF), barrier-maintained cats have lower immunoglobulin levels than cats in the general population (Table 6–1). Conventional cats reared in catteries have the highest immunoglobulin levels (Table 6–1), presumably because of greater incidence of disease in catteries. The higher immunogobulin levels of cattery-reared cats has been previously described (Kristensen and

**Table 6–2 IgG, IgA, and IgM Levels in Colostrum, Milk, and Blood of a Lactating Queen**

| SAMPLE | IMMUNOGLOBULIN CLASS | 0* | 2* | 5* | 9 | 13 | 16 | 21 | 26 | 30 | 31 | 44 | 55 |
|---|---|---|---|---|---|---|---|---|---|---|---|---|---|
| **Milk** | IgG | 44.0 | 32.50 | 7.25 | 4.40 | 3.60 | 3.90 | 3.00 | 3.15 | 4.40 | 5.40 | 1.00 | 1.50 |
| | IgA | 3.4 | 1.50 | 0.78 | 0.44 | 0.20 | 0.20 | 0.20 | 0.24 | 0.62 | 0.24 | 0.24 | 0.24 |
| | IgM | 0.58 | 0.47 | 0.14 | 0.02 | 0† | 0 | 0 | 0 | 0 | 0 | 0 | 0 |
| **Blood (serum)** | IgG | 13.75 | | | | | | | | | | | |
| | IgA | 2.15 | | | | | | | | | | | |
| | IgM | 1.16 | | | | | | | | | | | |

*Colostral phase days 0–5.
†Nondetectable by assay used.

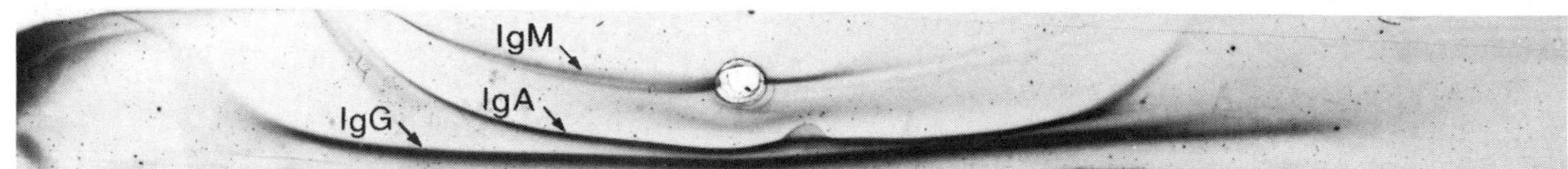


**Figure 6–6** Immunoelectrophoretic gel demonstrating the precipitin arcs formed by feline IgG, IgA, and IgM.

Barsanti, 1977). Household cats have immunoglobulin levels nearer to those of SPF cats (Table 6–1).

Hiraga and associates (1981) studied the development of humoral immunity in germ-free cats. Hysterectomy-derived, sterile-reared kittens were found to have no immunoglobulins in their serum on day 1, only IgG at day 10, and IgG, IgA, and IgM at day 60. After transfer from a germ-free to a specific-pathogen-free environment there was a pronounced increase in IgG levels and a slower rise in IgM and IgA levels. Lymphocyte counts in germ-free cats always exceeded neutrophil counts. The germ-free state seemed to decrease quantitative antibody responsiveness.

Because feline immunoglobulins are structurally similar to immunoglobulins of man and other mammals, some antisera to human or mammalian immunoglobulins cross react with corresponding classes of feline immunoglobulins. Neoh and coworkers (1973) found that certain sheep and rabbit antihuman IgM sera also precipitated feline IgM. They also found that chicken antihuman IgA and IgG reacted with cat IgA or IgG, although there was no reactivity with antisera to human IgD and IgE and any protein in cat serum.

Antisera to human IgA and IgM were also used by Vaerman et al. (1969) to precipitate feline IgM and IgA. Kehoe and coworkers (1972), by amino-acid sequencing a feline IgG myeloma protein, found a close relationship between the heavy chains of this protein and human $V_H$III heavy chains. Feline IgE was shown to be weakly reactive with human and bovine anti-IgE sera (Nielsen, 1977).

**IgG.** At least two subclasses of IgG exist in cat serum and have been designated $IgG_1$ and $IgG_2$ (Okoshi et al., 1967; Schultz et al., 1974). Cat IgG migrates electrophoretically to both the beta and the gamma regions (Fig. 6–6). Cats, like other species, possess both complement-fixing (CF′) and complement–nonfixing IgG. Cats infected with calicivirus produce complement–nonfixing IgG during the first three weeks after infection, while the CF′ IgG antibody titer steadily increases after this time (Olsen et al., 1974). Precipitating antibodies of the IgG class are also produced by cats. Cats respond with generally low titers of precipitating antibody when injected with heterologous serum proteins (Aitken et al., 1967; Aitken and McCusker, 1969). Lest it be inferred that cats are poor producers of precipitating antibodies to all antigen, Silberman-Ziv and coworkers (1968) reported that cats were particularly efficient producers of precipitating antibodies against human tissue proteins.

IgG antibodies are also found in secretions but, unlike IgA, in lower levels than in serum (Yamada et al., 1984). Beside IgA, Vaerman et al. (1969) found low or undetectable levels of IgG in cat tears and nasal secretions. Schultz and coworkers (1974) identified IgA and IgG in 80 per cent of the feline tears and nasal secretions that they assayed. The origin of this IgG is thought to be the same as described for man. Butler and coworkers (1970) found that over 50 per cent of the local IgG in man arises as a transudate from serum, while the rest is synthesized by plasma cells under mucous membranes. Where the membranes are inflamed, however, they found that much more IgG exudes from the blood.

The importance of IgG in membrane secretions has probably been underestimated. In calicivirus infection of cats, virtually all virus-neutralizing activity in nasal washings is of the IgG class (Johnson, 1980).

**IgA.** Cats secrete large amounts of IgA into saliva, intestinal and respiratory mucus, tears, and bile (Schultz et al., 1974; Vaerman et al., 1969; Yamada et al., 1984). It is present as a dimer linked to a secretory component and is the next most abundant immunoglobulin after IgG in the serum of cats (Table 6–1). Gel filtration studies indicate that serum IgA in the cat, like secretory IgA, is present mainly as a dimer (two units) (Fig. 6–7). In immunoelectrophoresis, feline IgA migrates mainly in the beta region but extends into the gamma region as well (Fig. 6–6).

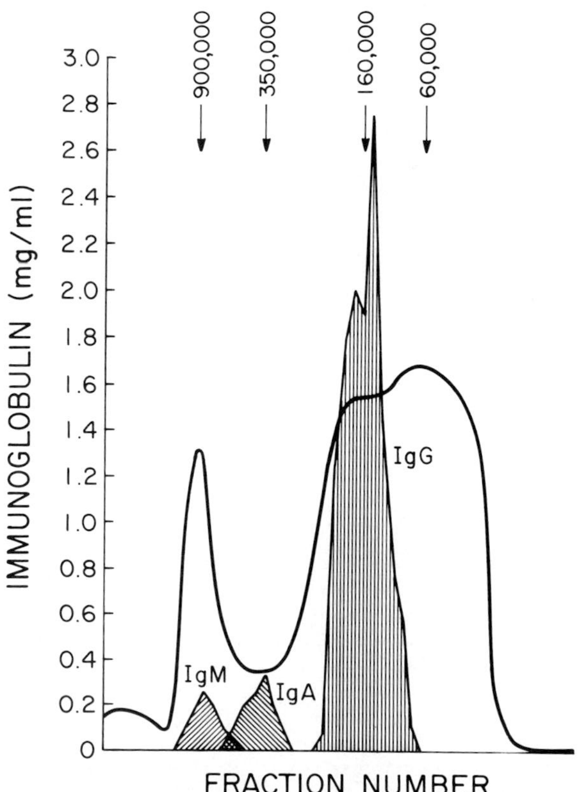


**Figure 6–7** Biogel 1.5 M separation of feline whole serum, demonstrating the different molecular sizes of feline IgM, IgA, and IgG. The arrows indicate the approximate molecular weight in daltons of proteins eluting from the column in that fraction.

The mechanisms of IgA secretion in the cat are similar to those in other species. Secretory IgA is produced mainly in plasma cells situated between the mucous epithelium and the lamina propria (Figs. 6–3 and 6–4). Although it has not been determined for cats, the IgA present in secretions of other animal species and man is usually locally produced. Some of the secretory IgA may come from dimeric IgA in the blood (Lamm, 1976). Plasma cells in the mucous membranes probably originate from precursor lymphocytes stimulated in diffuse lymphoid aggregates such as the tonsils, Peyer's patches, cecum, and other such tissues (Lamm, 1976).

Feline IgA, as in man (Butler et al., 1967), is secreted from the plasma cells as a dimer. The dimeric IgA is made up of two monomeric IgA molecules linked by a joining protein (J chain). The secreted immunoglobulin is abundant in the interstitial fluid bathing the mucosal cells, which have membrane receptors that bind the dimeric IgA and admit it into the cells. Within the cell the dimeric IgA molecule is linked with another protein ("secretory piece"). The entire molecule is then transported across the cell and is actively secreted by the brush border on the apical side of the cell (Figs. 6–4 and 6–8). Once in the lumen, the molecules tend to be trapped in the mucus. The secretory component protects the molecule from degradation by the intestinal contents.

**IgM.** IgM is relatively low in the serum of cats compared with IgG (Table 6–1). Like other animals, cats often produce considerable IgM during the primary response to certain antigens (Trainin et al., 1983) and during active infection with agents such as FeLV (Adams et al., 1979). Feline IgM, the molecular weight of which is nearly 900,000 daltons (Fig. 6–7), behaves in gel filtration like IgM of other animals. It migrates in immunoelectrophoresis as a beta globulin (Fig. 6–6).

IgM is also secreted into nasal mucus, tears, intestinal fluid, and bile (Schultz et al., 1974; Vaerman et al., 1969; Yamada et al., 1984). IgM is present in feline milk during the colostral phase of lactation but is not detectable after this time (Table 6–2). IgM can be secreted from mucous membranes by a process similar to IgA secretion.

**REAGINIC IMMUNOGLOBULIN (IgE).** An antibody analogous to IgE of other mammals probably exists in the cat, but whether this is structurally and antigenically similar to IgE of other species remains to be determined. McCusker and Aitken (1967) were able to induce a typical immediate hypersensitivity reaction in the skin of cats sensitized with bovine serum or bovine immunoglobulin. Serum from these cats would transfer this sensitivity to guinea pigs as measured by a reversed passive cutaneous anaphylaxis (PCA) test. This sensitivity could also be transferred to the skin of nonsensitized cats by a similar procedure. Gotschlich and Stetson (1960) induced reversed PCA in guinea pigs with cat antiserum to human C-reactive protein. Powell and coworkers (1980) transferred reaginic sensitivity to ear mites from infested to noninfested cats. Walton and associates (1968) were able to transfer bovine lactalbumin sensitivity by a reversed PCA test from a naturally sensitized to a nonsensitized cat. It would thus seem that cats possess a reaginic or mast cell–fixing antibody. Serologic evidence of the possible existence of feline IgE was described by Nielsen (1977), who was able to show a weak cross-reaction between human and bovine anti-IgE sera and a protein in cat blood.

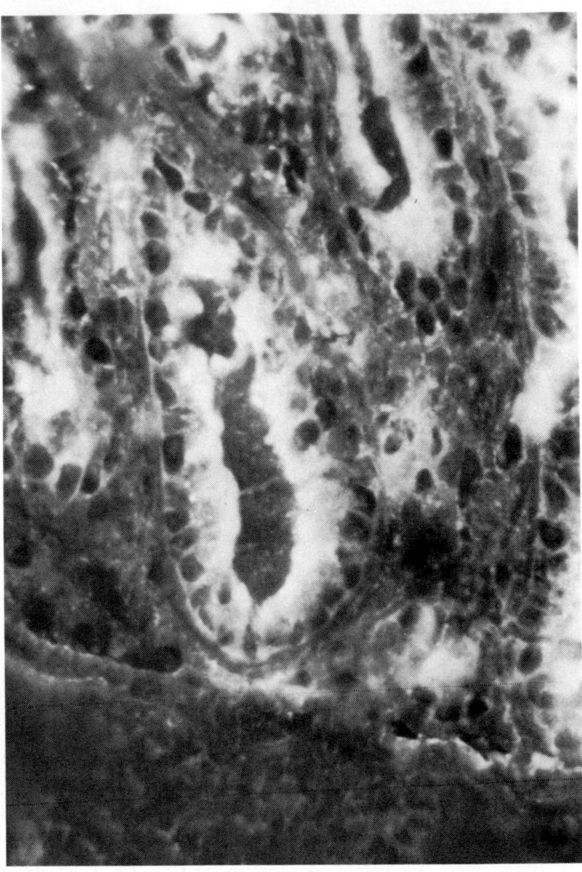

**Figure 6–8** Intestinal crypts in the jejunum of a cat. Fluorescent antibody staining is seen in the apices of mucosal cells. IgA and IgM antibodies are actively taken up and transported across the mucosal membrane by the epithelial cells and secreted by the brush border into the bowel lumen. Rabbit anti-cat IgA globulin–FITC stain, × 800.

Reaginic antibodies, or IgE, probably evolved as a mechanism to combat certain parasitic infections. In all species in which it has been studied, IgE levels are always greatly elevated in cases of heavy parasitism. Because the interface between parasite and host is usually skin or mucous membrane, IgE-mediated immunity, not surprisingly, is also concentrated in these areas.

IgE is produced by plasma cells in the membranes, and once it is secreted, it does not circulate in the body for long. The complement-binding (Fc) region of the IgE molecule has a high degree of affinity for receptors on the surface membranes of mast cells. Mast cells, like IgE-producing plasma cells, are abundant under the epithelium of skin and mucous membranes. In cats the lungs (Riley and West, 1953) and skin (McCusker and Aitken, 1967) contain numerous mast cells. Once coated with specific IgE, they are sensitized to subsequent antigen exposure. If a specific antigen (allergen) later binds with the corresponding membrane-bound IgE, a sequence of events is triggered that leads to degranulation of the mast cells and release of vasoactive amines, including histamine, serotonin, slow reactive substance of anaphylaxis, bradykinin, eosinophil chemotactic factor, and probably other compounds. The role of these substances in parasite immunity is not understood. Perhaps they have a deleterious effect on parasite migration or well-being, or facilitate the influx and phagocytic activity of inflammatory cells.

## Cell-Mediated Immunity

Cell-mediated immunity involves the interaction of a subset of thymus-derived, T-effector lymphocytes (or macrophages) with a specific antigen. As a consequence of antigen binding, the lymphocyte releases substances called lymphokines. Lymphokines have the effect of killing cells that the lymphocyte contacts (cytotoxins), inhibiting macrophage and leukocyte migration from the site (macrophage and leukocyte migration-inhibition factors), inducing blastogenesis of lymphocytes (blastogenic factors), and perform numerous other functions. Interferons are lymphokines that can be produced by T-lymphocytes.

The specificity of the lymphocyte attack is determined in several ways. In the first, a subset of T-effector lymphocytes are induced to divide in response to appropriate antigens. These antigens may be cells infected with viruses, bacteria, or fungi or foreign tissue such as tumor cells or cells from other individuals (grafts). The T-effector lymphocytes produced by this stimulus express receptors on their surface membranes that recognize and bind specifically with the foreign substance that initially triggered the lymphocyte proliferation. These small T-effector lymphocytes recirculate throughout the body and, on contact with antigen, bind to it and release lymphokines. If the antigen is present on the surface of a cell, the cell may be destroyed. Macrophages brought into the area are held there by the effect of macrophage and leukocyte migration-inhibition factors, and more lymphocytes proliferate in response to the blastogenic stimulation factors. Interferons are also released as well as other mediators.This type of reaction is called antibody-independent, cell-mediated immunity because antibody is not involved in the response.

As well as antibody-independent, cell-mediated immunity, there is an antibody-dependent, cell-mediated reaction. Specific antibody binds to the target cell or protein, and T-effector lymphocytes nonspecifically bind to the antibody by virtue of their cell surface receptors to the Fc portion of the antibody. Null lymphocytes may also participate in this type of reaction. Antibody-mediated binding also leads to release of lymphokines by the participating lymphocytes. In this reaction it is antibody and not the lymphocyte that determines the specific target to be attacked.

The domestic cat possesses both antibody-independent and antibody-dependent cell-mediated immunity. During the rejection of sarcoma virus-induced tumors, for instance, cytotoxic lymphocytes of both types appear in the blood (Johnson et al., 1985). Their appearance also corresponds to the detection of cytolytic antibodies and to the regression of the tumor (Fig. 6–9). The simultaneous appearance of humoral and cellular immunity is expected, because the cat like other animals responds to an antigenic challenge with its full immunologic armamentarium whenever possible.

**DELAYED HYPERSENSITIVITY.** The delayed hypersensitivity reaction is a local dermal manifestation of systemic cell-mediated immunity. It is mediated entirely by the interaction of T-effector lymphocytes and the specific foreign substance to which they are sensitized.

The delayed hypersensitivity reaction must be differentiated from IgE-mediated (allergic) and Arthus-type reactions, each of which is mediated by different immune responses (McCusker and Aitken, 1967). If specific IgE-coated mast cells are present, an almost immediate edematous response occurs, reaching its peak in one-half to two hours and then subsiding. If precipitating antibody (IgG) is present, an Arthus reaction evokes the formation of antigen-antibody complexes in and around vessel walls in the area of the injection. This reaction reaches its peak in about 24 hours. The IgE-mediated reaction is typified

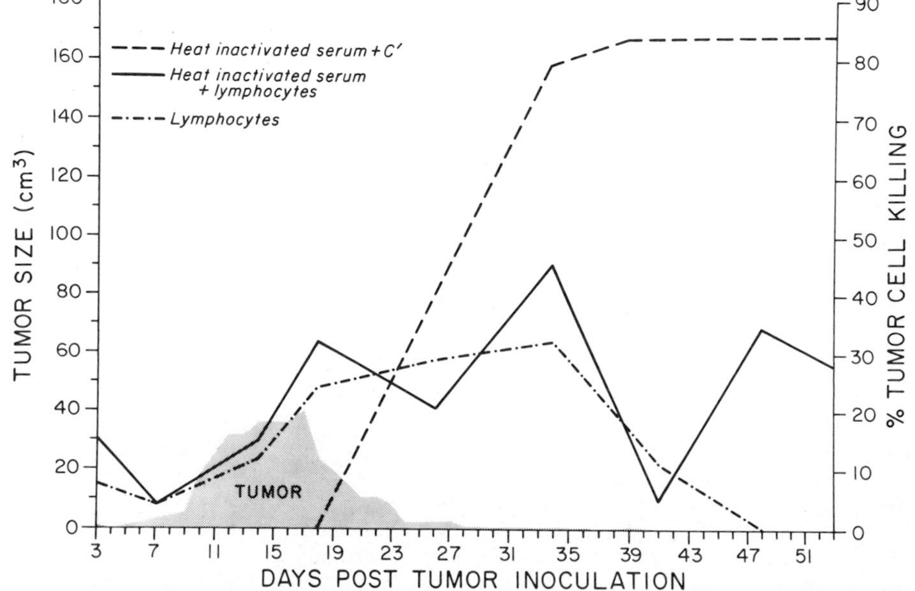


**Figure 6–9** The appearance of cytolytic antibody and cytotoxic lymphocytes in the blood of a cat inoculated with feline sarcoma virus. The resulting tumor (shaded area) grew rapidly but was eventually destroyed by the host's immune response. Antibody-dependent and antibody-independent lymphocyte-mediated cytotoxicity, as well as cytolytic antibody, was demonstrable at the time the tumor began to regress.

by edema, mast cell degranulation, and an eosinophil infiltrate (Parish, 1965), whereas the Arthus reaction is distinguished by vasculitis, edema, and a dense neutrophil infiltrate. Lymphocytes are not seen in the tissue surrounding either reaction. By contrast, if the cat has cell-mediated immunity, lymphocytes begin migrating into the site within 24 hours and reach maximal numbers in 48 to 72 hours. Associated with this infiltrate are inflammatory changes.

There has been a general feeling that delayed hypersensitivity reactions cannot be induced in cats (Akcasu, 1963). Cats infected with tuberculosis respond poorly and erratically to intradermally administered tuberculin (Francis, 1958; Hawthorne and Lauder, 1962; Snider et al., 1971), and a delayed hypersensitivity reaction to bovine serum albumin cannot be induced by techniques that induce such reactivity in guinea pigs (McCusker and Aitken, 1967). Hence the assumption that the immunity of cats to diseases like tuberculosis does not involve delayed hypersensitivity (Legendre et al., 1977; Scott, 1980). These studies, however, could give rise to unjustified conclusions. Cats can develop delayed hypersensitivity to foreign protein, and this sensitivity can be transferred to nonimmune cats with lymphocytes (Aitken and McCusker, 1969). Although it was difficult to demonstrate delayed hypersensitivity in the skin or footpads of cats, it could be readily elicited in the cornea. Even so, the reaction was much less intense and of shorter duration than the reaction in guinea pigs. These findings suggest that the cat's skin may not give a reliable indication of cell-mediated immunity. Even this, however, may be an overstatement, for good delayed reactions to bacillus Calmette-Guérin (BCG) vaccinations in cats have been elicited with either purified protein derivative (PPD) or old tuberculin (OT) injected intradermally in the ears (Pedersen, 1983). This distant sensitivity did not persist after the local BCG reaction subsided. Others have shown poor dermal reactions with PPD 60 days after BCG vaccination (Legendre et al., 1977). In their cats the macrophage-inhibition test result was positive when peripheral blood lymphocytes were reacted with PPD 7 to 30 days after BCG vaccination, but not thereafter. In addition, the in-vitro blastogenic response to tuberculin is greatly increased after natural infection of cats with tuberculosis (Guelfi et al., 1974).

Clinical and laboratory studies indicate that cats have a very well developed cell-mediated immunity. Schultz and Maguire (1982) were able to evoke delayed hypersensitivity in the skin of cats with dinitrochlorobenzene. Cats also respond like other animals in naturally occurring diseases in which cell-mediated immunity is thought to be important, e.g., rhinotracheitis (herpes), salmonellosis, coccidioidomycosis, and tuberculosis. They do not respond, however, with delayed hypersensitivity to some proteins such as bovine serum albumin (McCusker and Aitken, 1967). Delayed hypersensitivity reactions in cats are not so intense or consistent as those in guinea pigs. The guinea pig, however, appears to be somewhat atypical in the severity of its skin reactivity when compared with most other animals, whose reactions more often resemble the cat's. Finally, the granulomatous reactions occurring in lymph nodes regional to BCG injections are characteristic of reactions occurring in other species in which delayed hypersensitivity to tuberculin or PPD is well developed (Legendre et al., 1977). So also are the granulomatous lesions of tuberculosis in cats, which are indistinguishable from tuberculin responses in other animals and man (Jennings, 1949; Snider, 1971).

## The Phagocytic System

Cats resemble other mammals in the anatomy of their phagocytic system. Fixed tissue histiocytes are common around small blood vessels, particularly under mucous and serous membranes, skin, and meninges, and are present in hepatic sinusoids (Kupffer cells). The spleen and medullary areas of lymph nodes are also rich in phagocytic cells. Pleural and peritoneal macrophages can be obtained in small numbers by washing the pleural and abdominal cavities with physiologic saline solution. When substances such as potato starch or oyster shell glycogen are placed in these cavities, there is a rapid influx of neutrophils within 12 to 36 hours, followed by a larger influx of macrophages (Pedersen, 1983). The macrophages actively ingest large amounts of the starch or glycogen. Alveolar macrophages line the smaller airways of the lungs.

Monocytes make up less than 5 per cent of the white cells in the circulation. Their numbers increase in chronic infections, as they are drawn from the bone marrow to sites of disease. Once they leave the blood and enter tissues, they are transformed into macrophages.

Blood neutrophils of cats are highly phagocytic and have a pronounced bactericidal activity. They kill bacteria in vitro as do those of other species (Pedersen, 1983).

## Eosinophil-Mediated Immunity

The role of eosinophils in immunity is a matter of debate. The most widely held belief, that they moderate the effects of anaphylactic reactions, is supported by the finding that mast cells, which release histamine and other vasoactive amines, simultaneously release eosinophil-chemotactic factors. The hallmark of IgE- and mast cell-related immunity is eosinophilia and an eosinophil infiltrate at the site of reactions. Eosinophils may do more than correct the damage done by mast cells. David and coworkers (1980) have shown that eosinophils from humans with schistosomiasis kill larval *Schistosoma* in vitro in the presence of specific antibody. Schistosomal killing was associated with immune adherence of the eosinophils to the organisms. Enthusiasm for such an eosinophil function, however, has been tempered by Samter (1980).

## Blood Complement

Complement is not a single protein but consists of many substances. Eleven are concerned with activation, while others inactivate the system. The 11 activating proteins are designed C1q, C1r, C1s, and C2 through C9. The first three are loosely held together by a calcium-dependent bond. The individual proteins are produced in various tissues such as the liver (C3, C5 through C9), epithelial cells (C1), macrophages (C2, C4), and kidney, spleen, and lung (C7, C8) (Colten, 1976). C1 through C4, present in the serum in an inactive form, must be activated if the complement reaction is to take place. In their active forms each of these components functions as a specific proteolytic enzyme that has the subsequent component as its substrate. Once C5 is generated, the remaining complement components are bound molecule to molecule and have no enzyme activity.

The binding of antibody to antigen activates the complement reaction. Some IgG antibodies and all IgM antibodies cause complement binding, starting with C1 and ending with C9, this reaction being termed the "classical pathway" (Müller-Eberhard, 1968). Certain types of IgG antibodies, IgA and IgE antibodies, some bacterial polysaccharides and lipopolysaccharides, nucleated foreign cells, enveloped viruses, and some parasites activate complement beginning with C3 rather than with C1. This triggering, which occurs because of some property of the eliciting particle, involves properdin, factors B and D, and native C3 to form C3b (Müller-Eberhard and Schreiber, 1980). C3b is in turn bound to the biologic particle that is the target of the attack. C3b inactivator and $\beta_1$H protein are inhibitors of the reaction.

Although antibody determines the target of the immune attack, complement determines the effect of that attack. Fragments of low molecular weight (anaphylatoxins), derived from the activation of native C3 and C5, can cause contraction of smooth muscle and increased capillary permeability. Phagocyte chemotaxis toward the site of complement binding is caused by these fragments and by the activated C567 complex. Phagocytosis of antibody-coated antigen is stimulated by the binding of C3. Immune lysis, which has been seen with foreign cells, bacteria, and some enveloped viruses, is caused by the binding of C8 and C9.

Cats possess all the complement components recognized in other animals (Barta and Hubbert, 1978; Kobilinsky et al., 1979; Nelson, 1966). Hemolytic assays indicate that the levels of each component in cat serum are comparable, with a few variations, to those in other species (Kobilinsky et al., 1979; Nelson, 1966; Table 6–3). Nelson (1966), using guinea pig components, found that the greatest variation between cat and man was in the measurable levels of C8 (Table 6–3). He believed that cat serum possessed an inhibitor of C8 when guinea pig components were used to provide all the other factors. This is not apparent when human components are used (Table 6–3). Kobilinsky and associates (1979), however, showed C8 levels in cat serum to be comparable to man's. The only difference in the assay procedures in these two studies was in the use of human C4 by Kobilinsky and coworkers (1979).

Cat complement is not as hemolytic as rabbit, dog, or guinea pig complement in systems utilizing rabbit anti-sheep red cell serum and sheep red cells (Barta and Oyekan, 1981). Similar results can be obtained, however, if sheep red cells are coated with a 20-fold higher concentration of the hemolysin than would be used for assaying complement in these other species (Pedersen, 1983). Other researchers have claimed good success in assaying cat complement when they used cat sera directed against rabbit or chicken red cells (Schultz, 1977) or against guinea pig red cells (Barta and Oyekan, 1981). It would seem that in some antigen systems homologous antibody will fix only cat complement, whereas with other antigens cat complement is fixed very well by both homologous and heterologous antibody (Perryman et al., 1973).

Using hemolytic assays, we found that normal cat serum contains 40 to 80 total complement hemolytic 50 per cent ($CH_{50}$) units per ml (Pedersen, 1983). Others have reported 22 to 68 $CH_{50}$ units per ml. (Kitzmiller et al., 1972) and 92 ± 27 $CH_{50}$ units per ml (Kobilinsky et al., 1979). Barta and Oyekan (1981), using guinea pig red cells and cat hemolysin, obtained values of 70 to 150 $CH_{50}$ units per ml. In a study using cat antibody to feline oncornavirus-associated cell membrane antigen (FOCMA) and tissue-cultured, FeLV-infected lymphoblastoid cells as the target, it was found that normal cats had 31 ± 6 complement lytic 50 per cent units per ml of serum (Grant et al., 1979).

Comparing classical and alternative pathways of complement activation, Kobilinsky and coworkers (1979) found that many FeLV-infected cats had low complement levels, and measurement of serum levels of C1q and factor B showed that this depletion was caused by activation of the classical, not the alternative, pathway. Their study also showed normal cats to have factor B levels similar to man's (236 ± 82 units per ml).

## Interferons

Interferons are proteins of low molecular weight produced by cells after viral infection, chemical exposure, or antigenic stimulation. Three types of interferon (IFN) are presently recognized: IFN-α, IFN-β, and IFN-γ (Stewart et al., 1980). The first two were known previously as viral or type I interferons, IFN-α being produced by leukocytes and IFN-β by fibroblasts. Interferon-γ, immune interferon, is produced by antigenically stimulated lymphocytes. Future studies will undoubtedly identify other types or subtypes of interferons.

Interferons in some way activate a repressed cellular system that blocks the synthesis of viral proteins by the cell. They also enhance cell-mediated cytotoxic activity against infected or tumorous cells by null lymphocytes (Bloom, 1980) and suppress some antibody responses.

Interferon synthesis can be induced in cats with Newcastle disease virus (NDV), synthetic polyribonucleic acids

**Table 6–3 Complement Levels in Normal Cat Serum**

| $TCH_{50}$ | C1 | C4 | C2 | C3 | C5 | C6 | C7 | C8 | C9 | COMPLEMENT SOURCE* | REFERENCE† |
|---|---|---|---|---|---|---|---|---|---|---|---|
| 92 ±27 | 71,700 ±17,700 | 16,745 ±9,661 | 649 ±244 | 615 ±90 | 1,385 ±345 | 904 ±388 | 669 ±165 | 11,344 ±2,650 | 18,432 ±6,506 | C1gp,C4hu, C3–C9gp | 1 |
| — | 12,000 | 25,000 | 2,000 | 5,000 | 200,000 | 25,000 | 150,000 | 2,000 | 20,000 | C1–C9gp | 2 |
| 48 | 6,000 | 12,000 | 1,600 | 300 | 1,500 | 32,000 | 48,000 | 8,000 | 12,000 | C1–C9hu | 3 |
| 48 | 48,000 | 8,000 | 300 | 3,200 | 96,000 | 32,000 | 192,000 | 8,000 | 32,000 | C1–C9gp | 3 |

*hu = human; gp = guinea pig, sheep red blood cells, rabbit hemolysin.
†1. Kobilinsky et al., 1979.
2. Nelson, 1966.
3. Cordis Laboratories, Hialeah, FL.

such as poly I:C (McCullough, 1972; Stringfellow and Weed, 1977), and pyrimidinol compounds (Stringfellow and Weed, 1977). Poly I:C, however, is toxic to cats at the levels needed to induce a good response (McCullough, 1972; Stringfellow and Weed, 1977). Newcastle disease virus and poly I:C induce high levels of interferon in all cats, whereas levels induced by pyrimidinol compounds may be high in some cats and low in others (Stringfellow and Weed, 1977).

Feline interferons seem to resemble those of other mammals and man in their chemical and biologic properties (McCullough, 1972; Yamamoto et al., 1986). Cat interferon produced in vitro by NDV-stimulated, Crandell feline fetus cells renders cells resistant to infection with vesicular stomatitis virus and feline leukemia virus (FeLV) (Rodgers et al., 1972). Feline calicivirus and feline rhinotracheitis (herpes) virus are also sensitive in vitro to interferon. Unfortunately cat interferon administered in an aerosol has not been effective in vivo in reducing the clinical signs of experimental rhinotracheitis virus infection of cats (Kahn, 1973). Orally administered bovine IFN-β has been reported to be effective in reversing the anemia seen in some FeLV-infected cats (Tompkins and Cummins, 1982). Human IFN-α, which effectively reduced FeLV replication in vitro, had no in-vivo effect on FeLV levels when given intravenously to cats (Pedersen, 1983).

## Membrane Immunity

The mucous membranes and skin, the main barriers against microbial invasion, are protected by innate defense mechanisms, as well as more complex immune processes. The skin's cornified layer and sebum excretion constitute a formidable hindrance to pathogens. The normal microbial flora also tends to crowd out pathogenic inhabitants. The mucosa of the respiratory tract has cilia that sweep foreign material and microbes upward to the orpharynx, whereas if the mucosa is damaged, they can move downward into the lower airways. Gastric acid, enzymes in the small bowel, and normal peristalsis serve to restrict bacteria to the lower bowel. In addition, the mucous film of the mucous membranes contains bacteriostatic and virustatic substances.

Fixed phagocytes abound in mucosal surfaces and under the skin and when needed proliferate locally. In addition, monocytes and neutrophils can be rapidly recruited from the blood.

The mucous membranes are continuously bathed by immunoglobulins produced locally by plasma cells or derived from the serum. If a membrane is inflamed, serum exudation can add to the local immunoglobulin. Reaginic immunity is present in the skin and mucous membranes to combat parasite invasion.

Cell-mediated immunity is also active in membranes and skin. Lymphocytes can be drawn to areas of need, to participate locally in cell-mediated immune processes. Many pathogens of skin and mucosae are protected from humoral attack by their residence within phagocytes or epithelial cells. Cytotoxic lymphocytes, however, can often recognize and destroy infected cells, eliminating the pathogen's sanctuary.

Finally, interferon secreted actively by epithelial cells is important in containing a virus infection until other immune mechanisms join battle. Interferon secreted by an infected cell can render adjacent cells resistant to virus attack and enhance destruction of infected cells by cytotoxic lymphocytes. Some bacteria may bind complement by the alternate pathway without need for specific antibodies. Complement binding in turn facilitates phagocytosis and may lead to actual lysis of the bacteria. In these ways infection can be rapidly suppressed during the first few days, before more specific humoral and cell-mediated immunity is established.

Membrane immunity is of particular interest because of its apparent vulnerability to stress. Stress stimulates release of adrenal glucocorticoids, which impair almost all defense mechanisms involved in membrane immunity. The influence of various stresses on disease is discussed in the section on infection and immunity.

## Maternal Immunity

Maternal immunity is of two types, systemic and lactogenic.

**SYSTEMIC IMMUNITY.** Kittens absorb antibodies from colostrum during the first 24 hours of life (Scott et al., 1970). The colostral phase of lactation, during which abundant immunoglobulin is secreted, occurs during the first five days (Table 6–2). Early in this period more IgG and IgA are present in the milk than in the queen's serum, indicating active transport of these proteins. In contrast, levels of IgM lower than in the serum suggest that it enters the milk in a passive manner. IgM is not detectable in the milk after the first week of lactation, whereas IgG and IgA are secreted throughout lactation, although at decreasing levels (Table 6–2).

The serum immunoglobulin levels of kittens from 12 hours to 14 weeks of life are given in Figure 6–10. There is a rapid uptake of all classes of immunoglobulins during

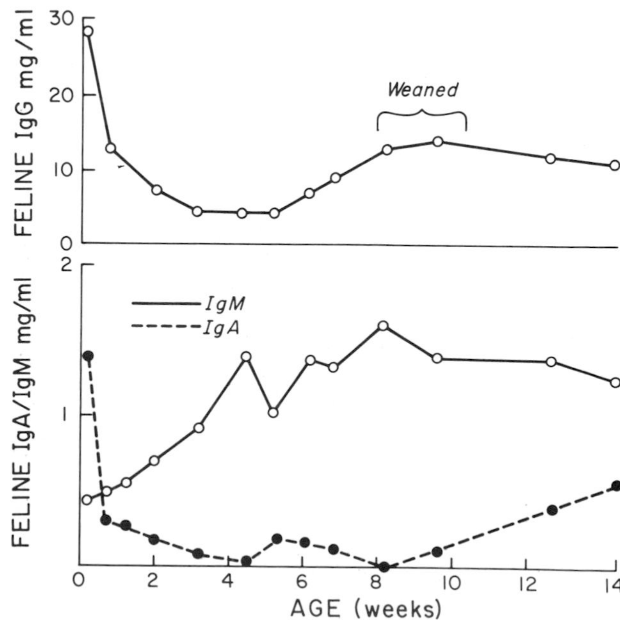


**Figure 6–10** The mean IgG, IgA, and IgM levels in the sera of four sibling kittens at intervals over the first 14 weeks of life. The initial measurements were made 12 hours after birth, at which time all the kittens had nursed.

the first 12 hours of nursing. IgG levels fall for five weeks and then rise. IgM levels increase steadily from birth, whereas IgA levels remain low for the entire nursing period and rise after weaning.

Although some researchers believe that cats get all their circulating maternal antibodies in colostrum (Okoshi et al., 1967), it appears that some kittens also receive a small amount of IgG through the placenta. Schultz and coworkers (1974) found that 33 per cent of kittens had some IgG in their precolostral sera, while Harding and associates (1961) found that 20 per cent of maternally derived anti-*Salmonella* antibodies in kittens were transferred through the placenta. Johnson (1980) found that the presuckling serum of kittens contained 3 per cent of the level of feline calicivirus antibodies possessed by their mothers. Scott and coworkers (1970) found kittens' presuckling titers to feline panleukopenia virus to be 1 per cent of their mother's titers.

Maternally derived IgG in the serum has a half-life of 7.0 to 18.5 days. Maternal antibodies to panleukopenia virus have a half-life of 9.7 days (Scott et al., 1970). This is, however, considerably shorter than the reported half-life of 15 days for maternally derived FeLV antibodies (Jarrett et al., 1977), 18.5 days for feline viral rhinotracheitis virus antibodies (Gaskell, 1975), and 15 days for feline calicivirus antibodies (Johnson, 1980). Antibodies to feline enteric coronavirus have a half-life of 7 days (Pedersen et al., 1981b).

Assuming a half-life of 14 days, only about 1 per cent of maternal antibody would be left at 12 weeks of age. The tremendous growth of kittens from birth to 12 weeks further dilutes the concentration of the remaining immunoglobulins. By 12 weeks, maternal antibody interference with most vaccines has disappeared (Scott et al., 1970). Nevertheless, in some queens with high titers of panleukopenia virus antibody, antibody interference may extend to 14 weeks of age or more, necessitating vaccination at 16 weeks (Scott et al., 1970).

The level of maternal antibodies in kittens is not necessarily correlated with the queen's titer. Gillespie and Scott (1973) reported a direct correlation between levels of panleukopenia virus antibody in the serum of queens and passive antibody titers in their kittens. This does not appear to be the case with maternal antibodies to rhinotracheitis virus (Gaskell, 1975), and the final titers that kittens obtain to calicivirus from their mothers vary greatly (Johnson, 1980), ranging in a large group of kittens, a week after nursing, from 30 to 100 per cent (± 69 per cent) of their mothers' titers at the time of birth.

Levels of maternal antibodies in kitten serum do not necessarily parallel protection. In the case of panleukopenia, there is good correlation between passive antibody titers and protection (Gillespie and Scott, 1973). In contrast, some kittens with high maternal titers to rhinotracheitis virus become infected, while others with low or undetectable titers resist challenge (Gaskell, 1975). Similarly with calicivirus infection, a number of kittens become infected at four to six weeks of age despite considerable levels of maternal antibody (Gillespie and Scott, 1973; Johnson, 1980).

As in other species (Roitt, 1977), maternal antibody depresses humoral immune responses of kittens to both live and killed antigens. Maternal antibodies interfere with both parenteral and intranasal attenuated live rhinotracheitis vaccines for at least the first 9 or 10 weeks of life (Slater and York, 1976), delay and lower the peak antibody response to oronasal inoculation with live calicivirus (Johnson, 1980), and interfere with the immunizing ability of both live and inactivated panleukopenia virus (Fastier, 1968; Gillespie and Scott, 1973; O'Reilly et al., 1969; Scott et al., 1970). Scott (1971) found that whereas 89 per cent of kittens without maternal panleukopenia virus antibodies responded to vaccination, only 73 per cent, 52 per cent, and 12 per cent of kittens with titers of, respectively, <1:10, 1:2 to 1:10, and >1:10 responded. He also found that modified live-virus panleukopenia vaccine was more likely to overcome a low maternal titer than inactivated-virus vaccines. The mechanisms of maternal antibody interference are not precisely known, although existing antibody appears to inhibit the proliferation of specific antibody-forming cells in other species (Fitch, 1975). Antibody-mediated depression of the immune response may be caused by natural feedback mechanisms that prevent overproduction of antibody (Uhr and Moeller, 1968).

**LACTOGENIC IMMUNITY.** Antibodies in the milk protect the newborn against intestinal pathogens ingested within the first few weeks of life, when active local immunity is not yet fully developed. Lactogenic immunity, to be effective, must be specific for the pathogens encountered and must be provided continuously and in adequate levels. Secretory IgA, because it is relatively resistant to degradation by gastric and intestinal contents, is the most important antibody in milk. IgG may function importantly in preventing infection higher in the digestive tract, as in the oropharynx. The presence of IgM in milk during the first five days of lactation may also be significant. IgM antibodies appear to be important in local immunity to pathogenic bacteria, and the neonatal period is the time when most fatal septicemias occur in animals. Table 6–2 shows the levels of IgG, IgA, and IgM in maternal serum, colostrum, and milk.

## Red-Cell and Lymphocyte Antigens

Holmes (1953) described three blood groups in cats, which he designated O, F, and EF. E and F were designated as the isoantigens present on cat red cells; isoantibodies against the antigens not present on the red cells were also found in the serum. In a small group of cats typed with anti-EF and anti-F sera, 95.15 per cent were EF, 0.97 per cent F, and 3.8 per cent O.

Using naturally occurring antibodies in cats' plasma, Eyquem and Podliachouk (1954) and Eyquem and associates (1962) distinguished two major red-cell antigens, which they designated A and B. Group A was found to be present in 85 per cent of cats and group B in 15 per cent. Braend and Andersen (1979) found that bovine anti-J blood group serum with rabbit complement would hemolyze red cells of cats with a blood group that they called A. Eyquem and Podliachouk (1954) considered their group A to be identical to Holmes' group EF and their group B to be identical to Holmes' groups O and F. They also described antigens that they designated C and D, often associated with B.

Cat red-cell antigens have also been studied in detail by Auer and Bell (1979). Analyzing the red cells of 1895 domestic cats in Brisbane, Australia, they found that 73.3 per cent of cats had blood group A, 26.3 per cent group B, and 0.4 per cent group AB. They postulated that the

A gene was dominant to B in most cats, while the rare AB blood group occurred when the A gene did not show dominance over B, possibly because of some other modifier gene. Their studies also showed that the 95 per cent of cats with blood type B also had antibodies to type A red cells, while only 25 per cent of cats with type A red cells had antibodies to type B. In this regard, the A-B system of cats resembles the human ABO system. Cats, however, do not secrete A-B blood group substance in their saliva as do humans, and there was no evidence of any serologic relationship between the cat A-B antigens and the human ABO antigens (Auer and Bell, 1979).

The importance of the feline A-B red-cell antigens and the frequent presence of antibodies to the opposite blood group has not been determined. It has always been assumed that the blood of one cat could be transfused into another without crossmatching, but in light of the findings of Auer and Bell (1979) and of Auer and coworkers (1982), it would seem that transfusions into a cat with natural antibodies to the transfused red cells could cause some clinical problems. At the least, the life span of the mismatched transfused cells is greatly shortened (Marion and Smith, 1983).

A transfusion with mismatched blood may also sensitize a cat to a subsequent transfusion with red cells of the same type. In practice, however, multiple transfusions from random donors have not been associated with violent hemolytic reactions in cats (Cotter, 1982; Hayes et al., 1982).

A review of the literature failed to discover any descriptions of lymphocyte antigens (histocompatibility antigens) in cats. Allograft rejection, well developed in cats (Perryman et al., 1972), suggests that the cat has a functional histocompatibility antigen system like that of other animals.

## IMMUNOLOGIC DISORDERS

### Type I Reactions (Anaphylaxis)

#### Anaphylactic Shock

Although an early report stated that anaphylaxis could not be induced in cats (Wilson and Miles, 1964), anaphylactic shock was induced by intravenous injection of 22 mg of bovine gamma globulin into two cats that had shown a local cutaneous anaphylactic reaction to the same protein (McCusker and Aitken, 1966). Within a few seconds the cats reacted with vigorous head scratching, labored respiration, salivation, vomiting, incoordination, and collapse, and one cat died. One of the cats also had blood-tinged froth around the mouth and nose.

On histologic examination the arterioles of the lungs were seen to be packed with white cells and the lung tissue was completely devoid of mast cells. It was concluded that the lungs were the primary target organ of anaphylactic shock in cats, a finding supported by studies of Riley and West (1953) that show cat lungs to be rich in mast cells. The cat lung, however, is about 200 times more sensitive to serotonin than to histamine (Austen and Humphrey, 1963), a phenomenon suggesting that serotonin released from mast cells is an important mediator of anaphylaxis in the cat. Anaphylactic reactions, manifested in mild cases by restlessness, head scratching, dyspnea, tachycardia, and urination, and in severe cases by exophthalmos, pupillary dilatation, convulsions, salivation, vomiting, defecation, cyanosis, and prostration, have also been induced in cats with intravenous injections of BCG (Jankovic et al., 1969).

The occurrence of anaphylactic shock in cats under natural conditions has apparently not been reported. The cat seems to be more resistant than other species, because the dose of protein (22 mg) used by McCusker and Aitken (1966) greatly exceeds that needed to induce anaphylactic shock in guinea pigs and rabbits.

#### Urticaria and Facioconjunctival Edema

Focal wheal and flare reactions of the skin (hives, urticaria), although common in dogs, are rare in cats, as is facioconjunctival (angioneurotic) edema. Reactions of this type are usually due to injections of vaccines and drugs or to insect bites. Local anaphylactic reactions usually take place one-half to two hours after the insult and persist for 10 to 24 hours. An injection of glucocorticoid often hastens their disappearance.

#### Atopic Skin Disease

Flea bite dermatitis is the most common allergic reaction of the skin of cats, representing both cutaneous anaphylaxis and cell-mediated immune responses (Gorham et al., 1971). Allergic dermatitis of cats can be caused by both dietary and inhaled allergens. Skin lesions due to food allergies are usually multiple and of miliary type. Walton (1966, 1967) described allergic dermatoses in 18 cats with focal exfoliations and edema of the skin associated, in a few cats, with diarrhea and vomiting. He determined the cause of the allergic reaction by using a controlled diet. Canned cat food, cow's milk, meat of rabbit, beef, whale, or, chicken, and penicillin were incriminated in individual cats. Baker (1975) reported on four cats, three of which developed skin disorders from commercial cat food and one from eggs. He suggested that food allergy could be diagnosed in most cats if signs disappeared or abated within five days after institution of a controlled diet such as chicken and rice. Cooked turkey is another excellent hypoallergenic test diet (Pedersen, 1983). Food allergy manifested by skin disease has also been described in two cats by Stogdale and coworkers (1982).

Allergic dermatitis associated with inhalant grass, weed, and tree pollens has been described by Reedy (1982). Unlike dietary allergic dermatitis, the offending allergens in these cats were identified by intradermal allergen testing. Reedy (1982) was successful in about two thirds of the cases in hyposensitizing these animals with injections of allergen extracts.

#### Allergic Conjunctival and Respiratory Disorders

Allergic rhinitis is rarely recognized in cats. Chronic allergic follicular conjunctivitis with episcleritis has been seen in a few cats and responds well to ophthalmic ointments containing glucocorticoids. Allergic disease of the trachea and bronchi seems to be uncommon.

Allergic disease of the small airways (bronchioles) may be more prevalent in cats than other allergic respiratory conditions. A condition of possible allergic etiology has been called bronchial asthma (Carpenter, 1974). The disease exists in two forms: an episodic disease manifested by transient periods of acute respiratory distress and a more chronic condition characterized by more or less persistent coughing and wheezing (Moise and Spaulding, 1981). There are no persistent radiographic changes with the first form, which is most similar to human asthma. The second form in cats is associated radiographically with peribronchiolar fibrosis and is more akin to chronic bronchitis, alveolitis, or so-called pulmonary infiltrate with eosinophila of man and dogs. Signs can be seasonal or consistent. Corticosteroids, along with bronchial dilators such as theophylline or beta-adrenergic blockers, have been used to treat the condition (Moise and Spaulding, 1981). The cause of this disorder is unknown. As presently described, it may embrace several unresolved entities of similar or diverse etiology.

## Allergic Enteritis

Allergic reactions can occur in the stomach, small intestine, or colon. Colitis is probably the most common form of allergic bowel disease in cats. It is most often manifested by the intermittent appearance of fresh blood and mucus in the stool. More severe generalized bowel involvement can lead to chronic diarrhea and weight loss. Eosinophilia is most apt to be observed in cats with more widespread bowel involvement.

Allergenic substances in the cat's diet are usually responsible. Treatment is with a carefully controlled diet, usually one containing a high proportion of a single type of meat protein. A combination of chicken and rice has been a good basic diet with which to start (Baker, 1975). If this is not effective, horsemeat and rice should be tried. Turkey is even better because most cats have not been exposed to it in their diet (Pedersen, 1983). Beef and milk products should be avoided until they are eliminated as a cause. If the controlled diet is successful, new foods can be introduced slowly, one at a time. Low-dosage corticosteroid therapy is used only when dietary control fails. An excellent review of dietary allergies in dogs, which is applicable to cats as well, is that of Baker (1974). This information is supported by case reports of allergic enteritis in cats, which provide an immunopathologic and pathologic description of the disorder (Parish, 1965; Walton et al., 1968).

# TYPE II REACTIONS (CYTOTOXIC ANTIBODIES)

## Neonatal Isoerythrolysis

Neonatal isoerythrolysis has been recognized at the Veterinary Medical Teaching Hospital, Davis, California, in several litters of kittens, offspring of two cattery queens and a household queen (Cain and Suzuki, 1985). The queens had serum hemolysins against red cells of the toms. Unlike natural hemolysins in the blood of many cats, these antibodies were apparently passed to the kittens in the colostrum. The kittens became lethargic 24 to 48 hours after birth and died within 12 to 24 hours. Hemoglobinuria was often severe. The tissues of the kittens were pale and jaundiced at autopsy, and the spleens and livers enlarged. Histologic examination of tissues disclosed pronounced erythrophagocytosis and hemosiderosis.

The blood group incompatibility responsible for this disorder has not yet been identified. The queens were responding to a blood group factor present in 75 per cent of randomly selected cats (group A). Sensitization occurred during the first pregnancy in some queens. Once the condition is recognized, subsequent kittens should be fostered to other queens before they nurse.

Of academic interest is Ditchfield's (1968) report on the occurrence of isoimmunization of pregnant queens with now obsolete homologous tissue-origin panleukopenia vaccine. Isoantibodies transferred to the kittens resulted in neonatal isoerythrolysis.

## Autoimmune Hemolytic Anemia

Autoimmune hemolytic anemia has been recognized in cats (Faircloth and Montgomery, 1981; Heise et al., 1973; Lubberink et al., 1971; Scott et al., 1973; Sodikoff and Custer, 1965, 1966), and may be more prevalent than previously estimated. Like the condition in man, it is often secondary to some underlying disease such as FeLV infection (Scott et al., 1973; Werner and Gorman, 1984). It may often be a prelude to some lymphoreticular or myeloproliferative neoplasm in FeLV-positive or -negative cats, preceding overt disease by several months (Werner and Gorman, 1984). *Haemobartonella felis* infection can lead to a Coombs'-positive hemolytic anemia (Maede and Hata, 1975), the antibodies being directed against *Haemobartonella* antigens on the parasitized red cells. Autoimmune hemolytic anemia has also been associated with systemic lupus erythematosus in the cat (Faircloth and Montgomery, 1981; Heise et al., 1973).

Signs include depression, pallor, usually reticulocytosis, and sometimes hepatosplenomegaly. The marrow may show erythroid hyperplasia, dysplasia, or rarely hypoplasia. Spherocytosis is difficult to recognize in cat blood, probably because cat red cells tend to be naturally spherocytic (Scott et al., 1973). The direct Coombs' test can be used to detect immunoglobulin-coated red cells (Scott et al., 1973; Werner and Gorman, 1984). This test, however, should be interpreted with caution in cats with no clinical or laboratory evidence of autoimmune hemolytic anemia (Dunn et al., 1984). Because of the frequent association of the anemia with some other condition, an effort should be made to identify predisposing causes by FeLV testing, examination of blood films for *Haemobartonella*, antinuclear antibody tests, and a careful search for lymphoreticular and myeloid neoplasms.

The treatment is prednisone or prednisolone 2 to 4 mg/kg daily until the packed cell volume is in the normal range, then 1 to 2 mg/kg daily for another week or so, and finally 1 mg/kg every day for four to eight weeks. There is a conflict of opinion as to whether evening administration is preferable for cats. Splenectomy was ineffective in one cat treated by this procedure (Faircloth and Montgomery, 1981).

## Autoimmune Thrombocytopenia

Like autoimmune hemolytic anemia, autoimmune thrombocytopenia may be primary or secondary. At the

Veterinary Medical Teaching Hospital, Davis, two cats with this disorder were studied, one in which thrombocytopenia was primary and one in which it was secondary to systemic lupus erythematosus. In a report concerning primary disease, the cat had circulating antiplatelet antibodies (Joshi et al., 1979). The treatment is the same as for autoimmune hemolytic anemia.

## Cold Agglutinin Disease

Cold agglutinins are autoantibodies, usually of the IgM class, that bind with red blood cells at body temperatures lower than normal. During bouts of low ambient temperature, the temperature of blood in the peripheral capillaries is lower than normal, and cold agglutinins combine with their corresponding red cell antigens. This process can lead to agglutination of red cells in peripheral capillaries and to vascular occlusion and gangrene of the extremities (ear tips, eyelids, digits, tip of tail). In uncommon cases, hemolytic anemia can also occur. Cold agglutinins are present in low titers (0 to 1:16) in some normal cats (Dunn et al., 1984; Schrader and Hurvitz, 1983). Titers in the thousands were observed in one cat with this disorder (Schrader and Hurvitz, 1983). Cold agglutinins may be associated with a preceding viral infection, as in the case reported by Schrader and Hurvitz (1983), but more often the eliciting cause is unknown.

## Bullous Dermatitides

Pemphigus vulgaris, pemphigus foliaceus, and pemphigus erythematosus have been recognized in the cat (Brown and Hurvitz, 1979; Faircloth and Montgomery, 1982; Manning et al., 1982; Scott, 1980; Scott et al., 1980). These uncommon conditions are associated with the development of antibodies against the intercellular cement holding the epidermal cells together.

## Eosinophilic Granuloma Complex

Two thirds of cats with eosinophilic granulomas were found to have circulating antibodies to normal cat epithelium (Gelberg et al., 1985). Similar antibodies were seen, however, in 1/16 (6 per cent) of normal cats. The authors concluded that either the antibodies participated in the disease process or they were merely secondary to the release of sequestered autoantigens from the lesions.

## Myasthenia Gravis

Acquired myasthenia gravis has been described in cats (Dawson, 1970; Indrieri et al., 1983; Mason, 1976). In man and dogs, it is caused by development of autoantibodies directed against the acetylcholine receptors of the myoneural junctions (Indrieri et al., 1983; Lennon, 1978).

# TYPE III REACTIONS (IMMUNE-COMPLEX DISEASE)

Diseases in this group are caused by deposition of circulating antigen-antibody complexes around the basement membrane of small blood vessels. These complexes, along with complement factors, elicit an inflammatory reaction in or around the vessels. Clinical signs develop when organ function is compromised by this reaction and vary greatly depending on the target tissue.

Immune-complex disease occurs when there is a continuing source of antigen, a persistent antibody response to that antigen, and resulting antigen-antibody complexes that are not so large that they are phagocytosed or so small that they pass freely out of blood vessels with other serum proteins. The complexes must also be of the appropriate physical charge and chemical composition. Under these conditions, the complexes pass between the endothelial cells, but are trapped on one side or the other of the basement membranes.

## Glomerulonephritis (Immune-Complex Type)

Glomerulonephritis occurs when antigen-antibody complement complexes are deposited around the basement membranes of the glomerular capillaries, causing the basement membrane to become irregularly thickened. These immune complexes can be detected with fluoresceinated anti-IgG or C3 globulins (Fig. 6–11). These complexes eventually interfere with the nutrition of the nephron. Death of nephrons can ultimately lead to renal failure and azotemia. Proteinuria is not a serious complication of glomerulonephritis in cats as it is in dogs. The

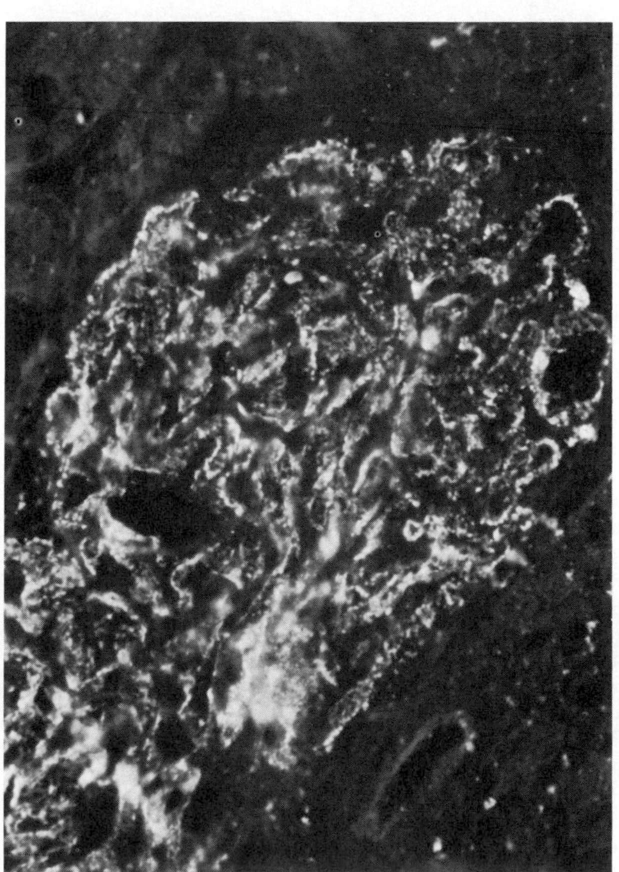

**Figure 6–11** Renal glomerulus in an FeLV-infected cat that died of lymphosarcoma. Diffuse granular deposits of IgG were found in the glomerular basement membranes. Rabbit anti-cat IgG globulin–FITC stain, × 250.

nephrotic syndrome, i.e., proteinuria, hypoproteinemia, and edema, is uncommon in cats.

Glomerulonephritis in cats is either idiopathic or secondary. The origin of the antigen in the idiopathic form is unknown, but in the secondary form it derives from some concurrent infectious or neoplastic disorder. Azotemia and the nephrotic syndrome are predominant manifestations of idiopathic glomerulonephritis. In contrast, secondary glomerulonephritis is often only a minor aspect of the total disease, and uremia is uncommon as the presenting complaint.

Secondary glomerulonephritis, the usual form of the disease in cats, is associated most often with FeLV infection and its related manifestations, e.g., anemia, myeloproliferative disease, and lymphoma (Anderson and Jarrett, 1971). In one FeLV-enzootic household, glomerulonephritis was a leading cause of death in chronically infected cats (Francis et al., 1980). In a series of 13 cats, membranous glomerulonephritis occurred without recognizable predisposing causes of FeLV infection (Nash et al., 1979). Other cases of idiopathic glomerulonephritis in cats have been described (Bown, 1971; Farrow et al., 1969; Saegusa et al., 1975; Scott et al., 1975; Slauson et al., 1971). Secondary glomerulonephritis has also been reported in cats with feline infectious peritonitis (Jacobse-Geels et al., 1980), non-FeLV related neoplasms, chronic infections, heartworm disease, and systemic lupus erythematosus.

## Amyloidosis

Amyloidosis results from deposition of a complex protein (in a β-pleated or fibrillar configuration) around vascular basement membrane, especially in the kidney. The chemical composition of amyloid varies with the underlying cause (Glenner, 1980). Amyloid can be made up of polymerized fragments of immunoglobulin light chains (amyloid L) or other protein constituents (amyloid A). The distinction between amyloid L and A (AL, AA) is not clear-cut, however, because some AA contains immunoglobulin light chains as well. The precursor proteins and their catabolic products ultimately result from some disease process.

Amyloidosis in man has been classified as primary or secondary. Primary amyloidosis (AL) in man is usually associated with benign or malignant plasma cell dyscrasias that result in increased production of immunoglobulin or immunoglobulin subunits, especially light chains. Secondary amyloidosis (AA) is associated with a wide range of chronic infectious and neoplastic, immunologic, or metabolic disorders.

The literature contains many references to amyloidosis in cats (e.g., Clark and Seawright 1968, 1969; Crowell et al., 1972; Hartigan et al., 1980, Hjärre and Morgan, 1933; Jakob, 1971; Nakamatsu et al., 1966; Saegusa et al., 1979; Seawright et al., 1967). Amyloidosis reported by Seawright and coworkers (1967) and Clark and Seawright (1968, 1969) was associated with hypervitaminosis A in Queensland cats fed predominantly raw liver. The inciting cause of amyloidosis in the other cases was unknown, although Jakob (1971) mentioned several associated diseases. At the Veterinary Medical Hospital, Davis, cats with amyloidosis were suffering from neoplasia and chronic infections. A familial type of progressive renal amyloidosis has also been described in Abyssinian cats (Chew et al., 1982). It is apparent, therefore, that amyloidosis in cats, as in other species (Jakob, 1971), is caused by a number of different mechanisms, some of which are clearly immunologic and others are not.

Although amyloid may be deposited in the liver, spleen, intestine, and the adrenal, thyroid, and parathyroid glands in cats, it is the kidney that is most consistently and severely involved, and chronic renal failure is the most frequent cause of death in cats with amyloidosis. Amyloid deposits are common in the pancreatic islets of aged cats, but usually have no clinical significance (Jakob, 1971); however, if diffuse and dense, they may cause diabetes mellitus (Carpenter, 1983).

Dehydration, emaciation, uremic breath, oral ulcers, and vomiting are the usual presenting signs and worsen over a period of weeks or months. Proteinuria, conspicuous in dogs, may not be pronounced or even consistent in feline renal amyloidosis, perhaps because the medulla is often more severely involved than the glomeruli in the cat (Clark and Seawright, 1969; Lucke and Hunt, 1965).

## Systemic Lupus Erythematosus

Systemic lupus erythematosus is a combination of immune complex disease and cytotoxic antibody reactions. The immune complexes are made up in part of nucleic acid and antinuclear antibody. This antibody, however, is probably not the ultimate cause of the disease, because antinuclear antibody in man is not pathologic by itself when transfused into normal individuals. Some underlying disorder is probably involved in bringing about the release of nucleic acids so that antibodies can have access to them. In the human disease there is generalized enhancement of antibody responses to many different viral and self antigens and a deficiency in T-lymphocytes of the suppressor type. A latent and unknown viral disease has been postulated as the cause of the disease in man and dog (Lewis, 1980). A lupus-like syndrome has also been described in hyperthyroid cats treated with propylthiouracil (Peterson et al., 1984).

Immune complex deposition commonly occurs in skin, synovial membranes, meninges, and glomeruli, causing dermatitis, polyarthritis, meningitis, or glomerulonephritis. Associated manifestations may include autoimmune hemolytic anemia or thrombocytopenia (Gabbert, 1983), which probably reflect an underlying disorder of immunoregulation and heightened antibody responsiveness.

Systemic lupus erythematosus is uncommon in cats but resembles the human and canine disease in its clinical form. Two cases of diffuse skin disease with systemic lupus erythematosus have been described in cats (Scott et al., 1979). Five cats with the disease have been observed at the teaching hospital of the University of California. The sole manifestation was autoimmune hemolytic anemia in one cat and autoimmune thrombocytopenia in the second. In the third, the disease was typical of classic fulminating systemic lupus erythematosus in man, with low-grade fever, nonerosive polyarthritis, meningitis, and glomerulonephritis. The meningitis was manifested by hyperesthesia, dementia, and convulsions. Blood tests showed neutropenia and hypocomplementemia. The fourth cat developed a low-grade, persistent lymphadenopathy and leukopenia at two years of age. Over the next three years it suffered from vague, transient episodes of depression and ultimately died of renal failure resulting from progressive glomerulonephritis. The fifth cat developed progressive renal failure and suffered from intermittent bouts of depression and anorexia. It was also neutropenic and leukopenic over the entire two-year course of illness.

The main diagnostic criterion for systemic lupus erythematosus, besides the diverse clinical signs of illness, is a positive serum test for antinuclear antibody. All seven cats just referred to had antinuclear antibody titers ranging from 1:10 to 1:320. IgG and C3 deposits in the basement membrane of the skin or glomeruli are added features. Hypocomplementemia was present in some of the cats studied at the University of California. Tests for FeLV infection were negative. Leukopenia and neutropenia were frequent.

Antinuclear antibody titers should be interpreted with care in cats, since about 10 per cent normally have low titers (1:2 to 1:10). The antibody can appear shortly after persistent infection with FeLV and may remain detectable for several months or more (Table 6–4). Very high titers (>1:50) are frequent in cats with cholangiohepatitis and biliary stasis, probably because of slow hepatic cell death and release of nucleic acid.

Systemic lupus erythematosus in cats is treated initially with prednisone or prednisolone. If a remission cannot be achieved, cyclophosphamide, chlorambucil, or azathioprine is included in the regimen.

## Polyarteritis (Periarteritis) Nodosa

Necrotizing angiitis of animals is believed to be due to hypersensitivity reactions in the vessel walls (Easley, 1979) and is thought in most cases to be immune-complex mediated. Polyarteritis (periarteritis) nodosa is an entity in this group of disorders. One cat with this disease presented with weight loss, weakness, glossitis, and stomatitis, which progressed into shock (Curtis et al., 1979). Autopsy disclosed necrotizing angiitis in large vessels such as the aorta and the carotid and pulmonary arteries. The lesions appeared grossly as discrete, confluent, nodular swellings 1 to 3 mm in diameter. Other cases of polyarteritis in cats have been described. Lesions were found in small and medium-sized arteries in the heart, thyroid, joints, and pancreas (Altera and Bonasch, 1966), renal arteries (Lucke, 1968), and arteries of the lungs, colon, pancreas, urinary bladder, joints, and leptomeninges (Lewis et al., 1965). Clinical signs in these cats included arthritis, uveitis, and renal failure. The phlebitis of feline infectious peritonitis may also be an immune-mediated vasculitis (Pedersen and Boyle, 1980; Weiss and Scott, 1981). Indeed, Carpenter (1983) reviewed tissue sections from several published cases of polyarteritis nodosa in cats and found that the animals actually had feline infectious peritonitis.

## Type IV Reactions (Disorders Involving Cell-Mediated Immune Phenomena)

Cell-mediated immune reactions are uncommon in cats. Noneffusive feline infectious peritonitis may result from a cell-mediated reaction against intracellular virus. Flea bite dermatitis may also involve, in part, a reaction of this type (Gorham et al., 1971; Scott, 1980). Contact dermatitis is uncommon in cats (Scott, 1980). Allergic encephalomyelitis was described in a cat as a postvaccinal reaction to phenolized heterologous brain-tissue rabies vaccine (Holzworth, 1966). In other species, such an encephalitis results from a delayed hypersensitivity reaction directed against shared nervous-tissue antigen (Paterson, 1966).

## Immunodeficiency Diseases

### Phagocytic Abnormalities

Deficiencies in phagocytosis occur when phagocytic cells (neutrophils, monocytes, tissue macrophages) are decreased in number, when the level of opsonizing antibodies or complement is depressed, or when the functions (e.g., chemotaxis, ingestion, intracellular killing of microbes) of the phagocyte are abnormal. Signs of deficiency are increased susceptibility to bacterial infections of the skin and of the respiratory and gastrointestinal tracts. These infections respond poorly to antibiotics.

Phagocytic deficiencies may be either congenital or acquired. Acquired deficiencies usually result from conditions that profoundly depress white cell formation, e.g., FeLV infection, panleukopenia, and cancer treatment with potent myelosuppressive drugs.

Congenital abnormalities that impair phagocytosis are well documented in man—deficiencies of opsonins, complement factors, chemotaxis, and intracellular lysosomal enzymes—but have not been recognized in cats. It has been reported, but not well documented, that cats with mucopolysaccharidosis (Langweiler et al., 1978) and Chédiak-Higashi syndrome (Collier et al., 1979; Kramer et al., 1977) are abnormally susceptible to infection. In both these disorders circulating white cells are abnormal, and in man phagocyte function is impaired and susceptibility to bacterial infections increased.

**Table 6–4 The Appearance of Antinuclear Antibody in the Serum of Cats After the Development of Persistent FeLV Infection**

| Cat Number | ANTINUCLEAR ANTIBODY TITER* (DAYS AFTER FeLV INFECTION) | | | | | | | | | | | | | | | | | | | | | | |
|---|---|---|---|---|---|---|---|---|---|---|---|---|---|---|---|---|---|---|---|---|---|---|---|
| | 0 | 20 | 40 | 60 | 80 | 100 | 120 | 140 | 160 | 180 | 200 | 220 | 240 | 260 | 280 | 300 | 320 | 340 | 360 | 380 | 400 | 420 | 440 |
| 1953 | Neg. | Neg. | 100 | 100 | 25 | — | — | Neg. | — | Neg. | — | Neg. | — | — | — | — | Neg. | — | — | — | — | — | — |
| 1892 | Neg. | Neg. | 100 | — | — | 100 | — | — | Neg. | — | — | — | Neg. | — | — | — | — | — | — | — | — | — | — |
| 1902 | Neg. | Neg. | — | — | Neg. | — | 10 | — | 10 | — | — | — | — | 10 | — | — | — | — | — | 10 | — | — | 10 |
| 1940 | Neg. | Neg. | — | — | Neg. | — | Neg. | 100 | — | — | — | — | 100 | — | 25 | 10 | — | 25 | — | 25 | — | — | 25 |

*Determined by an indirect fluorescent antibody procedure using cryostat-microtome–prepared, acetone-fixed cat liver substrate.

## Immunoglobulin Deficiencies

Immunoglobulin deficiencies may be acquired or congenital. Acquired deficiencies occur in newborns that fail to get adequate maternal antibodies and in older animals with disorders that decrease active immunoglobulin synthesis. Failure of passive transfer occurs when the young do not nurse properly during the first few days of life, or when the mother's colostrum contains low levels of specific antibodies. Kittens with this disorder fail to thrive and often succumb during the second week of life to *E. coli* infection (Griesemer, 1971) or to other pathogens.

Acquired hypogammaglobulinemia in man may be associated with a greater than normal number of circulating T-lymphocytes that suppress immunoglobulin production. A similar depression of immunoglobulins may occur in some cats with generalized lymphoma. Immunoglobulin-secreting lymphoid or plasma cell tumors are associated with a marked elevation of abnormal immunoglobulin but a pronounced decrease in normal immunoglobulin.

Congenital hypogammaglobulinemia has been recognized in man and some animal species, either alone or with deficiencies in cell-mediated immunity. The hypogammaglobulinemia may involve all immunoglobulin classes (total immunoglobulin deficiency) or only IgA, IgM, or subclasses of IgG. It has not so far been reported in cats but probably exists, since it occurs in other species, predisposing to skin, respiratory, and intestinal infections. Certain infections may be greatly increased in severity, while disease caused by other pathogens may not be influenced. Transient congenital hypogammaglobulinemia has not yet been recognized in animals. In children it is manifested by delayed development of active humoral immunity, which predisposes to skin, ear, respiratory, and intestinal infection until normal production of immunoglobulins begins.

Pure deficiencies in cell-mediated immunity and combined immunodeficiencies (humoral and cell-mediated) are relatively uncommon in man and animals and have not yet been recognized in cats. Such deficiencies usually lead to early death from viral and bacterial infections and could conceivably be involved in kitten mortality.

## Complement Deficiency

Congenital deficiencies of complement components have not been recognized in cats but occur in man and some laboratory animals. Deficiencies are most often associated with an increased incidence of bacterial infections. Acquired complement deficiencies have been recognized in cats with FeLV infection (Kobilinsky et al., 1979), lymphoreticular neoplasms, and systemic lupus erythematosus.

# GAMMOPATHIES

## Polyclonal Gammopathies

Polyclonal gammopathies, involving an increase in all major immunoglobulin classes, occur in cats with chronic, antigenically stimulating diseases, such as pyodermas, abscesses, fungal infections, feline infectious peritonitis, and parasitisms (e.g., occult dirofilariasis), and with immunologic diseases such as systemic lupus erythematosus and chronic progressive polyarthritis. In many cases the cause cannot be ascertained.

## Monoclonal Gammopathies

A monoclonal gamma globulin is a homogeneous protein produced by the progeny (clone) of a single antibody-forming cell. Monoclonal gamma globulins (M-proteins) can be produced by tumors arising from a single cell (plasma cell myeloma or lymphoproliferative neoplasm).

The incidence of immunoglobulin-producing tumors of cats is unknown, because at present proteins associated with tumors are infrequently studied. Engle and Brodey (1969) reported only one myeloma among 395 feline neoplasms.

Myeloma proteins of the cat are usually IgG or Bence Jones protein (immunoglobulin light chains), less often IgM or IgA. Multiple myeloma has been reported in cats by Drazner (1982), Engle and Brodey (1969), Farrow and Penny (1971), Hay (1978), Holzworth and Meier (1957), Hurvitz (1975), Kehoe et al. (1972), MacEwen and Hurvitz (1977), Mills et al. (1982), and Saar et al. (1973). Lymphoproliferative malignant disease (lymphoma, lymphocytic leukemia, reticulum cell sarcoma) may also be associated with monoclonal gammopathy, e.g., two cases of lymphoma with IgG (Hurvitz, 1975; MacEwen and Hurvitz, 1977) and a lymphoma producing IgM (Williams and Goldschmidt, 1982).

A rarer cause of monoclonal gammopathy is macroglobulinemia, reported by Saar et al. (1973) and also diagnosed by MacEwen and Hurvitz (1977) in a cat with an elevated IgM level and Bence Jones proteinuria.

Over 30 additional cases of multiple myeloma and other plasma cell tumors are on record at the Angell Memorial Animal Hospital (see the chapter on tumors) and at The Animal Medical Center (Hurvitz, 1982), and more than 20 cases of cats with immunoglobulin-producing tumors are in the files of the University of California Veterinary Medical Teaching Hospital.

General conclusions from both the published reports and the unpublished cases available to me are that in the majority of cats in which the immunoglobulin was classified, the monoclonal protein was identified as IgG. IgA, IgM, and Bence Jones proteinuria were less often present. The majority of cats were over 7 years old (range, 6 months to 17 years), with males predominating. Most presented with anorexia and weight loss, and the abnormal protein was detected during investigation of the high level of serum protein or globulin. The total protein level averaged about 10 gm/dl (7.3 to 16.5). All cats tested were FeLV-negative. Skeletal lesions were recognized in relatively few cats, which were lame or evidenced pain when handled. One had skin tumors and one had nosebleed (Hay, 1978). The hyperviscosity syndrome was seen in only one cat (Williams and Goldschmidt, 1982), probably because most of the cats had IgG or Bence Jones protein rather than IgA or IgM monoclonal protein.The hyperviscosity syndrome in this cat was manifested by depression, anorexia, hepatosplenomegaly, retinal hemorrhage, distended retinal veins, and coagulopathy. The tumor was of the IgM type, and the serum viscosity was over 10 times greater than normal.

At autopsy, tumors were often disseminated, most involving bone marrow, liver, kidney, and spleen. Epidural masses, skin infiltrates, and bone lesions were less common.

Treatment of these tumors has not been successful. Cats do not respond well to the regimen of prednisolone and phenylalanine mustard that produces a good response in many dogs and humans (Hurvitz, 1975).

Rarely monoclonal gammopathies are encountered in which none of the foregoing conditions can be diagnosed. In five such cases seen at The Animal Medical Center, four of the cats had feline infectious peritonitis; in one the source of the abnormal protein was not determined (MacEwen and Hurvitz, 1977). Polyclonal gammopathy is characteristic of feline infectious peritonitis, but in occasional cases the protein has been observed to convert to a monoclonal form (Hurvitz, 1982).

## INFECTION AND IMMUNITY

### Factors Influencing the Course of Infectious Diseases in Cats

It has been said that there is something peculiar about the cat's immune system that predisposes it to so many infectious diseases. It is highly unlikely, however, that cats have evolved as immunologic cripples. As a family, the Felidae are among the most evolutionarily successful carnivores. Why are cats plagued with so many infectious diseases? Most infectious disease problems of cats appear to reflect their environment and not any inherent immunologic weakness.

The ancestors of the domestic cat lived in the deserts of North Africa, and cats are still desert animals in their physiology. They can survive without water and at high temperature and low humidity for many days. Their resiliency and adaptability to varied environments is legend, as indicated by the tales of "nine lives."

In their original habitat, cats were solitary, territorial creatures. Contact among them was limited to brief encounters at night, when they do most of their roaming, and to the activities of the breeding season. The young were raised in seclusion mainly by the queen and had little contact with other cats until they began to feed and socialize on their own, usually after 12 to 16 weeks of age.

In contrast, consider the modern cat. With growing environmental pollution by animal wastes, increased urbanization and "apartmentalization" of humans, and the desire for cleaner, more economical pets, the cat has been slowly replacing the dog as the most popular companion animal. The cat is clean, fastidious, and reasonably free of objectionable habits. Waste disposal, thanks to the relatively recent introduction of litter, is simple. Cats lend themselves to apartment life and the mobile life style of their owners. They are quiet and can be left with food, water, and a litter pan for a weekend while their owners go away. Their aloof and self-sufficient personality meshes well with that of modern city dwellers.

Growing popularity has expanded the feline population in cities and suburbs. With increased neutering of household cats, kittens must be provided more and more by catteries. Developing interest in the showing and breeding of purebreds also favors proliferation of catteries and encourages inbreeding to create new breeds and to perpetuate certain traits.

The cattery provides an environment totally alien to that in which cats evolved. A solitary, territory-loving animal must now exist in a few rooms with many other animals and is forced to share food, water, litter, and perch space. Ventilation and sanitation are often poor, especially when compared with wide-open spaces with plenty of free-moving air and clear ground in which to bury excreta.

With this introduction, we can better understand how environmental and host factors influence the severity of infectious diseases in cats.

#### Inbreeding

Inbreeding greatly impairs disease resistance in some species, such as cats, whereas in others, such as dogs and mice, it has less influence. Through inbreeding, new breeds of cats are developed and older breeds are constantly altered to meet changing concepts of desirability. These alterations often lead to a high incidence of lethal and sublethal genetic defects and produce cats that are much smaller than outbred cats of the same age (Fig. 6–12). Such cats are often deliberately selected as breeders, despite their susceptibility to many infections and peculiar ailments.

Many breeders deny that they inbreed and insist that their cats are products of line breeding. It must be remembered, however, that many breeds and color types of cats originated from single mutations or from a small number of foundation cats introduced into the country. Therefore many breeders are already dealing with a highly inbred population. Line breeding within such a restricted gene pool does not necessarily improve breeding stock. Improper genetic manipulation of modern cats may represent man's greatest insult to the species.

#### Maternal Immunity

Maternal immunity is essential to help the very young combat disease while their immune systems are maturing, but contrary to popular belief, it does not give absolute protection for a defined period. The higher the dose or virulence of a microbe, the earlier in life maternal immunity can be overcome.

#### Age Resistance

Kittens are not as immunologically competent as adult cats. Age resistance approaches adult levels at 12 to 16 weeks of age. Nature provides maternal immunity up to this time. The younger a cat is when infected with a microbe, the more apt it is to develop severe illness, die, or be left with chronic complications. Exposure to infection should therefore be delayed as long as possible to minimize mortality and chronic complications. Like maternal immunity, age resistance is not absolute but can be overcome by an increased dose of the pathogen or by stress.

#### Pathogen Dose and Virulence

As another general rule, the greater the dose of a pathogen, the more severe the disease. Morbidity and mortality in rhinotracheitis, calicivirus infection, panleukopenia, feline infectious peritonitis, feline leukemia, and feline sarcoma can all be shown to be dose-influenced. The morbidity-mortality curves obtained from a range of doses of the pathogen can be shifted to either side by altering the age of the cats being infected.

Virulence is defined as the propensity of a given unit of a pathogen to produce clinical disease. The caliciviruses

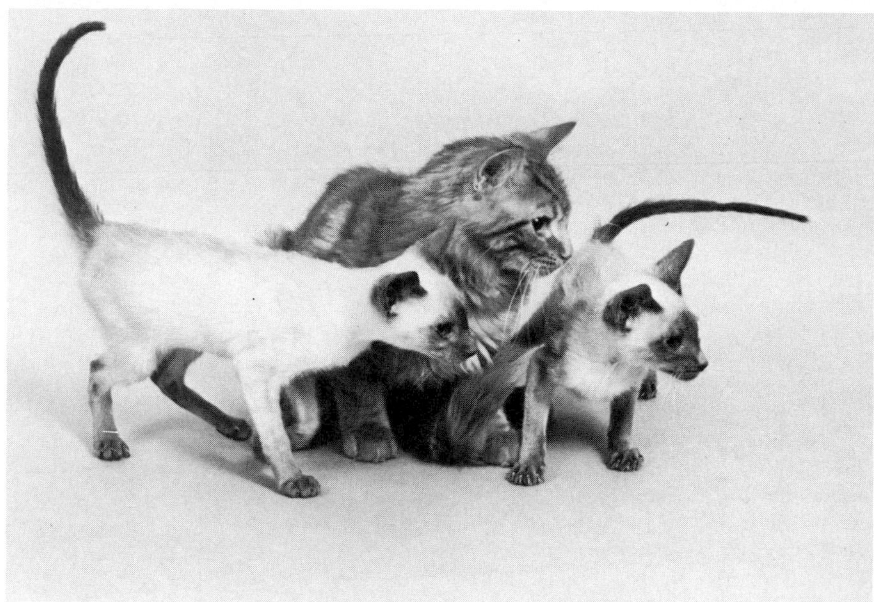

**Figure 6–12** Two purebred sibling male Siamese cats and an unrelated male domestic cat. Although all three were six months old, the purebred kittens were only a third the size of the domestic kitten. The Siamese kittens were from "show quality" parents and were the only two kittens to survive from a litter of five. They ate well and appeared normal in activity but failed to grow normally and suffered from chronic, low-grade upper respiratory disease. Routine laboratory tests and subsequent histologic examination of tissues failed to demonstrate any abnormalities. Their condition is due to the deleterious effects of inbreeding.

of cats, for example, exist in many serotypes ranging in virulence from producers of severe disease to virtual nonpathogens.

## Population Density

The more cats in an area, the greater the likelihood that a susceptible animal will contract infection and—probably more important—the greater the stress imposed on the animal. As aptly stated by Wolski (1981):

> A typical rural [cat] population may be closer to 25 cats per square kilometer, as opposed to a typical urban density of 1,000 cats or more. The low rural density allows each cat a comfortable range of territory exclusively his or her own, in which to hunt and reign. . . . The relatively recent trend of taking cats into houses as pets, with the outcome of high density, limited movement, and population instability, sometimes puts excessive stress on the cat's social makeup. This stress erupts into a variety of social behaviors. . . . Social stress [also] works as any physical stress does in lowering the immunologic competence of the animal.

The effect of population density on disease incidence can be seen with many diseases but is best documented for FeLV infection. At the lowest extreme are the farm cats of rural Scotland, only 6 per cent of which show evidence of having been infected (Rogerson et al., 1975). The infection rate gradually increases as the human (and feline) population increases and peaks in FeLV-enzootic catteries, where almost all the cats will be antibody-positive and 30 per cent will be chronic carriers (Hardy et al., 1973). An exception to this relationship occurs in New York City (Hardy et al., 1973) and Boston cats (Essex et al., 1975). Boston, where the human population is less dense, has a much higher level of FeLV infection. A possible reason is that New York City cats are isolated from each other in high-rise buildings, and few roam the streets and alleys where they can contact other cats. In Boston, low-level dwellings and apartments allow more opportunity for cats to contact each other at ground level, there are many more stray cats, and territories are less defined. Another reason for the contrast in incidence is that the New York study dealt with owned pets and the Boston study with strays.

## Sanitation and Ventilation

Good ventilation is needed to dilute air-borne pathogens, while good sanitation of the ground, perches, litter pans, and food and water dishes is essential to dilute agents in feces, saliva, and urine. Twelve to 20 air changes per hour are recommended to minimize problems from air-borne pathogens in a cattery (Povey, 1977)—a costly standard far beyond the reach of most catteries, which, in fact, are often rooms in private homes. Sanitation is also a difficult problem, because it is physically impossible for many cattery owners to clean thoroughly with the number of cats they possess.

## Housing Together Cats of Different Ages

With large animals, the disease-enhancing potential of housing animals of different ages together is well known. The same principle applies to catteries. Older cats harbor and shed many pathogens such as corona-, rota-, rhinotracheitis, and caliciviruses, *Chlamydia, Mycoplasma,* pathogenic bacteria, and ecto- and endoparasites. In most cases, however, these agents are shed in relatively low numbers. Kittens born in catteries resist this low level of exposure until their maternal and lactogenic immunity reaches a low level at about 6 to 12 weeks of age. When they do become infected, they develop a mild disease because of their greater age resistance and the smaller exposure dose, but shed considerably more of the pathogen than the adult carriers. If there are kittens several weeks younger, they are in turn exposed to this greater amount of the pathogen, which will overcome their maternal immunity at a younger age. These kittens develop a more serious disease because they are younger and infected with a larger dose of the pathogen. They in turn shed considerably more of the pathogen than the kittens from which they got the infection. In this way the cycle of disease revolves downward to involve even younger kittens.

## Stress

Stress results from physical, environmental, and psychological insults. Involving, in part, excessive adrenal stimulation and steroid hormone release, it can be mimicked to some extent by injections or by administration of glucocorticoids. Stress most affects local immunity and therefore potentiates diseases that involve the mucous membranes during some period of infection. Enteric, respiratory, and conjunctival diseases are thus most apt to be influenced. In diseases such as rhinotracheitis (Gaskell and Wardley, 1978), feline leukemia (Rojko et al., 1979, 1982), hemobartonellosis (Harvey and Gaskin, 1978), and toxoplasmosis (Dubey and Frenkel, 1974), glucocorticoids have been shown to convert latent to active infection, and transient to permanent infection.

Cats undergo many stresses, especially in catteries and multiple-cat households. Pregnancy, parturition, and lactation can activate rhinotracheitis virus infections in queens (Gaskell, 1975; Gaskell and Wardley, 1978). The stress of weaning at six to eight weeks of age is especially serious because maternal antibody levels and lactogenic immunity are declining. Weather and humidity changes often evoke flare-ups of respiratory disease in cats under natural conditions, although Gaskell (1975) could not provoke shedding of rhinotracheitis (herpes) virus in latent carriers by artificially created climatic stress. Cat shows involving travel and excessive grooming and handling inflict stress. Overcrowding in itself is stressful for animals that prefer solitary lives. When cats live together, a social order of dominance is established. Reshuffling of cats disrupts this pattern and places cats under great strain for several days or more while a new social order is created. Cats often develop upper respiratory and enteric disease after such events. Under experimental conditions, shedding of rhinotracheitis virus can be induced in carriers merely by reshuffling cats from one room to another (Gaskell, 1975).

## Nutrition

Malnutrition, even if minimal, is a potent cause of both stress and specific immunosuppression. The effects of specific dietary deficiencies on various aspects of the immune response have been well documented for animals (Sheffy and Schultz, 1978). Malnutrition is particularly harmful to young animals. Kittens require many more calories per unit of body weight than adults, and their need for specific nutrients is also greater. In households with many cats and a limited food budget, the ration is often substandard for animals at the lower level of social dominance—often the sickly, the young, and the pregnant or lactating queens.

## Concurrent Disease

With the high exposure and stresses in catteries, simultaneous diseases are common in kittens. Ascariasis, ringworm, ear mite infestation, chlamydial and mycoplasmal conjunctivitis, and infection with rhinotracheitis virus, calicivirus, coronavirus, and rotavirus all occur at about the same age in many cattery kittens. Some of these infections have additive or synergistic effects. Enzootic FeLV leads to a higher incidence of feline infectious peritonitis and a number of other diseases. *Mycoplasma, Chlamydia,* and other bacteria often complicate viral infections of the mucous membranes.

## The Cattery and Multiple-Cat Household

Outside such environments, cats generally handle infections well. Most disease is mild or inapparent and chronic complications the exception. Within catteries, kittens and even adult cats do not fare so well. Many catteries have too many cats and produce too many kittens at too close intervals. Ventilation is usually bad, and sanitation is difficult to maintain. New cats are frequently introduced, bringing with them a new set of microorganisms, and in turn they are exposed to a myriad of new microorganisms. Cats are continuously stressed by overcrowding. Kittens are exposed to massive levels of microbes from birth. The consequence is severe disease, deaths, and a high incidence of chronic sequelae. To these problems are added the insults of multiple infections, decreased resistance due to inbreeding, and weaning stresses. It is not surprising, therefore, that veterinarians see the cattery or multiple-cat household not only as a hotbed of acute and chronic disease but also as one of their most frustrating clinical dilemmas.

In conclusion, the immune system does not operate in a vacuum but is influenced at many points and in subtle ways by environmental, host, and pathogen-related factors. The cat is not an immunologic cripple; its great problem with infectious diseases is largely due to the practices of man, not to its own deficiencies.

# IMMUNE PHENOMENA IN SOME FELINE INFECTIONS

The importance of the host's immune mechanisms in the establishment, pathogenesis, and elimination or containment of infectious diseases cannot be underestimated. It is in the study of infectious diseases that one gains a true appreciation of the immune system and immune phenomena. Virtually every infectious disease of cats has some interesting immunologic twist to it. What follows, therefore, is a brief survey of the immunologic aspects of a variety of feline microbial and parasitic diseases.

## Salmonellosis

The main serotype isolated from cats is *S. typhimurium,* and clinical disease is most apt to occur in younger animals. Cats can also be infected with numerous other serotypes, including some pathogenic for man (Shimi and Barin, 1977). In areas of endemic human salmonellosis, cats carry and shed *Salmonella* twice as often as dogs (Shimi and Barin, 1977).

In its severe form salmonellosis causes gastroenteritis with vomiting and diarrhea and often ends fatally in septicemia. After clinical or inapparent infection, many cats shed *Salmonella* for months. Little is known about the carrier state in cats, except that antibody levels and bacterial shedding are not closely related (Timoney et al., 1978), a situation suggesting that cell-mediated immunity is important in eliminating the organism, as in man and other animals.

The clinical disease is difficult to re-create in cats. Cats could be infected experimentally with virulent *Salmonella* but shed the organisms without ever becoming ill, although the same isolate was originally responsible for a severe outbreak of illness among hospitalized cats (Timoney et al., 1978), stress perhaps affecting local immunity. Fatal salmonellosis has also occurred in FeLV-infected cats, which tend to be immunologically suppressed.

## Tuberculosis

Tuberculosis in cats, as in man, is a less serious problem than in the past. Cats are highly resistant to *Mycobacterium tuberculosis,* but very susceptible to *M. bovis* (Glover, 1949). Infection with *M. avium* is uncommon (Hix et al., 1969). In areas of high incidence of bovine infection in humans and animals, the incidence in cats is also high. The infection in cats resembles that in man in its propensity to cause well circumscribed granulomas. The major route of infection is oral, and lesions are often situated along and adjacent to the digestive tract, including the oropharynx (Jennings, 1949; Snider et al., 1971).

Cats develop delayed hypersensitivity to the tubercle bacillus but respond erratically to skin testing with PPD (Francis, 1958; Hawthorne and Lauder, 1961; Snider et al., 1971). Griffith (1926), however, reported that six of 11 cats responded when tested by the subcutaneous route. As in mice, delayed hypersensitivity to BCG vaccination continues only about as long as the primary inoculation lesion is active. Thus it may be concluded that, as in man, a persistent skin response parallels the persistence of organisms in the body.

## Tyzzer's Disease

Tyzzer's disease is caused by *Bacillus piliformis,* a normal inhabitant of the environment and only sporadically a pathogen. Most often affecting rodents, the disease is principally a bacteremia with the liver and intestine the main target organs. In the few feline cases reported, the disease took a similar form and was associated with FeLV infection (Bennett et al., 1977). (See also the chapter on bacterial diseases.)

## Other Bacterial Infections

Cats suffer less often than dogs from *Staphylococcus aureus, Proteus,* and *Pseudomonas* infections of the skin and ear canal, perhaps because they have fewer seborrheic disorders. A normal level of sebum has a bacteriostatic function; too much or too little leads to changes in the microenvironment of the skin and overgrowth of more pathogenic and invasive flora (Ihrke, 1979; Ihrke et al., 1978).

Bacterial abscesses and infections of the skin, oral cavity, and digestive and respiratory tracts, as well as septicemias, are more frequent in immunologically suppressed cats. Cats infected with FeLV are more susceptible to such infections early in the disease when there is a transient drop in the white cell count and terminally when the bone marrow is often depressed by myeloproliferative disorders or hypoplasia of stem cells. Bacterial infection, not neoplasia, is the major killer of such cats.

Omphalophlebitis occasionally affects young kittens, often causing death at one or two weeks of age from septicemia, usually due to *Pasteurella,* streptococci, or coliforms. The umbilical stump often becomes infected when the queen chews the cord off too short, inoculating bacteria under the skin, where a small abscess can form adjacent to the still patent umbilical vein.

*Bordetella bronchiseptica* is a common upper respiratory pathogen of many species. Its disease-causing potential in kittens is probably unappreciated (Pedersen, 1983). Infection with *Bordetella* usually takes the form of fatal pneumonia. Occasional concurrent infection with hemolytic *E. coli* may result in coliform septicemia. *Bordetella* infection occurs immediately after weaning, often striking an entire litter, but sparing others in the same environment. These observations suggest that the duration and level of maternal immunity and postweaning stresses are factors in the infection. Because we have seen it in specific pathogen–free cats, it appears that respiratory virus infections are not necessary predisposing causes.

## Hemobartonellosis

*Haemobartonella felis,* an obligate rickettsial blood parasite of cats, is taxonomically related to bacteria because it possesses a nucleus with RNA and DNA and cytoplasmic enzyme systems. It differs from most bacteria, however, in its dependence on a living cell for sustenance. After primary infection, there may be several waves of red-cell parasitism. Anemia may occur if large numbers of cells are parasitized and results from increased red-cell fragility and destruction of parasitized red cells by the spleen and other phagocytic tissue (Meade and Hata, 1975). This process is aided by the production of antibodies directed against the parasite. The antibody coating of parasitized red cells can be detected by a positive direct Coombs reaction (Maede and Hata, 1975).

Other immunologic phenomena are involved in feline hemobartonellosis. Of great clinical importance is the existence of a carrier state in the face of immunity. After initial infection and parasitemia, the spleen becomes very active in removing the organisms from the red-cell membrane (Maede, 1979). This "reconditioning" of parasitized red cells is done by phagocytes that trap the parasitized red cell and by opsonization remove the organisms. With time, the host's immune mechanisms contain the infection and parasitemia subsides. A previous exposure does not induce immunity against reinfection, and subsequent clinical episodes may occur. In inapparent carriers, in certain immunosuppressive situations, the organisms can replicate in large numbers and red cells become heavily parasitized, with recurrence of anemia. Recrudescence of parasitemia cannot be induced by cyclophosphamide, 6-mercaptopurine, or experimentally created abscesses but can be stimulated by glucocorticoids (Harvey and Gaskin, 1978).

Under natural conditions about 60 to 80 per cent of the cases of hemobartonellosis are secondary to some debilitating or immunosuppressive disease, most often feline leukemia virus infection. In FeLV-associated cases, red-cell parasitism often occurs when the bone marrow is already suppressed—directly from stem-cell infection with FeLV, from a preleukemic marrow dysplasia, or from overt myeloproliferative disease. Other malignant diseases, cat fight abscesses, chronic renal failure, and feline infectious peritonitis also predispose to flare-ups of hemobartonellosis.

## Chlamydial Infection (Pneumonitis)

*Chlamydia psittaci* is a common inhabitant of the mucous membranes of the eye, nasal passages, and possibly urogenital passages of cats. In cats, as in other species, it causes mainly conjunctivitis (Cello, 1971; Hoover et al., 1978), but in cats it does not usually spread systemically from local sites of infection to the joints, lungs, and gravid uterus as it does in other domestic animals.

Chlamydial conjunctivitis of cats can occur as early as 7 to 10 days of age (Shewen et al., 1978), causing the unopened lids to bulge forward because of the underlying purulent exudate. Certain queens repeatedly produce such litters because they fail to provide adequate maternal immunity or because they harbor the organism in high numbers. Infection of the newborn probably occurs through the nasolacrimal duct during birth. Much oftener kittens develop conjunctivitis in about 8 to 12 weeks; apparently they are provided with adequate maternal immunity up to this time. The disease at this age is often associated with concurrent mycoplasmal or bacterial infection. Although *Chlamydia* alone can cause disease, *Mycoplasma* is a poor pathogen by itself. The conjunctivitis may begin in one eye, proceed in several days or weeks to the other, and still later involve both. The initial attack may last up to six weeks.

After the primary disease disappears, many cats remain asymptomatic carriers, subject throughout life to flare-ups of conjunctivitis precipitated by corticosteroids, stresses such as weather and humidity changes, disturbances in living arrangements, surgical procedures, shows, parturition, and heavy lactation.

Cats vaccinated with attenuated chlamydial vaccines develop incomplete resistance to challenge (Shewen, 1979). Although clinical signs are diminished, two thirds of vaccinates shed virulent organisms for 21 to 35 days after challenge and one third for 61 days or more.

Corticosteroids given 40 to 44 days after infection can increase the severity of chlamydial conjunctivitis, an effect that lasts for four to five days after administration (Shewen, 1979). Unlike their effect on latent rhinotracheitis virus infection, corticosteroids increase the shedding of *Chlamydia* only in cats still culture-positive at the time of treatment (Shewen, 1979).

It is apparent that local membrane immunity is important in resistance to chlamydial infection. Continuous and adequate levels of IgA antibody may help to keep it from spreading. Cell-mediated immunity also appears to be related to resistance (Shewen, 1979). Serum CF antibody titers bear no relationship to protection (Cello, 1971).

## Mycoplasmosis

*Mycoplasma, Acholeplasma,* and T-mycoplasma are common inhabitants of the mucous membranes of the throat, nasal passages, and urogenital tract of normal cats (see also the chapter on bacterial infections). *Mycoplasma felis* is the only important pathogen in this group. In experimental infection, events occurring during the first 10 days seem important in determining whether the infection will persist (Blackmore and Hill, 1973).

By themselves, mycoplasmas are not severe pathogens in cats (Blackmore and Hill, 1973), but when there is a primary disease of the respiratory epithelium, they can become secondary invaders. *M. felis* could be isolated from cats with viral upper respiratory disease 26 times oftener than from normal cats (Tan and Miles, 1971).

*M. felis* has been isolated as the sole pathogen from the eyes of cats with conjunctivitis (Tan and Markham, 1971) but is not often isolated from the conjunctiva of normal cats (Tan and Miles, 1973). Conjunctivitis could be induced in normal cats with *Mycoplasma* isolated from inflamed conjunctivas (Tan and Miles, 1973). Earlier work by Cello (1957) demonstrated that pretreatment of the conjunctiva with cortisone injections will greatly enhance infectivity, suggesting that stress may play a role in the natural disease.

Like *Chlamydia, Mycoplasma* rarely spreads systemically in the cat, but a cat treated with radiation for advanced oropharyngeal squamous cell carcinoma developed acute suppurative arthritis in both carpal joints. The debilitation of the cat, together with irradiation, was probably responsible for the flare-up and systemic spread of the mycoplasmosis. Fatal mycoplasmal pneumonia has also been seen in a litter of kittens at the University of California clinic (Pedersen, 1983).

## Rhinotracheitis (Feline Herpes)

Feline rhinotracheitis (herpes) virus infection is usually manifested as rhinitis, pharyngitis, and, to a lesser extent, conjunctivitis in adolescent and older cats. It may cause fatal pneumonia in four-week-old kittens and fetal death (Hoover and Griesemer, 1971a). Maternal immunity usually suffices for at least the first 9 to 10 weeks of life. Overwhelming rhinotracheitis infection in young kittens is often associated with certain queens that apparently either infect their young early in life or fail to provide adequate maternal immunity. Fetal infection may result from systemic spread of virus during pregnancy.

About 80 per cent of cats with neutralizing antibodies to feline rhinotracheitis are latent or active carriers. In latent carriers the virus apparently persists in an inactive state in nerve ganglia under the nasal turbinates and mucous membranes (Gaskell and Povey, 1979). These cats do not ordinarily shed virus in the nasal and conjunctival secretions but do so for one to three weeks when treated with corticosteroids or stressed. The activation of latent infection suggests the importance of local immunity and stress as factors in feline rhinotracheitis.

Vaccination for feline rhinotracheitis is with killed virus, virulent virus given intramuscularly, or attentuated virus given intranasally. Parenteral vaccination with killed or virulent virus gives good systemic immunity and weak local immunity, which lessens the severity of clinical signs after a vigorous challenge with virulent virus; it will not, however, prevent the establishment of the virulent virus as a latent infection (Orr et al., 1980a). The intranasal vaccine reportedly induces sufficient local immunity to prevent the establishment of a latent infection by the virulent virus (Orr et al., 1980a). It is doubtful from what is known about natural immunity that this protection is long-lived.

The exact nature of feline rhinotracheitis virus immunity is not known; cell-mediated as well as humoral mechanisms are probably involved in cats as with herpes infection in other species (Russell, 1973). Walton and Gillespie (1970b) showed that cats were solidly immune to rechallenge with feline rhinotracheitis virus for at least 21 days but often developed a brief, mild disease if rechallenged 150 days later. They also found that the immunity present at 21 days was not always associated with detectable levels of virus-neutralizing antibodies in the serum. This finding suggests the importance of other types of immunity in feline rhinotracheitis.

The possibility that the virus may be a cause of chronic sinusitis in cats is supported by the observations that it causes turbinate necrosis and atrophy and damage to the mucosal linings (Hoover and Griesemer, 1971b; Lindt, 1965). Permanent damage to mucosa and turbinates in turn may render the nasal passages permanently susceptible to chronic bacterial and mycoplasmal invasion.

## Feline Infectious Peritonitis

Feline infectious peritonitis is caused by a coronavirus that is virtually indistinguishable in structure from a common enteritis-causing agent, feline enteric coronavirus (Pedersen, 1983a, b; Pedersen et al., 1981b). The lesions of the effusive form of feline infectious peritonitis are due to an Arthus-like reaction involving small veins and triggered by the interaction of serum antibody and complement with antigen produced by infected phagocytes (Pedersen and Boyle, 1980; Pedersen et al., 1981a). The infection seems to occur only in certain predisposed cats in which the virus infects the mucosal cells of the intestinal and respiratory tracts. After initial infection, humoral antibodies are produced. In some cats these are protective and eliminate internally disseminated virus (Pedersen et al., 1981a), but in others they actually appear to facilitate virus uptake by phagocytic cells (Pedersen and Boyle, 1980). The virus grows abundantly in the phagocytes, producing more virus and viral proteins, which ultimately contribute, along with antibody and complement, to the Arthus-like response.

The lesions in noneffusive feline infectious peritonitis are granulomatous. The disease in these cats begins, however, with a brief episode of effusive disease, after which granulomas appear in many organs. It has been postulated that immunity is entirely cell-mediated and that noneffusive disease is due to the development of only partial cell-mediated immunity (Pedersen, 1983a, b; Pedersen and Black, 1983).

## Feline Leukemia

Feline leukemia virus infection can be transient or persistent, latent or active. Latent infection often follows a transient active infection (Pedersen et al., 1984). The outcome of FeLV infection depends on age at exposure, maternal immunity, genetic susceptibility, dose of virus, and stress factors. Maternal immunity, when present, totally prevents infection for up to 16 weeks (Jarrett et al., 1977). Not only can the cat not be infected, it will not even react to the challenge with an active antibody response. Once the maternal antibody level falls, however, the cat becomes susceptible to infection and will mount an active immune response.

The course of disease after experimental infection depends on the age when the cat is exposed (Hoover et al., 1976). Persistent active infections develop in almost all newborn kittens, 50 per cent of 12-week-olds, 30 per cent of 18-week-olds, and fewer older cats (Pedersen, 1983). About 50 to 70 per cent of the cats that do not become actively infected become latently infected (Pedersen et al., 1984). Grant and coworkers (1980) showed that although 95 per cent of kittens exposed continuously to FeLV carriers became infected within a year, only 61 per cent of adults exposed in the same environment became infected within one and one-half years. They were unable to discover any immunologic basis for this age resistance. It can be overcome to some extent by increasing the dose of virus and can be abolished by corticosteroids (Rojko et al., 1979). Exposure coinciding with weekly injection of 10 mg/kg of methylprednisolone causes 80 to 100 per cent of adult cats to become persistently and actively viremic. Because corticosteroid administration mimics severe stress, stress is assumed to play an important role in FeLV infection. Weaning, malnutrition, concurrent disease, surgical procedures, and overcrowding at the time of exposure may also unfavorably influence the outcome of infection.

About three fourths of cats that become aviremic after initial FeLV infection retain the virus in the bone marrow and lymphoid tissue in a hidden or latent form (Madewell and Jarrett, 1983; Pedersen et al., 1984; Post and Warren, 1980; Rojko et al., 1982). The viral genome is present in cells of these tissues in a masked form, and virus is not actively expressed and shed as it is in active carriers. When bone marrow cells are cultured in vitro, away from the host's immune system, virus expression occurs in 1 to 12 weeks. Infection in latent carriers can be activated with glucocorticoid treatment (Pedersen et al., 1984; Post and Warren, 1980; Rojko et al., 1982). The percentage of latently infected cats in which infection can be activated with glucocorticoids varies greatly, depending on the strain of the virus (Pedersen et al., 1984). Latent infections with Rickard-FeLV, a commonly used experimental strain, are easily activated with glucocorticoids, whereas latent infections with most other strains are activated with greater difficulty. A small proportion of kittens born to latently infected queens are born with active infection, presumably caused by fetal contamination with maternal leukocytes (Pedersen et al., 1984).

The latent carrier state appears to be relatively stable. It is uncommon for a latent FeLV infection to activate spontaneously during aging or because of concurrent illnesses (Pedersen et al., 1984a). Latent carriers do not suffer from any unique illnesses but do develop a higher rate of virus-negative lymphomas (Pedersen et al., 1984). They do not shed and are noninfectious to susceptible cats that they contact (Madewell and Jarrett, 1983; Pedersen et al., 1984).

Once established, active infection can have a damaging immunopathologic effect on the host (Cockerell, 1978; Hardy, 1982). Very young kittens develop thymic atrophy, as do kittens infected in utero (Anderson et al., 1971). Such kittens fade away and die young from many causes, secondary infectious disease being an important one. Because of the thymic atrophy, actively infected kittens retain allogeneic skin grafts longer than normal (Perryman et al., 1972). In kittens 8 to 16 weeks old, transient bone marrow suppression and leukopenia often precede establishment of the chronic carrier state (Pedersen et al., 1977). This transient lack of white cells can temporarily render them much more susceptible to secondary respiratory or enteric infections.

Cats with chronic active infection demonstrate a number of immunologic defects in vivo and in vitro. Chronic active infection often terminates in bone marrow hypoplasia or myeloproliferative disease. These cats have very low white-cell counts and often succumb to secondary bacterial infections of the skin, intestinal tract, and respiratory system (Barrett et al., 1975; Cotter, 1976; Cotter et al., 1973, 1975; Hardy, 1981, 1982). In addition to such prominent defects, more subtle abnormalities can be detected in a number of in-vivo immune functions. Some are more pronounced in ill than in healthy actively infected cats, making it sometimes difficult to determine what is due to the virus infection itself and what is due to the more general debilitating effects of illness. About 25 per cent of actively infected cats have significant decreases in total white-cell counts, and 66 per cent have decreased numbers of lymphocytes (Hardy, 1982). Although total lymphocyte numbers are often decreased, the B-lymphocyte fraction in healthy actively infected cats is actually increased (Hardy, 1982). Ill cats, however, have a decreased number of B-lymphocytes. Actively infected cats make significantly fewer antibodies than normal cats after antigenic stimulation with sheep red cells (Hardy, 1982) and synthetic polypeptides (Trainin et al., 1983). Likewise, their antibody response to bacterial lipopolysaccharide antigens is depressed, especially in the secondary response (Pedersen, 1983). Primary responses to BCG vaccine and the delayed hypersensitivity response to tuberculin are normal in healthy, actively infected cats but greatly depressed in those that are ill (Pedersen, 1983). The acquired antibody response to feline rhinotracheitis virus is similar in FeLV-infected and noninfected cats (Pedersen, 1983). Similarly, bacterial functions of the blood neutrophils of FeLV-infected cats are normal, as are the absolute levels of IgG, IgM, and IgA (Pedersen, 1983). Complement levels of healthy, actively infected cats are usually normal (Pedersen, 1983), although others have found them to be sometimes depressed (Kobilinsky et al., 1979). Complement levels, however, are generally depressed in ill, actively infected cats. Interferon production in such cats, as stimulated by Newcastle disease virus, has been found to be normal (Hardy, 1982).

Actively infected cats also demonstrate abnormalities in the in-vitro function of their lymphoid cells. Blood lymphocyte mitogen reactivity of such cats appears to be depressed (Cockerell et al., 1976a). Lymphocyte responsiveness to mitogens can be specifically depressed by the p15E component of the virus (Mathes et al., 1979). This protein also appears to be immunosuppressive in vitro (Mathes et al., 1979).

Several other immune phenomena occur in infected cats. Shortly after the establishment of persistent active infection, antinuclear antibody often appears. The titers often reach 1:10 to 1:100 and persist for several months or longer (Table 6–4). The clinical significance of this is unknown. Glomerulonephritis, uveitis, hemolytic anemia, and other disorders such as neuritis or myositis also occur as immunologic sequelae of the FeLV-carrier state.

## Syncytium-Forming Virus Infection

Feline syncytium-forming virus (FeSFV) causes a common inapparent infection among cats (see chapter on viral diseases). The mode of transmission is not precisely known, but the infection is apparently acquired both horizontally in older cats and in utero. Not all kittens in a litter born to an infected queen themselves become infected; the reason is not known.

The infection is unique because virus is present in the blood despite high levels of virus-neutralizing antibodies. Even though virus can be readily isolated by cocultivation of blood platelets and white cells with cat cells in vitro, the virus is not identifiable in the blood or tissue by electron microscopy. This situation suggests that the viral genome is present in the tissue but that intact virions are not produced (latent infection). Virus is shed actively, however, from the oropharynx. Both active and latent infections exist, therefore, in the same host. FeSFV has been etiologically linked to chronic progressive polyarthritis of cats (Pedersen et al., 1980), a disease of apparent immunopathologic origin that resembles Reiter's syndrome and rheumatoid arthritis in man.

## Panleukopenia

Feline panleukopenia virus causes peracute to acute enterocolitis and bone marrow suppression. It has an affinity for cells of high mitotic rate so that the crypt epithelium of the intestine and the bone marrow stem cells are primary targets. Germ-free cats are relatively resistant to the effects of the virus because the germ-free bowel has a lower mitotic rate, and the virus therefore has fewer target cells to infect (Carlson and Scott, 1977).

After infection, the white-cell count drops precipitously because of bone marrow destruction and endotoxin absorption from the bowel. The cause of death in most cats is endotoxemia or septicemia or both. The septicemia is usually due to coliform bacterial invasion of the damaged mucosa and the lack of phagocytic cells. Systemic fungal infections have also been associated with panleukopenia (Fox et al., 1978; see also the chapter on mycotic diseases).

Mortality can be enhanced by concurrent infections. In one study, concurrent calicivirus and panleukopenia virus infections killed 82 per cent of inoculated kittens, while panleukopenia alone killed 10 per cent and calicivirus alone killed 5 per cent (Bittle et al., 1961).

Feline panleukopenia virus injected into 35-day fetuses depresses T-lymphocyte-mediated immunity, as measured by the prolonged survival of allogeneic skin grafts placed on the fetus later in gestation (Schultz et al., 1976). Virus infection at 45 days of gestation has no effect. Infection of adult cats transiently decreases the response of blood lymphocytes to concanavalin A and phytohemagglutinin-induced mitogenesis, but the response to pokeweed mitogen is unaffected (Schultz et al., 1976). This phenomenon also suggests a greater dpression of T-cell activity, but its clinical significance is not clear.

## Calicivirus Infection

The numerous isolates of feline calicivirus (FCV) vary greatly in pathogenicity. In its mildest form, the infection is inapparent, while in severe cases lingual and palatine ulcers and pneumonia may be prominent signs. Adult cats usually develop mild signs (Wardley and Povey, 1977b), while three-week-old kittens exposed to the same strain develop severe disease (Povey and Hale, 1974).

The virus persists in the oropharynx of many recovered cats (Walton and Gillespie, 1970a; Wardley, 1976; Wardley and Povey, 1977b). These carriers can be classified as low-, medium-, or high-level virus shedders. High shedders can infect susceptible cats within two to three days, while 11 to 13 days must pass for infection by low shedders (Wardley, 1976). Shedding, unlike that of feline rhinotracheitis (herpes) virus, is not influenced by natural or artificial stress (Wardley, 1976).

The various FCV isolates form an antigenic mosaic, and antibodies to one strain vary in degree of cross-reactivity with other strains. One isolate, F9, induces antibodies that cross-react with a majority of isolates. Another, M3, is neutralized by antibodies to most of the other isolates. By sequentially immunizing cats against three isolates, Povey (1974) produced an antiserum that neutralized over 80 isolates.

After immunization of cats with isolates such as F9, antibodies that react most specifically with F9 are at first produced, but after several weeks antibodies of much greater cross-reactivity begin to appear in higher titer (Kahn et al., 1975; Povey and Ingersoll, 1975), a phenomenon helpful in immunization.

Maternal immunity to FCV appears to be incomplete (Gaskell and Wardley, 1978; Gillespie and Scott, 1973; Johnson, 1980). Kittens with maternal immunity can often be infected as young as four to eight weeks of age (Johnson, 1980; Walton and Gillespie, 1970a). Although virus can be isolated from the oropharynx, clinical signs and an active humoral immune response do not occur until the maternal immunity decreases several weeks later (Johnson, 1980). At this point, clinical signs are either inapparent or relatively mild, and the resultant primary immune response develops slowly and reaches lower levels than would be present in kittens free of maternal immunity when exposed. In contrast, if kittens with very low maternal titers are affected, the disease develops rapidly and is more severe than in the previous situation (Johnson, 1980). Furthermore, the immune response comes on very quickly after infection and reaches higher levels.

Johnson (1980) has postulated that maternal immunity may lessen the severity of disease in situations in which the exposure is high and occurs earlier in life. He followed the course of disease caused by the highly pathogenic F255 strain in a small cattery where many of the cats were FCV carriers. In this environment, the kittens showed few signs of illness although infected early in life.

## Cryptococcosis

Cryptococcosis is caused by the yeast *Cryptococcus neoformans* (perfect form *Filobasidiella neoformans).* The organism is apparently inhaled in many cases, and an inapparent or mild respiratory infection results. Almost all cats recover, but in some, dissemination occurs with localization of infection in the nasal cavity and sinuses, choroid, meninges of the brain, or less commonly in bone, joints, skin, or other sites.

In sites of localization, the organism multiplies to massive numbers but with surprisingly little tissue reaction, probably because of the yeast's thick capsule of polysaccharides that are either weakly antigenic or tolerogenic.

High levels of capsular polysaccharide are present in the blood during infection, and free antibody is difficult or impossible to detect. If recovery occurs, the levels of capsular antigen decrease, and eventually free antibody becomes detectable at higher and higher levels. The disappearance of free antigen is monitored to evaluate the effect of therapy (Gordon and Vedder, 1966).

In man, chronic disseminated infection can signal immune incompetence, as in patients with debilitating cancers or other immunosuppressive conditions. Some humans may be predisposed to the infection as a result of a more specific lack of responsiveness to the organism, and the same may be true of cats. About 30 to 40 per cent of cats with cryptococcosis at the School of Veterinary Medicine, Davis, California, were found to be FeLV-infected, and cryptococcosis has occurred with lymphoma (Madewell et al., 1979).

## Coccidioidomycosis

Inhalation of spores of *Coccidioides immitis* causes an atypical pneumonia and in some cases disseminated granulomatous disease. In the United States, the infection is enzootic in the southwestern deserts and central valley of California. Cats seem to be far more resistant to infection than dogs. During a large California outbreak caused by a dust storm, thousands of cases occurred in man and dogs, but none was recognized in cats. Cats are not, however, completely resistant to infection, for rare cases of disseminated granulomatous disease resembling the disease in dogs are on record (Ontario Veterinary College; University of California, Davis).

Arthrospores introduced by penetrating wounds have caused lymphangitis and regional lymphadenitis in man, dogs, and a cat (Wolf, 1979). Infection by this route is usually self-limiting. Although precipitating antibodies are produced, CF antibodies, which indicate dissemination, do not develop to any extent. This serologic pattern is also true with localized cutaneous disease in the cat.

## Ringworm

*Microsporum canis* is the principal agent of ringworm in cats. The infection is enzootic in many catteries and is transmitted by spores in the environment, as well as by contact with actively infected cats or chronically infected asymptomatic carriers. Kittens born in catteries where the infection is enzootic seem to be resistant for the first weeks or so of life. Whether this is the time required for clinical signs to develop or whether there is a maternal immunity of this duration is not known. The most severe cases often occur in kittens debilitated by concurrent respiratory and enteric infection. Drug-resistant *Microsporum* infections have also been observed in a chronically uremic cat with polycystic kidney disease and in kittens with debilitating congenital heart defects or cardiomyopathy (Pedersen, 1983). Severe recurrence of ringworm occurred in a group of adolescent kittens treated weekly for three weeks with methylprednisolone (10 mg/kg) (Pedersen, 1983).

## Other Fungal Infections

Symptomatic infections of cats with ordinarily nonpathogenic or minimally pathogenic fungi have been described, in most cases associated with a concurrent debilitating and presumably immunosuppressive disorder. Skin granuloma caused by *Phialophora gougerotii* was reported in a cat with nasal squamous cell carcinoma (Haschek and Kasali, 1977), as were systemic infections with fungi such as *Candida, Aspergillus,* and phycomycetes in cats with panleukopenia (Fox et al., 1978; see also the chapter on mycotic diseases).

## Coccidian Infections

The immune phenomena involved in *Toxoplasma gondii, Isospora,* and *Hammondia* infections of cats constitute a fascinating area of study. These are coccidian parasites with sexual stages in the intestinal epithelium of cats and asexual stages sometimes in the cat but more often in herbivores or omnivores.

Cats acquire *T. gondii* infection by ingesting oocysts shed in the feces by other cats or by eating prey or raw or undercooked meat containing encysted forms. Transplacental transmission can also occur, in which case the kitten may be born diseased (Dubey and Johnstone, 1982). Sexual multiplication occurs in the intestinal epithelium, culminating a week or so later in the shedding of oocysts for 4 to 16 days (Dubey et al., 1977). Shedding is probably terminated by local immune phenomena. Although oocyst production ceases, some organisms appear to remain in the epithelium. Interestingly, male cats shed more oocysts after ingesting infected mice than do females, and cats under a year of age shed more than do older cats, in which shedding is variable (Dubey et al., 1977).

During the initial intestinal phase of infection some organisms may escape from the bowel and infect vascular endothelium in other organs. Asexual reproduction occurs and the host cells rupture, releasing more organisms. Within several days systemic immunity develops, in response to which the extraintestinal organisms form into cystlike structures. The severity of extraintestinal spread is age-dependent; cysts were isolated by mouse inoculation from the tissues of only 2 of 21 cats infected after eight weeks of age, but more frequently from those infected younger (Dubey et al., 1977).

After infection and in correlation with the end of oocyst shedding, cats develop some sort of immunity to reinfection. This immunity is somewhat age-dependent: about 60 per cent of cats younger than 13 weeks when infected again shed oocysts when fed infected mice, whereas immunity in cats infected after 13 weeks is much stronger (Dubey and Frenkel 1974). This reshedding after challenge occurs after a longer latent period than after primary infection and is much briefer in duration (Dubey and Frenkel, 1974). The level of serum antibody at the time of challenge is not related to the degree of immunity (Dubey and Frenkel, 1974).

With immunosuppression, such as that produced by large doses of corticosteroids, dissemination after the primary intestinal infection is more apt to take place (Dubey and Frenkel, 1974). Furthermore, reactivation of extraintestinal and intestinal infection, resulting in oocyst shedding and even clinical disease, can follow corticosteroid administration (Dubey and Frenkel, 1974). Such immunosuppression can also result from FeLV infection and indeed many cats with disseminated toxoplasmosis are FeLV-positive. Pregnancy may also cause some degree of cyst activation in some cats, for there have been queens that produced infected kittens at every pregnancy. Asexual spread during gestation presumably accounts for fetal infection. This mode of transmission has not, however, been reproduced experimentally (Dubey and Hoover, 1976).

Certain manipulations may activate the sexual stages of the organism. If a cat has not been previously infected with *Isospora, Isospora* infection will cause a transient reshedding of *T. gondii* oocysts (Dubey, 1976, 1978), apparently because infections with *Isospora* interfere with the established local immunity to *T. gondii.* Fortunately, because *Isospora* spp are much more prevalent in nature, the *Isospora* infection probably occurs first. This prevents reinfection with *Isospora;* hence activation of *T. gondii* oocyst production will not occur.

*Hammondia hammondi* infection produces a less stable immunity than *T. gondii* (Dubey, 1975). Furthermore, this immunity, unlike that to *T. gondii,* is not affected by age or sex. Immunity to reinfection may occur as early as two to four days after exposure. However, cats may subsequently reshed *H. hammondi* oocysts spontaneously or after injections of hydrocortisone.

## Ascariasis

*Toxocara cati* infection of kittens occurs by way of the mother's colostrum and milk. Larvae encysted in somatic tissue of the queen are activated during pregnancy and migrate to the mammary glands (Swerczek et al., 1971). Larvae ingested in the milk do not undergo a somatic migration but pass through all developmental states in the bowel. If, however, eggs from some contaminated source are swallowed, an extensive visceral migration occurs. This results in eosinophilia and also tissue damage along the migration path, e.g., intestine, lungs, and walls of pulmonary vessels. Some of this damage is caused by immune attack on the migrating larvae. A degree of immunity to further visceral migration develops with time and may explain why ascarids are more frequent in cats under six months of age than in older ones (Visco et al., 1978). It was also found that neutered cats appeared to have only about half the ascarid load of intact cats, perhaps because of some hormonal influence on ascarid immunity.

## Dirofilariasis

Parasitism with the heartworm *Dirofilaria immitis* is perhaps a greater problem in cats than previously thought and has been extensively reviewed by Ader (1979). The cat appears to have a greater immune reactivity to heartworms than the dog, which is the major definitive host. Early studies by Fowler and coworkers (1972) showed that this immunity in cats was a response to the migrating larvae, because only 0 to 8 per cent of infectious larvae developed into adults, as compared with 42 per cent in dogs (Wong and Suter, 1979). The immunity, however, seems to involve the microfilarial stages as well. In one study, microfilaremia was seen in only 8 of 15 cats given 4 to 400 infectious larvae, and it persisted in only 2 (Donahoe, 1975). Even in the eight cats that showed patent infection during at least one stage, the numbers of circulating microfilariae were low. Although only two cats remained microfilaremic, 12 had 1 to 19 living or dead adult worms 6 to 16 months after receiving infectious-stage larvae. The end result of the feline immunity to heartworm is that cats, in comparison with dogs, have fewer and less severe infections with adult worms and are less likely to exhibit microfilaremia.

Infection with adult worms in the absence of a detectable microfilaremia (occult infection) results from the presence of worms of only one sex or from destruction of microfilariae by the host's immunity. Occult infections in the dog are usually associated with gravid female worms and high levels of microfilarial antibodies (Wong and Suter, 1979). These antibodies cause immune trapping of microfilariae in the arterial bed (end arterioles) of the lungs and resultant immune-mediated endarteritis and perivascular inflammation. Occult dirofilariasis is therefore a more serious clinical disorder in dogs than patent infection.

Heartworm infection is more likely to be occult in cats than in dogs because fewer larvae reach adulthood and worms of both sexes are therefore less likely to be present. Also cats are more likely to mount an immune response to the microfilariae. Microfilarial antibodies can be detected in the serum of cats with occult dirofilariasis, provided gravid female worms are present (Wong, 1981).

Severe changes in the lungs, pulmonary arteries, and right heart are seen in occult feline dirofilariasis (Donahoe et al., 1976), as they are in dogs. In experimental infections, Donahoe and coworkers (1976) observed that lung lesions were more frequent in male cats than in females and were more severe in cats that developed microfilaremia at some stage of the infection. The lung lesions could not always be correlated with the presence of microfilariae, for the changes sometimes appeared before the worms reached maturity in the heart and in one cat were associated with only a single adult worm. These findings suggest that products of immature or sterile adults may also cause disease in the pulmonary vasculature and lung parenchyma.

Although the disease in cats is similar to that in dogs, clinical signs are more apt to go unobserved in cats, so that the infection is diagnosed only at autopsy. One cat presented with acute dyspnea (Hawe, 1979), and sudden death is frequent (Todd et al., 1976). Not all cats, however, succumb to infection, but, unlike dogs, apparently often recover. Donahoe and associates (1976) found that most radiographic and hematologic changes (eosinophilia) occurred three to nine months after inoculation with infectious larvae, and that these changes frequently disappeared by 6 to 14 months after inoculation.

A significant number of reports describe the finding of adult worms in unusual sites—the vena cava, central nervous system, spinal canal, and subcutaneous tissues (Ader, 1979; Cusick et al., 1976; Donahoe, 1975; Faries et al., 1974; Lindquist and Winters, 1981; Todd et al., 1976). It is tempting to speculate that these aberrant parasitisms are due in part to the greater immune response of the cat to migrating larvae, which are prevented from reaching the heart to complete their development. Two cats experimentally infected with heartworms developed chylothorax (Donahoe, 1974), and although the etiology of the condition was not indicated, it might have resulted from an aberrant worm migration to the thoracic lymphatic duct.

## Otoacariasis

*Otodectes cynotis* is a mite that infests the ear canal of cats, where it feeds on the epithelial debris, sebum, lymph, and whole blood resulting from its presence (Powell et al., 1980). Intact males seem to have greater mite infestations than females. Very young kittens born to some queens appear to have more resistance for the first two months of life than kittens of other queens (Pedersen, 1983). In addition, levels of mite infestation in our colony appear to reach a peak in adolescent kittens and decline after that (Pedersen, 1983), a phenomenon also noted by other researchers (Weisbroth et al., 1974). In infested catteries some cats are more heavily parasitized than others, and some debilitated, FeLV-infected cats harbor more mites than other cats (Pedersen, 1983). All these observations suggest some immune control mechanism.

The possible nature of mite immunity has been studied by Weisbroth and coworkers (1974) and Powell and associates (1980). Infected cats respond to the mite by producing precipitating (Weisbroth et al., 1974) and reaginic antibodies (Powell et al., 1980), the latter identified by a reverse passive cutaneous anaphylaxis type of reaction and therefore presumably IgE. An immediate hypersensitivity reaction can also be elicited in diseased cats by intradermal injections of mite antigen.

Eliciting an immediate skin reaction may be one way that the feeding mite assures its food supply. Histopathologic studies of skin where mites are feeding show hypertrophy of squamous epithelial cells, acanthosis, hyperplasia of sebaceous glands, and hyperemia and edema of the dermis associated with infiltration of mast cells, lymphocytes, and plasma cells (Weisbroth et al., 1974). It is this inflammatory exudate that the mites feed on.

Immunologic influence on mite populations could occur by two means. First, those cats that are most apt to develop an immune-mediated dermal reaction may provide the mite population with a greater food supply and therefore favor growth of the mites, whereas less sensitized cats provide mites with less food. A second possibility is that the mites are damaged by ingestion of lymph (presumably containing antibodies), as well as by the host's immunocytes and macrophages.

## Acknowledgment

Some of the original work presented in this chapter was supported by grants from the Save Our Cats and Kittens (SOCK) Corporation, Walnut Creek, CA, and the Winn Foundation of the Cat Fanciers' Association.

## REFERENCES

Aarden LA, Brunner TK, Cerottini J-C, et al: Revised nomenclature for antigen-nonspecific T cell proliferation and helper factors. [Letter to the editor.] J Immunol 123 (1979) 2928–2929.

Adams PW, Olsen RG, Mathes LE: Characterization of IgG and IgM response to feline oncornavirus-associated cell membrane antigen in cats exposed to feline oncornavirus. Abst Ann Mtg Am Soc Microbiol 79, E62 (1979) 65.

Ader P: Heartworm (Dirofilaria immitis) in the brain of a cat—review and case report. Calif Vet 33 (Nov) (1979) 23–28, 32.

Aitken ID, McCusker HB: Immunological studies in the cat. III. Attempts to induce delayed hypersensitivity. Res Vet Sci 10 (1969) 208–213.

Aitken ID, Olatsdottir E, McCusker HB: Immunological studies in the cat. I. The serological response to some foreign proteins. Res Vet Sci 8 (1967) 234–246.

Akcasu A: Why cats cannot be sensitized to foreign proteins. Int Arch Allergy Appl Immunol 22 (1963) 85–86.

Altera KP, Bonasch H: Periarteritis nodosa in a cat. J Am Vet Med Assoc 149 (1966) 1307–1311.

Anderson LJ, Jarrett WFH: Membranous glomerulonephritis associated with leukemia in cats. Res Vet Sci 12 (1971) 179–180.

Anderson LJ, Jarrett WFH, Jarrett O, Laird HM: Feline leukemia-virus infection of kittens: mortality associated with atrophy of the thymus and lymphoid depletion. J Natl Cancer Inst 47 (1971) 807–817.

Auer L, Bell K: The A-B blood group system in the domestic cat. *In* Programme Abstracts, XVII Conference on Animal Blood Groups and Biochemical Polymorphisms, The Int Soc for Animal Blood Group Research. Wageningen, The Netherlands, July 28–Aug 2, 1979, 106. (Abstr also in Animal Blood Groups and Biochemical Genetics 11 [1980] Suppl 1, 63.)

Auer L, Bell K, Coates S: Blood transfusion reactions in the cat. J Am Vet Med Assoc 180 (1982) 729–730.

Austen KF, Humphrey JH: *In vitro* studies of the mechanism of anaphylaxis. Adv Immunol 3 (1963) 1–96.

Baker E: Food allergy. Symposium on allergy in small animal practice. Vet Clin North Am 4 (1974) 79–90.

Baker E: Food allergy in the cat. Feline Pract 5 (3) (1973) 18–26.

Baker RD: The cellular content of chyle in relation to lymphoid tissue and fat transportation. Anat Rec 55 (1932–1933) 207–219.

Barrett RE, Post JE, Schultz RD: Chronic relapsing stomatitis in a cat associated with feline leukemia virus infection. Feline Pract 5 (6) (1975) 34–38.

Barta O, Hubbert NL: Testing of hemolytic complement components in domestic animals. Am J Vet Res 39 (1978) 1303–1308.

Barta O, Oyekan PP: Feline (cat) hemolytic complement optimal testing conditions. Am J Vet Res 42 (1981) 378–381.

Bennett AM, Huxtable CR, Love DN: Tyzzer's disease in cats experimentally infected with feline leukaemia virus. Vet Microbiol 2 (1977) 49–56.

Betton GR: Natural cell-mediated cytotoxicity in the canine. *In* Shifrine M, Wilson FD (eds): The Canine as a Biomedical Model: Immunological, Hematological, and Oncological Aspects. Springfield, Virginia, Technical Information Center/US Department of Energy, DOE/TIC-10191, 1980, 99–126.

Bittle JL, Emery JB, York CJ, McMillen JK: Comparative study of feline cytopathogenic viruses and feline panleukopenia virus. Am J Vet Res 22 (1961) 374–378.

Blackmore DK, Hill A: The experimental transmissions of various mycoplasmas of feline origin to domestic cats. *(Felis catus)*. J Small Anim Pract 14 (1973) 7–13.

Bloom BR: Interferons and the immune system. Nature 284 (1980) 593–595.

Bown P: A case of feline membranous glomerulonephritis. Vet Rec 89 (1971) 557–558.

Braend M, Andersen AE: Blood polymorphism in cats. *In* Programme Abstracts, XVII Conference on Animal Blood Groups and Biochemical Polymorphisms, The Int Soc for Animal Blood Group Research. Wageningen, The Netherlands, July 28–Aug 2, 1979, 105. (Abstr also in Animal Blood Groups and Biochemical Genetics 11 [1980] Suppl 1, 63.)

Brown N, Hurvitz AI: A mucocutaneous disease in a cat resembling human pemphigus. J Am Anim Hosp Assoc 15 (1979) 25–28.

Butler WT, Rossen RD, Waldmann TA: The mechanism of appearance of immunoglobulin A in nasal secretions in man. J Clin Invest 46 (1967) 1883–1893.

Butler WT, Waldmann TA, Rossen RD, Douglas RG Jr, Couch RB: Changes in IgA and IgG concentrations in nasal secretions prior to the appearance of antibody during viral respiratory infection in man. J Immunol 105 (1970) 584–591.

Cain GR, Suzuki Y: Presumptive neonatatal isoerythrolysins in cats. J Am Vet Med Assoc 187 (1985) 46–48.

Carlson JH, Scott FW: Feline panleukopenia. II. The relationship of intestinal mucosal cell proliferation rates to viral infection and development of lesions. Vet Pathol 14 (1977) 173–181.

Carpenter JL: Bronchial asthma in cats. *In* Kirk RW (ed): Current Veterinary Therapy V. Philadelphia, WB Saunders Company, 1974, 208–209.

Carpenter JL: Personal observation, 1983.

Cello RM: Association of pleuropneumonialike organisms with conjunctivitis of cats. Am J Ophthalmol 43 (1957) 296–297.

Cello RM: Microbiological and immunologic aspects of feline pneumonitis. J Am Vet Med Assoc 158 (1971) 932–938.

Chew DJ, DiBartola SP, Boyce JT, Gasper PW: Renal amyloidosis in related Abyssinian cats. J Am Vet Med Assoc 181 (1982) 139–142.

Clark L, Seawright AA: Skeletal abnormalities in tthe hindlimbs of young cats as a result of hypervitaminosis A. Nature 217 (1968) 1174–1176.

Clark L, Seawright AA: Generalised amyloidosis in seven cats. Pathol Vet 6 (1969) 117–134.

Cockerell GL: Naturally occurring acquired immunodeficiency diseases of the dog and cat. Vet Clin North Am 8 (1978) 613–628.

Cockerell GL, Hoover EA, LoBuglio AF, Yohn DS: Phytomitogen- and antigen-induced blast transformation of feline lymphocytes. Am J Vet Res 36 (1975) 1489–1494.

Cockerell GL, Hoover EA, Krakowka S, Olsen RG, Yohn DS: Lympyhocyte mitogen reactivity and enumeration of circulating B- and T-cells during feline leukemia virus infection in the cat. J Natl Cancer Inst 57 (1976a) 1095–1099.

Cockerell L, Krakowka S, Hoover EA, Olsen RG, Yohn DS: Characterization of feline T- and B-lymphocytes and identification of an experimentally induced T-cell neoplasm in the cat. J Natl Cancer Inst 57 (1976b) 907–911.

Collier LL, Bryan GM, Prieur DJ: Ocular manifestations of the Chédiak-Higashi syndrome in four species of animals. J Am Vet Med Assoc 175 (1979) 587–590.

Colten HR: Biosynthesis of complement. Adv Immunol 22 (1976) 67–118.

Cotter SM: Feline leukemia virus induced disorders in the cat. Vet Clin North Am 6 (1976) 367–378.

Cotter SM: Blood transfusion reactions in cats. [Letter to the editor.] J Am Vet Med Assoc 181 (1982) 5–6.

Cotter SM, Gilmore CE, Rollins C: Multiple cases of feline leukemia and feline infectious peritonitis in a household. J Am Vet Med Assoc 162 (1973) 449–454.

Cotter SM, Hardy WD, Essex M: Association of feline leukemia virus with lymphosarcoma and other disorders in the cat. J Am Vet Med Assoc 166 (1975) 449–454.

Crouch JE: Text-Atlas of Cat Anatomy. Philadelphia, Lea & Febiger, 1969, 260–262.

Crowell WA, Goldston RT, Schall WD, Finco DR: Generalized amyloidosis in a cat. J Am Vet Med Assoc 161 (1972) 1127–1133.

Curtis R, Bell WJ, Laing PW: Polyarteritis in a cat. Vet Rec 105 (1979) 354.

Cusick PK, Todd KS Jr, Blake JA, Daly WR: *Dirofilaria immitis* in the brain and heart of a cat from Massachusetts. J Am Anim Hosp Assoc 12 (1976) 490–491.

David JR, Vadas MA, Butterworth AE, DeBrito PA, Carvalho EM, David RA, Bina JC, Andrade ZA: Enhanced helminthotoxic capacity of eosinophils from patients with eosinophilia. N Engl J Med 303 (1980) 1147–1152.

Dawson JRB: Myasthenia gravis in a cat. Vet Rec 86 (1970) 562–563.

Ditchfield J: Newer information on viral diseases of the dog and cat. I. Viral infections of the cat. Southwest Vet 21 (1968) 125–129.

Donahoe JMR: Experimental infection of cats with *Dirofilaria immitis*. J Parasitol 61 (1975) 599–605.

Donahoe JM, Kneller SK, Thompson PE: Chylothorax subsequent to infection of cats with *Dirofilaria immitis*. J Am Vet Med Assoc 164 (1974) 1107–1110.

Donahoe JMR, Kneller SK, Lewis RE: Hematologic and radiographic changes in cats after inoculation with infective larvae of *Dirofilaria immitis*. J Am Vet Med Assoc 168 (1976) 413–417.

Drazner FH: Multiple myeloma in the cat. Compend Contin Ed 4 (1982) 206–210.

Dubey JP: Immunity to *Hammondia hammondi* infection in cats. J Am Vet Med Assoc 167 (1975) 373–377.

Dubey JP: Reshedding of *Toxoplasma* oocysts by chronically infected cats. Nature 262 (1976) 213–214.

Dubey JP: Effect of immunization of cats with *Isospora felis* and BCG on immunity and reexcretion of *Toxoplasma gondii* oocysts. J Protozool 25 (1978) 380–382.

Dubey JP, Frenkel JK: Immunity to feline toxoplasmosis: modification by administration of corticosteroids. Vet Pathol 11 (1974) 350–379.

Dubey JP, Hoover EA: Attempted transmission of *Toxoplasma gondii* infection from pregnant cats to their kittens. J Am Vet Med Assoc 170 (1976) 538–540.

Dubey JP, Hoover, EA, Walls KW: Effect of age and sex on the acquisition of immunity to toxoplasmosis in cats. J Protozool 24 (1977) 184–186.

Dubey JP, Johnstone I: Fatal neonatal toxoplasmosis in cats. J Am Anim Hosp Assoc 18 (1982) 461–467.

Easley JR: Necrotizing vasculitis: an overview: J Am Anim Hosp Assoc 15 (1979) 207–211.

Engle GC, Brodey RS: A retrospective study of 395 feline neoplasms. J Am Anim Hosp Assoc 5 (1969) 21–31.

Essex, M, Cotter SM, Carpenter JL, Hard, WD Jr, Hess P, Schaller J, Yohn DS: Feline oncornavirus associated cell membrane antigen. II. Antibody titers in healthy cats from household and laboratory colony environments. J Natl Cancer Inst 54 (1975) 631–635.

Eyquem A, Podliachouk L: Les groupes sanguins des chats. Ann Inst Pasteur (Paris) 87 (1954) 91–94.

Eyquem A, Podliachouk L, Millot P: Blood groups in chimpanzees, horses, sheep, pigs, and other mammals. Ann NY Acad Sci 97 (1962) 320–328.

Faircloth JC, Montgomery JK: Systemic lupus erythematosus in a cat presenting with autoimmune hemolytic anemia. Feline Pract 11 (2) (1981) 22–26.

Faircloth JC, Montgomery JK Jr: Pemphigus erythematosus in a cat. Feline Pract 12(5) (1982) 31–33.

Faries FC, Mainster ME, Martin PW: Incidental findings of *Dirofilaria immitis* in domestic cats. Vet Med Small Anim Clin 69 (1974) 599–600.

Farrow BRH, Huxtable CR, McGovern VJ: Nephrotic syndrome in the cat due to diffuse membranous glomerulonephritis. Pathology 1 (1969) 67–72.

Farrow BRH, Penny R: Multiple myeloma in a cat. J Am Vet Med Assoc 158 (1971) 606–611.

Fastier LB: Feline panleucopenia—a serological study. Vet Rec 83 (1968) 653–655.

Fearon DT, Austen KF: The alternative pathway of complement—a system for host resistance to microbial infection. N Engl J Med 303 (1980) 259–263.

Fitch FW: Selective suppression of immune responses. Regulation of antibody formation and cell-mediated immunity by antibody. Prog Allergy 19 (1975) 195–244.

Fowler JL, Matsuda K, Fernau RC: Experimental infection of the domestic cat with *Dirofilaria immitis*. J Am Anim Hosp Assoc 8 (1972) 79–80.

Fox JG, Murphy JC, Shalev M: Systemic fungal infections in cats. J Am Vet Med Assoc 173 (1978) 1191–1195.

Francis DP, Essex M, Jakowski RM, Cotter SM, Lerer TJ, Hardy WD Jr: Increased risk for lymphosarcoma and glomerulonephritis in a closed population of cats exposed to feline leukemia virus. Am J Epidemiol 111 (1980) 337–346.

Francis J: Tuberculosis in Man and Animals. A Study in Comparative Pathology. London, Cassell and Company, Ltd., 1958, 222.

Gabbert NH: Systemic lupus erythematosus in a cat with thrombocytopenia. Vet Med Small Anim Clin 78 (1983) 77–79.

Gaskell RM: Studies on feline viral rhinotracheitis with particular reference to the carrier state. PhD dissertation, Department of Veterinary Medicine, University of Bristol, UK, 1975.

Gaskell RM, Povey RC: Feline viral rhinotracheitis: sites of virus replication and persistence in acutely and persistently infected cats. Res Vet Sci 27 (1979) 167–174.

Gaskell RM, Wardley RC: Feline viral respiratory disease: A review with particular reference to its epizootiology and control. J Small Anim Pract 19 (1978) 1–16.

Gelberg HB, Lewis RM, Felsburg PJ, Smith CA: Antiepithelial autoantibodies associated with the feline eosinophilic granuloma complex. Am J Vet Res 46 (1985) 263–265.

Gillespie JH, Scott FW: Feline viral infections. Adv Vet Sci Comp Med 17 (1973) 163–200.

Glenner GG: Amyloid deposits and amyloidosis: The B-fibrilloses. N Engl J Med 302 (1980) 1283–1292.

Glover RE: Tuberculosis in animals other than cattle. Vet Rec 61 (1949) 875–878.

Gordon MA, Vedder DK: Serologic tests in diagnosis and prognosis of cryptococcosis. J Am Med Assoc 197 (1966) 961–967.

Gorham JR, Henson JB, Dodgen CP: Basic principles of immunity in cats. J Am Vet Med Assoc 158 (1971) 846–856.

Gotschlich E, Stetson CA: Immunologic cross-reactions among mammalian acute phase proteins. J Exp Med 111 (1960) 441–451.

Grant CK, Essex M, Gardner MB, Hardy WD Jr: Natural feline leukemia virus infection and the immune response of cats of different ages. Cancer Res 40 (1980) 823–829.

Grant CK, Pickard DK, Ramaika C, Madewell BR, Essex M: Complement and tumor antibody levels in cats, and changes associated with natural feline leukemia virus infection and malignant disease. Cancer Res 39 (1979) 75–81.

Griesemer RA: *In* York CJ: Comments or immunology of the cat. J Am Vet Med Assoc 158 (1971) 856.

Griffith AS: Tuberculosis of the cat. J Comp Pathol Ther 39 (1926) 71–79.

Guelfi J-F, Florio R, Berland HM: Sur une méthode possible de diagnostic allergique de la tuberculose des carnivores domestiques: Le test de transformation lymphoblastique. Premières investigations. Rev Méd Vét 125 (1974) 351–354.

Harding SK, Bruner DW, Bryant IW: The transfer of antibodies from the mother cat to her newborn kittens. Cornell Vet 51 (1961) 535–539.

Hardy WD Jr: Feline leukemia virus non-neoplastic diseases. J Am Anim Hosp Assoc 17 (1981) 941–949.

Hardy WD Jr: Immunopathology induced by the feline leukemia virus. Springer Seminars Immunopathol 5 (1982) 75–106.

Hardy WD Jr, Old LJ, Hess PW, Essex M, Cotter S: Horizontal transmission of feline leukaemia virus. Nature 244 (1973) 266–269.

Hartigan PJ, Tuite M, McAllister H: Generalized amyloidosis in the domestic cat. Ir Vet J 34 (1980) 1–6.

Harvey JW, Gaskin JM: Feline haemobartonellosis: attempts to induce relapses of clinical disease in chronically infected cats. J Am Anim Hosp Assoc 14 (1978) 453–456.

Haschek WM, Kasali OB: A case of cutaneous feline phaeohyphomycosis caused by *Phialophora gougerotti*. Cornell Vet 67 (1977) 467–471.

Hawe RS: The diagnosis and treatment of occult dirofilariasis in a cat. J Am Anim Hosp Assoc 15 (1979) 577–582.

Hawthorne VM, Lauder IM: Tuberculosis in man, dog, and cat. Am Rev Respir Dis 85 (1962) 858–869.

Hay JB, Murphy MJ, Morris B, Bessis MC: Quantitative studies on the proliferation and differentiation of antibody-forming cells in lymph. Am J Pathol 66 (1972) 1–24.

Hay LE: Multiple myeloma in a cat. Aust Vet Pract 8 (1978) 45–48.

Hayes A, Mastrota F, Mooney S, Hurvitz A: Safety of transfusing blood in cats. [Letter to the editor.] J Am Vet Med Assoc 181 (1982) 4–5.

Heise SC, Smith RC, Schalm OW: Lupus erythematosus with hemolytic anemia in a cat. Feline Pract 3 (3) (1973) 14–19.

Hiraga C, Kanki T, Ichikawa Y: Immunoglobulin characteristics of germfree and specific pathogen-free cats. Lab Anim Sci 31 (1981) 391–396.

Hix JW, Jones TC, Karlson AG: Avian tubercle bacillus infection in the cat. J Am Vet Med Assoc 138 (1961) 641–647.

Hjärre JR, Morgan AD: Uber das Vorkommen der Amyloid-degeneration bei Tieren. Acta Pathol Microbiol Scand Suppl 16 (1933) 132–162.

Holmberg CA, Manning JS, Osburn BI: Feline malignant lymphomas: comparison of morphologic and immunologic characteristics. Am J Vet Res 37 (1976) 1455–1460.

Holmes R: The occurrence of blood groups in cats. J Exp Biol 30 (1953) 350–357.

Holzworth J: Immunology of feline virus diseases. Cornell Vet 56 (1966) 306–315.

Holzworth J: Unpublished observations, 1982.

Holzworth J, Meier H: Reticulum cell myeloma in a cat. Cornell Vet 47 (1957) 302–316.

Hoover EA, Griesemer RA: Experimental feline herpesvirus infection in the pregnant cat. Am J Pathol 65 (1971a) 173–188.

Hoover EA, Griesemer RA: Bone lesions produced by feline herpesvirus. Lab Invest 25 (1971b) 457–464.

Hoover EA, Kahn DE, Langloss JM: Experimentally induced feline chlamydial infection (feline pneumonitis). Am J Vet Res 39 (1978) 541–547.

Hoover EA, Olsen RG, Hardy WD Jr, Schaller JP, Mathes LE: Feline leukemia virus infection: age-related variation in response of cats to experimental infection. J Natl Cancer Inst 57 (1976) 365–369.

Hu J-N, Starkey JR, Prieur DJ: A lack of natural killer cell activity in domestic cats. Fed Proc 41 (1982) 802 (abstr).

Hurvitz AI: Immunology. *In* Ettinger SJ (ed): Textbook of Veterinary Internal Medicine, Philadelphia, WB Saunders Company, 1975, Vol 2, 1708.

Hurvitz AI: Unpublished data, 1980, 1982.

Ihrke PJ: Canine seborrheic disease complex. Vet Clin North Am 9 (1979) 93–106.

Ihrke PJ, Schwartzman RM, McGinley K, Horwitz LN, Marples RR: Microbiology of normal and seborrheic canine skin. Am J Vet Res 39 (1978) 1487–1489.

Indrieri RJ, Creighton SR, Lambert EH, Lennon VA: Myasthenia gravis in two cats. J Am Vet Med Assoc 182 (1983) 57–60.

Jacobse-Geels HEL, Daha MR, Horzinek MC: Isolation and characterization of feline C3 and evidence for the immune complex pathogenesis of feline infectious peritonitis. J Immunol 125 (1980) 1606–1610.

Jakob W: Spontaneous amyloidosis of mammals. Vet Pathol 8 (1971) 292–306.

Jankovic BD, Rakic L, Veskov R, Horvat J: Anaphylactic reaction in the cat following intraventricular and intravenous injections of antigen. Experientia 25 (1969) 864–865.

Jarrett O, Russell PH, Stewart MF: Protection of kittens from feline leukaemia virus infection by maternally-derived antibody. Vet Rec 101 (1977) 304–305.

Jennings AR: The distribution of tuberculous lesions in the dog and cat, with reference to the pathogenesis. Vet Rec 61 (1949) 380–384.

Johnson L, Pedersen NC, Theilen GH: The nature of immunity to Snyder-Theilen fibrosarcoma virus–induced tumors in cats. Vet Immunol Immunopathol 9 (1985) 283–300.

Johnson RP: Immunity to feline calicivirus in kittens. PhD dissertation, University of Guelph, Guelph, Ontario, Canada, 1980.

Joshi BC, Raplee RG, Powell AL, Hancock F: Autoimmune thrombocytopenia in a cat. J Am Anim Hosp Assoc 15 (1979) 585–588.

Kahn DE: Unpublished data, 1973.

Kahn DE, Hoover EA, Bittle JL: Induction of immunity to feline caliciviral disease. Infect Immun 11 (1975) 1003–1009.

Kehoe JM, Hurvitz AI, Capra JD: Characterization of three feline paraproteins. J Immunol 109 (1972) 511–516.

Kitzmiller JL, Lucas WE, Yelenosky PF: The role of complement in feline endotoxin shock. Am J Obstet Gynecol 112 (1972) 414–421.

Klotz FW, Gathings WE, Cooper MD: Development and distribution of B lineage cells in the domestic cat: analysis with monoclonal antibodies to cat $\mu$-, $\gamma$-, $\kappa$- and $\lambda$-chains and heterologous anti $\alpha$-antibodies. J Immunol 134 (1985) 95–100.

Kobilinsky L, Hardy WD Jr, Day NK: Hypocomplementemia associated with naturally occurring lymphosarcoma in pet cats. J Immunol 122 (1979) 2139–2142.

Kramer JW, Davis WC, Prieur DJ: The Chédiak-Higashi syndrome of cats. Lab Invest 36 (1977) 554–562.

Kristensen F, Barsanti JA: Analysis of serum proteins in clinically normal pet and colony cats, using agarose electrophoresis. Am J Vet Res 38 (1977) 399–402.

Lamm ME: Cellular aspects of immunoglobulin A. Adv Immunol 22 (1976) 223–290.

Langweiler M, Cockerell GL: Generation of concanavalin A-induced suppressor cells in the cat. Int Arch Allerg Appl Immunol 69 (1982) 148–155.

Langweiler M, Haskins ME, Jezyk PF: Mucopolysaccharidosis in a litter of cats. J Am Anim Hosp Assoc 14 (1978) 748–751.

Legendre AM, Mallmann VH, Michel RL: Migration-inhibition response of peripheral leukocytes to tuberculin in cats sensitized with viable *Mycobacterium bovis* (BCG). Am J Vet Res 38 (1977) 819–822.

Lennon VA: Myasthenia gravis in dogs. acetylcholine receptor deficiency with and without anti-receptor antibodies. *In* Rose NR, Bigazzi PE, Warner NL (eds): Genetic Control of Autoimmune Disease. New York, Elsevier/North Holland Biomedical Press, 1978, 295–306.

Lewis RM: Systemic lupus erythematosus. *In* Shifrine M, Wilson FD (eds): The Canine as a Biomedical Research Model: Immunological, Hematological, and Oncological Aspects. Springfield, VA. Technical Information Center/U.S. Department of Energy, DOE/TIC-10191, 1980, 244–263.

Lewis RM, Schwartz RS, Gilmore CE: Autoimmune diseases in domestic animals. Ann NY Acad Sci 124 (1965) 178–200.

Lindquist WD, Winters KD: Cerebral feline dirofilariasis. Feline Pract 11 (2) (1981) 37–40.

Lindt S: Zur Morphologie und Ätiologie der Erkrankungen des oberen Respirationstraktes bei Katzen. Schweiz Arch Tierheilkd 197 (1965) 196–203.

Lubberink AAME, van Ooyen PG, Mieog WHW: Haemolytic anaemia in a cat. Results of prednisone therapy and splenectomy. Tijadschr Diergeneeskd 96 (1971) 261–264.

Lucke VM: Renal polyarteritis nodosa in the cat. Vet Rec 82 (1968) 622–624.

Lucke VM, Hunt AC: Interstitial nephropathy and papillary necrosis in the domestic cat. J Pathol Bacteriol 89 (1965) 723–728.

MacEwen EG, Hurvitz AI: Diagnosis and management of monoclonal gammopathies. Vet Clin North Am 7 (1977) 119–132.

Madewell BR, Holmberg CA, Ackerman N: Lymphosarcoma and cryptococcosis in a cat. J Am Vet Med Assoc 175 (1979) 65–68.

Madewell BR, Jarrett O: Recovery of feline leukaemia virus from non-viraemic cats. Vet Rec 112 (1983) 339–342.

Maede Y: Sequestration and phagocytosis of *Haemobartonella felis* in the spleen. Am J Vet Res 40 (1979) 691–695.

Maede Y, Hata R: Studies on feline haemobartonellosis. II. The mechanism of anemia produced by infection with *Haemobartonella felis*. Jpn J Vet Sci 37 (1975) 49–54.

Manning TO, Scott DW, Smith CA, Lewis RM: Pemphigus diseases in the feline: seven case reports and discussion. J Am Anim Hosp Assoc 18 (1982) 433–443.

Marion RS, Smith JE: Survival of erythrocytes after autologous and allogeneic transfusion in cats. J Am Vet Med Assoc 183 (1983) 1437–1440.

Mason KV: A case of myasthenia gravis in a cat. J Small Anim Pract 17 (1976) 467–472.

Mathes LE, Olsen RG, Hebebrand LC, Hoover EA, Schaller JP, Adams PW, Nichols WS: Immunosuppressive properties of a virion polypeptide, a 15,000 dalton protein, from feline leukemia virus. Cancer Res 39 (1979) 950–955.

McCullough B: Interferon response in cats. J Infect Dis 125 (1972) 174–177.

McCusker HB, Aitken ID: Anaphylaxis in the cat. J Pathol Bacteriol 91 (1966) 282–285.

McCusker HB, Aitken ID: Immunological studies in the cat. II. Experimental induction of skin reactivity to foreign proteins. Res Vet Sci 8 (1967) 265–271.

Miller-Ben Shaul D: The immunological response of the neonatal and suckling cat to various antigens administered parenterally and orally. Isr J Med Sci 1 (1965) 563–568.

Mills JN, Eger CE, Robinson WF, Penhale WJ, McKenna RP: A case of multiple myeloma in a cat. J Am Anim Hosp Assoc 18 (1982) 79–82.

Moise NS, Spaulding GL: Feline bronchial asthma. Pathogenesis, pathophysiology, diagnostics, and therapeutic considerations. Compend Contin Ed 3 (1981) 1091–1102.

Müller-Eberhard HJ: Chemistry and reaction mechanisms of complement. Adv Immunol 8 (1968) 1–80.

Müller-Eberhard HJ, Schreiber RD: Molecular biology and chemistry of the alternate pathway of complement. Adv Immunol 29 (1980) 2–53.

Murphy MJ, Hay JB, Morris B, Bessis MC: Ultrastructural analysis of antibody synthesis in cells from lymph and lymph nodes. Am J Pathol 66 (1972) 25–42.

Nakamatsu M, Goto M, Morita M: A case of generalized amyloidosis in the cat. Jpn J Vet Sci 28 (1966) 259–265.

Nash AS, Wright NG, Spencer AJ, Thompson H, Fisher EW: Membranous nephropathy in the cat: a clinical and pathological study. Vet Rec 105 (1979) 71–77.

Nathan CF, Murray HW, Cohn ZA: The macrophage as an effector cell. N Engl J Med 303 (1980) 622–626.

Nelson RA: A new concept of immunosuppression in hypersensitivity reactions and in transplantation immunity. Surv Ophthalmol 11 (1966) 498–505.

Neoh SH, Jahoda DM, Rowe DS: Immunoglobulin classes of various mammalian species identified by cross-reactivity with antisera to human immunoglobulin. Immunochemistry 10 (1973) 805–813.

Nielsen KH: Bovine reaginic antibody III. Cross-reaction of antihuman IgE and antibovine reaginic immunoglobulin antisera with sera from several species of mammals. Can J Comp Med 41 (1977) 345–348.

Okoshi S, Tomoda I, Makimura S: Analysis of normal cat serum by immunoelectrophoresis. Jap J Vet Sci 29 (1967) 337–346.

Olsen RG, Kahn DE, Hoover EA, Saxe NJ, Yohn DS: Differences in acute and convalescent-phase antibodies of cats infected with feline picornaviruses. Infect Immun 10 (1974) 375–380.

O'Reilly KJ, Paterson JS, Harriss ST: The persistence in kittens of maternal antibody to feline infectious enteritis (panleucopenia). Vet Rec 84 (1969) 376–378.

Orr CM, Gaskell CJ, Gaskell RM: Interaction of an intranasal combined feline viral rhinotracheitis, feline calicivirus vaccine and the FVR carrier state. Vet Rec 106 (1980a) 164–166.

Orr CM, Kelly DF, Luke VM: Tuberculosis in cats. A report of two cases. J Small Anim Pract 21 (1980b) 247–253.

Parish WE: The manifestation of anaphylactic reactions in the skin of different species. *In* Rook AJ, Walton GS (eds): Comparative Physiology and Pathology of the Skin. Oxford, Blackwell Scientific Publications, 1965, 471–475.

Paterson PY: Experimental allergic encephalomyelitis and autoimmune disease. Adv Immunol 5 (1966) 131–208.

Pedersen NC: Personal observations, 1983.

Pedersen NC: Feline infectious peritonitis and feline enteric coronavirus infections. Part 1: Feline enteric coronaviruses. Feline Pract 13 (4) (1983a) 13–19.

Pedersen NC: Feline infectious peritonitis and feline enteric coronavirus infections. Part 2: Feline infectious peritonitis. Feline Pract 13 (5) (1983b) 5–20.

Pedersen NC, Black JW: Attempted immunization of cats against feline infectious peritonitis, using avirulent live virus or sublethal amounts of virulent virus. Am J Vet Res 44 (1983) 229–234.

Pedersen NC, Boyle JF: Immunologic phenomena in the effusive form of feline infectious peritonitis. Am J Vet Res 41 (1980) 868–876.

Pedersen NC, Boyle JF, Floyd K: Infection studies in kittens utilizing feline infectious peritonitis virus propagated in cell culture. Am J Vet Res 42 (1981a) 363–367.

Pedersen NC, Boyle JF, Floyd K, Fudge A, Barker J: An enteric coronavirus infection of cats and its relationship to feline infectious peritonitis. Am J Vet Res 42 (1981b) 368–377.

Pedersen NC, Meric SM, Ho E, Johnson L, Plucker S, Theilen GH: The clinical significance of latent feline leukemia virus in cats. Feline Pract 14 (2) (1984) 32–48.

Pedersen NC, Pool RR, O'Brien T: Feline chronic progressive polyarthritis. Am J Vet Res 41 (1980) 522–535.

Pedersen NC, Theilen G, Keane MA, Fairbanks L, Mason T, Orser B, Chen C-H, Allison C: Studies of naturally transmitted feline leukemia virus infection. Am J Vet Res 38 (1977) 1523–1531.

Perryman LE, Hoover EA, Yohn DS: Immunologic reactivity of the cat. Immunosuppression in experimental feline leukemia. J Natl Cancer Inst 49 (1972) 1357–1365.

Perryman LE, Olsen RG, Yohn DS: Comparison of the serologic response in cats to various antigens, using homologous and heterologous complement. Am J Vet Res 34 (1973) 1529–1532.

Peterson ME, Hurvitz AI, Leib MS, Cavanagh PG, Dutton RE: Propylthiouracil-associated hemolytic anemia, thrombocytopenia, and antinuclear antibodies in cats with hyperthyroidism. J Am Vet Med Assoc 184 (1984) 806–808.

Post JE, Warren L: Reactivation of latent feline leukemia virus. *In* Hardy WD Jr, Essex M, McClelland AJ (eds): Feline leukemia virus. New York, Elsevier/North Holland, 1980, 151–155.

Povey RC: Serological relationships among feline caliciviruses. Infect Immun 10 (1974) 1307–1314.

Povey RC: Differential diagnosis and control of infectious respiratory disease in cats. Small Animal Veterinary Medicine Update Series 1 (1977) 1–5.

Povey RC, Hale CJ: Experimental infections with feline caliciviruses (picornaviruses) in specific-pathogen-free kittens. J Comp Pathol 84 (1974) 245–256.

Povey RC, Ingersoll J: Cross-protection among feline caliciviruses. Infect Immun 11 (1975) 877–885.

Powell MB, Weisbroth SH, Roth L, Wilhelmsen C: Reaginic hypersensitivity in *Otodectes cynotis* infestation of cats and mode of mite feeding. Am J Vet Res 41 (1980) 877–882.

Prieur DJ, Collier LL, Bryan GM, Meyers KM: The diagnosis of feline Chédiak-Higashi syndrome. Feline Pract 9 (5) (1979) 26–32.

Reedy LM: Results of allergy testing and hyposensitization in selected feline skin diseases. J Am Anim Hosp Assoc 18 (1982) 618–623.

Reinhardt WO: Some factors influencing the thoracic duct output of lymphocytes. Ann NY Acad Sci 113 (1964) 844–866.

Riley JF, West GB: The presence of histamine in tissue mast cells. J Physiol (Lond) 120 (1953) 528–537.

Rodgers R, Merigan TC, Hardy WD Jr, Old LJ, Kassel R: Cat interferon inhibits feline leukaemia virus infection in cell cultures. Nature [New Biol] 237 (1972) 270–271.

Rogerson P, Jarrett W, Mackey L: Epidemiological studies of feline leukaemia virus infection. I. A serological survey in urban cats. Int J Cancer 15 (1975) 781–785.

Roitt IM: Essential Immunology. Oxford, Blackwell Scientific Publications, 1977, 86–88.

Rojko JL, Hoover EA, Mathes LE, Krakowka S, Olsen RG: Influence of adrenal corticosteroids on the susceptibility of cats to feline leukemia virus infection. Cancer Res 39 (1979) 3789–3791.

Rojko JL, Hoover EA, Quackenbush SL, Olsen RG: Reactivation of latent feline leukaemia virus infection. Nature 298 (1982) 3789–3791.

Russell AS: Cell-mediated immunity to herpes simplex virus in man. Am J Clin Pathol 60 (1973) 826–830.

Saar C, Saar U, Opitz M, Burow H, Teichert G: Paraproteinämische Retikulosen bei der Katze (Bericht über je einen Fall von Plasmazellenretikulose und Makroglobulinämie). Berl Münch Tierärztl Wochenschr 86 (1973) 11–15, 21–24.

Saegusa S, Shimizu F, Kasegawa A, Usui K: Some clinical and immunological aspects on contracted kidney in cats. Jpn J Exp Med 45 (1975) 403–413.

Saegusa S, Shimizu F, Nagase M, Kasegawa A: Concurrent feline immune-complex nephritis. Tubular antigen-positive and renal amyloidosis. Arch Pathol Lab Med 103 (1979) 475–478.

Samter M: Eosinophils—nominated but not elected. N Engl J Med 303 (1980) 1175–1176.

Schrader LA, Hurvitz AI: Cold agglutinin disease in a cat. J Am Vet Med Assoc 183 (1983) 121–122.

Schultz KT, Maguire HC: Chemically-induced delayed hypersensitivity in the cat. Vet Immunol Immunopathol 3 (1982) 585–590.

Schultz RD: Laboratory diagnosis of immunologic disorders. *In* Kirk RW (ed): Current Veterinary Therapy VI. Philadelphia, WB Saunders Company, 1977, 453–463.

Schultz RD, Adams LS: Immunologic methods for the detection of humoral and cellular immunity. Vet Clin North Am 8 (1978) 721–768.

Schultz RD, Mendel H, Scott FW: Effect of feline panleukopenia virus infection on development of humoral and cellular immunity. Cornell Vet 66 (1976) 324–332.

Schultz RD, Scott FW, Duncan JR, Gillespie JH: Feline immunoglobulins. Infect Immun 9 (1974) 391–393.

Scott DW: Feline dermatology 1900–1978: a monograph. J Am Anim Hosp Assoc 16 (1980) 331–459.

Scott DW, Haupt KH, Knowlton BF, Lewis RM: A glucocorticoid-responsive dermatitis in cats, resembling systemic lupus erythematosus in man. J Am Anim Hosp Assoc 15 (1979) 157–171.

Scott DW, Miller WH, Lewis RM, Manning TO, Smith CA: Pemphigus erythematosus in the dog and cat. J Am Anim Hosp Assoc 16 (1980) 815–823.

Scott DW, Schultz RD, Post JE, Bolton GR, Baldwin CA: Autoimmune hemolytic anemia in the cat. J Am Anim Hosp Assoc 9 (1973) 530–539.

Scott FW: Comments on feline panleukopenia biologics. J Am Vet Med Assoc 158 (1971) 910–915.

Scott FW, Csiza CK, Gillespie JH: Maternally derived immunity to feline panleukopenia. J Am Vet Med Assoc 156 (1970) 439–453.

Scott RC, Hurvitz AI, Ehrenreich T, Derr JW: Idiopathic membranous glomerulonephritis in a cat. J Am Anim Hosp Assoc 11 (1975) 53–59.

Seawright AA, English PB, Gartner RJW: Hypervitaminosis A and deforming cervical spondylosis of the cat. J Comp Pathol 77 (1967) 29–39.

Sheffy BE, Schultz RD: Nutrition and the immune response. Cornell Vet 68 (Suppl 7) (1978) 48–61.

Shewen PE: Feline chlamydial infection. PhD dissertation, Ontario Veterinary College, University of Guelph, Guelph, Ontario, Canada, 1979.

Shewen PE, Povey RC, Wilson MR: Feline chlamydial infection. Can Vet J 19 (1978) 289–292.

Shimi A, Barin A: Salmonella in cats. J Comp Pathol 87 (1977) 315–318.

Silberman-Ziv G, Chiu SY, Buoen LC, Brand I, Brand KG: Antibody response patterns in various animal species to human cell and tissue antigens. Z Immunitätsforsch 134 (1968) 23–31.

Slater E, York C: Comparative studies on parenteral and intranasal inoculation of an attenuated feline herpes virus. Dev Biol Stand 33 (1976) 410–416.

Slauson DO, Russell SW, Schechter RD: Naturally occurring immune-complex glomerulonephritis in the cat. J Pathol 103 (1971) 131–133.

Smith JB, Pedersen NC, Morris B: The role of the lymphatic system in inflammatory responses. Ser Haematol 3 (1970a) 17–61.

Smith JB, Cunningham AJ, Lafferty KJ, Morris B: The role of the lymphatic system and lymphoid cells in the establishment of immunological memory. Aust J Exp Biol Med Sci 48 (1970b) 57–70.

Snider WR: Tuberculosis in canine and feline populations. Review of the literature. Am Rev Respir Dis 104 (1971) 877–887.

Snider WR, Cohen D, Reif JS, Stein SC, Prier JE: Tuberculosis in canine and feline populations. Study of high risk populations in Pennsylvania, 1966–1968. Am Rev Respir Dis 104 (1971) 866–876.

Sodikoff CH, Custer MA: Autoimmune hemolytic anemia in a cat. Anim Hosp 1 (1965) 261–262.

Sodikoff CH, Custer MA: Secondary autoimmune hemolytic anemia in cats. Anim Hosp 2 (1966) 20–23.

Stewart WE II, Blalock JE, Burke DC, et al: Interferon nomenclature. [Letter to the editor.] J Immunol 125 (1980) 2353.

Stogdale L, Bomzon L, van den Berg PB: Food allergy in cats. J Am Anim Hosp Assoc 18 (1982) 188–194.

Stringfellow DA, Weed SD: Feline interferon response to 2-amino-5-bromo-6-methyl-4-pyrimidinol (U-25, 166). Am J Vet Res 38 (1977) 1963–1967.

Swerczek TW, Nielsen SW, Helmboldt CF: Transmammary passage of *toxocara cati* in the cat. Am J Vet Res 32 (1971) 89–92.

Tan RJS, Markham J: Isolation of mycoplasma from cats with conjunctivitis. [Letter] NZ Vet J 19 (1971) 28.

Tan RJS, Miles JAR: Further studies of feline respiratory virus diseases. 2. Immunodiffusion tests. NZ Vet J 19 (1971) 15–18.

Tan RJS, Miles JAR: Characterization of mycoplasmas isolated from cats with conjunctivitis. NZ Vet J 21 (1973) 27–32.

Taylor D, Hokama Y, Perri SF: Differentiating feline T and B lymphocytes by rosette formation. J Immunol 115 (1975) 862–865.

Taylor DW, Siddiqui WA: Responses of enriched populations of feline T and B lymphocytes to mitogen stimulation. Am J Vet Res 38 (1977) 1969–1971.

Tham KM, Studdert MJ: Nylon wool column fractionation and characterization of feline-lymphocyte subpopulations. Vet Immunol Immunopathol 8 (1985) 3–13.

Timoney JF, Neibert HC, Scott FW: Feline salmonellosis. A nosocomial outbreak and experimental studies. Cornell Vet 68 (1978) 211–219.

Todd KS, Byerly CS, Small E, Krone JV: Heartworm infections in Illinois cats. Feline Pract 6 (2) (1976) 41–44.

Tompkins MB, Cummins JM: Response of feline leukemia virus-induced nonregenerative anemia to oral administration of an interferon-containing preparation. Feline Pract 12 (3) (1982) 6–15.

Tompkins MB, Huber K, Tompkins WAF: Natural cell-mediated cytotoxicity in the domestic cat: properties and specificity of effector cells. Am J Vet Res 44 (1983) 1525–1529.

Trainin Z, Wernicke D, Ungar-Waron H, Essex M: Suppression of the humoral antibody response in natural retrovirus infections. Science 220 (1983) 858–859.

Uhr JW, Moeller G: Regulatory effect of antibody on the immune response. Adv Immunol 8 (1968) 81–127.

Unanue ER: Cooperation between mononuclear phagocytes and

lymphocytes in immunity. N Engl J Med 303 (1980) 977–985.
Vaerman JP, Heremans JF, Van Kerckhoven G: Communications. Identification of IgA in several mammalian species. J Immunol 103 (1969) 1421–1423.
Visco RJ, Corwin RM, Selby LA: Effect of age and sex on the prevalence of intestinal parasitism in cats. J Am Vet Med Assoc 172 (1978) 797–800.
Walton GS: Symposium on allergic and endocrine dermatoses in the dog and cat—I. Allergic dermatoses in the dog and cat. J Small Anim Pract 7 (1966) 749–754.
Walton GS: Skin responses in the dog and cat to ingested allergens. Observations on 100 confirmed cases. Vet Rec 81 (1967) 709–713.
Walton GS, Parish WE, Coombs RRA: Spontaneous allergic dermatitis and enteritis in a cat. Vet Rec 83 (1968) 35–41.
Walton TE, Gillespie JH: Feline viruses. VI. Survey of the incidence of feline pathogenic agents in normal and clinically-ill cats. Cornell Vet 60 (1970a) 215–232.
Walton TE, Gillespie JH: Feline viruses. VII. Immunity to the feline herpesvirus in kittens inoculated experimentally by the aerosol method. Cornell Vet 60 (1970b) 232–239.
Wardley RC: Feline calicivirus carrier state: a study of the host/virus relationship. Arch Virol 52 (1976) 243–249.
Wardley RC, Povey RC: Aerosol transmission of feline caliciviruses. An assessment of its epidemiological importance. Br Vet J 133 (1977a) 504–508.
Wardley RC, Povey RC: The clinical disease and patterns of excretion associated with three different strains of feline caliciviruses. Res Vet Sci 23 (1977b) 7–14.
Weisbroth SH, Powell MB, Roth L, Scher S: Immunopathology of naturally occurring otodectic otoacariasis in the domestic cat. J Am Vet Med Assoc 165 (1974) 1088–1093.
Weiss RC, Scott FW: Pathogenesis of feline infectious peritonitis: nature and development of viremia. Am J Vet Res 42 (1981) 382–390.
Werner LL, Gorman NT: Immune-mediated disorders of cats. Vet Clin North Am 14 (1984) 1039–1064.
Williams DA, Goldschmidt MH: Hyperviscosity syndrome with IgM monoclonal gammopathy and hepatic plasmacytoid lymphosarcoma in a cat. J Small Anim Pract 23 (1982) 311–323.
Wilson GS, Miles AA: Anaphylactic shock in other animals. *In* Topley and Wilson's Principles of Bacteriology and Immunology, 5th ed. Baltimore, The Williams & Wilkins Company, 1964, Vol 2, 1397.
Wolski TR: Feline behavioral problems: social causes and practical solutions. Cornell Feline Health Center News 3 (1981) 1–2, 4–6.
Wolf AM: Primary cutaneous coccidioidomycosis in a dog and cat. J Am Vet Med Assoc 174 (1979) 504–506.
Wong MM: Unpublished data, 1981.
Wong MM, Suter PF: Indirect fluorescent antibody test in occult dirofilariasis. Am J Vet Res 40 (1979) 414–420.
Yamada T, Tomoda I, Usuik: Immunoglobulin compositions of the feline body fluids. Jpn J Vet Sci 46 (1984) 791–796.
Yamamoto JK, Ho E, Pedersen NC: A feline retrovirus induced T-lymphoblastoid cell-line that produces an atypical alpha type of interferon. Vet Immunol Immunopathol 11 (1986) 1–19.
Yoffey JM, Courtice FC: Lymphatics, Lymph, and the Lymphomyeloid Complex. New York, Academic Press, Inc., 1970.

# 7
## CHAPTER
# VIRAL DISEASES

## PANLEUKOPENIA

FREDRIC W. SCOTT

Feline panleukopenia is a highly contagious viral disease characterized by sudden onset, leukopenia, fever, anorexia, depression, vomiting and diarrhea, dehydration, and often a high mortality rate. In unvaccinated populations panleukopenia is the most devastating disease of cats. In all likelihood it was the offender in the great plagues that are said in early references to have almost wiped out the cat population in various parts of the world (Buniva, 1800; Fairweather, 1876; Hall, 1801). It has been and still is known by many names: cat distemper, cat fever, cat plague, maladie du jeune âge du chat, viral enteritis, infectious enteritis or gastroenteritis, typhus, typhoid, colibacillosis, croupous or pseudomembranous enteritis, laryngoenteritis, agranulocytosis, and feline parvovirus.

With the first knowledge of bacterial disease in humans, there was a tendency to assume that the disease in cats was related to epidemics in man, and it was sometimes likened to, or said to be identical to, typhoid, diphtheria, or cholera. From the turn of the century there were many attempts to discover the infectious agent involved in the cat disease, and coliform, *Salmonella, Pasteurella*, and influenza-like organisms were isolated (Milks and Goldberg, 1920).

In 1928, Verge and Cristoforoni first isolated a virus from a French case of "gastro-entérite infectieuse." Their discovery set off a great wave of research, and within a few years similar isolations were made in many parts of the world—in England (Dalling, 1934; Hindle and Findlay, 1932), France (Lombard, 1934; Urbain, 1933), Hungary (Jarmai, 1934), the United States (Leasure et al., 1934), Italy (Bisbocci, 1936), and Scandinavia (Momberg-Jorgensen, 1938; Thorshaug, 1939).

Leasure and colleagues (1934) first reported the successful immunization of cats against "feline infectious enteritis" using formalized tissue suspensions of spleen, brain, and kidneys from infected cats. They were also successful in immunizing cats using a simultaneous injection of virulent virus and homologous feline antiserum. For some 30 years this formalized tissue vaccine was used in cats and was considered to be one of the best biologic products available. Kittens vaccinated after weaning with two doses of this vaccine one to two weeks apart were considered immune for life.

Enders and Hammon (1940) proposed that passive immunity to panleukopenia was transferred from immune queens to their kittens across the placenta. They believed that this immunity lasted for only a few months but protected the kittens against feline panleukopenia virus (FPV). They further postulated that when exposure to virus occurred as this passive immunity waned, an active immunity resulted without clinical signs of panleukopenia being observed.

In 1938 the first of a group of papers was published that gave rise to a controversy that long divided American-trained veterinarians from those educated elsewhere. The first of these papers was by Lawrence and Syverton (1938), who isolated from cats in a laboratory colony at the University of Rochester a virus that produced an acute febrile disease, a conspicuous feature of which, in addition to an inflammation of the intestine, was a profound agranulocytosis. The following year a similar virus-caused disease, christened malignant panleukopenia, was reported by Hammon and Enders (1939a,b) from a laboratory colony at Harvard University. As a result of their work, antiserum harvested from mature donors was introduced at the Angell Memorial Animal Hospital to protect hospitalized cats.

Some time passed before it was agreed that the two laboratory outbreaks at Rochester and Harvard were caused by the same virus. A larger question remained: was this virus the same as that of infectious enteritis? Lawrence and his group (1943) did work that led them to believe that it was but acknowledged that some doubt might well remain, since blood and marrow examinations had not been performed by the earlier workers. An excellent summary of panleukopenia was presented by Arlein (1940).

Until the mid 1960s all experimental work with panleukopenia had been limited to inoculation of susceptible kittens with tissue suspensions from infected cats owing to the lack of a susceptible laboratory animal or an in-vitro test. Slater and Kucera (1962) were the first to isolate the virus in vitro. They isolated and adapted FPV (PR strain) to feline kidney cells, then attenuated this isolate to produce the first modified live virus (MLV) vaccine for panleukopenia. In England, Johnson (1964, 1965) was successful in isolating a virus from a leopard with a disease identical to panleukopenia. This virus produced Cowdry type A intranuclear inclusions (Fig. 7–1) in feline kidney cell cultures. With the isolation and propagation of FPV in vitro, a method was available for study of the agent as well as the development of a serum neutralization (SN) test. King and Croghan (1965) developed an immunofluorescence test for this agent that enabled both isolation and SN tests to be performed.

Studies by Kilham and Margolis (1966) and Kilham and coworkers (1967, 1971) showed that spontaneous feline ataxia, long presumed familial, was caused by a virus. Later studies identified this virus as FPV (Csiza et al., 1972; de Lahunta, 1971; Johnson et al., 1967; Margolis et al., 1968).

## Etiology

Panleukopenia is caused by a small (20 to 24 nm), highly stable, nonenveloped, single-stranded DNA virus classified as a parvovirus. This virus is one of the hardiest animal viruses known, being resistant to many chemicals including alcohol, ether, and chloroform. This resistance is due to the absence of a lipid envelope, which plays an important role in the stability or lability of a virus to acids and alkalis. Formalin inactivates FPV if sufficient concentration and time are employed (Johnson, 1966). This sensitivity is utilized to produce inactivated-virus vaccines and occasionally to decontaminate infected cages and equipment.

FPV is resistant to most environmental temperatures so that the clinician cannot rely upon time to decontaminate an infected cage or premise. The virus will persist longer than a year at room temperature with little if any decrease in infectivity (Poole, 1972). It is resistant to freezing and drying and will survive for many years under these conditions.

FPV is resistant to most commercial disinfectants, including those containing alcohols, iodines, phenols, and quaternary ammonium compounds; it is, however, destroyed by a 1:32 dilution of commercial sodium hypochlorite (5.6 per cent as household bleach, e.g., Clorox) (Scott, 1980a). Sodium hypochlorite may be combined with certain detergent/disinfectants, although caution must be used in such combinations to avoid toxic chlorine fumes. FPV is also inactivated by 2 per cent glutaraldehyde and 4 per cent formaldehyde (10 per cent formalin). Preliminary studies in our laboratory indicate that Alcide* may be an effective and nontoxic disinfectant for animal areas and examination rooms.

FPV is partially deficient and requires an actively dividing cell to complete its replicative cycle. This property limits the number of cells that can be infected in vivo and thus the clinical disease produced (Carlson and Scott, 1977b).

There is only one serotype of FPV, but there is variation in virulence among various strains. The virus that causes mink enteritis (MEV) is antigenically identical to FPV (Gorham et al., 1965; Wills, 1952). Canine parvovirus (CPV) is closely related to FPV serologically but has distinct biologic properties. CPV first appeared in dogs in 1977 in Europe and in 1978 in the United States and then spread rapidly throughout the world. To date CPV has not been shown to produce illness in the cat, although cats may be infected experimentally.

*Alcide Corporation, 125 Main St., Westport, CT 06880.

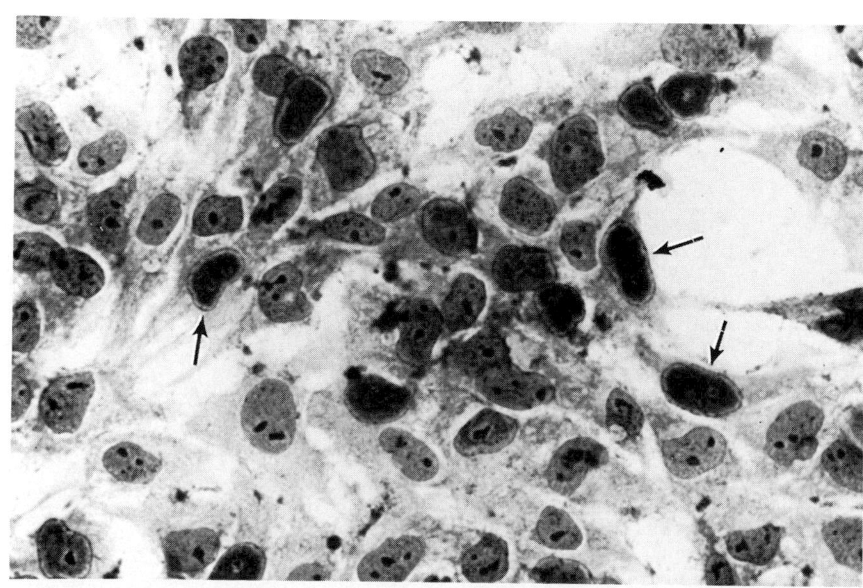

**Figure 7–1** Cell culture infected with feline panleukopenia virus (leopard virus strain) showing characteristic Cowdry type A intranuclear inclusions in several cells (arrows). Note the single, large, dark-staining intranuclear mass; the margination of chromatin to give a dark-staining nuclear membrane; and the light-staining halo inside the nuclear membrane. The cytoplasm is not affected until the latter stages of cytolysis.

## EPIZOOTIOLOGY

### Incidence

The incidence of clinical panleukopenia varies with the percentage of immune cats in the population, the virulence of the particular strain of virus, and the virulence of intestinal bacteria in the infected cats.

There tends to be a seasonal incidence (Reif, 1976) that coincides with the buildup of a suseptible population as young kittens lose their protective maternally derived immunity. The exact time of the year when this higher incidence occurs depends on the breeding season for that locality; however, panleukopenia can and does occur at any time of the year.

Although penleukopenia is predominantly a disease of young kittens two to four months of age, it can affect cats of all ages. Older cats, however, are more likely to develop subclinical or mild infections rather than the more severe disease afflicting kittens.

### Hosts

**FELIDAE.** The domestic cat is the primary host of FPV, but all members of the family Felidae are believed to be susceptible to FPV. Although it has been studied extensively in the domestic cat, only limited studies of panleukopenia in nondomestic cats have been reported. Cockburn (1947) summarized several outbreaks in a zoologic garden that caused high mortality in young cats (5 tigers, 17 leopards, 8 wild cats, 2 lynxes, 2 servals, 4 leopard cats, 7 tiger cats, 6 ocelots, 1 lyra cat, and 4 cheetahs). FPV has been isolated from fatal cases in lions (Johnson and Halliwell, 1968; Scott, unpublished data; Studdert et al., 1973), snow leopards (Johnson, 1964; Scott, unpublished data), tigers (Gray, 1972; Johnson and Halliwell, 1968; Theobald, 1978), and panthers (Johnson and Halliwell, 1968). Torres (1941) reported an outbreak of panleukopenia in wild felines in a zoo in Brazil, from which he experimentally transmitted panleukopenia to domestic cats. Species involved were *Felis maracaja, F. pardalis, F. concolor, F. onca*, and *Felis* sp.

**MUSTELIDAE.** Mink are highly susceptible to the mink strain of virus (MEV) but have subclinical infections with the cat strains of FPV. Ferrets can be infected in utero or neonatally (Kilham et al., 1967). Little information is available concerning the susceptibility to FPV of other Mustelidae such as skunks, otters, weasels, and badgers. Barker and coworkers (1983) were unable to produce clinical disease or establish infection in shunks inoculated with FPV.

**PROCYONIDAE.** The raccoon is highly susceptible to FPV (Barker et al., 1983), with outbreaks occurring on fur farms (Waller, 1940) and in raccoons in urban areas (Scott, unpublished data). FPV has been isolated from fatal cases in the coatimundi (Johnson and Halliwell, 1968; Scott, unpublished data).

**VIVERRIDAE.** Nair and associates (1964) reported an outbreak of gastroenteritis, presumably panleukopenia, in a group of 14 captive civet cats in India, with a 50 per cent mortality.

**CANIDAE.** Until the worldwide pandemic of CPV in 1977 and 1978, Canidae were generally believed to be resistant to FPV; however, Phillips (1943) reported an outbreak of hemorrhagic enteritis in the arctic blue fox from which he transmitted panleukopenia to experimental cats. Red foxes are susceptible to infection but may not show clinical disease (Barker et al., 1983).

### Transmission

Transmission is usually by direct contact between susceptible cats and infected cats, since virus is shed during the acute phase of the illness in all body secretions and excretions. Contaminated feed and water dishes, cages, bedding, litter boxes, rugs, and soil can serve as sources of virus capable of infecting a susceptible cat for many months and perhaps years. Virus can also be transmitted on contaminated clothing, shoes, and hands of humans. The rapid transmission of the related CPV throughout the world probably occurred in this way.

Aerosol transmission may occur, especially if the cat is coinfected with respiratory viruses so that it is sneezing. Insects and parasites, especially fleas, can transmit the virus as mechanical vectors (Torres, 1941).

## PATHOGENESIS

In newborn kittens nearly every tissue in the body contains virus after intranasal or oral inoculation (Csiza et al., 1971b). By 18 hours after inoculation, the virus has established itself, probably first in the oropharynx, and then a viremia develops. The virus is present in the thymus, heart, mesenteric lymph nodes, kidney, small intestine, and cerebellum. By two days after inoculation essentially every tissue has significant amounts of virus. High titers of virus remain in most tissues through seven days after inoculation. As circulating antibodies appear, titers gradually decrease until 14 days after inoculation when most tissues lose their virus. Although small quantities of virus may persist up to one year in certain tissues such as the kidney (Csiza et al., 1971a), the high titer of antibody effectively neutralizes the virus as it leaves infected cells so that most cats that have recovered from panleukopenia do not remain viral shedders for more than three weeks.

The most severely affected tissues in the newborn cat are those with cells undergoing rapid mitosis, namely the thymus and the external granular layer of the cerebellum. The small intestine, which has slow mitotic activity in the newborn, is not grossly or microscopically involved, although virus is present. At approximately nine days of age the cerebellum is no longer involved since the mitotic activity of its granular layer cells is reduced (Csiza et al., 1971b).

In older kittens, the pathogenesis also depends on the state of mitotic activity of the various tissues (Carlson et al., 1977a,b, 1978). Virus enters by the mouth, and infection occurs primarily in the lymphoid tissues of the oropharynx. The regional lymph nodes then become infected. Within 24 hours after ingesting virus the animal is viremic, and the virus is distributed throughout the body. The epithelial cells of the ileum and jejunum are particularly susceptible to FPV. Cytolytic replication of the virus in these cells destroys the epithelial lining of the crypts, producing ballooned, debris-filled crypts and shortened, blunted villi. If the mitotic rate of the crypt cells is low, as in germ-free kittens, the virus only destroys an occasional crypt cell and does not produce gross or microscopic lesions of the intestine (Carlson et al., 1977a,b, 1978). Other tissues with rapidly dividing cells (thymus, bone marrow, lymph nodes) are affected by the cytolytic replication of the virus.

Virus persists in the blood of the infected cat until about seven days after exposure (approximately the third day of illness), at which time circulating neutralizing antibodies appear (Fig. 7–2). The antibody titer increases rapidly and reaches its maximum by about 14 days after inoculation. With the appearance of antibody the virus in the various tissues gradually disappears. The virus may persist intracellularly where it is protected from antibodies for periods of several weeks, months, or years in certain tissues such as the kidney (Csiza et al., 1971b). However, shedding of virus is not common in cats that have recovered from panleukopenia. Generally, by three weeks after the illness, cats no longer shed infectious virus in the feces or urine; however, virus has been isolated from feces of a small percentage of recovered cats for several weeks after recovery.

Virus infecting a pregnant cat readily invades the uterus and crosses the placenta to infect the fetus (Csiza et al., 1971c). Infection then occurs throughout the fetus and crosses the blood-brain barrier to infect the cerebellum and other tissues within the central nervous system. The teratologic changes that result depend on the stage of gestation at the time of infection. Intrauterine infection may result in abortion, stillbirths, early neonatal deaths, or cerebellar hypoplasia or other teratologic changes. Evidence suggests that hydrocephalus may be a result of FPV infection during midgestation (Csiza et al., 1971c), similar to what has been described for mumps virus in rodents (Johnson and Johnson, 1968). Viral infection of the ependymal cells lining the aqueductus cerebri (aqueduct of Sylvius) and the third ventricle may result in loss of cells and subsequent healing with decreased diameter or closure of the lumen of the aqueduct. The caudal flow of cerebrospinal fluid (CSF) is impaired so that increased CSF pressure rostral to the lesion produces hydrocephalus.

In-utero or neonatal infection can result in cell damage in the retina, leading to retinal dysplasia but without loss of visual acuity (MacMillan, 1974; Percy et al., 1975). MacMillan (1974) reported focal retinal lesions in 31 per cent of kittens with naturally occurring cerebellar degeneration and ataxia due to FPV compared with less than 2 per cent in the general feline population.

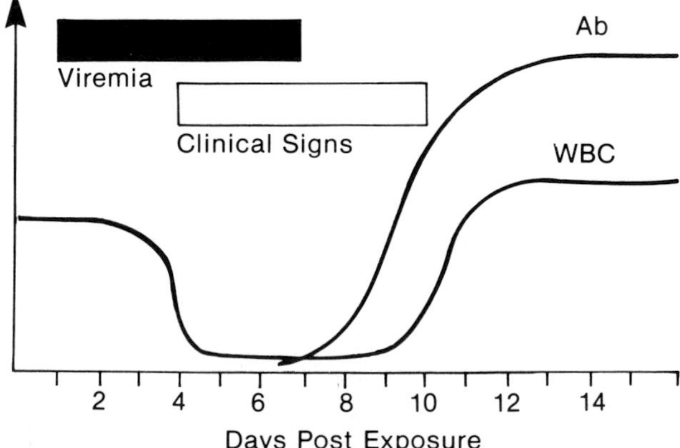


**Figure 7–2** Time line for feline panleukopenia. Note that cats are viremic by day 1, that clinical signs are concurrent with leukopenia, and that there is a rapid rebound in total leukocyte (WBC) count shortly after the appearance of humoral serum neutralizing antibodies (Ab).

Infection of queens during the first half of gestation can result in death of one or more fetuses with total resorption of dead fetuses and placental membranes if abortion does not occur. Later in gestation resorption of fluids from the dead fetus results in a dehydrated or mummified fetus and placenta, which may be retained until term. Queens infected during the latter half of gestation may give birth to litters containing normal healthy kittens, stillborn kittens, partly autolyzed fetuses, and mummified fetuses.

## Clinical Features

The incubation period can vary from two to seven days but usually is four or five days. In some natural cases it is longer. The illness varies from no outward signs to a rapidly fatal disease resembling an acute poisoning. For convenience, clinical signs will be discussed under five headings.

**PERACUTE.** Panleukopenia may progress so rapidly that an owner will state, "The cat was O.K. last night and dead this morning." Such cases are frequently presented as "poisonings." Illness develops rapidly with severe depression progressing within hours to coma and death. The cat may vomit but usually dies before diarrhea or dehydration has time to develop. Mortality in the peracute form of panleukopenia approaches 100 per cent.

**ACUTE OR TYPICAL FORM.** In the typical case of panleukopenia there is a sudden onset of clinical signs. The cat may have a temperature of 40 C (104 F) or higher and may show severe depression and complete anorexia. Vomiting is usual, and a severe fetid diarrhea may develop in 24 to 48 hours. Often the stool is blood-streaked or hemorrhagic and may contain stringy casts of fibrin-rich exudate. If the vomiting and diarrhea continue, severe dehydration and electrolyte imbalances occur.

Cats with panleukopenia often assume a typical attitude as exemplified in Figure 7–3. They crouch with their heads between their paws and often hang their heads over a water or feed dish. They frequently act as if they would like to drink and may even take a lap or two of milk or water but are unable or reluctant to swallow. The haircoat becomes rough and dull, and there is a loss of elasticity of the skin due to the dehydration. The third eyelid often appears prominent. The abdomen is tender, and abdominal palpation elicits signs of pain. The mesenteric nodes are enlarged, and the gastrointestinal tract contains excess gas and liquid.

Less common signs in natural infections have been described by Carpenter (1971) and are due to the depressed white-cell count and lowered resistance: purulent otitis, ulcerative and necrotic oral lesions, and cutaneous hemorrhage, infection, and "sloughs" at injection sites. Other occasional signs are mild jaundice and iritis with aqueous flare. A rare event is necrosis of the ear tips, perhaps owing to compromised circulation from fibrin thrombi (DIC). Areas of depigmentation occasionally develop on the brown masks of Siamese. Occasional cats are left with intestinal malabsorption due to fusing of villi and scarring of the mucosa.

Terminally, the temperature is subnormal, indicating a grave prognosis. Coma and death follow in a few hours.

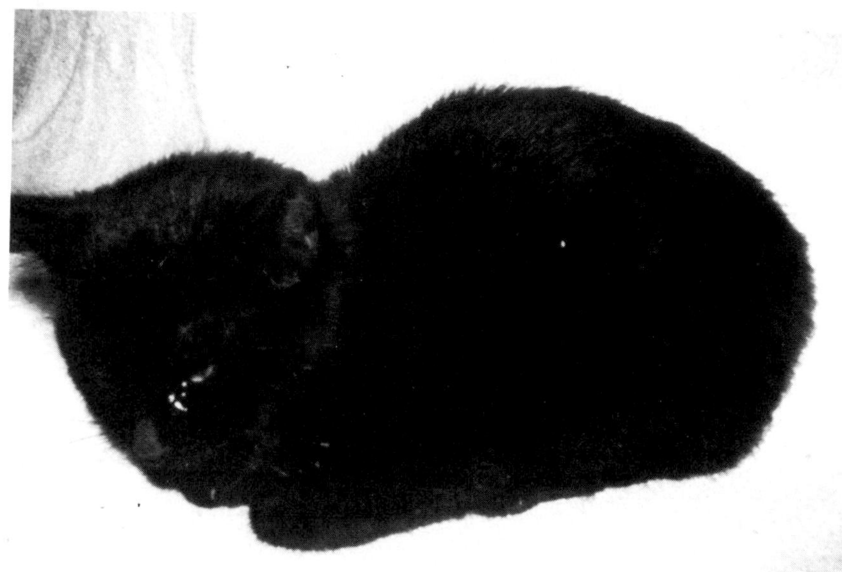

**Figure 7–3** Characteristic attitude of a kitten with typical panleukopenia. Note the hunched-up appearance with the head down between the paws. The chin may rest on the floor. The third eyelids usually are prominent.

The mortality in the acute form of panleukopenia may vary from 25 to 90 per cent in various outbreaks. Death may occur within the first five days of illness in uncomplicated cases or later in complicated cases. If the cat survives approximately five days of illness and secondary complications such as bacterial infections, dehydration, and chronic enteritis do not occur, then recovery should be fairly rapid. It is usually several weeks before the cat regains its lost weight and condition.

**SUBACUTE OR MILD FORM.** This form presents with a cat that is mildly depressed and not eating. Temperature may be slightly elevated, and abdominal palpation usually reveals gas in the intestines. Illness lasts for one to three days and recovery is usually rapid and uncomplicated.

**SUBCLINICAL.** FPV infections can occur without clinical signs of illness. Pregnant cats may show no signs of illness yet may later abort or give birth to kittens with neonatal panleukopenia in one or more of its many forms. Serologic and experimental studies indicate that subclinical infection is common in certain outbreaks. This is the usual form of the disease in germ-free kittens and kittens reared in extremely clean situations such as isolation units where pathogenic intestinal flora are absent.

**IN-UTERO INFECTION.** The clinical signs in kittens infected during late gestation or in the first few days after birth are either sudden death without any particular signs or the development of ataxia at two or three weeks of age when the kittens start to walk. The ataxia is a symmetric incoordination, evidenced by rolling or tumbling as the cat tries to walk, an involuntary twitching of the head, or swaying of the body. The stance is basewide with the tail held high and stiff for balance. The gait is hypermetric with the feet raised unusually high. These ataxic kittens are alert and strong. If they are coordinated enough to eat they will grow, but the ataxia will persist throughout life with little if any improvement or compensation.

Infection earlier in gestation with or without clinical signs of panleukopenia in the queen may result in fetal death with subsequent resorption, abortion, fetal mummification, or stillbirth.

**"CHRONIC" FP.** Although this diagnosis has been made by clinicians and pathologists, the author is not convinced that such a form of panleukopenia exists aside from the intestinal complications such as mycotic enteritis (Bolton and Brown, 1972; Schiefer, 1965). Each case of so-called chronic panleukopenia that has been investigated in the author's laboratory has turned out to be something other than panleukopenia. Most cases of chronic, persistent leukopenia, usually with anemia and often with enteritis, have been due to leukemia virus infection.

## Pathologic Features

The pathologic changes in panleukopenia have been described by many (e.g., Carlson et al., 1977a; Jubb and Kennedy, 1970; Langheinrich and Nielsen, 1971; Leasure et al., 1934; Riser, 1946; and Rohovsky and Griesemer, 1967). Except after peracute infections, cats that die appear gaunt, and dehydration is evidenced by sticky, dry tissues and sunken, soft eyes. There is usually evidence of vomiting and diarrhea.

The gross pathologic changes, if mild, may not be evident to the casual observer; if severe they are readily apparent, usually in the small intestine, primarily the ileum and jejunum (Fig. 7–4), less often in the duodenum and colon. The serosal and mucosal surfaces are often hyperemic or petechiated or both. The feces are yellowish gray, scant, and watery, with a fetid odor. Sometimes mural and intraluminal hemorrhage is present, and one or more casts of fibrin may be found. The mesenteric lymph nodes are edematous and may be hemorrhagic. The gastric mucosa is sometimes bile-stained and hemorrhagic. The esophagus is occasionally eroded or ulcerated, and in a few cats a tablet given as medication has been found adhering to the ulcerated mucosa. Oral ulcers and hyperemia and sloughing of the palate are occasionally present. Inflammation of the larynx, occurring in some cases, gave the disease one of its names, laryngo-enteritis.

Histopathologic changes are primarily restricted to tissues undergoing active cell mitosis. The most consistent and striking lesions are in the epithelium of the crypts of

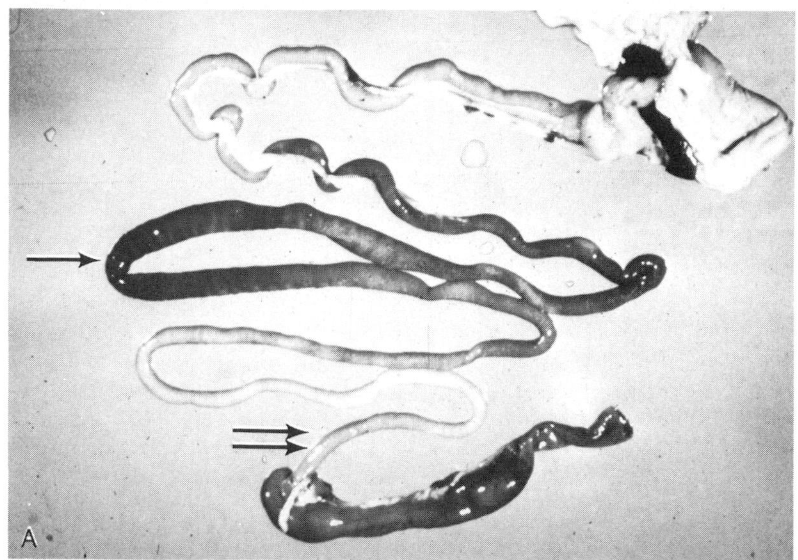


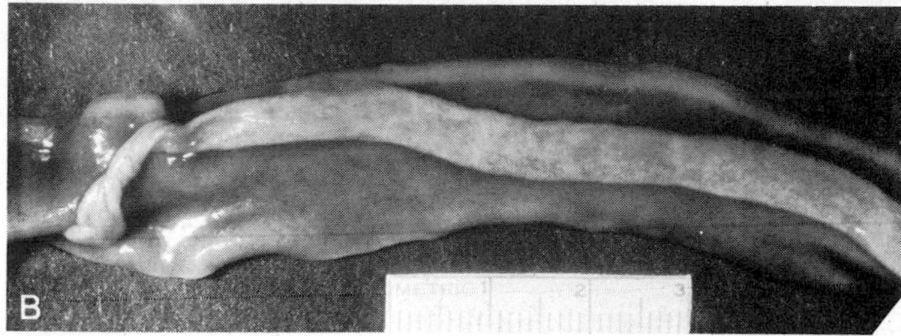


**Figure 7–4** *A,* Gross pathologic changes in the intestinal tract of a cat with panleukopenia. Note the turgid, hose-like appearance of the intestine and the dark, hemorrhagic jejunum (arrow). The ileum (double arrow) often shows extensive lesions as well. *B,* Fibrin cast in the small intestine of a cat with panleukopenia (Courtesy Angell Memorial Animal Hospital.)

the small intestine. Especially in the jejunum and ileum, the crypts are ballooned and filled with debris. The epithelial cells lining the crypts are in varying stages of degeneration or regeneration or may be sloughed off entirely so that the villi are shortened (Fig. 7–5). Intranuclear inclusions may be observed, especially in the crypt epithelial cells of the small intestine early in the disease. Bacteria are frequently found within the crypts and the lamina propria, as well as in other organs. The absence of an appropriate cellular response in the intestinal mucosa, owing to depressed numbers of white cells, is striking and characteristic. Vessels in all organs are usually devoid of leukocytes.

The liver often exhibits dissociation of hepatic cells and some degree of retention of bile pigment in hepatocytes and canaliculi.

The bone marrow and lymphoid tissues, such as the mesenteric nodes, spleen, and thymus, have a marked reduction in cellular elements and may have hemorrhages or red cells, or both, in the sinuses.

Bacterial culturing of affected tissues suggests that secondary infection with a variety of intestinal organisms, notably *E. coli,* is often the immediate cause of death. Fungal opportunists such as *Candida* and *Aspergillus* spp may also become involved. (See chapter on mycotic diseases.)

Disseminated intravascular coagulation (DIC) has been reported in some cases of panleukopenia in domestic cats and *Felis sylvestris* (Hoffman, 1973). Numerous microthrombi were present in peripheral blood vessels in renal medulla and cortex, liver, heart, lungs, and occasionally other organs. In another study 25 of 31 cats with panleukopenia had coagulation disturbances due to DIC (Kraft, 1973).

In kittens suffering from ataxia due to FPV, there is a gross reduction in the size of the cerebellum (Csiza et al., 1971c; de Lahunta, 1971; Kilham et al., 1971) (Fig. 7–6). Histologically, damage to the mitotic external germinal layer results in hypoplasia of the granular layer. The Purkinje cells are decreased in number and scattered. There may or may not be a correlation between the degree of hypoplasia and the clinical signs exhibited.

Kittens with FPV-induced hydrocephalus have an enlarged cranium with enlarged cerebral hemispheres due to dilated lateral and third ventricles. The cerebral cortex is thinned from increased pressure of the cerebrospinal fluid. The degree of disability and cerebellar abnormality may vary among kittens of the same litter. Some may be normal.

Newborn kittens that die from panleukopenia usually have minimal gross pathologic changes. The main lesion is a degeneration of the thymus. Hemorrhagic encephalopathy may be observed occasionally. Histologic examination reveals intranuclear inclusions in many tissues, especially the heart (Csiza et al., 1971b).

## Diagnosis

Panleukopenia is both overdiagnosed and underdiagnosed. To diagnose panleukopenia in all seriously ill cats with leukopenia is to overdiagnose the disease. On the other hand, panleukopenia may be misdiagnosed, especially in the peracute and mild forms. The diagnosis

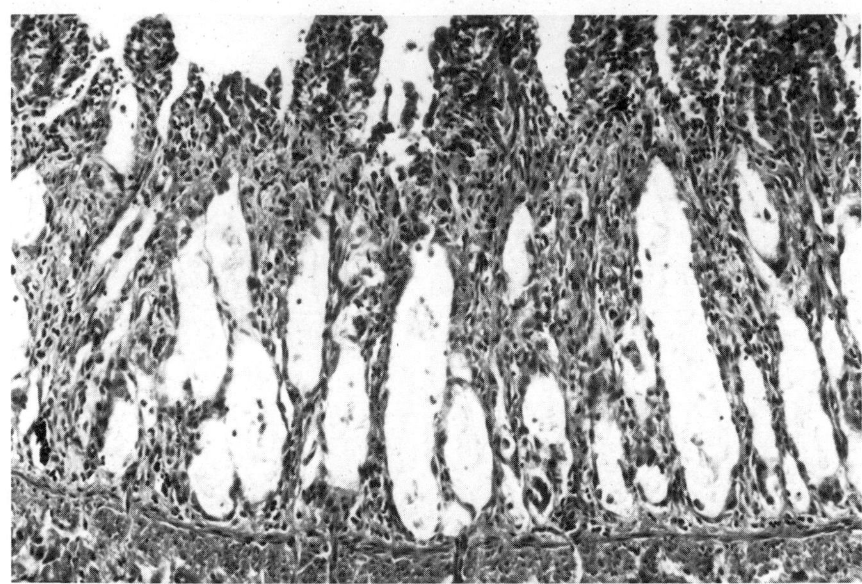

**Figure 7–5** Histopathologic appearance of the small intestine of a cat with panleukopenia. Note the enlarged, ballooned crypts devoid of epithelial cells and the shortened, blunted, fused villi.

is based on history, clinical signs, and the presence of leukopenia and may be confirmed by gross and microscopic changes and various laboratory tests.

## History

The history is very important, especially as regards age, vaccination record, and contact with strange cats within the previous two weeks (for example, in a boarding kennel, hospital, or adoption shelter). A sick, unvaccinated cat less than one year of age is highly suspect. A history of vaccination does not, however, rule out the possibility of panleukopenia. Maternally derived immunity can interfere with vaccination and leave a kitten susceptible after the maternally derived immunity has waned (Scott et al., 1970). This is more likely to occur if the kitten was last vaccinated when less than 12 weeks of age. An older cat vaccinated as a kitten without periodic revaccinations may lose its immunity after a few years. How often this happens is unknown.

## Hematology

The most characteristic laboratory finding in panleukopenia is the leukopenia, which is present in almost all infected cats even if they do not show clinical signs. There is usually a direct correlation between the severity of the leukopenia and the severity of the disease (Scott et al., 1970). A progressive drop in circulating white cells occurs one to two days before the development of clinical signs with a precipitous drop on the day of the crisis (see Fig. 7–2). The white-cell count usually is 4000 to 8000/$\mu$l in subclinical infections and less than 4000/$\mu$l in clinical infections. Counts below 2000/$\mu$l warrant a guarded prognosis. Owing to the extreme reduction in neutrophils, a relative lymphocytosis may occur, but as the disease progresses the lymphocytes may disappear also. A white-cell count of 0 to 200/$\mu$l is not unusual (Lawrence et al., 1940). If the cat survives for approximately five days after the onset of signs there is a dramatic rebound in the white-cell count (with a marked left shift), often exceeding

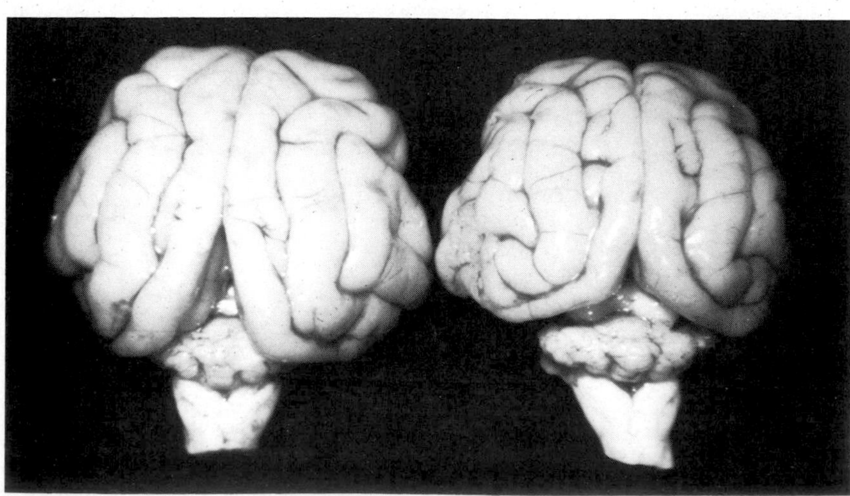

**Figure 7–6** Cerebellar hypoplasia of two 8-week-old littermates. The kittens had shown ataxia since they began to walk.

the upper normal limit in another three to four days (Riser, 1947; Schalm et al., 1975; Scott et al., 1970).

The course of typical infection is so rapid that there is no significant fall in PCV. Anemia may develop; however, if there is hemorrhage into the intestine, or if recovery is prolonged.

## Viral Isolation and Serology

Diagnosis of panleukopenia can be confirmed by viral isolation, serologic tests, or pathologic changes. Viral isolation can be done in cell cultures or by immunofluorescence. Swabs may be taken from the pharynx or the rectum, placed in viral transport medium or frozen, and submitted to a diagnostic laboratory equipped to do feline viral isolations. The best tissues to submit for viral isolation from autopsied animals are spleen, thymus, ileum, and mesenteric lymph node. These samples should be placed in sterile vials and either transmitted directly to the laboratory or frozen and submitted under dry ice refrigeration. For immunofluorescence, tissues from autopsied animals should be snap-frozen in liquid nitrogen and submitted for sectioning and staining. Impression films can also be taken of the spleen or mesenteric lymph node and fixed in cold acetone; the dried slide is then submitted to the diagnostic laboratory. Electron microscopic examination of fecal samples for typical parvovirus will also confirm the diagnosis.

For the serologic diagnosis of panleukopenia, paired serum samples (1 ml) are required. One blood specimen is taken during the acute phase of the disease and a second sample two weeks later. The serum samples are frozen until submitted to the laboratory, but they may be shipped by regular mail without refrigeration. Paired serum samples are required since results of a single sample are meaningless in establishing a diagnosis. Hemolysis does not affect the validity of the test.

## Differential Diagnosis

**FELINE LEUKEMIA VIRUS (FeLV) INFECTION.** FeLV infection can be differentiated from panleukopenia by the persistent, unresponsive leukopenia and anemia (not usually seen in panleukopenia) in a cat six months to two years of age with a good panleukopenia vaccination history. A blood film for IFA or serum for ELISA, if tested and found positive for FeLV antigen, provides a positive diagnosis of FeLV infection.

**SEVERE RESPIRATORY INFECTION.** Acute, severe respiratory infections can cause cats to be seriously depressed and dehydrated. While the respiratory infection is obvious, whether or not the cat also has panleukopenia is not so obvious. The total white-cell count is usually normal or elevated if panleukopenia is not present.

**TYZZER'S DISEASE.** Tyzzer's disease, caused by *Bacillus piliformis*, can produce symptoms identical to those of panleukopenia and can only be differentiated at autopsy by liver necrosis and the presence of the characteristic organisms on histologic examination of liver and small intestine (Kovatch and Zebarth, 1973). This infection probably occurs secondarily to panleukopenia in some cases.

**SEVERE BACTERIAL INFECTION.** Severe infections can result in a toxic leukopenia. Careful examination will usually reveal the source of the bacterial infection. *Salmonella* has been reported to produce a fatal gastroenteritis in cats (Timoney et al., 1978).

**OTHER VIRAL ENTERITIDES.** Several intestinal viruses have recently been identified in cats. In addition to FPV and FeLV, feline calicivirus can produce enteritis. One or more intestinal coronaviruses in addition to infectious peritonitis virus have been identified (Hoshino and Scott, 1980; Pedersen et al., 1981). A feline rotavirus and an astrovirus have also been isolated. The exact role of these intestinal viruses as intestinal pathogens awaits further study (Hoshino et al., 1981).

**INTESTINAL FOREIGN BODY.** The presence of intestinal foreign bodies such as string, cellophane, or broom straws can result in diagnostic challenges and can be confused with panleukopenia (Carpenter, 1971). A thorough physical examination, a complete blood count, and, if needed, a barium series will differentiate the two conditions.

**ACUTE POISONING.** Acute poisoning, such as with thallium, can mimic peracute panleukopenia (Carpenter, 1971).

**ACUTE TOXOPLASMOSIS.** Toxoplasmosis involving liver, pancreas, or intestine is occasionally misdiagnosed as panleukopenia. Both conditions are characterized by high fever and leukopenia. In toxoplasmosis, however, the fever tends to remain consistently or intermittently high and jaundice usually develops. Iritis is frequent. Terminal bronchopneumonia is characteristic of toxoplasmosis.

# TREATMENT

Panleukopenia usually has a high mortality rate, but with diligent treatment and good nursing care the fatalities can be reduced. The main object in treatment is to support the cat in reasonably good condition until the natural defenses take over, that is, the rebound in white cells and the appearance of antibody. Serum antibodies usually appear about three to four days after the first signs of the disease, and two to three days later a sharp rebound in total white cells occurs (see Fig. 7–2). If the cat can be maintained without complications for five to seven days the chances of recovery are usually good.

More specifically, the object of treatment is to correct and prevent the symptomatic abnormalities such as vomiting, diarrhea, and dehydration and to prevent secondary bacterial infections (Cotter, 1980; Ott, 1975; Scott, 1971b). The only specific treatment available is antiserum, and there are conflicting opinions as to its benefit once clinical signs have appeared. Some clinicians believe that antiserum is beneficial early in the disease.

The most important aspect of treatment is maintenance of fluid and electrolyte balances. To prevent the loss of fluids, parenteral administration of antiemetics and anticholinergic drugs may be indicated. For fluid replacement, 5 per cent dextrose in saline solution, lactated Ringer's solution, or 5 per cent dextrose in electrolyte replacer solution formulated for replacement of electrolytes lost in vomiting and diarrhea is indicated. These fluids should be administered intravenously (or subcutaneously as a poor second choice) at the rate of 5 to 15 ml/lb of body weight every 12 hours. Whole-blood transfusions, 10 ml/lb of body weight, have been reported to be highly beneficial (Kowall, 1974; Kraft, 1973; Ott, 1975; Scott, 1971b), especially if a cat is hypoproteinemic or hemorrhaging from the intestine.

Kraft (1973) reported that cats with severe DIC responded best when treated with heparin (100 units/kg) IV b.i.d. or t.i.d. in combination with whole blood transfusions or IV electrolyte solutions. (See also DIC, in chapter on the hematopoietic system.)

Broad-spectrum antibiotics are used in all cases since secondary bacterial infections are common. These antibiotics are administered parenterally until the gastroenteritis is controlled. Then they may be administered orally for a total of five days.

B-complex vitamins should be supplied parenterally until the cat is again eating well. Appetite may be stimulated by diazepam injections (0.01 mg/kg IV every eight hours for two or three days). All food should be withheld until the gastroenteritis is controlled. Then strained baby foods can be fed in small quantities several times a day.

Secondary viral respiratory infections are common complications, since the stress of panleukopenia may trigger a latent respiratory virus infection, or there may have been dual infections from simultaneous exposure to two or more viruses. This dual viral infection is more severe than if either of the viruses alone had infected the cat. The secondary viral infections should be treated as indicated.

There is no treatment for cats showing ataxia.

## PREVENTION

Several excellent vaccines are available for immunization. They are effective and inexpensive and confer long-lasting immunity. Panleukopenia vaccines are usually combined with feline viral rhinotracheitis (FVR) and feline calicivirus (FCV) vaccines and sometimes with feline pneumonitis vaccine. Since panleukopenia is entirely preventable with proper immunization, clinicians should emphasize the importance of proper vaccination. Considerable information has been published evaluating the types of vaccines and various vaccination recommendations (Bittle et al., 1970; Davis et al., 1970; Gorham et al., 1965; Povey, 1973; Sampson et al., 1972; Scott, 1971a, 1972, 1980b; Scott and Gillespie, 1971). Immunization against panleukopenia should be started at the first visit or at eight to nine weeks of age, whichever comes first. Tissue culture–origin vaccines, either inactivated or modified live (MLV), should be used. Vaccines should be repeated at four-week intervals until the kitten is at least 12 weeks of age. If the kitten is 12 weeks of age or older when the first vaccination with MLV is given, a second vaccination is not necessary. In rare instances, however, a kitten's level of maternal antibody may be high enough to prevent effective immunization for longer than 12 weeks, and later the cat may be susceptible to infection (Fig. 7–7).

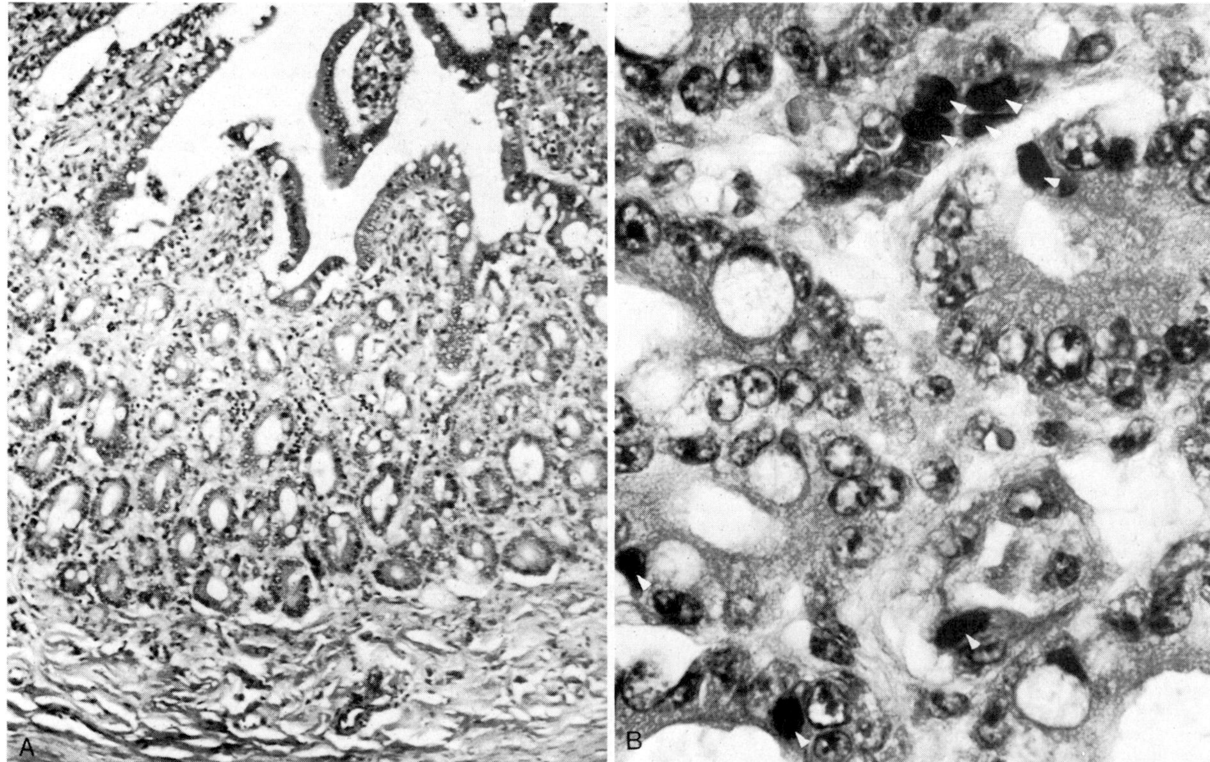


**Figure 7–7** *A,* Duodenal mucosa from a five-month-old kitten that was presented moribund after only six hours of abdominal discomfort. The kitten had received MLV vaccinations at 9 and 12 weeks of age but became ill several days after visiting the hospital clinic for treatment of coccidiosis. The epithelium, almost intact, contains numerous intranuclear inclusion bodies in the cells at the middle and lower portions of the crypts. H & E, × 120. *B,* Same kitten. The white arrows point to basophilic intranuclear inclusions in the crypt epithelium. H & E × 760. (Photomicrographs courtesy Dr. Joseph Alroy and Angell Memorial Animal Hospital.)

The choice of inactivated or MLV vaccine depends on the clinician's preference and any special circumstances. Inactivated vaccines are safe and can be given to any cat, even pregnant queens. Two doses are usually required initially, with annual or biannual revaccinations. The MLV vaccines produce high titers with a single vaccination after maternally derived immunity has been lost and theoretically should produce a longer period of protection. It is clear that MLV vaccines produce faster protection, usually within one or two days (Davis et al., 1970; Scott, 1980b). They definitely are indicated where exposure to FPV is likely, as in adoption shelters or veterinary hospitals. MLV vaccines definitely should not be given to pregnant queens.

Both types of vaccines produce immunity for long periods of time. Since the exact duration of immunity is not known, annual revaccinations are recommended for maximum protection. This is especially pertinent for apartment cats that usually are not exposed to street viruses. Cats that have recovered from FPV infection (clinical disease or subclinical infection) are immune for life.

Maternally derived immunity must be considered when establishing a vaccination program, since it is the most common cause of vaccine failure (Scott et al., 1970). There is a direct correlation between the titer of the queen at the time of parturition and the duration of passive immunity acquired via the colostrum by the kitten. This passive immunity, if present in sufficient quantities, not only will protect the kitten against virulent virus but also will interfere with vaccination. Thus vaccination must be done after the kitten has lost all or the majority of its maternally derived immunity.

The use of antiserum to passively immunize cats against panleukopenia is indicated for unvaccinated cats that have been exposed or probably will be exposed to virus before there is sufficient time to develop an immune response after vaccination. Antiserum should be given to such exposed cats at the rate of 2 ml/kg of body weight. Antiserum is also indicated for colostrum-deprived or orphaned kittens as soon after birth as possible. The routine use of antiserum for unexposed kittens is not recommended. Instead, these kittens should be vaccinated at their first visit to the veterinarian's office, regardless of age, and revaccinated as indicated. In the absence of specific antiserum, commercial feline homologous or normal serum usually contains adequate titers of panleukopenia antibodies. If neither is available, effective serum can be obtained from healthy hospital blood donor cats (FeLV- and coronavirus-negative) that have been vaccinated with a MLV panleukopenia vaccine at least two weeks previously.

Exotic Felidae should be vaccinated on the same vaccination schedule as domestic cats. Contrary to earlier recommendations, MLV vaccines should be used. For as yet unknown reasons, some large cats do not respond adequately when vaccinated with inactivated panleukopenia vaccines. The author has isolated FPV from lions and snow leopards that had received multiple vaccinations with inactivated vaccines yet had died of panleukopenia during an outbreak in the zoologic park. Exotic cats develop protective antibody titers following MLV vaccines without adverse reactions to vaccination (Fowler and Theobald, 1978; Gray, 1972; Laughlin, 1980).

## Public Health Significance

FPV does not infect man and thus has no public health significance. However, with the apparent mutations of the parvoviruses to cause new diseases in mink and dogs, one cannot help but wonder if these parvoviruses have a predilection to mutate, and if so, could one of these mutate to infect man.

## REFERENCES


Arlein MS: So-called infectious feline enteritis or panleucopenia. North Am Vet 21 (1940) 733–737.

Barker IK, Povey RC, Voight DR: Response of mink, skunk, red fox and raccoon to inoculation with mink virus enteritis, feline panleukopenia and canine parvovirus and prevalence of antibody to parvovirus in wild carnivores in Ontario. Can J Comp Med 47(1983) 188–197.

Bisbocci G: Ricerche batteriologiche sui germi d'irruzione secondaria nella gastro-enterite infettiva dei gatti. Boll Ist Sieroter Milan 15 (1936) 501–507.

Bittle JL, Emrich SA, Gauker FB: Safety and efficacy of an inactivated tissue culture vaccine for feline panleukopenia. J Am Vet Med Assoc 157 (1970) 2052–2056.

Bolton GR, Brown TT: Mycotic colitis in a cat. Vet Med Small Anim Clin 67 (1972) 978–981.

Buniva: Observations et expériences sur la maladie épizootique des chats, qui règne depuis quelques années en France, en Allemagne, en Italie et en Angleterre. Rec Périod Soc Méd 7 (1800) 269–292.

Burger D: The relationship of mink virus enteritis to feline panleukopenia virus. Pullman, Washington State University, Thesis, 1961.

Burger D, Gorham JR, Ott RL: Protection of cats against feline panleucopenia following mink virus enteritis vaccination. Small Anim Clin 3 (1963) 611–614.

Carlson JH, Scott FW, Duncan JR: Feline panleukopenia. I. Pathogenesis in germfree and specific pathogen-free cats. Vet Pathol 14 (1977a) 79–88.

Carlson JH, Scott FW: Feline panleukopenia. II. The relationship of intestinal mucosal cell proliferation rates to viral infection and development of lesions. Vet Pathol 14 (1977b) 173–181.

Carlson JH, Scott FW, Duncan JR: Feline panleukopenia. III. Development of lesions in the lymphoid tissues. Vet Pathol 15 (1978) 383–392.

Carpenter JL: Feline panleukopenia: clinical signs and differential diagnosis. J Am Vet Med Assoc 158 Suppl 2 (1971) 857–859.

Cockburn A: Infectious enteritis in the Zoological Gardens, Regent's Park. [Br] Vet J 103 (1947) 261–262.

Cotter SM: Feline panleukopenia. *In* Kirk RW (ed): Current Veterinary Therapy VII. Philadelphia, W B Saunders Company, 1980, 1286–1288.

Csiza CK, Scott FW, de Lahunta A, Gillespie JH: Immune carrier state of feline panleukopenia virus–infected cats. Am J Vet Res 32 (1971a) 419–426.

Csiza CK, de Lahunta A, Scott FW, Gillespie JH: Pathogenesis of feline panleukopenia virus in susceptible newborn kittens. II. Pathology and immunofluorescence. Infect Immun 3 (1971b) 838–846.

Csiza CK, Scott FW, de Lahunta A, Gillespie JH: Feline viruses. XIV. Transplacental infections in spontaneous panleukopenia of cats. Cornell Vet 61 (1971c) 423–439.

Csiza CK, de Lahunta A, Scott FW, Gillespie JH: Spontaneous feline ataxia. Cornell Vet 62 (1972) 300–322.

Dalling T: Distemper of the cat. Vet Rec 14 (1934) 1137–1148.

Davis EV, Gregory GG, Beckenhauer WH: Infectious feline panleukopenia (developmental report of a tissue culture origin formalin-inactivated vaccine). Vet Med Small Anim Clin 65 (1970) 237–242.

de Lahunta A: Comments on cerebellar ataxia and its congenital transmission in cats by feline panleukopenia virus. J Am Vet Med Assoc 158 Suppl 2 (1971) 901–906.

Enders JF, Hammon WD: Active and passive immunization against the virus of malignant panleucopenia of cats. Proc Soc Exp Biol Med 43 (1940) 194–200.

Fairweather J: Epidemic among cats in Delhi resembling cholera. Lancet 2 (1876) 115–117, 148–150.

Findlay GM: Cat distemper. [Br] Vet J 89 (1933) 17–20.

Fowler ME, Theobald J: Immunizing procedures. *In* Fowler ME (ed): Zoo and Wild Animal Medicine. Philadelphia, W B Saunders Company, 1978, 613–617.

Gillespie JH, Scott FW: Feline viral infections. Adv Vet Sci Comp Med 17 (1973) 163–200.

Gorham JR, Hartsough GR, Burger D, Lust S, Sato N: The preliminary use of attenuated feline panleukopenia virus to protect cats against panleukopenia and mink against virus enteritis. Cornell Vet 55 (1965) 559–566.

Goss LJ: Species susceptibility to the viruses of Carré and feline enteritis. Am J Vet Res 9 (1948) 65–68.

Gray C: Immunization of the exotic felidae for panleukopenia. J Zoo Anim Med 3 (1972) 14–15.

Hall R: Observations respecting an epidemic disease among cats which prevailed in the neighborhood of Jedburgh. Ann Med 5 (1801) 481–482.

Hammon WD, Enders JF: A virus disease of cats, principally characterized by aleucocytosis, enteric lesions and the presence of intranuclear inclusion bodies. J Exp Med 69 (1939a) 327–352.

Hammon WD, Enders JF: Further studies on the blood and the hematopoietic tissues in malignant panleucopenia of cats. J Exp Med 70 (1939b) 557–564.

Hindle E, Findlay GM: Studies on feline distemper. J Comp Pathol Ther 45 (1932) 11–26.

Hoffman R: [Consumption coagulopathy in spontaneous panleukopenia in domestic and wild cats]. Berl Münch Tierärztl Wochenschr 86 (1973) 72–74.

Hoshino Y, Scott FW: Coronavirus-like particles in the feces of normal cats. Arch Virol 63 (1980) 147–152.

Hoshino Y, Baldwin CA, Scott FW: Isolation and characterization of feline rotavirus. J Gen Virol 54 (1981) 313–323.

Jarmai K: Über die durch ein filtrierbares Virus versursachte Magen- und Darmentzündung der Katzen. Dtsch Tierärztl Wochenschr 42 (1934) 401–403; Allatorv Lapok 57 (1934) 43–45.

Johnson RH: Isolation of a virus from a condition simulating feline panleucopaenia in a leopard. Vet Rec 76 (1964) 1008–1013.

Johnson RH: Feline panleucopaenia. I. Identification of a virus associated with the syndrome. Res Vet Sci 6 (1965) 466–471.

Johnson RH: Feline panleucopenia virus. III. Some properties compared to a feline herpes virus. Res Vet Sci 7 (1966) 112–115.

Johnson RH: Feline panleukopenia. Vet Rec 84 (1969) 338–340.

Johnson RH, Halliwell REW: Natural susceptibility to feline panleucopenia of the coati-mundi. Vet Rec 82 (1968) 582.

Johnson RH, Margolis G, Kilham L: Identity of feline ataxia virus with feline panleucopenia virus. Nature 214 (1967) 175–177.

Johnson RT, Johnson KP: Hydrocephalus following viral infection: the pathology of aqueductal stenosis developing after experimental mumps virus infection. J Neuropathol Exp Neurol 27 (1968) 591–606.

Jubb KVF, Kennedy PC: Pathology of Domestic Animals, 2nd ed., vol 2. New York, Academic Press, 1970, 131–134.

Kilham L, Margolis GM: Viral etiology of spontaneous ataxia of cats. Am J Pathol 48 (1966) 991–1011.

Kilham L, Margolis G, Colby ED: Congenital infections of cats and ferrets by feline panleukopenia virus manifested by cerebellar hypoplasia. Lab Invest 17 (1967) 465–480.

Kilham L, Margolis G, Colby ED: Cerebellar ataxia and its congenital transmission in cats by feline panleukopenia virus. J Am Vet Med Assoc 158 Suppl 2 (1971) 888–901.

King DA, Croghan DL: Immunofluorescence of feline panleucopenia virus in cell culture: determination of immunological status of felines by serum neutralization. Can J Comp Med Vet Sci 29 (1965) 85–89.

Kovatch RM, Zebarth G: Naturally occurring Tyzzer's disease in a cat. J Am Vet Med Assoc 162 (1973) 136–138.

Kowall NL: Feline panleukopenia. *In* Kirk RW (ed): Current Veterinary Therapy V. Philadelphia, W B Saunders Company, 1974, 957–959.

Kraft W: [Thromboelastogram of healthy domestic cats and the treatment of disseminated intravascular coagulation in panleukopenia]. Berl Münch Tierärztl Wochenschr 86 (1973) 394–396.

Krembs J, Seifried O: Untersuchungen über die Laryngoenteritis infectiosa der Katzen. I Mitteilung. Arch Wissensch Prakt Tierheilkd 70 (1936) 259–277.

Langheinrich KA, Nielsen SW: Histopathology of feline panleukopenia: a report of 65 cases. J Am Vet Med Assoc 158 Suppl 2 (1971) 863–872.

Laughlin DC: Immunization of exotic cats. *In* Kirk RW (ed): Current Veterinary Therapy VII. Philadelphia, W B Saunders Company, 1980, 1258–1261.

Lawrence JS, Syverton JT: Spontaneous agranulocytosis in the cat. Proc Soc Exp Biol Med 38 (1938) 914–918.

Lawrence JS, Syverton JT, Shaw JS Jr, Smith FP: Infectious feline agranulocytosis. Am J Pathol 16 (1940) 333–354.

Lawrence JS, Syverton JT, Ackart RJ, Adams WS, Ervin DM, Haskins AL Jr, Saunders RH Jr, Stringfellow MB, Wetrich RM: The virus of infectious feline agranulocytosis. II. Immunological relation to other viruses. J Exp Med 77 (1943) 57–64.

Leasure EE, Lienhardt HF, Taberner FR: Feline infectious enteritis. North Am Vet 15 (7) (1934) 30–44.

Lombard C: Contribution à l'étude anatomopathologique de la gastro-entérite infectieuse des chats. Rev Vét 86 (1934) 268–270.

Lucas AM, Riser WH: Intranuclear inclusions in panleukopenia of cats. A correlation with the pathogenesis of the disease and comparison with inclusions of herpes, B-virus, yellow fever, and burns. Am J Pathol 21 (1945) 435–465.

Lupu A: Gastro-enterita contagiosa a pisicilor. Arhiva Vet 26 (1934) 189–215.

MacMillan AD: Retinal dysplasia and degeneration in the young cat: feline panleukopenia virus as an etiological agent. University of California–Davis, PhD Thesis, 1974.

MacPherson LW: Feline enteritis virus—its transmission to mink under natural and experimental conditions. Can J Comp Med 20 (1956) 197–202.

Margolis G, Kilham L, Johnson RN: Ataxia, panleucopenia and enteritis: change of viral target with maturation of host. J Neuropathol Exp Neurol 27 (1968) 133–135.

Milks HJ, Goldberg SA: Infectious enteritis of cats. Cornell Vet 10 (1920) 189–202.

Momberg-Jorgensen HC: Kattesyge [Cat distemper]. Maanedsskr Dyrlaeg 49 (1938) 685–695.

Nair KPD, Iyer RP, Venugopalan A: An outbreak of gastroenteritis in civet cats. Indian Vet J 41 (1964) 763–765.

Ott RL: Viral diseases. *In* Catcott EJ (ed): Feline Medicine and Surgery, 2nd ed. Santa Barbara, American Veterinary Publications Inc, 1975, 17–62.

Pedersen NC, Boyle JF, Floyd K, Fudge A, Barker J: An enteric coronavirus infection of cats and its relationship to feline infectious peritonitis. Am J Vet Res 42 (1981) 368–377.

Percy DH, Scott FW, Albert DM: Retinal dysplasia due to feline panleukopenia virus infection. J Am Vet Med Assoc 167 (1975) 935–937.

Phillips CE: Haemorrhagic enteritis in the arctic blue fox caused by the virus of feline enteritis (preliminary report). Can J Comp Med J (1943) 33–35.

Poole GM: Stability of a modified, live panleucopenia virus stored in liquid phase. Appl Microbiol 24 (1972) 663–664.
Povey RC: Feline panleukopenia—which vaccine? J Small Anim Pract 14 (1973) 399–406.
Reif JS: Seasonality, natality and herd immunity in feline panleukopenia. Am J Epidemiol 103 (1976) 81–87.
Riser WH: The histopathology of panleucopenia (agranulocytosis) in the domestic cat. Am J Vet Res 7 (1946) 455–465.
Riser WH: The behavior of the peripheral blood elements in panleucopenia (agranulocytosis) of the domestic cat. Am J Vet Res 8 (1947) 82–90.
Rohovsky MW, Griesemer RA: Experimental feline infectious enteritis in the germfree cat. Pathol Vet 4 (1967) 391–410.
Sampson GR, Counter FT, Schlegel BF, Rathmacher, RP: Antibody response of cats vaccinated with an inactivated cell culture feline panleukopenia vaccine. J Am Vet Med Assoc 160 (1972) 1619–1621.
Schalm OW, Jain NC, Carroll EJ: Veterinary Hematology, 3rd ed. Philadelphia, Lea & Febiger, 1975, 679–682.
Schiefer B: Zur Histopathologie der durch Candida-, Aspergillus- und Mucor-Arten verursachten Darmmykosen bei Katzen mit Panleukopenie. Dtsch Tierärztl Wochenschr 72 (1965) 73–76.
Scott FW, Csiza CK, Gillespie JH: Maternally derived immunity to feline panleukopenia. J Am Vet Med Assoc 156 (1970) 439–453.
Scott FW: Comments on feline panleukopenia biologics. J Am Vet Med Assoc 158 (1971a) 910–915.
Scott FW: Feline panleukopenia. *In* Kirk RW (ed): Current Veterinary Therapy IV. Philadelphia, W B Saunders Company, 1971b, 644–649.
Scott FW, Gillespie JH: Immunization for feline panleukopenia. Vet Clin North Am 1 (1971) 231–240.
Scott FW: Feline panleukopenia vaccinations. Feline Pract 2 (2) (1972) 10–13.
Scott FW, Gillespie JH: Feline viral diseases. Vet Scope 17(1) (1973) 2–11.
Scott FW: Virucidal disinfectants and feline viruses. Am J Vet Res 41 (1980a) 410–414.
Scott FW: Update on feline immunization. *In* Kirk RW (ed): Current Veterinary Therapy VII. Philadelphia, W B Saunders Company, 1980b, 1256–1258.
Slater EA, Kucera CJ: Panleukopenia Vaccine. US patent #3293130. Filed Nov. 27, 1962, dated Dec. 20, 1966.
Studdert MJ, Kelly CM, Harrigan KE: Isolation of panleucopenia virus from lions. Vet Rec 93 (1973) 156–158.
Syverton JT, Lawrence JS, Ackart RJ, Adams WS, Ervin DM, Haskins AL Jr, Saunders RH Jr, Stringfellow MB, Wetrich RM: The virus of infectious feline agranulocytosis. I. Characters of the virus: Pathogenicity. J Exp Med 77 (1943) 41–56.
Theobald J: Felidae. *In* Fowler ME (ed): Zoo and Wild Animal Medicine. Philadelphia, W B Saunders Company, 1978, 650–667.
Thorshaug K: "Kattepest." Infektios gastro-enteritis hos katt. Norsk Vet-Tidsskr 51 (1939) 397–415.
Timoney JF, Neibert HC, Scott FW: Feline salmonellosis. A nosocomial outbreak and experimental studies. Cornell Vet 68 (1978) 211–219.
Torres S: Infectious feline gastroenteritis in wild cats. North Am Vet 22 (1941) 297–299.
Urbain A: Contribution à l'étude de la gastro-entérite infectieuse des chats. Ann Inst Pasteur 51 (1933) 202–214.
Verge J, Cristoforoni N: La gastro-entérite infectieuse des chats est-elle due à un virus filtrable? Compt Rend Soc Biol 99 (1928) 312–314.
Waller EF: Infectious gastro-enteritis in raccoons (Procyon lotor). J Am Vet Med Assoc 96 (1940) 266–268.
Wills CG: Notes on infectious enteritis of mink and its relationship to feline enteritis. Can J Comp Med Vet Sci 16 (1952) 419–420.

# CORONAVIRUS DISEASES (CORONAVIRUS ENTERITIS, FELINE INFECTIOUS PERITONITIS)

NIELS C. PEDERSEN

Coronaviruses are being isolated with increasing frequency from cats with a variety of conditions. In general, however, all the current isolates can be divided into two groups: (1) those that cause feline infectious peritonitis (FIP), i.e., FIP virus (FIPV), and (2) those that are associated with a transient and infrequently fatal enteritis, i.e., feline enteric coronavirus (FECV) (Pedersen et al., 1981a,b; Pedersen and Black, 1983). These various isolates are closely related to the transmissible gastroenteritis virus (TGEV) of swine and canine coronavirus (CCV) (Pedersen et al., 1978). A possible exception is the FECV isolate described by Dea and coworkers (1982), which is antigenically related to bovine coronavirus. The close antigenic relationship of various FIPV, FECV, TGEV, and CCV isolates has led some researchers to conclude that they are all strains of a single virus (Horzinek et al., 1982).

## CLASSIFICATION OF FELINE CORONAVIRUSES

Feline coronaviruses have been tentatively classified according to their antigenic relationships to either of two related groups of mammalian coronaviruses, the type of disease they cause, their growth characteristics in cell culture, and their similarity to CCV (Pedersen et al., 1984a). With such a classification scheme, the various feline coronavirus isolates can be categorized as follows:

A. Virus isolates related to mouse hepatitis virus, bovine coronavirus, human coronavirus OC43, and hemagglutinating encephalomyelitis virus of swine (Pedersen et al., 1978). With the possible exception of the FECV isolate of Dea and associates (1982), there are no characterized feline isolates in this group at the present time.

B. Virus isolates related to TGEV, human coronavirus 229E, and CCV (Pedersen et al., 1978).

Type I: difficult to grow in cell culture, grows best in selective macrophage-like cell lines, level of virus production in cell culture is low, antiserum to these strains reacts weakly in virus neutralization with heterologous strains such as CCV.

- FIP-inducing strains:
  - FIPV-UCD1
  - FIPV-UCD3
  - FIPV-UCD4
  - FIPV-TN406 (Black)
- enteritis-inducing strain:
  - FECV-UCD

Type II: easily isolated in cell culture, grows in many different cell lines, produced in large amounts in cell culture, cytopathic effect resembles that of CCV, antiserum to these strains reacts strongly in virus neutralization with CCV.

- FIP-inducing strains:
  - FIPV-79-1146
  - FIPV-UCD2
- enteritis-inducing strain:
  - FECV-79-1683

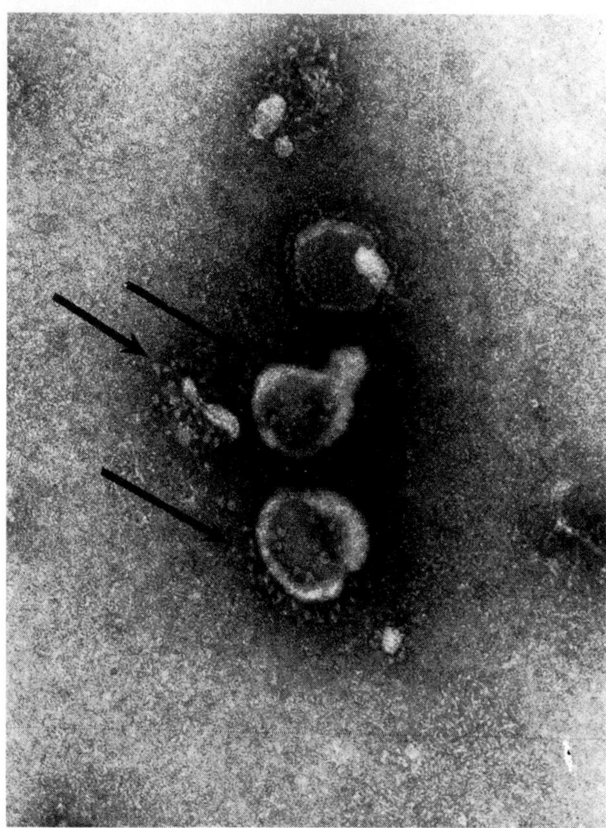

**Figure 7–8** Feline enteric coronavirus virions (arrows). Particles have numerous envelope projections called peplomers. The crown-like appearance produced by the peplomers gives the virus its name (crown = corona). Phosphotungstic acid stain, × 110,000.

## CORONAVIRUS ENTERITIS

Feline enteric coronaviruses causes inapparent or mild intestinal infections in kittens between birth and 12 weeks of age. Although they are morphologically and antigenically similar to FIPV, FECV strains do not cause FIP. To date, two different strains of FECV have been characterized. The first isolate, designated FECV-UCD, was described by Pedersen and coworkers (1981b). A second isolate was identified by McKeirnan and associates (1981) and has been designated FECV-79-1683 (Pedersen et al., 1984a, 1984b). FECV-79-1683 was isolated from a fatal case of peracute hemorrhagic enteritis in an adult cat. Like FECV-UCD, this strain produces a mild or inapparent enteritis in specific pathogen–free cats (Pedersen et al., 1984b). Coronavirus particles identical to those described for FECV-UCD have been identified in the stools of a cat with diarrhea by Dea and coworkers (1982). This isolate shared some antigens with calf diarrhea coronavirus. Hayashi and coworkers (1982) also observed a coronavirus in the intestine of a cat with diarrhea. This virus was antigenically similar to FIPV and was probably another FECV. Hoshino and Scott (1980a) have demonstrated coronavirus-like particles in the stool of normal cats, but they appeared morphologically and antigenically different from other FECV isolates.

Repeated attempts to grow FECV-UCD in cell culture have failed. The virus is currently maintained by in-vivo passage in kittens. FECV-79-1683 grows readily in cell culture, and it is similar to FIPV-79-1146 with regard to cytopathic effect, cell tropism, and level of free virus production (Pedersen et al., 1984a). It also seems to be more closely related to CCV than does FECV-UCD.

### Etiology

The feline enteric coronavirus is similar to other coronaviruses. On negative staining, surface projections radiate from the envelope (Fig. 7–8). These resemble a crown, hence the name coronavirus. The particles are very pleomorphic in stool specimens, ranging from 75 to 150 nm or more in diameter. The particle is virtually indistinguishable from FIP virus (compare Horzinek et al., 1977; Hoshino and Scott, 1980b; Pedersen et al., 1981b). Although its nucleic acid content has not been determined, it probably contains single-stranded RNA like other coronaviruses (Tyrrell et al., 1970). Serum antibodies to the enteric coronavirus cross-react in indirect fluorescent antibody, ELISA, and virus neutralization tests with FIPV, CCV, and TGEV of swine (Boyle et al., 1984; Pedersen et al., 1981b). Although they are morphologically and antigenically similar, prior infection with enteric coronaviruses does not render cats resistant to oral challenge with FIPV. In fact, heterotypic immunity to feline enteric coronavirus often renders cats more susceptible to parenteral FIPV challenge (Pedersen and Boyle, 1980; Pedersen et al., 1984b).

## Epizootiology

Earlier serologic studies of FIPV infection (Horzinek and Osterhaus, 1979a; Loeffler et al., 1978; Pedersen, 1976a) probably measured mainly the incidence of FECV rather than FIPV infection (Pedersen et al., 1981b). Feline enteric coronavirus infection appears, therefore, to be worldwide and infects 25 per cent or more of free-roaming cats. The infection is present within most catteries and multiple-cat households (Pedersen et al., 1981b), indicating that these types of environment are more conducive to disease. As many as 80 to 90 per cent of the cats within individual catteries and multiple-cat households will be seropositive (Pedersen et al., 1981b). The infection may recur throughout life in some cats and is manifested by waxing and waning of the coronavirus titers at intervals of several months to several years (Pedersen et al., 1981b).

### Source of Virus in Nature

Many antibody-positive cats shed feline enteric coronavirus (Pedersen et al., 1981b). Cats with higher coronavirus antibody titers, however, seem to be more infectious than cats with lower titers. Carrier cats shed the virus in their stools, and it can be readily transmitted from one animal quarter to another on caretakers' clothing.

## Pathogenesis

The pathogenesis of FECV infection is similar to that of CCV (Appel et al., 1979) and porcine TGE (Bohl, 1975) infections. This is not surprising, considering the close antigenic relationship of these viruses (Pedersen et al., 1981a,b). As in the porcine and canine diseases, enteritis occurs mainly in young animals. The queens pass on IgG antibodies in their colostrum (Pedersen et al., 1981b) and presumably IgA antibodies in their milk. These antibodies appear to have a protective function because kittens are not usually infected until some time between the fifth and tenth weeks of life.

The most accurate description of FECV infection has been acquired from studies with specific pathogen–free kittens (Pedersen et al., 1981b, 1984b). The disease in cattery-reared kittens is often inapparent. A mild or moderately severe diarrhea may persist for two to five days in some cats. The severity of the disease in specific pathogen–free kittens is somewhat age-dependent. Five-week-old kittens that are infected orally frequently develop clinical disease. The illness varies from moderately severe to inapparent depending on the individual. The infection in 12-week-old kittens is mild or inapparent but in adult cats is usually inapparent, although in isolated instances it can be severe or even fatal. Clinical disease is manifested by a low-grade fever beginning on the third to sixth day after infection. Just before fever develops, bowel movements may become more frequent and there may be intermittent vomiting. Within a day or so the stools become progressively more fluid and mucus-laden. Fresh blood sometimes appears in the stool. Kittens with clinical disease may become anorectic and lethargic for two or three days. If the enteritis is severe, they become dehydrated. Mortality, however, is extremely low. Fatal coronavirus enteritis in newborn kittens has been documented only once (McKeirnan et al., 1981). TGE virus, a closely related agent, is notorious for causing fatal disease in piglets several days to two weeks of age (Bohl, 1975), so neonatal disease cannot be excluded.

With the onset of diarrhea, the WBC often drops transiently to 50 per cent or less of normal (Pedersen et al., 1981b). The leukopenia is mainly due to a decrease in the absolute numbers of neutrophils. Antibodies appear in the serum from 10 to 14 days after infection, and titers reach levels of 1:32 to 1:1024 or greater as determined by the IFA procedure (Pedersen et al., 1981b, 1984b).

Gross lesions are not usually observed at autopsy. We have, however, seen one adolescent cat with naturally occurring disease that had pronounced mesenteric lymphadenopathy, edema of the bowel, and mucus-laden diarrheic stool.

The target tissue for the virus is the mature columnar epithelium of the intestinal tract from the mid-duodenum to the terminal ileum and cecum (Pedersen et al., 1981b, 1984b). The lesions are most severe in the jejunum and ileum. Except in severe cases, the infection tends to be patchy throughout the length of the involved intestine. Microscopically, lesions evolve as follows: vacuolation and syncytium formation of the mature epithelial cells on the tips of the intestinal villi; fusion of adjacent villi; sloughing of the infected epithelium and retraction of the villi (villous atrophy); covering of the denuded tips of villi with immature columnar epithelium; hyperplasia of the crypt epithelium; regeneration of the mature columnar epithelium; and re-establishment of normal villous architecture (Pedersen et al., 1981b). Diarrhea probably results from alterations in the transport of fluid and nutrients caused by the temporary loss of absorptive epithelium. A few small foci of infected epithelial cells can often be detected in the small bowel and cecum of recovered cats.

## Treatment

Food and water should be withheld during the more severe stages of the disease, and a balanced electrolyte solution should be administered parenterally if dehydration occurs. Systemic and intestinal antibiotic therapy is not necessary.

## Prevention

There is no way to prevent the infection in cats nor is there a need to do so in most situations. Nature limits the severity of the infection by providing most kittens with passive maternal protection during the critical first few weeks of life. Furthermore, the severity of disease is somewhat age-dependent and by weaning time the infection is often inapparent. The severity of the disease can be minimized by preventing as many postweaning stresses as possible and by keeping litters segregated by age. Newly weaned kittens are more likely to develop a severe disease if they are exposed to massive amounts of virus shed by other diseased kittens.

## FELINE INFECTIOUS PERITONITIS

Feline infectious peritonitis (FIP) is a generally fatal disease of domestic and some wild Felidae. Isolated cases of the disease were first described in the early 1960s (Feldman and Jortner, 1964; Holzworth, 1963). Earlier references to a disease that may have been FIP were made by Joshua (1960) and Smith and Jones (1961). The disease was recognized as a distinct entity and its infectious nature discovered several years later by Wolfe and Griesemer (1966), who gave it the name "feline infectious peritonitis." Ultrastructural evidence for a viral etiology was subsequently presented by Zook and coworkers (1968). The similarity of the FIP agent to viruses of the family Coronaviridae was first reported by Ward (1970).

### ETIOLOGY

Feline infectious peritonitis is caused by a coronavirus (Pedersen, 1976c; Ward, 1970). The virus is morphologically (compare Horzinek et al., 1977 and Pedersen et al., 1981b) and antigenically (Boyle et al., 1984; Pedersen et al., 1981a,b) similar to the FECV. It is also antigenically related to TGEV of swine and CCV (Pedersen et al., 1978; Reynolds et al., 1977, 1980; Witte et al., 1977; Woods and Pedersen, 1979; Woods et al., 1981) and HCV-229E (Pedersen et al., 1978a).

Feline infectious peritonitis virus is seen mainly in macrophages within lesions, where it replicates by budding from internal profiles of smooth endoplasmic reticulum (Beesly and Hitchcock, 1982; Pedersen, 1976c; Ward, 1970). It is easily identified in tissues of experimentally infected cats but has rarely been identified in spontaneously infected animals (Eugster and Liauw, 1979; Hayashi et al., 1978). As are other coronaviruses, the FIPV is about 100 nm in diameter, with 15 nm petal-shaped envelope projections called peplomers (Horzinek et al., 1977; Hoshino and Scott, 1980b). The nucleic acid is probably single-stranded RNA. The virus is relatively unstable outside the body, ether- and heat-labile, and very susceptible to most commonly used disinfectants (Pedersen, 1976c).

The FIPV was first propagated in vitro in macrophage cultures (Pedersen, 1976c) and later in whole-organ ring cultures of intestine and trachea (Hoshino and Scott, 1980b). More recently, it has been propagated in continuous and primary cultures of feline fetal cells (Black et al., 1980; Evermann et al., 1981; McKeirnan et al., 1981; O'Reilly et al., 1979; Pedersen et al., 1981a). It has also been adapted to grow in the brains of suckling mice, rats, and hamsters (Horzinek et al., 1978; Osterhaus et al., 1978).

#### Strains of Virus

A number of isolations of FIPV have been made throughout the world. Unfortunately, early isolates could be propagated only in vivo by serial passage in cats, so comparisons of isolates were difficult to make. Within the last several years, however, at least eight FIPV isolates have been cultivated in tissue culture: the isolate of O'Reilly and coworkers (1979), the NW1 (UCD1) strain (Pedersen et al., 1981a), the TN-406 (Black) strain (Black, 1980), the Nor-15 isolate (Evermann et al., 1981), the 79-1146 virus (McKeirnan et al., 1981; Pedersen et al., 1984b), and the UCD2, UCD3, and UCD4 strains (Pedersen and Floyd, 1985) (Table 7–1).

The UCD1, UCD3, and Black strains are very similar in their cytopathic effect (cpe), low virus yields in cell culture, pathogenicity, and comparative neutralization by antiserum to various strains of FECV, FIPV, TGEV, and CCV (Pedersen et al., 1983). The 79-1146 and UCD2 strains, however, are clearly different in growth characteristics in tissue culture, in pathogenicity, and in their greater resemblance to CCV (Boyle et al., 1984; Pedersen, 1983a; Pedersen et al., 1984a).

### EPIZOOTIOLOGY

#### Geographic Distribution

The earliest confirmable report of FIP was from the United States (Holzworth, 1963). FIP was subsequently recognized in England (Ishmael and Howell, 1968), Japan (Konishi et al., 1971), Canada (Stevenson et al., 1971), the Netherlands (Mieog and Richter, 1971), Ireland (Hartigan and Wilson, 1972), Mexico (DeAluja, 1971), South Africa (Colly, 1971), Switzerland (Stünzi and Grevel, 1973), Australia (Jones, 1974), Germany (Tuch et al., 1974), Belgium (Pastoret et al., 1974), Senegal (Chantal

**Table 7–1 Designation, Origin, Infectivity, and Pathogenicity of Various Feline Coronavirus Strains**

| STRAIN | DISEASE OF ORIGIN | INFECTIVITY BY ORAL ROUTE | SEROCONVERSION AND FIP INDUCTION AFTER: Oral Inoculation | | Intraperitoneal Inoculation | |
|---|---|---|---|---|---|---|
| | | | SEROCONVERSION | FIP | SEROCONVERSION | FIP |
| FECV-UCD1 | enteritis | strong | yes | no | yes | no |
| FECV-79-1683 | enteritis | strong | yes | no | yes | no |
| FIPV-TN406 (low passage) | FIP | weak | yes | yes | yes | yes |
| FIPV-TN406 (high passage) | FIP | weak | yes | no | yes | no |
| FIPV-79-1146 | neonatal pneumonia | strong | yes | yes | yes | yes |
| FIPV-Nor15 | FIP | strong | yes | yes | yes | yes |
| FIPV-UCD1 | FIP | weak | yes | yes | yes | yes |
| FIPV-UCD2 | FIP | weak | yes | no | yes | no |
| FIPV-UCD3 | FIP | strong | yes | no | yes | yes |
| FIPV-UCD4 | FIP | strong | yes | no | yes | yes |

**Table 7–2 The Age Incidence of FIP in the Total Feline Autopsy Population, University of California, 1969 to 1979**

| AGE IN YEARS | NO. OF CATS IN AUTOPSY POPULATION | NO. OF CATS DYING OF FIP | PER CENT |
|---|---|---|---|
| 0–½ | 331 | 22 | 6.6 |
| ½–1 | 206 | 36 | 17.5 |
| 1–2 | 396 | 67 | 16.9 |
| 2–3 | 293 | 34 | 11.6 |
| 3–4 | 240 | 32 | 12.9 |
| 4–5 | 154 | 12 | 7.8 |
| 5–6 | 124 | 6 | 4.8 |
| 6–7 | 114 | 6 | 5.3 |
| 7–8 | 82 | 1 | 1.2 |
| 8–9 | 79 | 4 | 5.1 |
| 9–10 | 57 | 2 | 3.5 |
| 10–11 | 61 | 0 | 0.0 |
| 11–12 | 39 | 3 | 7.7 |
| 12–13 | 50 | 0 | 0.0 |
| 13–14 | 38 | 1 | 2.6 |
| 14–15 | 36 | 5 | 13.9 |
| 15–16 | 25 | 0 | 0.0 |
| 16–17 | 13 | 0 | 0.0 |
| 17–18 | 9 | 0 | 0.0 |
| 18–19 | 10 | 0 | 0.0 |
| 19–20 | 3 | 0 | 0.0 |
| 20–21 | 3 | 0 | 0.0 |

and Deschamps, 1974), France (Auclair-Semere and Groulade, 1975), Denmark (Mortensen and Steensborg, 1976), Austria (Heider, 1979), New Zealand (Horzinek and Osterhaus, 1979a), and Finland (Mannonen et al., 1979).

## Hosts

The disease has been recognized in lions (Colby and Low, 1970; Colly, 1971), mountain lions (Theobald, 1978), leopards (Colly, 1971; Tuch et al., 1974), jaguars (Colly, 1971; Fransen, 1974), and cheetah (Pfeifer et al., 1983). Smaller cats that have been infected with FIP virus (FIPV) include the lynx and caracal (Poelma et al., 1974), sand cat (Theobald, 1978), and pallas cat (Pedersen, 1983a).

## Incidence

The incidence of FIP is difficult to determine. The disease was diagnosed in less than 1 per cent of the cats presented to the teaching hospital at the University of California, Davis. The incidence in the autopsy population at this institution was around 1 per cent in the early 1960s and increased progressively until 1973, when it was the cause of death in 16.1 per cent of cats autopsied. The autopsy incidence fluctuated between 5.5 and 13.9 per cent between 1974 and 1979. In catteries as well as in the general population, losses appear to be sporadic and unpredictable. Under the worst conditions, the morbidity of FIP in cattery-reared cats rarely exceeds 10 per cent and in most cases ranges from 0 to 5 per cent. A 3 to 49 per cent yearly infection rate was observed, however, in kittens raised in one cattery over a four-year period (Potkay et al., 1974). The author has also known a similar high incidence in two other catteries (Pedersen, 1983a). The disease has a predilection for several siblings in a litter (Potkay et al., 1974). Deaths in such litters can occur over a period of 6 to 12 months. The disease often affects the smaller and more sickly kittens, and the mortality rate among clinically ill cats approaches 100 per cent.

**Table 7–3 Sex Incidence of FIP in the Total Feline Autopsy Population, University of California, 1969 to 1979**

| SEX | TOTAL AUTOPSY POPULATION | FIP CASES |
|---|---|---|
| Male | 1454/2534 (57.4%) | 162/267 (60.7%) |
| Female | 1080/2534 (42.6%) | 105/267 (39.3%) |

**Table 7–4 Breed Incidence of FIP in the Total Feline Autopsy Population, University of California, 1969 to 1979**

| BREED | FIP CASES | PER CENT |
|---|---|---|
| Domestics | 155/1776 | 8.7 |
| Siamese | 56/461 | 12.1 |
| Persian | 9/82 | 11.0 |
| Burmese | 9/43 | 20.9 |
| Miscellaneous purebreds | 13/106 | 12.3 |
| Average | 242/2468 | 9.8 |

Feline infectious peritonitis occurs mainly in cats between six months and five years of age, with the highest incidence between six months and two years (Table 7–2). In one cattery, however, deaths were almost always in cats less than one year of age, with the mean incidence at 5.8 months (Potkay et al., 1974). We have recognized FIP in stillborn and weak newborn kittens of a queen that had effusive abdominal FIP during the later stages of pregnancy. Effusive FIP has also occurred in a 23-day-old kitten (Norsworthy, 1974). There is a decreased incidence in cats between the ages of 5 and 13 years followed by an increased incidence in cats 14 to 15 years of age (see Table 7–2).

The incidence of FIP in males and females is probably comparable to the sex ratio in the general population at risk (Table 7–3). Earlier reports, however, suggested that the disease was more prevalent in males (Potkay et al., 1974); Robison et al., 1971; Schalm, 1979; Wolfe and Griesemer, 1966). Feline infectious peritonitis occurs more frequently in purebred than in domestic cats (Robison et al., 1971; Table 7–4), probably because purebred cats are often raised in catteries and multiple-cat households. Such environments are more conducive to disease in general (Pedersen, 1978), and cats from these environments often have more problems with FeLV infection, which is a potentiator of FIP (Cotter et al., 1973).

## Source of Virus in Nature

The source of FIPV in nature is unknown. Cats that are ill with FIP are not highly infectious and are relatively uncommon. Since there is frequently no known contact between cats developing FIP and cats that have had the

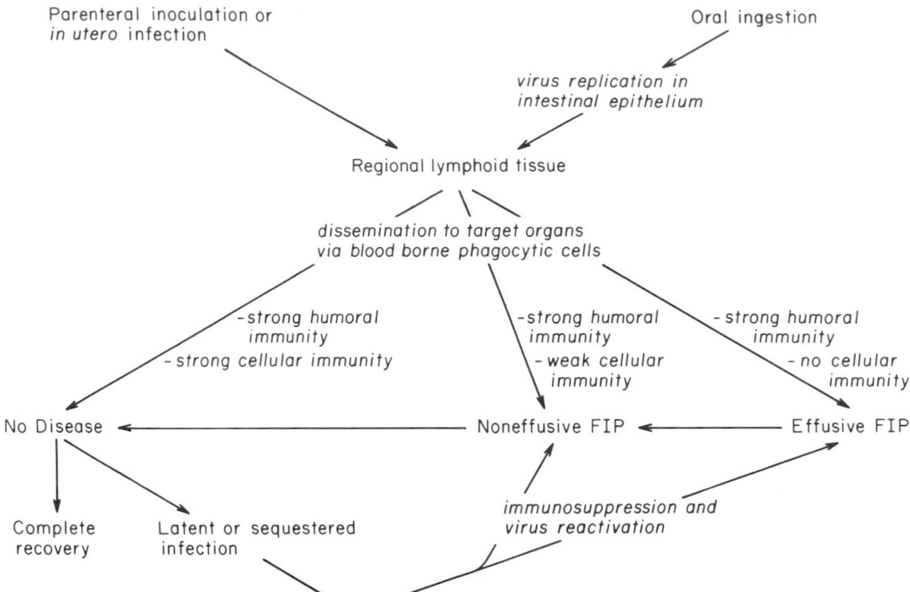


**Figure 7–9** The proposed pathogenesis of FIP based on current knowledge.

disease, it can also be assumed that ill cats are not the major source of virus. Asymptomatic carrier cats undoubtedly exist, but the epizootiology of the infection indicates either that they are uncommon or that they shed very low amounts of virus at any given time. Virus is probably shed in the stools. Urine shedding has also been suggested by the studies of Hardy and Hurvitz (1971). In-utero transmission may also be important and will be discussed in the following section.

A novel mode of transmission has been postulated by Pedersen and associates (1981a). They suggested that FIPV can arise as a mutant of FECV and that FECV carriers might be a reservoir for FIPV. This postulate, however, remains to be verified by experimental studies.

## Pathogenesis

The pathogenesis of FIPV infection is complex and incompletely understood. Enough is known about the disease, however, to hypothesize its pathogenesis (Fig. 7–9).

Healthy carriers of FIPV have not been identified. It is not known, therefore, how the virus is spread. The disease can be reproduced experimentally by intraperitoneal (IP), intratracheal, or oronasal routes of inoculation. The behavior of the disease after infection by these routes is not, however, typical of the behavior of natural infection. The role of in-utero transmission from latently infected queens to their kittens is currently under study, and preliminary evidence indicates that in-utero transmission may be more important than previously believed. In one experiment, a group of specific pathogen–free cats was infected IP with FIPV-UCD3 or -UCD4 (Pedersen and Floyd, 1985). About half became seropositive without ever developing FIP and were completely resistant to reinfection. Females from this group were later bred and their kittens studied. Healthy FIPV-recovered queens kept completely isolated from other cats gave birth to healthy kittens, and the size of their litters was normal. The kittens passively acquired coronavirus antibodies from their mothers immediately after birth, and the titers of these antibodies dropped during the first few weeks of life. At about five weeks, however, the antibody titers suddenly began to rise. When the kittens were 12 to 16 weeks of age they were experimentally infected by the IP route with highly virulent FIPV-UCD1. All the kittens were resistant to the infection. The immunity that these kittens demonstrated could have resulted only from a preceding asymptomatic infection with virulent FIPV. This infection had to come from the queen, either horizontally during neonatal life or in utero. The pattern of seroconversion in these kittens was very similar, however, to the situation following in-utero infection of kittens with feline syncytium-forming virus (FeSFV) infection (see section on FeSFV).

In support of in-utero infection, McKeirnan and associates (1981) isolated an FIPV (FIPV-79-1146) from a four-day-old kitten that had died of pleural pneumonia and hepatitis. The lesions in this kitten were too chronic to have occurred after birth. Interestingly, neither the mother nor a surviving littermate showed any signs of illness. This observation, combined with those from previous experimental studies, indicated that carrier mothers may infect their young in utero. Many kittens are born healthy and remain that way, whereas others apparently can become sick before or after birth.

The importance of postnatal horizontally acquired infection has not been determined. This form of infection, however, has been studied extensively in the laboratory (Evermann et al., 1981; Pedersen et al., 1981a, 1984b). Unlike the naturally occurring disease, which seems to be associated with a high rate of infection but a low mortality, the disease created by oronasal or IP inoculation is associated with high morbidity and high mortality. The morbidity figures vary greatly, however, depending on the strain of FIPV used for the study (Table 7–1). Some strains of FIPV, such as UCD1, TN406 (low passage), 79-1146, and Nor15, cause FIP by both oronasal and IP routes. Among these strains, the first two are of low infectivity, whereas the second two are highly infectious.

Other strains, such as UCD3 and UCD4, are unique because they behave as FECVs when given orally but as FIPVs when given IP, i.e., they cause seroconversion but no disease by the oronasal route and seroconversion and disease by the IP route. To further complicate matters, FIPV-UCD2, which was isolated from a cat with FIP, behaves as an FECV by both oronasal and IP routes (Pedersen and Floyd, 1985). These findings once again indicate the complex relationship between FIPVs and FECVs.

After IP inoculation, FIPV probably replicates within phagocytic cells in the peritoneal cavity and regional lymph nodes. After oral inoculation, however, virus replication is initially observed in the mature apical epithelium of the small intestine (Hayashi et al., 1982). In support of this latter finding, orally administered FIPV infects the intestinal epithelium of neonatal pigs in a manner identical to TGEV (Woods et al., 1981). This intestinal tropism of FIPV probably reflects its close relationship to FECV and similar intestinal viruses of pigs and dogs. Unlike these intestinal viruses, however, FIPV does not cause demonstrable intestinal disease after oronasal inoculation. In fact, regardless of the route of infection, no clinical signs develop until 8 to 14 days or more after infection when serum antibodies began to appear.

At about the time that immunity begins to develop, the virus is disseminating from regional lymphoid structures to other target tissues in the body. This dissemination is associated with blood-borne phagocytes (Weiss and Scott, 1981a) and is another essential difference between FIPV and FECV. FECV does not spread farther than the intestinal epithelium and regional lymph nodes (Pedersen et al., 1981b, 1984b). Target tissues for disseminated virus are usually rich in small venules and phagocytic cells and include the liver, visceral peritoneum and pleura, uvea, and the meninges and ependyma of the brain and spinal cord.

Feline infectious peritonitis occurs in two clinical forms (Holmberg and Gribble, 1973; Pedersen, 1976b). The first, or effusive, form of the disease is characteristically a peritonitis or pleuritis or both. Target tissues include the visceral peritoneum and pleura and the omentum. Inflammation in these tissues results in a great outpouring of fluid into either or both of the body cavities, hence the name "wet" or "effusive" FIP. Central nervous system and ocular involvement are not usually of clinical significance in the effusive form of FIP. Effusive FIP is characterized by a pyogranulomatous reaction around small venules in the target organs (Feldman and Jortner, 1964; Hayashi et al., 1977; Montali and Strandberg, 1972; Ward et al., 1968, 1974). This vasculitis is responsible for the outpouring of protein- and fibrin-rich fluid into the body cavities.

The second, or noneffusive, form of FIP was first described by Montali and Strandberg (1972). Lesions in this form of the disease are of a more classic granulomatous appearance and are localized in tissues or organs such as lymph nodes, kidneys, uvea, and the meninges and ependyma of the brain and spinal cord. There is usually no exudation associated with the lesions, hence the name "dry" or "noneffusive" FIP. Noneffusive FIP is only about one fourth as common as effusive FIP in both field and experimental situations.

The effusive form of FIP occurs in cats that develop humoral but not cellular immunity (Fig. 7–9). The lesions of effusive FIP develop simultaneously with the appearance of humoral antibodies (Pedersen et al., 1981a). Humoral immunity in the absence of protective cellular immunity appears to potentiate the infection. It has been postulated that antibody enhances the uptake of coated virus by phagocytic cells. Because FIPV prefers to grow in such cells, the net effect is to enhance the level of virus replication and to aid dissemination of the virus to other sites by wandering phagocytes. Antibody might also react with antigen and complement and result in a localized Arthus-like response (Pedersen and Boyle, 1980; Weiss et al., 1980; Weiss and Scott, 1981a,b,c). The presence of circulating immune complexes is also suggested by the fluctuating complement levels and the development of glomerulonephritis in cats with FIP (Jacobse-Geels et al., 1980, 1982). Complement-mediated activation of terminal clotting factors, together with vascular lesions that consume platelets and clotting factors, causes a coagulopathy in cats with effusive FIP (Weiss et al., 1980).

Noneffusive FIP is thought to occur in cats that develop partial cellular immunity (Pedersen and Black, 1983) (Fig. 7–9). This incomplete immunity limits the level of virus replication and dissemination. The granulomatous lesions of noneffusive FIP occur around small foci of virus-laden macrophages. The lesions of noneffusive FIP are equivalent, therefore, to similar lesions in diseases such as tuberculosis.

Recovery from FIPV infection is presumably due to a strong cellular immunity (Pedersen and Black, 1983). Such immunity may not, however, always lead to complete elimination of the virus. It appears that FIPV persists in some animals as a latent or sequestered infection. Anything that interferes with this established immunity has the potential to cause reactivation of disease. This probably explains why FeLV infection, surgical stresses, and pregnancy have a greater than expected temporal relationship to clinical cases of FIP.

Immunity is discussed in more detail later in this section.

## Clinical Features of Effusive FIP

Effusive FIP is most frequently manifested by a fluctuating fever lasting one to five weeks or more, progressive weight loss, decreasing appetite, malaise, and abdominal distention with fluid (Fig. 7–10; Table 7–5). The amount of fluid varies from 25 to 700 ml or more. The abdomen

**Table 7–5 Variability in the Presenting Clinical Signs of Effusive FIP**

| PRESENTING CLINICAL SIGNS REFERABLE TO INVOLVEMENT OF: | NO. OF CATS |
|---|---|
| Peritoneal cavity | 62 |
| Peritoneal and pleural cavities | 24 |
| Pleural cavity | 12 |
| Peritoneal cavity and eyes | 3 |
| Peritoneal cavity and CNS | 2 |
| Peritoneal and pleural cavities, CNS | 1 |
| Peritoneal and pleural cavities, CNS, eyes | 1 |
| Pleural cavity and CNS | 1 |
| Peritoneal cavity, CNS, eyes | 1 |
| TOTAL | 107 |

(From Pedersen NC: Feline Pract 13 [5][1983] 5–20.)

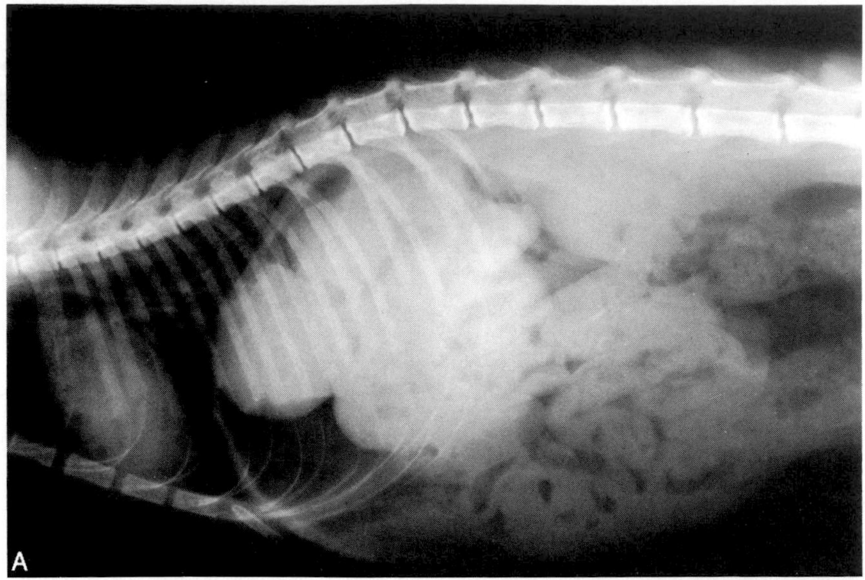


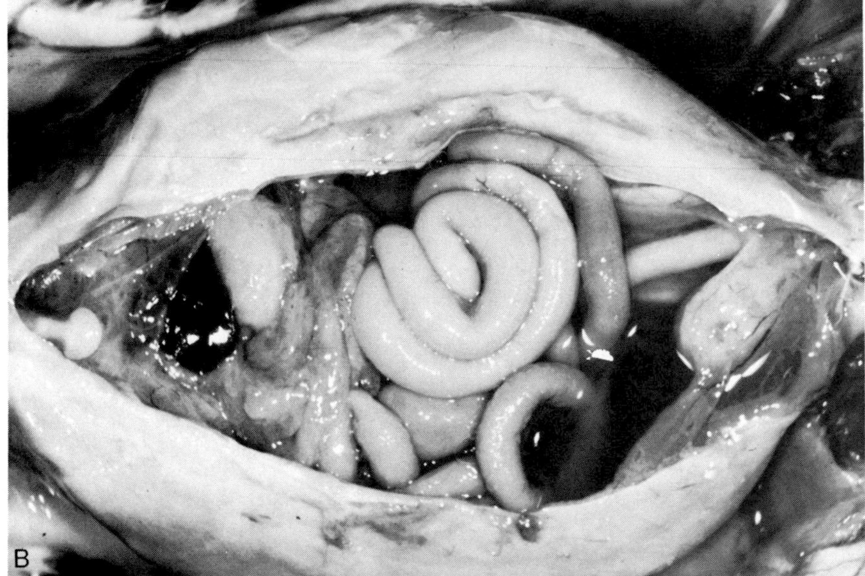


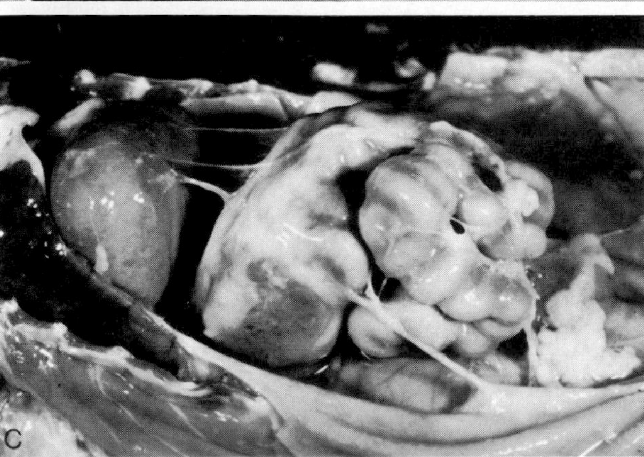


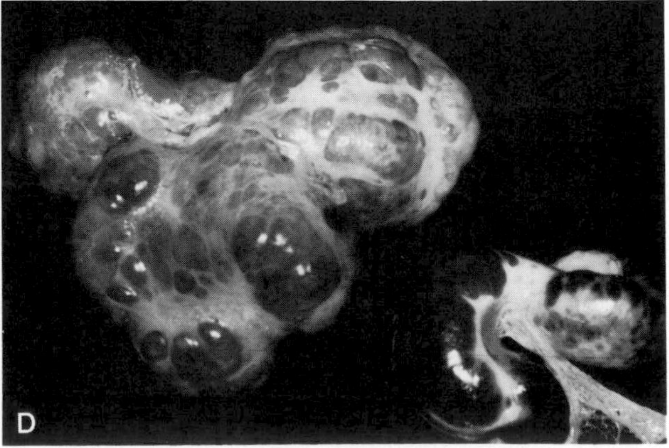


**Figure 7–10** *A,* Abdomen, effusive FIP in a seven-month-old kitten autopsied at the Angell Memorial Hospital in 1954. After removal of all fluid, the liver appeared remarkably abnormal. It was compressed and distorted by a thick fibrous coating and the omentum was tightly bunched by adhesions caudal to the stomach. *B,* Abdominal cavity, effusive FIP. The abdomen is filled with a deep yellow, protein-rich exudate. The omentum is thickened and retracted into a compact mass behind the liver and stomach. Fibrin coats the stomach and urinary bladder, and adhesions are present. *C,* Thorax and abdomen, effusive FIP. After a prolonged course, fibrin deposited on the pericardium and on the abdominal viscera has become organized into a pale, tough, fibrous coating that constricts and deforms the organs. Many cord-like adhesions have developed. *D,* Chronic effusive FIP, perihepatitis and perisplenitis in an 11-year-old cat autopsied at the Angell Memorial Animal Hospital in 1954. The liver and spleen are compressed and distorted by a thick fibrous covering that developed as the earlier fibrinous coating became organized. (Courtesy Angell Memorial Animal Hospital.)

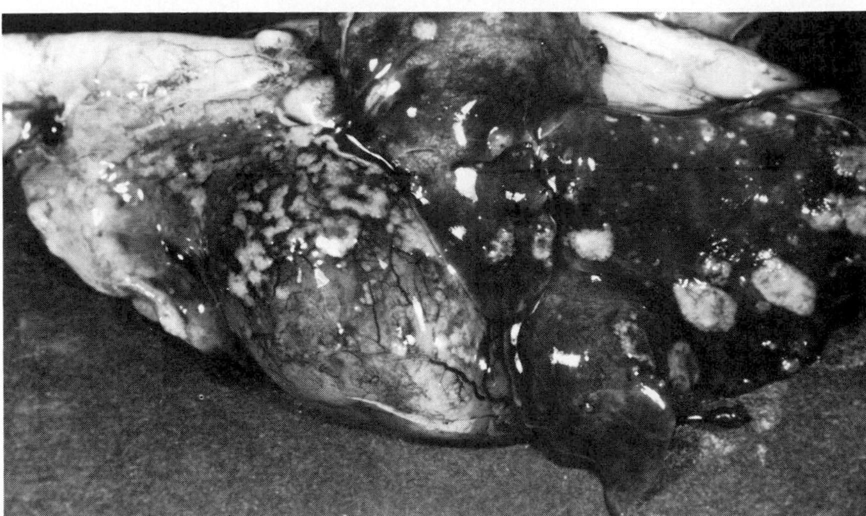

**Figure 7–11** Heart and lungs, effusive FIP. Granulomatous plaques stud the pericardium and the pulmonary pleura. Tiny granulomas on the epicardium are visible under the pericardium. (Courtesy Angell Memorial Animal Hospital.)

is usually doughy and painless on palpation, except early in the disease when it can be somewhat sensitive and in rare cases intensely painful. Some cats may not appear ill even though abdominal distention is pronounced. In such instances, the owner may mistake the abdominal distention for pregnancy. Intact male cats with peritonitis often have scrotal and testicular enlargement, due largely to the extension of peritoneal disease into the tunics surrounding the testes. Mild jaundice is common in cats with effusive abdominal FIP.

Occasionally peritoneal lesions of incipient FIP are found at spaying. Castration has "triggered" peracute abdominal FIP in cats presumably incubating or carrying latent infection.

Dyspnea, due to pleuritis and inflammatory effusion, occurs in about one third of cats with effusive FIP (Fig. 7–11; Table 7–5). Pericarditis and epicarditis are common in cats with thoracic cavity involvement but do not usually lead to clinical signs. Occasionally, however, pericarditis causes a massive pericardial effusion and cardiac tamponade (Fig. 7–12).

Ocular and central nervous system (CNS) involvement occurs in effusive FIP but is seldom of clinical significance (Table 7–5). Signs referable to the CNS and eyes are far more common in the noneffusive form of FIP (Table 7–6).

## Clinical Features of Noneffusive FIP

Cats with noneffusive FIP are usually presented with a chronic fluctuating fever, malaise, and weight loss extending over weeks or months. In addition, specific signs reflect involvement of various abdominal organs, chest, CNS, or eyes (Table 7–6).

The abdominal cavity is involved in more than one third of the cats with noneffusive FIP. The kidneys (Fig. 7–13), mesentery (Fig. 7–14), mesenteric lymph nodes, liver, spleen, pancreas, omentum, and surfaces of the bowels are the most frequent sites of lesions. The abdominal lesions of effusive FIP are surface-oriented but extend

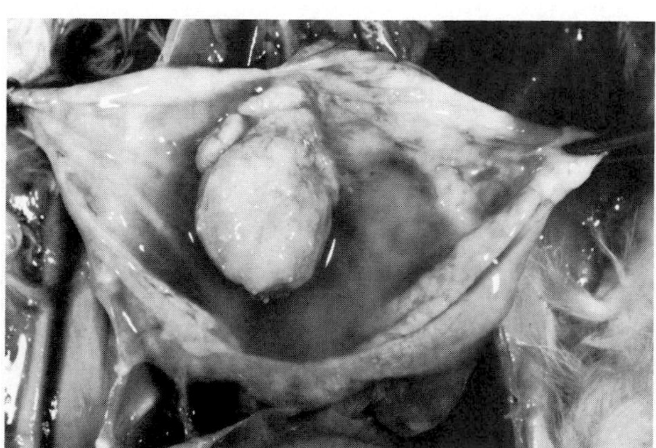

**Figure 7–12** Granulomatous pericarditis and epicarditis, FIP. (Courtesy Angell Memorial Animal Hospital.)

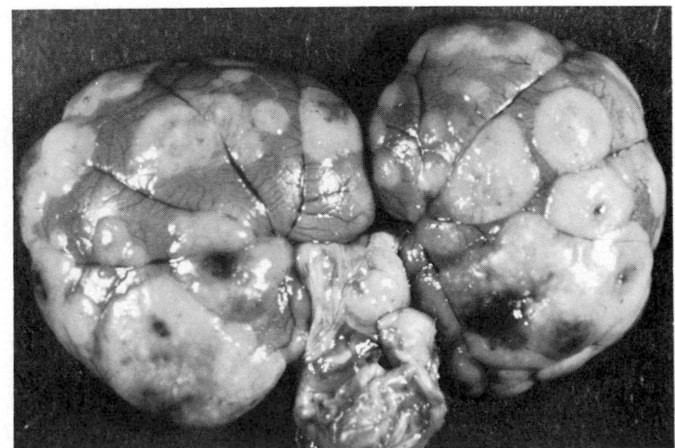

**Figure 7–13** Kidney, noneffusive FIP. Multiple granulomas of varying size bulge above the kidney surface. (Courtesy Angell Memorial Animal Hospital.)

**Table 7–6 Variability in the Presenting Clinical Signs of Noneffusive FIP**

| PRESENTING CLINICAL SIGNS REFERABLE TO INVOLVEMENT OF: | NO. OF CATS |
|---|---|
| Peritoneal cavity | 30 |
| CNS | 22 |
| Eyes | 14 |
| CNS and eyes | 8 |
| Peritoneal cavity and eyes | 7 |
| Peritoneal and pleural cavities | 4 |
| Peritoneal and pleural cavities, CNS | 3 |
| Peritoneal and pleural cavities, eyes | 2 |
| Peritoneal cavity, CNS, eyes | 2 |
| Pleural cavity | 1 |
| Pleural cavity, CNS, eyes | 1 |
| TOTAL | 94 |

(From Pedersen NC: Feline Pract 13 [5] [1983] 5–20.)

into the parenchyma and range from less than 1 mm to 10 cm or more in diameter. Lesions within abdominal viscera are frequently palpable as somewhat painful and irregular masses. Although the granulomas are sometimes very large, they seldom interfere totally with organ function. On occasion, however, signs of hepatic, renal, or pancreatic endocrine malfunction are present. Infrequently, extensive lesions in the bowel wall may lead to vomiting or diarrhea.

Chest cavity lesions occur in the noneffusive form of FIP but are not usually of clinical importance (Table 7–6). Involvement of the nasal passages and the oral cavity (Fig. 7–15) has been observed on rare occasions.

Central nervous system involvement is varied in its clinical expression. Spinal signs such as posterior paresis and brachial, trigeminal, and sciatic nerve palsies have been described (Kornegay, 1978; Holliday, 1971; Legendre and Whitenack, 1975; Pedersen, 1976b; Pedersen et al., 1974; Slauson and Finn, 1972). Hydrocephalus, secondary to disease of the choroid and ependyma, has also been reported (Fankhauser and Fatzer, 1977; Hayashi et al., 1980; Krum et al., 1975). Cerebral involvement (Fig. 7–16) can lead to dementia, personality changes (shyness or rage), and convulsions (Feldman, 1974). Cerebellar-vestibular signs, such as nystagmus, head tilt, and circling, have all been associated with noneffusive FIP.

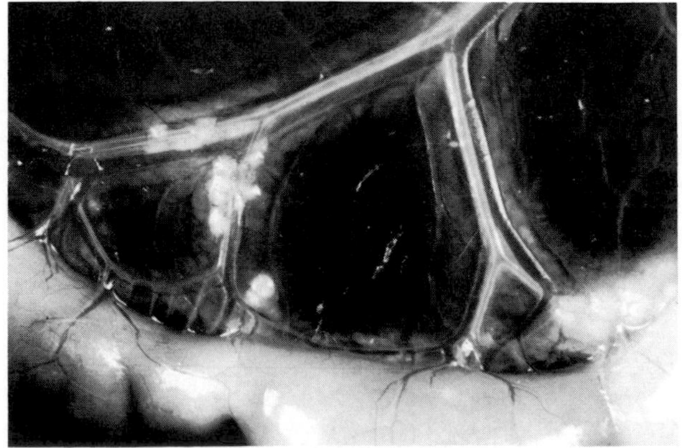

**Figure 7–14** Granulomatous beading along mesenteric vessels, noneffusive FIP. (Courtesy Angell Memorial Animal Hospital.)

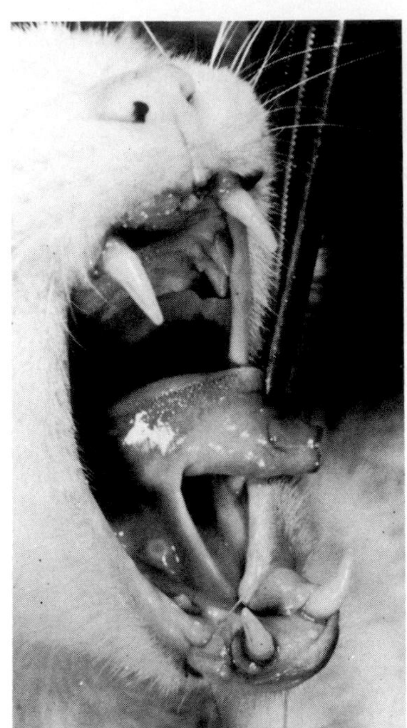

**Figure 7–15** Small granuloma on the frenulum of the tongue, noneffusive FIP. (Courtesy Angell Memorial Animal Hospital.)

The ocular lesions of FIP have been well documented (Campbell and Reed, 1975; Campbell and Schiessl, 1978; Doherty, 1971; Gelatt, 1973; Krebiel et al., 1974; Pedersen et al., 1974; Slauson and Finn, 1972). Eye disease can occur with CNS or peritoneal involvement or alone (Table 7–6). Ocular FIP is characterized by necrotizing and pyogranulomatous inflammation in the iris and ciliary body. This can cause a slight clouding of the aqueous humor or a more exudative process involving the anterior and posterior chambers. Keratic precipitates (Fig. 7–17) and hyphema are common, as are sheathing of the retinal blood vessels with exudate and retinal hemorrhages. Retinal hemorrhages may appear as flame- or keel-shaped lesions. Vascular involvement can be manifested by engorgement of scleral vessels and decreased intraocular pressure. (See also the chapter on the eye.)

## DIAGNOSIS

### Clinicopathologic Features

The hemograms are similar in both the effusive and noneffusive forms of the disease (Pedersen, 1976b). The leukocyte count is frequently elevated, with an absolute neutrophilia and normal or low lymphocyte counts. In some cats, however, the leukocyte count is low—usually cats with fulminating effusive FIP or FeLV-related illnesses. Anemia is mild or moderately severe in many cats with FIP and may result from hematopoietic suppression

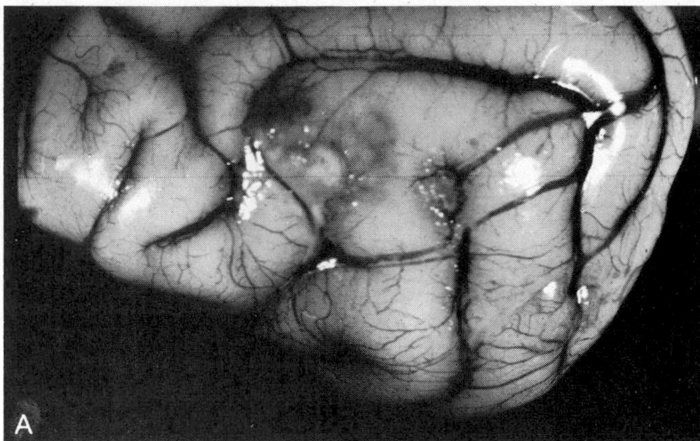


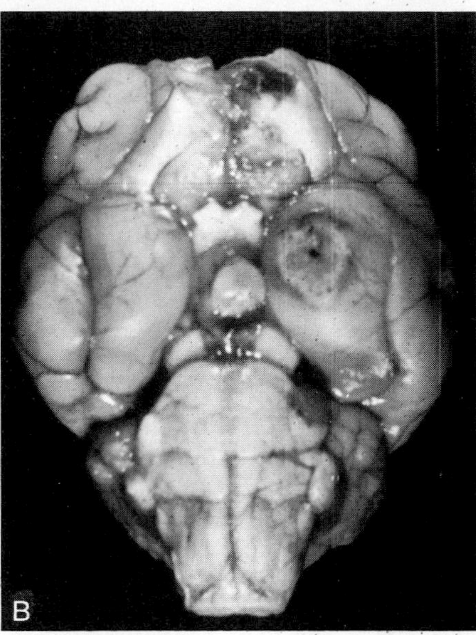


**Figure 7–16** *A,* Superficial granuloma in the frontoparietal area of the cerebrum, noneffusive FIP. *B,* Granuloma, left piriform lobe of the brain, noneffusive FIP. (Courtesy Angell Memorial Animal Hospital.)

associated with chronic illness or from concurrent FeLV or *Haemobartonella* infection.

Inclusion bodies within circulating neutrophils have been described in a small proportion of cats with FIP (Ward et al., 1971). The origin of these inclusions is unknown; it has been suggested that they may represent immune complexes (Horzinek and Osterhaus, 1979b).

Serum fibrinogen levels are elevated above 400 mg/dl in 45 per cent of the cats with FIP (Pedersen, 1976b; Schalm, 1979). This is of little diagnostic specificity and merely indicates the inflammatory nature of the disease. Plasma proteins are elevated above 7.8 gm/dl in about half the cats with effusive FIP and three fourths of those with noneffusive FIP (Pedersen, 1976b). Elevations in the plasma proteins are due to variable increases in the alpha-2, beta, and gamma globulins (Pedersen, 1976b). The alpha-2 globulin elevation is due in part to an increase in the level of serum haptoglobin (Harvey and Gaskin, 1978). This electrophoretic pattern of globulin elevation is not pathognomonic for FIP but rather reflects chronic inflammation and elevated levels of antibody production. Serum IgG, apparently of monoclonal type, is increased in some cats with noneffusive FIP.

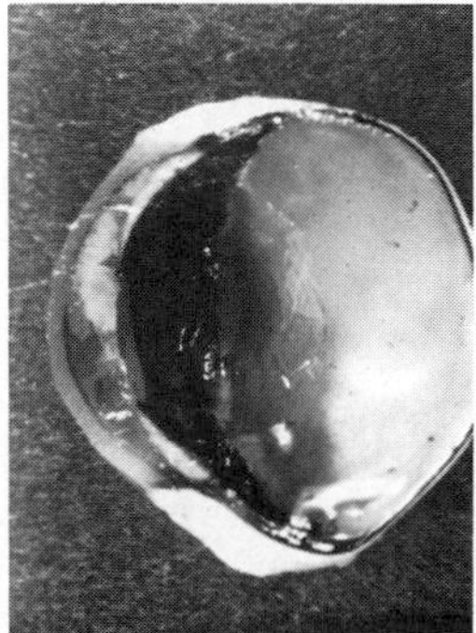

**Figure 7–17** Eye, sectioned, noneffusive FIP. Pale "mutton-fat" keratic precipitates adhere to the inner surface of the cornea. They are composed of fibrin and inflammatory cells exuding from the inflamed uveal tract. (Courtesy Angell Memorial Animal Hospital.)

A disseminated intravascular coagulopathy has been described in cats with experimentally induced effusive FIP (Weiss et al., 1980), and similar coagulopathy occurs in natural cases of effusive FIP. This is associated with increased prothrombin and partial thromboplastin times, increased levels of fibrin degradation product, increased activated clotting time, and decreased levels of intrinsic clotting factors. The coagulopathy may result from widespread vascular damage or from activation of clotting factors by the activation of terminal complement components (Pedersen and Boyle, 1980).

The peritoneal and pleural fluid of effusive FIP is characteristic (Pedersen, 1976b; Robison et al., 1971; Ward and Pedersen, 1969). Light to dark yellow and of a sticky viscous consistency, the exudate is high in protein (near serum levels) and contains from 1,600 to 25,000 or more leukocytes/μl. Neutrophils, lymphocytes, macrophages, and mesothelial cells are present but not in great numbers.

Cerebrospinal fluid (CSF) is abnormal in cats with extensive meningeal involvement; however, if the disease is focal or localized in the subependymal areas the CSF may be normal. Abnormal CSF has an elevated protein content of 90 to 2000 mg/dl and leukocyte counts (mainly neutrophils) of 90 to 9250 cells/μl.

The aqueous humor is abnormal in eyes with involvement of the anterior uveal tract. The aqueous humor protein content is elevated and the leukocyte numbers increased (Feldman, 1974). Neutrophils and large and small mononuclear cells predominate in the fluid.

A mild proteinuria with or without concurrent elevation in the blood urea nitrogen or serum creatinine level occurs in some cats with renal involvement. The icterus index and total bilirubin are often mildly to moderately elevated, especially in cats with the peritoneal form of effusive FIP or with granulomatous hepatitis. Liver enzyme levels may be mildly to moderately elevated in such cases.

In the past, tests for FeLV infection were positive in 40 to 50 per cent of cats with either effusive or noneffusive FIP. Not surprisingly, therefore, FIP can occur concurrently with lymphoma, reticulum cell sarcoma, or myeloproliferative disease. Presently, however, an increasing proportion of cats with FIP are FeLV-negative, probably

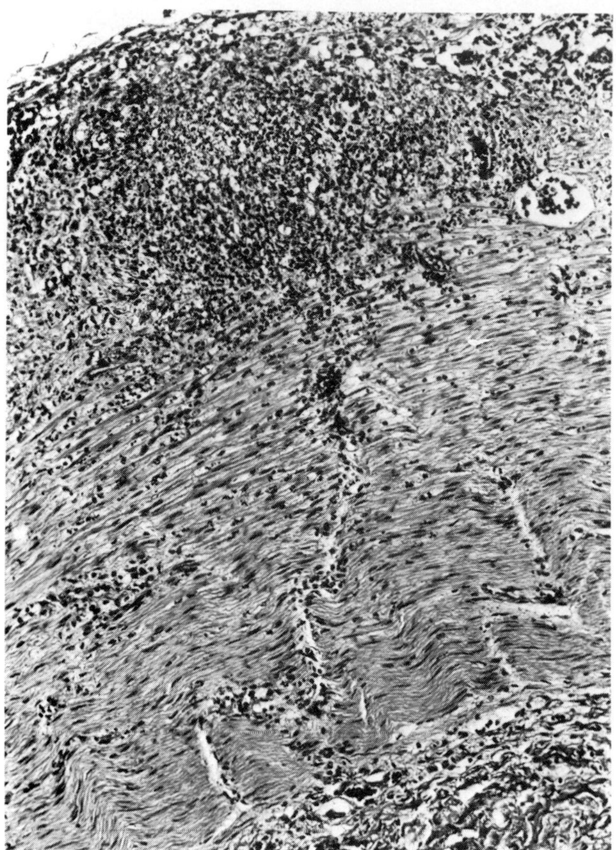

**Figure 7–18** A pyogranuloma in the serosa of the intestine of a cat with effusive FIP. The center of the lesion consists of a few neutrophils and dead and dying cells. A zone of inflammatory cells, mainly macrophages and occasional lymphocytes and plasma cells, surrounds this area. H & E, × 100. (From Pedersen NC: *In* Greene CE: Clinical Microbiology and Infectious Diseases of the Dog and Cat. Philadelphia, WB Saunders Company, 1983.)

because of elimination of FeLV infection from many catteries.

Serologic testing and the limitations of its usefulness for diagnosis are discussed in the section on serologic studies.

Biopsy is the only definitive diagnostic procedure for FIP, the specimen being obtained by endoscopy or exploratory surgery.

## Differential Diagnosis

Noneffusive FIP and lymphoma are most often confused: both diseases may present with palpable masses, both are frequently associated with FeLV infection, and both involve the same organ systems. Effusive FIP is most often mistaken for diseases in which there is transudation or exudation of fluid into the chest or abdominal cavity. Chylothorax, pyothorax, cancers associated with effusion, heart failure, cirrhosis of the liver with abdominal transudate, and bacterial peritonitis must all be differentiated from FIP. Bacterial peritonitis is often chronic in cats, and the clinical presentation is virtually identical to that of effusive abdominal FIP. Bacterial peritonitis can follow rupture of the small intestine in kittens with massive ascarid infestation and has been caused by penetrating foreign bodies. Broom straws are a particularly common penetrating object (see also Smith and Jones, 1966). Chronic bacterial peritonitis of unknown origin occurs in some cats with FeLV infection. The correct diagnosis of disorders that involve fluid accumulations in the chest and abdomen is greatly aided by careful analysis of the fluid.

With ocular involvement, toxoplasmosis, lymphosarcoma, and the mycoses must be considered in differential diagnosis.

Pansteatitis can mimic both effusive and noneffusive FIP (Summers et al., 1982). The abdominal and ventral subcutaneous fat is most often involved. Thickened and inflamed fat in the omentum, mesenteries, and perirenal

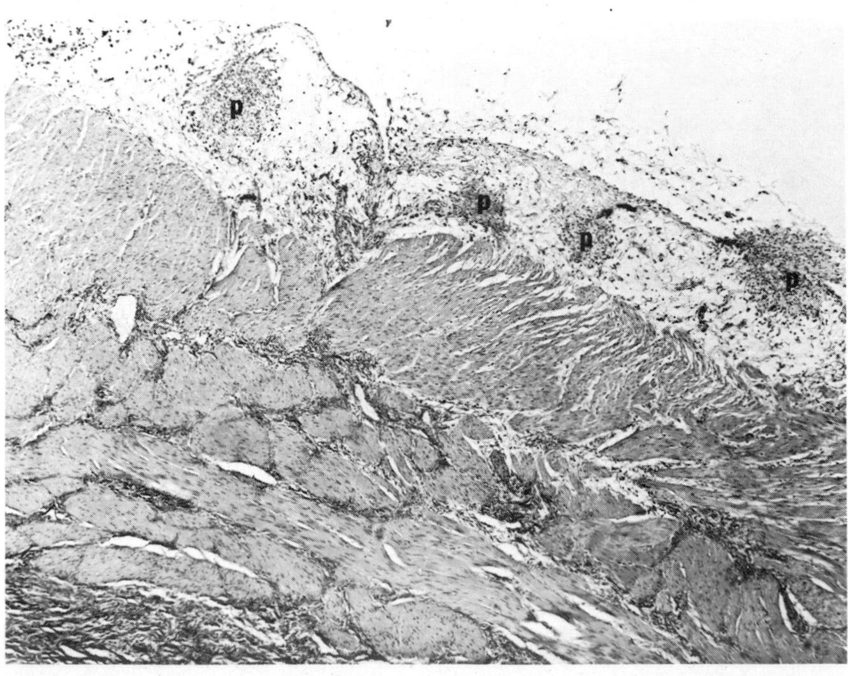


**Figure 7–19** Urinary bladder in a cat with effusive FIP. Numerous pyogranulomas (p) can be seen within the serosa. The serosal membrane is edematous and thickened. The underlying muscularis is uninvolved in this section. H & E, × 40. (From Pedersen NC: *In* Greene CE: Clinical Microbiology and Infectious Diseases of the Dog and Cat. Philadelphia, WB Saunders Company, 1983.)

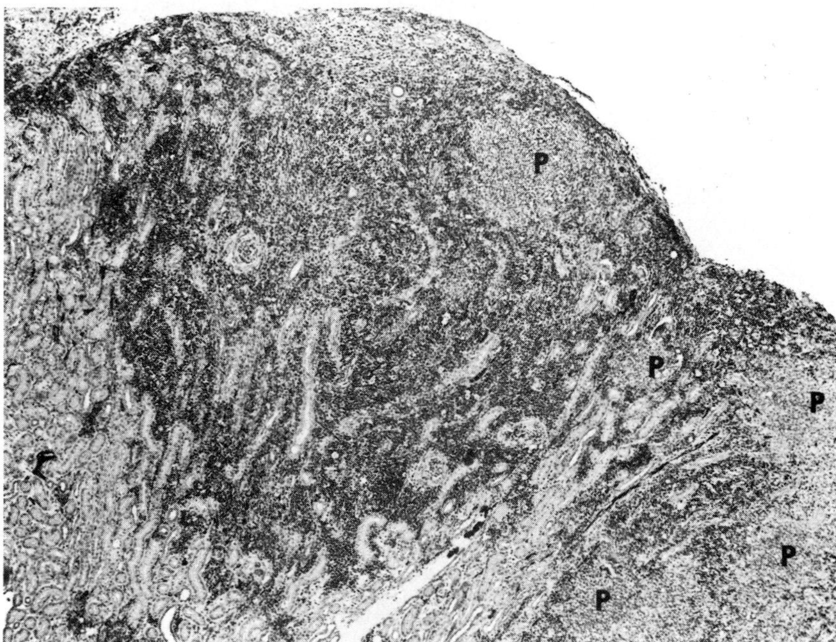


**Figure 7–20** Kidney in a cat with noneffusive FIP. Several pyogranulomas (P) of varying sizes are present in the subcapsular area. A dense plasmacytic-lymphocytic infiltrate dissects between renal tubules. H & E, × 40. (From Pedersen NC: *In* Greene CE: Clinical Microbiology and Infectious Diseases of the Dog and Cat. Philadelphia, WB Saunders Company, 1983.)

areas can be mistaken for lesions of FIP. In addition, there may be an effusion of fluid into the abdomen associated with fat necrosis. The yellow color of the involved fat and the nodular consistency of the ventral subcutaneous tissue strongly suggest pansteatitis.

## Pathologic Features

The characteristic lesion of FIP is the pyogranuloma (Holmberg and Gribble, 1973; Wolfe and Griesemer, 1971; Weiss and Scott, 1981c). In the effusive form, pyogranulomas appear as distinct or coalescing serosal plaques 0.5 to 2.0 mm or more in diameter. The visceral serosa of the chest and abdomen is more likely to be involved, the omentum often being thickened, edematous, and retracted into a compact mass (Fig. 7–10*B,C*). The pyogranulomatous reactions of noneffusive FIP vary in size depending on the organ involved (Holmberg and Gribble, 1973; Montali and Strandberg, 1972; Slauson and Finn, 1972). Lesions in the CNS and eyes range from microscopic to 1.0 or 2.0 mm in diameter, the larger lesions being most noticeable in the meninges. Serosal, mesenteric, and omental lesions consist mainly of small whitish plaques or nodules. Kidney lesions are often very large, sometimes exceeding 5.0 cm in diameter, and are

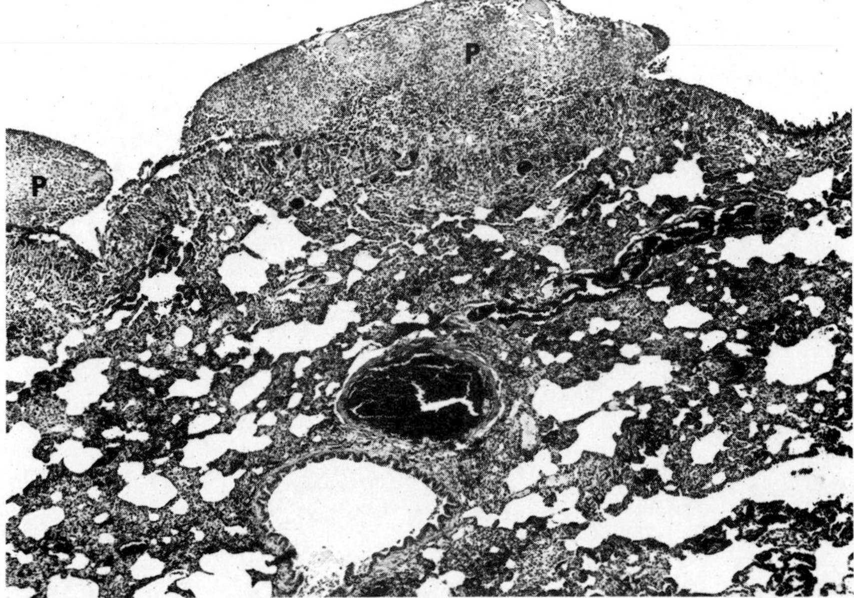


**Figure 7–21** Lung in a cat with noneffusive FIP. The pleura contains several well-delineated, raised plaques (P) made up of fibrin, macrophages, neutrophils, and a few lymphocytes and plasma cells. The disease process has broken through the pleura at one point to involve the underlying pulmonary parenchyma. H & E, × 40.

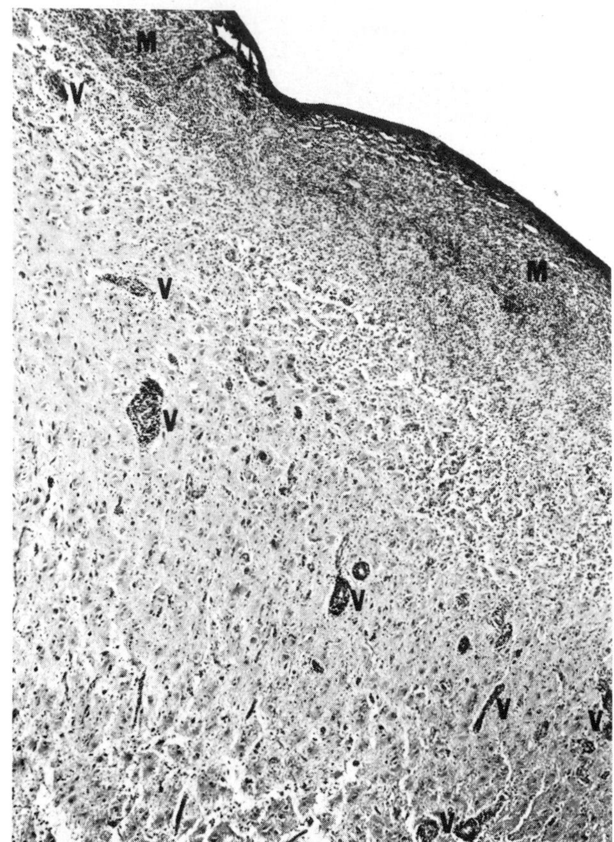


**Figure 7–22** Brain in a cat with noneffusive FIP. The meninges (M) are greatly thickened and infiltrated with inflammatory cells. The superficial inflammatory response extends down into the parenchyma along penetrating veins (V). H & E, × 40. (From Pedersen NC: *In* Greene CE: Clinical Microbiology and Infectious Diseases of the Dog and Cat. Philadelphia, WB Saunders Company, 1983.)

more numerous in the subcapsular tissues (Fig. 7–13). Similarly, mesenteric lymph node lesions tend to be large.

Pyogranulomas are often oriented around small veins (Fig. 7–14), and phlebitis and periphlebitis can be intense (Weiss and Scott, 1981c). In effusive FIP, the pyogranuloma consists of necrotic debris and neutrophils, surrounded by a dense accumulation of phagocytic cells interspersed with a few lymphocytes and plasma cells (Figs. 7–18 and 7–19). There is an accumulation of fibrin- and protein-rich exudate in the lesion and surrounding tissue. In the noneffusive form, the outer zone is characteristically more fibrous, and the numbers of plasma cells and lymphocytes are much greater (Fig. 7–20); edema, hyperemia, and fibrin and protein exudation are also not as pronounced.

Although the pyogranulomatous process is usually surface-oriented (Figs. 7–21 and 7–22), a similar inflammatory process may extend into underlying tissues along penetrating veins (Fig. 7–22). Focal lesions, often associated with phlebitis, may be seen deep in underlying muscle or organ parenchyma and are characterized by mixed cell inflammatory infiltrates. Such lesions occur commonly in kidney and liver, less often in lung and heart, and only occasionally in the intestines.

Lesions in lymphoid organs are common in both effusive and noneffusive forms of FIP. Splenic enlargement may be due to histiocytic and plasmacytic infiltration of the red pulp, hyperplasia of the lymphoid elements in the white pulp, necrotizing splenitis with fibrin deposition and polymorphonuclear cell infiltrates, or more organized pyogranulomatous reactions. Gross lymph node involvement is usually limited to thoracic and abdominal nodes. Their enlargement is due to a range of lesions resembling those described for the spleen (Fig. 7–23).

Fluorescent antibody staining of tissue sections from cats with both forms of FIP demonstrates virus in lesions. In effusive FIP, a large amount of viral antigen is contained in phagocytic cells that make up the periphery of the pyogranulomas (Fig. 7–24), in Kupffer cells within and adjacent to hepatic sinusoids, and in parenchymal lesions in the liver (Weiss and Scott, 1981c). There is less virus antigen in the lesions of noneffusive FIP, and it is usually found within a few macrophages adjacent to venules in the center of the lesions (Fig. 7–25).

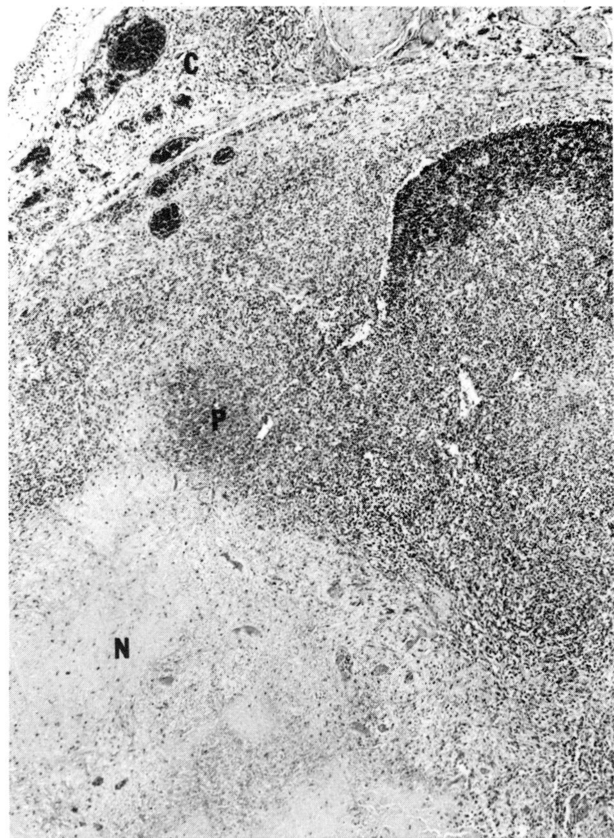


**Figure 7–23** Mesenteric lymph node in a cat with noneffusive FIP. A large area of necrosis is present within the node (N). A small pyogranuloma is seen adjacent to the necrotic focus (P). The capsule (C) of the node is infiltrated with inflammatory cells. The remainder of the node shows lymphoid hyperplasia. H & E, × 40.

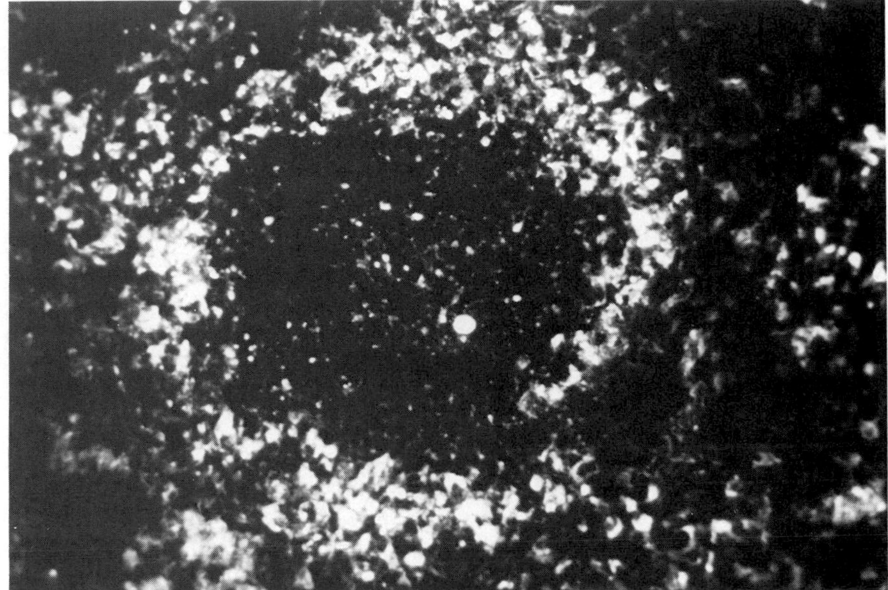

**Figure 7–24** Omentum in a cat with effusive FIP. A large amount of viral antigen is detected in macrophages in the periphery of a pyogranuloma. Cat anti-FIPV serum, rabbit anti-cat IgG–fluorescein isothiocyanate, Evan's blue counterstain, × 750.

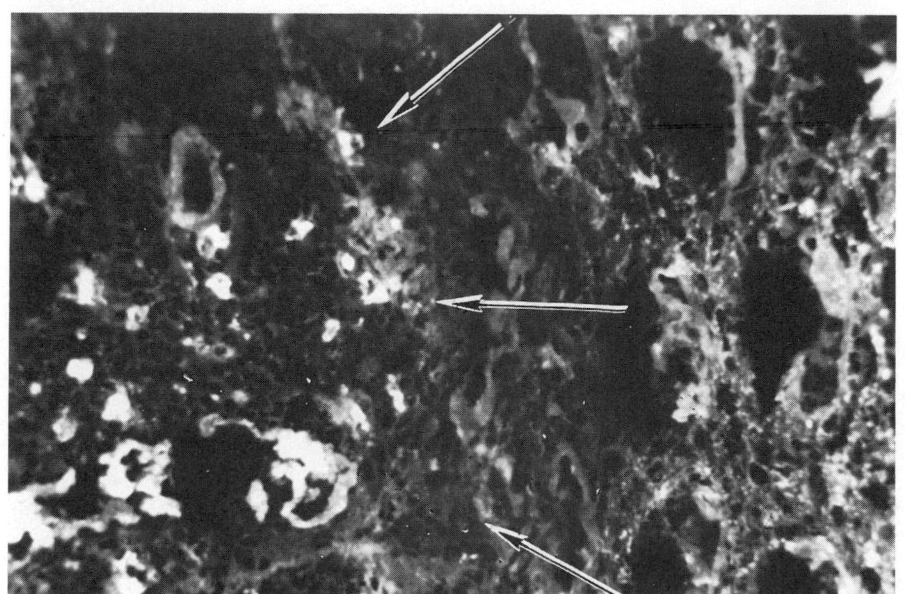

**Figure 7–25** Kidney in a cat with noneffusive FIP. The arrows outline the periphery of a pyogranuloma. Normal kidney parenchyma lies to the right of the arrows. Several mononuclear cells in the center of the pyogranuloma contain viral antigen. Cat anti-FIPV serum, globulin-fluorescein isothiocyanate, Evan's blue counterstain, × 750.

## Immunity

Immunity to FIPV infection is especially interesting because it is involved in both disease and disease resistance. The incidence of FIPV-immune cats in nature is not known. From 25 to 90 per cent or more of cats, depending on the environment, have been infected with a coronavirus as evidenced by serum antibodies (Pedersen, 1976a). Most of these cats, however, succumb if challenged with FIPV (Pedersen, 1983a). This means that most cats with coronavirus antibodies have been infected orally with either FECV or a strain of FIPV such as UCD3 or UCD4 that usually does not cause FIP by natural routes of infection (Pedersen and Floyd, 1985). Some seropositive cats, however, resist challenge with virulent FIPV. These cats have presumably undergone a previous systemic infection with a strain of coronavirus that causes FIP (Pedersen and Floyd, 1985).

Cats that are naturally or experimentally infected with FECV or orally infected with certain strains of FIPV develop antibodies that cross-react with all known feline coronavirus isolates (Boyle et al., 1984). These antibodies, however, are not protective. In fact, cats with such serum antibodies are often more sensitive to intraperitoneal infection with FIPV (Pedersen and Boyle, 1980; Pedersen et al., 1981a,b). Cats with pre-existing sensitizing coronavirus antibodies develop effusive FIP within 24 to 72 hours after FIPV infection, as contrasted with 8 to 14 days or more for cats without such antibodies. This enhancement occurs most consistently when the challenge strain is FIPV-UCD1 or TN406; FIPV-79-1146 infection is not influenced in one way or another by prior coronavirus exposure (Pedersen et al., 1984b). Aerosol inoculation with FIPV-UCD1 of cats with prior coronavirus exposure can cause a fulminating pneumonia (Weiss et al., 1980; Weiss and Scott, 1981a,b,c). The enhancement of illness caused by prior exposure to an antigenically related strain of virus is reminiscent of dengue hemorrhagic shock syndrome of man (Horzinek and Osterhaus, 1979b; Pedersen and Boyle, 1980; Weiss and Scott, 1981b).

Cats infected parenterally (or orally in the case of some strains) with FIPV either seroconvert without developing disease or seroconvert and die of FIP. Strains such as FIPV-UCD1, TN406 (low passage), and especially 79-1146 and Nor15 cause fatal FIP in from 75 to 90 per cent of the cats that become seropositive after infection. Strains such as UCD3 and UCD4 are much less lethal, inducing FIP in only 30 to 50 per cent of the cats that become seropositive after IP inoculation. Cats that become seropositive after IP inoculation and do not show signs of illness are solidly immune to reinfection with virulent FIPV. This immunity is usually, but not inevitably, non–strain-specific. FIP strains such as UCD2 and TN406 (high passage) have lost their ability to cause FIP by oronasal or IP route of inoculation. Unfortunately, the immunity that they induce is not protective but rather is immunoenhancing for virulent FIPV infection. Similarly, the immunity induced by oronasal inoculation with FIPV UCD3 and UCD4 is not always protective and may be immunoenhancing for infection with FIPV-UCD1 (Pedersen and Floyd, 1985).

Immunity to FIPV infection may also vary according to the route of inoculation and age at exposure. As mentioned previously, kittens born to FIPV-recovered queens seem to have a high degree of immunity to infection with virulent FIPV. Regardless of how this immunizing infection was acquired (in utero or neonatally), infection at a very early age appears to lead to a much higher rate of immunity than later infection.

Immunity to FIP does not involve humoral antibodies. High-titered serum from FIPV-recovered cats renders specific pathogen–free cats more susceptible to infection (Pedersen and Black, 1983). Immunity induced by attenuated live FIPV is also nonprotective and in many cases immunoenhancing (Pedersen and Black, 1983). The failure of attenuated strains of FIPV to evoke protective immunity indicates that protective immunity is a product of infection with virulent virus only. It has been suggested that this protective immunity is cell-mediated and that development of such immunity requires persistence of living virus in the body (Pedersen and Black, 1983). Attenuated virus might fail to provide protection because it fails to persist long enough in the body.

Most cats die after the appearance of clinical signs of FIP. A small percentage, however, develop signs of disease and recover. In the experimental situation, recovery always involves a progression from effusive through noneffusive disease. In keeping with this pattern, noneffusive FIP is always preceded by a brief episode of effusive disease. This is taken as indirect evidence for the theory that noneffusive FIP is an intermediate stage between effusive disease and complete immunity.

## FIP and FeLV Infection

The relationship of FIP to concurrent FeLV infection may have an immunologic basis. In the past, 40 to 50 per cent of the field cases of FIP occurred in cats also infected with FeLV (Cotter et al., 1973). We have observed 16 cats with FIP that had been raised in a single cattery (Pedersen, 1983). Fourteen of the 16 infections occurred in cats that were experimentally infected with FeLV, and FIP occurred in all within 2 to 12 weeks of the time that they became persistently infected with FeLV. Sibling cats not exposed to FeLV never developed FIP. Twelve of the 14 cats were actively FeLV-infected at the time they contracted FIP, and two were aviremic after having been actively infected several weeks earlier. In one study, six cats that had been previously "immunized" against FIPV with sublethal amounts of virulent virus were infected with FeLV (Pedersen and Floyd, 1985). All six developed FIP 6 to 16 weeks after they became persistently viremic with FeLV. It appeared that FeLV infection in some way activated a latent or sequestered FIPV infection. FIP immunity in some cats may therefore be one of premunition, resulting from the persistence of FIPV as a latent or walled-off infection. In support of this, vaccination with attenuated live FIPV does not protect cats against the virulent virus, probably because the attenuated virus does not persist in the body (Pedersen and Black, 1983). The relationship between virus persistence and immunity has precedents in other infectious diseases, not surprisingly infections in which cell-mediated immunity is also important. Immunity in diseases such as tuberculosis, histoplasmosis, and blastomycosis often involves the presence of organisms sequestered in the body, sometimes for life. FeLV infection is known to be immunosuppressive in cats (Anderson et al., 1971; see also chapter on immunology), and this may explain the apparent deterioration of established FIPV immunity.

## Serologic Studies

The diagnosis of FIP solely by serology is at present impossible. Initially, when FIP was thought to be an uncommon secondary manifestation of a common self-limiting enteric infection, the presence of FIPV antibodies in healthy cats was understandable (Pedersen, 1977). Now that antigenically similar FIP-inducing and non–FIP-inducing viruses have been discovered, the meaning of a positive FIPV indirect immunofluorescent antibody (IFA) titer is questionable (Pedersen, 1983b,c). Serologic tests must be interpreted in light of what is currently known about experimentally induced FIP and non–FIP-causing coronavirus infections.

Specific pathogen–free kittens infected by oral or intratracheal instillation of FIPV can be expected to react serologically in one of several ways (Pedersen et al., 1981a). Some cats do not develop any signs of infection after prolonged exposure and remain antibody-negative. Presumably the dose of virus that these cats were exposed to was insufficient to cause infection. Infected cats that do not develop illness demonstrate a plateau-shaped IFA antibody response, whereas cats that develop illness usually show a progressive titer rise (Fig. 7–26). The ultimate IFA titer in ill cats may exceed 1:25,000. Virus-neutralizing antibodies tend to correlate with the IFA titers in both groups of animals. Uncommonly, however, an infected cat will develop only virus-neutralizing antibodies and its IFA titers will be negligible.

If the cats have been previously infected with the enteric coronavirus (heterotypic immunity), the serologic response to FIPV challenge is more difficult to determine. Exposed cats that do not become ill do not show an increase in the baseline coronavirus antibody titer. The IFA titer of cats that develop FIP often rises above the background enteric coronavirus titer (Fig. 7–27).

Although antibody titers of experimentally infected cats are easy to interpret, the interpretation of serologic tests in natural disease is much more difficult. In clinical practice, antibody titers are measured at one point in time and without previous knowledge of the background enteric coronavirus antibody levels. It was not possible at the time this discussion was written to differentiate the background enteric coronavirus antibody titers from the titers that are specific for FIPV. The substrates used for the antibody tests (FIPV, TGEV or swine, canine coronavirus) detect antibodies to both FIPV and the feline enteric coronavirus. This is true of IFA, enzyme-linked immunosorbent assay (ELISA), and virus neutralization tests. In addition to this lack of specificity, the coronavirus antibody titer in a cat with FIP can be low. These low IFA titers (0 to 1:100) are most commonly seen in kittens with fulminating effusive FIP and less frequently in older cats with noneffusive disease.

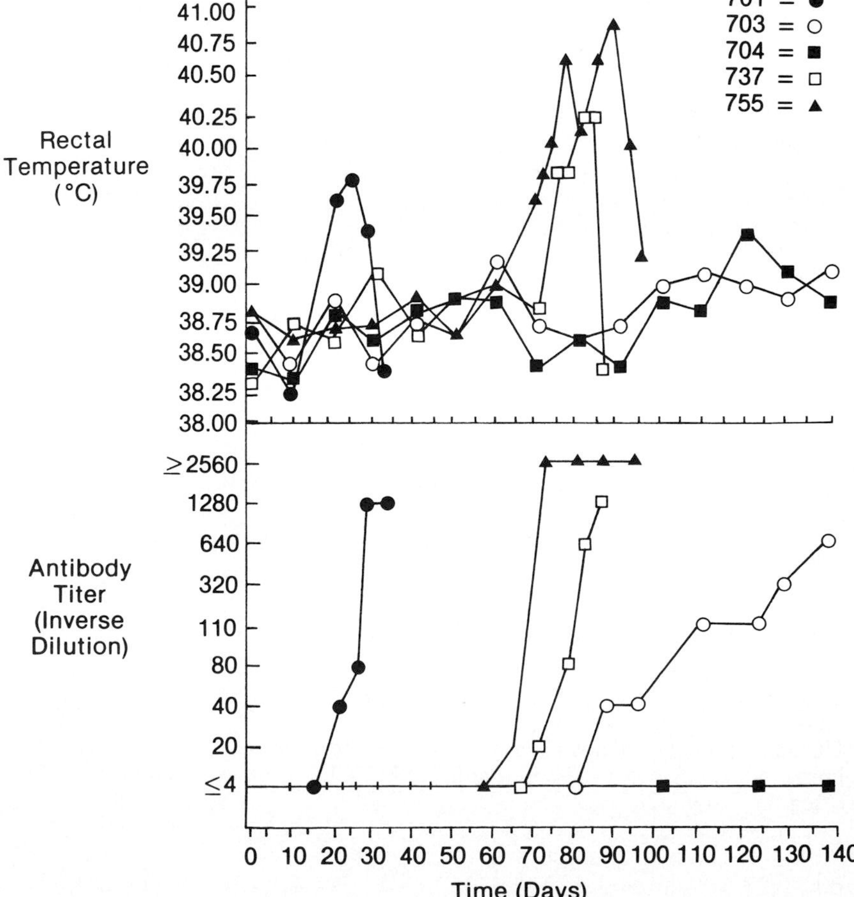


**Figure 7–26** The serologic response of antibody-negative cats that were fed FIPV daily for several months. Rectal temperatures of cats that develop FIP are elevated. Cats 701, 737, and 755 developed FIP and died several weeks later. Cat 703 developed serum antibodies without ever becoming ill. Cat 704 showed no clinical or serologic signs of infection.

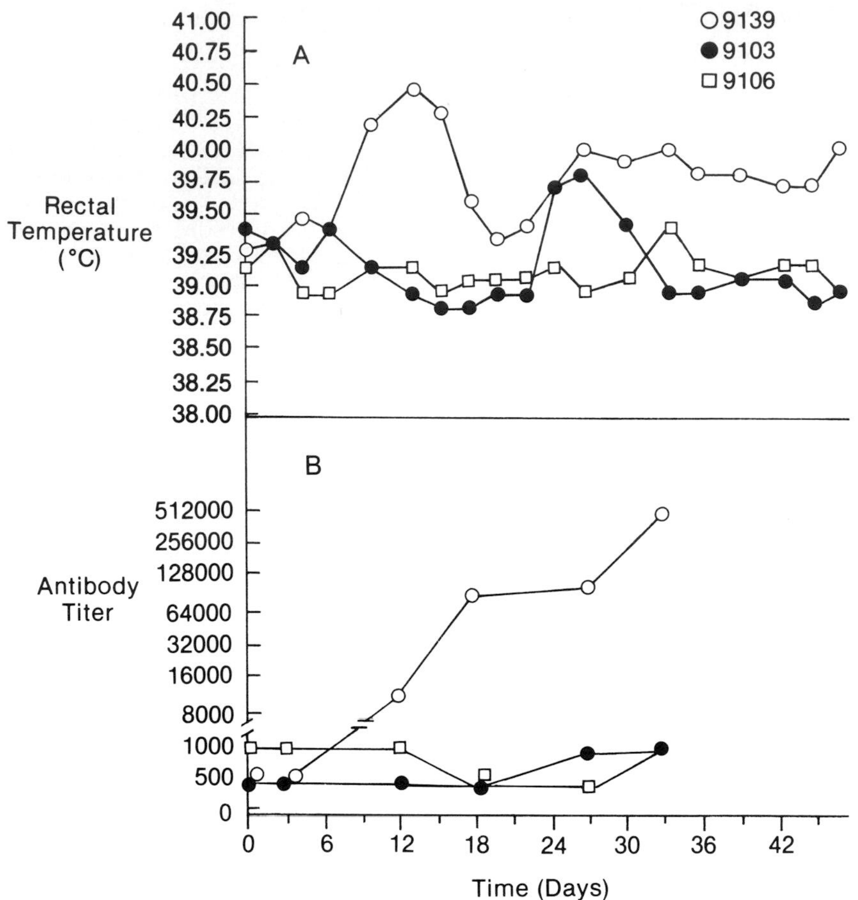


**Figure 7–27** The serologic responses of enteric coronavirus–positive cats that were fed FIPV for several months. Cat 9139 developed a fever several days after exposure to the virus and died over a month later of FIP. With the development of fever there was a progressive rise in the anti-FIPV titer in the serum. Cats 9103 and 9106 did not become ill, and their antibody titers to coronavirus did not rise above the initial levels.

Currently practiced serologic procedures can nonetheless help in diagnosing FIP. IFA antibody titers greater than 1:3200 are usually associated with FIP, frequently of the noneffusive type. This titer is generally above the titers resulting from the enteric coronavirus infection. IFA antibody titers of 1:100 to 1:3200 are common in cats with effusive FIP and in some cats with noneffusive disease. Because IFA titers of 1:25 to 1:3200 are also found in cats that have undergone the enteric coronavirus infection, the diagnosis of FIP in cats with titers in this range depends on a careful review of the entire clinical and clinicopathologic picture. A positive titer should alert a clinician to the possibility of FIP, whereas a negative titer may help to rule out the disease. Tests are needed that specifically measure antibodies to FIPV and not to other coronaviruses as well.

## Treatment

Once it is clinically manifest, FIPV infection is usually fatal. Remission from disease has been documented on only a few occasions, usually after the use of glucocorticoids with or without drugs such as cyclophosphamide or phenylalanine mustard (Colgrove and Parker, 1971; Madewell et al., 1978; Pedersen, 1976b). Successfully treated cats had several things in common. They usually had milder signs of illness, and they were still eating and not overly debilitated at the time treatment was undertaken. In addition, the owners were willing to expend considerable time on symptomatic nursing care. Treatment is invariably futile in debilitated animals and may shorten survival time. Even in selected cases successful remission is achieved in only a small percentage.

A complicating factor in evaluating apparently successful treatment is the occurrence of spontaneous remissions. Not every cat with FIP dies. Autopsies of older cats without signs of overt FIP have occasionally demonstrated fibrous lesions on the spleen and liver that indicate a past FIP infection. Cats with ocular disease and very high FIP virus antibody titers have occasionally gone into remission with just topical treatment, and the antibody titers have decreased. Finally, cats with small quiescent lesions in their spleens and mesenteric lymph nodes have been discovered during the course of routine oophorohysterectomies.

## Prevention

### Immunization

Initial attempts to immunize cats with TGE virus of swine have been unsuccessful (Toma et al., 1979; Woods and Pedersen, 1979). Experiments with attenuated live FIPV have also been unsuccessful (Pedersen and Black, 1982). Kittens immunized oronasally with attenuated live FIPV-TN406 (high passage) developed both IFA and virus-neutralizing antibodies. After challenge with virulent FIPV-TN406 (low passage), however, the infection rate was enhanced, latency period reduced, and disease severity increased in vaccinated kittens compared with nonvaccinates. The same phenomena have been observed in cats infected oronasally with virulent FIPV-UCD3 or -UCD4 (Pedersen and Floyd, 1985). Apparently, avirulent virus does not confer a protective immunity but may have elicited humoral immunity that was actually deleterious. Cats can be immunized against FIP with very small amounts of virulent FIPV (Pedersen and Black, 1982). This finding is not of clinical value, however, because the dose required to immunize some cats was sufficient to cause fatal FIP in others.

### Husbandry and Breeding Practices

The incidence of FIP in a cattery often parallels the incidence of other infectious diseases, including infections with *Chlamydia, Mycoplasma*, herpes, enteric coronavirus, calicivirus, and of course FeLV. Environmental manipulations to eliminate overcrowding and decrease the number of young kittens reared at any one time, increased ventilation and cleanliness, isolation of queens with litters from other cats until after their kittens are weaned, and segregating kittens of different ages from one another all help to lower the incidence of these diseases. Such measures should be combined with a sound breeding program in which replacement cats are selected because they were free of kittenhood disease. Queens should also be selected for their good mothering instincts and for a record of raising large healthy litters rather than for more esoteric qualities. If these practices are implemented, FIP and other cattery diseases may be to a great extent controlled.

## FIPV AND KITTEN MORTALITY

Scott and coworkers (1979) described a syndrome of fetal death, weak fading kittens, and cardiomyopathy. Since many of the affected catteries had cats seropositive for FIPV antibodies, they postulated that FIPV might be the cause of what they called the "kitten mortality complex." Their argument is weakened, however, by the facts that all conventional catteries have indigenous coronavirus infections and that not all catteries have problems with kitten mortality. Moreover, cardiomyopathy, fetal death, and abortions have been observed in two specific pathogen–free catteries that were free of coronavirus infection (Pedersen, 1983a). The presence of FIPV antibodies does not indicate that there is an FIP-inducing coronavirus infection on the premises. In most cases, the FIPV antibodies are induced by non–FIP-inducing enteric coronaviruses that are antigenically similar to FIPV.

Coronaviruses, including both enteric and FIP viruses, cannot be excluded, however, as causes of kitten mortality. Transmissible gastroenteritis virus (TGEV) of swine is notorious for causing sporadic but explosive outbreaks that kill neonatal pigs. FIPV and enteric coronaviruses are merely serologic variants of TGEV (Horzinek et al., 1982), and FIPV can actually cause a TGE-like syndrome in neonatal pigs (Woods et al., 1981). Coronavirus-like agents have also been implicated in cardiomyopathy in rabbits (Small et al., 1979) and humans (Riski et al., 1980). The most convincing evidence for the role of FIPV in abortion and kitten mortality comes from the studies of McKeirnan and associates (1981). They isolated a coronavirus designated 79-1146 from a four-day-old fading kitten, one of three born to a queen that had produced two normal litters followed by two consecutive abortions. One of the kittens was born with a cleft palate, whereas the third kitten remained healthy. Histopathologic examination of the liver of the fading kitten revealed congestion, hemorrhage, and necrosis. The alveolar walls of the lung were moderately infiltrated by macrophages and lymphocytes. The coronavirus isolated from tissues of this kitten grew readily in tissue cultures of feline cells and caused FIP when given oronasally to specific pathogen–free kittens (Pedersen et al., 1984b). The chronicity of the lung lesions suggested that the infection occurred in utero, indicating that the queen was probably a carrier of FIPV. Lesions similar to those in this kitten were not seen, however, in kittens that succumbed to the "kitten mortality complex" that is so prevalent in catteries.

To more directly study the role of FIPV in kitten mortality, FIPV-recovered queens have been bred and their kittens observed for disease (Pedersen and Floyd, 1985). Among eight such queens, three have produced a total of five litters. The litter sizes have been normal, and the kittens have all been healthy.

In conclusion, there is insufficient evidence at this time to implicate FIPV or other feline coronaviruses as major causes of kitten mortality. There is no question, however, that they are involved to some degree.

### Acknowledgment

Some of the work reported in this section was supported by grants from the Robert L. Winn Foundation for cat research of the Cat Fanciers Association, Red Bank, NJ, Save Our Cats and Kittens Organization, Walnut Creek, CA, and the Laurence Skewes estate for feline health–related research.

### REFERENCES

Anderson LJ, Jarrett WFH, Jarrett O, Laird HM: Feline leukemia-virus infection of kittens: mortality associated with atrophy of the thymus and lymphoid depletion. J Natl Cancer Inst 47 (1971) 807–817.

Appel MJG, Meunier P, Greisen H, Carmichael LE, Glickman L: Enteric viral infections of dogs. Proc 19th Gaines Vet Symp, Gainesville, Florida, Oct 17, 1979, 3–8.

Auclair-Semere G, Groulade P: Péritonite infectieuse chez une chatte. Bull Acad Vét (Toulouse) 48 (1975) 289–292.

Beesley JE, Hitchcock LM: The ultrastructure of feline infectious peritonitis virus in feline embryonic lung cells. J Gen Virol 59 (1982) 23–28.

Black JW: Recovery and *in vitro* cultivation of a coronavirus from laboratory-induced cases of feline infectious peritonitis (FIP). Vet Med Small Anim Clin 75 (1980) 811–814.

Bohl EH: Transmissible gastroenteritis. *In* Dunne HW, Leman AD (eds): Diseases of Swine, 4th ed. Ames, Iowa State University Press, 1975, 168–188.

Boyle JF, Pedersen NC, Evermann JF, McKeirnan AJ, Ott RL, Black JW: Plaque assay, polypeptide composition and immunochemistry of feline infectious peritonitis virus and feline enteric coronavirus. Adv Exp Med Biol 173 (1984) 133–147.

Campbell LH, Reed C: Ocular signs associated with feline infectious peritonitis in two cats. Feline Pract 5(3) (1975) 32–35.

Campbell LH, Schiessl MM: Ocular manifestations of toxoplasmosis, infectious peeritonitis and lymphosarcoma in cats. Mod Vet Pract 59 (1978) 761–764.

Chantal J, Deschamps B: Un cas de pleuro-péritonite sérofibrineuse chronique chez un chat. Rev Méd Vét (Paris) 125 (1974) 1208–1209.

Colby ED, Low RJ: Feline infectious peritonitis. Vet Med Small Anim Clin 65 (1970) 783–786.

Colgrove DJ, Parker AJ: Feline infectious peritonitis. J Small Anim Pract 12 (1971) 225–232.

Colly LP, Johannesburg, South Africa, cited in Robison RL et al.: J Am Vet Med Assoc 158 (1971) 981–986.

Cotter SM, Gilmore CE, Rollins C: Multiple cases of feline leukemia and feline infectious peritonitis in a household. J Am Vet Med Assoc 162 (1973) 1054–1058.

Dea S, Roy RS, Elazhary MASY: Coronavirus-like particles in the feces of a cat with diarrhea. Can Vet J 23 (1982) 153–155.

DeAluja AS: Peritonitis infecciosa felina (informe de un caso). Veterinaria (Mexico City) 3 (1972) 106–108.

Doherty MJ: Ocular manifestations of feline infectious peritonitis. J Am Vet Med Assoc 159 (1971) 417–424.

Evermann JF, Baumgartener L, Ott RL, Davis EV, McKeirnan AJ: Characterization of a feline infectious peritonitis virus isolate. Vet Pathol 18 (1981) 256–265.

Eugster AK, Liauw H: Detection of antibodies to feline infectious peritonitis (FIP) virus in cats using transmissible gastroenteritis virus as antigen and an electron microscopic search for FIP virus. Southwest Vet 32 (1979) 109–112.

Fankhauser R, Fatzer R: Meningitis und Chorioependymitis granulomatosa der Katze; mögliche Beziehungen zur felinen infektiösen Peritonitis (FIP). Kleintierpraxis 22 (1977) 19–22.

Feldman BF: Feline infectious peritonitis: A case report of a variant form. Feline Pract 4(5) (1974) 32–37.

Feldmann BM, Jortner BS: Clinicopathologic conference [Feline systemic proliferative and exudative vasculitis]. J Am Vet Med Assoc 144 (1964) 1409–1420.

Fransen DR: Feline infectious peritonitis in an infant jaguar. Proc Annu Meeting, Am Assoc Zoo Veterinarians, 1972, Houston, Texas, 1973, Columbus, Ohio, 1974, 261–264.

Gelatt KN: Iridocyclitis-panophthalmitis associated with feline infectious peritonitis. Vet Med Small Anim Clin 68 (1973) 56–57.

Hardy WD Jr, Hurvitz AI: Feline infectious peritonitis: Experimental studies. J Am Vet Med Assoc 158 (1971) 994–1002.

Hartigan PJ, Wilson P: Feline infectious peritonitis. Ir Vet J 26 (1972) 8–10.

Harvey JW, Gaskin JM: Feline haptoglobin. Am J Vet Res 39 (1978) 549–553.

Hayashi T, Goto N, Takahashi R, Fujiwara K: Systemic vascular lesions in feline infectious peritonitis. Jpn J Vet Sci 39 (1977) 365–377.

Hayashi T, Goto N, Takahashi R, Fujiwara K: Detection of coronavirus-like particles in a spontaneous case of feline infectious peritonitis. Jpn J Vet Sci 40 (1978) 207–212.

Hayashi T, Utsumi F, Takahashi R, Fujiwara K: Pathology of non-effusive type feline infectious peritonitis and experimental transmission. Jpn J Vet Sci 42 (1980) 197–210.

Hayashi T, Watabe Y, Nakayama H, Fujiwara K: Enteritis due to feline infectious peritonitis virus. Jpn J Vet Sci 44 (1982) 97–106.

Heider E: Zum Vorkommen der felinen infektiösen Peritonitis in Österreich. Wien Tierärztl Monatsschr 66 (1979) 203–206.

Holliday TA: Clinical aspects of some encephalopathies of domestic cats. Vet Clin North Am 1 (1971) 367–378.

Holmberg CA, Gribble DH: Feline infectious peritonitis: Diagnostic gross and microscopic lesions. Feline Pract 3(4) (1973) 11–14.

Holzworth J: Some important disorders of cats. Cornell Vet 53 (1963) 157–160.

Horzinek MC, Osterhaus ADME, Ellens DJ: Feline infectious peritonitis virus. Zentralbl Veterinärmed [B] 24 (1977) 398–405.

Horzinek MC, Osterhaus ADME, Wirahadiredja RMS, de Kreek P: Feline infectious peritonitis (FIP) virus. III. Studies on the multiplication of FIP virus in the suckling mouse. Zentralbl Veterinärmed [B] 25 (1978) 806–815.

Horzinek MC, Osterhaus ADME: Feline infectious peritonitis: A worldwide serosurvey. Am J Vet Res 40 (1979a) 1487–1492.

Horzinek MC, Osterhaus ADME: The virology and pathogenesis of feline infectious peritonitis. Brief review. Arch Virol 59 (1979b) 1–15.

Horzinek MC, Lutz H, Pedersen NC: Antigenic relationships among homologous structural polypeptides of porcine, feline, and canine coronaviruses. Infect Immun 37 (1982) 1148–1155.

Hoshino Y, Scott FW: Coronavirus-like particles in the feces of normal cats. Brief report. Arch Virol 63 (1980a) 147–152.

Hoshino Y, Scott FW: Immunofluorescent and electron microscopic studies of feline small intestine organ cultures infected with feline infectious peritonitis virus. Am J Vet Res 41 (1980b) 672–681.

Ishmael J, Howell J McC: Observations on the pathology of the spleen of the cat. J Small Anim Pract 9 (1968) 7–13.

Jacobse-Geels HEL, Daha MR, Horzinek MC: Isolation and characterization of feline C3 and evidence for the immune complex pathogenesis of feline infectious peritonitis. J Immunol 125 (1980) 1606–1610.

Jacobse-Geels HEL, Daha MR, Horzinek MC: Antibody, immune complexes, and complement activity fluctuations in kittens with experimentally induced feline infectious peritonitis. Am J Vet Res 43 (1982) 666–670.

Jones BR: Feline infectious peritonitis—clinical findings, clinical diagnosis and epidemiological aspects. Vict Vet Proc 32 (1974) 31–33.

Joshua JO: Vomiting in the cat. Mod Vet Pract 41(22) (1960) 36–42.

Konishi S, Takahashi E, Ogata M, Ishida K: Studies on feline infectious peritonitis (FIP). I. Occurrence and experimental transmission of the disease in Japan. Jpn J Vet Sci 33 (1971) 327–333.

Kornegay JN: Feline infectious peritonitis: The central nervous system form. J Am Anim Hosp Assoc 14 (1978) 580–584.

Krebiel JD, Sanger VL, Ravi A: Ophthalmic lesions in feline infectious peritonitis: Gross, microscopic and ultrastructural changes. Vet Pathol 11 (1974) 443–444.

Krum S, Johnson K, Wilson J: Hydrocephalus associated with the noneffusive form of feline infectious peritonitis. J Am Vet Med Assoc 167 (1975) 746–748.

Legendre AM, Whitenack DL: Feline infectious peritonitis with spinal cord involvement in two cats. J Am Vet Med Assoc 167 (1975) 931–932.

Loeffler DG, Ott RL, Evermann JF, Alexander JE: The incidence of naturally occurring antibodies against feline infectious peritonitis in selected cat populations. Feline Pract 8(1) (1978) 43–47.

Madewell BR, Crow SE, Nickerson TR: Infectious peritonitis in a cat that subsequently developed a myeloproliferative disorder. J Am Vet Med Assoc 172 (1978) 169–172.

Mannonen J, Nikander S, Rimaila-Pärnänen E: [Feline infectious peritonitis (FIP), a case report.] Suomen Eläinlääkärilehti 85 (1979) 292–294.

McKeirnan AJ, Evermann JF, Hargis A, Miller LM, Ott RL: Isolation of feline coronaviruses from two cats with diverse disease manifestations. Feline Pract 11(3) (1981) 16–20.

Mieog WHW, Richter JHM: Feline infectious peritonitis. Tijdschr Diergeneeskd 96 (1971) 585–598.

Montali RJ, Strandberg JD: Extraperitoneal lesions in feline infectious peritonitis. Vet Pathol 9 (1972) 109–121.

Mortensen VA, Steensborg K: Infektiøs peritonitis hos katte (FIP). Dansk Vet Tidsskr 59 (1976) 761–764.

Norsworthy GD: Neonatal feline infectious peritonitis. Feline Pract 4(6) (1974) 34.

O'Reilly KJ, Fishman B, Hitchcock LM: Feline infectious peritonitis: Isolation of a coronavirus [short communication]. Vet Rec 104 (1979) 348.

Osterhaus ADME, Horzinek MC, Wirahadiredja RMS, Kroon

A: Feline infectious peritonitis (FIP) virus. IV. Propagation in suckling rat and hamster brain. Zentralbl Veterinärmed [B] 25 (1978) 816–825.

Pastoret PP, Gouffaux M, Henroteaux M: Description et étude expérimentale de la péritonite infectieuse féline. Ann Méd Vét 118 (1974) 479–492.

Pedersen NC: Serologic studies of naturally occurring feline infectious peritonitis. Am J Vet Res 37 (1976a) 1449–1453.

Pedersen NC: Feline infectious peritonitis: Something old, something new. Feline Pract 6(3) (1976b) 42–51.

Pedersen NC: Morphologic and physical characteristics of feline infectious peritonitis virus and its growth in autochthonous peritoneal cell cultures. Am J Vet Res 37 (1976c) 567–572.

Pedersen NC: Feline infectious peritonitis test results: What do they mean? Feline Pract 7(3) (1977) 13–14.

Pedersen NC: Feline infectious disease. Proc Am Animal Hosp Assoc, 1978, 125–146.

Pedersen NC: Personal observation, 1983a.

Pedersen NC: Feline infectious peritonitis and feline enteric coronavirus infections. Part 1: Feline enteric coronavirus. Feline Pract 13(4) (1983b) 13–19.

Pedersen NC: Feline infectious peritonitis and feline enteric coronavirus infections. Part 2: Feline infectious peritonitis. Feline Pract 13(5) (1983c) 5–19.

Pedersen NC, Black JW: Attempted immunization of cats against feline infectious peritonitis using either avirulent live virus or sublethal amounts of virulent virus. Am J Vet Res 44 (1983) 229–234.

Pedersen NC, Floyd K: Experimental studies with three new strains of feline infectious peritonitis virus: FIPV-UCD2, FIPV-UCD3, and FIPV-UCD4. Compend Contin Ed 7 (1985) 1001–1011.

Pedersen NC, Black JW, Boyle JF, Evermann JF, McKeirnan AJ, Ott RL: Pathogenesis of feline coronaviruses. Adv Exp Biol Med 173 (1984a) 365–380.

Pedersen NC, Boyle JF: Immunologic phenomena in the effusive form of feline infectious peritonitis. Am J Vet Res 41 (1980) 868–876.

Pedersen NC, Boyle JF, Floyd K: Infection studies in kittens utilizing feline infectious peritonitis virus propagated in cell culture. Am J Vet Res 42 (1981a) 363–367.

Pedersen NC, Boyle JF, Floyd K, Fudge A, Barker J: An enteric coronavirus infection of cats, and its relationship to feline infectious peritonitis. Am J Vet Res 42 (1981b) 368–377.

Pedersen NC, Evermann JF, McKeirnan AJ, Ott RL: Pathogenicity studies of feline coronavirus isolates 79-1146 and 79-1683. Am J Vet Res 45 (1984b) 2580–2585.

Pedersen NC, Holliday TA, Cello RM: Feline infectious peritonitis. Proc Am Anim Hosp Assoc, 1974, 147–153.

Pedersen NC, Ward J, Mengeling WL: Antigenic relationship of the feline infectious peritonitis virus to coronaviruses of other species. Arch Virol 58 (1978) 45–53.

Pfeifer ML, Evermann JF, Roelke ME, Gallina AM, Ott RL, McKeirnan AJ: Feline infectious peritonitis in a captive cheetah. J Am Vet Med Assoc 183 (1983) 1317–1319.

Poelma FG, Peters JC, Mieog WHW, Zwart P: Infektiöse Peritonitis bei Karakal (*Felis caracal*) und Nordluchs (*Felis lynx lynx*). Erkrankungen der Zootiere 13th Int Symp, Helsinki, 1974, 249–253.

Potkay S, Bacher JD, Pitts TW: Feline infectious peritonitis in a closed breeding colony. Lab Anim Sci 24 (1974) 279–289.

Reynolds DJ, Garwes DJ, Gaskell CJ: Detection of transmissible gastroenteritis virus neutralising antibody in cats. Arch Virol 55 (1977) 77–86.

Reynolds DJ, Garwes DJ, Lucey S: Differentiation of canine coronavirus and porcine transmissible gastroenteritis virus by neutralization with canine, porcine and feline sera. Vet Microbiol 5 (1980) 283–290.

Riski H, Hovi T, Frick MH: Carditis associated with coronavirus infection [letter]. Lancet 2 (1980) 100–101.

Robison RL, Holzworth J, Gilmore CE: Naturally occurring feline infectious peritonitis: signs and clinical diagnosis. J Am Vet Med Assoc 158 (1971) 981–986.

Schalm OW: Feline infectious peritonitis vital statistics and laboratory findings. Calif Vet 25(10) (1979) 6–9.

Schalm OW, Jain NC, Carroll EJ: Veterinary Hematology, 3rd ed. Philadelphia, Lea & Febiger, 1975.

Scott FW, Weiss RC, Post JE, Gilmartin JE, Hoshino Y: Kitten mortality complex (neonatal FIP). Feline Pract 9(2) (1979) 44–56.

Slauson DO, Finn JP: Meningoencephalitis and panophthalmitis in feline infectious peritonitis. J Am Vet Med Assoc 160 (1972) 729–734.

Small JD, Aurelian L, Squire RA, Strandberg JD, Melby EC Jr, Turner TB, Newman B: Rabbit cardiomyopathy associated with a virus antigenically related to human coronavirus strain 229E. Am J Pathol 95 (1979) 709–729.

Smith HA, Jones TC: Veterinary Pathology, 2nd ed. Philadelphia, Lea & Febiger, 1961, 846–848.

Smith HA, Jones TC: Veterinary Pathology, 3rd ed. Philadelphia, Lea & Febiger, 1966, 953.

Stevenson RG, Tilt SE, Purdy JG: Feline infectious peritonitis and pleurisy. Can Vet J 12 (1971) 97–99.

Stünzi H, Grevel V: Die ansteckende fibrinöse Peritonitis der Katze. Vorläufige Mitteilung über die ersten spontanen Fälle in der Schweiz. Schweiz Arch Tierheilkd 115 (1973) 579–586.

Summers BA, Sykes G, Martin ML: Pansteatitis mimicking infectious peritonitis in a cat. J Am Vet Med Assoc 180 (1982) 546–549.

Theobald J: Felidae. *In* Fowler ME (ed): Zoo and Wild Animal Medicine. Philadelphia, W B Saunders Company, 1978, 650–667.

Toma B, Duret C, Chappuis G, Pellerin B: Échec de l'immunisation contre la péritonite infectieuse féline par injection de virus de la gastroentérite transmissible du porc. Recl Méd Vét 155 (1979) 799–803.

Tuch K, Witte KH, Wüller H: Feststellung der felinen infektiösen Peritonitis (FIP) bei Hauskatzen und Leoparden in Deutschland. Zentralbl Veterinärmed [B] 21 (1974) 426–441.

Tyrrell DAJ, Alexander DJ, Almeida JD, Cunningham CH, Easterday BC, Garwes DJ, Hierholzer JC, Kapikian A, McNaughton MR, McIntosh K: Coronaviridae. Second report. Intervirology 10 (1978) 321–328.

Ward BC, Pedersen N: Infectious peritonitis in cats. J Am Vet Med Assoc 154 (1969) 26–35.

Ward JM: Morphogenesis of a virus in cats with experimental feline infectious peritonitis. Virology 41 (1970) 191–194.

Ward JM, Gribble DH, Dungworth DL: Feline infectious peritonitis: Experimental evidence for its multiphasic nature. Am J Vet Res 35 (1974) 1271–1275.

Ward JM, Munn RJ, Gribble DH, Dungworth DL: An observation of feline infectious peritonitis. Vet Rec 83 (1968) 416–417.

Ward JM, Smith R, Schalm OW: Inclusions in neutrophils of cats with feline infectious peritonitis. J Am Vet Med Assoc 158 (1971) 348.

Weiss RC, Dodds WJ, Scott FW: Disseminated intravascular coagulation in experimentally induced feline infectious peritonitis. Am J Vet Res 41 (1980) 663–671.

Weiss RC, Scott FW: Pathogenesis of feline infectious peritonitis: Nature and development of viremia. Am J Vet Res 42 (1981a) 382–390.

Weiss RC, Scott FW: Antibody-mediated enhancement of disease in feline infectious peritonitis: Comparisons with dengue hemorrhagic fever. Comp Immunol Microbiol Infect Dis 4 (1981b) 175–189.

Weiss RC, Scott FW: Pathogenesis of feline infectious peritonitis: Pathologic changes and immunofluorescence. Am J Vet Res 42 (1981c) 2036–2048.

Witte KH, Tuch K, Dubenkropp H, Walther C: Untersuchungen über die Antigenverwandtschaft der Viren der felinen infektiösen Peritonitis (FIP) und der transmissiblen Gastroenteritis (TGE) des Schweines. Berl Münch Tierärztl Wochenschr 90 (1977) 396–401.

Wolfe LG, Griesemer RA: Feline infectious peritonitis. Pathol Vet 3 (1966) 255–270.

Wolfe LG, Griesemer RA: Feline infectious peritonitis: review of gross and histopathologic lesions. J Am Vet Med Assoc 158 (1971) 987–993.

Woods RD, Pedersen NC: Cross-protection studies between feline infectious peritonitis and porcine transmissible gastroenteritis viruses. Vet Microbiol 4 (1979) 11–16.

Woods RD, Cheville NF, Gallagher JE: Lesions in the small intestine of newborn pigs inoculated with porcine, feline, and canine coronaviruses. Am J Vet Res 42 (1981) 1163–1169.

Zook BC, King NW, Robison RL, McCombs HL: Ultrastructural evidence for the viral etiology of feline infectious peritonitis. Pathol Vet 5 (1968) 91–95.

# VIRAL RESPIRATORY DISEASES AND CHLAMYDIOSIS

EDWARD A. HOOVER

Diagnosis of feline upper respiratory diseases must often be based on clinical observations since identification of the causative agent is usually impractical. Presumptive diagnosis of specific infections, however, is frequently possible. This discussion will emphasize information obtained through experimental and clinical investigations of the major pathogens of the feline respiratory tract and conjunctiva. The distinctive signs and lesions will be stressed.

## FELINE VIRAL RHINOTRACHEITIS

Feline viral rhinotracheitis (FVR), the most prevalent and most severe respiratory infection of cats, is caused by feline rhinotracheitis virus (FRV), a feline herpesvirus (Crandell and Maurer, 1958; Ditchfield and Grinyer, 1965). FVR is representative of upper respiratory herpesvirus infections of several animal species (e.g., infectious bovine rhinotracheitis, equine viral rhinopneumonitis, porcine pseudorabies, avian laryngotracheitis) and shares with these diseases the properties of viral latency, reactivation, and tropism for the gravid uterus (Crandell, 1971). FVR occurs enzootically throughout the world and can be induced experimentally in conventional, specific pathogen–free (SPF), and gnotobiotic cats (Bürki et al., 1964; Crandell et al., 1961; Hoover et al., 1970). Several reviews of FRV and FVR have been published (Crandell, 1971, 1973; Gillespie and Scott, 1973; Povey, 1976).

### Characteristics of the Virus

Crandell (1971) reviewed the properties of the virus in detail. In vivo, it infects only Felidae. In vitro, it replicates in various feline cell cultures including alveolar and peritoneal macrophages, pneumocytes, and tracheal explants (Crandell, 1971; Langloss et al., 1978a; Milek et al., 1976). FRV replication has also been induced in rabbit kidney cells (Ditchfield and Grinyer, 1965), and abortive viral infection, marked by inclusion body formation in the absence of viral synthesis, has been produced in human embryonic lung cells artificially fused by Sendai virus after absorption of FRV (Abraham and Tegtmeyer, 1970). The species-specific susceptibility of cells to FRV, therefore, is presumably a reflection of appropriate receptors for viral entry into cells (Abraham and Tegtmeyer, 1970).

FRV cytopathic effect in feline cell cultures occurs in 24 to 48 hours and consists of increased cell refractility, cytoplasmic retraction and fusion, formation of acidophilic intranuclear inclusion bodies, and subsequent cell lysis (Crandell and Despeaux, 1959) (Fig. 7–28). FRV also forms plaques in cell cultures, and viral infectivity titers can be expressed as plaque-forming units or 50 per cent tissue culture infectious doses, the latter being more common (Crandell, 1971). In addition to upper respiratory epithelial cells, FRV has been shown to replicate in vivo in feline endothelial cells, osteoblasts, osteoclasts, endometrial epithelium, trophoblast, adrenal cells, hepatocytes, oral mucosa, corneal cells, and alveolar cells (Bistner et al., 1971; Hoover and Griesemer, 1971a,c; Karpas and Routledge, 1968; Langloss et al., 1978a; Love, 1971).

The structure and replication of FRV are typical of herpesviruses. Nonenveloped icosahedral virions approximately 100 nm in diameter are assembled in the nucleus and are associated with clumping and margination of chromatin and accumulation of focal aggregates of dense viral nucleoid material (Fig. 7–29). Mature virions approximately 150 nm in diameter become enveloped by budding from invaginations of the nuclear membrane (Fig. 7–29) into cytoplasmic channels that communicate with the cell surface (Abraham and Tegtmeyer, 1970; Ditchfield and Grinyer, 1965).

Isolates of FRV appear to be antigenically homogeneous by serum neutralization and hemagglutination inhibition assays (Crandell et al., 1960a,b; Mochizuki, 1977c). The C-27 isolate of Crandell and Maurer (1958) is considered the FRV prototype. FRV induces hemagglutination of feline erythrocytes and hemadsorption of feline erythrocytes to FRV-infected cells (Mochizuki et al., 1977a,b).

FRV infectivity is sensitive to lipid solvents, low pH,

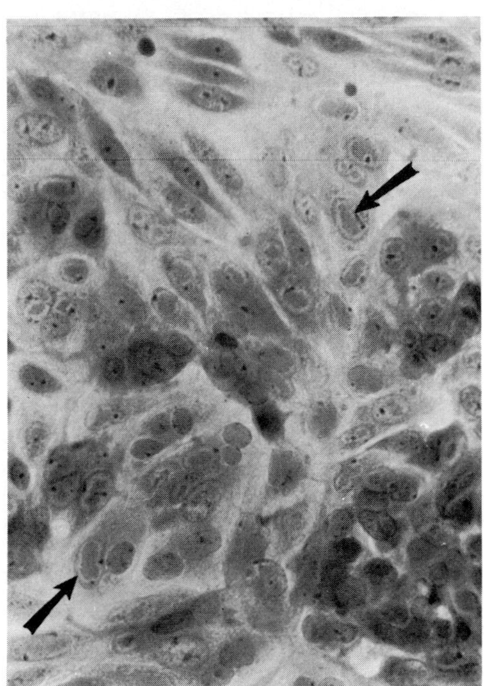

**Figure 7–28** FVR: Intranuclear inclusion bodies (arrows) in feline cell culture; unaffected cells are at top of field. H & E.

desiccation, detergents, common disinfectants, and fixatives (Miller and Crandell, 1962; Wardley and Povey, 1977). Virus survival is favored by fluid medium, neutral pH, and low temperatures (in cell culture medium, survival is three hours at 37 C, less than one month at 25 C, several months at 4 C, and several years at −70 C) (Miller and Crandell, 1962). Transmission of FRV among cats appears to depend primarily on direct contact or short-distance aerosolization through sneezing (Gaskell and Povey, 1982; Povey, 1976). Opportunity for contagion is maximized in environments such as pet shops, shelters, and catteries. Fomite transmission probably is of little consequence owing to the sensitivity of FRV to desiccation and chemical inactivation (Donaldson and Ferris, 1976; Gaskell and Povey, 1982; Wardley and Povey, 1977). Protective maternal immunity is transferred with passive antibody to suckling kittens; this antibody declines to negligible levels by 6 to 10 weeks of age (Edwards et al., 1977a; Gaskell and Povey, 1982).

## Clinical Features, Pathogenesis, Lesions

### Respiratory Disease

FRV is transmitted most efficiently by contact or short-distance (6 feet or less) macrodroplet aerosol transfer of oronasal secretions from virus-shedding cats (Gaskell and

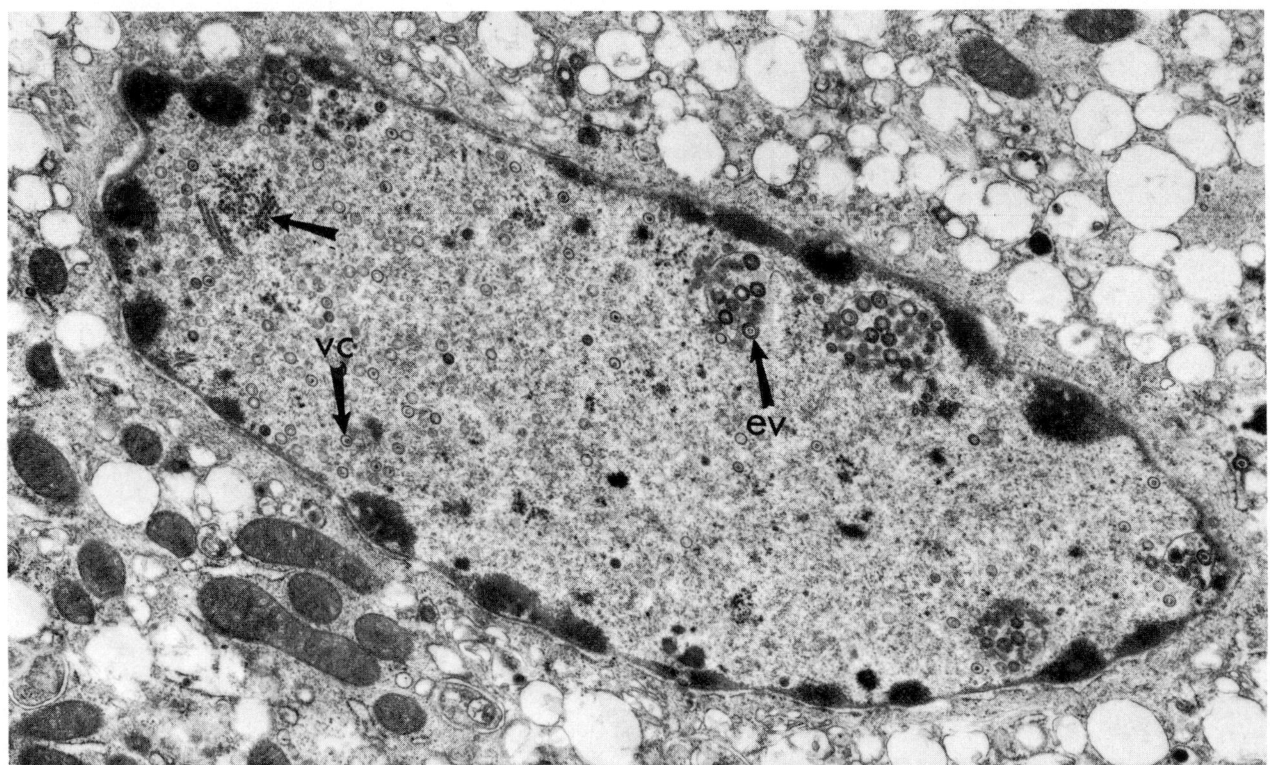


**Figure 7–29** FVR: Intranuclear viral development. Scattered viral nucleocapsids (VC) and clusters of enveloped virions (ev) that acquire envelopes from invaginations of the nuclear membrane. Electron micrograph. (From Hoover EA, Griesemer RA: Lab Invest 25 [1971] 457–464.)

Povey, 1973, 1982; Povey, 1976). Clinical signs of respiratory disease appear one to three days after aerosol or intranasal inoculation: fever, blepharospasm, paroxysmal sneezing, coughing, shaking of the head, serous then mucopurulent nasal and conjunctival exudates, excessive salivation, anorexia, and malaise (Bürki et al., 1964; Crandell et al., 1961; Hoover et al., 1970) (Figs. 7–30 through 7–32). Clinical illness usually lasts 7 to 14 days. Mortality is low. Death in cats with severe, protracted FVR is related to inanition, dehydration, bacterial infection, or immunosuppression due to concurrent viral infection (such as feline leukemia virus infection). The disease is mild in cats with immunity resulting from previous exposure to FRV and in cats exposed to minimal infectious doses of virus (Gaskell and Povey, 1979b; Walton and Gillespie, 1970b).

FVR is an upper airway disease. Pneumonia is uncommon, although the virus has been recovered from the lungs of experimentally infected kittens six to nine days after exposure (Hoover et al., 1970). Virus recovered from pulmonary tissue usually reflects viral replication in bronchioles (Hoover et al., 1970); however, both alveolar pneumocytes and macrophages are susceptible to FRV (Langloss et al., 1978a), and viral pneumonia has been observed in kittens with severe FVR (Love, 1971). Because FRV is the principal cause of damage to the epithelium of the nasal sinuses, it is considered a major antecedent to chronic bacterial sinusitis in cats.

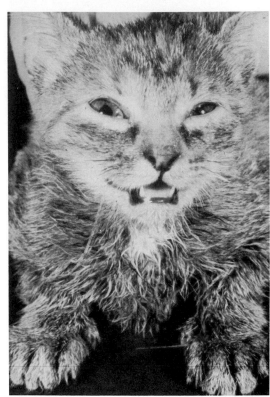

**Figure 7–31** FVR: Seromucoid nasal and conjunctival discharges, excessive salivation, oral respiration, and wiping of secretions on medial forepaws. Four days after FRV exposure.

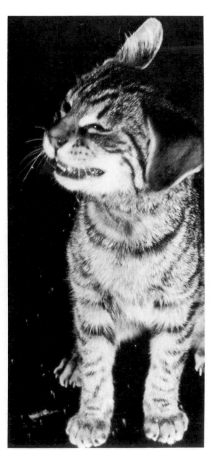

**Figure 7–30** FVR: Paroxysmal sneezing is a cardinal sign often signaling the onset of clinical disease. Two days after experimental aerosol exposure to FRV.

The pathogenesis of FVR involves cytolytic viral infection of the mucosal epithelium of the nasal passages, trachea, and conjunctiva (Crandell et al., 1961; Hoover et al., 1970). Within 48 hours after intranasal inoculation,

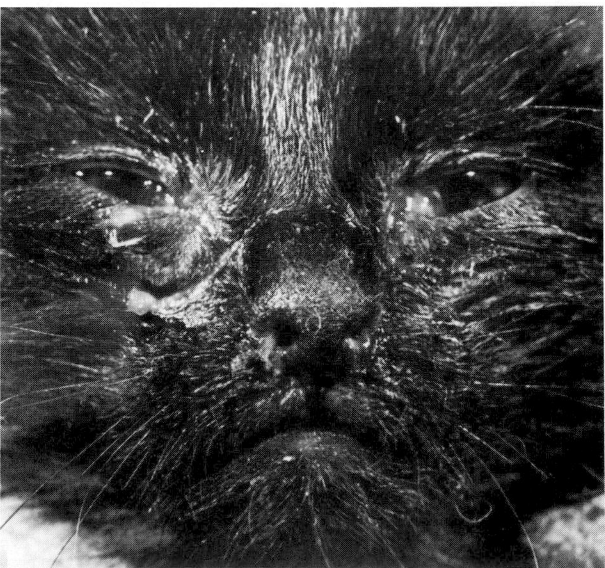

**Figure 7–32** FVR: Extensive mucopurulent ocular and nasal exudates, partial occlusion of the nostrils seven days after FVR exposure. (From Hoover EA, Rohovsky MW, Griesemer RA: Am J Pathol 58 [1970] 269–282.)

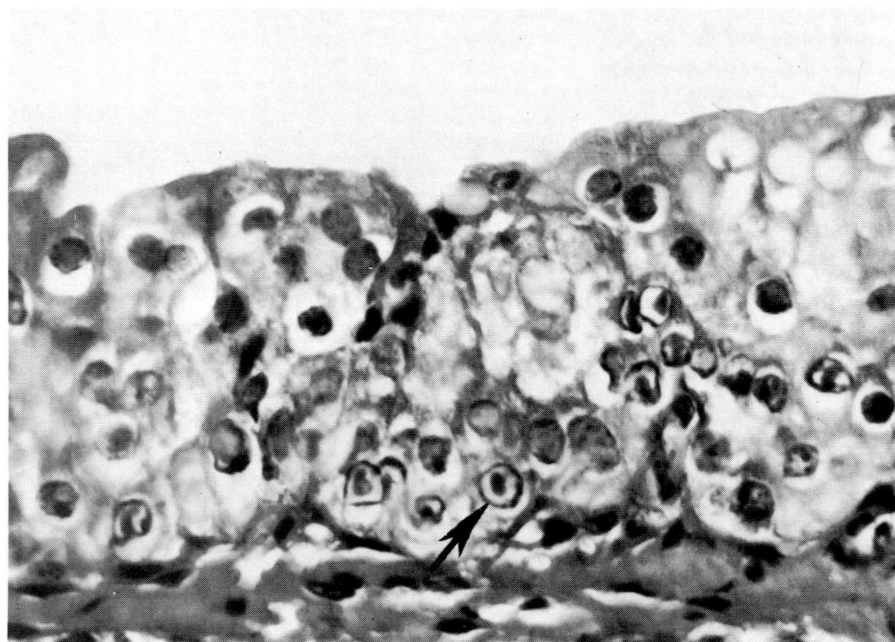

**Figure 7–33** FVR: Early focus of nasal epithelial cell infection characterized by margination of chromatin, cytoplasmic vacuolation, and formation of intranuclear inclusion bodies (arrow). H & E.

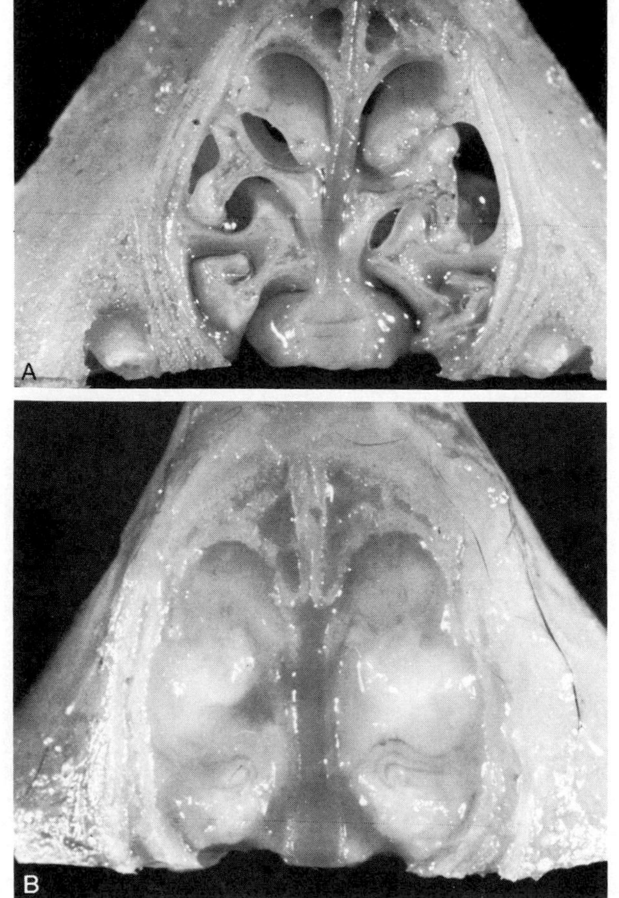


**Figure 7–34** FVR: Cross sections of the anterior nasal turbinates of a normal cat (*A*) and of a cat with severe FVR (*B*) eight days after exposure. Extensive necrosis of nasal mucosa and suppurative inflammation have occluded the nasal passages and obliterated profiles of nasal turbinate bones.

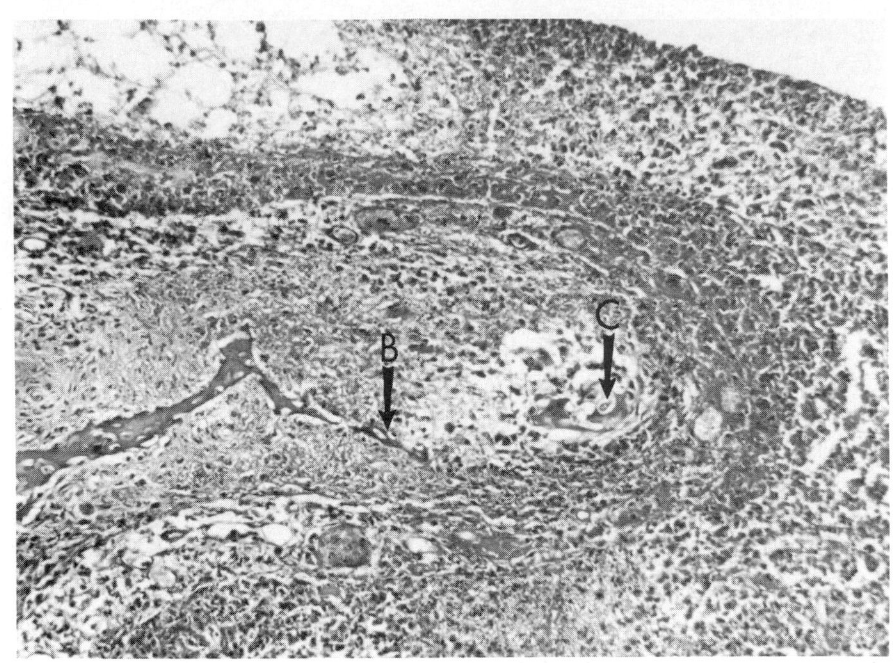


**Figure 7–35** FVR: Nasal turbinate. Extensive necrosis and sloughing of nasal mucosa, dissolution of central nasal turbinate bone (B) and cartilage (C). (From Hoover EA, Rohovsky MW, Griesemer RA: Am J Pathol 58 [1970] 269–282.)

multifocal degeneration and intranuclear inclusion bodies are evident in nasal epithelium (Fig. 7–33), and virus is present in nasal secretions (Crandell et al., 1961; Hoover et al., 1970). Epithelial necrosis is associated with intense leukocytic infiltration, and the nasal passages become occluded by necrotic epithelial cells and mucopurulent exudate (Fig. 7–34). The necrotizing process may involve the nasal turbinate bone itself in growing cats (Fig. 7–35) (Hoover et al., 1970; Hoover and Griesemer, 1971b). Inclusion bodies are no longer detectable from days 10 through 21, when mononuclear leukocytic infiltration and epithelial regeneration are the dominant histologic changes. Mucociliary epithelium is replaced promptly, but olfactory epithelium of the ethmoidal turbinates may regenerate incompletely (Hoover et al., 1970).

Viral titers in nasal and pharyngeal fluids are high between days 3 and 10, and viral shedding ceases 14 to 21 days after infection (Crandell et al., 1961; Gaskell and Povey, 1979a; Hoover et al., 1970). Viremia is rarely detectable in cats with FVR except after experimental intravenous inoculation (Hoover and Griesemer, 1971a, 1971c; see further on).

## Abortion and Fetal Infection

Abortion and fetal resorption are proven consequences of FVR in pregnant cats. Intravenous inoculation of queens with FRV during the sixth week of gestation produced abortion, intrauterine fetal death, and congenital fetal infection associated with placental infarction due to viral-induced vasculitis and thrombosis (Figs. 7–36 through 7–39) (Hoover and Griesemer, 1971c). FRV replication has been demonstrated in uterine and maternal placental vessels, endometrial epithelium, and fetal trophoblast in the junctional zone of the placenta. In queens in which early abortion did not occur and maternal viral antibody developed, congenital fetal infection occurred (see Figs. 7–37 through 7–39 (Hoover and Griesemer, 1971c).

Abortion has been observed in pregnant cats inoculated intranasally with FRV; however, neither viral antigen nor infectious virus was demonstrable in the placentas or fetuses of these cats (Hoover and Griesemer, 1971c). Viremia, detected on days 2 and 3 after intravenous inoculation of pregnant cats, was not detected after intranasal inoculation (in agreement with other studies of FVR in weanling kittens and adult cats) (Crandell et al., 1961; Gaskell and Povey, 1979a; Hoover et al., 1970; Povey, 1976). Intravaginal inoculation of pregnant cats with FRV produced vaginitis and respiratory signs of FVR in the queens and signs and lesions indicative of congenital FRV infection in 18 of 22 kittens born 1 to 24 days after maternal FRV inoculation (Bittle and Peckham, 1971). Thus it appears that the abortifacient action of FRV in pregnant queens may occur in concert with, or independent of, clinical signs of FVR.

Reactivation and shedding of FVR by latently infected, convalescent queens has been demonstrated at 3 to 52 days post partum (Gaskell and Povey, 1982). Although postnatal transfer of virus from shedding queens to kittens may occur in such instances, congenital infection of fetuses in convalescent, latently infected queens has not been detected (Gaskell and Povey, 1982). Additional information concerning the relationship of FVR to reproductive disease is needed, since other viral infections associated with fetal death and resorption, notably feline leukemia virus (Cotter et al., 1975; Hoover et al., 1983) are also common in catteries in which interrupted pregnancies occur habitually.

## Keratitis

FRV-associated ulcerative, dendritic keratitis has been described (Bistner et al., 1971; Roberts et al., 1972). All cats had clinical disease typical of FVR one to two weeks previously. Diagnosis was established by immunofluorescent staining, virus isolation, or both from corneal and conjunctival cells. FRV replication was demonstrated in

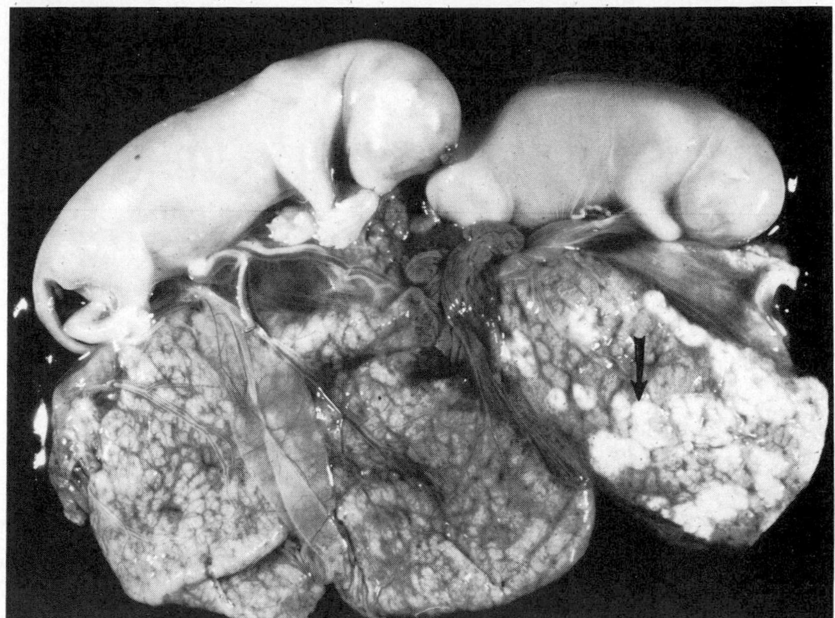

**Figure 7–36** FVR: Areas of infarction (arrow) due to virus-induced vasculitis and thrombosis in the placenta of a fetus aborted six days after maternal intravenous inoculation with FRV. (From Hoover EA, Griesemer RA: Am J Pathol 65 [1971] 173–188.)

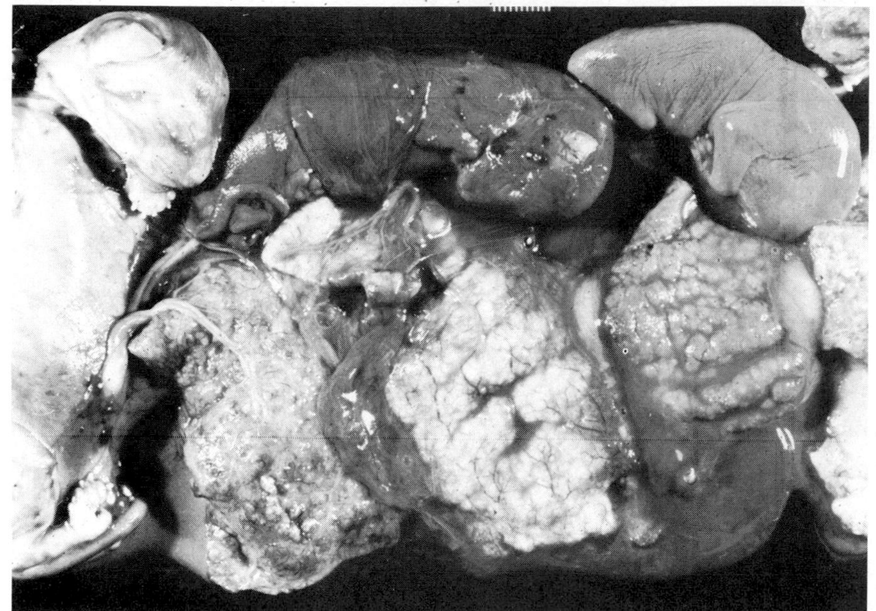

**Figure 7–37** FVR: Virus-induced placental necrosis, fetal death, and congenital fetal infection 26 days after intravenous maternal FRV inoculation. (From Hoover EA, Griesemer RA: Am J Pathol 65 [1971] 173–188.)

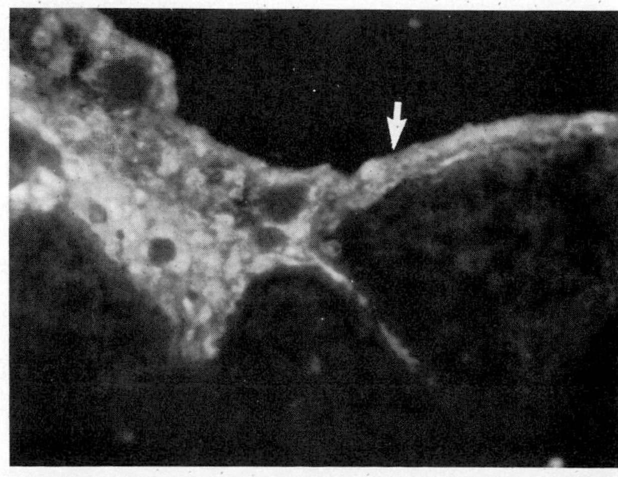

**Figure 7–38** Transplacental FRV infection involving the chorioallantoic membrane (arrow) of the placenta 26 days after maternal inoculation with FRV. Immunofluorescence.

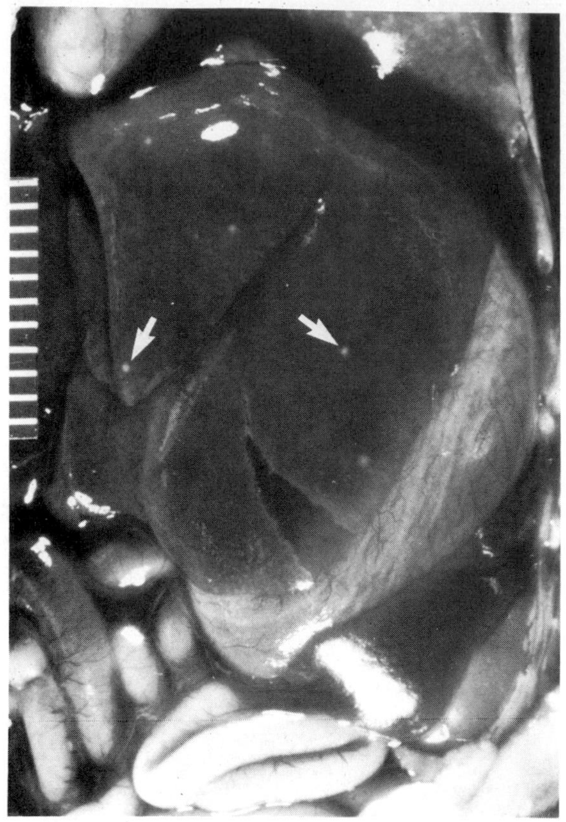

**Figure 7–39** FVR: Liver of fetus with congenital FRV infection 26 days after maternal inoculation with FRV. Foci of necrosis (arrows) in which viral antigen was demonstrable.

corneal epithelium by electron microscopy, and treatment of one cat with iododeoxyuridine and dexamethasone resulted in improvement (Roberts et al., 1972). Keratitis could not be reproduced by experimental inoculation of the intact or scarified corneas of kittens with FVR, although conjunctivitis and typical FVR developed in all cats (Bistner et al., 1971). Neither the factors responsible for the induction of FRV dendritic keratitis in certain cats nor the relationship of latent FRV infection to keratitis have been established. Nevertheless, FRV, like herpes simplex virus in man, is established as a corneal pathogen and is a primary consideration in the diagnosis and therapy of dendritic corneal lesions in cats.

## Glossitis

Ulcerative glossitis is a primary feature of feline calicivirus infection but may be caused by FRV, although less often. Lingual ulcers have been induced after experimental inoculation of FRV onto the scarified lingual mucosa (Karpas and Routledge, 1968) and by experimental induction of FVR infection in SPF cats in which concomitant FCV infection could be excluded (Fig. 7–40) (Hoover, E. A., Kahn, D. E., unpublished data). In the latter cats, FRV-induced lingual lesions involved the anterior perimeter of the tongue, developed after respiratory signs of FVR had been present for several days, and were associated with intranuclear inclusion bodies in lingual epithelium. FRV-induced glossitis occurs in cats with severe FVR. Lingual ulcers in cats without concurrent signs of severe upper respiratory disease are more likely to be caused by feline calicivirus.

## Dermatitis

FRV has been isolated from cats with ulcerative cutaneous and oral lesions and signs of concomitant FVR (Flecknell et al., 1979; Johnson and Sabine, 1971). Cutaneous lesions have not been produced by experimental infection of cats with FRV; the potential role of FRV as a feline dermal pathogen awaits further definition.

## Generalized Infection

Particularly in young kittens infected postnatally or congenitally (Hoover and Griesemer, 1971a, 1971c; Love, 1971) and occasionally in adults (Shields and Gaskin, 1977), FVR may be associated with systemic viral infection and visceral lesions. Recognized systemic FRV infections have been fatal and are characterized by multifocal necrosis associated with intranuclear inclusion bodies in liver, adrenal, lung, and bone (see Fig. 7–39). Cats with generalized feline herpesvirus usually have severe respiratory FVR.

## Bone Lesions

Osteolytic lesions confined to sites of osteogenesis (e.g., metaphyses of long bones) have been induced in kittens inoculated intravenously with FRV (Hoover and Griesemer, 1971a, 1971b). Viral replication was demonstrated

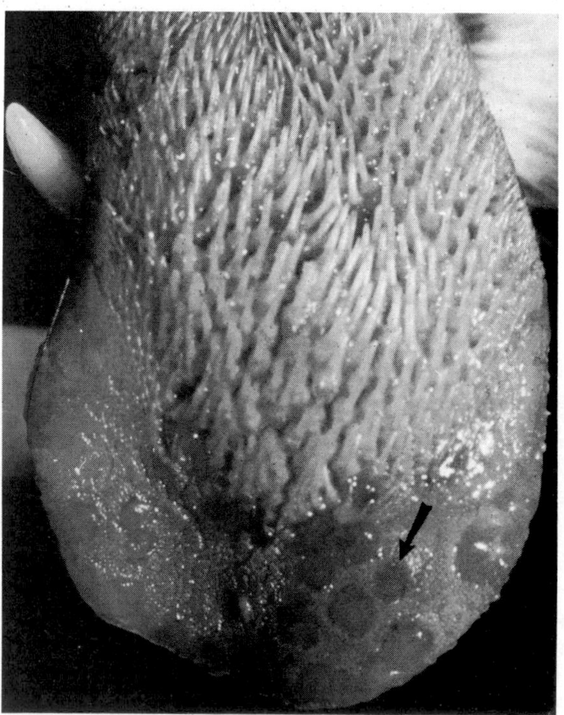

**Figure 7–40** FVR: FRV-induced lingual ulceration (arrow) in a cat 11 days after aerosol exposure to FRV. Typical respiratory signs of FVR also were present.

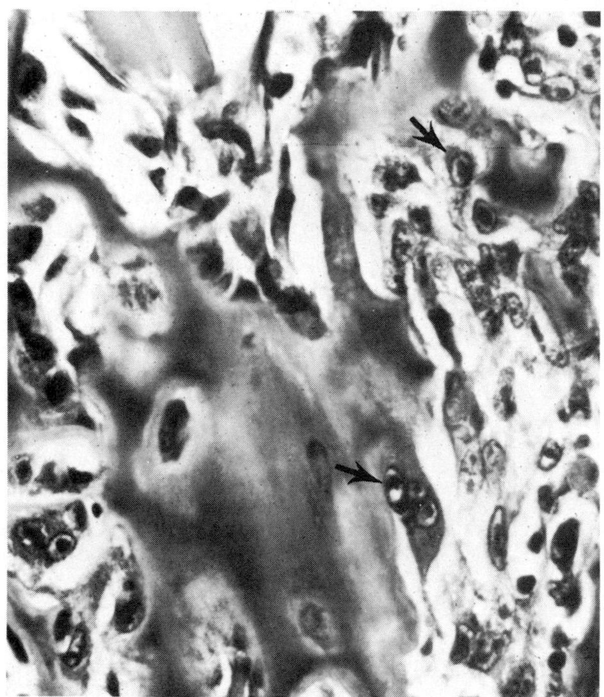

**Figure 7–41** FVR: Viral infection and inclusion bodies (arrows) in osteoblasts in the metaphysis of the femur of a kitten two days after intravenous inoculation of FRV. Viral bone lesions in experimentally infected kittens are restricted to sites of osteogenesis. (From Hoover EA, Greisemer RA: Lab Invest 25 [1971] 457–464.)

in endothelium, osteoblasts, and osteoclasts (Fig. 7–41). Lesions in nasal turbinates began at sites of osteogenesis and secondarily affected the overlying mucosal epithelium (Fig. 7–42).

## Neurologic Disease

Although convulsions have been described in moribund cats with FVR (Povey and Johnson, 1967), neither lesions nor virus have been detected in the nervous system of cats infected experimentally apart from damage to the olfactory epithelium and associated nerve fibers during necrotizing rhinitis (Hoover et al., 1970). However, latent FRV has been recovered from the trigeminal ganglia of 1 of 47 cats and the olfactory bulb of one of four cats convalescent from experimental FRV infection (Gaskell and Povey, 1979a). Thus, apart from latent ganglionic infection, neurotropism has not been associated with feline herpesvirus.

### Hematologic Response

Moderate neutrophilic leukocytosis and mild lymphopenia are typical (Crandell et al., 1961; Hoover et al., 1970). Neither leukopenia nor anemia is a feature of uncomplicated FVR, although either may occur in natural infections in which intercurrent infection or prolonged anorexia is a factor or when intercurrent feline leukemia virus infection is present.

### Immune Response

FRV characteristically elicits modest titers of viral neutralizing antibody (1:4 to 1:32) (Bartholomew and Gillespie, 1968; Crandell et al., 1961; Gaskell and Povey, 1979b; Hoover et al., 1970; Povey and Johnson, 1967; Walton and Gillespie, 1970b; others). Titers decline to minimal detectable levels within two months (Walton and Gillespie, 1970b). Re-exposure of convalescent cats to FRV provokes either no disease or mild signs of FVR and elicits an anamnestic antibody response. Cats with little or no humoral antibody to FRV may nevertheless be resistant to viral inoculation (Walton and Gillespie, 1970b). Cats with persistent high FRV antibody titers may be carriers of latent viral infection and subject to periodic reactivation of viral replication (Gaskell and Povey, 1973, 1977, 1979a, 1982). Colostral transfer of maternal FRV antibody has been demonstrated; immunity of kittens declines between five and eight weeks of age (Gaskell and Povey, 1982; Povey, 1976). Neither cell-mediated immune mechanisms nor secretory antibody levels have been studied in FVR.

### Latent Viral Infection and the Carrier State

FRV reactivation and excretion by convalescent cats occurs spontaneously and can be triggered experimentally by administration of corticosteroids or epinephrine, by stress associated with transfer to new surroundings, and

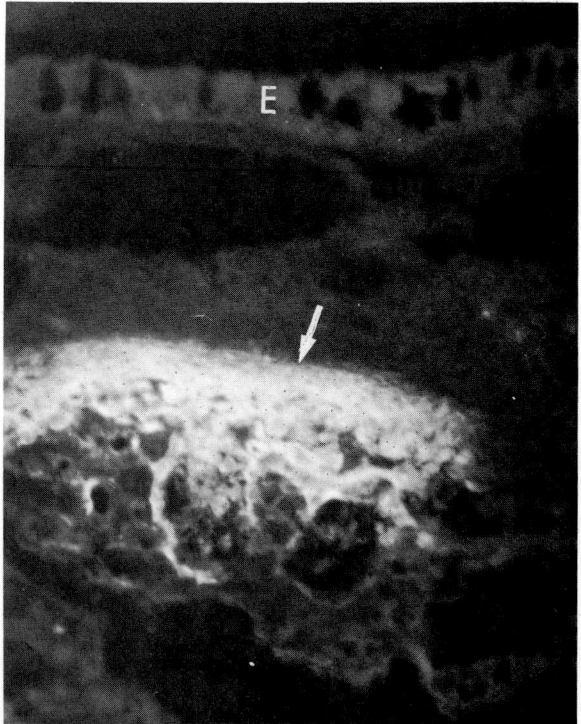


**Figure 7–42** FVR: Nasal turbinate of kitten five days after intravenous inoculation of FRV. Immunofluorescent demonstration of FRV replication in ossifying region of turbinate bone (arrow). E = mucosal epithelium.

perhaps by parturition (Gaskell and Povey, 1973, 1977, 1979a, 1982; Plummer et al., 1970). FRV has been isolated from the nasopharyngeal secretions, nasal turbinates, and oropharyngeal mucosa of convalescent cats reshedding virus. The specific cells involved in persistence of FRV in cats have yet to be identified. With one exception, trigeminal ganglia of latently infected cats have failed to yield virus (Gaskell and Povey, 1979a).

Cats convalescent from FVR, as with other herpesvirus infections, must be considered potential latently infected carriers subject to intermittent shedding of virus in oronasal secretions even though clinical signs are absent and serum antibody is present. Such latently infected viral carriers probably play a significant role in the epizootiology of FVR. Whether vaccination of cats with attenuated FRV strains will prevent establishment of latent infection (by either virulent or vaccinal virus) is a question relevant to the control of FVR in cats. One investigation indicated that re-excretion of FRV could not be elicited by corticosteroid treatment of cats vaccinated intranasally with attenuated virus or cats vaccinated and then challenged with virulent FRV (Orr et al., 1980). Steroid-induced reshedding of virus could, however, be demonstrated in nonvaccinated, FRV-convalescent cats (Orr et al., 1980).

### TREATMENT

Therapy of FVR is supportive and designed to counteract bacterial infection, dehydration, respiratory distress, and inanition. Ampicillin or tetracycline, lactated Ringer's solution, vitamins, manual removal of exudates, and placement of the cat in an atmosphere with a saturated humidity (such as that created by a steam vaporizer in an enclosure) will aid materially in recovery of cats with severe FVR. Use of large doses of vitamin C has been advocated but has not been studied under controlled conditions.

Assiduous nursing care, provided at home whenever possible, is important. Use of antibiotic eye and nose drops and ointments and careful cleaning of nasal and conjunctival exudates have considerable value. Intake of soft, highly nutritious foods with high olfactory appeal should be encouraged and is best accomplished in the home environment (Holzworth, 1971). If chronic symptoms of rhinitis or sinusitis develop, intensive antibiotic treatment based on culture and sensitivity testing may be tried; however, surgical drainage of the nasal sinuses may ultimately be required. FRV-induced dendritic keratitis has been treated successfully with topical iododeoxyuridine (Roberts et al., 1972). Neither exogenous interferon, interferon inducers, nor systemic 6-azauridine have been found effective in ameliorating the signs of FVR even when these agents were initiated early in the course of experimentally induced infections (Kahn, 1976; Steffenhagen et al., 1976).

### IMMUNOPROPHYLAXIS

Attenuated strains of FRV have been produced by prolonged cell culture passage at reduced temperatures or by other methods (Bittle and Rubic, 1974, 1975; Davis and Beckenhauer, 1976; Edwards et al., 1977a,b; Povey, 1979). FRV-neutralizing antibody and a significant degree of protection have been induced by parenteral (Bittle and Rubic, 1974; Scott, 1975) or intranasal (Davis and Beckenhauer, 1976; Gaskell and Povey, 1979b) administration of these FRV vaccines. Vaccination has been effective in preventing or ameliorating the severity of disease when cats were exposed to virulent FRV challenge. As is the case in cats immunized by natural exposure to FRV, vaccination does not protect all cats from limited viral replication and mild clinical signs of FVR after experimental challenge with virulent virus (Povey, 1979; Scott, 1975).

Intranasally administered attenuated FRV replicates in the nasal mucosa; intramuscularly administered vaccine virus does not. No evidence has been obtained to indicate that vaccine virus establishes latent infection or is re-shed after the initial immunizing phase of replication has occurred (Orr et al., 1980). Nevertheless, these considerations remain reasonable possibilities that will bear continued appraisal.

The efficacy of vaccine administration as therapy for cats with active disease has not been studied.

## FELINE CALICIVIRUS INFECTION

Feline caliciviruses (FCV) (formerly termed picornaviruses) were recognized as cytopathic agents in 1957 (Bolin, 1957; Fastier, 1957) and as feline pathogens in 1960 (Crandell and Madin, 1960; Crandell et al., 1960b). Subsequently, FCV have been isolated from cats with various signs of respiratory disease and from clinically normal cats (for reviews see Povey, 1967, and Studdert, 1978). Overall, the pathogenicity of FCV is less than that of FRV. Asymptomatic FCV infections are common among cats (Hoover and Kahn, 1975; Kahn and Gillespie, 1970, 1971; Povey and Hale, 1974; Povey et al., 1973; Wardley, 1976). The virulence of individual FCV isolates varies substantially and correlates with the degree of viral pneumotropism. Under experimental conditions, most FCV isolates induce a mild disease characterized by oral ulcers and modest serous nasal or conjunctival discharges (Hoover and Kahn, 1975; Love, 1975; Ormerod et al., 1979; Povey and Hale, 1974). Virulent FCV isolates induce pneumonia, especially if cats are exposed to aerosolized virus (Holzinger and Kahn, 1970; Hoover and Kahn, 1973; Kahn and Gillespie, 1970; Ormerod et al., 1979).

### CHARACTERISTICS OF THE VIRUS

FCV are small (35 to 40 nm), nonenveloped, single-stranded RNA viruses. Caliciviruses are closely related to picornaviruses and rhinoviruses but differ in capsid structure and possess a single structural polypeptide of 65,000 to 68,000 daltons (Black and Brown, 1977; Burroughs and Brown, 1974; Komolafe et al., 1980; Peterson and Studdert, 1970). Other caliciviruses of animals include porcine vesicular exanthema virus and San Miguel sea lion virus. Caliciviruses have icosahedral structure with cup-like depressions between projections of capsomers (Peterson and Studdert, 1970). FCV replicate in the cytoplasm, do not form inclusion bodies, and are resistant to acid pH and lipid solvents. They form plaques and are not protected from heat inactivation (50 C) by $Mg^{++}$ ions as are rhinoviruses (Crandell, 1967).

Cytopathic effects evoked by FCV in feline monolayer cell cultures are rapid and consist of increased cell refractility, retraction of cytoplasmic processes, and rapid de-

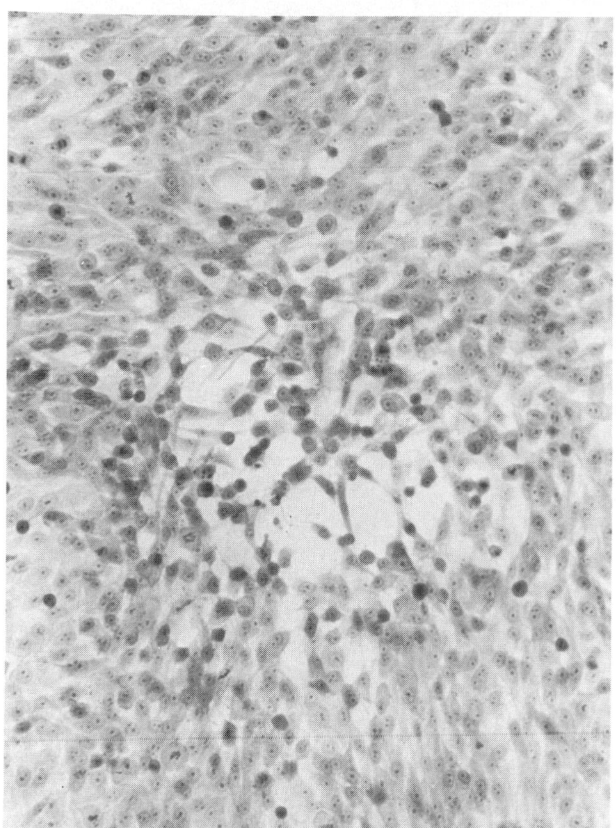

**Figure 7–43** FCV: Viral cytopathic effect in feline cell culture. Cell retraction, pyknosis, and detachment occur; no inclusion bodies form. H & E.

tachment from the growth surface in 12 to 14 hours (Crandell et al., 1960b; Crandell, 1967; Kahn and Gillespie, 1970; Spradbrow et al., 1970a; Studdert et al., 1970; others). Changes in stained cells are pyknosis and increased cytoplasmic acidophilia (Fig. 7–43). FCV are synthesized and assembled in the cytoplasm and are discernible either as aggregates of virions in paracrystalline arrays (Figs. 7–44 and 7–45) or as small clusters of virions that are distinguished from free ribosomes only by their slightly larger size (Langloss et al., 1978b; Peterson and Studdert, 1970). Degenerative changes in FCV-infected cells are dilation and invagination of the rough endoplasmic reticulum and dense intracytoplasmic masses of nucleoprotein-like material (Peterson and Studdert, 1970). Relatively few of the degenerate cells observed in infected cell cultures contain discernible virions. Similarly, in FCV lesions induced in vivo it appears that cytopathic effect can occur before or independent of viral synthesis (Langloss et al., 1978a; Peterson and Studdert, 1970).

In contrast to FRV, FCV isolates differ considerably in serologic reactivity (Bittle et al., 1960; others). Common antigenic sites also occur among FCV isolates, however, and are the basis for successful cross-protective immunization against FCV infections (Kahn et al., 1975; Povey, 1974). Serum neutralization by $TCID_{50}$ or plaque reduction assay is the standard serologic assay for determining antigenic relationships among FCV (Kalunda et al., 1975). Differences in FCV antibody class and specificity have been demonstrated in the acute and convalescent phases of FCV infection in cats by complement fixation (Olsen et al., 1974).

FCV are more resistant to inactivation in the environment and by detergents and disinfectants than is FRV (Crandell, 1967). However, infection of cats appears to depend principally upon close contact; aerosol transmission over distances greater than several feet is inefficient and probably of little importance (Wardley and Povey, 1977).

## Clinical Findings, Pathogenesis, Lesions

The cardinal signs of FCV infection are fever, anorexia, and mucosal ulceration or vesiculation affecting the tongue (Fig. 7–46), hard palate (Fig. 7–47), nasal philtrum (Fig. 7–48), lip (Fig. 7–49), or periodontal gingiva (Hoover and Kahn, 1975; Kahn and Gillespie, 1970, 1971; Ormerod et al., 1979; Povey and Hale, 1974; others). With FCV isolates of low or moderate virulence, small oral ulcers may be the only manifestation of infection (Hoover and Kahn, 1975; Love, 1972; Povey and Hale, 1974; others). Mild to moderate serous nasal or conjunctival discharge, musculoskeletal soreness, and hyperesthesia may accompany the oral lesions (Pedersen et al., 1983; Studdert, 1978). One instance of recovery of FCV from ulcerative skin lesions has been reported (Cooper and Sabine, 1972). Dyspnea and severe depression in cats with FCV-like oral lesions may indicate FCV-induced pneumonia (Figs. 7–50 and 7–51) (Hoover and Kahn, 1975; Kahn and Gillespie, 1970; Ormerod et al., 1979). Death due to FCV infection is uncommon. Fatal infections are most frequent in kittens and are often associated with pneumonia (Hoover and Kahn, 1975; Ormerod et al., 1979).

Signs of upper airway disease in cats infected with FCV are variable but generally less severe than those in cats with FVR (Hoover and Kahn, 1975; Love, 1972; Ormerod et al., 1979; Povey and Hale, 1974). The greater frequency of upper respiratory signs (i.e., sneezing, blepharospasm, nasal and conjunctival discharges) in natural versus experimental FCV infections may reflect greater impact of synergistic bacterial infections in the former (Povey, 1976; Povey and Hale, 1974). Experimental infection of cats with most of the FCV isolates tested results primarily in fever, anorexia, and ulcerative lesions in the epithelium of the nostril, tongue, and palate. Although induction of significant upper respiratory disease has been reported with some FCV isolates (Bartholomew and Gillespie, 1968; Flagstad, 1974), this appears to be the exception under experimental conditions.

An FCV-induced nonrespiratory syndrome characterized by fever, small glossal and palatine ulcers, malaise, joint or muscle soreness, hyperesthesia, and limping in postweanling kittens has been described and reproduced experimentally with two FCV isolates (Pedersen et al., 1983). These viral isolates were serologically related yet were significantly divergent from the broadly cross-reactive virus strains used in present FCV vaccines—which failed to protect immunized cats from the pathogenic effects of these newer FCV isolates (Pedersen et al., 1983). Neither lesions nor evidence of FCV replication could be detected in neuromusculoskeletal tissues of acutely infected cats. The pathogenesis of this interesting syndrome remains enigmatic.

*Text continued on page 228*

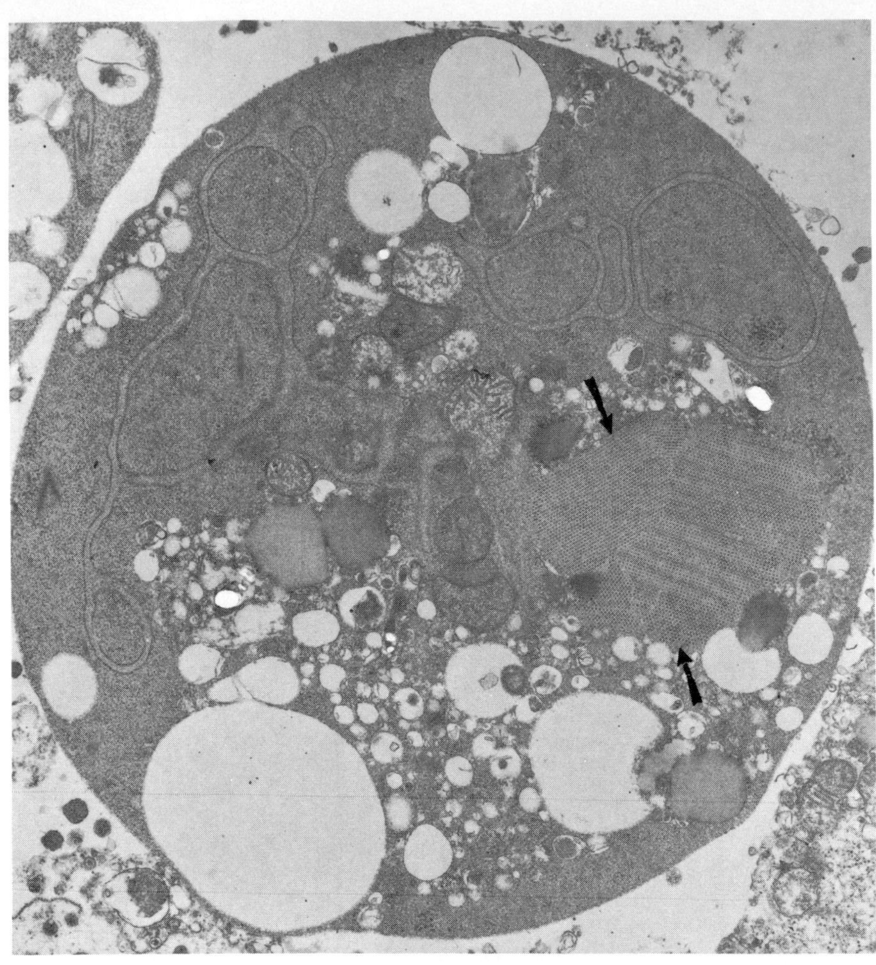

**Figure 7–44** FCV: FCV-infected cell containing cytoplasmic paracrystalline aggregate of virions (arrows) and vacuolar degenerative changes in the cytoplasm. Electron micrograph.

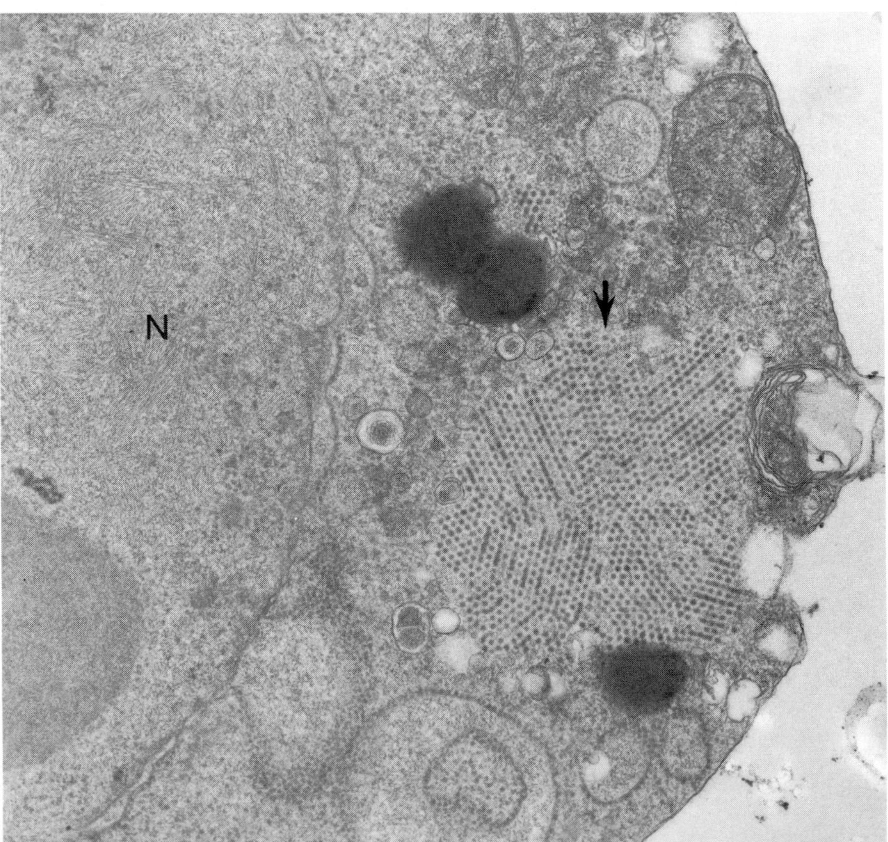


**Figure 7–45** FCV: Paracrystalline array of virions in cytoplasm (arrow). N = nucleus. Electron micrograph.

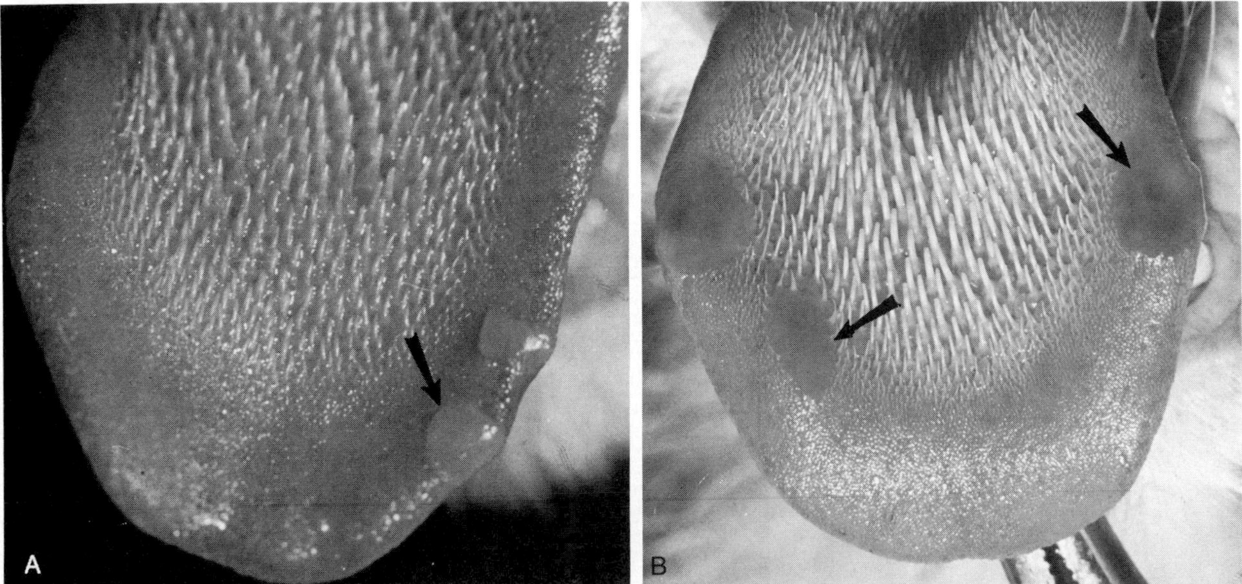


**Figure 7–46** FCV: Tongue lesions. Vesicle formation (*A*, arrow) and subsequent ulceration (*B*, arrows) of lingual epithelium.

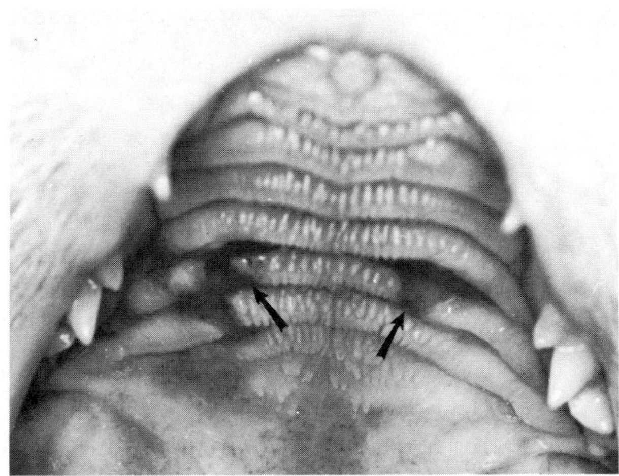

**Figure 7–47** FCV: Palatine lesions. Bilateral ulceration (arrows). (From Hoover EA, Kahn DE: Vet Pathol 10 [1973] 307–322.)

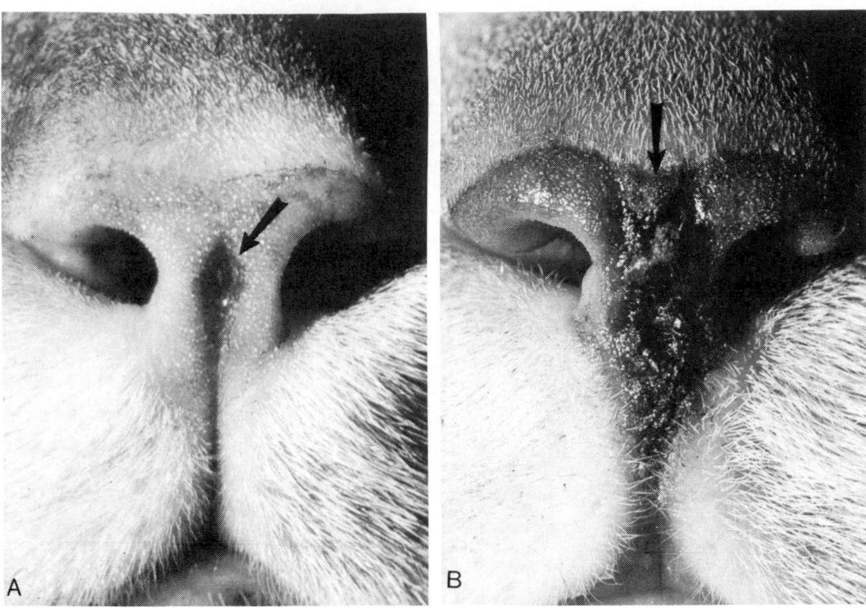


**Figure 7–48** FCV: Nostril lesions. Ulceration (*A*) and accumulation of crusted exudate (*B*) in philtrum of the nostril. (From Hoover EA, Kahn DE: J Am Vet Med Assoc 166 [1975] 464–468.)

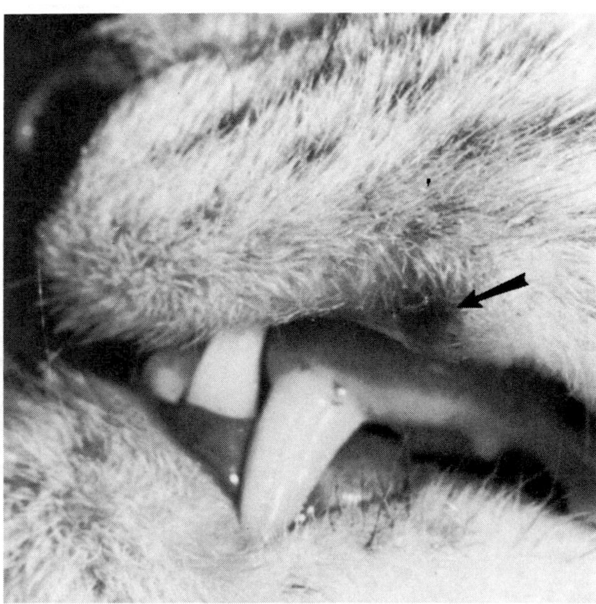

**Figure 7–49** FCV: Small ulcerative lesion (arrow) at mucocutaneous junction of the upper lip.

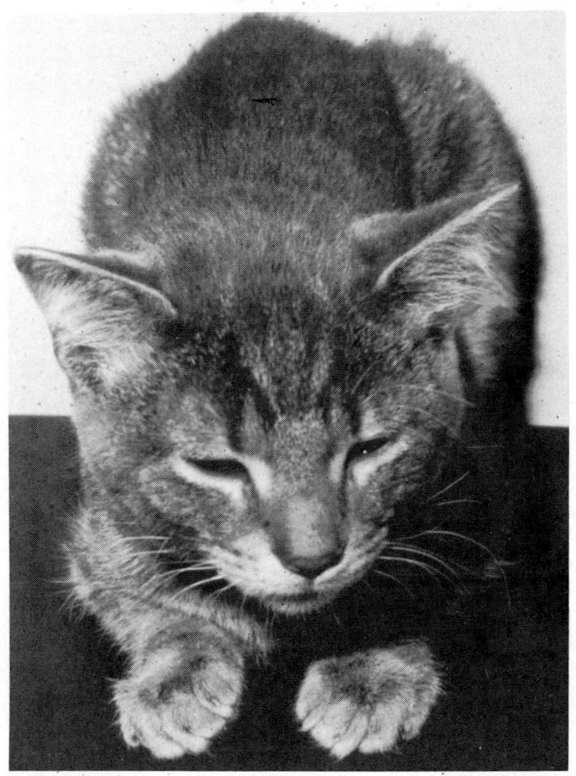

**Figure 7–50** FCV: Appearance of a cat with FCV-induced pneumonia three days after aerosol exposure to virulent pneumotropic virus strain. Depression, dyspnea, and fever are present; sternal posture is preferred.

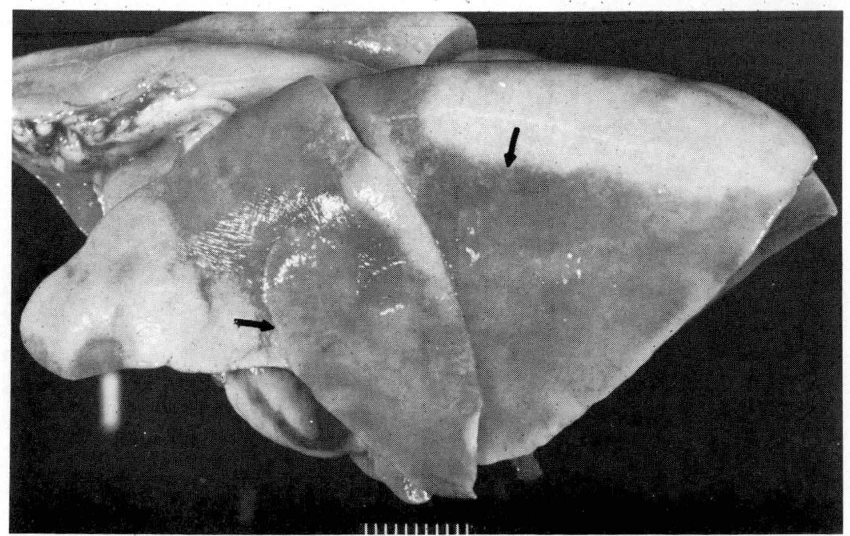

**Figure 7–51** FCV: Pneumonia. Regions of pulmonary consolidation (arrows) due to severe exudative pneumonia are present in the right lobes of the lung seven days after aerosol exposure to virulent FCV strain FPV-255.

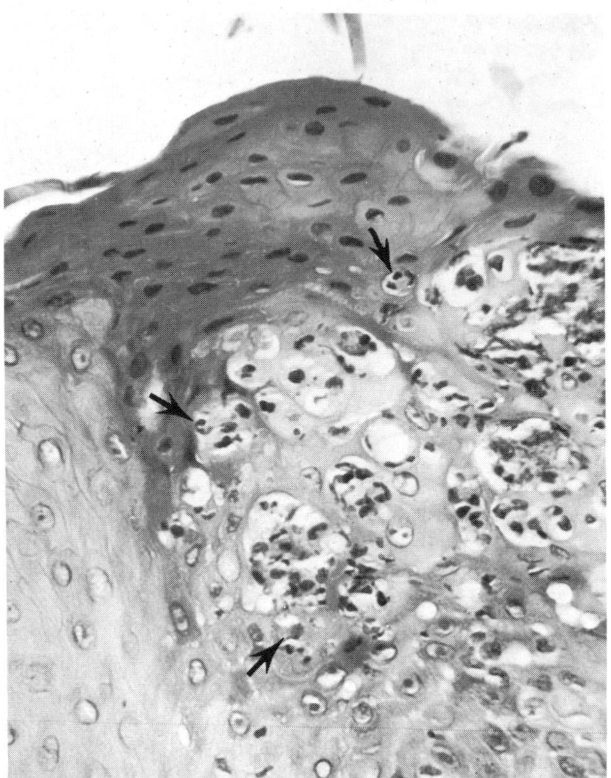

**Figure 7–52** FCV: Focal early lesion in stratified squamous epithelium of the palate. Focus of epithelial cell degeneration and intraepithelial neutrophil infiltration (area delineated by arrows). No inclusion bodies form. H & E.

The principal known target cells for FCV replication are the stratified squamous mucosal cells of the tongue, pharynx, tonsil, and nostril, although FCV antigen or virus has been identified in spleen, blood, skin, and mucociliary upper respiratory epithelium (Hoover and Kahn, 1973; Kahn and Gillespie, 1971; others). In mucosal epithelial cells, cytolytic viral replication results in necrosis, sloughing, neutrophil infiltration, and ulceration. Infected cells become pyknotic, acidophilic, and retracted, but no inclusion bodies form (Fig. 7–52). Although FCV antigen has been demonstrated in nasal and tracheal epithelium and infectious virus can be isolated from these tissues (Kahn and Gillespie, 1970, 1971; Love, 1972; Love and Baker, 1972; Love and Donaldson-Wood, 1975; Povey and Hale, 1974), lesions in the conjunctiva and upper respiratory mucosa of cats infected experimentally with FCV were either absent or confined to moderate neutrophil infiltration, edema, and necrosis of individual epithelial cells (Hoover and Kahn, 1973, 1975; Ormerod et al., 1979). Specific visceral or neuromusculoskeletal lesions could not be detected in the acute phase of infection by FCV isolates that produced a hyperesthesia "limping" syndrome (Pedersen et al., 1983).

Pneumotropic strains of FCV replicate cytolytically in alveolar type I pneumocytes and initiate an acute exudative viral pneumonia (Figs. 7–53 and 7–54) (Holzinger and Kahn, 1970; Hoover and Kahn, 1973; Kahn and Gillespie, 1970, 1971; Langloss et al., 1977, 1978b). Necrosis of pneumocytes results in denudation of the alveolar lining and exudation of serous fluid, fibrin, and neutrophils into alveoli (Langloss et al., 1978b). Resolution of pulmonary lesions occurs over a two- to three-week period and involves exudation of macrophages, regenerative hyperplasia to type II pneumocytes, and infiltration of lymphoid cells (Fig. 7–55) (Holzinger and Kahn, 1970; Hoover and Kahn, 1973; Langloss et al., 1978b). Pneumocytes, but not alveolar macrophages, are susceptible to productive, lytic FCV replication in vitro (Langloss et al., 1978a). The resistance of alveolar macrophages to FCV infection demonstrated in vitro may account for the limitation of viral replication in the peripheral lung.

Although pneumotropic FCV produce pneumonia when cats are exposed to aerosols of virus, oronasal inoculation (the dominant natural route) is much less efficient in inducing pulmonary lesions and results in a milder disease (Ormerod et al., 1979). Under natural conditions, mortality due to FCV infection is associated with pneumonia and occurs chiefly in kittens in catteries or colonies where presumably large infective doses are generated or other synergistic factors are involved (Kahn and Gillespie, 1970).

Although FCV have been isolated occasionally from urine, feces, blood, and visceral tissues of cats (Kahn and Gillespie, 1971; Ormerod et al., 1979; Pichler and Bürki, 1970; Povey, 1976), evidence that these viruses induce

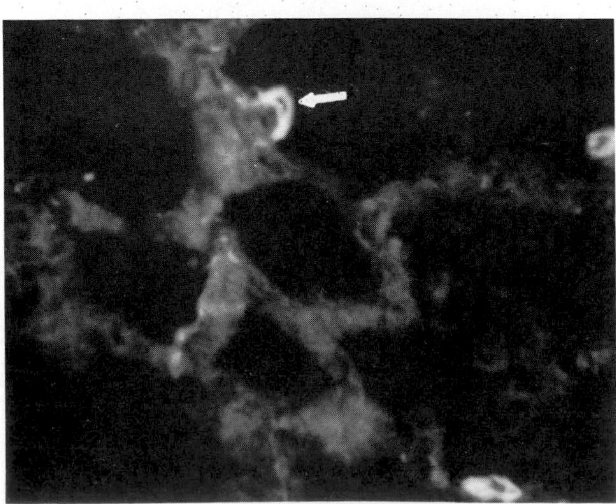

**Figure 7–53** FCV: Viral antigen in alveolar type I pneumocytes (arrow) in early pulmonary lesion induced by aerosol exposure to virulent strain FPV-255. Immunofluorescence. (From Langloss JM, Hoover EA, Kahn DE: Am J Vet Res 39 [1978] 1577–1583.)

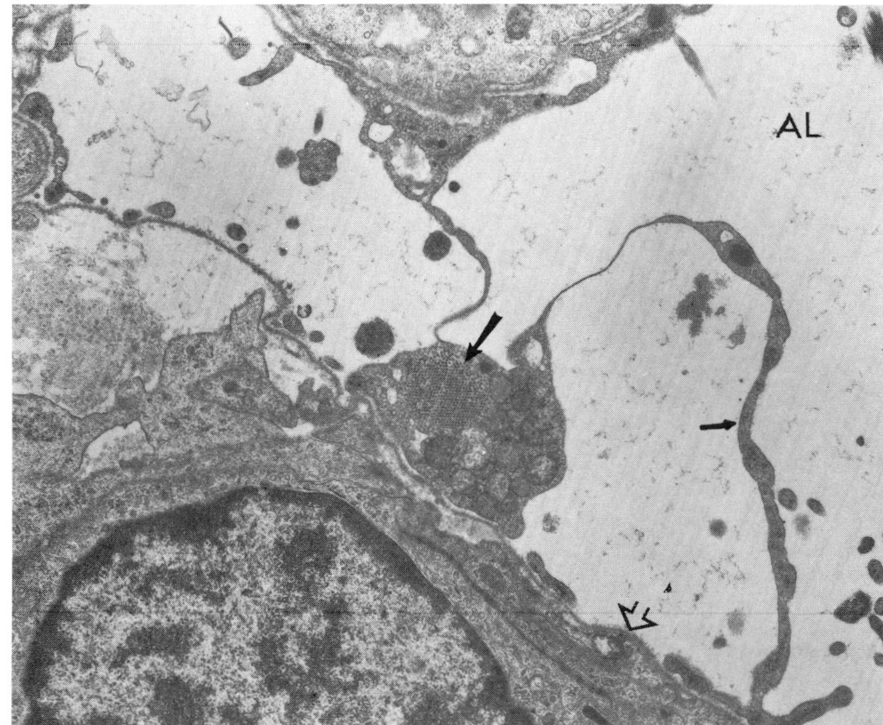


**Figure 7–54** FCV: FCV replication (large arrow) in alveolar type I pneumocyte in an early pulmonary lesion induced by FCV strain FPV-255. Pneumocyte has become separated from alveolar basement membrane (open arrow). Displaced and elevated cytoplasm of pneumocyte (small arrow). AL = alveolar lumen. Electron micrograph. (From Langloss JM, Hoover EA, Kahn DE: Am J Vet Res 39 [1978] 1577–1583.)

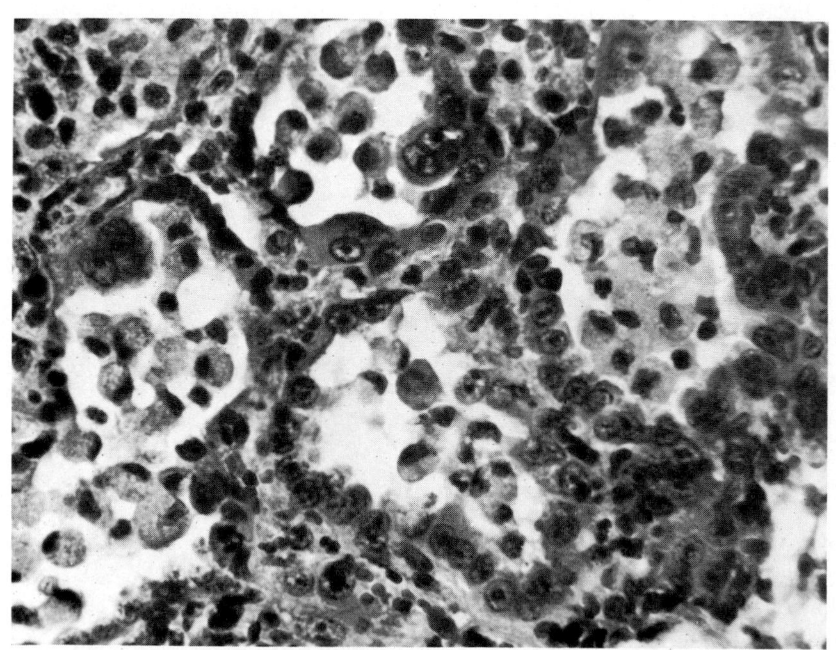

**Figure 7–55** FCV: Resolving lung lesion—day 10. Exudation of alveolar macrophages and regenerative hyperplasia of type II pneumocytes and terminal bronchiolar cells. (From Hoover EA, Kahn DE: Vet Pathol 10 [1973] 307–322.)

lesions in tissues other than the oropharyngeal or respiratory mucosa is sparse (Hoover and Kahn, 1975; Ormerod et al., 1979; Povey and Hale, 1974). Excretion of FCV in oropharyngeal fluids of cats usually persists for 10 to 14 days; however, virus has been recovered from oral swabbings or tonsils of some convalescent cats for up to six weeks (Kahn and Walton, 1971; Povey et al., 1973; Wardley, 1976).

### Hematologic Response

Neutrophilic leukocytosis or leukocyte numbers within normal limits are typical. Neither leukopenia nor alterations in erythrocyte values are features of FCV disease (Hoover and Kahn, 1975; Kahn and Gillespie, 1970).

### Immune Response

FCV induce neutralizing antibody within 10 days after exposure (Kahn et al., 1975; Olsen et al., 1974; Povey, 1974; Povey and Hale, 1974). The degree to which antibody to one FCV isolate will neutralize infectivity of other isolates varies considerably (Kahn et al., 1975; Olsen et al., 1974). Antibody produced early after infection is non-complement-fixing and relatively strain-specific, whereas antibodies appearing at three to five weeks are complement-fixing and more broadly reactive (Olsen et al., 1974). Vaccination against FCV disease is based on use of viral isolates with high degrees of antigenic cross-reactivity (Kahn and Hoover, 1976a; Povey, 1974). As with FRV, cats with low antibody titers against a given virulent FCV isolate may possess substantial resistance to viral challenge and produce a secondary antibody response after challenge (Kahn et al., 1975; Olsen et al., 1974). Cell-mediated immunity to FCV has not been studied.

### Immune Carrier State

Asymptomatic infection and shedding of FCV in oropharyngeal fluids are well documented (Kahn and Walton, 1971; Povey et al., 1973; Wardley, 1976) and constitute the principal reasons why FCV infection is difficult to eliminate from cat populations except by Caesarean derivation or establishment of closed breeding colonies originating from cats selected by rigorous virologic and serologic testing to ensure freedom from FCV infection. The site of chronic FCV infection appears to be the tonsil or the associated pharyngeal mucosa (Kahn and Gillespie, 1970; Povey et al., 1973). Factors governing the FCV carrier state and viral shedding have not been studied.

### Treatment

Therapy of FCV disease is supportive and designed to combat bacterial infections, dehydration, and inanition as described for FVR. Mild FCV infection marked only by oral ulcers does not require treatment. Cats with FCV-induced pneumonia should receive antibiotic therapy and be managed as befits acute pneumonia with pulmonary edema.

### Immunoprophylaxis

Commercial vaccines consist of attenuated FCV strains with minimal virulence and wide serologic reactivity (Bittle and Rubic, 1975; Davis and Beckenhauer, 1976; Edwards et al., 1977a,b; Povey, 1976). Inactivated FCV has also been employed for immunization (Povey and Wilson, 1978). The vaccines are administered either parenterally or intranasally and are usually combined with FRV and panleukopenia vaccines. FCV are stronger immunogens than FRV and elicit a stronger antibody response. FCV immunization provides a significant degree of protection from pulmonary and mucosal lesions induced by virulent FCV challenge strains (Kahn et al., 1975; Kahn and Hoover, 1976). Annual revaccinations are recommended for FCV and FRV vaccines.

The efficacy of vaccine as a therapeutic agent has not been investigated.

## CHLAMYDIOSIS ("PNEUMONITIS")

Feline *Chlamydia psittaci* is a bacterium rather than a virus and is principally a conjunctival pathogen. Although the feline pneumonitis agent was described in 1942 (Baker, 1942), it is probable that the majority of cases of "feline pneumonitis" diagnosed clinically since that time have been due to FRV or FCV infections (Cello, 1971; Ott, 1971). The occurrence and pathogenicity of feline *C. psittaci* in the cat population are uncertain (Ott, 1971; Povey and Johnson, 1971; Walton and Gillespie, 1970a). Experimental aerosol or intranasal exposure of cats to *C. psittaci* produces conjunctivitis but not significant pulmonary lesions (Cello, 1971; Hoover et al., 1978).

*C. psittaci* has also been isolated from one cat with peritonitis (Dickie and Sniff, 1980). Organisms morphologically identified as *Chlamydia* spp have been demonstrated by light and electron microscopy in the gastric epithelium of 12 cats necropsied for various reasons (Hargis et al., 1983). The chlamydiae were not associated with a gastric lesion or with disease.

### Characteristics of Etiologic Agent

The feline pneumonitis agent, a feline strain of *C. psittaci*, is an obligate intracellular bacterium formerly known as *Miyagawanella felis* and later *Bedsonia felis* (Cello, 1967, 1971; Schachter, 1978; Schachter and Caldwell, 1980). Chlamydiae are Gram-negative, have cell walls, contain both DNA and RNA, and replicate by binary fission in the cytoplasm of host cells. They can be propagated in embryonated eggs, mice, or cell cultures. Two species of *Chlamydia* are recognized: *C. psittaci* and *C. trachomatis*. *C. psittaci* forms intracytoplasmic inclusion bodies that stain with Wright-Giemsa stains but not with iodine (Schachter, 1978). The chlamydial replication cycle in cells is initiated by the elementary body form of the organism, a 0.3 to 0.5 μ coccoid bacterium, which is the only chlamydial form capable of extracellular survival (Schachter and Caldwell, 1980). Elementary body adsorption and penetration of cells by endocytosis depend on compatible host cell receptors (Schachter, 1978). Elementary bodies reorganize into larger reticulate bodies, which divide by binary fission and differentiate into new generations of elementary bodies. Intracellular chlamydiae are contained within phagosomes where the entire chlamydial replication cycle occurs (Schachter and Caldwell, 1980). Chlamydial replication interrupts cell metabolism to varying degrees. Eventually, most parasitized cells degenerate, detach, and liberate infectious elementary bodies onto mucosal surfaces.

## Clinical Features, Pathogenesis, Lesions

Cats are infected with *C. psittaci* by contact with elementary bodies in oculonasal secretions. The degree of contagiousness probably is similar to that of feline calicivirus. Replication in conjunctival and nasal epithelial cells leads to cell degeneration, detachment, and sloughing, which peak 7 to 10 days after exposure (Hoover et al., 1978). Conjunctivitis appears 5 to 10 days after exposure and is characterized by blepharospasm, congestion, chemosis, and increased lacrimation (Fig. 7–56) (Cello, 1967; Hoover et al., 1978; Mitzel and Strating, 1977). Conjunctivitis often is initially unilateral, but both eyes ultimately become involved. Ocular exudates become mucopurulent, and follicular hyperplasia of lymphoid tissue in the palpebrae and nictitating membrane becomes a prominent feature within seven days (see Fig. 7–56) (Cello, 1967; Hoover et al., 1978).

Signs of rhinitis are mild to moderate, i.e., intermittent sneezing and serous nasal discharge. Fever occurs several days after the onset of conjunctivitis (between 11 and 15 days after experimental *C. psittaci* infection) (Hoover et al., 1978). Neither severe rhinitis nor ulceration of the tongue, palate, nostril, or cornea has been induced by feline *C. psittaci* infection (Cello, 1971; Hoover et al., 1978; Mitzel and Strating, 1977).

Conjunctival lesions evoked by the feline pneumonitis agent are characterized by early intense infiltration of neutrophils superseded by lymphocytes and plasma cells. Regenerative hyperplasia and prominent nodular lymphoid cell infiltrations dominate the microscopic lesions by 10 days after infection (Cello, 1971; Hoover et al., 1978). Chlamydial inclusion bodies in conjunctival cells are inconspicuous in H & E–stained sections; staining with Giemsa or other stains is usually required for their detection. Consequently, histologic examination is an insensitive and impractical method of detecting *C. psittaci* infection (see further on).

Nasal and pulmonary lesions in cats exposed by aerosol to *C. psittaci* are mild to moderate neutrophilic rhinitis and occasional mild, focal, interstitial pneumonia (Hoover et al., 1978). Hyperplasia of the splenic lymphoid follicles and peribronchiolar lymphoid nodules occurs two to seven weeks after exposure to *C. psittaci* (Hoover et al., 1978). No other visceral lesions have been attributed to *C. psittaci* infection, although the organism has been isolated from the spleen and liver of some experimentally infected cats for up to 27 days after inoculation (Mitzel and Strating, 1977).

Examination of Wright- or Giemsa-stained conjunctival smears can be used clinically to identify chlamydial inclusions for up to two weeks after *C. psittaci* infection (Cello, 1971; Hoover et al., 1978). Superficial conjunctival epithelium is collected by rotation of a moistened swab against the palpebral mucosa and inner surface of the nictitating membrane. The cells obtained on the swab are transferred to a glass slide by similar rotation of the swab and are then stained. Usually, many neutrophils and other leukocytes will be present in conjunctival smears, but chlamydial inclusions are best sought in conjunctival epithelial cells. The latter are identified by the large round nuclei and abundant, lightly staining cytoplasm. Clusters of blue coccoid intracytoplasmic bodies (Figs. 7–57 and 7–58) approximately 0.5 μ in diameter detected by oil immersion microscopy indicate *C. psittaci* infection. Green or brown melanin granules are common in feline conjunctival epithelium. Chlamydiae are distinguished from these by their blue staining, their larger size, and their occurrence in tight clusters (Hoover et al., 1978).

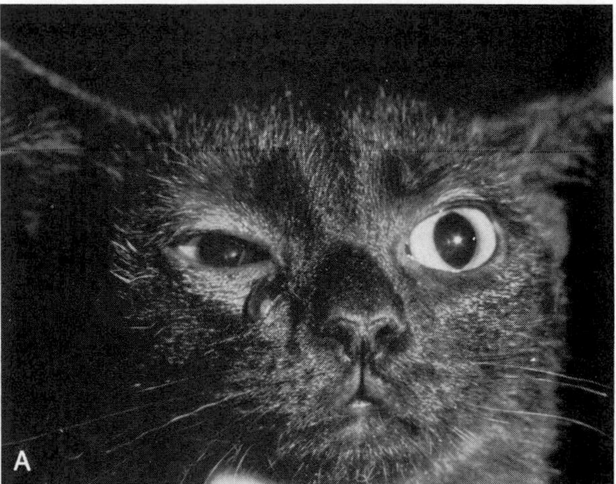


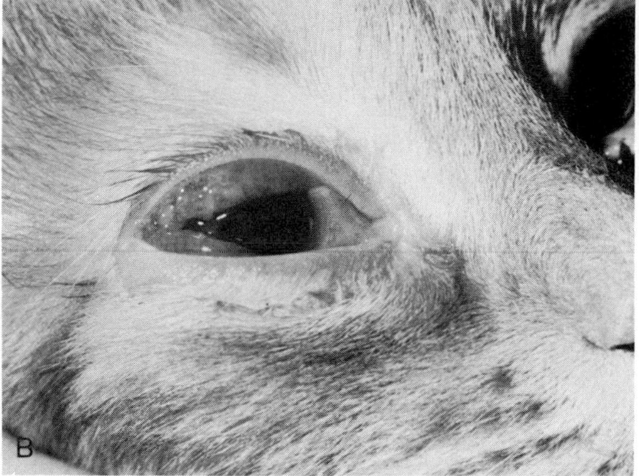


**Figure 7–56** Chlamydial infection: stages of conjunctivitis in experimentally infected cats. *A*, Acute unilateral blepharospasm and seromucoid discharge seven days after exposure. *B*, Follicular conjunctivitis with severe chemosis 20 days after exposure. (From Hoover EA, Kahn DE, Langloss JM: Am J Vet Res 39 [1978] 541–547.)

Chlamydiae not demonstrable by conventional stains may sometimes be detected by immunoperoxidase staining (Dr. Frances Moore, unpublished data).

Feline chlamydiae have been propagated in the chorioallantoic membrane of embryonated eggs, the only

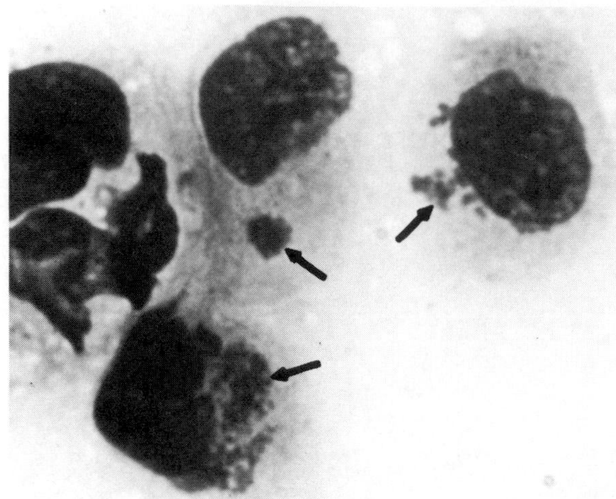

**Figure 7–57** Chlamydial infection. Giemsa-stained conjunctival smear seven days after experimental exposure. Intracytoplasmic replicative forms of *C. psittaci* (arrows) arranged in various patterns. (From Hoover EA, Kahn DE, Langloss JM: Am J Vet Res 39 [1978] 541–547.)

method currently available for isolation of feline *C. psittaci*. Technical difficulties associated with these cultivation procedures have limited both diagnostic utility and investigation of the incidence of *C. psittaci* infection in cats.

## Hematologic Response

A leukocyte count within normal limits or mild neutrophilic leukocytosis is typical. Erythrocyte data remain normal (Hoover et al., 1978).

## Immune Response

Antibody to *C. psittaci* can be detected by complement fixation, although the antibody titers appear to have limited relevance to the resistance of cats to induction of chlamydial conjunctivitis after challenge exposure (McKercher, 1952; Mitzel and Strating, 1977). A neutralizing antibody assay for feline *C. psittaci* has not been developed. Immunity conferred by chlamydial infection is transient. Reinfection results in milder signs of shorter duration and an anamnestic antibody response (Cello, 1971; Mitzel and Stating, 1977).

## Immune Carrier State

Latency of *C. psittaci* infection has been documented in birds and humans but has not been investigated in cats. Fecal excretion appears to be the major route of dissemination of avian *C. psittaci* infection (Schachter and Caldwell, 1980). Human *C. trachomatis* infection can remain latent for years and can be activated by corticosteroid administration (Schachter, 1978). Neither the specific host cell involved in latent chlamydial infections nor the nature of the host-parasite relationship has been determined. Although chlamydial replication does not always lead to cell death, no evidence has been obtained that chlamydiae persist intracellularly in a nonreplicating form (Schachter, 1978).

## Treatment

Chlamydiae are bacteria and therefore are sensitive to antibiotics, tetracycline being the most effective. Therapy at standard dosages should be continued for 14 days to

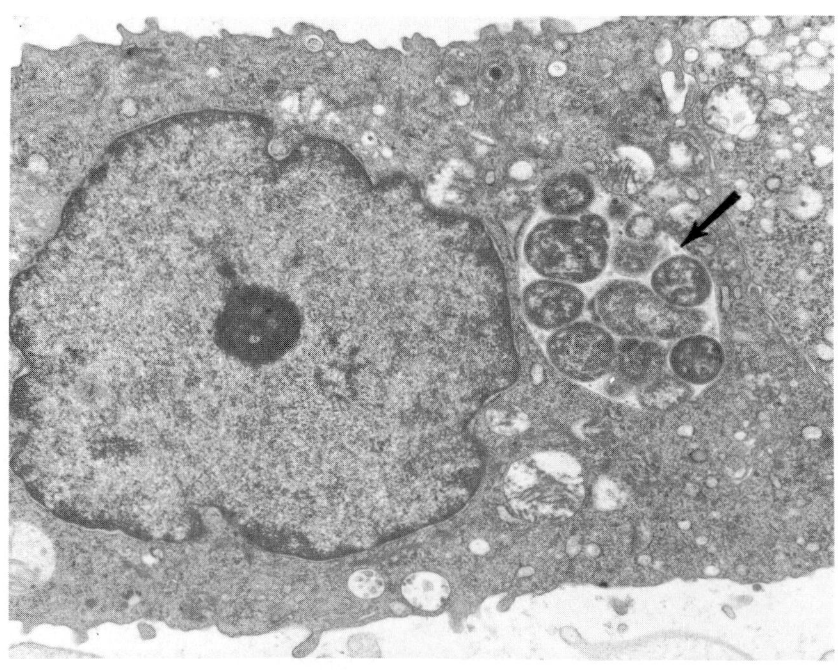

**Figure 7–58** Chlamydial infection. Conjunctival cell containing *C. psittaci* replicative forms (arrow) within phagosome. Electron micrograph. (From Hoover EA, Kahn DE, Langloss JM: Am J Vet Res 39 [1978] 541–547.)

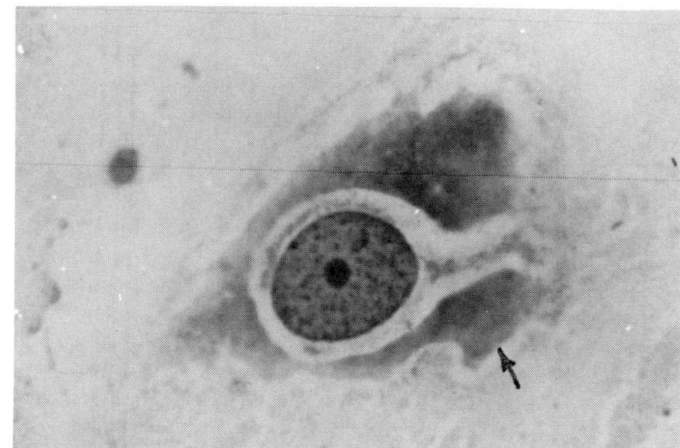

**Figure 7–59** Reovirus infection. Large, intracytoplasmic basophilic inclusion body (arrow) occupies much of the cytoplasm. Infection cell culture, Giemsa stain. (From Scott FW, Kahn DE, Gillespie JH: Am J Vet Res 31 [1970] 11–20.)

minimize the possibility of recurrence or chronic latent infection. *C. psittaci* is sensitive also to sulfonamides but less so to penicillin, ampicillin, and streptomycin (Schachter, 1978).

### IMMUNOPROPHYLAXIS

Feline pneumonitis vaccines produced from attenuated organisms propagated in embryonated eggs have been available for many years (McKercher, 1952). Vaccination has been shown to reduce significantly the duration and severity of conjunctivitis, rhinitis, and fever in vaccinated as compared with control cats (McKercher, 1952; Mitzel and Stating, 1977). As with FRV and FCV vaccines, vaccination ameliorated but did not completely prevent chlamydial infection (Mitzel and Strating, 1977). In vaccination programs for feline respiratory disease, immunization against chlamydial infection must be considered less important than that against FRV and FCV infections. The vaccine is available as a monovalent product or in combination with FRV, FCV, and panleukopenia vaccines.

## FELINE REOVIRUS INFECTION

Feline reovirus was isolated from intestinal tissue of cats in 1970 (Scott et al., 1970) and produces a disease characterized by mild conjunctivitis with little or no effect on the nasal passages or lower respiratory tract (Scott et al., 1970).

Reoviruses are double-stranded RNA, nonenveloped viruses that replicate in the cytoplasm. Feline reovirus replicates in feline cell cultures where it produces a slowly developing cytopathic effect associated with Giemsa-staining intracytoplasmic inclusion bodies (Scott, 1971) (Figs. 7–59 and 7–60). Ultrastructural features of feline reovirus are identical to those described for prototype reoviruses. Serologic characteristics indicate that the feline virus isolates resemble the type 3 class of reoviruses (Scott, 1971), which infects mice, humans, and other species.

Clinical disease produced by intranasal inoculation or contact exposure of cats is limited to serous conjunctivitis, lacrimation, and blepharospasm between 4 and 19 days after exposure (Scott et al., 1970). No significant nasal discharge or other signs of respiratory disease occurred. Virus was isolated (in descending order of frequency)

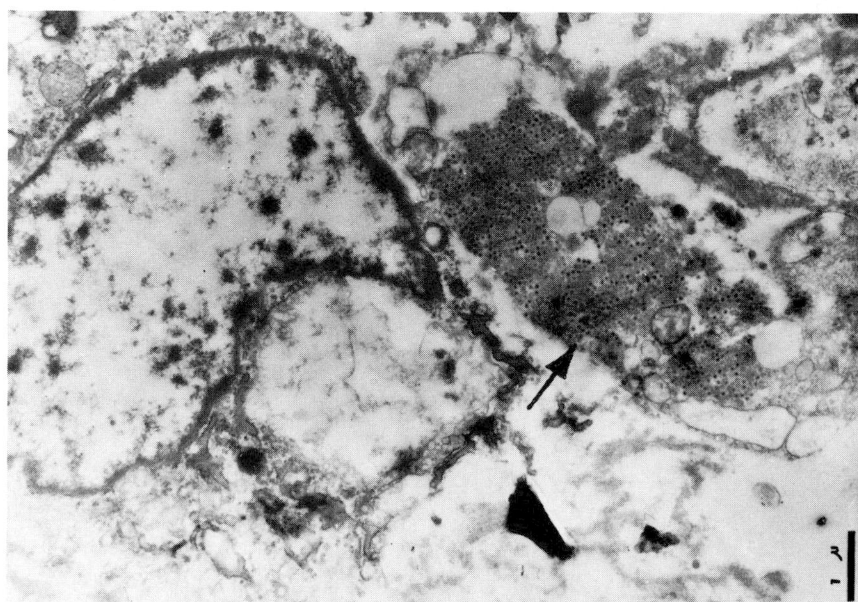

**Figure 7–60** Reovirus infection. Reovirus particles (arrow) in the cytoplasm of an infected cell. Electron micrograph. (From Scott FW, Kahn DE, Gillespie JH: Am J Vet Res 31 [1970] 11–20.)

from rectal, pharyngeal, nasal, and ocular swabbings 6 to 10 days after exposure.

No hematologic alterations of diagnostic significance have been detected (Scott et al., 1970).

Infected cats produce neutralizing antibody titers ranging from 1:30 to 1:60. Low antibody titers were detected in 50 per cent of 110 cats surveyed in the Ithaca, N. Y., area (Scott, 1971).

Treatment of feline reovirus conjunctivitis is neither specific nor essential.

Reoviruses are known to exist as latent infections in several species and are occasional contaminants of cell cultures prepared from normal animals. The same may be surmised for the feline reovirus, although this subject has not been studied.

No vaccine for feline reovirus is available nor does present information indicate a need for vaccination of cats against this virus.

## OTHER MICROBIAL RESPIRATORY PATHOGENS

*Bordetella bronchiseptica, Staphylococcus epidermidis*, and nonhemolytic *Streptococcus* spp have been isolated from nasal and conjunctival exudates of cats with upper respiratory disease (Povey, 1976; Scott, 1977; Shewen et al., 1980). It appears that primary bacterial infection can be responsible for moderate rhinitis or conjunctivitis in cats (Hoover, E. A., Kahn, D. E., unpublished data; Snyder et al., 1973). Ancillary pathogenetic factors, however, such as inadequate ventilation, poor sanitation, elevated ambient atmospheric ammonia, or immunosuppression, may be required.

*Mycoplasma* spp have been isolated from the conjunctiva of cats with conjunctivitis and from conjunctiva of normal cats (Campbell et al., 1973; Cello, 1971; Heyward et al., 1969; Hill, 1971; Kotani et al., 1980; Tan, 1974; Tan and Miles, 1974a). The characteristics of feline mycoplasmal infection are discussed in greater detail in the chapter on bacterial diseases. Experimental inoculation of cats with feline *Mycoplasma* isolates has rarely resulted in conjunctivitis or other disease (Heyward et al., 1969; Hill, 1971; Tan, 1974). Thus it appears that *Mycoplasma* organisms act principally in a secondary or synergistic role in the pathogenesis of feline respiratory disease (Campbell et al., 1973; Cello, 1971; Shewen et al., 1980).

Fungi that may involve the respiratory tract are discussed in the chapter on mycotic diseases.

## DIFFERENTIAL DIAGNOSIS OF FELINE UPPER RESPIRATORY INFECTIONS

The following conclusions can be drawn concerning the diagnosis of respiratory infections in cats and are presented in Table 7–7.

1. Severe rhinitis and conjunctivitis, abortion, and keratitis are features of FRV infection.
2. Ulcerations of the tongue, gingiva, or nostril in the absence of severe rhinitis are features of FCV infection.
3. Chronic follicular conjunctivitis without severe rhinitis, oral ulcers, or keratitis is characteristic of feline chlamydial infection.
4. Signs of mild rhinitis, conjunctivitis, or both have little value in presumptive diagnosis.
5. Lingual ulcers are most frequently associated with FCV but can also be produced in severe FRV infections.
6. Virulent strains of FCV and large aerosol exposures produce primary acute pneumonia.
7. FVR rarely induces pneumonia or generalized visceral infection; kittens and immunosuppressed cats are most susceptible.
8. FCV infections sometimes are associated with severe rhinitis or conjunctivitis; synergistic bacterial infection may be implicated in these instances.
9. The possibility of concurrent immunosuppressive viral infection (notably feline leukemia virus infection) should be considered. Concomitant nonregenerative anemia, leukopenia, diarrhea, and weight loss are principal indicators that leukemia virus infection might be involved.

## MANAGEMENT AND CONTROL

The immune carrier state occurs with all the feline upper respiratory pathogens. Elimination of enzootic infections, especially in a colony or cattery environment, should entail removal of all infected cats and vaccination of all exposed or newly introduced cats. Transmission of respiratory pathogens occurs principally by contact; aerosol transmission over an air space of more than 10 feet is minimal (Gaskell and Povey, 1977; Wardley and Povey, 1977). Fomite transmission probably is of minor importance in the epizootiology of feline upper respiratory infections (Wardley and Povey, 1977).

Vaccination programs for FVR, FCV, and chlamydial infection decrease the population of susceptible cats and thereby the incidence of clinical disease. Vaccines for

**Table 7–7 Guidelines for Presumptive Diagnosis of Feline Upper Respiratory Infections**

| LESION OR SIGN | MOST CHARACTERISTIC OF: | LESS CHARACTERISTIC OF: | LEAST CHARACTERISTIC OF: |
|---|---|---|---|
| Rhinitis, severe, exudative | FVR | FCV, FCh | |
| Conjunctivitis, severe, sensitive | FVR, FCh* | FCV | |
| Ulcers—tongue, gingiva, nostril | FCV | FVR | FCh |
| Sneezing, coughing, salivation | FVR | FCV, FCh | |
| Pneumonia—dyspnea | FCV | FVR | FCh |
| Keratitis | FVR | FCh | FCh |
| Abortion | FVR | | FCV, FCh |

Modified from Kahn DE, Hoover EA: Vet Clin North Am 6 (1976) 399–413.
*FCh = chlamydial infection (pneumonitis).

FRV, FCV, and chlamydial infection provide a significant degree of protection against challenge with virulent organisms. Although the level of immunity to these respiratory pathogens declines more rapidly than with strong immunogens such as feline panleukopenia virus, a significant degree of residual immunity remains and can be augmented by revaccination or subsequent natural exposure.

## REFERENCES


Abraham A, Tegtmeyer P: Morphological changes in productive and abortive infection by feline herpesvirus. J Virol 5 (1970) 617–623.

Baker JA: A virus obtained from a pneumonia of cats and its possible relation to the cause of atypical pneumonia in man. Science 96 (1942) 475–476.

Bartholomew PT, Gillespie JH: Feline viruses. I. Characterization of four isolates and their effect on young kittens. Cornell Vet 58 (1968) 248–265.

Bistner SI, Carlson JH, Shively JN, Scott FW: Ocular manifestations of feline herpesvirus infection. J Am Vet Med Assoc 159 (1971) 1223–1237.

Bittle JL, York CJ, Newberne JW, Martin M: Serologic relationship of new feline cytopathogenic viruses. Am J Vet Res 21 (1960) 547–550.

Bittle JL, Emery JB, York CJ, McMillen JK: Comparative study of feline cytopathogenic viruses and feline panleukopenia virus. Am J Vet Res 22 (1961) 374–378.

Bittle JL, Peckham JC: Comments: Genital infection induced by feline rhinotracheitis virus and effects on newborn kittens. J Am Vet Med Assoc 158 (1971) 927–928.

Bittle JL, Rubic WJ: Studies of feline viral rhinotracheitis vaccine. Vet Med Small Anim Clin 69 (1974) 1503–1505.

Bittle JL, Rubic WJ: Immunogenic and protective effects of the F-2 strain of feline viral rhinotracheitis virus. Am J Vet Res 36 (1975) 89–91.

Bittle JL, Rubic WJ: Immunization against feline calicivirus infection. Am J Vet Res 37 (1976) 275–278.

Black DN, Brown F: Proteins induced by infection with caliciviruses. J Gen Virol 38 (1978) 75–82.

Bolin VS: The cultivation of panleucopenia virus in tissue culture. Virology 4 (1957) 389–390.

Brehaut L, Jones RH, McEwan PJ, Miles JAR: Viruses associated with feline respiratory disease in Dunedin. N Z Vet J 17 (1969) 82–86.

Bürki F: Picornaviruses of cats. Arch Ges Virusforsch 15 (1965) 690–696.

Bürki F: Zur Organaffinität feliner Picornaviren. Zentralbl Bakteriol (Orig) 200 (1966) 281–289.

Bürki F: Virologic and immunologic aspects of feline picornaviruses. J Am Vet Med Assoc 158 (1971) 916–919.

Bürki F, Lindt S, Freudiger U: Enzootischer virusbedingter Katzenschnupfen in einem Tierheim. 2. Mitteilung: Virologischer und experimenteller Teil. Zentralbl Veterinärmed [B] 11 (1964) 110–118.

Burroughs JN, Brown F: Physico-chemical evidence for the reclassification of the calciviruses. J Gen Virol 22 (1974) 281–286.

Campbell LH, Snyder SB, Reed C, Fox JG: *Mycoplasma felis*-associated conjunctivitis in cats. J Am Vet Med Assoc 163 (1973) 991–995.

Cello RM: Ocular infections in animals with PLT (Bedsonia) group agents. Am J Ophthalmol 63 Suppl (1967) 1270–1274.

Cello RM: Microbiological and immunologic aspects of feline pneumonitis. J Am Vet Med Assoc 158 (1971) 932–938.

Cole BC, Golightly L, Ward JR: Characterization of mycoplasma strains from cats. J Bacteriol 94 (1967) 1451–1458.

Cooper LM, Sabine M: Paw and mouth disease in a cat [letter]. Aust Vet J 48 (1972) 644.

Cotter SM, Hardy WD Jr, Essex M: Association of feline leukemia virus with lymphosarcoma and other disorders in the cat. J Am Vet Med Assoc 166 (1975) 449–454.

Crandell RA, Maurer FD: Isolation of a feline virus associated with intranuclear inclusion bodies. Proc Soc Exp Biol Med 97 (1958) 487–490.

Crandell RA, Despeaux EW: Cytopathology of feline viral rhinotracheitis virus in tissue cultures of feline renal cells. Proc Soc Exp Biol Med 101 (1959) 494–497.

Crandell RA, Madin SH: Experimental studies on a new feline virus. Am J Vet Res 21 (1960) 551–556.

Crandell RA, Ganaway JR, Niemann WH, Maurer FD: Comparative study of three isolates with the original feline viral rhinotracheitis virus. Am J Vet Res 21 (1960a) 504–506.

Crandell RA, Niemann WH, Ganaway JR, Maurer FD: Isolation of cytopathic agents from the nasopharyngeal region of the domestic cat. Virology 10 (1960b) 283–285.

Crandell RA, Rehkemper JA, Niemann WH, Ganaway JR, Maurer FD: Experimental feline viral rhinotracheitis. J Am Vet Med Assoc 138 (1961) 191–196.

Crandell RA: A description of eight feline picornaviruses and an attempt to classify them. Proc Soc Exp Biol Med 126 (1967) 240–245.

Crandell RA: Virologic and immunologic aspects of feline viral rhinotracheitis virus. J Am Vet Med Assoc 158 (1971) 922–926.

Crandell RA: Feline viral rhinotracheitis (FVR). Adv Vet Sci Comp Med 17 (1973) 201–224.

Crandell RA, Fabricant CG, Nelson-Rees WA: Development, characterization, and viral susceptibility of a feline (*Felis catus*) renal cell line (CRFK). In Vitro 9 (1973) 176–185.

Davis EV, Beckenhauer WH: Studies on the safety and efficacy of an intranasal feline rhinotracheitis—calicivirus vaccine. Vet Med Small Anim Clin 7 (1976) 1405–1410.

Dickie CW, Sniff ES: Chlamydial infection associated with peritonitis in a cat. J Am Vet Med Assoc 1976 (1980) 1256–1259.

Ditchfield J, Grinyer I: Feline rhinotracheitis virus: A feline herpesvirus. Virology 26 (1965) 504–506.

Donaldson AI, Ferris NP: The survival of some air-borne animal viruses in relation to relative humidity. Vet Microbiol 1 (1976) 413–420.

Edwards BG, Buell DJ, Acree WM, Payne JB: Evaluation of feline rhinotracheitis/feline panleukopenia combination vaccines by consecutive virulent challenge. Feline Pract 7(4) (1977a) 45–50.

Edwards BG, Buell DJ, Acree WM: Evaluation of a new feline rhinotracheitis virus vaccine. Vet Med Small Anim Clin 72 (1977b) 205–209.

Fastier LB: A new feline virus isolated in tissue culture. Am J Vet Res 18 (1957) 382–389.

Flagstad A: Isolation and classification of feline picornavirus and herpesvirus in Denmark. Acta Vet Scand 13 (1972) 462–471.

Flagstad A: Experimental picornavirus infection in cats. Acta Vet Scand 14 (1974) 501–510.

Flecknell PA, Orr CM, Wright AI, Gaskell RM, Kelly DF: Skin ulceration associated with herpesvirus infection in cats. Vet Rec 104 (1979) 313–315.

Gaskell RM, Povey RC: Re-excretion of feline viral rhinotracheitis virus following corticosteroid administration. Vet Rec 93 (1973) 204–205.

Gaskell RM, Povey RC: Experimental induction of feline viral rhinotracheitis virus re-excretion in FVR-recovered cats. Vet Rec 100 (1977) 128–132.

Gaskell RM, Povey RC: Feline viral rhinotracheitis: Sites of virus replication and persistence in acutely and persistently infected cats. Res Vet Sci 27 (1979a) 167–174.

Gaskell RM, Povey RC: The dose response of cats to experimental infection with feline viral rhinotracheitis virus. J Comp Pathol 89 (1979b) 179–191.

Gaskell RM, Povey RC: Transmission of feline viral rhinotracheitis. Vet Rec 111 (1982) 359–362.

Gillespie JH, Judkins AB, Scott FW: Feline viruses. XII. Hemagglutination and hemadsorption tests for feline herpesvirus. Cornell Vet 61 (1971a) 159–171.

Gillespie JH, Judkins AB, Kahn DE: Feline viruses. XIII. The use of the immunofluorescent test for the detection of feline picornaviruses. Cornell Vet 61 (1971b) 172–179.

Gillespie JH, Scott FW: Feline viral infections. Adv Vet Sci Comp Med 17 (1973) 163–200.

Hargis AM, Prieur DJ, Gaillard ET: Chlamydial infection of the gastric mucosa in twelve cats. Vet Pathol 20 (1983) 170–178.

Hersey DF, Maurer FD: Immunological relationship of selected feline viruses by complement fixation. Proc Soc Exp Biol Med 107 (1961) 645–646.

Heyward JT, Sabry MZ, Dowdle WR: Characterization of mycoplasma species of feline origin. Am J Vet Res 30 (1969) 615–622.

Hill A: Further studies on the morphology and isolation of feline mycoplasmas. J Small Anim Pract 12 (1971) 219–223.

Holzinger EA, Kahn DE: Pathologic features of picornavirus infections in cats. Am J Vet Res 31 (1970) 1623–1630.

Holzworth J: Naturally occurring upper respiratory infection in cats. J Am Vet Med Assoc 158 (1971) 964–968.

Hoover EA, Rohovsky MW, Griesemer RA: Experimental feline viral rhinotracheitis in the germfree cat. Am J Pathol 58 (1970) 269–282.

Hoover EA, Griesemer RA: Bone lesions produced by feline herpesvirus. Lab Invest 25 (1971a) 457–464.

Hoover EA, Griesemer RA: Pathogenicity of feline viral rhinotracheitis virus and effect on germfree cats, growing bone, and the gravid uterus. J Am Vet Med Assoc 158 (1971b) 929–931.

Hoover EA, Griesemer RA: Experimental feline herpesvirus infection in the pregnant cat. Am J Pathol 65 (1971c) 173–188.

Hoover EA, Kahn DE: Lesions produced by feline picornaviruses of different virulence in pathogen-free cats. Vet Pathol 10 (1973) 307–322.

Hoover EA, Kahn DE: Experimentally induced feline calicivirus infection: Clinical signs and lesions. J Am Vet Med Assoc 166 (1975) 463–468.

Hoover EA, Kahn DE, Langloss JM: Experimentally induced feline chlamydial infection (feline pneumonitis). Am J Vet Res 39 (1978) 541–547.

Hoover EA: Feline pneumonitis. *In* Kirk RW (ed): Current Veterinary Therapy VIII. Philadelphia, W B Saunders Company, 1980.

Hoover EA, Rojko JL, Quackenbush SL: Congenital feline leukemia virus infection. Leuk Rev Int 1 (1983) 7–8.

Johnson RH, Thomas RG: Feline viral rhinotracheitis in Britain. Vet Rec 79 (1966) 188–190.

Johnson RP, Sabine M: The isolation of herpesviruses from skin ulcers in domestic cats. Vet Rec 89 (1971) 360–362.

Johnson RP, Povey RC: Transfer and decline of maternal antibody to feline calicivirus. Can Vet J 24 (1) (1983) 6–9.

Kahn DE, Gillespie JH: Feline viruses. X. Characterization of a newly isolated picornavirus causing interstitial pneumonia and ulcerative stomatitis in the domestic cat. Cornell Vet 60 (1970) 669–683.

Kahn DE, Gillespie JH: Feline viruses: pathogenesis of picornavirus infection in the cat. Am J Vet Res 33 (1971) 521–531.

Kahn DE, Walton TE: Epizootiology of feline respiratory infections. J Am Vet Med Assoc 158 (1971) 955–959.

Kahn DE: Unpublished data, 1976.

Kahn DE, Hoover EA, Bittle JL: Induction of immunity to feline caliciviral disease. Infect Immun 11 (1975) 1003–1009.

Kahn DE, Hoover EA: Infectious respiratory diseases of cats. Vet Clin North Am 6 (1976a) 399–413.

Kahn DE, Hoover EA: Feline caliciviral disease: experimental immunoprophylaxis. Am J Vet Res 37 (1976b) 279–283.

Kalunda M, Lee KM, Holmes DF, Gillespie JH: Serologic classification of feline caliciviruses by plaque-reduction neutralization and immunodiffusion. Am J Vet Res 36 (1975) 353–356.

Kamizono M, Konishi S, Ogata M, Kobori S: Studies on cytopathogenic viruses isolated from cats with respiratory infections. I. Jpn J Vet Sci 30 (1968) 197–206.

Karpas A, Routledge JK: Feline herpesvirus: Isolations and experimental studies. Zentralbl Veterinärmed [B] 15 (1968) 599–606.

Komolafe OO, Jarrett O, Neil JC: Feline calicivirus induced polypeptides. Microbios 27 (1980) 185–192.

Kotani H, Harasawa R, Yamamoto K, Ogata M: Serological studies with feline ureaplasmas. Microbiol Immunol 24 (1980) 83–86.

Langloss JM, Hoover EA, Kahn DE: Diffuse alveolar damage in cats induced by nitrogen dioxide or feline calicivirus. Am J Pathol 89 (1977) 637–648.

Langloss JM, Hoover EA, Kahn DE, Kniazeff AJ: In vitro interaction of alveolar macrophages and pneumocytes with feline respiratory viruses. Infect Immun 20 (1978a) 836–841.

Langloss JM, Hoover EA, Kahn DE: Ultrastructural morphogenesis of acute viral pneumonia produced by feline calicivirus. Am J Vet Res 39 (1978b) 1577–1583.

Lee KM, Kniazeff AJ, Fabricant CG, Gillespie JH: Utilization of various cell culture systems for propagation of certain feline viruses and canine herpesvirus. Cornell Vet 59 (1969) 539–547.

Lindt S, Mühlethaler E, Bürki F: Enzootischer, virusbedingter Katzenschnupfen in einem Tierheim. 1. Mitteilung: Klinik, Patho-Histologie, Ätiologie und Epizootiologie. Schweiz Arch Tierheilkd 107 (1965) 91–101.

Love DN: Feline herpesvirus associated with interstitial pneumonia in a kitten. Vet Rec 89 (1971) 178–181.

Love DN, Baker KD: Sudden death in kittens associated with a feline picornavirus. Aust Vet J 48 (1972) 643.

Love DN: Pathogenicity of a strain of feline calicivirus for domestic kittens. Aust Vet J 51 (1975) 541–546.

Love DN, Donaldson-Wood C: Replication of a strain of feline calicivirus in organ culture. Arch Virol 47 (1975) 167–175.

MacLachlan NJ, Burgess GW: A survey of feline viral upper respiratory tract infections. N Z Vet J 26 (1978) 260–261.

McEwan PJ, Miles JAR: An electron microscope study of viruses associated with upper respiratory tract infections in cats. Proc Univ Otago Med Sch 45 (1967) 21–23.

McKercher DG: Feline pneumonitis. I. Immunization studies in kittens. Am J Vet Res 13 (1952) 557–561.

Milek M, Wooley RE, Blue JL: Replication of feline herpesvirus and feline calicivirus in cell and organ cultures. Am J Vet Res 37 (1976) 723–724.

Miller GW, Crandell RA: Stability of the virus of feline viral rhinotracheitis. Am J Vet Res 23 (1962) 351–353.

Mitzel JR, Strating A: Vaccination against feline pneumonitis. Am J Vet Res 38 (1977) 1361–1363.

Mochizuki M, Konishi S, Ogata M: Studies on cytopathogenic viruses from cats with respiratory infections, III. Isolation and certain properties of feline herpesviruses. Jpn J Vet Sci 39 (1977a) 27–37.

Mochizuki M, Konishi S, Ogata M: Studies on cytopathogenic viruses from cats with respiratory infections. IV. Properties of hemagglutinin in feline herpesvirus suspensions and receptors on feline erythrocytes. Jpn J Vet Sci 39 (1977b) 389–395.

Mochizuki M, Konishi S, Ogata M: Sero-diagnostic aspects of feline herpesvirus infection. Jpn J Vet Sci 39 (1977c) 191–194.

Olsen RG, Kahn DE, Hoover EA, Saxe NJ, Yohn DS: Differences in acute and convalescent-phase antibodies of cats infected with feline picornaviruses. Infect Immun 10 (1974) 375–380.

Ormerod E, McCandlish IAP, Jarrett O: Diseases produced by feline caliciviruses when administered to cats by aerosol or intranasal instillation. Vet Rec 104 (1979) 65–69.

Orr CM, Gaskell CJ, Gaskell RM: Interaction of an intranasal combined feline viral rhinotracheitis, feline calicivirus vaccine and the FVR carrier state. Vet Rec 106 (1980) 164–166.

Ott RL: Comments on feline pneumonitis. J Am Vet Med Assoc 158 (1971) 939–941.
Pedersen NC, Laliberte L, Ekman S: A transient febrile "limping" syndrome of kittens caused by two different strains of feline calicivirus. Feline Pract 13(1) (1983) 26–35.
Peterson JE, Studdert MJ: Feline picornavirus. Structure of the virus and electron micoscopic observations on infected cell cultures. Arch Ges Virusforsch 32 (1970) 249–260.
Pichler L, Bürki F: Zur Pathogenese der felinen Picornavirusinfection. Wien Tierärztl Monatsschr 57 (1970) 256–249.
Plummer G, Hollingsworth DC, Phuangsab A, Bowling CP: Chronic infections by herpes simplex viruses and by the horse and cat herpesviruses. Infect Immun 1 (1970) 351–355.
Povey RC, Johnson RH: Further observations on feline viral rhinotracheitis. Vet Rec 81 (1967) 686–689.
Povey RC, Johnson RH: A standardized serum neutralization test for feline viral rhinotracheitis. I. Virus assay. J Comp Pathol 79 (1969a) 379–385.
Povey RC, Johnson RH: A standardized serum neutralization test for feline viral rhinotracheitis. II. The virus-serum system. J Comp Pathol 79 (1969b) 387–392.
Povey RC, Johnson RH: Observations on the epidemiology and control of viral respiratory disease in cats. J Small Anim Pract 11 (1970) 485–494.
Povey RC, Johnson RH: A survey of feline viral rhinotracheitis and feline picornavirus infection in Britain. J Small Anim Pract 12 (1971) 233–247.
Povey RC, Wardley RC, Jessen H: Feline picornavirus infection: the *in vivo* carrier state. Vet Rec 92 (1973) 224–229.
Povey RC, Hale CJ: Experimental infections with feline caliciviruses (picornaviruses) in specific-pathogen-free kittens. J Comp Pathol 84 (1974) 245–256.
Povey RC: Serological relationships among feline caliciviruses. Infect Immun 10 (1974) 1307–1314.
Povey RC, Ingersoll J: Cross-protection among feline caliciviruses. Infect Immun 11 (1975) 877–885.
Povey RC: Feline respiratory infections—a clinical review. Can Vet J 17 (1976) 93–100.
Povey RC, Wilson MR: A comparison of inactivated feline viral rhinotracheitis and feline caliciviral disease vaccines with live-modified viral vaccines. Feline Pract 8 (3) (1978) 35–42.
Povey RC: The efficacy of two commercial feline rhinotracheitis calicivirus-panleukopenia vaccines. Can Vet J 20 (1979) 253–260.
Prydie J: Viral diseases of cats. Vet Rec 79 (1966) 729–738.
Roberts SR, Dawson CR, Coleman V, Togni B: Dendritic keratitis in a cat. J Am Vet Med Assoc 161 (1972) 285–289.
Sabine M, Hyne RHJ: Isolation of a feline picornavirus from cheetahs with conjunctivitis and glossitis. Vet Rec 87 (1970) 794–796.
Schachter J: Chlamydial infections. N Engl J Med 298 (1978) 428–435, 490–495, 540–549.
Schachter J, Caldwell HD: Chlamydiae. Ann Rev Microbiol 34 (1980) 285–309.
Schachter J, Ostler HB, Meyer KF: Human infection with the agent of feline pneumonitis. Lancet 1 (1969) 1063–1065.
Scott FW: Feline reovirus. J Am Vet Med Assoc 158 (1971) 944–945.
Scott FW: Evaluation of a feline viral rhinotracheitis vaccine. Feline Pract 5 (1) (1975) 17–22.
Scott FW: Evaluation of a feline viral rhinotracheitis-feline calicivirus disease vaccine. Am J Vet Res 38 (1977) 229–234.
Scott FW, Kahn DE, Gillespie JH: Feline viruses: Isolation, characterization, pathogenicity of a feline reovirus. Am J Vet Res 31 (1970) 11–20.
Shewen PE, Povey RC, Wilson MR: A survey of the conjunctival flora of clinically normal cats and cats with conjunctivitis. Can Vet J 21 (1980) 231–233.
Shields RP, Gaskin JM: Fatal generalized feline viral rhinotracheitis in a young adult cat. J Am Vet Med Assoc 170 (1977) 439–442.
Snyder SB, Fisk SK, Fox JG, Soave OA: Respiratory tract disease associated with *Bordetella bronchiseptica* infection in cats. J Am Vet Med Assoc 163 (1973) 293–294.
Spradbrow PB, Bagust TJ, Burgess G, Portas B: The isolation of picornaviruses from cats with respiratory disease. Aust Vet J 46 (1970a) 105–108.
Spradbrow PB, Marley J, Portas B, Burgess G: The isolation of mycoplasmas from cats with respiratory disease. Aust Vet J 46 (1970b) 109–110.
Spradbrow PB, Carlisle C, Watt DA: The association of a herpesvirus with generalised disease in a kitten. Vet Rec 89 (1971) 542–544.
Steffenhagen KA, Easterday BC, Galasso GJ: Evaluation of 6-azauridine and 5-iododeoxyuridine in the treatment of experimental viral infections. J Infect Dis 133 (1976) 603–612.
Studdert MJ, Martin MC: Virus diseases of the respiratory tract of cats. 1. Isolation of feline rhinotracheitis virus. Aust Vet J 46 (1970) 99–104.
Studdert MJ, Martin MC, Peterson JE: Viral diseases of the respiratory tract of cats: Isolation and properties of viruses tentatively classified as picornaviruses. Am J Vet Res 31 (1970) 1723–1732.
Studdert MJ: Caliciviruses. Brief review. Arch Virol 58 (1978) 157–191.
Takahashi E, Konishi S, Ogata M: Studies on cytopathogenic viruses from cats with respiratory infections. II. Characterization of feline picornaviruses. Jpn J Vet Sci 33 (1971) 81–87.
Tan RJS: Serological comparisons of feline respiratory viruses. Jpn J Med Sci Biol 23 (1970) 419–424.
Tan RJS, Miles JAR: Further studies on feline respiratory virus diseases. 1. Vaccination experiments. NZ Vet J 19 (1971a) 12–15.
Tan RJS, Miles JAR: Further studies on feline respiratory virus diseases. 2. Immunodiffusion tests. NZ Vet J 19 (1971b) 15–18.
Tan RJS: Susceptibility of kittens to *Mycoplasma felis* infection. Jpn J Exp Med 44 (1974) 235–240.
Tan RJS, Miles JAR: Incidence and significance of mycoplasmas in sick cats. Res Vet Sci 16 (1974a) 27–34.
Tan RJS, Miles JAR: Possible role of feline T-strain mycoplasmas in cat abortion. Aust Vet J 50 (1974b) 142–145.
Tegtmeyer P, Enders JF: Feline herpesvirus infection in fused cultures of naturally resistant human cells. J Virol 3 (1969) 469–476.
Torlone V: Agente citopatogeno isolato da una forma rinocongiuntivale del gatto. Vet Ital 11 (1980) 915–928.
Walton TE, Gillespie JH: Feline viruses. VI. Survey of the incidence of feline pathogenic agents in normal and clinically-ill cats. Cornell Vet 60 (1970a) 215–232.
Walton TE, Gillespie JH: Feline viruses VII. Immunity to the feline herpesvirus in kittens inoculated experimentally by the aerosol method. Cornell Vet 60 (1970b) 232–239.
Wardley RC: Feline calicivirus carrier state. A study of the host/virus relationship. Arch Virol 52 (1976) 243–249.
Wardley RC, Povey RC: Aerosol transmission of feline caliciviruses. An assessment of its epidemiological importance. [Br] Vet J 133 (1977) 504–508.
Wardley RC, Gaskell RM, Povey RC: Feline respiratory viruses–their prevalence in clinically healthy cats. J Small Anim Pract 15 (1974) 579–586.
Yerasimides TG: Isolation of a new strain of feline pneumonitis virus from a domestic cat. J Infect Dis 106 (1960) 290–296.

# RABIES

MELVIN K. ABELSETH

Rabies is an encephalomyelitis caused by a virus with a special affinity for nervous tissue. The virus contains RNA and is classified in the rhabdovirus group. The virion is cylindrical, measuring about 75 by 180 nm. It is easily inactivated in saliva by heat and a variety of chemicals and survives only a few hours in dried saliva. The disease is endemic in all the United States, except Hawaii, and in most of the rest of the world. Most islands, both large and small, are successful in maintaining a disease-free status because of their natural isolation and their greater success in enforcing quarantine regulations.

## Epizootiology

Exposure is most often from the bite of a rabid animal, since the virus multiplies in the salivary gland. Salivary contamination of an open scratch or abrasion is also considered exposure. Once the virus is deposited in striated muscle tissue it multiplies in myocytes, whence it is shed into extracellular spaces; neuromuscular tendons and neurotendinal spindles are next involved, and later the peripheral nerves (Murphy et al., 1973). From these the virus travels to the spinal cord and brain and then spreads centrifugally to peripheral tissues. If one can compare the pathogenicity of the disease in the cat with that in the naturally infected fox, it is likely that virus can be found in practically all tissues of the body (Debbie and Trimarchi, 1970). Virus may be present in the cat's saliva for at least a day before clinical signs appear and for several days after (Vaughn et al., 1963). Other evidence indicates that saliva may be infectious up to five days before overt disease appears (Vaughn, 1975)—a possibility to be considered in evaluating the need for human treatment. Rabies does not, however, invariably result from the bite of every rabid animal, because virus is not always present in its salivary gland.

Transmission by ingestion and aerosol is possible but infrequent.

Rabies in man and animals, except in rare instances, is fatal. Chronic or recrudescent rabies has been observed in experimentally infected cats (Gardner et al., 1978; Murphy et al., 1980; Perl et al., 1977) and could conceivably occur under natural conditions.

Cats are considered highly susceptible to rabies (WHO, 1973), but the incidence of rabies in the cat, as in other domestic animals, is closely correlated with the incidence among wild animals. The relationship of feline infection to epizootics in wildlife in various parts of the world is discussed in detail by Vaughn (1975). Although the relative incidence in dogs in the United States appears to be decreasing, that in cats, as in the wild animal population, seems to be rising according to data from the U.S. Communicable Disease Center. The reduction of canine cases is no doubt due in part to the availability of safe and effective vaccines and, especially, extensive vaccination programs. Less attention has been paid to vaccination of cats, which do not seem to be an important reservoir of infection in nature. Wherever rabies in foxes, dogs, or other species is eradicated, rabies in cats disappears spontaneously. Cat-to-cat transmission is believed to be rare.

Of particular concern is the possibility of rabies transmission to cats from bats. Rabies is present among bats throughout the United States and in many other countries, and it is not uncommon for cats to catch bats and possibly to be bitten during the encounter or to eat them, thereby abrading the alimentary mucosa. Bats can have high titers of virus in their salivary glands. Although it has been suggested (Constantine, 1967) that bats are nonclinical carriers, it is more likely that they become exposed and eventually die, as do other animals. In a number of cases, bats have been found acting atypically, sometimes aggressive, sometimes ill, and have been proven to be rabid (Trimarchi et al., 1979). Cases of rabies in animals where terrestrial rabies is not known to occur are difficult to explain other than by bat exposure. In 1980 a case occurred in a cat in the Boston area where rabies other than in bats had not occurred for many years. Rabies was also diagnosed in very young indoor kittens in Florida where no exposure other than through the mother's introduction of infected prey (possibly bats) was likely (Scatterday et al., 1960). Other feline cases without epidemiologic explanation have occurred in Arizona (Morb. Mortal. Rep., 1964) and New York.

Bats are considered rabies-positive until proven negative by laboratory examination. Any bat caught by a cat should be considered as rabid and should be submitted for testing.* If a cat becomes involved with a bat that escapes or is not examined in a laboratory, the cat must be considered exposed. In this situation, quarantine for six months is necessary, unless the cat has been vaccinated against rabies within the previous 12 months, in which case it need only receive a "booster" vaccination.

Skunks are also considered a principal reservoir of rabies in many areas and have been suggested as possible sources of feline disease, the two species being similar in their habits and perhaps more compatible socially than is usual between cats and other animals (Bolin, 1952; Price et al., 1961).

The incubation period of natural rabies varies from 10 days to 6 months or longer, but in the relatively few feline cases for which date of exposure is known it usually falls between two weeks and two months (Ott, 1975). In experimental infection of a sizable group of cats the incubation period was similar, varying between 9 and 51 days, with a median of 18 days (Vaughn, 1975).

## Clinical Features

With minor differences, the clinical pattern of rabies is the same in the cat and the dog. Three stages of development can usually be discerned in the cat, although they

*Living animals should never be submitted to a rabies diagnostic laboratory. This is especially the case with bats, since they may be subdued by the shipping ice and later revive and bite.

are perhaps less sharply defined than in the dog. During a prodromal phase of one or two days, the cat exhibits a change in mien. It may be restless or depressed and may eat more or less than usual. It may be more than ordinarily affectionate and eager for companionship, or it may be apathetic and seek solitude. Sometimes it cries a lot or scratches the ground. There may be slight fever (but 105 F in one case, Erlewein, 1981), dilatation of the pupils (occasionally unequal), and sluggish corneal reflexes. It has been suggested that some feline cases are never diagnosed because a cat seeks a hiding place and dies there (Ott, 1975).

In many cases, subtle changes in personality and behavior escape notice and the illness appears to begin as posterior weakness or ataxia, which develops into a progressive ascending paralysis. In this case the clinician would be far more likely at the outset to suspect lymphoma or noneffusive feline infectious peritonitis involving the spinal cord.

The stage of excitation, of gradual or sudden onset, is prominent in feline rabies, and cats often develop the furious form of the disease. "Furious" well describes the actions of some rabid cats, which become a serious menace to humans because of their natural facility with teeth and claws. Seizing or chewing at foreign objects may come first, then biting at the legs or face of humans and even dogs—for which species the rabid cat loses its customary respect. Farm cats may bite cows (Lewis, 1965). Hyperesthesia may lead to violent spasms when the cat is touched. Sometimes the cat chews at the site of exposure (e.g., Erlewein, 1981). Heavy leather gloves are recommended for handling such suspects. Some cats become frankly maniacal, hurtling from an open cage, attacking attendants, and battering themselves against wall and furniture until they collapse from sheer exhaustion (Cushing, 1960).

With the onset of paralysis of the throat muscles, the cat drools and cannot swallow water or food. Because of progressive paralysis of the vocal cords, its voice assumes an unnatural quality. Some cats may purr until shortly before death (Blenden, 1961).

Sometimes death occurs during seizures, but often a final "dumb" or paralytic stage develops. This is heralded by paralysis of the limbs, usually first affecting the hindquarters and eventually involving the whole body. Clonic tetany has been observed (Blenden, 1961). Apathy progresses into coma, and death occurs usually in from two to five days from the onset of illness. One cat is known to have lived 11 days from the first signs of disturbance (Blenden, 1961), but in a reported case of a 48-day course of illness (Schieler, 1959) it seems probable that the early signs described were those of coexisting juvenile osteoporosis, also confirmed at autopsy. In a case of vaccine-associated rabies, 15 days passed between the earliest signs and euthanasia (Erlewein, 1981).

Postvaccinal rabies is reported from time to time in cats vaccinated with modified live virus vaccine. The first sign is usually lameness in the hindleg where the vaccine was given. In cases of vaccine-induced rabies, virus may appear in the saliva, and therefore exposed humans should be evaluated for postexposure prophylaxis.

Cats infected experimentally have survived for over two years but eventually died or were destroyed because of progressive paresis (Perl et al., 1977; Murphy et al., 1980).

## Diagnosis

A tentative diagnosis of rabies depends on the possibility of exposure, the incidence of rabies in the area, and characteristic clinical signs. If the cat is a stray or is unowned or unwanted and has exposed humans, it may be destroyed immediately, but the head must be submitted to a diagnostic laboratory proficient in performing the direct fluorescent antibody test (DFA) (Dean and Abelseth, 1973).

The basis of this recommendation is that, if the cat was shedding virus at the time of the bite owing to multiplication in the salivary gland, virus would be detectable in the brain by the DFA test, since rarely, if ever, is virus detected in the salivary gland but not the brain. Laboratory examination should be required even if human exposure has not been reported, for it is not unusual to learn belatedly, once a positive laboratory diagnosis is reported, that human exposure may have occurred.

Common sense and humanity dictate that not every biting cat be suspected of rabies. Many a frightened, harassed, or injured cat or dog bites a person trying to handle it, and some have been destroyed unnecessarily on a very unlikely suspicion of rabies.

If a suspect cat is to be observed, it must be quarantined for 10 days, in a manner in which it cannot endanger humans or other animals. If it is healthy at the end of the period, there need be no concern that it was shedding virus before quarantine. If the cat dies during quarantine, the head must be submitted to a laboratory immediately.

### Differential Diagnosis

Among disorders that may be or have been misinterpreted as rabies are feline infectious peritonitis, toxoplasmosis, encephalitic pasteurellosis, lymphoma of the central nervous system, thiamine deficiency, lead and other poisonings, parasitism, aortic embolism, injuries, and a variety of organic troubles (Mitchell and Monlux, 1962).

## Pathologic Features

Self-mutilation may be evident, and the stomach may contain foreign matter, but there are no pathognomonic gross lesions in rabies. A positive diagnosis is most rapidly and reliably made by the DFA test. When this test is performed in laboratories that have good equipment, high quality conjugate, and experienced laboratory diagnosticians, it is essentially 100 per cent accurate. Technicians must be aware of the so-called cat bodies (Szlachta and Habel, 1953) that appear with the DFA test (as well as with older methods of histologic examination), but an experienced reader utilizing the inhibition test can differentiate these structures from fluorescing particles typical of rabies virus.

Some laboratories still perform diagnosis by examining for Negri bodies. This procedure is less accurate than the DFA test and is not used by progressive institutions. If this is the only test available, a suspect animal should not be destroyed before 10 days or before advanced symptoms are evident, since Negri bodies may not yet be present and it would be necessary to inoculate mice.

If there is any question about the results of DFA testing or examination for Negri bodies, mouse inoculation is required. Isolation in tissue culture is as accurate as mouse inoculation and more rapid (Rudd, Trimarchi, and Abelseth, 1980).

The DFA technique has recently been adapted for skin testing (Blenden, 1979) and could be used to evaluate a pet that has bitten someone but has a record of up-to-date vaccination and is exhibiting no abnormal signs. A negative-testing biopsy specimen does not, however, constitute proof that virus is not present elsewhere. Therefore, while the biopsy result might be grounds for recommending further observation of the animal, it should not be regarded as a contraindication for prophylactic treatment of an exposed human.

## Management After Exposure

An unvaccinated cat that is bitten by a known rabid animal should be destroyed immediately or else quarantined for at least six months and vaccinated one month before release. If a vaccinated cat is bitten by a suspected or known rabid animal it should have an immediate "booster" vaccination and be confined for 90 days. Regulations vary locally, and a veterinarian should apply those in effect in the locality of the occurrence. A healthy pet that bites a person should be observed for 10 days.

## Treatment

No data are available as to the effectiveness of prophylactic treatment of exposed animals or even regular vaccination at that time. The World Health Organization (WHO) does not advise treatment of exposed animals, as it may create a false sense of security for the owner and hence a public health hazard.

## Prevention

Vaccination of cats has never been widely practiced. In 1927, the First International Congress on Rabies decreed that cats should never receive vaccine for either prevention or treatment. In the years that followed, feline rabies was recognized as a substantial problem in certain Moslem areas of the Mediterranean region where, for religious reasons, cats enjoyed a favored status. A colorful episode in which a pet cat, dislodged forcibly from its hiding place under a sofa in a Turkish bath, attacked and bit 15 persons stimulated research on the possibility of preventive vaccination for this species (Remlinger and Bailly, 1934).

In the light of present knowledge, vaccination of "outdoor" cats should be mandatory wherever rabies is endemic in wildlife. The association with bats, already discussed, suggests that bat-to-cat transmission, although rare, is possible. It is recognized that cats, especially those in rural areas, roam freely and thus could be exposed if rabies exists in wildlife. Under these circumstances, it is quite possible that the cat could be exposed without the knowledge of its owner and eventually transmit the disease.

Inactivated virus and modified live-virus (MLV) vaccines providing solid immunity for cats for at least one year have long been available, and some vaccines are now effective for three years. All but one of the MLV vaccines have now been withdrawn for use in cats because of occasional instances in which they have caused vaccine-induced rabies. Some practitioners advocate that, for maximum safety, cats be vaccinated only with inactivated virus vaccine (e.g., Erlewein, 1981). Vaccination may be started at three months of age. A cat vaccinated between 3 and 12 months should be revaccinated one year later. The National Association of State Public Health Veterinarians, Inc., publishes and updates yearly a Compendium of Animal Rabies Vaccines. The Compendium provides manufacturers' names and recommendations for the administration of all vaccines licensed for use in the United States as of January 1 of each year. These recommendations, together with the package leaflet supplied with the vaccine, provide the necessary information for vaccination programs.

In countries where vaccines of nervous tissue origin may still be in use, the veterinarian should inform the owner of the occasional occurrence of postvaccinal damage to the nervous system.

## Requirements for Travel

In regard to international transfer of pets, the WHO suggests that countries free of rabies either prohibit importation of dogs and cats or quarantine them for six months. Where quarantine is impractical or rabies already exists, a cat should be vaccinated at least one month before but within one year of departure for another country. A certificate signed by an appropriate veterinary authority should accompany the cat stating the country of origin and the countries visited during the previous year, together with dates. Details should also be given as to the type of vaccine used, manufacturer's lot number, and dose.

Within the United States, many states require that a cat being brought into the state be accompanied by a certificate of rabies vaccination. It is important that owners retain a certificate of a cat's annual or triennial vaccination, for in the event that the cat bites a person or animal the date of the last vaccination determines the course of action to be followed.

## Handling of Specimens

It is essential that material submitted for diagnosis be handled properly. If a cat dies, the head must be sent promptly to a laboratory qualified to do rabies diagnosis. (Most laboratories refuse whole carcasses except those of small animals, such as a bat.) The head is severed far enough back on the neck so that the salivary glands are undamaged and may be examined if necessary.

If it is not possible to hand-deliver the specimen, it should be packed so as to assure its prompt and safe delivery to the laboratory.

The head (or, as in the case of a small animal, the whole body) should be wrapped in several layers of newspaper or paper towels, securely enclosed in a heavy plastic bag, and placed with protective packing and at least two cans of prefrozen "cooler" in a styrofoam or metal container. This, in turn, is placed in an outer corrugated carton labelled "Rabies Specimen—Perishable. Keep Away from Heat."

The postal service accepts only brains that have been removed from the head. This procedure is hazardous for the prosector, so it is best to ship a head by some other form of public transportation. Health departments often provide shipping containers and instructions. It is essential that the stated mandated procedures be followed. Freezing from the use of dry ice, decomposition, and preservation in glycerine or formalin cause delays in processing the tissues or may interfere with the DFA test. Shipping specimens by postal service should be discouraged owing to the possibility of delay or loss and possible deterioration. Where public carriers are utilized one must ascertain delivery time and notify the laboratory by telephone to expect the specimen.

## Human Exposure

Obviously, if a human is exposed by a suspect cat, the attending physician should determine the course to be followed. Immediate treatment with serum (Human Rabies Immune Globulin) and vaccine (Human Diploid Cell) provides the best regimen for protection. However, owing to the availability of fast, accurate diagnostic methods, many physicians choose to withhold treatment until laboratory results are available. In this case, it is essential that the specimen reach the laboratory quickly.

Proper management of a rabies suspect is a serious responsibility, for the lives of humans and other animals may be at stake. When a rabies suspect is under veterinary care, public health officials should be notified immediately. Although the owner may deny that human exposure occurred, this should be verified by the public health authorities.

## REFERENCES


Blenden DC: Rabies in the domestic cat. Vet Med 56 (1961) 339–341.

Blenden DC: Immunofluorescence examination of skin biopsy specimens for rabies diagnosis and the evaluation of biting animals (Abstr). J Am Vet Med Assoc 175 (1979) 618.

Bolin FM: The domestic cat and the rabies problem. Proc North Dakota Acad Sci 6 (July 1952) 11–16.

Constantine DG: Bat rabies in the southwestern United States. Public Health Rep 82 (1967) 867–888.

Cushing ER: Personal communication to J Holzworth, 1960.

Dean DJ, Abelseth MK: The fluorescent antibody test. *In* Kaplan MM, Koprowski H (eds): Laboratory Techniques in Rabies, 3rd ed. WHO Monograph, Unisante, Geneva, 1973, 73–84.

Debbie JG, Trimarchi CV: Pantropism of rabies virus in free-ranging rabid red fox *Vulpes fulva*. J Wildlife Dis 6 (1970) 500–506.

Erlewein DL: Post-vaccinal rabies in a cat. Feline Pract 11 (2) (1981) 16–17, 19–21.

Gardner JJ, Bauer SP, Moore GL, Stewart SJ, Bell JF, Murphy FA: Chronic rabies infection in the cat (Abstr). J Neuropathol Exp Neurol 37 (1978) 615.

Lewis A: Personal communication to J Holzworth, 1965.

Mitchell FE, Monlux WS: Diagnosis and incidence of rabies in a selected group of domestic cats. Am J Vet Res 23 (1962) 435–442.

Morbidity and Mortality Weekly Report (USPHS) 13 (32) Aug 15, 1964, 273–275.

Morbidity and Mortality Weekly Report (US DHEW CDC) 29 (23) June 13, 1980, 265–280.

Murphy FA, Bauer SP, Harrison AK, Winn WC Jr: Comparative pathogenesis of rabies and rabies-like viruses. Viral infection and transit from inoculation site to the central nervous system. Lab Invest 28 (1973) 361–376.

Murphy FA, Bell JF, Bauer SP, Gardner JJ, Moore GJ, Harrison AK, Coe JE: Experimental chronic rabies in the cat. Lab Invest 43 (1980) 231–241.

Ott RL: Viral diseases. *In* Catcott EJ (ed): Feline Medicine and Surgery, 2nd ed. Santa Barbara, American Veterinary Publications Inc, 1975.

Perl DP, Bell JF, Moore GJ, Stewart SJ: Chronic recrudescent rabies in a cat. Proc Soc Exp Biol Med 155 (1977) 540–548.

Price ER, Blenden DC, Logue JT: Rabies in Missouri 1950–1960. Mo Med 58 (1961) 460–466.

Remlinger P, Bailly J: La vaccination du chat contre la rage. Presse Méd 42 (1934) 907–908.

Rudd RR, Trimarchi CV, Abelseth MK: Tissue culture technique for routine isolation of street strain rabies virus. J Clin Microbiol 12 (1980) 590–593.

Scatterday JE, Schneider NJ, Jennings WL, Lewis AL: Sporadic animal rabies in Florida. Public Health Rep 75 (1960) 945–953.

Schieler W: Beitrag zur Klinik der Tollwut des Hundes und der Katze. Tierärztl Umsch 14 (1959) 370–372.

Szlachta HL, Habel RE: Inclusions resembling Negri bodies in the brains of nonrabid cats. Cornell Vet 43 (1953) 207–212.

Trimarchi CV, Abelseth MK, Rudd RJ: Aggressive behavior in rabid big brown bats (*Eptesicus fuscus*). Rabies Information Exchange 1 (1979) 34–35.

Vaughn JB: Cat rabies. *In* Baer GM (ed): The Natural History of Rabies, Vol 2. New York, Academic Press, 1975, 139–154.

Vaughn JB, Gerhardt P, Paterson JCS: Excretion of street rabies virus in saliva of cats. J Am Med Assoc 184 (1963) 705–708.

World Health Organization: WHO Expert Committee on Rabies, Sixth Report, WHO, Geneva, 1973, 1–55.

# PSEUDORABIES (AUJESZKY'S DISEASE, MAD ITCH, INFECTIOUS BULBAR PARALYSIS)

DONALD P. GUSTAFSON

Pseudorabies, caused by *Herpesvirus suis*, is a widely distributed neurologic disease of many animal species. First described in Hungary in cattle, dogs, and cats (Aujeszky, 1902), it occurs in all continents except Australia. There is strong evidence that the disease has been present in North America since the early nineteenth century (Hanson, 1954). The reservoir for pseudorabies virus (PrV) is the domestic pig, the most resistant but most often affected of the susceptible species (Gustafson, 1981). After recovery from disease, pigs may remain latently infected, and, under undefined circumstances, viral replication resumes without recurring disease but with release of virus into the environment. Thus cats living on swine farms are much more likely to become infected and develop disease than those having no contact with swine. Early signs of pseudorabies in swine are often difficult to distinguish for diagnostic purposes; concurrent fatal neurologic disease in cats and dogs strongly suggests that the disease in the pigs is pseudorabies.

Herpesviruses characteristically have very limited host ranges. In contrast, PrV infection may occur naturally in nearly all mammals with the notable exception of tailless nonhuman primates and humans. Avian species are susceptible, but natural infections have not been proven. Thus there is a broad spectrum of potentially PrV-infected animal tissues that cats might eat with resulting fatal infection. It had been accepted that rats were important to the spread of PrV among swine and constituted a reservoir for the virus (Shope, 1935), until others in more definitive efforts found that infected rats invariably get sick, go into their burrows, and die. Furthermore, those rats that remain do not develop antibodies and are fully susceptible to the virus (Ulbrich, 1969; McFerran and Dow, 1970; Maes et al., 1979). Rats are not an important source of PrV for swine or cats. All available reports indicate that cats become infected by ingesting the virus; none have shown that lateral transmission among cats or other animals has occurred.

## Etiology

Pseudorabies virus, a prototype herpesvirus, contains a single molecule of double-stranded DNA in an icosahedral capsid containing 162 capsomeres covered by an envelope composed of glycoprotein and lipid, acquired by passage of the capsid through virally modified areas of the nuclear membrane of infected cells. The enveloped form is the complete infectious virion. The capsid and the nucleic acid are not infectious together or separately. The core of the virus measures 75 nm in diameter, the nucleocapsid 105 nm, and the virion about 180 nm. The infective cycle, from attachment of the virus to the end of virus production and lysis of the cell, requires 15 to 19 hours. The replicative cycle of the virus also begins with attachment to the cell but ends with the first release of mature virions from the cell six to nine hours later. The morphologic and biochemical particulars have been studied in considerable detail (Ben-Porat and Kaplan, 1973; Watson, 1973).

The envelope of the virion contains important structural lipids, and consequently the virus can be inactivated by lipid solvents such as chloroform and ethyl ether (Kaplan and Vatter, 1959). The virus is also sensitive, because of effects on the envelope, to enzymes such as trypsin (Kaplan, 1969). Fluorocarbon effects on the envelope have also been found to inactivate PrV (Ivanicŏvá, 1961). Chemicals that disrupt the whole virion include detergents, urea, and dithiothreitol (Kaplan, 1969; Gainer et al., 1971). Common disinfectants (0.5 per cent NaOH, 5 per cent phenol, and 0.5 per cent formaldehyde) have been suggested (Ott, 1975). We have found that common household solutions of chlorine are very effective for decontaminating surfaces and instruments. Roizman (1969) summarized much data on the topic.

Pseudorabies virus may be inactivated by heat; at 44 C (111.2 F) in cell culture fluids 28 per cent of infectivity remained after five hours. The terminal portion of the survival curve declined at $2 \times 10^{-1}$ per hour (Kaplan and Vatter, 1959). However, it is possible to stabilize herpesviruses against heat inactivation by a number of cationic agents such as 1 M $NaSO_4$ and $Na_2HPO_4$ (Wallis and Melnick, 1965). Although the inactivation curve appears to follow first-order kinetics (Scott et al., 1961), it has been suggested that a second element of the degradation curve is due to clumping of virus or that more than one step is required for heat inactivation (Kaplan, 1969). Conversely, PrV can be stored for 15 years without significant loss of titer at −70 C (−94 F) in cell culture fluids containing 10 per cent bovine serum or skim milk.

## Pathogenesis

After oral exposure, primary virus replication takes place in the epithelium of the tonsils and the pharyngeal mucosa. Virus has been isolated from the turbinate mucosa 24 hours after exposure (Hagemoser et al., 1980). It invades the vagus (X), trigeminal (V), and glossopharyngeal (IX) nerves and travels in the epineurial lymph centripetally to the ganglia of these cranial nerves and into the brainstem, cerebellum, and cerebrum. Virus may be found in the cervical spinal cord as early as 24 hours after exposure and in the thoracic cord from 72 hours (Hagemoser et al., 1980). As crucial nerve cell aggregations become progressively involved and are destroyed, neural functions are increasingly impaired until death occurs (Sabó et al., 1968; Hagemoser et al., 1980).

Non-neural tissues also yielding virus included retropharyngeal lymph nodes, salivary glands, lung, mesenteric lymph nodes, and adrenal glands. Virus was not obtained from other organs, the intestinal tract, or its contents (Hagemoser et al., 1980). Efforts to transmit the infection to other cats with blood failed (Horvath and Papp, 1967). These observations in cats partially parallel the findings made in swine (Gustafson and Mitchell, 1970) that viremia is at least of low titer and intermittent. It may be that virus-induced necrosis of the highly vascular tonsils permits virus to enter the blood intermittently as the lesions develop and resolve.

Investigation of the pathophysiology of pruritus (Saiko, 1960a,b) suggested that itching is caused by changes in the balance of acetylcholine and cholinesterase in the skin. These changes disrupt the afferent nerve system involving receptor and motor nerve elements. Cholinergic processes in the CNS are depressed by the virus and toxic materials due to its presence, so that functional capacity to analyze is diminished and esthetic sensitivity is therefore altered.

## Clinical Features

Early descriptions of the disease in cats were provided largely by European investigators (Schmiedhoffer, 1910; Remlinger and Bailly, 1933; Ercegovac et al., 1958; Ercegovac and Ciric, 1963). These reports documented the association of the disease in urban cats with the consumption of infected pig viscera and also described significant differences in the clinical signs present in some cases.

The course and manifestations of the disease have some common aspects in most mammals: anorexia, excessive salivation, depression, muscular tremors, opisthotonos, convulsions, and coma ending in death. The disease progresses rapidly and is of short duration in most species, usually lasting four to seven days.

Many veterinarians believe that cats suffering from pseudorabies always have an intense pruritus, usually involving the head. Actually, its occurrence in cats, and in most other species as well, depends on a break in the skin or the mucosa of a body opening, which allows the virus to establish local infection and invade neural pathways to the central nervous system (CNS). Although pruritus is considered typical, a study of 58 naturally infected cats found that only 58.7 per cent had pruritus (Horvath and Papp, 1967), which is a less consistent clinical feature of the disease in cats than in dogs. Experimental infections have not resulted in pruritus (Sabó et al., 1968; Vandeputte and Pensaert, 1979; Hagemoser et al., 1980).

In experimental infections signs commonly appear about 40 to 48 hours after oral exposure, beginning with decreased activity. This is followed by inappetence, discomfort marked by agitation, and drooling of saliva because of difficulty in swallowing. The fur about the face becomes matted with saliva and tears. Salivation increases with time and may be accompanied by vomiting. Mewing is almost constant and often of low timbre. Temperature is nearly normal during the disease. As the affected cat becomes increasingly depressed (Fig. 7–61), it emits deep, low-pitched growling sounds (Hagemoser, 1979). Eventually the severely affected cat is unable to maintain balance and lies on one side. Convulsions precede the terminal coma.

In naturally occurring disease in cats, anisocoria occurs in less than 10 per cent of cases. It may be associated with unilateral pruritus of the head. Spasms of facial muscles and paralysis of an eyelid or the lower lip may occur. A light touch may cause erection of the hair, especially of the lumbar area and tail (Remlinger and Bailly, 1933). Breathing becomes labored late in the disease with a pulse of 130 to 140 per minute (Horvath and Papp, 1967). Reduced food and water intake results

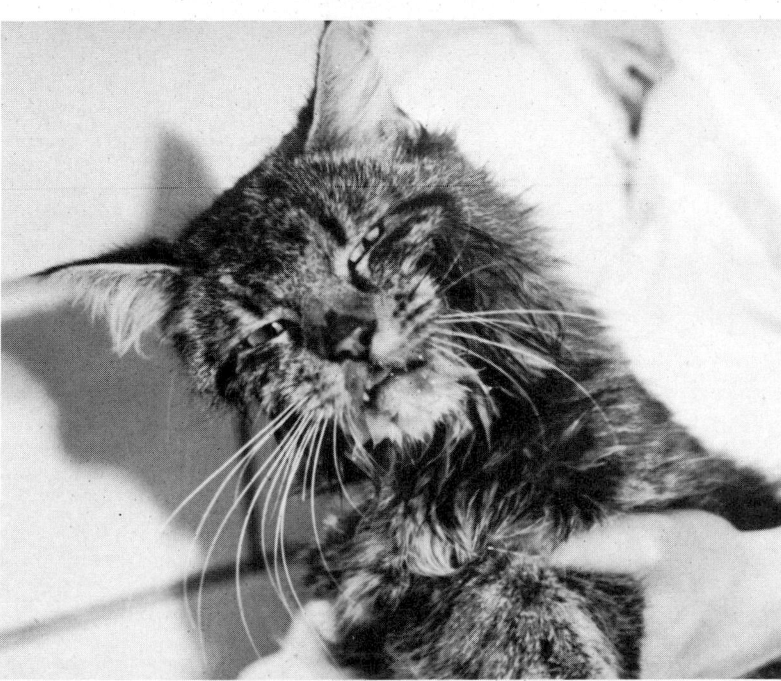

**Figure 7–61** Cat, 70 hours after eating pseudorabies virus–contaminated food. Note fur matted with saliva and depressed attitude.

in dehydration and hemoconcentration. However, qualitative erythrocyte and leukocyte cell counts remain in the normal range. Urine may be expressed from a distended urinary bladder when a cat is lifted. Erection of the penis is frequent in male cats, and the abdomen may be slightly distended owing to intestinal gas (Horvath and Papp, 1967). Experimental infections (Ercegovac et al., 1958) have revealed that leukocytosis occurs during the incubation period and continues. Similarly, sugar levels increase in the CSF, blood, and urine as the disease progresses.

A less common course in cats is one in which deep depression develops swiftly. They stop eating, salivate excessively, and become weak as apparently painful efforts to swallow are made. The head is held low and may be canted to one side, and the tail is flailed from side to side. Other signs are muted or absent, and death follows in a day or so. Infected cats have not been found to be aggressive toward objects or living things during the illness.

The duration of the disease from experimental infection to death varies somewhat. The prodromal period usually lasts 40 to 48 hours with termination after five to seven days. Less often cats may live for as long as nine days after exposure (Hagemoser, 1979). In natural infection the duration of clinical disease is usually from 24 to 36 hours.

## Pathologic Features

### Gross Lesions

Gross lesions of pseudorabies in all species are meager, and none are considered diagnostic. Some cats dying of pseudorabies did not have gross lesions (Sabó et al., 1968; Hagemoser et al., 1980). The most common observable change is reddened meninges, a constant finding in swine but also seen in many cats.

### Microscopic Lesions

Histopathologic changes are generally confined to the oro- or nasopharynx, tonsils, and CNS, but, as reported by Hagemoser and coworkers (1980), there is often an inflammatory response in the interstitial tissue of the lungs (30/33 cats). Usual lesions in the CNS are neuronal death, neuronophagia, lymphocytic perivascular cuffing, and focal and diffuse gliosis in the nucleus of the tractus solitarius, trigeminal ganglion, and vagus nerve. In affected trigeminal ganglia, eosinophilic intranuclear inclusions may be found in rare cases, such as reported by Dow and McFerran (1963) and by Sabó and others (1968), as contrasted with none among 33 experimental infections reported by Hagemoser and associates (1980). The lesions are not bilaterally symmetric (Dow and McFerran, 1963; Sabó et al., 1968; Knösel, 1968; Hagemoser et al., 1980) and are not so common or severe in the thoracic spinal cord, cerebellum, or cerebrum.

## Diagnosis

Pseudorabies may be diagnosed by a variety of methods (in increasing order of specificity): characteristic signs and autopsy findings, animal inoculation, immunofluorescence, and virus isolation with identification.

### Signs and Autopsy Findings

The signs of illness often strongly suggest pseudorabies, but depression, anorexia, and salivation alone are insufficient evidence for diagnosis. However, even in these cats, the normal temperature, normal hematologic values, and accelerated pulse are suggestive of pseudorabies. The meager autopsy findings and the presence of meningitis and tonsillitis are supportive, as is histopathologic evidence of nonsuppurative meningitis and encephalitis. The medulla oblongata and pons are the tissues of choice for microscopic evaluation.

### Animal Inoculation

Inoculation of rabbits with extracts of suspect tissue has been used in diagnosis since the earliest studies of pseudorabies (Aujeszky, 1902). Half a ml of material (nasal swab fluid, 10 per cent wt/vol tonsil extract or brainstem extract) is inoculated subcutaneously in the flank of a rabbit. With samples positive for virus, rabbits are expected to develop pruritus at the site of inoculation and die in three to five days. Intracranial inoculations of two-week-old mice with 0.03 ml of test fluid are also useful for diagnosis. If mice become infected with PrV, depression, excessive grooming activity, and pruritus characterize the syndrome, which ends in death usually within four to seven days after inoculation.

### Virus Isolation

A specific diagnosis can be made by virus isolation in cell cultures and identification of the virus by FA procedures or virus neutralization with specific anti-pseudorabies serum. The tissues of choice for virus isolation from infected cats are tonsil, brainstem, nasal mucosa, and subcutis from scratched areas.

Blood samples taken from cats for viral isolation procedures should not contain heparin. Heparin, a sulfated polyanion, blocks the absorption of virus to host cells. Some diagnostic efforts have failed because of ignorance of this reaction.

Occasionally one is presented with serum from a cat believed to have recovered from PrV infection for virus neutralization testing for determination of its immunologic status. The envelope of the virus contains four immunologically important glycoprotein antigens. Serologically strong cross-neutralization relationships with other herpesviruses do not exist. Thus the test is specific.

### Fluorescent Antibody Tests

Fluorescent antibody (FA) tests are very reliable and specific diagnostic procedures. The direct test is especially useful for fresh, virus-rich tissues such as tonsil or medulla oblongata (Kanitz et al., 1974). The indirect FA technique, more specific than the direct (Leslie et al., 1977), is used when the tissues to be tested are from animals that have been dead for some time before collection or when the tissues are likely to have small concentrations of viral antigens. The FA tests are often more sensitive than virus isolation, because they demonstrate the presence of antigen even when virus isolation procedures may be negative owing to absence of viable virus or because it is present in such low concentration as to be below threshold values for cell cultures.

## Prognosis

Once a cat develops the disease the outcome is invariably death. Serologic evidence of recovery has not been reported.

## Treatment

A variety of regimens were used without success for the treatment of affected cats (Horvath and Papp, 1967) in both prodromal and late stages of the disease. Heterologous antisera, antibiotics (streptomycin, chloramphenicol, oxytetracycline), cortisone preparations, and a "cholinesterase paralyzer" were found to be ineffective.

Two reports of success in treatment of affected cats are available (Breter, 1962, 1970). The diagnosis of the disease in both was made on the basis of symptoms and the fact that raw pig meat was part of the diet, but the reports were without verification through serologic or virus identification data. Consequently such an exciting prospect is severely diminished.

## Prevention

Both inactivated and attenuated vaccines are available in the United States for swine. They have not been approved by the U.S.D.A. for use in cats, but approval has not been sought. The most appropriate immunizing agent for cats would be an inactivated one. Antiserum from swine is available in a few research organizations but has not been shown to be effective in prevention (Horvath and Papp, 1967). However, one might extrapolate from experience in swine and suggest that a minimum of 5 ml and an additional ml per pound of body weight over 5 lb to a maximum of 12 ml given intraperitoneally to asymptomatic cats may be beneficial in prevention.

The best means of prevention is to avoid the disease. Cats should not be fed raw pork. Throat, lung, brain, and spinal cord should be especially avoided, as these tissues generally have the highest concentration of PrV. When the disease is present in swine or other livestock, cats should be removed from the virus-contaminated environment and kept away for at least three weeks after the last signs of disease have disappeared from swine or for one week after other livestock have died and the carcasses have been removed.

## Interspecies Transmission and Public Health Significance

Cats are highly susceptible to pseudorabies virus and as such are essentially a terminal host. They may be infected experimentally by several routes but acquire the virus in nature almost exclusively by eating or drinking virus-contaminated material. Cats in urban areas became infected after eating food that included uncooked porcine offal (Ercegovac et al., 1958; Haagsma and Rondhuis, 1967). Cats that drank milk contaminated with PrV became infected also (Sabó et al., 1968). However, pseudorabies is more common on farms where they may be exposed to infected swine, cattle, or sheep. Infected cats apparently are not a source of infection for swine, as attempts to transmit the disease to swine from cats were unsuccessful, although the cats had demonstrable virus in nasal and oral secretions (Vandeputte and Pensaert, 1979). The presence of virus in urine of affected cats has not been demonstrated, nor has lateral transmission among cats been reported, although the presence of virus in their skin lesions and oral secretions makes this theoretically possible.

Humans are evidently very resistant to infection. After 21 years of manipulation of the virus in several species of animal in our laboratory, no evidence has been obtained of illness or immunologic response in anyone of some 25 persons associated with the activity. None of 16 swine producers who worked with swine during episodes of pseudorabies developed antibodies against the virus. Investigators in Europe have not found any evidence of disease or seroconversion among hundreds of people in occupational association with PrV (Ercegovac and Ciric, 1963; Jentzsch and Apostoloff, 1970). However, in another survey (Khristov et al., 1972), two positive serums were found among 66 samples obtained from people, but the neutralization indices were very low (4.0 and 1.0) in these two samples. The hazard for humans, if any exists, is extremely low by the usual routes of exposure such as laboratory accidents resulting in puncture wounds, animal bites, aerosols containing PrV, and handling contaminated utensils. Nevertheless, the virus should be handled with reasonable care, since some species of nonhuman primates have been shown susceptible to infection (Hurst, 1936).

## REFERENCES


Aujeszky A: Ueber eine neue Infektionskrankheit bei Haustieren. Zentralbl Bakteriol Abt I Orig 32 (1902) 353–357.

Ben-Porat T, Kaplan AS: Replication—biochemical aspects. *In* Kaplan AS (ed): The Herpesviruses. New York, Academic Press, 1973, 163–200.

Breter M: Behandlung von Aujeszkyschen Krankheit bei Siamesischen Katzen mit Omnamycin. Blauen Hefte Tierarzt. 3/4 (1962) 36–37.

Breter M: Diagnose und Therapie der Aujeszkyschen Krankheit bei Katzen. Kleintierpraxis 15 (1970) 83–84.

Dow C, McFerran JB: Aujeszky's disease in the dog and cat. Vet Rec 75 (1963) 1099–1102.

Ercegovac D, Ciric V: [Aujeszky's disease in cats and investigation on transmissibility to man.] Vet Glasn 17 (1963) 499–501. Abstr Vet Bull 34 (1964) 1287.

Ercegovac D, Trumic P, Lapcevic E, Ciric AV: [An outbreak of Aujeszky's disease among cats.] Acta Vet Belgrade 8(3) (1958) 25–34. Abstr Vet Bull 30 (1960) 3890.

Gainer JH, Long J Jr, Hill P, Capps WI: Inactivation of the pseudorabies virus by dithiothreitol. Virology 45 (1971) 91–100.

Gustafson DP: Pseudorabies in dogs and cats. *In* Kirk RW (ed): Current Veterinary Therapy VII. Philadelphia, W B Saunders Company, 1980, 1296–1298.

Gustafson DP: Pseudorabies. *In* Leman AD, Glock RD, Mengeling WL, Penny RCH, School E, Straw B (eds): Diseases of Swine, 5th ed. Ames, Iowa State University Press, 1981, 209–223.

Gustafson DP, Mitchell MV: Pseudorabies infections in pregnant swine. Symposium Proceedings 70-0, Effect of disease and stress on reproductive efficiency in swine, University of Nebraska, College of Agriculture, November 1970.

Haagsma J, Rondhuis PR: [Aujeszky's disease in cats.] Tijdschr Diergeneeskd 92 (1967) 1245–1249. Abstr Vet Bull 38 (1968) 952.

Hagemoser WA: Studies on the pathogenesis of pseudorabies in domestic cats following oral exposure. Iowa State University, PhD Thesis, 1979.

Hagemoser WA, Kluge JP, Hill HT: Studies on the pathogenesis of pseudorabies in domestic cats following oral inoculation. Can J Comp Med 44 (1980) 192–202.

Hanson RP: The history of pseudorabies in the United States. J Am Vet Med Assoc 124 (1954) 259–261.

Horvath Z, Papp L: Clinical manifestations of Aujeszky's disease in the cat. Acta Vet Acad Sci Hung 17 (1967) 49–54. Abstr Vet Bull 37 (1967) 4188.

Hurst EW: Studies on pseudorabies (infectious bulbar paralysis, mad itch) III. The disease in the rhesus monkey, Macaca mulatta. J. Exp Med 63 (1936) 449–463.

Ivanicŏvá S: Inactivation of Aujeszky disease (pseudorabies) virus by fluorocarbon. Acta Virol 5 (1961) 328.

Jentzsch KD, Apostoloff E: [Susceptibility of man to Aujeszky's disease virus. 4. Serological findings in occupationally exposed persons.] Z Ges Hyg 16 (1970)692–696. Abstr Vet Bull 41 (1971) 3322.

Kanitz CL, Hand RB, McCrocklin SM: Pseudorabies in Indiana: current status, laboratory confirmation and epizootiologic consideration. Proc US Anim Health Assoc 78 (1974) 346–358.

Kaplan AS: Herpes simplex and pseudorabies viruses. Virology Monographs 5. New York, Springer-Verlag, Inc, 1969, 1–115.

Kaplan AS, Vatter AE: A comparison of herpes simplex and pseudorabies viruses. Virology 7 (1959) 394–407.

Khristov S, Karadzhov I, Genev Kh: [Tests for inapparent infection with Aujeszky's disease virus in animals and human beings.] Veterinarnomeditsinski Nauki (Sofia) 9(1) (1972) 19–25. Abstr Vet Bull 42 (1972) 5200.

Knösel H: Zur Histopathologie der Aujeszky'schen Krankheit bei Hund und Katze. Zentralbl Veterinärmed B 15 (1968) 592–598.

Leslie PF, Anson MA, McAdaragh JP: The virologic diagnosis of pseudorabies in terminal host species. Proc Am Assoc Vet Lab Diag 20 (1977) 11–16.

Maes RK, Kanitz CL, Gustafson DP: Pseudorabies virus infections in wild and laboratory rats. Am J Vet Res 40 (1979) 393–396.

McFerran JB, Dow C: Experimental Aujeszky's disease (pseudorabies) in rats. Br Vet J 126 (1970) 173–179.

Ott RL: Viral diseases. *In* Catcott EJ (ed): Feline Medicine and Surgery, 2nd ed. Santa Barbara, American Veterinary Publications Inc, 1975, 17–62.

Remlinger P, Bailly J: La maladie d'Aujeszky expérimentale du chat. CR Soc Biol Paris 112 (1933) 1274–1276.

Roizman B: The herpesviruses—a biochemical definition of the group. Curr Top Microbiol Immunol 49 (1969) 1–79.

Sabó A, Rajcáni J, Raus J, Karelová E: [Investigations on the pathogenesis of Aujeszky's disease of cats.] Arch Ges Virusforsch 25 (1968) 288–298.

Saiko AA: Pathogenesis of the itching associated with Aujeszky's disease. Part I: Role of the histidine decarboxylase and the histamine-histaminase systems. Sborn Trud Kharkov Vet Inst 24 (1960a) 186–192.

Saiko AA: Pathogenesis of the itching associated with Aujeszky's disease. Part II: Role of the acetylcholine-cholinesterase system in the skin. Sborn Trud Kharkov Vet Inst 24 (1960b) 193–202.

Schmiedhoffer J: Beiträge zur Pathologie der infektiösen Bulbarparalyse (Aujeszkyschen Krankheit). Z Infektionskr Haustiere 8 (1910) 383–405.

Scott TFMcN, McLeod DL, Tokumaru T: A biologic comparison of two strains of Herpesvirus hominis. J Immunol 86 (1961) 1–12.

Shope RE: Experiments on the epidemiology of pseudorabies. J Exp Med 62 (1935) 85–117.

Ulbrich F: Zur Rolle der Ratten in der Epizootiologie der Aujeszkyschen Krankheit. Arch Exp Veterinärmed (Leipzig) 24 (1969) 297–301.

Vandeputte J, Pensaert M: [Virus excretion in cats with Aujeszky's disease (pseudorabies) and their role in virus spread to piglets.] Vlaams Diergeneeskd Tijdschr 48 (1979) 140–150.

Wallis C, Melnick JL: Thermostabilization and thermosensitization of herpesvirus. J Bacteriol 90 (1965) 1632–1637.

Watson DH: Replication of the viruses—morphological aspects. *In* Kaplan AS (ed): The Herpesviruses. New York, Academic Press, 1973, 133–161.

# ONCOGENIC VIRUSES OF CATS: THE FELINE LEUKEMIA AND SARCOMA VIRUSES

WILLIAM D. HARDY, JR.

At the turn of this century, Rous (1911) showed for the first time that a virus caused tumors in chickens. Since then both DNA- and RNA- containing viruses have been shown to cause cancer in various species (Hardy, 1980b; Hardy and McClelland, 1981). Cancer viruses induce tumors by inserting their DNA (DNA viruses) or a DNA copy of their viral RNA (RNA viruses) into the host cell's chromosomes. Although this mechanism is not fully understood, the inserted DNA then induces neoplastic transformation either directly or by altering existing cellular genes, which in turn cause transformation.

RNA tumor virses are classified in the subfamily Oncovirinae (Oncoviruses) within the family Retroviridae (Retroviruses) because they contain the reverse transcrip-

**Table 7–8 Origin of Feline Oncoviruses**

| VIRUS | DISEASES INDUCED | SPECIES FROM WHICH VIRUS ORIGINATED | METHOD BY WHICH VIRUS IS TRANSMITTED |
|---|---|---|---|
| RD-114 | None | Baboon (Old World monkey) | Genetically |
| FeLV | Lymphosarcoma<br>Myeloproliferative malignancies<br>Non-neoplastic diseases | Rat ancestor | Contagiously |
| FeSV | Multicentric fibrosarcomas | FeLV recombination with cat cellular genes | Contagiously as FeLV<br>May be generated only de novo |

tase enzyme (Retro), which copies their single-stranded RNA genome into a complementary single strand of DNA (Fenner, 1976). Both endogenous and exogenous oncoviruses exist. Endogenous oncoviruses are present in the chromosomes of all uninfected cells of a host species as a DNA copy (provirus) and are transmitted from the parents to the offspring as genes in the egg or sperm. Exogenous oncoviruses, on the other hand, are not present in the chromosomes of uninfected cells and are transmitted contagiously among individuals of the host species (Benveniste and Todaro, 1974). During millions of years of evolution, some non-disease-producing endogenous oncoviruses escaped from the control of their hosts and infected other species, in which they become disease-producing (oncogenic) viruses (Todaro, 1980). The pet cat has three groups of retroviruses (Table 7–8): (1) the non–disease producing endogenous RD-114 virus, (2) the leukemogenic feline leukemia viruses (FeLVs), which also cause non-neoplastic diseases, and (3) the sarcoma-inducing feline sarcoma viruses (FeSVs), (Besmer, 1983; Hardy, 1980a, 1981a).

## RD-114 VIRUS

The RD-114 virus is an endogenous retrovirus of pet cats (Fischinger et al., 1973). DNA copies of the RD-114 viral RNA are present in all cat cells. Since the RD-114 viral gene is repressed or kept under control by the cat cell's genome, the virus does not replicate in cats or cause any known disease. In addition, pet cats do not produce antibodies to the RD-114 virus under natural conditions (Mandel et al., 1979). However, low levels of one RD-114 viral protein and of RD-114 RNA are found in stimulated normal lymphoid cells and in FeLV-positive and -negative lymphosarcoma cells (Niman et al., 1977). There is evidence that the RD-114 virus originated as an endogenous baboon virus, which, as a result of contagious trans-species transmission, infected the ancestors of the present-day cat and has since been transmitted genetically as an endogenous oncovirus in cats (Benveniste and Todaro, 1973).

## FELINE LEUKEMIA VIRUS

FeLV originated as an endogenous retrovirus of the ancestral rat. In some unknown manner, about 1 million to 10 million years ago the endogenous rat virus was activated and infected an ancestor of the present-day pet cat and became an exogenous cat virus that has been transmitted contagiously among cats ever since (Benveniste et al., 1975). FeLV was discovered in Scotland in 1964 in a cat with lymphosarcoma (LSA) that had lived with several other cats that had developed LSA (Jarrett et al., 1964).

### CHARACTERIZATION OF THE VIRUS

The FeLV genome consists of a single strand of RNA, containing the *gag* (group specific antigen) and the *env* (envelope) genes, which code for the structural viral proteins. In addition, the FeLV genome contains a gene known as the *pol* (polymerase) gene, which codes for the RNA-dependent DNA polymerase (reverse transcriptase) enzyme. This enzyme copies the viral RNA into complementary DNA, which is then inserted into the chromosomes (provirus) of the infected cell (Hardy, 1980b). The viral genome does not possess an oncogene (cancer-inducing gene) and thus induces leukemia by an indirect, as yet unknown, mechanism.

#### Structure of FeLV

FeLV is spherical and contains its RNA in the viral core (Fig. 7–62*A*) (Bolognesi et al., 1978). The envelope of FeLV contains protein spikes supporting knobs composed of glycoproteins. Antibodies against the envelope glycoproteins are neutralizing antibodies that inactivate the virus (Hardy, 1974).

#### Replication of FeLV

The first step in the replication cycle of FeLV is cell attachment and penetration. FeLV, therefore, can infect only cells with surface receptors that are complementary to proteins on its envelope (Jarrett et al., 1973a). After penetrating the cell membrane, the RNA is released, together with the reverse transcriptase that synthesizes a DNA copy (provirus) of the viral RNA (Baltimore, 1970). The provirus becomes incorporated into the DNA of the host's chromosomes at multiple sites and then may code for the synthesis of viral messenger RNA. Once messenger RNA is produced, the synthesis of viral proteins can take place, and new viral particles can then be assembled from the various viral components (RNA and proteins) in the cell cytoplasm. The final stage of the replicative cycle is budding, when the virus particle buds from the surface of the infected cell, where it acquires its surface (viral) envelope (Fig. 7–62 *B, C, D*).

### PATHOGENESIS OF FeLV INFECTION

The major vehicle of FeLV transmission is saliva, which can contain as many as 2 million infectious FeLV particles per ml (Francis et al., 1977; Gardner et al., 1971b; Hardy

*Text continued on page 250*

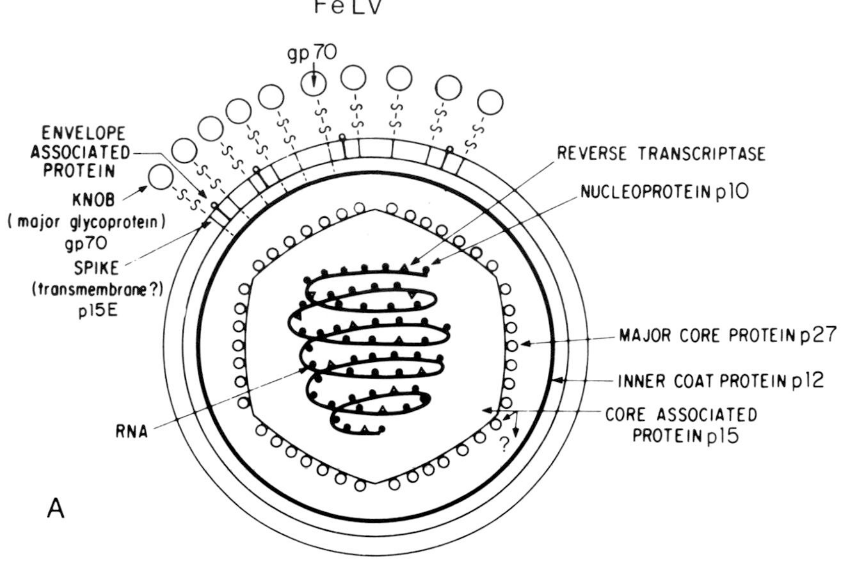


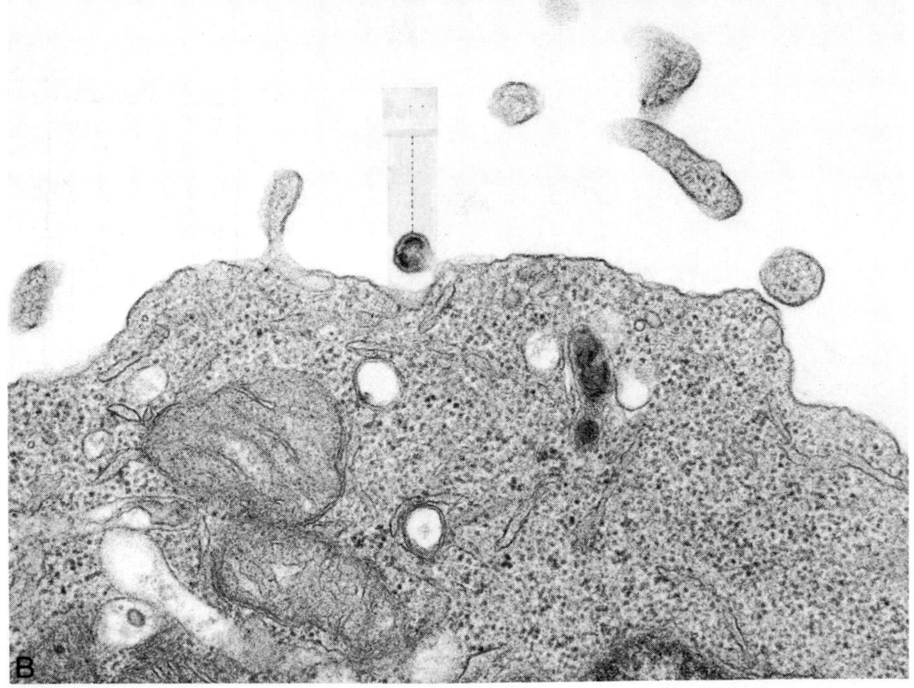


**Figure 7–62** The structure and replication of the feline leukemia virus. *A*, Diagram of the feline leukemia virus showing the relationship of the viral antigens, viral RNA, and the reverse transcriptase to the structure of the virus. *B*, A feline leukemia virus particle budding from the cell membrane of an infected cell. 71,500 ×.

*Illustration continued on opposite page*

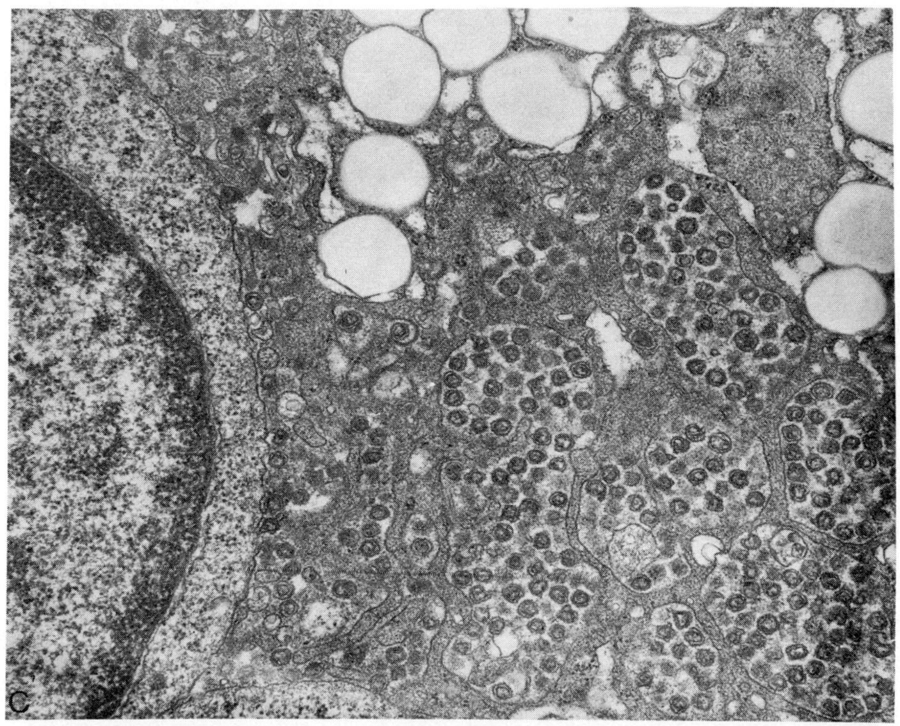


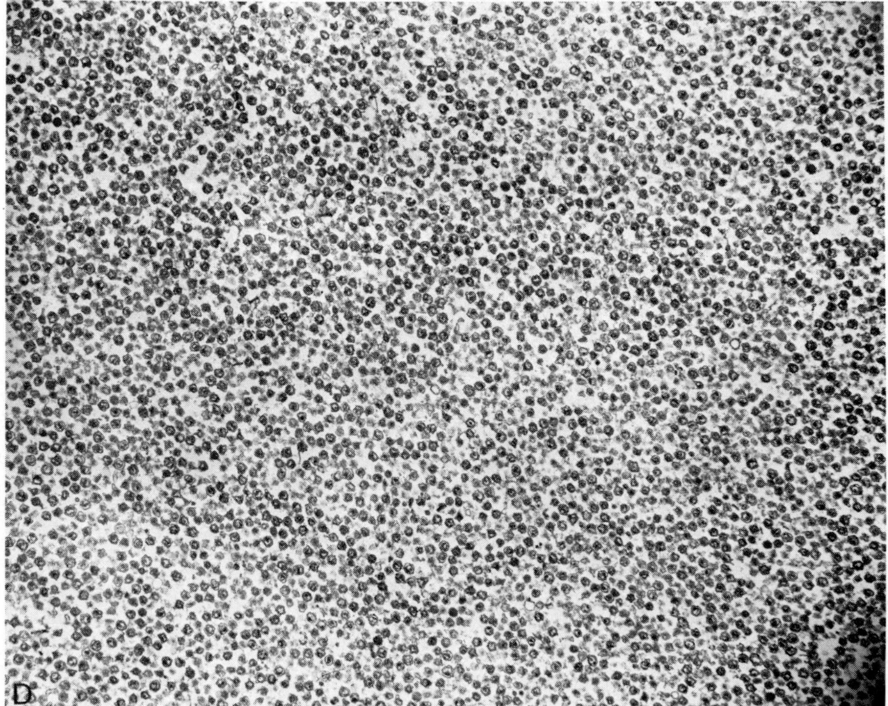


**Figure 7–62** *Continued C*, Spherical feline leukemia virus particles in the cytoplasmic vacuoles of a degenerated leukocyte. 42,000 ×. *D*, Purified feline leukemia virus particles for use in an FeLV subunit vaccine. 24,500 ×. (*A* adapted from Bolognesi DP, Montelaro RC, Frank H, et al.: Science 199 [1978] 183–186. Used by permission. Copyright 1978 by the American Association for the Advancement of Science.)

et al., 1969, 1973a). FeLV-infected cats transmit the virus to the ocular, oral, and nasal membranes of uninfected cats by licking or biting. The virus then penetrates these membranes and infects lymphocytes in the local lymph nodes of the head and neck (Rojko et al., 1979). Bite wounds that penetrate the skin are also important portals of infection. Most FeLV-infected pet cats reject FeLV at this early stage and become immune. FeLV requires rapidly dividing cells, such as lymphoid and bone marrow cells, to replicate, and in those cats that do not become immune the virus spreads from the lymphoid tissues of the head to the rapidly dividing cells of the bone marrow. There FeLV replicates to high titers and enters the blood both in infected leukocytes and as free virus in the plasma. At this stage the cat is viremic and is likely to remain persistently viremic for the rest of its life (Hardy, 1980b). Within a few weeks FeLV spreads to, and replicates in, the salivary gland and respiratory epithelial cells, whence it is shed into the environment. FeLV replicates in the cat's lymphocytes, neutrophils, megakaryocytes, and erythroblasts, in cells of the pancreas and intestinal mucosal cells, and in respiratory and urinary bladder cells and can cause proliferative or degenerative diseases in many of these cells (Hardy, 1980a). The period of FeLV disease development is highly variable, but 83 per cent of FeLV-infected healthy pet cats die within three and a half years (McClelland et al., 1980).

## IMMUNOLOGY OF FeLV INFECTION

### FeLV Antigens

There are three categories of FeLV antigens: (1) envelope antigens, (2) internal antigens, and (3) the reverse transcriptase. The FeLV envelope consists of two antigens, which are coded for by the *env* gene. The major envelope antigen is a glycoprotein with a molecular weight of 70,000 daltons (gp70), and the minor component is a 15,000 dalton protein (p15E) (see Fig. 7–62*B*). Based on the gp70 antigenic determinants, FeLV is classified into three subgroups—FeLV-A, -B, and -C (Jarrett et al., 1973a; Sarma and Log, 1973). FeLV-A is found in all cats naturally infected with the virus either alone (50 per cent of cats), in combination with FeLV-B (49 per cent), or with FeLV-B and FeLV-C (1 per cent) (Hardy et al., 1976a; Jarrett et al., 1978). Some cats can produce antibody to the gp70 antigen of the FeLV envelope and thus can neutralize or reject FeLV and become immune to infection (Hardy et al., 1976a; Russell and Jarrett, 1978; Sarma et al., 1974). Although all three subgroups of FeLV can replicate in cat cells, each subgroup differs in its ability to replicate in cells from species other than the cat (Hardy, 1980b; Jarrett et al., 1973a; Sarma et al., 1975). FeLV-A has the most limited host range and can only replicate in dog and some human cells, whereas FeLV-B has the widest host range and can replicate in dog, mink, hamster, pig, cattle, monkey, and human cells. Intermediate in host range between FeLV-A and FeLV-B, FeLV-C replicates in dog, mink, guinea pig, and human cells.

There are four internal FeLV structural antigens, all of which are coded for by the *gag* gene of FeLV. These antigens are proteins of 27,000, 15,000, 12,000, and 10,000 dalton molecular weight (p27, p15, p12, p10) and constitute the internal structural elements of the virus. The internal FeLV antigens are produced in great excess in the cytoplasm of infected cat cells and can be detected in infected leukocytes by the immunofluorescent antibody (IFA) test or as free soluble antigens in the plasma by the enzyme-linked immunosorbent assay (ELISA) test to determine the FeLV status of infected cats (Hardy et al., 1973b, 1974a; Kahn et al., 1980). Some cats can produce antibodies against the FeLV internal antigens—antibodies which are not beneficial to the cat in any way but which, in persistently infected cats, can cause the formation of immune complexes that may result in immunosuppression, immunologic damage, and immune-complex glomerulonephritis (Charman et al., 1976; Cotter et al., 1975; Snyder et al., 1982; Stephenson et al., 1977a; Weksler et al., 1975).

The RNA-dependent DNA polymerase (reverse transcriptase), which copies the viral RNA into complementary DNA, is also antigenic. Some FeLV-exposed cats produce antibodies to this enzyme, although no known beneficial or detrimental effect has been attributed to them (Jacquemin et al., 1978a).

### Feline Oncornavirus–Associated Cell Membrane Antigen (FOCMA)

FOCMA is an FeLV- and FeSV-induced tumor-specific antigen found on the cell membranes of FeLV-induced lymphosarcoma, erythroleukemia, and myelogenous leukemia cells and FeSV-induced fibrosarcoma cells (Fig. 7–63) (Essex et al., 1975, 1977b; Hardy et al., 1977). FOCMA is present on both FeLV-positive and -negative lymphosarcoma cells but is not found on normal cells, even those infected with FeLV-A and -B. Thus, although FOCMA is induced by FeLV and FeSV, it is not a structural component of FeLV-A or -B. Recently FOCMA has been shown to be a molecule composed of FeLV-C gp70 and another antigenic component (Snyder et al., 1983, Vedbrat et al., 1983). Thus FOCMA appears

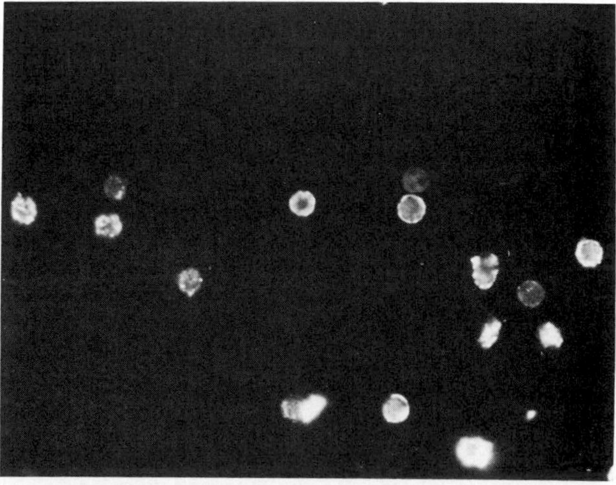

**Figure 7–63** The viable cell membrane immunofluorescent antibody test for FOCMA. The discrete punctate cell membrane fluorescence indicates the presence of FOCMA on these feline lymphosarcoma cells. FOCMA is an FeLV- and FeSV-induced tumor-specific antigen.

to be a recombinant molecule probably generated through recombination of FeLV-A and endogenous FeLV-C gp70-related sequences (genes) found in uninfected normal cat DNA (Snyder et al., 1983).

Those cats that produce antibody against FOCMA are protected from developing FeLV- and FeSV-induced tumors but not FeLV-induced non-neoplastic diseases (Essex et al., 1971a, b, 1975; Hardy et al., 1976a). Thus the presently available FOCMA antibody test for cats exposed to FeLV is of little or no use for practitioners in determining prognosis, since infected cats with high FOCMA antibody titers are still likely to develop the FeLV-induced non-neoplastic diseases (Hardy, 1980a, b).

## IMMUNE RESPONSE TO FeLV

Exposure to FeLV does not necessarily result in infection and subsequent disease. The consequences of exposure depend on the extent and period of exposure. Forty-two per cent of cats exposed to FeLV become immune to the virus, whereas 28 per cent become persistently infected (Hardy, 1980b). The remaining 30 per cent are neither immune nor infected, probably because of insufficient exposure. The immunologic response of cats to FeLV exposure determines their fate. We have found that healthy cats can be placed in one of six classes depending on their FeLV status and FOCMA and FeLV-neutralizing antibody titers (Hardy et al., 1976a): class 1, FeLV-uninfected cats susceptible to both FeLV infection and LSA; class 2, uninfected cats susceptible to FeLV infection but resistant to LSA; class 3, uninfected cats resistant to FeLV infection but susceptible to LSA; class 4, uninfected cats resistant to both FeLV and LSA; class 5, infected cats susceptible to LSA; and class 6, infected cats resistant to LSA development (FeLV-FeSV carrier cats). Pet cats belonging to each of these six classes have been found in household environments (Table 7–9).

Most unexposed cats or stray cats whose exposure to FeLV is unknown are class 1 cats; that is, they are not immune to FeLV or LSA and are thus susceptible to FeLV. In contrast, 42 per cent of exposed cats are class 4 cats; that is, they are immune to FeLV and LSA, whereas the remaining 58 per cent of exposed cats either are infected with the virus or are susceptible to FeLV infection (Hardy, 1980b). It should be remembered that this classification is dynamic; for example, a class 1 cat may become a class 3 cat, or a class 5 cat may become a class 6 cat, depending on the immune response of the cat.

Paradoxically, an effective immune response to FeLV does not always protect against the development of LSA. This is because the FeLV RNA genome can become integrated into the genome of the infected cells of an FeLV-exposed cat before the cat develops an effective immune response and rejects the virus infection. The integrated FeLV genome may transform the host cell at any time after integration, even without the production of infectious FeLV. Thus some transiently infected cats, even those that produce neutralizing antibody, can develop an FeLV-negative LSA (Francis et al., 1979a; Hardy et al., 1980). We have found that 30 per cent of cats with LSA are FeLV-negative (Hardy et al., 1978), and in an epidemiologic study we have shown that FeLV causes FeLV-negative LSA (Hardy et al., 1980). In this study, a total of 1612 FeLV-exposed and -unexposed pet cats from all regions of the United States were observed for the development of LSA. A cat was classified as unexposed if it was FeLV-negative and if, according to the owner, it had not lived with any FeLV–test-positive cat or with any cat that had an FeLV disease. The FeLV status of all cats was determined by the IFA test for FeLV antigens. Of the 1612 cats, 1074 living in 96 households had never been exposed to FeLV and were not infected with FeLV. None of these unexposed control cats developed LSA during the study. In contrast, the remaining 538 pet cats living in 23 households had been exposed to an FeLV-infected cat. Of these exposed cats, 389 were found to be uninfected and 149 were found to be FeLV-infected. During the period of the study 41 of the cats developed LSA: 30 of the 149 FeLV-infected cats developed FeLV-positive LSAs and 11 of the 389 FeLV-uninfected cats developed FeLV-negative LSAs. The difference in the occurrence of FeLV-negative LSA between the unexposed control cats and the exposed cats was highly significant by the $X^2$ test ($p < 0.0001$). Our finding that the development of FeLV-negative LSAs in pet cats is associated with exposure to FeLV suggested that FeLV is the etiologic agent for all feline LSAs. Recently FeLV has been reactivated from the bone marrow cells, but not the LSA cells, of four of five cats with FeLV-negative LSAs (Rojko et al., 1982). This finding is direct evidence for the etiologic role of FeLV in FeLV-negative LSAs.

## IMMUNOSUPPRESSION

As mentioned earlier, an immune response to FeLV may be detrimental to the health of a cat. The continuous production of viral antigens in persistently infected cats

**Table 7–9 Immune Classes of Healthy Cats***

| CLASS | HISTORY OF EXPOSURE | FeLV STATUS | PROTECTIVE ANTIBODY TO: FeLV | FOCMA | SUSCEPTIBILITY OR RESISTANCE TO: FeLV Infection | Lymphosarcoma Development |
|---|---|---|---|---|---|---|
| 1 | Unexposed | − | − | − | Susceptible | Susceptible |
| 2 | Exposed | − | − | + | Susceptible | Resistant |
| 3 | Exposed | − | + | − | Resistant | Susceptible |
| 4 | Exposed | − | + | + | Resistant | Resistant |
| 5 | Exposed | + | − | − | Infected | Very susceptible |
| 6 | Exposed | + | − | + | Infected | Resistant |

*Adapted from Hardy WD Jr: The virology, immunology, and epidemiology of the feline leukemia virus. *In* Hardy WD Jr, Essex M, McClelland AJ (eds): Feline Leukemia Virus. New York, Elsevier/North Holland Inc, 1980b, 33–78.

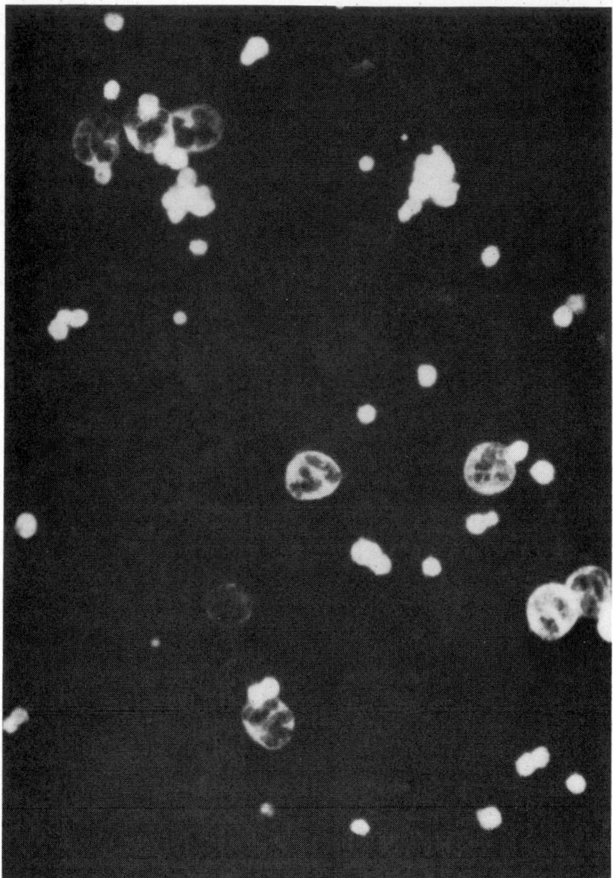

**Figure 7–64** The immunofluorescent antibody test for feline leukemia virus. A positive FeLV IFA test. Punctate granular cytoplasmic fluorescence represents FeLV antigens in the peripheral blood leukocytes and platelets and indicates that the cat is viremic and is shedding FeLV in the saliva. In a negative test no cytoplasmic fluorescence is present in the leukocytes.

and a continuing immune response to these antigens can result in the formation of immune complexes. These complexes can be detrimental in two ways. First, they are immunosuppressive and may therefore enable tumors to develop or allow other feline diseases to occur (Hardy, 1980a,b). Second, immune complexes are nephrotoxic and may damage the basement membrane of the renal glomeruli, causing inflammatory degeneration. We have found circulating FeLV-IgG immune complexes in six cats and fixed immune complexes in the glomeruli of three other cats (Hardy, 1980a,b, 1982). There is also preliminary clinical evidence that a relationship exists between FeLV infection and glomerulonephritis (Cotter et al., 1975; Hardy, 1980a; Jakowski et al., 1980).

Another way in which FeLV may be immunosuppressive is by exfoliating p15E from the viral envelope. Under experimental conditions p15E can abrogate feline lymphocyte functions and may be able to induce in persistently infected cats a lowered immune responsiveness that increases susceptibility to other infectious agents (Mathes et al., 1978).

**Table 7–10 Comparison of the FeLV Immunofluorescent Antibody (IFA) Test and Virus Isolation (VI) with ELISA-Positive Tests**

| REFERENCES | ELISA-POSITIVE CATS | IFA- OR VI-POSITIVE CATS | PER CENT AGREEMENT |
|---|---|---|---|
| Jarrett et al., 1982a, b | 682 | 465 | 68 |
| Hardy, 1981a | 405 | 135 | 33 |
| Lutz et al., 1980 | 210 | 146 | 69 |
| Kahn et al., 1980 | 43 | 38 | 88 |
| Gwalter, 1981 | 28 | 21 | 75 |
| Lazarowicz (Gwalter, 1981) | 48 | 30 | 38 |
| | 1416 | 835 | 58.9 |

## FeLV Testing Methods

In 1973 we developed a specific, sensitive, and rapid immunofluorescent antibody (IFA) test for the detection of FeLV antigens in leukocytes of the peripheral blood (Fig. 7–64) (Hardy et al., 1973b, 1974a). A positive IFA test indicates FeLV infection but is not diagnostic for LSA or any other disease. Positive IFA tests correlate (97.5 per cent) with recovery of FeLV in tissue culture and indicate that the positive cat is shedding FeLV (Hardy et al., 1973a; Hardy, 1980b). Ninety-seven per cent of IFA test–positive cats remain viremic for life and never reject the virus. However, 3 per cent of the IFA test–positive cats reject the virus and become test-negative and immune to FeLV.

An in-hospital enzyme-linked immunosorbent assay (ELISA) test for FeLV is also available (Kahn et al., 1980). Several comparative studies have evaluated the ELISA and IFA FeLV tests (Tables 7–10 and 7–11) (Gwalter, 1981; Hardy, 1981a; Jarrett et al., 1982a,b; Kahn et al., 1980; Lutz et al., 1980). In one study of 553 pet cats it was found that only 48 per cent of the ELISA and IFA test results were concordant (Hardy, 1981a). Only 33 per cent of the ELISA-positive cats were IFA test–positive, whereas 87 per cent of ELISA-negative cats were also IFA-negative. The most complete study of FeLV testing methods was done by Jarrett and coworkers (1982a,b). They compared virus isolation and results of IFA and ELISA tests in 1148 pet cats and found that

**Table 7–11 Comparison of the FeLV Immunofluorescent Antibody (IFA) Test and Virus Isolation (VI) with ELISA-Negative Tests**

| REFERENCES | ELISA-NEGATIVE CATS | IFA- OR VI-NEGATIVE CATS | PER CENT AGREEMENT |
|---|---|---|---|
| Jarrett et al., 1982a, b | 466 | 466 | 100 |
| Hardy, 1981a | 148 | 129 | 87 |
| Lutz et al., 1980 | 416 | 408 | 98 |
| Kahn et al., 1980 | 52 | 50 | 96 |
| Gwalter, 1981 | 93 | 93 | 100 |
| Lazarowicz (Gwalter, 1981) | 0 | 0 | 0 |
| | 1175 | 1053 | 89.6 |

**Table 7–12 Occurrence of FeLV in Healthy Pet and Stray Cats***

| ENVIRONMENT AND FeLV EXPOSURE HISTORY | PER CENT OF CATS PERSISTENTLY INFECTED WITH FeLV |
|---|---|
| Single-cat households (no known exposure to FeLV) | 0.7 |
| Multiple-cat households | |
| Exposed to FeLV | 28 |
| Not exposed to FeLV | 0 |
| Stray cats (unknown FeLV exposure) | 0.9 |

*Determined by the IFA test for FeLV.

FeLV could be isolated from only 68 per cent of the ELISA test-positive cats, whereas FeLV could be isolated from 98.5 per cent of the IFA test–positive cats. They concluded that the IFA test should be used for routine testing of cats for persistent FeLV infection and that ELISA test–positive cats should be tested by IFA before isolation or euthanasia is recommended.

## Epidemiology of FeLV in Pet Cats

Persistently FeLV-viremic cats are not common in the general healthy pet cat population. Viremic cats are found mainly in exposure environments such as multiple-cat households and catteries where other cats with FeLV or LSA have lived (Essex et al., 1977a; Gardner et al., 1977; Hardy et al., 1973a; Jarrett et al., 1973b). Approximately 30 per cent of healthy exposed cats are persistently infected, whereas only 1 to 2 per cent of cats with no known exposure are infected with FeLV (Table 7–12) (Hardy, 1980b). Stray cats are not often persistently viremic, and less than 1 per cent have been found to be infected (Hardy, 1980b). Surprisingly, we have found that 12 per cent of 852 hospital blood donor or potential blood donor cats were infected with FeLV (Hardy, 1980b). Accordingly, I suggest that donor cats be used only if they test FeLV-negative and that they be isolated from all other cats, especially hospitalized sick cats. Prolonged, intimate, cat-to-cat contact is needed for efficient transmission of FeLV, since the virus dies quickly outside the cat's body.

The prognosis for healthy FeLV-infected pet cats is not good. We have observed 96 infected cats for a period of three and one half years and found that 83 per cent died during this time, whereas only 16 per cent of the 513 uninfected cats living in the same households died during the same observation period (McClelland et al., 1980).

As mentioned earlier, only 28 per cent of FeLV-exposed cats become persistently infected, whereas the largest group, 42 per cent, become immune to FeLV, and 30 per cent remain neither immune nor infected (Table 7–13) (Hardy, 1980b).

**Table 7–13 Consequences of FeLV Exposure of Pet Cats**

| CONSEQUENCE OF FeLV EXPOSURE | FeLV STATUS | PER CENT OF EXPOSED PET CATS |
|---|---|---|
| Persistently FeLV-infected | Infected | 28 |
| Susceptible to FeLV (not infected with FeLV by contact) | Not infected | 30 |
| Immune to FeLV | Not infected | 42 |

## FeLV Control Measures

### Inactivation of FeLV

Although FeLV is transmitted contagiously, prolonged and intimate cat-to-cat contact, as when cats groom or bite one another, is required for infection to occur. Communal use of litter pans may pose some risk. FeLV is not transmitted by aerosol under natural household conditions. The virus dies quickly outside the cat's body, inactivation occurring in two to three minutes when the virus dries on environmental surfaces. Ordinary hospital or household detergents quickly kill FeLV by lysing its lipid envelope (Francis et al., 1979b; Hardy, 1980b). Thus veterinary hospital waiting rooms, examination rooms, and cages are not likely places where uninfected cats will become infected. However, infection is likely in multiple-cat households, and uninfected cats can be protected only by implementation of an FeLV test and removal program and by vaccination.

### FeLV Immunofluorescent Antibody Test and Removal Program

There is no effective treatment for the diseases caused by FeLV, but the spread of the virus and its related diseases in the natural environment can be prevented by the use of the FeLV immunofluorescent test and removal program (Hardy et al., 1974a, 1976b). In this program, all cats in a household are tested for FeLV and any infected cats are removed, by isolation or euthanasia, from contact with uninfected healthy cats. At present I do not recommend euthanasia or isolation of cats testing positive by hospital-performed ELISA tests until the discrepancies in the test results obtained by the ELISA test and the IFA test have been resolved (see section on disposition of FeLV-infected cats). After the infected cats have been removed, the uninfected cats are quarantined and retested three months later. If all the uninfected cats are still uninfected in the second test, the cats in the household are considered FeLV-free. If any of the initially uninfected cats are found to be infected in the second FeLV test, they are removed and a third test is done on the remaining cats three months after the second test. When all the cats in a household are negative in two consecutive FeLV tests done three months apart, the cats in the household are considered to be FeLV-free.

### Vaccination Against FeLV

From our knowledge of the natural immune response to FeLV, it was clear that pet cats can produce serum-neutralizing (SN) antibody and can reject FeLV, and it was therefore thought to be possible to develop a vaccine against the virus. There are three possible types of FeLV vaccines: (1) a live FeLV vaccine, (2) a killed FeLV vaccine, and (3) an FeLV envelope subunit vaccine that is free of the viral RNA. Several research groups have produced an effective live-FeLV vaccine that induces high (protective) titers of SN antibody (Hardy, 1980b; Jarrett et al., 1974; Pedersen et al., 1979). However, the ability of the FeLV RNA to integrate into the DNA of the host cell and possibly to produce FeLV-negative LSA indicates that a live-FeLV vaccine, no matter how effective, is too dangerous to the vaccinated cat to be feasible (Hardy, 1980b). Similarly, the ability of FeLV to grow in the cells of other species, including human cells, suggests that a live-virus vaccine could not be made commercially available because of the possible public health risk.

Killed-FeLV vaccines have not been found to be effective in two studies (Hardy, 1980b; Olsen et al., 1977). In fact, in one experiment, kittens immunized with a combination of killed FeLV and LSA cells were more susceptible to FeLV infection than those kittens given only the LSA cell vaccine (Olsen et al., 1977).

Subunit viral vaccines, which are composed of only the outer immunogenic envelope of the virus, have been used successfully against influenza and herpesviruses. In one study, cats immunized with the purified gp70 of FeLV were found not to produce protective titers of SN antibody (Salerno et al., 1978). However, in another study, LSA cell tissue culture fluid, free of infectious FeLV and containing FeLV gp70, gave 80 per cent protection to vaccinated cats (Mathes et al., 1980; Olsen et al., 1976, 1980). A tissue culture–origin FeLV vaccine, free of live FeLV, has been developed and became available to practitioners in 1985. It is not without side effects, and some questions have been raised as to its immunogenicity and effectiveness (Pedersen and Ott, 1985). The most effective and safe FeLV vaccine will most likely be produced through genetic engineering techniques where the FeLV envelope gp70 molecule will be made by bacteria or yeasts in which the cloned FeLV *env* genes have been inserted. Such a method should produce a plentiful and inexpensive supply of viral protein for vaccination.

## Public Health Significance

### Growth of FeLV in Human Cells

Until 1969 there was little concern about the ability of FeLV to induce disease in humans. However, in 1969 it was found that natural field isolates of FeLV could infect and grow in human tissue culture cells (Jarrett et al., 1969). It is now known that only the FeLV-B and -C subgroups (which occur in 50 per cent of infected pet cats) can infect human cells but that FeLV-A, the subgroup found in every infected pet cat either alone or in combination with FeLV-B or -C, or both, is unable to infect most, but not all, human cells (Jarrett et al., 1973a, 1978; Sarma and Log, 1973). More concern about the public health risks of FeLV arose when it was discovered that the virus is spread contagiously among cats (Hardy et al., 1973a; Jarrett et al., 1973b) and that the virus is shed by infected cats (Francis et al., 1977; Gardner et al., 1971b; Hardy et al., 1969). As a result of these observations and because FeLV is probably the only known animal tumor virus to which humans are frequently and intimately exposed (Essex and Hardy, 1977; Hardy et al., 1973a, 1974b; Levy, 1974), there is now greater concern about the public health aspects of FeLV.

### FeLV Oncogenicity in Other Species

FeLV can infect and replicate in dog cells in culture, and when the virus is inoculated into newborn puppies it can induce both FeLV-positive and -negative LSAs (Rickard et al., 1973). Similarly, since FeLV can infect and replicate and induce FOCMA in human lymphoid cultured cells, it seems possible that FeLV may be able to induce lymphoid tumors in humans (Azocar and Essex, 1979; Essex et al., 1972). Of course experimental challenge of humans with FeLV can never be done, and therefore the possible oncogenicity of FeLV in humans can only be determined by long-term observation of people living with infected cats, especially children who were exposed while in utero or early in life (Hardy, 1980b). Even if FeLV has not yet been shown to infect humans, there still seems, to this author, to be a possibility that the virus might be able to infect people in the future, especially as cats become more numerous as pets. It should be noted that several retroviruses have already been transmitted from one species to another under natural conditions. For example, FeLV originated in rats and spread to cats, the gibbon ape leukemia virus originated in Asian mice and spread to Asian apes, and the bovine leukemia virus originated from an as yet unidentified species and spread to cattle (Benveniste and Todaro, 1974; Todaro, 1980).

### Human Epidemiologic Studies

Because FeLV was shown to grow in human cells, because FeLV induced LSA in puppies, and because cats live in such close association with people, epidemiologic studies of veterinarians, children, and adults exposed to cats were done to determine if FeLV was associated with any human disease. Because of their occupation, veterinarians are considered the highest FeLV exposure group. Five mortality studies of a total of 23,149 United States veterinarians have been reported. Two of these studies involving 876 veterinarians concluded that there was no excess occurrence of any type of cancer in veterinarians compared with the general population (Botts et al., 1966; Schnurrenberger et al., 1977). In another study, an excess occurrence of skin melanoma was found among 1722 veterinarians (Fasal et al., 1966). Two recent studies of large numbers of veterinarians revealed an excess occurrence of lymphoid tumors. The first study, by Gutensohn and coworkers (1980), indicated an 80 per cent excess occurrence of lymphoid cancers in 19,000 veterinarians over 45 years of age. The second study, by Blair and Hayes (1980), found an excess occurrence of leukemia and Hodgkin's disease in 1551 male veterinarians in clinical practice. These last two studies are significant because they involved a large number of veterinarians and were performed by medical epidemiologists. However, the authors were not able to find the cause for the apparent excess risk of lymphoid cancers among veterinarians, and FeLV could not be conclusively associated or excluded as a possible causative factor.

Children are, in general, more susceptible to infectious agents than adults, and two retrospective studies have been done of 328 leukemic children who were exposed to cats. In a study in England, exposure to cats was found twice as often among London children with lymphoid cancers as among children with other forms of cancer (Penrose, 1970). Similarly, a study in the United States of 300 children with leukemia and 831 control children found that the relative risk among leukemic children exposed to "sick" cats was more than double that of the control children (Bross and Gibson, 1970).

Three retrospective studies of more than 1965 adults exposed to cats have been done. Hanes and coworkers (1970) found no excess occurrence of cancer in 530 people exposed to cats, and Schneider (1970) found no excess occurrence of cancer in an unstated number of people exposed to 675 cats with various types of cancer. More specifically, no excess occurrence of cancer was found among 760 people exposed to 221 cats with LSA (Schneider, 1972); however, using the same methodology, Schneider (1970) was unable to detect the contagious spread of FeLV among cats.

## Seroepidemiologic Studies

Serologic and virologic tests are more definitive than epidemiologic methods for detecting exposure of humans to FeLV. Eight studies to determine if antibody to FeLV occurred in 4069 people have been done and have yielded conflicting results. Half the studies reported antibody to one or more FeLV antigens in 224 of 2089 people (10.7 per cent) (Caldwell et al., 1976; Fink et al., 1971; Jacquemin et al., 1978b; Olsen et al., 1975). One study found that 70 per cent of people with LSA had antibody to FeLV compared with only 6 per cent of healthy people (Olsen et al., 1975). Caldwell and colleagues (1976), working at the Communicable Disease Center, found that 69 per cent of exposed people had antibody to FeLV. Workers at the National Cancer Institute found antibody to the FeLV reverse transcriptase enzyme on the tumor cell membrane in eight of nine people with chronic myelogenous leukemia in blast crisis but not on normal leukocytes from 29 healthy people (Jacquemin et al., 1978b). In the four other studies, no antibody to FeLV was found in 1538 healthy people, in 631 people with cancer, in 209 people with non-neoplastic diseases, or in 662 healthy veterinarians (Hardy et al., 1976a; Krakower and Aaronson, 1978; Sarma et al., 1974; Schneider and Riggs, 1973).

Four studies have attempted to detect FeLV antigens in humans. In one, FeLV antigens were found in the glomeruli of two people with acute myelogenous leukemia (Sutherland and Mardiney, 1973). In another, FeLV-related antigens were found on the leukemic cell surfaces of 43 of 53 (81 per cent) patients with myeloid leukemias and on 35 of 36 (97 per cent) patients with lymphoid cancers but not on normal lymphocytes of 12 healthy people (Metzger et al., 1976). In contrast, in studies done in my laboratory, we did not find FeLV antigens in any of the 439 people we examined (Hardy et al., 1976a), and Krakower and Aaronson (1978) did not find FeLV antigens in any of the 1324 people they studied.

## Disposition of FeLV-Infected Cats

At present there is no direct evidence that FeLV has caused any disease in humans, but as described above, some epidemologic studies suggest that exposure to cats increases the risk of development of lymphoid cancers in humans. In addition, several research groups have found either antibody to FeLV or FeLV antigens in people exposed to cats with the virus. At present we cannot conclude that there is any danger to humans from FeLV nor can we be certain that there is absolutely no risk. What then should veterinarians recommend to owners of FeLV-infected cats? This is a very emotional and important question that veterinarians must answer for themselves after carefully considering all aspects of our present knowledge about the virus. The following recommendation is that of this author alone and does not represent the recommendation of his research institution or of the National Cancer Institute.

I recommend that all FeLV-infected pet cats, sick or healthy, be destroyed. If the owner is unwilling, then I recommend isolation of the cat in a cage in a separate room away from all other cats and away from children, pregnant women, and people with known chronic or immunosuppressive diseases (Hardy et al., 1974b). I must qualify my recommendation, however, according to the FeLV test performed. Since there are now numerous laboratories using the FeLV ELISA test and various IFA tests for FeLV and since some practitioners are also using the ELISA in-hospital FeLV test, I wish to stress that my recommendation that infected cats be destroyed is made only for those cats that test positive in the IFA test for FeLV. This qualification is based on the finding that many cats that test positive in the ELISA test test negative in the IFA test. We have demonstrated that an IFA test–positive cat is viremic and is shedding FeLV in the saliva, whereas similar correlary studies have shown that cats that test positive in the ELISA FeLV test, but negative in the IFA test, do not have FeLV in their blood nor are they shedding the virus in their saliva (Francis et al., 1977; Hardy et al., 1973a, 1976b; Jarrett et al., 1982a,b; Kahn et al., 1980). I am not suggesting that the ELISA test should not be done but simply that practitioners follow the recommendation of the laboratory to which they submit samples for FeLV testing or the recommendation made for the ELISA FeLV test regarding disposition of FeLV test–positive cats. The manufacturers of the ELISA in-hospital FeLV test do not recommend that ELISA test–positive cats be destroyed (Kahn et al., 1980).

My recommendation that IFA test–positive cats be destroyed is based on the following considerations: (1) FeLV is very contagious among cats; (2) FeLV-positive sick cats have short survival times; (3) although FeLV-infected healthy cats have a poor prognosis, some can live for years and continuously shed high amounts of virus in their saliva; (4) FeLV has already crossed species barriers since it originated in rats; (5) FeLV can induce LSA in another species—the dog; (6) FeLV can infect and grow in human cells; (7) pet cats live in intimate contact with people; (8) FeLV is classified as a moderate-risk virus by the National Cancer Institute and must be handled with proper precautions in research laboratories (Biol. Safety Man. 1976); (9) there is evidence that antibodies against FeLV and FeLV antigens are found in some people; (10) some studies have shown that there is an increased risk of developing lymphoid cancers in children exposed to cats and in veterinarians; and, finally, (11) the feline sarcoma virus, a highly oncogenic virus, originates in cats by the recombination of FeLV and cat cellular genes (see next section), and it is remotely possible that FeLV may be able to produce a human sarcoma virus in a similar manner under the appropriate conditions.

Practitioners must be able to present the known facts about FeLV in an accurate, calm, and rational manner to enable an owner to decide the fate of an infected cat. Making strong recommendations to destroy infected cats will unduly alarm the cat owner, but, on the other hand, veterinarians who suggest that infected cats are absolutely no danger to humans are not being objective in considering all that is presently known about FeLV.

## FELINE SARCOMA VIRUS

The first sarcoma virus was discovered in 1911 in a spindle-cell sarcoma of a chicken (Rous, 1911). It was not until the early 1960s that the first mammalian sarcoma virus was found. The first feline sarcoma virus (FeSV) was discovered in 1969 in a two-year-old female domestic shorthair pet cat with multiple subcutaneous fibrosarcomas (Snyder and Theilen, 1969). Shortly thereafter, two other FeSVs were isolated from young cats with multiple fibrosarcomas (Gardner et al., 1970; McDonough et al., 1971), and since then several more isolates of FeSVs have been obtained (Table 7–14) (Besmer et al., 1983a,b, 1986a,b; Hardy, 1980c; Hardy et al., 1986; Irgens et al., 1973; Snyder, 1971).

### Characterization of the Virus

There are two major types of retroviruses: (1) chronic leukemia viruses, and (2) acute transforming leukemia and sarcoma viruses (Shih and Scolnick, 1980). The chronic leukemia viruses, such as FeLV, replicate to high titers in cats, cause monoclonal leukemia or lymphosarcoma only after long latent periods, and are called "replication-competent" helper viruses. The acute transforming leukemia and sarcoma viruses possess transforming genes or oncogenes (*onc* genes), induce polyclonal tumors shortly after infection, and are recombinant viruses, generated by the insertion of a cellular gene (protooncogene) into the helper chronic leukemia virus genome. An FeSV is formed by the insertion of a cat cellular gene into the FeLV RNA genome (Frankel et al., 1979), and thus FeSVs can be generated in any cat that is infected with FeLV. FeSVs are retroviruses because they contain an RNA genome and are identical in morphology to FeLV (Hardy, 1980c).

There are presently approximately 26 *onc* genes known in acute transforming retroviruses of birds and mammals, seven of which occur in different isolates of FeSVs. The retroviral *onc* genes have normal cellular counterparts called protooncogenes. Normal cells have one gene copy of each protooncogene, and these genes have been conserved in evolution and exist in yeast, fruit flies, mammals, and humans (Stehelin et al., 1976). The *onc* genes (Table 7–14) are responsible for the transforming properties of FeSVs (Fig. 7–65) (Duesberg and Vogt, 1979). When the FeLV genome acquires an *onc* gene and becomes an FeSV, it loses part of the *gag* gene, most of the *env* gene, and usually all of the *pol* gene. Without these necessary genes FeSV cannot replicate, since it cannot copy its viral RNA into complementary DNA or produce the proteins necessary for its envelope. FeSV acquires its envelope at the membrane of the infected cell from the components produced by the helper FeLV that replicates in the FeSV-transformed cell and that is always present in excess in all pet cats infected with FeSV. With the FeLV envelope and the FeSV RNA genome, the FeSV is able to infect and transform cells but can only replicate if the same cells are concurrently infected with FeLV. As with FeLV-transformed cells, FeSV-transformed cells express FOCMA (Sherr et al., 1978; Sliski et al., 1977; Stephenson et al., 1977b). FeSVs can transform nonfeline cells, such as mink, rat, bovine, and human cultured cells, with or without any FeLV or FeSV production (Hardy, 1980c; Sherr et al., 1980; Sliski et al., 1977; Stephenson et al., 1977b). Similarly, FeSVs can cause sarcomas in dogs, rabbits, sheep, and monkeys that do not produce FeLV or FeSV (Hardy, 1980c).

At present there are 10 well-characterized FeSV isolates (Table 7–14) that have transduced seven different oncogens, *v-fes, v-fms, v-sis, v-abl, v-fgr, v-rasK*, and *v-kit*. The viral oncogenes are designated by a "*v*" followed by a three-letter gene name, whereas the cellular counterpart is designated "*c*" followed by the gene (Coffin et al., 1981).

The first FeSV isolate, the Snyder-Theilen (ST)-FeSV, and the second isolate, the Gardner-Arnstein (GA)-FeSV, possess the *fes* oncogene (Gardner et al., 1970; Snyder and Theilen, 1969). Recently my laboratory has isolated the Hardy-Zuckerman 1 (HZ1)-FeSV, which also possesses the *fes* oncogene (Hardy et al., 1982; Snyder et al., 1984a). In 1980 the *v-fps* oncogene of the Fujinami avian sarcoma virus was found to be the same gene (homologous) as the *v-fes* oncogenes of the FeSVs (Fujinami et al., 1914; Shibuya et al., 1980). This discovery demon-

**Table 7–14 Isolates of Feline Sarcoma Viruses from Pet Cats**

| FeSV ISOLATE | | v-onc | MULTIPLE VERSUS SOLITARY FIBROSARCOMA | BREED | AGE (YEARS) | SEX |
|---|---|---|---|---|---|---|
| Snyder-Theilen | ST-FeSV | fes | Multiple | DSH | 2 | Female |
| Gardner-Arnstein | GA-FeSV | fes | Multiple | Siamese | 5½ | Male |
| Hardy-Zuckerman 1 | HZ1-FeSV | fes | Multiple | DSH | 4 | Male |
| Susan McDonough | SM-FeSV | fms | Multiple | DSH | 1½ | Female |
| Hardy-Zuckerman 5 | HZ5-FeSV | fms | Multiple | DSH | 3 | Male |
| Parodi-Irgens | PI-FeSV | sis | Multiple | DSH | 1½ | Female |
| Gardner-Rasheed | GR-FeSV | fgr | Solitary | DSH | 8 | Male |
| Hardy-Zuckerman 2 | HZ2-FeSV | abl | Multiple | Siamese | 4 | Male |
| Noronha-Youngren | NY-FeSV | rasK | Multiple | Siamese | 3 | Male |
| Hardy-Zuckerman 4 | HZ4-FeSV | kit | Multiple | DSH | 7 | Male |

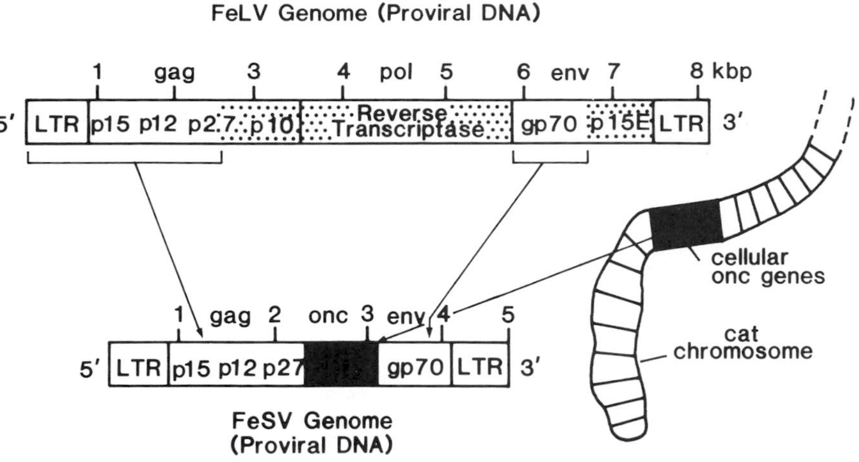


**Figure 7–65** Generation of the feline sarcoma virus. The feline sarcoma virus (FeSV) is generated by recombination of the feline leukemia virus (FeLV) genome (proviral DNA) with cat cellular genes designated cellular oncogenes (*onc*) or protooncogenes. The cellular *onc* is inserted into the FeLV genome, and part of the *gag* gene, most of the *env* gene, and all of the *pol* gene are lost in the recombinational event. Because of the loss of the viral genes, FeSVs require excess helper FeLVs in order to replicate. Adapted with permission from Hardy WD Jr, Essex M, McClelland AJ (eds): Feline Leukemia Virus. New York, Elsevier/North Holland, 1980.)

strates that acute transforming viruses originating de novo in different species are able to transduce the same gene and suggests that normal cells probably contain a limited number of protooncogenes (Besmer, 1983). The *fes* oncogene is the most prevalent acute transforming virus oncogene and is found in three FeSVs and five avian sarcoma viruses (Besmer, 1983). The Gardner-Arnstein FeSV, in addition to inducing fibrosarcomas, has induced melanomas when inoculated into the iris or intradermally (McCullough et al., 1972; Shadduck et al., 1981).

The Susan McDonough (SM)-FeSV and the Hardy-Zuckerman 5 (HZ5)-FeSV contain the unique *v-fms* oncogene (Besmer et al., 1986a; Hardy et al., 1986; McDonough et al., 1971). To date no other retrovirus from any other species has been found to possess the *v-fms* oncogene. The Hardy-Zuckerman 2 (HZ2)-FeSV was isolated from a Siamese cat with large multiple fibrosarcomas (Besmer et al., 1983a; Hardy et al., 1981). The HZ2-FeSV contains the *v-abl* oncogene, which is homologous to the *v-abl* of the Abelson murine leukemia virus (MuLV), the only mammalian leukemogenic retrovirus that possesses an oncogene (Abelson and Rabstein, 1970; Besmer et al., 1983a; Hardy et al., 1982). Since the *v-abl* in the Abelson MuLV induces leukemias in mice, it will be interesting to determine if the sarcomagenic HZ2-FeSV can also induce leukemias in cats.

The Parodi-Irgens (PI)-FeSV and the Noronha-Youngren-FeSV contain oncogenes that are homologous to the *v-sis* of the simian sarcoma virus and the *v-rasK* of the Kirsten murine sarcoma virus (Besmer et al., 1983b; Irgens et al., 1973; Youngren and Noronha, 1984). The protein product of the *sis* oncogene encodes a protein that is identical to the platelet-derived growth factor (PDGF), which stimulates fibroblast proliferation in wound healing (Doolittle et al., 1983; Robbins et al., 1983). Thus an excess production of PDGF by *v-sis*–transformed fibroblasts might lead to excessive proliferation of cells that have PDGF receptors and result in tumor formation.

The Gardner-Rasheed (GR)-FeSV and the Hardy-Zuckerman 4 (HZ4)-FeSV have unique oncogenes, *v-fgr* and *v-kit*, respectively, that have been found only in these viruses to date (Besmer et al., 1986b; Hardy et al., 1984b; Naharro et al., 1983; Rasheed et al., 1982).

## FeSV-Induced Tumors of Pet Cats

Fibrosarcomas account for between 6 and 12 per cent of all cat tumors (Hardy, 1980c, 1981b). FeSVs induce multiple fibrosarcomas of young cats (three years old or younger), whereas the more common solitary fibrosarcomas that occur in older cats (mean age of 10 years) are not caused by FeSVs (Hardy, 1981b). The FeSV-induced multiple fibrosarcomas are more anaplastic and more invasive and contain more mitotic figures and less collagen than the solitary non–FeSV-induced fibrosarcomas of old cats (Gardner et al., 1970; Hardy, 1980c; McDonough et al., 1971; Snyder and Theilen, 1969). It should be noted, however, that FeSV-induced fibrosarcomas occur very rarely in pet cats (Hardy, 1980c).

## Oncogenicity of FeSV in Other Species

Under experimental conditions, FeSV can induce fibrosarcomas and melanomas (a rare tumor of cats) in cats (Gardner et al., 1970; Hardy, 1980c; McCullough et al., 1972; McDonough et al., 1971; Snyder and Theilen, 1969). In addition, FeSV has been found to induce sarcomas in dogs (Gardner et al., 1971a; Theilen et al., 1970), rabbits (Theilen et al., 1970), sheep fetuses (Theilen, 1971), pigs (Pearson et al., 1973), and nonhuman primates (Deinhardt et al., 1970; Theilen et al., 1970; Wolfe et al., 1972). Many of the sarcomas induced in these nonfeline species do not contain detectable FeLV or FeSV (Hardy, 1980c). Tissue culture cells can be transformed by FeSV from various species including mouse, rat, mink, guinea pig, rabbit, cat, dog, cattle, tree shrew, and human (Hardy, 1980c).

The wide host range of FeSVs can be attributed to the fact that all FeSV isolates occur with excess FeLV-A and -B helper viruses (Sarma et al., 1971a,b, 1972). The FeLV-B subgroup can infect cells from many species, so that the FeSV genome contained within the FeLV-B envelope can infect and transform cells from many species (Jarrett et al., 1973a; Sarma et al., 1975). Since FeSV has such a wide host range, I regard it as a significant potential public health risk, although we are not sure if FeSV is spread contagiously or if each FeSV must be generated individually by FeLV in infected cats (Hardy, 1980c).

### Immunology of FeSV

The immunology of FeSV is essentially the same as that of FeLV. FeSV-transformed cells express FOCMA, and FOCMA antibody prevents the development of FeSV-induced fibrosarcomas (Essex et al., 1971a, 1977a; Essex and Snyder, 1973).

### FeSV Testing Methods

Since FeSV is always accompanied by excess FeLV, the tests for FeLV will detect FeSV-induced fibrosarcomas in cats.

### FeSV Control Measures

The same control measures recommended for FeLV apply to FeSV. An effective and safe FeLV vaccine will also protect cats from FeSV infection.

### Public Health Significance

The same concerns regarding the public health aspects of FeLV apply to FeSV. In addition, unlike FeLV, FeSV can induce tumors in many species, often without virus production, and can transform human cells in culture. Thus I strongly recommend that all cats with fibrosarcoma be tested for FeLV and that any IFA test–positive cats be destroyed. The National Cancer Institute has classified FeSV as a moderate-risk virus (Biol. Safety Man., 1976).

## FELINE LEUKEMIA VIRUS DISEASES

Collectively, the FeLV diseases are one of the leading causes of death among pet cats. As mentioned earlier, FeLV grows best in rapidly dividing cells and can cause fatal proliferative (neoplastic) and degenerative (blastopenic) diseases of various cell types (Table 7–15) (Cotter et al., 1975; Hardy, 1974, 1980a, 1981 a,b,c,d, 1982). For example, lymphosarcoma is a neoplastic disease of lymphocytes, usually thymic-derived (T cells), whereas thymic atrophy is a degenerative disease of thymic lymphocytes (Anderson et al., 1971; Hardy, 1981d). FeLV can also induce neoplastic diseases of precursor red blood cells (erythremic myelosis and erythroleukemia), whereas FeLV-induced degenerative red blood cell disease results in several types of anemia (Hardy, 1981d; see also chapter on the hematopoietic system). Granulocytic leukemia is an FeLV-induced malignant proliferation of granulocytes, whereas the FeLV panleukopenia-like disease (myeloblastopenia) is a degenerative disease of granulocytes (Hardy, 1980a, 1981d, 1982; Jarrett et al., 1971).

FeLV also causes immune-complex glomerulonephritis

**Table 7–15 Feline Leukemia Virus Diseases***

| CELL TYPE | PROLIFERATIVE DISEASES (NEOPLASTIC) | PER CENT FeLV-POSITIVE | DEGENERATIVE DISEASES (BLASTOPENIC) | PER CENT FeLV-POSITIVE BY IFA TEST |
|---|---|---|---|---|
| Lymphoid cells | Lymphosarcoma (507 cases studied) | 70 | Thymic atrophy† | 88 |
| | | | Immunosuppressive diseases† | 45 |
| Bone marrow cells (50 cases studied) | | | | |
| Primitive mesenchymal cell | Reticuloendotheliosis | 100 | — | — |
| Erythroblast | Erythremic myelosis | 100 | Erythroblastosis† | 15 |
| | Erythroleukemia | 100 | Erythroblastopenia† | 70 |
| | | | Pancytopenia† | ? |
| Myeloblast‡ | Granulocytic leukemia | 100 | Panleukopenia-like syndrome† | 80 |
| Megakaryocyte | Megakaryocytic leukemia | 100 | Thrombocytopenia† | ? |
| Fibroblast | Myelofibrosis | 100 | — | — |
| Osteoblast | Medullary osteosclerosis | 100 | — | — |
| | Osteochondromatosis | 100 | — | — |
| Kidney | — | — | FeLV immune complex glomerulonephritis | 100 |
| Uterus | — | | Abortions and resorptions† | 68 |
| Nerve cells | — | | Neurologic syndrome† | ? |
| Fibroblasts, skin | FeSV-induced multicentric fibrosarcomas (25 cases studied) | 100 | — | — |

*Adapted from Hardy WD Jr: Feline leukemia virus diseases. *In* Hardy WD Jr, Essex M, McClelland AJ (eds): Feline Leukemia Virus. New York, Elsevier/North Holland, 1980a, 3–31; and Hardy WD Jr: Hematopoietic tumors of cats. J Am Anim Hosp Assoc 17 (1981c) 921–940.

†This condition can be caused by infectious agents or factors other than FeLV. If FeLV causes this condition, the cat is FeLV-positive.

‡Basophilic, monocytic, and myelomonocytic leukemias have also occurred in FeLV-positive cats (Henness and Crow, 1977; Henness et al., 1977; Stann, 1979), and eosinophilic leukemia has resulted from inoculation with FeLV (Lewis et al., 1985).

(Cotter et al., 1975; Hardy, 1980a, 1981d, 1982; Jakowski et al., 1980; Weksler et al., 1975) and is thought to cause fetal abortions and resorptions and possibly a neurologic syndrome (Hardy, 1980a, 1981d). One of the most important effects of FeLV is the immunosuppression it causes in adult cats, enabling infectious diseases to develop (Hardy 1980a, 1981d, 1982; Perryman et al., 1972). Since illness in cats that develop secondary infectious disease due to FeLV-induced immunosuppression is so similar to that in humans with the acquired immune deficiency syndrome (AIDS), I have chosen to call this FeLV-induced syndrome the feline immune deficiency syndrome (FAIDS) (Centers for Disease Control, 1982; Hardy, 1984a,b). More pet cats die of FeLV-induced FAIDS than from any other FeLV-induced disease.

**Table 7–17 FeLV-Induced Feline Immune Deficiency Syndrome (FAIDS)**

I. Immune cell deficiencies
   A. Lymphoid depletions
      1. Thymic atrophy—kittens
      2. General lymphoid depletion—adult cats
   B. Myeloid depletion
      1. Neutropenias
II. Immune cell dysfunctions
   A. Deficient cell-mediated immune response
      1. Cutaneous anergy
   B. Deficient antibody-mediated immune response
      1. To threshold antigen stimulation
III. Pathogenic antibody immune-mediated disease
   A. Immune-complex glomerulonephritis
IV. Complement deficiency

## LYMPHOSARCOMA

One third of cat tumors are hematopoietic tumors, and 90 per cent of these are LSA (Dorn et al., 1968) (see also chapters on tumors and on the hematopoietic system). Pet cats develop LSA more frequently than any other animal, 200 cases occurring for every 100,000 cats at risk (Essex, 1980; Hardy, 1981a). Multicentric LSA is the most common anatomic form, in which the tumor localizes in internal organs and lymph nodes. According to two studies, only 30 per cent of cats with LSA have leukemic blood profiles (Crighton, 1969; Hardy, 1981c). In my experience, thymic LSA is the second most common form, followed by alimentary LSA, which is characterized by tumor localization in the gastrointestinal tract. The majority of cat LSAs are T-cell tumors, although B-cell LSAs occur in the gastrointestinal tract (Hardy et al., 1978, 1980). About two thirds of cats with LSA have nonregenerative anemias (Cotter, 1979; Hardy, 1981c; Hoover et al., 1974; Maggio, 1979).

Seventy per cent of cats with LSA are infected with FeLV, whereas 30 per cent have LSA with no detectable virus (Table 7–16) (Francis et al., 1979a; Hardy et al., 1969; 1980). In these cases, no FeLV antigens or infectious FeLV is present. However, the FeLV-induced tumor-specific FOCMA antigen is found on the cell membranes of both FeLV-positive and -negative LSA cells (Hardy et al., 1977; Hardy, 1981a,c). FeLV-negative cases of LSA are frequent in households where FeLV-infected cats have lived. In a study of 507 cats with LSA we found that cats with FeLV-positive LSAs are usually less than seven years old and have T-cell tumors, whereas cats with FeLV-negative LSAs are usually over seven years of age and have alimentary B-cell LSAs (Hardy et al., 1977; Hardy 1981a,c). We found that cats with FeLV-negative LSAs have the same degree of exposure to FeLV as do cats that develop FeLV-positive LSAs. Recently, two groups of researchers have been able to reactivate latent FeLV from the bone marrow, but not from the FeLV-negative LSA cells, of 80 per cent of the cats studied (Post and Warren, 1980; Rojko et al., 1982). Thus it is apparent that FeLV induces FeLV-negative LSAs in some cats. FeLV can also induce FeLV-negative LSAs in puppies (Rickard et al., 1973). Puppies developed FeLV-negative LSAs if they were inoculated with the virus during the first day of life, whereas those inoculated in utero developed FeLV-positive LSAs.

LSA can be diagnosed only by histologic or cytologic analysis. A positive FeLV test merely detects the virus and is not diagnostic for LSA or any other disease.

**Table 7–16 Comparison of FeLV-Positive and FeLV-Negative Feline Lymphosarcomas**

| CATEGORY | FeLV-POSITIVE LSAs | FeLV-NEGATIVE LSAs |
|---|---|---|
| Anatomic form | Multicentric form<br>Thymic form | Most often alimentary or skin form |
| T- or B-cell origin | Usually T cell | Usually B cell |
| Age | Young (under 7 yrs) | Old (over 7 yrs) |
| FeLV antigens | Present | Absent |
| Infectious FeLV | Present | Absent from LSA cells<br>Reactivatable from bone marrow cells |
| FOCMA | Present | Present |
| Exposure to FeLV | Exposed | Exposed |

## DEGENERATIVE LYMPHOID DISEASES

FeLV replicates in all feline lymphoid cells and often induces severe depletion or dysfunction of these cells (Table 7–17).

**THYMIC ATROPHY.** Thymic atrophy is a degenerative disease of the T-lymphocytes of the thymus gland of FeLV-infected kittens (Anderson et al., 1971; Hardy, 1980a, 1981d, 1982). The virus is usually transmitted to these kittens from their viremic queen while they are in utero or shortly after birth by the milk. FeLV damages the thymus (Figs. 7–66 and 7–67), causing a defective cell-mediated immune response that renders the kittens susceptible to secondary infectious diseases such as bronchopneumonia and enteritis. An FeLV-positive test of the kitten or its queen and the finding of an atrophic thymus at autopsy are required for a diagnosis of thymic atrophy.

**LYMPHOID ATROPHY.** Lymphoid atrophy and lymphoid hyperplasia are frequent in FeLV-infected cats (Hardy, 1982; Hoover et al., 1973). The lymph nodes are atrophied in infected cats that do not have opportunistic infections. These cats may also be lymphopenic and often die from opportunistic infections.

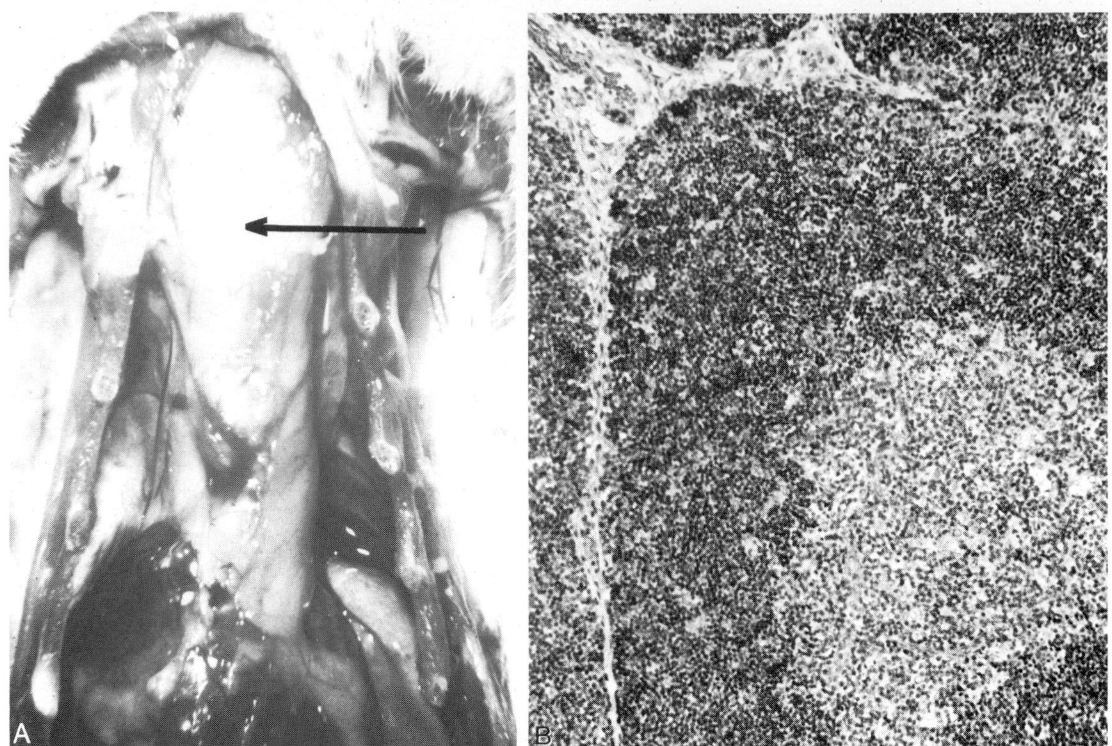


**Figure 7–66** Normal thymus. *A*, Normal large thymus in the thoracic cavity of a healthy, FeLV-negative kitten. *B*, Section of the thymus of a seven-week-old, FeLV-negative, healthy kitten, × 125. The cortical and medullary regions of a thymic lobule are clearly distinguishable. (Courtesy Dr. E. A. Hoover. Reprinted with permission from Cancer Research and Springer-Verlag [Hardy, 1982].)

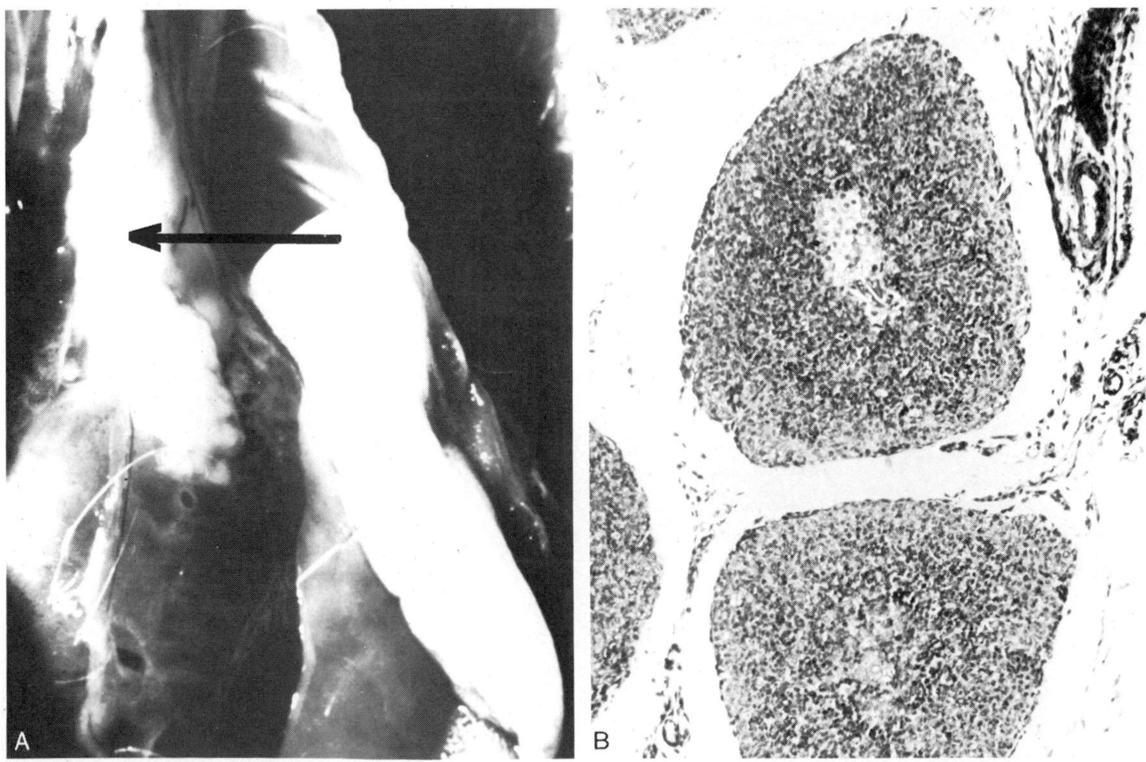


**Figure 7–67** Atrophic thymus. *A*, A small, atrophic thymus in an FeLV-infected kitten that died of FeLV-induced feline acquired immune deficiency syndrome (FAIDS) and opportunistic infection. *B*, Section of the thymus of an FeLV experimentally infected seven-week-old kitten, × 125. There are extreme thymic atrophy and depletion of the cortical thymocytes. (Courtesy, Dr. E. A. Hoover. Reprinted with permission from Cancer Research and Springer-Verlag [Hardy, 1982].)

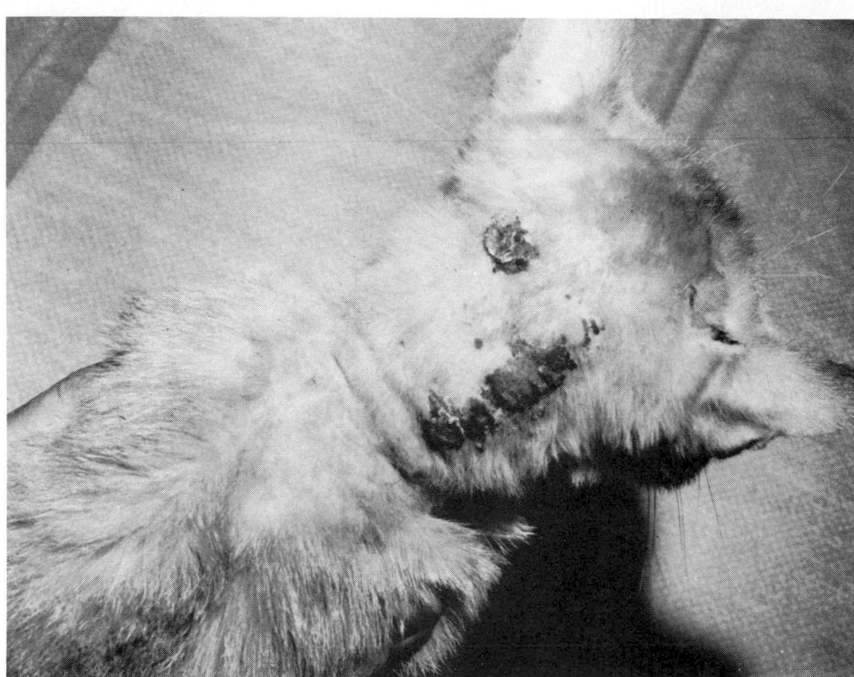

**Figure 7–68** Chronic, nonhealing skin lesions on the back of the neck of a cat with FeLV-induced feline acquired immune deficiency syndrome (FAIDS).

## FeLV-Induced Feline Acquired Immune Deficiency Syndrome (FAIDS)

Persistently FeLV-infected pet cats often develop severe immune-cell deficiencies, characterized by a drastic reduction in the numbers of lymphocytes and neutrophils (Hardy, 1981a,d, 1982; Hoover et al., 1980), as well as immune-cell dysfunctions including cutaneous anergy (Perryman et al., 1972), reduced T-cell blastogenic responsiveness (Cockerell et al., 1976); Cockerell and Hoover, 1977), and impaired antibody production (Hardy, 1982; Trainin et al., 1983). The impairment of immune functions renders these cats very susceptible to other infectious agents.

Many FeLV-infected, clinically healthy cats have immune-cell alterations. In one study, 25 per cent of FeLV-infected cats were leukopenic and 66 per cent lymphopenic (Hardy, 1982). Similarly, 32 per cent of pet cats with FAIDS and secondary opportunistic infectious diseases were leukopenic and 51 per cent were lymphopenic. B-cell dysfunctions have also been observed in infected cats. FeLV-infected cats were shown to be less able than uninfected cats to produce antibody (IgG) to low numbers of sheep red blood cells and a synthetic antigen (Hardy, 1982; Trainin et al., 1983).

More pet cats die from FeLV-induced FAIDS than from any other FeLV-induced disease (Hardy, 1981d, 1982). Almost 50 per cent of cats with feline infectious peritonitis, 33 per cent of cats with chronic abscesses or nonhealing lesions of the skin (Fig. 7–68), 50 per cent of cats with chronic upper respiratory disease and pneumonia, 50 per cent of cats with chronic infections such as septicemias and pyothorax, 50 per cent of cats with chronic stomatitis and gingivitis (Fig. 7–69), and 87 per cent of

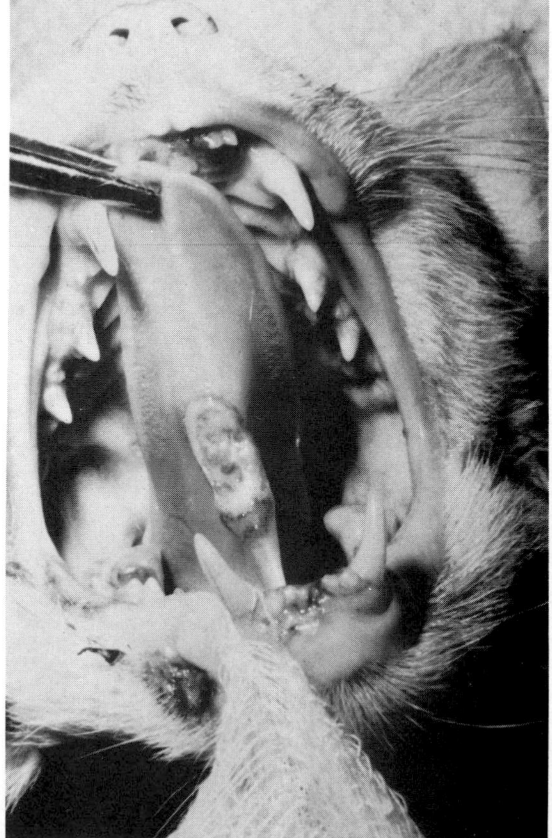

**Figure 7–69** Chronic oral ulcers in a pet cat with FeLV-induced feline acquired immune deficiency syndrome (FAIDS).

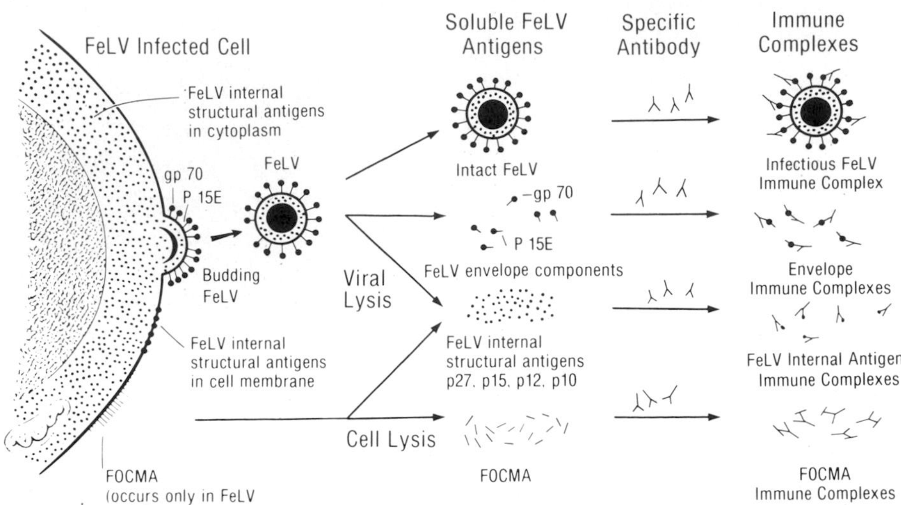


**Figure 7–70** A schematic representation of the generation of FeLV and FeLV structural-protein circulating immune complexes. (Reproduced with permission of Springer-Verlag [Hardy, 1982].)

kittens with thymic atrophy are infected with FeLV (Hardy, 1981d, 1982).

The mechanism by which FeLV induces FAIDS is not understood, but several possibilities exist. (1) FeLV may cause lysis of cells or may sensitize cells to cell-mediated immune destruction by viral replication and budding from cell membranes. (2) FeLV-soluble circulating proteins may be immunosuppressive. In this regard, FeLV p15E, the protein of the viral envelope spikes (see Fig. 7–62*A*), has been shown to decrease lymphocyte functions by 45 to 92 per cent (Cockerell and Hoover, 1977; Mathes et al., 1978). (3) Circulating immune complexes (CICs) are known to be immunosuppressive, and CICs composed of whole infectious FeLV, FeLV gp70, p27, p15, and p15E are present in infected cats (Fig. 7–70) (Day et al., 1980; Hardy, 1982; Snyder et al., 1982). In addition, therapeutic removal of FeLV CICs by ex vivo immunosorption on *Staphylococcus aureus* Cowans I columns resulted in marked improvement in two cats with FAIDS (Jones et al., 1980; Snyder et al., 1984b). (4) FeLV-infected cats with LSA and 50 per cent of FeLV-infected healthy cats are hypocomplementemic—a deficiency that probably contributes to the immunosuppression (Kobilinsky et al., 1979).

There are many similarities between FeLV-induced FAIDS of pet cats and human AIDS (Essex et al., 1983; Hardy, 1984; Hardy and Essex, 1986). Both syndromes are characterized by lymphopenia, reduced lymphocyte blastogenesis, cutaneous anergy, reduced numbers of T cells, impaired antibody response, and the occurrence of secondary infectious diseases. FAIDS is caused by a retrovirus that has an affinity for T cells, and recent evidence has shown that a similar virus, the human T-cell leukemia virus (HTLV) subgroup III, is the cause of human AIDS (Gallo et al., 1984; Popovic et al., 1984; Sarngadharan et al., 1984; Schüpbach et al., 1984).

## Erythroid Diseases

FeLV replicates in all nucleated erythroid cells in the bone marrow and thus can cause neoplastic (myeloproliferative) or degenerative (blastopenic) diseases (Hardy et al., 1973b; Hardy, 1981d) (see also chapter on the hematopoietic system).

**ERYTHROID NEOPLASTIC (MYELOPROLIFERATIVE) DISEASES.** In my experience, FeLV only rarely causes erythremic myelosis and erythroleukemia (Hardy et al., 1981c,d) (see, however, chapter on the hematopoietic system). Erythremic myelosis is characterized by the presence of abnormally high numbers of proliferating nucleated erythroid cells without concurrent proliferation of granulocytes. In erythroleukemia, myeloblasts (granulocytic leukocyte precursors) are present along with abnormal nucleated erythrocytes. Most cats with either disease have marked anemia.

**ERYTHROID DEGENERATIVE DISEASES.** Erythroid degenerative (blastopenic) diseases occur far more often in FeLV-infected pet cats than do neoplastic diseases (see chapter on the hematopoietic system). Three types of FeLV-induced anemias occur: (1) erythroblastosis (regenerative anemia), (2) erythroblastopenia (nonregenerative anemia), and (3) pancytopenia (Hardy, 1981d; Mackey et al., 1975; Maggio, 1979). FeLV subgroup A has been shown experimentally to induce nonfatal transient erythroblastosis, whereas several FeLV-C isolates induced fatal erythroblastopenias (Mackey et al., 1975; Onions et al., 1982).

## Myeloid Diseases

FeLV replicates in all precursor and differentiated neutrophils, basophils, and eosinophils in the bone marrow and thus can cause neoplastic or degenerative disease of these cell types.

**MYELOID NEOPLASTIC (MYELOPROLIFERATIVE) DISEASES.** FeLV has been found in pet cats with the following myeloid neoplastic (myeloproliferative) diseases: reticuloendotheliosis; neutrophilic, basophilic, monocytic, myelomonocytic, and megakaryocytic leukemia; myelofibrosis; and osteosclerosis (Hardy, 1981c; Henness and Crow, 1977; Henness et al., 1977; Stann, 1979). Recently, a case of eosinophilic leukemia was induced by inoculation with FeLV (Lewis et al., 1985). However, these diseases occur far less often in pet cats than the lymphoproliferative neoplasms.

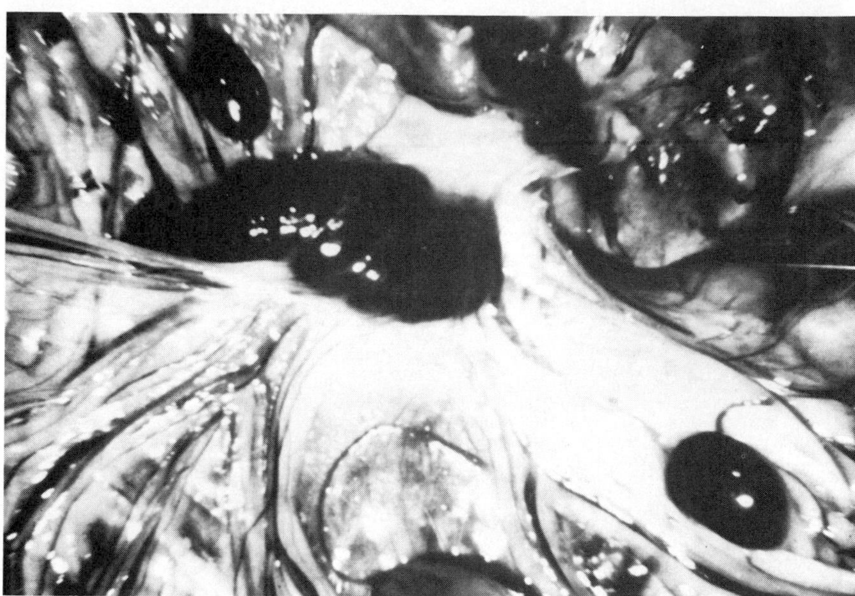

**Figure 7–71** Hemorrhagic lymphadenitis of the mesenteric lymph nodes in a cat with FeLV-induced myeloblastopenia (panleukopenia-like syndrome). (Reproduced with permission of Springer-Verlag [Hardy, 1982].)

**MYELOID DEGENERATIVE DISEASES.** Degenerative myeloid diseases are far more frequent in infected pet cats than myeloproliferative diseases. A specific disorder, FeLV-induced myeloblastopenia (panleukopenia-like syndrome), is fairly common and is characterized by severe dysentery, hemorrhagic lymphadenitis (Fig. 7–71), and a panleukopenia (Hardy, 1981d). Intestinal hemorrhaging is severe owing to erosion of the epithelium of the tips of the villi of the small bowel. Some cats lose so much blood from intestinal bleeding that they become severely anemic in one or two days. Opportunistic infections enter through the sites of intestinal erosion, resulting in septicemia and death. FeLV antigens and replicating virus are present in the intestinal epithelial cells and in lymphocytes in the lamina propria (Hardy, 1981d; Rojko et al., 1979).

## Other FeLV-Associated Diseases

**ABORTION AND RESORPTION.** FeLV has been detected in two thirds of 307 cats with a history of abortions or fetal resorptions and has been shown experimentally to induce these disorders (Hardy, 1981d; Hoover and Quackenbush, personal communication).

**FeLV NEUROLOGIC SYNDROME.** A neurologic syndrome occurs in FeLV-infected cats that is characterized by posterior paresis, paralysis, or tetraplegia (Hardy, 1981d). However, FeLV has not yet been proven to cause this disease under experimental conditions.

**FeLV IMMUNE-COMPLEX GLOMERULONEPHRITIS.** The lifelong viremia that occurs in FeLV-infected pet cats offers ideal conditions for the formation of immune complexes (CICs) (Fig. 7–70) (Hardy, 1981a,d), and they occur often in FeLV-infected cats (Day et al., 1980; Hardy, 1981d, 1982; Snyder et al., 1982, 1984). Two studies have shown that cats living in FeLV-exposure households have a high incidence of glomerulonephritis (Cotter et al., 1975; Jakowski et al., 1980). FeLV antigens, antibody (IgG), and complement have been found deposited in the glomeruli (Fig. 7–72) of 25 per cent of healthy FeLV-infected cats (Hardy, 1982). Although many pet cats are chronically infected with FeLV and develop CICs, immune complex glomerulonephritis is infrequent.

## REFERENCES

Abelson HT, Rabstein LS: Lymphosarcoma: virus-induced thymic-independent disease in mice. Cancer Res 30 (1970) 2213–2222.

Anderson LJ, Jarrett WFH, Jarrett O, Laird HM: Feline leukemia virus infection of kittens: mortality associated with atrophy of the thymus and lymphoid depletion. J Natl Cancer Inst 47 (1971) 807–817.

Azocar J, Essex M: Susceptibility of human cell lines to feline leukemia and feline sarcoma viruses. J Natl Cancer Inst 63 (1979) 1179–1184.

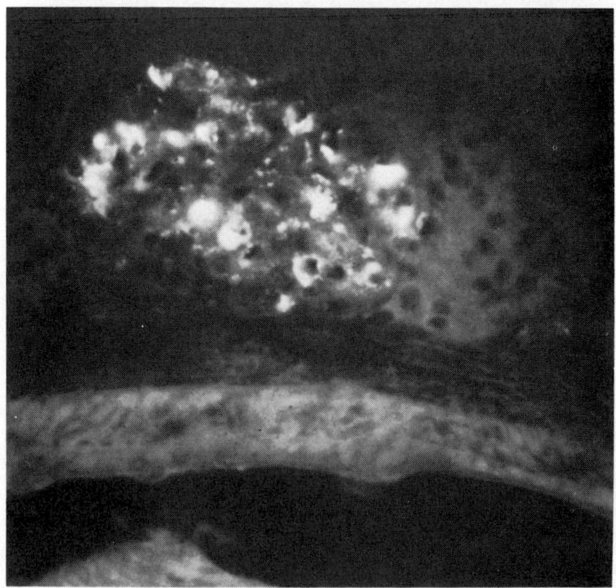

**Figure 7–72** Deposition of IgG, FeLV proteins, and complement in a glomerulus of an FeLV-infected cat. (Reproduced with permission of Springer-Verlag [Hardy, 1982].)

Baltimore D: RNA-dependent DNA polymerase in virions of RNA tumor viruses. Nature 226 (1970) 1209–1211.

Barrett RE, Post JE, Schultz RD: Chronic relapsing stomatitis in a cat associated with feline leukemia virus infection. Feline Pract 5 (6) 1975) 34–38.

Benveniste RE, Todaro GJ: Homology between type-C viruses of various species as determined by molecular hybridization. Proc Natl Acad Sci USA 70 (1973) 3316–3320.

Benveniste RE, Todaro GJ: Multiple divergent copies of endogenous C-type virogenes in mammalian cells. Nature 252 (1974) 170–173.

Benveniste RE, Sherr CJ, Todaro GJ: Evolution of type-C viral genes: origin of feline leukemia virus. Science 190 (1975) 886–888.

Besmer P: Acute transforming feline retroviruses. Curr Top Microbiol Immunol 107 (1983) 1–27.

Besmer P, Hardy WD Jr, Zuckerman EE, Bergold P, Lederman L, Snyder HW Jr: The Hardy-Zuckerman 2-FeSV, a new feline retrovirus with oncogene homology to Abelson-MuLV. Nature 303 (1983a) 825–828.

Besmer P, Snyder HW Jr, Murphy JE, Hardy WD Jr, Parodi A: The Parodi-Irgens feline sarcoma virus and simian sarcoma virus have homologous oncogenes, but in different contexts of the viral genomes. J Virol 46 (1983b) 606–613.

Besmer P, George PC, Snyder HW Jr, Zuckerman EE, Lederman L, Hardy WD Jr: Characterization of the *v-fms* oncogene from a new feline sarcoma virus, HZ5-FeSV. (1986a) Manuscript in preparation.

Besmer P, Murphy JE, George PC, Qui P, Bergold P, Lederman L, Snyder HW Jr, Brodeur D, Zuckerman EE, Hardy WD Jr: A new acute transforming feline retrovirus and its oncogene *v-kit* with the protein kinase gene family. Nature (1986b). In press.

Biological Safety Manual for Research Involving Oncogenic Viruses. US Dept of Health, Education and Welfare, National Institutes of Health, Washington DC NIH 76–1165, part 2, 1976.

Blair A, Hayes HM Jr: Cancer and other causes of death among US veterinarians, 1966–1977. Int J Cancer 25 (1980) 181–185.

Bolognesi DP, Montelaro RC, Frank H, Schäfer W: Assembly of type C oncornaviruses: a model. Science 199 (1978) 183–186.

Botts RP, Edlavitch S, Payne G: Mortality of Missouri veterinarians. J Am Vet Med Assoc 149 (1966) 499–504.

Bross IDJ, Gibson R: Cats and childhood leukemia. J Med 1 (1970) 180–187.

Caldwell GG, Baumgartener L, Carter C, Cotter S, Currier R, Essex M, Hardy W, Olson C, Olsen R: Seroepidemiologic testing in man for evidence of antibodies to feline leukemia virus and bovine leukemia virus. *In* Clemmesen J, Yohn DS (eds): Comparative Leukemia Research 1975. Basel, S. Karger, 1976, 238–241.

Centers for Disease Control: Report of the Centers for Disease Control task force on Kaposi's sarcoma and opportunistic infections. N Engl J Med 306 (1982) 248–252.

Charman HP, Kim N, Gilden RV, Hardy WD Jr, Essex M: Humoral immune responses of cats to feline leukemia virus: comparison of response to the major structural protein p30 and to a virus specific cell membrane antigen (FOCMA). J Natl Cancer Inst 56 (1976) 859–861.

Cockerell GL, Hoover EA, Krakowka S, Olsen RG, Yohn DS: Lymphocyte mitogen reactivity and enumeration of circulating B- and T-cells during feline leukemia virus infection in the cat. J Natl Cancer Inst 57 (1976) 1095–1099.

Cockerell GL, Hoover EA: Inhibition of normal lymphocyte mitogenic reactivity by serum from feline leukemia virus-infected cats. Cancer Res 37 (1977) 3985–3989.

Coffin JM, Varmus HE, Bishop JM, Essex M, Hardy WD Jr, Martin GS, Rosenberg NE, Scolnick EM, Weinberg RA, Vogt PK: Proposal for naming host cell-derived inserts in retrovirus genomes. J Virol 40 (1981) 953–957.

Cotter SM: Anemia associated with feline leukemia virus infection. J Am Vet Med Assoc 175 (1979) 1191–1194.

Cotter SM, Hardy WD Jr, Essex M: Association of feline leukemia virus with lymphosarcoma and other disorders in the cat. J Am Vet Med Assoc 166 (1975) 449–454.

Cotter SM, Essex M: Animal model of human disease: feline acute lymphoblastic leukemia and aplastic anemia. Am J Pathol 87 (1977) 265–268.

Crighton GW: Lymphosarcoma in the cat. Vet Rec 84 (1969) 329–331.

Day NK, O'Reilly-Felice C, Hardy WD Jr, Good RA, Witken SS: Circulating immune complexes associated with naturally occurring lymphosarcoma in pet cats. J Immunol 125 (1980) 2363–2366.

Deinhardt F, Wolfe LG, Theilen GH, Snyder SP: ST-feline fibrosarcoma virus: induction of tumors in marmoset monkeys. Science 167 (1970) 881.

Doolittle RF, Hunkapiller MW, Hood LE, Devare SG, Robbins KC, Aaronson SA, Antoniades HN: Simian sarcoma virus *onc* gene, v-*sis*, is derived from the gene (or genes) encoding a platelet-derived growth factor. Science 221 (1983) 275–277.

Dorn CR, Taylor DON, Schneider R, Hibbard HH, Klauber MR: Survey of animal neoplasms in Alameda and Contra Costa Counties, California. II. Cancer morbidity in dogs and cats from Alameda County. J Natl Cancer Inst 40 (1968) 307–318.

Duesberg PH, Vogt PK: Avian acute leukemia viruses MC29 and MH2 share specific RNA sequences: evidence for a second class of transforming genes. Proc Natl Acad Sci USA 76 (1979) 1633–1637.

Essex M: Feline leukemia and sarcoma viruses. *In* Klein G (ed): Viral Oncology. New York, Raven Press, 1980, 205–229.

Essex M, Klein G, Snyder SP, Harrold JB: Correlation between humoral antibody and regression of tumors induced by feline sarcoma virus. Nature 233 (1971a) 195–196.

Essex M, Klein G, Snyder SP, Harrold JB: Antibody to feline oncornavirus-associated cell membrane antigen in neonatal cats. Int J Cancer 8 (1971b) 384–390.

Essex M, Klein G, Deinhardt F, Wolfe LG, Hardy WD Jr, Theilen GH, Pearson LP: Induction of the feline oncornavirus associated cell membrane antigen in human cells. Nature 238 (1972) 187–189.

Essex M, Snyder SP: Feline oncornavirus associated cell membrane antigen. I. Serologic studies with kittens exposed to cell-free materials from various feline fibrosarcomas. J Natl Cancer Inst 51 (1973) 1007–1012.

Essex M, Sliski A, Cotter SM, Jakowski RM, Hardy WD Jr: Immunosurveillance of naturally occurring feline leukemia. Science 190 (1975) 790–792.

Essex M, Francis DP: The risk to humans from malignant disease of their pets: an unsettled issue. J Am Anim Hosp Assoc 12 (1976) 386–390.

Essex M, Hardy WD Jr: Transmissibility of animal cancer viruses. J Am Vet Med Assoc 171 (1977) 685, 688, 692.

Essex M, Cotter SM, Sliski AH, Hardy WD Jr, Stephenson JR, Aaronson SA, Jarrett O: Horizontal transmission of feline leukemia virus under natural conditions in a feline leukemia cluster household. Int J Cancer 19 (1977a) 90–96.

Essex M, Cotter SM, Stephenson JR, Aaronson SA, Hardy WD Jr: Leukemia, lymphoma and fibrosarcoma of cats as models for similar diseases of man. *In* Hiatt HH, Watson JD, Winsten JA (eds): Origins of Human Cancer. Cold Spring Harbor, New York, Cold Spring Harbor Laboratory, 1977b, 1197–1211.

Essex M, McLane MF, Lee TH, Falk L, Howe CWS, Mullins JI, Cabradilla C, Francis DP: Antibodies to cell membrane antigens associated with human T-cell leukemia virus in patients with AIDS. Science 220 (1983) 859–862.

Fasal E, Jackson EW, Klauber MR: Mortality in California veterinarians. J Chronic Dis 19 (1966) 293–306.

Fenner F: The classification and nomenclature of viruses. Virology 71 (1976) 371–378.

Fink MA, Sibal LR, Plata EJ: Serologic detection of feline leukemia virus antigens or antibodies. J Am Vet Med Assoc 158 (1971) 1070–1075.
Fischinger PJ, Peebles PT, Nomura S, Haapala DK: Isolation of RD-114–like oncornavirus from a cat cell line. J Virol 11 (1973) 978–985.
Francis DP, Essex M, Hardy WD Jr: Excretion of feline leukemia virus by naturally infected pet cats. Nature 269 (1977) 252–254.
Francis DP, Cotter SM, Hardy WD Jr, Essex M: Comparison of virus-positive and virus-negative cases of feline leukemia and lymphoma. Cancer Res 39 (1979a) 3866–3870.
Francis DP, Essex M, Gayagian D: Feline leukemia virus: survival under home and laboratory conditions. J Clin Microbiol 9 (1979b) 154–156.
Frankel AE, Gilbert JH, Porzig KJ, Scolnick EM, Aaronson SA: Nature and distribution of feline sarcoma virus nucleotide sequences. J Virol 30 (1979) 821–827.
Fujinami A, Inamoto K: Ueber Geschwülste bei japanischer Haushühnern insbesondere über einen transplantablen Tumor. Z Krebsforsch 14 (1914) 94–119.
Gallo RC, Salahuddin SZ, Popovic M, Shearer GM, Kaplan M, Haynes BF, Palker TJ, Redfield R, Oleske J, Safai B, White G, Foster P, Markham PD: Frequent detection and isolation of cytopathic retroviruses (HTLV-III) from patients with AIDS and at risk for AIDS. Science 224 (1984) 500–503.
Gardner MB, Rongey RW, Arnstein P, Estes JD, Sarma P, Huebner RJ, Rickard CG: Experimental transmission of feline fibrosarcoma to cats and dogs. Nature 226 (1970) 807–809.
Gardner MB, Arnstein P, Johnson E, Rongey RW, Charman HP, Huebner RJ: Feline sarcoma virus tumor induction in cats and dogs. J Am Vet Med Assoc 158 (1971a) 1046–1053.
Gardner MB, Rongey RW, Johnson EY, DeJournett R, Huebner RJ: C-type tumor virus particles in salivary tissue of domestic cats. J Natl Cancer Inst 47 (1971b) 561–568.
Gardner MB, Henderson BE, Estes JD, Rongey RW, Casagrande J, Pike M, Huebner RJ: The epidemiology and virology of C-type virus-associated hematological cancers and related diseases in wild mice. Cancer Res 36 (1976) 574–581.
Gardner MB, Brown JC, Charman HP, Stephenson JR, Rongey RW, Hauser DE, Diegmann F, Howard E, Dworsky R, Gilden RV, Huebner RJ: FeLV epidemiology in Los Angeles cats: Appraisal of detection methods. Int J Cancer 19 (1977) 581–589.
Gutensohn N, Essex M, Francis DP, Hardy WD Jr: Risk to humans from exposure to feline leukemia virus: epidemiological considerations. *In* Essex M, Todaro GJ, zur Hausen H (eds): Viruses in Naturally Occurring Cancers. Cold Spring Harbor, New York, Cold Spring Harbor Laboratory, 1980, 699–706.
Gwalter RH: FeLV testmethoden: IFA oder ELISA. Kleintierpraxis 26 (1981) 23–28.
Hanes B, Gardner MB, Loosli CG, Heidbreder G, Kogan B, Marylander H, Huebner RJ: Pet association with selected human cancers: a household questionnaire survey. J Natl Cancer Inst 45 (1970) 1155–1162.
Hardy WD Jr: Immunology of oncornaviruses. Vet Clin North Am 4 (1974) 133–146.
Hardy WD Jr: Feline leukemia virus diseases. *In* Hardy WD Jr, Essex M, McClelland AJ (eds): Feline Leukemia Virus. New York, Elsevier/North Holland, 1980a, 3–31.
Hardy WD Jr: The Virology, immunology and epidemiology of the feline leukemia virus. *In* Hardy WD Jr, Essex M, McClelland AJ (eds): Feline Leukemia Virus. New York, Elsevier/North Holland, 1980b, 33–78.
Hardy WD Jr: The biology and virology of the feline sarcoma viruses. *In* Hardy WD Jr, Essex M, McClelland AJ (eds): Feline Leukemia Virus. New York, Elsevier/North Holland, 1980c, 79–118.
Hardy WD Jr: The feline leukemia virus. J Am Anim Hosp Assoc 17 (1981a) 951–980.
Hardy WD Jr: The feline sarcoma viruses. J Am Anim Hosp Assoc 17 (1981b) 981–997.
Hardy WD Jr: Hematopoietic tumors of cats. J Am Anim Hosp Assoc 17 (1981c) 921–940.
Hardy WD Jr: Feline leukemia virus non-neoplastic diseases. J Am Anim Hosp Assoc 17 (1981d) 941–949.
Hardy WD Jr: Immunopathology induced by the feline leukemia virus. *In* Klein G (ed): Springer Semin Immunopathol 1982. New York, Springer-Verlag, 1982, 75–105.
Hardy WD Jr: Feline leukemia virus as an animal retrovirus model for the human T-cell leukemia virus. *In* Gallo RC, Essex M, Gross L (eds): Human T-Cell Leukemia/Lymphoma Viruses. Cold Spring Harbor, New York, Cold Spring Harbor Laboratory, 1984, 35–43.
Hardy WD Jr, Geering G, Old LJ, De Harven E, Brodey RS, McDonough S: Feline leukemia virus: occurrence of viral antigen in the tissues of cats with lymphosarcoma and other diseases. Science 166 (1969) 1019–1021.
Hardy WD Jr, Hurvitz AI: Feline infectious peritonitis: experimental studies. J Am Vet Med Assoc 158 (1971) 994–1002.
Hardy WD Jr, Old LJ, Hess PW, Essex M, Cotter SM: Horizontal transmission of feline leukaemia virus. Nature 244 (1973a) 266–269.
Hardy WD Jr, Hirshaut Y, Hess P: Detection of the feline leukemia virus and other mammalian oncornaviruses by immunofluorescence. *In* Dutcher RM, Chieco-Bianchi L (eds): Unifying Concepts of Leukemia. Basel, S. Karger, 1973b, 778–799.
Hardy WD Jr, McClelland AJ, Hess PW, MacEwen EG: Veterinarians and the control of feline leukemia virus. J Am Anim Hosp Assoc 10 (1974a) 367–372.
Hardy WD Jr, McClelland AJ, Hess PW, MacEwen EG: Feline leukemia virus and public health awareness. J Am Vet Med Assoc 165 (1974b) 1020–1021.
Hardy WD Jr, Hess PW, MacEwen EG, McClelland AJ, Zuckerman EE, Essex M, Cotter SM, Jarrett O: Biology of feline leukemia virus in the natural environment. Cancer Res 36 (1976a) 582–588.
Hardy WD Jr, McClelland AJ, Zuckerman EE, Hess PW, Essex M, Cotter SM, MacEwen EG, Hayes AA: Prevention of the contagious spread of the feline leukaemia virus and the development of leukaemia in pet cats. Nature 263 (1976b) 326–328.
Hardy WD Jr, Zuckerman EE, MacEwen EG, Hayes AA, Essex M: A feline leukaemia virus–and sarcoma virus–induced tumor-specific antigen. Nature 270 (1977) 249–251.
Hardy WD Jr, Zuckerman EE, Essex M, MacEwen EG, Hayes AA: Feline oncornavirus-associated cell membrane antigen: an FeLV- and FeSV-induced tumor-specific antigen. *In* Clarkson B, Marks, PA, Till JE (eds): Differentiation of Normal and Neoplastic Hematopoietic cells. Cold Spring Harbor Laboratory, Cold Spring Harbor, New York, 1978, 601–623.
Hardy WD Jr, McClelland AJ, Zuckerman EE, Snyder HW Jr, MacEwen EG, Francis D, Essex M: Development of virus non-producer lymphosarcomas in pet cats exposed to FeLV. Nature 288 (1980) 90–92.
Hardy WD Jr, McClelland AJ: Oncogenic RNA viral infections. *In* Steele JH, Beran G (eds): Viral Zoonoses. Boca Raton, CRC Press, 1981, 299–340.
Hardy WD Jr, Zuckerman E, Markovich R, Besmer P, Snyder HW: Isolation of feline sarcoma viruses from pet cats with multicentric fibrosarcomas. *In* Yohn DS, Blakeslee JR (eds): Advances in Comparative Leukemia Research. Elsevier/North Holland Inc, 1982, 205–206.
Hardy WD Jr, Essex M: FeLV-induced feline acquired immune deficiency syndrome (FAIDS): A model for human AIDS. *In* Klein E (ed): Acquired Immune Deficiency Syndrome. Basel, S. Karger, 1986.

Hardy WD Jr, Zuckerman EE, Besmer P, Markovich R, George PC, Lederman L, Snyder HW Jr: Isolation of a new feline sarcoma virus HZ5-FeSV containing the *v-fms* oncogene. (1986) Manuscript in preparation.

Henness AM, Crow SE, Anderson BC: Monocytic leukemia in three cats. J Am Vet Med Assoc 170 (1977) 1325–1328.

Henness AM, Crow SE: Treatment of feline myelogenous leukemia: Four case reports. J Am Vet Med Assoc 171 (1977) 263–266.

Hoover EA, Perryman LE, Kociba GJ: Early lesions in cats inoculated with feline leukemia virus. Cancer Res 33 (1973) 145–152.

Hoover EA, Kociba GJ, Hardy WD Jr, Yohn DS: Erythroid hypoplasia in cats inoculated with feline leukemia virus. J Natl Cancer Inst 53 (1974) 1271–1276.

Hoover EA, Rojko JL, Olsen RG: Host-virus interactions in progressive versus regressive feline leukemia virus infection in cats. *In* Essex M, Todaro G, zur Hausen H (eds): Viruses in Naturally Occurring Cancers. New York, Cold Spring Harbor Laboratory, 1980, 635–651.

Irgens M, Wyers M, Moraillon A, Parodi A, Fortuny V: Isolement d'un virus sarcomatogène félin à partir d'un fibrosarcome spontané du chat: étude du pouvoir sarcomatogène in vivo. CR Acad Sci (Paris) 276 (1973) 1783–1786.

Jacquemin PC, Saxinger C, Gallo RC, Hardy WD Jr, Essex M: Antibody response in cats to feline leukemia virus reverse transcriptase under natural conditions of exposure to the virus. Virology 91 (1978a) 472–476.

Jacquemin PC, Saxinger C, Gallo RC: Surface antibodies of human myelogenous leukaemia leukocytes reactive with specific type-C viral reverse transcriptases. Nature 276 (1978b) 230–236.

Jakowski RM, Essex M, Hardy WD Jr, Stephenson JR, Cotter SM: Membranous glomerulonephritis in a household cluster of cats persistently viremic with feline leukemia virus. *In* Hardy WD Jr, Essex M, McClelland AJ (eds): Feline Leukemia Virus. New York, Elsevier/North Holland Inc, 1980, 141–149.

Jarrett WFH, Crawford EM, Martin WB, Davie F: A virus-like particle associated with leukaemia (lymphosarcoma). Nature 202 (1964) 567–568.

Jarrett O, Laird HM, Hay D: Growth of feline leukaemia virus in human cells. Nature 224 (1969) 1208–1209.

Jarrett WFH, Anderson LJ, Jarrett O, Laird HM, Stewart MF: Myeloid leukaemia in a cat produced experimentally by feline leukaemia virus. Res Vet Sci 12 (1971) 385–387.

Jarrett O, Laird HM, Hay D: Determinants of the host range of feline leukaemia viruses. J Gen Virol 20 (1973a) 169–175.

Jarrett WFH, Jarrett O, Mackey L, Laird H, Hardy WD Jr, Essex M: Horizontal transmission of leukemia virus and leukemia in the cat. J Natl Cancer Inst 51 (1973b) 833–841.

Jarrett WFH, Mackey L, Jarrett O, Laird H, Hood C: Antibody response and virus survival in cats vaccinated against feline leukaemia. Nature 248 (1974) 230–232.

Jarrett O, Hardy WD Jr, Golder MC, Hay D: The frequency of occurrence of feline leukaemia virus subgroups in cats. Int J Cancer 21 (1978) 334–337.

Jarrett O, Golder MC, Stewart MF: Detection of transient and persistent feline leukaemia virus infections. Vet Rec 110 (1982a) 225–228.

Jarrett O, Golder MC, Weijer K: A comparison of three methods of feline leukaemia virus diagnosis. Vet Rec 110 (1982b) 325–328.

Jones FR, Yoshida LH, Ladiges WC, Kenny MA: Treatment of feline leukemia and reversal of FeLV by *ex vivo* removal of IgG. Cancer 46 (1980) 675–684.

Kahn DE, Mia AS, Tierney MM: Field evaluation of Leukassay F, an FeLV detection test kit. Feline Pract 10 (2) (1980) 41–45.

Kobilinsky L, Hardy WD Jr, Day NK: Hypocomplementemia associated with naturally occurring lymphosarcoma in pet cats. J Immunol 122 (1979) 2139–2142.

Krakower JM, Aaronson SA: Seroepidemiologic assessment of feline leukaemia virus infection risk for man. Nature 273 (1978) 463–464.

Levy SB: Cat leukemia: a threat to man? N Engl J Med 290 (1974) 513–514.

Lewis MG, Kociba GJ, Rojko JL, Stiff MI, Haberman AB, Velicer LF, Olsen RG: Retroviral-associated eosinophilic leukemia in the cat. Am J Vet Res 46 (1985) 1066–1070.

Lutz H, Pedersen NC, Harris CW, Higgins JS, Theilen GH: Detection of feline leukemia virus infection. Feline Pract 10 (4) (1980) 13–23.

Mackey L, Jarrett W, Jarrett O, Laird H: Anemia associated with feline leukemia virus infection in cats. J Natl Cancer Inst 54 (1975) 209–217.

Maggio L: Anemia in the cat. Compend Contin Ed 1 (1979) 114–122.

Mandel MP, Stephenson JR, Hardy WD Jr, Essex M: Endogenous RD-114 virus of cats: absence of antibodies to RD-114 envelope antigens in cats naturally exposed to the feline leukemia virus. Infect Immun 24 (1979) 282–285.

Mathes LE, Olsen RG, Hebebrand LC, Hoover EA, Schaller JP: Abrogation of lymphocyte blastogenesis by a feline leukaemia virus protein. Nature 274 (1978) 687–689.

Mathes LE, Lewis MG, Olsen RG: Immunoprevention of feline leukemia: efficacy testing and antigenic analysis of soluble tumor-cell antigen vaccine. *In* Hardy WD Jr, Essex M, McClelland AJ (eds): Feline Leukemia Virus. New York, Elsevier/North Holland, 1980, 211–216.

McClelland AJ, Hardy WD Jr, Zuckerman EE: Prognosis of healthy feline leukemia virus infected cats. *In* Hardy WD Jr, Essex M, McClelland AJ (eds): Feline Leukemia Virus. New York, Elsevier/North Holland Inc, 1980, 121–126.

McCullough B, Schaller J, Shadduck JA, Yohn DS: Induction of malignant melanomas associated with fibrosarcomas in gnotobiotic cats inoculated with Gardner feline fibrosarcoma virus. J Natl Cancer Inst 48 (1972) 1893–1896.

McDonough SK, Larsen S, Brodey RS, Stock ND, Hardy WD Jr: A transmissible feline fibrosarcoma of viral origin. Cancer Res 31 (1971) 953–956.

Metzger RS, Mohanakumar T, Bolognesi DP: Antigenic relationships between murine, feline and primate RNA tumor viruses and membrane antigens of human leukemic cells. *In* Clemmesen J, Yohn DS (eds): Comparative Leukemia Research 1975. Basel, S. Karger, 1976, 549–554.

Naharro G, Dunn CY, Robbins KC: Analysis of the primary translational product and integrated DNA of a new feline sarcoma virus, GR-FeSV. Virology 125 (1983) 502–507.

Niman HL, Stephenson JR, Gardner MB, Roy-Burman P: RD-114 and feline leukaemia virus genome expression in natural lymphomas of domestic cats. Nature 266 (1977) 357–360.

Olsen RG, Mathes LE, Yohn DS: Complement-fixation-inhibition as a test for antibodies in cats and humans to C-type RNA tumor virus antigen. *In* Ito Y, Dutcher RM (eds): Comparative Leukemia Research 1973. Basel, S. Karger, 1975, 419–429.

Olsen RG, Hoover EA, Mathes LE, Heding L, Schaller JP: Immunization against feline oncornavirus disease using a killed tumor cell vaccine. Cancer Res 36 (1976) 3642–3646.

Olsen RG, Hoover EA, Schaller JP, Mathes LE, Wolff LH: Abrogation of resistance to feline oncornavirus disease by immunization with killed feline leukemia virus. Cancer Res 37 (1977) 2082–2085.

Olsen RG, Lewis M, Mathes LE, Hause W: Feline leukemia vaccine: efficacy testing in a large multicat household. Feline Pract 10 (5) (1980) 13–16.

Onions D, Jarrett O, Testa N, Frassoni F, Toth S: Selective effect of feline leukaemia virus on early erythroid precursors. Nature 296 (1982) 156–158.

Pearson LD, Snyder SP, Aldrich CD: Oncogenic activity of feline fibrosarcoma virus in newborn pigs. Am J Vet Res 34 (1973) 405–409.

Pedersen NC, Ott RL: Evaluation of a commercial feline leukemia virus vaccine for immunogenicity and efficacy. Feline Pract 15(6) (1985) 7–20.

Pedersen NC, Theilen GH, Werner LL: Safety and efficacy studies of live- and killed- feline leukemia virus vaccines. Am J Vet Res 40 (1979) 1120–1126.

Penrose M: Cat leukemia. Br Med J 1 (1970) 755.

Perryman LE, Hoover EA, Yohn DS: Immunologic reactivity of the cat: immunosuppression in experimental feline leukemia. J Natl Cancer Inst 49 (1972) 1357–1365.

Popovic M, Sarngadharan MG, Read E, Gallo RC: Detection, isolation, and continuous production of cytopathic retroviruses (HTLV-III) from patients with AIDS and pre-AIDS. Science 224 (1984) 497–500.

Post JE, Warren L: Reactivation of latent feline leukemia virus. *In* Hardy WD Jr, Essex M, McClelland AJ (eds): Feline Leukemia Virus. New York, Elsevier/North Holland Inc, 1980, 151–155.

Rasheed S, Barbacid M, Aaronson S, Gardner MB: Origin and biological properties of a new feline sarcoma virus. Virology 117 (1982) 238–244.

Rickard CG, Post JE, Noronha F, Barr LM: Interspecies infection by feline leukemia virus: serial cell-free transmission in dogs of malignant lymphomas induced by feline leukemia virus. *In* Dutcher RM, Chieco-Bianchi L (eds): Unifying Concepts of Leukemia. Basel, S. Karger, 1973, 102–112.

Robbins KC, Antoniades HN, Devare SG, Hunkapiller MW, Aaronson SA: Structural and immunological similarities between simian sarcoma virus gene product(s) and human platelet-derived growth factor. Nature 305 (1983) 605–608.

Rojko JL, Hoover EA, Mathes LE, Olsen RG, Schaller JP: Pathogenesis of experimental feline leukemia virus infection. J Natl Cancer Inst 63 (1979) 759–768.

Rojko JL, Hoover EA, Quackenbush SL, Olsen RG: Reactivation of latent feline leukaemia virus infection. Nature 298 (1982) 385–388.

Rous P: A sarcoma of the fowl transmissible by an agent separable from the tumor cells. J Exp Med 13 (1911) 397–411.

Roussel M, Saule S, Lagrou C, Rommens C, Beug H, Graf T, Stehelin D: Three new types of viral oncogene of cellular origin specific for haematopoietic cell transformation. Nature 281 (1979) 452–455.

Russell PH, Jarrett O: The occurrence of feline leukaemia virus neutralizing antibodies in cats. Int J Cancer 22 (1978) 351–357.

Salerno RA, Lehman ED, Larson VM, Hilleman MR: Feline leukemia virus envelope glycoprotein vaccine: preparation and evaluation of immunizing potency in guinea pig and cat. J Natl Cancer Inst 61 (1978) 1487–1494.

Sarma PS, Baskar JF, Gilden RV, Gardner MB, Huebner RJ: *In vitro* isolation and characterization of the GA strain of feline sarcoma virus. Proc Soc Exp Biol Med 137 (1971a) 1333–1336.

Sarma PS, Log T, Theilen GH: ST feline sarcoma virus. Biological characteristics and *in vitro* propagation. Proc Soc Exp Biol Med 137 (1971b) 1444–1448.

Sarma PS, Sharar AL, McDonough S: The SM strain of feline sarcoma virus. Biologic and antigenic characterization of virus. Proc Soc Exp Biol Med 140 (1972) 1365–1368.

Sarma PS, Log T: Subgroup classification of feline leukemia and sarcoma viruses by viral interference and neutralization tests. Virology 54 (1973) 160–169.

Sarma PS, Sharar A, Walters V, Gardner M: A survey of cats and humans for prevalence of feline leukemia-sarcoma virus neutralizing serum antibodies. Proc Soc Exp Biol Med 145 (1974) 560–564.

Sarma PS, Log T, Jain D, Hill PR, Huebner R: Differential host range of viruses of feline leukemia-sarcoma complex. Virology 64 (1975) 438–446.

Sarngadharan MG, Popovic M, Bruch L, Schüpbach J, Gallo RC: Antibodies reactive with human T-lymphotropic retroviruses (HTLV-III) in the serum of patients with AIDS. Science 224 (1984) 506–508.

Schneider R: The natural history of malignant lymphoma and sarcoma in cats and their associations with cancer in man and dog. J Am Vet Med Assoc 157 (1970) 1753–1758.

Schneider R: Human cancer in households containing cats with malignant lymphoma. Int J Cancer 10 (1972) 338–344.

Schneider R, Riggs JL: A serologic survey of veterinarians for antibody to feline leukemia virus. J Am Vet Med Assoc 162 (1973) 217–219.

Schnurrenberger PR, Martin RJ, Walker JF: Mortality in Illinois veterinarians. J Am Vet Med Assoc 170 (1977) 1071–1075.

Schüpbach J, Popovic M, Gilden RV, Gonda MA, Sarngadharan MG, Gallo RC: Serological analysis of a subgroup of human T-lymphotropic retroviruses (HTLV-III) associated with AIDS. Science 224 (1984) 503–505.

Shadduck JA, Albert DM, Niederkorn JY: Feline uveal melanomas induced with feline sarcoma virus: Potential model of the human counterpart. J Natl Cancer Inst 67 (1981) 619–627.

Sherr CJ, Sen A, Todaro GJ, Sliski A, Essex M: Pseudotypes of feline sarcoma virus contain an 85,000-dalton protein with feline oncornavirus-associated cell membrane antigen (FOCMA) activity. Proc Natl Acad Sci 75 (1978) 1505–1509.

Sherr CJ, Fedele LA, Oskarsson M, Maizel J, Vande Woude G: Molecular cloning of Snyder-Theilen feline leukemia and sarcoma viruses: comparative studies of feline sarcoma virus with its natural helper virus and with Moloney murine sarcoma virus. J Virol 34 (1980) 200–212.

Shibuya M, Hanafusa T, Hanafusa H, Stephenson JR: Homology exists among the transforming sequences of avian and feline sarcoma viruses. Proc Natl Acad Sci USA 77 (1980) 6536–6540.

Shih TY, Scolnick EM: Molecular biology of mammalian sarcoma viruses. *In* Klein G (ed): Viral Oncology. New York, Raven Press, 1980, 135–160.

Sliski AH, Essex M, Meyer C, Todaro G: Feline oncornavirus-associated cell membrane antigen: expression in transformed nonproducer mink cells. Science 196 (1977) 1336–1339.

Snyder HW Jr, Jones FR, Day NK, Hardy WD Jr: Isolation and characterization of circulating feline leukemia virus-immune complexes from plasma of persistently infected pet cats removed by *ex vivo* immunosorption. J Immunol 128 (1982) 2726–2730.

Snyder HW Jr, Singhal MC, Zuckerman EE, Jones FR, Hardy WD Jr: The feline oncornavirus-associated cell membrane antigen (FOCMA) is related to, but distinguishable from, FeLV-C gp70. Virology 131 (1983) 315–327.

Snyder HW Jr, Singhal MC, Zuckerman EE, Hardy WD Jr: Isolation of a new feline sarcoma virus (HZ1-FeSV): Biochemical and immunological characterization of its translation product. Virology 132 (1984a) 205–210.

Snyder HW Jr, Singhal MC, Hardy WD Jr, Jones FR: Clearance of feline leukemia virus from persistently infected pet cats treated by extracorporeal immunoadsorption is correlated with an enhanced antibody response to FeLV gp70. J Immunol 132 (1984b) 1538–1543.

Snyder SP: Spontaneous feline fibrosarcomas: transmissibility and ultrastructure of associated virus-like particles. J Natl Cancer Inst 47 (1971) 1079–1085.

Snyder SP, Theilen GH: Transmissible feline fibrosarcoma. Nature 221 (1969) 1074–1075.

Stann SE: Myelomonocytic leukemia in a cat. J Am Med Assoc 174 (1979) 722–725.

Stehelin D, Varmus HE, Bishop JM, Vogt PK: DNA related to the transforming gene(s) of avian sarcoma viruses is present in normal avian DNA. Nature 260 (1976) 170–173.

Stephenson JR, Essex M, Hino S, Hardy WD Jr, Aaronson SA: Feline oncornavirus-associated cell membrane antigen (FOCMA). Distinction between FOCMA and the major virion glycoprotein. Proc Natl Acad Sci USA 74 (1977a) 1219–1223.

Stephenson JR, Khan AS, Sliski AH, Essex M: Feline oncornavirus-associated cell membrane antigen: evidence for an immunologically cross-reactive feline sarcoma virus-coded protein. Proc Natl Acad Sci USA 74 (1977b) 5608–5612.

Sutherland JC, Mardiney MR Jr: Immune complex disease in the kidneys of lymphoma-leukemia patients: the presence of an oncornavirus-related antigen. J Natl Cancer Inst 50 (1973) 633–644.

Theilen GH: Continuing studies with transmissible feline fibrosarcoma virus in fetal and newborn sheep. J Am Vet Med Assoc 158 (1971) 1040–1045.

Theilen GH, Snyder SP, Wolfe LG, Landon JC: Biological studies with viral induced fibrosarcomas in cats, dogs, rabbits and non-human primates. *In* Dutcher RM (ed): Comparative Leukemia Research 1969. Basel, S. Karger, 1970, 393–400.

Todaro GJ: Interspecies transmission of mammalian retroviruses. *In* Klein G (ed): Viral Oncology. New York, Raven Press, 1980, 291–309.

Trainin Z, Wernicke D, Ungar-Waron H, Essex M: Suppression of the humoral antibody response in natural retrovirus infections. Science 220 (1983) 858–859.

Vedbrat SS, Rasheed S, Lutz H, Gonda MA, Ruscetti S, Gardner MB, Prensky W: Feline oncornavirus-associated cell membrane antigen: A viral and not a cellularly coded transformation-specific antigen of cat lymphomas. Virology 124 (1983) 445–461.

Weksler ME, Ryning FW, Hardy WD Jr: Immune complex disease in cancer. Clin Bull 5 (1975) 109–113.

Wolfe LG, Smith RD, Hoekstra J, Marczynska B, Smith RK, McDonald R, Northrop RL, Deinhardt F: Oncogenicity of feline fibrosarcoma viruses in marmoset monkeys: pathologic, virologic, and immunologic findings. J Natl Cancer Inst 49 (1972) 519–539.

Youngren SD, Noronha F: Transmissible feline sarcoma virus containing sequences related to the K-ras *onc* gene. *In* Hardy WD Jr (ed): Proc Fourth Internat FeLV Mtg, 1984, 16.

***Supplemental References***

Barlough JE: Serodiagnostic aids and management practice for feline retrovirus and coronavirus infections. Vet Clin North Am 14 (1984) 955–969.

Jarrett O: Update—Feline leukaemia virus. In Practice 7 (1985) 125–126.

Jarrett O, Edney ATB, Toth S, Hay D: Feline leukaemia virus–free lymphosarcoma in a specific pathogen free cat. Vet Rec 115 (1984) 249–250.

Kociba GJ, Weiser MG, Olsen RG: Enhanced susceptibility to feline leukemia virus in cats with *Haemobartonella felis* infection. Leuk Rev Int 1 (1983) 88–89 (Abstr Vet Bull 55 [1985] 1021).

Liu WT, Engelman RW, Trang LQ, Hau K, Good RA, Day NK: Appearance of cytotoxic antibody to viral gp70 on feline lymphoma cells (FL-74) in cats during ex vivo immunoadsorption therapy: quantitation, characterization, and association with remission of disease and disappearance of viremia. Proc Natl Acad Sci USA 81 (1984) 3516–3520.

Liu WT, Good RA, Trang LQ, Engelmann RW, Day NK: Remission of leukemia and loss of feline leukemia virus in cats injected with staphyloccocus protein A: association with increased circulating interferon and complement-dependent cytotoxic antibody. Proc Natl Acad Sci USA 81 (1984) 6471–6475.

Lutz H, Pedersen NC, Thielen GH: Course of feline leukemia virus infection and its detection by enzyme-linked immunosorbent assay and monoclonal antibodies. Am J Vet Res 44 (1983) 2054–2059.

Pedersen NC, Meric SM, Ho E, Johnson L, Plucher S, Theilen GH: The clinical significance of latent feline leukemia virus infection in cats. Feline Pract 14 (2) (1984) 32–48.

Rojko JL, Perdzock ML, Cheney CM, Kociba GJ: The effects of concurrent viruses on the susceptibility of cats to the feline leukemia virus and disease. Feline Pract 15 (2) (1985) 30–31.

Ziemiecki A, Hennig D, Gardner L, Ferdinand F-J, Friis RR, Bauer H, Pedersen NC, Johnson L, Theilen GH: Biological and biochemical characterization of a new isolate of feline sarcoma virus: Theilen-Pedersen (TP1-FeSV). Virology 138 (1984) 324–331.

# FELINE SYNCYTIUM-FORMING VIRUS INFECTION

NIELS C. PEDERSEN

Feline syncytium-forming virus (FeSFV) was first isolated from domestic cats in 1969 (Kasza et al., 1969; Riggs et al., 1969). These and subsequent isolates were obtained from various cat tumors (Hackett et al., 1970; Jarrett et al., 1974; McKissick and Lamont, 1970; Whitman et al., 1975). The virus has also been isolated from a cat with feline infectious peritonitis (Low et al., 1971), from cats with respiratory disease (Mochizuki et al., 1977; Takahashi et al., 1971), and from some of a group of healthy and diseased cats in a study of experimentally induced cystitis (Fabricant et al., 1969). Although FeSFV has been recovered from the tissues of many diseased cats, it was not thought to be involved in any of the illnesses.

The virus has also been isolated from many normal cats (Chappuis and Tektoff, 1974; Ellis et al., 1979; Gillespie and Scott, 1973; Hackett et al., 1970; Jarrett et al., 1974; Mochizuki and Konishi, 1979; Pedersen et al., 1980; Riggs et al., 1969). Furthermore, cats experimentally infected with FeSFV have remained healthy, at least for the periods that they were observed (Gaskin and Gillespie,

1973; Hackett et al., 1970; Kasza et al., 1969; McKissick and Lamont, 1970; Pedersen et al., 1980). Isolation from the CNS has been reported (Wilcox et al., 1984).

## Etiology

The FeSFV is an enveloped, RNA-containing virus of the family Retroviridae, subfamily Spumavirinae (Fenner, 1976). The virus has been called feline syncytial virus, feline foamy virus, and feline syncytia-forming virus. It is included in an unnamed genus of serologically distinct bovine, hamster, simian, and human syncytial viruses and has been placed in the family Retroviridae because it possesses the reverse transcriptase or RNA-dependent DNA-polymerase enzyme (Parks and Todaro, 1972) and because infectious proviral DNA is found in infected cells (Chiswell and Pringle, 1977, 1978, 1979). Feline leukemia virus (FeLV) and feline sarcoma virus are also members of the family Retroviridae, but because of their oncogenic potential and budding morphology they are classified in the subfamily Oncornavirinae, genus *Oncornavirus C* (Fenner, 1976).

The FeSFV virion is about 100 nm in diameter, with a central core about 45 nm in diameter, and its envelope has many short, surface spikes. The virus buds from the plasma membrane as in oncornaviruses (Chiswell and Pringle, 1979; Hackett and Manning, 1971). In tissue culture, the virus causes fusion of adjacent cells into large, multinucleated cells or syncytia. Although it has been considered nononcogenic, FeSFV has been reported to cause malignant transformation of kidney cells in vitro (McKissick and Lamont, 1970). There appears to be one major serotype of FeSFV and possibly several minor ones (Hackett and Manning, 1971).

## Epizootiology

### Incidence

The incidence of FeSFV infection varies greatly with the geographic area and the environment in which cats live. Among cats in the general population in California it rises dramatically after one year of age and reaches 50 per cent or more by three or four years (Fig. 7–73). In New York City, however, the infection rate is nearer 25 per cent. The incidence of FeSFV infection in apparently healthy cats is about 4 per cent in Tokyo (Mochizuki and Konishi, 1979) and ranges from 0 to 6 per cent in Australia (Ellis et al., 1979; Sabine and Love, 1973). Unlike almost all other infectious diseases of cats, FeSFV infection does not occur at a higher rate where cats are confined (catteries). In a survey of over 40 California catteries, 55 of 532 cats (9.4 per cent) of all ages were found to be infected, as contrasted with 477 of 1398 (34.1 per cent) of a random population of noncattery cats.

FeSFV infection is present in many cats. Any cat with serum antibodies to the virus, as detected by virus neutralization (Jarrett et al., 1974; Mochizuki and Konishi, 1979), immunodiffusion (Gaskin and Gillespie, 1973), or immunofluorescence (Pedersen et al., 1980), is infected.

### Transmission

Cats become infected by several routes. Although earlier studies reported that in-utero infection was infrequent

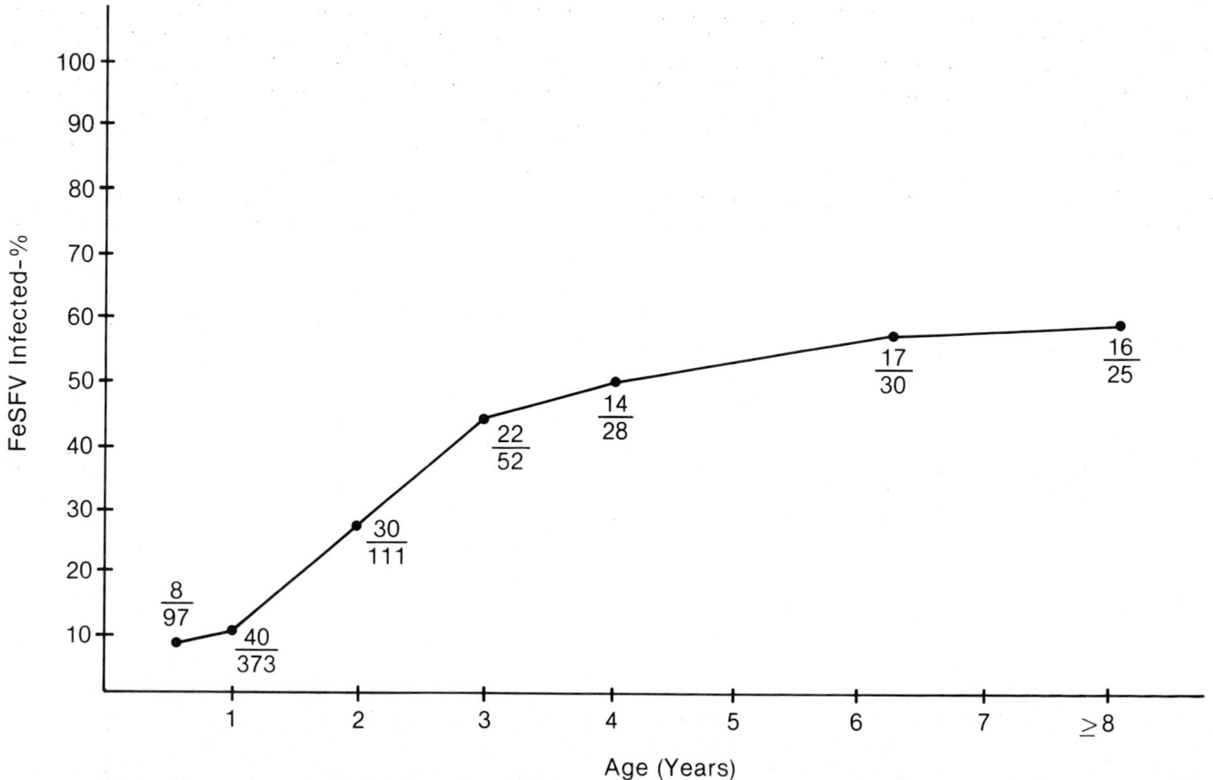


**Figure 7–73** The incidence with age of FeSFV infection among cats from Northern California.

(Gaskin and Gillespie, 1973), we have found that 25 to 50 per cent of kittens born to FeSFV-infected queens are infected at birth. Why some fetuses within the same litter are spared is not understood. Infected and uninfected kittens can be distinguished at birth by culturing the buffy coat of their blood. In addition, the uninfected siblings lose their maternal precipitating antibodies by two to four weeks of age (Gaskin and Gillespie, 1973) and their fluorescent antibody titers by six to eight weeks of age. In contrast, the maternal antibody titers in infected kittens drop during this same period but rise after 8 to 10 weeks. Gillespie and Scott (1973) suggested that infection could occur when newborn kittens nurse infected queens. I have found, however, that this route of exposure does not lead to infection.

Although in-utero exposure is one means of infection, it is apparently not the most important. Serologic studies in California demonstrated a progressive rise in the infection rate from one year of age onward (Fig. 7–73). The mechanism by which these cats are infected is not known. Although the virus is shed in high levels from the oropharynx, controlled cat-to-cat contact does not often lead to infection. In one experiment, I deliberately housed infected and uninfected cats together for six months to three years. Only one of five susceptible cats became infected and then only after being in contact with infected cats for two years. We have also housed infected cats with uninfected cats within a cattery and have not seen any spread of the virus from cat to cat. These observations seem inconsistent with the dramatic rise in the infection rate that occurs in outdoor cats.

Clues to the natural mode of transmission of FeSFV may be found by comparing confined cattery cats with cats that are allowed to roam more or less freely. We have noticed a much lower incidence of cat bites when cats are kept in catteries. Because virus is present in the oral secretions and is infectious mainly by parenteral inoculation, such a route of exposure seems plausible. It does not seem likely, however, that this could be the sole explanation for the rapid infection rate in free-roaming cats. There is also a greater exposure to rodents and birds, and mosquitoes are more apt to be a problem when cats are allowed outdoors.

## Pathogenesis

After infection the virus can be isolated from virtually any tissue. The virus is manifested only after growth of the tissue in culture for one to four cell passages. This feature makes the infection a nuisance to cell culturists attempting to establish cell lines from cat tissues. Within the body, the virus is found in a complete form only in the secretions of the oropharynx. It cannot be identified by electron microscopy in other tissues or in the blood. The virus is not present in the plasma or red cell pack of whole blood. The buffy coat from peripheral blood, however, is a rich source of infectious material (Shroyer and Shalaby, 1978). In the blood the viral genome apparently exists in white blood cells, even though virus replication is somehow suppressed in vivo. In this respect, FeSFV infection of cats resembles bovine leukemia virus infection (Miller et al., 1969). Cocultivation of blood cells with fetal cat cells in vitro appears to allow the virus to be expressed. Although the virus is latent in the blood and other tissues, cells within the oropharynx seem to be actively producing intact virus, as evidenced by the isolation of virus from oropharyngeal secretions (Ellis et al., 1979; Jarrett et al., 1974; Shroyer and Shalaby, 1978).

The infection is most easily reproduced by parenteral inoculation of cats with infectious tissue or tissue culture–propagated virus. The infection cannot be readily transmitted by the oral route. After parenteral inoculation, serum antibodies to FeSFV appear in about three weeks, at which time the virus can be isolated by cultivating buffy coat leukocytes and platelets with fetal cat cells or by exposing cells to oropharyngeal secretions. After parenteral inoculation, all cats become infected for life.

Serum antibodies in infected cats will neutralize FeSFV in vitro. The existence of latent FeSFV infection in blood and other tissues despite high virus-neutralizing antibody titers in the serum is a fascinating feature of syncytium-forming virus infections of many species of animals. Possible mechanisms for this phenomenon have been suggested by Hooks and coworkers (1976). The ability of the virus to spread between contiguous cells in the presence of neutralizing antibodies may result from the failure of antibody and complement to lyse infected cells or the relative resistance of the virus to the action of interferon.

## Clinical Features

After experimental infection, I have not observed any fever or outward signs of illness, and the hemograms have remained normal during an observation period of three years. In an attempt to link latent FeSFV infection statistically with specific diseases, I compared the incidence of FeSFV infection in healthy and ill cats in general and in healthy cats and cats with specific disorders. The incidence of FeSFV infection in a large, randomly selected group of ill cats (non–cancer-bearing) at the teaching hospital at the University of California was not significantly different from that in healthy, age-matched cats in the same population (Table 7–18). A study of a smaller number of cats from the New York City area also showed no relationship between illness in general and chronic FeSFV infection. It can be concluded, however, that FeSFV infection is not an important cause of noncancerous illnesses in cats.

Although there was no significant difference between the incidence of FeSFV infection and that of a broad

**Table 7–18 FeSFV Infection and Its Relationship to Non–Cancer-Associated Illnesses in Cats***

| AGE (YRS) | FeSFV-INFECTED/ TOTAL CATS | | | |
|---|---|---|---|---|
| | Normal Cats | Ill Cats† | $X^2$‡ | P§ |
| 3 | 22/52 | 32/62 | 0.98 | > 0.05 |
| 4 | 14/28 | 41/60 | 2.41 | > 0.05 |
| 5–7 | 17/30 | 73/114 | 0.55 | > 0.05 |
| >8 | 16/25 | 116/168 | 0.26 | > 0.05 |

*At the Veterinary Medical Teaching Hospital, University of California, Davis.

†Ill cats are cats with illnesses of all types except myeloproliferative disease, lymphosarcoma, and other types of cancer.

‡$X^2$ = chi square.

§P = probability, P > 0.05 not significantly different.

**Table 7–19 FeSFV Infection and Its Relationship to Myeloproliferative Disorders in Cats***

| AGE (YRS) | FeSFV-INFECTED/ TOTAL CATS: Normal Cats | Cats with Myeloproliferative Disorders | $X^2$† | P‡ |
|---|---|---|---|---|
| 2–8+ | 99/246 | 15/25 | 26.96 | < 0.001 |

*At the Veterinary Medical Teaching Hospital, University of California, Davis.
†$X^2$ = chi square.
‡P = probability, P > 0.05 not significantly different.

range of illnesses, we were interested in learning whether certain diseases were related to FeSFV infection at a higher incidence than could be accounted for by chance. Since FeSFV is a retrovirus and is present as a chronic infection, we were particularly interested in comparing the incidence of infection and cancer. In the California cat population, cats with myeloproliferative disease had a significantly higher incidence of FeSFV infection than age-matched healthy cats (Table 7–19). This could not be accounted for by a linkage between feline leukemia virus (FeLV) and FeSFV infections, as we observed that both infections occurred independently of one another. Cats with lymphosarcoma appeared also to have a higher rate of FeSFV infection than healthy cats of the same age, but this relationship was not statistically significant (Table 7–20). Likewise, no significant relationship was observed between FeSFV infection and a composite group of cats with non-FeLV-associated carcinomas and sarcomas (Table 7–21).

FeSFV infection has been statistically linked to chronic progressive polyarthritis of cats (Pedersen et al., 1980). This disorder occurs predominantly in males two to five years of age, either as a periosteal proliferative polyarthritis similar to Reiter's arthritis of man or as a more insidious, deforming condition resembling human and canine rheumatoid arthritis. In the initial series of cats with this disease, all were infected with FeSFV and two thirds with FeLV. Both viral infections occur at a much higher incidence in this disease than in age- and sex-matched normal cats from the same population. The disease has not been reproduced, however, in male cats inoculated with either or both viruses. It is possible that chronic progressive polyarthritis occurs only in certain genetically predisposed male cats infected with FeSFV. Feline leukemia virus may play a direct role in the pathogenesis, or it may potentiate FeSFV infection by altering the host's normal immune reaction.

**Table 7–20 FeSFV Infection and Its Relationship to Lymphosarcoma in Cats***

| AGE (YRS) | FeSFV-INFECTED/ TOTAL CATS: Normal Cats | Cats with Lymphosarcoma | $X^2$† | P‡ |
|---|---|---|---|---|
| 3–5 | 14/28 | 11/13 | 4.47 | < 0.05, > 0.02 |
| 5–7 | 17/30 | 21/25 | 0.72 | > 0.05 |
| > 8 | 16/25 | 21/26 | 1.80 | > 0.05 |

*At the Veterinary Medical Teaching Hospital, University of California, Davis.
†$X_2$ = chi square.
‡P = probability, P > 0.05 significantly different.

**Table 7–21 FeSFV Infection and its Relationship to Nonlymphoid and Nonmyeloid Cancers in Cats***

| AGE (YRS) | FeSFV-INFECTED/ TOTAL CATS: Normal Cats | Cats with Cancer | $X^2$† | P‡ |
|---|---|---|---|---|
| 3–6 | 53/110 | 9/25 | 5.05 | < 0.05, > 0.02 |
| 7–8+ | 16/25 | 30/48 | 0.02 | 0.99 |

*At the Veterinary Medical Teaching Hospital, University of California, Davis.
†$X^2$ = chi square.
‡P = probability, P > 0.05 not significantly different.

## Conclusion

Although the full significance of FeSFV infection of cats has not been determined, it seems to be statistically linked with myeloproliferative disease and chronic progressive polyarthritis. Although there may be a direct cause-and-effect relationship between infection and disease, it is also possible that both are related to yet other factors. The fact that FeSFV is actively shed from the oropharynx while at the same time it is present in a latent form in the tissues is unique to virus infections. If FeSFV does cause disease, it would be predicted that it would do so in a manner similar to other chronic and so-called slow virus infections, i.e., unusual diseases occurring at a low incidence over a long period of time.

## REFERENCES


Chappuis G, Tektoff J: Isolement et identification du virus syncytial félin. Ann Microbiol (Paris) 125A (1974) 371–386.

Chiswell DJ, Pringle CR: Infectious DNA from cells infected with feline syncytium-forming virus (Spumavirinae). J Gen Virol 36 (1977) 551–555.

Chiswell DJ, Pringle CR: Feline syncytium-forming virus proviral DNA: Time of synthesis and relationship to the host cell genome. Virology 90 (1978) 344–350.

Chiswell DJ, Pringle CR: Feline syncytium-forming virus: Identification of a virion-associated reverse transcriptase and electron microscopical observations of infected cells. J Gen Virol 43 (1979) 429–434.

Ellis TM, MacKenzie JS, Wilcox GE, Cook RD: Isolation of feline syncytia-forming virus from oropharyngeal swabs of cats. Aust Vet J 55 (1979) 202–203.

Fabricant CG, Rich LJ, Gillespie JH: Feline viruses. XI. Isolation of a virus similar to a myxovirus from cats in which urolithiasis was experimentally induced. Cornell Vet 59 (1969) 667–672.

Fenner F: Classification and nomenclature of viruses. Second report of the International Committee on Taxonomy of Viruses. Intervirology 7 (1976) 1–115.

Gaskin JM, Gillespie JH: Detection of feline syncytia-forming virus carrier state with a microimmunodiffusion test. Am J Vet Res 34 (1973) 245–247.

Gillespie JH, Scott FW: Feline viral infections. Am Vet Sci Comp Med 17 (1973) 163–200.

Hackett AJ, Pfiester A, Arnstein P: Biological properties of a syncytia-forming agent isolated from domestic cats (feline

syncytia-forming virus). Proc Soc Exp Biol 135 (1970) 899–904.
Hackett AJ, Manning JS: Comments on feline syncytia-forming virus. J Am Vet Med Assoc 158 (1971) 498–954.
Hooks JJ, Burns W, Hayashi K, Geis S, Notkins AL: Viral spread in the presence of neutralizing antibody: Mechanisms of persistence in foamy virus infection. Infect Immun 14 (1976) 1172–1178.
Jarrett O, Hay D, Laird HM: Infection by feline syncytium-forming virus in Britain. Vet Rec 94 (1974) 200–201.
Kasza L, Hayward AHS, Betts AO: Isolation of a virus from a cat sarcoma in an established canine melanoma cell line. Res Vet Sci 10 (1969) 216–218.
Low RJ, Colby ED, Covington HJ, Benirschke K: Report on the isolation of an agent from cell cultures of kidneys from domestic cats. Vet Rec 88 (1971) 557–559.
McKissick GE, Lamont PH: Characteristics of a virus isolated from a feline fibrosarcoma. J Virol 5 (1970) 247–257.
Miller JM, Miller LD, Olson C, Gillette KG: Virus-like particles in phytohemagglutinin-stimulated lymphocyte cultures with reference to bovine lymphosarcoma. J Natl Cancer Inst 43 (1969) 1297–1305.
Mochizuki M, Konishi S, Ogata M: Studies on cytopathogenic viruses from cats with respiratory infections. III. Isolation and certain properties of feline herpesviruses. Jpn J Vet Sci 39 (1977) 27–37.
Mochizuki M, Konishi S: Feline syncytial virus spontaneously detected in feline cell cultures. Jpn J Vet Sci 41 (1979) 351–362.
Parks WP, Todaro GJ: Biological properties of syncytium-forming ("foamy") viruses. Virology 47 (1972) 673–683.
Pedersen NC, Pool RR, O'Brien T: Feline chronic progressive polyarthritis. Am J Vet Res 41 (1980) 522–535.
Riggs IL, Oshiro LS, Taylor DON, Lennette EH: Syncytium-forming agent isolated from domestic cats. Nature 222 (1969) 1190–1191.
Sabine M, Love DN: Feline "foamy" viruses: Incidence in Australia. Arch Ges Virusforsch 43 (1973) 397–400.
Scott FW: Feline syncytial virus. J Am Vet Med Assoc 158 (1971) 946–948.
Shroyer EL, Shalaby MR: Isolation of feline syncytia-forming virus from oropharyngeal swab samples and buffy coat cells. Am J Vet Res 39 (1978) 555–560.
Takahashi E, Konishi S, Ogata M: Studies on cytopathogenic viruses isolated from cats with respiratory infections. II. Characterization of feline picornaviruses. Jpn J Vet Sci 33 (1971) 81–87.
Whitman JE Jr, Cockrell KO, Hall WT, Gilmore CE: An unusual case of feline leukemia and an associated syncytium-forming virus. Am J Vet Res 36 (1975) 873–880.
Wilcox GE, Flower RLP, Cook RD: Recovery of viral agents from the central nervous system of cats. Vet Microbiol 9 (1984) 355–366.

# FELINE UROLITHIASIS

CATHERINE G. FABRICANT

Infection has been considered a major cause of urolithiasis in cats and humans (Krabbe, 1949; Scardino et al., 1963; Vermeulen et al., 1955). However, others (Dorn et al., 1973; Fabricant and Rich, 1971; Foster, 1967; Hogle, 1970; Holzworth, 1966; Rich, 1969; Schechter, 1970) reported that urines of obstructed cats were free of bacteria. The bacteria (enteric) isolated from occasional urine specimens could be characterized as secondary invaders (Fabricant, 1973). Given the location of the urinary orifice, these bacteria might easily be introduced accidentally during the course of the disease by therapeutic or diagnostic catheterization (Fabricant, 1979b).

## Studies Leading to Recognition of a Viral Etiology

Rich (1969) was the first to suspect a possible viral etiology. He induced urinary obstruction in conventionally reared (CR) male cats by inoculating them with a filtrate of urine from obstructed cats (Rich and Fabricant, 1969). Our isolation of a calicivirus from urine of an obstructed Manx cat supported such a hypothesis, particularly since three of four CR male cats developed urinary obstruction following inoculation with the virus (Rich and Fabricant, 1969). This virus was called the Manx virus only for purposes of identification. The virus is antigenically similar to some of the other feline caliciviruses associated with respiratory disease. In serum neutralizing tests, the Manx virus was found to be partially neutralized by antisera to some of these caliciviruses.

The results of a more extensive experiment with the Manx virus in CR male cats did not define its role in the pathogenesis of urolithiasis (Fabricant and Rich, 1971). Twelve of 15 cats in this experiment developed the disease following inoculation or exposure to aerosols of the virus (Rich et al., 1971). The Manx virus was found to persist in the urinary tract for only four days (Fabricant and Rich, 1971). Furthermore, a second virus, identified as the feline syncytium-forming virus (FeSFV), was isolated from the bladders and kidneys of all 12 obstructed cats (Fabricant et al., 1969).

These results suggested that the viral etiology of urolithiasis was more complicated than the initial experiment with the Manx virus in CR cats had indicated. Although the Manx virus appeared to have a role in inducing the disease in the latter experiment, it did not seem to be a primary one. We speculated that the Manx virus might act as an inciter—reactivating a latent virus (such as the FeSFV) of the urinary tract (Fabricant and Rich, 1971).

The reactivated virus might then proliferate in the urinary tract, causing cellular damage and disease (as suggested by Jensen, 1967). We speculated further that two or more viruses might act synergistically to induce the disease (Fabricant and Rich, 1971).

The source and peculiar cytopathic effects (CPE) in infected cell cultures of a third virus isolated from feline urinary tract tissues supported these hypotheses (Fabricant et al., 1971). This virus was characterized as a herpesvirus (Fabricant and Gillespie, 1974). It was found to be antigenically distinct from the feline rhinotracheitis herpesvirus (FRV) associated with feline respiratory disease. This herpesvirus had not been described previously. Not only was the virus antigenically different from FRV, but it was also much more strongly cell-associated than the latter virus. That is, little or no infectious virus was released from infected tissues or cell cultures. Even at present, primary isolation attempts require that cell cultures be explanted from tissues. These cell cultures are subpassaged and held for prolonged periods of time (months) before virus isolation may be made.

The source of the cell-associated herpesvirus (CAHV) was of particular interest. It was first isolated from pooled kidney tissues of apparently normal five-week-old kittens. Another isolation of CAHV was made from kidney tissue of a four and a half-month-old kitten and was considered especially significant. This kitten had died of acute urolithiasis one month after contracting a respiratory disease caused by a calicivirus (Fabricant et al., 1971).

In addition, the peculiar CPE observed in CAHV-infected cell cultures suggested that this virus might have a role in feline urolithiasis. The virus induced not only the expected herpesvirus cytopathic effects (i.e., intranuclear inclusions, syncytia, and cytomegalic cells in these cultures) but also changes that had not been described previously, including (1) a variety of intracellular and extracellular chemical crystalline formations; (2) intracellular and extracellular lipid droplets; and (3) structures in the supernatant cell culture fluids that closely resembled the obstructing urethral plugs found in cats. These latter structures were designated tissue culture (TC) calculi for purposes of reference. When examined histologically they were found to consist of crystals, dead cells, and amorphous proteinaceous materials (Fabricant et al., 1971). One of the CAHV-induced chemical crystalline types was identified as cholesterol by structure, polarized light microscopy, and mass spectroscopy (Fabricant et al., 1973).

It was clear that further experimental studies required specific pathogen–free (SPF)* cats to establish the potential roles of the three isolated viruses in urolithiasis. These SPF cats not only had to be free of the three viruses, but they had to be from a colony without a history of "spontaneous" cases of urinary obstruction. Fortunately cats from such a colony were available to us. The colony was established by the Department of Pathology at the New York State College of Veterinary Medicine, Cornell University, under contract with the National Institutes of Health to study feline leukemia. Since 1975, the colony has been maintained at the College by the Division of Laboratory Animal Services.

*The SPF status is frequently misunderstood. It does not imply that animals are germ-free or free of *all* microbes. It does signify that the animals come from a closed colony maintained in isolation and that they are known to be free of those microbial pathogens that have been tested for and found to be absent.

## SPF Cat Studies Establishing a Primary Etiologic Role for Herpesvirus

A preliminary experiment with eight SPF male cats under one year of age was performed. Four of the cats were inoculated with the Manx virus and four with both the CAHV and Manx viruses. The experimental cats were housed in separate Horsfall-type isolation cages and fed the moist Prescription Diet (P/D Diet*) throughout the experiment (Fabricant, 1975). In this experiment, three of the cats developed urinary obstructions. Two cats had been inoculated with both viruses, and the third cat had been inoculated with the Manx virus alone. Herpesvirus isolations were made from cell cultures explanted from the kidneys and bladders of the three cats. This finding indicated that the cat inoculated with the Manx virus alone must have been accidentally infected with the CAHV.

The results of this experiment supported several theories. (1) A CAHV played a role in feline urolithiasis, since this virus was isolated from the urinary tract tissues of the three obstructed cats. (2) There was a Manx calicivirus–herpesvirus interaction in the disease. (3) Indirect evidence from this experiment indicated that the FeSFV did not have a primary role in feline urolithiasis, since the disease was induced in its absence. (No antibodies to FeSFV were detected in either pre- or postinoculation urine or serum samples.)

The results of a second SPF experiment were unequivocal. In this experiment 18 SPF cats between three and four and a half months of age were divided into three groups of six cats each. One group (all males) was inoculated with the Manx virus, a second group (five males and one female accidentally included) was inoculated with CAHV, and a third group (all males) was inoculated with both viruses (Fabricant, 1977). The cats were housed in Horsfall-type isolation cages and fed the moist Clinicare Diet (C/D Diet†) during the experiment.

Five of the cats inoculated with the CAHV alone developed clinical signs of urolithiasis. The sixth cat, the female, did not develop clinical signs of the disease. Four of the cats with clinical signs were found to have cystitis and two of these also had urethral obstruction. The herpesvirus was reisolated from cell cultures of urinary tract tissues of all six cats and from the ovarian tissue of the female cat. Serum-neutralizing (SN) antibodies against the CAHV were found only in postinoculation (PI) serum samples of the six cats (Fabricant, 1981).

One cat, in the group inoculated with Manx virus alone, developed clinical signs of the disease late in the experiment. It was found to have both cystitis and a bladder stone. Since only herpesvirus was isolated from the kidney cell cultures of this cat, we concluded that this cat must have been accidentally infected with CAHV. Manx virus was not isolated from any of the cell cultures explanted from urinary tract tissues of these cats. SN antibodies against the Manx, but not the CAHV, were detected only in PI serum samples (Fabricant, 1981).

All six cats inoculated with both Manx virus and CAHV developed clinical signs of the disease. Six were found to have cystitis, and four were also found to have urethral obstruction. CAHV (but not Manx virus) was reisolated

*Hills Division of Riviana Foods, Inc, Topeka, KS.
†Agway, Inc, Syracuse, NY.

from cell cultures of the urinary tract tissues of the six cats. SN antibodies against both CAHV and Manx virus were detected only in PI serum samples of all these cats (Fabricant, 1981).

Several conclusions could be drawn from this experiment: (1) infection with the CAHV alone induced all the manifestations of feline urolithiasis; (2) infection with the Manx virus alone did not induce the disease, since the only cat in this group that developed the disease was accidentally infected with CAHV; (3) the results suggested that the Manx virus might act as a secondary complicating factor, since all six cats in this group had signs of clinical disease and cystitis, whereas four also had urethral obstruction; (4) since the disease was induced in the absence of the FeSFV, we surmised either that this virus does not have a role in the disease or that it may act as a secondary complicating factor in dual infections with CAHV.

## Further SPF Cat Studies

Unpublished experimental data indicate that (SPF) queens infected with the herpesvirus may transmit the virus either in utero (vertically) or by contact (horizontally). Potential horizontal transmission was indicated by the accidental infection with CAHV of one cat in each of the SPF cat experiments previously discussed. That the CAHV might also be transmitted vertically was suggested by isolations of the virus from ovarian tissues of infected queens (Fabricant, 1977, 1979b). In later experiments, in utero transmission was indicated when CAHV was isolated from fetuses of a queen infected with the virus during gestation. Data from these experiments also indicate that, once infected, a queen may continue to transmit the virus to succeeding litters. Further, a queen may transmit the virus to other cats by contact (Fabricant, 1984).

Experiments on the effects of a dry diet on the urinary tract of (SPF) cats do not support an etiologic role in the pathogenesis of urolithiasis in these cats (Fabricant and Lein, 1984).

## Discussion

Experimental studies in SPF cats have demonstrated that infection with CAHV causes urolithiasis (Fabricant, 1975, 1977, 1979b). All the manifestations of the disease were reproduced in cats after infection with the herpesvirus (Fabricant, 1977).

Other viruses, including herpesvirus, are known to cause diseases of the urinary tract in humans and animals (Fabricant, 1979a). For example herpes simplex, herpes zoster, and cytomegalovirus were respectively reported to cause urethritis (Jensen, 1967; Smith and Aquino, 1971), cystitis (Jensen, 1967; Meyer et al., 1959), and interstitial nephritis (Morrison and Wright, 1977) in humans. Gernert and coworkers (1967) also reported that herpes zoster caused urine retention in humans. Jensen (1967) and Smith and Aquino (1971), in their reviews, reported that canine herpesvirus infections caused tubular necrosis and multiple cortical hemorrhages in puppy kidneys.

Defining the etiologic role of a herpesvirus in disease is particularly difficult because these viruses are known to establish persistent inapparent infections (Rapp and Jerkofsky, 1973). Studies of such infections in urinary tract disease may be further complicated by secondary adventitious infections or transient viruses excreted through the kidneys (Fabricant, 1979a).

Although herpesvirus infections may be acquired early in life with a high incidence of infection, they do not necessarily produce clinical disease at the same time (Rapp and Jerkofsky, 1973). These infections, however, persist for life with the viral DNA integrated within infected cells and replicated during cell division. Occasionally a cell may be "turned on" to produce a complete virus without development of overt clinical disease. However, if the host-parasite equilibrium is disturbed by lowered resistance due to secondary infections or other factors, the silent herpesvirus may be reactivated to cause clinical disease (Rapp and Jerkofsky, 1973). Further, the interval between infection and development of clinical disease may be prolonged, making it exceedingly difficult to establish a relationship between an etiologic agent and the disease. An example of this is shingles in adults, which was found to be the disease caused by reactivated herpes zoster acquired with chicken pox during childhood.

The feline herpesvirus causing urolithiasis has all these characteristics. As mentioned in the discussion of experimental studies, this virus may be transmitted in utero from an infected queen. Clinical disease may not be evident, since the first isolation of the virus was made from kidney tissues of apparently normal kittens. Thus infection may occur long before clinical disease is manifested.

## Conclusions

The herpesvirus etiology of feline urolithiasis is supported by the following experimental evidence:

1. SPF cats infected with CAHV developed the disease.
2. All the manifestations of the disease were reproduced in the infected cats (straining to urinate, hematuria, cystitis, and urethral obstruction).
3. The disease was induced in cats infected with the CAHV alone.
4. The disease was induced in CAHV infected cats fed moist diets (either P/D or C/D prescription diets).
5. Koch's postulates were fulfilled: CAHV was reisolated from urinary tract tissues of cats that developed the disease.

## References

Dellers RW: Infectious bovine rhinotracheitis virus induced abortion in cattle. Ithaca, Cornell University, PhD Thesis, 1975.

Dorn CR, Saueressig S, Schmidt DA: Factors affecting risk of urolithiasis-cystitis-urethritis in cats. Am J Vet Res 34 (1973) 433–436.

Fabricant CG: Urolithiasis: A review with recent viral studies. Feline Pract 3(1) (1973) 22–25, 28–30.

Fabricant CG: Feline urolithiasis. *In* Nutrition and Management of Dogs and Cats. St. Louis, Ralston Purina, 1975, 1–5.

Fabricant CG: Herpesvirus-induced urolithiasis in specific pathogen–free male cats. Am J Vet Res 38 (1977) 1837–1842.

Fabricant CG: Viruses associated with diseases of the urinary tract. Vet Clin North Am 9 (1979a) 631–644.

Fabricant CG: Herpesvirus induced feline urolithiasis—a review. Comp Immunol Microbiol Infect Dis 1 (1979b) 121–134.

Fabricant CG: Serological responses to the cell associated herpesvirus and the Manx calicivirus of SPF male cats with herpesvirus induced urolithiasis. Cornell Vet 71 (1981) 59–68.
Fabricant CG: The feline urologic syndrome induced by infection with a cell-associated herpesvirus. Vet Clin North Am 14 (1984) 493–502.
Fabricant CG, Gillespie JH: Identification and characterization of a second feline herpesvirus. Infect Immun 9 (1974) 460–466.
Fabricant CG, Lein DH: Feline urolithiasis neither induced nor exacerbated by feeding a dry diet. J Am Anim Hosp Assoc 20 (1984) 213–220.
Fabricant CG, Rich LJ: Microbial studies of feline urolithiasis. J Am Vet Med Assoc 158 (1971) 976–980.
Fabricant CG, Gillespie JH, Krook L: Intracellular and extracellular mineral crystal formation induced by viral infection of cell cultures. Infect Immun 3 (1971) 416–419.
Fabricant CG, Krook L, Gillespie JH: Virus-induced cholesterol crystals. Science 181 (1973) 566–567.
Fabricant CG, Rich LJ, Gillespie JH: Feline viruses. XI. Isolation of a virus similar to a myxovirus from cats in which urolithiasis was experimentally induced. Cornell Vet 59 (1969) 667–672.
Foster SJ: The "urolithiasis" syndrome in male cats; a statistical analysis of the problems, with clinical observations. J Small Anim Pract 8 (1967) 207–214.
Gernert JE, Bischoff AJ, Bors E: Herpes zoster as a cause of urinary retention. Urol Int (Basel) 22 (1967) 222–226.
Hogle RM: Antibacterial-agent sensitivity of bacteria isolated from dogs and cats. J Am Vet Med Assoc 156 (1970) 761–764.
Holzworth J: Urolithiasis is cats. *In* Kirk RW (ed): Current Veterinary Therapy. Philadelphia, W B Saunders Company, 1966, 410–412.
Jensen MM: Viruses and kidney diseases. Am J Med 43 (1967) 897–911.
Krabbe A: Urolithiasis in dogs and cats. Vet Rec 61 (1949) 751–775.
Meyer R, Brown HP, Harrison JH: Herpes zoster involving the urinary bladder. N Engl J Med 260 (1959) 1062–1065.
Morrison WI, Wright NG: Viruses associated with renal disease of man and animals. Prog Med Virol 23 (1977) 22–50.
Rapp F, Jerkofsky MA: Persistent and latent infections. *In* Kaplan AS (ed): The Herpesviruses. New York, Academic Press, 1973, 271–289.
Rich LJ: Feline urethral obstruction: Etiologic factors and pathogenesis. Ithaca, Cornell University, PhD Thesis, 1969.
Rich LJ, Fabricant CG: Urethral obstruction in male cats: transmission studies. Can J Comp Med 33 (1969) 164–165.
Rich LJ, Fabricant CG, Gillespie JH: Virus induced urolithiasis in male cats. Cornell Vet 61 (1971) 542–553.
Scardino PL, Prince CL, Su TC: An aftermath of pyelonephritis. J Urol 90 (1963) 516–520.
Schechter RD: The significance of bacteria in feline cystitis and urolithiasis. J Am Vet Med Assoc 156 (1970) 1567–1573.
Smith RD, Aquino J: Viruses and the kidney. Med Clin North Am 55 (1971) 89–106.
Vermeulen CW, Miller GH, Sawyer JB: Some nonsurgical aspects of urolithiasis. Med Clin North Am 39 (1955) 281–295.

# OTHER VIRUS INFECTIONS

JEAN HOLZWORTH

## CATPOX

Infection with a virus of the pox family was first recognized in exotic zoo cats in Moscow, and since the late 1970s sporadic infections among domestic cats have been reported in Britain and continental Europe.

Lesions appearing first on the face and limbs may ultimately involve the whole body. Measuring 3 to 6 mm in diameter, the lesions may be flat, red, and hairless, or they may take the form of thick scabs covering red areas or purulent ulcers. Mild ocular inflammation and lung infection occur in some cats. A striking sign may be edema of the head, neck, and distal extremities.

Characteristic intracytoplasmic inclusion bodies are demonstrable histologically in affected tissues. The infection is also diagnosed by virus isolation and serologic testing of paired samples obtained in the acute and convalescent stages of an illness.

Pox infection of domestic cats is discussed in more detail in the chapter on skin disorders.

## ENTERIC VIRUSES

Diarrheas for which the cause cannot be identified by procedures available in routine veterinary practice are commonplace in cats. The viruses of panleukopenia and feline infectious peritonitis, as well as less pathogenic coronaviruses, reovirus, and calicivirus, may cause diarrhea of varying degrees of severity. Still other viruses have been seen in, or recovered from, feces of normal or diarrheic cats (Baldwin, 1983).

Rotavirus, measuring about 60 to 70 nm and characterized by a wheel-like structure, is an important cause of diarrhea in the young of many species, especially human infants and calves. The upper parts of the villous epithelial cells of the small intestine are the principal site of replication, and destruction of the tips of the villi leads to malabsorption and diarrhea.

Rotavirus has been seen by electron microscopy and has also been isolated from cats with diarrhea (Chrystie et al., 1979; Hoshino et al., 1981a; Snodgrass et al., 1979).

When passed to a colostrum-deprived kitten, the isolate caused diarrhea (Snodgrass et al., 1979).

Because rotavirus is unenveloped, it is resistant to commonly used disinfectants and might become a troublesome inhabitant if it became established in a cattery, shelter, or laboratory where young kittens are present. For symptomatic infection, maintenance of hydration until the intestinal villi regenerate is the most important measure of treatment.

Astrovirus, measuring about 28 nm in diameter and taking the form of a five- or six-pointed star when negatively stained, has been seen by electron microscopy in feces of humans and several animal species. The virus multiplies in the mature villous epithelium of the small intestine and has been shown by transmission studies to cause mild constitutional signs. Astrovirus has been seen in the feces of a four-month-old kitten with diarrhea (Hoshino et al., 1981b).

A noncultivable enteric virus (about 29 nm in diameter) was seen in a sample from a young adult cat with no signs of gastrointestinal illness. The virus, larger than that of panleukopenia but smaller than feline calicivirus, was spherical, with no characteristic surface configuration (Hoshino and Scott, unpublished data).

Further study is needed to determine whether these agents have a pathogenic role, but practitioners confronted with a recalcitrant diarrhea, especially if it occurs in a young kitten, should be aware of their existence. Many laboratories now have the capability for examining fecal specimens by electron microscopy and for attempting isolation of viruses that are observed. A practitioner wishing to submit a specimen for such study should ascertain from the laboratory the best way to obtain and transmit material.

## "MUMPS" (PAROTITIS)

The susceptibility of the domestic cat to mumps virus was demonstrated experimentally by Wollstein (1916, 1918). Occasional natural infections with mumps virus are reported to take the form of parotitis in household cats and dogs exposed to human cases (Gillespie and Timoney, 1981).

## ENCEPHALITIS AND MYELITIS OF POSSIBLE VIRAL ETIOLOGY

Inflammations of the brain and spinal cord, with lesions suggestive of viral etiology, have been reported sporadically.

A localized outbreak of rapidly fatal encephalitis of cats was reported from Italy (Magrassi et al., 1951; Scanu, 1951). Bacteria could not be cultured from the brains, but the infection was transmitted by intracerebral inoculation.

Encephalomyelitis or myelitis with many clinical features in common and lesions of viral type has been reported from cats in Morocco (Martin and Hintermann, 1952), Ceylon (McGaughey, 1953, 1954), Australia (Borland and McDonald, 1965), Scandinavia (Kronevi et al., 1974), and, more recently, the United States (Vandevelde and Braund, 1979) and Switzerland (Hoff and Vandevelde, 1981). It is a matter of speculation whether any of the cases represent a single disease entity.

Young, mature, and aged cats have been affected. In the majority the signs were slowly progressive, most often taking the form of disturbances in locomotion: muscular weakness, impaired reactions in the limbs, ataxia, and paresis. Less frequent signs were behavioral changes, hyperesthesia, atony of the bladder, and seizures. Some cats have survived but without complete recovery.

The lesions of nonsuppurative encephalomyelitis or meningoencephalomyelitis were considered suggestive of viral infection: neuronal degeneration, mononuclear perivascular cuffing, and gliosis. The only successful transmission attempts were reported by Martin and Hintermann (1952) and McGaughey (1954).

A paramyxovirus-like agent was isolated from the central nervous system of cats naturally affected with demyelinating lesions of the optic nerves associated with inclusion body formation (Cook, 1979; Cook and Wilcox, 1981).

## FELINE SUSCEPTIBILITY TO SOME VIRUS DISEASES OF OTHER SPECIES

**CANINE DISTEMPER.** Inapparent infection can be produced in young kittens by intranasal and intracerebral inoculation (Appel et al., 1974). Virus can spread from infected dogs to cats but not from infected cats to dogs or cats. Serum samples from 14 to 150 cats had neutralizing antibody to canine distemper virus.

**CANINE HEPATITIS.** Although cats have been said to be resistant to the virus of fox encephalitis (e.g., Lawrence et al., 1943), serologic evidence has been reported of a feline antigen pointing to the existence of a type of contagious canine hepatitis virus infective for the cat (Lehnert, 1948), and kittens have been infected experimentally, with the production of eye lesions (Parry et al., 1951). Rubarth (1953) reported that he was unable to infect cats by intraperitoneal injection but had encountered several spontaneous cases of contagious canine hepatitis in cats.

**PARVOVIRUS INFECTIONS.** Although the virus of feline panleukopenia, a parvovirus, is closely related antigenically to canine parvovirus and is indistinguishable serologically from mink enteritis virus, cats do not develop symptomatic infection with these viruses and do not transmit them to the natural hosts.

**EQUINE INFLUENZA-ABORTION.** Experimental inoculation of day-old kittens, by the intranasal or intraperitoneal route, produces signs and lesions of acute encephalitis as well as inflammatory changes in the thoracic and abdominal viscera (Hatziolos and Reagan, 1960).

**FOOT-AND-MOUTH DISEASE.** Experimentally induced infections indicate that cats have a degree of susceptibility to this virus of cloven-footed animals (Galloway, 1931; Lotti, 1941; Nagel, 1952). Several cases of clinical infection have been described in which the signs resembled those seen in commonly infected species, but the diagnoses were unsupported by isolation of the virus (Curtze, 1932; Estor-Crefeld, 1899; Hauptmann, 1926; Höve, 1929).

**NEWCASTLE DISEASE.** This infection of poultry is reported to have occurred spontaneously in a laboratory cat, producing severe nervous signs. The infection was also successfully transmitted to experimental cats (Nakamura and Iwasa, 1942). Both natural exposure and experimental inoculation may produce demonstrable antibodies. Some workers observed no signs of clinical illness and were unable to recover virus (Moses et al., 1957; Orlandella, 1954; Reagan et al., 1954a,b); others produced encephalitis and described myoclonus resulting from lesions in the brainstem or spinal cord (Luttrell and Bang, 1958). A case of natural infection was confirmed by inoculation of both fowls and kittens (Tozzini and Mani, 1973).

**HUMAN INFLUENZA.** Cats were reported to be susceptible to infection with $A_2$ Hong Kong influenza virus by intranasal inoculation and by contact with an infected cat or human influenza patient (Paniker and Nair, 1970). The cats developed no clinical illness but shed the virus from the throat for one week and developed hemagglutination-inhibiting antibodies. Sera from 6 of 28 normal cats inhibited hemagglutination.

**RIFT VALLEY FEVER.** This virus disease causes hepatitis in sheep, cattle, and humans in Africa and the Middle East. Kittens and puppies 8 to 10 weeks old were demonstrated to be susceptible to inapparent infection by the respiratory route (Keefer et al., 1972). Neutralizing antibody was the criterion for infection, but some animals were viremic.

**YELLOW FEVER.** Experimental infections of cats usually result only in serologic immunity (Linhares, 1943) but can produce transient episodes of fever and apathy (Monteiro, 1930) or typical paralytic symptoms (da Fonseca and Artigas, 1938).

## REFERENCES


Baldwin S: Feline enteric viruses. *In* Kirk RW: Current Veterinary Therapy VIII. Philadelphia, W B Saunders Company, 1983.

Borland R, McDonald N: Feline encephalomyelitis. Br Vet J 121 (1965) 479–482.

Chrystie IL, Goldwater PN, Banatvala JE: Rotavirus infection in a domestic cat. Vet Rec 105 (1979) 404–405.

Cook RD: Observations on focal demyelinating lesions in cat optic nerves. Neuropathol Appl Neurobiol 5 (1979) 395–404.

Cook RD, Wilcox GE: A paramyxovirus-like agent associated with demyelinating lesions in the CNS of cats. J Neuropathol Exp Neurol 40 (1981) 328.

Gillespie JH, Timoney JF: Hagan and Bruner's Infectious Diseases of Domestic Animals, 7th ed. Ithaca, Comstock Publishing Associates, Cornell University Press, 1981.

Hoff EJ, Vandevelde M: Nonsuppurative encephalomyelitis suggestive of a viral origin. Vet Pathol 18 (1981) 170–180.

Hoshino Y, Baldwin CA, Scott FW: Isolation and characterization of feline rotavirus. J Gen Virol 54 (1981a) 313–323.

Hoshino Y, Zimmer JF, Moise NS, Scott FW: Detection of astroviruses in feces of a cat with diarrhea. Arch Virol 70 (1981b) 373–376.

Kronevi T, Nordström M, Moreno W, Nilsson PO: Feline ataxia due to nonsuppurative meningoencephalomyelitis of unknown aetiology. Nord Vet-Med 26 (1974) 720–725.

Magrassi F, Leonardi G, Scanu A: Osservazioni su un' encefalopatia virale del gatto. Boll Soc Ital Biol Sper 27 (1951) 1233.

Martin L-A, Hintermann J: Sur l'existence, au Maroc, d'une maladie contagieuse du chat, non encore décrite: la myélite infectieuse. Bull Acad Vét Fr 25 (1952) 387–392.

McGaughey CA: Infectious myelitis of cats: preliminary communication. Ceylon Vet J 1 (1953) 38–40.

McGaughey CA: Infectious myelitis of felines. A note on two cases in young leopards in Ceylon [and five more in cats]. Ceylon Vet J 2 (1954) 18–21.

Scanu A: Osservazioni di ordine epidemiologico relative ad una encefalopatia virale del gatto. Boll Soc Ital Biol Sper 27 (1951) 1236–1238.

Snodgrass DR, Angus KW, Gray EW: A rotavirus from kittens. Vet Rec 104 (1979) 222–223.

Vandevelde M, Braund KG: Polioencephalomyelitis in cats. Vet Pathol 16 (1979) 420–427.

Wollstein M: An experimental study of parotitis (mumps). J Exp Med 23 (1916) 353–375.

Wollstein M: A further study of experimental parotitis. J Exp Med 28 (1918) 377–385.


**Feline Susceptibility to Some Virus Diseases of Other Species**


Appel M, Sheffy BE, Percy DH, Gaskin JM: Canine distemper virus in domesticated cats and pigs. Am J Vet Res 35 (1974) 803–806.

Curtze W: Ein Fall von Maul- und Klauenseuche, bei der Katze. Tierärztl Rundsch 38 (1932) 40–41.

da Fonseca F, Artigas P: Sensibilité du chat au virus amaril neurotrope. C R Soc Biol (Paris) 129 (1938) 1143–1145.

Estor-Crefeld: Maul- und Klauenseuche bei einer Katze. Dtsch Tierärztl Wochenschr 7 (1899) 266.

Galloway IA: Detailed report of work at the National Institute for Medical Research, Hampstead, Fourth Progress Report of the Foot and Mouth Disease Research Committee, Ministry of Agriculture and Fisheries, Great Britain, 1931, 341–344.

Hatziolos BC, Reagan RL: Neurotropism of equine influenza-abortion virus in infant experimental animals. Am J Vet Res 21 (1960) 856–861.

Hauptmann: Die Aphthenseuche bei Katzen. Berl Tierärztl Wochenschr 42 (1926) 590.

Höve KR: Die Maul- und Klauenseuche bei Katzen. Arch Wissensch Prakt Tierheilk 60 (1929) 123–148.

Keefer GV, Zebarth GI, Allen WP: Susceptibility of dogs and cats to Rift Valley fever by inhalation or ingestion of virus. J Infect Dis 125 (1972) 307–309.

Lawrence JS, Syverton JT, Ackart RJ, Adams WS, Ervin DM, Haskins AL, Saunders RH, Stringfellow MB, Wetrich RM: The virus of infectious feline agranulocytosis. II. Immunological relation to other viruses. J Exp Med 77 (1943) 57–64.

Lehnert E: Der Wert der Komplementbindungsmethode bei der Hepatitis contagiosa canis. Skand Vet Tidskr 38 (1948) 94–107.

Linhares H: Inoculacao de virus amarilico em gatos jovens. Mem Inst Cruz 28 (1943) 201–207.

Lotti L: Studio dell' azione patogena del virus aftoso nel gatto. Clin Vet 64 (1941) 427–439.

Luttrell CN, Bang FB: Newcastle disease encephalomyelitis in cats. I. Clinical and pathological features. Arch Neurol Psychiatr 79 (1958) 647–657.

Monteiro JL: Sobre vivencia do virus amarillico no organismo de certos animaes domesticos. Arch Soc Biol Montevideo 6 (1930) 1681–1695; Brasil-Med 44 (1930) 1087–1093.

Moses HE et al.: Cats and Newcastle disease virus. J Am Vet Med Assoc 119 (1951) 213.

Nagel HC: Das Verhalten des Maul- und Klauenseuchevirus in neugeborenen Laboratoriumstieren. Zentralbl Bakteriol Abt I [Orig] 159 (1952) 40–46.

Nakamura J, Iwasa T: On the fowl pest infection in cat. Jpn J Vet Sci 4 (1942) 522–523.

Orlandella V: Ricerche sulla sensibilita del gatto all' infravirus della pseudopeste aviare. Nuova Vet 30 (1954) 262–265 (Abstr Vet Bull 25 [1955] 1366).

Paniker CKJ, Nair CMG: Infection with $A_2$ Hong Kong influenze virus in domestic cats. Bull WHO 43 (1970) 859–862.

Parry HB, Larin NM, Platt H: Studies on the agent of canine virus hepatitis (Rubarth's disease). II. The pathology and pathogenesis of the experimental disease produced by four strains of virus. J Hyg 49 (1951) 483–496.

Reagan RL, Delaha EC, Cook SR, Brueckner AL: Response of kittens to the California strain of Newcastle disease virus (NDV) after oral and nasal routes of exposure. Poultry Sci 33 (1954a) 1275–1276.

Reagan RL, Delaha EC, Cook SR, Brueckner AL: The response of kittens to three strains of Newcastle disease virus. Vet Med 49 (1954b) 488–489.

Rubarth S: Die Epizootologie und Virologie der Hepatitis contagiosa canis. Arch Exp Veterinärmed 6 (1953) 105–109.

Tozzini F, Mani P: Isolamento del virus di Newcastle dalla milza di un gatto. Annali Fac Med Vet Pisa 25 (1973) 189–195 (Abstr Vet Bull 44 [1974] 1585).

# 8
CHAPTER
# BACTERIAL DISEASES

ERNST L. BIBERSTEIN and JEAN HOLZWORTH

CONTRIBUTING AUTHORS:
ERWIN SMALL, MIODRAG RISTIC, and NIELS C. PEDERSEN

Cats suffer less often than other animals from specific bacterial diseases, whereas bacteria in combination with other agents, both infectious and noninfectious, play an important role in many feline disorders. In the main section of this chapter we discuss first the specific infections to which cats are subject and then other bacteria that have roles of varying importance in illnesses of cats.

Hemobartonellosis and mycoplasmal infections are described in separate sections. Chlamydial infection ("pneumonitis") is discussed in the chapter on viral infections, together with the viral respiratory infections with which it is often associated.

## ACTINOMYCETIC INFECTIONS

Actinomycetes are Gram-positive bacteria with certain distinctive cell wall characteristics. Their taxonomy has been in a perpetual state of turmoil and the nomenclature notoriously loose. Terms like streptothricosis, actinomycosis, nocardiosis, oösporosis, and pseudoactinomycosis have been used indiscriminately to designate the filamentous forms, making the older literature often impossible to interpret. Medically important genera include *Corynebacterium, Mycobacterium, Actinomyces, Nocardia, Dermatophilus,* and *Streptomyces.* The last four grow as branching filaments, a trait formerly interpreted as indicating a link with fungi. This interpretation is unjustified. Filamentous actinomycetes are bacteria in every essential respect, an all-important feature from the therapeutic viewpoint.

### ACTINOMYCOSIS

Members of the genus *Actinomyces* are normal inhabitants of mammalian oral mucous membranes and dental surfaces. Actinomycosis is interpreted as the result of a breakdown in the integrity of normal host protective mechanisms on a local or systemic level.

The incidence of actinomycotic infection in cats is difficult to define. If every instance of *Actinomyces* sp in a pathologic specimen is considered a case of actinomycosis, we have seen 33 such cases at the Veterinary Medical Teaching Hospital, University of California, during a 10-year period among an estimated 6000 feline samples submitted (Table 8–1).

Actinomycosis is assumed to begin with introduction of the agent through the skin or mucous membrane into tissue already debilitated, possibly by previous infection. An inflammatory focus is established, which develops into a pyogranuloma or abscess. Formation of fistulous tracts to the body surface is common. Pus obtained from actinomycotic lesions often contains small yellowish gray agglomerations called sulfur granules, consisting of bacterial colonies and tissue debris. Sulfur granules and solid tissue lesions show the filamentous organisms arranged radially in a ring pattern. These are covered by acidophilic "clubs," the products of host-parasite interaction. Inflammation around this "rosette" results in abscesses encased by granulation tissue.

Although the lesion described is accepted as diagnostic

**Table 8–1 *Actinomyces* spp from Cats (Veterinary Medical Teaching Hospital, University of California, Davis, 1971–1980)**

| | |
|---|---|
| Subcutaneous abscesses | 9 |
| Serous membranes | 8 |
| Pulmonary | 2 |
| Central nervous system | 2 |
| Bones | 2 or 3 |
| Diverse types* | 10 or 11 |

*Include two from eye, two ear canal, three oral infections, three upper respiratory tract, one sinus tract on forearm (possible osteomyelitis).

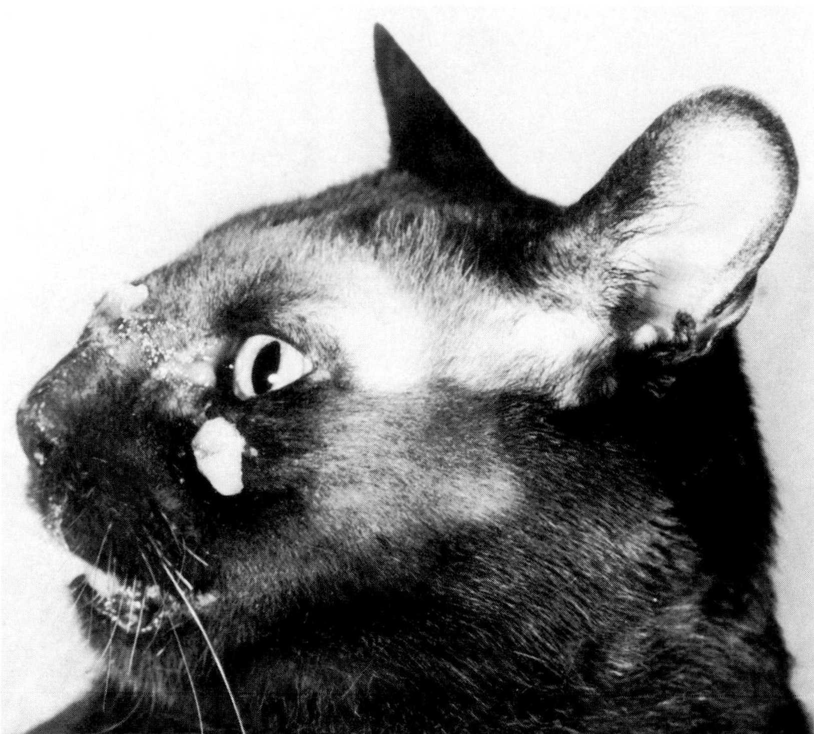

**Figure 8–1** Actinomycosis of the face, six-year-old male Burmese. The bridge of the nose is swollen, and pus exudes from fistulae on the nose, at the medial canthus of the eye, and in the maxillary area. The infection responded to surgical drainage and to penicillin flushed directly into the fistulae and also administered systemically. (Angell Memorial Animal Hospital.)

of actinomycosis, the vast majority of such infections are mixed. *Pasteurella multocida* and non–spore-forming, Gram-negative anaerobes are the most frequent admixtures.

An early discussion of feline actinomycosis (Brion, 1939) mentions six disease patterns: (1) cutaneous-subcutaneous (Fig. 8–1), (2) serosal (Fig. 8–2), (3) pulmonary, (4) central nervous system, (5) osseous (Fig. 8–3), and (6) diverse types including granulomas and mycetomas. The author thought cats to be particularly susceptible to the first type. Pattern 2 includes the pleural effusion and pyothorax syndrome. Most case reports in the older literature concern one of the five specific categories (McGaughey, 1952). Some of the more recent ones point to the oral mucous membranes as the first primary loci of infection (Chestain et al., 1977; Libke and Walton, 1974; Lotspeich, 1974). Signs obviously depend on the localization of the infection and its extent.

A diagnosis of actinomycosis can be established only by laboratory examination, since other agents may cause, or participate in, all the disease processes named (Prévot et al., 1961). In a Gram stain of a direct smear, *Actinomyces* classically appears as branching slender filaments. Often the staining is intermittent, giving the filaments a beaded elusive appearance (Fig. 8–4). At the other extreme, some *Actinomyces* appear as very short filaments resembling corynebacteria. Culturing requires rich media (e.g., blood agar). *Actinomyces* spp are anaerobic or microaerophilic and catalase-negative (except *A. viscosus*). Most strains can be identified as *Actinomyces* sp by a competent clinical laboratory, but feline isolates rarely fit current species descriptions.

The main problems in differential diagnosis concern nocardiosis (see following section) and mixed infections with non–spore-forming Gram-negative anaerobes, e.g., *Bacteroides* and *Fusobacterium* spp. Differentiation requires laboratory study.

*Actinomyces* species have been uniformly susceptible to penicillin. Several case studies report on the efficacy of lincomycin, chloramphenicol (Chastain et al., 1977; Lotspeich, 1974; Stowater et al., 1978), and tetracycline (Attleberger, 1980). Accessible lesions should be treated surgically like other suppurative processes. Systemic and surgically inaccessible infections may not respond satisfactorily to antimicrobial drugs despite in-vitro susceptibility to the agent: the nature of the lesion may preclude efficient drug delivery to infected foci. Prolonged therapy is indicated and may still be unsuccessful.

Actinomycosis is considered an endogenous nontransmissible disease: individuals develop infections with strains previously carried as harmless commensals. In cats, the occurrence of apparently primary cutaneous lesions has suggested to some (Wilkinson, 1983a) that transmission by biting may be important. In a paraplegic cat, a suppurative and granulomatous skin infection of the base of the tail, associated with *A. viscosus,* ultimately penetrated into the epidural space (Bestetti et al., 1977). Such an infection could well have originated in a cat bite wound. Chastain et al. (1977) consider extra-oral infections a rarity, however.

There appears to be no transmission to other species, including humans.

## NOCARDIOSIS

*Nocardia* is the other filamentous actinomycete capable of causing serious disease in cats. In our experience (E.B.), nocardiosis is much rarer than actinomycosis: during the 10 years when 33 isolations of *Actinomyces*

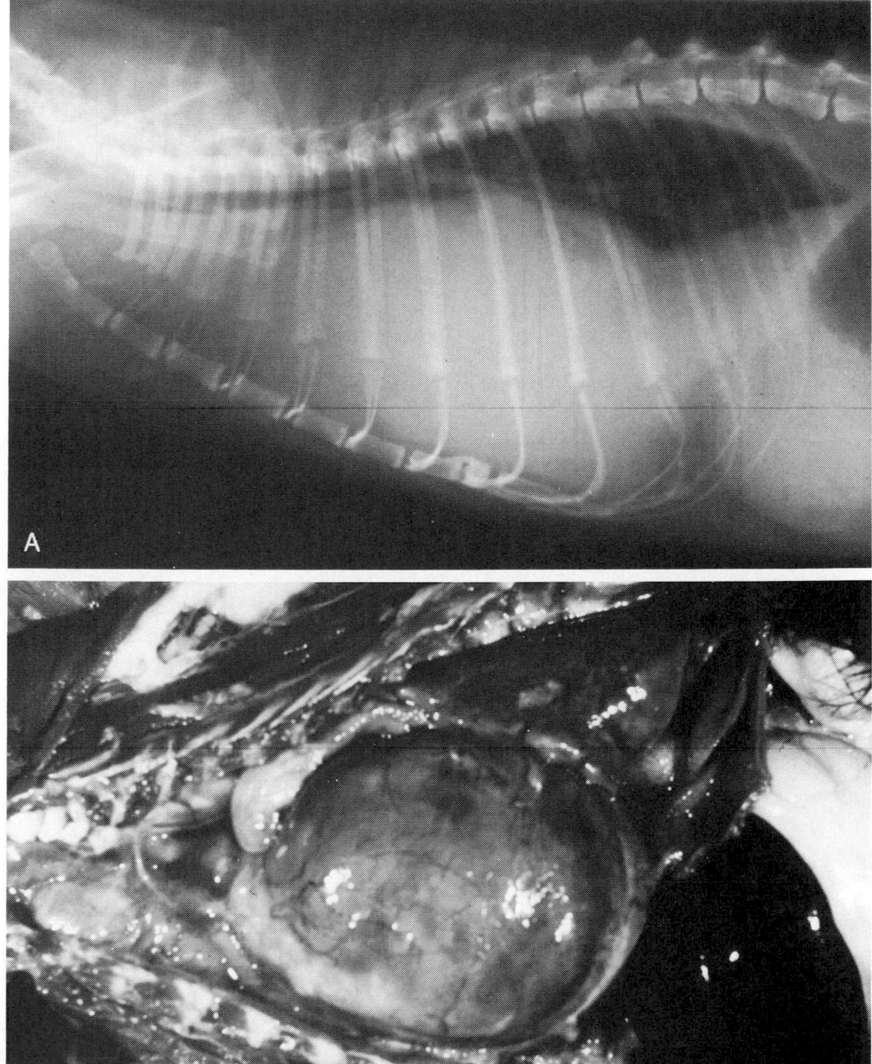

**Figure 8–2** *A*, Actinomycosis of the pleural cavity and pericardium, associated with lung abscesses, 12-year-old female domestic shorthair. Fluid is present in the thoracic cavity, the cardiac silhouette is greatly enlarged, and the trachea is elevated. *B*, Same cat. The opaque and thickened pericardium is distended with 160 ml of pink-tan pus containing "sulfur granules." The right lung is collapsed, as is the left cranial lung lobe except for its emphysematous tip. The pericardium probably became involved by extension of infection from the adherent right lung. Severe dental disease may have given rise to the infection. (Angell Memorial Animal Hospital.)

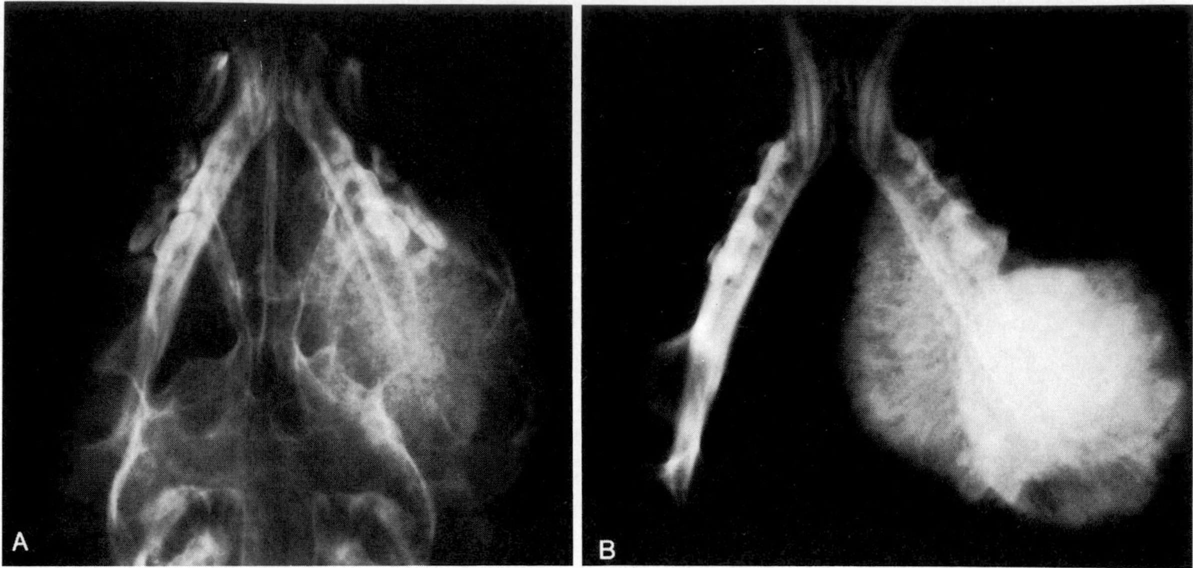


**Figure 8–3** *A* and *B*, Actinomycosis of the mandible, two-year-old male cat. There is lysis of bone as well as a tremendous bony proliferative reaction characterized by a "sunburst" appearance resembling that of osteosarcoma or squamous cell carcinoma. (Angell Memorial Animal Hospital.)

were made, *Nocardia* was encountered twice. The pathogenic patterns of nocardiosis are similar to those of *Actinomyces* and include infections of skin (Marder et al., 1973; Wilkinson, 1983b; Fig. 8–5*A*), serous cavities, lungs, central nervous system, bone, and miscellaneous sites (Attleberger, 1983). Neutered males aged three to six years have been predominantly affected, according to a review of reported cases (Beaman and Sugar, 1983).

A soil saprophyte, *Nocardia* is introduced by inhalation or wound infection (Akün, 1952). In contrast with *Actinomyces, Nocardia* evokes reactions more suppurative than pyogranulomatous, and lymph nodes are commonly involved. While the exudate may contain granules, they are smaller than, and lack the substructure of, actinomycotic "sulfur granules." The microscopic lesion is typically a tangle of filaments surrounded by pus and granulation tissue. Rosette formation is not seen (Fig. 8–5*B*).

There are no specific clinical characteristics of nocardiosis. In disseminated cases or serositis with empyema, the cat presents a picture of chronic debilitating illness. Discharging fistulous tracts would suggest an actinomycotic or fungal infection or possibly tuberculosis. A definitive diagnosis requires laboratory identification of the agent. Lacking this, case reports, especially in the older literature, deserve to be viewed with some skepticism.

In a Gram-stained smear, *Nocardia* spp closely resemble *Actinomyces.* Most strains encountered in systemic disease are at least partially acid-fast (Kinyoun stain). They grow on the simplest media (e.g., Sabouraud's agar), are obligate aerobes, and are catalase-positive. Of the three common species, *N. asteroides, N. brasiliensis,* and *N. caviae,* the first two have caused disease in cats (Ajello et al., 1961; Campbell and Scott, 1975; Langham et al., 1959).

The sulfonamides with or without trimethoprim are the drugs of choice for medical treatment of nocardiosis in humans and animals (Attleberger, 1980). Although some physicians choose to combine these with various antibiotics, there is little evidence of benefit (Lerner, 1979). Drainage of abscesses and relief of empyema, combined with long-term sulfonamide treatment, offer the best hope of cure in local-regional processes (Campbell and Scott, 1975). The outlook in systemic cases is extremely guarded.

*Nocardia* is a common soil saprophyte, to which animals are probably continuously exposed. The factors rendering them susceptible to clinical infection by a nontraumatic route are not understood. A predisposing failure of host defenses, which can often be correlated with human (Lerner, 1979) and equine nocardiosis, has not been documented in cats.

Like other zoonoses caused by saprophytes, nocardiosis is not known to be transmitted by infected animals.

## *Dermatophilus congolensis* INFECTION

*Dermatophilus congolensis* is an actinomycete with an unusual growth cycle, which includes branching filamentous proliferation by cell division in both a transverse and a longitudinal direction resulting in thickening as well as elongation of the filaments (Fig. 8–6). Eventually the filaments break up into flagellated motile zoospores—the reproductive units of *Dermatophilus*.

*D. congolensis* causes an exudative epidermatitis in several species, e.g., horses, sheep, cattle, and, rarely, humans. In cats, the agent was described in granulomas in a lymph node (Jones, 1976), the tongue (Baker et al., 1972; O'Hara and Cordes, 1963), the bladder wall serosa (O'Hara and Cordes, 1963), and a forepaw (Carakostas et al., 1984). Traumatic origin was suggested in three cases. Understandably, *Dermatophilus* was not suspected and was confirmed culturally only once. Surgical removal and penicillin therapy appear to be effective treatments.

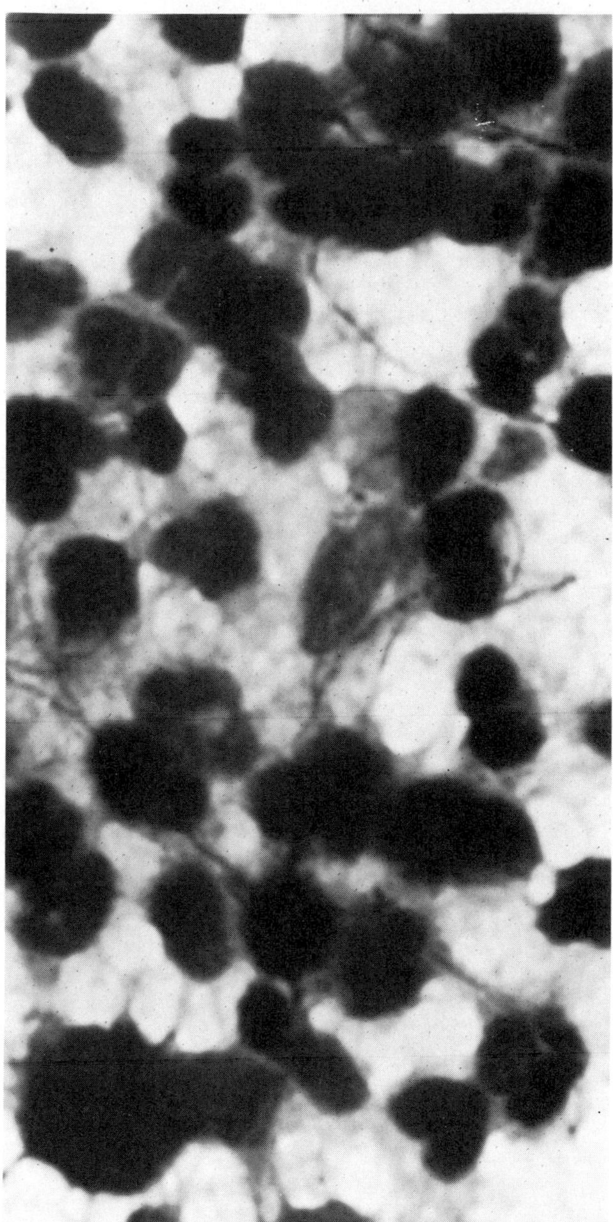

**Figure 8–4** Actinomycosis in a cat. Smear of thoracic aspirate containing degenerate neutrophils and branching, often beaded filaments of *Actinomyces* sp. Gram stain, approximately × 2000. (University of California, Davis.)

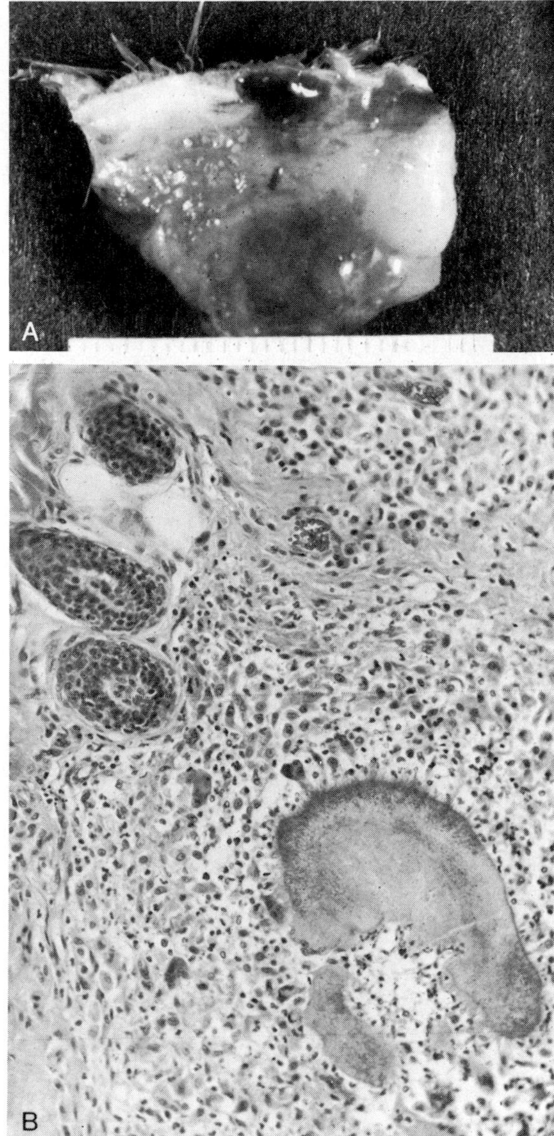


**Figure 8–5** *A*, Nocardiosis, section of skin and subcutis of the lumbar area and groin, 10-year-old castrated male domestic longhair. Pockets of dark red exudate lie within the dermis and extend into the subcutis. Numerous "sulfur granules" are seen as pale or highlighted foci in much of the inflamed subcutis. *B*, Nocardiosis, same lesion. Deep dermal pyogranulomatous inflammation centered about a "sulfur granule" (lower right). Adjacent neutrophils and more distant epithelioid and multinucleate cells form a wide zone about the bacteria and the associated Hoeppli-Splendore phenomenon. H & E, × 200. (Angell Memorial Animal Hospital.)

The agent is not thought to multiply in the nonliving environment, but its long persistence in the soil makes transmission through inanimate objects a possibility.

## ACTINOMYCETIC MYCETOMAS

Actinomycetic mycetomas are pyogranulomatous masses containing granular pus. In humans, the agents responsible include *Actinomyces, Nocardia, Actinomadura,* and *Streptomyces* spp. Since all are either soil saprophytes or oral bacteria, the condition is presumably initiated by wound infection. A case of mycetoma due to a *Streptomyces* sp was described in a cat in which the lesion at first appeared as a subcutaneous mass over one scapula but recurred six months after surgical removal, invading underlying muscles and the axilla (Lewis et al., 1972).

The outlook for mycetomas is poor. Radical surgery may succeed in early cases. Appropriate antimicrobial drugs have some effect. (See *Actinomyces* and *Nocardia*

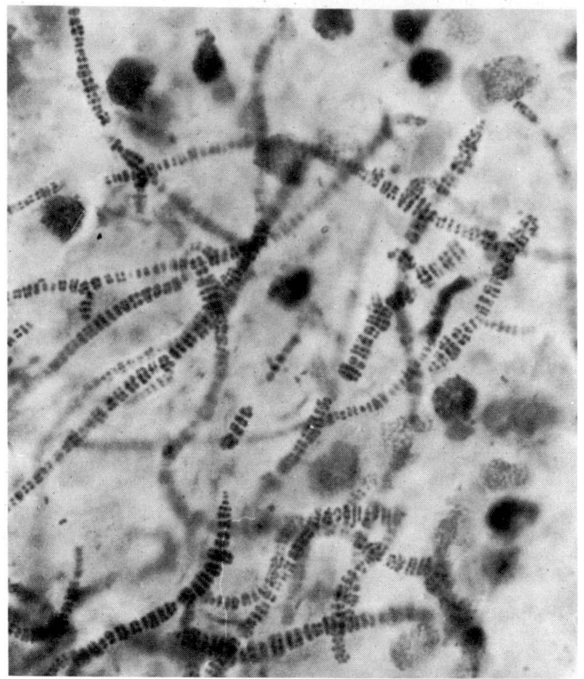

**Figure 8–6** *Dermatophilus congolensis.* Typical banded filaments, granuloma, cat's forepaw. × 2000. (From Carakostas MC, Miller RI, Woodward MG: J Am Vet Med Assoc 185 [1984] 675–676.)

infections.) *Actinomadura* and *Streptomyces* infections have responded to streptomycin (Rippon, 1982). The reported case ended in euthanasia following relapse.

## TUBERCULOSIS

While tuberculosis of cats has been ascribed to all four species of tubercle bacilli, the main cause has been *Mycobacterium bovis*, and the disease has been closely linked to tuberculosis in cattle, particularly dairy cows (Francis, 1958, 1961). By contrast, confirmed cases due to *M. tuberculosis* (human type) are rare (Verge and Senthille, 1942), as are proven natural cases of avian tuberculosis *(M. avium)* (Buergelt et al., 1982; Hix et al., 1961; Suter et al., 1984). Feline tuberculosis due to the vole bacillus *(M. microti)* has been described in the Netherlands (Huitema and van Vloten, 1960; van Dorssen, 1960).

Prevalence figures relating to feline tuberculosis vary widely and mostly antedate the general decline of the disease in technically advanced countries. A relatively recent compilation from Switzerland gives a rate of 0.2 per cent in 3621 feline autopsies. According to the authors, it stood at 7 per cent before the eradication of bovine tuberculosis (Isler and Lott-Stolz, 1978). Feline tuberculosis may still occur, however, even in countries where control measures have been long and vigorously pursued (e.g., Grossman, 1983; Isaac et al., 1983; Orr et al., 1980; Willemse and Beijer; 1979), and it remains a serious possibility in underdeveloped countries where cats have access to unpasteurized milk or to livestock offal.

### Pathogenesis and Lesions

While tuberculosis in cats can be acquired by the alimentary, respiratory, and percutaneous routes, the most common pathway is by ingestion (Francis, 1961; Snider, 1971; Stableforth, 1929; Stünzi, 1954). Colonization can occur anywhere along the gastrointestinal tract, with predilections for the pharyngotonsillar and ileocecal regions (Innes, 1940). The primary complex in the intestine is often incomplete because lesions found at autopsy may be limited to the local lymph nodes. Only occasionally do ulcerated Peyer's patches or submucosal tubercles mark the point of entry (Snider, 1971).

When infection has occurred by the respiratory tract, a primary lesion usually forms in the lung parenchyma, followed by prompt lymphatic involvement and tubercle formation in a hilar node (Ghon's complex) (Snider, 1971). A third method of infection peculiar to cats is percutaneous. The transmission is credited to bites or scratches by infected cats (Smith, 1964). Two cases of apparently primary infection of the genital tract (metritis) are on record (Berthelon, 1943).

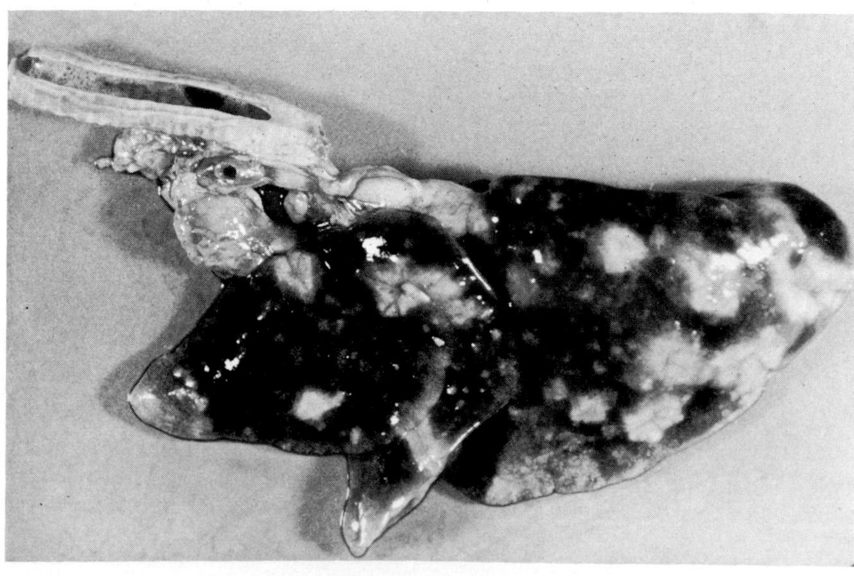

**Figure 8–7** Tuberculosis of the lung and tracheobronchial lymph nodes, six-year-old spayed female Swiss cat. Pale, firm nodules varying greatly in size are scattered throughout the parenchyma and extend to the pleura. (Courtesy Dr. H.-R. Luginbühl, University of Bern, Switzerland.)

Feline tuberculosis is often progressive and disseminating (Snider, 1971). Affected lymph nodes enlarge and may rupture, producing tuberculous serositides (peritonitis, pleuritis) (Innes, 1940) or fistulous tracts discharging on the skin or a mucous surface, depending on the location of the affected node. The female genital tract may be infected by such extension. Lymphohematogenous dissemination appears to seed the lung first from a primary enteromesenteric focus (Innes, 1940). Other organs found infected include parotid glands (Mason, 1924), kidneys (Orr et al., 1980; Seren, 1936), adrenals (Blähser, 1962), liver (Cobbett, 1926; Dobson, 1930; Jennings, 1949; Jensen, 1891; Stableforth, 1929), spleen (Cobbett, 1926; Dobson, 1930; Griffith, 1926; Jennings, 1949; Jensen, 1891), pancreas (Stableforth, 1929), testicle (Pezzoli, 1954; Robin and Fontaine, 1954), bones and joints (Cella, 1942; Collet, 1942; Douville, 1922; Robin and Lesbouyries, 1926), myocardium (Blähser, 1962), eye (Hancock and Coats, 1911; Matthias and Niemand, 1943), meninges (Methner, 1957; Teuscher, 1954, 1955; Walzl, 1956), cerebrum (Methner, 1957), and cerebellum (Collet and Lucam, 1941). Hypertrophic pulmonary osteoarthropathy, a rarity in cats, has been reported with tuberculosis (Houdemer, 1928).

At autopsy, enlarged lymph nodes contain foci of caseation and liquefaction (Snider, 1971). Depending on the route of infection and the degree of generalization, pleuritis, peritonitis, and pericarditis may be present. Lesions in the lungs tend to be multicentric (Fig. 8–7), an observation supporting the view that they are usually metastatic (Stünzi, 1954). Calcification is absent. Cavitation and miliary patterns are unusual (Innes, 1940). Lesions in other organs resemble those in lymph nodes and lungs.

Microscopically, the lesions differ from classic tubercles. They consist largely of macrophages surrounding areas of necrosis. Lymphocytes, sometimes a few neutrophils, and, peripherally, fibroblasts are present. Epithelioid cells and Langhans-type giant cells are not seen (Innes, 1940).

## Clinical Features

Experimental infections suggest an incubation period of about three weeks (Kuwabara, 1938). Since a parenteral route and large numbers of organisms are usual in these cases, this figure may be assumed to be low. Presenting signs, although variable, are suggestive of a chronic systemic disorder: weight loss, dehydration, irregular appetite, fluctuating or persistent low-grade fever, and occasional diarrhea or vomiting or both (Wolff, 1966). In the thoracic form, coughing, respiratory difficulty, and rales may be noticed. With significant pleural exudate, the least exertion or struggle by the cat may lead to death from respiratory failure on the examining table. In the abdominal form, the mesenteric lymph nodes may be sufficiently enlarged to be palpable through the abdominal wall (Snider, 1971). An inflammatory effusion is common with abdominal tuberculosis, but acid-fast bacilli are only rarely isolated.

Tuberculous infection of the eyes appears to be a specialty of the cat (e.g., Hancock and Coats, 1911; Matthias and Niemand, 1943). Blindness or abnormality in pupillary responses is sometimes the first sign noted. In the experience of many, both eyes are more often affected than one. Presumably blood-borne, the infection may begin as a granulomatous proliferation in the choroid, which results in detachment of the retina and sometimes the appearance of webs of exudate in the vitreous. Later the anterior parts of the eye are involved, the iris becomes thickened and discolored, lacework appears on the anterior surface of the lens, and finally pericorneal congestion and vascularization and conjunctivitis develop. In some cases the eyeball shrinks; in others it is enlarged. Eye involvement of this type may occur in young kittens and sometimes on a litter basis. Abscesses of periorbital tissues may be tuberculous (Hobday, 1953).

Tuberculosis of the skin, also frequent in cats, is likely to manifest itself as a soft swelling or flat ulcer, most often involving the face, neck, and shoulders, less often the underside of the chest, base of the tail, forearms, and genitals. Although in some cases a skin lesion may result from hematogenous dissemination or an underlying focus of infection (Snider, 1971), many cases are believed to arise from bites or scratches received in fights or from licking or washing after ingestion of infected milk or meat. The eyelids, lips, and nose are often the site of unresponsive ulcers with necrotic floors and hard peripheries—lesions not to be confused with eosinophilic granuloma. Sometimes the infection takes the form of a draining fistula under the eye or a tract from a cervical node. Often the trouble starts as a deformity of the forehead or bridge of the nose ("parrot's beak"). Later the infection breaks through to the surface and ultimately exposes and destroys the bones of the nose and face. In one cat a lump on the forehead proved to be associated with tuberculous frontal sinusitis (Foresti, 1936).

## Diagnosis

Diagnosis in the live cat depends on clinical signs, radiographic findings, and demonstration of the causative agent. The latter should be attempted by direct smears or biopsy specimens stained with the appropriate version of the Ziehl-Neelsen stain. Cultures should also be attempted, but the slow growth rate of the agent reduces the practical value of this procedure, which lies mostly in epidemiologic information that it may supply. The intradermal tuberculin test is considered unreliable. In a relatively recent study employing old tuberculin, second strength PPD, and standard mammalian tuberculin, not one of 24 cats infected with bovine tuberculois reacted (Snider et al., 1971). The intradermal use of BCG for detection of tuberculosis in carnivores has been described. The test consists of injections of 0.1 ml of the standard vaccine into the shoulder region. A reaction proceeding to ulceration not later than the fourteenth day constitutes a positive test result (Hawthorne and Lauder, 1962). Another group of investigators injected the antigen into the medial aspect of the thigh. A swelling occurring no sooner than 24 hours after injection constituted a positive test result. The ulceration two weeks later was considered a side reaction. Although the test was reported to be accurate in dogs, it was considered unreliable in cats (Parodi et al., 1965).

A subcutaneous thermal test has been favored by some; others reported frequent false-positive results (Christoph, 1963). A complement fixation test also has its advocates (Francis, 1961) and critics (Nowacki, 1967).

In summary, diagnosis of feline tuberculosis must rest on clinical observations and laboratory procedures, none of which is totally dependable. It is not surprising that most reports on feline clinical tuberculosis are derived from post-mortem observations.

### Treatment

Successes in treating feline tuberculosis with isoniazid (Monti, 1953; Smith, 1964) and streptomycin (Collinot, 1953) have been reported. These usually represented clinical improvements but not bacteriologic cures (Christoph, 1963; Monti, 1953). On consideration of public health, the advisability and defensibility of treating tuberculous cats can be disputed. Such concerns, the prospects of long-term medication, and the often advanced state of disease tend to discourage attempts at treatment.

### Epidemiology

Feline tuberculosis has no age or sex predilection (Francis, 1958). A predisposition among Siamese cats is apparent (Stünzi, 1954).

The high incidence of tuberculosis in cats has been related to uncontrolled bovine tuberculosis (Diehl, 1971; Reif, 1969). In a study of infected dairy farms representing islands of tuberculosis in a nearly tuberculosis-free environment, almost half the cats (24 of 52) were infected (Snider et al., 1971). Most had lesions, and many were shedding *M. bovis* by the oronasal or intestinal route. In this and other instances, they were thought to perpetuate the infection among successive populations of cattle (Milbradt and Römmele, 1960).

Spread among cats presumably occurs by the respiratory and cutaneous routes. With the decline of bovine tuberculosis, some authors have described a change from the alimentary-abdominal forms due to *M. bovis* to respiratory-thoracic infections by *M. tuberculosis* (Parodi et al., 1965). The very few documented infections by *M. avium* and *M. microti* point toward either a respiratory (van Dorssen, 1960; Hix et al., 1961) or an alimentary route of infection (Huitema and van Vloten, 1960). The sources of infection were not known in these cases.

Tuberculous cats, regardless of clinical status, can shed tubercle bacilli from natural orifices and discharging sinuses. Despite the frequently intimate association between humans and cats, transmission between these species has only rarely been documented. Nonetheless it would seem dubious practice to retain tuberculous cats as house pets, particularly around children or individuals of otherwise uncertain immunocompetence.

## CAT LEPROSY

Since 1962 a chronic nodular, often ulcerative, granulomatous dermatitis of cats has been reported sporadically from Australia, New Zealand, Britain, the Netherlands, and western North America. Histologic and clinical features and the presence of acid-fast bacteria that defied attempts at cultivation suggested the name "cat leprosy." The responsible agent was believed to be the rat leprosy bacillus, *Mycobacterium lepraemurium* (Lawrence and Wickham, 1963; Leiker and Poelma, 1974), which has since been reported to have been cultivated on artificial media (Pattyn and Portaels, 1980). Attempts to produce the feline disease with *M. lepraemurium,* however, failed, although material from cases of cat leprosy reproduced the infection in recipient cats and caused disseminated disease in rats (Schiefer and Middleton, 1983). How natural feline infection is acquired is unknown.

### Pathogenesis and Pathologic Features

The lesions begin as single or multiple nodules in the dermis and subcutis, enlarging rapidly and attaining sizes from 1.0 to 3.5 cm (Fig. 8–8). They are freely movable. Eventual ulceration is common. Regional lymph nodes are sometimes enlarged, and dissemination to spleen, liver, and lungs has been observed (Brown et al., 1962; McIntosh, 1982; Poelma and Leiker, 1974; Wilkinson, 1977).

Foamy histiocytes or epithelioid cells predominate, with fewer neutrophils, plasma cells, and lymphocytes and rare giant cells (Brown et al., 1962; Gee et al., 1975; Poelma and Leiker, 1974; Fig. 8–9). Caseation necrosis occurs irregularly, and encapsulation is usually inconspicuous.

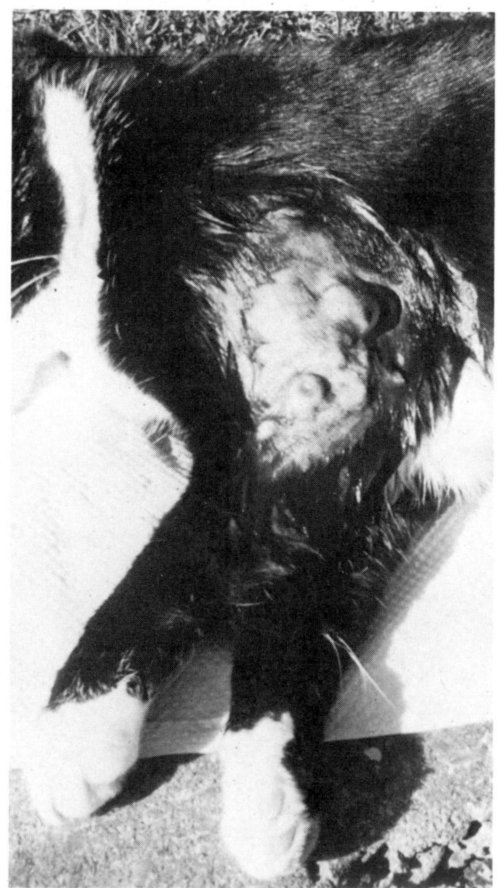

**Figure 8–8** Cat leprosy. Several nodules, one ulcerated, on the shaved area of the left foreleg. (Courtesy Dr. Ian Mayhew. *In* White SD, et al.: J Am Vet Med Assoc 182 [1983] 1218–1222.)

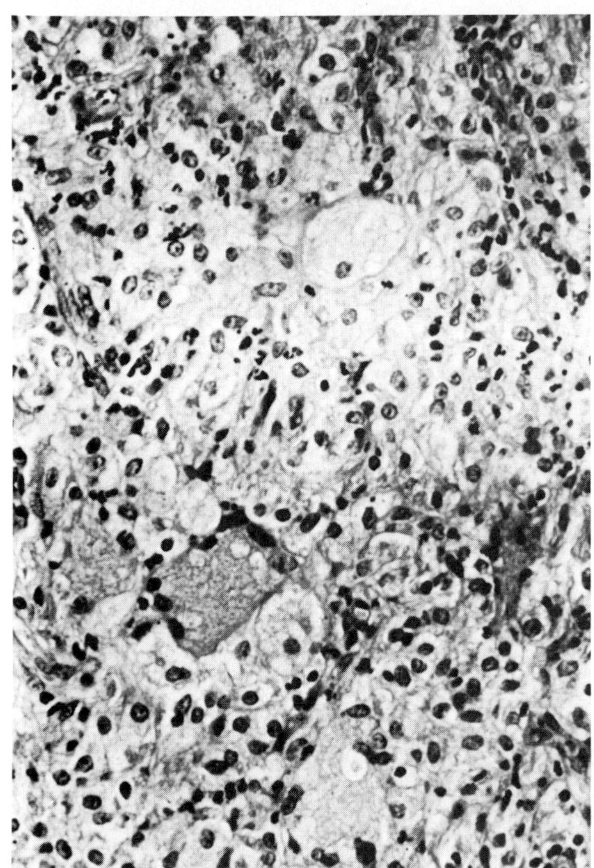

**Figure 8–9** Cat leprosy. Section of lesion showing histiocytes with foamy cytoplasm and giant cells. H & E, × 160. (From Schiefer B, Gee BR, Ward GE: J Am Vet Med Assoc 165 [1974] 1085–1087.)

Neural invasion has been observed (Schiefer et al., 1974). The abundance of beaded, slender, acid-fast bacilli may vary (Brown et al., 1962). Within the histiocytes, bacteria tend to be arranged in parallel bundles (Fig. 8–10), a feature, along with reported neurotropism, characteristic of human but not murine leprosy (Schiefer et al., 1974). Glomerulonephritis was mentioned in an earlier report (Lawrence and Wickham, 1963).

## Clinical Features

Field observations suggest an incubation period of two weeks to several months (Frye et al., 1974; Poelma and Leiker, 1974; Wilkinson, 1964). The nodulo-ulcerative lesions may occur on any part of the body and are nonpruritic, painless, and typically nonfluctuant. Most cats are otherwise in good general health.

In a curious case of mycobacteriosis in an Idaho cat with diffuse dorsolateral alopecia and non-nodular skin thickening, specimens had microscopic changes and acid-fast bacilli suggestive of feline leprosy (Matthews and Liggitt, 1983). There was also dissemination to lymph nodes, bone marrow, spleen, perithyroidal tissue, and certain skeletal and cutaneous muscles.

## Diagnosis

Feline leprosy is recognized by the nature of the lesions, combined with the finding of acid-fast bacilli intracellularly in smears stained with Ziehl-Neelsen stain. Since the bacilli are not always abundant (Brown et al., 1962), biopsy is advisable. The differential diagnosis includes neoplastic, parasitic, and possibly mycotic conditions. Tuberculosis characteristically results in flattened circular areas firmly adherent to underlying tissues; acid-fast bacteria are always few, and caseation is more prominent than in feline leprosy (Wilkinson, 1977). Moreover, the tuberculosis organism is readily cultivable. (So-called atypical mycobacteria that have been found associated with similar ulcerative dermatitides are discussed separately.)

Infection of experimental animals may be helpful. Mice and rats are susceptible to cat leprosy, although fatal infections require over six months to develop. Guinea pigs develop inapparent and self-limiting infections unlike those produced by *M. tuberculosis* and *M. bovis.* Interfeline transmission attempts have yielded variable results (Lawrence and Wickham, 1963; Poelma and Leiker, 1974). No allergic or serologic diagnostic tests are available.

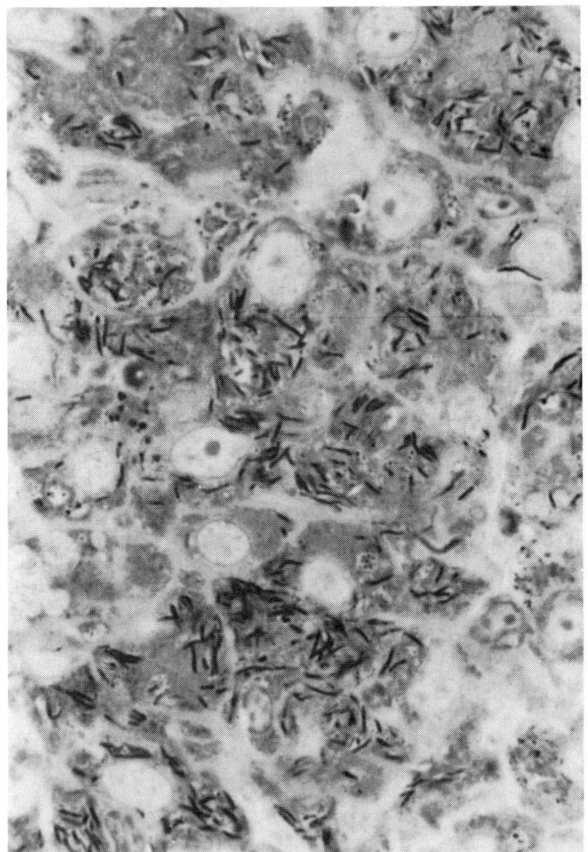

**Figure 8–10** Cat leprosy. Acid-fast bacteria frequently arranged in parallel within the cytoplasm of macrophages, especially of giant cells. Semithin section. Toluidine-blue and safranin stains, × 2000. (From Schiefer B, Gee BR, Ward GE: J Am Vet Med Assoc 165 [1974] 1085–1087.)

### TREATMENT

Excision is the preferred treatment, especially of solitary lesions (Muller et al., 1983), and is sometimes curative. Recurrences at the same or other sites are frequent. Frye and colleagues (1974) reported four relapses within 12 months after the first excision. Among medical treatments, local infiltration of streptomycin has been recommended. For systemic therapy, oral administration of dapsone or rifampin has been suggested (Wilkinson, 1977). Dapsone has given equivocal results and at a dose of 50 to 100 mg daily for an adult cat for one or two weeks has been suspected of causing hemolytic anemia and neurotoxicity (Allan and Wickham, 1976). Experience with dogs suggests that the dose should be limited to 1 mg/kg t.i.d. (Scott, 1984).

### EPIDEMIOLOGY

Cats of all ages and either sex appear to be susceptible. The inconsistent results of interfeline transmission experiments suggest as a source a common (? rodent) reservoir rather than infected cats. Nothing is known of predisposing factors.

There are no known public health implications associated with feline leprosy.

## CUTANEOUS ATYPICAL MYCOBACTERIOSIS

Since 1976 sporadic reports from Australia, Europe, and North America have described ulcerative cutaneous pyogranulomatous lesions from which were isolated acid-fast organisms belonging to Runyon's "atypical mycobacteria," usually group IV ("rapid growers"). Although some observers distinguished differences between these infections and feline leprosy, many of these differences have turned out to be less than clearcut as additional cases have been described. The species implicated include *Mycobacterium xenopi* (Tomasovic et al., 1976), *M. fortuitum* (Dewèvre et al., 1977; Kunkle et al., 1983; White et al., 1982), *M. smegmatis* (Wilkinson et al., 1982), *M. phlei* (White et al., 1983), and unidentified mycobacteria (Kunkle et al., 1983; White et al., 1983). Abscess infections with *M. chelonei* have been reported from France, one with no details (Toma et al., 1979), the other thoroughly studied (Thorel and Boisvert, 1974).

*Mycobacterium avium* serotype II was the causative organism in an "atypical mycobacterium granuloma" that took the form of a localized skin nodule on the hindfoot of a seven-month-old female cat (Suter et al., 1984).

### PATHOGENESIS AND PATHOLOGIC FEATURES

Although the portal and method(s) of infection have not been established, indications point to trauma or, at any rate, exposure of the skin. Because the most frequently implicated agents are free-living saprophytes, acquisition from the soil directly by casual exposure or indirectly by bites or other septic trauma (including veterinary procedures) is likely (Kunkle et al., 1983). The ventral aspect of the body is preferentially although not exclusively affected (Kunkle et al., 1983; White et al., 1983). The development of palpable lesions appears to require a few weeks, as judged by the reappearance of nodules after surgical excision (Wilkinson et al., 1978). The lesions vary from nodules, up to 3 cm in diameter, to large masses, many centimeters in diameter. Ulceration and sinus formation are common (Fig. 8–11). Lymph node involvement seems to be rare. There is no other organ involvement, although in one of the reported cases, a splenic pyogranuloma containing unidentified acid-fast organisms was discovered and removed, after which the cat recovered (Kunkle et al., 1983).

Microscopically, the lesions are best described as pyogranulomas. Acid-fast bacteria, when seen in section, often occupy circular vacuoles surrounded by suppuration. Neutrophils ring the bacterial colonies and are in turn surrounded by macrophages and epithelioid cells (Fig. 8–12). Often no organism can be demonstrated visually in the lesions (Dewèvre et al., 1977; Wilkinson et al., 1978; White et al., 1983).

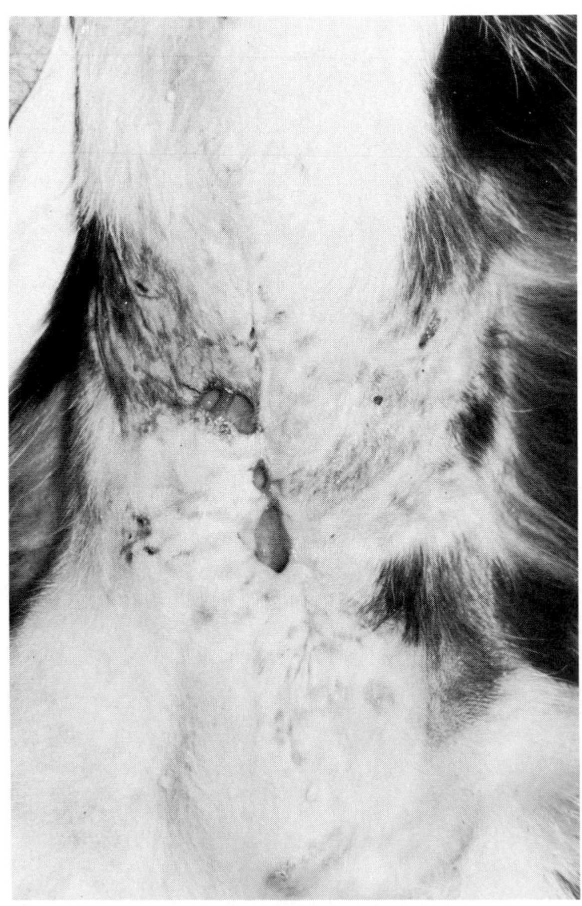

**Figure 8–11** Cutaneous atypical mycobacteriosis, three and one half-year-old spayed female domestic longhair. Subcutaneous nodules and fistulous tracts on the ventral abdomen were present for over two years, failed to respond to treatment with a variety of antibiotics, but eventually resolved. (From White SD, et al.: J Am Vet Med Assoc 182 [1983] 1218–1222.)

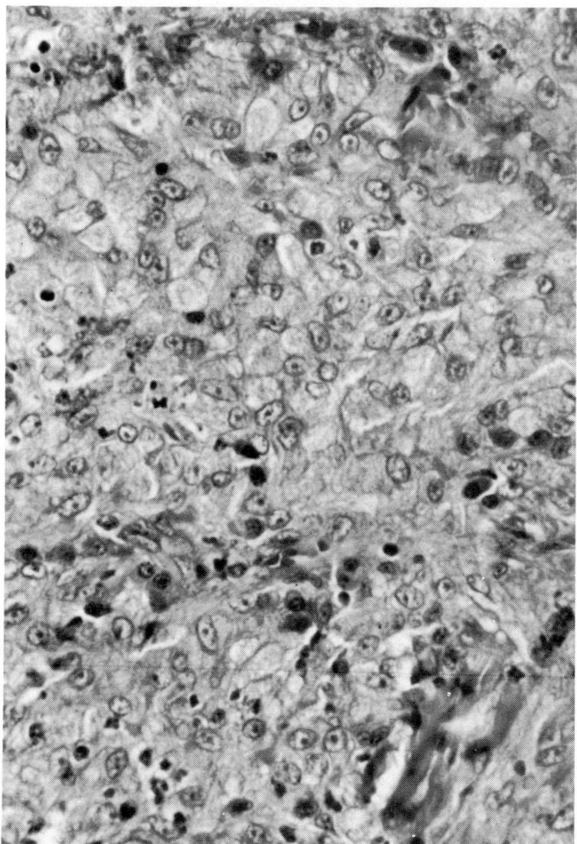

**Figure 8–12** Cutaneous atypical mycobacteriosis caused by *M. fortuitum.* The granuloma is characterized mainly by epithelioid macrophages and fewer scattered neutrophils and plasma cells. H & E, × 300. (From Scott DW: J Am Anim Hosp Assoc 16 [1980] 331–459.)

### Clinical Features

The incubation period of the natural disease is not known, but it must be weeks or months, and the lesions have often been noticed for several months before first consultation. History and findings usually include recurring swellings in or under the skin of chest, abdomen, and inguinal region, with abscesses, ulcers, and fistulous tracts. Improvement occurs with a variety of medical and surgical treatments, and sometimes without treatment, but recrudescences at the original or other sites are extremely common. Temperature and leukocyte counts may or may not be elevated. The nodular lesions are often, although not always, painless, and the general condition of the cat is usually unchanged.

### Diagnosis

Although clinical signs may be suggestive, any diagnosis must be tentative until results of culture are known. A biospy may be helpful but not definitive. The only feature distinguishing this infection from feline leprosy with certainty is the presence of atypical mycobacteria, especially "rapid growers," and their presence can be established only by culture and subsequent identification of the agent. Repeated attempts may be necessary, since not every sample is positive even in eventually proven cases. Most of the organisms implicated can grow well on blood agar at 37 C within less than a week. Suggestive growth should be submitted to a laboratory versed in the identification of mycobacteria (a state public health laboratory or the National Jewish Hospital, Denver, CO).

The most obvious consideration in differential diagnosis is feline leprosy, in which lesions tend to be more generally distributed and sinus tracts are not typical. Some clinicians decline to attempt a distinction and question its validity. Tuberculosis, however, must be ruled out. White et al. (1983) further list "neoplasia, foreign body granuloma, mycotic infection, nodular panniculitis, pansteatitis, and chronic abscesses secondary to feline leukemia or other causes of immunosuppression."

### Treatment

*Mycobacterium fortuitum* and other mycobacteria found in cutaneous granulomas are susceptible in vitro to several antimicrobial drugs, particularly kanamycin, gentamicin, and amikacin, although most of the antituberculous drugs, (except ethambutol) are ineffective (Kunkle et al., 1983; Wilkinson et al., 1978). Tetracycline and chloramphenicol have been most often used, with some encouraging results. One case of infection with *M. chelonei* appeared to respond to treatment with rifampin (Thorel and Boisvert, 1974). Surgical excision sometimes seems effective. The important caveat is that untreated cases of such infections in humans have regressed spontaneously, while "successfully" treated cases have relapsed (Dewèvre et al., 1977). Experience with the feline disease is too limited to allow any definitive conclusions.

### Epidemiology

Since infection with atypical mycobacteria in humans is often associated with immunologic defects, feline leukemia might be suspected as a predisposing condition (Wilkinson et al., 1978). Yet, so far, tests of affected cats for feline leukemia virus (FeLV) have turned out to be negative (Kunkle et al., 1983; White et al, 1983). The agents are widely distributed in the inanimate environment. Although only a minority of reported cats had a history of trauma, the hypothesis of skin and wound contamination remains, in the absence of contrary evidence, the most acceptable one.

## SALMONELLOSIS

*Salmonella,* a Gram-negative, usually motile bacterium of the family Enterobacteriaceae, is a universally distributed pathogen of vertebrates. The genus is divided into well over 1000 serotypes ("species"), of which about 50 have been identified in cats—*S. typhimurium* with perhaps the greatest frequency. Domestic carnivores are relatively resistant to *Salmonella*-related disease, and most of the isolations recorded were from apparently healthy animals. Although epidemics of clinical salmonellosis occur, especially in kittens, the chief interest in *Salmonella* in cats concerns the possible epidemiologic significance, especially to humans. Estimates of the prevalence of *Salmonella* in cats have varied from less than 1 per cent (van der Gulden and Janssen, 1970) to over 20 per cent (Khan, 1970). The higher figures reflect cultures of mesenteric lymph nodes rather than of intestinal contents, feces, or rectal swabs. In general, there are fewer reports of either asymptomatic or clinical infection in cats than in other domestic animals (Wilkinson, 1983).

## PATHOGENESIS AND PATHOLOGIC FEATURES

Clinical salmonellosis in cats follows mostly three possible patterns: gastrointestinal, septicemic, or local-regional. In the first two, the portal of entry seems to be the gastrointestinal tract (Wilkinson, 1983). Cases destined to develop into clinical infections presumably begin, as in other host species, with colonization of the lower small intestine. Proliferation and invasion of the enteric mucosa often lead to gastrointestinal manifestations, particularly diarrhea. Feline *Salmonella* infection may also develop into septicemia with or without gastroenteritis, with colonization of organs, including liver, spleen, lymph nodes, and bone marrow. The organism may be recovered from the blood by appropriate culture. Lesions include catarrhal or hemorrhagic enteritis, enlarged spleen and lymph nodes, necrotic foci in the liver, fibrin deposits on the abdominal viscera, and fluid in the serous cavities (Ingham and Brentnall, 1972; Timoney, 1976, 1977). Widespread hemorrhages and thrombosis consistent with disseminated intravascular coagulation have been reported (Krum et al., 1977).

## CLINICAL FEATURES

Vomiting, diarrhea, or both are usually present as early signs. Cachexia and dehydration develop in cases of several days' duration. Fluctuating temperatures reaching as high as 41 C (106 F) are common. Inappetence, depression, and uncertain gait occur in various combinations (Madewell and McChesney, 1975; Timoney, 1976, 1977). Mucous membranes are pale. Blood studies reveal leukopenia, low hemoglobin levels, and hypoproteinemia. Occasional infections have been found to be localized in the conjunctivae (Fox and Beaucage, 1979), uterus (Hemsley, 1956; Mera, 1941; Messow and Hensel, 1960, 1961), and pleural cavity.

In an adult cat at the Angell Memorial Animal Hospital (AMAH), leukopenia, anemia, and terminal *S. typhimurium* septicemia were associated with a chronic gastric ulcer in which colonies of bacteria were numerous. In a cat with pyothorax, *S. choleraesuis* was isolated twice, but despite an initial response to drainage of the chest and chloramphenicol therapy, progressive interstitial pneumonia developed, and at autopsy the organism was recovered from the lungs.

## DIAGNOSIS

Neither clinical nor pathologic manifestations of salmonellosis include reliable pathognomonic features. Diagnosis is based on the isolation of a *Salmonella* in numbers consistent with infection. Isolations from stools may be misleading: they may reveal a presence of the agent unrelated to the cause of illness, or, in *Salmonella* septicemia, the agent may not be present in the feces. Serologic tests are not available, nor would they help in acute cases since antibody will not be demonstrable in time for useful therapeutic decisions.

For differential diagnosis, viral infections must be ruled out. Although neutropenia characterizes both panleukopenia and Gram-negative septicemias, the absence of neutrophils is virtually complete in panleukopenia, while some neutrophils can usually be found in salmonellosis and colibacillosis (Timoney, 1976).

## TREATMENT

Simple gastroenteritis and diarrhea should be treated symptomatically and not with antibiotics, for these reasons:

1. Antimicrobial drugs rarely eliminate the offending agent and prolong shedding (Carpenter, 1978).
2. They eliminate the normal flora, which preempts attachment areas targeted by pathogens and has other protective functions.
3. They cause emergence of resistant variants, complicating the case and contributing to the reduced usefulness of antimicrobial drugs in their legitimate sphere of application.

Systemic illness calls for antimicrobial therapy based on the results of susceptibility tests. Under optimal conditions these should be completed 36 to 48 hours after sample collection. Meanwhile therapy should be instituted. The drug of first choice is chloramphenicol. Trimethoprim has also been recommended (Timoney, 1976). Ampicillin and amoxicillin should not be chosen unless they are shown to be effective by susceptibility testing, since the majority of *Salmonella* isolates have been resistant to these. When effective in vitro, however, they have been shown, in contrast to chloramphenicol, to be capable of eliminating the carrier state in humans (Hirsh and Enos, 1980).

The correlation between in-vitro susceptibility and in-vitro response to therapy is often poor in salmonelloses. Aminoglycosides, although commonly showing good activity in vitro, are not recommended for treatment (Gardner and Provine, 1975). Their inability to penetrate promptly into cells may be related to this discrepancy. Specific antimicrobial treatment aside, fluid and electrolyte replacement should be a main concern when diarrhea and vomiting have been prolonged. Shock due to endotoxemia needs to be counteracted (Timoney, 1976).

## EPIDEMIOLOGY

The ultimate source of *Salmonella* is the intestinal tract of another animal. Birds and rodents are frequent carriers of *Salmonella* spp and presumably constitute a ready source of infection for cats. Infected milk, eggs, and meat are other possible sources (Wilkinson, 1983).

In general, only very young and stressed cats are affected clinically by salmonellosis. Attack rates of 32 per cent and a case fatality rate of 61 per cent were reported in a pet hospital outbreak (Timoney et al., 1978). Infection—not disease—was readily produced and transmitted to contact controls. Shedding of the agent was observed for up to four weeks.

Cats have been involved in outbreaks of salmonellosis that also included human cases, and circumstantial evidence sometimes suggested transmission from animals to people (Wollenweber et al., 1937). Often the route of dissemination is unclear, and the infection may originate from a common source (Madewell and McChesney, 1975). Owners concerned about possible *Salmonella*-shedding cats should submit periodic stool samples to a qualified laboratory. Test results should be negative for three successive weeks (Kraft, 1978).

## PSEUDOTUBERCULOSIS

Pseudotuberculosis is essentially an infection of wild rodents and birds. Humans and domestic animals are rarely infected (if so, presumably through interaction with one of the primary hosts). The causative agent, *Yersinia pseudotuberculosis,* is a Gram-negative motile bacterium, which, along with the plague bacillus, *Y. pestis,* and several human pathogens (formerly combined under the name *Y. enterocolitica*), is now considered part of the family Enterobacteriaceae. Previously it was classified as a *Pasteurella.* A number of serotypes exist, type I being most often identified in cats.

Among the domestic mammals, the cat is the main target of *Y. pseudotuberculosis* infection, probably as a result of its preying habits. The fact that most cases on record have been fatal may be more a reflection of the difficulty of clinical diagnosis than of the intractability of the infection.

As for incidence, pseudotuberculosis of cats has been described variously as "extremely rare" (Stünzi, 1957) and "common," i.e., more than 20 per cent (Jarmai, 1936). Mollaret (1965) believed that, owing to its nondistinctive manifestations, it is probably underdiagnosed. Without citing specific figures, Isler and Lott-Stolz (1978) described the incidence as undergoing a "considerable increase." A Japanese survey revealed a carrier incidence of 3.2 per cent among 373 cats (as well as 2.9 per cent carriers of *Y. enterocolitica*, an organism that can be isolated from feces of many normal domestic and wild animals) (Yanagawa et al., 1978).

### Pathogenesis and Lesions

All indications are that pseudotuberculosis of cats is acquired by ingestion. Except in an acute septicemic form with no localizing signs, manifestations and eventually lesions point to a gastrointestinal infection, which may begin with a catarrhal, nonulcerative inflammation of the stomach and intestine (Aubert, 1945; Chappuis, 1943; Communal, 1945; Leblois, 1920; Pallaske and Meyn, 1932). Involvement of the mesenteric lymph nodes need not be preceded by clinical or pathologic changes in the intestine. The nodes may be hemorrhagic and undergo striking enlargement up to three times normal size. The organ most consistently affected is the liver. Typically it is enlarged, often to twice or more its normal size, and presents an irregular, nodular surface. It is covered or permeated randomly by gray or yellowish white nodules measuring from a few millimeters to over a centimeter in diameter (Fig. 8–13). When incised, they yield a caseous material. They may or may not be readily separable from the liver parenchyma, which becomes friable and fatty, presenting a yellowish appearance.

The spleen is not as consistently affected as the liver. Its lesions resemble those of the liver. Other organs occasionally involved include kidney (Blähser, 1962), lung (Blähser, 1962), various lymph nodes (Aubert, 1945; Chappuis, 1943; Communal, 1945), and uterus (Labie, 1962).

Microscopically, the lesions begin with bacterial colonization of capillaries, e.g., of the hepatic lobules, evoking a modest mononuclear response and degenerative changes in adjacent hepatocytes. Eventually frank necrosis of liver parenchyma develops, appearing in stained sections as an acidophilic zone surrounded by bacteria. The cellular exudate enveloping this focus consists of macrophages and lymphocytes with admixtures of neutrophils and epithelioid cells (Drieux, 1970; Rahko and Saloniemi, 1969). The absence of giant cells and the abundance of bacteria constitute notable differences between *Y. pseudotuberculosis* lesions in cats and those in other species. Although usually called abscesses, their granulomatous features suggest the term pyogranuloma as more appropriate. Similar processes occur in the spleen where lesions begin in the malpighian corpuscles (Mollaret, 1965). Interstitial infiltration of inflammatory cells accounts for the enlargement of affected organs.

### Clinical Features

Estimates of the incubation period range from four days to several months, with a mean of three weeks (Mollaret, 1965). Specific signs are few. In acute cases inappetence, vomiting, and other signs of acute gastroenteritis may be present (Allard, 1975; Hubbert, 1972; Mair et al., 1967; Rahko and Saloniemi, 1969). Diarrhea may develop in some cases, constipation in others. Depending on the acuteness of the illness, depression will be followed by prostration at variable rates (Mollaret, 1965; Robinson, 1972). Weight loss is sometimes rapid. Fever may occur. Polyuria and urinary incontinence were described in one cat (Mair et al., 1967).

On physical examination, the mucous membranes are very pale or slightly yellow. Jaundice may, in fact, be the only presenting sign suggesting the nature of the condition. According to Mollaret (1965), four of five cases of feline jaundice seen in Lyons were ascribed to *Y. pseudotuberculosis* infection. Deep palpation sometimes reveals increased size and firmness and surface irregularities of the liver. Pain may be evinced on palpation, especially in the costolumbar fossa and right hypogastrium. Other possible findings are an enlarged, hardened spleen and palpable mesenteric lymph nodes. None of the changes described are dependably consistent. Auscultation and percussion reveal no abnormalities.

The course, almost invariably fatal, ranges from three days to as long as three months. Terminal signs are severe jaundice, subnormal temperature, complete constipation, and anorexia. Death may be preceded by convulsions or coma (Mollaret, 1965).

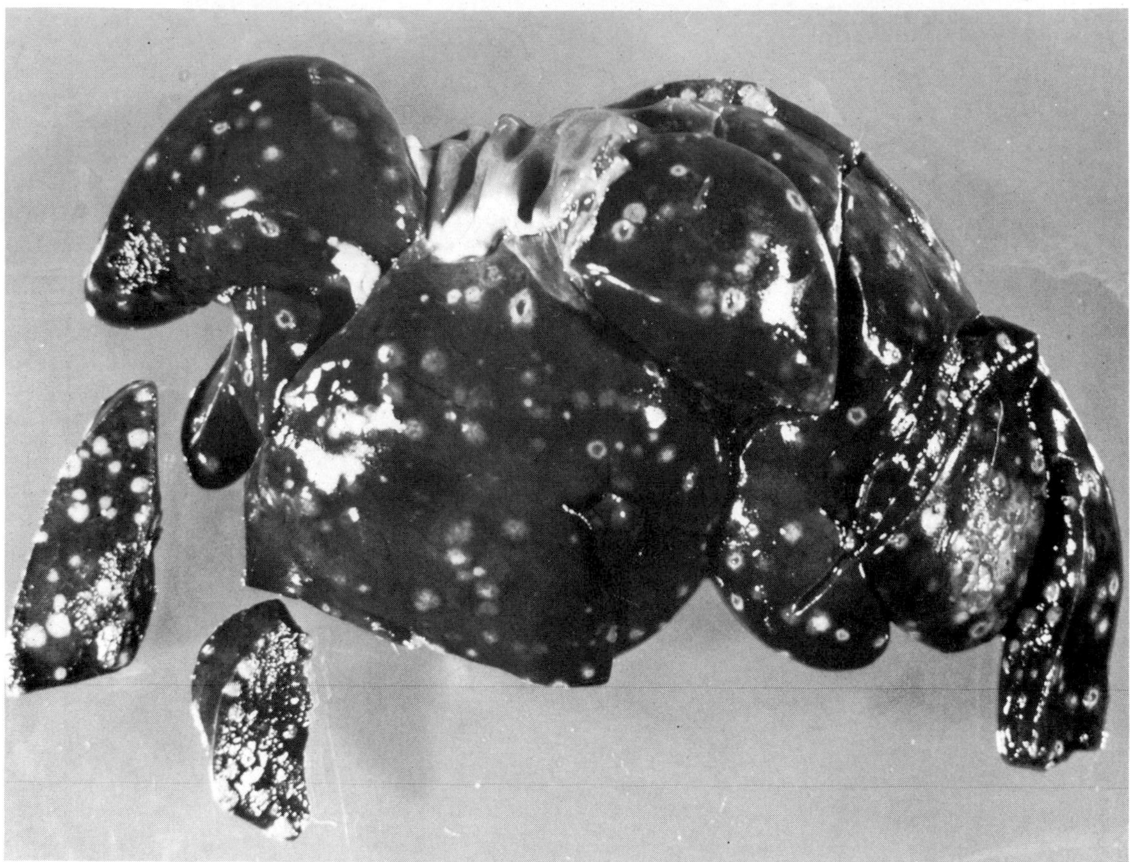

**Figure 8–13** Pseudotuberculosis, lynx. Numerous pale lesions widely disseminated on the liver surface and throughout the parenchyma are characteristic. (Department of Veterinary Pathology, University of California, Davis.)

## Diagnosis

The signs described, particularly if in an adult cat, should suggest pseudotuberculosis. Most helpful are the pale, faintly yellow mucous membranes and the abdominal pain, if present. Among the differential diagnoses are panleukopenia, which usually has a more rapid course and is attended by a greater degree of dehydration, tuberculosis, hepatic tumors, and chronic nephritis (Mollaret, 1965).

No dependable hematologic abnormalities have been described, nor is a routine diagnostic test available. Blood and feces should be cultured. Spearman et al. (1979) diagnosed a case by liver biopsy utilizing both histologic examination and culture.

## Treatment

Although the agent is generally susceptible in vitro to chloramphenicol, kanamycin, streptomycin, and tetracycline (Mollaret, 1965), proven cases of successfully treated *Y. pseudotuberculosis* infection are few. One cat was reported cured by injections of 100 mg tetracycline t.i.d. for 10 days (Allard, 1979). The case was atypical in that the main presenting sign was swelling of the mandibular lymph nodes, from which the agent was isolated. Constitutional manifestations, apart from occasional vomiting, were lacking. Another infection resolved after 20 days of oral hetacillin therapy (110 mg b.i.d.) and three months of supportive nursing and dietary care (Spearman et al., 1979).

## Epidemiology

*Yersinia pseudotuberculosis* infection is typically a disease of young adult and mature cats. Both sexes seem to be equally affected. The disease has been recorded mainly in continental Europe (Mollaret, 1965) but also in Great Britain (Robinson, 1972) and North America (Allard, 1979; Hubbert, 1972; Spearman et al., 1979). Most cases occur in winter or spring. Its limitation to active hunters and its absence in confined urban cats correlate with the presumed sources of infection, i.e., rodent and avian prey. Since the experimental feeding of pure cultures rarely reproduces the disease, Mollaret (1965) suggested the need for accessory etiologic factors, e.g., cold, intestinal injury, and humidity.

*Yersinia pseudotuberculosis* is pathogenic for humans. Actual evidence of feline-to-human dissemination is circumstantial (Paul and Weltmann, 1934), but families in which cats have been shown to be infected should be alerted and advised to consult their physicians concerning possible prophylactic measures.

## CAMPYLOBACTERIOSIS

Campylobacteriosis, both asymptomatic and diarrheic, is recognized increasingly in many species of pets and livestock as well as in humans, and much of the interest in infection in animals is focused on their possible role as reservoirs for human infection. The organism, *Campylobacter (Vibrio) jejuni*, a Gram-negative, S- or comma-shaped, flagellated rod, can now be cultured easily on selective media (for method see Fox et al., 1983b). With the current population explosion among pets and their growing concentration, especially in the limited confines of urban homes, it is likely that *Campylobacter* infection will be recognized with increasing frequency.

Infection is by the oral route, and sources include feces from infected animals and contaminated water, unpasteurized milk, and raw or undercooked poultry and meat.

Reports of feline infection were extensively reviewed by Fox et al. (1983a) and by Weber et al. (1983), and additional findings were presented by the latter group. Infections in cats have been reported in the United States, Great Britain, the European continent, and Australia. Prevalence is low among household pets, both healthy and diarrheic, but in shelters, pounds, and laboratory colonies incidences of infection as high as 45 per cent have been reported. In a survey at AMAH, of 21 normal cats and 23 diarrheic cats aged from four months to over a year, none proved to be infected (Moore, 1984). In both cats and dogs, infection is more frequent in young animals originating in pet shops and adoption organizations, but the prevalence of infection is consistently lower in cats than in dogs.

Cats, especially kittens with diarrhea, have been implicated as sources of human infection, although not nearly so often as dogs (Blaser et al., 1982; Skirrow et al., 1980; Svedhem and Norkrans, 1980). Antibody titers have been used to confirm suspected cat-human transmission (Blaser et al., 1982). However, in evaluating cases in which both human and pet are affected, the possibility of a common source should also be considered (Weber et al., 1983).

The picture is confusing because the agent can be found in the absence of diarrhea (Blaser et al., 1982) or in its presence when other possible causes have not been excluded (Fox et al., 1983a). In view of the diagnostic uncertainties of proven campylobacteriosis, clinical description must be interpreted with caution. Watery diarrhea, sometimes with vomiting, has been described in kittens (Skirrow et al., 1980; Svedhem and Norkrans, 1980). In dogs, mucus-laden or watery diarrhea, sometimes with blood and white cells, of three to seven days' duration, partial inappetence, occasional vomiting, and slight fever have been reported (Fox et al., 1983a). Why some animals develop diarrhea and others remain clinically normal is unclear.

What little is known of the pathologic changes points to a catarrhal enteritis affecting the colon. Dogs with both natural and experimental infections have exhibited stunting of intestinal villi, inflammatory cell infiltration of the lamina propria, and enlarged Peyer's patches (Fox et al., 1983a).

The duration of shedding by cats and dogs is not known, but in certain other species it may be as long as several months (Fox et al., 1983a; Weber et al., 1983).

In man the disease is often self-limiting and is usually not treated; however, antibiotic administration may be desirable to eliminate the infection and prevent relapses (Fox et al., 1983a). Although in-vitro studies indicate sensitivity to several antibiotics, erythromycin is considered the drug of choice for man. It has been reported to eliminate infection in dogs when given orally at the rate of 40 mg/kg for five days (Holt, 1980).

## PASTEURELLOSIS

Having over 100 mammalian and avian hosts, *Pasteurella multocida* is one of the most widely distributed microorganisms of animals (Biberstein, 1979). A small Gram-negative coccobacillus, it is a common inhabitant of the oral and upper respiratory mucous membranes in cats. The carrier rate is over 30 per cent (Oudar et al., 1972; Soltys, 1951; van Dorssen et al., 1964).

Numerous reports in the older literature described feline pasteurellosis, sometimes in cattery or laboratory outbreaks, as a septicemic disease in which the manifestations were predominantly respiratory (taking the form of pneumonia and pleurisy) or enteric (sometimes with vomiting and diarrhea) (Frohböse, 1926; Gaertner, 1909; Harms, 1939; Krembs, 1937; Pospischil, 1920; Ruppert, 1912, Spalatin, 1940). It is possible that in the latter type the primary pathogen may sometimes have been the panleukopenia virus.

One cat died of septicemic pasteurellosis within 18 hours after eating an infected duck (Palmeiro, 1942).

Occasionally *Pasteurella* has localized in the brain, producing signs suggestive of rabies or toxoplasmosis (Calaprice, 1959; Wachnik and Jasinska, 1958). Extension of an abscess into the spinal canal resulted in posterior paresis (Mitrovic, 1949).

In more recent experience, *P. multocida* appears to have little pathogenic activity in cats by itself, unless introduced into deeper tissue. Under these circumstances, as in bite wounds, the infectious process rarely yields *P. multocida* in pure culture. Typically *P. multocida* participates in mixed infections, its common associates being non–spore-forming anaerobic bacteria, e.g., *Bacteroides* spp, *Fusobacterium* spp, *Peptostreptococcus* sp, and *Actinomyces* spp. The infections tend to be purulent and necrotizing and include, apart from bite wounds and their sequelae (Balk et al., 1974), necrotic glossitis, pharyngitis, laryngitis, pyothorax, pulmonary abscesses, and pneumonia. Many of them require surgical relief as well as antimicrobial treatment (see also staphylococcal and streptococcal infections). In our experience, *P. multocida* infection in cats has generally been susceptible to penicillin and broad-spectrum antibiotics (as determined by the Kirby-Bauer method). Arnbjerg (1978) reported 100 per cent susceptibility to chloramphenicol, 50 per cent to tetracycline, and considerable resistance to penicillin, but did not state the testing method.

Feline *Pasteurella* infections are endogenous or transmitted by bites and scratches. The latter two mechanisms account for some human infections (Biberstein, 1979). Attempts to ascribe human pasteurellosis of nontraumatic origin to animal (especially feline) contacts (Atin and Beetham, 1957) have little solid support at present.

*Pasteurella pneumotropica,* a related agent often found in rodents, also occurs as a commensal in the throat of cats (van Dorssen et al., 1964) and has been found in cases of pneumonia or pleuropneumonia (Haagsma, 1964).

## PLAGUE

The susceptibility of cats to the plague bacillus, *Yersinia pestis,* has long been recognized (De Souza et al., 1910). Feline plague is of concern mainly as a possible source for human plague. Some of the more recent cases in cats were discovered in connection with human plague and implicated as sources of human infection in bite, scratch, airborne, and undetermined routes of transmission (Barnes and Poland, 1983; Ettenger et al., 1982; Goethals et al., 1981; Heaton et al., 1977; Thornton et al., 1975).

### Pathogenesis and Lesions

The known contact of cats with rodents recognized as plague carriers affords ample opportunity for transmission through flea bites, ingestion of infected rodents, or possibly inhalation of infected material. In one instance, kittens may have been infected by nursing an infected queen (Thornton et al., 1975). Pathologic evidence suggests ingestion and inhalation as means of infection, since most affected cats have had lesions related to the alimentary and respiratory tracts, including edema around head and neck, suppurative lymphadenitis, necrotic tonsillitis, and pneumonia.

### Clinical Features

Illness in cats may be signaled by dullness, inactivity, fever (41.5 C, 107 F) and inappetence (Fitch et al., 1977). Incoordination and quadriplegia have been described (Thornton et al., 1975). Swellings around the head, neck, and eyes with enlargement of the mandibular lymph nodes are particularly common. There may be sneezing of purulent material (Fitch et al., 1977) and hemoptysis (Green et al., 1977).

The prognosis is guarded. In a group of five kittens from two litters, four died within four to seven days (Thornton et al., 1975).

### Diagnosis

In view of their public health implications, all suspected cases of plague should be subjected to exhaustive attempts at laboratory confirmation. These should be carried out under the instructions and close supervision of appropriate public health personnel (see section on special precautions). From the living animal, samples of affected lymph nodes and edematous tissues, transtracheal aspirates, and nasal swab specimens should be obtained. Blood should be cultured. If neural signs are present, cerebrospinal fluid should also be collected. All specimens should be forwarded promptly to a laboratory experienced in, and equipped for, plague diagnosis. The direct examination of smears by immunofluorescence techniques as well as cultures should be requested. Serum or clotted blood should also be submitted for antibody determination, the first sample accompanying the samples for culture. If the cat survives, another sample should be submitted about two weeks later. The appearance of antibody or a rise in antibody titer in the second sample would be strong indication of the presence of plague.

Among the differential diagnoses to be considered, tularemia would rank high and call for the same laboratory diagnostic measures applicable in plague. Nonspecific local infections around the head and neck, especially in cats with systemic manifestations, would have to be differentiated by culture.

### Treatment

Successful treatment with tetracycline was reported in one case (Fitch et al., 1977). Streptomycin is the drug of choice in human plague, and chloramphenicol is another alternative.

### Epidemiology

The likely sources and routes of feline infection have already been considered. The disease has been reported only in known endemic areas, including South Africa (Isaäcson et al., 1973) and the western United States (Arizona, California, Colorado, and New Mexico) (Fitch et al., 1977; Green et al., 1977; Heaton et al., 1977; Rollag et al., 1980, 1981). Cats of all ages have apparently been involved. Apart from being possible sources of flea- and airborne plague, infected cats have been suspected of passing the infection to humans by bites and scratches, neither of which figure significantly in the transmission of plague from other hosts (Weniger et al., 1984). Cat-to-cat transmission has been implied only once (Thornton et al., 1975).

### Special Precautions

The Centers for Disease Control have made the following recommendations concerning the handling of feline plague suspects:

1. Consult local and state public health officials immediately to arrange for laboratory testing and measures for prevention of spread and contamination.
2. Strictly isolate all cats under suspicion of infection.
3. When handling a suspect cat, wear mask, gown, and gloves.
4. Treat all suspected cats for fleas, "whether or not fleas are apparent . . . using a product with residual effect such as 5 per cent carbaryl dust" (Rollag et al., 1980).

## TETANUS

Although the cat is estimated to be at least 2000 times more resistant to the toxin of *Clostridium tetani* than the horse (Fildes et al., 1929, 1931), the disease develops occasionally in animals with contaminated wounds—most often castration wounds (Bateman, 1931; Hopson, 1932), trap injuries (Fildes et al., 1929; Goetz, 1976; Groulade, 1947; Killingsworth et al., 1977; Lettow, 1955), lacerations (Ludins, 1939), or deep punctures (Kodituwakku and Wijewanta, 1958; Miller, 1949). Most affected cats are young males, but posthysterectomy and postpartum cases have been reported (Loeffler et al., 1962; Nam, 1956; Saranta, 1977).

In natural infections, clinical signs appear over a period varying from a few days to two weeks, most often at about 10 days. Since the diagnosis is invariably clinical and confirmed bacteriologically in only exceptional cases and, further, since the time of relevant exposure is an assumption by the diagnostician, reports of unusually short incubation periods (Nam, 1956) should perhaps be accepted with some reserve.

A stiff gait and rigidity of the tail are first signs, with hypersensitivity to sound and touch. The tail may be drawn forward over the back, and the ears adducted. Later the head is drawn back, and the limbs are so stiffly extended that the cat is unable to walk. Consciousness is not impaired. A spasm of the masticatory muscles may develop in some cats, some manifesting trismus, but others continue to be able and eager to eat (Killingsworth et al., 1977). Defecation and urination may be suspended. The temperature varies, being elevated in some cats, subnormal in others. In some, there is prolapse of the nictitating membrane. Death is usually due to exhaustion or respiratory failure.

If the disease is not too far advanced, it may be treated successfully. Prompt administration of antitoxin in a single dose of 100 to 500 units/kg is more effective if given intravenously than by the intramuscular or subcutaneous route. A test dose of 0.1 to 0.2 ml should be given subcutaneously 30 minutes before the intravenous dose to test for an allergic reaction. The intravenous dose should be given slowly over five to 10 minutes. Antitoxin (1000 units) may also be injected intramuscularly about the wound. Penicillin G (10,000 to 15,000 units/kg) should be given every 12 hours as long as clinical signs continue; it may be injected intramuscularly close to the wound site.

After administration of antitoxin, an infected wound may be débrided and flushed with hydrogen peroxide.

In early cases, recovery may occur overnight; in others, some days or even weeks elapse before the cat returns to normal. The cat must be kept in a quiet, darkened room, observed constantly, and handled as little as possible. Good nursing is essential. Chlorpromazine may be administered for hyperexcitability and barbiturates (pentobarbital, phenobarbital) or diazepam for controlling spasms and seizures. Narcotics and parasympatholytic drugs (e.g., atropine) are contraindicated. Tracheostomy is sometimes required for maintenance of an airway, and the urinary bladder may have to be expressed or catheterized. Because of the exhausting nature of the disease, electrolyte, fluid, and caloric needs must be met by parenteral administration or tube feeding if a cat cannot eat or drink.

Treatment has been described in detail by Greene (1983).

## LISTERIOSIS

*Listeria monocytogenes,* a motile, non–spore-forming, Gram-positive rod with a broad host range and impressive capacity to survive and probably multiply apart from any host, has occasionally been encountered in cats. Of the two forms of listeriosis recognized in animals, the central nervous system and the visceral, most of the feline cases reported have involved visceral lesions. Depression, inappetence, and abdominal pain have been common signs, with diarrhea or vomiting usually present (Decker et al., 1976; Held, 1958; Nilsson and Karlsson, 1959; Turner, 1962). Autopsy usually reveals enlarged livers, spleens, and lymph nodes. An instance of isolation from a cat brain is on record (McIlwain et al., 1966).

Listeriosis appears to be extremely rare in cats. Except for isolation from a skin wound (Jones et al., 1984), it has never been diagnosed in a living animal. Should it be suspected, the penicillins, erythromycin, tetracycline, and chloramphenicol should be tried, for they have been found effective in other species (Armstrong, 1979).

## TYZZER'S DISEASE

Tyzzer's disease was originally described as a necrotizing enterohepatitis of mice caused by a Gram-negative, spore-bearing bacterium, *Bacillus piliformis*, which has not been propagated on lifeless media. It has since been diagnosed in a variety of other mammals (Hall and Van Kruiningen, 1974; Qureshi et al., 1976). Four of five reports of Tyzzer's disease in cats have concerned laboratory animals.

The disease begins with anorexia and depression. There is constipation in some cats (Kobokawa et al., 1973), diarrhea in others (Kovatch and Zebarth, 1973; Schneck, 1975), followed by death within two weeks. Jaundice was reported by Jones et al. (1985). Focal hepatic necrosis and necrotizing ileocolitis are consistent findings. Enlarged mesenteric lymph nodes and adrenal hypertrophy have been seen (Kobokawa et al., 1973). A diagnostic feature is the presence of bundles of filamentous bacteria within hepatocytes near the periphery of the necrotic foci and within intestinal epithelial cells. The bacteria are demonstrable by Giemsa (Kovatch and Zebarth, 1973) and silver stains (Warthin-Starry, Gomori methenamine silver [Bennett et al., 1977]). Myocarditis was observed by Jones et al. (1985). The predominance of the reported cases in laboratory cats may reflect less on stress factors implicit in laboratory situations than on the availability of diagnostic services. No treatment is known for the feline infection. Tetracycline has shown some effectiveness in experimental mouse infections (Schneck, 1969).

## BRUCELLOSIS

Clinical infections with *Brucella* organisms appear to be rare in the cat, those few reported taking the form of orchitis (Reinhardt, 1952) and of abortion due to *B. suis* (Frei, 1932), *B. abortus* (Koegel, 1924), and *B. melitensis* (Hirchert et al., 1967). Only rarely do serologic surveys turn up a cat with a suspicious or positive reaction (Menchaca, 1959; Pallaske, 1938; Poelma et al., 1933; Shaw, 1907; Valla, 1933).

Resistance extends to experimental infections (Jørgensen, 1943). Except for rare instances of abortion or arthritis (Nechayeva, 1952), most cats remain asymptomatic, and the antibody response is irregular. In one instance only, when cats were inoculated parenterally with cultures of *B. melitensis* or *B. abortus,* some developed chronic illness manifested by weight loss, conjunctivitis, cough, and arthritis, while one died in 10 days with septicemic signs (Makhawejsky and Karkadinowskaya, 1932). The agents were recovered from lesions of internal organs, joints, or urine at autopsy, and antibody titers ranged from negative to 1:32,000.

Although no natural clinical infections with *B. canis* are on record, cats are described as moderately susceptible (Pickerell and Carmichael, 1972). Bacteremia was shown to occur after experimental exposure in 3 of 14 animals but with a much slower onset than in dogs. No abortions were induced, and the mortality among kittens of exposed queens was comparable to that among control litters (Pickerell, 1970). The serologic response appears to be as erratic as to the classic *Brucella* spp, and the significance of titers detected in random field samples could not be determined (Randhawa et al., 1977).

## TULAREMIA

Clinical infection of cats with *Francisella tularensis* is apparently rare. The few reports suggest a close association with rodent epidemics and die-offs inviting massive exposure of predators through ingestion of infected tissues (Ditchfield et al., 1960; Schuller and Erdmann, 1943). Affected cats showed anorexia, uncontrolled vomiting, and rapid weight loss. Death occurred within two to five days. White foci on the liver and spleen were the predominant autopsy finding. Although no successfully treated cases of feline tularemia have been reported, streptomycin would be the drug of choice.

Cats have been circumstantially implicated as sources of human tularemia (Packer et al., 1982).

## ANTHRAX

Carnivores have considerable resistance to infection with the Gram-positive, spore-forming anthrax bacillus. A few cases traceable to the ingestion of infected meat have been reported in cats (Cripps and Young, 1960; Reinhardt, 1952). Signs were inappetence; uneasiness; apathy; local hemorrhagic inflammation of the lips, tongue, and throat; carbuncle-like lesions in the digestive tract; and swelling of the spleen, liver, and kidneys. Blood films stained with methylene blue teemed with organisms.

An anthrax-like bacillus, *B. cereus,* which has been implicated in human food poisoning, was reported to be the agent of enteritis and septicemia in a cat (Niléhn, 1958).

## GLANDERS

Large zoo cats and rarely domestic cats develop glanders after being fed on the flesh of infected horses. Nodules and ulcers appear on the mucous membranes of the palpebral conjunctivae, nostrils, larynx, trachea, and bronchi. A purulent discharge, at first gray-yellow but later bloody, flows from the nose. Owing to swelling of lymph nodes about the esophagus and respiratory passages, breathing becomes difficult. Death occurs in 8 to 14 days (Reinhardt, 1952). With the disappearance of equine glanders from the developed countries, it is unlikely to cause a problem in cats. Its main importance would be as a public health threat.

## LEPTOSPIROSIS

Leptospirae are the most slender of spirochetes, measuring about 0.1 μm in width and 10 μm in length. Of the two species, *L. biflexa* and *L. interrogans,* only the latter is of medical interest. It is made up of many serotypes ("serovars"), which were formerly considered species, e.g., *L. icterohaemorrhagiae, L. canicola,* and *L. pomona.* Although serotypes are bacteriologically indistinguishable, they differ in their pathogenicity patterns and epidemiologic aspects. In contrast with humans and most domestic animals, cats are rarely affected by clinical leptospirosis and even demonstrable subclinical leptospiral infections. In susceptible hosts, leptospiral disease begins, like other acute systemic infections, with a febrile reaction. This may be followed by localizing signs referable to liver and kidney malfunction, e.g., jaundice, urinary abnormalities, and an elevated blood urea nitrogen level. In surviving animals, the organisms localize in the renal tubules whence they are excreted for variable periods and where they may possibly contribute to eventual chronic renal failure.

Most animals exposed to leptospirae develop no clinical disease but, like those surviving the first 7 to 10 days of clinical leptospirosis, develop antibodies.

Information about feline leptospirosis rests largely on serologic surveys, which demonstrated reactor rates from about 5 per cent (Murphy et al., 1958) to over 20 per cent (Modrić, 1978). Their relationship to disease in cats or to leptospirosis in other species has not been persuasively established. Nor have leptospirae been convincingly implicated as a significant cause of jaundice (Carlos, 1971; Mason et al., 1972) or renal lesions in cats (Hamilton, 1966; Lucke and Crowther, 1965), rare exceptions notwithstanding (Hemsley, 1956; Rees, 1964). Experimental infections have produced no clinical disease and negligible pathologic changes, but a temporary carrier state for periods up to three months (Fessler and Morter, 1964; Klaarenbeek and Winsser, 1938; Otten et al., 1954). Cats occasionally have been shown to be carriers under natural conditions (Harkness et al., 1970).

Available evidence argues against feline leptospirosis as either a significant clinical or public health problem.

## NONSPECIFIC INFECTIONS

### *Escherichia coli*

Apart from sporadic involvement in mixed opportunistic infections and secondary bacteremias, *E. coli* has been implicated mainly in three kinds of syndromes: gastrointestinal, urinary, and genital.

The evidence for a significant etiologic role in gastroenteritis is circumstantial: certain serotypes of the agent, e.g., 06 and 042 described as potentially enteropathogenic in other hosts, have been found repeatedly in diarrheal disease of cats. Normal cats also carry these and other serotypes, as well as untypable strains (Langman, 1964; Månsson and Lindblad, 1962; Rhoades et al., 1971). Most reports antedate the recognition of the *E. coli* enterotoxins and of dysenteric types. They are therefore, at most, tentative evidence of pathogenicity of *E. coli.*

Bacterial urinary tract infection in cats is a relative rarity compared with that in dogs and nonbacterial urinary tract problems in cats (Schechter, 1970). When bacterial cystitis occurs, *E. coli* is the agent most frequently identified (Wilkinson, 1966). It has also been implicated in pyelonephritis (Hara et al., 1976). Most isolates are hemolytic and tend to be resistant to many antimicrobial drugs as determined by the Kirby-Bauer tests. Since this test ignores the penicillin and tetracycline levels attained in urine, these findings may not rule out these drugs for treating urinary tract infections.

*Escherichia coli* is often found in pyometra (endometritis, cystic hyperplasia), although other bacteria (β-hemolytic streptococci) or no bacteria may accompany this condition (Wilkinson, 1966). Almost all isolates are hemolytic, and a diversity of serotypes has been encountered (Choi and Kawata, 1975). Their primary etiologic significance in the condition is questionable, but they may possibly complicate the disease and contribute to toxic manifestations (Finco et al., 1975).

Possibly *E. coli* is implicated in the "fading kitten" syndrome, since hemolytic *E. coli* has been isolated occasionally from dead kittens (Langman, 1964; Scott et al., 1979). In view of current evidence, *E. coli* seems unlikely to be the only or even chief cause of the problem (Scott et al., 1979).

Antimicrobial treatment of *E. coli* infections is becoming increasingly complicated by the rise in prevalence of antimicrobial resistance (e.g., Moss and Prost, 1984). Ampicillin and tetracycline are no longer likely to be effective. Chloramphenicol and the newer aminoglycosides are usually effective, but a properly performed susceptibility test should be done for best results. Lacking data on antimicrobial urinary levels in cats, we may perhaps extrapolate from human and canine studies and assume that trimethoprim-sulfonamide and ampicillin levels will be adequate for the elimination of *E. coli* from the urinary tract (Ling, 1980).

Little is known about the epidemiology of potentially pathogenic *E. coli* in cats. In one study, 40 per cent of a sample of 103 normal animals proved to be carriers of suspect serotypes (Mackel et al., 1960). The criteria of enteropathogenicity have become more rigorous, and it is uncertain how many of such strains would qualify as pathogens. No relationship between feline carriers and human disease (infant diarrhea) has ever been established (Mackel et al., 1960).

## Staphylococcal Infections

*Staphylococcus intermedius* and *Staphylococcus aureus,* including types affecting humans, have been isolated from the nostrils of apparently normal cats (Daigo, 1973; Hearst, 1967; Raus and Love, 1983). The public health significance of this finding is uncertain. Among 827 staphylococcal species isolated from seven anatomic sites on 113 clinically healthy cats, *S. simulans* and *S. intermedius* predominated (Cox et al., 1985); both organisms have also been isolated from pathologic conditions in cats. Another study found *S. simulans* to be the most frequent species on the healthy skin and in the nares of cats, while *S. aureus* and *S. epidermidis* were most often associated with lesions (Devriese et al., 1984). Staphylococci participate in many pyogenic processes in cats, e.g., wound abscesses, otitis, and pyothorax. Usually such infections respond to surgical drainage and appropriate antibiotic therapy. A California survey found 21 of 40 *S. aureus* strains in cats resistant to at least one of eight common antibiotics, most often penicillin (40 per cent), tetracycline (27 per cent), and streptomycin (20 per cent) (Biberstein et al., 1974). All cultures were susceptible to chloramphenicol.

An acute and often intractable dermatitis occurs in cats in which staphylococci and streptococci have been implicated. The lesions, usually on the head or forelegs near the flexure of the elbow, are raw and weeping, often with a plaque-like, thickened periphery. The cat's licking may lead to a chronic course (Wilkinson, 1966). Irrespective of in-vitro susceptibility, response to antimicrobial drugs is usually discouraging. Wilkinson recommended applying 1 per cent aqueous gentian violet and restraint from licking (Elizabethan collar). Macdonald et al. (1972) reported success with autogenous bacterin in treating a previously refractory case of chronic dermatitis associated with staphylococcal infection.

Staphylococcal granuloma ("botryomycosis") appears to be uncommon in cats, but a cutaneous process (Walton et al., 1983) and a pneumonia of this type have been reported (Nielsen, 1957). The term "botryomycosis" was also applied to a generalized infection with *Micrococcus ascoformans,* an organism of the same family as the staphylococci (Habermann and Williams, 1956). The agent was isolated from granulomas of the lung, esophagus, stomach, spleen, colon, and abdominal cavity.

## Streptococcal Infections

Beta-hemolytic streptococci, most commonly of Lancefield group G, are often recovered from lesions of the skin and upper respiratory and lower genital tracts. Their significance as primary causes of disease is often uncertain, but descriptions of a highly contagious, experimentally reproducible cervical lymphadenitis in laboratory cats suggest parallels with the transmissible streptococcal infections in humans (group A), horses (group C), and swine (group E) (Goldman and Moore, 1973; Swindle et al., 1980; Tillman et al., 1982). Isolates have been uniformly susceptible to penicillin.

## *Bordetella bronchiseptica*

This Gram-negative, motile, nonfermentative rod is implicated in several respiratory infections of animals, including occasionally laboratory cats (Snyder et al., 1973). Normal carriers have been identified and mentioned as potential threats for other, more susceptible laboratory species (Fisk and Soave, 1973). The disease in kittens responded to chloramphenicol therapy, and the agent has shown in-vitro susceptibility to gentamicin, kanamycin, tetracycline, carbenicillin, erythromycin, neomycin, and polymyxin (Roudebush and Fales, 1981). Success was also claimed for immunization with autogenous bacterin (Paterson, 1963).

### *Haemophilus* SPP

*Haemophilus* spp, resembling most closely *H. parainfluenzae,* have been associated with conjunctivitis in successive litters of cattery kittens (Wilkinson, 1966) and also with chronic rhinitis (Wilkinson, 1983). We (E.B.) have made repeated isolations of this kind from cats of varying ages. Of eight such cases, *Haemophilus* sp was the single isolate in two. One further strain was recovered from cerebrospinal fluid. Detailed bacteriologic studies of isolates have yet to be done. The suggestion that these originate in humans (Wilkinson, 1966, 1983) is conjectural and, in view of the usual host specificity of *Haemophilus* spp, unlikely.

### CLOSTRIDIA OTHER THAN *C. tetani*

Botulism is an intoxication usually due to the ingestion of food in which *C. botulinum* has been proliferating. No clinical descriptions of the disease in cats exist. In other species, flaccid paralysis of skeletal muscles is the predominant sign. Death results from respiratory failure. The sole interest in botulism in connection with cats stems from the observation that the agent can proliferate and elaborate toxin in cat carcasses, which, under farm conditions, have been implicated as a source of botulism in livestock (Prévot and Sillioc, 1955).

There is a reference to the death of two cats in the course of an outbreak of human botulism (Haugaard and Jørgensen, 1974). The carcass of one of them, exhumed after four days, was shown to contain toxin and organisms of the homologous type.

Natural wound infections and gas gangrene have been reported in cats in association with *C. septicum* (Soltys, 1963), *C. chauvoei–C. septicum* (Poonacha et al., 1982), and *C. sporogenes* (Mansfield et al., 1984). A new species, *C. villosum,* has been isolated from subcutaneous abscesses of cats (Love et al., 1979).

*C. perfringens,* an organism widespread in nature and part of the intestinal flora in normal warm-blooded animals, has been recovered in pure culture from the intestine and feces of cats with acute enteric disorders, but its role as a pathogen is uncertain (Wilkinson, 1983).

### EUGONIC FERMENTER-4 (EF-4)

Strains of EF-4, a Gram-negative bacterium, have been associated with a rapidly fatal, necrotizing pneumonia in several outdoor, domestic-breed cats (Jang et al., 1973; McParland et al., 1982). One cat, apparently in good health before disappearing for two days, was found dead. Severe dyspnea was the outstanding sign in three others. Blood studies in two disclosed moderate anemia and depressed white-cell counts. Pale nodules scattered diffusely throughout the lungs were the characteristic autopsy finding and proved microscopically to be multiple colonies of Gram-negative bacteria associated principally with mononuclear white cells.

### *Serratia marcescens*

This Gram-negative enteric bacterium was long believed to be a harmless saprophyte but has been increasingly identified as a pathogen in a variety of infections in humans and in domestic and wild animals. In some cases it has been implicated as a contaminant of parenteral solutions or associated with use of intravenous catheters (Armstrong, 1984).

In one cat it was isolated from an intravenous catheter and from the liver at autopsy (Fox et al., 1981). In another cat severe bruising from a car accident resulted in systemic infection with *S. marcescens* sensitive to chloramphenicol and gentamicin, as well as an *Enterobacter* sp with a similar pattern of antibiotic resistance (Armstrong, 1984). The cat recovered after two weeks' treatment with chloramphenicol. In many cases, however, resistance to antibiotics is a serious problem, and synergistic combinations may be required.

### *Klebsiella* SPP

These Gram-negative encapsulated rods are common environmental saprophytes and also commensals in the gastrointestinal tract of healthy animals. They are important offenders in nosocomial disease and often give rise to secondary respiratory and genitourinary infections. They can be a special hazard in intensive care units where seriously ill and debilitated animals may be subjected to numerous invasive procedures over protracted periods.

For example, a cat hospitalized intermittently at AMAH for acute episodes of what was believed to be feline infectious peritonitis ultimately succumbed to meningitis from which a *Klebsiella* sp was recovered.

### OTHER INFECTIONS

Isolated encounters with bacteria in feline disease include cases of meningitis associated with a bacterium resembling *Flavobacterium meningosepticum* (Sims, 1974); a cattery outbreak of conjunctivitis due to *Moraxella lacunata* (Withers and Davies, 1961); a thoracic pyogranuloma and a leg abscess associated with *Corynebacterium equi* (Jang et al., 1975; Higgins and Paradis, 1980); and a uterine infection involving a *Campylobacter fetus*–like agent (Vallée et al., 1961).

#### Mixed Purulent-Necrotic Infections

Paradoxically perhaps, the most prevalent bacterial infections of cats cannot be ascribed to the activity of single bacterial species, but to the combined effect of several, all members of normal flora. These processes include skin and subcutaneous abscesses, pyothorax, and the various forms of "fusospirochetal disease." Many are probably traumatic in some aspect of their origin, a circumstance consistent with the orogastrointestinal flora colonizing them. The oral forms are sometimes related to pre-existing dental problems. The microbes most commonly involved are *Pasteurella multocida,* non–spore-forming anaerobes like *Bacteroides* spp, *Fusobacterium* spp, *Peptostreptococcus anaerobius, Actinomyces* spp, *Treponema* spp, *Leptotrichia buccalis,* and Enterobacteriaceae, including *E. coli* and *Proteus mirabilis* (Fig. 8–14). Culturing for anaerobes is relatively costly but has demonstrated the important role of a variety of these agents in suppurative processes in cats—bite wound infection, pyothorax, osteomyelitis, and peritonitis (e.g., John-

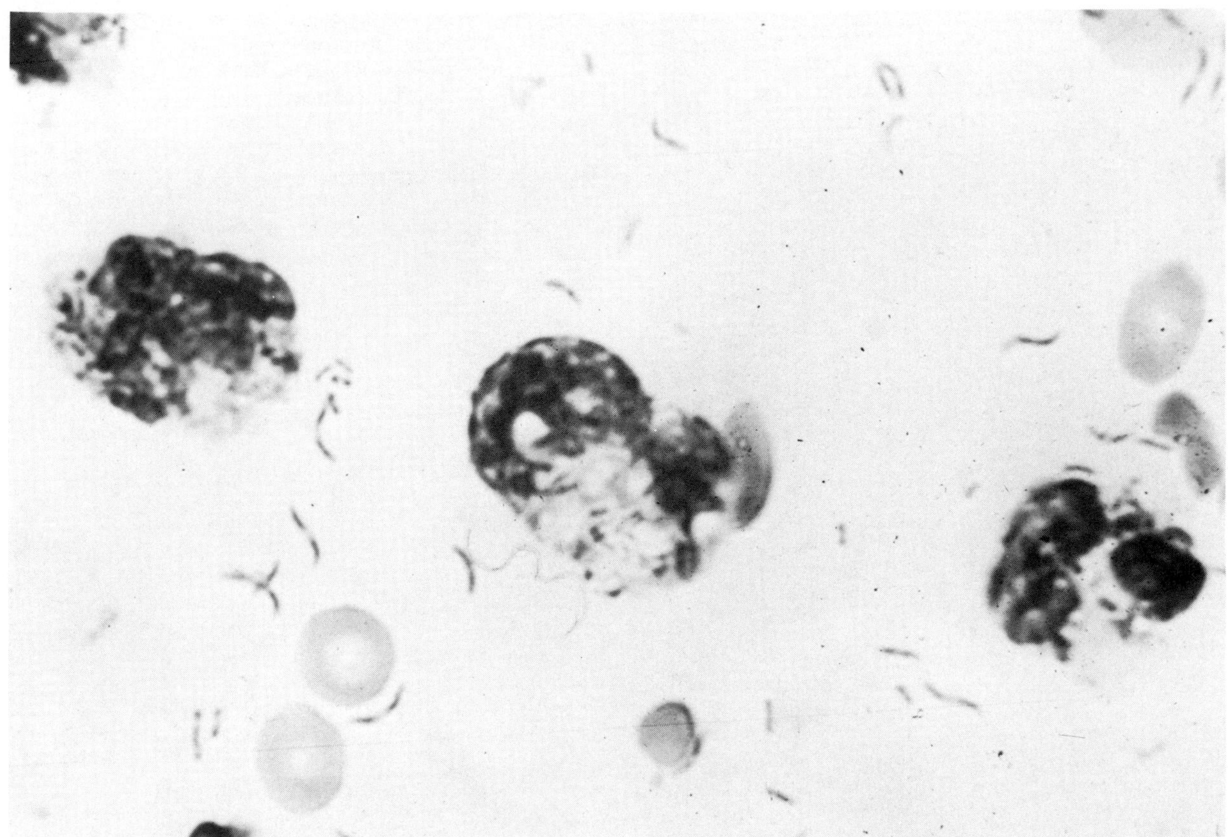

**Figure 8–14** Pyothorax in a cat, direct smear. At least three bacterial forms are distinguishable: crescentic, fusiform, presumably anaerobic bacteria; bipolar rods of varying length, consistent with *Pasteurella* sp; and a spirochete (center) suggestive of *Treponema* sp. Giemsa stain, approximately × 2000. *Bacteroides* and *Pasteurella* spp were isolated. (University of California, Davis.)

son et al., 1984; Love et al., 1982; Scott et al., 1984). Staphylococci, α- or β-hemolytic streptococci, and corynebacteria, often unidentifiable as to species, are also found (Dickie, 1979). Love et al. (1982) have identified, in addition to some of the foregoing, a hitherto undescribed *Clostridium villosum* as a frequent participant.

Many of the infections caused by these organisms require primarily a surgical approach for draining the pus and removing necrotic debris and fibrinous deposits (e.g., Creighton and Wilkins, 1980). Nursing and supportive care are all-important. Antimicrobial treatment calls for either a broad-spectrum drug like chloramphenicol or penicillin, which will be effective against most of the anaerobes, in combination with an aminoglycoside (e.g., kanamycin) for control of enteric Gram-negative agents. Clindamycin is effective against the non–spore-forming anaerobes and is preferable to penicillin when *Bacteroides fragilis* is present. Gentamicin by itself, despite its broad range, would not be a good choice because of its ineffectiveness against anaerobic bacteria (Rosenblatt, 1980). A clindamycin-gentamicin combination is used in human medicine for the control of mixed aerobe-anaerobe infections (Chow et al., 1974). A claim of clindamycin-aminoglycoside antagonism raises some question concerning the validity of this practice (Zinner et al., 1976). Metronidazole has been used with apparent success for enteric anaerobic infection (Carwardine, 1983). There is some evidence for changes in prevalence and susceptibility of obligate anaerobes obtained from domestic animals, but all isolates were susceptible to chloramphenicol, tetracycline (except for penicillin-resistant *Bacteroides*), clindamycin, and metronidazole (Hirsh et al., 1985).

## "Fusospirochetal" Infections

Although it is possible that the primary etiologic significance of spiral forms seen in direct smears may be overestimated, for the clinician certain feline infections in which spirochetes and fusiform bacilli are seen in great numbers constitute rather characteristic entities. Presumably lowered resistance permits these commensals of the mouth to act as pathogens.

Fusospirochetal stomatitis, sometimes referred to as "trench mouth," varies in its manifestations, depending on whether it is acute or chronic, but consistently betrays itself by its characteristic foul odor. Dental disease in the form of accumulated tartar and retained deciduous or loose teeth is often present, but sometimes no predisposing cause is apparent. Some affected cats are leukopenic and anemic, and a deficiency in these defenses may permit organisms that are ordinarily harmless to become pathogenic. Some affected cats are carriers of the feline leukemia virus.

Fusospirochetal stomatitis may occur in cats of any age. Signs are a strong, sweetish, foul odor from the mouth, reluctance to eat, sometimes drooling of thick, odorous

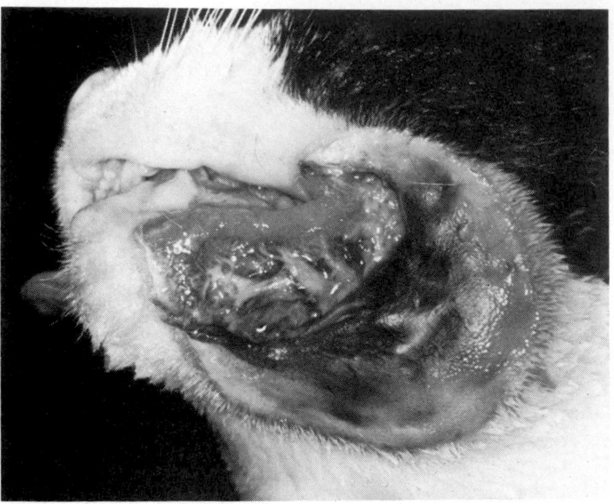

**Figure 8–15** Fulminating fusospirochetal infection extending from the gingiva to the face and underside of the jaw, five-year-old male domestic shorthair. Spirochetes and fusiform bacilli were numerous in smears of necrotic gum and cheek. Thrombosis of a submaxillary vein probably was responsible for the sharply demarcated necrosis and loss of tissue. (Angell Memorial Animal Hospital.)

saliva, and a chattering movement of the lower jaw. Early in the infection the veterinarian may find nothing except the characteristic odor and slimy saliva. Often, however, the margins of the gums have begun to redden and occasionally the lips are swollen. Ulceration and necrosis follow. The lesions are at first tiny and confined to the gum line but gradually enlarge, involving more and more tissue until the underlying bone is denuded of flesh and the necrotizing process extends to the inside of the cheeks, the lips, and even the skin of the face (Fig. 8–15). Occasionally there are ulcers of the tip or lateral edges of the tongue. In severe infections of this sort, the cats usually have high fevers (to 41.5 C, 107 F) and, if the disease goes unchecked, become apathetic and even prostrate.

In most cases, the response to administration of penicillin and B-complex vitamins is swift. If a cat is not eating or is dehydrated, parenteral administration of fluids is required. Flushing the mouth several times a day with physiologic saline solution prevents accumulation of slime and debris. This may be followed by swabbing with a mild antiseptic such as 2 per cent sodium perborate. Rarely an advanced infection proves refractory, involving more and more tissue despite all measures; the fever remains high, and the cat becomes more and more depressed. In some such cases, a blood transfusion is lifesaving.

More frequent than fulminating stomatitis is a mild chronic infection that does not seem to affect the cat's general health but betrays itself by a consistently foul odor and excessive saliva. The gum line is stubbornly inflamed and teeth loosen prematurely. A course of antibiotic treatment brings about a temporary remission, but, in the experience of one of the authors (J.H.), only when most or all of the teeth are removed, will the cat have a healthy mouth.

In occasional cases of pyothorax, spirochetes and fusiform bacilli are present in great numbers in a thin, pinkish tan pus with the same odor as in the mouth infection. Cats seem sicker with this variety of empyema than with any other and often die despite prompt drainage of the chest, medication with antibiotics, and supportive measures. A bizarre histologic finding in a fatal case of fusispirochetal empyema at the AMAH was the presence of spirochetes in the adventitial fat of the intestine.

Bite wound infections in which smears of pus show a predominance of fusospirochetal organisms are occasionally encountered (e.g., Prévot et al., 1951). They differ from the usual bite abscess in that they do not localize and become walled off but undermine large areas of skin. Subcutaneous tissue and superficial muscle layers become necrotic and liquefy, until an extensive fluctuating swelling is formed. The overlying skin becomes thin and weak and ultimately breaks down and sloughs away. So debilitating is such an infection that some cats die before drainage and antibiotic treatment can produce results. Anemia and leukopenia, sometimes present, retard recovery, the wound fails to granulate, and efforts to close it by suturing result in further sloughing.

Rarely spirochetes and fusiform bacilli are found to be numerous in the nasal exudate associated with chronic purulent rhinitis, and they have been reported in ulcers and fistulae of the face and in a suborbital abscess associated with dental disease (Velu et al., 1941).

## FELINE ASSOCIATION WITH CERTAIN HUMAN DISEASES

### Cat Scratch Disease

Cat scratch disease (benign lymphoreticulosis) is not a disorder of cats at all, but of man. It is mentioned here chiefly for the convenience of veterinarians, who for no good reason are expected by both laymen and the medical profession to have a special expertise on the subject. This regional lymphadenitis is usually associated with a history of a scratch or bite by a cat, but because the initiating wounds have in some cases been inflicted by other agencies, both animate and inanimate, the cat is usually considered no more than a mechanical vector of the agent, the ultimate source of which is unknown. In support of this hypothesis it is pointed out that the great majority of cats responsible for the disease in man have themselves been in good health, have failed to react to the skin test antigen, and have not given any evidence for harboring the infective agent. Virtually the only evidence for the possibility that cats may themselves suffer from the disease is embodied in an Italian report of cases of human disease caused by two cats in which lymphadenopathy was generalized but especially prominent in the cervical region (Citterio, 1955). Sections stained with Giemsa and other stains demonstrated bipolar organisms 0.2 to 0.5 μ wide and 1 to 1.4 μ long. They were seen in both the periphery and the parenchyma of the node, always associated with the larger vessels. Similar organisms were demonstrated in the nodes of the ill humans. In respect to other pathologic changes, the feline and human nodes were rather different, except for one common feature, the presence of great numbers of basophilic cells. Although attempts were made to transmit the disease, by inoculation of human pus, to a number of animal species including the cat, there was success only with the albino mouse.

It is now believed that the causative agent of cat scratch disease is a tiny pleomorphic Gram-negative rod ranging from 0.3 to 0.5 μ in diameter and 0.5 to 1.0 μ in length;

it is best demonstrated in involved lymph nodes or other tissue by Warthin-Starry stain (Hadfield et al., 1985; Wear et al., 1983). Attempts at isolation by cultivation on a variety of media and by animal inoculation have been unsuccessful.

The problem of what to do with a cat whose scratches produce cat scratch disease could in most instances be satisfactorily solved by having the cat declawed. This, however, is a procedure that should be resorted to only with indoor cats that do not need their claws for self-defense or climbing trees.

### Coxiellosis (Q-Fever)

Q-fever is a human disease caused by *Coxiella burnetii,* a rickettsial organism transmitted by certain ticks. The cat may serve as one of the animal reservoirs of infection, while not developing clinical illness (Gillespie and Baker, 1952). A pet cat in a large family was implicated in a household outbreak of Q-fever pneumonia (Kosatsky, 1984). The cat had just given birth to kittens. The organism is excreted in birth fluids and placenta, and parturition is known to cause airborne transmission.

# HEMOBARTONELLOSIS

ERWIN SMALL and MIODRAG RISTIC

Feline hemobartonellosis (feline infectious anemia) is an acute or chronic disease of domestic cats characterized by initial high temperature, depression, anorexia, often weight loss, macrocytic hemolytic anemia, and the presence of the causative agent, *Haemobartonella felis,* on the erythrocytes.

The disease was first recognized in 1942 in South Africa by Clark, who described the organism from postmortem material only and thought that it represented a new species, for which he proposed the name *Eperythrozoon felis.* A similar organism, tentatively designated *Bartonella felis,* was observed in cats in Leningrad in 1946–1947 (Kolabskii and Melnikova, 1951). In the United States, Flint and Moss (1953) described an infectious anemia of cats associated with erythrocyte parasites that appeared to Dr. David Weinman of Yale University to be either *Haemobartonella* or *Eperythrozoon.* Subsequently Flint and McKelvie (1955) proposed the name *Haemobartonella felis.* English, Australian, and European authors, on the other hand, generally supported the name *E. felis* (Harbutt, 1963; Seamer and Douglas, 1959; Thomsett, 1960; Wilkinson, 1963).

## Etiology

According to the 9th edition of Bergey's *Manual of Determinative Bacteriology, H. felis* is a member of the genus *Haemobartonella,* family Anaplasmataceae, order Rickettsiales (Ristic and Kreier, 1984). *Haemobartonella felis* is unique among members of the genus, because it is the only species that produces patent parasitemia and severe, sometimes fatal anemia in intact (spleen in situ) animals under natural conditions.

### Light Microscopic Examination

In Wright- and Giemsa-stained blood films, *H. felis* organisms stain deep violet and appear as pleomorphic small round dots, short rods, or coccoids. The latter sometimes occur in chains. The coccoids are 0.1 to 0.8 μ in diameter, and the rods are 0.2 to 0.5 μ by 0.9 to 1.5 μ. Ring-like forms are seen occasionally. The parasites occur singly, in pairs, or in groups in shallow or deep indentations on the surface of the erythrocytes. The most common shape is a small dot or short rod adhering to the erythrocytic surface (Kreier and Gothe, 1976; Kreier and Ristic, 1968). The organism may also be seen free in the plasma (Flint and McKelvie, 1955).

Living organisms can be stained with brilliant cresyl blue. Small (1965) and Small and Ristic (1967) stained the parasite with acridine orange. Organisms stained in this way and illuminated by ultraviolet light fluoresced bright orange with an undertone of yellow-green, indicating a high ribonucleic acid content and the possible presence of deoxyribonucleic acid. These workers also used fluorescent antibody techniques to demonstrate the organisms in blood films of infected cats (Small, 1965; Small and Ristic, 1971). They believed that acridine orange staining and fluorescent antibody techniques detected parasites that routine staining procedures failed to reveal.

### Electron Microscopic Examination

Both transmission and scanning electron microscopic techniques have been used for subcellular definition of the structural features of *H. felis.* The nature of the association between the organism and the host erythrocyte also has been investigated by these techniques.

Demaree and Nessmith (1972) examined ultra-thin sections of erythrocytes from a cat with clinical signs of hemobartonellosis. They observed rod, coccoid, and ring-shaped forms of the organism. All forms were surrounded by a single membrane. Occasionally an amorphous cell coat was seen external to the plasmalemma. At the point of attachment, parasites appeared to have caused identation of the erythrocyte membrane. It appeared that the parasite's membrane typically attached to the host cell membrane at several points and was separated at other

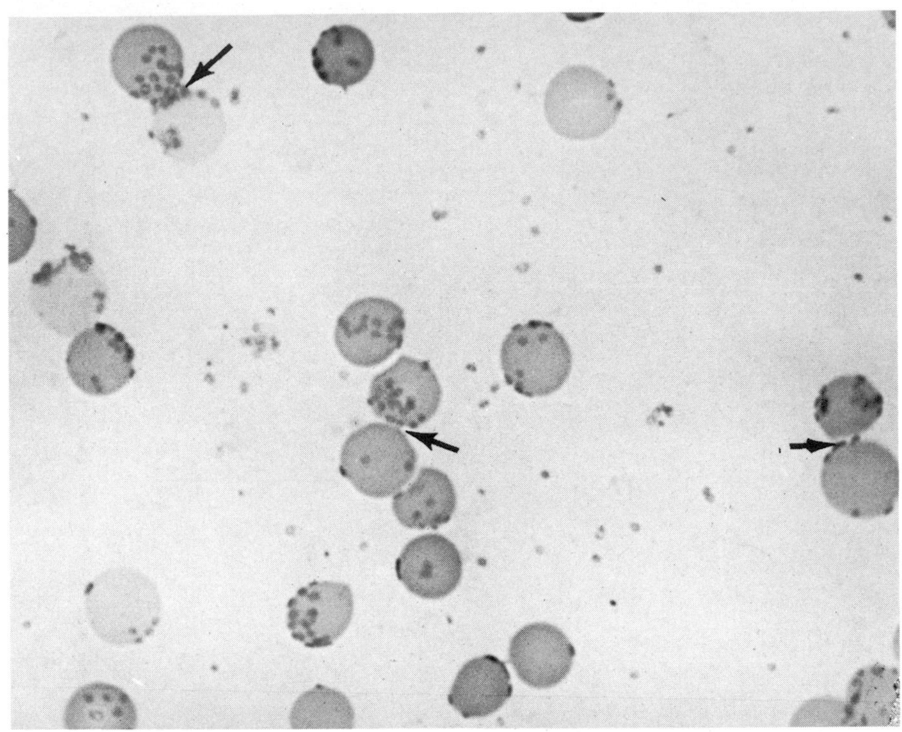

**Figure 8–16** Adjacent erythrocytes are attached by intervening organisms (arrows). There also are free organisms between erythrocytes. Giemsa stain, × 1250. (From Simpson CF, Gaskin JM, Harvey JW: J Parasitol 64 [1978] 504–511.)

points. There was an indication of two types of possible division of the parasite, budding and binary fission.

Simpson et al. (1978) conducted electron microscopic studies of *H. felis* using blood from three experimentally infected cats. They reported structural features generally similar to those found by Demaree and Nessmith (1972) (Figs. 8–16 to 8–18) but also described large crystalloid inclusions in about 10 per cent of erythrocytes of infected cats, whereas less than 0.01 per cent of the erythrocytes of a control cat contained such inclusions (Figs. 8–19 and 8–20). They concluded that *H. felis* infection enhances the propensity of feline hemoglobin to form intraerythrocytic crystalloids.

Another interesting feature described by Simpson et al. (1978) was the joining of erythrocytes due to binding of common organisms on their surfaces (Figs. 8–19 and 8–21). Such a phenomenon may enhance sequestration of erythrocytes in narrow vascular spaces and potentiate their phagocytosis by macrophages of the reticuloendothelial system (Fig. 8–18).

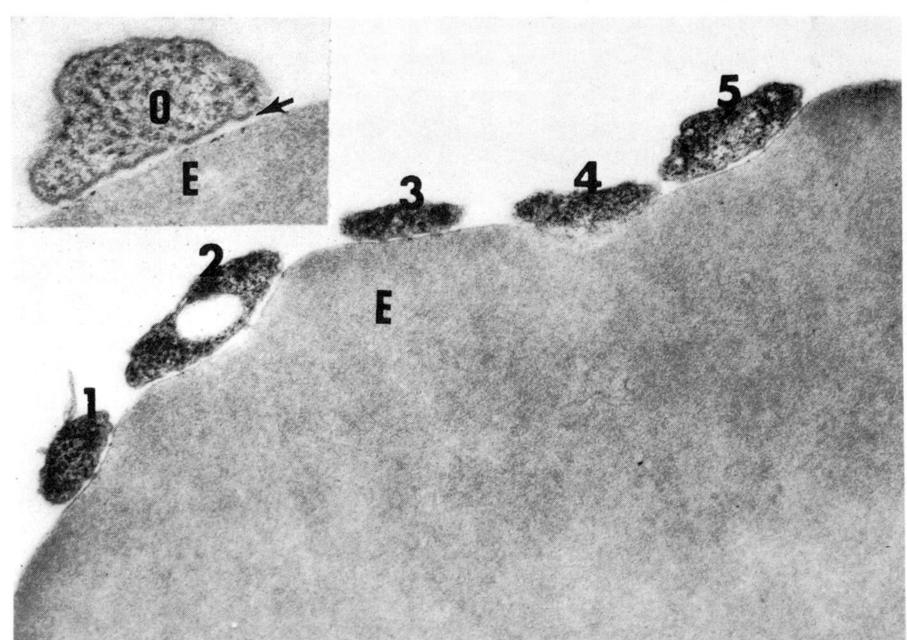


**Figure 8–17** Ultrastructure of erythrocytes parasitized by *Haemobartonella felis*. Five organisms (1–5) are in intermittent contact with the plasmalemma of an erythrocyte (E). × 25,000. Inset: An organism (O) is separated (arrow) from the plasmalemma of an erythrocyte (E). × 40,000. (From Simpson CF, Gaskin JM, Harvey JW: J Parasitol 64 [1978] 504–511.)

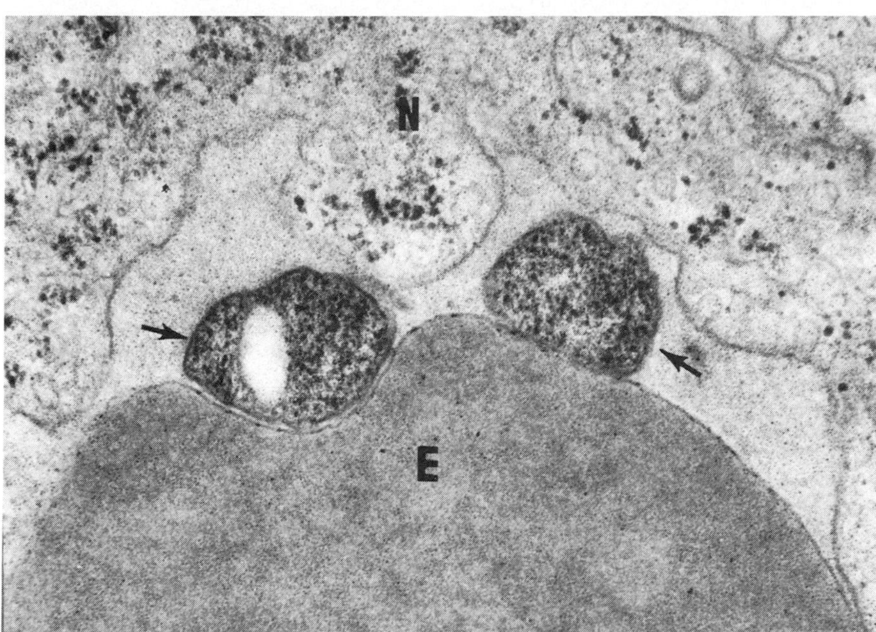


**Figure 8–18** The parasites (arrows) on an erythrocyte (E) in a capillary of the lung are in contact with or close to endothelial cells (N). × 40,000. (From Simpson CF, Gaskin JM, Harvey JW: J Parasitol 64 [1978] 504–511.)

Jain and Keeton (1973) were the first investigators to study three-dimensional features of *H. felis* in association with erythrocytes by the scanning electron microscopic technique. They confirmed morphologic features of the organism, its epicellular location, and its manner of attachment as reported by Demaree and Nessmith (1972) by use of transmission electron microscopy. They also demonstrated that the organisms were partly buried in the erythrocytes, with a substantial portion projecting beyond the surface of the cell. The area of attachment was slightly depressed. An erosion seemed to develop on the erythrocyte surface at sites previously occupied by the parasites. The authors concluded that hemolysis, a common feature in feline hemobartonellosis, results from development of a lesion at the site of the parasite's attachment on the erythrocyte surface. Major injuries of the cell surface that do not permit immediate escape of the hemoglobin may, however, create ionic imbalances that lead to osmotic fragility of the erythrocytes.

In another study of *H. felis* using scanning electron microscopy, Maede and Sonoda (1975) showed that the organisms are 0.5 to 0.6 μ in diameter, mostly discoid with a shallow central concavity. The erythrocytes of an infected cat were described as having small, shallow pockmarks, thought to represent lesions produced by the parasite's adherence. Most of the organisms appeared to

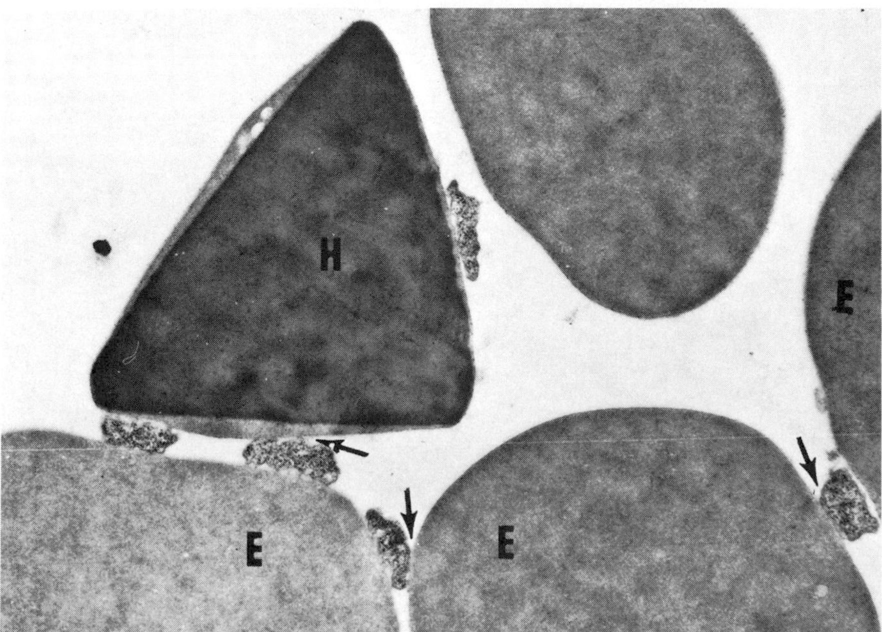


**Figure 8–19** A crystalloid inclusion is shaped like an arrowhead (H). The crystalloid erythrocyte and three others (E) are attached by organisms (arrows). × 15,000. (From Simpson CF, Gaskin JM, Harvey JW: J Parasitol 64 [1978] 504–511.)

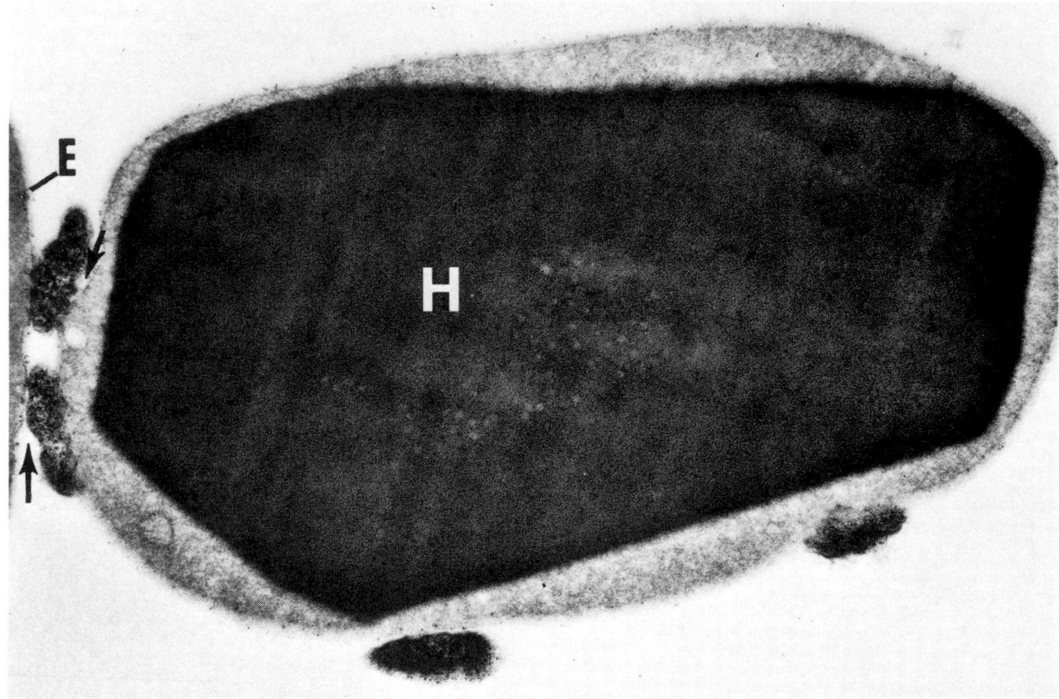


**Figure 8–20** The shape of the inclusion (H) is irregular. Organisms (arrows) bind the crystalloid erythrocyte to a second erythrocyte (E). × 20,000. (From Simpson CF, Gaskin JM, Harvey JW: J Parasitol 64 [1978] 504–511.)

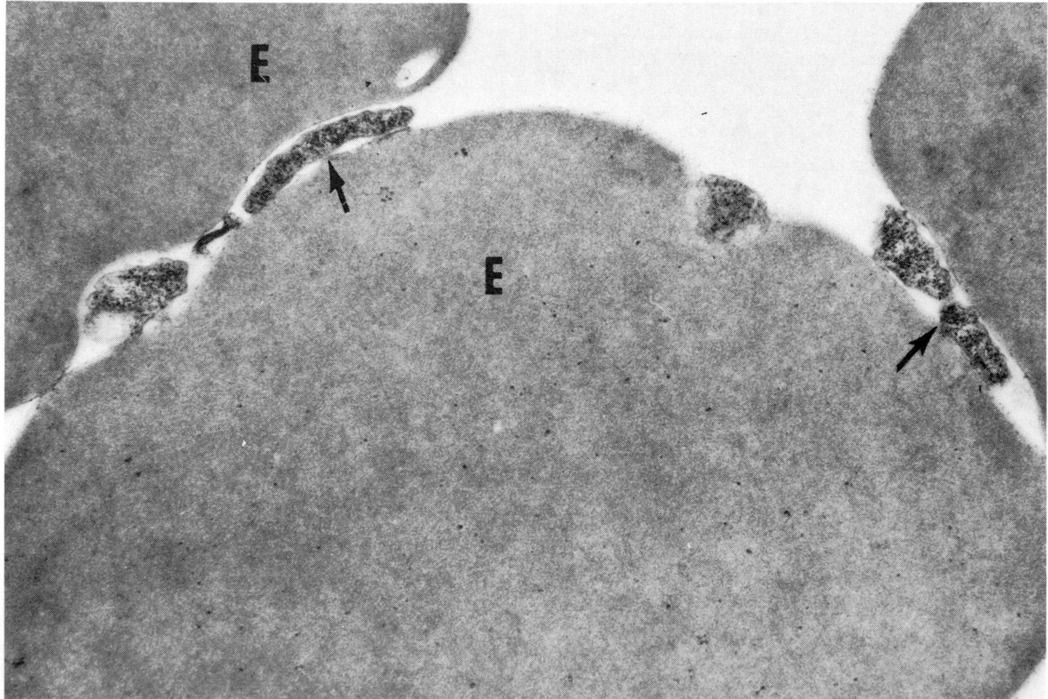


**Figure 8–21** Erythrocytes (E) are attached because of contact with common organisms (arrows). × 20,000. (From Simpson CF, Gaskin JM, Harvey JW: J Parasitol 64 [1978] 504–511.)

be attracted to the erythrocyte in pairs. Some seemed to be at a stage of binary fission on the erythrocyte surface. Affected erythrocytes tended to lose their usual biconcave shape and became spherocytes.

## Pathogenesis

### Transmission

The mode of transmission of *H. felis* has not been established. Experimentally the infection has been transmitted by the intraperitoneal route (Flint and Moss, 1953; Flint et al., 1958) and by the intravenous and oral routes (Flint et al., 1959). Flint et al. (1959) observed cases of the disease among cats with various types of abscesses and suggested the possibility of transmission by the bite of an infected cat. Edwards (1960) speculated that blood-sucking ectoparasites may be vectors of *H. felis* and suggested that fleas probably claim first place among such possible vectors because of their mobility, ubiquity, and nonspecificity. Other investigators, however, were unable to find any ectoparasites on naturally infected cats despite careful search (Wilkinson, 1969). Doubt that fleas were a major factor in transmission of hemobartonellosis was also voiced by Flint et al. (1959), who reported many cases of the disease in Salt Lake City, Utah, where fleas are virtually unknown. These workers caged infected and noninfected cats together for months without any evidence of spread of the infection.

The possibility of intrauterine infection as one mode of transmission was proposed by Harbutt (1963), who found parasites in kittens less than a day old. Not all positive cats studied by Harbutt were related, but all were subjected to the same environment. Experimentally, infection can be transmitted from clinically affected queens to newborn kittens in the absence of arthropod vectors (Harvey and Gaskin, 1977), but whether in utero, during birth, or by nursing is unknown.

The risk of transmission by blood transfusions is very real. Potential blood donors should be carefully screened by examination of blood films on several different days.

### Stress and Other Disease-contributing Factors

It is the general opinion of those who have had extensive experience with hemobartonellosis that many mature cats are carriers of the disease as a result of earlier exposure. The infection can apparently remain latent for long periods until some immunosuppressive event disturbs the immune balance between host and parasite. Flint et al. (1958) suggested that stress such as pregnancy, abscesses, other intercurrent infections, and debilitating conditions such as neoplasia could lower resistance to dormant hemobartonellosis.

All efforts to test this hypothesis experimentally have failed, however, including attempts to induce relapses of clinical disease in chronically infected cats by treatment with immunosuppressive drugs (cyclophosphamide and 6-mercaptopurine) (Harvey and Gaskin, 1978a).

Histories of 3741 cases of hemobartonellosis in clinics of 11 veterinary schools revealed that the risk for the disease increased with age, the risk for males was two and a half times that for females, spring was the likeliest time of the year for clinical hemobartonellosis to develop, and transmission appeared to be horizontal, probably by direct contact between cats (Hayes and Priester, 1973).

An increased incidence of leukemia as a sequel to hemobartonellosis has been reported by Priester and Hayes (1973), who suggested that the close relationship between the diseases results from the activation of one by the other. It was further suggested that FeLV-positive cats were most likely to acquire other diseases, owing to the immunosuppressive nature of the virus (Cotter et al., 1975).

### Experimental Studies

Experimental infections in susceptible cats seldom result in acute illness; more often, inoculated animals develop subclinical infection (Splitter et al., 1956). These workers reported the initial detection of parasites 3 to 20 days (average, seven) after intraperitoneal injection of 0.1 to 0.2 ml of infectious blood. Schwartzman and Besch (1958) detected parasites as early as 2 days and as late as 69 days after inoculation. Flint et al. (1959) found an average incubation period of about 15 to 16 days, whether or not cats were splenectomized.

The pathogenesis of the disease and the cycle of development of *H. felis* are poorly understood. In some cases, when the blood from individual infected cats is injected into susceptible recipient cats, no evidence of infection may result. On the contrary, if samples of pooled blood from random-source adult cats are injected into susceptible recipients, variable degrees of disease resembling natural infections may develop, sometimes followed by a carrier state (Splitter et al., 1956). The cyclical course of the infection is well described by these authors.

A characteristic feature of hemobartonellosis is sudden disappearance of the parasite from the peripheral circulation, sometimes followed by a rapid increase in packed cell volume. Studies by Simpson et al. (1978) and Maede and Murata (1978) may in part explain the mechanism of removal of *H. felis* from the circulation. According to Simpson et al. (1978), the attachment of erythrocytes to one another (formation of erythrocytic aggregates) is due to binding by common organisms attached to the surface coat of adjacent erythrocytes. The resulting sequestration of erythrocytes in narrow vascular spaces in turn potentiates their phagocytosis by macrophages of the reticuloendothelial system.

By electron microscopic study of splenic samples from infected cats, Maede and Murata (1978) demonstrated that *H. felis* was detached from parasitized erythrocytes by reticular cells in the spleen. This removal of the organism from the erythrocytes took place by a process of pitting that did not destroy the host cell (Maede, 1979). Accordingly, at least some of the parasitized erythrocytes sequestered in the spleen returned to the circulation after removal of the organism. This phenomenon may explain the rapid increase in packed cell volume often observed after the clearance of organisms from the peripheral blood.

Maede (1978) studied the role of the spleen in protection against an *H. felis* infection. He infused $^{51}$Cr-labeled parasitized erythrocytes into intact and splenectomized cats. In intact cats, he showed remarkable changes corresponding to the appearance and disappearance of the organism on the erythrocytes during the observation period, and demonstrated that the splenic radioactivity in infected cats, even very early in infection, was six times that in normal cats. In splenectomized cats, radioactivity of liver, lung, and bone marrow doubled but only after prolonged infection.

## Clinical Features

The outstanding sign of naturally occurring hemobartonellosis is anemia. According to Flint et al. (1958), any cat with a hemoglobin level of 7 gm/dl (PCV, 20) or less should be considered as possibly having hemobartonellosis. Hemoglobin levels as low as 2 gm/dl (PCV, 5 or 6) and red cell counts of less than 2 million/dl are not unusual.

Clinical infection is most often recognized in young adult males, although it may occur in cats of any age or either sex. It is an acute or chronic disease with a fever initially as high as 40 C (104 to 105 F) that may subsequently fluctuate in a lower range. The development of a macrocytic, hemolytic anemia is accompanied by anorexia, depression, weakness, and eventual loss of body condition. Skin, sclera, mucosae, and tongue are usually very pale and occasionally mildly jaundiced. Rapid respiration and cardiac murmurs are consequences of the hypoxia resulting from severe anemia. The spleen is often moderately, and occasionally greatly, enlarged. Microscopic examination of stained blood films at this time usually reveals the presence of *H. felis*.

Cats in which the onset of illness is sudden are often in good body condition but suffer most severely from the rapid development of anemia. They may be too weak to walk or stand, and are sometimes presented on the verge of death, with subnormal temperatures.

In chronic or relapsing infections, cats may be presented thin or emaciated, with a history of gradual weight loss, and often with concurrent infections or other disorders. Such cats have often adapted to a state of chronic anemia and are apt to show fewer *Haemobartonella* organisms than cats with acute infection. They may or may not be febrile.

Latent or opportunistic infection is often discovered in cats with other primary disorders, and it is a common experience to see occasional *Haemobartonella* organisms in nonregenerative anemias. Occasionally a rare *Haemobartonella* organism is seen in the blood of an apparently normal cat.

## Clinicopathologic Features

Typical of acute hemobartonellosis is a regenerative macrocytic anemia with erythrocytes varying in size and shape, the largest being basophilic (reticulocytes). Cells containing Howell-Jolly bodies (larger than *Haemobartonella*) and metarubricytes may be numerous. Occasional prorubricytes and rubricytes may also be present. As part of the marrow response, neutrophilic leukocytes and platelets may be increased in number. In some cases there is a monocytosis. Erythrophagocytosis by mononuclear cells or rarely by neutrophils is observed shortly after the first appearance of *H. felis* in the peripheral blood films (Maede and Hata, 1975) (Fig. 8–22).

Erythrocytic fragility is markedly increased immediately after appearance of *H. felis*, with no recovery even after disappearance of the parasites, presumably because the erythrocytes may have been damaged by the parasite on their surface so that their life span was impaired, even when the parasite was released.

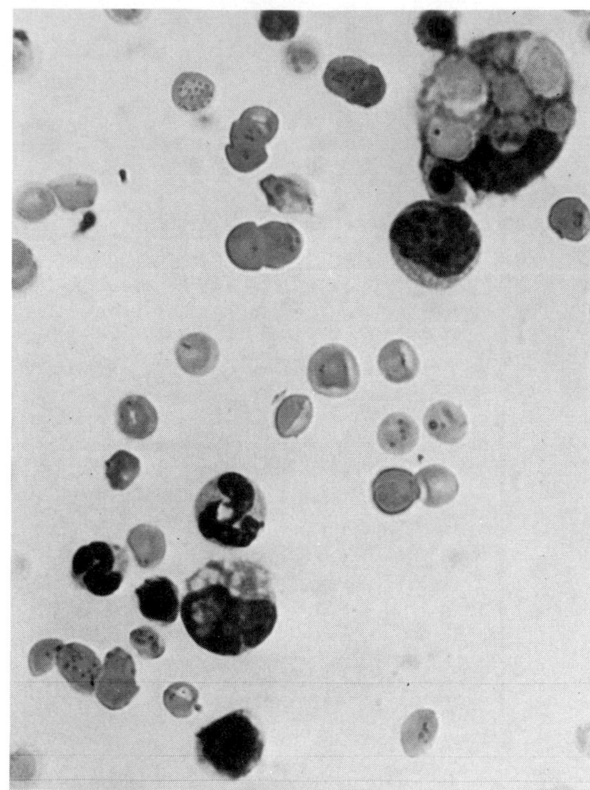

**Figure 8–22** Acute hemobartonellosis in a naturally infected young cat. Organisms are numerous on the red cells. Erythrophagocytosis by monocytes is a prominent feature. Giemsa stain, × 950. (Courtesy, Angell Memorial Animal Hospital.)

The direct Coombs test result likewise usually becomes positive in all cats shortly after the appearance of the parasite.

When hemolysis is severe enough to cause jaundice, the urine may be slightly bile-tinged. Hemoglobinuria is a rare occurrence (Holzworth, 1956).

## Diagnosis

Hemobartonellosis is most reliably diagnosed by identification of *H. felis* in stained blood films, but this method has the limitation that the parasite is not always detectable during either acute or chronic stages of the disease, especially if a transfusion or other treatment has been given. Films must sometimes be examined on several consecutive days.

Among the histochemical methods found most effective for staining *H. felis* for examination by light microscopy are the Giemsa and toluidine blue methods. Farrow (1976) recommends the following modification of the procedure for Giemsa staining because the conventional technique frequently results in deposition on the slide of precipitates that may confuse the diagnosis: thin blood films are air-dried, fixed in methyl alcohol for three minutes, and then stained overnight in a Coplin jar in a 6 per cent solution of stock Giemsa stain* made up in tap water of pH 6.8 to 7.0. When removed from the Coplin jar, the slide is flooded with tap water until all the staining solution is removed. It is next rinsed in methanol until the excess stain is removed (about 15 seconds), and is finally rinsed in water, air-dried, and examined under oil.

With the toluidine blue method, originally developed by Rogers and Wallace (1966) for staining *Anaplasma marginale* and adapted by Wilkinson (1969) for staining *H. felis,* stock solution is made from 1 gm each of toluidine blue and sodium borate in 100 ml of water. The solution is filtered and diluted 1:10 with 70 per cent ethyl alcohol. Freshly made blood films are air-dried (without fixation) and stained by dipping them two or three times into the solution, or by dropping the stain directly on the films and allowing them to be stained for 10 to 20 seconds. Excess stain is drained off and the film is air-dried without rinsing. Erythrocytes stain blue, and the parasites stain deep purple.

The acridine orange staining method increases the period of time during which visualization of the organism is possible (Small and Ristic, 1967). The organism stains intensely orange-red and when viewed by the fluorescence microscope is easily spotted because of the strong contrast between the dark greenish erythrocytes and the brilliant orange organism. For this test about 0.5 ml of venous blood is collected and immediately transferred into a vial containing 1 to 2 ml of formalin-saline mixture. The blood is fixed for at least one hour at room temperature and then thin slide films are made and air dried. The films are stained by immersion in a working acridine orange solution for 20 seconds. (The technique for preparation of the fixative and the acridine orange solution is given below.)† The films are thoroughly rinsed with distilled water, air dried, and examined under oil with an ultraviolet microscope. Typical *H. felis* structures, predominantly in pairs and chains on the erythrocytes, are easily distinguishable from Howell-Jolly bodies and other possible nuclear elements of immature erythrocytes.

Supravital staining with new methylene blue is unsatisfactory, since *H. felis* may be difficult to distinguish from punctate reticulocytosis.

The diagnosis of hemobartonellosis by serologic means is also possible. The most suitable method is the indirect fluorescent antibody (IFA) test. For this test to be functional and specific, the antigen-containing erythrocytes infected with *H. felis* must be properly prepared. Ristic and Holland (1979), on the basis of experience with *A. marginale* (Ristic and White, 1960), found that in infected cats there is an antibody that arises in response to infection with *H. felis*. This antibody blocks antigenic sites of this organism. Slides with such antibody-blocked antigens are not suitable for use in the IFA test. To prepare antigen slides with *H. felis* antigens free of antibodies, one must dissociate the blocking antibodies from the antigens before preparing slides to be used. The procedure is as follows: Whole blood is collected (with an anticoagulant) from a cat known to harbor *H. felis*. The erythrocytes are washed twice with phosphate buffered saline solution of pH 7.2, and the sedimented erythrocytes are resuspended in a physiologic saline solution having a pH of 4 to 5. The mixture is allowed to stand at room temperature for 15 minutes and is centrifuged again, after which the erythrocytes are again washed twice in phosphate buffered saline of pH 7.2. This final suspension is used to prepare antigen slides for the IFA test. The method used to store slides for future use and the procedure for conducting IFA tests are similar to those for the diagnosis of tropical canine pancytopenia or canine ehrlichiosis (Ristic et al., 1972).

Especially for the practitioner, a most important aid to diagnosis of clinical hemobartonellosis is the type of anemia revealed in blood films of infected cats. In most instances the anemia associated with hemobartonellosis is a responsive anemia (Norsworthy, 1976). Large basophilic erythrocytes (reticulocytes) and often younger nucleated erythrocytes in the peripheral circulation are indicators of the bone marrow's compensatory activity. By contrast, in the majority of feline anemias, and prominently so in feline leukemia, the bone marrow is depressed and nonresponsive, and even though nucleated red cells may be present, reticulocytes are absent.

### Differential Diagnosis

Other parasitisms of erythrocytes from which hemobartonellosis would have to be distinguished are cytauxzoonosis (in the southern United States) and babesiosis (in Africa).

A similar regenerative anemia is seen in hemolytic anemias due to noninfectious causes, e.g., autoimmune hemolytic anemia and those caused by toxins such as methylene blue. In the recovery phase from bone marrow depression caused by infections or other agents, there may be a similar picture of regenerative response.

There should be no difficulty in differentiating hemobartonellosis and panleukopenia, since the latter is rarely characterized by anemia and is typified by a low white cell count, in contrast with the leukocytosis characteristic of hemobartonellosis.

## Pathologic Features

There are no specific gross or microscopic lesions in hemobartonellosis. The tissues are usually pale and sometimes moderately jaundiced. The blood is watery. The spleen is variably enlarged and the liver often yellow. Sometimes the lymph nodes are slightly or moderately enlarged.

Microscopically there is reactive hyperplasia of lymphoid tissue. In the spleen hemosiderin deposits are common, and reticuloendothelial cell proliferation may be so severe as to suggest neoplasia. The centrilobular areas of the liver exhibit fatty change, congestion, and ultimately central and paracentral necrosis—all resulting from hypoxia. Hepatocellular and canalicular cholestasis vary in degree of severity.

*Stock Giemsa solution consists of 7.6 gm of Giemsa powder, 250 ml of glycerine, and 750 ml of methanol. These reagents are mixed in a flask and placed in an incubator at 37 C for 10 days until the solution is polychrome. The solution is agitated daily to remove the sediment.

†Preparation of reagents for the acridine orange staining method: (a) Formalin solution is prepared by mixing 1 volume of formaldehyde solution with 9 volumes of physiologic saline; (b) Acridine orange stain consists of 1 part concentrated stock acridine orange to 8 parts of diluent (physiologic saline containing 0.856 per cent concentrated HCl).

### Treatment

No satisfactorily controlled evaluations of treatment for hemobartonellosis are available. An immediate blood transfusion may be lifesaving in an apparently moribund cat. Cats with hemoglobin values of 6 gm/dl or below and hematocrit levels under 10 or 15 per cent usually need blood transfusions, although with chronic infections cats adapt amazingly to severe degrees of anemia provided that they are not stressed. According to Flint et al. (1959), a number of cats with both clinical and experimental infections recovered uneventfully after two or more transfusions. Transfusions usually range from 40 to 50 ml. If there is a need to repeat blood transfusion, one must consider possible differences in blood types between donor and recipient in order to avoid hypersensitivity reactions due to the earlier immunologic stimulation. There are three blood groups in the cat, and transfusion of heterologous blood type may evoke an unfavorable reaction (Auer et al., 1982).

*Haemobartonella felis,* like other rickettsiae, is sensitive to broad-spectrum antibiotics. Oxytetracycline is preferred, at a dose of 25 mg/kg t.i.d. for three weeks. Chloramphenicol is effective in about half the cases. The dosage is 10 to 15 mg/kg twice a day for 10 to 14 days. Arsenicals have been recommended for *H. felis* infections, but are not known to be more effective than oxytetracycline. These drugs, moreover, must be given intravenously and have a potential for causing toxicity (depression, vomiting, and diarrhea).

A positive Coombs test result is evidence of immune-mediated hemolysis, but opinion is divided as to steroid treatment. One view is that in hemobartonellosis this treatment may suppress the immune response (Cotter, 1983), whereas others recommend it to inhibit erythrophagocytosis (Harvey and Gaskin, 1978b).

### Prognosis

Relapses after apparently successful antibiotic treatment suggest that antibiotics suppress infection rather than permanently eliminating it. Some cats, however, appear to make complete and lasting recoveries.

Since about half the cats with hemobartonellosis are FeLV-positive, every cat exhibiting *Haemobartonella* in a blood film should be tested. The prognosis for FeLV-negative cats is good, and some of those that are FeLV-positive respond favorably to treatment with oxytetracycline, at least for a time, although they are likely ultimately to succumb to some FeLV-induced disease.

# MYCOPLASMAL INFECTIONS

NIELS C. PEDERSEN

*Mycoplasma* and related genera are small, coccoid, cell wall–deficient, bacteria-like organisms that inhabit the mucous membranes of the nasal passages, oropharynx, and genitourinary tract of many species of animals. The domestic cat is not unique therefore in having its own resident flora of mycoplasmal organisms. Mycoplasmas were formerly called pleuropneumonia-like organisms (PPLO).

### Etiologic Agents

*Mycoplasma* and *Mycoplasma*-like organisms of domestic cats belong to three basic groups: *Mycoplasma,* T-mycoplasmas or ureaplasmas, and acholeplasmas. *Mycoplasma felis* and *Mycoplasma gateae* are the two most common mycoplasmas of cats (Blackmore and Hill, 1973; Blackmore et al., 1971; Heyward et al., 1969; Tan and Miles, 1973). *M. felis* is antigenically unrelated to other mammalian mycoplasmas, while *M. gateae* is antigenically related to *M. arthritidis, M. salivarium, M. hominis* (type 1), and *M. orale* (types 1, 2) (Cole et al., 1967). These two strains also differ in their capacity to cleave egg yolk lipids, produce ammonia from arginine, reduce methylene blue, and lyse avian or sheep red blood cells, as well as in their sensitivity to neomycin and novobiocin (Cole et al., 1967). The most apparent gross differences are in their colony morphology on agar. *M. felis* forms a prominent colony with a dense periphery that browns with age and has a distinct brown central pore, while colonies of *M. gateae* appear vacuolated or lacy and the central pore is much less conspicuous (Hill, 1971).

In addition to the two major strains of *Mycoplasma, M. arginini* and *M. feliminutum* have been isolated from domestic cats (*M. feliminutum* on only a single occasion) (Heyward et al., 1969). Tan and Miles (1973) suggested that this strain represented a spurious isolation of an organism that lived naturally in another species of animal. *M. arginini* is not specific to domestic cats and is also commonly isolated from captive wild Felidae (Blackmore and Hill, 1973; Hill, 1975), as well as from other species of animals (Tan et al., 1977a,b). Similarly, Wilkinson (1980) has described the occasional isolation of *M. pulmonis, M. arthritidis,* and *M. gallisepticum* from cats.

T-mycoplasmas or ureaplasmas are the second type of *Mycoplasma*-like organisms commonly isolated from cats (Harasawa et al., 1977; Tan and Markham, 1971; Tan and Miles, 1974b). T-mycoplasmas produce minute colonies and can utilize urea to produce ammonia. They can be isolated from a majority of normal cats, where they inhabit the oral cavity and less commonly the prepuce or vagina (Harasawa et al., 1977). The feline strains of T-mycoplasma have no serologic relationship to human T-mycoplasma strains (Harasawa et al., 1977).

*Acholeplasma laidlawii* is the major strain of *Acholeplasma* found in cats. It is widespread in nature and can be isolated from many other animals, such as cattle, swine, and poultry (Tan and Miles, 1972).

## INCIDENCE

Mycoplasmas, T-mycoplasmas, and acholeplasmas are ubiquitous in domestic cats. Tan and Miles (1974a) isolated *M. felis* from 4.4 per cent, *M. gateae* from 62.2 per cent, and *M. arginini* from 6.7 per cent of normal cats. Heyward and coworkers (1969) made 149 isolations of *Mycoplasma* from 90 healthy cats—29 of which were *M. felis,* 118 *M. gateae,* and one *M. feliminutum.* Campbell and associates (1973b) cultured the conjunctival sac of 120 normal cats and isolated 12 mycoplasmal strains, seven of which proved to be *M. felis.*

T-mycoplasmas, first isolated from cats by Tan and Markham (1971), are also common inhabitants of normal cats. Harasawa and associates (1977) isolated T-mycoplasmas from 25 of 36 normal cats. The most common sites of infection were the oral cavity (60 per cent) and the vagina or prepuce (15 per cent).

The incidence of *Acholeplasma laidlawii* infection in normal domestic cats varies with the environment. Farm or rural cats have a higher incidence because of contact with other carrier species (Tan and Miles, 1974a). Tan and Miles (1974a) isolated *A. laidlawii* from 22.2 per cent of normal cats. In an earlier study, the same researchers isolated 45 strains of *Mycoplasma* from 32 normal cats, and 10 of these isolates were *A. laidlawii* (Tan and Miles, 1972).

## PATHOGENICITY

As with mycoplasmas in other species, there is some controversy about their relationship to disease. Tan and Miles (1974a), who studied the frequency of isolation of mycoplasmas from sick and diseased cats, concluded that only *M. felis* could be statistically linked with illness. In their study population, *M. felis* was isolated seven to eight times more often from sick than from normal cats. Many of the sick cats were suffering from respiratory disorders. *M. arginini* was isolated slightly more frequently from sick than from healthy cats. Later studies by Tan and coworkers (1977b), however, failed to show any disease-causing potential for *M. arginini* in cats. *Acholeplasma laidlawii* is not believed to be pathogenic for cats, but rather is thought to be picked up as a saprophyte from other animals (Tan and Miles, 1974a). *M. gateae* was actually isolated from normal cats more frequently than from sick cats and was therefore assumed by Tan and associates (1977b) to be nonpathogenic for cats. Recently, however, *M. gateae* has been associated with arthritis and tenosynovitis in cats (Moise et al., 1983).

If mycoplasmas of cats can cause disease similar to that in other species, the following disease states are worthy of note: conjunctivitis, respiratory infections, arthritis, urethritis and cystitis, abortions and fetal loss, and chronic abscesses. Some of the evidence for the role of mycoplasmas and related organisms in several of these disorders is quite strong, some is circumstantial, and some is speculative.

## CLINICAL FEATURES

### Conjunctivitis

Although there was early skepticism about the role of mycoplasmas in conjunctivitis of cats, it is now generally conceded that they are important in this condition. Cello (1957), one of the early investigators, reported the association of mycoplasmas with conjunctivitis in three cats. More important, he showed that while his *Mycoplasma* isolates would not produce conjunctivitis in normal cats, conjunctivitis was readily inducible if the normal eye was first treated with an intrapalpebral injection of corticosteroid. Subsequent reports also linked conjunctivitis with mycoplasmas (Colegrave et al., 1964; Laborde, 1971; Tan and Markham, 1971; Wilkinson, 1966). Most of these early studies were based on the observation that mycoplasmas, especially *Mycoplasma felis,* were isolated much more commonly from inflamed than from normal eyes (Campbell et al., 1973a,b; Tan and Miles, 1973). Some of these studies could be criticized because they failed to adequately exclude the presence of other potential pathogens, such as *Chlamydia* and feline respiratory viruses (Blackmore et al., 1971; Povey and Wardley, 1973). Indeed Blackmore and coworkers (1971), recognizing the extremely high incidence of mycoplasmas in normal cats from three unrelated cat colonies, suggested that there was no evidence that mycoplasmas caused disease. Subsequent experimental studies, however, have shown fairly conclusively that mycoplasmas can cause conjunctivitis in cats (Tan, 1974).

Naturally occurring mycoplasmal conjunctivitis of cats is caused predominantly by *M. felis.* As mentioned previously, *M. felis* is a frequent inhabitant of the normal oropharynx, but it is not often isolated from normal conjunctiva. Tan and Miles (1973) isolated *M. felis* 26 times more often from cats with "snuffles" (conjunctivitis, rhinitis) than from normal cats.

Mycoplasmal conjunctivitis is much more frequent in catteries and multiple-cat households than in single-cat homes or among outdoor cats. In kittens, it usually develops shortly after weaning at 10 to 14 weeks of age. The earliest sign is acute swelling and reddening of the conjunctivia, usually in one eye, associated with some squinting and photophobia. The conjunctival swelling is sometimes so severe that the cornea is barely visible. Within one or two weeks the other eye may become similarly involved (Fig. 8–23). Early in the course of the disease the ocular discharge is usually serous, but it can soon become cloudy. Sneezing is a minor complication, whereas it is prominent in calicivirus infection and rhinotracheitis. When present, sneezing is due both to low-grade rhinitis and to increased lacrimal fluid drainage into the nasal cavity. The primary infection lasts two to six weeks. After recovery, the organisms tend to disappear from the conjunctival sac but often persist in the oro-

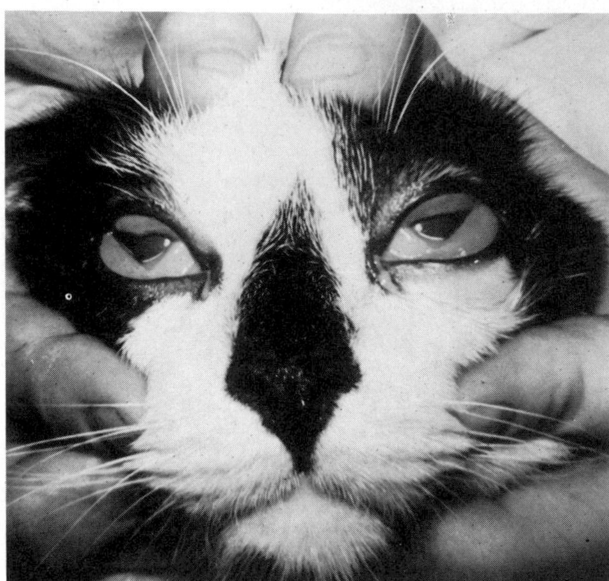

**Figure 8–23** Mycoplasmal conjunctivitis in a kitten. The swollen conjunctiva bulges over the eyeballs, and a serous discharge wets the hair below the lower eyelids.

pharynx. Bouts of conjunctivitis may recur throughout life, but they are usually not so severe or long-lasting as the initial infection.

Mycoplasmal conjunctivitis can occur by itself, but in colonies and multiple-cat households, it is often associated with chlamydial infection (Cello, 1967, 1971). Indeed chlamydial conjunctivitis appears virtually identical to mycoplasmal conjunctivitis. Both tend to begin in one eye, untreated infections can last two to six weeks, and conjunctival scrapings taken from cats with either infection show a predominance of neutrophils and epithelial cells (Cello, 1971). The two infections are best differentiated by Giemsa- or Macchiavello-stained smears. Mycoplasmas appear as small coccoid rods present in large numbers on the cell membrane of epithelial cells and free in the surrounding fluid (Fig. 8–24), whereas chlamydiae occur as intracytoplasmic inclusions.

The major complication of conjunctivitis in cats is corneal ulcer. Less often, adhesions may develop between the conjunctiva and the cornea. These lesions are more apt to occur in severe infections complicated by bacteria such as staphylococci or *Pseudomonas*. Improper use of steroid ointments in inflamed eyes may prolong the infection and can predispose the cornea to ulceration.

Mycoplasmal conjunctivitis is treated most effectively with eye ointments containing tetracycline or oxytetracycline. The addition of gentamicin ophthalmic drops provides a greater range of effectiveness against both mycoplasmas and secondary bacterial invaders. Medication is instilled into the eyes a least three or four times a day and continued for several days after all signs of conjunctivitis have disappeared. Deep corneal ulcers are most effectively treated by sewing the third eyelid to the upper eyelid—a common procedure for the treatment of corneal ulcers in small animals. The third-eyelid flap is left in place for 5 to 10 days while antibiotics are frequently

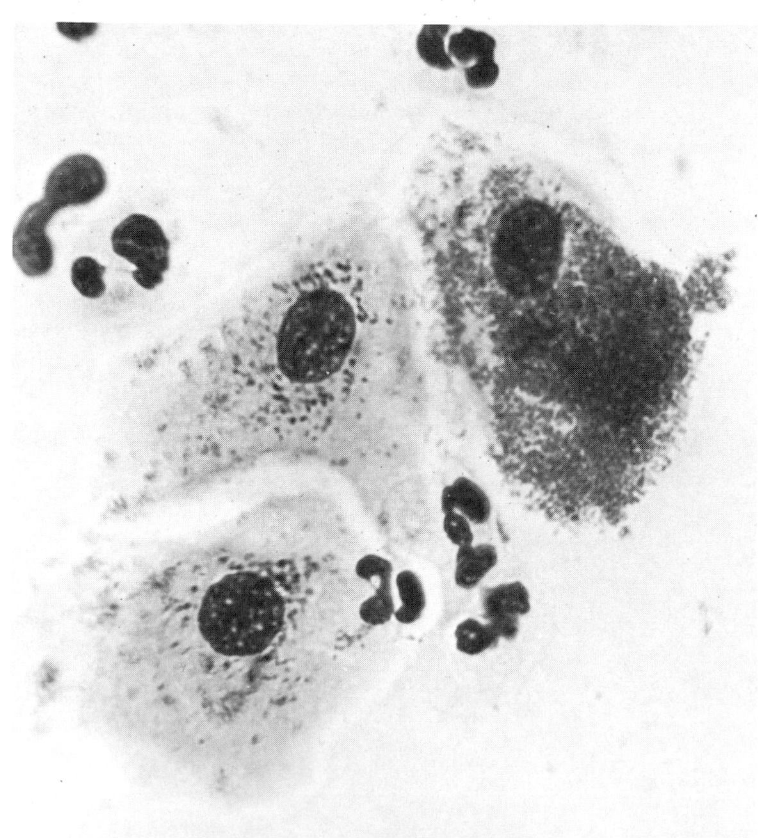

**Figure 8–24** Conjunctival scraping from a cat with mycoplasmal conjunctivitis. There are numerous small coccoid bodies associated with epithelial cells. Giemsa stain, × 2000.

instilled into the conjunctival sac. Systemic antibiotic treatment is not necessary in most cases, because the infection is usually limited to the conjunctiva. If there is evidence of concurrent rhinitis or possible pneumonitis, systemic treatment with gentamicin, lincomycin, or tylosin is used. Tetracycline should not be used in young cats as a systemic treatment because of the danger of discoloration of the teeth.

## Respiratory Disease

Pneumonia is a well recognized feature of mycoplasmal infections in other animals, such as poultry, cattle, sheep, and goats. There is little evidence, however, that these organisms are important causes of respiratory disease in cats. Colegrave and coworkers (1964) isolated mycoplasmas from many cats with what they termed "snuffles," presumably rhinitis and conjunctivitis. Wilkinson (1966) also suggested that mycoplasmas could be associated with both upper respiratory infection and conjunctivitis. Switzer (1967) reported isolation of a mycoplasma from the lung of a kitten with pneumonia. I have also observed a litter of four-week-old kittens that died of what seemed, on the basis of culture and histopathologic findings, to be mycoplasmal pneumonia. Tan (1974), in a study of experimentally induced conjunctivitis, observed one kitten that developed mild pneumonia after experimental infection with *M. felis*. Schneck (1972) observed that mycoplasmas were more commonly isolated from colony cats than from outdoor cats and postulated a synergistic role of mycoplasmas and viruses in respiratory disease. Most of these observations are anecdotal, however, and there is no overwhelming evidence that mycoplasmas are a major cause of respiratory disease in cats. In this regard, Spradbrow and associates (1970) cultured specimens from the nasal cavity, conjunctiva, tonsils, and lungs of cats with respiratory disease and found that although mycoplasmas were commonly isolated from the upper respiratory passages and tonsils, they were not isolated from lung suspensions.

## Arthritis

Mycoplasmas commonly cause arthritis in young animals such as calves, foals, lambs, kids, and chicken and turkey poults. The arthritis in these species results from the dissemination of organisms from localized sites of infection in the upper respiratory tract. Young kittens, however, do not develop arthritis as a consequence of localized mycoplasmal conjunctivitis. Cats appear, therefore, to have a high degree of resistance to systemic mycoplasmosis.

Mycoplasmal arthritis of cats is an infrequent problem of aged cats. Moise and coworkers (1983) recovered *M. gateae* from the synovium of an eight-year-old cat with severe generalized fibrinopurulent tenosynovitis of two months' duration. This cat had a history of recurrent upper respiratory infection and was hypogammaglobulinemic at the time of illness. The role of immunosuppression in the disease of this cat was not determined. The mycoplasma isolated from the cat was pathogenic and caused mild transient polyarthritis in adult cats. The experimental disease was much more severe and chronic, however, when the cats were immunosuppressed with azathioprine before being infected.

Mycoplasmal arthritis was also observed in two aged cats at the Veterinary Medical Teaching Hospital, University of California, Davis. Both were suffering from advanced cancer and were probably also immunologically compromised. The arthritis involved one or two limb joints, which were acutely swollen and reddened and contained a thin, cloudy synovial fluid with large numbers of nondegenerative neutrophils. The arthritis in these cats responded promptly to systemic tetracycline therapy.

## Urethritis and Cystitis

Mycoplasmas and T-mycoplasmas have been shown to cause urethritis in humans. They have also been isolated from dogs with cystitis. Little attention has been devoted to their possible role in the urolithiasis syndrome in cats, but limited culture studies suggest that they are not involved. Nonetheless, because they are known to cause urinary tract disease in other species, they should not be dismissed without more thorough research.

## Abortion and Fetal Death

Mycoplasmas have been shown to be a cause of sporadic abortions and fetal death in humans, cattle, and sheep. Tan and Miles (1974b) demonstrated experimentally that feline T-mycoplasmas (ureaplasmas) might be involved in fetal losses in catteries. Three pregnant T-mycoplasma-free queens were inoculated intranasally and intravaginally with the T-385 strain of T-mycoplasma. One queen aborted her fetuses nine days later, and the T-385 organism was isolated from the endometrium. The uterus and ovaries were also observed to be inflamed at the time of culture. The other two queens developed transient fever 13 to 36 days after inoculation. Six kittens were born to these two queens. Those in one litter were small and died at 17 days of age; the two in the other litter were born normal-sized but died at 10 days. T-385 T-mycoplasma was isolated from the heart blood of the only kitten that was cultured. Noninfected pregnant control queens did not abort and produced healthy kittens. Moise and associates (1983) caused one queen to abort three days after infection with *M. gateae*. In a naturally occurring case of pleuritis and peritonitis from which a pure culture of a *Mycoplasma* sp was isolated, the cat had aborted two months before (Lindley, 1966).

In light of the high incidence of mycoplasmal infection in catteries and the higher than normal incidence of fetal deaths in cattery cats, the role of these organisms in fetal losses in cats should be further studied.

## Chronic Abscesses

An organism resembling mycoplasma was isolated from chronic, antibiotic-resistant, subcutaneous abscesses in three cats presented to the Ontario Veterinary College (Keane, 1983). Microscopic examination and culturing of the nonodorous, reddish brown discharge present in all three cases gave no evidence of bacteria, yeasts, or fungi. Treatment with tetracycline was successful.

## REFERENCES


**Actinomycetic Infections**

Ajello L, Walker WW, Dungworth DL, Brumfield GL: Isolation of Nocardia brasiliensis from a cat, with a review of its prevalence and geographic distribution. J Am Vet Med Assoc 138 (1961) 370–376.

Akün RS: Nokardiose bei zwei Katzen in der Türkei. Dtsch Tierärztl Wochenschr 59 (1952) 202–204.

Attleberger MH: Subcutaneous and opportunistic mycoses, the deep mycoses, and the actinomycetes. *In* Kirk RW (ed): Current Veterinary Therapy VII. Philadelphia, WB Saunders Company, 1980, 477–486.

Attleberger MH: Systemic mycoses. *In* Pratt RW (ed): Feline Medicine. Santa Barbara, American Veterinary Publications Inc, 1983.

Baker GJ, Breeze RG, Dawson CO: Oral dermatophilosis in a cat: a case report. J Small Anim Pract 13 (1972) 649–654.

Beaman BL, Sugar AM: *Nocardia* in naturally acquired and experimental infections in animals. J Hyg 91 (1983) 393–419.

Bestetti G, Bühlmann V, Nicolet J, Fankhauser R: Paraplegia due to Actinomyces viscosus infection in a cat. Acta Neuropathol (Berl) 39 (1977) 231–235.

Brion A: L'actinomycose du chien et du chat. Rev Méd Vét 91 (1939) 121–159.

Campbell B, Scott DW: Successful management of nocardial empyema in a dog and cat. J Am Anim Hosp Assoc 11 (1975) 769–773.

Carakostas MC, Miller RI, Woodward MG: Subcutaneous dermatophilosis in a cat. J Am Vet Med Assoc 185 (1984) 675–676.

Chastain CB, Greer RL, Mitten RW, Hogle RM: Actinomycotic periodontitis in a cat. J Am Anim Hosp Assoc 13 (1977) 65–67.

Jones RT: Subcutaneous infection with *Dermatophilus congolensis* in a cat. J Comp Pathol Ther 86 (1976) 415–421.

Langham RF, Schirmer RG, Newman JP: Nocardiosis in the dog and cat. Mich State Univ Vet 19 (1959) 102–107.

Lerner PI: *Nocardia* species. *In* Mandell GL, Douglas RG, Bennett JE (eds): Principles and Practice of Infectious Diseases. New York, John Wiley & Sons, 1979, Vol 2, 1962–1969.

Lewis GE, Fidler WJ, Crumrine MH: Mycetoma in a cat. J Am Vet Med Assoc 161 (1972) 500–503.

Libke KG, Walton AM: Actinomycosis-like infection in the mandible of a cat. Mod Vet Pract 55 (1974) 201–202.

Lotspeich M: Actinomycosis in a cat. Vet Med Small Anim Clin 69 (1974) 571.

Marder MW, Kantrowitz MD, Davis T: Clinical pathological conference [Nocardiosis, cutaneous, *N. asteroides*]. Feline Pract 3 (5) (1973) 20–31.

McGaughey CA: Actinomycosis in carnivores. A review of the literature. Br Vet J 108 (1952) 89–92.

O'Hara PJ, Cordes DO: Granulomata caused by *Dermatophilus* in two cats. NZ Vet J 11 (1963) 151–154.

Prévot AR, Joubert L, Goret P: Le syndrome "actinomycose" des carnivores. Ann Inst Pasteur 101 (1961) 771–792.

Rippon JW: Medical Mycology. The Pathogenic Fungi and the Pathogenic Actinomycetes. Philadelphia, WB Saunders Company, 1982.

Stowater JL, Codner EC, McCoy JC: Actinomycosis in the spinal canal of a cat. Feline Pract 8 (1) (1978) 26–27.

Wilkinson GT (ed): Diseases of the Cat and Their Management. Melbourne, Blackwell Scientific Publications, 1983a, 431.

Wilkinson GT: Cutaneous nocardia infection in a cat. Feline Pract 13 (4) (1983b) 32–34.

**Tuberculosis**

Berthelon M: Observations sur la tuberculose utérine de la chatte. Recl Méd Vét 119 (1943) 5–7.

Blähser S: Über nicht alltägliche Todesursachen und einige plötzliche Todesfälle bei der Katze. Kleintierpraxis 7 (1962) 192–201.

Buergelt CD, Fowler JL, Wright PJ: Disseminated avian tuberculosis in a cat. Calif Vet 36 (10) (1982) 13–15.

Cella F: Di un caso di carpite tubercolare primitiva in un gatto. Clin Vet (Milano) 65 (1942) 412–423.

Christoph HJ: Klinik der Katzenkrankheiten. Jena, Gustav Fischer VEB, 1963, 291.

Cobbett L: The type of tubercle bacillus found in tuberculosis of the cat. J Comp Pathol Ther 39 (1926) 142–148.

Collet P: Les localisations osseuses de la tuberculose chez le chat. Bull Soc Sci Vét Lyon 43 (1942) 112–117.

Collet P, Lucam F: Tuberculose du cervelet chez un chat. Bull Soc Sci Vét Lyon 42 (1941) 52–60.

Collinot M: Contribution à l'étude de la tuberculose des carnivores domestiques. Traitement par la streptomycine. Thesis. Alfort, 1953.

Diehl KE: An epizootic of bovine tuberculosis traced from slaughter. J Am Vet Med Assoc 158 (1971) 1888–1889.

Dobson N: Tuberculosis of the cat. J Comp Pathol Ther 43 (1930) 310–316.

Dorssen CA van: Infectie met Mycobacterium microti bij een kat. Tijdschr Diergeneeskd 85 (1960) 404–412.

Douville [no init]: Sur le diagnostic et la nature des lésions cutanées ulcéreuses chez le chat (Tuberculose cutanée et arthrite tuberculeuse. Erythème papulo-érosif. Sarcome et épithéliome). Rev Vét 74 (1922) 209–217.

Foresti C: Su di un caso di tubercolosi del seno frontale. Nuova Vet 14 (1936) 321–324.

Francis J: Tuberculosis in Animals and Man. A Study in Comparative Pathology. London, Cassell and Company, 1958, 217ff.

Francis J: Tuberculosis in small animals. Mod Vet Pract 42 (18) (1961) 39–42.

Griffith AS: Tuberculosis of the cat. J Comp Pathol Ther 39 (1926) 71–82.

Grossman A: Mycobacterial hepatitis associated with long-term steroid therapy. Feline Pract 13 (6) (1983) 37–38, 40–41.

Hancock WI, Coats G: Tubercle of the choroid in the cat. Vet Rec 23 (1911) 433–436.

Hawthorne VM, Lauder IM: Tuberculosis in man, dog, and cat. Am Rev Respir Dis 85 (1962) 858–869.

Hix JW, Jones TC, Karlson AG: Avian tubercle bacillus infection in the cat. J Am Vet Med Assoc 138 (1961) 641–647.

Hobday's Surgical Diseases of the Dog and Cat, 7th ed. London, Baillière Tindall and Cox, 1953.

Houdemer [no init]: Sur quelques cas de tuberculose observés chez les animaux domestiques ou sauvages du Tonkin. Bull Acad Vét Fr 81 (1928) 40–42.

Huitema H, van Vloten J: Murine tuberculosis in a cat. Antonie van Leeuwenhoek 26 (1960) 235–240.

Innes JRM: The pathology and pathogenesis of tuberculosis in domesticated animals compared with man. Br Vet J 96 (1940) 96–105.

Isaac J, Whitehead J, Adams JW, Barton MD, Coloe P: An outbreak of *Mycobacterium bovis* in cats in an animal house. Aust Vet J 60 (1983) 243–245.

Isler D, Lott-Stolz G: Die wichtigsten Krankheits- und Todesursachen der Katze. Sektionsfälle 1965–1976. Kleintierpraxis 23 (1978) 333–334, 336–337.

Jennings AR: The distribution of tuberculous lesions in the dog and cat, with reference to the pathogenesis. Vet Rec 61 (1949) 380–385.

Jensen CO: Tuberkulose beim Hund und bei der Katze. Dtsch Z Tiermedizin 17 (1891) 295–324.

Kuwabara T: Susceptibility of cats to tubercle bacilli. Kitasato Arch Exp Med 15 (1938) 318–329; 16 (1939) 275–284.

Mason JH: Tuberculosis in a cat. Br Vet J 80 (1924) 370–371.

Matthias D, Niemand HG: Augentuberkulose bei einer Katze. Z Infektionskr Haustiere 59 (1943) 203–210.

Methner U: Beitrag zur Tuberkulose des Hundes und der Katze. Tierärztl Umschau 12 (1957) 85–89.

Milbradt H, Roemmele O: Tuberkulöse Katze infiziert Rinderbestand. Dtsch Tierärztl Wochenschr 67 (1960) 17.

Monti F: Saggi terapeutici nella tubercolosi spontanea dei carnivori domestici (steptomicina-pas-idrazide dell' acido isonicotinico). Zooprofilassi 8 (1953) 321–360.

Nowacki J: [Haemagglutination, haemolysis and complement fixation tests in the diagnosis of experimental tuberculosis of cats]. Medycyna Wet 23 (1967) 484–487 (Abstr Vet Bull 38 [1968] 1766).

Orr CM, Kelly DF, Lucke VM: Tuberculosis in cats. A report of two cases. J Small Anim Pract 21 (1980) 247–253.

Parodi A, Fontaine M, Brion A, Tisseur H, Goret P: Mycobacterioses in the domestic carnivora—Present-day epidemiology of tuberculosis in the cat and dog. J Small Anim Pract 6 (1965) 309–326.

Pezzoli G: La tubercolosi del testicolo nel gatto. Zooprofilassi 9 (1954) 289–298.

Reif JS: Solitary pulmonary lesions in small animals. J Am Vet Med Assoc 155 (1969) 717–722.

Robin V, Fontaine M: Tuberculose génitale du chat. Recl Méd Vét 130 (1954) 213–216.

Robin V, Lesbouyries G: Les ostéo-arthrites tuberculeuses des carnivores domestiques. Rev Gén Méd Vét 35 (1926) 177–183.

Seren E: Contributo clinico, radiografico, anatomo-isto-patologico e batteriologico allo studio della tubercolosi renale del gatto. Nuova Vet 14 (1936) 177–189.

Smith JE: Symposium on diseases of cats III. Some pathogenic bacteria of cats with special reference to their public health significance. J Small Anim Pract 5 (1964) 517–523.

Snider WR: Tuberculosis in canine and feline populations. Review of the literature. Am Rev Respir Dis 104 (1971) 877–887.

Snider WR, Cohen D, Reif JS, Stein SC, Prier JE: Tuberculosis in canine and feline populations. Study of high risk populations in Pennsylvania, 1966–1968. Am Rev Respir Dis 104 (1971) 866–876.

Stableforth AW: A bacteriological investigation of cases of tuberculosis in five cats, sixteen dogs, a parrot, and a wallaby. J Comp Pathol Ther 42 (1929) 163–188.

Stünzi H: Zur Pathologie der Katzentuberkulose. Schweiz Arch Tierheilk 96 (1954) 604–612.

Suter MM von, Rotz A von, Weiss R, Mettler Ch: Atypisches mykobakterielles Hautgranulom bei einer Katze in der Schweiz. Zentralbl Veterinärmed A31 (1984) 712–718.

Teuscher E: Hirntuberkulose bei Hund und Katze. Schweiz Z Allg Pathol Bakteriol 17 (1954) 776–779.

Teuscher E: Hirntuberkulose bei Hund und Katze. Schweiz Med Wochenschr 85 (1955) 18.

Verge J, Senthille F: Recherches sur la fréquence des différents types de bacilles tuberculeux dans l'infection spontanée du chat. Ann Inst Pasteur 68 (1942) 114–117.

Walzl H: Zur Tuberkulose des Zentralnervensystems bei der Katze. Monatsh Tierheilk Die Rindertuberkulose 5 (1956) 199–205.

Willemse A, Beijer EGM: Bovine tuberculose bij een Kat (Bovine tuberculosis in a cat). Tijdschr Diergeneeskd 104 (1979) 717–721.

Wolff A: Tuberculosis in a domestic cat. Vet Med Small Anim Clin 61 (1966) 553.

**Cat Leprosy**

Allan GS, Wickham N: Mycobacterial granulomas in a cat diagnosed as leprosy. Feline Pract 6 (5) (1976) 33–36.

Brown LR, May CD, Williams SE: A nontuberculous granuloma in cats. NZ Vet J 10 (1962) 7–9.

Frye FL, Carney JD, Loughman WD: Feline lepromatous leprosy. Vet Med Small Anim Clin 69 (1974) 1273–1274.

Gee BR, Schiefer B, Ward GE: Disease resembling feline leprosy. Can Vet J 16 (1975) 30.

Lawrence WE, Wickham N: Cat leprosy: infection by a bacillus resembling *Mycobacterium lepraemurium*. Aust Vet J 39 (1963) 390–393.

Leiker DL, Poelma FG: On the etiology of cat leprosy. Int J Lepr 42 (1974) 312–315.

Matthews JA, Liggitt HD: Disseminated mycobacteriosis in a cat. J Amer Vet Med Assoc 183 (1983) 701–702.

McIntosh DW: Feline leprosy: A review of forty-four cases from western Canada. Can Vet J 23 (1982) 291–295.

Muller GH, Kirk RW, Scott DW: Small Animal Dermatology, 3rd ed. Philadelphia, WB Saunders Company, 1983, 227–229.

Pattyn SR, Portaels F: In vitro cultivation and characterization of *Mycobacterium lepraemurium*. Int J Lepr 48 (1980) 7–14.

Poelma FG, Leiker DL: Cat leprosy in the Netherlands. Int J Lepr 42 (1974) 307–311.

Schiefer B, Gee BR, Ward GE: A disease resembling feline leprosy in western Canada. J Am Vet Med Assoc 165 (1974) 1085–1087.

Schiefer B, Middleton DM: Experimental transmission of a feline mycobacterial skin disease (feline leprosy). Vet Pathol 20 (1983) 460–471.

Scott DW: Personal communication, 1984.

Wilkinson GT: A non-tuberculous granuloma of the cat associated with an acid-fast bacillus. Vet Rec 76 (1964) 777–778, 833–834.

Wilkinson GT: Feline leprosy. *In* Kirk RW (ed): Current Veterinary Therapy VI. Philadelphia, WB Saunders Company, 1977, 569–571.

**Cutaneous Atypical Mycobacteriosis**

Dewevre PJ, McAllister HA, Schirmer RG, Weinacker A: *Mycobacterium fortuitum* infection in a cat. J Am Anim Hosp Assoc 13 (1977) 68–70.

Kunkle GA, Gulbas NK, Fakok V, Halliwell REW, Connelly M: Rapidly growing mycobacteria as a cause of cutaneous granulomas: report of five cases. J Am Anim Hosp Assoc 19 (1983) 513–521.

Suter MM von, Rotz A von, Weiss R, Mettler Ch: Atypisches mykobakterielles Hautgranulom bei einer Katze in der Schweiz. Zentralbl Veterinärmed A 31 (1984) 712–718.

Thorel MF, Boisvert H: Abcès du chat à *Mycobacterium chelonei*. Bull Acad Vét 47 (1974) 415–422.

Toma B, Gaumont R, Paris-Hamelin A: La tuberculose féline et son danger pour l'homme. Comp Immunol Microbiol Infect Dis 1 (1979) 185–192.

Tomasovic AA, Rac R, Purcell DA: *Mycobacterium xenopi* in a skin lesion of a cat. Aust Vet J 52 (1976) 103.

White SD, Ihrke PJ, Stannard AA, Cadmus C, Griffin C, Kruth SA, Rosser EJ Jr, Reinke SI, Jang S: Cutaneous atypical mycobacteriosis in cats. J Am Vet Med Assoc 182 (1983) 1218–1222.

Wilkinson GT, Kelly WR, O'Boyle D: Cutaneous granulomas associated with *Mycobacterium fortuitum* infection in a cat. J Small Anim Pract 19 (1978) 357–362.

Wilkinson GT, Kelly WR, O'Boyle D: Pyogranulomatous panniculitis in cats due to *Mycobacterium smegmatis*. Aust Vet J 58 (1982) 77–78.

**Salmonellosis**

Carpenter CC: Infectious diarrheas. *In* Cluff LE, Johnson JE (eds): Clinical Concepts of Infectious Diseases, 2nd ed. Baltimore, The Williams & Wilkins Company, 1978, 292.

Fox JG, Beaucage CM: The incidence of *Salmonella* in random-source cats purchased for use in research. J Infect Dis 139 (1979) 362–365.

Gardner P, Provine HT: Manual of Acute Bacterial Infections: Early Diagnosis and Treatment. Boston, Little, Brown & Company, 1975, 233ff.

Gulden WJI van der, Janssen FCI: Salmonellen bij voor experimenten aangekochte honden en katten. Tijdschr Diergeneeskd 95 (1970) 495–497.

Hemsley LA: Abortion in two cats, with the isolation of *Salmonella cholera* (sic) *suis* from one case. Vet Rec 68 (1956) 152.

Hirsh DC, Enos LR: The use of antimicrobial drugs in the treatment of gastrointestinal disorders. *In* Kirk RW (ed): Current Veterinary Therapy VII. Philadelphia, WB Saunders Company, 1980, 913–914.

Ingham B, Brentnall DW: Acute peritonitis in a kitten associated with *Salmonella typhimurium* infection. J Small Anim Pract 13 (1972) 71–74.

Khan AQ: Salmonella infections in dogs and cats in the Sudan. Br Vet J 126 (1970) 607–612.

Kraft W: Infektionskrankheiten. *In* Kraft W, Dürr UM (eds): Katzenkrankheiten. Klinik und Therapie. Hannover, M & H Schaper, 1978, 93.

Krum SH, Stevens DR, Hirsh DC: *Salmonella arizonae* bacteremia in a cat. J Am Vet Med Assoc 170 (1977) 42–44.

Madewell BR, McChesney AE: Salmonellosis in a human infant, a cat, and two parakeets in the same household. J Am Vet Med Assoc 167 (1975) 1089–1090.

Mera AF: Un caso de infeccion a paratifico "A" en gato. Rev Med Vet (B. Aires) 23 (1941) 421–425.

Messow C, Hensel L: Die Salmonellose der Karnivoren. Dtsch Tierärztl Wochenschr 67 (1960) 623–626, 678–682; 68 (1961) 51–53.

Timoney JF: Feline salmonellosis. Vet Clin North Am 6 (1976) 395–398.

Timoney JF: Feline salmonellosis. *In* Kirk RW (ed): Current Veterinary Therapy VI. Philadelphia, WB Saunders Company, 1977, 1313–1315.

Timoney JF, Neibert HC, Scott FW: Feline salmonellosis. A nosocomial outbreak and experimental studies. Cornel Vet 68 (1978) 211–219.

Wilkinson GT (ed): Diseases of the Cat and Their Management. Melbourne, Blackwell Scientific Publications, 1983, 441.

Wollenweber N, Wüstenberg J, König F: Ueber das Vorkommen von Enteritisinfektionen bei Katzen und ihre Uebertragung auf den Menschen. Zentralbl Bakteriol Abt I [Orig] 139 (1937) 169–172.

**Pseudotuberculosis**

Allard AW: *Yersinia pseudotuberculosis* in a cat. J Am Vet Med Assoc 174 (1979) 91–92.

Aubert JM: Contribution à l'étude anatomopathologique de la pseudotuberculose des carnivores et rongeurs domestiques. Thesis. Lyon, 1945.

Blähser S: Über nicht alltägliche Todesursachen und einige plötzliche Todesfälle bei der Katze. Kleintierpraxis 7 (1962) 192–201.

Chappuis C: La pseudotuberculose due chat par le coccobacille de Malassez et Vignal. Thesis. Lyon, 1943.

Communal R: La pseudotuberculose du chat à bacille de Vignal et Malassez. Thesis. Alfort, 1945.

Drieux H: Milz. *In* Dobberstein J, Pallaske G, Stünzi H (eds): Joest E: Handbuch der Speziellen Pathologischen Anatomie der Haustiere, 3rd ed. Berlin, Paul Parey, 1970, Vol II, 511–583.

Hubbert WT: Yersiniosis in mammals and birds in the United States. Am J Trop Med Hyg 21 (1972) 458–463.

Isler D, Lott-Stolz G: Die wichtigsten Krankheits- und Todesursachen der Katze. Sektionsfälle 1965–76. Kleintierpraxis 23 (1978) 333–334.

Jarmai K: Über Pseudotuberkulose bei Katzen. Allatorv Lapok 59 (1936) 295–297 (Abstr Jahresber Veterinärmed 61 [1937] 80).

Labie C: Cited by Blähser, op cit, 192.

Leblois C: La pseudo-tuberculose zoogléïque chez le chat. Recl Méd Vét 96 (1920) 307–310.

Mair NS, Harbourne JF, Greenwood MT, White G: Pasteurella pseudotuberculosis infection in the cat: two cases. Vet Rec 81 (1967) 461–462.

Mollaret HH: L'infection à bacille de Malassez et Vignal chez le chat. I: La maladie naturelle. Recl Méd Vét 141 (1965) 1079–1094.

Pallaske G, Meyn A: Ueber die Pseudotuberkulose (Bact. pseudotub. rodentium) bei Katzen. Dtsch Tierärztl Wochenschr 40 (1932) 577–581.

Paul F, Weltmann O: Pseudotuberkulose beim Menschen. Wien Klin Wochenschr 47 (1934) 603–604.

Rahko T, Saloniemi H: Beobachtungen über die Pathologie der natürlichen *Yersinia pseudotuberculosis*-infektion bei der Katze. Dtsch Tierärztl Wochenschr 76 (1969) 611–613.

Robinson M: Pasteurella pseudotuberculosis infection in the cat. Vet Rec 91 (1972) 676–677.

Spearman JG, Hunt P, Nayar PSG: *Yersinia pseudotuberculosis* infection in a cat. Can Vet J 20 (1979) 361–364.

Stünzi H: Discussion of paper by Riniker P: Über die enterale Pseudotuberkulose. Schweiz Z Allg Pathol 20 (1957) 52–58.

Yanagawa Y, Maruyama T, Sakai S: Isolation of *Yersinia enterocolitica* and *Yersinia pseudotuberculosis* from apparently healthy dogs and cats. Microbiol Immunol 22 (1978) 643–646.

**Campylobacteriosis**

Blaser MJ, Weiss SH, Barrett TJ: *Campylobacter* enteritis associated with a healthy cat. J Am Med Assoc 247 (1982) 816.

Fox JG, Moore R, Ackerman JI: Canine and feline campylobacteriosis: Epizootiology and clinical and public health features. J Am Vet Med Assoc 183 (1983a) 1420–1424.

Fox JG, Moore R, Ackerman JI: *Campylobacter jejuni*–associated diarrhea in dogs. J Am Vet Med Assoc 183 (1983b) 1430–1433.

Holt PE: Incidence of campylobacter, salmonella and shigella infections in dogs in an industrial town. Vet Rec 107 (1980) 254.

Moore R: Personal communication, 1984.

Murtaugh RJ, Lawrence AE: Feline *Campylobacter jejuni*–associated enteritis. Feline Pract 14 (5) (1984) 37–40, 42.

Skirrow MB, Turnbull GL, Walker RE, Young SEJ: Campylobacter jejuni enteritis transmitted from cats to man [corresp]. Lancet I (8179) (1980) 1188.

Svedhem A, Norkrans G: Campylobacter jejuni enteritis transmitted from cat to man [corresp]. Lancet I (8166) (1980) 713–714.

Weber A, Schäfer R, Lembke C, Seifert U: Untersuchungen zum Vorkommen von Campylobacter jejuni bei Katzen. Berl Münch Tierärztl Wochenschr 96 (1983) 48–50.

**Pasteurellosis**

Arnbjerg J: Pasteurella multocida from canine and feline, with a case report of glossitis calcinosa in a dog caused by P. multocida. Nord Vet Med 30 (1978) 324–332.

Atin HL, Beetham WP: *Pasteurella multocida* empyema. N Engl J Med 256 (1957) 979–981.

Balk MW, Hughes HC. Lang CM: Ascending meningomyelitis resulting from a bite wound in a cat. J Am Vet Med Assoc 164 (1974) 1126.

Biberstein EL: The pasteurelloses. *In* Steele JH (ed): CRC Handbook Series in Zoonoses. Boca Raton, CRC Press, 1979, 495–514.

Calaprice A: Sulla pasteurellosi del gatto a sintomatologia nervosa. Zooprofilassi 14 (1959) 767–773.

Dorssen CA van, Smidt AC de, Stam JWE: Over het voorkommen van Pasteurella pneumotropica bij katten. Tijdschr Diergeneeskd 89 (1964) 674–682.

Frohböse H: Beitrag zum biochemischen Verhalten der bipolaren Bakterien der hämorrhagischen Septikämie. Zentralbl Bakteriol Abt I [Orig] 100 (1926) 213–218.

Gaertner A: Eine neue Katzenseuche. Zentralbl Bakteriol Abt I [Orig] 51 (1909) 232–249.

Haagsma J: Een studie over urease bezittende Pasteurella multocida-stammen bij de kat in Nederland. Tijdschr Diergeneeskd 89 (1964) 1225–1233.

Harms F: Hämorrhagische Septikämie bei Katzen. Dtsch Tierärztl Wochenschr 47 (1939) 436–437.

Krembs J: Hämorrhagische Septikämie bei einer Katze. Münch Tierärztl Wochenschr 8 (1937) 361–362.
Mitrovic M: Un caso di pasteurellosi del gatto. Studio dello stipite di pasteurella isolato. Clin Vet(Milano) 72 (1949) 97–107.
Oudar J, Joubert L, Prave M, Dickelé C, Munoz Trana J-C: Le portage buccal de *Pasteurella multocida* chez le chat. Étude épidémiologique, biochimique, et sérologique. Bull Soc Sci Vét Méd Comp Lyon 74 (1972) 353–357.
Palmeiro JM: Um caso de pasteurelose aviário no gato. Repos Trab Lab Central Patol Vet (Lisboa) 5 (1942) 105–108; Rev Med Vet (Lisboa) 37 (1942) 168–170.
Pospischil E: Eine hämorrhagische Septikämie bei Katzen. Deutschösterr Tierärztl Wochenschr 2 (1920) 1–2.
Ruppert F: Bipolare Bakterien als Erreger einer Katzenseuche. Dtsch Tierärztl Wochenschr 29 (1912) 441–442.
Soltys MA: *Pasteurella septica* in cats and the action of aureomycin and chloromycetin on experimental pasteurellosis. Vet Rec 63 (1951) 689–691.
Spalatin J: [Fatal pasteurellosis in a cat]. Jugoslav Vet Glaznik 20 (1940) 201–202 (Abstr Jahresb Vet Med 68 [1941] 369).
Wachnik Z, Jasinska S: Przypadek pasterelozy u kota [A case of pasteurellosis in a cat]. Med Weter 14 (1958) 331–333.

**Plague**

Barnes AM, Poland JD: Plague in the United States. Morb Mort Weekly Rep 32 No. 3SS (1983) 19ss–24ss.
De Souza A, Arruda J, Pinto M: Report on experiments undertaken to discover whether the common domesticated animals of Terceira Island [Azores] are affected by plague. J Hyg 10 (1910) 196–208.
Ettenger MM, Porvoznik J, Skeels MR, Mann JM, Leedom J, Heseltine P, Fannin SL, Chin J, Emerson JK, Hopkins RS, Williams LP, Sacks JJ: Human plague—United States. Morb Mort Weekly Rep 31 (1982) 74–76.
Fitch R, Smith L, Christensen SL, Bayer EV, Nygaard G, Werner SB: Feline plague—California. Morb Mort Weekly Rep 26 (1977) 362.
Goethals RM, Hildreth B, Wilson RL, Smith K, Weidmer C, Nygaard GS, Werner SB, von Rueden, R, Johnson C, Emerson J, Hopkins R: Human plague associated with domestic cats—California, Colorado. Morb Mort Weekly Rep 30 (1981) 265–266.
Green W, Gorman G, Counts JM, Marks F, Vernon TM, Mann JM: Plague—Arizona, Colorado, New Mexico. Morb Mort Weekly Rep 26 (1977) 215.
Heaton F, Gaskin J, Marchiando K, Hughes L, Graves G, Mann J, Matzner P, Montman C, Pressman A, Weeks K, Counts JM, Werner SB, Vernon TM, Googins JA: Plague—United States. Morb Mort Weekly Rep 26 (1977) 337.
Isaäcson M, Levy D, Pienaar BJ te WN, Bubb HD, Louw JA, Genis DK: Unusual cases of human plague in southern Africa. S Afr Med J 47 (1973) 2109–2113.
Rollag OJ, Mann JM, Hibbs C, Skeels M, Nims L: Feline plague—New Mexico. CDC Vet Public Health Notes (Nov 1980) 5–7.
Rollag OJ, Skeels MR, Nims LJ, Thilsted JP, Mann JM: Feline plague in New Mexico: report of five cases. J Am Vet Med Assoc 179 (1981) 1381–1383.
Thornton DJ, Tustin RC, Pienaar BJ te WN, Bubb HD: Cat bite transmission of *Yersinia pestis* infection to man. J S Afr Vet Assoc 46 (1975) 165–169.
Weniger BG, Warren AJ, Forseth V, Shipps GW, Creelman T, Gorton J, Barnes AM: Human bubonic plague transmitted by a domestic cat scratch. J Am Med Assoc 251 (1984) 927–928.

**Tetanus**

Bateman JK: Tetanus in a kitten. Vet Rec 11 (1931) 805.
Fildes P, Bullock W, O'Brien RA, Glenny AT: *Bacillus tetani. In* Fildes P, Ledingham JEG (eds): A System of Bacteriology. London, H.M. Stationery Office, 1929, Vol. 3, 298–372.
Fildes P, Hare T, Wright JG: Case of tetanus in a cat. Vet Rec 43 (1931) 731.
Goetz EF: Tetanus in a cat. J Am Vet Med Assoc 169 (1976) 174.
Greene CE: Tetanus. *In* Kirk RW (ed): Current Veterinary Therapy VIII. Philadelphia, WB Saunders Company, 1983.
Groulade M: Un cas de tétanos chez le chat. Bull Acad Vét 20 (1947) 254–255.
Hopson CG: Tetanus in a cat. Vet Rec 12 (1932) 302.
Killingsworth C, Chiapella A, Veralli P, de Lahunta A: Feline tetanus. J Am Anim Hosp Assoc 13 (1977) 209–215.
Kodituwakku GE, Wijewanta EA: Tetanus in a cat. Br Vet J 114 (1958) 48–50.
Lettow K: Tetanus bei einer Katze. Berl Münch Tierärztl Wochenschr 68 (1955) 197.
Loeffler K, Hensel L, Ehrlein HJ: Tetanus bei Hund und Katze. Dtsch Tierärztl Wochenschr 69 (1962) 476–479.
Ludins GH: Tetanus in a cat. J Am Vet Med Assoc 97 (1939) 231.
Miller ER: Tetanus in the cat. Vet Rec 61 (1949) 40.
Nam CC: Clinical communication: tetanus in a cat. J Malayan Vet Med Assoc 1 (1956) 56.
Saranta JT: Tetanus in a cat [letter]. J Am Vet Med Assoc 170 (1977) 3.

**Listeriosis**

Armstrong D: *Listeria monocytogenes. In* Mandell GL, Douglas RG, Bennett JE (eds): Principles and Practice of Infectious Diseases. New York, John Wiley & Sons, 1979, 1626–1633.
Decker RA, Rogers JJ, Lesar S: Listeriosis in a young cat. J Am Vet Med Assoc 168 (1976) 1025.
Held R: Listeriose bei einer Katze. Zentralbl Bakteriol I Abt [Orig] 173 (1958) 485–486.
Jones BR, Cullinane LC, Cary PR: Isolation of *Listeria monocytogenes* from a bite in a cat from the common tree weta *(Hemideina crassidens)* [letter]. NZ Vet J 32 (5) (1984) 79–80.
McIlwain PK, Andrews MF, Barnes RW, Bolin FM, Eveleth DF: Occurrence of *Listeria monocytogenes* in the brains of wild and domestic animals. Am J Vet Res 27 (1966) 1497–1499.
Nilsson A, Karlsson KA: Listeria monocytogenes isolations from animals in Sweden during 1948–57. Nord Vet Med 11 (1959) 305–315.
Turner T: A case of *Escherichia monocytogenes (Listeria monocytogenes)* in the cat [corresp]. Vet Rec 74 (1962) 778.

**Tyzzer's Disease**

Bennett AM, Huxtable CR, Love DN: Tyzzer's disease in cats experimentally infected with feline leukaemia virus. Vet Microbiol 2 (1977) 49–56.
Hall WC, Van Kruiningen HJ: Tyzzer's disease in a horse. J Am Vet Med Assoc 164 (1974) 1187–1189.
Jones BR, Johnstone AC, Hancock WS: Tyzzer's disease in kittens with familial primary hyperlipoproteinemia. J Small Anim Pract 26 (1985) 411–419.
Kobokawa K, Kubo M, Takasaki Y, Oghiso Y, Sato K, Lee YS, Goto N, Takahashi R, Fujiwara K: Two cases of feline Tyzzer's disease. Jpn J Exp Med 43 (1973) 413–421.
Kovatch RM, Zebarth G: Naturally occurring Tyzzer's disease in a cat. J Am Vet Med Assoc 162 (1973) 136–138.
Qureshi SR, Carlton WW, Olander HJ: Tyzzer's disease in a dog. J Am Vet Med Assoc 168 (1976) 602–604.
Schneck G: Therapieversuche gegen Tyzzer's Disease bei Mäusen. Wien Tierärztl Monatschr 56 (1969) 243–245.
Schneck G: Tyzzer's disease in an adult cat. Vet Med Small Anim Clin 70 (1975) 155–156.

**Brucellosis**

Frei W: Über eine Abortusenzootie bei Mutterschweinen mit Übergang von Bangbazillen auf den Menschen. Schweiz Arch Tierheilkd 74 (1932) 120–126.

Hirchert R, Lange W, Leonhardt H-G: Zum Vorkommen von Brucella melitensis bei Tieren in Syrien. Berl Münch Tierärztl Wochenschr 80 (1967) 45–47.

Jørgensen H: *Brucella abortus*-infektioner hos katten. Maanedsskr Dyrlaeger 55 (1943) 116–123.

Koegel A: Beiträge zur Abortusforschung. Münch Tierärztl Wochenschr 75 (1924) 73–78.

Makhawejsky WN, Karkadinowskaja IA: Ueber die Empfindlichkeit der Katzen gegen Brucella melitensis-abortus. Dtsch Tierärztl Wochenschr 40 (1932) 229–231.

Menchaca ES: Indice de infeccion brucelica en los gatos de la capital federal y de gran Buenos Aires. Rev Vet Med (B. Aires) 40 (1959) 5–12.

Nechayeva NM: [Susceptibility of cats to *Brucella abortus bovis, Br. suis, Br. melitensis*]. Veterinariya (Moscow) 29 (March) (1952) 30 (Abstr RE Habel, J Am Vet Med Assoc 121 [1952] 314).

Pallaske G: Zur Frage der Abortus-Bang-Infektion der Fleischfresser. Berl Münch Tierärztl Wochenschr (1938) 752–755.

Pickerell PA: Comments on epizootiology and control of canine brucellosis. J Am Vet Med Assoc 156 (1970) 1741–1742.

Pickerell PA, Carmichael LE: Canine brucellosis: control programs in commercial kennels and effect on reproduction. J Am Vet Med Assoc 160 (1972) 1607–1615.

Poelma LJ, Everson CL, Brueckner AL, Pickens EM: A study of the Brucella abortus titers of the various species of farm animals in Maryland. Cornell Vet 23 (1933) 344–347.

Randhawa AS, Dieterich WH, Hunter CC, Kelly VP, Johnson TC, Svoboda B, Wilson DF: Prevalence of seropositive reactions to *Brucella canis* in a limited survey of domestic cats. J Am Vet Med Assoc 171 (1977) 267–268.

Reinhardt R: Die Krankheiten der Katze. Hannover, M & H Schaper, 1952.

Shaw EA: Further observations on goats, cats, rats and ambulatory cases in connection with Mediterranean fever. Reports of the Royal Society of London, Mediterranean Fever Commission. London, Harrison & Sons, 1907.

Valla G: Sulla recettività del gatto alle brucellosi. Nuova Vet 11 (1933) 458–460.

**Tularemia**

Ditchfield I, Meads E, Julian R: Tularemia of muskrats in eastern Ontario. Can J Public Health 51 (1960) 474–478.

Packer RM, Harrison LR, Matthews CF, Halloway JT, Sikes RK, Pond AD, Schupbach T, Hibbs C, Brown S, Skeels M, Rollag OJ, Mann JM: Tularemia associated with domestic cats—Georgia, New Mexico. Morb Mort Weekly Rep 31 (1982) 39–41.

Schuller A, Erdmann B: Beobachtungen bei einer Tularämie-Epidemie. Z Hyg Infektkr 124 (1943) 624–635.

**Anthrax**

Cripps JHH, Young RC: A case of anthrax in a cat and in a monkey. Vet Rec 72 (1960) 1054.

Niléhn P: [Infections with anthrax-like bacilli *(B. cereus)*]. Nord Vet Med 10 (1958) 325–330.

Reinhardt R: Die Krankheiten der Katze. Hannover, M & H Schaper, 1952.

**Glanders**

Reinhardt R: Die Krankheiten der Katze. Hannover, M & H Schaper, 1952.

**Leptospirosis**

Carlos ER, Kundin WD, Watten RH, Tsai CC, Irving GS, Carlos ET, Directo AC: Leptospirosis in the Philippines: Feline studies. Am J Vet Res 32 (1971) 1455–1456.

Fessler JF, Morter RL: Experimental feline leptospirosis. Cornell Vet 54 (1964) 176–190.

Hamilton J: Nephritis in the cat. J Small Anim Pract 7 (1966) 445–449.

Harkness AC, Smith BL, Fowler GF: An isolation of *Leptospira* serotype *pomona* from a domestic cat. NZ Vet J 18 (1970) 175–176.

Hemsley LA: *Leptospira canicola* and chronic nephritis in cats. Vet Rec 68 (1956) 300–301.

Klaarenbeek A, Winsser J: De leptospirosen bij de kleine huisdieren. Een statistisch en experimenteel onderzook. Tijdschr Diergeneeskd 65 (1938) 666–670.

Lucke VM, Crowther ST: The incidence of leptospiral agglutination titres in the domestic cat. Vet Rec 77 (1965) 647–648.

Mason RW, King SJ, McLachlan NM: Suspected leptospirosis in two cats. Aust Vet J 48 (1972) 622–623.

Modrić Z: Prirodna i eksperimentalna leptospiroza u macke. Vet Arhiv 48 (1978) 147–156.

Murphy LC, Cardeilhac PT, Carr JW: The presence of leptospiral agglutinins in the sera of the domestic cat. Cornell Vet 48 (1958) 3–9.

Otten E, Henze S, Goethe H: Leptospireninfektionen bei der Hauskatze. Z Tropenmed Parasitol 5 (1954) 187–204.

Rees HG: Leptospirosis in a cat. NZ Vet J 12 (1964) 64.

***Escherichia coli***

Choi W-R, Kawata K: 0 group of *Escherichia coli* from canine and feline pyometra. Jpn J Vet Res 23 (1975) 141–143.

Finco DR, Kneller SK, Crowell WA: Diseases of the urinary system. *In* Catcott EJ (ed): Feline Medicine and Surgery, 2nd ed. Santa Barbara, American Veterinary Publications Inc, 1975, 272.

Hara M, Mutoh T, Kishikawa S, Nakazawa M, Ishizaka T: Characterization of *Escherichia coli* isolated from bacterial pyelonephritis of kittens. Bull Azabu Vet Coll 1 (1976) 81–98.

Langman BA: Bacterial gastro-enteritis in cats [letter]. Vet Rec 76 (1964) 190.

Ling GV: Choice of antimicrobial agents in the treatment of urinary tract infections. *In* Kirk RW (ed): Current Veterinary Therapy VII. Philadelphia, WB Saunders Company, 1980, 1162–1163.

Mackel DC, Weaver RE, Langley LF, DeCapito TM: Observations on the occurrence in cats of *Escherichia coli* pathogenic for man. Am J Hyg 71 (1960) 176–178.

Månsson I, Lindblad G: [Observations on haemolytic *Escherichia coli* in dogs and cats]. Nord Vet Med 14 Suppl 2 (1962) 67. Proc 9th Nordic Vet Congr, Copenhagen, 1962, Vol 11, 880–883 (Abstr Vet Bull 34 [1964] 764).

Moss S, Frost AJ: The resistance to chemotherapeutic agents of *Escherichia coli* from domestic dogs and cats. Aust Vet J 61 (1984) 82–84.

Rhoades HE, Saxena SP, Meyer RC: Serological identification of *Escherichia coli* isolated from cats and dogs. Can J Comp Med 35 (1971) 218–233.

Schechter RD: The significance of bacteria in feline cystitis and urolithiasis. J Am Vet Med Assoc 156 (1970) 1567–1573.

Scott FW, Weiss RC, Post JE, Gilmartin JE, Hoshino Y: Kitten mortality complex (neonatal FIP?). Feline Pract 9 (2) (1979) 44–56.

Wilkinson GT: Diseases of the Cat. Oxford, Pergamon Press, 1966, 134, 144.

**Staphylococcal Infections**

Biberstein EL, Franti CE, Jang SS, Ruby A: Antimicrobial sensitivity patterns in *Staphylococcus aureus* from animals. J Am Vet Med Assoc 164 (1974) 1183–1186.

Cox HU, Hoskins JD, Newman SS, Turnwald GH, Foil CS, Roy AF, Kearney MT: Distribution of staphylococcal species on clinically healthy cats. Am J Vet Res 46 (1985) 1824–1828.

Daigo Y: [Characterization of *Staphylococcus aureus* isolated from the nostrils of dogs and cats. I. Biological characters of the isolated strains.] Bull Azabu Vet Coll 26 (1973) 11–26 (Abstr Vet Bull 45 [1975] 592).

Devriese LA, Nzuambe D, Godard C: Identification and characterization of staphylococci isolated from cats. Vet Microbiol 9 (1984) 179–285.

Habermann RT, Williams FP: Metastatic micrococcic infection (botryomycosis) in a cat. J Am Vet Med Assoc 129 (1956) 30–33.

Hearst BR: Low incidence of staphylococcal dermatitides in animals with high incidence of *Staphylococcus aureus*. Part 1: preliminary study of cats. Vet Med Small Anim Clin 62 (1967) 475–477.

Macdonald KR, Greenfield J, McCausland HD: Remission of staphylococcal dermatitis by autogenous bacterin therapy. Can Vet J 13 (1972) 45–48.

Nielsen SW: Personal communication, 1957.

Raus J, Love DN: Characterization of coagulase-positive *Staphylococcus intermedius* and *Staphylococcus aureus* isolated from veterinary clinical specimens. J Clin Microbiol 18 (1983) 789–792.

Walton DK, Scott DW, Manning TO: Cutaneous bacterial granuloma (botryomycosis) in a dog and cat. J Am Anim Hosp Assoc 19 (1983) 537–541.

Wilkinson GT: Diseases of the Cat. Oxford, Pergamon Press, 1966, 193.

**Streptococcal Infections**

Goldman PM, Moore TD: Spontaneous Lancefield group G streptococcal infection in a random source cat colony. Lab Anim Sci 23 (1973) 565–566.

Swindle MM, Narayan O, Luzarraga M, Bobbie DL: Contagious streptococcal lymphadenitis in cats. J Am Med Vet Assoc 177 (1980) 829–830.

Tillman PC, Dodson ND, Indiveri M: Group G streptococcal epizootic in a closed cat colony. J Clin Microbiol 16 (1982) 1057–1060.

***Bordetella bronchiseptica***

Fisk SK, Soave OA: *Bordetella bronchiseptica* in laboratory cats from central California. Lab Anim Sci 23 (1973) 33–35.

Paterson JS: Cats. *In* Lane-Petter W (ed): Animals for Research. Principles of Breeding and Management. London, Academic Press, 1963.

Roudebush P, Fales WH: Antibacterial susceptibility of *Bordetella bronchiseptica* isolates from small companion animals with respiratory disease. J Am Anim Hosp Assoc 17 (1981) 793–797.

Snyder SB, Fisk SK, Fox JG, Soave OA: Respiratory tract disease associated with *Bordetella bronchiseptica* infection in cats. J Am Vet Med Assoc 163 (1973) 293–294.

***Haemophilus* spp**

Wilkinson GT: Diseases of the Cat. Oxford, Pergamon Press, 1966, 96, 204.

Wilkinson GT (ed): Diseases of the Cat and Their Management. Melbourne, Blackwell Scientific Publications, 1983.

***Clostridia* Other Than *C. tetani***

Haugaard P, Jørgensen IM: Et utbrud a fiskebaren type E botulisme hos mennesker og kat. Danske Dyrlaegerforening Medlemsblad 57 (1974) 361–367.

Love DN, Jones RF, Bailey M: *Clostridium villosum* sp. nov. from subcutaneous abscesses in cats. Int J Systematic Bacteriol 29 (1979) 241–244.

Mansfield PD, Wilt GR, Powers RD: Clostridial myositis associated with an intrathoracic abscess in a cat. J Am Med Assoc 184 (1984) 1150–1151.

Poonacha KB, Donahue JM, Leonard WH: Clostridial myositis in a cat. Vet Pathol 19 (1982) 217–219.

Prévot A-R, Sillioc R: Une énigme biologique: chat et botulisme. Ann Inst Pasteur 89 (1955) 354–357.

Soltys M: Bacteria and Fungi Pathogenic to Man and Animals. Baltimore, The Williams & Wilkins Company, 1963.

Wilkinson GT (ed): Diseases of the Cat and Their Management. Melbourne, Blackwell Scientific Publication, 1983.

**Infections with Other Bacteria**

Armstrong PJ: Systemic *Serratia marcescens* infections in a dog and cat. J Am Vet Med Assoc 184 (1984) 1154–1158.

Carwardine P: The use of metronidazole for the treatment of non-specific anaerobic infections in dogs and cats. Vet Res Commun 7 (1983) 261–262.

Chow AW, Ota J, Guze LB: Gentamicin-clindamycin therapy for suspected sepsis; a prospective study. Clin Res 22 (1974) 438A.

Creighton SR, Wilkins RJ: Pleural effusions. *In* Kirk RW (ed): Current Veterinary Therapy VII. Philadelphia, WB Saunders Company, 1980, 253–261.

Dickie CW: Feline pyothorax caused by a *Borrelia*-like organism and *Corynebacterium pyogenes*. J Am Vet Med Assoc 174 (1979) 516–517.

Fox JG, Beaucage CM, Folta CA, Thornton GW: Nosocomial transmission of *Serratia marcescens* in a veterinary hospital due to contamination by benzalkonium chloride. J Clin Microbiol 14 (1981) 157–160.

Higgins R, Paradis M: Abscess caused by *Corynebacterium equi* in a cat. Can Vet J 21 (1980) 63–64.

Hirsh DC, Indiveri MC, Jang SS, Biberstein EL: Changes in prevalence and susceptibility of obligate anaerobes in clinical veterinary practice. J Am Vet Med Assoc 186 (1985) 1086–1089.

Jang SS, Demartini JC, Henrickson RV, Enright FM: Focal necrotizing pneumonia in cats associated with a gram negative eugonic fermenting bacterium. Cornell Vet 63 (1973) 446–454.

Jang SS, Lock A, Biberstein EL: A cat with Corynebacterium equi lymphadenitis clinically simulating lymphosarcoma. Cornell Vet 65 (1975) 232–239.

Johnson KA, Lomas GR, Wood AKW: Osteomyelitis in dogs and cats caused by anaerobic bacteria. Aust Vet J 61 (1984) 57–61.

Love DN, Jones RF, Bailey M, Johnson RS, Gamble N: Isolation and characterisation of bacteria from pyothorax (empyaemia [sic]) in cats. Vet Microbiol 7 (1982) 455–461.

McParland PJ, O'Hagan J, Pearson GR, Neill SD: Pathological changes associated with group EF-4 bacteria in the lungs of a dog and a cat. Vet Rec 11 (1982) 336–338.

Prévot AR, Goret L, Joubert L, Tardieux P, Aladame N: Recherches bactériologiques sur une infection purulente d'allure actinomycosique chez le chat. [Subcutaneous phlegmon due to spiral organisms.] Ann Inst Pasteur 81 (1951) 85–88.

Rosenblatt JE: Antimicrobial susceptibility testing of anaerobes. *In* Lorian V (ed): Antibiotics in Laboratory Medicine. Baltimore, The Williams & Wilkins Company, 1980, 118–120.

Scott PC, Taylor TK, Gilmore JF, Hart AT: Suppurative peritonitis in cats associated with anaerobic bacteria. Aust Vet J 61 (1984) 367–368.

Sims MA: *Flavobacterium meningosepticum*: a probable cause of meningitis in a cat. Vet Rec 95 (1974) 567–569.

Vallée A, Le Cain A, Thibault P, Second L: Isolement chez la chatte d'un vibrion voisin de Vibrio-foetus. Bull Acad Vét Fr 34 (1961) 151–152.

Velu H, Lasserre R, Soulié P: Plaie grave de la face chez le chat et association fusospirochètienne. Bull Acad Vét Fr 14 (1941) 167–174.

Withers AR, Davies ME: An outbreak of conjunctivitis in a cattery caused by *Moraxella lacunatus* [sic]. Vet Rec 73 (1961) 856–857.

Zinner SH, Provonchee RB, Elias KS, Peter G: Effect of clindamycin on the *in vitro* activity of amikacin and gentamicin against gram-negative bacilli. Antimicrob Agents Chemother 9 (1976) 661–664.

**Feline Association with Certain Human Diseases**

Citterio L: Del microbo della linforeticulosi d' inoculazione (c.d. malattia da graffio di gatto. Boll Ist Sieroter (Milan) 34 (1955) 657–664.

Gillespie JH, Baker JA: Experimental Q fever in cats. Am J Vet Res 13 (1952) 91–94.

Hadfield TL, Schlagel C, Margileth A: Stalking the cause of cat-scratch disease. Diagnostic Med 8 (1985) 22–27.

Kosatsky T: Household outbreak of Q-fever pneumonia related to a parturient cat. Lancet II (8417/8) (1984) 1447–1449.

Wear DJ, Margileth AM, Hadfield TL, Fischer GW, Schlagel CJ, King FM: Cat scratch disease: a bacterial infection. Science 221 (1983) 1403–1405.

**Supplementary References, Bacterial Infections**

Berg JN, Fales WH, Scanlan CM: Occurrence of anaerobic bacteria in diseases of the dog and cat. Am J Vet Res 40 (1979) 876–881.

Biberstein EL, Jang SS, Hirsh DC: Species distribution of coagulase-positive staphylococci in animals. J Clin Microbiol 19 (1984) 610–615.

Love DN, Johnson JL, Jones RF, Bailey M: Comparison of *Bacteroides zoogleoformans* strains isolated from soft tissue infections in cats with strains from periodontal disease in humans. Infect Immun 47 (1985) 166–168.

Love DN, Jones RF, Bailey M: Isolation and characterization of bacteria from abscesses in the subcutis of cats. J Med Microbiol 12 (1979) 207–212.

Love DN, Jones RF, Bailey M: Characterization of *Fusobacterium* species isolated from soft tissue infections in cats. J Appl Bacteriol 48 (1980) 325–331.

Love DN, Jones RF, Bailey M: Characterization of *Bacteroides* species isolated from soft tissue infections in cats. J Appl Bacteriol 50 (1981) 567–575.

**Hemobartonellosis**

Auer L, Bell K, Coates S: Blood transfusion reactions in the cat. J Am Vet Med Assoc 180 (1982) 729–730.

Clark R: *Eperythrozoon felis* (Sp. Nov.) in a cat. J S Afr Vet Med Assoc 13 (1942) 15–16.

Cotter SM: Management of the anemic cat. *In* Kirk RW (ed): Current Veterinary Therapy VIII. Philadelphia, WB Saunders Company, 1983.

Cotter SM, Hardy WD Jr, Essex M: Association of feline leukemia virus with lymphosarcoma and other disorders in the cat. J Am Vet Med Assoc 166 (1975) 449–454.

Demaree RS Jr, Nessmith WB: Ultrastructure of *Haemobartonella felis* from a naturally infected cat. Am J Vet Res 33 (1972) 1303–1308.

Edwards FB: A new blood parasite in British cats. Vet Rec 72 (1960) 439.

Farrow BRH: Laboratory diagnosis of viral and other infectious diseases. Vet Clin North Am 6 (1976) 755–765.

Flint JC, McKelvie DH: Feline infectious anemia—diagnosis and treatment. Proc Am Vet Med Assoc 92 (1955) 240–242.

Flint JC, Moss LC: Infectious anemia in cats. J Am Vet Med Assoc 122 (1953) 45–48.

Flint JC, Roepke MH, Jensen R: Feline infectious anemia. I. Clinical aspects. Am J Vet Res 19 (1958) 164–168.

Flint JC, Roepke MH, Jensen R: Feline infectious anemia. II. Experimental cases. Am J Vet Res 20 (1959) 33–40.

Harbutt PR: A clinical appraisal of feline infectious anemia and its transmission under natural conditions. Aust Vet J 39 (1963) 401–404.

Harvey JW, Gaskin JM: Experimental feline haemobartonellosis. J Am Anim Hosp Assoc 13 (1977) 28–38.

Harvey JW, Gaskin JM: Feline haemobartonellosis: attempts to induce relapses of clinical disease in chronically infected cats. J Am Anim Hosp Assoc 14 (1978a) 453–456.

Harvey JW, Gaskin JM: Feline haemobartonellosis. Proc Am Anim Hosp Assoc 45 (1978b) 117–123.

Hayes HM, Priester WA: Feline infectious anemia. Risk by age, sex and breed; prior disease; seasonal occurrence; mortality. J Small Anim Pract 14 (1973) 797–804.

Holzworth J: Anemia in the cat. J Am Vet Med Assoc 128 (1956) 471–488.

Jain NC, Keeton KS: Scanning electron microscopic features of *Haemobartonella felis*. Am J Vet Res 34 (1973) 697–700.

Kolabskii NA, Melnikova AD: [Parasitic inclusions in the erythrocytes of the blood during an epizootic of cats.] Sborn Rabot Leningrad Vet Inst [Collected Works of the Leningrad Veterinary School] 12 (1951) 177–180.

Kreier JP, Gothe R: Aegyptianellosis, eperythrozoonosis, grahamellosis and haemobartonellosis. Vet Parasitol 2 (1976) 83–95.

Kreier JP, Ristic M: Haemobartonellosis, eperythrozoonosis, grahamellosis, and ehrlichiosis. *In* Weinman D, Ristic M (eds): Infectious Blood Diseases of Man and Animals. New York, Academic Press, 1968, Vol II, 387–472.

Maede Y: Studies on feline haemobartonellosis. V. Role of the spleen in cats infected with *Haemobartonella felis*. Jpn J Vet Sci 40 (1978) 141–146.

Maede Y: Sequestration and phagocytosis of *Haemobartonella felis* in the spleen. Am J Vet Res 40 (1979) 691–695.

Maede Y, Hata R: Studies of feline haemobartonellosis. II. The mechanism of anemia produced by infection with *Haemobartonella felis*. Jpn J Vet Sci 37 (1975) 49–54.

Maede Y, Murata H: Ultrastructural observation on the removal of *Haemobartonella felis* from erythrocytes in the spleen of a cat. Jpn J Vet Sci 40 (1978) 203–205.

Maede Y, Sonoda M: Studies on feline haemobartonellosis. III. Scanning electron microscopy of *Haemobartonella felis*. Jpn J Vet Sci 37 (1975) 209–211.

Norsworthy GD: Diagnosis of feline infectious anemia. Feline Pract 6 (1) (1976) 26–32.

Priester WA, Hayes HM: Feline leukemia after feline infectious anemia. J Natl Cancer Inst 51 (1973) 289–291.

Ristic M, Holland CJ: Unpublished data, University of Illinois, 1979.

Ristic M, Huxsoll DL, Weisiger RM, Hildebrandt, PK, Nyindo MBA: Serological diagnosis of tropical canine pancytopenia by indirect immunofluorescence. Infect Immun 6 (1972) 226–231.

Ristic M, Kreier JP: Family III. Anaplasmataceae. *In* Buchanan RE, Gibbons NE (eds): Bergey's Manual of Determinative Bacteriology, 9th ed. Baltimore, The Williams & Wilkins Company, 1984, 719–729.

Ristic M, White FH: Detection of an *Abaplasma marginale* antibody complex formed *in vivo*. Science 131 (1960) 987–988.

Rogers TE, Wallace WR: A rapid staining technique for *Anaplasma*. Am J Vet Res 27 (1966) 1127–1128.

Schwartzman RM, Besch ED: Feline infectious anemia. Vet Med 53 (1958) 494–500.

Seamer J, Douglas SW: A new blood parasite of British cats. Vet Rec 71 (1959) 405–408.

Simpson CF, Gaskin JM, Harvey JW: Ultrastructure of erythrocytes parasitized by *Haemobartonella felis*. J Parasitol 64 (1978) 504–511.

Small E: The morphology of *Haemobartonella felis* and the pathogenesis of infectious anemia caused by it. Master's Thesis, University of Illinois, 1965.

Small E, Ristic M: Morphologic features of *Haemobartonella felis*. Am J Vet Res 28 (1967) 845–851.

Small E, Ristic M: Haemobartonellosis. Vet Clin North Am 1 (1971) 225–230.

Splitter EJ, Castro ER, Kanawyer WL: Feline infectious anemia. Vet Med 51 (1956) 17–22.

Thomsett LR: *Eperythrozoon felis*: observations on incidence and relationship to external parasitism in the cat. Vet Rec 72 (1960) 397–399.

Wilkinson GT: Feline infectious anaemia: a case in a cat and its successful treatment. Vet Rec 75 (1963) 324–325.

Wilkinson GT: Feline infectious anaemia. Vet Rec 84 (1969) 331–333.

**Mycoplasmal Infections**


Blackmore DK, Hill A: The experimental transmission of various mycoplasmas of feline origin to domestic cats *(Felis catus)*. J Small Anim Pract 14 (1973) 7–13.

Blackmore DK, Hill A, Jackson OF: The incidence of mycoplasma in pet and colony maintained cats. J Small Anim Pract 12 (1971) 207–217.

Campbell LH, Snyder SB, Reed C, Fox JG: *Mycoplasma felis*-associated conjunctivitis in cats. J Am Vet Med Assoc 163 (1973a) 991–995.

Campbell LH, Fox JG, Snyder SB: Ocular bacteria and mycoplasma of the clinically normal cat. Feline Pract 3 (6) (1973b) 10–12.

Cello RM: Association of pleuropneumonia-like organisms with conjunctivitis of cats. Am J Ophthalmol 43 (1957) 296–297.

Cello RM: Ocular infections in animals with PLT (Bedsonia) group agents. Am J Ophthalmol 63 Suppl (1967) 1270–1274.

Cello RM: Clues to differential diagnosis of feline respiratory infections. J Am Vet Med Assoc 158 (1971) 968–973.

Cole BC, Golightly L, Ward JR: Characterization of mycoplasma strains from cats. J Bacteriol 94 (1967) 1451–1458.

Colegrave AJ, Ingham B, Inglis JM: Chronic rhinitis in cats. Vet Rec 76 (1964) 67–68.

Harasawa R, Yamamoto K, Ogata M: Isolation of T-mycoplasmas from cats in Japan. Microbiol Immunol 21 (1977) 179–181.

Heyward JT, Sabry MZ, Dowdle WR: Characterization of mycoplasma species of feline origin. Am J Vet Res 30 (1969) 615–622.

Hill A: Further studies on the morphology and isolation of feline mycoplasmas. J Small Anim Pract 12 (1971) 219–223.

Hill A: Comparison of mycoplasmas isolated from captive wild felines. Res Vet Sci 18 (1975) 139–143.

Keane DP: Chronic abscesses in cats associated with an organism resembling mycoplasma. Can Vet J 24 (1983) 289–291.

Laborde G: [Mycoplasmas of the cat: Isolation, identification and discussion of their role in feline respiratory diseases]. Thesis. Lyon, 1971, No. 5.

Lindley JW: A case of Mycoplasma sp. found in cats. Southwest Vet 19 (1966) 320–321.

Moise NS, Crissman JW, Fairbrother JF, Baldwin C: *Mycoplasma gateae* arthritis and tenosynovitis in cats: Case report and experimental reproduction of the disease. Am J Vet Res 44 (1983) 16–21.

Povey RC, Wardley RC: Mycoplasma species in a cat colony. Vet Rec 92 (1973) 27–28.

Schneck GW: Mycoplasma species in association with feline viruses. Vet Rec 91 (1972) 594–595.

Spradbrow PB, Marley J, Portas B, Burgess G: The isolation of mycoplasmas from cats with respiratory disease. Aust Vet J 46 (1970) 109–110.

Switzer WP: The Genus Mycoplasma. *In* Merchant IA, Packer RA (eds): Veterinary Bacteriology and Virology, 7th ed. Ames, Iowa State University Press, 1967, 531–548.

Tan RJS: Susceptibility of kittens to *Mycoplasma felis* infection. Jpn J Exp Med 44 (1974) 235–240.

Tan RJS, Lim EW, Ishak B: Ecology of mycoplasmas in clinically healthy cats. Aust Vet J 53 (1977a) 515–518.

Tan RJS, Lim EW, Ishak B: Significance and pathogenic role of *Mycoplasma arginini* in cat diseases. Can J Comp Med 41 (1977b) 349–354.

Tan RJS, Markham J: Isolation of mycoplasma from cats with conjunctivitis [letter]. NZ Vet J, 19 (1971) 28.

Tan RJS, Miles JAR: Mycoplasma isolations from clinically normal cats. Br Vet J 128 (1972) 87–90.

Tan RJS, Miles JAR: Characterization of mycoplasmas isolated from cats with conjunctivitis. NZ Vet J 21 (1973) 27–32.

Tan RJS, Miles JAR: Incidence and significance of mycoplasmas in sick cats. Res Vet Sci 16 (1974a) 27–34.

Tan RJS, Miles JAR: Possible role of feline T-strain mycoplasmas in cat abortion. Aust Vet J 50 (1974b) 142–145.

Wilkinson GT: Diseases of the Cat. Oxford, Pergamon Press, 1966, 273–274.

Wilkinson GT: Mycoplasms of the cat. Vet Annu 20 (1980) 145–150.

# 9
CHAPTER
# MYCOTIC DISEASES

JEAN HOLZWORTH

CONTRIBUTING AUTHORS:
PAULE BLOUIN and MICHAEL W. CONNER

The agents of mycotic infections belong to the fungi. The diseases that they produce may involve either the integument (hair, claws, epidermis, and dermis) or the deeper tissues and internal organs. In the first group are the dermophytoses (ringworm). They are almost never fatal but may be highly contagious, not only among cats but in other animals and man as well.

In the second group, the deeper or systemic mycoses, the agents are not primarily animal pathogens and the risk of contagion is negligible, but the diseases generally are graver and often end fatally. It behooves the practicing veterinarian to be alert to the general characteristics of these infections, for with more refined diagnostic methods they are being identified more readily. Also, with the widespread use of antibacterial antibiotics, steroids, immunosuppressants, and anticancer drugs, certain of these mycoses are appearing more frequently as secondary complications. Candidiasis, for instance, has caused relapses and death in cats recovering from panleukopenia, and pulmonary aspergillosis may be the final outcome in a cat treated for viral respiratory disease with a succession of antibiotics.

With the principal exception of ringworm due to *Microsporum canis*, fungus diseases cannot be accurately diagnosed without resort to laboratory procedures. The commercial availability of Sabouraud's medium and numerous modifications such as neopeptone-glucose agar with chloramphenicol as a bacterial inhibitor makes it an easy matter for the practicing veterinarian to culture whenever a fungus disease is suspected; however, for identification of fungus pathogens in either culture or tissues, he must usually seek the assistance of qualified mycologists and pathologists.*

Treatment of the mycoses is today far more promising than in the past, thanks to the development of antifungal antibiotics. The discovery of griseofulvin, a drug administered orally, has revolutionized and simplified the treatment of ringworm, and nystatin is available for topical and oral administration in candidiasis. In many of the deep and systemic mycoses, for which surgery and iodides long constituted the principal and often ineffective therapy, amphotericin B, 5-fluorocytosine and ketoconazole are now overcoming infections that would once have been fatal.

The diseases caused by *Actinomyces, Nocardia, Streptomyces,* and *Dermatophilus*, although closely resembling the mycoses, are discussed in the chapter on bacterial diseases.

*For a detailed and superbly illustrated discussion of the morphology and identification of the agents of mycotic disease, the reader is referred to Emmons et al., *Medical Mycology*, 3rd ed, 1977. Fungal diseases of the skin in the cat are most extensively described and pictured by Scott in *Feline Dermatology 1900–1978: A monograph* (1980).

## DERMATOPHYTOSES ("RINGWORM")

Although ringworm is never itself the cause of death, it is in one sense the most serious infectious disease of cats: it is highly contagious, not only for other cats but also for dogs and humans; treatment can be long and costly; and apparently recovered animals may suffer recurrences or become carriers.

Ringworm is caused by a group of closely related fungi, the dermatophytes, which infect the superficial keratinaceous tissues of the body—hair, skin, and nails—and very rarely invade deeper areas.

Ringworm in animals and its relationship to that in man has been thoroughly studied by mycologists of the U.S. Public Health Service. Their work has done much to unravel the tangle of nomenclature and establish the nature and incidence of infection produced by the various organisms.

### Etiology

#### *Microsporum canis*

Almost all ringworm infections in cats (about 98 per cent) (Kaplan and Ajello, 1959; Menges and Georg,

1955a) are caused by *Microsporum canis* (syn., *M. felineum, M. lanosum*). Although isolated first from a dog, this organism is actually much more common in cats (Menges and Georg, 1955b). The infection seems to be more frequent among purebreds, probably because they are reared in breeding establishments or sold in pet shops where it is easily spread and perpetuated. Longhaired cats, with coats that increase the difficulty of detection and treatment of lesions, are subject to infection more frequently than shorthairs.

Dermatophytosis occurs most often in temperate and tropical climates. In the United States, *M. canis* infections are said to be most numerous from late summer to early winter (Kaplan and Ivens, 1961).

The disease has been recognized in kittens under three weeks of age, presumably infected shortly after birth. From experimental infections it has been learned that fluorescence may appear within seven days and clinical signs of the disease in two to four weeks (Hill, 1956; Hoerlein, 1945). Eosinophils may be increased in the circulating blood (Petrak, 1962).

The lesions, seen most often in kittens, usually appear at first on the head as scaly areas, bare except for a few broken hairs. Tiny patches on the bridge of the nose, lips, chin, temples, or ears, they may easily escape notice at first but gradually enlarge in a generally circular, sharply demarcated pattern (Fig. 9–1). Where new lesions are developing, the hair pulls out easily, together with a thin, dry, white superficial layer of epithelium. Some lesions develop a thin, grayish white crust and others a thick, moist scab suggestive of bacterial infection. The cat's washing spreads the infection, especially to the feet and toes, and then here and there over all the body. In some cases, the patches enlarge and coalesce until large areas of the body surface are affected. The lesions are not always itchy. Secondary bacterial infection is uncommon. In advanced infections, lesions are seen in all stages—tiny incipient ones; large, bare, and scaly patches; and areas with new growth of short, velvety hair. Except in white cats, new hair is likely to be dark and contrasts sharply with the lighter and generally "motheaten" looking fur around it. In a chinchilla longhair treated at the Angell Memorial Animal Hospital (AMAH), the normally pink skin developed generalized dark pigmentation after two weeks' treatment with griseofulvin and sulfur dips.

In untreated cats, the infection regresses spontaneously after several weeks or even months, and a new coat grows in. Some recovered cats, however, remain carriers, although they are entirely free of lesions.

The claws should always be examined. Occasionally they are infected; their normal, pellucid, gray-white color is replaced by an opaque, whitish mottling, and the nail surface shreds (La Touche, 1955) (Fig. 9–2).

*M. canis* infection is occasionally the cause of external otitis (e.g., Dreisörner et al., 1964; Rose, 1976; and at AMAH).

Although young cats are most susceptible to ringworm, adult and even aged cats may acquire it in hospitals and catteries, and a few fluoresce or carry small, scabby lesions throughout life. Tomcats may contract the disease when they are scratched in fights by other cats having claw infections. Their lesions may at first be dismissed as simple scratches with scab formation, until spreading scaliness and loss of hair prompt a more thorough examination. Another form of ringworm occasionally affecting mature cats is loss of fur, reddening, and follicular infection limited to the chin. There is also a generalized chronic ringworm of adult cats in which the skin is covered with small brownish crusts through which the hair grows in clumps; alopecia is not present, but the coat is poor (Conroy, 1964).

It has been suggested that poor nutritional status may predispose to the development of clinical infection in carrier cats (de Almeida et al., 1950), but solid substantiating evidence is lacking.

So varied are the manifestations of ringworm that atypical lesions may easily escape diagnosis. The possibility should never be ignored in any feline skin disorder until specifically ruled out by skin scrapings and culture (Scott, 1980).

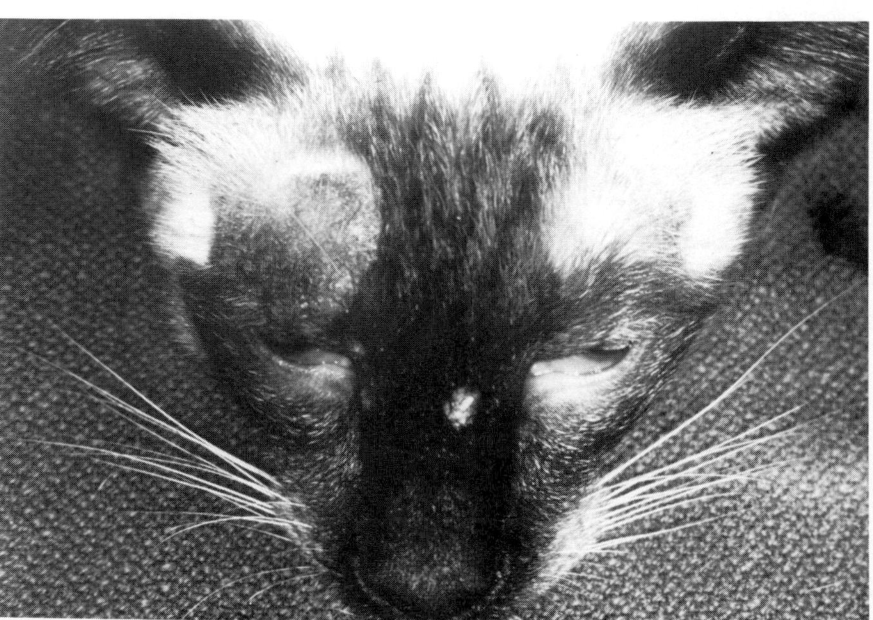

**Figure 9–1** *M. canis*. Circular, hairless, scaly patch above one eye; smaller lesion on the bridge of the nose.

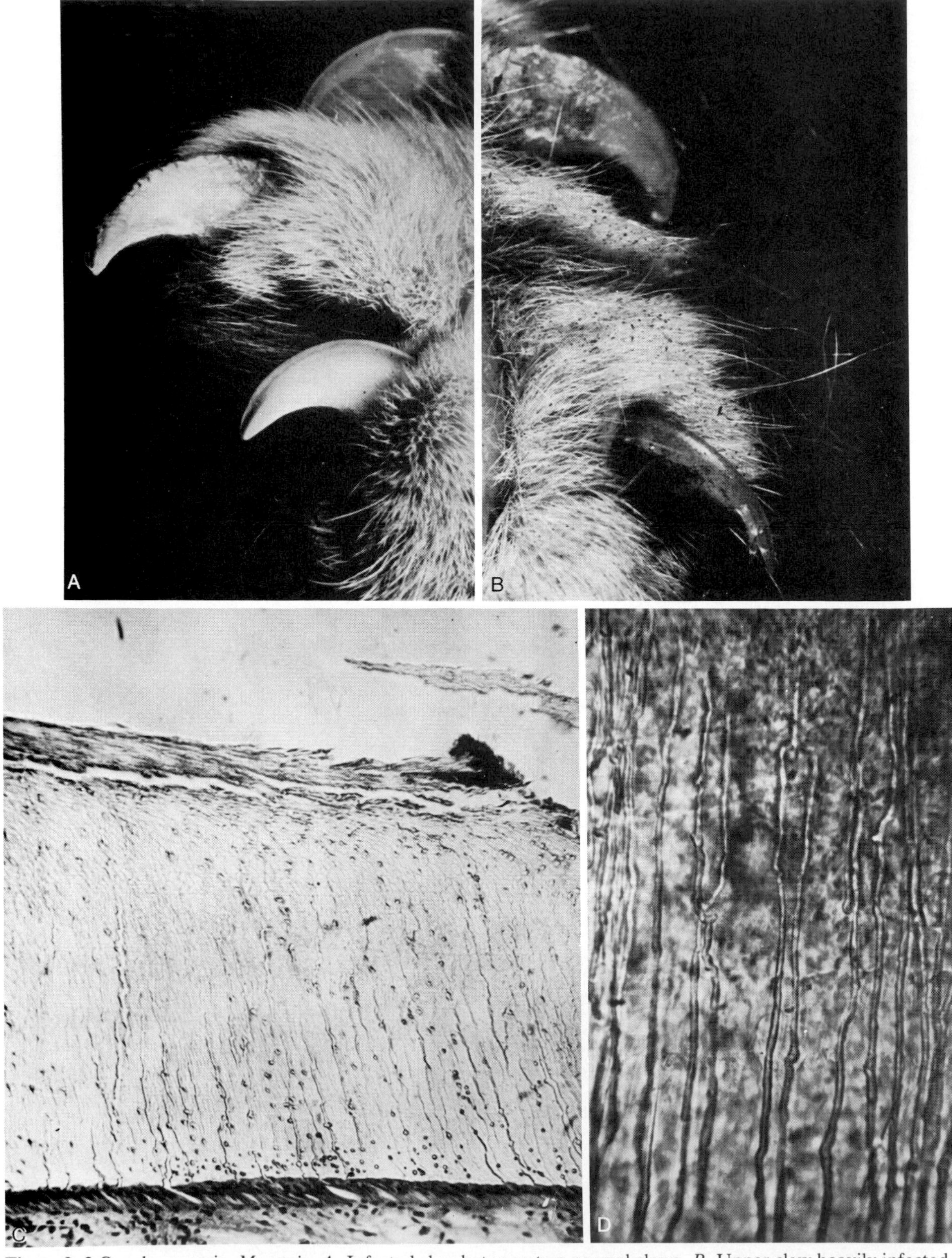


**Figure 9–2** Onychomycosis, *M. canis*. *A*, Infected claw between two normal claws. *B*, Upper claw heavily infected, lower claw slightly so. *C*, Hyphae in transverse section and cut obliquely, distributed throughout the keratinized part of the claw, × 200. *D*, Mycelium of *M. canis* in claw shaving. Unstained, × 514. (From LaTouche CJ: Vet Rec 67 [1955] 578–579.)

Very rarely *M. canis* causes deep granulomas (see Mycetomas).

The most serious aspect of *M. canis* infection is the ease with which it is spread. In catteries, especially those where longhairs are bred, the disease is often enzootic, and many breeders accept it as an unavoidable evil, treating the infection only enough to eliminate visible lesions or allowing it to run its course in each new litter of kittens, and showing and selling infected and carrier animals. Most cattery cats, after the initial episode of infection, either recover spontaneously within a few weeks or become normal-appearing carriers. Rarely, however, breeding cats show evidence of infection steadily into old age, despite repeated treatments. In such a cat, large areas of the coat, especially about the head and legs, simply appear thin and the skin scurfy, but examination with ultraviolet light reveals extensive fluorescence.

Cats obtained from breeders, shelters, or pet shops should be carefully examined. In laboratories, infection is introduced and important experiments disrupted when infected or carrier cats are obtained from pounds and dealers and introduced without thorough examination and quarantine.

Among pet owners, outbreaks involving cats, dogs, and humans are frequent and have been the subject of countless reports. The majority of such epidemics originate with infected or carrier kittens, but sometimes infection enters a household or school by way of a dog or child. Often it is first suspected in a pet when a physician diagnoses ringworm in an owner. Conversely, a veterinarian's discovery of ringworm in an animal may lead to the detection of round, itchy lesions in its human companions. Many adults have considerable resistance to *M. canis* infection, developing only one or two tiny spots that yield promptly to a few topical applications of a fungicide. In children, however, infection may be extensive and is especially difficult to eradicate if it involves the scalp.

Because a single infected hair may transmit the disease from one victim to another and transmission may even occur by way of inanimate objects (Milian and Karatchentzeff, 1935), early diagnosis and vigorous hygienic measures are essential.

Other forms of ringworm encountered less commonly in cats are due to *M. gypseum, Trichophyton mentagrophytes*, and *T. schoenleinii* (see references).

## *Microsporum gypseum*

Considering that *M. gypseum* is a common saprophyte of soil and has been cultured from the hair of apparently healthy animals (Fuentes et al., 1954), it is remarkable that clinical infections are not encountered more often in animals and man. From the reports of symptomatic infections in cats (e.g., Ajello, 1953; Kaplan et al., 1957; Scott, 1980; Trice and Shafer, 1951) it seems that lesions tend to be single and occur most often on the head or extremities, thick, adherent, gray crusts being typical (Scott, 1980). Some lesions resemble those of *M. canis* infection, comprising chiefly scaliness and alopecia; in others there may be suppuration and kerion formation. Since there is little or no fluorescence, a positive diagnosis may be made only by microscopic examination and culturing (Table 9–1).

## *Trichophyton mentagrophytes*

*Trichophyton mentagrophytes (syn. Achorion quinckeanum)*, which may cause ringworm of the beard in man and affects a variety of domestic and wild animals including the dog, fox, monkey, and certain rodents, is also rare in the cat. Although the lesions characteristically are purulent (e.g., Anderson, 1977), in two feline infections reported by Georg et al. (1957), circular areas of alopecia and scaliness were scattered on various parts of the body, chiefly the head, legs, and tail. In another instance, scutula were present on a cat's abdomen and ears (Zauder, cited by Blank, 1957); granulomatous lesions also have been seen (Fig. 9–3). Since fluorescence does not occur, definitive diagnosis requires microscopic and cultural study (Table 9–1). Rodents are frequently infected and have been suggested as a source of infection in pets. Cats may pass the infection to dogs or man (Blank, 1957). *T. mentagrophytes* has also been cultured from the hairs of apparently healthy cats (Fuentes et al., 1954).

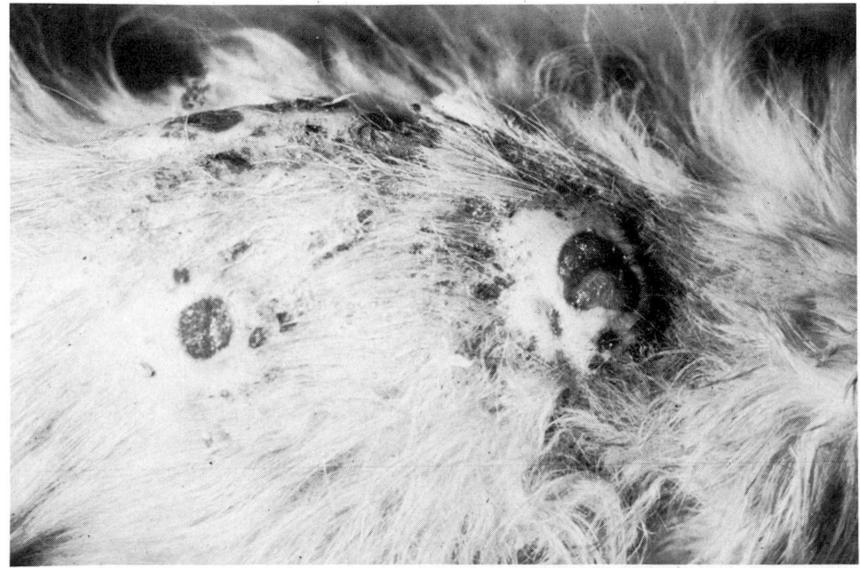

**Figure 9–3** Nodules, ulcers, and crusts in the granulomatous form of *Trichophyton* infection on a cat's back. (Courtesy Dr. Craig Griffin. *In* Scott DW: J Am Anim Hosp Assoc 16 [1980] 331–459.)

**Table 9–1 Ringworm Infections of the Cat***

| SPECIES | HOSTS AFFECTED | LESIONS | FLUORESCENCE | NAOH MOUNTS | CULTURE |
|---|---|---|---|---|---|
| *M. canis* (syn. *M. lanosum, M. felineum, M. equinum*) | Cat, dog, man; occasionally horse, monkey | Kittens and puppies: scaliness, breaking and loss of hair in irregular patches on face, neck, and feet, or diffusely over the body. Grown cats and dogs: well defined areas of scaliness and alopecia; claws may also be infected in cats. Some cats without lesions may be carriers; may show a few fluorescent hairs | Sometimes; yellow-green | Mosaic sheath of small spores entirely surrounding base of hair; mycelium in interior of hair | Growth rapid on Sabouraud's dextrose-agar; colonies flat with regular border; surface white to yellow-tan; at first, fine silky aerial growth, later fluffy with woolly areas; pigment on reverse bright yellow; many septate, spindle-shaped macroconidia, thick-walled with rough surface; few microconidia |
| *M. gypseum* (syn. *M. fulvum, Achorion gypseum*) | Occasionally cat, man; frequently dog, horse; common in soil | Often single lesion—head or feet; well defined patches with loss of hair and some scaliness in central area; dense scaling or crusts at edge; crusts may be thick, yellowish, moist; may vary from scaling and alopecia to inflammation and suppuration | Little or none | Sheath of small spores in mosaic or large spores in chains or irregular masses on surface of hairs; mycelium in interior of hair and in scales | Growth rapid on Sabouraud's dextrose agar; colonies flat, powdery, cinnamon brown with tannish pigment on reverse; many elliptical, multiseptate, rough-walled macroconidia; micronconidia not observed |
| *T. mentagrophytes* (syn. *T. granulosum, gypseum, asteroides, caninum, felineum, quinckeanum*) | Occasionally cat; commonly dog, horse, rodents; also monkey, opossum, fox; causes tinea barbae in man | In cat, circular area of hair loss and scaliness, various areas of body but chiefly head, legs, tail | None | Sheath or isolated chains of spores (3–5μ) on surface of hair; mycelium in interior of hair | Rapid growth on Sabouraud's dextrose agar; colonies flat or slightly raised at centers; surface white, cream, or tan; texture powdery or coarsely granular; reverse dull yellowish or deep red; masses of nearly round microconidia attached by delicate sterigmata or directly to the mycelium; clavate macrocondia occasionally |
| *T. schoenleinii* (syn. *Achorion schoenleinii*) | Occasionally cat, dog, mouse; causes favus in man | In cat, tends to localize on ears, sometimes invades external ear canal; skin lesions characterized by a raised yellow or gray, cuplike crust (scutulum), which may be pierced by hairs; reddish moist base beneath | None or dull gray | No spores on outside of hairs, mycelium inside hair running along its length; spores with air bubbles and fat droplets are characteristically seen in hair | Slow growth on Sabouraud's dexrose agar; colonies cream, yellow, or gray, with heaped irregular border; moist and smooth or fine, white, downy surface, no pigment on reverse; occasionally grows submerged in agar; mycelium irregular, thick branches ending in complex clubs; large irregular swellings common; occasionally a few microconidia |

*Adapted from Georg LK: The diagnosis of ringworm in animals, Vet Med 49(1954) 157–166, and from Kral and Schwartzman, 1964.

Varying percentages of asymptomatic cats have been found by culture of brushings to carry (perhaps only transiently or as contaminants) various dermatophytes, principally *M. canis, M. gypseum*, and *T. mentagrophytes* (Scott, 1980).

### Other Dermatophytes

A fourth agent isolated only occasionally in cats and mainly in the Mediterranean area is *T. schoenleinii*, the cause of favus in man, characterized by yellow-brown, cup-like, elevated crusts (scutula) under which is a moist base. In cats, the infection is likely to localize in the ears, sometimes invading the external canal (Kral, 1955).

Other dermatophytes are occasionally isolated from cats. *M. sapporense*, reported in 1952 as the agent in an epidemic in both children and cats on the island of Hokkaido, Japan, was said to differ culturally from any other species previously known (Komuro et al., 1952), although the clinical infection was very similar to that produced by *M. canis*.

Also of rare occurrence in cats are *M. cookei, M. distortum, T. rubrum, T. terrestre, T. tonsurans, T. verrucosum,* and *T. violaceum* (Fitzgerald et al., 1969; Refai and Miligy, 1968; Scott, 1980; Scott et al., 1980).

## Diagnosis

Because ringworm infection often fails to conform to the "textbook" clinical picture, the diagnosis should be confirmed by other methods. The Wood's light provides ultraviolet rays that cause infected hairs to give off a greenish yellow fluorescence. Inexperienced observers must not be misled by the lavender glow given off by scabs, dandruff, nails, and a variety of medicaments but must be satisfied with nothing less than definitely and brightly fluorescing hairs or hair stubs. This examination must be thorough, lest tiny incipient lesions be missed. Infected claws may fluoresce in their entirety owing to infiltration of both the superficial and the deep layers with mycelium (La Touche, 1955). Suspected carriers must be examined with particular care, as there may be only a few fluorescing hairs in the entire coat.

Because *M. canis* fluoresces in only a minority of feline infections (Menges and Georg, 1955b) and other dermatophytes causing ringworm rarely if ever do, a definite diagnosis often depends on microscopic examination and culturing of hairs and skin scales.

Successful identification requires careful procedure (Scott, 1980). Recently medicated lesions should be avoided. The area to be sampled should be soaked gently (not rubbed) with 70 per cent alcohol for 30 seconds and then allowed to dry. One should pull only a few obviously abnormal (broken, lusterless) hairs, especially ones that fluoresce. Large masses of hair and debris can lead to contaminating growth that overwhelms the true pathogen.

For microscopic examination, suspect material is placed on a clean slide in a drop of 10 per cent NaOH or KOH. A coverslip is added, and the preparation is permitted to stand for 15 or 20 minutes. The clearing process may be accelerated by gentle heating over a Bunsen burner. The preparation is examined under low and high power. Spores on or inside the hairs are evidence of ringworm infection. Unfortunately, even trained mycologists have found that hydroxide preparations are only 60 to 70 per cent successful in demonstrating the presence of fungi (Scott, 1980).

For culture, hairs should be removed carefully with a sterile forceps into a sterile envelope or tube or placed on a medium. Culturing is done on Sabouraud's medium or a variant thereof. Antibiotics may be added to inhibit saprophytic fungi (actidione) and bacteria (chloramphenicol). Such media are available commercially. Incubation is at room temperature. Tiny colonies may develop within two or three days (Hoerlein, 1945), but a week or so may be required, and cultures should not be discarded as negative until four weeks have passed. Dermatophyte Test Medium (Pitman Moore) includes a phenol red indicator that turns the medium from amber to red at about the same time that the small, white colonies of pathogenic dermatophytes become visible (within three to seven days). A red color appearing after seven days usually indicates the presence of a saprophyte (Muller et al., 1983; Scott, 1980).

The microscopic and cultural characteristics of the organisms most likely to be involved in feline ringworm are tabulated (Table 9–1).

Cats suspected of being asymptomatic carriers but showing no lesions occasionally have brilliantly fluorescing hairs throughout the coat. If no fluorescence is detected, a cat may be brushed with a sterile toothbrush, the bristles of which are then pressed directly onto the medium. This procedure is especially useful for detecting carriers in catteries and colonies.

Stained sections of biopsy specimens of skin are occasionally diagnostic when cultures are negative but are only about 80 per cent as accurate as cultures (Scott, 1980).

## Treatment

The treatment of ringworm was revolutionized by the development of griseofulvin, a metabolic product of a species of *Penicillium* and an effective oral fungistatic antibiotic. It alone often eliminates an infection in far less time than any topical treatment formerly did. Absorbed from the gastrointestinal tract into the blood, griseofulvin is deposited in the keratin of skin, hair, or nails, where it inhibits the growth of sensitive fungi. As the hair grows out, the downward infiltration of the fungus is checked so that the new basal hair or nail is free of infection. The organism remains viable, however, in the tissues previously affected, and thus treatment must be continued until fur or claws are grown out and shed or otherwise removed.

As experience with griseofulvin has increased and it has been produced in "micro" form, recommendations for dosage and frequency of administration have proliferated. It is Scott's belief (1980) that many reportedly resistant infections would have been overcome if treated long enough with sufficiently large doses. He recommends 110 to 132 mg/kg once a day, given with an oily or fatty meal to enhance absorption and prevent vomiting. Treatment should be continued for two weeks after the disappearance of lesions (average four to six weeks) or until culture is negative. Infection of claws may require treatment for five or six months, as well as daily soaks with lime sulfur solution or chlorhexidine. Declawing could even be considered for refractory onychomycosis.

Experience with "ultramicrosize" griseofulvin (Gris-Peg, Dorsey Laboratories) is limited. In a 5 kg (12 lb) cat, 125 mg (25 mg/kg) given daily for six weeks apparently eliminated multifocal infection with *T. mentagrophytes* (Anderson, 1977).

Because bone marrow depression has been observed in a few cats treated with griseofulvin, it is desirable that hemograms be performed before and during treatment or, at the very least, if untoward effects occur (Petrak, 1960). Generalized itching was a possible side reaction in one cat but stopped spontaneously in three days without interruption of treatment (Kaplan and Ajello, 1959). Some cats treated with griseofulvin at AMAH have lost their appetite and been nauseated. Diarrhea and ataxia have also been observed (Horne, 1975).

Griseofulvin should not be given to pregnant queens during the first half of pregnancy because of toxicity to the fetuses, which may be stillborn or affected with a variety of malformations of the skeleton, eyes, heart, and digestive and central nervous systems (Scott et al., 1975).

Ketoconazole (Janssen Pharmaceutica), although not approved for use in cats, is effective against a variety of fungus infections of animals and has been used successfully in the treatment of *M. canis* infection (Woodard, 1983). The 200 mg tablets were crushed in a liquid vitamin supplement so as to give a dose of 2 to 4 mg/lb for cats weighing 5 to 10 lb. This was added to the food daily, as the drug is less effective if administered on an empty stomach. By four weeks all lesions in a group of Persians and Himalayans had disappeared. Treatment was continued for eight weeks without recurrence of dermatophytosis in any cats of the cattery.

Studies so far have revealed few adverse side effects with ketoconazole. Transient increases in SGOT levels have been noted in a few subjects, and there have been reports of symptomatic hepatocellular malfunction (Woodard, 1983).

Although griseofulvin or ketoconazole alone may effect a cure, close clipping of affected areas at least and, with longhairs, of the whole cat is highly desirable, even though damaging to the cat's appearance and morale. It brings to light lesions that might otherwise be missed, facilitates topical treatment and bathing, and lessens the hazard of reinfection or contamination of the environment by loose fur. Many veterinarians clip at the start of treatment but might better defer this until griseofulvin has been given for a few days, so that the basal hair is free of fungi. In a cat with fluorescing *M. canis* infection, the appearance of nonfluorescing hair roots indicates that the time is ripe for clipping.

The complete clipping of a cat with ringworm is time-consuming but should be done by the veterinarian himself unless a conscientious and meticulous assistant is available. The chore requires general anesthesia and takes 30 to 45 minutes if the fur is completely removed from the feet and nail sheaths, as it should be. The person doing the clipping should wear a gown, cap, and gloves that can be sterilized or burned after the procedure. The clipping should be done in an isolated, draft-free room, with the cat lying in a shallow box to prevent scattering of loose fur. The clippers must be sterilized after use, and the box and fur burned. Stubborn infections may require repeated clipping. It is inadvisable to follow the clipping with a dip while the cat is still under anesthesia, as the body temperature may be lowered to a dangerous degree.

Topical treatment is not essential but may shorten the period during which griseofulvin must be given. It also reduces the hazards of reinfection or contamination of the environment by infected hairs.

The most effective aqueous topical agents are 2 per cent lime sulfur, a 1:200 dilution of 45 per cent captan (Ortho-Tack-Wash), "tamed" iodines (as in iodine soaps), and sodium hypochlorite 5.25 per cent (Clorox 1 part to 20 parts water). Cats should not be rinsed, but be allowed to dry after antifungal dips, because such medications are beneficial only if they remain on the skin and fur. For paronychia, daily 10- to 15-minute soaking with lime sulfur or chlorhexidine (Nolvasan, Fort Dodge) is recommended (Scott, 1980).

For "spot" treatment of localized lesions, clotrimazole, cuprimyxin, miconazole, and thiabendazole are often effective. Topical miconazole may, however, precipitate drug eruptions (Scott, 1980). Tincture of iodine should be applied to localized lesions with caution, since cats are especially sensitive to iodine. Topical tolnaftate, although sensationally successful in some human dermaphytoses, is of little value in feline infections (Scott, 1980). Griseofulvin in dimethylsulfoxide may be effective (Levine et al., 1971). A glass-marking pencil is useful to outline fluorescent areas for topical treatment (Sternfels, 1958). "Spot" treatment with radiofrequency current hyperthermia has been described (Lucker and Kainer, 1981).

Treatment of feline dermatophytosis with vaccine is an approach that remains to be further evaluated (Mosher et al., 1977).

Cats should be hospitalized only when adequate isolation facilities are available so that other animals are not endangered. Because attendants cannot always be relied on to observe the necessary sanitary precautions, and because they may worry too much about the possible danger to themselves to do a thorough job of caring for infected animals, it may be necessary for the veterinarian himself to treat the cat. If it is clipped, care must be taken not to let fur fly about, and a special clipper should be kept for use in ringworm only.

Hospitalization is especially to be desired when there are children in a household. If adults only will be exposed to the cat, they may usually give the necessary treatment without becoming infected.

## HYGIENIC MEASURES

Hygienic measures are important. Hairs shed by an infected animal may remain infective and contaminate the environment for over a year (Keep, 1960). If a cat is treated at home, it should be restricted to one small area that is easily cleaned or, better yet, it should be confined in a roomy cage. Vacuuming of all areas and objects with which a cat has been in contact is the most effective method of getting rid of infected hairs. In fact, the cat itself may be vacuumed. Floors, certain furniture, utensils, bedding, and some of an owner's garments may be disinfected in a solution of Clorox, Lysol, or ammonia (10 per cent) or boiled for 20 minutes in water (Conroy, 1964). A 1:200 dilution of 45 per cent technical captan (Ortho-Tack-Wash) may also be used for disinfection in situations (e.g., cages) in which there is no objection to the white deposit that it leaves on surfaces (Kaplan, 1965, 1968). Instruments such as scissors and clipper blades may be sterilized with 10 per cent formalin, alcohol, or steam. Other pets that have been exposed may be given two weeks' preventive treatment with griseofulvin and fungicidal rinses.

Outbreaks of ringworm originating in pet shops and catteries and resulting in human infections should be reported to local public health authorities.

A discussion of superficial fungus infection would not be complete without mention of the confusions that can be caused by the presence on the skin of fungal "saprophytes" or "contaminants." Every clinician has had the experience of culturing material from skin disorders highly suggestive of ringworm, only to receive a laboratory report of the isolation of a "nonpathogenic fungus," often not named but sometimes designated, for example, as a species of *Aspergillus, Alternaria, Chaetonium, Hormodendrum*, or *Penicillium*. As these are frequently found on healthy skins, one is instructed to regard them as harmless. Nonetheless, in occasional animals such organisms seem to be associated with itching or dermatitis (Bone and Jackson, 1971; Senser, 1966).

## ASPERGILLOSIS

*Aspergillus* spp grow worldwide on decaying vegetation and are frequent laboratory contaminants. Man and animals inevitably inhale conidia, but with few exceptions invasive or systemic infection is secondary to other infections or chronic disease (e.g., panleukopenia, diabetes mellitus, malignancy, especially leukemia) or develops in patients with defenses weakened by treatment with corticosteroids, a variety of antibiotics, or immunosuppressant drugs.

### Etiology and Diagnosis

In exudates and sputum the characteristic septate hyphae (forked, branching) and club-like conidiophores can usually be recognized by direct inspection of wet mounts. In tissues, *Aspergillus* is usually easily identified by its hyphae, which measure about 4 $\mu$ in diameter and tend to branch repeatedly in the same direction. They often stain adequately with hematoxylin and eosin, but the Gridley stain best demonstrates their morphology and may pick up an infection that would otherwise be missed.

Culturing on fungus media produces firm, woolly colonies with long aerial hyphae. Most frequently isolated is *A. fumigatus*, the pigmented spores of which impart a gray-green hue to the growth. The mycelium of *A. niger* is at first white, then yellow, and finally black.

### Clinical Features

After cryptococcosis, aspergillosis is probably the "deep" fungus most often recognized in cats. In the majority of cases it has been considered secondary to panleukopenia or, less often, upper respiratory infection, especially in cats that have been treated with antibiotics or corticosteroids or both (Bolton and Brown, 1972; Fox et al., 1978; Köhler et al., 1978; McCausland, 1972; Nielsen, 1956; Pakes et al., 1967; Sautter et al., 1955; Schiefer, 1965; Stokes, 1973; Vogler and Wagner, 1976; Weiland, 1970). Most often involved are the lungs or intestine or both. Pulmonary infection takes the form of granulomatous pneumonia. In the intestine there is infiltration of the wall. Invasion and thrombosis of vessels are characteristic.

As in man and dog, *Aspergillus* spp may assume a pathogenic role in chronic sinusitis of cats. *A. flavus* was isolated in sinusitis in colony cats at Harvard University (Buckley, 1977) and a species of *Aspergillus* in a cat with frontal sinusitis, orbital cellulitis, and proptosis of both eyeballs (Wilkinson et al., 1982).

In addition to infections observed at AMAH secondary to panleukopenia, *Aspergillus* pneumonia has developed in leukemic cats receiving antibiotics, steroids, and cyclophosphamide (Cotter et al., 1973) (Fig. 9–4). In another cat, mycotic esophagitis and pneumonia appeared to be superimposed on lipid pneumonia caused by mineral oil administration for hairballs. In a cat dying with diabetes mellitus and chronic active pancreatitis, the trachea was found to be infected with both *Aspergillus* and bacteria.

The urinary bladder was the site of bacterial infection and *Aspergillus* granulomas in a cat at AMAH that had a history of chronic cystitis, had had bladder stones removed two months before, and died of septicemia. Fungus "balls" yielding a pure growth of *A. fumigatus* were found in the bladder of a cat with chronic hemorrhagic cystitis (Kirkpatrick, 1982). After a month's treatment of the cystitis with methenamine the fungus was no longer present in the urine.

A chronic sublingual lesion characterized by a large, white, cheesy, submucosal focus and refractory to a variety of treatments yielded *A. nidulans* and finally responded to curettage (De Wailly, 1967).

Of two cases of mycotic keratoconjunctivitis (Schmidt, 1974), one developed as a sequel of upper respiratory infection and treatment with antibiotics and steroids. Cultures of scrapings yielded *A. fumigatus* in addition to normal bacterial flora. It was treated successfully with a "third-lid" flap and chloramphenicol ophthalmic ointment, but no antifungal drug.

*Aspergillus* spp may also be responsible for dermal and pulmonary allergies in man. The fungus has been isolated at AMAH from skin scrapings in cats with small, itchy areas of dermatitis much like those in ringworm—whether as a contaminant or allergen is not clear.

### Treatment

Unfortunately, most cases of aspergillosis will be recognized only at autopsy. In treatment, iodides have long been used but often with little or no effect. Iodide irrigation of canine nasal aspergillosis has resulted in fatal inhalation pneumonia (AMAH). Aerosols of nystatin are used for human patients with pneumonia due to *Aspergillus* spp. Amphotericin B and 5-fluorocytosine are currently the drugs of choice. (For their use in cats, see section on cryptococcosis.) Thiabendazole has been recommended for nasal aspergillosis in dogs (Lane, 1977).

## BLASTOMYCOSIS

Blastomycosis is a chronic suppurative and granulomatous infection that involves predominantly the skin, inter-

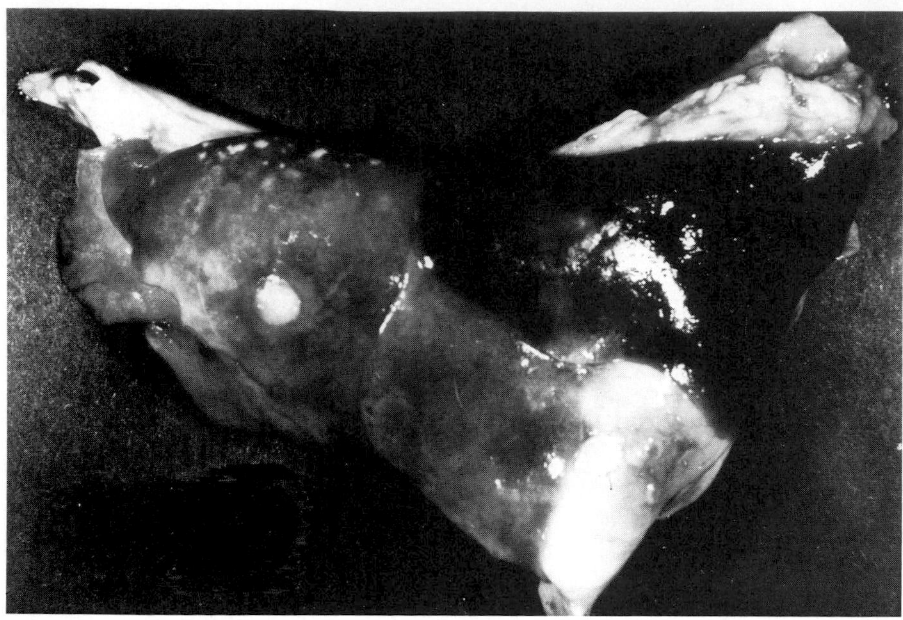

**Figure 9–4** Aspergillosis. Granulomatous pneumonia and thrombosis of a lung lobe (right) in a cat treated for lymphoma with cyclophosphamide and prednisone.

nal organs, and bones. It has been reported in southern Canada, the United States, notably the southeast, Central and South America, and Africa. In areas where it is endemic, human and canine cases may occur in the same locale, but there is no evidence of transmission among living creatures. Airborne infection from a common natural source, e.g., soil, is suspected.

## Etiology and Diagnosis

*Blastomyces dermatitidis* appears in exudates and tissues as spherical, yeast-like bodies, 8 to 20 μ across. The wall is thick and the inner and outer contours so well defined that it often has the appearance of being double (Fig. 9–5). The organism reproduces by buds that have a broad attachment, and the connection is so persistent that a second or third bud may be put forth before the first is shed. *Blastomyces* differs from *Histoplasma* and *Cryptococcus* in having multiple nuclei. It is so large and characteristic in appearance that it may be identified in unstained wet mounts of exudate. Lacking a capsule, it does not, like *Cryptococcus*, ordinarily stain in tissue sections with mucicarmine. On fungus media at room temperature or 30 C, *B. dermatitidis* grows in less than two weeks as a white, cottony mold with short, slim conidiophores bearing spherical or ovoid conidia 2 to 10 μ in diameter. Later the growth becomes tan or brown. Isolation by mouse inoculation requires three or four weeks. Culture specimens must be handled carefully, as spores from mycelium are infectious.

In man, at least, infection appears usually to start in

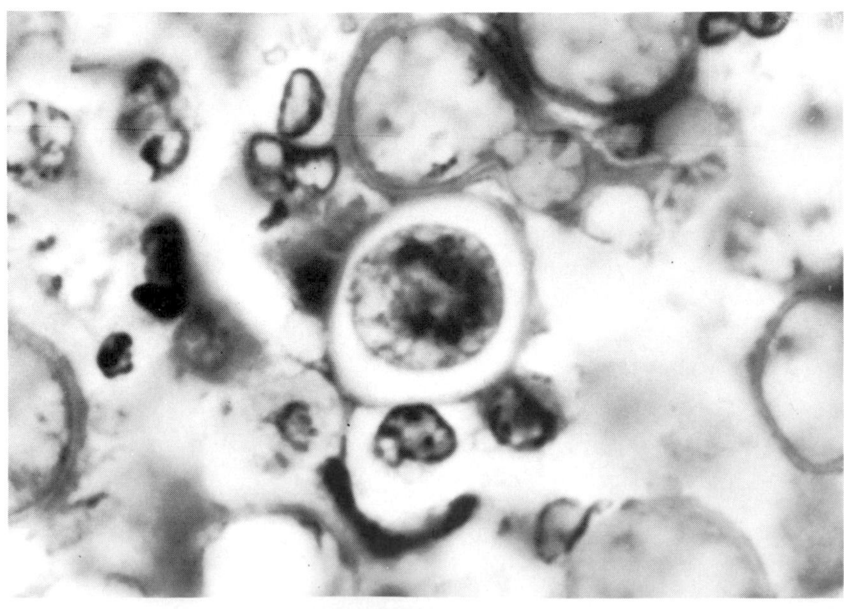

**Figure 9–5** *Blastomyces dermatitidis.* A typical organism (center) and a budding form above it. H&E; Bauer's, × 2000. (Courtesy Dr. R. T. Habermann.)

the lungs, presumably from inhalation of conidia, and may disseminate to skin, bone, central nervous system, and other sites. Skin lesions are likely to develop as nodules or pustules that eventually break down into ulcers containing tiny abscesses in their indurated borders. Underlying bone lesions may open to the outside by suppurating fistulae. Radiographically and grossly, lesions in the lungs and bones are indistinguishable from those of many other granulomatous and neoplastic diseases, but microscopically they are characterized by tiny foci of suppuration or by epithelioid and giant cell granulomas. A diagnosis of blastomycosis can usually be made by microscopic examination of pus, sputum, spinal fluid, or tissues, but culturing is desirable for positive identification. Dermal and serologic tests are available but do not always give conclusive results. There may be cross reactions between *Blastomyces* and *Histoplasma*.

## Clinical Features

Only a few feline infections have been reported. Fever may or may not be present, and hematologic findings are not significant.

Cutaneous disease was described from Canada in a Siamese with a painful paronychial infection of one toe (Easton, 1961). The lesion was a red papule with a serosanguineous discharge, and the claw was reduced to half its normal length. There was no lymphadenopathy, and radiographs revealed no involvement of bone or lung. The organism was cultured from pus obtained by incising the lesion. Histoplasmin and blastomycin skin tests and complement-fixation tests for histoplasmosis and blastomycosis were negative. The lesion healed when the cat was treated with potassium iodide, 5 grains IV for four days, then 3 grains IV for seven days, and finally 5 grains orally for seven days.

In another cat, a three-year-old male in North Carolina, a foreleg infection that started with a puncture wound proved refractory to treatment with penicillin, and the leg enlarged to three times normal diameter, with development of fistulous tracts (Campbell et al., 1980). Fungal culture yielded no growth, but as *Aerobacter* was isolated another antibiotic was tried. When the leg continued to enlarge and the cat became lethargic and inappetent, amputation was performed. Tissue examination disclosed a granulomatous reaction with numerous *B. dermatitidis* organisms. As the cat made an excellent recovery after surgery, and radiographs gave no evidence of lung involvement, treatment with amphotericin, the preferred drug, was not advised. An infection of a hind toe and lip was reported but without further details (McDonough and Kuzma, 1980).

Such localized cutaneous infections appear to be the exception, the majority of feline cases involving the lungs, often with spread to a variety of sites.

Miliary granulomas of the lungs with involvement of bronchial lymph nodes were found in an adult male cat from a research laboratory in Kentucky (Sheldon, 1966) (Fig. 9–6) and in a four-year-old male Arkansas cat with a history of several weeks' inappetence, weight loss, intermittent nonproductive cough, and fever (Breshears, 1968). Both cats were dyspneic, and radiographs of the second disclosed scattered small pulmonary densities and an enlarged bronchial mode. Two Mississippi cases of pyogranulomatous pneumonia and pleuritis, one of which presented as pyothorax, were reported by Hatkin et al. (1979). Immunodiffusion tests conducted on sera from other healthy cats in the household of the second victim revealed no antibodies to *B. dermatitidis, H. capsulatum*, or *C. immitis*.

In a cluster of cases reported from a Florida cattery, four Siamese acquired from various areas of Florida or from California and having a history of previous illness and respiratory disease developed signs including nasal and ocular discharge, pulmonary rales, abdominal effusion (three), and central nervous disturbance (one) (Jasmin et al., 1969; personal communication from owner). *B. dermatitidis* was recovered from nasal and throat swabs. Autopsy findings among the four included varying degrees of pneumonia and an exudative peritonitis (three), and pleuritis and encephalitis (one). Special stains revealed the organism in the lesions.

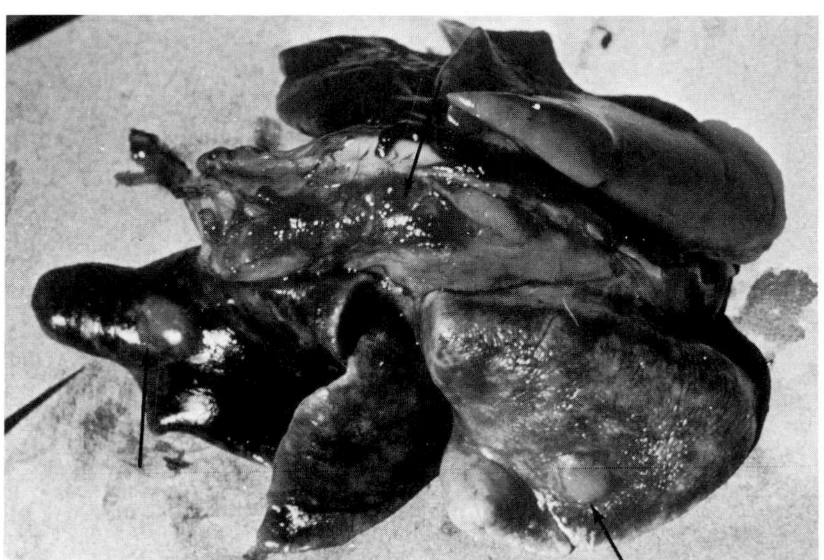

**Figure 9–6** Blastomycosis of the lung in an adult cat. The lower arrows point to granulomas and the upper arrow to enlarged bronchial lymph nodes. (From Sheldon WG: Lab Anim Care 16 [1966] 280–285.)

In Tennessee, blastomycosis is notoriously frequent in dogs, but cats apparently suffer less often from clinical infection. In one reported case, bilateral chorioretinitis and dyspnea were the presenting signs in a three-year-old castrated male domestic shorthair that proved on autopsy to have disseminated disease (Nasisse et al., 1985).

Panophthalmitis and ataxia, as well as labored respirations and abnormal lung sounds, were the signs in a seven-year-old female domestic cat in Ohio (Alden and Mohan, 1974). Autopsy examination of the eyes disclosed pyogranulomatous inflammation and retinal detachment, with *B. dermatitidis* in macrophages and giant cells and free in exudate. The organisms were also identified in impression smears and sections of the lungs, which contained multiple pyogranulomas with central caseation necrosis. Granulomas were also present in the cerebellum, pons, and medulla oblongata. Pulmonary and central nervous infections have also been encountered by McGrath (1958). Lesions in a Wisconsin cat involved the lungs and ear (McDonough and Kuzma, 1980).

The manifestations in a North Carolina cat further illustrate the protean forms that blastomycosis may assume (Neunzig, 1983). Presented with a complaint of blindness, the cat also had an open sore on one shoulder. Because of poor response to treatment the cat was destroyed, and autopsy revealed a large brain abscess containing *Blastomyces*. The organism was also present in granulomatous reactions in the skin, in the subcutis around the trachea, and in lymph nodes. The eyes had been spared, blindness probably resulting from degeneration in the optic centers of the brain.

### Treatment

For treatment, amphotericin B has been considered the drug of choice. Recently ketoconazole has been used with success in canine blastomycosis. By extrapolation from experience with management of blastomycosis in dogs, it is suggested that in disseminated or fulminating infection treatment be started with amphotericin B for prompt effect and then continued with ketoconazole, which may be given orally on a long-term outpatient basis (Legendre, 1984). (For dosage regimens, see sections on cryptococcosis and histoplasmosis.)

## CANDIDIASIS (MONILIASIS)

In man, species of *Candida*, notably *C. albicans (Monilia albicans, Oidium albicans)*, are normally present in the mouth, upper respiratory tract, and intestine but frequently assume a pathogenic role in cutaneous, oral, respiratory, or systemic disease. Chronic debilitating illness and prolonged antibiotic, immunosuppressive, or steroid therapy predispose to candidiasis.

### Etiology and Diagnosis

*Candida* is a simple, yeastlike fungus that forms septate mycelia (pseudohyphae) and produces spores by the successive budding of special egg-shaped cells at the ends of hyphae or at nodes in the filaments. Both yeastlike cells, 2 to 4 μ in width, and mycelia may be seen in scrapings, exudates, and tissues. As *Candida* is Gram-positive, a Gram stain, as well as special fungus stains, can be useful in identification. *Candida* is cultured at room temperature or 37 C on Sabouraud's agar with an antibiotic added to inhibit bacterial contaminants. Creamy colonies with a yeasty odor appear in two to four days (Emmons et al., 1977), but a "serum tube" test discloses filamentous pseudohyphae several hours after inoculation of suspect material into serum and incubation at 37 C (Small, 1974). Serologic tests and animal inoculation are not useful in diagnosis (Emmons et al., 1977).

### Clinical Features

In the cat, *Candida* has been recognized as a pathogen most often in the esophagus and intestine in association with panleukopenia and other types of enteritis (Langheinrich and Nielsen, 1971; McCausland, 1972; Schiefer, 1965; also at AMAH). (Two intestinal mycoses originally believed by Schiefer and Weiss [1959] to be candidiasis were restudied and diagnosed as aspergillosis and mucormycosis.)

Oral infections occasionally follow treatment with broad-spectrum antibiotics. In a six-month-old cat at AMAH, an episode of upper respiratory infection treated for 12 days with tetracycline was followed two weeks later by severe vesicular and ulcerative inflammation of the tip of the nose, lips, gums, tongue, and soft palate. Patches of whitish pseudomembrane were present in the mouth. The infection was spread by the cat's licking to the preputial and anal mucosae, which were swollen, cracked, ulcerated, and bleeding (Fig. 9–7). A species of *Candida* was isolated from the mouth lesions. Treatment with a multivitamin preparation and nystatin (50,000 units Mycostatin, Squibb) every six hours resulted in complete disappearance of the lesions within four days. Nystatin was continued for eight days longer as a precautionary measure.

*Candida albicans* was one of several agents isolated from a case of pyothorax (McCaw et al., 1984). Treatment included ketoconazole as well as antibacterial drugs.

As in man, this fungus may also be a secondary invader in chronic debilitating or neoplastic diseases. It was cultured in an adult cat from a granulomatous-appearing growth involving the palate and nasal passages. The lesion proved on microscopic examination to be a reticulum cell sarcoma (AMAH). *Candida* was also present in a terminal bronchopneumonia in an elderly cat with diabetes mellitus (AMAH).

### Treatment

For topical treatment, 1 per cent solutions of gentian violet or iodine (Small, 1974) or potassium permanganate 1:4000 may be effective. Nystatin, too, is used topically and also by mouth for candidiasis of the alimentary tract. In man, oral administration of potassium iodide may eliminate *Candida* from the sputum. Amphotericin B is used in systemic infections. Ketoconazole and 5-fluorocytosine are also effective against certain forms of candidiasis.

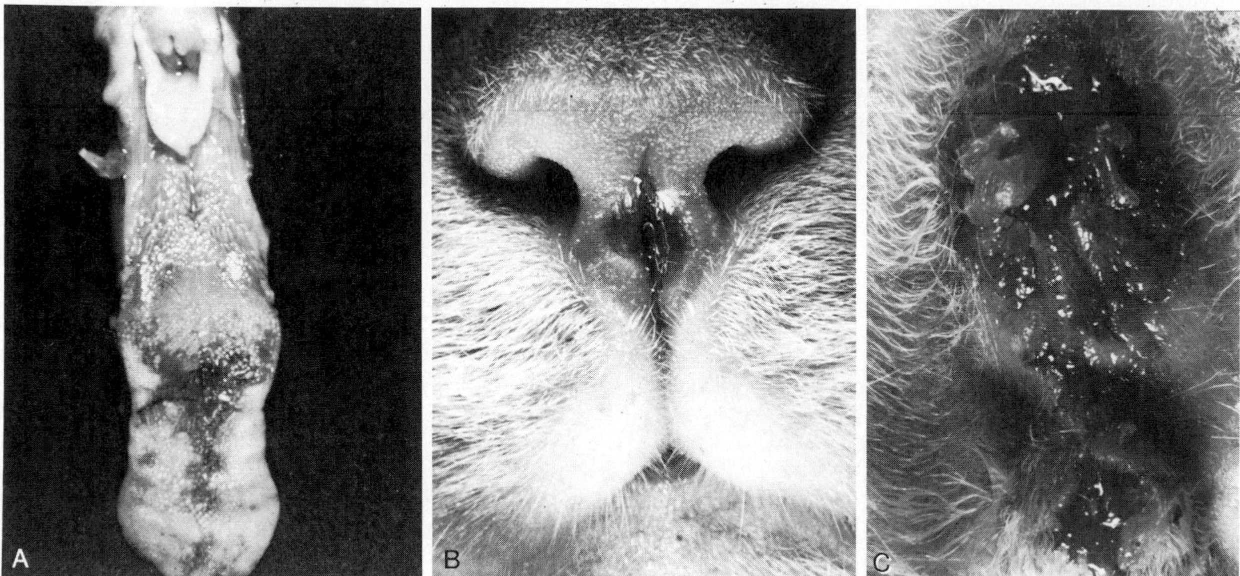


**Figure 9–7** Candidiasis. Upper respiratory infection treated with an antibiotic was followed by candidiasis of (*A*) the tongue, (*B*) the nasal philtrum, and (*C*) the anus and prepuce.

## COCCIDIOIDOMYCOSIS

Coccidioidomycosis is endemic in the dry southwest of the United States, where in certain areas as many as three quarters of the human population may react positively to the coccidioidin skin test. Infections are not infrequent in dogs and have been recognized in many other domestic and wild animals. Cats are either relatively insusceptible or have not been adequately examined. The infection also occurs in Central America and parts of South America.

### Etiology and Diagnosis

The agent, *Coccidioides immitis*, a thick-walled spherule varying in diameter from 10 to 80 μ, reproduces in tissues by endosporulation, endospores even in the hundreds sometimes appearing in the parent organism. It may live in the soil whence it is inhaled or finds its way into wounds. Direct host-to-host transmission has not been established. The great size of some of the spheres and the reproduction by endospores distinguish *Coccidioides* from *Cryptococcus neoformans*, *Blastomyces dermatitidis*, and *Histoplasma capsulatum*. *Coccidioides* may be identified in unstained preparations of body fluid, exudates, or scrapings from lesions. The organism is easily cultured, the mycelia growing in small, white, fluffy colonies.

### Clinical and Pathologic Features

The infection, which is benign in most humans, is extensively discussed in a classic monograph by Fiese (1958). In both man and animals many localized pulmonary infections remain asymptomatic, but others result in a chronic granulomatous disease with clinical and radiographic signs much like those of tuberculosis or blastomycosis. In certain victims the infection generalizes to bones, joints, skin, viscera, or central nervous system, and many organs may exhibit grayish nodular or purulent foci. Healed lesions may undergo calcification. Infections entering through breaks in the skin are rare; they produce swellings and refractory discharging lesions from which the agent may be isolated.

Three cases of coccidioidomycosis have been reported in cats in Arizona (Reed et al., 1963) and one in California (Wolf, 1979). One of the Arizona cats, a four-year-old spayed female, had an abscess over one hip that yielded only *Aspergillus* on culture and failed to respond to five months' treatment with antibiotics (Reed et al., 1963). At the end of this time the cat ceased to eat and, despite forced feeding, died a week later, having at no time had fever or respiratory difficulty. There was a discrete white oval lesion 6 mm long in the caudal lobe of one lung and a friable white hilar granuloma; the cranial mediastinal nodes were enlarged. *Coccidioides* was identified microscopically in the pulmonary lesions and nodes and tissue from the subcutaneous tract over the hip.

Another Arizona cat, a three-year-old tom with a history of prolonged lameness, cough, and progressive weight loss, had an abscess over the left hip, and a radiograph of the left elbow disclosed a smooth enlargement of the lower humerus, as well as demineralization of cortical bone and rough periosteal bone deposition in the olecranon and upper radius. An intradermal injection of undiluted coccidioidin, 0.1 ml, resulted at 48 and 72 hours in a firm 3 mm swelling but no reddening. At autopsy the right cranial lung lobe was found to be solidified, and irregular or circular yellow-white lesions 0.5 to 3 mm in diameter were found on and throughout the rest of the lung tissue. Below the trachea was a firm, pale yellow, enlarged node and above it just cranial to the bifurcation a firm, fibrous mass, white on cut section but with several yellow foci. On the spleen was a spherical tan mass 4 mm in diameter and in the cortex of one kidney a yellow streak 1 mm wide. Microscopic examination disclosed characteristic spherules in the lungs, kidneys, liver, and subcutaneous lesion. Changes in the spleen and bone were typical of coccidioidal infection, but organisms could not be demonstrated.

*Coccidioides* was cultured from the thoracic granulomas of both cats and recovered from mice inoculated with culture material. Complement-fixation and precipitin tests performed with serum from the second cat were negative.

*Coccidioides* was the cause of chronic pyogranulomatous endophthalmitis in one eye of a 12-year-old Persian in Arizona (Angell et al., 1985). Two years after removal of the eye the cat had no evidence of disease. Latex particle agglutination, agar gel diffusion, and complement fixation tests gave negative results.

The California cat, a one and a half-year-old castrated male domestic longhair, had had an abscess opened on the left hind foot four months before, but subsequently draining tracts developed on the medial side of the foot and in the left popliteal and ischial areas (Wolf, 1979). A coccidioidin precipitin test was positive, a complement-fixation test negative. An aspirate from the left popliteal area contained PAS-positive spherules, which when cultured on blood agar at 37 C yielded a pure culture of *C. immitis*. As radiographs indicated no involvement of bone or lungs, no treatment was given, and at the end of two months the draining tracts had closed and the popliteal swelling decreased. On the basis of the clinical course and the absence of complement-fixing antibodies, which are elevated with disseminated disease, the cat was presumed to have had a primary and self-limiting cutaneous infection.

In a Texas cat, involvement of the lungs and hilar lymph nodes caused severe dyspnea (Schwartz, 1981).

### Treatment

For disseminated coccidioidomycosis, amphotericin B has been the treatment of choice, but ketoconazole has been used with success in dogs and has the advantage of oral administration and relatively few side effects (Attleberger, 1983).

## CRYPTOCOCCOSIS (TORULOSIS, EUROPEAN BLASTOMYCOSIS)*

Cryptococcosis is the most frequently diagnosed systemic mycosis of cats. Usually manifested as a subacute or chronic disease, it appears to have a worldwide distribution, having been described in Australia, Austria, Canada, Hawaii, Japan, New Zealand, Papua New Guinea, the United Kingdom, and the United States (Wilkinson, 1979). Since the first published report by Curtis in 1951, at least 60 cases of feline cryptococcosis have been described in the veterinary literature (Brown et al., 1978; Duckworth et al., 1975; Legendre et al., 1982; Madewell et al., 1979; McDonald, 1968; Moore, 1982; Prevost et al., 1982; Rosenthal et al., 1981; Ryer and Ryer, 1981; Thrall et al., 1976; Wilkinson, 1979; Wilkinson et al., 1983). The works of Barrett and Scott (1975) and of Wilkinson (1979) give excellent reviews of previous reports. Eighteen additional cases were also seen at the Veterinary Medical Teaching Hospital, University of California, Davis (VMTH, UCD) during a 10½-year period (Blouin, 1979), while 34 cases were diagnosed at the Angell Memorial Animal Hospital (AMAH) in Boston over a 29-year period. One of the University of California cases was published by Madewell et al. (1979).

Cryptococcosis can thus no longer be considered a rare disease of cats, and its importance is enhanced by the uniformly fatal nature of the infection when left untreated. Even though the treatment is often unsuccessful, better methods of diagnosis and newer drugs have contributed to an improved prognosis.

### Etiology

Cryptococcosis is caused by the encapsulated yeast *Cryptococcus neoformans*. Although the organism has been isolated from numerous natural sources, it has been most frequently associated with the presence of pigeon excreta, presumably because of favorable growth conditions afforded by bird droppings, including creatinine, which *C. neoformans* can utilize as a sole source of nitrogen (Ajello, 1967; Pappagianis, 1967; Rippon, 1982).

The cultural characteristics of the yeast form are well recognized. The cells are round or oval, thin-walled, and surrounded by a mucinous capsule of variable thickness forming a clear or refractile halo. The cell diameter varies from 2.5 to 8.0 μ under laboratory conditions, while it can reach up to 15 μ in tissues. This is in contrast to the much smaller dimensions of the yeast cells found in pigeon excreta (Powell et al., 1972) or incubated in soil (Neilson et al., 1977). Asexual reproduction occurs by single or multiple budding. *C. neoformans* can grow on most culture media at both 20 C (68 F) and 36 C (96.8 F) but not at 39 C (102.2 F). Opaque, creamy, yeastlike colonies usually appear within two to five days, and production of the polysaccharide capsular material gives the growth a mucoid appearance and consistency. The organism produces urease and starchlike compounds and is unable to assimilate nitrate or ferment sugars. It can assimilate glucose, maltose, sucrose, and galactose but not lactose or melibiose. Pathogenicity for animals is an important characteristic of *C. neoformans* and helps to differentiate it from other yeasts. Virulence is greatest for chick embryos and mice, and less so for rats, guinea pigs, and rabbits (Benham, 1955; Emmons et al., 1977; Kreger–van Rij, 1964; Littman and Zimmerman, 1956; Lodder, 1970; Rippon, 1982).

The ability of the yeast to form a capsule has been associated with virulence and is considered by most investigators to be an essential requirement for production of disease; this may be related to the immunosuppressive properties of the capsular polysaccharide, particularly the inhibition of phagocytosis (Bennett and Hasenclever, 1965; Bulmer and Sans, 1968; Swenson and Kozel, 1978). There are four distinct serotypes (A, B, C, and D) of *C. neoformans*, which may be associated with differences in pathogenicity and geographic location. Serotype A is the most prevalent in the United States (Bennett et al., 1977).

Although *C. neoformans* was long considered to exist exclusively as a yeast, it has recently been discovered to have a sexual reproductive phase under critical laboratory conditions. The fungus is now classified as a basidiomycete bearing the name *Filobasidiella neoformans* or *bacillospora Kwon-Chung*, depending on the serotype (Kwon-Chung, 1975, 1976). The mycelial form of the organism

*By Paule Blouin and Michael W. Conner.

is not usually involved in the production of clinical disease. In contrast with other dimorphic fungi, such as *Coccidioides immitis* and *Blastomyces dermatitidis*, the yeast phase is found both in tissues and under laboratory conditions.

## Immunosuppression and Cryptococcosis

In man, an important factor predisposing to cryptococcosis is a pre-existing immunosuppressive condition, such as Hodgkin's disease, lymphoma, sarcoidosis, or prolonged corticosteroid treatment (Emmons et al., 1977; Littman, 1959; Littman and Walter, 1968; Pappagianis, 1967; Rippon, 1982). While such a relationship has not been described in the feline disease, it is conceivable that infection with the feline leukemia virus (FeLV) makes cats more susceptible to cryptococcosis. This virus is known to have immunosuppressive properties, particularly on cell-mediated immune responses (Essex, 1975; Perryman et al., 1972), and since the host defense against *C. neoformans* is thought to be provided by cell-mediated immunity rather than antibody production (Graybill and Drutz, 1978; Monga et al., 1979), FeLV infection may in some cases be the immunosuppressive factor allowing the development of cryptococcal disease.

It is impossible to draw valid conclusions on the relationship between FeLV infection and cryptococcosis from reported cases, since very few cats were tested for the presence of FeLV, but it is interesting to note that one cat had both renal lymphoma and cryptococcosis (Madewell et al., 1979), while in the case published by Barrett and Scott (1975), the animal was successfully treated even though it was FeLV-positive. The influence of FeLV is supported by experimental studies (Blouin, 1979) and by the VMTH and AMAH cases. In the VMTH series, 5 of 11 cats were positive for the presence of FeLV antigen (Blouin, 1979). This is much higher than the incidence found either in the general feline population (0.31 per cent) or in healthy cats exposed to animals with leukemia (33 per cent) as reported by Hardy et al. (1976). In the AMAH cases, three of four cats tested for FeLV were positive, including one with myeloproliferative disease and one with lymphosarcoma of the jejunum and mesenteric lymph nodes. In addition, a second diagnosis unrelated to FeLV infection was made in 6 of 21 autopsied cases: three animals had cardiomyopathy, and three cats had a renal adenoma, a renal adenocarcinoma, and a congenital renal malformation, respectively.

## Clinical Features

Cryptococcosis can affect cats of any age, but the majority are between three and seven years of age (average five). While the human disease is more prevalent in males than in females (Pappagianis, 1967), a sex predisposition does not appear to be present in cats, possibly because of the influence of neutering. A strong breed predisposition is not apparent, with the possible exception of the Siamese breed. Fever is an inconsistent finding and can be related to a superimposed bacterial infection.

### Upper Respiratory Involvement

Cryptococcal infection can affect many different organ systems, alone or in combination. The cases reported and those at VMTH show that the upper respiratory system is most commonly involved. Many cats present with a uni- or bilateral chronic rhinitis or sinusitis characterized by sneezing, snorting or snoring sounds, respiratory difficulties, and a mucopurulent or sanguineous nasal discharge (see Fig. 9–16). The condition responds poorly to antibacterial treatment and gradually worsens over a period of weeks or months. A frequent and important diagnostic finding is the presence of polyp-like masses protruding from one or both nostrils (Fig. 9–8). These are usually small, fleshy, and granulomatous in appearance. Auscultation seldom reveals pulmonary involvement, and the cervical lymph nodes may be enlarged. Mouth lesions are occasionally associated with this form of the disease. They

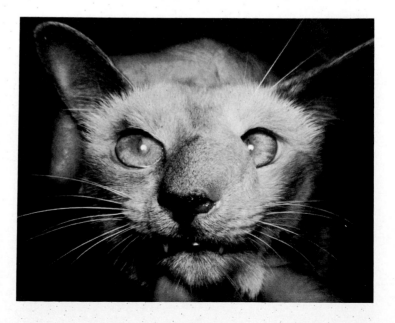

**Figure 9–8** Extensive cryptococcal lesions involving both nostrils and the dorsal aspect of the nose in a five-year-old female Siamese cat. (From Palumbo NE, Perri S: Vet Med Small Anim Clin 70 [1975] 553–557.)

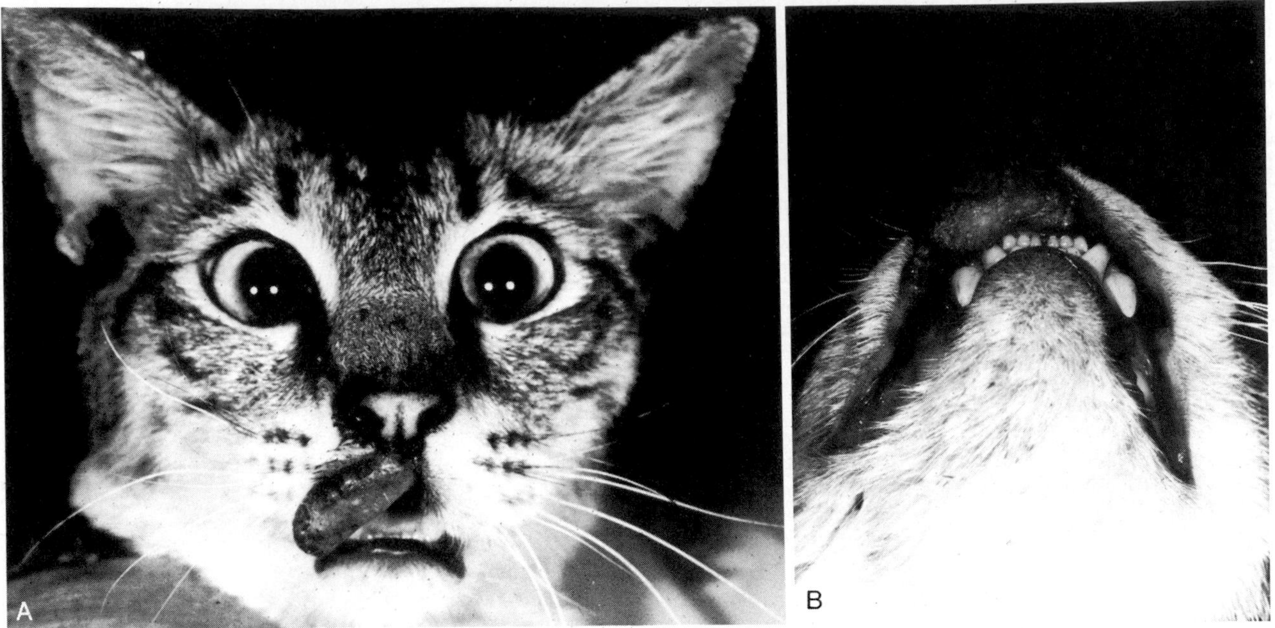

**Figure 9–9** *A* and *B*, Fleshy mass extending from the upper lip of a cat and mimicking an eosinophilic granuloma. A diagnosis of cryptococcosis was obtained from a biopsy specimen. (Courtesy Angell Memorial Animal Hospital.)

can involve the tongue, the gingiva, or the palate and can be either ulcerative or proliferative.

The first case published in America by Holzworth in 1952 is a good illustration of this type of clinical presentation. The cat was a six-year-old male of domestic breed with a one-month history of ocular and nasal discharge, coughing, and respiratory difficulty. Physical examination revealed a fever, a sanguineous nasal discharge, and small proliferating masses in both nostrils. The cat also had a purulent discharge from the right eye, small ulcerated masses in the mouth, enlarged tonsils and cervical lymph nodes, and increased vesicular lung sounds with occasional rales. Autopsy disclosed generalized cryptococcal involvement.

## Facial Involvement

The presence of facial lesions is the second most common clinical finding. A firm, nodular swelling can be found anywhere on the head but most frequently over the bridge of the nose, the side of the face, the upper lip, or the nostril (Figs. 9–8 to 9–10). Most lesions appear to be subcutaneous, but some will ulcerate and be covered with a viscous exudate. The lesions can be single or multiple, they elicit little pruritus, and they can mimic a neoplasm. The adjacent lymph nodes are usually firm and enlarged. Facial lesions frequently occur in combination with upper respiratory involvement or generalized cryptococcal skin disease.

The article by Rutman et al. (1975) describes a three-year-old domestic longhair with two ulcerated, tumor-like masses on the forehead. The first nodule had been noted three months previously, the second two months later. Both masses had been enlarging for a month and were associated with mild edema of the upper lids and epiphora. The cat was otherwise normal, as were the hematologic values. Surgery was attempted, but when cryptococcosis was diagnosed histologically, the cat was destroyed. Autopsy revealed involvement of the brain, skin of the forehead, periorbital tissues, nasal turbinates, and lungs.

## Central Nervous System Involvement

Infection of the central nervous system is the third most common clinical presentation. It is one of the most difficult to diagnose, since it may occur alone and can mimic the

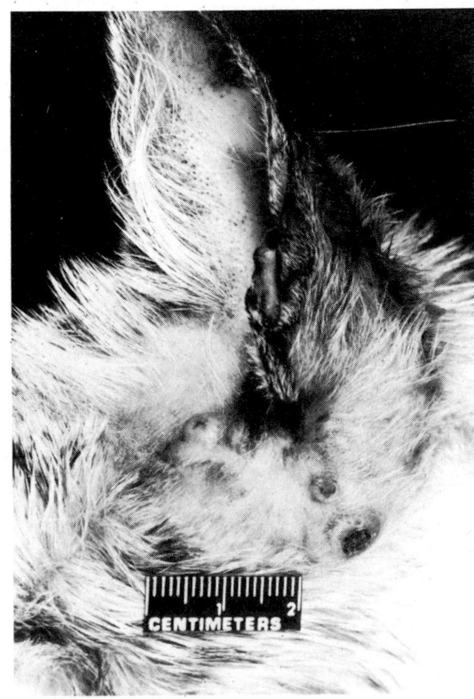


**Figure 9–10** Nodular and ulcerated skin lesions located at the base of the left ear in a cat with cryptococcosis. (Courtesy Angell Memorial Animal Hospital.)

neural form of other disorders such as trauma, feline infectious peritonitis (FIP), toxoplasmosis, lymphosarcoma, and other less common conditions. The neurologic manifestations can appear abruptly, or be mild at first and progress over a few weeks. Brain involvement is most common, although the spinal cord is occasionally affected (Wilkinson, 1979).

Signs vary greatly from case to case and range from the mildest to the most severe. Some cats have only a change in temperament, while others show ataxia, circling, head pressing, convulsions, or paresis. The cat may also be blind with or without abnormal pupillary responses. In a particularly unusual AMAH case, the only clinical sign was marked sleepiness of sudden onset in a cat that seemed otherwise healthy. The animal was hospitalized for observation but died a few hours later. Cryptococcal meningoencephalitis was documented at autopsy.

A good example of cryptococcal meningoencephalitis is provided by the case of Beauregard and Malkin (1970). A three-year-old neutered female was presented for circling and blindness of a few days' duration. At the time of physical examination, the cat showed loss of balance, light spasmodic convulsions, and dilated, fixed pupils. It became semiconscious during the next day, and the convulsions became more severe. The cat was then destroyed, and autopsy examination of the head revealed cryptococcal meningoencephalitis.

## Skin Involvement

Skin infection, less common than other clinical presentations, is usually manifested by multiple cutaneous or subcutaneous nodules. The head is often affected. The nodules can be fluctuant or firm and many eventually become ulcerated, oozing a gelatinous or mucosanguineous exudate. While the lesions can be limited to the skin (e.g., the feet, Thrall et al., 1976), they are usually associated with involvement of other organ systems, such as the upper respiratory tract.

In the sixth case reported by Wilkinson in 1979, a four-year-old neutered male domestic shorthair was presented with skin nodules over all the body. Present for two months, some had become ulcerated, and the peripheral lymph nodes were enlarged. A nodule was also present on the tip of the tongue. Cryptococcosis was diagnosed from impression smears of the ulcerated lesions, and the cat was destroyed. Involvement of skin, lymph nodes, tongue, and left nasal cavity and turbinates was found at autopsy.

## Unusual Presentations

Cryptococcosis can occasionally manifest itself in a most unusual manner and mimic other diseases. For instance, one of the VMTH cats was admitted with compulsive pacing and circling of a few days' duration, bilateral mydriasis, and marked protrusion of the left eye thought to be caused by an orbital abscess or tumor. Ten months earlier the cat had been found to be an FeLV carrier. While cultures of the cerebrospinal fluid were negative, *C. neoformans* was isolated from the specimen obtained by needle aspiration of the retrobulbar mass.

In another VMTH case, a six-year-old spayed female domestic shorthair was presented with lameness of the left hindleg associated with a painful, distended stifle. Radiographs showed destruction of the distal femur thought to be due to a tumor, but a biopsy revealed cryptococcal osteomyelitis.

Squire and Bush (1971) mentioned a cat with a huge anterior mediastinal mass and hydrothorax diagnosed clinically as lymphoma, but subsequently proven to be a cryptococcal granuloma. Chiba et al. (1967) described a cat with an abdominal mass suggestive of a peritoneal neoplasm but likewise shown microscopically to be a cryptococcal granuloma.

In a cat at AMAH in which a nasopharyngeal infection was intermittently controlled by 5-fluorocytosine, one recurrence took the form of a polyp in the external ear canal.

## Disseminated Cryptococcosis

Cryptococcosis can be manifested clinically by involvement of more than one organ or anatomic area, including in rare instances the long bones. Such cases are usually shown at autopsy to be the result of disseminated, overwhelming infection, as in the first case of Wilkinson's report (1979).

An eight-year-old neutered male Siamese was presented for multiple skin lesions of six months' duration, accompanied by malaise and weight loss of five weeks. Physical examination revealed painless, occasionally ulcerated nodules in the skin of the trunk, serous discharge from the left nostril, swelling over the left side of the bridge of the nose, peripheral lymph node enlargement, and spastic extension of the left hindleg. *Cryptococcus* was recovered from both skin lesions and nasal exudate. Sporadic treatment with amphotericin B over a period of 12 weeks resulted in only transient improvement, and the cat was destroyed. Autopsy disclosed cryptococcal involvement of the skin, nasal turbinates, lumbar spinal cord, and kidneys.

An unusual finding in a case of disseminated infection at AMAH was an intestinal polyp that proved to be a cryptococcal granuloma.

## Ocular Involvement

The intraocular manifestations of cryptococcosis can range from optic neuritis to panophthalmitis. In many cases, the lesions affect the fundus without causing a detectable visual deficit, and since the majority of published case reports do not state whether a fundic examination was performed, it is difficult to evaluate the true incidence of ocular involvement in feline cryptococcosis. Fifteen of the 18 cats in the VMTH series had an ophthalmoscopic examination, and nine of these were shown to have ocular involvement (Blouin, 1979). Single or multifocal chorioretinal lesions were detected in a total of seven cats (Fig. 9–11). They were circular, ranging in size between ¼ and 1½ disc diameters. Many of the lesions located in the tapetal fundus gave the impression of being almost transparent. The larger lesions were elevated, as evidenced by distortion of the overlying retinal vessels. They had the appearance of small, focal, serous retinal detachments with minimal inflammatory reaction. Histologic examination disclosed subretinal accumulation of yeast cells with variable numbers of inflammatory cells in the retina, choroid, and subretinal space (Fig. 9–12).

Similar lesions were consistently reproduced experimentally by the intracarotid inoculation of live yeast cells (Blouin, 1979; Blouin and Cello, 1980). In the majority of eyes, the lesions had a characteristic appearance: they started as multifocal pinpoint opacities and enlarged to reach the circular, transparent stage. In some cases, the lesions eventually became dark and indistinct as the

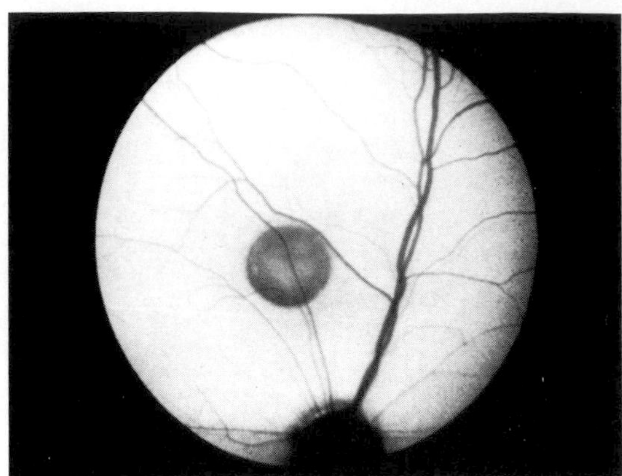

**Figure 9–11** Single, circular cryptococcal chorioretinal lesion located superotemporally to the optic nerve head.

inflammatory reaction became more intense. In severely affected eyes, the whole fundus was involved, the retina was detached, and a marked iridocyclitis was present even though organisms could usually not be recovered from the aqueous humor. The fundic lesions appear to be the consequence of hematogenous dissemination. They indicate systemic involvement and can easily be used to monitor the effects of antifungal therapy.

Inflammation of the optic nerve head (papillitis) was detected in five of the VMTH cases but could usually not be reproduced experimentally by intracarotid inoculation. In contrast to the chorioretinal lesions, papillitis appears to be associated with brain involvement, with subsequent optic nerve meningitis. It may or may not be accompanied by chorioretinitis. Papillitis is manifested by congestion of the optic nerve head, increased tortuosity of the retinal vessels, peripapillary retinal hemorrhages, and occasionally inflammation or serous detachments of the retina immediately surrounding the optic nerve head.

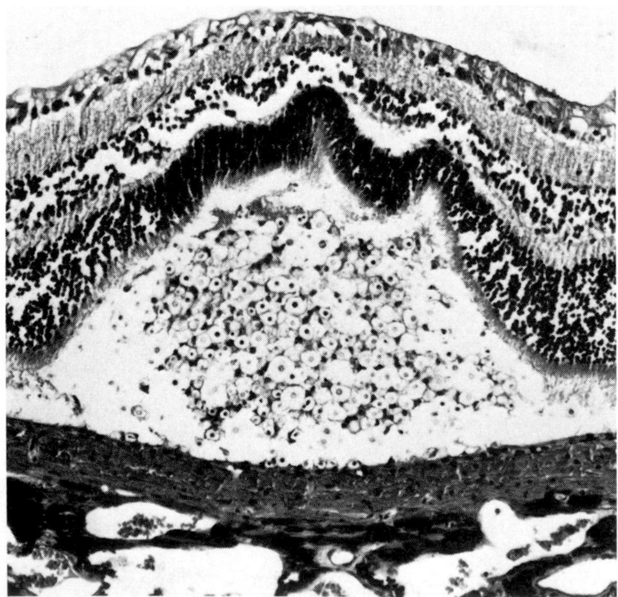

**Figure 9–12** Focal chorioretinal lesion in the tapetal area in a cat with cryptococcosis. The retina is separated from the retinal pigment epithelium by cryptococci and mononuclear inflammatory cells. The tapetal layers contain scattered lymphocytes. H&E, × 125.

Iridocyclitis usually occurs in conjunction with fundic lesions and varies from mild to very severe. Signs include keratic precipitates, a fibrinous, occasionally blood-tinged clot in the anterior chamber, and posterior synechiae. The iridocyclitis is not pathognomonic of cryptococcosis, since similar findings can be present in FIP, toxoplasmosis, and occasionally lymphosarcoma.

It is interesting that in two of the published cases, bilateral ocular involvement occurred without other detectable lesions at autopsy (Fischer, 1971; Gwin et al., 1977). More often, though, the ocular lesions are accompanied by involvement of other organs, as in the second case published by Fischer (1971).

A seven-year-old female Siamese showed progressive neurologic signs for seven months. At the time of examination, both pupils reacted normally to light. Lesions were detected only in the fundus of the left eye, where a large cystic retinal detachment was observed. Dark areas corresponding to subretinal granulomas and evidence of retinal inflammation were also observed. Cultures of cerebrospinal fluid were negative. The cat was destroyed and autopsy revealed cryptococcal involvement of the tonsils, submandibular lymph nodes, and cerebral meninges. Ocular lesions were confined to the posterior segment of the left eye and consisted of peripapillary retinitis associated with large numbers of intraretinal organisms but without involvement of the optic nerve or meninges. In addition, a portion of the inferior retina was detached by subretinal fluid, organisms, and inflammatory cells. The underlying choroid contained inflammatory cells.

## Diagnosis

Cryptococcosis should always be considered in cats with chronic upper respiratory disease, focal or generalized skin nodules, or signs of meningoencephalitis. Multifocal chorioretinitis or papillitis in such cases is always an indication for an aggressive diagnostic study to eliminate the possibility of cryptococcal infection.

Whether hematologic or biochemical blood values are abnormal depends on the severity of infection and on the organs involved. Even when changes are present, they are not diagnostic of cryptococcal infection. Anemia, occasionally present, may be associated with concurrent *Haemobartonella felis* or FeLV infection. Secondary bacterial infections can also influence the total and differential white-cell counts, evoking an absolute neutrophilia.

Radiographs can aid in determining the extent of infection, but the radiologic changes are not pathognomonic. In cats with upper respiratory infection, there usually is increased soft tissue density in the nasal passages or sinuses, with occasional evidence of bone destruction (Fig. 9–13). Facial lesions are sometimes associated with underlying osteomyelitis. Thoracic radiographs appear normal in the majority of cases, even when lung involvement is later demonstrated at autopsy. When present, radiographic pulmonary changes are not specific and only seldom suggest granulomatous mycotic disease. Radiologic examination is mostly helpful in assessing the extent of the disease and the response to the treatment.

Definitive diagnosis of cryptococcosis is by positive identification of the organism. Swabs of nasal or skin

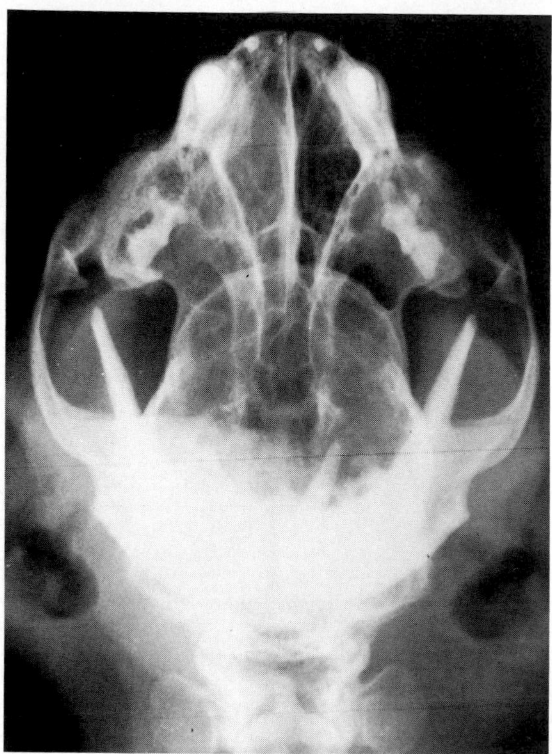

**Figure 9–13** Soft tissue density involving nasal cavity on one side. A smear of exudate from the nostril yielded cryptococci.

exudate, fresh specimens of cutaneous nodules obtained by biopsy, and a sample of cerebrospinal fluid (if neurologic signs are present) should be submitted to the laboratory for direct examination and culture. Rarely, *Cryptococcus* may be identified in, and cultured from, urine (AMAH).

Examination of an India ink preparation of the material is the fastest and easiest way to make the diagnosis, and has the advantage that it can be performed immediately with very little equipment. A drop of the liquid specimen or a smear of swabs or cut tissues is mixed with a drop of India ink on a glass slide. Microscopic examination at 400 × under a coverslip reveals the striking picture of typical round or oval yeast cells, each surrounded by a clear halo corresponding to the capsule. Budding can usually be demonstrated (Fig. 9–14). Other stains such as Gram and Wright-Giemsa can also be used (Fig. 9–15), but the India ink is usually readily available and provides the most contrast with the clear capsule because of the very dark background. *C. neoformans* is readily differentiated from *B. dermatitidis* by its mucinous capsule and thin wall.

Even though the morphology of the organism is typical, all specimens should be cultured to confirm the diagnosis. *C. neoformans* will usually grow on blood agar, but the best culture medium is Sabouraud's dextrose agar without cycloheximide, an inhibitor often used to prevent the growth of saprophytic fungi. The plates are placed in the incubator and at room temperature. Final identification of the organism is provided by sugar assimilation tests, production of urease, and pathogenicity for mice.

Serologic tests are valuable both in making or supporting a diagnosis of the disease and in monitoring its course (Bennett et al., 1964; Bindschadler and Bennett, 1968; Drouhet et al., 1979; Gordon and Vedder, 1966; Kaufman and Blumer, 1968; Prevost and Newell, 1978). The presence of antibodies can be determined by complement fixation, immunodiffusion, enzymatic techniques, indirect fluorescent antibodies, or tube agglutination, the last two methods being the most useful. Antibody testing has limited applications, however, since positive titers cannot differentiate between a previous subclinical infection and active disease. In addition, a positive antibody titer is seldom found in clinical cases of cryptococcosis, probably because *C. neoformans* produces a large amount of capsular polysaccharide that is released in the blood and other body fluids. Circulating antibodies are then likely

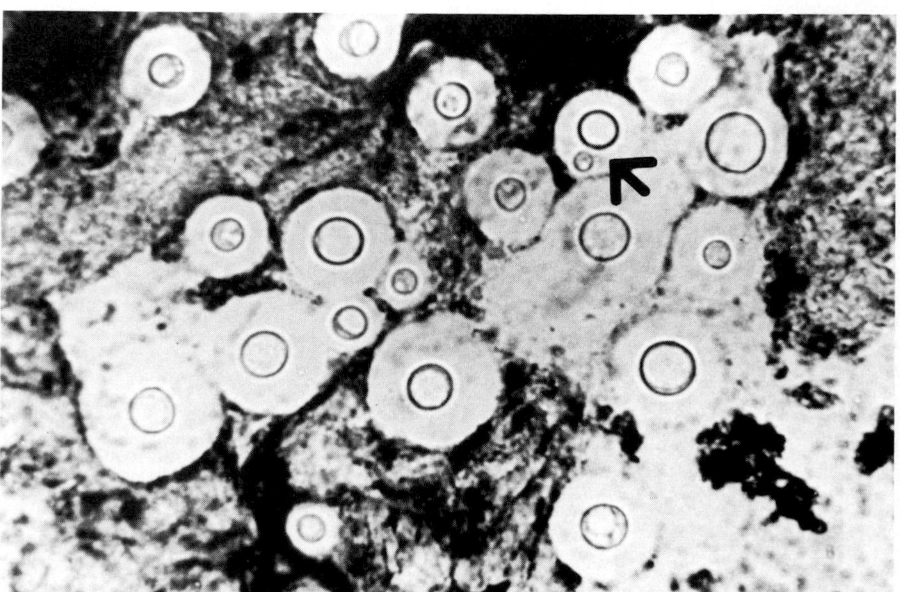

**Figure 9–14** India ink smear prepared from the brain of an experimentally infected mouse. The average yeast cell diameter is 7.1 μ and the mean capsule width is 5.0 μ. Proliferation of the organism is demonstrated by the presence of budding (arrow). × 400.

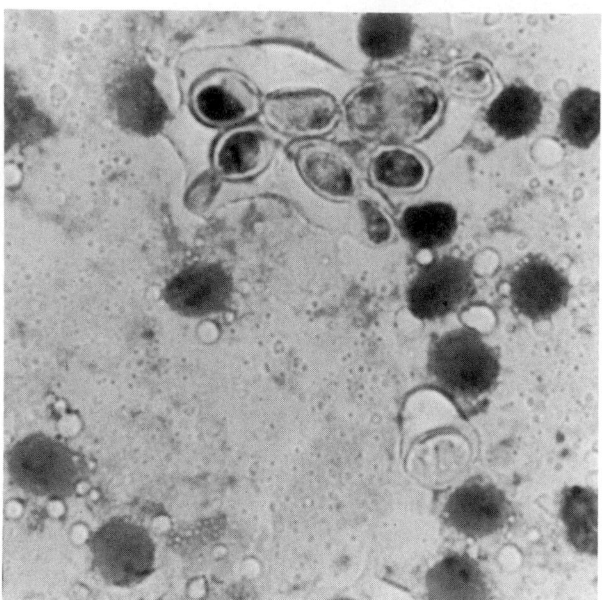

**Figure 9–15** Smear of the nasal exudate in a case of feline cryptococcosis demonstrating numerous yeast cells. Wright-Giemsa, × 1000.

to be bound to this antigen, becoming unavailable for laboratory detection. This disadvantage has led to the development of techniques such as complement fixation, immunodiffusion, and latex particle agglutination for detection of cryptococcal antigen. The latex agglutination test is the most sensitive and provides an excellent index of the severity of infection, since the height of the titer is proportional to the antigenic load. False positive reactions are rare if appropriate controls are run for the presence of rheumatoid factor. A commercial kit is now available,* but since it has been reported to be less sensitive and specific than the test performed by reference laboratories, duplicate samples should be sent out for confirmation of the diagnosis (MacKinnon et al., 1978). Antigen titers can be negative if the infection is localized in the lung as demonstrated in man by Prevost and Newell in 1978, or limited to the eyes in experimental feline cryptococcosis (Blouin, 1979; Blouin and Cello, 1980). Six of the 18 VMTH cats were tested for the presence of cryptococcal antigen. All had positive titers ranging from 1:2 to 1:8192. A positive cryptococcal antigen titer in a cat showing signs compatible with cryptococcosis is probably strong enough evidence of the disease to justify a therapeutic trial, even if cultures are negative.

Several recent reports have demonstrated the usefulness of serologic procedures in managing feline infections (Brewer, 1980; Moore, 1982; Prevost et al., 1982; Weir et al., 1979).

## Autopsy Findings

Autopsy findings vary with the extent of dissemination of the infection. Macroscopic lesions can occur anywhere in the body. Most frequent are a viscous exudate in the nasal passages and sinuses (Fig. 9–16), small gelatinous nodules scattered in the thoracic and abdominal viscera (Fig. 9–17), congestion of the meninges with a scanty mucoid exudate resembling soap bubbles, and brain or spinal cord abscesses (Fig. 9–18).

Histologically, the lesions usually have a spongy appearance with hematoxylin and eosin stain because the large capsule fails to retain the stain. Yeast cells appear to be surrounded by clear vacuoles, and they can be in sufficient numbers to completely distort the architecture of the infected tissue (Fig. 9–17). The best stain for identifying *C. neoformans* in tissue sections is Mayer's mucicarmine, which gives the capsule a bright magenta color over a brownish background. Other stains such as Gomori's methenamine silver (Fig. 9–19) and periodic acid–Schiff also demonstrate the organism nicely but may not give as characteristic an appearance as the mucicarmine stain.

An interesting feature of *C. neoformans* is the variability in the extent of the inflammatory reaction it induces, as described by Littman and Zimmerman (1956) in their superb monograph on cryptococcosis:

> Frequently the relative paucity of both cellular and humoral reactions is impressive, especially in the nervous system. Great masses of cryptococci and an overabundance of their mucinous capsular material distend the meninges and fill cystoid spaces within the parenchyma of brain and spinal cord. On casual examination it may seem that within these lesions inflammatory cells are virtually absent. Scrutiny under greater magnification, however, will usually reveal many of the fungus cells within macrophages, the cytoplasm of which is so pale and distended by the mucinous material that they are barely visible. Lesions of the thoracic and abdominal viscera, notably those removed surgically, are more often obviously granulomatous than are those of the brain or meninges. Nevertheless, any tissue may reveal lesions that appear to be essentially acellular or that are densely infiltrated with chronic inflammatory cells. . . . Early lesions are gelatinous (mucinous) while older lesions are granulomatous. Cryptococci are initially inert in tissues and form masses of organisms with but little surrounding inflammatory response; later they are engulfed by giant cells and macrophages.

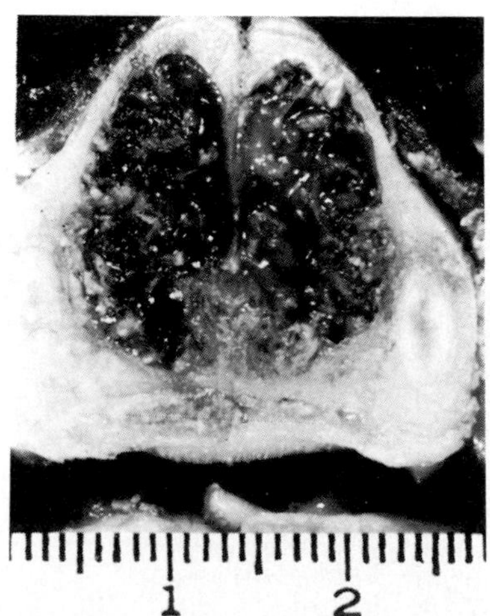


**Figure 9–16** Vertical section through the nasal cavities and sinuses of a cat with cryptococcosis. Bilateral abundant gelatinous exudate is present. (Courtesy Angell Memorial Animal Hospital.)

*Crypto LA Kit, International Biological Laboratories, Inc.

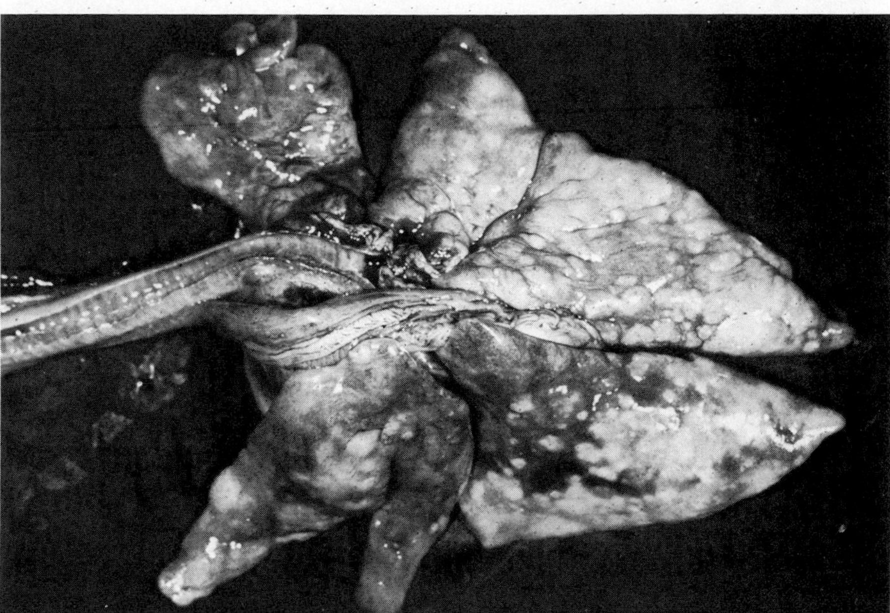

**Figure 9–17** Multiple nodular cryptococcal lesions protruding from the surface of the lungs.

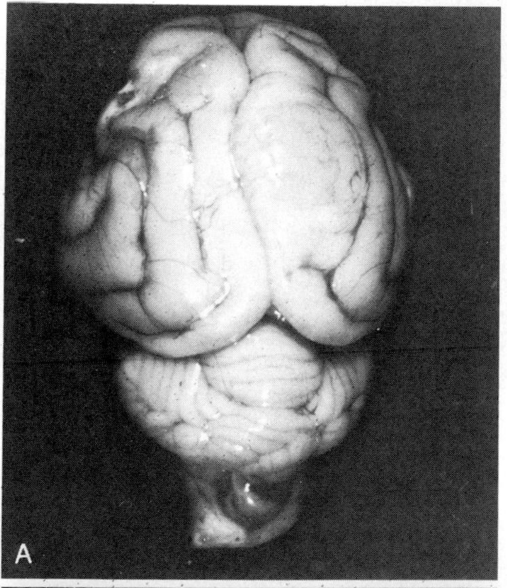

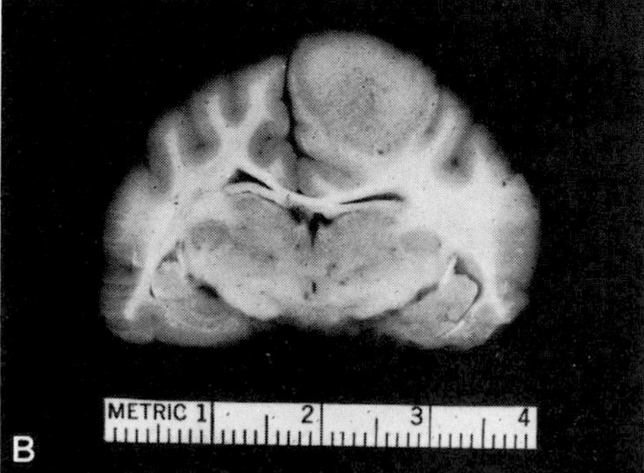


**Figure 9–18** *A* and *B*, Large brain abscess in a cat with cryptococcal meningoencephalitis.

## Prognosis

Cryptococcosis always has a poor or, at best, uncertain prognosis. Untreated cases of clinical infection are fatal in cats, and treatment is by no means always successful. The prognosis is worse in debilitated animals with widespread disease, or if the central nervous system is involved. The height of the antigen titer can help to determine the severity of an infection but should not be used as the only criterion for prognosis. A positive FeLV antigen test result may alter the prognosis and the decision whether to treat or destroy the cat.

## Treatment

Resection of affected tissues has occasionally been attempted but rarely achieves a cure, probably because the disease is seldom so localized that all organisms can be eliminated surgically. The case reported by Olander et al. (1963) is most unusual in this respect, since resection of a lesion involving the subcutaneous tissues of the bridge of the nose resulted in a cure lasting for more than seven years. Another cat from which a nasal granuloma was excised was in good health two and a half years later (Medleau et al., 1985).

### Amphotericin B

The availability of amphotericin B (Fungizone, Squibb) in 1956 was followed by a major breakthrough in the treatment of human cryptococcosis (Edwards et al., 1970). Amphotericin B is a polyene antibiotic that binds to certain sterols found in fungal cell membranes, causing altered permeability and loss of intracellular components. Toxicity to mammalian cells is probably due to attachment of the drug to cholesterol in cell membranes. The major side effects are impairment of renal and hepatic functions,

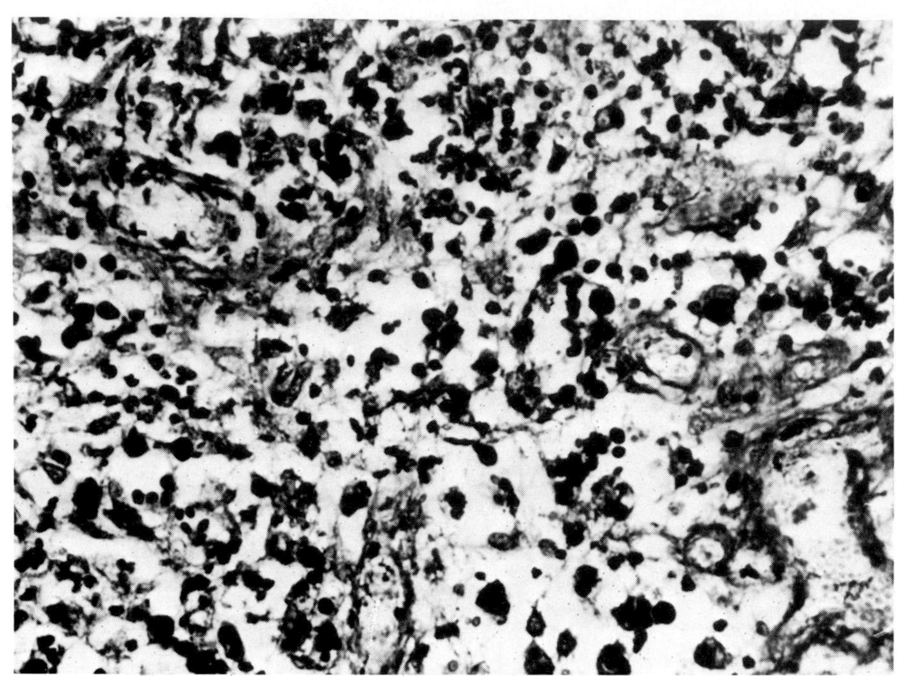

**Figure 9–19.** Biopsy specimen of a nasal mass demonstrating large numbers of cryptococcal yeast cells. Gomori's methenamine silver, × 250.

anemia, electrolyte disturbances (especially hypokalemia), severe falls in blood pressure, and various neurologic symptoms (Meyers et al., 1980). The water-soluble methyl ester preparation is reported to cause less toxicity in mice but unfortunately also appears to be less effective (Gadebusch et al., 1976); its effects have yet to be evaluated in cats.

Topical or intralesional administration of amphotericin B usually fails to cure the animal, effective therapy requiring intravenous administration. The drug is extremely irritant, and accidental perivascular injection can result in severe tissue sloughing. Flushing of the nasal cavity and sinuses with amphotericin B is poorly tolerated in cats and cannot be recommended. Intrathecal administration of the drug is advocated for the treatment of human cryptococcal meningitis but has not yet been tried in cats. Treatment of feline cryptococcosis with systemic amphotericin B has been attempted in seven cases, with successful results in two animals (Duckworth and Taylor 1975; Gwin et al., 1977; Palumbo and Perri, 1975; Thrall et al., 1976; Wilkinson, 1979).

## 5-Fluorocytosine

5-Fluorocystosine (5-FC) (Ancobon, Roche) is a fluorinated pyrimidine that acts by inhibiting nucleic acid synthesis. It can be administered orally and is much less toxic than amphotericin B. Its main disadvantage is the development of resistance by initially susceptible organisms (Meyers et al., 1980).

Successful treatment with 5-fluorocytosine alone has been reported in feline infections of the nasal passages and skin (Brewer, 1980; Moore, 1982; Wilkinson et al., 1983). Dosages variously recommended are 100 to 200 mg/kg divided into three or four doses daily or 100 mg/kg b.i.d. Treatment may have to be continued for several months before the latex particle agglutination titer falls to a level indicating that the infection has probably been eradicated. In two of the cases reported by Wilkinson et al. (1983) an autogenous vaccine was used as adjunctive treatment.

The treatment of feline cryptococcosis with 5-FC alone was attempted in eight of the VMTH cases with only one cure. Some of the other treated cats improved initially but later gradually worsened (Blouin, 1979).

The one survivor was a three-year-old neutered male domestic shorthair presented with massive facial involvement of a month's duration. Radiographs showed proliferative and osteolytic changes in the maxilla and tibia as well as extensive pulmonary infiltrates. Multifocal circular areas of chorioretinitis were detected in both eyes. Oral treatment with 5-FC for 10 months induced a gradual but complete regression of all lesions. The cat remained asymptomatic three years after cessation of treatment. The serum cryptococcal antigen titer was positive at a 1:8192 dilution after one month of treatment, but was negative six months and three years later.

## Combination of 5-Fluorocytosine and Amphotericin B

The renal toxicity of amphotericin B and the development of resistance to 5-FC have led investigators to look for safer and more effective treatments. Experimental studies in mice (Graybill et al., 1978) and clinical trials in man (Bennett et al., 1979; Jimbow et al., 1978) have convincingly shown that combined treatment with amphotericin B and 5-FC has a synergistic effect, resulting in more and faster cures. Renal toxicity was also decreased, since the shorter treatment allowed the administration of a smaller cumulative dose of amphotericin B. In the feline case reported by Barrett and Scott (1975), the drugs were administered sequentially. 5-FC was first given with marked improvement for five weeks, followed by gradual recurrence of the nasal lesions. Acquired resistance to the drug was demonstrated in vitro. A total dose of 8.5 mg/kg of amphotericin B was then administered intravenously over a period of 12 weeks for a complete recovery. Simultaneous administration of 5-FC and amphotericin B in a cat was reported by Weir et al. (1979).

A 7½-year-old neutered female Siamese was presented with a history of sneezing for two months and recurrence for one month of a mass over the left nostril that had been removed surgically. Examination revealed a soft, fluctuant swelling over the right nostril and bilateral mucopurulent nasal discharge with marked nasal congestion. Skull radiographs showed an increased soft tissue density within the left nasal cavity with loss of trabecular pattern. Thoracic radiographs were normal. Cryptococcosis was diagnosed histologically and by culture. The cat was treated for 32 days with 0.5 mg/kg of amphotericin B administered intravenously three times weekly, and with 100 mg/kg/day of oral 5-FC divided in three doses. Blood urea nitrogen and creatinine levels were monitored every two to four days, and the treatment was stopped when these reached values of 70 and 4.8 mg/dl, respectively. The lesions had regressed by the time treatment was stopped, and the cat was still asymptomatic 11 months later. The serum cryptococcal antigen titer was 1:16 at the beginning of the treatment and gradually decreased to 1:1 6 and 10 months later.

Four months of similar combination therapy was apparently successful in another case of nasal cryptococcosis also monitored by serologic procedures (Prevost et al., 1982).

The combination of oral doses of 5-FC and intravenous administration of amphotericin B thus seems to have great potential in the treatment of feline cryptococcosis. 5-FC should be administered orally at a dosage of 100 to 200 mg/kg/day divided in three or four doses. Amphotericin B is given intravenously at a dosage of 0.3 to 0.5 mg/kg, repeated three times a week. Because of the high cost and instability of the drug, Palumbo and Perri (1975) recommend the following procedure: 10 ml of sterile water for injection is added to a vial containing 50 mg of amphotericin B to obtain a concentration of 5 mg/ml. The drug is then stored in 1.5 ml aliquots at −20 C (−4 F), and one of these is thawed weekly. For each treatment, 0.5 ml is withdrawn and diluted with 2.0 ml of sterile 5 per cent dextrose in water (final concentration, 1 mg/ml). The appropriate dose is then administered intravenously over three to five seconds with a 25-gauge needle. The unused portion of the aliquot should be stored in the dark at 4 C (39.2 F) for the rest of the week.

The manufacturer of amphotericin B recommends a weekly BUN determination and urinalysis, with withdrawal of the drug if the BUN rises above 40 mg/dl. Treatment is resumed with a lower dose when renal function returns to normal. Periodic monitoring of SGPT, SGOT, and alkaline phosphatase is advisable during treatment with 5-FC, and patients with impaired renal function or bone marrow depression should be given a lower dose.

The total duration of treatment varies with individual cases. Drug administration should probably be continued for at least two weeks after complete remission of clinical signs and until the serum antigen titer has decreased to 1:1 or 1:2. It would be advisable to monitor the serum antigen titer for a few months after cessation of treatment.

### Other Treatments

Ketoconazole, an imidazole administered orally for a variety of fungal infections, was used successfully after surgical curettage of a nasal granuloma in an FeLV-positive cat (Legendre et al., 1982). The drug was given at a dosage of 10 mg/kg/day in two courses of 60 and 30 days. The cat was normal six months after completion of therapy. There were no side effects of treatment in the cat, although ketoconazole may induce increased liver enzyme activity in man.

Ketoconazole was used alone in treatment of a cat with multiple cutaneous lesions (10 mg/kg once daily for five months) (Medleau et al., 1985). All the lesions had resolved within four months, and the cat was still asymptomatic eight months after treatment was stopped.

Miconazole is another antifungal agent that may eventually be useful in the treatment of feline cryptococcosis, since it has been reported to be effective in vitro (Graybill et al., 1978). Although this drug had no effect on experimental cryptococcosis in mice (Graybill et al., 1978), it cured a human patient affected with meningitis refractory to amphotericin B (Graybill and Levine, 1978). Miconazole cream was used as adjunctive treatment in a feline skin infection (Wilkinson et al., 1983).

Stimulation of the immune system is likely to become increasingly popular for the treatment of many animal and human diseases. The successful treatment of a human patient with cryptococcal meningitis refractory to amphotericin B and 5-FC has been reported with the use of transfer factor (Gross et al., 1978). It is to be hoped that effective ways to potentiate the feline immune system will eventually be found.

## Prevention

Because no vaccine is available for cryptococcosis, the only way to prevent the disease is to avoid contact with the organism. Since the yeast is found in greatest concentrations in pigeon feces (Ajello, 1967; Pappagianis, 1967; Rippon, 1982), cats should theoretically be prevented from going to places where bird droppings are abundant. There are no other practical preventive measures at this time.

## Public Health Significance

Transmission of the disease from animal to animal or animal to man has yet to be documented. The only known case of man-to-man transmission occurred in unusual circumstances, when an infected corneal button was accidentally used to perform a penetrating corneal transplant, causing cryptococcal endophthalmitis (Beyt and Waltman, 1978). Because of the severity of the disease, precautions should still be taken when handling affected cats, particularly if they have open, draining lesions. A mask and gloves should be used, and the cage and litter box should be disinfected regularly and thoroughly. Treatment is best performed in the hospital until the signs begin to resolve, particularly if the household of the owner includes persons with impaired immune mechanisms such as pregnant women, infants, old people, cancer patients, diabetics, and people receiving immunosuppressive treatment. Such precautions are warranted even though cryptococcosis does not appear to be contagious.

## Cryptococcosis in Other Species

Cryptococcosis has been diagnosed in man and in a large number of animal species including the horse, cow, pig, dog, fox, cheetah, civet, monkey, guinea pig, ferret, gazelle, goat, koala, mink, wallaby, dolphin, fennec, and pigeon (Ajello, 1967; Griner and Walch, 1978; Migaki et al., 1978; Saez et al., 1978). While the relative incidence of the disease among the various species is difficult to determine from the veterinary literature, cats do appear to be more susceptible to the infection than dogs: in the VMTH series, there were 18 cases of feline cryptococcosis among 18,900 admissions (0.095 per cent), while only two cases were diagnosed in dogs in a total of 61,910 admissions (0.003 per cent) during a similar period. More cats than dogs were also affected at AMAH. A possible explanation is the prevalence of FeLV in the cat population, since it is conceivable that even transient viremia could impair the immune system sufficiently to allow establishment of a cryptococcal infection.

Differences in life style could also affect the incidence of the disease. The cat is a notoriously fastidious animal, and when allowed to go outdoors, it regularly digs in the soil before urinating or defecating. Its feet are thus likely to be in contact with most soil organisms, including *C. neoformans*. A further and possibly crucial habit peculiar to the cat is the frequency with which it grooms its head by licking its forepaws and rubbing them along its face. It could then directly inoculate some parts of its head with cryptococci much more often than the dog, in which this behavior is much less common. Lastly, feline nasal tissue may be particularly predisposed to cryptococcal infection—a possibility supported by results obtained after intracarotid inoculation of organisms, since all three cats infected with a large number of cryptococci ($8.0 \times 10^8$ colony-forming units) developed ipsilateral nasal lesions (Blouin and Cello, 1980). It is then tempting to speculate that not all nasal lesions found in the naturally occurring disease are due to a primary infection following direct inoculation, but that at least some are the consequence of hematogenous dissemination from another nidus of infection, for instance, a pulmonary lesion caused by inhalation of the organism.

## GEOTRICHOSIS

Geotrichosis is an uncommon disease in man but important because it may be misdiagnosed as blastomycosis unless differentiated by culture. Usually mild and chronic, it may take an oral, intestinal, bronchial, pulmonary, or cutaneous form. *Geotrichum*, species of which are saprophytes in nature and also inhabit the alimentary tract in many normal humans and animals, including the cat (Shields and Gaskin, 1977), appears in fresh preparations and tissues as striking barrel-shaped or cylindrical cells (arthrospores) 4 μ wide and 8 μ long, or as large subspherical cells 4 to 10 μ in diameter, the latter resembling *Blastomyces*. In mild human infections, iodides, neomycin, and nystatin have been reported to be effective; amphotericin B is recommended for severe cases (Martin and Nichols, 1960).

In a feline case, the organism was isolated at the Massachusetts State Laboratory from a nonhealing infection on the cat's back, from its stool, and also from a granulomatous infection of the skin and subcutis in its owner. The infection responded in both owner and cat to amphotericin B (Gray, 1958).

## HISTOPLASMOSIS

Histoplasmosis, first recognized in man in Panama in 1906, occurs in temperate and tropical climates throughout the world, predominantly in man and dogs but also in many other animals including the cat, opossum, fox, raccoon, and a number of rodents. In the United States, certain river valleys are areas of endemic infection, and states with high incidence are Arkansas, Indiana, Kansas, Kentucky, Missouri, Ohio, Tennessee, and Virginia. Surveys in those areas indicate a high rate of infection in both man and animals, but the vast majority of cases, being asymptomatic, go unrecognized and unreported. Since sporadic cases occur elsewhere, however, the physician and veterinarian cannot afford to overlook histoplasmosis as a possibility in certain types of illness.

Epidemiology is not a matter of host-to-host transmission but of a common environment in which both man and animals are exposed to the organism (e.g., Menges et al., 1954). The distribution of lesions and the occurrence of "epidemics" in which the disease was apparently acquired by inhalation of contaminated dust suggest that infection is most often by the respiratory route.

### Etiology and Epidemiology

*Histoplasma capsulatum* is a dimorphic fungus that grows naturally in soil or other sites where there is decayed manure of chickens, birds, and bats. Both in soil and on culture media (blood agar or Sabouraud's), on which it grows within about a month at temperatures below 35 C, it develops as a white or brown mold, producing two kinds of spores, spherical microconidia 3 to 4 μ in diameter and spherical or, rarely, club-shaped macroconidia 8 to 12 μ in diameter with finger-like projections. Yeast forms developing from these spores in mammalian hosts appear as delicate, budding, spherical or egg-shaped bodies, 2 or 3 μ wide and 3 or 4 μ long, in the cytoplasm of the cells of the reticuloendothelial system or lying free after rupture of the host cells. In fresh material, they stain with Giemsa's or Wright's stain. In tissue section stained with hematoxylin and eosin, they appear as central bodies surrounded by an unstained zone in turn encircled by a thin wall. With special fungus methods (PAS, Gridley, or Bauer stain), the wall only is stained, giving the appearance of an empty ring.

The prominent feature of the infection in man and animals generally is proliferation of reticuloendothelial tissue, the organism appearing in varying numbers in the cytoplasm of microphages and monocytes. In benign involvement, lesions tend to be focal and encapsulated. Thus "coin dot" shadows may be discovered in routine lung radiographs, and lymph nodes, particularly those draining the thoracic region, may contain walled-off nodules from which *Histoplasma* can be isolated.

In disseminated infections, which may be acute or subacute but are far more often chronic, clinical signs vary tremendously with the organs affected but commonly include fever, respiratory difficulty, diarrhea, wasting, anemia, jaundice, and ascites. Common organic changes are uniform enlargement of nodes, liver, and spleen due to reticuloendothelial proliferation, granulomatous bronchopneumonia, and chronic rugose or nodular enteritis, sometimes with ulceration. Central nervous symptoms occasionally result from brain involvement.

While substantial proportions of the cat population in areas surveyed in the United States have been shown, both by isolation of the organism and by microscopic lesions, to be infected (Emmons, 1949, 1950; Emmons et al., 1955; Rowley, 1956; Rowley et al., 1954), clinical disease is not often recognized. Those instances reported in North America occurred in Kansas (Gabbert et al., 1984; Mahaffey et al., 1977), Missouri (Breitschwerdt et al., 1977; Burk et al., 1978; Noxon et al., 1982; Peiffer and Belkin, 1979), New York (Bentinck-Smith et al., 1952; Weissman and Acampado, 1975), Ohio (Gwin et al., 1980), Oklahoma (Buckner, 1966; Quinn, 1982), Pennsylvania (McGrath, 1958), Texas (Blass, 1982; Goad and Roenick, 1983; Hall and Hurst, 1964; Stark, 1982), and Ontario (Nielsen, 1952; Percy, 1981; Soltys and Sumner-Smith, 1971). Information was not reported as to the place of origin or travels of the cats, except for the New York State cats, one born and reared in the state, the other taken briefly to Florida, and one of Buckner's patients, which had been purchased from a Texas farm that had chickens. Histoplasmosis was also recognized in a cat in Ankara, Turkey, where the disease occurs in man as well (Akün, 1950).

Incomplete data on breed, sex, and age indicate that of 13 cats, 4 were Siamese and 1 Abyssinian; of 12 in which sex was specified, 8 were male and 4 female; and in 18 cases ages ranged from three months to seven years.

## Clinical and Pathologic Features

Cats appear to be resistant to *Histoplasma* infection. In the handful of clinical cases described, respiratory involvement predominates. Signs of illness most often noted include inappetence, depression, weight loss, anemia, fever, nasal discharge, coughing, and dyspnea. Pulmonary involvement is not always evident radiographically but may be indicated by focal or miliary densities (Fig. 9–20). In most cases, the lungs were described at autopsy as having a gross appearance suggestive of bronchopneumonia. Focal, pale, firm areas or nodules are characteristic (Fig. 9–21). Typical microscopic changes are focal granulomatous pneumonia with proliferation of reticuloendothelial elements, diffuse infiltration with giant and round cells, areas of necrosis and liquefaction, and *Histoplasma* intracellularly in macrophages and also free within the alveoli. Tracheobronchial nodes, liver, spleen, and small intestine are frequently involved in disseminated disease, less often small intestine and kidneys. Watery feces flecked with fresh blood were associated in an emaciated febrile cat, with nodules and thickening of the terminal ileum and colon, involvement of mesenteric nodes, and peritoneal effusion (Stark, 1983). In a cat having a third episode of abortion and uterine hemorrhage, infection was present in the placenta as well as other organs (Buckner, 1966).

Less frequent accompaniments of disseminated disease are skin nodules that may ulcerate (Fig. 9–22), and swellings of several joints with draining tracts and sometimes underlying destruction of bone (Mahaffey et al., 1977). In another disseminated infection, swelling, edema, and lytic changes in the limbs were the prominent clinical feature (Goad and Roenick, 1983). Other complications of systemic infection are chorioretinitis and retinal detachment (Gwin et al., 1980; Mahaffey et al., 1977; Peiffer and Belkin, 1979; Quinn, 1982).

Rarely there may be suggestions of involvement of the nervous system (Mahaffey et al., 1977) or lesions in the brain (Buckner, 1966).

## Diagnosis

The diagnosis of histoplasmosis may sometimes be made ante mortem by biopsy of nodes or other tissues, and examination of Wright- or Giemsa-stained films of blood, marrow, exudates, sputum, transtracheal aspirate, or saline wash of chest or abdominal cavity (Weissman and Acampado, 1975), *Histoplasma* appearing in the mononuclear cells (Fig. 9–23). For blood examination, it is recommended that a sample be centrifuged and a film made from the white-cell layer, to increase the chances

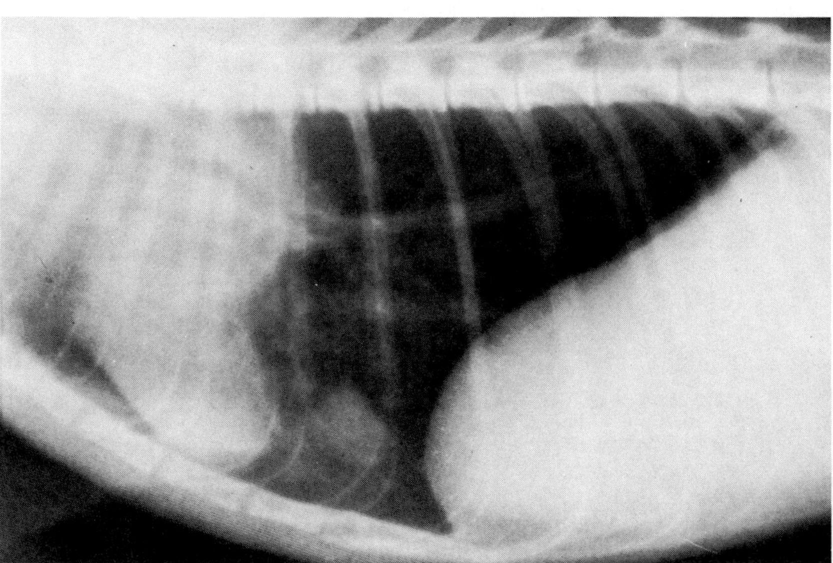

**Figure 9–20** Histoplasmosis of the lung in an adult cat in Oklahoma. A focal granuloma is evident as well as enlargement of the bronchial lymph nodes. (Courtesy Dr. R. Buckner.)

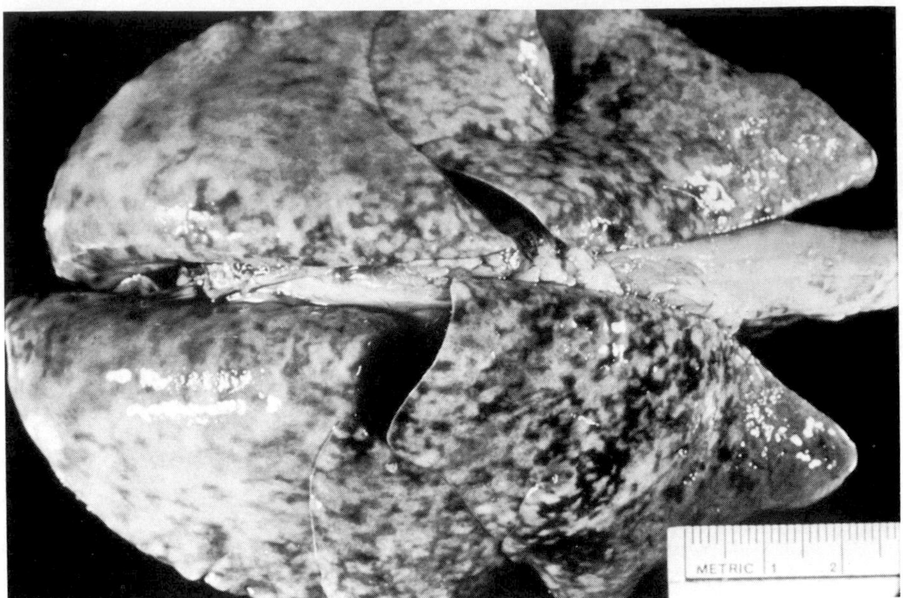


**Figure 9–21** Miliary granulomas of the lung in a cat with histoplasmosis. (From Breitschwerdt EB, Halliwell WH, Burk RL, et al.: J Am Anim Hosp Assoc 13 [1977] 216–222.)

of finding parasitized monocytes (Bentinck-Smith et al., 1952). To judge from surveys of cats in *Histoplasma* environments and from the experience in some clinical cases the serologic and histoplasmin skin tests cannot be relied on to give positive results in cats carrying infection (Breitschwerdt et al., 1977; Wolf and Belden, 1984). Few cats tested have been FeLV-positive.

For cultural isolation the organism grows well on blood-agar slants and certain other media (Emmons et al., 1977). The mouse is the choice for animal inoculation.

### Treatment

In treatment of human cases of disseminated histoplasmosis some successes have been reported with amphotericin B, and it appeared to be effective in a cat with pulmonary infection (Soltys and Sumner-Smith, 1971). Ketoconazole was reported to be successful in treatment of a case of disseminated infection (Noxon et al., 1982). Two courses of treatment were required (over six months total). The dose found to be effective was 20 mg/kg b.i.d. on alternate days. Response to treatment was monitored by determination of the complement fixation titer (a titer of 1:16 or over being considered evidence of active infection) and by lymph node aspirates and biopsy.

In the group of cats reported by Wolf and Belden (1984) many were too ill to be considered for treatment. Of four treated with amphotericin B, three were destroyed because of failure to improve; one of two treated with ketoconazole apparently recovered.

## PAECILOMYCOSIS

*Paecilomyces*, a genus of soil-inhabiting fungi morphologically resembling *Penicillium*, is sometimes found as a contaminant of skin and sputum of man. It has occasionally assumed a pathogenic role in both man and animals.

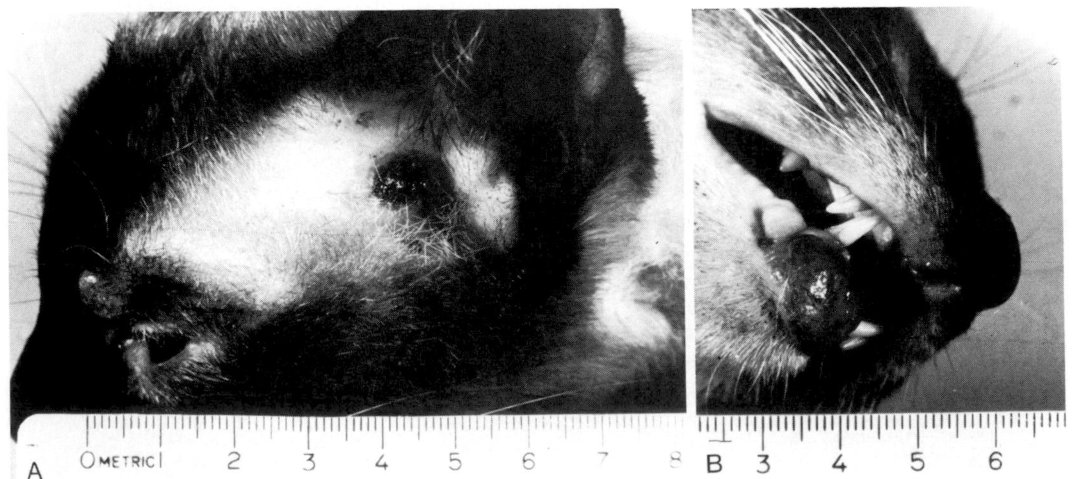


**Figure 9–22** Histoplasmosis of the skin: nodules on the face (*A*) and chin (*B*). (From Mahaffey E, Gabbert N, Johnson D, et al.: J Am Anim Hosp Assoc 13 [1977] 46–51.)

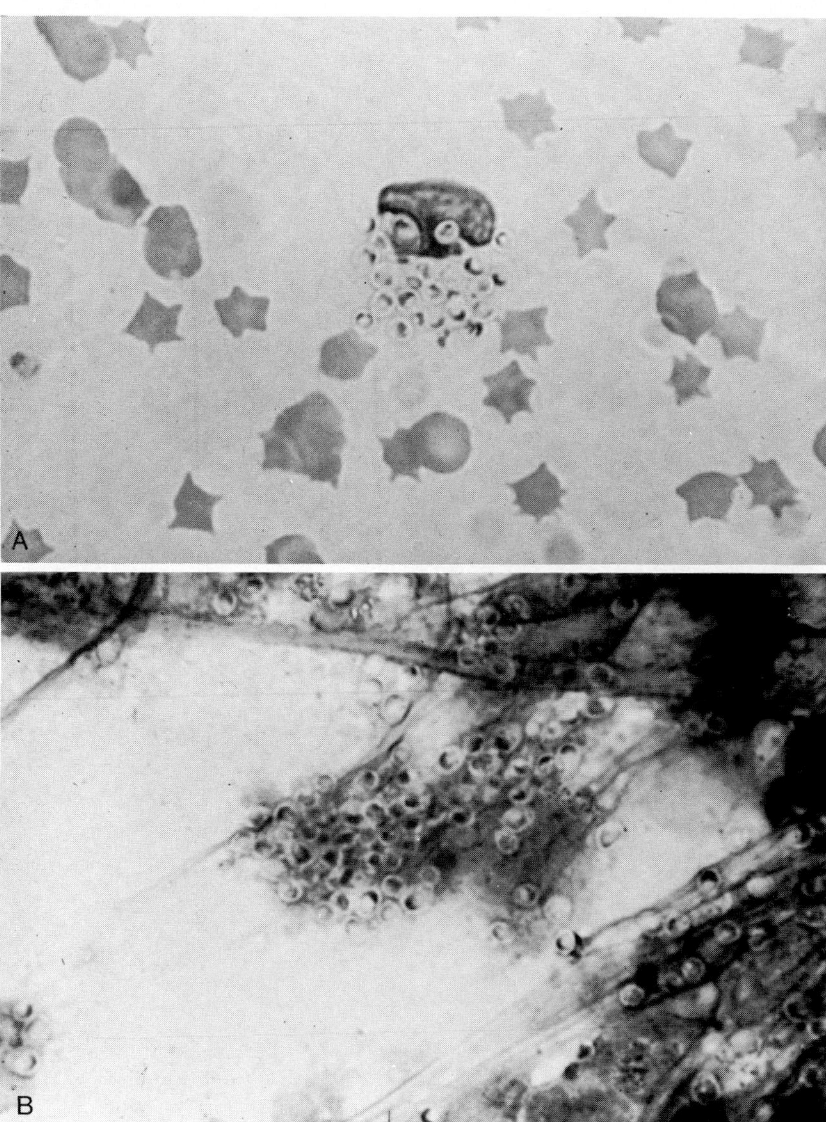


**Figure 9–23** *A*, *Histoplasma capsulatum* released from a ruptured monocyte in the blood of a cat. Wright-Giemsa, × 1000. *B*, Masses of organisms in the bone marrow of the same cat. (Courtesy Dr. R. Buckner.)

In an adult spayed female domestic shorthaired cat, *P. fumosoroseus* was the causal agent in a digital granuloma and subsequent nasal infection (Elliott et al., 1984). Surgical treatment and several months' medication with ketoconazole were ineffective. At autopsy, granulomas caused by the same organism were found in the liver and mesenteric lymph nodes.

## PENICILLIOSIS

Because of the ubiquity of species of *Penicillium* as contaminants, their isolation is often regarded as insignificant or incidental. Occasionally, however, they assume the role of serious pathogens by invading tissue, as in a middle-aged cat exhibiting protrusion of the third eyelids, progressive exophthalmos, facial edema, and finally sinusitis and rarefaction of the zygomatic arch (Peiffer et al., 1980). Autopsy disclosed paranasal, orbital, and pulmonary granulomas from which a species of *Penicillium* was cultured (Fig. 9–24).

## PHAEOHYPHOMYCOSIS

The term phaeohyphomycosis is applied to granulomatous nodules and abscesses usually single, usually involving only skin and subcutis, and caused by species of soil- and wood-dwelling fungi (e.g., *Phialophora, Drechslera*, and *Cladosporium* species) that produce dark (dematiaceous) hyphae and spores. These fungi are recognizable in both fresh preparations and fixed tissues stained with hematoxylin and eosin or fungus stains, but mycotic culture is required for definitive species identification. A characteristic draining, subcutaneous nodule is pictured by Muller et al. (1983). Typically, the lesions are walled off by connective tissue, and giant cells and epithelioid cells are numerous.

These infections are distinguished from mycetoma by absence of granule formation.

Such an infection was reported in a three-year-old Texas cat with an enlarged and ulcerated paw, from which *Brachycladium* (now *Drechslera*) *spiciferum* was repeatedly isolated (Bridges and Beasley, 1960). As there was

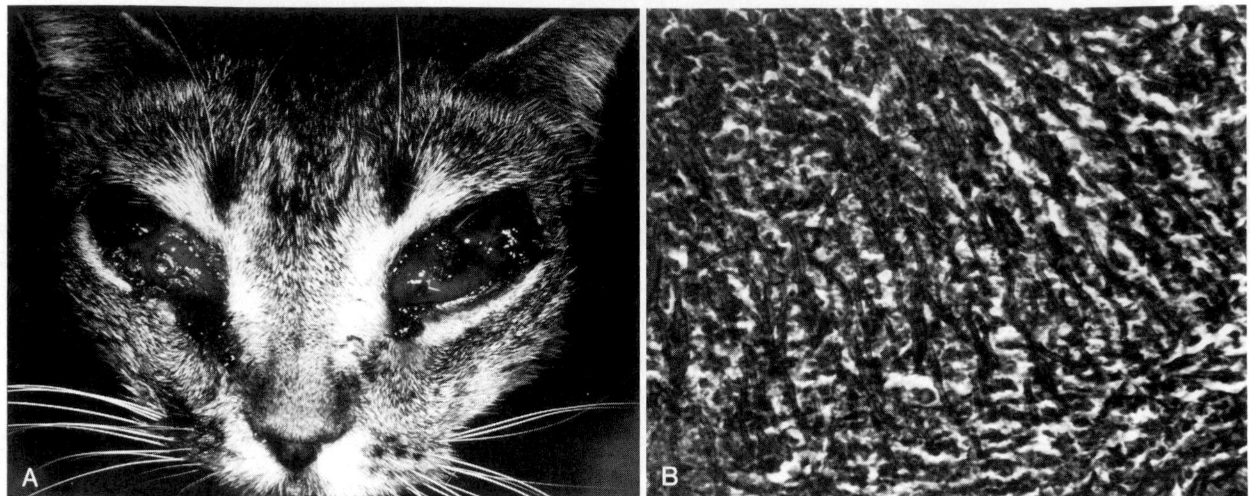


**Figure 9–24** *A*, *Penicillium* infection of nasal cavities and orbit resulted in bilateral exophthalmos, prolapsed and thickened third eyelids, and keratitis from exposure. *B*, Hyphae were observed at the margins of the orbital granulomas. (From Peiffer RL Jr, Belkin PV, Jenke BH: J Am Vet Med Assoc 176 [1980] 449–450.)

no response to a variety of agents, the cat was destroyed after three years. Another cat, a domestic neutered male with a thoracic nodule caused by the same agent and recurring over a six-year period despite surgery, was finally cured by total excision (Fig. 9–25; Muller et al., 1975).

Surgical excision was also successful in two other domestic cats, an adult female and a 10-year-old neutered male, with granulomas on the dorsal aspect of a foreleg. In both cases, *Phialophora* spp were identified on the basis of color and morphology in tissue sections (Fig. 9–26) (Haschek and Kasali, 1977; Hill et al., 1978). A granuloma from which *P. verrucosa* was cultured was excised from a cat's muzzle but recurred at the same site (Dion et al., 1982). In another cat a similar nasal mass from which *Exophiala jeanselmei* (formerly *Phialophora gougerotii*) was cultured was successfully removed by wide excision and cauterization (Bostock et al., 1982).

*Cladosporium bantianum*, a species closely related to *C. trichoides*, was isolated from a subcutaneous abscess

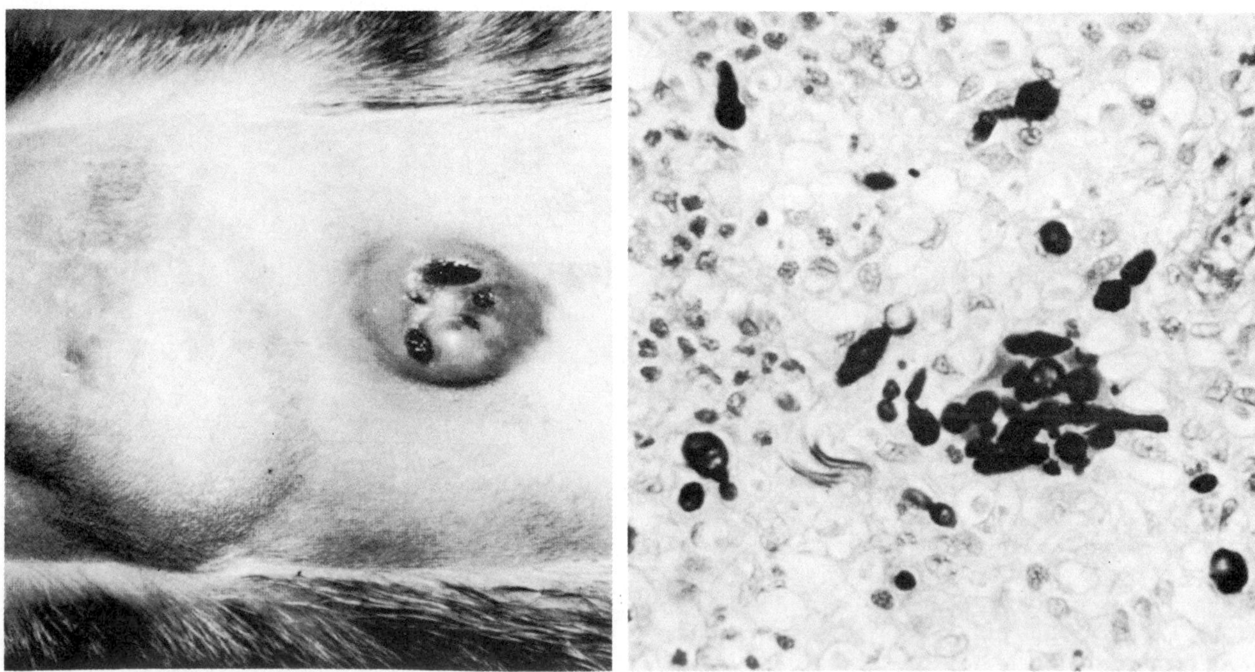

**Figure 9–25** Phaeohyphomycosis. *A*, Subcutaneous granulomas on the thorax and abdomen of a cat. *B*, Hyphae and chlamydospores of *Drechslera spicifera*. Gomori—H&E, × 500. (From Muller GH, Kaplan W, Ajello J, Padhye AA: Phaeohyphomycosis caused by *Drechslera spicifera* in a cat. J Am Vet Med Assoc 166 [1975] 150–153.)

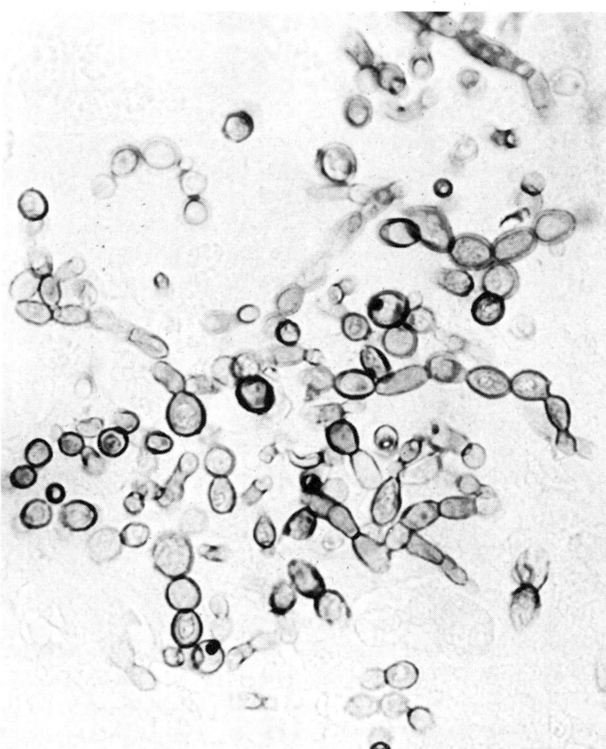

**Figure 9–26** *Phialophora* sp from a granuloma of the foreleg. Unstained, × 705. (From Hill JR, Migaki G, Phemister RD: Vet Pathol 15 [1978] 559–561.)

in a cat, but no clinical details were given (Kwon-Chung and deVries, 1983).

Simultaneous infection with two mycoses has been described (Sisk and Chandler, 1982). Small, deeply pigmented nodules containing pigmented septate mycelium compatible histologically with phaeohyphomycosis were removed from the upper lip of a cat with bilaterally enlarged mandibular lymph nodes. The cat was anorexic, anemic, and dyspneic, but post-mortem examination was permitted only for the lymph nodes, which contained cryptococci.

Surgical removal is clearly the treatment of choice whenever possible, but antifungal drugs have also achieved cures. Ketoconazole was used effectively for infection with a species of *Phialophora* on a cat's paw (Walton, cited by Muller et al., 1983). Satellite nodules developing on a cat's metatarsus after amputation of a toe infected with *P. verrucosa* were eliminated by combination treatment with amphotericin B and 5-fluorocytosine (5-FC). Over a 22-day period, amphotericin totalling 3.75 mg (0.5 mg/kg) was given IV on five occasions, as determined by levels of serum urea nitrogen, and 5-FC 95 mg orally t.i.d. (80 mg/kg) for 42 doses (McKeever et al., 1983).

In an otherwise healthy cat with a series of four skin masses that were excised from distal sites on the limbs, one yielded a species of *Stemphylium* and another a species of *Cladosporium*, isolated on potato flake agar (Sousa et al., 1984). The cat was treated with ketoconazole 50 mg b.i.d. for one month, then three times a week for another month. Eighteen months later there had been no recurrence of infection.

Rarely, fungi of these species affect deeper tissues. *Cladosporium trichoides* was reported from the kidney of a leukemic cat (Reed et al., 1974).

Phaeohyphomycosis of nervous tissue has been caused in man by several species of *Cladosporium* and *Phialophora* and has a predilection for the cerebrum.

Two cases of brain abscess caused by *C. trichoides* were reported in young male domestic shorthaired California cats (Jang et al., 1977). One had had fight injuries and a foreign body of the right eye a year before; the other had had a seizure several days before admission. Depression and other signs of central nervous disturbance were present in both. Autopsy disclosed areas of discoloration and softening in both brains, with histologically similar inflammation affecting meninges and both white and gray matter (Fig. 9–27). Fungal hyphae were found in vessel walls. Gram-stained impression smears disclosed occasionally branched septate hyphae and chains of dark-walled cells. On Sabouraud's medium, the fungal colonies were at first olive-colored, then brown, and finally black.

5-FC has been used in treatment of cladosporial brain abscesses in humans.

A pigmented corneal mass that eventually invaded the anterior chamber and iris in a six-year-old castrated male cat was shown by touch-impressions, sections, and cultures to be caused by a dematiaceous fungus tentatively identified as a species of *Cladosporium* (Miller et al., 1983). Treatment with miconazole was ineffective.

## PHYCOMYCOSIS-MUCORMYCOSIS

Mucormycosis includes infections caused by species of *Absidia, Mortierella, Mucor,* and *Rhizopus*. A more inclu-

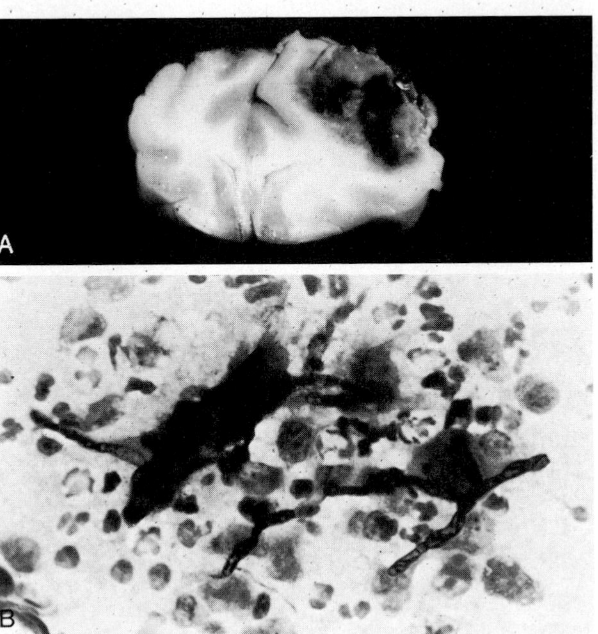


**Figure 9–27** *Cladosporium trichoides. A*, Darkly mottled abscess in the brain of a cat. *B*, Branched septate hyphae and dark-walled cells in a Gram-stained impression smear. × 400. (From Jang SS, Biberstein EL, Rinaldi ME, Henness AM, Boorman GA, Taylor RF: Sabouraudia 15 [1977] 115–123.)

sive term, phycomycosis, has sometimes been used to designate infections with these and other phycomycetes as well (Emmons et al., 1977).

In mucormycosis of man, especially diabetics, fulminating infections of sinuses, orbit, and brain may end in death, even before a diagnosis can be made. The lungs and gastrointestinal tract may be involved in disseminated disease. Chronic lesions of the skin and subcutis also occur. Other illness and treatment with antibiotics, corticosteroids, and anticancer drugs may be predisposing factors.

Species identification requires culture, but most cases of mucormycosis are recognizable in tissue sections because of the very broad, haphazardly branching and rarely septate hyphae that stain excellently with hematoxylin but often poorly with special fungus stains. Neutrophilic reaction, necrosis, and vascular invasion and thrombosis are characteristic.

Mucormycosis, most often involving the intestine, has been reported in a number of cats, mostly young and in several of which panleukopenia was considered to be the primary disease (Fox et al., 1978; König et al., 1967; Nielsen, 1962; Schiefer, 1965). Most of the cats had received treatment with antibiotics or antibiotics and steroids. One cat was FeLV-positive and one leukopenic (Ader, 1979). *Absidia corymbifera* was cultured from an intestinal ulcer in one of the panleukopenia cases (Nielsen, 1962).

At AMAH two young cats that may have had panleukopenia died as a result of mucormycosis with perforation at the ileocolic junction, and jejunal mucormycosis was diagnosed in another cat with subleukemic leukemia.

Diabetes, as evidenced by significantly elevated blood or urine sugar has, in several cats, been associated with mucormycosis. In one, a hemorrhagic infarct of the cardiac lobe of the right lung was caused by a large thrombus, containing masses of hyphae, in a branch of the pulmonary artery (Loupal, 1982). At AMAH, mucormycosis of the intestine was found at autopsy of a diabetic cat, and mucormycosis of the retropharyngeal node in a cat that died with leukopenia, anemia, and a 4+ urine sugar after a month's treatment of unilateral conjunctivitis with antibiotics and a corticosteroid.

In another cat at AMAH, the infection took a limited superficial form, being localized in a mass that was excised from a footpad.

Disseminated disease is apparently uncommon, but was reported, in a nine-month-old cat that was ill for four months, as involving all visceral organs and the central nervous system (Ader, 1979).

*Mortierella parasitica* was isolated from the trachea of a cat dying of asphyxia (Costantin, 1892), and *Mucor pusillus* from the brain of a cat suspected of rabies when it died soon after biting its owner during a vaccination (Ravisse et al., 1978).

## SPOROTRICHOSIS

Sporotrichosis is a fungus disease affecting both man and animals, the horse most frequently among the latter. Distribution is worldwide in tropical and temperate zones; the Missouri and Mississippi river valleys are areas of endemic infection.

### Etiology and Epidemiology

The causative organism, *Sporothrix (Sporotrichum) schenckii*, occurs naturally in soil and on plants and is believed to gain entrance into the host by way of an injury to the skin. In man, a number of cases have resulted from handling salt hay or peat moss. A nodule develops at the site of the wound, and additional nodules may form along lymphatic trunks. Sometimes the nodules ulcerate, releasing a creamy pus. Infections persist indefinitely, unless treated systemically. Rarely the disease generalizes to skin, viscera, bones, joints, and nervous system. Open lesions are potentially infectious to man (Read and Sperling, 1982; Singer and Muncie, 1952) and to other animals and should be handled with suitable precautions.

The organism is usually Gram-positive. In pus or tissue it occurs as a spindle- or cigar-shaped body about 3 to 5 μ long and reproduces by budding at one end (Fig. 9–28). Frequently it is situated in polymorphonuclear leukocytes. As the agent often escapes detection in exudates or in tissue sections, even when the latter are stained with PAS or Gridley techniques, cultures are of more diagnostic value than smears or histopathologic methods. Cells in tissue may be identified by the fluorescent antibody technique (Werner et al., 1971).

*Sporothrix schenckii* is easily grown from pus from young lesions on Sabouraud's dextrose agar, brain-heart broth, or Emmon's glucose-neopeptone agar at 25 to 35 C. The colonies are at first small, white, and shiny, resembling those of bacteria. There is a short, aerial, cotton-like mycelium. As growth continues, the color of the colonies becomes cream, tan, coffee-brown, or black. Mice and rats are preferred for animal inoculation.

Sporotrichosis appears to be rare in cats, but an increasing number of published and word-of-mouth reports suggest that serious efforts at diagnosis might reveal a higher incidence of infection than has hitherto been recognized.

### Clinical and Pathologic Features

The first report of feline infection, from Long Island, New York, described leg ulcers in two cats that played in a pile of peat moss (Singer and Muncie, 1952). After eight months of ineffective remedies the diagnosis was finally made by cultures. The owner, who cared for the cats for some months, herself acquired the infection. The fate of the cats was not described, but the owner's infection eventually responded to treatment with potassium iodide. In similar cases persons handling cats with open lesions became infected (Nusbaum et al., 1983; Read and Sperling, 1982).

Sporotrichosis was also reported in a six-year-old Brazilian cat, in which nodules appeared at first in the skin of one foreleg but ultimately involved much of the body. There were extensive areas of ulceration, some of which were crusted. The cat had a fever, neutrophilia, and anemia, and all palpable nodes were enlarged. An autopsy was not obtained, but terminal loss of appetite, wasting, and dyspnea suggested that the condition might have generalized (Freitas et al., 1956). The diagnosis was made by culturing of pus. Subsequently, eight more feline infections were encountered in Brazil (Freitas et al., 1965).

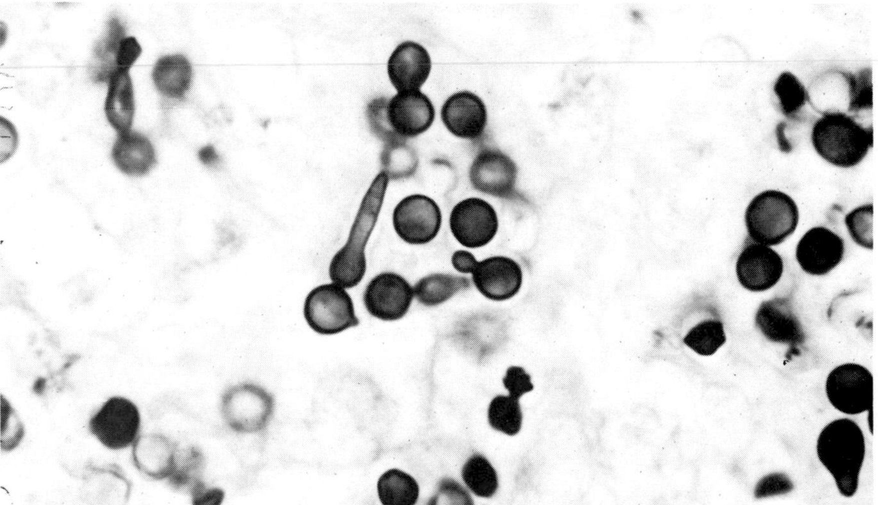

**Figure 9–28** *Sporotrichum schenckii* budding forms and pseudohyphae in the dermis of a cat. Gomori's methenamine silver, × 1000. (From Werner RE, Levine BG, Kaplan W, Hall WL, Nilles BJ, O'Rourke MD: J Am Vet Med Assoc 159 [1971] 407–411.)

Cutaneous infection with multiple lesions has been reported in two Siamese cats, an adult in which an initial head lesion had been treated unsuccessfully as a dermatophyte with topical and systemic antifungal medication (Werner et al., 1971) and a one-year-old castrated male in which a digit was first involved (Anderson et al., 1973). The first cat was destroyed without an attempt at specific treatment, the second after it reacted poorly to potassium iodide. In a luckier cat, treatment was successful (Fig. 9–29).

Disseminated infection developed in a three-year-old intact male domestic shorthair in which a granulomatous lesion on a toepad of the right forepaw had failed to respond to topical antibiotic and antifungal medication and oral antibiotics (Kier et al., 1979). After a month all pads of the foot were involved and the lesion had extended proximally for 3 cm. In biopsy sections stained with PAS and Grocott's stain the characteristic cigar-shaped, single-budded organisms of *S. schenckii* were easily detected, a method of identification ordinarily said to be unreliable. Given a poor prognosis, the owner surrendered the cat for further study. It was not reported to have a fever and a hemogram was unremarkable, but within three weeks it became weak, failed to eat, and died. At autopsy the fungus was found in the enlarged right axillary node and in the lung and liver. The organism was isolated on Sabouraud's agar and blood agar, and the infection was reproduced by animal inoculation (cat, mouse). The organism was also studied in detail by electron microscopy (Garrison et al., 1979).

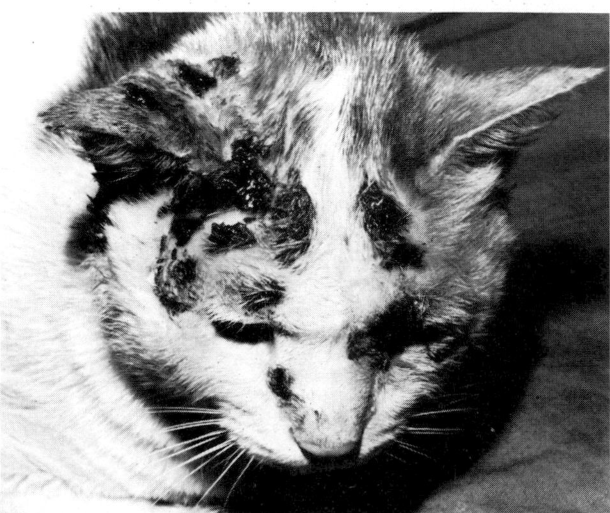

**Figure 9–29** Sporotrichosis. Multiple cutaneous granulomas of the head responded to oral treatment with potassium iodide, 20 per cent, three drops twice daily, for five weeks. (Personal communication and photograph courtesy Dr. G. H. Muller.)

## Treatment

As treatment of cutaneous infection, oral administration of iodides is often very effective. Potassium iodide in aqueous solution is generally used (Emmons et al., 1977), but Scott (1980) recommends a 20 per cent aqueous sodium iodide solution at a dosage of 0.1 ml/kg every 12 to 24 hours. It may be given in milk or food. Cats are highly sensitive to iodine in any form and must be watched for signs of toxicity, such as depression, inappetence, vomiting, muscular twitching, subnormal temperature, and cardiovascular collapse. At the first sign of unfavorable reaction, treatment should be halted. It should be resumed at a lower dose when the cat returns to normal and should be continued for three or four weeks after apparent recovery (Emmons et al., 1977).

Cutaneolymphatic sporotrichosis in a cat with multiple open ulcers was treated successfully by a sequential regimen of ketoconazole and sodium iodide (Burke et al., 1983). Ketoconazole given for two months at 5 mg/kg b.i.d. brought about only partial resolution of the lesions, but subsequent treatment for about five weeks with oral doses of sodium iodide (20 mg/kg b.i.d.) brought about apparently complete resolution of this infection.

Treatment of experimental sporotrichosis with ketoconazole and with potassium iodide indicated that both drugs are effective, but the cats did not take to the "food ball" method of administration so that it was uncertain how much of the drugs they actually consumed, and residual infection was found in lymph nodes of some clinically asymptomatic cats (Raimer et al., 1983). In several cats in which the experimentally induced lesions regressed with no treatment, administration of methylprednisolone reactivated the lesions (MacDonald et al., 1980; Raimer et al., 1983). The results of this work suggest that either drug must be given in adequate dosage and continued for some time after all clinical signs have resolved.

Disseminated infection has responded dramatically in some human cases to amphotericin B, but its use for this purpose was unsuccessful in one instance (Nusbaum et al., 1983).

## MYCETOMAS (MADURAMYCOSIS)

A mycetoma is a localized swelling involving skin, subcutis, and bone, with abscesses and granulomas discharging granule-containing pus through fistulous tracts (Emmons et al., 1977). The granules vary in color and size according to the bacterium or fungus that produces them. Mycetomas caused by *Actinomyces, Streptomyces*, and *Nocardia* are described in the chapter on bacterial infection. Fungi associated with mycetoma include species of *Madurella, Allescheria, Cephalosporium, Curvularia,* and *Aspergillus* (Emmons et al., 1977).

Such infections are not contagious; whatever the part of the body involved, the infection results from injury to the skin and inoculation of the organism by way of the wound. Most of the agents are believed to come from soil, plants, or decaying organic matter. Mycetomas occur in temperate and tropical areas about the world but, in man at least, are most frequent in India and Africa.

Examination of the granules may suggest to an experienced mycologist the identity of the agent in a given infection, but culturing is required for positive identification. To avoid contamination, material is best obtained from deep tissues.

Although mycetomas most often affect the limbs, *Cephalosporium potronii*, a member of the group of Fungi Imperfecti, was reported to be the causative agent in a tumor-like swelling on the underside of the tongue and floor of a cat's mouth (van den Akker, 1952).

In a middle-aged spayed female domestic shorthair first presented to a California veterinarian in 1957 (Craige, 1957–1961), a bulbous swelling in the subcutis over the bridge of the nose seemed to respond to thorough curettage but recurred early in 1958. A smear showed a branched fungus resembling *Candida*. Local treatment with nystatin brought only transient improvement. In January 1959 the cat received two intravenous doses of amphotericin B 48 hours apart. As the second dose evoked a severe reaction, this form of treatment was not repeated. The lesion remained inactive for almost two years but flared up again in December 1960, when the organism was finally identified by culture as *Madurella grisea* (Emmons, 1961). A solution of amphotericin B injected two or three times directly into the lesion caused it to regress, but another appeared nearby and two on the hind feet, presumably because of the cat's scratching its face. These lesions also were apparently cleared up by local infiltration with amphotericin, but the cat became listless, inappetent, and progressively wasted, finally dying in September 1961. An autopsy was not permitted.

A polypoid mycetoma in which an unidentified fungus was associated with bluish granules was removed from the ear canal of a four-year-old domestic male cat at AMAH.

In two extraordinary and strikingly similar cases, *Microsporum canis* was the cause of mycetomas. In a case spanning nine years, a three-year-old male tabby Persian was first admitted at AMAH in 1957 from a cattery where the infection was endemic. The cat also had soft masses on its back under an old scar, where it had been clawed by a rival stud. During examination, the scar broke down, discharging a tan, granular, gelatinous material (Fig. 9–30). Biopsy of the skin and subcutis disclosed a granulomatous reaction to a fungus. This was identified by culture at both AMAH and the Massachusetts State Laboratory as *M. canis* (Gray, 1957). After extensive débridement and treatment with griseofulvin, the lesion appeared to heal.

During the following eight years the cat was treated intermittently with griseofulvin for generalized cutaneous ringworm but would become leukopenic and anemic, so that a full course of the drug could never be given. The owner would then treat the cat with prednisone as a "tonic and conditioner."

The mycetomas recurred at least five times, once as a mass in an ear that grossly resembled a ceruminous gland tumor (Fig. 9–31). The fungus, examined on two occasions by Dr. Chester Emmons at the National Institutes of Health, was characterized by him as *M. canis* of atypical morphology, perhaps owing to chronicity and the unusual subcutaneous location.

At the time of the cat's death in 1966, shortly after removal of an intestinal leiomyoma, mycetomas, 0.5 to 3 cm in diameter, were widespread over the body. One, in the groin (Fig. 9–32), was associated with an enlarged inguinal node in which the same dermatophyte was recognized microscopically.

A strong predisposing factor in the persisting mycosis was probably the owner's lavish use of corticosteroids as an appetite stimulant and general conditioner.

In 1975 a mycetoma caused by *M. canis* was reported in a French cat, also a Persian male, treated for ringworm in 1966 and scratched one year later at the base of the tail by another cat (Boudin et al., 1975). In 1970 a swelling diagnosed microscopically as a fatty cyst had been removed from the base of the tail, but in 1971 and 1972 pea-sized swellings recurring at the same site were removed and diagnosed at the veterinary school at Alfort as "dermal mycotic granuloma of maduromycotic type." Late in 1973 new swellings appeared, this time with ulcerations and granules. In 1974 the Institut Pasteur cultured *M. canis* from the granules. Two months' treatment with griseofulvin caused the suppuration and discharge of granules to cease, and scar formation was under way when the cat died of chronic nephritis.

Two other cases of deep dermatophytosis have been reported by Tuttle and Chandler (1983). In the first, the agent was identified as *M. canis* and at the time of writing surgical excision had apparently been succesful.

The term "pseudomycetoma" has been suggested for these dermatophyte aggregates (Ajello et al., 1980).

## PROTOTHECOSIS

Protothecosis is a cutaneous or disseminated disease of man and animals included by courtesy among the mycoses,

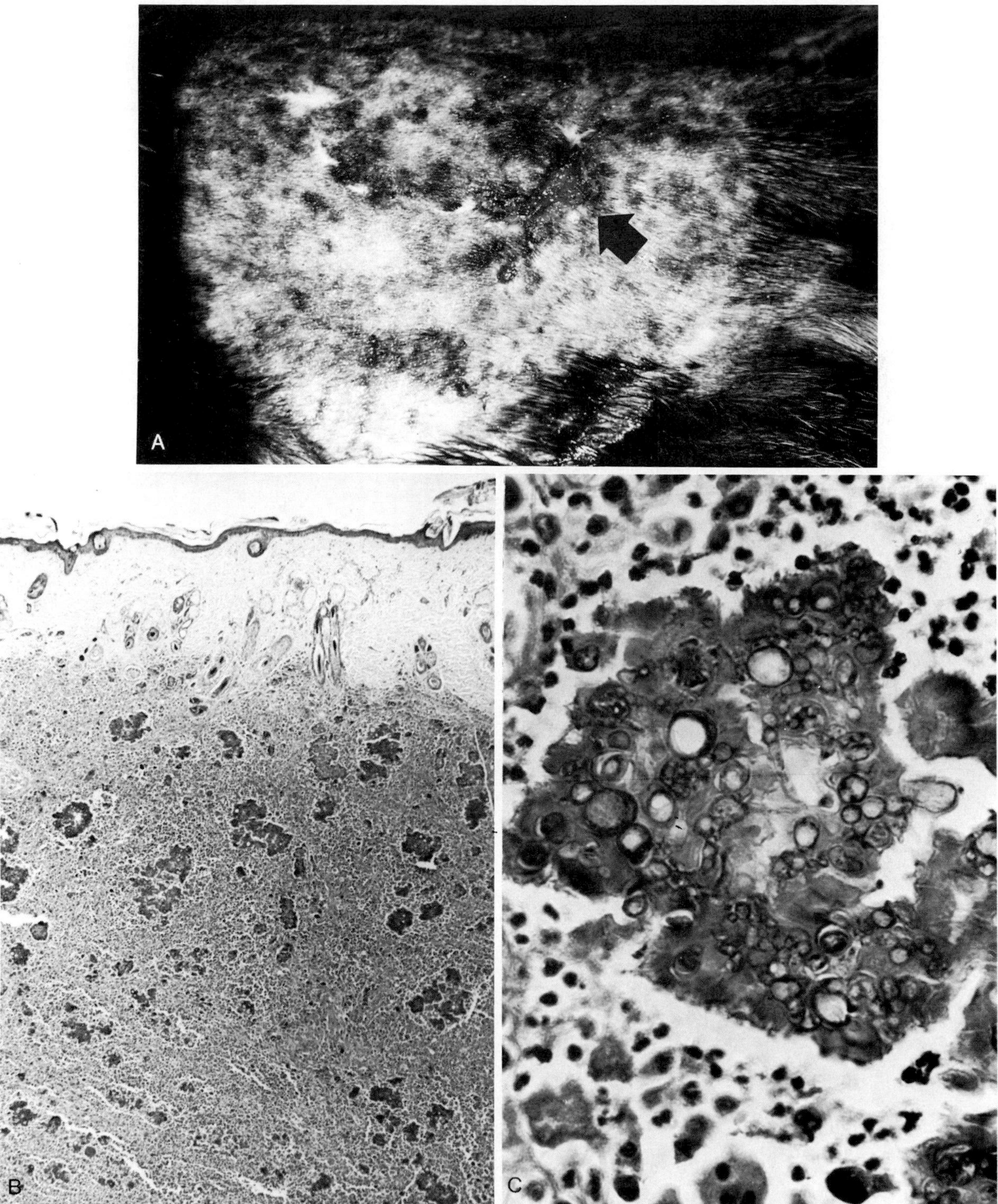

**Figure 9–30** *A*, *M. canis* mycetoma, three-year-old Persian male with patchy dermatomycosis and an old scar on its back from which gelatinous, fungus-containing material (arrow) broke out from time to time. *B*, Granulomatous inflammation of dermis and subcutis of the back. Numerous dark-staining fungal colonies are scattered throughout. PAS, × 30. *C*, Pyogranuloma having in its center multiple hyphae cut at various angles. PAS, × 500.

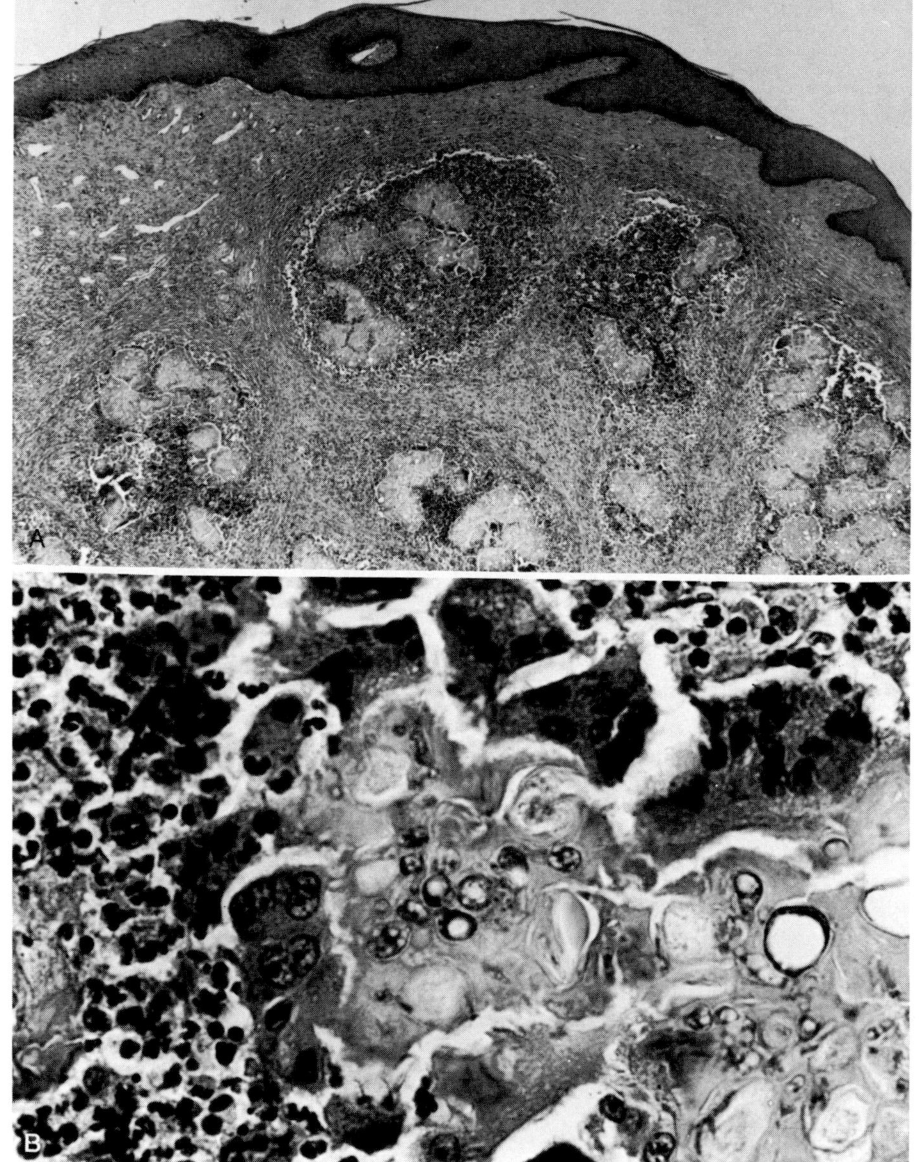


**Figure 9–31** *A*, *M. canis* mycetoma. Under the epithelium of the ear canal are multiple mycotic granulomas. H&E, × 200. *B*, Numerous multinucleated giant cells characteristic of a mature granuloma surround a focus of hyphae. PAS, × 500.

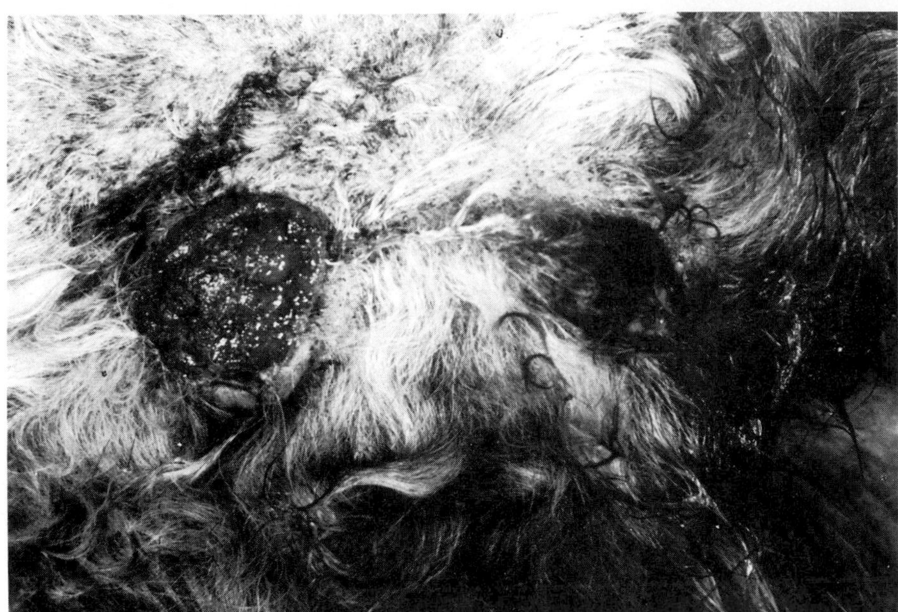

**Figure 9–32** *M. canis* mycetoma of the groin appearing cranial to the prepuce (right) as a proliferative cutaneous mass.

although *Prototheca* is actually a colorless alga. It is a saprophyte in moist areas of the environment.

*Prototheca* occurred as a pathogen in a soft, subcutaneous mass on the left tarsus of an elderly Georgia cat. Involving arteries and nerves, the mass could not be completely excised but when it recurred did not affect the cat's general health adversely (Kaplan et al., 1976). Microscopically, granulomatous inflammation was associated with numerous spherical, oval, and crescent-shaped, nonbudding organisms, many in epithelioid or giant cells, but not within blood vessels. The organisms measured 2 to 20 μ in diameter and were multiplying by endosporulation. Their structures stained best with Gridley stain and they were identified specifically as *P. wickerhamii* by cultural tests and immunofluorescence.

A similar infection with *P. wickerhamii* was reported in an eight-year-old Australian cat with a soft, pliable mass involving a tarsal pad and infiltrating among the metatarsal bones and adjacent tendons. Organisms were present in the associated popliteal lymph node (Coloe and Allison, 1982).

A third case of protothecosis was recognized by histologic examination in a 16-mm nodule removed from the skin of the forehead of a 16-year-old male domestic Australian cat and stained with Grocott-Gomori methenamine silver (Finnie and Coloe, 1981). Cultural identification of the organism was impossible, as the specimen was submitted in formalin.

## REFERENCES

### Mycotic Diseases—General


Ainsworth GC, Austwick PKC: Fungal Diseases of Animals, 2nd ed. Commonwealth Agricultural Bureau. Farnham Royal, England, 1973.

Conant NF, Smith DT, Baker RD, Calloway JL, Martin DS: Manual of Clinical Mycology, 3rd ed. Philadelphia, WB Saunders Company, 1971.

Emmons CW, Binford CH, Utz JP, Kwon-Chung KJ: Medical Mycology, 3rd ed. Philadelphia, Lea & Febiger, 1977.

Horne RD: Feline systemic mycoses: an up-to-date review. Mod Vet Pract 45(1) (1964) 39–46.

Jungerman PF, Schwartzman RM: Veterinary Medical Mycology. Philadelphia, Lea & Febiger, 1972.

Kaplan W: Epidemiology of the principal systemic mycoses of man and lower animals and the ecology of their etiologic agents. J Am Vet Med Assoc 163 (1973) 1043–1047.

Köhler H, Kuttin E, Kaplan W, Burtscher H, Grünberg W, Swoboda R: Einige Beobachtungen über das Auftreten von System-Mykosen in Österreich. Zentralblatt Veterinärmed B25 (1978) 785–799.

Kral F, Schwartzman RM: Veterinary and Comparative Dermatology. Philadelphia, JB Lippincott Company, 1964.

Muller GH, Kirk RW, Scott DW: Small Animal Dermatology, 3rd ed. Philadelphia, WB Saunders Company, 1983.

Nielsen SW: Infectious granulomas. *In* Joest E: Handbuch der Speziellen Pathologischen Anatomie der Haustiere, 3rd ed. Berlin, Paul Parey, 1962, Vol 2, 590–632.

Rippon JW: Medical Mycology: The Pathogenic Fungi and the Pathogenic Actinomycetes, 2nd ed. Philadelphia, WB Saunders Company, 1982.

Scott DW: Feline dermatology 1900–1978: a monograph. J Am Anim Hosp Assoc 16 (1980) 331–459.

Vanbreuseghem R (transl J Wilkinson): Mycoses of Man and Animals. Springfield, IL, Charles C Thomas, 1959.


### Dermatophytoses (Ringworm)


Ajello L: The dermatophyte, *Microsporum gypseum,* as a saprophyte and parasite. J Invest Dermatol 21 (1953) 157–171.

Anderson RK: Dermatomycosis in a cat [*T. mentagrophytes*]. Feline Pract 7 (4) (1977) 19–20, 23.

Blank F: Favus of mice. Can J Microbiol 3 (1957) 885–896.

Bone WJ, Jackson WF: Pathogenic fungi in dermatitis: Incidence in two small animal practices in Florida. Vet Med Small Anim Clin 69 (1971) 140–142.

Connole MD: Keratinophilic fungi on cats and dogs. Sabouraudia 4 (1965) 45–48.

Conroy JD: *Microsporum* infections in cats. J Am Vet Med Assoc 145 (1964) 115–121.

de Almeida F, da Silva AC, Brandao CH, Monteiro EL, Moura RA: Saprofitismo do *Microsporum canis* em gatos. Rev Inst Adolfo Lutz 10 (1950) 49–52.

Dreisörner H, Refai M, Rieth H: Otitis externa durch Microsporum canis bei Katzen. Kleintierpraxis 9 (1964) 230–234.

Fitzgerald NW, McCarthy MD, Taylor BB: Isolation of Microsporum distortum from skin lesions of humans and cats in Otago. NZ Med J 70 (1969) 320–321.

Fuentes CA, Bosch ZE, Boudet CC: Occurrence of *Trichophyton mentagrophytes* and *Microsporum gypseum* on hairs of healthy cats. J Invest Dermatol 23 (1954) 311–313.

Georg LK: The diagnosis of ringworm in animals. Vet Med 49 (1954) 157–166.

Georg LK, Roberts CS, Menges RW, Kaplan W: *Trichophyton mentagrophytes* infections in dogs and cats. J Am Vet Med Assoc 130 (1957) 427–432.

Hill BNR: Ringworm diseases affecting the cat. NZ Vet J 4 (1956) 157–160.

Hoerlein AR: Studies on animal dermatomycoses. I. Clinical studies. II. Cultural studies. Cornell Vet 35 (1945) 287–298, 299–307.

Horne RD: Mycotic diseases. *In* Catcott EJ (ed): Feline Medicine and Surgery, 2nd ed. Santa Barbara, American Veterinary Publications Inc, 1975.

Kaplan W: Personal communication, 1965.

Kaplan W: Dermatophytosis (ringworm, dermatomycosis). *In* Kirk RW (ed): Current Veterinary Therapy III. Philadelphia, WB Saunders, 1968.

Kaplan W, Ajello L: Oral treatment of spontaneous ringworm in cats with griseofulvin. J Am Vet Med Assoc 135 (1959) 253–261.

Kaplan W, Georg LK, Bromley CL: Ringworm in cats caused by *Microsporum gypseum.* Vet Med 52 (1957) 347–349.

Kaplan W, Ivens MS: Observations on the seasonal variations in incidence of ringworm in dogs and cats in the United States. Sabouraudia 1 (1961) 91–102.

Keep JM: The viability of *Microsporum canis* on isolated cat hair. Aust Vet J 36 (1960) 277–278.

Komuro S, Aoki Y, Odashima S: On *Microsporon sapporense.* Sapporo Med J 3 (1952) 1–13.

Kral F: Classification, symptomatology, and recurrent treatment of animal dermatomycoses (ringworm). J Am Vet Med Assoc 127 (1955) 395–402.

La Touche CJ: Some clinical and microscopic features of *Microsporum canis* Bodin infection of the skin and its appendages as it occurs in the cat. Vet Rec 65 (1953) 680–681.

La Touche CJ: Onychomycosis in cats infected by *Microsporum canis* Bodin. Vet Rec 67 (1955) 578–579.

Levine HB, Cobb JM, Friedman RH: Griseofulvin in dimethyl sulfoxide: Penetration into guinea pig skin and clinical findings in feline ringworm. Sabouraudia 9 (1971) 43–49.

Lueker DC, Kainer RA: Hyperthermia for the treatment of dermatomycosis in dogs and cats. Vet Med Small Anim 76 (1981) 658.

Menges RW, Georg LK: Animal ringworm study. Vet Med 50 (1955a) 293–297.

Menges RW, Georg LK: Observations on feline ringworm caused by *Microsporum canis* and its public health significance. Proc Am Vet Med Assoc (1955b) 471–474.

Milian and Karatchentzeff: Epidémie de trichophytie propagée par un chat. Bull Soc Fr Derm Syphilol 42 (1935) 944–945.

Mosher CL, Langendoen K, Stoddard P: Treatment of ringworm *(Microsporum canis)* with inactivated fungal vaccine. Vet Med Small Anim Clin 72 (1977) 1343–1345.

Petrak M: Griseofulvin in the treatment of ringworm in cats. Proc Am Anim Hosp Assoc, 1960, 149–151.

Petrak M: Personal communication, 1962.

Refai M, Miligy M: Trichophyton rubrum infection in a family transmitted from a cat. Mykosen 11 (1968) 191–194.

Rose WR: Small animal clinical otology: Otitis externa—4: Otomycosis. Vet Med Small Anim Clin 71 (1976) 1025–1026, 1029.

Scott DW, Kirk RW, Bentinck-Smith J: Dermatophytosis due to *Trichophyton terrestre* infection in a dog and cat. J Am Anim Hosp Assoc 16 (1980) 53–59.

Scott FW, de Lahunta A, Schultz RD, Bistner SI, Riis RC: Teratogenesis in cats associated with griseofulvin therapy. Teratology 11 (1975) 79–86.

Senser F: *Penicillium martensii* Biourge als Erreger einer Mycose. Zentralblatt Bakt I (Orig) 200 (1966) 519–524.

Sternfels M: Ringworm—an effective treatment in cats. North Am Vet 39 (Feb 1, 1958) 48.

Trice ER, Shafer JC: Occurrence of Microsporum gypseum (M. fulvum) infection in the District of Columbia area. Arch Dermatol Syphilol 64 (1951) 309–313.

Woodard DC: Ketoconazole therapy for *Microsporum* spp. dermatophytes in cats. Feline Pract 13 (5) (1983) 28–29.


**Aspergillosis**


Bolton GR, Brown TT: Mycotic colitis in a cat. Vet Med Small Anim Clin 67 (1972) 879–891.

Buckley H: Seminar on Fungus Diseases given at Angell Memorial Animal Hospital, 1977.

Cotter SM, Gilmore CE, Rollins C: Multiple cases of feline leukemia and feline infectious peritonitis in a household. J Am Vet Med Assoc 162 (1973) 1054–1058.

DeWailly PH: Personal communication, 1967.

Fox JG, Murphy JC, Shalev M: Systemic fungal infections in cats. J Am Vet Med Assoc 173 (1978) 1191–1195.

Kirkpatrick RM: Mycotic cystitis in a male cat. Vet Med Small Anim Clin 77 (1982) 1365–1371.

Köhler H, Kuttin E, Kaplan W, Burtscher H, Grünberg W, Swoboda R: Einige Beobachtungen über das Auftreten von System-Mykosen in Österreich. Zentralblatt Veterinärmed B25 (1978) 785–799.

Lane JG: Rhinitis and sinusitis in the dog. *In* Kirk RW (ed): Current Veterinary Therapy VI. Philadelphia, WB Saunders Company, 1977.

McCausland IP: Systemic mycoses of two cats. NZ Vet J 20 (1972) 10–12.

Nielsen SW: Personal communication, 1956.

Pakes SP, New AE, Benbrook SE: Pulmonary aspergillosis in a cat. J Am Vet Med Assoc 151 (1967) 950–953.

Sautter JH, Steele DS, Henry JF: Aspergillosis in a cat. Symposium on granulomatous disease—Part 2. J Am Vet Med Assoc 127 (1955) 515–523.

Schiefer B: Zur Histopathologie der durch Candida-, Aspergillus- und Mucor-Arten verursachten Darmmykosen bei Katzen mit Panleukopenie. Dtsch Tierärztl Wochenschr 72 (1965) 73–76.

Schmidt GM: Mycotic keratoconjunctivitis. Vet Med Small Anim Clin 69 (1974) 1177–1179.

Stokes R: Intestinal mycosis in a cat. Can Vet J 49 (1973) 499–500.

Vogler GA, Wagner JE: What's your diagnosis? [Aspergillosis, lung, colon, secondary to panleukopenia.] Lab Anim 5(5) (1976) 14, 16.

Weiland F: Darmmykosen bei einer Katze. Dtsch Tierärztl Wochenschr 77 (1970) 232–237.

Wilkinson GT, Sutton RH, Grono LR: *Aspergillus* spp infection associated with orbital cellulitis and sinusitis in a cat. J Small Anim Pract 23 (1982) 127–131.


**Blastomycosis**


Alden CL, Mohan R: Ocular blastomycosis in a cat. J Am Vet Med Assoc 164 (1974) 527–528.

Breshears DE: What is your diagnosis? [Blastomycosis of lungs and mediastinal lymph node in a cat.] J Am Vet Med Assoc 152 (1968) 1555–1556.

Campbell KL, Humphrey JA, Ramsey GH: Cutaneous blastomycosis. Feline Pract 10(3) (1980) 28, 30, 32.

Easton KL: Cutaneous North American blastomycosis in a Siamese cat—case report. Can Vet J 2 (1961) 350–351.

Hatkin JM, Phillips WE, Utroska WR: Two cases of feline blastomycosis. J Am Anim Hosp Assoc 15 (1979) 217–220.

Jasmin AM, Carroll JM, Baucom JN, Beusse DO: Systemic blastomycosis in Siamese cats. Vet Med Small Anim Clin 64 (1969) 33–37.

Legendre AM: Personal communication, 1984.

McDonough ES, Kuzma JF: Epidemiological studies on blasto-

mycosis in the state of Wisconsin. Sabouraudia 18 (1980) 173–183.
McGrath JT: Personal communication, 1958.
Nasisse MP, van Ee RT, Wright B: Ocular changes in a cat with disseminated blastomycosis. J Am Vet Med Assoc 187 (1985) 629–631.
Neunzig RJ: Epidemiology, diagnosis, and treatment of canine and feline blastomycosis. Vet Med Small Anim Clin 78 (1983) 1081–1085, 1088.
Sheldon WG: Pulmonary blastomycosis in a cat. Lab Anim Care 16 (1966) 280–285.

**Candidiasis**

Langheinrich KA, Nielsen SW: Histopathology of feline panleukopenia: A report of 65 cases. J Am Vet Med Assoc 158 (1971) 863–872.
McCausland IP: Systemic mycoses of two cats. NZ Vet J 20 (1972) 10–12.
McCaw D, Franklin R, Fales W, Stockham S, Lattimer J: Pyothorax caused by *Candida albicans* in a cat. J Am Vet Med Assoc 185 (1984) 311–312.
Schiefer B: Zur Histopathologie der durch Candida-, Aspergillus- und Mucor-Arten verursachten Darmmykosen bei Katzen mit Panleukopenie. Dtsch Tierärztl Wochenschr 72 (1965) 73–76.
Schiefer B, Weiss E: Soormykose des Darmes bei Katzen. Dtsch Tierärztl Wochenschr 66 (1959) 275–277.
Small E: Candidiasis (Moniliasis). *In* Kirk RW (ed): Current Veterinary Therapy VI. Philadelphia, WB Saunders Company, 1974.

**Coccidioidomycosis**

Angell JA, Shively JN, Merideth RE, Reed RE, Jamison KC: Ocular coccidioidomycosis in a cat. J Am Vet Med Assoc 187 (1985) 167–169.
Attleberger MH: Systemic mycoses. *In* Kirk RW (ed): Current Veterinary Therapy VIII. Philadelphia, WB Saunders Company, 1983.
Fiese MJ: Coccidioidomycosis. Springfield, IL, Charles C Thomas, 1958.
Reed RE, Hoge RS, Trautman RJ: Coccidioidomycosis in two cats. J Am Vet Med Assoc 143 (1963) 953–956.
Schwartz W: *Coccidioides immitis* infection in a cat. Southwest Vet 34 (1981) 94.
Wolf AM: Primary cutaneous coccidioidomycosis in a dog and a cat. J Am Vet Med Assoc 174 (1979) 504–506.

**Cryptococcosis**

Ajello L: Comparative ecology of respiratory mycotic disease agents. Bacteriol Rev 31 (1967) 6–24.
Barrett RE, Scott DW: Treatment of feline cryptococcosis: literature review and case report. J Am Anim Hosp Assoc 11 (1975) 511–518.
Beauregard M, Malkin KL: Cryptococcosis in a cat: a case report. Can J Public Health 61 (1970) 547–549.
Benham RW: The genus of *Cryptococcus*: the present status and criteria for the identification of the species. Trans NY Acad Sci 17 (1955) 418–429.
Bennett JE, Dismukes WE, Duma RJ, Medoff G, Sande MA, Gallis H, Leonard J, Fields BT, Bradshaw M, Haywood H, McGee ZA, Cate TR, Cobbs CG, Warner JF, Alling DW: A comparison of amphotericin B alone and combined with flucytosine in the treatment of cryptococcosis. N Engl J Med 301 (1979) 126–131.
Bennett JE, Hasenclever HF: *Cryptococcus neoformans* polysaccharide: studies of serologic properties and role in infection. J Immunol 94 (1965) 916–920.
Bennett JE, Hasenclever HF, Tynes BS: Detection of cryptococcal polysaccharide in serum and spinal fluid; value in diagnosis and prognosis. Trans Assoc Am Physicians 77 (1964) 145–150.
Bennett JE, Kwon-Chung KJ, Howard DH: Epidemiologic differences among serotypes of *Cryptococcus neoformans*. Am J Epidemiol 105 (1977) 582–586.
Beyt BE Jr, Waltman SR: Cryptococcal endophthalmitis after corneal transplantation. N Engl J Med 298 (1978) 825–826.
Bindschadler DD, Bennett JE: Serology of human cryptococcosis. Ann Intern Med 69 (1968) 45–52.
Blouin P: Experimental feline cryptococcosis: characteristics and pathogenesis of ocular lesions. PhD thesis, University of California (Davis), 1979.
Blouin P, Cello RM: Experimental ocular cryptococcosis: preliminary studies in cats and mice. Invest Ophthalmol Vis Sci 19 (1980) 21–30.
Brewer WG Jr: Treatment of cryptococcosis in a cat with 5-fluorocytosine. Sci Proc Am Coll Vet Int Med, 1980, 111.
Brown RJ, Nowlin CL, Taylor DR, O'Neill TP: Dermal cryptococcosis in a cat. Mod Vet Pract 59 (1978) 447.
Bulmer GS, Sans MD: *Cryptococcus neoformans*. III. Inhibition of phagocytosis. J Bacteriol 95 (1968) 5–8.
Chiba T, Kato Y, Nonogaki M: Cryptococcosis in a cat mistakingly [sic] diagnosed as a peritoneal neoplasm. J Jpn Vet Med Assoc 20 (1967) 287–288.
Curtis AF: A case of torulosis in a domestic cat. Australas J Med Technol 1 (1951) 71–74.
Drouhet E, Othman T, Guesdon JL, Dupont B: Humoral immunity in cryptococcosis: study of serum antibodies by enzymatic immunological techniques as compared with classical techniques. Bull Soc Fr Mycol Med 8 (1979) 41–44.
Duckworth RH, Taylor DES, Julian AF: *Neoformans* infection in a cat. Vet Rec 96 (1975) 48.
Edwards VE, Sutherland JM, Tyrer JH: Cryptococcosis of the central nervous system. Epidemiological, clinical, and therapeutic features. J Neurosurg Psychiatr 33 (1970) 415–425.
Emmons CW, Binford CH, Utz JP, Kwon-Chung KJ: Medical Mycology. Philadelphia, Lea & Febiger, 1977.
Essex M: Horizontally and vertically transmitted oncornaviruses of cats. Adv Cancer Res 21 (1975) 175–248.
Fischer CA: Intraocular cryptococcosis in two cats. J Am Vet Med Assoc 158 (1971) 191–198.
Gadebusch HH, Pansy F, Klepner C, Schwind R: Amphotericin B and amphotericin B methyl ester ascorbate. I Chemotherapeutic activity against *Candida albicans, Cryptococcus neoformans,* and *Blastomyces dermatitidis* in mice. J Infect Dis 134 (1976) 423–427.
Gordon MA, Vedder DK: Serologic tests in diagnosis and prognosis of cryptococcosis. J Am Med Assoc 197 (1966) 961–967.
Graybill JR, Craven PC, Mitchell LF, Drutz DJ: Interaction of chemotherapy and immune defenses in experimental murine cryptococcosis. Antimicrob Agents Chemother 14 (1978) 659–667.
Graybill JR, Drutz DJ: Host defense in cryptococcosis: II. Cryptococcosis in the nude mouse. Cell Immunol 40 (1978) 263–274.
Graybill JR, Levine HB: Successful treatment of cryptococcal meningitis with intraventricular miconazole. Arch Intern Med 138 (1978) 814–816.
Graybill JR, Mitchell L, Levine HB: Treatment of experimental murine cryptococcosis: a comparison of miconazole and amphotericin B. Antimicrob Agents Chemother 13 (1978) 277–283.
Griner LA, Walch HA: Cryptococcosis in columbiformes at the San Diego Zoo. J Wildl Dis 14 (1978) 389–394.
Gross PA, Patel C, Spitler LE: Disseminated *Cryptococcus* treated with transfer factor. J Am Med Assoc 240 (1978) 2460–2462.
Gwin RM, Gelatt KN, Hardy R, Peiffer RL Jr, Williams LW: Ocular cryptococcosis in a cat. J Am Anim Hosp Assoc 13 (1977) 680–684.
Hardy WD JR, McClelland AJ, Zuckerman EE, Hess PW, Essex M, Cotter SM, MacEwen EG, Hayes AA: Prevention of the contagious spread of feline leukemia virus and the development of leukemia in pet cats. Nature 263 (1976) 326–328.

Holzworth J: Cryptococcosis in a cat. Cornell Vet 42 (1952) 12–15.

Jimbow T, Tejima Y, Ikemoto H: Comparison between 5-fluorocytosine, amphotericin B and the combined administration of these agents in the therapeutic effectiveness for cryptococcal meningitis. Chemotherapy 24 (1978) 374–389.

Kaufman L, Blumer S: Value and interpretation of serological tests for the diagnosis of cryptococcosis. Applied Microbiol 16 (1968) 1907–1912.

Kreger–van Rij NJW: The genus *Cryptococcus*. Ann Soc Belge Med Trop 44 (1964) 601–610.

Kwon-Chung KJ: A new genus, *Filobasidiella,* the perfect state of *Cryptococcus neoformans*. Mycologia 67 (1975) 1197–1200.

Kwon-Chung KJ: A new species of *Filobasidiella,* the sexual state of *Cryptococcus neoformans* B and C serotypes. Mycologia 68 (1976) 942–946.

Legendre AM, Gompf R, Bone D: Treatment of feline cryptococcosis with ketoconazole. J Am Vet Med Assoc 181 (1982) 1541–1542.

Littman ML: Cryptococcosis (torulosis). Current concepts and therapy. Am J Med 27 (1959) 976–998.

Littman ML, Walter JE: Cryptococcosis: current status. Am J Med 45 (1968) 922–932.

Littman ML, Zimmerman LE: Cryptococcosis, Torulosis, or European Blastomycosis. New York, Grune & Stratton, Inc, 1956.

Lodder J: The Yeasts, a Taxonomic Study. Amsterdam, North-Holland Publishing Company, 1970.

MacKinnon S, Kane JG, Parker RH: False-positive cryptococcal antigen test and cervical prevertebral abscess. J Am Med Assoc 240 (1978) 1982–1983.

Madewell BR, Holmberg CA, Ackerman N: Lymphosarcoma and cryptococcosis in a cat. J Am Vet Med Assoc 175 (1979) 65–68.

McDonald A: Case report of three mycotic infections. Southwest Vet 21 (1968) 239–240.

Medleau L, Hall EJ, Goldschmidt MH, Irby N: Cutaneous cryptococcosis in three cats. J Am Vet Med Assoc 187 (1985) 169–170.

Meyers FH, Jawetz E, Goldfien A: Review of Medical Pharmacology, 7th ed. Los Altos, Lange Medical Publications, 1980.

Migaki G, Gunnels RD, Casey HW: Pulmonary cryptococcosis in an Atlantic bottlenosed dolphin (*Tursiops truncatus*). Lab Anim Sci 28 (1978) 603–606.

Monga DP, Kumar R, Mohapatra LN, Malaviya AN: Experimental cryptococcosis in normal and B-cell-deficient mice. Infect Immun 26 (1979) 1–3.

Moore R: Treatment of feline nasal cryptococcosis with 5-flucytosine. J Am Vet Med Assoc 181 (1982) 816–817.

Neilson JB, Fromtling RA, Bulmer GS: *Cryptococcus neoformans:* size range of infectious particles from aerosolized soil. Infect Immun 17 (1977) 634–638.

Olander HJ, Reed H, Pier AC: Feline cryptococcosis. J Am Vet Med Assoc 142 (1963) 138–143.

Palumbo NE, Perri S: Amphotericin B therapy in two cases of feline cryptococcosis. Vet Med Small Anim Clin 70 (1975) 553–557.

Pappagianis D: Epidemiological aspects of respiratory mycotic infections. Bacteriol Rev 31 (1967) 25–34.

Perryman LE, Hoover EA, Yohn DS: Immunologic reactivity of the cat: immunosuppression in experimental feline leukemia. J Nat Cancer Inst 49 (1972) 1357–1365.

Powell KE, Dahl BA, Weeks RJ, Tosh FE: Airborne *Cryptococcus neoformans:* particles from pigeon excreta compatible with alveolar deposition. J Infect Dis 125 (1972) 412–415.

Prevost E, McKee JM, Crawford P: Successful medical management of severe feline cryptococcosis. J Am Anim Hosp Assoc 18 (1982) 111–114.

Prevost E, Newell R: Commercial cryptococcal latex kit: clinical evaluation in a medical center hospital. J Clin Microbiol 8 (1978) 529–533.

Rippon JW: Medical Mycology. The Pathogenic Fungi and the Pathogenic Actinomycetes, 2nd ed. Philadelphia, WB Saunders Company, 1982.

Rosenthal JJ, Heidgerd J, Peiffer RL Jr: Ocular and systemic cryptococcosis in a cat. J Am Anim Hosp Assoc 17 (1981) 307–310.

Rutman MA, Rickards DA, Chandler FW: Feline cryptococcosis. Feline Pract 5(3) (1975) 36–43.

Ryer K, Ryer J: A case of feline mycotic rhinitis caused by *Cryptococcus neoformans*. Vet Med Small Anim Clin 76 (1981) 1150–1151.

Saez H, Rinjard J, Battesti MR: Cryptococcosis in a fennec, *Fennecus zerda:* characteristics and differentiation of *Cryptococcus neoformans*. Bull Soc Fr Mycol Med 7 (1978) 69–72.

Squire RA, Bush M: Comments on treatment of leukemia in the cat. J Am Vet Med Assoc 158 (1971) 1134–1136.

Swenson FJ, Kozel TR: Phagocytosis of *Cryptococcus neoformans* by normal and thioglycolate-activated macrophages. Infect Immun 21 (1978) 714–720.

Thrall MA, Rich LJ, Freemyer FG: Feline cryptococcosis treatment with amphotericin B. Feline Pract 6(3) (1976) 15–28.

Weir EC, Schwartz A, Buergelt CD: Short-term combination chemotherapy for treatment of feline cryptococcosis. J Am Vet Med Assoc 174 (1979) 507–510.

Wilkinson GT: Feline cryptococcosis: a review and seven case reports. J Small Anim Pract 20 (1979) 749–768.

Wilkinson GT, Bate MJ, Robins GM, Croker A: Successful treatment of four cases of feline cryptococcosis. J Small Anim Pract 24 (1983) 507–514.

**Geotrichosis**

Gray J: Personal communication, 1958.

Martin WJ, Nichols DR: Current practices in general medicine 15. The mycoses. Proc Staff Meet, Mayo Clin 35 (1960) 149–161.

Shields RP, Gaskin JM: Total generalized rhinotracheitis in a young adult cat. J Am Vet Med Assoc 170 (1977) 439–441.

**Histoplasmosis**

Akün RS: Histoplasmosis in a cat. J Am Vet Med Assoc 117 (1950) 43–44.

Bentinck-Smith J, Kennedy PC, Saunders LZ: Histoplasmosis in a dog. Cornell Vet 42 (1952) 61–66.

Blass CE: Histoplasmosis in a cat. J Am Anim Hosp Assoc 18 (1982) 468–470.

Breitschwerdt EB, Halliwell WH, Burk RL, Schmidt DA: Feline histoplasmosis. J Am Anim Hosp Assoc 13 (1977) 216–221.

Buckner G: Personal communication, 1966.

Burk RL, Corley EA, Corwin LA Jr: The radiographic appearance of pulmonary histoplasmosis in the dog and cat: A review of 37 case histories. J Am Vet Radiol Soc 19 (1978) 2–7.

Emmons CW: Histoplasmosis in animals. Trans NY Acad Sci Ser II 2 (1949) 248–254.

Emmons CW: Histoplasmosis: animal reservoirs and other sources in nature of the pathogenic fungus, histoplasma. Am J Publ Health 40 (1950) 436–440.

Emmons CW, Rowley DA, Olson BJ, Mattern CFT, Bell JA, Powell E, Marcy EA: Histoplasmosis. Proved occurrence of inapparent infection in dogs, cats and other animals. Am J Hyg 61 (1955) 40–44.

Gabbert NH, Campbell TW, Beiermann RL: Pancytopenia associated with disseminated histoplasmosis in a cat. J Am Anim Hosp Assoc 20 (1984) 119–122.

Goad MEP, Roenick WJ: Osseous histoplasmosis in a cat. Feline Pract 13 (2) (1983) 32–36.

Gwin RM, Makley TA Jr, Wyman M, Werling K: Multifocal

ocular histoplasmosis in a dog and cat. J Am Vet Med Assoc 176 (1980) 638–642.

Hall JE, Hurst HL: Personal communication, 1964.

Mahaffey E, Gabbert N, Johnson D, Guffy M: Disseminated histoplasmosis in three cats. J Am Anim Hosp Assoc 13 (1977) 46–51.

McGrath JT: Personal communication, 1958.

Menges RW: The histoplasmin skin test in animals. J Am Vet Med Assoc 119 (1951) 69–71.

Menges RW, Furcolow ML, Habermann RT: An outbreak of histoplasmosis involving animals and man. Am J Vet Res 15 (1954) 520–524.

Nielsen SW: Personal communication, 1952.

Noxon JO, Digilio K, Schmidt DA: Disseminated histoplasmosis in a cat: Successful treatment with ketoconazole. J Am Vet Med Assoc 181 (1982) 817–820.

Peiffer RL, Belkin PV: Ocular manifestations of disseminated histoplasmosis in a cat. Feline Pract 9 (4) (1979) 24–29.

Percy DH: Feline histoplasmosis with ocular involvement. Vet Pathol 18 (1981) 163–169.

Quinn AJ: Granulomatous chorioretinitis of disseminated histoplasmosis. Proc Am Soc Vet Ophthalmol Int Soc Ophthalmol, Las Vegas, 1982, 159–163.

Rowley DA: Pathological studies of histoplasmosis; preliminary report on fifty cats and fifty dogs from Loudoun County, Virginia. Publ Health Monogr 39 (1956) 268–271.

Rowley DA, Habermann RT, Emmons CW: Histoplasmosis: pathologic studies of fifty cats and fifty dogs from Loudoun County, Virginia. J Infect Dis 95 (1954) 98–108.

Soltys MA, Sumner-Smith G: Systemic mycoses in dogs and cats. Can Vet J 12(10) (1971) 191–199.

Stark DR: Primary gastrointestinal histoplasmosis in a cat. J Am Anim Hosp Assoc 18 (1982) 154–156.

Weissman S, Acampado EE: Primary pulmonary histoplasmosis in a cat. Feline Pract 5(5) (1975) 28.

**Paecilomycosis**

Elliott GS, Whitney MS, Reed WM, Tuite JF: Antemortem diagnosis of paecilomycosis in a cat. J Am Vet Med Assoc 184 (1984) 93–94.

**Penicilliosis**

Peiffer RL, Belkin PV, Jenke BH: Orbital cellulitis, sinusitis, and pneumonitis caused by *Penicillium* sp in a cat. J Am Vet Med Assoc 176 (1980) 449–450.

**Phaeohyphomycosis-Chromomycosis**

Bostock DE, Coloe PJ, Castellani A: Phaeohyphomycosis caused by *Exophiala jeanselmei* in a domestic cat. J Comp Pathol 92 (1982) 479–482.

Bridges C, Beasley JN: Maduromycotic mycetomas in animals—*Brachycladium spiciferum* Bainier as an etiologic agent. J Am Vet Med Assoc 137 (1960) 192–201.

Dion WM, Pukay BP, Bundza A: Feline cutaneous phaeohyphomycosis caused by *Phialophora verrucosa.* Can Vet J 23 (1982) 48–49.

Haschek WM, Kasali OB: A case of cutaneous feline phaeohyphomycosis caused by *Phialophora gougerotii.* Cornell Vet 67 (1977) 467–471.

Hill JR, Migaki G, Phemister RD: Phaeomycotic granuloma in a cat. Vet Pathol 15 (1978) 559–561.

Jang SS, Biberstein EL, Rinaldi MG, Henness AM, Boorman GA, Taylor RF: Feline brain abscesses due to *Cladosporium trichoides.* Sabouraudia 15 (1977) 115–123.

Kwon-Chung KJ, de Vries GA: Comparative study of an isolate resembling Banti's fungus with *Cladosporium trichoides.* Sabouraudia 21 (1983) 59–72.

McKeever PJ, Caywood DD, Perman V: Chromomycosis in a cat: Successful medical therapy. J Am Anim Hosp 19 (1983) 533–536.

Miller DM, Blue JL, Winston SM: Keratomycosis caused by *Cladosporium* sp in a cat. J Am Vet Med Assoc 182 (1983) 1121–1122.

Muller GH, Kaplan W, Ajello J, Padhye AA: Phaeohyphomycosis caused by *Drechslera specifera* in a cat. J Am Vet Med Assoc 166 (975) 150–153.

Muller GH, Kirk RW, Scott DW: Small Animal Dermatology, 3rd ed. Philadelphia, WB Saunders Company, 1983.

Reed C, Fox JG, Campbell LH: Leukaemia in a cat with concurrent *Cladosporium* infection. J Small Anim Pract 15 (1974) 55–62.

Sisk DB, Chandler FW: Phaeohyphomycosis and cryptococcosis in a cat. Vet Pathol 19 (1982) 554–556.

Sousa CA, Ihrke PJ, Culbertson R: Subcutaneous phaeohyphomycosis (*Stemphylium* sp and *Cladosporium* sp) infections in a cat. J Am Vet Med Assoc 185 (1984) 671–673.

**Phycomycosis-Mucormycosis**

Ader PL: Phycomycosis in fifteen dogs and two cats. J Am Vet Med Assoc 174 (1979) 1216–1223.

Costantin [no init]: Note sur un cas de pneumomycose observé sur un chat par M. Neumann. Bull Soc Mycol Fr 8 (1892) 57–59.

Fox JG, Murphy JC, Shalev M: Systemic fungal infections in cats. J Am Vet Med Assoc 173 (1978) 1191–1195.

König H, Nicolet J, Lindt W, Raaflaub W: Einige Mucormykosen bei Rind, Schwein, Katze, Reh und Flamingo. Schweiz Arch Tierheilk 109 (1967) 260–268.

Loupal G: Hämorrhagischer Lungeninfarkt infolge Mukormykose bei einer Katze mit Diabetes mellitus. Dtsch Tierärztl Wochenschr 89 (1982) 104–107 (Abstr Vet Bull 1982, 6210).

Nielsen SW: Infectious granulomas. *In* Joest E (ed): Handbuch der Speziellen Pathologischen Anatomie der Haustiere, 3rd ed. Berlin, Paul Parey, 1962, Vol 2, 590–632.

Ravisse P, Fromentin H, Destombes P, Mariat F: Mucormycose cérébrale du chat due à Mucor pusillus. Sabouraudia 16 (1978) 291–298.

Schiefer B: Zur Histopathologie der durch Candida-, Aspergillus- und Mucor-Arten verursachten Darmmykosen bei Katzen mit Panleukopenie. Dtsch Tierärzl Wochenschr 72 (1965) 73–76.

**Sporotrichosis**

Anderson NV, Ivoghli D, Moore WE, Leipold HW: Cutaneous sporotrichosis in a cat: A case report. J Am Anim Hosp Assoc 9 (1973) 526–529.

Burke MJ, Grauer GF, Macy DW: Successful treatment of cutaneolymphatic sporotrichosis in a cat with ketoconazole and sodium iodide. J Am Anim Hosp Assoc 19 (1983) 542–547.

Freitas DC, Migliano MF, Zani Neto L: Esporotricose: observacao de caso espontaneo em gato domestico (F. catus, L.). Rev Sao Paulo, U Fac Med Vet 5 (1956) 601–604.

Freitas DC, Moreno G, Saliba AM, Bottino JA, Mos EN: Esporotricose em caes e gatos. Rev Sao Paulo, U Fac Med Vet 7 (1965) 381–387.

Garrison RG, Boyd KS, Kier AB, Wagner JE: Spontaneous feline sporotrichosis: A fine structural study. Mycopathologia 69 (1979) 57–62.

Kier AB, Mann PB, Wagner JE: Disseminated sporotrichosis in a cat. J Am Vet Med Assoc 175 (1979) 202–204.

MacDonald E, Ewert A, Reitmeyer JC: Reappearance of *Sporothrix schenckii* lesions after administration of Solu-Medrol[R] to infected cats. Sabouraudia 18 (1980) 295–300.

Nusbaum BP, Gulbas N, Horwitz SN: Sporotrichosis acquired from a cat. J Am Acad Dermatol 8 (1983) 386–391.

Raimer SS, Ewert A, MacDonald EM, Reitmeyer JC, Dotson AD, Mader JT: Ketoconazole therapy of experimentally induced sporotrichosis infections in cats: a preliminary study. Curr Ther Res 33 (1983) 670–680.

Read SI, Sperling LC: Feline sporotrichosis transmission to man. Arch Dermatol 118 (1982) 429–431.

Singer JI, Muncie JE: Sporotrichosis: etiologic considerations and report of additional cases from New York. NY State J Med 52 (1952) 2147–2153.

Werner RE, Levine BG, Kaplan W, Hall WL, Nilles BJ, O'Rourke MD: Sporotrichosis in a cat. J Am Vet Med Assoc 159 (1971) 407–411.

**Mycetomas**

Ajello L, Kaplan W, Chandler FW: Dermatophyte mycetomas: Fact or fiction? Proc 5th Internat Conf Mycoses, Pan Am Health Organ Sci Publ 396 (1980) 135–140.

Bourdin M, Destombes P, Parodi AL, Drouhet E, Segretain G: Première observation d'un mycétome à *Microsporum canis* chez un chat. Recl Méd Vét 151 (1975) 475–480.

Craige JE: Personal communication, biopsy, and culture, 1957–1961.

Emmons CW: Personal communications, 1959, 1961.

Gray J: Personal communication, 1957.

Tuttle PA, Chandler FW: Deep dermatophytosis in a cat. J Am Vet Med Assoc 183 (1983) 1106–1108.

van den Akker S: Een Schimmelinfectie *(Cephalosporium potronii)* in de mondholte van een kat. Tijdschr Diergeneeskd 77 (1952) 515–516.

**Protothecosis**

Coloe PJ, Allison JF: Protothecosis in a cat. J Am Vet Med Assoc 180 (1982) 78–79.

Finnie JW, Coloe PJ: Cutaneous protothecosis in a cat. Aust Vet J 57 (1981) 307–308.

Kaplan W, Chandler FW, Holzinger EA, Plue RE, Dickinson RO: Protothecosis in a cat: First recorded case. Sabouraudia 14 (1976) 281–286.

# 10
CHAPTER
# PROTOZOAN DISEASES

J. K. FRENKEL, ANN B. KIER, JOSEPH E. WAGNER, and JEAN HOLZWORTH

Protozoa are single-celled animals consisting of one or more large basophilic nuclei and acidophilic cytoplasm. Many are motile, the more primitive extruding pseudopodia, others moving by means of cilia or flagella. Multiplication may be by binary fission, budding, or schizogony. In some, there is a phase of sexual reproduction.

Protozoa live in vast numbers as saprophytes of vegetation, soil, and water. Coprozoic protozoa are common contaminants of stool samples and must be carefully distinguished from potentially pathogenic species. Some protozoa are parasitic. Of these, a small number are known to cause disease; that others may also be pathogenic is possible but not always certain. Many protozoa, especially the parasites, form cysts, which, while not particularly resistant to heat, are at least more resistant to drying than the vegetative form. Because of the ubiquitous distribution of protozoa, accurate identification is necessary, lest harmless organisms be mistaken for pathogens.

Blood protozoa may often be detected in fresh wet unstained smears, but for precise study, films should be dried and stained with Wright's, Giemsa's, or some specialized stain. The thinner the film and the more rapidly it is dried, the less the distortion.

For direct microscopic examination of feces, a bit of stool is mixed with a drop of physiologic saline solution on a microscope slide and a coverslip is applied. The concentration of feces is right if one can read newsprint through the preparation. Both low and high dry powers should be used for the examination. Staining with Lugol's solution diluted 1:4 with distilled water brings out details not visible in the living organisms.

Techniques for fixing and staining fecal smears, for examination of intestinal mucosa, and for concentrating protozoan cysts have been described by Levine (1973).

## THE COCCIDIA

J. K. FRENKEL and JEAN HOLZWORTH

Coccidia are parasitic sporozoa of the suborder Eimeriorina (Levine, 1973a) infecting the intestine. They form oocysts, resistant stages, which are passed in the feces and infect new hosts. In birds and most mammals, all propagative and sexual stages of the coccidia occur in one and the same host; these coccidia are grouped in the family Eimeriidae. However, in cats coccidia develop sexual stages in the gut, and the oocysts passed in the feces are infectious to a second, intermediate host (e.g., the mouse), in which tissue cysts develop. These two-host coccidia are grouped in the family Sarcocystidae. Typically, fecal-oral transmission of oocysts from cats to intermediate hosts alternates with carnivorous transmission of tissue cysts from intermediate host to cat. In a few genera, the archetypal transmission of oocysts from cat to cat remains. In others, transmission of tissue cysts occurs from one to another carnivorous intermediate host (Fig. 10–1).

## SARCOCYSTIDAE

The sarcocystid coccidia in cats (Table 10–1) fall into three subfamilies, the Cystoisosporinae, the Toxoplasmatinae, and the Sarcocystinae (Frenkel et al., 1979).

The Cystoisosporinae, with the genus *Cystoisospora* Frenkel, 1977 and two species, *C. felis* (Wenyon, 1923) and *C. rivolta* (Grassi, 1879), spend most of their life cycle in the intestine of cats, where they may cause *coccidiosis*, the disease, or *coccidiasis*, an asymptomatic infection (Levine, 1973b). Oocysts are shed unsporulated. Optional intermediate hosts are mice and other mammals in which tissue cysts containing one zoite are formed (Fayer and Frenkel, 1979; Frenkel and Dubey, 1972a).

The Toxoplasmatinae comprise three genera transmitted by cats: *Toxoplasma* Nicolle and Manceaux, 1909,

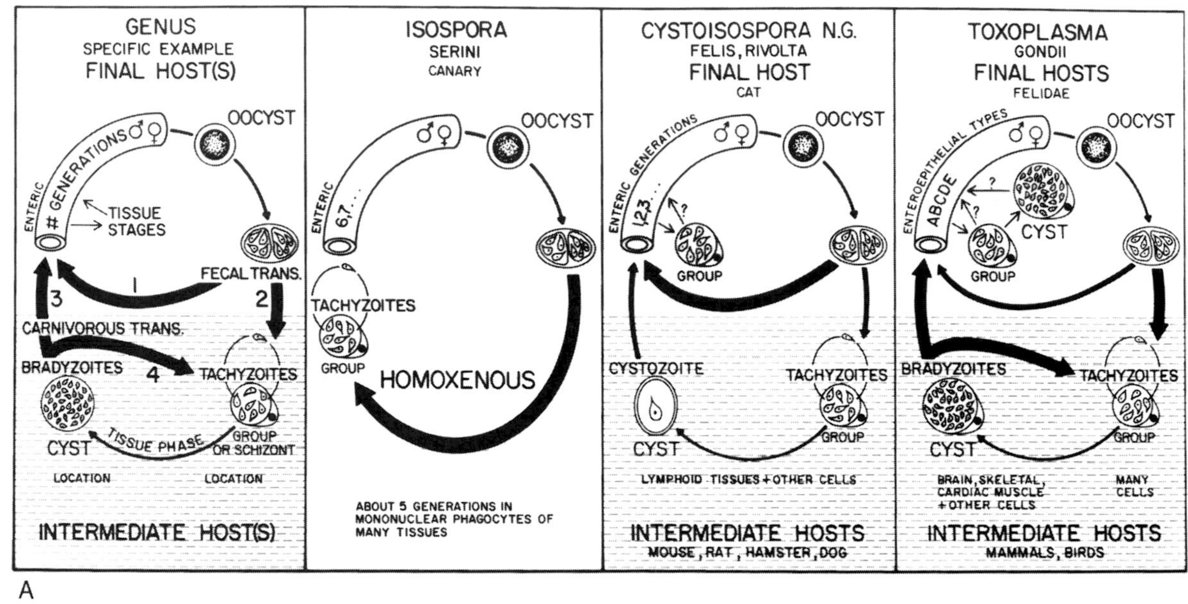


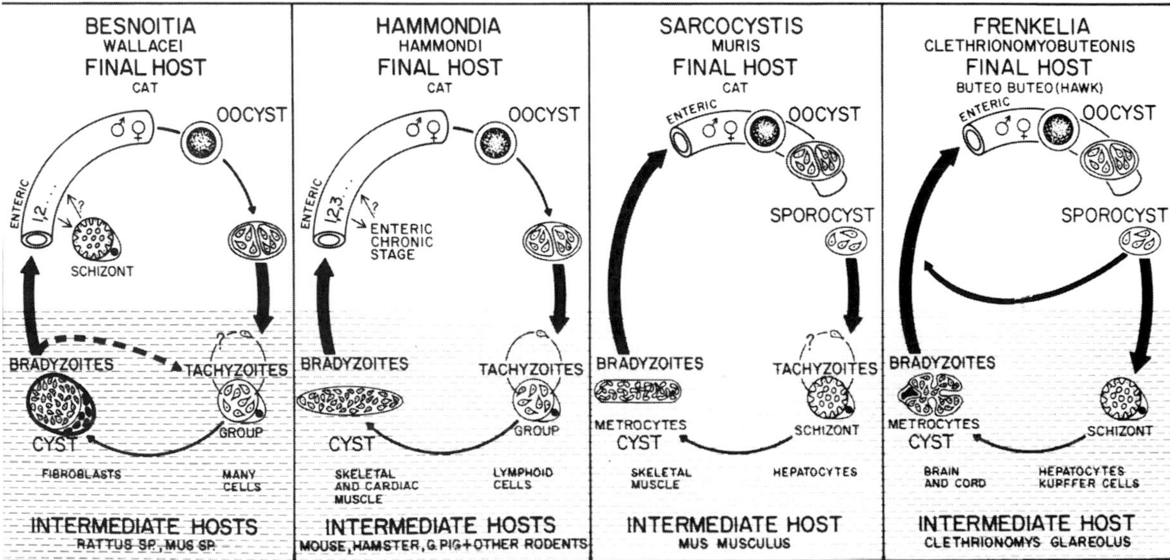


**Figure 10–1** *A* and *B,* Life cycle patterns of seven genera of isosporoid coccidia, most of which are transmitted by cats. The left panel serves as a legend and identifies the four arrows describing transmission routes: 1, oocyst to same host (homoxenous, fecal); 2, oocyst to intermediate host (heteroxenous, fecal); 3, cyst to final host (heteroxenous, carnivorous); 4, cyst to intermediate host (homoxenous, carnivorous). The more important the transmission route, the heavier the arrow. *Isospora serini* is an example of a single-host coccidium. All the other genera involve two hosts. The final host, usually cats, is shown in the upper panel, indicating the types of stages found in the intestine and elsewhere. The intermediate host is given in the lower panel. (From Frenkel JK: J Parasitol 63 [1977a] 611-628.)

with cysts developing within the cytoplasm of many cells; *Besnoitia* Henry, 1913, with cysts probably in fibroblasts and the cyst wall including the entire cell and with hyperplasia of host cell nuclei; and *Hammondia* Frenkel and Dubey, 1975, with cysts in cytoplasm mainly of striated muscle (Table 10–1). Part of the life cycle takes place in the cat's intestine with unsporulated oocysts being shed. The other part of the life cycle occurs in tissues of the intemediate host; however, with *Toxoplasma*, tissues of the cat are also infected. Disease was first recognized in the intermediate hosts, and we speak of toxoplasmosis of sheep, dogs, and humans; besnoitiosis of cattle, sheep, and horses; and, by analogy, hammondiosis of mice and cattle. Disease may also occur in cats, especially with *Toxoplasma*. Most cycles of *Besnoitia* and *Hammondia* are obligatorily heteroxenous, alternating between cats and intermediate hosts. *Toxoplasma* is facultatively heteroxenous with transmission between intermediate hosts by carnivorism, between cats by fecal-oral transmission, or with fecal-oral transmission to intermediate hosts alternating with carnivorism by cats (Fig. 10–1).

The Sarcocystinae comprise two genera: *Sarcocystis* Lankester, 1882, with some species transmitted by cats and by other carnivorous mammals, birds, and reptiles; and *Frenkelia* Biocca, 1968, transmitted as far as we know only by birds of prey. All known species are obligatorily heteroxenous. Species of *Sarcocystis* transmitted by cats give rise to muscle cysts in intermediate hosts such as sheep, cattle, mice, rats, European rabbits, and cottontail rabbits (Table 10–1). The intestine of cats suffers a minimum of lesions because there is no proliferation. After formation of gametocytes and fertilization, oocysts develop, which sporulate in the lamina propria of the intestine. Sporocysts with four sporozoites are shed (Fig. 10–1).

The cycles are illustrated in Figure 10–1, which indicates the extent of multiplication in cats and intermediate hosts and the usual modes of transmission.

Oocysts in the feces of cats that are shed unsporulated and develop two sporocysts, each with four sporozoites, outside the host could belong to the genus *Cystoisospora*, *Toxoplasma*, *Hammondia*, or *Besnoitia*. Only oocysts of *Cystoisospora* can be differentiated by size, *C. felis* measuring 27 to 39 (mean 31) × 38 to 51 (mean 42) μ, and *C. rivolta* measuring 20 to 26 (mean 23) × 23 to 29 (mean 25) μ (all sporulated). *Isospora novocati* (Pellerdy 1974a) is considered synonymous with *C. rivolta*. Oocysts shed unsporulated and measuring about 9 × 12 μ could be *Toxoplasma*, *Hammondia*, or *Besnoitia*, and mice need to be inoculated to determine the genus from the character of the cyst (Table 10–1). For practical purposes, pending identification, they are best regarded as *Toxoplasma*.

In the fresh stool of a cat, single sporocysts containing four sporozoites suggest *Sarcocystis*. The meat from an intermediate host eaten by the cat was infected, and the cat's feces would be infectious to the same intermediate host. *Sarcocystis* does not appear to be pathogenic in the cat's intestine, although oocysts remain for a long time in the lamina propria and gradually enter the intestinal lumen by unknown means. Some of the *Sarcocystis* are pathogenic in intermediate hosts infected with cat feces.

Contrary to reports before 1975, there are no known oocysts common to cats and dogs. Most coccidia studied are host-specific, although cattle and buffalo share some coccidia. Of what used to be called *Isospora bigemina* in cats, the "large race" is now recognized as sporulated sporocysts of *Sarcocystis* (Frenkel et al., 1979); oocysts that were shed unsporulated, or "the small race," belong to the genus *Toxoplasma*, *Besnoitia*, or *Hammondia*. Not until the two-host cycles of these genera were recognized could the identity of oocysts be determined. In addition, cross-infectivity studies were done between the large oocysts of *Cystoisospora* of dogs and cats (Shah, 1970).

The coccidia of cats, with dimensions of oocysts and sporocysts, are listed in Table 10–1. From their size, one can determine the possible genera and for definitive identification determine whether cats or intermediate hosts should be inoculated. Representative oocysts are illustrated in Figure 10–2. Possibly there are some unrecognized species, especially outside the United States.

Several surveys in the United States indicate that most common oocysts from cats are *Cystoisospora* spp (up to 20 per cent), followed by *Toxoplasma-Hammondia* (up to 1.5 per cent) and *Sarcocystis* (up to 0.8 per cent) (Dubey, 1976a). The frequency of antibody to *Toxoplasma* in weaned kittens is less than 10 per cent and varies in adult populations between 30 and 60 per cent. An inverse relationship between *Toxoplasma* antibody and oocyst shedding was observed (Ruiz and Frenkel, 1980b). No serologic surveys of cats for the other infections are available.

## COCCIDIOSIS

Young kittens may become infected with *C. felis* or *C. rivolta*, or both, often while nursing. Some infections are asymptomatic; in others manifestations vary from transient catarrhal diarrhea to severe hemorrhagic enteritis. The latter may be accompanied by dehydration, anorexia, weakness, weight loss, fever, anemia, and depression and may sometimes end in death. In most such instances concomitant panleukopenia has not been excluded. A stringy, gelatinous stool is sometimes found during the recovery phase of coccidiosis. Adult cats are usually resistant. They may shed a few oocysts from time to time, either as asymptomatic carriers or after reinfection.

### LIFE CYCLE AND EXPERIMENTAL INFECTION

The cycles of *C. felis* and *C. rivolta* are similar. The intestinal cycle of *C. felis* was described by Shah (1971) and that of *C. rivolta* by Dubey (1979). Stages mainly in lymph nodes but also in other organs of kittens infected with *C. felis* and *C. rivolta* were found by Dubey and Frankel (1972a). It is possible that these stages are the source of the chronic, persistent oocyst shedding. The identification of tissue infections in mice, rats, and hamsters and the formation of unizoic cysts (Frenkel and Dubey, 1972a) were the reasons for moving these species from the genus *Isospora* (comprising one-host species) to a newly created genus, *Cystoisospora* (Frenkel, 1977a).

In experimental studies in which sheep as well as rabbits and rats were infected with oocysts of *C. felis* and *C. rivolta*, cats were infected by way of the infected meat (Suten, 1983). It thus appears that sheep as well as rodents can serve as transport hosts involved in indirect transmission of feline coccidiosis (Suten, 1983).

**Table 10–1 Genera and Species of Cyst-Forming Coccidia Reported from Cats**

| | OOCYSTS (μ) (After Sporulation) | SPOROCYSTS (μ) | OOCYST INFECTIVITY TO: Cats | OOCYST INFECTIVITY TO: Intermediate Host | LOCATION OF CYST IN INTERMEDIATE HOST | DISTRIBUTION | KEY REFERENCE FOR IDENTIFICATION |
|---|---|---|---|---|---|---|---|
| | UNSPORULATED OOCYSTS ARE SHED | | | WIDE RANGE | | | |
| *Cystoisospora felis* | 27–39(31) × 38–51(42) | 18.4 × 22.6 | Yes | Mice et al. | Lymphoid tissue | Worldwide | Shah, 1971<br>Frenkel and Dubey, 1972a |
| *C. rivolta* | 20–26(23) × 23–29(25) | 15 × 17.2 | Yes | Mice et al. | Lymphoid tissue | Worldwide | Dubey, 1979<br>Frenkel and Dubey, 1972a |
| *Toxoplasma gondii* | 10–11(11) × 11–15(12.5) | 6 ×8.5 | Yes | All mammals, birds | Central nervous system, muscle, other organs, (cysts also in cats) | Worldwide | Frenkel, 1973 |
| *Hammondia hammondi* | 10.0–10.7(10.6) × 12.6–13.8(13.2) | 6.5 × 9.8 | No | Mice, rats | Skeletal muscle | U.S., Hawaii, Europe | Frenkel and Dubey, 1975 |
| *H.* (?) *pardalis* | 25–35(28.5) × 36–46(40.8) | 16 × 22 | No | Mice | Cyst not described | Panama | Hendricks et al., 1979 |
| *Besnoitia wallacei* | 12–15(13) × 15–18(16) | 8 × 11 | No | Rats | Many tissues | Hawaii, Pacific, Japan | Frenkel, 1977a |
| *B. darlingi* | 9.6–11.2(10.3) × 11.2–12.8(12) | 5.4 × 7.9 | No | Opossum | Many tissues | Central U.S. to Panama | Smith and Frenkel, 1977 |
| *B. besnoiti* | 11.6–14.2(13) × 14.2–16.0(15) | ? | ? | Cattle, goat (rabbit) | Many tissues | S. Europe, Asia, S. Africa | Peteshev et al., 1974<br>Pols, 1960 |
| *B. tarandi* | Felines suspected as final hosts | | ? | Mice, marmot, reindeer, caribou | | Alaska, Canada | Choquette et al., 1967 |

| Sporulated Sporocysts Are Shed | | | Narrow Range | | | |
|---|---|---|---|---|---|---|
| *Sarcocystis muris* | 7.5–9(8.5) × 8.7–11.7(10.3) | No | House mouse | Skeletal muscle | Worldwide | Ruiz and Frenkel, 1976 |
| *S. bovifelis* | 6.9–9.3(7.8) × 10.8–13.9 (12.5) | No | Cattle | Skeletal muscle | Worldwide | Heydorn and Rommel, 1972a,b |
| *S. ovifelis* | 7.7–9.3(8.1) × 10.8–13.9 (12.4) | No | Sheep | Skeletal muscle | Worldwide | Romel et al., 1972 |
| *S. porcifelis* | 7–8(8) × 13–14(14) | No | Pigs | Skeletal muscle | Worldwide | Dubey, 1976a |
| *S. leporuum* | 9.3–11.1(9.4) × 13–16.7 (13.6) | No | Cottontail rabbit (*Sylvilagus floridanus*) | Skeletal muscle | U.S. | Fayer and Kradel, 1977<br>Crum and Prestwood, 1977 |
| *S. fusiformis* | 12–14(13) × 7–9(7) | No | Water buffalo (*Bubalus bubalus*) | Skeletal muscle | Africa, Asia | Dissanaike et al., 1977 |
| *S. cymruensis* | 10.5 × 7.9 | No | Norway rat | Skeletal muscle | England | Ashford, 1978 |
| *S. cuniculi* | 8.7–10.0(9.5) × 11.6–14.5 (12.8) | No | European hare (*Oryctolagus cuniculus*) | Skeletal muscle | Europe, Australia | Munday et al., 1980 |
| *Sarcocystis* sp | 8.4–12.0(9.2) × 10.8–15.6 (13.2) | No | Grant's gazelle (*Gazella granti*) | Skeletal muscle | Tanzania | Janitschke et al., 1976 |
| Small 5–6 μ oocysts, without sporocysts, are shed, resembling large yeast; sporulation state not easily determined. | | | | | | |
| *Cryptosporidium felis* 5–6 μ | — | Yes | Probably infects many species | All known stages in gut | Worldwide | Iseki, 1979 |

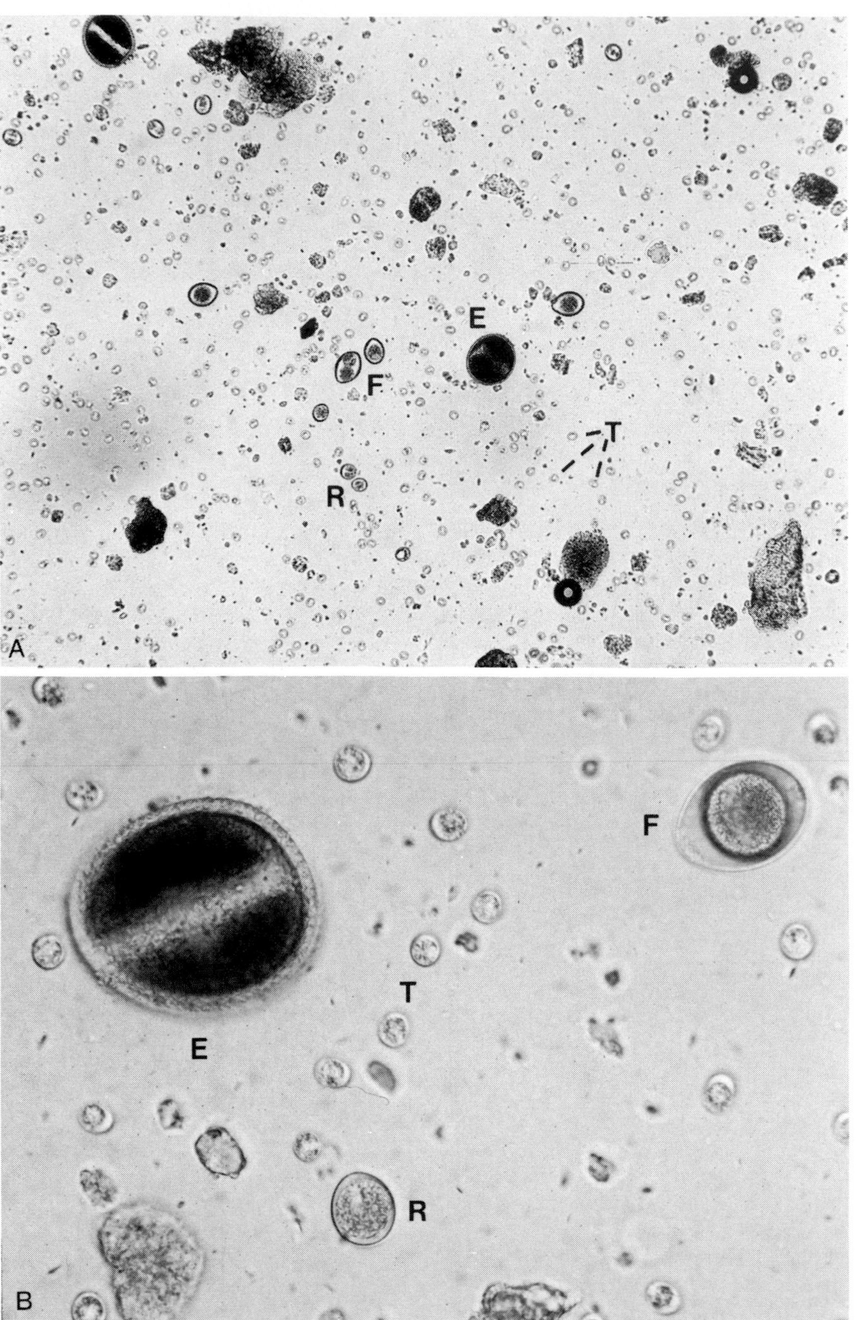


**Figure 10–2** Representative oocysts from cats. *A* and *B,* Unsporulated oocysts of *Cystoisospora felis* (F), *C. rivolta* (R), and *Toxoplasma gondii* (T) are compared with a *Toxocara* egg (E). Unstained, × 100 (*A*), × 430 (*B*).
*Illustration continued on opposite page*

In both species asexual stages consist of three morphologic types and possibly "generations," which are found in the epithelial cells of the small intestine, cecum, and colon. Since the epithelial cells turn over naturally about every two to three days in cats (McMinn, 1954), coccidiosis adds but little to the normal attrition of intestinal epithelium. The propagative stages are followed by male and female gametes and formation of oocysts, which are shed with the feces to sporulate outside the host. Diarrhea developed in nursing kittens three to four days after they were fed 100,000 oocysts of *C. rivolta* or infected mouse tissues. Shedding usually began after four to seven days, depending on the dose and the age of the cat; it occurred earlier after the administration of mice (mean 5.3 days) than after ingestion of oocysts (mean 5.8 days). When infected with *C. felis*, nursing young kittens developed soft stools or diarrhea eight to nine days after ingesting 100,000 oocysts or more (Shah, 1971). Oocyst shedding started five to six days (mean 5.3) after infected mice were given, and eight to ten days (mean 9.0) after infection with oocysts of *C. felis* (Frenkel and Dubey, 1972a).

Unsporulated oocysts can be used for diagnosis; those of *C. rivolta* measured 18 to 25 (mean 22.3) × 16 to 23 (mean 19.7) μ. Sporulation was usually complete within 24 hours at 22 to 26 C (72 to 79 F) (Dubey, 1979). Unsporulated oocysts of *C. felis* measured 12 to 14 (mean 13) × 9 to 10.5 (mean 9.9) μ. Sporulation was usually

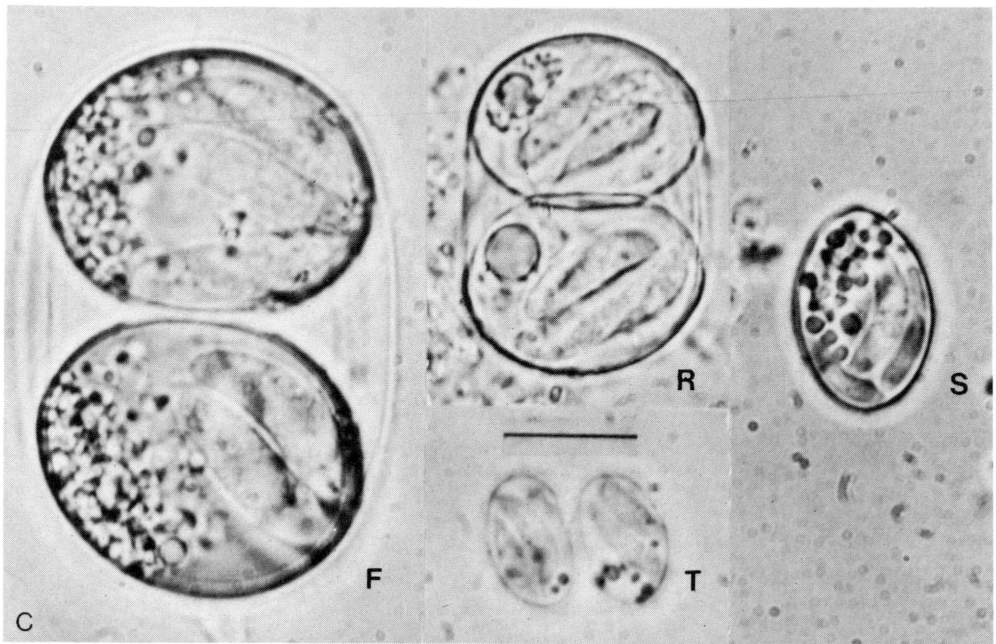


**Figure 10–2** *Continued C,* Sporulated oocysts of *Cystoisospora felis* (F), *C. rivolta* (R), and *Toxoplasma gondii* (T), and a sporulated sporocyst from a cat, probably a *Sarcocystis* (S) sp. Unstained, × 1600. (*A* and *B* from Dubey JP: J Am Vet Med Assoc 162 [1973] 873–877. *C* from Frenkel JK: *In* Hammond DM, Long PL [eds]: The Coccidia. *Eimeria, Isospora, Toxoplasma,* and Related Genera. Baltimore, University Park Press, 1973.)

complete within 12 to 24 hours. Measurements of sporulated oocysts are shown in Table 10–1.

## IMMUNITY

In both *C. felis* and *C. rivolta* infections, immunity develops slowly, as evidenced by the low-grade shedding of oocysts, which may be continuous or intermittent (Dubey, 1979; Shah, 1971). The quality of immunity to *C. felis*, *C. rivolta*, and *Toxoplasma gondii* was compared in groups of weanling and adult cats by challenge at intervals; 15 were challenged after two to six weeks, five after 8 to 26 weeks, and two after 32 weeks (Dubey and Frenkel, 1974). With each challenge fewer cats shed oocysts. The stability of immunity was tested in 29 cats by the injection or feeding of corticosteroids 2 to 23 weeks after primary infection. Of 11 of these cats injected with methylprednisolone (10 to 80 mg/kg/body weight per week) until death, usually between two and four weeks, four reshed *C. felis* and four, *C. rivolta* oocysts—probably owing to reactivation, although reinfection could not be wholly excluded. The decline in immunity against toxoplasmosis was far greater; 50 per cent reshed oocysts and 20 of 21 cats relapsed and died with numerous *Toxoplasma* in many tissues, but with only relatively few stages of *Cystoisospora* in the gut (Dubey and Frenkel, 1974).

## DIAGNOSIS

The finding of $10^4$ to $10^7$ *C. felis* or *C. rivolta* oocysts in daily stools of kittens suggests that coccidiosis may be the cause of the illness observed. However, panleukopenia may be present concomitantly with coccidiosis and account for the severe and fatal illness. In experimental infections, *C. felis* and *C. rivolta* gave rise to little illness (Dubey, 1979; Shah, 1971). The presence of a small number of oocysts may be interpreted as coccidiasis.

Stool examination is carried out by mixing 1 part of fecal material with 10 parts of a sucrose solution of 1.15 specific gravity (53 gm cane sugar, 1 dl water, 0.8 gm phenol) and filtering through gauze (to remove large particles) into a test tube. The filtrate is centrifuged for 10 minutes at 3000 rpm, and a drop from the surface is examined. For quantitation, the top few milliliters of the centrifuged solution are removed, diluted with a 10-fold quantity of water, and recentrifuged. The fluid is discarded except for about 1 ml, which is agitated to disperse the sediment. The oocysts are then counted in an exactly measured portion. No systematic study of the optimal specific gravity to recover *C. felis* and *C. rivolta* has apparently been published. Solutions of sodium nitrate, sodium chloride, zinc sulfate, and magnesium sulfate with specific gravity between 1.15 and 1.30 have also been used.

Only by histopathologic examination can one definitively relate signs of illness to lesions, distinguish coccidiasis from coccidiosis, and detect confounding infections such as panleukopenia.

## TREATMENT

Coccidiostatic drugs have not been systematically studied for cats. In symptomatic infections, triple sulfonamides (sulfamethazine, sulfamerazine, sulfadiazine) are administered orally at a dose of 50 mg/kg b.i.d. (Kirk, 1980).

Sulfadimethoxine is reported to be effective at an initial dose of 50 mg/kg and continued for at least two weeks at a level of 25 mg/kg (Fish, 1964; Wilkinson, 1977). Also used is nitrofurantoin, 4 mg per kg t.i.d. (Kirk, 1980). Amprolium (Corid, Merck) is said to eliminate oocysts from the stool of dogs in 7 to 12 days and has been used in dogs and cats at a dose of 60 to 80 mg/kg daily for five consecutive days (Vogt and Weber, 1973). In a study with sulfadiazine-trimethoprim (Tribrissen, Burroughs Wellcome) given at a dose of 30 to 60 mg/kg daily (divided into four doses) for six days, feces of 19 of 27 kittens were free of coccidia after one treatment; the others required a second or third (Dürr, 1976). Fluid and electrolyte balance should be maintained. In directing treatment at coccidiosis, one should never overlook possible participation of another etiologic agent. None of the drugs completely eliminates the shedding of oocysts, because drugs usually retard only the proliferative part of the cycle. The occasional schizonts reaching the gametocyte stage are no longer affected.

### Prevention

Moist conditions prolong survival of oocysts. Objects can be disinfected by heat, but there is no practical way to chemically disinfect a house or areas outside. Cockroaches and possibly flies can carry oocysts (Smith and Frenkel, 1978).

### Uncertain Coccidia of Cats

Single occurrences of infections with *Eimeria* have been reported: *E. felina* from a cat in the Netherlands (Nieschulz, 1924) and *E. cati* from a domestic cat in the Leningrad Zoo (Yakimoff, 1933). Unsporulated *Eimeria* oocysts were found in the feces of 4 of 1000 cats examined in an Ohio animal shelter (Christie et al., 1976), but neither of two cats subsequently fed the sporulated oocysts shed oocysts within 30 days. These are apparent examples of pseudoparasitism, in which the coccidia of prey may be found in the feces of predators. If, for example, a cat ate a rabbit infected with *E. perforans* ($26 \times 16$ μ), it would shed oocysts similar in size to those of *E. felina* ($24 \times 16$ μ), and if it ate entrails from a goose infected with *E. anseri* ($21 \times 17$ μ), its feces would contain oocysts of the same size as described for *E. cati* ($21 \times 17$ μ).

An atypical coccidium of uncertain genus was observed in a fatal case of coccidiosis in an adult cat (Pospischil et al., 1984). Asexual and sexual stages appeared simultaneously in macrophages of the intestinal lamina only.

For comprehensive descriptions of coccidia, see Hammond and Long (1973), Levine (1973a), Long (1982), and Pellerdy (1974b); for coccidia of carnivores, see Levine and Ivens (1981).

## CRYPTOSPORIDIOSIS

### Etiology

Small coccidian oocysts with four sporozoites have been described in cats (Iseki, 1979), mice (Hampton and Rosario, 1966), guinea pigs (Vetterling et al., 1971), cattle (Pohlenz et al., 1978), and humans (Stemmerman et al., 1980). Histologically, they resemble large cocci or small yeasts projecting beyond the surface of the intestinal epithelium to which they are affixed by an "attachment organ" (Fig. 10–3).

The endogenous stages were described from touch preparations (Heine and Boch, 1981; Iseki, 1979) and electron micrographs (Pohlenz et al., 1978). Infection is maintained not only by schizogony, as in other coccidia, but also by sporozoites liberated from thin-walled oocysts giving rise to endogenous reinfection (Current and Long, 1983). Cryptosporidia may cause acute or prolonged diarrhea and, with heavy infections, malabsorption in calves and humans. Cryptosporidia appear to be unique among coccidia in their lack of host specificity; the agent from cows has been transferred to sheep, goats, rabbits, rats, mice, guinea pigs, and chickens, and by contact to man (Reese et al., 1982; Tzipori et al., 1980). Cats were found inapparently infected (Fig. 10–3), and the organism was described as *C. felis* by Iseki (1979). Levine (1984) reviewed the nomenclature and cross-transmission experiments and considered *C. muris* to be the valid species in mammals.

In a group of 31 kittens infected experimentally at the veterinary school in Munich, the prepatent period was 2 to 11 days and shedding lasted from 2 to 25 days without any sign of illness (Augustin-Bichl et al., 1984). Reinfection evoked only a minor degree of shedding. Six control kittens acquired infection from positive littermates. The cecum proved to be involved as well as the small intestine. In a survey of fecal specimens from 300 Munich cats aged from 4 weeks to 13 years, cryptosporidia were found in four cats aged from seven months to two years.

### Clinical Features

Symptomatic infection appears to be uncommon in cats, perhaps because the organism is so small that it easily escapes detection or is interpreted as a yeast.

Anorexia, weight loss, and persistent diarrhea for two and a half months in a five-year-old domestic longhair cat were attributed to cryptosporidiosis by Poonacha and Pippin (1982). Two other cats, both six months old, had a history of persistent diarrhea and weight loss (Bennett et al., 1984). In one, which tested negative for feline leukemia virus (FeLV), but on one occasion excreted *Campylobacter*, oocyst shedding ceased after a further six weeks, at which time the stools were much firmer, and no recurrence of diarrhea was reported. The other cat was inappetent, anemic, and dehydrated, with extensive buccal ulceration. It tested negative for FeLV but had a complement fixation titer of 1:64 to feline calicivirus. Because of its poor condition the cat was destroyed. No gross changes were seen in the gastrointestinal tract, but histologic examination disclosed endogenous stages of *Cryptosporidium* in and adjacent to the jejunal brush border.

Unless fecal specimens are carefully examined, symptomatic cryptosporidiosis may be diagnosed only histologically after autopsy, as was the case with an FeLV-positive cat with chronic unresponsive diarrhea and weight loss (Greene and Prestwood, 1984).

Two instances of infection shared by a cat and its immunodeficient owner have been reported. Foul-smell-

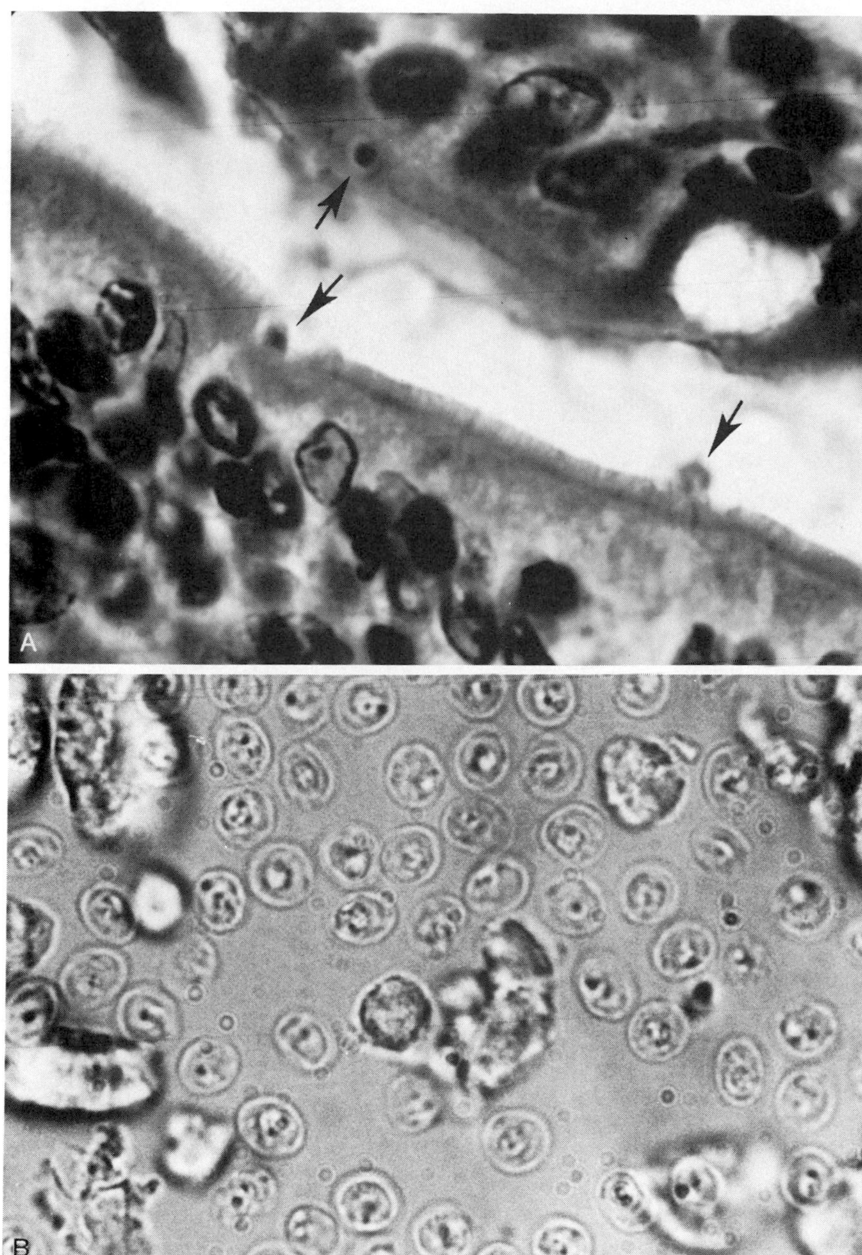

**Figure 10–3** *A, Cryptosporidium* (arrows) from the small intestine of a two-year-old Persian cat. Three organisms are embedded in the microcrovilli; they stain with hematoxylin and eosin, but detail is visible only by electron microscopy. × 1600. *B,* Oocysts from feces concentrated by flotation. × 1500.
*Illustration continued on following page*

ing stools resembling pudding were associated with cryptosporidia in a cat that was given to a patient with AIDS (Koch et al., 1983). The man, who cleaned the litterbox and often held and slept with his cats, developed diarrhea, with cryptosporidia identified in the stool. He failed to respond to treatment with furazolidone and died three months later. Autopsy disclosed cryptosporidiosis in the small intestine and colon, as well as disseminated candidiasis and cytomegalovirus pneumonia.

In the other case, oocysts were found in the feces of a four-month-old kitten after the diagnosis of cryptosporidiosis in its owner, a five-year-old boy under treatment for leukemia (Bennett et al., 1985). No oocysts were found in subsequent samples from the cat or in those of the child after withdrawal of immunosuppressive drugs. Two months later both child and cat again excreted oocysts. The cat was healthy throughout and tested negative for the feline leukemia virus.

## Diagnosis

Cryptosporidia are identified in fecal smears either directly or after flotation and washing; they appear as 5 μ, round to slightly oval oocysts best seen under reduced light or by phase contrast microscopy (Fig. 10–3). After drying and staining with Giemsa stain, they appear as negatively staining bodies (Anderson, 1981), or four sporozoites may be visible. Histologically, they can be recognized by their characteristic position (Fig. 10–3). No sporocysts are formed. Cryptosporidial oocysts stain red with Kinyoun's carbol fuchsin, whereas fungi stain light green (Ma and Soave, 1983).

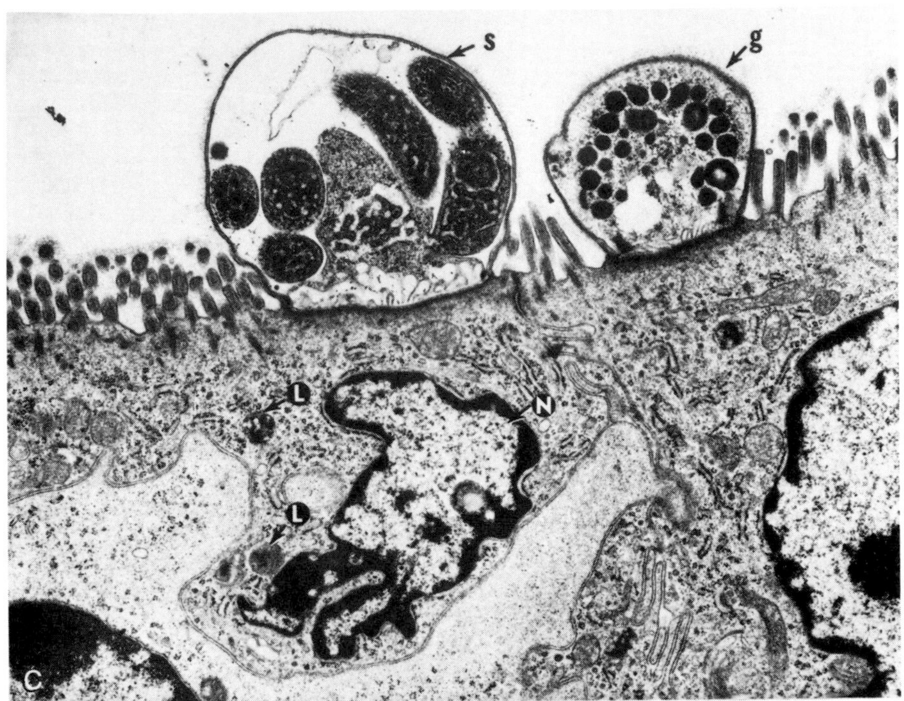


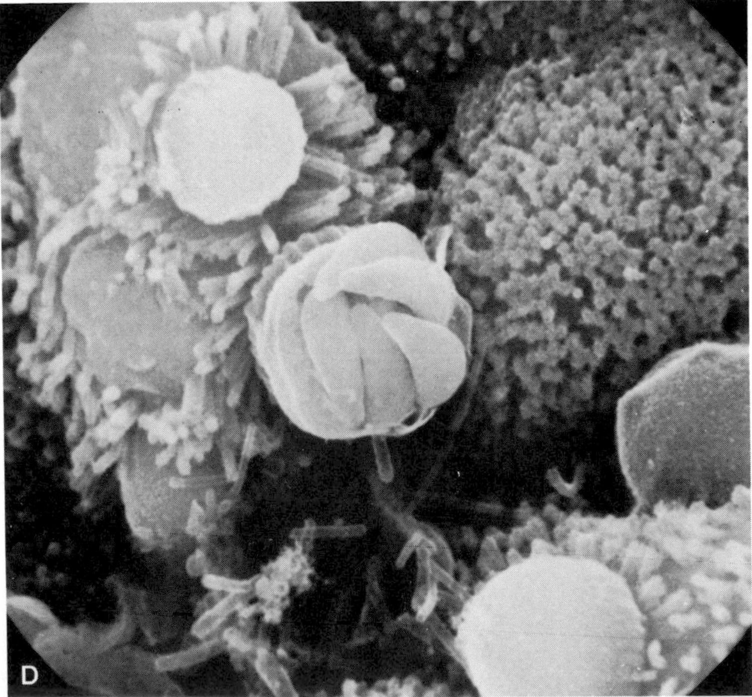


**Figure 10–3** *Continued* Transmission and scanning electron micrographs of bovine *Cryptosporidium*. *C,* Schizont (s) and gamete (g) in brush border adhering to two different epithelial cells. The attachment zone of both parasites is differentiated into a vacuolated and tubulated "feeder organelle," which is more developed in s than in g. Four merozoites are visible inside the schizont; one is umbilicated. Note internal electron-dense "polysaccharide granules" of different sizes, typical of gametes. The nucleus (N) of one epithelial cell is lobulated. L = lysosome. × 12,000. *D,* Scanning electron micrograph. Opened schizont (eight merozoites) in center of figure. Upper left: parasite deep in brush border surrounded by elongated microvilli. × 11,600. (*A* courtesy Dr. J. B. Phaneuf: Université de Montreal. *B* from Heine J, Boch J: Berl Münch Tierärztl Wochenschr 94 [1981] 289–292. *C* and *D* from Pohlenz J, Bemrick WJ, Moon HW, Cheville NF: Vet Pathol 15 [1978] 417–427.)

### TREATMENT

Therapy with several drugs active against other coccidia was not successful in calves; however, lasalocid was effective, although at a dose that was toxic (Moon et al., 1982). Spiramycin or quinine and clindamycin have been used in treatment of human infection (Greene and Prestwood, 1984).

### PUBLIC HEALTH SIGNIFICANCE

Because of the high risk of interspecies transmission and the resistance of *Cryptosporidium* to chemical disinfectants, animal infections must be managed with caution. Oocysts are inactivated by 10 per cent formalin solution or 5 per cent ammonia (Campbell et al., 1982); undiluted Clorox is also effective.

## TOXOPLASMOSIS

*Toxoplasma gondii* has evolved from a classic one-host coccidian of cats to infect many mammals and birds and to invade many organs other than the intestine. The tissue stages are clinically most important, as shown by the 60-year history of toxoplasmosis known only as a disseminated infection or disease (Frenkel, 1973). However, recognition of the coccidial stages explained the transmission to noncarnivores. Infection is transmitted not only fecally-orally by the oocyst, but also carnivorously by the tissue cyst, and even transplacentally by the tachyzoite.

### ETIOLOGY AND CYCLES

Because of the elaborate life cycle of *Toxoplasma*, it is necessary to define the various growth and infectious stages. As in the classic one-host coccidia, oocysts, sporocysts, and sporozoites are developed. When ingested by a cat, the definitive host, the sporozoites invade and multiply in the intestinal wall and various organs, but no oocysts are formed until after three weeks or longer. However, after the ingestion of tissue cysts from the intermediate host, the typical coccidian enteroepithelial cycle begins directly and leads to production of oocysts in as few as three to five days. There are several propagative divisions, and five morphologic types of organisms, A to E, can be identified. These stages are followed by male (micro- ) and female (macro- ) gametocytes and by gametes that form a zygote, which develops a wall and becomes the oocyst. These are shed for one to two weeks and sporulate outside the host (Fig. 10–4).

When oocysts are ingested by cats, other mammals, or birds, the sporozoites enter the gut wall and multiply by endodyogeny (internal generation of two daughter cells) in the epithelial, mucosal, and submucosal cells as tachyzoites (rapidly multiplying forms), groups of which accumulate in a cytoplasmic vacuole (Fig. 10–5). Tachyzoites are banana-shaped and about $7 \times 2$ μ in size when fresh; in sections they may appear spherical and 3 μ in diameter owing to poor fixation. The cell disintegrates after the tachyzoites reach numbers greater than it can sustain, and they enter adjacent cells, the lymphatics, and the blood, becoming disseminated to other organs and cells. The proliferation of tachyzoites continues either until the animal dies or until immunity appears.

Tissue cysts develop usually by the end of a week and become more numerous and larger in the next two to three weeks. They are characterized by argyrophilic cyst walls and by bradyzoites (slowly multiplying organisms). Bradyzoites measure about $8 \times 2$ μ when fresh but appear smaller in sections. As bradyzoites multiply toward 100 to 1000 in number, the cysts enlarge slowly within the host cell, up to 200 μ in diameter, taking a spherical form in neurons and an elongated shape in muscle (Fig. 10–6). Generally the host cell nucleus is present, but some cysts probably persist even after the nucleus has degenerated. These tissue cysts persist for months to years. The contained bradyzoites accumulate amylopectin, a glycogen-like polysaccharide staining brilliantly with the periodic acid–Schiff technique. Biologically, bradyzoites are resting stages waiting to be reingested by a predator. If they are transferred to another mammal or bird, tachyzoites will again be formed. If they are eaten by a cat, the enteroepithelial cycle is initiated (Fig. 10–4); at the same time tachyzoites start to multiply in the mucosa and in other tissues, where cysts will eventually be formed. *Toxoplasma gondii* is the only one of the heteroxenous coccidia in which the tachyzoites and bradyzoites of the intermediate host also develop in the final host. The cat is not merely the definitive host; it is the complete host.

### EPIDEMIOLOGY

In nature, numerous species of mammals and birds are commonly infected with *Toxoplasma*. Cats account directly for the infection of herbivores and indirectly for the infection of predators (Fig. 10–7). After the first infection of a cat, millions of oocysts are produced in a two-week period. After sporulation, usually in a day or two, the oocysts are highly infectious for all mammals, birds, and humans ingesting them. Oocysts remain viable in moist and shaded garden soil or sand for many months. They have been observed for up to 18 months (Frenkel et al., 1975). Epidemiologically, soil contact is more important than contact with cats. Sheep, goats, and other herbivores are thought to become infected by eating grass with roots contaminated by soil. Ground-feeding birds are highly exposed. In Costa Rica, where climate favors persistence of oocysts and human and animal populations coexist closely, barnyard chickens rapidly acquire a high rate of infection, and sparrows, rats, and house mice are also significantly infected (Ruiz and Frenkel, 1980a). Infection of stray cats starts early and reaches 100 per cent by the time they are full-grown (Ruiz and Frenkel, 1980b).

As soon as a mother cat brings prey to her kittens, infection can occur. The prevalence of infection in intermediate hosts is important. When environmental conditions are favorable and prey available, the rate of infection depends on the concentration of cats in an area, which in turn determines the degree of saturation of the soil with oocysts that intermediate hosts can ingest. Man becomes infected from cats mostly during the crawling and dirt-playing ages and in cities where cats live close to houses and where soil for defecation may be limited (Frenkel and Ruiz, 1980). Pet cats fed noncontaminated food (dry, canned, cooked) consume less prey and have a lower infection rate. In the United States, few children are

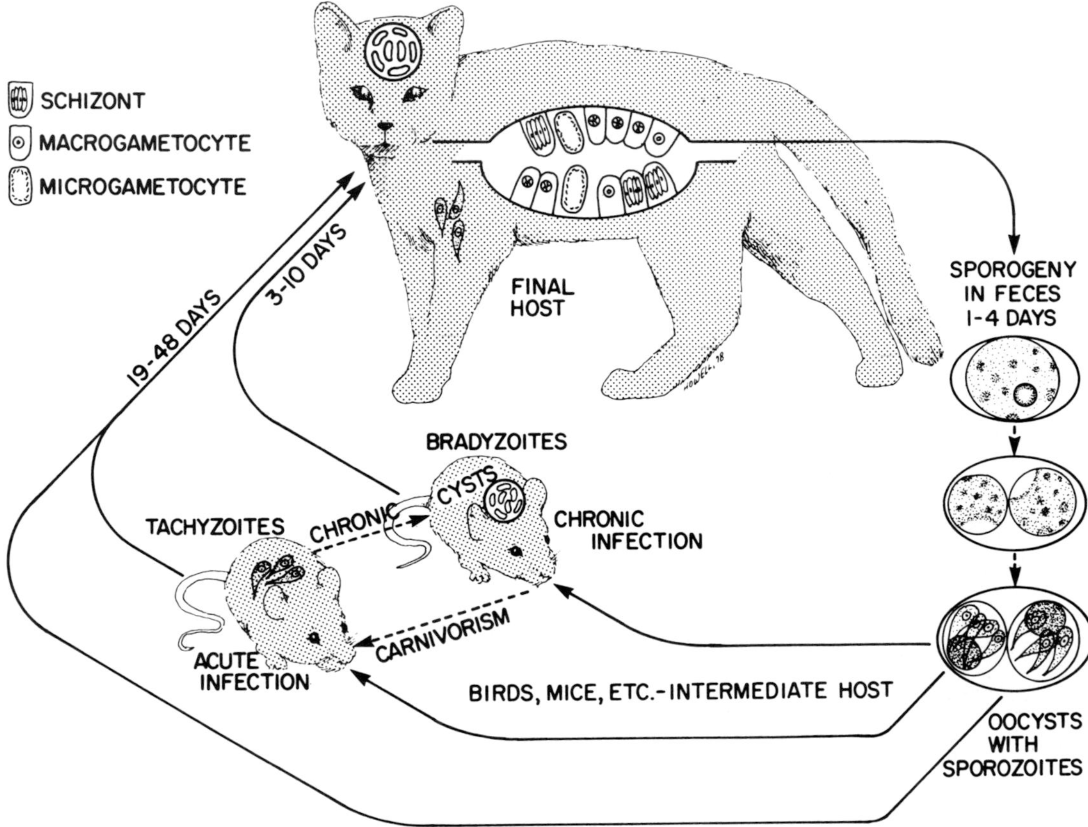


**Figure 10–4** Life cycle of *Toxoplasma gondii.* Cats, as the final host, shed oocysts in their feces, which undergo sporulation within one to four days. These oocysts can infect other cats directly. Shedding of oocysts begins 19 to 48 days after infection of the cat. Oocysts can also infect many mammals and birds as intermediate hosts (symbolized by two mice), in which first tachyzoites and later bradyzoites develop. When a cat is infected with bradyzoites from a chronically infected animal, the cycle is shorter, and oocysts start to appear three to ten days after infection. The cat can also be considered a complete host because it supports the growth of intestinal propagative, sexual stages and also of tachyzoites and bradyzoites. (From Frenkel JK: *In* Montali RJ, Migaki G [eds]: Proceedings of the Symposium on the Comparative Pathology of Zoo Animals. Washington, DC, Smithsonian Institution Press, 1980, 329-342.)

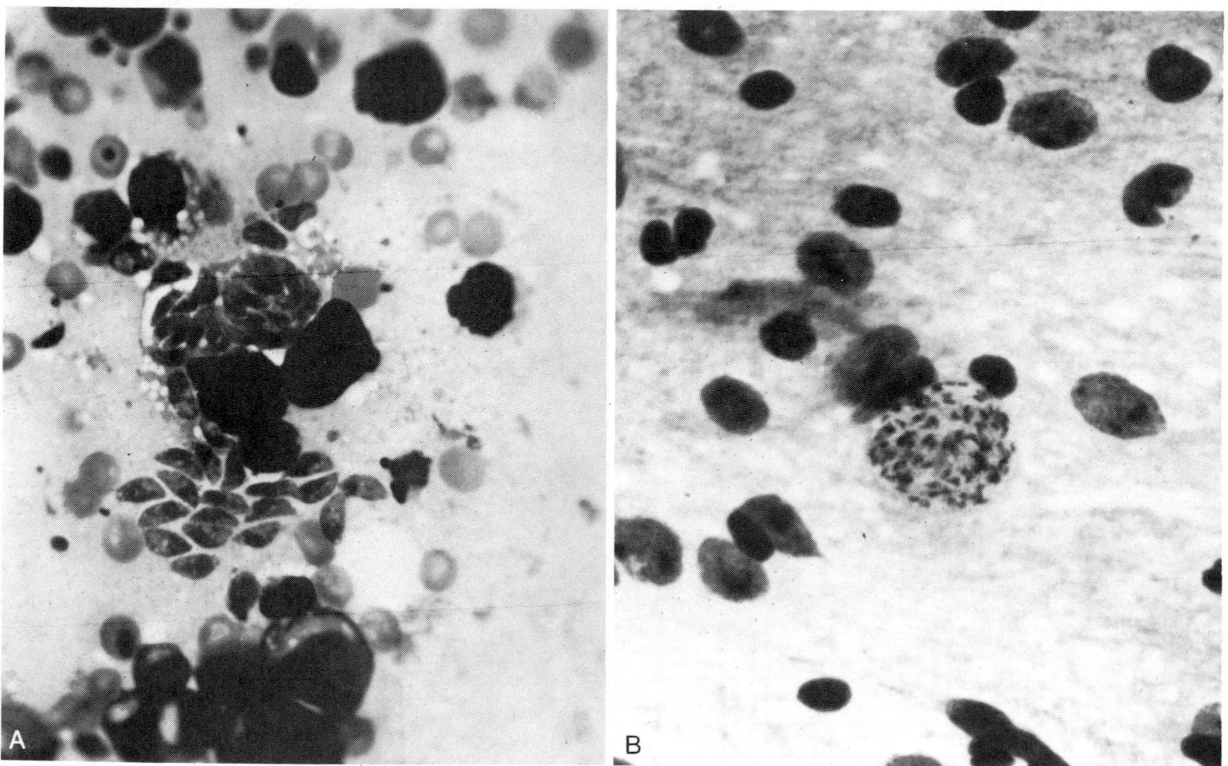


**Figure 10–5** *A*, A group of elongate tachyzoites of *Toxoplasma* showing nucleus and cytoplasm; from a tissue impression print. Giemsa, × 1000. (Figures 10–11*B*, 10–15, and 10–16 show tachyzoites in sections.) *B*, Small cyst containing densely packed bradyzoites from an impression print from brain. Giemsa, × 800. (From Frenkel JK, Ruiz A: Acta Med Costarric 16 [1973] 5–73.)

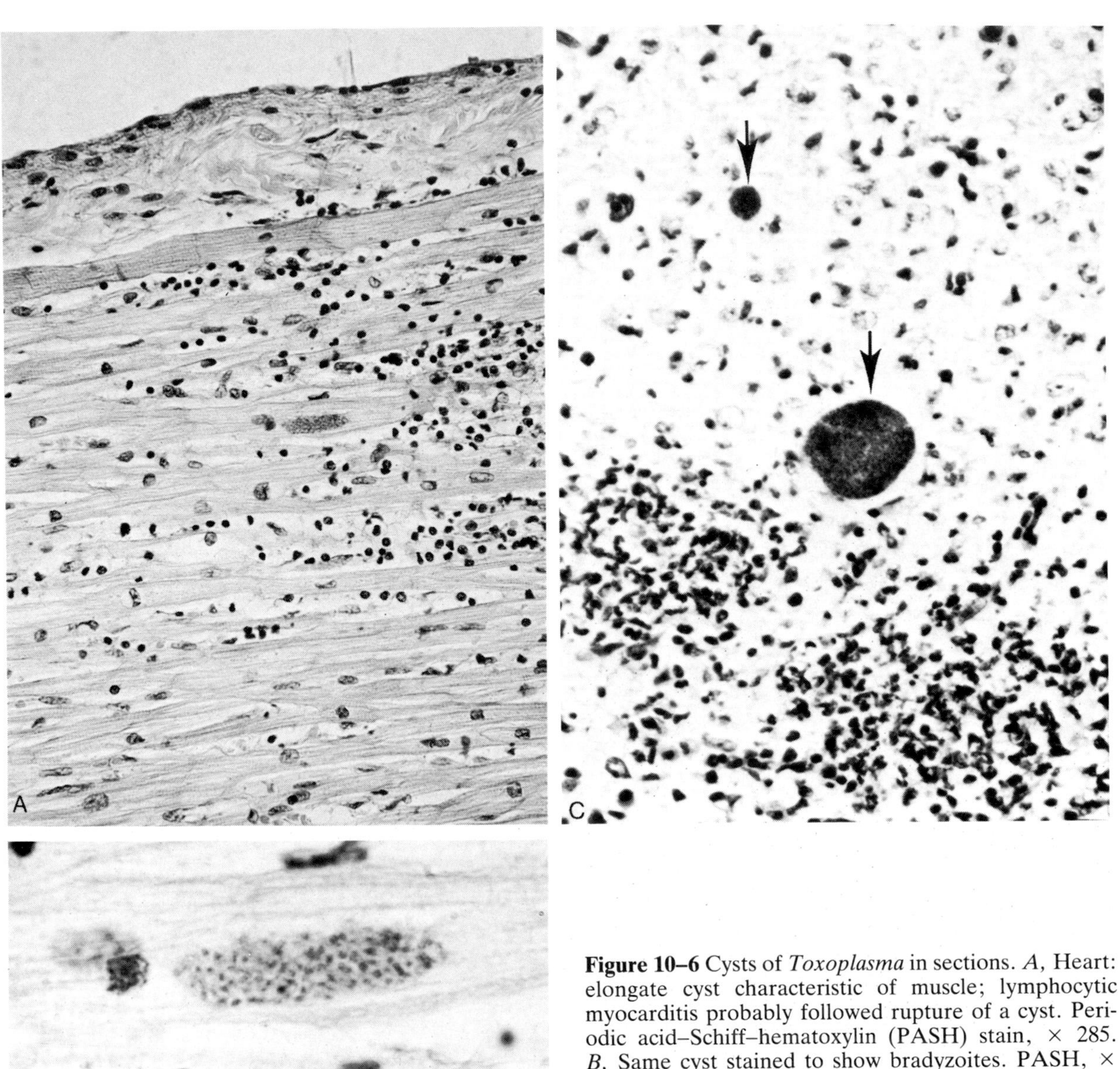


**Figure 10–6** Cysts of *Toxoplasma* in sections. *A,* Heart: elongate cyst characteristic of muscle; lymphocytic myocarditis probably followed rupture of a cyst. Periodic acid–Schiff–hematoxylin (PASH) stain, × 285. *B,* Same cyst stained to show bradyzoites. PASH, × 1140. *C,* Two spherical cysts in brain next to a focus of encephalitis. PASH, × 400.

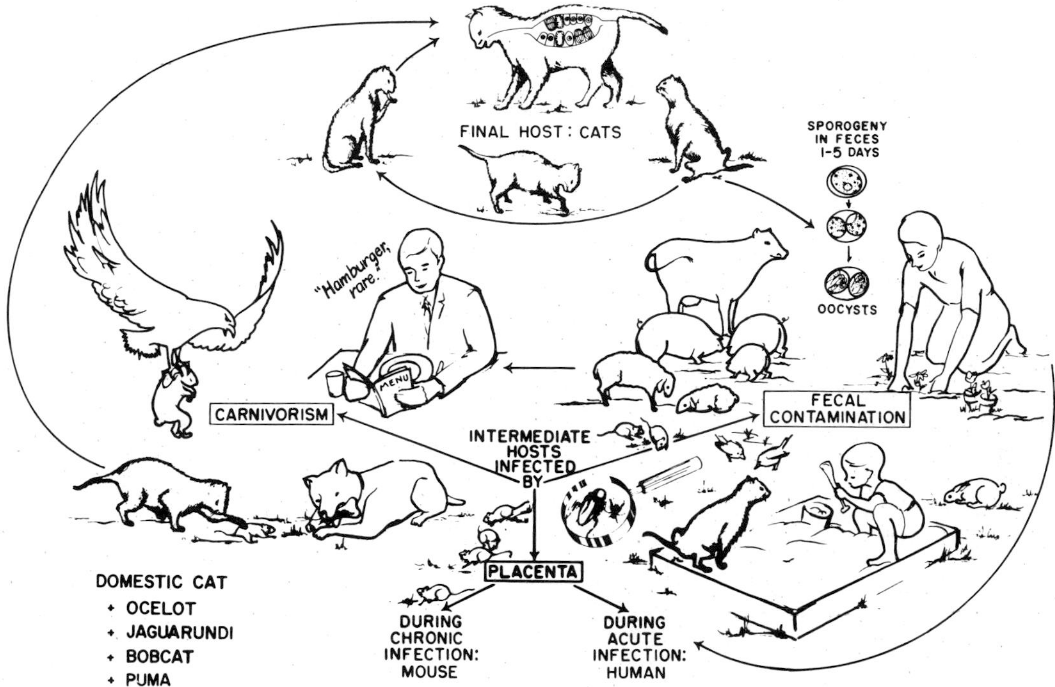


**Figure 10–7** Transmission of toxoplasmosis. Domestic cats and other Felidae shed oocysts, which, after sporulation, can infect man, mammals, and birds. Fecal contamination may be direct or through flies and cockroaches (right). Carnivorism transmits zoites from cysts in muscles of chronically infected meat animals. Transplacental infection in humans, sheep, and mice is epidemiologically rare. (From Frenkel JK: *In* Marcial-Rojas R [ed]: Pathology of Protozoal and Helminthic Diseases. Baltimore, The Williams & Wilkins Company, 1971.)

infected by oocysts (Stagno et al., 1980). Except in the South, most of the transmission occurs in adults from ingesting undercooked infected meat (Frenkel and Ruiz, 1981). On islands without cats, toxoplasmosis is usually absent (Munday, 1972; Wallace, 1969).

## Fetal Transmission

Attempts to induce in-utero toxoplasmosis in kittens of acutely or chronically infected females have been inconclusive (Dubey, 1977a; Dubey and Hoover, 1977). When young kittens of a naturally ill or serologically positive mother develop toxoplasmosis, it may likewise be uncertain whether infection has occurred pre- or postnatally. In case 1 of Meier et al. (1957), when the mother died with toxoplasmosis proven at autopsy, its nine-week-old kitten was in good health without antibody by dye test. Four days later, when fever and loose stools developed, the titer was 1:256. Three days after that the titer had risen to 1:1024, where it remained for at least five months after the kitten recovered from its mild three-week illness, which was treated principally with sulfadiazine and pyrimethamine. Among cases reported by Hirth and Nielsen (1969), two unrelated kittens died at three weeks, both with focal hepatitis, one also with encephalitis and interstitial pneumonia and the other with myocarditis.

To date, the most likely instance of congenital infection was encountered in a litter of seven Abyssinians in which the first sign of illness appeared at five days, three kittens dying or being destroyed on days 16, 18, and 32 (Dubey and Johnstone, 1982). Three of the four remaining healthy kittens, as well as the queen, had indirect fluorescent antibody (IFA) titers ranging from 1:256 (the queen) to 1:2048. The most persuasive evidence for transplacental infection was the finding of *T. gondii* cysts in kittens 1 and 2, on which autopsies were performed at 16 and 18 days of age, whereas in experimentally infected cats, well-developed cysts are not seen before the fourth week after inoculation (Dubey, 1977c).

Fetal or neonatal infection was suspected in two pallas cats (*Felis manul*) that died at 16 and 58 days of age (Riemann et al., 1974b). The mother was known to have had antibodies to *Toxoplasma* for almost a year.

Transplacental transmission, although clinically important, is so rare as to be epidemiologically unimportant in man. It is, however, important in sheep and goats. An appreciable percentage of lambs may become infected, and the placenta and stillborn lambs may be sources of infection of carnivores, including cats (Dubey, 1982; Dubey et al., 1981; Waldeland, 1976, 1977).

## Toxoplasmosis in Cats

Prevalence rates for *Toxoplasma* antibody in the United States were 38 per cent in domiciled cats and 58 per cent in strays, according to one study (Dubey, 1973); up to

100 per cent of 3- to 4 kg cats had antibody in Costa Rica (Ruiz and Frenkel, 1980b). These figures indicate that populations of cats coexist well with *Toxoplasma gondii*. If at one time there existed highly pathogenic strains of *Toxoplasma* leading to fatal infections, cats would have been selected for resistance over the millennia that they presumably coexisted with *Toxoplasma*. The finding of severe toxoplasmosis in snow leopards (Riemann et al., 1974a) and pallas cats (Riemann et al., 1974b) suggests that *Toxoplasma* is not a selection factor in the native habitat of these cats.

## Experimental Infection

During a study of the *Toxoplasma* cycle, 73 cats of various ages were infected with *Toxoplasma* cysts by mouth and observed for shedding of oocysts (Dubey and Frenkel, 1972b). All newborn kittens developed severe diarrhea five to six days after infection, became dehydrated, and died or were moribund by nine days. Autopsy showed disseminated toxoplasmosis and no evidence of panleukopenia. Infection of two-week-old kittens led to diarrhea in four of eight kittens, occurring simultaneously with the shedding of oocysts. Histologic studies between 12 and 19 days showed widespread toxoplasmal lesions. Weanling kittens (6 to 12 weeks old) appeared well during the peak of oocyst shedding, seven to eight days after infection, and none of 27 developed diarrhea. Some lost appetite and weight after the tenth day, and nine died "suddenly" between 16 and 30 days; at autopsy acute *Toxoplasma* encephalitis was found in all. None of 39 adult cats developed clinical illness after the ingestion of cysts, although all shed oocysts and most developed antibody (Dubey and Frenkel, 1972b). This experience has been confirmed over the succeeding years.

Later, studying oral infection with cysts, we found 21 per cent mortality in 33 kittens weighing under 1 kg, 4 per cent mortality in 25 kittens weighing between 1.0 and 1.5 kg, and no mortality in 21 cats over 1.5 kg (Frenkel and Smith, 1982a). In closed colonies of specific pathogen–free (SPF) cats, lower mortality rates have been reported (Parker et al., 1981). Although clinically unimportant, it is of interest that parenteral infection, often used experimentally, leads to more severe illness than oral infection, the natural route. This is probably because the lung is involved by direct spread from the parenteral infection site. In contrast, after natural infection, less vital tissues, gut and liver, are first infected, and by the time substantial numbers of organisms reach the lungs, some immunity has developed.

The course of infection and resulting organ involvement may be appreciated from a study of 50 kittens whose tissues were examined histologically for lesions between 2 and 30 days after administration of tissue cysts (Table 10–2). In those killed on days 2 and 3 intestinal stages were found, and the rest shed oocysts between days 3 and 19. At autopsy, 80 per cent showed stages of *Toxoplasma* in the intestinal epithelium. The mesenteric lymph nodes usually showed lesions during the first two to three weeks, as did the liver and heart. The lungs became involved in a third of the kittens, but not until after nine days, and not severely. Brain lesions started to appear six days after infection and were found in routine sections of 89 per cent of the kittens examined from 9 to 16 days. All eyes were examined, but neither gross nor microscopic lesions were seen.

## Natural Disease

Feline toxoplasmosis was first recognized by Olafson and Monlux (1942) in a year-old cat acutely ill with inappetence, fever, cough, and enlarged mesenteric nodes. Numerous case reports illustrating the protean nature of the infection have since appeared, but the principal studies of the signs and lesions of the natural disease are those of Meier et al. (1957), Petrak and Carpenter (1965), and Hirth and Nielsen (1969). A review of 93 cases at the Angell Memorial Animal Hospital (AMAH) (Andrews, 1981) contributed significant additional data. While the course and lesions of experimental

**Table 10–2 Location of *Toxoplasma* and Related Lesions in 50 Kittens Killed Between 2 and 30 Days After Ingestion of Bradyzoites in Tissue Cysts***

| | KITTENS WITH *TOXOPLASMA* LESIONS IN RELATION TO DURATION OF INFECTION | | | DAYS ON WHICH *TOXOPLASMA* WERE PRESENT IN LESIONS |
|---|---|---|---|---|
| Total number (50) | 20 | 18 | 12 | 50 |
| Age at infection (weeks) | 0–1 | 1–2 | 6–10 | 0–10 |
| Duration of infection (days) | 2–8 | 9–16 | 17–30 | 2–30 |
| Oocysts in rectal feces† | 17 | 18 | 2 | 3–19 |
| Gut† | 20 + 0§ | 15 + 0 | 5 + 0 | 1–27 |
| Mesenteric lymph node | 6 + 11 | 6 + 6 | 1 + 1 | 5–19 |
| Liver | 7 + 4 | 7 + 5 | 0 + 2 | 3–16 |
| Lung | 0 + 0 | 5 + 1 | 1 + 2 | 9–19 |
| Heart | 8 + 2 | 8 + 5 | 0 + 2 | 5–16 |
| Skeletal muscle | 1 + 1 | 5 + 5 | 0 + 3 | 6–14 |
| Adrenal | 3 + 0 | 3 + 1 | 0 | 6–16 |
| Brain | 7 + 0 | 14 + 2 | 4 + 2 | 6–23 |
| Eye | 0 | 0 | 0 | 0 |

*Summarized from Dubey and Frenkel, 1972b.
†All kittens killed between 3 and 30 days had shed oocysts; those killed before 3 days had not.
§*Toxoplasma* with lesion + lesions only.

**Table 10–3 Clinical Signs in 35 Cats with Acute Toxoplasmosis**

| SIGN | PETRAK AND CARPENTER, 1965 (12 cats) | MEIER ET AL., 1957 (10 cats) | HIRTH AND NIELSEN, 1969 (13 cats) | TOTAL NO. | TOTAL % |
|---|---|---|---|---|---|
| Dyspnea, polypnea, abdominal respiration | 9 | 11 | 9 | 29 | 83 |
| Anorexia | 12 | 10 | 5 | 27 | 77 |
| Lethargy, apathy, depression | 9 | 5 | 6 | 20 | 57 |
| Fever (typically about 40 C, 104 F) | 9 | 8 | 3 | 20 | 57 |
| Pallor, anemia | 5 | 4 | 0 | 9 | 26 |
| Vomiting | 2 | 3 | 1 | 6 | 17 |
| Icterus, brown urine | 2 | 4 | 0 | 6 | 17 |
| Diarrhea | 2 | 1 | 1 | 4 | 11 |
| CNS signs: tremors, ataxia, paralysis, opisthotonos, convulsions, personality changes | 1 | 1 | 2 | 4 | 11 |
| Thirst | 0 | 4 | 0 | 4 | 11 |
| Palpably enlarged mesenteric lymph nodes | 3 | 1 | 0 | 4 | 11 |
| Ocular signs: iritis, hyphema, hypopyon, mydriasis, blindness | 3 | 1 | 0 | 4 | 11 |
| Dehydration | 0 | 2 | 0 | 2 | 6 |
| Pharyngitis | 1 | 0 | 0 | 1 | 3 |
| Abortion | 1 | 0 | 0 | 1 | 3 |
| Submandibular edema | 1 | 0 | 0 | 1 | 3 |
| Cachexia | 0 | 1 | 0 | 1 | 3 |
| Splenomegaly | 0 | 1 | 0 | 1 | 3 |
| Hepatomegaly | 0 | 1 | 0 | 1 | 3 |
| Abdominal distention | 0 | 1 | 0 | 1 | 3 |
| Hypothermia | 0 | 0 | 1 | 1 | 3 |
| Coma | 0 | 1 | 0 | 1 | 3 |

toxoplasmosis presented in the foregoing discussion and in Table 10–2 provide a solid basis for understanding of the pathogenesis of infection, naturally occurring illness principally involves sites other than the intestine and is more varied and complex in its manifestations (Table 10–3).

**AGE**. As illustrated by the experimental infections, toxoplasmosis, which is uniformly fatal in week-old kittens, becomes manageable immunologically by an increasing percentage of cats as they get older, and no mortality was observed in 21 cats weighing over 1.5 kg (Frenkel and Smith, 1982a). In the much larger general population, with its diversity in living conditions and in life span, natural disease occurs sporadically in cats of all ages, ranging in clinical reports from less than 3 weeks (Dubey and Johnstone, 1982; Hirth and Nielsen, 1969) to 17 years (Andrews, 1981). In the 93 cats studied by Andrews (1981) the age distribution, parallelling that in earlier reports, was as follows:

| | | |
|---|---|---|
| 35 | <1 year | 69% 1 month to 2 years |
| 20 | 1 to 2 years | |
| 25 | 2 to 10 years | |
| 13 | >10 years | |

Although the disease clearly occurs preponderantly in kittens and young adult cats, it must be recognized as a real possibility in middle-aged and old cats. As epidemiologic studies suggest, primary infection must occur in many or most of these cats at an early age, illness in older animals most often representing reactivation of latent infection.

**BREED**. Breed does not appear to be a factor in incidence. Endemic infection, manifested in several Siamese and Abyssinian catteries by sudden death of kittens, acute fatal pneumonias, and abortions, more likely results from inadequate handling of litter, heavy exposure, and possibly transplacental transmission than from a genetic predisposition.

**SEX**. In combined figures from the four studies cited, males outnumbered females by more than 2 to 1; but in the absence of accurate data on sex distribution in the cat population at large and among hospitalized cats, it is uncertain whether the predominance of males is significant.

## Course and Features of Natural Disease

In duration, illness in cats may be characterized as acute (typically two to three days), subacute (two to three weeks), or chronic (months or years). It is difficult, however, to correlate signs and lesions with length of illness. Although systemic disease, and thus a wider spectrum of signs, may occur more often in acute and subacute cases, all the signs listed for acute disease in Table 10–3 may also occur in chronic cases.

Acute and subacute illness affects predominantly cats from a few weeks to several years of age. Early signs are apathy and fever, a temperature of about 104 F (40 C) being typical and persisting with some fluctuations despite treatment with a variety of antibacterial drugs. Most cats stop eating. The single most striking sign of feline toxoplasmosis, present almost from onset in a majority of cats or developing terminally in many caes of acute and chronic illness, is dyspnea, with respirations of increasing depth and rapidity as pneumonia progresses. There may be an expiratory grunt. In contrast with the dyspnea accompanying conditions in which air, fluid, or an abnormal mass partly fills the thorax, loud pulmonary sounds are heard over the entire chest. Coughing and pleural effusion are uncommon. Cats with severe respiratory embarrassment do not survive, even with specific treatment.

In some cats, signs of toxoplasmosis mimic those of a severe systemic disease such as panleukopenia, or suggest an acute abdominal disorder such as hepatitis, pancreatitis, or if the mesenteric nodes are greatly enlarged, intestinal obstruction by foreign body, intussusception, or tumor. Prostration, occasional vomiting, diarrhea, abdominal tenderness, liver enlargement, and mild jaundice characterize severe liver involvement. Pancreatitis, of which toxoplasmosis has been found at AMAH to be the most frequent cause (Andrews, 1981), may be associated with abdominal tenderness, palpable masses of necrotic fat, peritoneal effusion, vomiting, and loose, greasy feces.

Eye involvement, a frequent and sometimes principal feature in both acute and chronic infection, should always lead to consideration of toxoplasmosis. The retina and often the choroid as well are first involved, so that fundic examination reveals generalized retinitis or irregular foci, which may be reddish, dark, or pale, and sometimes raised. Retinal vessels may be congested, with hemorrhage and exudate clouding the vitreous humor. The retina may be focally or extensively detached. When infection extends to the ciliary body and iris, the iris becomes reddened and fuzzy and the aqueous cloudy, with hypopyon, hyphema, and fibrinous precipitates that sometimes attach to the lens or cornea and lead to synechiae. Rarely, the conjunctiva and nictitating membranes are affected (Dubey and Johnstone, 1982). Neural involvement may cause abnormalities of pupillary size and reflexes, blinking, nystagmus, and blindness. Occasionally a prolonged, smouldering infection leads to opacity of the cornea, glaucoma, and panophthalmitis. In one such case at AMAH, the final phase of illness, developing four months after the onset of eye lesions, involved the brain, and the cat was destroyed because of violent signs associated with meningoencephalitis. Residual inactive retinal lesions appear as sharply demarcated, pale or pigmented focal scars. Ocular toxoplasmosis has been well described and illustrated by Vainisi and Campbell (1969) and Campbell (1974). (See also the chapter on the eye.)

Disturbances of the central nervous system may occur in very young kittens (e.g., Dubey and Johnstone, 1982) but are more frequent in mature or elderly cats, in which they may result from subacute infection or the reactivation of a latent infection. Signs are protean, depending on the site of lesions—convulsions, restlessness, sleepiness, head pressing, grinding of the teeth, personality changes such as excessive affection or viciousness, atypical cries, hyperesthesia, incoordination, somersaulting, episodes of trembling, opisthotonos, circling, twitching of the ears, slackness of the jaw, and difficulty in seizing, chewing, and swallowing food. With spinal cord involvement, placing reflexes may be depressed and the bladder and rectum paralyzed (Bolle, 1952; Verlinde and Makstenieks, 1950; Wickham and Carne, 1950).

In an elderly cat treated at AMAH for tapeworm, administration of arecoline-acetarsol (Drocarbil) was followed within minutes by acute pulmonary effusion and respiratory and cardiac arrest. Although the cat was resuscitated, it exhibited the "dummy" signs that typically result from cerebral anoxia. Surprisingly, however, these were followed within a couple of days by hyperirritability and convulsions, ending in exhaustion and death. Microscopic examination of the brain disclosed a severe cellular reaction to *Toxoplasma* cysts that had ruptured, it was speculated, because of the episode of anoxia.

Enteric signs, of principal importance in experimental infection of young kittens (see Table 10–2), are infrequent in natural disease (Table 10–3). Diarrhea is the principal manifestation. In two cases, one acute and one chronic, numerous "coccidia" were present in the loose or watery stool (Meier et al., 1957). Rarely, a palpable granuloma of the small intestine, grossly resembling lymphoma or mast cell tumor, is associated with diarrhea and with vomiting due to obstruction. Most lesions of this type occur in elderly cats (Hulland, 1956; Lieberman, 1955; Meier et al., 1957), but one was reported in a seven-month-old kitten (Hirth and Nielsen, 1969).

Pallor is often a presenting sign (e.g., Meier et al., 1957), but anemia is more severe in protracted infections, e.g., with prolonged diarrhea. In two chronic cases, in which anemia was the prominent presenting sign, other signs were extreme fatigability, cardiac enlargement, and episodes of tenderness and stiffness of the limbs, associated in one cat with severe pain in certain joints. Both cats were sometimes too weak to rise or take food but were helped temporarily by blood transfusions. Severe myocardial involvement was found in both at autopsy (Holzworth, 1982).

If pregnant, a cat may abort and develop acute metritis. With lymphadenopathy of the cervical region, there may be edema of the head and neck.

Skin lesions are an infrequent feature in chronic infections (Guilhon et al., 1957). At AMAH a two-year-old cat with fever, lameness, and painful swellings of the forelegs localized about the carpus and elbow ultimately developed firm nodules in the skin of the forelegs. The cat died of pneumonia. As well as systemic toxoplasmosis, autopsy disclosed periarthritis, myositis, and necrotizing dermatitis with *Toxoplasma*.

## Differential Diagnosis

Although some cases of toxoplasmosis assume suggestive clinical patterns, numerous conditions more common in cats must be excluded.

The principal respiratory disorders from which pneumonic toxoplasmosis must be differentiated are "coldlike" infections, other pneumonias, and abnormal conditions of the thoracic cavity in which lung expansion is limited. The common viral and chlamydial infections predominantly involve the upper respiratory tract, with conspicuous salivation, sneezing, and ocular and nasal discharge. In disorders of the pleural cavity (diaphragmatic hernia, pneumothorax, hemothorax, chylothorax, pyothorax, and effusions associated with tumors and heart disease), lung and heart sounds are muffled to varying degrees, and breathing is slow and of labored abdominal type. Radiographs (the lateral view preferably made with the cat standing) and study of any fluid aspirated from the thorax usually establish a diagnosis in these conditions. Pneumonias of varying etiology—aspiration, bacterial, mycotic, and helminthic—present more serious differential diagnostic problems, for which fecal examination and transtracheal aspiration or needle biopsy with culture are indicated.

Cases of toxoplasmosis characterized by fever, leukopenia, and mesenteric node enlargement may be confused with panleukopenia, salmonellosis, and other overwhelming bacterial infections, as well as with leukemia and feline infectious peritonitis, all of which sometimes produce leukopenia. Moderate jaundice is sometimes present in all these conditions.

Significantly enlarged mesenteric nodes or an intestinal granuloma must be differentiated from an intestinal foreign body, fecal mass, intussusception, or tumor.

The ocular lesions previously described should always suggest toxoplasmosis but cannot be differentiated with certainty from those occurring in feline infectious peritonitis, leukemia, or some of the mycoses.

When the central nervous system is involved, a host of disorders must be considered—injury, epilepsy, cerebellar hypoplasia, tumor, and infections such as feline infectious peritonitis, cryptococcosis, rabies, pasteurellosis, actinomycosis, nocardiosis, tuberculosis, coccidioidomycosis, and microsporidiosis due to either *Nosema* or *Encephalitozoon*.

## Diagnostic Procedures

The total white-cell count ranges from leukopenia to moderate leukocytosis, but as toxoplasmosis progresses, the white cells usually decrease in numbers. Even when leukopenia is present, neutrophils usually outnumber lymphocytes.

Anemia is rarely severe when a cat is first seen but often develops as the disease progresses.

In cats in which the outstanding clinical sign is respiratory distress, radiographs taken early disclose diffuse pulmonary congestion. Later, spotty areas of increased density appear, notably in the dependent portions of the lungs, but increasingly involve the dorsal areas as the disease progresses (Fig. 10–8). Although suggestive of toxoplasmosis, these features may be seen in pneumonias of other etiologies.

In cats with greatly enlarged mesenteric nodes or necrosis of the pancreas and adjacent mesenteric and omental fat, radiographs may show irregular abdominal masses. Annular intestinal granulomas may appear as elongated densities consisting of a thickened wall with a constricted lumen (Fig. 10–9).

Cerebrospinal fluid, in cases of involvement of the nervous system, can be expected to have increased protein and increased numbers of both neutrophils and mononuclear cells. In both of two feline cases studied, the serum creatine phosphokinase was increased (Wilson, 1977).

A definitive diagnosis of toxoplasmosis can be made only by a fecal examination, microscopic examination of infected material, isolation by animal inoculation, and serologic testing.

Fecal examination of fresh feces from a cat ill with suspected toxoplasmosis would, if it revealed *Toxoplasma*-like oocysts (unsporulated, about 10 × 12 μ; see Table 10–1), establish a cat's communicability and strongly support the clinical diagnosis. Definitive differentiation from oocysts of a similar size (*Hammondia* and *Besnoitia*) would, however, necessitate submitting a fecal specimen (preservative and refrigeration unnecessary) to a qualified laboratory for inoculation of appropriate intermediate hosts.

Various techniques of fecal flotation routinely used by veterinarians are satisfactory, but small *Toxoplasma*-like oocysts should be searched for at magnifications of 250 to 500 ×; measuring with an ocular micrometer is highly recommended. A simplified method of fecal flotation that can be followed by animal inoculation has been described (Frenkel, 1977b). Probably because few cases of clinical disease occur at the time of oocyst shedding, fecal examination has only rarely (Dubey and Johnstone, 1982) disclosed *Toxoplasma*-like oocysts.

A definitive diagnosis of symptomatic toxoplasmosis is most often made by microscopic identification of *Toxoplasma* in autopsy material, or in biopsy specimens or aspirated fluid from the living animal.

Isolation of *Toxoplasma*, if required as a last resort, is by inoculation of mice with tissue or exudate from suspect cats in which microscopic examination was negative, or with fecal oocysts or sporocysts for which differentiation from *Hammondia* or *Besnoitia* is desired. Intraperitoneal inoculation of mice may provide a diagnosis within 4 to 10 days for the peritoneal exudate. If not, mice inoculated by any route can be used for studies of tissues and serologic confirmation.

**Serology.** For several reasons tests for antibody are of limited use in the diagnosis of illness in cats due to *Toxoplasma*: First, acute toxoplasmosis in young kittens may be fatal before antibody develops; second, antibody titers in cats with chronic disease are similar to titers found in the normal population of cats, an increasing proportion of which become infected with increasing age; and third, the rate of antibody titer rise in cats is usually slow and is not related to acute disease. However, serologic tests can be useful to exclude toxoplasmosis or to confirm infection in a young kitten not likely to have been infected previously (e.g., Meier et al., 1957, Table 2).

Two serum specimens should be obtained a week or more apart and tested simultaneously in the same serologic test "run." Only by such a comparison can one avoid day-to-day variations in a given test and the greater variation in different tests. To be significant, a titer change of two to three tubes must be present. If a twofold dilution series is used, this change would be an increase from 1:2 to 1:16, and if a fourfold dilution series is used, to be significant the titer would have to increase from 1:4 to 1:256. For proper interpretation, the dilution interval must be known and whether the two sera were compared in the same test run. If one sends two serum specimens to a laboratory at different times, they will probably be tested on different days, and for proper interpretation one would need to know the day-to-day variation, preferably on the days when these tests were performed. It is preferable, therefore, to send the two specimens together or to request retesting of the first specimen together with the second.

The dye test is the standard antibody test (Sabin and Feldman, 1948). It measures lysis of *Toxoplasma* as a function of antibody concentration, in the presence of a constant amount of human complement or "accessory factor" (Schreiber and Feldman, 1980). Methylene blue dye (hence the name of the test) is added to facilitate reading. The test is sensitive and specific. It is read with

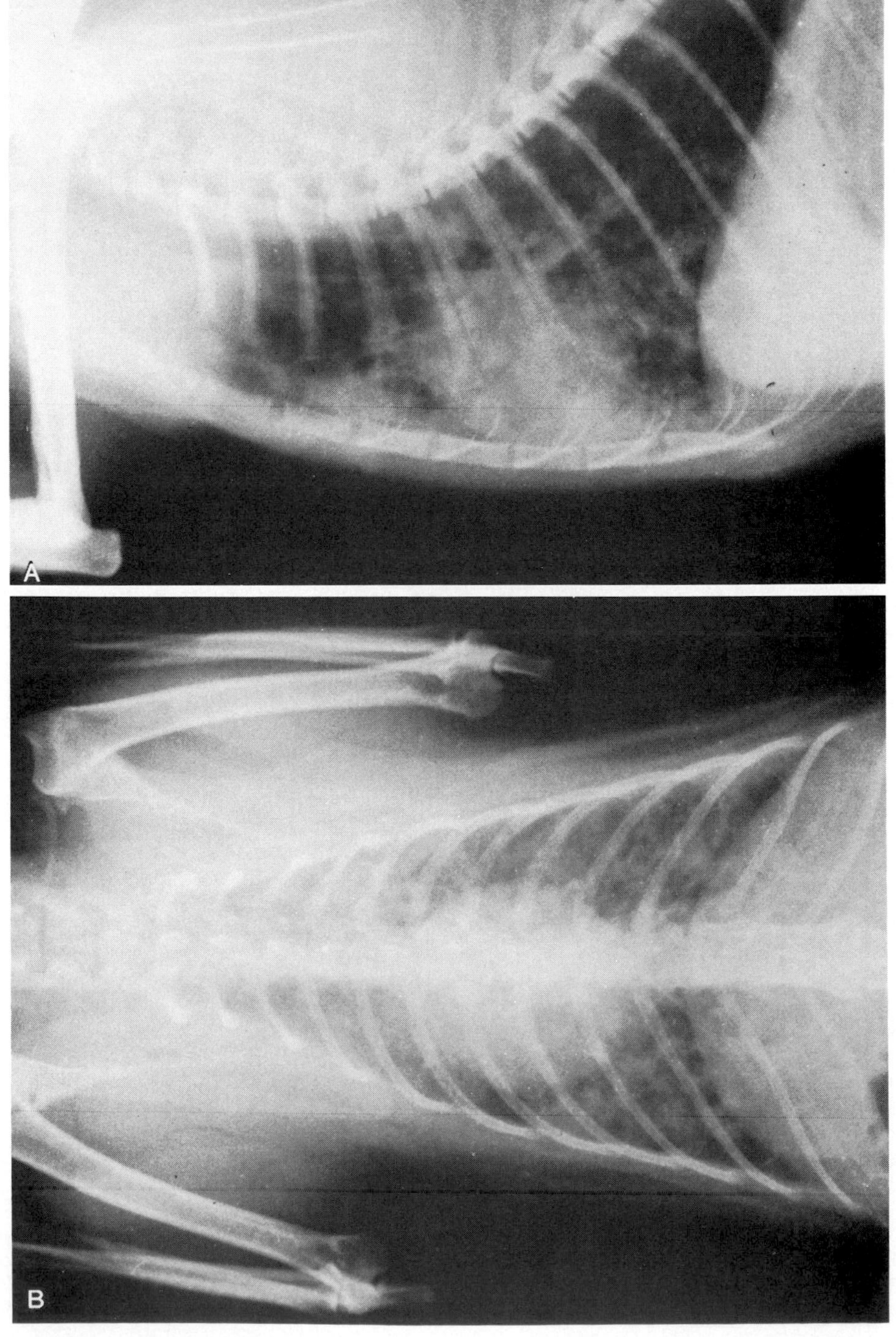


**Figure 10–8** Acute toxoplasmal pneumonia. Fluffy to dense focal infiltrates result from hematogenous dissemination and local extension around each focus. (From Meier H, Holzworth J, Griffiths RC: J Am Vet Med Assoc 131 [1957] 395–414.)

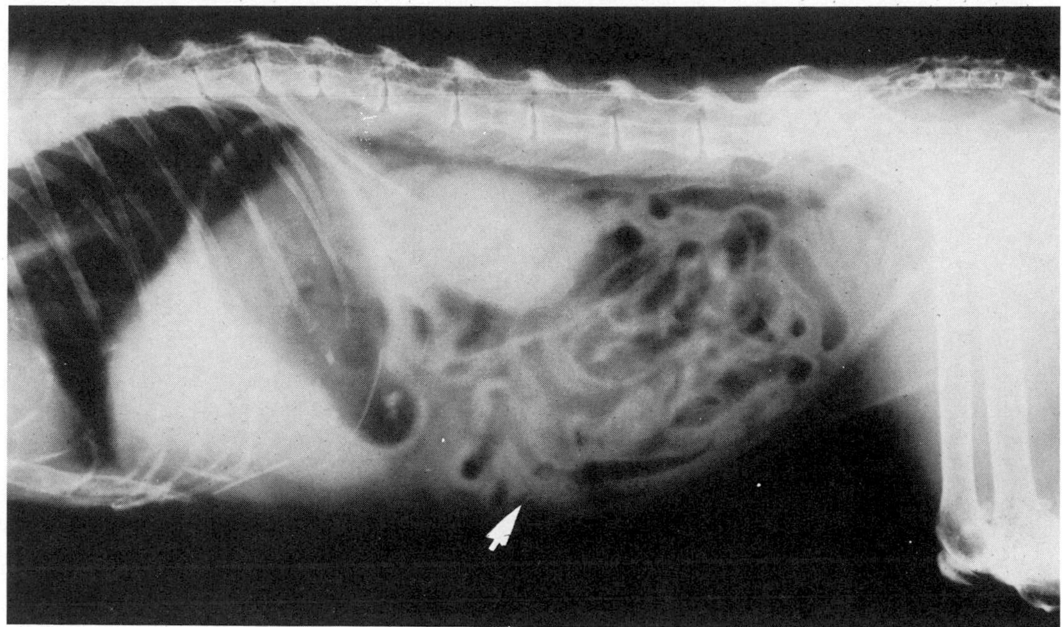

**Figure 10–9** Chronic intestinal toxoplasmosis. Thickening of the wall of a segment of small intestine can be recognized in the lower abdomen (arrow). Radiographically, such a granuloma is indistinguishable from an annular lymphoma. (From Meier H, Holzworth J, Griffiths RC: J Am Vet Med Assoc 131 [1957] 395–414.)

an ordinary microscope. Because antibody-mediated lysis is thought to be immunologically important in most animals, the dye test provides the most useful information. However, since it requires living *Toxoplasma* and human serum without antibody, the test is performed by few laboratories. Details of the technique were described by Frenkel and Jacobs (1958).

The indirect fluorescent antibody (IFA) test is as sensitive and specific as the dye test, although the titer reported is not always identical with that of a dye test. It measures the attachment of antibody to *Toxoplasma* affixed to a slide, as indicated by fluorescent antispecies serum. The slides are washed after the addition of each serum; if the patient's serum is free of antibody, it is washed off, and the fluorescent antispecies serum will not adhere to *Toxoplasma*. Often a red counterstain is used to facilitate recognition of the unstained organisms. Sera submitted to a laboratory accepting veterinary specimens must be clearly identified as to whether from cat, dog, cattle, and so forth, so that the specific antispecies serum conjugated with fluorescein will be used. Each antispecies serum needs to be shown to be free of antibody to *Toxoplasma*, since, if it were present, a false positive reaction would result. If one wished to measure antibody against other coccidia of cats, the antispecies serum would need to be tested for freedom of antibody against the particular organism. Some cross-reactions have been observed. Although it is relatively easy to set up the appropriate controls, the referring clinician cannot easily be sure that no error has occurred. While the IFA test is easier to set up and maintain in the laboratory, it is more complex and offers more potential sources of error than the dye test. A fluorescence microscope is required. A detailed description of the technique is available (Palmer et al., 1977).

The enzyme-linked immunoassay (ELISA) is a new test of potential promise, which, however, requires further testing in practice before it can be recommended for routine use. Like the IFA test, the ELISA test employs antispecies sera, which, however, are linked to an enzyme that can impart color to a substrate added as an indicator. If the patient's serum has antibody, it will adhere to the *Toxoplasma* antigen previously adsorbed to the inside wall of a polystyrene tube; if not, it is washed off. If the patient's serum attaches to the *Toxoplasma* antigen, the correct antispecies serum will also attach; if not, it is washed off. Finally, the colorless substrate is added; it is colored brown with the enzyme linked to the antispecies antibody, the patient's serum, and the *Toxoplasma* antigen on the wall of a tube. The reaction is read in a colorimeter or qualitatively by direct inspection. The technique has been detailed by Walls et al. (1977) and by Voller et al. (1976). The day-to-day variations in results with the ELISA test tend to be great; therefore controls must always be used.

The indirect hemagglutination (IHA) test described by Jacobs and Lunde (1957) utilizes tannic acid–treated red blood cells to which *Toxoplasma* antigen is adsorbed. They are agglutinated by antiserum to *Toxoplasma*. This test avoids the problems of antispecies serum and of complement, as well as the need to maintain a strain of *Toxoplasma*, which is required for the dye test. However, it measures a different kind of antibody from the preceding three tests, and not enough information is available about the interpretation of titers from cats. Difficulties include reproducible adsorption of antigen to the tanned red blood cells, lack of reactivity in human babies and some animals, and nonspecific agglutination of cells by heterophilic antibody to sheep cells. Hence in humans 1:64 is the lowest titer that can be considered specific.

Sensitivity is sacrificed to avoid nonspecificity, and the test is useful only when high titers can be expected. If heterophilic antibody titers do not occur in cats, the sensitivity of the test could be improved by utilizing low serum dilutions.

Other tests, including the complement-fixation, latex (Remington et al., 1983), agglutination (Desmonts and Remington, 1980), lymphocyte transformation (Wilson et al., 1980), and skin tests (Rougier and Ambrose-Thomas, 1985), are useful in certain circumstances but are not developed at present for clinical study of illness in cats.

An IgM fluorescent antibody test would probably aid in the differentiation of antibody from chronic or recent infection. This awaits the preparation of an antibody against IgM of cats. A sensitive double-sandwich sequence to avoid competition of IgG with IgM was described by Naot and Remington (1980). First, anti-cat IgM is applied to the test well, followed by the feline patient's serum, then *Toxoplasma* antigen, then anti-*Toxoplasma* serum linked to enzyme, and finally the colorless substrate.

A carbon immunoassay provides a simple and economical means for serologic testing of cats (Pakes and Lai, 1985). Suspensions of *Toxoplasma* tachyzoites are dried on slides, and serum of the feline patient is added, incubated, washed, and dried. The slides are then flushed with a special India ink, which attaches to *Toxoplasma* coated with antibody but leaves *Toxoplasma* exposed to negative serum unstained.

Kits for the serologic diagnosis of toxoplasmosis appear on the market from time to time. The IFA and ELISA tests require reagents specific for the host to be tested. Of the kits available for the diagnosis of human toxoplasmosis, only kits for IHA, carbon immunoassay, and skin tests can be used for cats. Kits are usually designed for 40 to 100 tests and furnish positive and negative control sera for 5 to 10 test runs. If used in this manner, they may be useful; however, they are not suitable for the performance of occasional tests, two sera at a time, in which case maintenance of proficiency is also a problem. The shelf life of the antigen may also be a limiting factor. Some kits are suitable only for a qualitative screening test, not for diagnosis.

## Pathologic Features of Natural Disease

In a survey of 93 cases at AMAH (Andrews, 1981), tissues involved in order of frequency were lung, liver, central nervous system, heart, lymph nodes, digestive tract, pancreas, spleen, adrenal, eye, and rarely kidney, urinary bladder, stomach, esophagus, skeletal muscle, skin, and joints. It is likely that if eyes and skeletal muscle had been examined more often, they would have appeared higher on the list.

The intestine is not a common site of infection in naturally occurring disease. However, if a cat dies or is destroyed because of known or suspected toxoplasmosis, and particularly if $9 \times 12$ μ oocysts have been found in the feces, autopsy should be performed as promptly as possible to obtain tissue from the intestine, especially the ileum, before autolysis of the epithelial cells in which the characteristic intestinal stages are found. The first step in the autopsy should be to perfuse the lumen with fixative. Segments can first be removed if one wishes to scrape the musosa for fresh examination or impression films, to be dried and stained with Giemsa stain. Later the segments are flushed and then immersed in fixative. Ten per cent formalin is adequate, although better preparations can be obtained with Zenker-formol or Bouin's fixative. After a few minutes the segments are cut down to 4 to 8 mm lengths and fixed for at least 24 hours. In an advanced infection, the terminal portion of the ileum usually contains the most organisms.

Pulmonary lesions, as emphasized by Petrak and Carpenter (1965), are the most frequent and grossly the most characteristic lesions of naturally occurring toxoplasmosis—edema and small pale areas, often with red centers. Owing to the edema, the lungs have a glistening appearance and a rubbery consistency, failing to collapse normally and oozing pale fluid when sectioned (Fig. 10–10).

Giemsa-stained impression prints of sectioned tissue often reveal *Toxoplasma* organisms free or within macrophages, providing a rapid diagnosis.

Microscopically, accumulation of inflammatory exudate and cells in the alveolar septa produces interstitial pneumonia. The alveoli contain exudate, fibrin, and desquamated cells. In some cases hyperplasia and hyptertrophy of alveolar cells progress to produce a proliferative "adenomatous" pattern (Fig. 10–11). Tachyzoites occur in alveolar walls, segments of which may be necrotic, and in pneumocytes, macrophages, and bronchial epithelium. Secondary invaders such as *Bordetella bronchiseptica*, *Pasteurella multocida*, and streptococci may give rise to bronchopneumonia and abscesses.

In a two-year-old cat at AMAH, routine administration of a teniacide evoked within hours a rapidly progressive and fatal pneumonia complicated by an unsuspected *Aelurostrongylus* infection.

Significant pleural effusion is rare in cats.

The liver may be moderately swollen, with rounded edges, and there may be small red or yellow foci or mottling. Microscopically, areas of necrosis are distributed irregularly throughout the parenchyma. Tachyzoites may be found extracellularly or, more often, in hepatic and Kupffer cells. In long-standing infections, organisms may be few, with healing by regeneration at the periphery of necrotic foci. Enteric-type stages may be found in bile duct epithelium (e.g., Smart et al., 1973).

In brain and spinal cord, which are infected by the vascular route, the earliest change is vasculitis, followed by extension to nervous tissue, which exhibits small areas of focal necrosis with free and intracellular tachyzoites and microglial reaction (Fig. 10–12). Sometimes there is perivascular cuffing. Rarely a necrotic lesion is large enough to be visible grossly (Hirth and Nielsen, 1969). As immunity develops (in the second and third weeks in experimentally infected kittens), these lesions subside. *Toxoplasma* cysts remain, however, usually without glial reaction. Intact cysts, although destroying the neuron, are asymptomatic. When cysts disintegrate, they evoke an inflammatory reaction. In the immunocompetent, most bradyzoites are destroyed, and a few form new cysts. Clinical signs are related to necrosis and associated glial reaction. In the presence of immunosuppression, the liberated bradyzoites enter new cells and multiply as tachyzoites, destroying the parasitized cells. Because the liberated tachyzoites enter adjacent cells and destroy these in turn, small necrotic foci accompanied by numerous tachyzoites may be formed.

The heart may appear grossly normal or in acute infection may exhibit hemorrhage and focal pallor of the

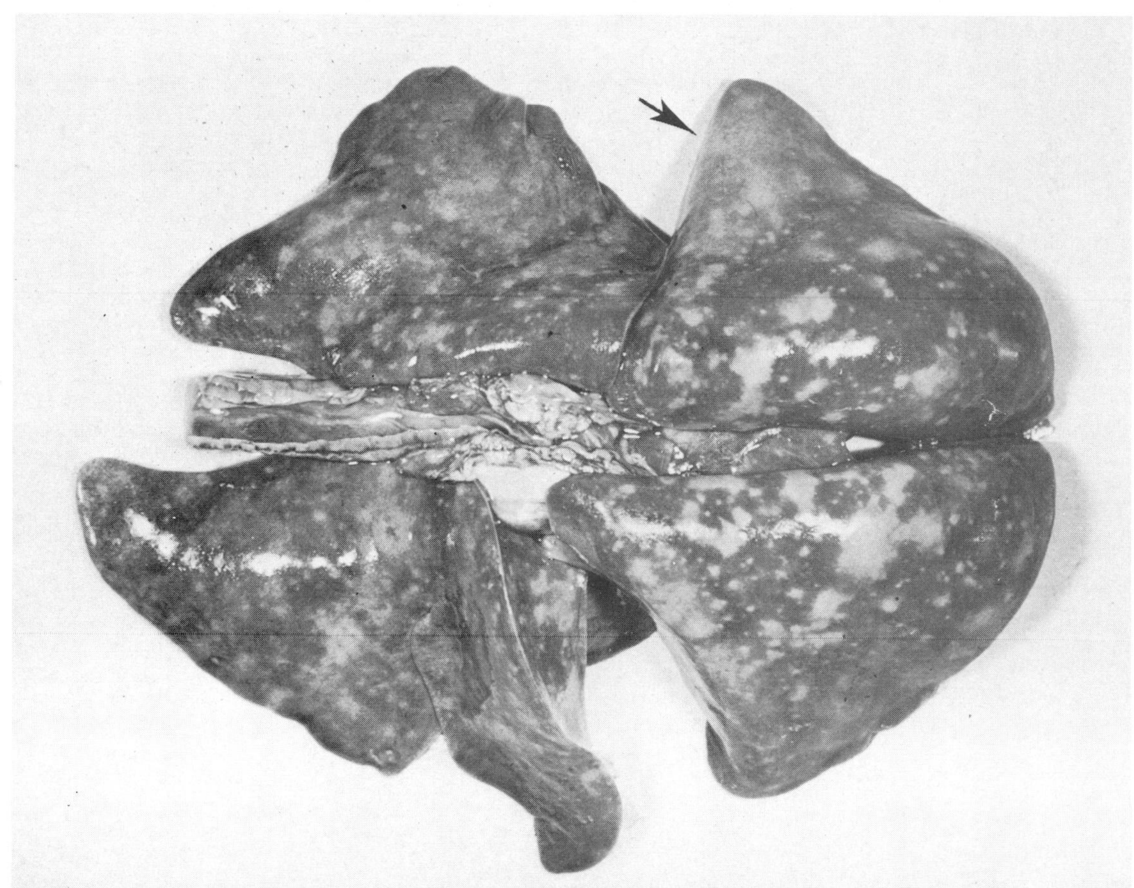

**Figure 10–10** Diffuse focal pneumonia due to *Toxoplasma* (dorsal view). The foci of consolidation vary in density and color; near the arrow the consolidation is early and diffuse; the whitish areas are older lesions. (From Meier H, Holzworth J, Griffiths RC: J Am Vet Med Assoc 131 [1957] 395–414.)

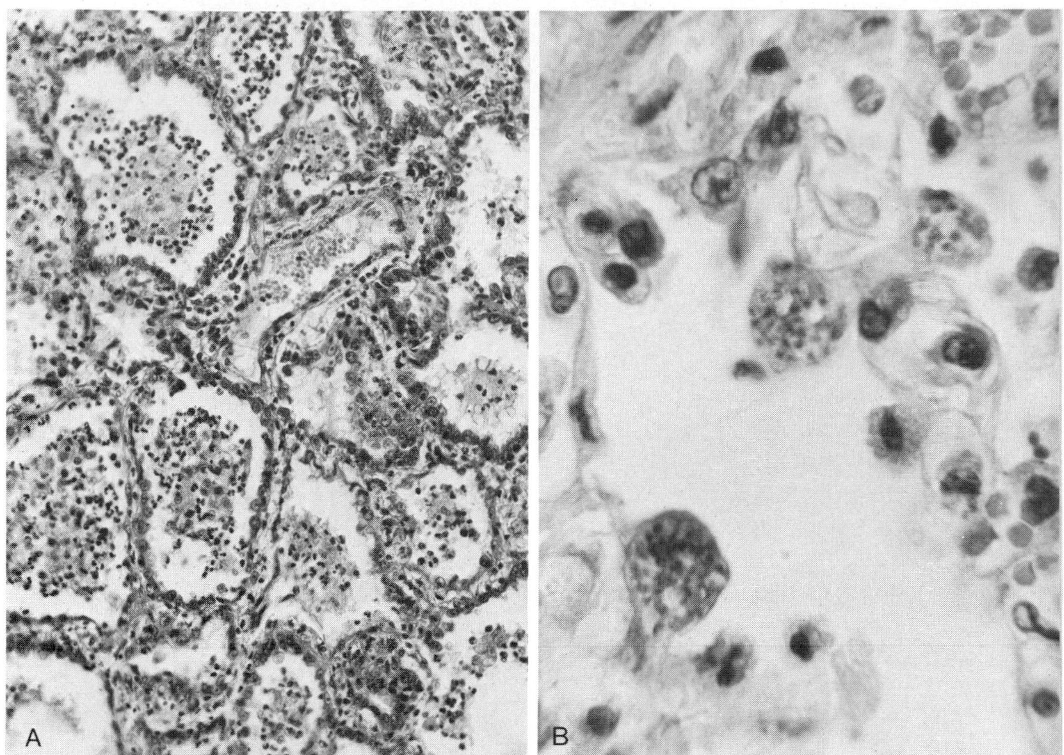


**Figure 10–11** *A*, "Adenomatous" pneumonia in a cat with acute toxoplasmosis. The alveolar and bronchial epithelia are hyperplastic and hypertrophied, the interstitium is edematous, and there is alveolar exudate. H&E, × 200. *B*, Groups of *Toxoplasma* tachyzoites in alveolar lining cells. H&E, × 1100. (From Meier H, Holzworth J, Griffiths RC: J Am Vet Med Assoc 131 [1957] 395–414.)

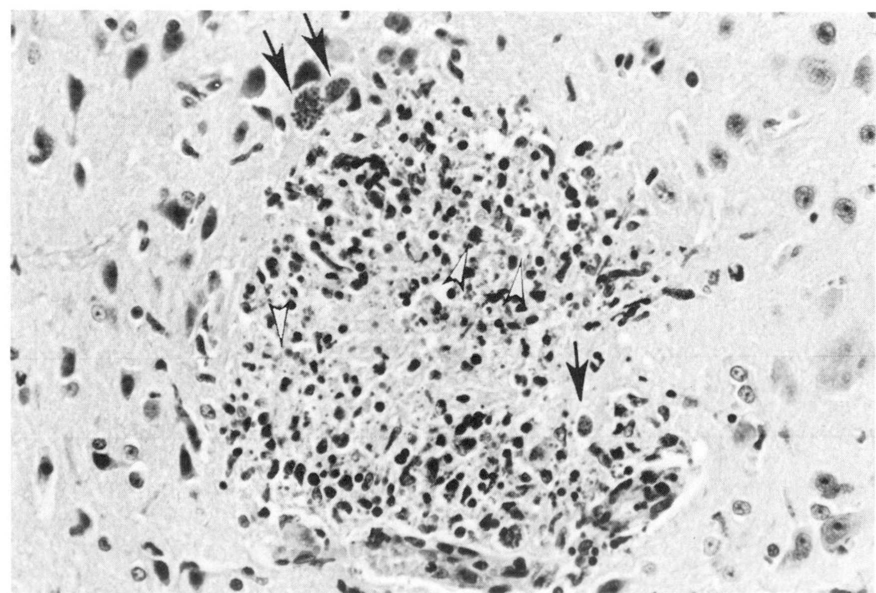

**Figure 10–12** Focal encephalitis with central necrosis due to *Toxoplasma* tachyzoites, which are numerous in the lesion (arrowheads). Three cysts are also shown (arrows). H&E, × 400. (From Dubey JP, Frenkel JK: Vet Pathol 11 [1974] 350–379.)

myocardium, while similar pale areas of necrosis or fibrosis may be seen in chronic infection. Microscopically, foci of tachyzoites in myocardial fibers and mononuclear inflammatory cells are typical of acute infection. Later these lesions heal, but hundreds of encysted bradyzoites may remain, staining a deep red wth periodic acid–Schiff stain, and usually unaccompanied by inflammation. Valvular involvement, with tachyzoites, has been described in acute infection of young kittens (Dubey and Johnstone, 1982). Pericardial edema or effusion occasionally occurs.

Lymph nodes are variably enlarged and reddened, most often in the thorax and abdomen. When not draining an infected area, a node may contain few organisms, but it is nonetheless diagnostic if removed as a biopsy specimen. Reticular cell hyperplasia is the most consistent feature, but extensive necrosis is not uncommon. Lymphocytic depletion is usual in prolonged fatal infections.

Intestinal lesions are not among the most frequent in natural disease (Fig. 10–13). Rarely in acute infection of very young kittens, muscular necrosis may be associated with tachyzoites (Dubey and Johnstone, 1982), and in a litter of three-month-old kittens with loose stools, in which *Toxoplasma* was identified morphologically ante mortem, heavy parasitization of the epithelium by schizonts and occasional tachyzoites was recognized microscopically at AMAH. An unusual lesion in a four-month-old kitten at AMAH was a mass involving the hepatopancreatic ampulla and obstructing the bile duct, which was thickened and dilated; microscopically, severe inflammation characterized by tachyzoites was found to have virtually destroyed the ampulla and extended into both common bile duct and pancreatic duct as well as the pancreas. Most often, organisms evoking little or no reaction are found in cats with principal lesions elsewhere. Occasionally, as described in the section on symptomatology, chronic infection takes the form of granulomas grossly resembling lymphoma or mast cell tumor (Fig. 10–14). Chronic enteritis with ulcers or papillary or polypoid proliferation is associated with such granulomas, and cysts and tachyzoites are seen microscopically in the muscle and mucosa. In one such cat, aged 15 years, scrapings throughout the intestine revealed structures characterized at the time as "coccidia" (Meier et al., 1957) but actually perhaps *Toxoplasma* oocysts shed in a reactivated infection.

The pancreas and adjacent mesenteric and omental fat may be so extensively involved as to be palpable as an abdominal mass. Microscopically, acute infection is characterized by inflammatory edema and necrosis, with tachyzoites most numerous within acinar cells but also in ductal epithelium and islets and free in the interstitium (Fig. 10–15). The peripancreatic fat necrosis results from the action of pancreatic enzymes with no *Toxoplasma* present. Fibrosis is characteristic of relapsing and chronic infection. Inflammatory effusion may accompany acute and subacute pancreatitis, and jaundice may result from compression of the common bile duct.

The spleen is sometimes moderately enlarged and may show pale or hemorrhagic foci. If there is peritoneal effusion, the splenic capsule may be covered with fibrin. Microscopically, reticular cell hyperplasia is common, lymphocytes usually being depleted. Infected reticular cells are common, giving rise to smaller or larger foci of necrosis. Tachyzoites and bradyzoites may also be found in smooth muscle cells of capsule and trabeculae. Erythrophagocytosis is sometimes present. Extramedullary hematopoiesis is often seen in cats with chronic infection.

The adrenals, which may be involved in acute or chronic infection in cats of any age, exhibit necrotic foci of varying size, most often in the medulla. Fibrous tissue replaces the medulla in some acute cases (Petrak and Carpenter, 1965).

Ocular lesions visible to the naked eye or by ophthalmoscopy have been described in the section on symptomatology. Microscopic changes are those of necrotizing and, later, granulomatous inflammation with infiltration by plasma cells, large mononuclear cells, and epithelioid cells. The retina and often the choroid are primarily involved; in many cases infection progresses to the anterior eye, causing iridocyclitis (e.g., Piper et al., 1970). Both tachyzoites and encysted organisms may be found in the retina and choroid, less often in the anterior eye. Near the center of a retinal lesion the pigment epithelium is disturbed or destroyed, while peripherally there is hyperplasia of pigment cells (Campbell, 1974; Vainisi and Campbell, 1969). Lesions and organisms are occasionally recognized in the optic nerve, extraocular muscles, and orbital fat. Exudate may be found in either chamber of the eye. Conjunctival involvement was an unusual feature of natural illness in a month-old kitten (Dubey and Johnstone, 1982) but has been seen in experimentally infected cats only after administration of large doses of methylprednisolone (Dubey and Frenkel, 1974).

Kidney infection is infrequently reported (Dubey and Johnstone, 1982; Groulade et al., 1956; Smart et al., 1973). It was recognized in 4 of 93 cases at AMAH (Andrews, 1981). In three Abyssinian littermates under a month of age with generalized disease, Dubey and Johnstone (1982) described focal necrosis of glomeruli, tubules, and capillaries and infiltration with mononuclear cells; both tachyzoites and cysts were present in glomeruli and tubular epithelium. Similar changes were observed at AMAH in the kidneys of an Abyssinian aged four and a half months with an acute fulminating infection that killed several littermates (Fig. 10–16). Organisms were observed, unassociated with lesions, in a year-old Siamese with systemic toxoplasmosis (Smart et al., 1973) and together with changes of chronic mononuclear fibrosing nephritis in an eight-year-old domestic cat dying of acute generalized toxoplasmosis.

The urinary bladder wall was the site of mural hemorrhages, together with *Toxoplasma* organisms, in two cases of systemic illness at AMAH (Andrews, 1981).

The stomach is occasionally affected with hemorrhage, necrosis, ulceration, and desquamation of gastric mucosa (AMAH). Esophagitis with mononuclear infiltration and the presence of *Toxoplasma* is a rare lesion (Andrews, 1981).

Skeletal muscle is occasionally found in autopsies to be the site of encysted *Toxoplasma* without a cellular reaction (Ward et al., 1971). In severe systemic illness in a month-old kitten, focal necrosis and arteritis associated with encysted *Toxoplasma* were found in the tongue, and necrosis, mononuclear infiltration, and cysts in extraocular muscles and in smooth muscle of the third eyelid (Dubey and Johnstone, 1982). In experimental infection, tachyzoites, evoking an intense inflammatory reaction, have also been found in smooth muscle of the uterus. In both skeletal and smooth muscle, cysts persist into the asymptomatic, chronic phase of infection.

Skin involvement, as already noted, is uncommon (Guilhon et al., 1957). In the one case recognized at AMAH it was associated, in a two-year-old domestic cat,

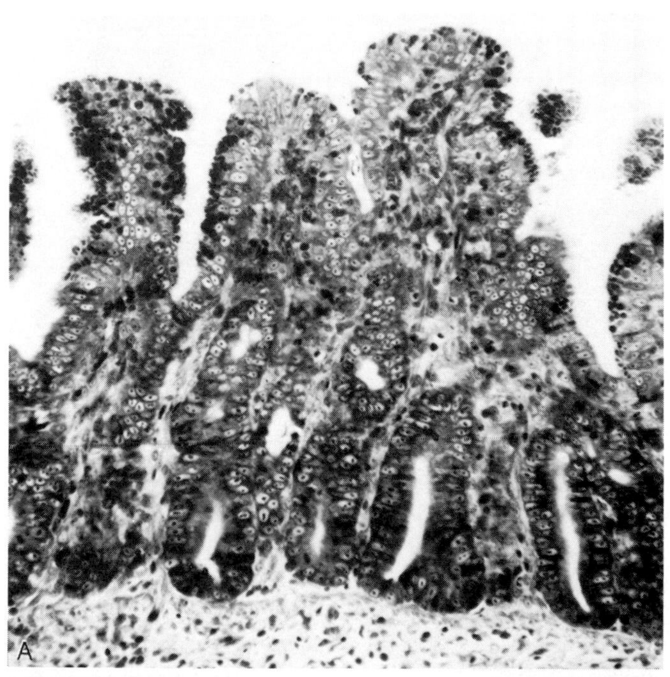


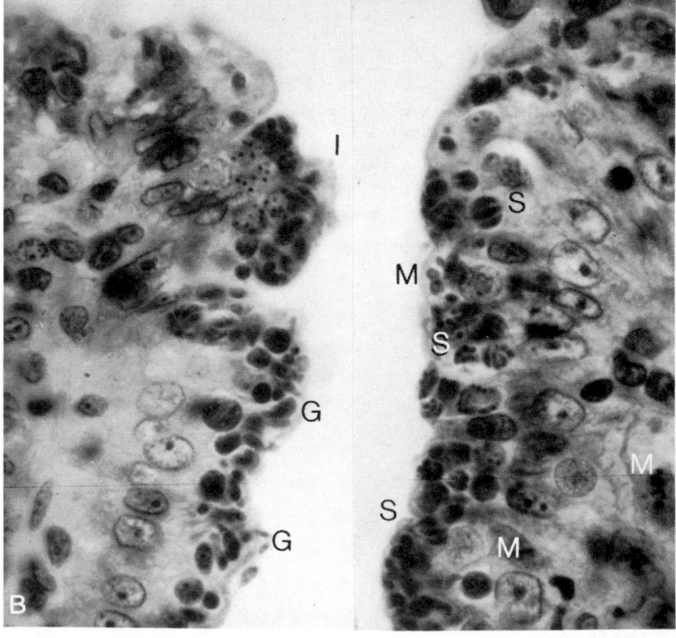


**Figure 10–13** *A,* Ileum of kitten heavily parasitized with *Toxoplasma* seven days after infection with bradyzoites. The organisms are located between the vesicular nuclei and the tips of the epithelial cells, and stain darkly with Giemsa. × 200. *B,* Schizonts (S), young gametes (G), macrogametes (M), and microgametes (I) of *Toxoplasma* in distal end of epithelial cell, the base of which is indicated by a row of vesicular nuclei. Giemsa, × 800. (Same animal and section.)

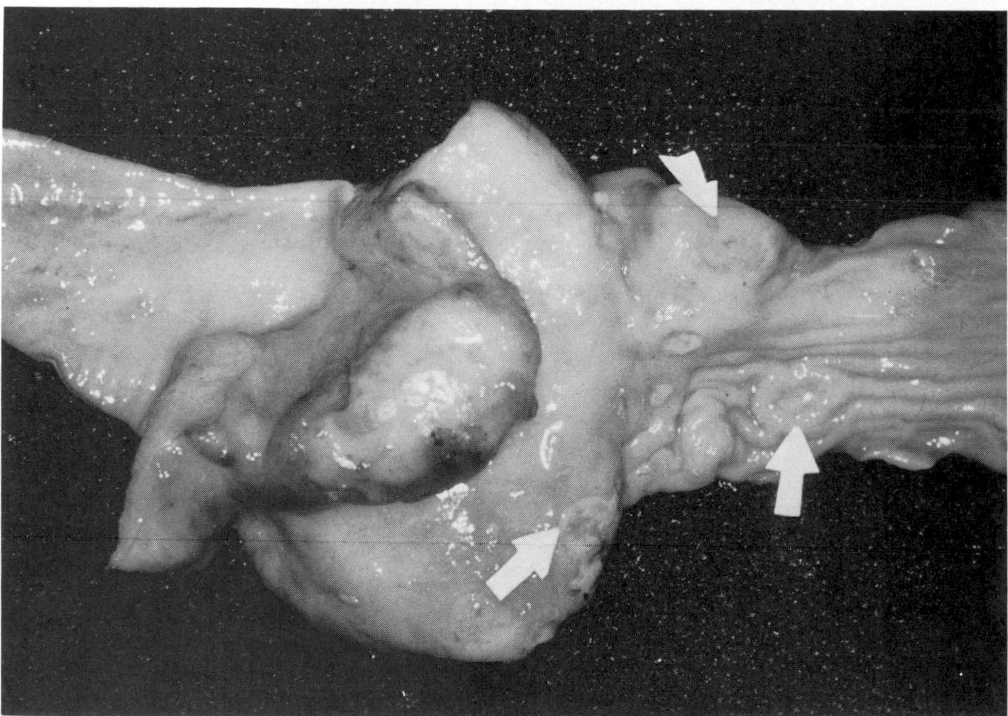

**Figure 10–14** A granulomatous mass containing *Toxoplasma* cysts projects into the lumen of the terminal ileum. There are superficial ulcerations (arrows) of the colon (right). In this and another aged cat, papillary or polypoid growths also projected from the mucosa of the small intestine. (From Meier H, Holzworth J, Griffiths RC: J Am Vet Med Assoc 131 [1957] 395–414.)

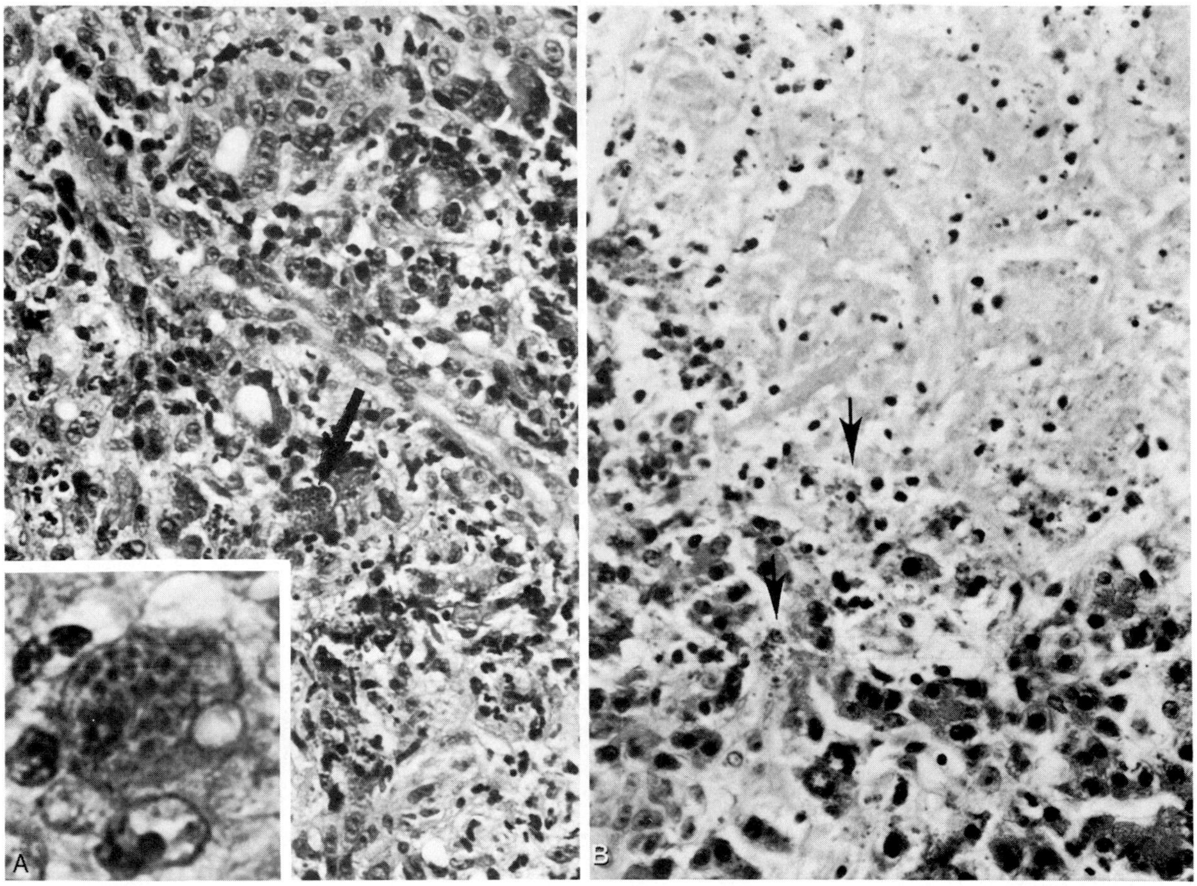

**Figure 10–15** *A,* Pancreatitis due to *Toxoplasma* organisms (arrow). Purulent mononuclear and necrotizing inflammation has destroyed all but a few tubules (top center). H&E, × 330. The inset shows a group of organisms apparently in a cyst (same animal), × 1200. *B,* Pancreatic necrosis due to *Toxoplasma* tachyzoites (arrows) in a cat that was injected IM with massive doses of 6-methylprednisolone acetate (40 mg/kg body weight/week) and died 25 days after the first injection. H&E, × 400. (*A* courtesy Angell Memorial Animal Hospital. *B* From Dubey JP, Frenkel JK: Vet Pathol 11 [1974] 350–379.)

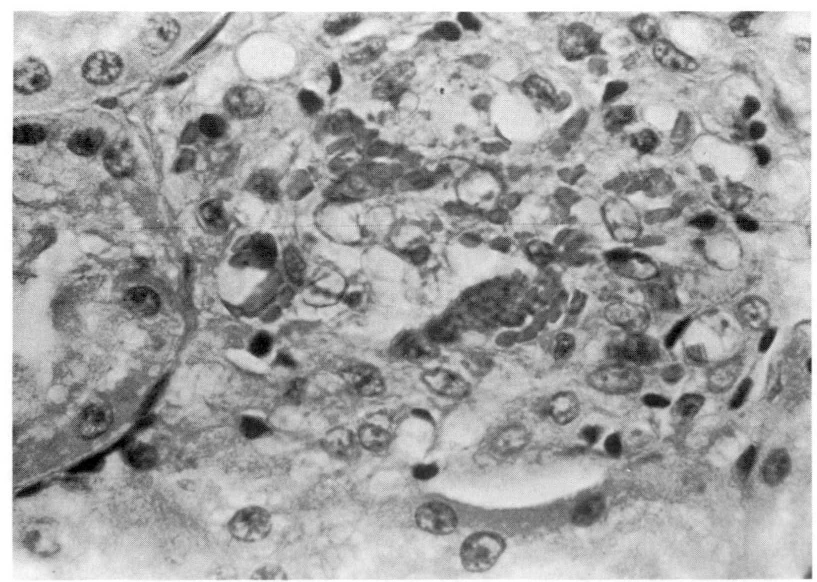

**Figure 10–16** Kidney. A cluster (center) of *Toxoplasma* tachyzoites in an altered and hemorrhagic glomerulus of a cat with disseminated toxoplasmosis. Organisms were present in many renal endothelial cells. Renal tubules (left) were unaffected. H&E, × 600. (Courtesy Angell Memorial Animal Hospital.)

with painful swelling of the forelegs. In addition to systemic toxoplasmosis, autopsy disclosed *Toxoplasma* in impression prints from the joints, as well as necrotizing dermatitis (Fig. 10–17), fibrositis, and myositis associated with *Toxoplasma*.

## Immunity

The quality of immunity that cats develop is more important to human than to feline well-being. The frequency of oocyst shedding and the numbers shed determine how many other animals and people are exposed to infection. However, we will first examine clinical immunity and antibody development before focusing on the role of immunity in transmission and epidemiology.

After experimental oral infection with cysts, newborn and nursling kittens generally sicken and sometimes die, but in kittens three to four months of age, illness and death are rare even though most cats still acquire a generalized infection. As do some other species, cats exhibit increased natural resistance with age.

**Premunition.** As in most animals, acute infection with *Toxoplasma* is followed by chronic infection, and infection-immunity (premunition) is common in cats. The finding of *Toxoplasma* cysts in routine autopsies of normal cats has already been mentioned (Ward et al., 1971), and the organism can be isolated from cats with antibody, either by inoculation of mice or by feeding tissues to cats and recovering oocysts after a few days (Dubey and Frenkel, 1976).

**Relapse.** Recrudescence of chronic infection occurs in seropositive cats and kittens given very large doses of anti-inflammatory corticosteroids (Dubey and Frenkel, 1974). Anti-inflammatory and immunosuppressive activity are closely related. That therapeutic administration of cortisol or its more potent analogues may reactivate latent toxoplasmosis or accentuate lesser levels of clinical activity has, however, been suggested by only one case report (Smart et al., 1973).

**Predisposing Factors.** In the cat as in other species, including man, it is likely that immunologic defects or suppression of immunity predispose to activation of what might otherwise have been an asymptomatic infection. Because testing for the feline leukemia virus (FeLV) is increasingly used as a diagnostic aid in illness of uncertain etiology, instances are coming to light of association of the FeLV carrier state with clinical toxoplasmosis. Indeed, in one cat followed at AMAH for four months for typical subacute toxoplasmosis with rising dye test titers despite specific chemotherapy, lesions of lymphoma were actually found at autopsy. Latent infections with coronavirus and syncytium-forming virus might also be predisposing factors.

The immunosuppressive effect of corticosteroid administration on latent experimental infection does not, however, seem to be duplicated under natural conditions;

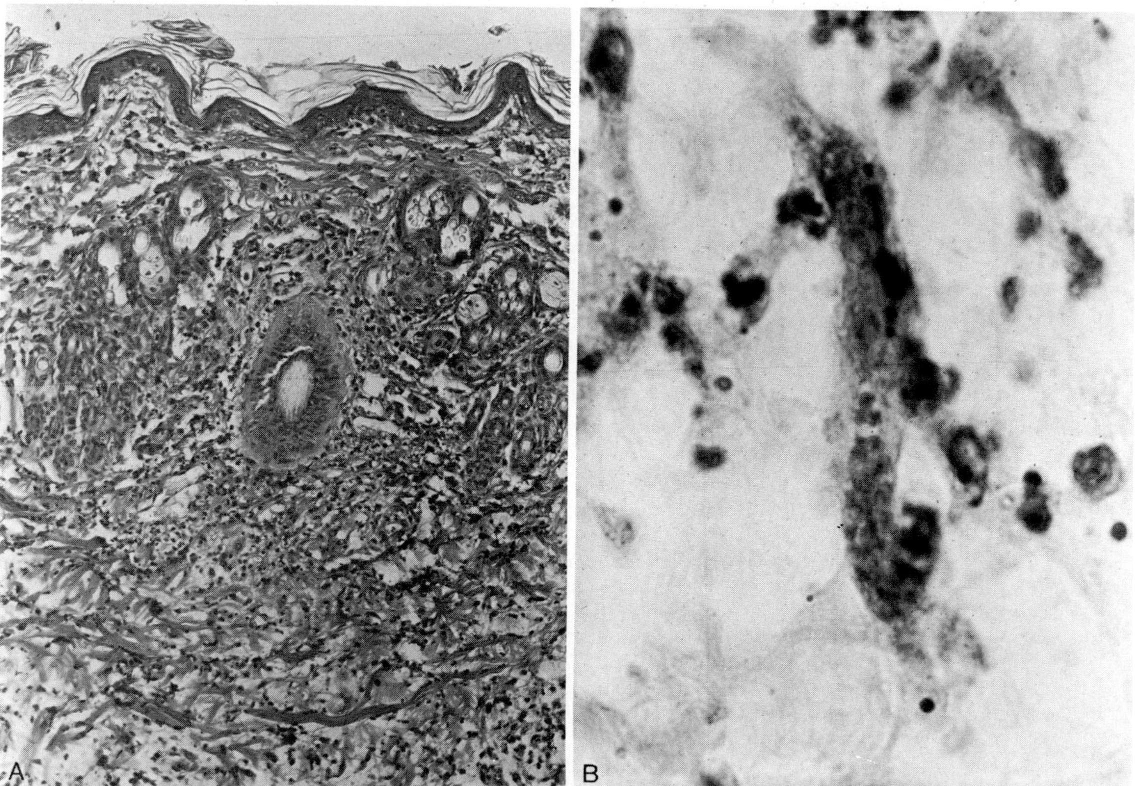


**Figure 10–17** *A*, Skin of the forearm of a cat with generalized toxoplasmosis. There is purulent, hemorrhagic, and necrotizing inflammation of the subcutis and deep dermis. Vascular damage led to necrosis and ulceration (not illustrated). H&E, × 125. *B*, *Toxoplasma* tachyzoites in a capillary of the subcutis of the forearm of the same cat. H&E, × 1000. (Courtesy, Angell Memorial Animal Hospital.)

doses that led to recrudescence of toxoplasmosis within a week in experimental cats were at least twice the maximal doses recommended clinically (Kirk, 1980). For a variety of feline disorders, steroids are administered in therapeutic, occasionally massive doses, sometimes for long periods, yet there appears to be only one published report (Smart et al., 1973) suggesting that 13 days of steroid treatment might have reactivated a latent *Toxoplasma* infection associated with cholangitis and pancreatitis. Because immunosuppression often is multicausal, with participation of genetic predisposition, underlying illness, accompanying infections, and therapy, the addition of corticosteroids might sometimes be the "last straw" that converts subclinical toxoplasmosis into disease.

**Role of Antibody and Its Relationship to Clinical Immunity in Cats.** Antibodies (measured by the dye test) appear toward the end of primary infection, and the end of oocyst shedding is taken to be one indicator of developing immunity. After infection of kittens with cysts, oocyst shedding started between four and five days, peaking at five to eight days, after which it declined and had ceased by day 15 in spite of reinfections (Frenkel and Dubey, 1972b). Antibody titers of 1:8 and 1:16 were measured in two of seven kittens by day 9 and in three kittens by day 12, but one kitten was still seronegative at day 25, although it had stopped shedding oocysts between days 12 and 15. This and the result of reinfection indicate that the clinical immunity instrumental in terminating oocyst shedding developed earlier than measurable antibody.

Just as immunity can appear in the absence of measurable antibody, so may immunity be absent or incomplete or may wane in the presence of antibody. For example, kittens born to a mother with antibody will, for two to three months, have passively transferred antibody, without being infected, yet show no evidence of immunity. Young kittens that develop antibody after primary infection may reshed oocysts when reinfected (Dubey and Frenkel, 1974, Table 1). After administration of large doses of methylprednisolone, three cats with antibody titers between 1:16 and 1:1024 reshed oocysts, and two died with disseminated recrudescent toxoplasmosis (Dubey and Frenkel, 1974, Fig. 1, Table 4). Interestingly, antibody titers decreased during this hypercorticoid period, a phenomenon not observed in hamsters or humans with fatal recrudescent toxoplasmosis.

Antibody titers in cats over two to three months of age indicate past and possibly persistent infection. The latter is not altogether certain, because *Toxoplasma* cannot be isolated from every cat with antibody; whether because of insufficient sample or loss of infection is not certain in most cases. Although some cats develop high antibody titers, the many low titers found are in contrast to those in chronic toxoplasmosis of dogs, mice, and hamsters; in humans presumably infected, titers may be similarly low. Rarely, after experimental infection, no antibody titers develop; on reinfection, antibody appears but no oocysts are shed (Dubey et al., 1970, Table 2). Several cats in which no antibody developed after primary infection were also free of chronic infection (Frenkel and Smith, unpublished study).

**Intestinal Immunity and the Effect on Oocyst Shedding.** The period of oocyst shedding ended 14 to 15 days after infection, irrespective of whether a single infection or eight infections were given at intervals of two days (Dubey and Frenkel, 1974). This finding was interpreted as indicating intestinal immunity, since if the duration of shedding depended merely on the endogenous cycle, oocysts should have been present for a month. However, administration of immunosuppressive doses of methylprednisolone, started on day 14 of infection, did prolong oocyst shedding until day 29, when the cats died (Dubey and Frenkel, 1974, Fig. 3).

The duration of shedding has never aroused as much interest as the onset of shedding. From a perusal of experiments in the author's laboratory in a population that is heterogeneous genetically and in age, 85 to 90 per cent of the cats ceased shedding by day 15 of infection; 10 to 15 per cent shed for 23 to 27 days.

How solid is immunity after a single infection and oocyst shedding cycle? Of kittens younger than 13 weeks when first infected, only 40 per cent were immune, and 60 per cent reshed oocysts on challenge after two to six weeks; all 15 cats older than 13 weeks when first infected were immune on challenge (Dubey and Frenkel, 1974, Table 1). The level of antibody present at the time of challenge played no role in the immunity exhibited: Six kittens with titers of 1:2 to 1:64 did not reshed on challenge, whereas 10 of 23 kittens with titers of 1:128 or over shed oocysts when challenged with the same strain of tissue cyst. All kittens challenged a second and third time were immune (Dubey and Frenkel, 1974, Table 2). Reinfection with different isolates of *Toxoplasma* resulted in more frequent reshedding, although this was not statistically significant. When immunity was not complete, most kittens, except the youngest, shed fewer oocysts after reinfection, and intervals between infection and shedding were longer than after primary infection.

This brings us to the role of a cat's immunity in the transmission of toxoplasmosis. When first infected at about six months of age, kittens shed once and are immune thereafter. When first infected while nursing or soon after weaning, kittens may shed a second time (usually fewer oocysts) and are immune thereafter. How long cats are immune thereafter is not known with certainty. Six to 12 months seems a safe assumption, based on a year's observation of a few cats (the cost of holding many cats for such long periods is prohibitive).

**Complicating Malnutrition and Coccidial Infections.** Since cats may not find sufficient food during the dry season in the tropics and may lose weight, this situation was simulated with kittens challenged at six to eight week intervals. Only one of seven reshed a moderate number of oocysts; its weight dropped from 2.0 to 1.6 kg, its hematocrit level from 37 to 24 per cent, and the antibody titer from 1:16 to 0 (Ruiz and Frenkel, 1980b). Similar reshedding on challenge was observed in six to 12 per cent of well-nourished kittens. Infection with *C. felis* and *C. rivolta* was reported to result in reshedding of *Toxoplasma* (Dubey, 1976b). However, in the experiments reported, gnotobiotic kittens, after weaning, were first infected with *Toxoplasma* and later with *C. felis* and *C. rivolta*, an unlikely situation in nature, where kittens are usually infected with *C. felis* and *C. rivolta*, often while nursing, and *Toxoplasma* infection occurs later. In previous studies (Dubey and Frenkel, 1974), *Toxoplasma* oocysts were not reshed by older kittens reinfected with *C. felis*, *C. rivolta*, and *T. gondii*. Six of 11 reshed on first challenge but were immune subsequently.

**Cellular Immunity.** How is immunity against *Toxo-*

*plasma* mediated? Most of the detailed information comes from studies of hamsters, mice, and humans. Antibody lyses *Toxoplasma* in the presence of accessory factor contained in normal human and certain animal sera (Sabin and Feldman, 1948). Recently the accessory factor system was shown to be identical to the classical complement pathway (Schreiber and Feldman, 1980). Antiserum with accessory factor reduces the number of extracellular *Toxoplasma* in a suspension to one-hundredth (Sulzer et al., 1967); they do not affect intracellular *Toxoplasma*. Transfusion of antiserum prolongs the survival time of hamsters with a fatal infection. It probably inactivates extracellular *Toxoplasma* without, however, affecting the total number of *Toxoplasma*, most of which are intracellular.

Intracellular immunity is mediated by lymphoid cells. Cells from spleen and lymph nodes of immune hamsters specifically protect immunologically naive hamsters against either *Toxoplasma* or *Besnoitia* (Frenkel, 1967). In-vitro analysis has shown that lymphocytes from immune donors mediate this immunity in macrophages (Hoff and Frenkel, 1974). A potential role of activated macrophages has been indicated by Remington and collaborators (1972). Cortisol interfered with lymphocyte mediation and to a lesser degree with mediation of immunity by macrophages (Lindberg and Frenkel, 1977a).

The role of thymic lymphocytes was shown with congenitally athymic nude mice. They develop immunity to *Toxoplasma* only if they have received transplants of thymic cells from syngeneic donors (Lindberg and Frenkel, 1977b). Soluble mediators of lymphocytes from immune donors do not kill *Toxoplasma* but inhibit its multiplication within cells. Such lymphocyte products have been described in mice, humans, and hamsters. The mediator from lymphocytes of hamsters conferred a measure of protection also on kidney cells and fibroblasts of hamsters and partially protected intact hamsters (Chinchilla and Frenkel, 1978). *Toxoplasma* mediator is specifically induced and expresses immunity specifically against *Toxoplasma* but not against *Besnoitia*, an organism used for specificity control, and only in the host of origin, the hamster. Its molecular weight is close to 4000 to 5000 daltons, and it resembles transfer factor in some respects.

Whether cellular immunity operates similarly in cats is not known. A mediator as described might be effective in the parenchymatous organs. Whether it also mediates intestinal immunity is doubtful. The possible role of IgA has not yet been studied. From a practical point of view, immunity protecting the vital organs of the cat and immunity preventing the shedding of oocysts should be differentiated.

## Treatment

Since the course of clinical toxoplasmosis is often rapid and fatal, treatment should be started as soon as the diagnosis appears probable, without a delay for laboratory confirmation.

The most effective treatment combines a sulfonamide, usually sulfadiazine or sulfamerazine, and pyrimethamine (Daraprim, Burroughs Wellcome). The combination inhibits multiplication of *Toxoplasma* but does not usually eradicate an established tissue infection. The drugs act synergistically by interfering sequentially with the biosynthesis of folinic acid by *Toxoplasma* (Eyles and Coleman, 1955; Summers, 1953). Sulfonamides prevent the conversion of para-aminobenzoic acid to dihydrofolate, and diaminopyridines (pyrimethamine, trimethoprim) suppress dihydrofolate reductase. Pyrimethamine is superior to trimethoprim in the latter function. If pyrimethamine is not on hand, sulfadiazine-trimethoprim (Tribrissen, Burroughs Wellcome), stocked by most veterinary practitioners may be used, although it may be no more effective than the sulfonamide alone.

Used alone, the more effective sulfonamides are sulfadiazine, sulfamerazine, sulfamethazine (singly or combined as "triple sulfa"), and sulfamethoxazole. All these reach a relatively high intracellular concentration where *Toxoplasma* multiplies. Some other sulfonamides (e.g., sulfisoxazole, sulfadimetine) are dissolved mainly in extracellular space and should not be used. Sulfathalidine and sulfasuxidine are not absorbed and are therefore ineffective.

The sulfonamide is given as a dose of 60 mg/kg body weight/day (divided into four doses) and pyrimethamine, 0.5 to 1.0 mg/kg (in a single daily dose). A loading dose of the latter (double dose for three days) is advocated for humans but has never been proven superior and could be hazardous to cats, in which the risk of marrow suppression appears to be high. If a cat is uncooperative about oral medication (especially with pyrimethamine and trimethoprim, which taste bitter), the drugs can be injected intramuscularly. The sodium salts of the sulfonamides are soluble in water; pyrimethamine can be dissolved in 85 per cent lactic acid (or 5 per cent acetic acid), refrigerated, and diluted with saline solution as needed (Sheffield and Melton, 1976). A soluble form of pyrimethamine may be available from Burroughs Wellcome. If a cat will eat, one may try mixing the drugs with food. Treatment should be given for one or two weeks and continued for a few days after improvement is certain.

A hemogram should be performed before treatment is started and repeated at intervals as dictated by an individual cat's hematologic reaction. In case of a significant fall in white cells (to 3000), platelets (to 100,000), or hematocrit, if the cat's condition is improving, pyrimethamine may be stopped and the sulfonamide continued at 120 mg/kg/day; otherwise folinic acid (leucovorin calcium, Lederle) should be given by injection or by mouth (1.0 mg daily for three days, the ampule with the remaining 2 mg being refrigerated). An alternative, cheaper source of folinic acid less easily administered to cats is bakers' yeast—a third of a package (100 mg/kg) daily by mouth or, if the cat is eating, in food. If the cat develops excessive gas, the amount should be reduced. Both leucovorin and yeast can be given together with therapy, without impairing its effect (Frenkel and Hitchings, 1957).

**Suppression of Oocyst Shedding.** Shedding of oocysts may be largely suppressed by sulfadiazine 60 to 120 mg/kg body weight daily, and by the combination of sulfadiazine 15 mg and pyrimethamine 0.2 to 2 mg/kg body weight daily (Frenkel, 1975). Clindamycin has been less effective and 2-sulfamoyl-4,4-diaminodiphenylsulfone clearly unreliable (Dubey and Yeary, 1977).

In the rather unlikely situation of starting treatment before anticipated infection, sulfadiazine (60 mg/kg) and pyrimethamine (0.5 mg/kg) divided into two to four daily doses or mixed with food effectively suppresses the cycle and prevents oocyst shedding (Frenkel and Smith, 1982a). Monensin (Coban, Eli Lilly), 0.02 per cent in food, use of which must be carefully supervised to avoid toxicity, prevents oocyst shedding even when started one to two days after an infectious meal, and could be used if for some compelling reason it were considered necessary to treat a cat that had consumed raw meat or had got out of doors for a possible meal of prey (Frenkel and Smith, 1982b).

## Public Health Significance

Modes of transmission to man as well as to a wide variety of animals have been described and illustrated in the section on epidemiology. Cats are of central importance in transmission. Although they clean themselves fastidiously and are therefore likely to carry few oocysts on fur or paws, they may, if infected, briefly shed in their feces vast numbers of oocysts potentially infectious for similar numbers of animals and humans. Man contracts infection directly by ingesting oocysts (e.g., from contaminated soil) or indirectly by handling (e.g., butchers, cooks) or eating raw or undercooked meat of animals (goats, sheep, pigs, cattle) that have been infected by oocysts (Penkert, 1973; Plant et al., 1974). Although infection is least likely in cattle, owing to early development of high antibody titers and sterile immunity (Fayer and Frenkel, 1979), a taste for raw beef and veal, as in France (Desmonts et al., 1965), entails a high risk of infection. So also may raw pork or "rare" lamb for ethnic societies or uninformed gourmets who consider these a delicacy.

Most human infections are asymptomatic or accompanied only by a febrile influenza-like illness, but serious disease of varied type is possible if immune potential is undeveloped or impaired, as in fetuses, infants, occasional adults, and patients imunosuppressed by corticosteroids or cytostatic drugs.

Sensationalist reporting in the lay press from time to time evokes extreme reactions such as irrational fear of cats, sometimes leading to their unnecessary destruction, as well as unrealistic bureaucratic schemes such as mass serologic surveillance of pregnant women, of pigs to be slaughtered, or even of pet cats. About half the United States population escapes infection without any special effort, and with available information and at small cost all persons can minimize the risk to themselves (and their cats) by a few simple hygienic precautions that protect against many other infections as well (Frenkel, 1973, 1974, 1981).

## Prevention

Meat should be heated to at least 66 C (150 F), or until the color changes throughout; freezing, salting, pickling, and smoking do not reliably destroy cysts. Hands should be washed before touching the face or eating and after contact with raw meat or soil. Children's sandboxes should be covered when not in use, and contaminated sand replaced. Flies and cockroaches should be controlled.

As for cats, they should be fed only commercial cat food or cooked or canned meat, with the possible exception of necks of commercially raised chickens, which are unlikely to be infected. Outdoor cats are less apt to consume prey if well-fed, and success in hunting is somewhat reduced if a cat wears a bell. Cat feces should be flushed down the toilet or burned within 24 hours, before oocysts, if present, become infective. Litter pans should be cleaned with boiling water, since no disinfectant is dependably active against *Toxoplasma* oocysts. A pregnant woman, unless known to be seropositive, should wear disposable gloves when handling a litter pan or should delegate the chore to someone else.

If for some special reason serologic testing appears desirable for a pregnant woman or a cat, informed interpretation of the result is essential. An antibody titer of 1:8 or over in the woman is reassuring, since it indicates immunity that will protect the unborn child from infection. A positive serologic test in a cat over two or three months of age is also evidence of immunity, but if reinfected or immunologically impaired, the cat might briefly reshed oocysts.

In the apparently rare event that oocysts in the size range of *Toxoplasma* (9 to 12 μ) are found in a cat's feces, the practical course, whether the cat is well or ill, is to isolate it for two to three weeks and handle feces and litter pan with maximal care. Treatment with drugs, as discussed earlier, may if desired be used as a further precaution, to suppress oocyst shedding, and would certainly be indicated in a cat suspected of symptomatic toxoplasmosis.

**VACCINATION.** Vaccination of cats, especially those going out of doors, would be desirable, less to prevent uncommon instances of illness than to avoid seeding of oocysts in litter pans and soil. Vaccines utilizing killed organisms and non–oocyst-producing laboratory strains of *Toxoplasma* do not immunize against oocyst shedding (Frenkel and Smith, 1982a). The only procedure so far developed is to infect cats by feeding viable tissue cysts and then inhibit oocyst shedding by administration of drugs (Frenkel and Smith, 1982b). Reshedding could still occur under certain circumstances. Research toward a possible vaccine for humans and meat animals is in progress with a strain of *Toxoplasma* that is immunogenic but does not persist in experimental animals (Elwell and Frenkel, 1984; Waldeland and Frenkel, 1983).

# CYTAUXZOONOSIS

ANN B. KIER and JOSEPH E. WAGNER

Cytauxzoonosis is a fatal blood protozoan disease of cats first reported in southwestern Missouri (Wagner, 1976). The infection has since been reported in cats in other areas of the United States—Texas (Bendele et al., 1976), Arkansas (Wagner et al., 1976), Georgia (Doster, 1976), Florida (Rubin, 1977), Mississippi (Conroy, 1979), Oklahoma (Glenn and Stair, 1984), and Louisiana (Hauck and Snider, 1982).

Although the life cycle of *Cytauxzoon felis* (Kier, 1979) has not been elucidated, both red-cell and tissue phases are observed. The red-cell phase is associated with hemolytic anemia, while the tissue phase may cause severe circulatory impairment or toxemia.

## Etiology

The genus *Cytauxzoon* of the family Theileriidae was first proposed by Neitz and Thomas (1948) in describing a fatal protozoan disease of African duikers. Cytauxzoonosis has since been described in other African ungulates—kudu (Neitz, 1957), eland (Martin and Brocklesby, 1960), sable and roan antelopes (Wilson et al., 1974), giraffe (McCully et al., 1970), and springbok (McCully, 1975). The report of the disease in cats in the United States was the first in other than African ruminants.

Some taxonomists believe that the genus *Cytauxzoon* should be incorporated into the genus *Theileria* in the family Theileriidae (Burridge, 1978; Levine, 1971). Members of this family have red-cell and tissue phases. Members of the genus *Cytauxzoon* have a prominent tissue phase in which schizonts develop in reticuloendothelial-like cells or macrophages mostly lining the walls of blood vessels. In contrast, the protozoans of the genus *Theileria* have a tissue phase primarily within lymphocytes. The red-cell phase of the two genera is identical, characterized by round, oval, "signet ring," and anaplasmoid-shaped bodies (piroplasms) about 1 μ in diameter within red cells.

## Clinical Features

Cats first become depressed and do not eat. Their temperature may rise to about 41.5 C (106 to 107 F), and anemia, jaundice, and dehydration may develop rapidly during the period of fever. Marked enlargement of the spleen and occasionally of the liver may be palpable. Changes in the hemogram are not consistent, but red- and white-cell counts may fall to half the normal levels. The number of nucleated red cells may rise slightly. Liver and kidney function test results and bilirubin values may be elevated in febrile or comatose animals but are not elevated earlier in the course of the disease. Hemoglobinuria and bilirubinuria are rare. After the period of fever, the temperature may become subnormal, and the cat may have difficulty in breathing. Cats usually die two or three days after the temperature peak, and the entire course of clinical illness is usually less than a week. Experimentally infected cats die 14 to 20 days after inoculation (Wagner et al., 1980).

## Diagnosis

Cytauxzoonosis should be considered in the differential diagnosis when a cat develops acute anemia, jaundice, and high fever. Diagnosis is made by demonstrating the red-cell phase (piroplasms) in Wright- or Giemsa-stained thin blood films (Fig. 10–18) and the tissue phase in Wright- or Giemsa-stained impression smears of spleen (Fig. 10–19), in H&E-stained paraffin sections (Fig. 10–20), or in Lee's methylene blue, basic fuchsin-stained plastic sections.

The piroplasms within red cells are round "signet ring"-shaped bodies 1 to 1.5 μ in diameter, bipolar oval "safety pin" forms 1 by 2 μ, or anaplasmoid round "dots" less than 1 μ in diameter. All forms may be observed in one blood film. The cytoplasm of the piroplasm stains light blue, the nucleus dark red or purple. The number of parasitized red cells varies from cat to cat and with the

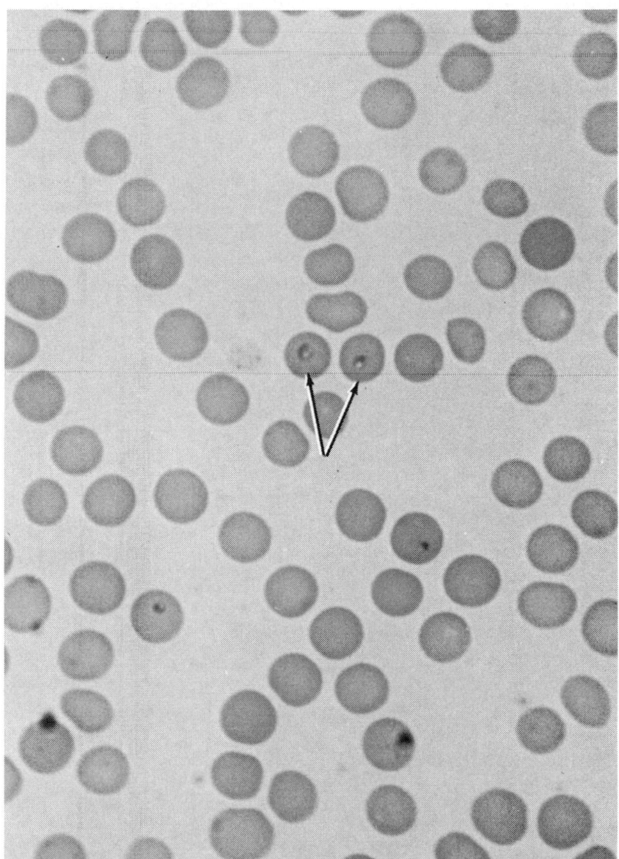

**Figure 10–18** Feline red blood cells infected with *Cytauxzoon* piroplasms: ring forms (arrows). Giemsa-Triton.

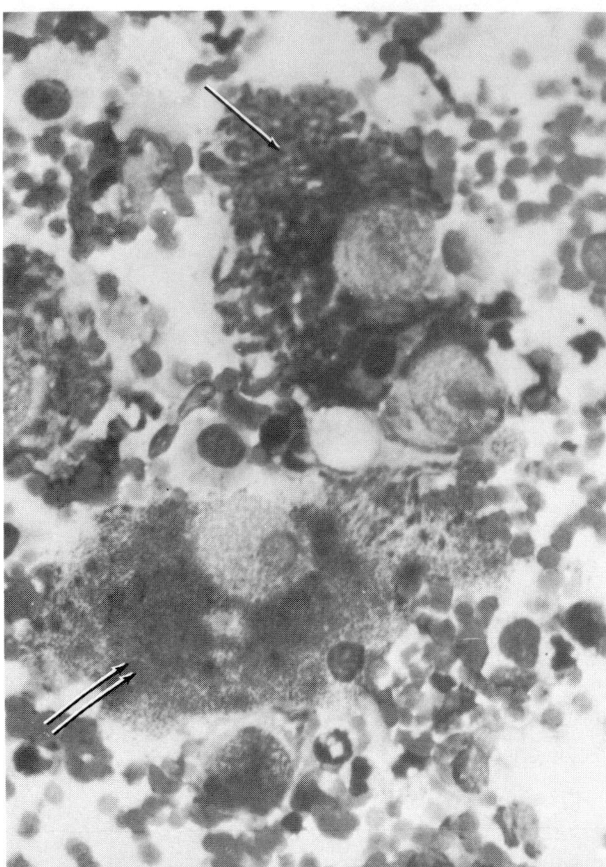

**Figure 10–19** Mature schizonts (arrow) and small merozoites (arrows) filling the cytoplasm of two macrophages (mononuclear phagocytes). Spleen impression smear, Giemsa-Triton.

stage of the disease. In experimental inoculations, piroplasms first appear with the onset of fever, and infected red cells may range from only a few per film to 25 per cent before death (Kier, 1979). A single red cell usually contains only one parasite, but pairs and tetrads (Maltese crosses) are observed occasionally.

At autopsy, veins in the abdominal cavity are greatly distended, and the spleen is dark and very large. The lungs may be diffusely red (congested) and edematous, often with petechiae throughout. Various lymph nodes may be large, edematous, and also often petechiated.

Microscopic examination of fixed tissue or tissue impression films is necessary to differentiate *Cytauxzoon* from *Babesia*, because their red-cell phases may appear identical (Riek et al., 1968). *Babesia felis* infection does not have a tissue phase, whereas the histopathologic lesions of *C. felis* infection are prominent. Large numbers of parasitized macrophages line the walls mostly of veins and venous channels in virtually all organs. Spleen, lungs, liver, and lymph nodes are the most heavily parasitized and are the organs of choice for histopathologic examination. Spleen should be used for tissue impression films, which should be stained with Wright's or Giemsa's stain.

An indirect fluorescent antibody (IFA) test was developed for the detection of feline cytauxzoonosis by Shindel et al. (1978) at the Plum Island Foreign Animal Disease Center.

## Pathogenesis and Ultrastructural Features

Success in the experimental isolation, passage, and cryopreservation of *C. felis* (Wagner et al., 1980) provides an opportunity for detailed study of the infection. Light microscopic and electron microscopic serial studies reveal that schizonts first appear as indistinct vesicular structures within the cytoplasm of infected macrophages and later in the course of the disease as distinct nucleated schizonts (macroschizonts) that divide by schizogony and binary fission. Late in the disease, buds develop on the macroschizonts and separate to become merozoites, filling the cytoplasm of the host cell. The host macrophage, filled with merozoites, probably ruptures and releases the organisms into the blood or tissue fluid. Merozoites appear in macrophages at about the same time that piroplasms are observed in red cells (Fig. 10–18), usually one to three days before the cat dies (Kier, 1979).

Details of the ultrastructure of the intraerythrocytic and schizont stages of a similar parasite from bobcats have been described (Simpson et al., 1985a, b).

## Transmission

The cat is most likely an accidental or dead-end host because of the relatively short course of illness and the

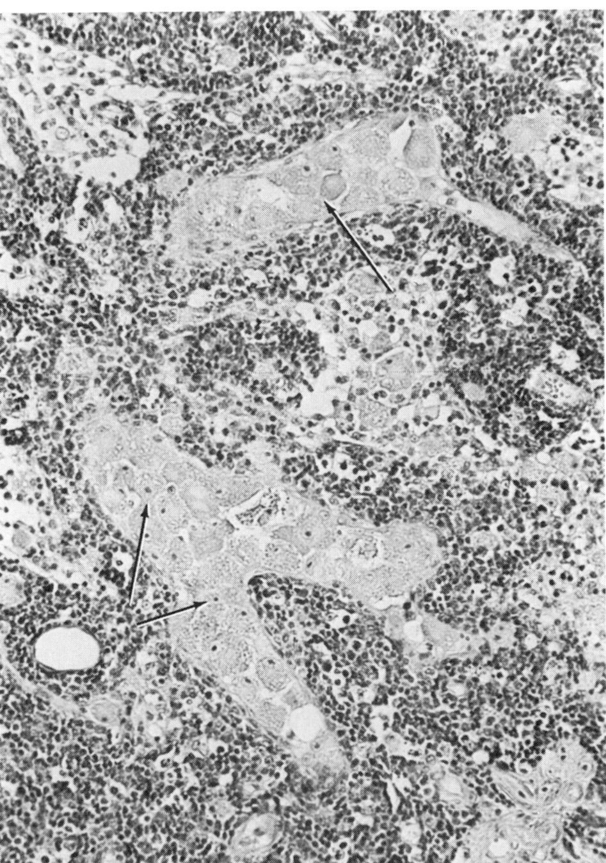

**Figure 10–20** Numerous infected mononuclear phagocytes filling the lumen and lining the walls of veins (arrows) within a lymph node from a cat infected with cytauxzoonosis. H&E.

uniformly fatal outcome of the disease. The mechanism of natural transmission of *C. felis* in cats or African ruminants is unknown. The disease can be experimentally transmitted by parenteral injection of fresh or frozen blood or tissue homogenates from an infected cat showing clinical signs. Contact with infected animals and inoculation by gavage with similar fresh or frozen material has failed to produce infection (Wagner et al., 1980). *Theileria* species in the same family (Theileriidae) as *Cytauxzoon* are transmitted by ixodid ticks. An arthropod vector remains the most likely mechanism of transmission (Wightman, 1978), and tick transmission of infection from bobcats to domestic cats has been demonstrated experimentally (Blouin et al., 1984).

Attempts to infect numerous domestic, laboratory, and wildlife species have been unsuccessful except in the bobcat, *Lynx rufus* (Kier et al., 1982a). Experimental infection of two bobcats produced in one, *Lynx rufus floridanus*, a fatal infection typical of that in domestic cats, while a long-lasting (four and a half years), nonfatal parasitemia developed in the other, *Lynx rufus rufus*. Inoculation of parasitemic blood from the latter bobcat into domestic cats resulted in nonfatal parasitemias of long duration (Kier et al., 1982b). The parasitemic domestic cats died when challenged with fresh-frozen ground spleen from cats succumbing to the fatal form of the disease. Asymptomatic infection occurs in the bobcat, which may serve as a biologic reservoir of cytauxzoonosis in the wild (Glenn et al., 1982).

### Prognosis, Treatment, and Preventive Measures

Preliminary attempts to treat cats with natural and experimentally induced disease have failed. Rapid multiplication of the tissue phase of the parasite may cause mechanical obstruction of blood flow, especially through the lungs (Wightman, 1978). By-products of tissue parasites may be toxic, pyrogenic, and vasoactive, while the blood phase may induce destruction and phagocytosis of red cells (Kier, 1979). Infected cats appear to die from a shocklike state in which supportive therapy with fluids and broad-spectrum antibiotics (e.g., tetracyclines) may prolong the course of illness but do not effect a cure.

A conscientiously applied ectoparasite control program and confinement of cats indoors could be beneficial in preventing cytauxzoonosis, since all naturally occurring cases have involved cats free to roam in rural, wooded, tick-infested areas.

## Acknowledgments

This work was supported in part under terms of a Memorandum of Agreement with the Animal Plant Health Inspection Service (APHIS) of the USDA and cooperative studies by UMC and the PIADC (USDA ARS 12-14-1001-811), by the Foreign Animal Disease Laboratory of the Agricultural Research Service, USDA (Greenport, New York 11944), and by NIH grants RR00471 and RR00506.

# OTHER PROTOZOAN DISEASES

JEAN HOLZWORTH

## BABESIOSIS (PIROPLASMOSIS, NUTTALLIOSIS, BILIARY FEVER, TICK BITE FEVER)

The Babesiae are parasitic protozoa occurring in the red blood cells and transmitted by ticks. They are tiny, pear-shaped bodies usually arranged in twos in the red cells. With Giemsa's stain, the cytoplasm is bluish and the nucleus red. Reproduction is by binary fission, which takes place both in the vertebrate host's red cells and in ticks that transmit the disease by injecting the organism into the host when they suck blood.

Babesiosis has been reported in members of the cat family, both wild and domestic, in Africa and India. Although found in pumas imported into Egypt from California and in American lynx in the London zoo, its occurrence in Felidae in North America is uncertain (Levine, 1973). A species of *Babesia* was identified in a jaguarundi originating in South America (Dennig, 1967).

*Babesia felis* was first recognized in a Sudanese wild cat (Davis, 1929). It appears to be specific for members of the cat family. It is not infectious for dogs, rodents, or ruminants (Davis, 1929), nor can cats, on the other hand, be infected by *Babesia canis* (Thomas and Brown, 1934). Davis found that the infection could be passed by any route to domestic cats, in which the incubation period was about one to three weeks, depending on the dose of infective blood. The organism measured 1.0 to 2.24 μ. Its cytoplasm stained faint blue, its chromatin dark red. The bodies were pear-shaped, ameboid, or round, many appearing ring-shaped owing to central vacuolation. When division occurred, there was the appearance of four individuals arranged in a cruciform manner.

Although the hemoglobin level dropped and there was a tendency to leukocytosis, clinical signs were absent despite the indefinite persistence of a slight fluctuating infection. In a cat splenectomized after inoculation, hemoglobinuria developed, but death occurred only in the one cat splenectomized before infection.

Naturally occurring infection in domestic cats was first recognized in South Africa in 1937. Futter and coworkers (1980, 1981) reviewed the literature on feline infection and reported their findings in 70 natural and 20 experimental cases.

In the domestic cat, babesiosis is encountered almost exclusively in the Republic of South Africa, where it is an infectious disease of great importance. Single cases of infection of domestic cats with *Babesia* species of uncertain identification have been reported in Zimbabwe (Stewart et al., 1980) and India (Mangrulkar, 1937). The infection is presumed to be tick-borne, although the vector has never been identified.

### Clinical Features

A majority of clinical infections occur in cats two years old or younger (Futter and Belonje, 1980b). Immunity from exposure appears to develop after that age, and affected older cats usually have some concurrent illness. In some cats the infection is asymptomatic, being discovered in routine blood examination, as when a cat is presented for spaying.

Characteristic signs in overt infection are lethargy, weakness, partial or complete inappetence, weight loss, and pallor. Unlike humans and dogs with babesiosis, cats are rarely febrile. The feces are typically bright orange, and occasionally there is diarrhea. Jaundice is present in about 18 per cent of cases (13 of 70, Futter and Belonje, 1980b). Tachycardia and dyspnea are present in severe cases, with low tolerance for handling and exertion. Terminally cats may cry out as though in pain, and temperatures become subnormal.

Among experimental cases, the general course of the infection was similar in the splenectomized and nonsplenectomized cats, although the latter were less severely affected.

### Diagnosis

Blood films should be checked routinely in examination of any cat in endemic areas. In contrast with hemobartonellosis, parasitemia is consistently present in cats with babesiosis. Fifty per cent or more of the red cells may be parasitized. Giemsa's stain is favored, but less time-consuming methods give satisfactory results in practice. Single signet-ring or round forms with varying dispositions of chromatin were the most frequent forms of *Babesia* (Futter and Belonje, 1980b). Single and double pear-shaped forms were also common. The typical Maltese-cross forms were not always seen.

The red cells exhibit the characteristics of a regenerative anemia: polychromasia, increased anisocytosis, Howell-Jolly bodies, and nucleated red cells. Many red cells may be macrocytic and hypochromic. Anemia is considered to be severe when the PCV falls to 9 to 12 per cent. No consistent alteration in the total white-cell count is observed. Erythrophagocytosis, of both parasitized and non-parasitized cells, by monocytes is frequent.

Blood films taken from the kittens of a parasitized mother shortly after birth showed no organisms (Futter and Belonje, 1980b).

Total serum protein levels in a large group of natural cases were in general unchanged, but $\gamma$-globulin levels were significantly increased, while $\alpha$- and $\beta$-globulin levels were decreased (Futter et al., 1981). Total bilirubin was elevated in about half the clinical cases, indirect bilirubin values exceeding the direct in the most anemic cats. The SGPT (ALT) was elevated in less than half of 37 naturally infected cats tested; these cats were receiving primaquine phosphate in treatment. Renal function was unimpaired.

### Pathologic Features

Autopsy findings were nonspecific (Futter et al., 1981). Icterus was uncommon, but the liver was often enlarged and yellow or dark brown, sometimes with mottling. The mesenteric nodes were occasionally enlarged. Microscopically, the most consistent changes in the liver were varying degrees of centrilobular necrosis, bile stasis, and extramedullary hematopoiesis. Pigment presumed to be hemosiderin was found in livers and an unidentified pigment in kidneys.

### Treatment

In treatment a variety of agents have been used with varying success: trypan blue, acriflavine, phenamidine, oxytetracycline, tetracycline, cephaloridine, quinuronium sulfate (Acaprin, Bayer), diminazene (Berenil, Hoechst), and primaquine phosphate. Primaquine (0.5 mg/kg IM) appears to be the most effective (Potgieter, 1981; Stewart et al., 1980). With gentle handling and prompt treatment the prospects of recovery are good (e.g., in 40 of 70 clinical cases, Futter and Belonje, 1980a). Occasional relapses occur and also occasional cases of toxicity from primaquine. Severely anemic cats are sometimes given a blood transfusion before drug treatment is started.

In human babesiosis and in experimental babesiosis of hamsters, clindamycin has been found to be effective (Rowin et al., 1982).

## GIARDIASIS

*Giardia*, a protozoan parasite of the small intestine of many vertebrates worldwide, has provided recreation for taxonomists for over a century. Some have recognized but a single species, others three principal types, and still others as many as 40 more or less host-specific species.

### Etiology

*G. lamblia* (*G. intestinalis*) of man was first described in detail in 1859, and a similar parasite was observed in the domestic cat in Italy as early as 1881 (Grassi, 1881) and subsequently elsewhere in Europe and in South America. The species of the domestic cat, however, was not named or carefully described until 1925, when studies appeared simultaneously in France and the United States (Deschiens, 1925; Hegner, 1925). Deschiens' term *G. cati* received precedence over Hegner's *G. felis*. (*G. felis* was assigned to the species Hegner recovered from the North American bay lynx, a species since considered to be the same as *G. cati*). It has been suggested that *G. cati* may also be the same species as *G. canis* of the dog, but Deschiens was unable to infect dogs with the feline species (Deschiens, 1926).

Pending thorough restudy for comparative morphology and specificity, it was suggested in 1978 that traditional specific names be retained (Kulda and Nohynkova, 1978). As the result of a subsequent review, however, the pendulum has swung back to the view that all forms described may be but variants of a single species, *Giardia lamblia* (Levine, 1979). Numerous studies of interspecies transmission have shown that there are indeed many isolates of *Giardia* that are not host-specific. *Giardia* of man has, for example, been transmitted to cats (Kessel, 1929), and feline *Giardia* can infect Mongolian gerbils (Belosevic et al., 1984; Kirkpatrick and Farrell, 1984). There is also immunologic evidence of interspecies susceptibility, preliminary experiments indicating that *Giardia* of the human, the cat, and the guinea pig are antigenically isologous (Visvesvara et al., 1980).

## Morphology

*Giardia* occurs in two forms—trophozoites and cysts (Fig. 10–21). Trophozoites are most likely to be seen in diarrheic feces; cysts occur in both loose and formed stools. The trophozoite is bilaterally symmetric, rounded anteriorly, pointed posteriorly, and convex dorsally, with two nuclei, a pair of dark median bodies, and eight paired flagella. The trophozoite has been likened in outline to a longitudinally split pear (Wenyon, 1926) or a tennis racket (Georgi, 1980), but the eyelike nuclei and liplike median bodies just below also give it the appearance of a face. Seen from the side it has a crescent shape. These comparisons, however, apply to fixed, stained specimens. When *Giardia* is moving rapidly in fresh preparations, its distinguishing features are not so easily recognized.

The trophozoites are 10 to 18 μ long and 6.5 μ wide and attach to the intestine by a sucking disc that interdigitates between the microvilli of the epithelial cells (Kulda and Nohynkova, 1978). Unlike trophozoites of most other species, those of the cat have been found not only in the small intestine, principally the jejunum, but also in the cecum and colon (Hitchcock and Malewitz, 1956). The trophozoites feed by imbibition of intestinal fluids containing products from the host's epithelial cells (Kulda and Nohynkova, 1978). They multiply by binary fission, and some encyst. Binary fission may also occur in cysts. The oval cysts, measuring about 10 × 7 μ, may thus contain two or four nuclei.

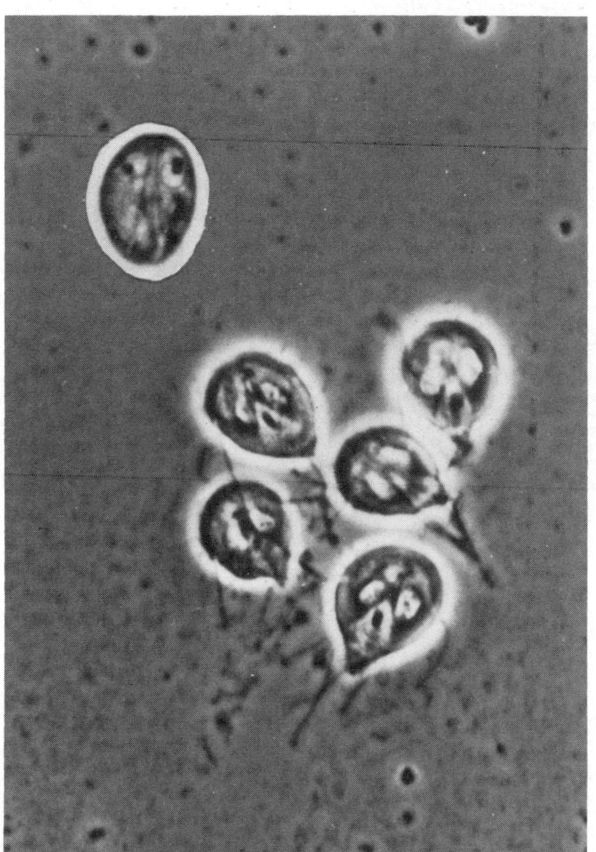

**Figure 10–21** *Giardia.* A group of trophozoites (center) and a cyst (inset, upper left). *Giardia* trophozoites and cysts are commonly found in mice. Bona fide infections occur in cats but must be distinguished from cases of spurious parasitism arising from carnivorism. × 1700. (From Georgi JR: Parasitology for Veterinarians, 4th ed. Philadelphia, WB Saunders Company, 1985.)

## Epizootiology

The cysts, excreted in stool, may survive for months in cold water (even in chlorinated drinking water) but are quickly destroyed by drying or by boiling water. Freezing at −13 C for two weeks does not completely inactivate them (Kirkpatrick and Farrell, 1982). They infect new hosts by contamination of food or water, by coprophagy, or by direct fecal spread. In the cat the prepatent period between exposure and the appearance of *Giardia* in the feces has been variously reported as 11 to 13 days (Belosevic et al., 1984) and 5 to 16 days (mean 9.6) (Kirkpatrick and Farrell, 1984). Shedding of cysts is usually intermittent.

English cats were found to be commonly infected (Wenyon, 1926), but information as to prevalence is sparse. In a study of parasitism in a group of 147 Michigan kittens, *Giardia* was found in 5 per cent (Hitchcock, 1953); in a Minnesota study of 291 fecal samples, in 3 per cent (Bemrick, 1961); and in 2.4 per cent of 757 stray cats in New Jersey (Burrows and Hunt, 1970). Among 90 cats examined in Milan by intestinal scrapings, 5.6 per cent yielded *Giardia* (De Carneri and Castellino, 1963); among 100 similarly examined in Valdivia, Chile, 7 per cent (Torres et al., 1972); and among 500 in a Belgian survey, 10.8 per cent (Vanparijs and Thienpont, 1973). A survey in Zurich identified only six infections among 927 cats (Wolff and Eckert, 1979).

## Pathogenesis and Clinical Features

*Giardia* varies greatly in pathogenicity. Heavy infections, with discharge of numerous cysts, may be asymptomatic, while in some severe cases of diarrhea trophozoites may be recovered only with difficulty. The mechanism by which *Giardia* causes diarrhea is a matter of debate. Diarrhea is most often chronic or intermittent.

Typically stools are light-colored and soft or loose, with much mucus. Blood is rarely present, but in some cases there is excessive fat, suggesting pancreatic insufficiency or malabsorption. Experimental findings indicate that the trophozoites directly inhibit lipolysis by pancreatic lipase; they also damage the brush border of the intestinal epithelium, causing a deficiency of some disaccharidases, especially lactase (Kirkpatrick and Farrell, 1982). Not surprisingly, the resulting digestive impairment leads to weight loss even in a host that is eating well. Young animals are most often affected, suggesting that a degree of immunity may develop with age.

Reports of symptomatic infections in cats are uncommon. Craige (1963) encountered a few cases in which he judged the organism to be the cause of diarrhea, which ceased after treatment with quinacrine hydrochloride (Atabrine 5 mg/kg b.i.d. orally for two or three days, repeated after several days if necessary).

The majority of clinical cases have occurred in cattery or colony groups. Five cases in which *Giardia* was apparently the pathogen were reported by Brightman and Slonka (1976). Four of the cats were young Persian littermates, the fifth a three-year-old spayed female Birman. Weight loss and soft, sometimes mucoid stools were the principal signs. The youngest cat also had a rectal prolapse. Feline leukemia tests and fecal cultures for *Salmonella* were negative in all. Slight eosinophilia in four cats and increased levels of split and unsplit fecal fat were the only significant laboratory findings, in addition to the demonstration, by a standard flotation technique, of moderate to heavy infection with *Giardia* cysts. In one case it was only on a third fecal examination that the cysts were found; in another, two examinations were needed. Twelve days' treatment with quinacrine hydrochloride (10 mg/kg daily) resulted in normal stools and weight gain, although only one cat was entirely free of cysts at the end of treatment.

In a cattery where diarrhea had been a continuous or intermittent problem for several years, 7 of 14 Persians were found to be infected in the course of three testings. The infection mainly involved cats under three years of age. The cats were treated with apparent success with furazolidone suspension, and the cages were cleaned with detergent and soaked with 1 per cent bleach (sodium hypochlorite) (Kirkpatrick and Laczak, 1985).

An outbreak of giardiasis in a small laboratory colony was traced to introduction of a stud cat that infected two females during breeding contact (Belosevic et al., 1984). Two other cats that had no contact with the stud remained uninfected. The stud cat had diarrhea, but the stools of the other two cats appeared normal, although they were passing large numbers of cysts. The stud cat was treated successfully with metronidazole.

Individual cases of natural infection were recorded by Kirkpatrick and Farrell (1984), Nesvadba (1979), and Wolff and Eckert (1979). Only a few cases of giardiasis have been recognized at AMAH. A notable feature in one kitten was prominent protrusion of the third eyelids; after five days' treatment with metronidazole (50 mg/kg once a day), the diarrhea had ceased and the eyelids had returned to normal.

## Diagnosis

If giardiasis is suspected, several fecal examinations may be required. It is likely that many *Giardia* infections are not diagnosed, because the organisms are not continuously present and also because routine methods of fecal examination are unsuitable for detection of the parasite.

Diagnostic procedures are well described by Kirkpatrick and Farrell (1982). Trophozoites can be demonstrated only in wet mounts of direct smears of fresh feces. One slide is left unstained and a second is stained with a drop of Lugol's iodine solution, which accentuates the characteristic internal features of the trophozoites, although stopping their motility.

For concentrating *Giardia* cysts in a fecal sample, the favored method is the zinc sulfate centrifugation technique, because sugar solution or other salts render the cysts unrecognizable. Preparation of the solution and the steps in the technique are described by Kirkpatrick and Farrell (1982), as well as in laboratory manuals. An alternative method is the formalin–ethyl acetate sedimentation technique.

If a fecal specimen cannot be examined at once, refrigeration in a tightly closed container will preserve cysts for several days (Kirkpatrick, 1984). Otherwise the specimen may be preserved at room temperature by addition of three volumes of 2 to 5 per cent formalin or polyvinyl alcohol. Fixed smears stained with iron-hematoxylin or trichrome are desirable for study of the finer details of morphology. Tissue sections are adequately stained with hematoxylin and eosin, but Giemsa staining gives superior results.

Giardiasis may also be diagnosed by intestinal aspirates or mucosal impression smears of biopsy specimens obtained by an endoscope. In dogs duodenal aspiration has revealed more than twice as many infections as detected by a single zinc sulfate fecal flotation (Pitts et al., 1983).

## Treatment

Quinacrine, metronidazole, and furazolidone have all been used for treatment of giardiasis in cats, although not approved by the Food and Drug Administration for veterinary use. Metronidazole has been used most often and has been reported effective at doses varying from 10 to 25 mg/kg b.i.d. Furazolidone (4 mg/kg b.i.d. for five days) was found to be equally effective, with the advantages that it is less costly and can be easily administered as a suspension (Kirkpatrick and Laczak, 1985). Quinacrine is given at 10 mg/kg daily for five days and repeated if necessary.

## Public Health Significance

In view of the evidence of interspecies transmission of many strains of *Giardia* it must clearly be regarded as a possible public health hazard. In fact, infected cats have been found in households of persons with giardiasis (Davies and Hibler, 1979).

Preventive measures should take into account that infection occurs by fecal contamination of water, food, and the environment. Prompt disposal of cat litter and thorough cleaning of sanitary pans are important measures for prevention and elimination of giardial infection. It is of interest that most of the cases reported (Brightman and Slonka 1976; Kirkpatrick and Laczak, 1985) involved purebred cats, for catteries or laboratory colonies would provide the environment most conducive to infection.

## LEISHMANIASIS

Leishmaniasis, a disease predominantly of man and dogs but also occasionally of the cat, occurs in the Mediterranean basin, the Middle East and Far East, and South America. Visceral and superficial forms of the disease are distinguished, although the two may coexist. In the former (kala-azar, dumdum fever), the signs are fever, wasting, anemia, and leukopenia, and the spleen, liver, and lymph nodes are enlarged. The parasite, *Leishmania donovani*, is found in these organs and the bone marrow as well.

In cutaneous leishmaniasis, "oriental sore," the agent of which is *L. tropica*, the lesion is a chronic ulcer elevated at the borders and covered with a crust. Histologically, there is a diffuse infiltration of plasma cells and lymphocytes. Healing is slow and leaves a depressed scar. With recovery comes permanent immunity. In the South American form of leishmaniasis (espundia), caused by *L. braziliensis*, there are ulcers both of the skin and of the oral and nasal mucosa.

Infection is by the bite of *Phlebotomus* sandflies and may also occur, in cutaneous infections, by direct contact or self-inoculation (e.g., through scratching or wounds). In the insect, the organism exists in a flagellate form; in the mammalian host, where it parasitizes and multiplies in the reticuloendothelial cells, it is without flagella.

In the visceral disease, the agent is rarely found in the blood, and the diagnosis is usually made by biopsy punctures of marrow, spleen, liver, or lymph nodes. In superifical infections, *Leishmania* is usually found in smears of the lesions. In Wright- or Giemsa-stained preparations, it appears as a round or ovoid body, 2 to 5 μ long and 1 to 2 μ wide; the cytoplasm is light blue and the prominent spherical nucleus, eccentric and red. The tiny, rod-shaped kinetoplast, staining red or violet, is situated near the nucleus. In diagnosis, culturing on a rabbit-blood medium and inoculation of mice or hamsters must sometimes be resorted to.

Wild rodents are the main reservoir of the agent; humans, dogs, and occasionally cats suffer from symptomatic infection. In cats, the cutaneous form of the disease, recognized in the Far and Middle East, Algeria, and South America, usually takes the form of crusty ulcers on the lip, nose, eyelids, and edge of the ears (Bergeon, 1927; Bosselut, 1948; Machattie et al., 1931; Mello, 1940). The occurrence of most of the lesions on the head suggests that they may result from *Phlebotomus* bites or possibly from scratches inflicted by the victim itself or by other cats.

Clinical cases of visceral disease appear to be uncommon in cats, but in a case reported from Indochina, the organism was found both in a stubborn ulcer on the skin of the thorax and in the spleen (Bergeon, 1927).

It would seem that although cats in the Mediterranean area and in South America may occasionally be found to harbor the agent of visceral leishmaniasis without showing clinical signs of illness (Ferreira et al., 1938; Gimeno Ondovilla, 1933; Sergent et al., 1912), this is perhaps an unusual occurrence, inasmuch as a Sicilian survey conducted in an area and at a season of high incidence in man failed to discover a single infected cat (Giordano, 1933).

Treatment of clinically infected cats does not seem to have been reported. Leishmaniasis in man and the dog is treated with antimony compounds and the aromatic diamidines (Levine, 1973). Cutaneous infections may also be treated with amphotericin B (Fungizone, Squibb), metronidazole (Flagyl, Searle), and cycloguanil pamoate.

## TRICHOMONIASIS

Trichomonads are occasionally found in the stool of cats, mostly as asymptomatic commensals but sometimes in association with illness and diarrhea. Whether they are the cause of the diarrhea or are stimulated by it to proliferate has long been the subject of varying opinions.

Trichomonads are variably ellipsoid or pear-shaped protozoans, rounded in front and pointed behind, with a group of anterior flagella, an axostyle constituting a central longitudinal axis, and a posterior flagellum passing back along an undulating membrane that contributes an asymmetric appearance to the organism. Trichomonads reproduce by longitudinal binary fission. In fresh suspensions of feces in physiologic saline solution they exhibit a rapid, jerky, swimming movement.

The trichomonad of the cat's large intestine, also found occasionally in the stomach and small intestine (Brumpt, 1925; Wagner and Hees, 1935), was named *Trichomonas felis* when it was first recognized in a Brazilian cat sick with diarrhea (da Cunha and Muniz, 1922), but this organism, as well as those reported from the monkey, dog, and rat, has been shown experimentally to be identical with *Pentatrichomonas hominis* (*Trichomonas intestinalis*) of man, and the cat may be an accidental rather than natural host (e.g., Kessel, 1926; Wenrich, 1944). Experimental evidence indicates that infection may occur among cats by contact (Hegner and Eskridge, 1935).

The trichomonads of the cat's intestine vary in length from 6 to 14 μ, with a mean of 7.5 μ and are 4 to 6 μ wide (Brumpt, 1925; da Cunha and Muniz, 1922; Wenrich, 1944). They have three, four, or, most often, five anterior flagella. An additional posterior flagellum extends along the outer margin of the undulating membrane and trails free behind.

Instances of naturally occurring infection have been reported, usually in young cats—in the United States in Georgia (Jordan, 1956), Maryland (Hegner and Eskridge, 1935), Michigan (Hitchcock, 1953), and Missouri (Visco et al., 1978) and also in Brazil (da Cunha and Muniz, 1922), France (Brumpt, 1925), Germany (Wagner and Hees, 1935), Yugoslavia (Simic, 1932), and China (Kessel, 1926, 1928).

### DIAGNOSIS

Diagnosis is by several methods. The simplest is microscopic examination of direct smears made from stool freshly passed or obtained by a rectal swab and diluted with physiologic saline solution. Identification is facilitated if fresh stool is fixed and stained with Giemsa, by the Schaudinn iron-hematoxylin method, or by the use of picric acid and formaldehyde fixative (Burroughs, 1967) and thionin or azure A stain. For detection of light infection the stool may have to be examined several times, and culture may even be required.

### Clinical Features and Treatment

Not all the infected cats showed signs of illness, and even when they did, there was sometimes a possibility that another parasite or agent was the primary cause of trouble. In 3 of 10 cats harboring intestinal trichomonads, the organisms were also found in the blood (Wagner and Hees, 1937).

In what was believed to be a primary clinical infection, signs of illness in some kittens were diarrhea, with a yellow-brown stool, and wasting, leading to death in a week. Autopsy disclosed a catarrhal inflammation of the intestine with necrosis and ulceration of the superficial layer of the mucosa. Trichomonads were found in the necrotic areas, between the cells of the mucosa, and within the lumen of enlarged glands (Kessel, 1926, 1928).

Infections in which trichomonads appeared to be the cause of illness have been encountered by Fishler (1979) and at AMAH. In one of Fishler's cases, the cat, a depressed six-month-old, 3-kg male, had a fever of 39.8 C (103.5 F), no appetite, and severe diarrhea with a gray-brown, semiliquid stool. High-power microscopic examination disclosed numerous motile flagellates identical with those seen in cases of canine trichomoniasis. Treatment with metronidazole was started (125 mg orally t.i.d.), and even before the second dose the cat acted better, its fever started down, and diarrhea ceased. Within a day the cat resumed eating. Metronidazole treatment was continued at home for 10 days, at the end of which the owner reported the cat was in excellent heatlh.

In the case at AMAH, a six-month-old male longhair acquired from a pet store had passed a chalky white, watery stool five or six times a day for eight weeks. The cat was small for its age, thin, ataxic, and disoriented, with a fever of 39.9 C (103.8 F). The total WBC was 82,390/μl, with 90 per cent segmented neutrophils; the PCV was 40. Stool culture was negative for *Salmonella*, but on the third day's microscopic examination, numerous trichomonads were seen. Although the cat's general condition and ataxia improved with administration of electrolytes and vitamins, the diarrhea had been unaffected by chloramphenicol and neomycin. However, quinacrine (Atabrine), 50 mg daily for five days, brought about prompt cessation of diarrhea and return of the temperature to normal.

Trichomonads were eliminated from experimentally infected cats with carbarsone (Lilly), 150 mg/kg by mouth daily for five days (Hegner and Eskridge, 1935). Carbarsone enemas eliminated the trichomonads from a chronically ill, three-year-old Georgia cat also parasitized with hookworms, but the animal subsequently died of a hemorrhagic diarrhea, with autopsy findings suggestive of acute systemic disease, possibly the result of the hookworm treatment (Jordan, 1956)

At present metronidazole, administered as for giardiasis, is the drug of choice.

*T. felistomae*, an oral trichomonad, was found in 2 of 28 Maryland cats, in which it seemed to be causing no trouble (Hegner and Ratcliffe, 1927). It measured 6 to 11 μ in length and 3 to 4 μ in width. It had four anterior flagella and a free posterior flagellum. This trichomonad may be similar to or identical with *T. tenax*, a natural inhabitant of the mouths of man and some nonhuman primates, in which it is believed capable, under certain unfavorable conditions, of assuming a pathogenic role.

## ENCEPHALITOZOONOSIS

*Encephalitozoon*, a genus of the class Microsporidia, obligate intracellular protozoans, was once considered to be identical with *Nosema*, but electron microscopy now permits differentiation of the two genera. Spores of *Nosema* are binucleated, whereas *Encephalitozoon* has a uninucleated spore (Cali, 1970; Canning, 1977).

Transmission is believed to be by infective spores that are shed in the urine and contaminate the environment, whence they are ingested by new hosts. Dogs and cats may possibly acquire the infection from latently infected prey.

*E. cuniculi* is a parasite of many rodents and occasionally of man, other mammals, and birds. It is encountered most often as a cause of asymptomatic infection of laboratory animals. Under stressful conditions, kittens infected experimentally showed no clinical signs (Szabo et al., 1984) *E. cuniculi* is capable of producing overt disease, most often encephalitis. It has been observed in spontaneous meningoencephalitis in the cat (Meier et al., 1957); Schuster, 1925). In another report of infection of one of four Siamese kitten littermates, all of which showed nervous system signs, autopsy disclosed nonpurulent meningoencephalitis and interstitial nephritis with organisms present in brain, kidney, spleen, lymph nodes, and the tunica media of some blood vessels (van Rensburg and du Plessis, 1971).

*Encephalitozoon* infection of the eye has been described in an adult domestic cat (Buyukmihci et al., 1977). Numerous superficial opacities of the right cornea that were refractory to topical treatment were excised and shown to contain spores similar to those of *Encephalitozoon*. A year later there had been no recurrence.

*E. cuniculi* may be mistaken in tissues for *Toxoplasma gondii* and, like *Toxoplasma*, may be assumed to be responsible for signs of nervous system disturbance in a given case when actually it is merely an incidental finding. *Encephalitozoon* can usually be distinguished from *Toxoplasma* by differences in morphology and staining reactions.

## AMEBIASIS

*Entamoeba histolytica*, the agent of amebic dysentery in man, is highly pathogenic for the kitten, which is the preferred experimental animal, but natural infections seem to be rare (Faust, 1929; Kessel, 1928). Spontaneous amebic dysentery occurring in the cat at the same time as an epidemic in man was reported in Italy (Franchini, 1920). Since *E. histolytica* never forms cysts in cats, infection cannot be disseminated by way of their feces nor can they serve as carriers (Wenyon, 1926). For this reason, the report of *E. histolytica* in a kitten with diarrhea (Nestle, 1963) must be regarded with skepticism.

Amebae indistinguishable from *E. gingivalis* of man have been recognized in pyorrheic mouth ulcers of the cat (Goodrich and Mosely, 1916). In man these organisms, harmless commensals associated with diseased gums, are frequently found between the teeth and in tartar.

## HEPATOZOONOSIS

A blood protozoan, *Hepatozoon felis* (Patton, 1908) (syn *Haemogregarina felis*, *Leucocytozoon felis*), was reported in India in the leukocytes of the domestic cat and also in Nigeria (Leeflang and Ilemobade, 1977). This organism is considered by some to be identical with *H. canis*, a well-known blood parasite of dogs and other carnivores in the Orient, Africa, and Italy (Levine, 1973), as well as in South America and Texas. Dogs are known to be infected by ingesting a vector tick.

*Hepatozoon*-like schizonts have been described in the myocardium in a large proportion of apparently healthy cats in Israel. The organisms appeared to be located in the lumen of capillaries. No parasites were observed in peripheral blood, lymph nodes, or spleen (Klopfer et al., 1973; Nobel et al., 1974). Similar schizonts also caused granulomatous cholangiohepatitis in a California cat originating in Hawaii (Ewing, 1977).

Hepatozoonosis in a cat was successfully treated with a combination of oxytetracycline and primaquine (van Amstel, 1979).

## *PNEUMOCYSTIS CARINII* INFECTION

*Pneumocystis carinii* has been described as occurring in the lungs of normal cats as well as of other animals (Carini and Maciel, 1915; Gajdusek, 1957; Zavala and Rosado, 1972). Formerly encountered mostly in Europe and the tropics, but recognized increasingly in North America as a significant pathogen in very young, old, debilitated, or immunosuppressed humans, this organism may cause acute or subacute plasma-cell pneumonia.

## TRYPANOSOMIASIS

Both natural and experimental feline infections with many of the pathogenic trypanosomes of Africa, Asia, and South America have been reported, but in the vast majority the cat appears to harbor the infection without exhibiting signs of illness (e.g., Andrews and Sanders, 1928; Brumpt, 1939; Carmichael, 1934; Davis, 1931; Launoy, 1934; Mazza, 1934; Mazza et al., 1940; Mettam, 1933; Mott et al., 1978; Panisset, 1905).

Clinical disease is most likely to occur in Africa in cats and dogs infected with *Trypanosoma brucei*, to which they are especially sensitive. The infection is usually acute and fatal unless treated. Signs are fever, anemia with the presence of the parasite in the blood, inappetence, depression, muscle weakness, weight loss, and edema. Involvement of the ciliary body of the eye is a striking feature, with milky turbidity and increased pressure in the anterior chamber, and finally blindness (Stephen, cited by Mortelmans and Neetens, 1975).

Typical signs were described in a one-year-old female cat in Nigeria: listlessness, inappetence, pallor, edema of the head, photophobia, lacrimation, conjunctivitis, keratitis, pannus, hypopyon, and finally blindness (Hill, 1955). A blood film disclosed heavy parasitism with *T. brucei*. The condition of the eyes improved at once with a subcutaneous injection of quinapyramine (antrycide methylsulfate, 6 mg/kg in a 5 per cent solution), but the cat suffered two relapses and was destroyed.

Although most infections occur as a result of the bite of carrier flies, a report from Somaliland concerned a cat assumed to be infected with *T. brucei* by eating raw viscera of an infected camel. Signs were typical—pallor, depression, purulent conjunctivitis, and ulcerative keratitis. Two treatments, eight days apart, with quinapyramine (antrycide methyl sulfate), 1.5 ml of a 1 per cent solution SC) brought about recovery (Gongiu, 1953).

When infected with *T. congolense*, cats show few signs of illness, but virulent strains may result in lack of appetite, loss of hair and weight, and death in a few weeks (Soltys and Woo, 1977).

Fatal natural infection with *T. evansi* was reported in India in a two-year-old domestic male cat presented because of lethargy, inappetence, and incoordination. Symptomatic treatment was ineffective. Blood films obtained at autopsy contained numerous *T. evansi* organisms. Pathologic changes were present in the heart, liver, lungs, and brain; the spleen showed reticular hyperplasia (Paikne and Dhake, 1974).

Experimental feline infection with *T. evansi* characterized by cyclical peaks of fever and facial inflammation was described by Choudhury and Misra (1972).

In South America, natural feline infections with *T. cruzi*, the agent of Chagas' disease, have long been known, but only very rarely are signs of illness recognized—fever, edema, weight loss, and neurologic disturbances such as convulsions and paresis (Neveu-Lemaire, 1952; Talice, 1938).

African trypanosomiasis is treated in man with suramin and with melarsoprol, a trivalent arsenical; there is no satisfactory treatment for Chagas' disease (Merck Manual, 1982).

## REFERENCES

**General References**

Index-Catalogue of Medical and Veterinary Zoology, United States Department of Agriculture. Washington, DC, US Government Printing Office, 1932–1982; publication continued by Oryx Press..

Jones TC, Hunt RD: Veterinary Pathology, 5th ed. Philadelphia, Lea & Febiger, 1983.

Kreier JP (ed): Parasitic Protozoa. New York, Academic Press, Inc, 1977–1978, Vols 1–4.

Levine ND: Protozoan Parasites of Domestic Animals and of Man, 2nd ed. Minneapolis, Burgess Publishing Company, 1973.

Levine ND, Corliss JO, Cox FEG, et al.: A newly revised classification of the protozoa. J Protozool 27 (1980) 37–58.

Morgan BB: Veterinary Protozoology, rev ed. Minneapolis, Burgess Publishing Company, 1952.

Neveu-Lemaire M: Traité de Protozoologie Médicale et Vétérinaire. Paris, Vigot Frères, 1943.

Reichenow E: Lehrbuch der Protozoenkunde, 6th ed. Jena, Gustav Fischer, 1949–1953, Vols 1–3.

Rothstein N: Vital staining of blood parasites with acridine orange. J. Parasitol 44 (1958) 588–595.

Stiles CW, Baker CE: Key-Catalogue of Parasites Reported for Carnivora (Cats, Dogs, Bears, etc.) with their Public Health Importance. National Institute of Health, Bull. No. 163. Washington, DC, US Government Printing Office, 1935.

Von Prowazek S: Handbuch der Pathogenen Protozoen. Leipzig, Johann Ambrosius Barth, 1912.

Wenyon CM: Protozoology. London, Baillière, Tindall and Cox, 1926.

**The Coccidia, including *Toxoplasma***

Anderson BC: Patterns of shedding of cryptosporidial oocysts in Idaho calves. J Am Vet Med Assoc 178 (1981) 982–984.

Andrews LK: A survey of 93 cases of feline toxoplasmosis at the Angell Memorial Animal Hospital, Boston, 1981. Unpublished study.

Ashford RW: *Sarcocystis cymruensis* n. sp., a parasite of rats *Rattus norvegicus* and cats *Felis catus*. Ann Trop Med Parasitol 72 (1978) 37–43.

Augustin-Bichl G, Boch J, Henkel G: Kryptosporidien-Infektionen bei Hund und Katze. Berl Münch Tierärztl Wochenschr 97 (1984) 179–181.

Bennett M, Baxby D, Blundell N, Gaskell CJ, Hart CA, Kelly DF: Cryptosporidiosis in the domestic cat. Vet Rec 116 (1985) 73–74.

Bolle W: Zur vergleichenden Pathologie der Toxoplasmenenzephalitis. Zentralbl Allg Pathol 89 (1952) 313–318.

Campbell I, Tzipori S, Hutchison G, Angus KW: Effect of disinfectants on survival of cryptosporidium oocysts. Vet Rec 111 (1982) 414–415.

Campbell LH: *Toxoplasma* retinitis in a cat. Feline Pract 4(3) (1974) 36–39.

Chinchilla M, Frenkel JK: Mediation of immunity to intracellular infection (*Toxoplasma* and *Besnoitia*) within somatic cells. Infect Immun 19 (1978) 999–1012.

Choquette LPE, Broughton E, Miller FL, Gibbs HC, Cousineau JG: Besnoitiosis in barren-ground caribou in northern Canada. Can Vet J 8 (1967) 282–287.

Christie E, Dubey JP, Pappas PW: Prevalence of *Sarcocystis* infection and other intestinal parasitisms in cats from a humane shelter in Ohio. J Am Vet Med Assoc 168 (1976) 421–422.

Crum JM, Prestwood AK: Transmission of *Sarcocystis leporum* from a cottontail rabbit to domestic cats. J Wildl Dis 13 (1977) 174–175.

Current WL, Long PL: Development of human and calf *Cryptosporidium* in chicken embryos. J Infect Dis 148 (1983) 1108–1113.

Desmonts G, Remington JS: Direct agglutination test for diagnosis of *Toxoplasma* infection: method for increasing sensitivity and specificity. J Clin Microbiol 11 (1980) 562–568.

Desmonts G, Couvreur J, Alison F, Baudelot J, Gerbeaux J, Lelong M: Étude épidémiologique sur la toxoplasmose: de l'influence de la cuisson des viandes de boucherie sur la fréquence de l'infection humaine. Rev Franc Études Clin Biol 10 (1965) 952–958.

Dissanaike AS, Kan SO, Retnasabapathy A, Baskavar G: Developmental stages of *Sarcocystis fusiformis* (Railliet, 1897) and *Sarcocystis* sp., of water buffalo, in the small intestines of cats and dogs, respectively. Southeast Asian J Trop Med Public Health 8 (1977) 417.

Dubey JP: Feline toxoplasmosis and coccidiosis: A survey of domiciled and stray cats. J Am Vet Med Assoc 162 (1973) 873–877.

Dubey JP: A review of *Sarcocystis* of domestic animals and of other coccidia of cats and dogs. J Am Vet Med Assoc 169 (1976a) 1061–1078.

Dubey JP: Re-shedding of *Toxoplasma* oocysts by chronically infected cats. Nature 262 (1976b) 213–214.

Dubey JP: Attempted transmission of feline coccidia from chronically infected queens to their kittens. J Am Vet Med Assoc 170 (1977a) 541–543.

Dubey JP: Persistence of *Toxoplasma gondii* in the tissues of chronically infected cats. J Parasitol 63 (1977b) 156–157.

Dubey JP: *Toxoplasma*, *Hammondia*, *Besnoitia*, *Sarcosystis* and other tissue cyst-forming coccidia of man and animals. *In* Kreier JP (ed): Parasitic Protozoa. New York, Academic Press, Inc, 1977c, Vol 3, 101–237.

Dubey JP: Life cycle of *Isospora rivolta* (Grassi, 1879) in cats and mice. J Protozool 26 (1979) 433–443.

Dubey JP: Repeat transplacental transfer of *Toxoplasma gondii* in goats. J Am Vet Med Assoc 180 (1982) 1220–1221.

Dubey JP, Frenkel JK: Extra-intestinal stages of *Isospora felis* and *I. rivolta* (Protozoa: Eimeriidae) in cats. J Protozool 19 (1972a) 89–92.

Dubey JP, Frenkel JK: Cyst-induced toxoplasmosis in cats. J Protozool 19 (1972b) 155–177.

Dubey JP, Frenkel JK: Immunity to feline toxoplasmosis; modification by administration of corticosteroids. Vet Pathol 11 (1974) 350–379.

Dubey JP, Frenkel JK: Feline toxoplasmosis from acutely infected mice and the development of *Toxoplasma* cysts. J Protozool 23 (1976) 537–546.

Dubey JP, Hoover EA: Attempted transmission of *Toxoplasma gondii* infection from pregnant cats to their kittens. J Am Vet Med Assoc 170 (1977) 538–540.

Dubey JP, Johnstone I: Fatal neonatal toxoplasmosis in cats. J Am Anim Hosp Assoc 18 (1982) 461–467.

Dubey JP, Yeary RA: Anticoccidial activity of 2-sulfamoyl-4,4-diaminodiphenylsulfone, sulfadiazine, pyrimethamine and clindamycin in cats infected with *Toxoplasma gondii*. Can Vet J 18 (1977) 51–57.

Dubey JP, Miller NL, Frenkel JK: Characterization of the new fecal form of *Toxoplasma gondii*. J Parasitol 56 (1970) 447–456.

Dubey JP, Sundberg JP, Matiuck SW: Toxoplasmosis associated with abortion in goats and sheep in Connecticut. Am J Vet Res 42 (1981) 1624–1626.

Dürr UM: Klinische Erfahrungen mit Trimethoprim-Sulfadiazin (Tribrissen) bei der Kokzidiose bei Hund and Katze. Tierärztl Umschau 31 (1976) 177–178. Abstr Vet Bull 46 (1976) 5084.

Elwell MR, Frenkel JK: Immunity to toxoplasmosis in hamsters. Am J Vet Res 45 (1984) 2668–2674.

Ettinger SJ (ed): Textbook of Veterinary Medicine, 2nd ed. Philadelphia, WB Saunders Company, 1982.

Eyles DE, Coleman N: An evaluation of the curative effects of pyrimethamine and sulfadiazine, alone and in combination, on experimental mouse toxoplasmosis. Antibiot Chemother 5 (1955) 529–538.

Fayer R, Frenkel JK: Comparative infectivity for calves of oocysts of feline coccidia: *Besnoitia*, *Hammondia*, *Cystoisospora*, *Sarcocystis*, and *Toxoplasma*. J Parasitol 65 (1979) 756–762.

Fayer R, Kradel D: *Sarcocystis leporum* in cottontail rabbits and its transmission to carnivores. J Wildl Dis 13 (1977) 170–173.

Fish JG: Sulfadimethoxine: an effective drug for the control of coccidiosis and enteric infections in small animals. Auburn Vet 20 (1964) 111–112.

Frenkel JK: Adoptive immunity to intracellular infection. J Immunol 98 (1967) 1309–1319.

Frenkel JK: *Toxoplasma* in and around us. BioScience 23 (1973) 343–352.

Frenkel JK: Breaking the transmission chain of *Toxoplasma*: a program for the prevention of human toxoplasmosis. Bull NY Acad Sci 50 (1974) 228–235.

Frenkel JK: Toxoplasmosis in cats and man. Feline Pract 5 (1) (1975) 28–41.

Frenkel JK: *Besnoitia wallacei* of cats and rodents: with a reclassification of other cyst-forming isosporoid coccidia. J Parasitol 63 (1977a) 611–628.

Frenkel JK: Toxoplasmosis. *In* Kirk RW (ed): Current Veterinary Therapy VI. Philadelphia, WB Saunders Company, 1977b, 1318–1324.

Frenkel JK: Congenital toxoplasmosis: Prevention or palliation? Am J Obstet Gynecol 141 (1981) 359–361.

Frenkel JK, Dubey JP: Rodents as vectors for feline coccidia, *Isospora felis* and *Isospora rivolta*. J Infect Dis 125 (1972a) 69–72.

Frenkel JK, Dubey JP: Toxoplasmosis and its prevention in cats and man. J Infect Dis 126 (1972b) 664–673.

Frenkel JK, Dubey JP: *Hammondia hammondi* gen. nov., sp. nov., from domestic cats, a new coccidian related to *Toxoplasma* and *Sarcocystis*. Z Parasitenkd 46 (1975) 3–12.

Frenkel JK, Hitchings GH: Relative reversal by vitamins (p-aminobenzoic, folic, and folinic acids) of the effects of sulfadiazine and pyrimethamine on *Toxoplasma*, mouse and man. Antibiot Chemother 7 (1957) 630–638.

Frenkel JK, Jacobs L: Ocular toxoplasmosis: pathogenesis, diagnosis and treatment. AMA Arch Ophthalmol 59 (1958) 260–279.

Frenkel JK, Ruiz A: Human toxoplasmosis and cat contact in Costa Rica. Am J Trop Med Hyg 29 (1980) 1167–1180.

Frenkel JK, Ruiz A: Endemicity of toxoplasmosis in Costa Rica: transmission between cats, soil, intermediate hosts and humans. Am J Epidemiol 13 (1981) 254–269.

Frenkel JK, Smith DD: Immunization of cats against shedding of *Toxoplasma* oocysts by cats. J Parasitol 68 (1982a) 744–748.

Frenkel JK, Smith DD: Inhibitory effects of monensin on shedding of *Toxoplasma* oocysts by cats. J Parasitol 68 (1982b) 851–855.

Frenkel JK, Heydorn AO, Mehlhorn H, Rommel M: Sarcocystinae: *Nomina dubia* and available names. Z Parasitenkd 58 (1979) 115–139.

Frenkel JK, Ruiz A, Chinchilla M: Soil survival of *Toxoplasma* oocysts in Kansas and Costa Rica. Am J Trop Med Hyg 24 (1975) 439–443.

Greene CE, Prestwood AK: Coccidial infections. *In* Greene CE (ed): Clinical Microbiology and Infectious Diseases of the Dog and Cat. Philadelphia, WB Saunders Company, 1984.

Groulade P, Sergent G, Béquignon R: Formes cliniques de la toxoplasmose chez les carnivores domestiques. Bull Acad Vét Fr 29 (1956) 49–56.

Guilhon J, Simitch T, Fankhauser R, Béquignon R, Groulade P, Constantin A: Colloque sur les toxoplasmes et les toxoplasmoses animales. Rec Méd Vét 133 (1957) 715–794.

Hammond DM, Long PL (eds): The Coccidia. *Eimeria*, *Isospora*, *Toxoplasma*, and Related Genera. Baltimore, University Park Press, 1973.

Hampton JC, Rosario B: The attachment of protozoan parasites to intestinal epithelial cells of the mouse. J Parasitol 52 (1966) 939–949.

Heine J, Boch J: Kryptosporidien-Infektionen beim Kalb. Nachweis, Vorkommen und experimentelle Übertragung. Berl Münch Tierärztl Wochenschr 94 (1981) 289–292.

Hendricks LD, Ernst JV, Courtney CH, Speer CA: *Hammondia pardalis* sp. n. (Sarcocystidae) from the ocelot, *Felis pardalis*, and experimental infection of other felines. J Protozool 26 (1979) 39–43.

Heydorn AO, Rommel M: Beiträge zum Lebenszyklus der Sarkosporidien. II. Hund und Katze als Überträger der Sarkosporidien des Rindes. Berl Münch Tierärztl Wochenschr 85 (1972a) 121–123.

Heydorn AO, Rommel M: Beiträge zum Lebenszyklus der Sarkosporidien. IV. Entwicklungsstadien von *S. fusiformis* in der Dünndarmschleimhaut der Katze. Berl Münch Tierärztl Wochenschr 85 (1972b) 333–336.

Hirth RS, Nielsen SW: Pathology of feline toxoplasmosis. J Small Anim Pract 10 (1969) 213–221.

Hoff RL, Frenkel JK: Cell-mediated immunity against *Besnoitia* and *Toxoplasma* in specifically and cross-immunized hamsters and in cultures. J Exp Med 139 (1974) 560–580.

Holzworth J: Personal communication, 1982.

Hulland TJ: Toxoplasmosis in Canada. J Am Vet Med Assoc 128 (1956) 74–79.

Iseki, M: *Cryptosporidium felis* sp. n. (Protozoa: Eimeriorina) from the domestic cat. Jpn J Parasitol 28 (1979) 285–307.

Jacobs L, Lunde M: A hemagglutination test for toxoplasmosis. J Parasitol 43 (1957) 308–314.

Janitschke K, Protz D, Werner H: Beitrag zum Entwicklungszyklus von Sarkosporidien der Grantgazelle (*Gazella granti*). Z Parasitenkd 48 (1976) 215–219.

Kirk RW (ed): Current Veterinary Therapy VII. Philadelphia, WB Saunders Company, 1980.

Koch KL, Shankey TV, Weinstein GS, Dye RE, Abt AB, Current WL, Eyster ME: Cryptosporidiosis in a patient with hemophilia, common variable hypogammaglobulinemia, and the acquired immunodeficiency syndrome. Ann Intern Med 99 (1983) 337–340.

Levine ND: Introduction, history, and taxonomy. *In* Hammond DM, Long PL (eds): The Coccidia. *Eimeria*, *Isospora*, *Toxoplasma*, and Related Genera. Baltimore, University Park Press, 1973a.

Levine ND: Protozoan Parasites of Domestic Animals and of Man, 2nd ed. Minneapolis, Burgess Publishing Company, 1973b.

Levine ND: Taxonomy and review of the coccidian genus *Cryptosporidium* (Protozoa, Apicomplexa). J Protozool 31 (1984) 94–98.

Levine ND, Ivens V: The Coccidian Parasites (Protozoa, Apicomplexa) of Carnivores. Illinois Biol Monogr 51. Champaign, University of Illinois Press, 1981.

Lieberman L: Intestinal toxoplasmosis in a cat. North Am Vet 36 (1955) 43–45.

Lindberg RE, Frenkel JK: Cellular immunity to *Toxoplasma* and *Besnoitia* in hamsters: specificity and the effects of cortisol. Infect Immun 15 (1977a) 855–862.

Lindberg RE, Frenkel JK: Toxoplasmosis in nude mice. J Parasitol 63 (1977b) 219–221.

Long PL: The Biology of the Coccidia. Baltimore, University Park Press, 1982.

Ma P, Soave R: Three-step stool examination for cryptosporidiosis in 10 homosexual men with protracted watery diarrhea. J Infect Dis 147 (1983) 824–828.

McMinn RM: The rate of renewal of intestinal eptihelium in the cat. J Anat 88 (1954) 527–533.

Meier H, Holzworth J, Griffiths RC: Toxoplasmosis in the cat—fourteen cases. J Am Vet Med Assoc 131 (1957) 395–414.

Moon HW, Woode GN, Ahrens FA: Attempted chemoprophylaxis of cryptosporidiosis in calves. Vet Rec 110 (1982) 181.

Munday BL: Serological evidence of *Toxoplasma* infection in isolated groups of sheep. Res Vet Sci 13 (1972) 100–102.

Munday BL, Smith DD, Frenkel JK: *Sarcocystis* and related organisms in Australian wildlife: IV. Studies on *Sarcocystis cuniculi* in European rabbits (*Oryctolagus cuniculus*). J Wildl Dis 16 (1980) 201–204.

Naot Y, Remington JS: An enzyme-linked immunosorbent assay for detection of IgM antibodies to *Toxoplasma gondii*: use for diagnosis of acute acquired toxoplasmosis. J Infect Dis 142 (1980) 757–766.

Nieschulz O: Over oon geval van Eimeria infektie bij een kat (*Eimeria felina* n. sp.). Tijdschr Diergeneeskd 51 (1924) 129–131.

Olafson P, Monlux WS: *Toxoplasma* infection in animals. Cornell Vet 32 (1942) 176–190.

Pakes SP, Lai WC: Carbonimmunoassay—a simple and rapid serodiagnostic test for feline toxoplasmosis. Lab Anim Sci 35 (1985) 370–372.

Palmer DF, Cavallaro JJ, Herrmann K, Stewart JA, Walls KW: Serodiagnosis of: Toxoplasmosis, Rubella, Cytomegalic Inclusion Disease, Herpes simplex. Immunology Series No. 5, Procedural Guide. Atlanta, Centers for Disease Control, 1977.

Parker GA, Langloss JM, Dubey JP, Hoover EA: Pathogenesis of acute toxoplasmosis in specific pathogen free cats. Vet Pathol 18 (1981) 786–803.

Pellerdy LP: Studies on the coccidia of the domestic cat. *Isospora novocati* sp. n. Acta Vet Acad Sci Hung 24 (1974a) 127–131.

Pellerdy LP: Coccidia and Coccidiosis, 2nd ed. Budapest, Akademiai Kiado, 1974b.

Penkert RA: Possible spread of toxoplasmosis by feed contaminated by cats. J Am Vet Med Assoc 162 (1973) 924.

Peteshev VM, Galuzo IG, Polomoshnov AP: [Cats—definitive hosts of *Besnotia* (*Besnoitia besnoiti*)]. Izvest Akad Nauk Kazakh SSR, Ser Biol 1974 (1974) 33–38.

Petrak M, Carpenter J: Feline toxoplasmosis. J Am Vet Med Assoc 146 (1965) 728–734.

Piper RC, Cole CR, Shadduck JA: Natural and experimental ocular toxoplasmosis in animals. Am J Ophthalmol 69 (1970) 662–668.

Plant JW, Richardson N, Moyle GG: *Toxoplasma* infection and abortion in sheep associated with feeding of grain contaminated with cat feces. Aust Vet J 50 (1974) 19–21.

Pohlenz J, Bemrick WJ, Moon HW, Cheville NF: Bovine cryptosporidiosis: a transmission and scanning electron microscopic study of some stages in the life cycle and of the host-parasite relationship. Vet Pathol 15 (1978) 417–427.

Pols JW: Studies on bovine besnoitiosis with special reference to the aetiology. Onderstepoort J Vet Res 28 (1960) 265–356.

Poonacha KB, Pippin C: Intestinal cryptosporidiosis in a cat. Vet Pathol 19 (1982) 708–710.

Pospischil A, Goebel E, Schafer M, Geisel O: A fatal case of an unusual coccidiosis in a cat: asexual and sexual development of parasites in macrophages. Zentralbl Veterinärmed B31 (1984) 141–150.

Powell EC, McCarley JB: A murine *Sarcocystis* that causes an *Isospora*-like infection in cats. J Parasitol 61 (1975) 928–931.

Reese NC, Current WL, Ernst JV, Bailey WS: Cryptosporidiosis of man and calf: A case report and results of experimental infections in mice and rats. Am J Trop Med Hyg 31 (1982) 226–229.

Remington JS, Efron B, Cavanaugh E, Simon HJ, Trejos A: Studies on toxoplasmosis in El Salvador. Prevalence and incidence of toxoplasmosis as measured by the Sabin-Feldman dye test. Trans R Soc Trop Med Hyg 64 (1970) 252–267.

Remington JS, Eimstad WM, Araujo FG: Detection of immunoglobulin in antibodies with antigen-tagged latex particles in an immunosorbent assay. J Clin Microbiol 17 (1983) 939–941.

Remington JS, Krahenbuhl JL, Mendenhall JW: A role for activated macrophages in resistance to infection with *Toxoplasma*. Infect Immun 6 (1972) 829–834.

Riemann HP, Behymer DE, Fowler ME, Schulz T, Lock A, Orthoefer JG, Silverman S, Franti CE: Prevalence of antibodies to *Toxoplasma gondii* in captive exotic animals. J Am Vet Med Assoc 165 (1974a) 798–800.

Riemann HP, Fowler ME, Schulz T, Lock A, Thilsted J, Pulley LT, Henrickson RV, Henness AM, Franti CE, Behymer DE: Toxoplasmosis in pallas cats. J Wildl Dis 10 (1974b) 471–477.

Rommel M, Heydorn AO, Gruber F: Beiträge zum Lebenszyklus der Sarkosporidien. I. Die Sporozyste von *S. tenella* in den Fäzes der Katze. Berl Münch Tierärztl Wochenschr 85 (1972) 101–105.

Rougier D, Ambrose-Thomas P: Detection of toxoplasmic immunity by multipuncture skin test with excretory-secretory antigen. Lancet 1985 (July 20) 121–123.

Ruiz A, Frenkel JK: Recognition of cyclic transmission of *Sarcocystis muris* by cats. J Infect Dis 133 (1976) 409–418.

Ruiz A, Frenkel JK: Intermediate and transport hosts of *Toxoplasma gondii* in Costa Rica. Am J Trop Med Hyg 29 (1980a) 1161–1166.

Ruiz A, Frenkel JK: *Toxoplasma gondii* in Costa Rican cats. Am J Trop Med Hyg 29 (1980b) 1150–1160.

Sabin AB, Feldman HA: Dyes as microchemical indicators of a new immunity phenomenon affecting a protozoon parasite (*Toxoplasma*). Science 108 (1948) 660–663.

Schreiber RD, Feldman HA: Identification of the activator system for antibody to *Toxoplasma* as the classical complement pathway. J Infect Dis 141 (1980) 366–369.

Shah HL: Sporogony of the oocysts of *Isospora felis* Wenyon, 1923 from the cat. J Protozool 17 (1970) 609–614.

Shah HL: The life cycle of *Isospora felis* Wenyon, 1923, a coccidium of the cat. J Protozool 18 (1971) 3–17.

Sheffield HG, Melton ML: Effects of pyrimethamine and sulfadiazine on the intestinal development of *Toxoplasma gondii* in cats. Am J Trop Med Hyg 25 (1976) 379–383.

Smart ME, Downey RS, Stockdale PHG: Toxoplasmosis in a cat associated with cholangitis and progressive pancreatitis. Can Vet J 14 (1973) 313–316.

Smith DD, Frenkel JK: *Besnoitia darlingi* (Protozoa: Toxoplasmatinae): cyclic transmission by cats. J Parasitol 63 (1977) 1066–1071.

Smith DD, Frenkel JK: Cockroaches as vectors of *Sarcocystis muris* and of other coccidia in the laboratory. J Parasitol 64 (1978) 315–319.

Stagno S, Dykes AC, Amos CS, Head RA, Juranek DD, Walls K: An outbreak of toxoplasmosis linked to cats. Pediatrics 65 (1980) 706–712.

Stemmermann GN, Hayashi T, Glober GA, Oishi N, Frenkel RI: Cryptosporidiosis. Report of a fatal case complicated by disseminated toxoplasmosis. Am J Med 69 (1980) 637–642.

Sulzer AJ, Leaverton PE, Gogel RH: Comparison of reactions of human antisera in the methylene blue dye test for toxoplasmosis using bioassay procedures. Exp Parasitol 20 (1967) 1–8.

Summers WA: The chemotherapeutic efficacy of 2,4-diamino-5-p-chlorophenyl-6-ethyl-pyrimidine (Daraprim) in experimental toxoplasmosis. Am J Trop Med Hyg 2 (1953) 1037–1044.

Suteu E: [Study of the life cycles of some Isospora species transmitted via sheep meat.] *In* Lucrarile celui de al 8-lea seminar ameliorarea tehnologia si patologia rumegatoarelor, Cluj-Napoca, 11–12 Noiembrie 1983. Sectia de Patologie. Cluj-Napoca, Romania; Institutul Agronomic "Dr. Petru Groza" (1983) 171–175. Abstr Vet Bull 54 (1984) 6405.

Tzipori X, Angus KW, Campbell I, Gray EW: *Cryptosporidium*: Evidence for a single-species genus. Infect Immun 30 (1980) 884–886.

Vainisi SJ, Campbell LH: Ocular toxoplasmosis in cats. J Am Vet Med Assoc 154 (1969) 141–152.

Verlinde JD, Makstenieks O: Een geval van hydrocephalie in verband met toxoplasmose bij een kat? Maandschr Kindergeneesk 17 (1950) 360–365.

Vetterling JM, Takeuchi A, Madden PA: Ultrastructure of *Cryptosporidium wrairi* from the guinea pig. J Protozool 18 (1971) 248–260.

Vogt F, Weber H: [Coccidiosis of dogs and cats and use of Amprolvet as a specific coccidiostat.] Praktischer Tierarzt 54 (1973) 444–445. Abstr Vet Bull 44 (1974) 1081.

Voller A, Bidwell DE, Bartlett A, Fleck DG, Perkins M, Oladehin B: A microplate enzyme-immunoassay for *Toxoplasma* antibody. J Clin Pathol 29 (1976) 150–153.

Waldeland H: Toxoplasmosis in sheep. The relative importance of the infection as a cause of reproductive loss in sheep in Norway. Acta Vet Scand 17 (1976) 412–425.

Waldeland H: Toxoplasmosis in sheep. Epidemiological studies in flocks with reproductive loss from toxoplasmosis. Acta Vet Scand 18 (1977) 91–97.

Waldeland H, Frenkel JK: Live and killed vaccines against toxoplasmosis in mice. J Parasitol 69 (1983) 60–65.

Wallace GD: Serologic and epidemiologic observations on toxoplasmosis on three Pacific atolls. Am J Epidemiol 90 (1969) 103–111.

Wallace GD: The role of the cat in the natural history of *Toxoplasma gondii*. Am J Trop Med Hyg 22 (1973) 313–322.

Walls KW, Bullock SL, English DK: Use of the enzyme-linked immunosorbent assay (ELISA) and its micro-adaptation for the serodiagnosis of toxoplasmosis. J Clin Microbiol 5 (1977) 273–277.

Ward JM, Nelson N, Wright JR, Berman E: Chronic nonclinical cerebral toxoplasmosis in cats. J Am Vet Med Assoc 159 (1971) 1012–1014.

Wickham N, Carne HR: Toxoplasmosis in domestic animals in Australia. Aust Vet J 26 (1950) 1–3.

Wilkinson GT: Coccidial infection in a cat colony. Vet Rec 100 (1977) 156–157.

Wilson CB, Desmonts G, Couvreur J, Remington JS: Lymphocyte transformation in the diagnosis of congenital *Toxoplasma* infection. N Engl J Med 302 (1980) 785–788.

Wilson JW: Clinical application of cerebrospinal fluid creatine phosphokinase determination. J Am Vet Med Assoc 171 (1977) 200–202.

Yakimoff WL: Zur Frage der Eimeriose der Katzen. Arch Protistenk 80 (1933) 172–176.

**Cytauxzoonosis**

Barnett SF: Theileria. *In* Kreier JP (ed): Parasitic Protozoa. New York, Academic Press, Inc, 1977, Vol IV, 77–144.

Bendele RA, Schwartz WL, Jones LP: Cytauxzoonosis-like disease in Texas cats. Southwest Vet 29 (1976) 244–246.

Blouin EF, Kocan AA, Glenn BL, Hair JA: Transmission of *Cytauxzoon felis* (Kier, 1979) from bobcats, *Felis rufus* (Schreber), to domestic cats by *Dermacentor variabilis* (Say). J Wildl Dis 20 (1984) 241–242.

Brocklesby DW: *Cytauxzoon taurotragi*, Martin and Brocklesby, 1960, a piroplasm of the eland (*Taurotragus oryx pattersonianus* Lydekker, 1906). Res Vet Sci 3 (1962) 334–344.

Burridge MJ: Personal communication, 1978.

Conroy J: Personal communication, 1979.

Doster AR: Personal communication, 1976.

Glenn BL, Stair EL: Cytauxzoonosis in domestic cats: report of two cases in Oklahoma, with a review and discussion of the disease. J Am Vet Med Assoc 184 (1984) 822–825.

Glenn BL, Rolley RE, Kocan AA: *Cytauxzoon*-like piroplasms in erythrocytes of wild trapped bobcats in Oklahoma. J Am Vet Med Assoc 181 (1982) 1251–1252.

Hauck WN, Snider TG III, Lawrence JE: Cytauxzoonosis in a native Louisiana cat. J Am Vet Med Assoc 180 (1982) 1472–1474.

Kier AB: The etiology and pathogenesis of feline cytauxzoonosis. University of Missouri, PhD thesis, 1979.

Kier AB, Morehouse LG, Wagner JE: Feline cytauxzoonosis: an update. Mo Vet 29 (1979) 15–18.

Kier AB, Wagner JE, Morehouse LG: Experimental transmission of *Cytauxzoon felis* from bobcats (*Lynx rufus*) to domestic cats (*Felis domesticus*). Am J Vet Res 43 (1982a) 97–101.

Kier AB, Wightman SF, Wagner JE: Interspecies transmission of *Cytauxzoon felis*. Am J Vet Res 43 (1982b) 102–105.

Kier AB, Wightman SF, Wagner JE, Morehouse LG: Diagnostic features of a newly described blood protozoan disease in domestic cats—a *Cytauxzoon* species. Am Assoc Vet Lab Diagnosticians, 20th Annual Proceedings, 1977, 123–130.

Levine ND: Taxonomy of the piroplasms. Trans Am Microsc Soc 90 (1971) 2–33.

Martin H, Brocklesby DW: A new parasite of the eland. Vet Rec 72 (1960) 331–332.

McCully RM: Personal communication, 1975.

McCully RM, Keep ME, Basson PA: Cytauxzoonosis in a giraffe, *Giraffa camelopardalis* (Linnaeus, 1758) in Zululand. Onderstepoort J Vet Res 37 (1970) 7–10.

Neitz WO: Theileriosis, gonderiosis and cytauxzoonosis. A review. Onderstepoort J Vet Res 27 (1957) 275–415.

Neitz WO, Thomas AD: *Cytauxzoon sylvicaprae* gen. nov., spec. nov., a protozoon responsible for a hitherto undescribed disease in the duiker *Sylvicapra grimmia* (Linne). Onderstepoort J Vet Sci Anim Industry 23 (1948) 63–76.

Riek RF: Babesiosis. *In* Weinman D, Ristic M (eds): Infectious Blood Diseases of Man and Animals. New York, Academic Press, Inc, 1968, Vol II, 220–265.

Rubin HL: Personal communication, 1977.

Shindel N, Dardiri AH, Ferris DH: An indirect fluorescent antibody test for the detection of cytauxzoon-like organisms in experimentally infected cats. Can J Comp Med 42 (1978) 460–465.

Simpson CF, Harvey JW, Carlisle JW: Ultrastructure of the intraerythrocytic stage of *Cytauxzoon felis*. Am J Vet Res 46 (1985a) 1178–1180.

Simpson CF, Harvey JW, Lawman MJP, Murray J, Kocan AA, Carlisle JW: Ultrastructure of schizonts in the liver of cats with experimentally induced cytauxzoonosis. Am J Vet Res 46 (1985b) 384–390.

Wagner JE: A fatal cytauxzoonosis-like disease in cats. J Am Vet Med Assoc 168 (1976) 585–588.

Wagner JE, Ferris DH, Kier AB, Wightman SR, Maring E, Morehouse LG, Hansen RD: Experimentally induced cytauxzoonosis-like disease in domestic cats. Vet Parasitol 6 (1980) 305–311.

Wagner JE, Kier AB, Morehouse LG: Feline cytauxzoonosis, a newly reported blood protozoan disease from Southwestern Missouri. Mo Vet 26 (1976) 12–13.

Wightman SR: Clinical features, interspecies susceptibility, and biological transmission of experimentally induced feline cytauxzoonosis. University of Missouri, MS thesis, 1978.

Wightman SR, Kier AB, Wagner JE: Feline cytauxzoonosis: clinical features of a newly described blood parasite disease. Feline Pract 7 (3) (1977) 23–26.

Wilson DE, Bartsch RC, Bigalke RD, Thomas SE: Observations on mortality rates and disease in roan and sable antelope on nature reserves in the Transvaal. J South Afr Wildl Mgmt Assoc 4 (1974) 203–206.

**Babesiosis**

Davis LJ: On a piroplasm of the Sudanese wild cat (*Felis ocreata*). Trans R Soc Trop Med Hyg 22 (1929) 523–534.

Dennig HK: Eine unbekannte Babesienart beim Jaguarundi (*Herpailurus yaguarundi*). Kleintierpraxis 12 (1967) 146–152.

Futter GJ, Belonje PC: Studies on feline babesiosis 1. Historical review. J S Afr Vet Assoc 51 (1980a) 105–106.

Futter GJ, Belonje PC: Studies on feline babesiosis 2. Clinical observations. J S Afr Vet Assoc 51 (1980b) 143–146.

Futter GJ, Belonje PC, van den Berg A: Studies on feline babesiosis 3. Haematologic findings. J S Afr Vet Assoc 51 (1980) 271–280.

Futter GJ, Belonje PC, van den Berg A, van Rijswijk AW: Studies on feline babesiosis 4. Chemical pathology; macroscopic and microscopic *post mortem* findings. J S Afr Vet Assoc 52 (1981) 5–14.

Levine ND: Protozoan Parasites of Domestic Animals and of Man, 2nd ed. Minneapolis, Burgess Publishing Company, 1973.

Mangrulkar MY: On a piroplasm of the Indian cat (*Felis domesticus*). Ind J Vet Sci 7 (1937) 243–246.

Potgieter FT: Chemotherapy of *Babesia felis* infection: efficacy of certain drugs. J S Afr Vet Assoc 52 (1981) 289–293.

Rowin KS, Tanowitz HB, Wittner M: Therapy of experimental babesiosis. Am Intern Med 97 (1982) 556–558.

Stewart CG, Hackett KJW, Collett MG: An unidentified *Babesia* of the domestic cat (*Felis domesticus*). J S Afr Vet Assoc 51 (1980) 219–221.

Thomas AD, Brown MHV: An attempt to transmit canine biliary fever to the domestic cat. J S Afr Vet Assoc 5 (1934) 179–181.

**Giardiasis**

Belosevic M, Faubert GM, Guy R, MacLean JD: Observations on natural and experimental infections with *Giardia* isolated from cats. Can J Comp Med 48 (1984) 241–244.

Bemrick W: A note on the incidence of three species of *Giardia* in Minnesota. J Parasitol 47 (1961) 87–89.

Brightman AH, Slonka GF: A review of five clinical cases of giardiasis in cats. J Am Anim Hosp 12 (1976) 492–497.

Burrows RB, Hunt GR: Intestinal protozoan infections in cats. J Am Vet Med Assoc 157 (1970) 2065–2067.

Craige JE: Personal communication, 1963.

Davies RB, Hibler CP: Animal reservoirs and cross-species transmission of *Giardia*. *In* Jakubowski W, Hoff JC (eds): Waterborne Transmission of Giardiasis. Cincinnati, USEPA, 1979, 104–125.

De Carneri L, Castellino S: Bassa incidenza di *Giardia cati* Deschiens 1925 e assenza de protozoi orali nei gatti a Milano. Riv Parassitol 24 (1963) 1–4.

Deschiens R: *Giardia cati* (n. sp.) du chat domestique. CR Soc Biol (Paris) 92 (1925) 1271–1272.

Deschiens R: *Giardia cati* R. Deschiens, 1925, du chat domestique (*Felis domestica*). Ann Parasitol Hum Comp 4 (1926) 33–48.

Georgi JR: Parasitology for Veterinarians, 3rd ed. Philadelphia, WB Saunders Company, 1980.

Grassi B: Di un nuovo parassita dell'uomo, *Megastoma entericum* (mihi). Prima nota. Gazzetta degli Ospitali 2 (1881) 577–580.
Hegner RW: *Giardia felis*, n. sp., from the domestic cat and giardias from birds. Am J Hyg 5 (1925) 258–273.
Hitchcock DJ: Incidence of intestinal parasites in some Michigan kittens. North Am Vet 34 (1953) 428–429.
Hitchcock DJ, Malewitz TD: Habitat of *Giardia* in the kitten. J Parasitol 42 (1956) 286.
Kessel JF: Experimental giardiasis in kittens and puppies. J Parasitol 16 (1929) 99–100.
Kirkpatrick CE: Enteric protozoal infections. *In* Greene CE (ed): Clinical Microbiology and Infectious Diseases of the Dog and Cat. Philadelphia, WB Saunders Company, 1984.
Kirkpatrick CE, Farrell JP: Giardiasis. Compend Contin Ed 4 (1982) 367–377.
Kirkpatrick CE, Farrell JP: Feline giardiasis: Observations on natural and induced infections. Am J Vet Res 45 (1984) 2182–2188.
Kirkpatrick CE, Laczak JP: Giardiasis in a cattery. J Am Vet Med Assoc 187 (1985) 161–162.
Kulda J, Nohynkova E: Intestinal flagellates. *In* Kreier JP: Parasitic Protozoa. New York, Academic Press, Inc, 1978, Vol. II.
Levine ND: Protozoan Parasites of Domestic Animals and of Man, 2nd ed. Minneapolis, Burgess Publishing Company, 1973.
Levine ND: *Giardia lamblia*: Classification, structure, identification. *In* Jakubowski W, Hoff JC (eds): Waterborne transmission of Giardiasis. Proceedings of a Symposium September 18–20, 1978, US Environmental Protection Agency, 600/9—001, June 1979 (Natl Technical Information Service, Springfield, VA 22151).
Nesvadba J: Giardiabefall bei einer Katze. Kleintierpraxis 24 (1979) 177–179.
Pitts RP, Twedt DC, Mallie KA: Comparison of duodenal aspiration with fecal flotation for diagnosis of giardiasis in dogs. J Am Vet Med Assoc 182 (1983) 1210–1211.
Torres P, Hott A, Boehmwald H: Protozoos, helmintos y artropodos en gatos de la ciudad de Valdivia [Chile] y su importancia para el hombre. Arch Med Vet 4 (2) (1972) 20–29.
Vanparijs OFJ, Thienpont DC: Canine and feline helminths and protozoan infections in Belgium. J Parasitol 59 (1973) 327–330.
Visvesvara GS, Healy GR, Meyer EA: Comparative antigenic analysis of *Giardia* from the human, the cat, and the guinea pig (abstract). J Protozool 27 (1980) 38A.
Wenyon CM: Protozoology. New York, William Wood and Company, 1926.
Wolff K, Eckert J: Giardia-Befall bei Hund und Katze und dessen mögliche Bedeutung für den Menschen. Berl Münch Tierärztl Wochenschr 92 (1979) 484–490.

**Leishmaniasis**

Bergeon P: Un cas de leishmaniose chez le chat. Bull Soc Sci Vét Lyon 30 (1927) 92–93.
Bosselut H: Un cas de leishmaniose générale du chat. Arch Inst Pasteur Algér 26 (1948) 14.
Ferreira LC, Mangabeira O, Deane L, Chagas AW: Notas sobre a transmissao da leishmaniose visceral americana. Hosp Rio de Jan 14 (5) (1938) 1077–1087.
Gimeno Ondovilla [no init]: Contribución a la epidemiología del kala azar. Trabajos. Madrid 2 (1933) 26–27. Abstr Trop Dis Bull 30 (1933) 752.
Giordano A: Le chat dans la transmission de la leishmaniose viscérale de la méditerranée. Bull Sez Ital Soc Internaz Microbiol 5 (1933) 330–332. Abstr Vet Bull 4 (1934) 722.
Levine ND: Protozoan Parasites of Man and of Animals, 2nd ed. Minneapolis, Burgess Publishing Company, 1973.
Machattie C, Mills EA, Chadwick CR: Naturally occurring oriental sore of the domestic cat in Iraq. Trans R Soc Trop Med Hyg 25 (1931) 103–106.
Mello GB: Verificacao da infeccao natural do gato (*Felix domesticus*) por um protozoario do genero Leishmania. Brasil-Med 54 (1940) 180.
Sergent EE, Lombard, Quilichini: La leishmaniose à Alger. Infection simultanée d'un enfant, d'un chien et d'un chat dans la même habitation. Bull Soc Pathol Exot 5 (1912) 93–98.

**Trichomoniasis**

Brumpt E: Recherches morphologiques et expérimentales sur le *Trichomonas felis* da Cunha et Muniz, 1922, parasite du chat et du chien. Ann Parasitol Hum Comp 3 (1925) 239–251.
Burroughs RB: A new fixative and techniques for the diagnosis of intestinal parasites. Tech Bull Reg Med Techn 37 (1967) 208–212.
da Cunha A, Muniz J: Sobre um flagellado parasito do gato (Nota previa). Brasil-Med 36 (1) (1922) 285–286.
Fishler JJ: Personal communication, 1979.
Hegner R, Eskridge L: Absence of pathogenicity in cats infected with *Trichomonas felis* from cats and *Trichomonas hominis* from man. Am J Hyg 22 (1935) 322–325.
Hegner R, Ratcliffe H: Trichomonads from the vagina of the monkey, from the mouth of the cat and man, and from the intestine of the monkey, opossum and prairie-dog. J Parasitol 14 (1927) 27–35.
Hitchcock DJ: Incidence of intestinal parasites in some Michigan kittens. North Am Vet 34 (1953) 428–429.
Jordan HE: Trichomonas spp. in feline: A case report. Vet Med 51 (1956) 23–24.
Kessel JF: Trichomoniasis in kittens. Proc Soc Exp Biol Med 24 (1926) 200–202.
Kessel JF: Trichomoniasis in kittens. Trans R Soc Trop Med Hyg 22 (1928) 61–80.
Simic T: Étude biologique et expérimentale du *Trichomonas intestinalis*, infectant spontanément l'homme, le chat et le chien. Ann Parasitol Hum Comp 10 (1932) 209–224.
Visco RJ, Corwin RM, Selby LA: Effect of age and sex on the prevalence of intestinal parasitism in cats. J Am Vet Med Assoc 172 (1978) 797–800.
Wagner O, Hees E: Der kulturelle Nachweis von Trichomonas vaginalis und anderen Trichomonasarten. Zentralbl Bakteriol I [Orig] 135 (1935) 310–317.
Wagner O, Hees E: 156 positive Trichomonasblutbefunde bei Mensch and Tier. Zentralbl Bakteriol I [Orig] 138 (1937) 273–290.
Wenrich DH: Morphology of the trichomonad flagellates in man and of similar forms in monkeys, cats, dogs and rats. J Morphol 74 (1944) 189–211.

**Other Protozoan Infections**

Andrews J, Sanders EP: Changes in the blood of cats infected with *Trypanosoma equiperdum*. Am J Hyg 8 (1928) 947–962.
Brumpt E: Quelques faits épidémiologiques concernant la maladie de C. Chagas. Presse Méd 47 (2) (1939) 1081–1085.
Buyukmihci N, Bellhorn RW, Hunzicker J, Clinton J: *Encephalitozoon* (*Nosema*) infection of the cornea in a cat. J Am Vet Med Assoc 171 (1977) 355–357.
Cali A: Morphogenesis in the Genus *Nosema*. Proc IV Int Colloq Insect Pathol, Aug 1970, 431–438.
Canning EU: Microsporidia. *In* Kreier JP (ed): Parasitic Protozoa. New York, Academic Press, Inc, 1977, Vol IV.
Carini A, Maciel J: Ueber *Pneumocystis carinii*. Zentralbl Bakteriol Abt 1 [Orig] 77 (1915) 46–50.
Carmichael J: [Experimental *T. brucei* infection in kittens]. Annual Report, 1933, of the Veterinary Pathologist, Entebbe, Uganda Protectorate Ann Rep Vet Dept (1933), 1934) 29–45.
Choudhury A, Misra KK: Experimental infection of *T. evansi* in the cat. Trans R Soc Trop Med Hyg 66 (1972) 672–673.
Davis LJ: Experimental feline trypanosomiasis with especial reference to the effect of splenectomy. Ann Trop Med Parasitol 25 (1931) 79–89.

Ewing GO: Granulomatous cholangiohepatitis in a cat due to a protozoan parasite resembling *Hepatozoon canis*. Feline Pract 7 (6) (1977) 37–40.

Faust EC: The animal parasites of the dog and cat in China. Lingnan Sci J 8 (1929) 27–44.

Franchini F: Dissenteria amebica spontanea nel gatto concomitante ad una circonscritta epidemia di dissenteria nell'uomo in un commune del bolognese (Nota preventiva). Giorn Clin Med 1 (1920) 352–355. (Cited by Wenyon, 1926.)

Gajdusek DC: *Pneumocystis carinii*—etiological agent of interstitial plasma cell pneumonia of premature and young infants. Pediatrics 19 (1957) 543–565.

Gongiu S: Transmissione naturale per via digerente del T. brucei nel gatto. Zooprofilassi 8 (1953) 412–414.

Goodrich HP, Mosely M: On certain parasites of the mouth in cases of pyorrhoea. J R Micr Soc 37 (1916) 513–527.

Hill DH: *Trypanosoma brucei* in the cat. Br Vet J 111 (1955) 77–80.

Kessel JF: Amoebiasis in kittens infected with amoebae from acute and "carrier" human cases and with the tetranucleate amoebae of the monkey and of the pig. Am J Hyg 8 (1928) 311–355.

Klopfer U, Nobel TA, Neumann F: Hepatozoon-like parasite (schizonts) in the myocardium of the domestic cat. Vet Pathol 10 (1973) 185–190.

Launoy L: Maladie inapparente à *Trypanosoma annamense* chez le chat. Bull Soc Pathol Exot 27 (1934) 848–850.

Leeflang P, Ilemobade AA: Tick-borne diseases of domestic animals in northern Nigeria. Trop Anim Health Prod 9 (1977) 211–218.

Levine ND: Protozoan Parasites of Domestic Animals and of Man, 2nd ed. Minneapolis, Burgess Publishing Company, 1973.

Mazza S: Hallazgo del gato como portador natural del *Schizotrypanum cruzi* en la provincia de Jujuy, Rev Med-Cir Brasil 42 (1934) 309–310.

Mazza S, Lovaglio J, Cornejo A: Investigaciones sobre enfermedad de Chagas. Publ Mision Estud Patol Reg Argent 45 (1940) 3–35, 36–40, 97–105.

Meier H, Holzworth J, Griffiths RC: Toxoplasmosis in the cat—fourteen cases. J Am Vet Med Assoc 133 (1957) 395–414.

Merck Manual of Diagnosis and Therapy, 14th ed. Rahway, NJ, Merck Sharp & Dohme Research Laboratories, 1982.

Mettam RWM: *T. congolense* in the domestic cat. Uganda Protectorate Ann Rep Vet Dept (1933) 39–40.

Mortelmans J, Neetens A: Ocular lesions in experimental Trypanosoma brucei infection in cats. Acta Zool Pathol Antverp 62 (1975) 149–172.

Mott KE, Mota EA, Sherlock I, Hoff R, Muniz TM, Oliveira TS, Draper CC: *Trypanosoma cruzi* infection in dogs and cats and household seroreactivity to *T. cruzi* in a rural community in northeast Brazil. Am J Trop Med Hyg 27 (1978) 1123–1127.

Nestle AS: Amoebic dysentery in a kitten. Vet Med 58 (1963) 341.

Neveu-Lemaire M: Précis de Parasitologie Vétérinaire, 2nd ed. Paris, Vigot Frères, 1952.

Nobel TA, Neumann F, Klopfer U: Histopathology of the myocardium in 50 apparently healthy cats. Lab Ans 8 (2) (1974) 119–125.

Paikne DL, Dhake PR: Trypanosomiasis in a domestic cat (*Felis catus*). Indian Vet J 51 (1974) 387.

Panisset L: Le surra du chat. C R Soc Biol (Paris) 58 (1905) 15–16.

Patton WS: The haemogregarines of mammals and reptiles. Parasitology 1 (1908) 318–321.

Schuster J: Über eine spontan bei Kaninchen auftretende encephalitische Erkrankung. Klin Wochenschr 4 (1) (1925) 550.

Soltys M, Woo PTK: Trypanosomes producing disease in livestock in Africa. *In* Kreier JP: Parasitic Protozoa. New York, Academic Press, Inc, 1977, Vol I.

Szabo JR, Pang V, Shadduck JA: Encephalitozoonosis. *In* Greene CE (ed): Clinical Microbiology and Infectious Diseases of the Dog and Cat. Philadelphia, WB Saunders Company, 1984.

Talice RV: Primeros observaciones en el Uruguay de gatos espontaneamente infectados por el *Trypanosoma cruzi*. Arch Urug Med 13 (1938) 61–64.

van Amstel S: Hepatozoönose in 'n kat. J S Afr Vet Assoc 50 (1979) 215–216.

van Rensburg IBJ, du Plessis JL: Nosematosis in a cat: A case report. J S Afr Vet Med Assoc 42 (1971) 327–331.

Wenyon CM: Protozoology. New York, William Wood and Company, 1926.

Zavala J, Rosado R: *Pneumocystis carinii* en animales domesticos de la ciudad de Merida, Yucatan. Salud Publica Mex 14 (1) (1972) 103–106.

# 11 CHAPTER

# Tumors and Tumor-like Lesions

JAMES L. CARPENTER, LAURA K. ANDREWS, and JEAN HOLZWORTH

CONTRIBUTING AUTHORS:
DAMON R. AVERILL, MARGARET L. HARBISON, and FRANCES M. MOORE

The study of tumors in animals is of tremendous interest to the veterinary clinician, surgeon, pathologist, and scientific researcher both in their professional and in their personal lives. Cancer, still enshrouded in many mysteries, affects both animal and plant species and awaits elucidation and control. About one in four persons in the United States dies of cancer (Robbins et al., 1984). Although the incidence of tumors in general appears to be lower in cats than in man, the relatively high proportion of malignant tumors warrants a detailed study and description of feline tumors. Tumor incidences in cats of 188.3 and 470 per 100,000 have been reported (Dorn et al., 1968b; MacVean et al., 1978). These rates would almost certainly be higher if a greater proportion of the cat population received veterinary attention.

The percentage of feline tumors that are malignant is more alarming than the tumor incidence. Tumors of cats, unlike those of dogs, are far more often malignant than benign. Surveys have shown that malignant neoplasms constitute 75 or 83 per cent of all feline tumors (Wilkinson, 1966; MacVean et al., 1978). A review of a two-year (1975–1976) sample of feline tumors at Angell Memorial Animal Hospital (AMAH) composed of autopsy and surgical specimens revealed that the proportion of malignancy was 80 per cent. The veterinary clinician and surgeon should be aware of this fact, and their medical approach and surgical procedures should be governed by it.

Even the smallest of masses should be examined. For example, what is to an owner a tiny "wart" has proved on microscopic examination to be a highly malignant mast cell tumor. It should also be remembered that such a tiny tumor may already have given rise to metastatic lesions that are many times larger. Another important reason for examination is that not all masses are neoplasms, often to the surprise of the clinician and surgeon. For example, an otic or nasal tumor may prove to be an inflammatory polyp or a cryptococcal granuloma.

When multiple similar-appearing masses are present, each, or at least two, should be examined by paraffin section, imprint, or aspiration (whichever allows for identification) before it is concluded that all growths either are or probably are similar.

Whenever a malignancy is suspected and an enlarged regional node is accessible, the regional node should be removed to permit tumor detection and staging, so that a more precise prognosis can be given and the most appropriate management chosen.

The veterinarian should remember that to the cat owner, as well as to the human patient, words such as tumor, neoplasm, and cancer evoke fear and confusion. Neoplasm (G. neos, new + plasma, thing formed) and tumor (L. tumor, a swelling) are often used synonymously. A neoplasm is an abnormal mass of tissue, virtually autonomous, useless, and often harmful; its growth is by cellular division that continues after the stimulus that initiated the new growth ceases.

Those neoplasms called cancer or malignant have uncontrollable growth and may invade and destroy normal tissue, disseminate (metastasize), recur after apparently complete removal, and cause death of the host unless treated early and adequately. Benign tumors will not metastasize but may recur if not completely excised or destroyed. The so-called benign tumor, although unable to spread to distant sites, can still kill by local interference with vital body functions owing to its location, size, or late detection.

The following discussion of feline tumors is based primarily on the review of surgical and autopsy material and case records collected over a 35-year period at AMAH. It should be emphasized that the tumors reported represent only a small part of the total number of tumors of cats presented there, because many cats die or are euthanatized without biopsies or autopsies being obtained. A significant and valuable portion of the tumors in the latter five years were submitted by practitioners principally from New England.

An extensive but certainly incomplete review of the literature on feline tumors constitutes a lesser component of the chapter. Citations from the literature, of value for historical and comparative purposes, cannot be exhaustive in a single chapter of a book, but we have tried to include the most significant surveys and reports, and many themselves review earlier work. For uncommon tumors we have often cited vintage reports, even though their terminology is sometimes obscure and there may be some question as to whether a pathologist today would concur in the diagnosis. We have learned "never to say never" and never to feel certain that we are reporting the first instance of a tumor. Many able pathologists in many countries have been increasingly interested in feline tumors for more than a century, and there are doubtless "first" reports that are now gathering dust in remote corners of "the literature." Especially when searches are limited to those performed by computer only since the 1960s, much excellent earlier work may escape notice.

Unfortunately, a cat population survey or a tumor registry does not exist in the northeastern United States. Accurate epidemiologic evaluation is therefore impossible.

Seventeen per cent (5777) of the 33,396 surgical specimens examined at AMAH over the 35-year period surveyed were obtained from cats. A small percentage of those specimens were selected tissues from incomplete autopsies. Of the 14,989 autopsies, 30 per cent (4520) were performed on cats. Several different tumors were occasionally found in a single autopsy. A few recent tumors of unusual interest have been included in the total studied (3248) (Table 11–1).

A regrettable shortcoming of the records at AMAH is the lack of complete and accurate data on the breed and color of cats. We have settled for breed and colors, insofar as they were recorded, in a somewhat arbitrary and inconsistent manner. Incomplete as our data were, however, we have a strong impression that breed and color may sometimes be factors in predisposition or resistance to certain tumors. To cite only a few examples, cats with white fur on the ears and face are most subject to actinic squamous cell carcinoma of the skin, while Siamese appear to be underrepresented for skin tumors and for oral carcinoma. On the other hand, Siamese seem, according to some surveys and our own experience, to suffer disproportionately from mammary and intestinal adenocarcinomas and from lymphocytic malignancies. Finally, in a number of instances, our data suggest that tricolor cats may be more subject than others to certain tumors. Veterinarians could contribute importantly to the understanding of the epidemiology of feline tumors if they would familiarize themselves with the breeds and colors of cats, note them accurately in their records, and include them in surgical and autopsy requisitions.

The microscopic diagnoses of tumors on file at AMAH represent the conclusions and points of view of a number of veterinary pathologists. There has not always been unanimous agreement as to diagnosis of a difficult tumor, and a few tumors for which no diagnosis could be reached with confidence have been omitted. We have occasionally revised the diagnosis of a predecessor or disagreed with that of a worker elsewhere who was kind enough to allow us to review a section. In general we have adopted the classification and terminology recommended by the World Health Organization.

We are greatly indebted to former directors of the Department of Pathology at AMAH: Dr. David Coffin, its founder, Dr. T. Carl Jones, Dr. Charley E. Gilmore, and Dr. Irwin Leav, and to the many residents and trainees whose labors are also represented. In the early years valuable interpretation and consultation were obtained at New England Deaconess Hospital from Dr. Shields Warren, Dr. Olive Gates, Dr. Edna Tompkins, and others. Some cases were submitted to the Armed Forces Institute of Pathology for consultation. Assistance in interpreting melanomas and nevi was obtained from Dr. Daniel Albert and Dr. Michael Olmstead. Our diagnoses of tumors of bones were reviewed by Dr. Scott Schelling.

## TUMORS OF THE SKIN AND SUBCUTIS

As indicated by many studies, after hematopoietic malignancies, tumors of the skin are next in frequency in cats, and the majority are malignant (e.g., Priester and McKay, 1980; Scott, 1980). Except for lymphocytic and mast cell tumors, which may occur in young cats, affected animals are typically middle-aged or elderly. According to one study, Siamese were significantly underrepresented among cases of skin cancer other than melanoma (Dorn et al., 1968b).

Four hundred and thirty skin tumors of cats were on file at AMAH. This total does not include mammary tumors, tumors of ceruminous glands of the ear, or lymphomas, which are discussed separately.

Skin tumors in cats are far less varied than those of dogs. Basal cell tumors, only rarely malignant, are the most frequent. Squamous cell carcinomas hold second place in exceedingly sunny climates, but in recent years have been edged out by mast cell tumors in some other geographic regions. Fibrosarcomas appear to be third in frequency, followed by glandular tumors. Fibromas, fatty tumors, melanomas, and hemangiosarcomas occur occasionally. Trichoepitheliomas, hair-matrix tumors, histiocytomas, and hemangiopericytomas are rare in cats.

### Basal Cell Tumor

In the experience of a majority of investigators, basal cell tumors are the most numerous of feline skin neoplasms. At AMAH they were second only to mammary tumors among primary neoplasms of the skin and adnexa.

**BREED, AGE, AND SEX.** Twenty of the 97 basal cell tumors (21 per cent) occurred in Siamese, although this breed represents no more than 5 per cent of hospital

**Table 11–1 3248 Feline Tumors and Tumor-like Lesions Diagnosed at the Angell Memorial Animal Hospital in a 35-Year Period***

| | |
|---|---|
| **SKIN AND SUBCUTIS** | |
| Basal cell tumor | 97 |
| Mast cell tumor | 89 |
| Fibrosarcoma | 68 |
| Hemangiosarcoma | 25 |
| Apocrine adenoma | 24 |
| Lipoma | 23 |
| Squamous cell carcinoma | 20 |
| Neurofibroma | 18 |
| Apocrine adenocarcinoma | 16 |
| Sebaceous nodular hyperplasia | 12 |
| Melanoma | 10 |
| Lymphangiosarcoma | 9 |
| Hemangioma | 7 |
| Fibroma | 5 |
| Melanogenic nevi | 5 |
| Sebaceous adenoma | 2 |
| Sebaceous adenocarcinoma | 2 |
| Liposarcoma | 2 |
| Leiomyosarcoma | 1 |
| Aggressive fibromatosis | 1 |
| Apocrine adenocarcinoma of anal sac | 1 |
| Hair matrix tumor | 1 |
| Lipomatosis | 1 |
| Merocrine adenocarcinoma | 1 |
| Papilloma | 1 |
| Plasmacytoma | 1 |
| Sebaceous epithelioma | 1 |
| Trichoepithelioma | 1 |
| **HEMATOPOIETIC SYSTEM** | |
| **General** | |
| Leukemias | See chapter on the hematopoietic system |
| Lymphoma | 1329 |
| Mast cell tumor (all sites) | 176 |
| Plasma cell myeloma and plasmacytoma | 4 |
| **Spleen** | |
| Mast cell tumor | 35 |
| Hemangiosarcoma | 10 |
| Nodular hyperplasia | 6 |
| Myelolipoma | 4 |
| Lipoma | 1 |
| **Thymus** | |
| Thymoma | 17 |
| **MUSCULOSKELETAL SYSTEM** | |
| **Bone** | |
| Osteosarcoma | 50 |
| Osteochondroma | 13 |
| Osteochondromatosis | 6 |
| Chondrosarcoma | 4 |
| Fibrodysplasia ossificans | 3 |
| Aneurysmal bone cyst | 2 |
| Fibrosarcoma | 1 |
| Angioma | 2 |
| Ossifying fibroma | 1 |
| **Tendon Sheath** | |
| Synoviosarcoma | 1 |
| **Skeletal Muscle** | |
| Rhabdomyoma/sarcoma | 0 |
| **RESPIRATORY SYSTEM** | |
| **Nose** | |
| Carcinoma | 12 |
| Inflammatory polyp (nasal origin) | 7 |
| Osteosarcoma | 4 |
| Fibrosarcoma | 3 |
| Squamous cell carcinoma | 3 |
| Osteochondromatosis | 2 |
| Melanoma | 2 |
| Melanogenic nevus | 2 |
| Hemangiosarcoma | 2 |
| Hemangioma | 1 |
| Chondrosarcoma | 1 |
| Carcinosarcoma | 1 |
| **Larynx** | |
| Squamous cell carcinoma | 1 |
| **Trachea** | 0 |
| **Lung** | |
| Adenocarcinoma | 34 |
| Adenocarcinoma, bronchial gland origin (?) | 8 |
| Squamous cell carcinoma | 3 |
| Adenosquamous carcinoma | 1 |
| **CARDIOVASCULAR SYSTEM** | |
| **Heart and Blood Vessels** | |
| Hemangiosarcoma | 56 |
| Hemangioma | 8 |
| Angioma | 2 |
| **Lymphatic Vessels** | |
| Lymphangioma/sarcoma | 9 |
| **ALIMENTARY SYSTEM** | |
| **Mouth** | |
| Squamous cell carcinoma | 72 |
| Fibrosarcoma | 5 |
| Melanoma | 4 |
| Epulis | 3 |
| Hemangiosarcoma | 2 |
| Leiomyosarcoma | 1 |
| **Tonsils** | |
| Squamous cell carcinoma | 8 |
| **Salivary Glands** | |
| Adenocarcinoma | 11 |
| Adenoma | 2 |
| **Esophagus** | |
| Squamous cell carcinoma | 4 |
| **Stomach** | |
| Polyp | 3 |
| **Intestine** | |
| Adenocarcinoma | 112 |
| Small intestine | 90 |
| Colon | 16 |
| Cecum | 4 |
| Rectum | 2 |
| Mast cell tumor | 46 |
| Polyp | 11 |
| Small intestine | 4 |
| Colon | 3 |
| Rectum | 3 |
| Cecum | 1 |
| Plasmacytoma | 1 |
| Leiomyoma | 1 |

*In a few instances, the same tumor is listed for more than one anatomic location, e.g., basal cell tumors of skin and eyelid, or squamous cell carcinomas of skin and ear. For this reason the total of tumors listed in the table does not accord exactly with that for the text. Leukemias are not included in this list.

*Table continued on opposite page*

**Table 11–1 3248 Feline Tumors and Tumor-like Lesions Diagnosed at the Angell Memorial Animal Hospital in a 35-Year Period** *Continued*

| | |
|---|---|
| **LIVER** | |
| Hepatocellular carcinoma | 18 |
| Adenoma of intrahepatic bile ducts | 18 |
| Adenocarcinoma of intrahepatic bile ducts | 14 |
| Adenocarcinoma of extrahepatic bile ducts | 4 |
| Hemangiosarcoma | 4 |
| Adenocarcinoma of gallbladder | 2 |
| Myelolipoma | 2 |
| Adenoma of gallbladder | 1 |
| Hemangioma | 1 |
| Mesothelioma | 1 |
| **PANCREAS** | |
| **Exocrine** | |
| Adenocarcinoma | 58 |
| Adenoma | 1 |
| Nodular hyperplasia | Not counted |
| **Endocrine** | |
| Islet cell tumor | 1 |
| **URINARY SYSTEM** | |
| **Kidney** | |
| Transitional cell carcinoma | 8 |
| Renal cell carcinoma | 6 |
| Sarcoma, poorly differentiated | 2 |
| Nephroblastoma | 1 |
| Squamous cell carcinoma | 1 |
| **Ureter** | 0 |
| **Bladder** | |
| Transitional cell carcinoma | 23 |
| Polyp | 6 |
| Leiomyosarcoma | 2 |
| **Urethra** | 0 |
| **MALE REPRODUCTIVE SYSTEM** | |
| **Testis** | |
| Sertoli cell tumor | 2 |
| **Prostate** | |
| Adenocarcinoma | 3 |
| **FEMALE REPRODUCTIVE SYSTEM** | |
| **Ovary** | |
| Granulosa cell tumor | 3 |
| **Uterus** | |
| Leiomyoma | 8 |
| Adenocarcinoma | 4 |
| Leiomyosarcoma | 3 |
| **Vagina** | |
| Fibroleiomyoma | 2 |
| Leiomyosarcoma | 1 |
| Squamous cell carcinoma | 1 |
| **MAMMARY GLAND** | |
| Simple adenocarcinoma | 180 |
| Adenosquamous carcinoma | 40 |
| Fibroepithelial hyperplasia | 30 |
| Adenoma | 13 |
| Malignant mixed tumor | 4 |
| Complex adenocarcinoma (?) | 3 |
| Benign mixed tumor | 1 |
| **ENDOCRINE SYSTEM** | |
| **Pituitary** | |
| Adenoma | 18 |
| **Adrenal** | |
| Adenoma, cortex | 2 |
| Pheochromocytoma, medulla | 4 |
| **Thyroid** | |
| Multinodular adenomatous hyperplasia | 138 |
| Carcinoma | 10 |
| **Parathyroid** | |
| Adenoma | 9 |
| Carcinoma | 1 |
| **Pancreatic Islets** | |
| Islet cell tumor | 1 |
| **Paraganglia** | |
| Retroperitoneal paraganglioma | 2 |
| Carotid body tumor | 1 |
| **CENTRAL NERVOUS SYSTEM** | |
| **Brain** | |
| Meningioma | 64 |
| Ependymoma | 6 |
| Primitive lymphoreticular tumor | 4 |
| Astrocytoma | 3 |
| Esthesioneuroblastoma (nose) | 2 |
| Cerebellar medulloblastoma | 1 |
| Capillary telangiectasia | 1 |
| **Spinal Cord** | |
| Astrocytoma | 3 |
| Angioma | 2 |
| Meningioma | 2 |
| Ependymoma | 1 |
| **EYE** | |
| **Globe** | |
| Intraocular melanoma | 19 |
| Adenoma of ciliary body | 3 |
| Ocular nevus | 2 |
| **Eyelid** | |
| Squamous cell carcinoma | 4 |
| Basal cell tumor | 3 |
| Melanoma | 3 |
| Melanogenic nevus | 1 |
| Epithelioma of meibomian gland | 1 |
| **EAR** | |
| Inflammatory polyp, ear, nasopharynx | 104 |
| Ceruminous adenocarcinoma | 30 |
| Ceruminous adenoma | 22 |
| Squamous cell carcinoma | 7 |
| Mast cell tumor | 7 |
| Fibrosarcoma | 4 |
| Sebaceous nodular hyperplasia | 3 |
| Melanoma | 2 |
| Melanogenic nevus | 1 |
| Adenosquamous carcinoma, middle ear | 1 |
| Basal cell tumor | 1 |
| **MESOTHELIOMA** | 1 |

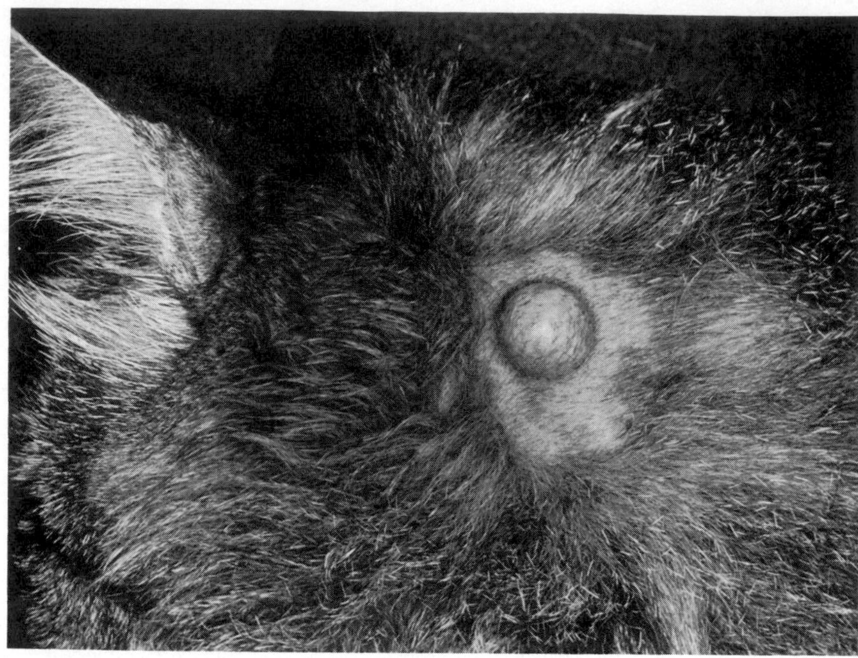

**Figure 11–1** Benign cystic basal cell tumor of apocrine gland origin in the cervical skin of a 10-year-old tabby. A similar soft but slightly larger cystic tumor was present over the right temple (not shown). Some of the cystic and usually unpigmented basal cell tumors are of apocrine gland rather than epidermal origin.

admissions. Fifty-four cats were females, 36 spayed; 43 were males, 14 castrated. A similar ratio of males to females (10:17) was reported by Priester and McKay (1980). The age range of cats at AMAH was 5 to 18 years (mean 10.8); only nine cats were less than seven years old.

**GROSS FEATURES.** About 75 per cent of the tumors occurred on the cranial half of the body: neck, 31 (Fig. 11–1); thorax, 16; head, 13; lumbar area, 7; hind leg, 7; shoulders, 6; abdomen, 6; foreleg, 5; tail, 3; paws, 2. The location of one tumor was not recorded. Only one cat had more than one tumor at a given time.

Basal cell tumors, oval or round and sharply circumscribed, are intradermal, except for large ones that extend into the subcutis. They elevate the overlying epidermis, which is often hairless or ulcerated. They ranged in size from 0.2 to 10.9 cm. Because of their firmness 10 per cent were detected when as small as 0.2 to 0.5 cm. About 9 per cent were pedunculated. Half the tumors were pigmented, a third ulcerated, and a quarter cystic. The fluid in some cysts was gray, brown, or black; in others, clear and colorless or pale yellow. The solid tumors appeared lobulated on cut surface, about half being white or pink, the rest tan, gray, or black.

**MICROSCOPIC FEATURES.** Patterns, in decreasing order of frequency, were solid (compact), cystic, adenoid, medusoid, and garland (ribbon). Combinations of patterns, with or without melanin pigmentation, were common. Over half the tumors were of the solid type, formed of lobules having compact groups of cells and fine eosinophilic stroma. Some groups had a peripheral layer of palisading cells. The lobules were most often composed of pleomorphic cells with nuclei varying from fusiform to round; in some lobules the cells were monomorphic with round nuclei. There were foci in which the configuration of cells suggested attempts at follicle or duct formation. Rare foci of differentiation into sebaceous glands were seen in two tumors, one of which also had apocrine gland formation. Squamoid cells with prominent desmosomes were common in the center of lobules, but keratinization was rare.

Many basal cell tumors had a central, fluid-filled cyst lined by nonkeratinizing squamoid cells (Fig. 11–2). The solid part of the tumor consisted of squamoid and fusiform cells, a few clefts, and a few empty spaces lined by a single row of more basophilic cells forming glands of apocrine type. Melanin was often present in melanocytes and in the epithelial cells. Glandular differentiation (adenoid pattern) occurred to varying degree in nearly 30 per cent of the tumors, medusoid differentiation in 7 per cent, and garland patterns in 5 per cent. Mitotic figures were surprisingly numerous for benign growths (up to five, with an average of two, per high-power field [HPF]). Necrosis in the center of solid lobules gave a comedo appearance to 20 per cent of the solid tumors. Mineralization in necrotic areas was rare.

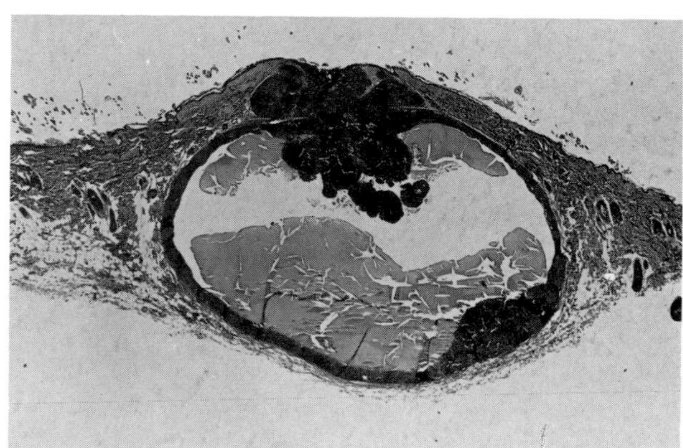

**Figure 11–2** Cystic basal cell tumor from the back of a 15-year-old Siamese. The clearly demarcated tumor, which arose from the epidermis, is pigmented and has papillary proliferations into a central cyst with melanin-containing gray fluid. H & E, × 10.

The tumors were routinely examined in only one microscopic section, but even so, one or more points of origin in the epidermis were seen in 16 per cent of the growths. Up to five points of tumor origin from the overlying epidermis were seen in one section. Only one tumor was observed to arise from a follicle. It is the opinion of one of the authors (JLC) that some of the cystic tumors with clear mural spaces and spindle cell and squamoid differentiation are of apocrine gland origin.

The benign basal cell tumors were sharply demarcated but not well encapsulated. Ten of the 97 tumors were malignant (carcinomas), characterized by stromal invasion, fibroplasia, high mitotic index, and foci of necrosis (Fig. 11–3). All were of a solid pattern, two with a lesser glandular component. Half invaded vessels, and one metastasized to the regional node (Fig. 11–4). Melanin, present in over half the benign tumors, was not observed in the malignant ones.

**MANAGEMENT.** Since about 10 per cent of basal cell tumors in cats may be malignant, the veterinarian should be alert for enlargement of regional nodes. Wide surgical excision is indicated whenever the site permits. Cryosurgery, topical treatment with 5-FU ointment, and systemic chemotherapy with cyclophosphamide are other possibilities (Theilen and Madewell, 1979).

## Squamous Cell Carcinoma

Squamous cell carcinoma (epidermoid carcinoma) has been reported to constitute from 9 to 25 per cent of the skin tumors of cats (Cotchin, 1961; Engle and Brodey, 1969; Macy and Reynolds, 1981; Nielsen, 1964; Patnaik et al., 1975). A relationship between solar exposure and the development of squamous cell carcinoma in cats was first recognized in Italy and North Africa (e.g., Ciampi, 1949; Ottani, 1923) and later in the United States, especially in Florida and California, where the incidence is high (Foley, 1977; Theilen and Madewell, 1979). Cats having skin areas thinly covered by white fur or unpigmented areas of skin, such as eyelids, nose, and lips, are at greater risk for squamous cell carcinoma, especially in sunny climates; however, white-furred, outdoor cats in temperate climates, and even white-furred indoor cats that sun themselves in picture windows, are occasional victims.

**BREED, AGE, AND SEX.** At AMAH 20 cases of cutaneous squamous cell cancer were diagnosed. Of the four totally white cats in the group, two had lesions on both ear tips and two had eyelids affected on one side. No breed or sex predisposition has been reported for cutaneous squamous cell carcinoma. No purebred was affected in the group at AMAH. The mean age was 12.4 years with a range of 7 to 24. Females outnumbered the males 3:2 for cutaneous squamous cell carcinoma at AMAH, where females constitute about 47 per cent of the total hospital population. The higher incidence of squamous cell carcinoma in females at AMAH may be related to a longer life than that of males. The average age at time of tumor diagnosis was 11.6 years for males and 12.6 for females.

**GROSS FEATURES.** Squamous cell carcinoma most often arises from skin of the head, particularly the ears, nose and eyelids, and also from the digits. Of 20 cats at AMAH, seven had tumors of the ears. One or both ear tips were involved in five; two had growths in an ear canal. (See discussion and photographs in the chapter on the ear.) All these cats were white or partly white, and tumor may have developed from sites of solar keratoses. Four cats had tumors of the eyelids. In five cats a digit was involved, and one each had a tumor on the top of the head, near an ear, over a tibia, and near a lip. In a survey by Priester and McKay (1980), 21 squamous cell carcinomas of the skin arose from the external ear and 20 from the eyelid, conjunctiva, or lacrimal gland.

The squamous cell carcinomas were firm or hard as the result of accompanying fibrosis. The skin surface was ulcerated in nearly half the tumors and appeared granular, friable, umbilicated, or necrotic, often resembling granulation tissue. Rarely the tumor formed a proliferative, cauliflower-like mass. Cut surfaces of the tumors were often nodular, granular, necrotic, dry, and white with yellow foci. Because the tumor infiltrated surrounding tissue, its margins were usually poorly demarcated.

Some tumors were misdiagnosed from gross appearance as draining abscesses, as infected wounds, or, in cases of digital involvement, as osteomyelitis. Several years of erythema and crusty dermatitis of a white ear may precede the transformation into tumor. With continued neglect, the tumor may disfigure the ear extensively before veterinary care is sought and a correct diagnosis is made.

Distant metastasis is uncommon. A white cat with suspected solar-induced carcinoma of one auricle had excisional surgery and three months later had a front digit removed because of destructive metastatic tumor. After another three months, two digits on a rear paw also had bone lesions. At autopsy metastatic tumor was found in the two digits and in the lungs and kidneys.

**MICROSCOPIC FEATURES.** Compact groups of epithelial cells (some with desmosomes), individual cells with keratin in their cytoplasm (often in laminar form), and groups of keratinizing cells forming keratin "pearls" are the diagnostic features of squamous cell carcinoma. Fibrous connective tissue may surround nests of cells, and lymphocytes, plasma cells, macrophages, and neutrophils often form a cellular cuff. Lymphatic invasion may be difficult to identify, because the tightly joined epithelial cells form occlusive thrombi.

**PROGNOSIS AND TREATMENT.** Most squamous cell carcinomas of the skin are highly invasive but usually slow to metastasize. The tumor spreads by invading thin-walled lymphatic vessels; less often, it invades veins. Desmosomes, which hold the tumor cells tightly together, probably delay spread to regional nodes even after vascular invasion has occurred.

Wide excision, when possible, is the preferred treatment. Involved digits should be amputated. The veterinarian can better determine the extent of tumor and predict its behavior if he also removes regional nodes and submits them for histologic examination. Radiation therapy is the treatment of choice for those tumors in which total excision is impossible (e.g., Carlisle and Gould, 1982). Cryosurgery and hyperthermia are other possible methods of treatment for tumors that cannot be excised (Grier et al., 1980; Muller et al., 1983). Bleomycin has been used systemically (Theilen and Madewell, 1979).

In a 17-year-old female cat with long-standing crusting of both white ear tips, confinement indoors and application of lanolin brought about complete healing of one ear, but the lesion on the other progressed to cancer, which was successfully excised.

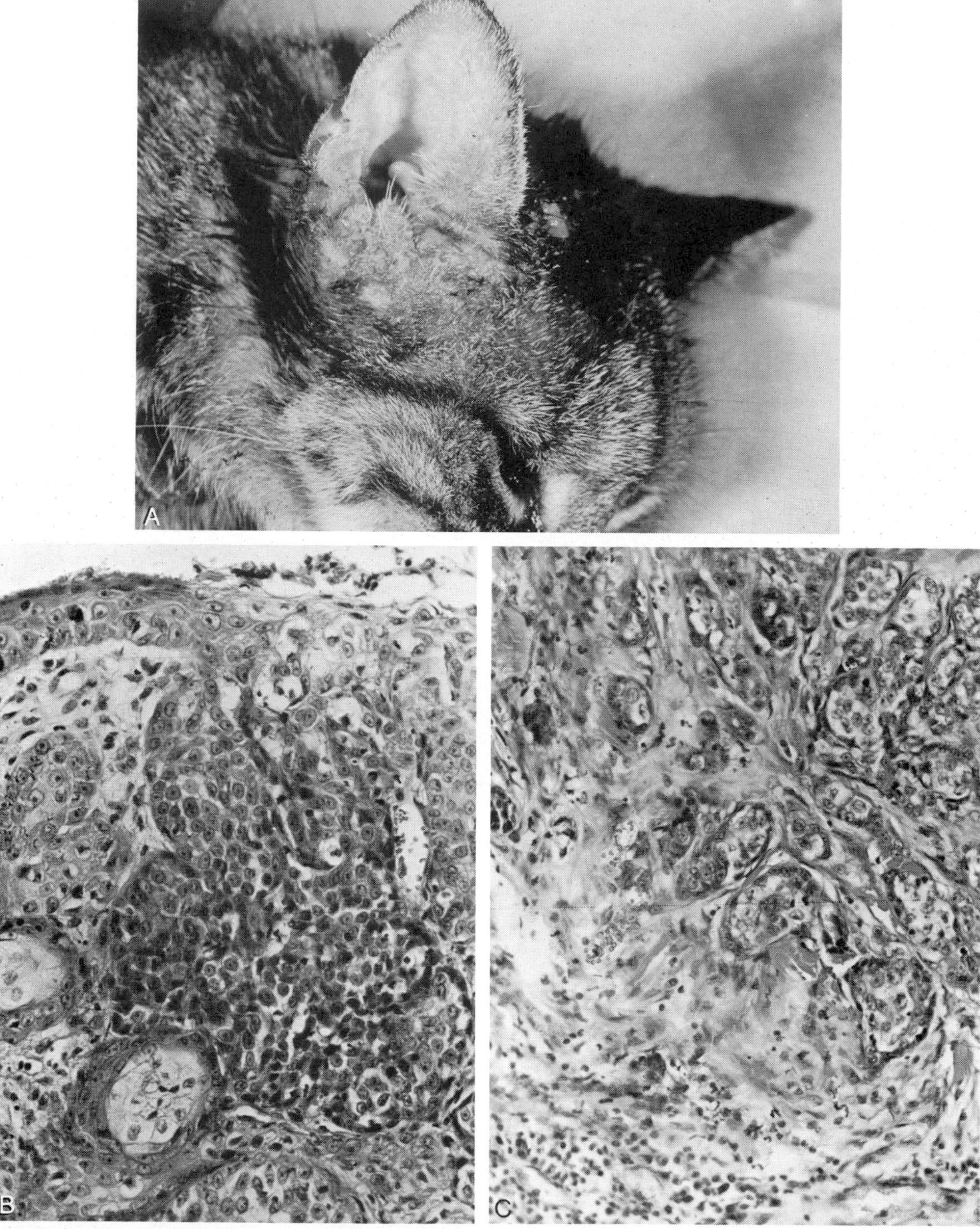

**Figure 11–3** *A*, Malignant basal cell tumor at the base of an ear, eight-year-old female tabby. Skin at the base of the pinna and below the ear is thickened and irregular and has small ulcerated foci of tumor over the tragus. *B*, Malignant basal cell tumor, same cat. An aggregate of intensely stained neoplastic basal cells (center and right) arises from the epidermis (upper right). H & E, × 300. *C*, Same malignant basal cell tumor in the subcutis. Deep infiltration, desmoplasia, lack of encapsulation, and inflammatory response (bottom) are features suggesting malignant behavior. Vascular invasion (not shown) caused edema and diffuse thickening of the skin at the base of the ear. H & E, × 250.

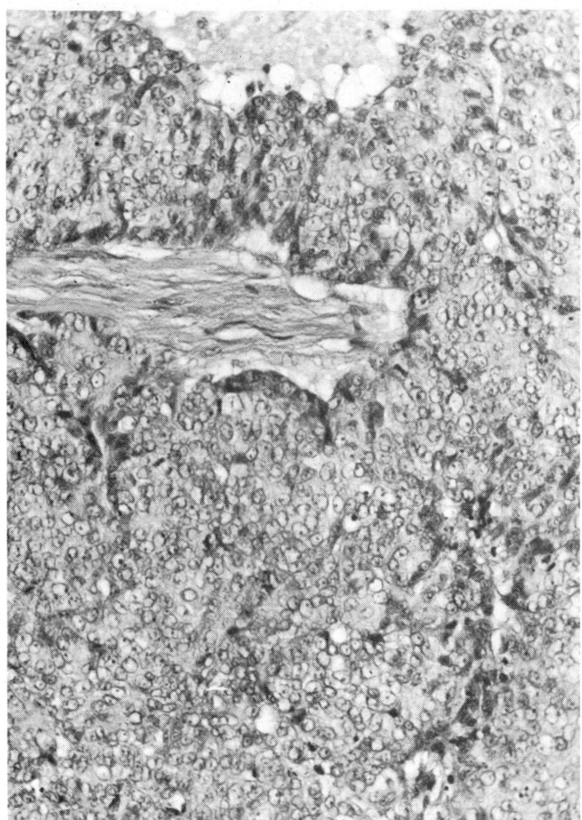

**Figure 11–4** Malignant basal cell tumor located below the ear, 20-year-old tricolor cat. The solid tumor has hyperchromatic cells that border on fibrous stroma (center), suggesting a basal cell origin. The tumor arose from basal cells of the epidermis (not shown) and metastasized to the prescapular node. H & E, × 180.

Application of a sun-screen lotion containing para-aminobenzoic acid has been suggested as a preventive measure (Hayes et al., 1976), as well as confinement indoors during the hours of most intense sunlight. Tattooing is also effective (Foley, 1977).

The reader is referred to the chapter on tumor management for further detail.

## Papilloma

Few papillomas have been reported in cats (Engle and Brodey, 1969; Macy and Reynolds, 1981; Mugera, 1968; Mulligan, 1951; Priester and McKay, 1980; Sedlmeier and Weiss, 1963). Papillomatosis near the external acoustic meatus in a one and a half-year-old Persian has been pictured by Austin (1975). The lesion was removed by hyfrecation.

At AMAH, a single case of papilloma was on record on the ear tip of a 10-year-old castrated male domestic longhaired tabby. Microscopically, it appeared to arise from a hair follicle.

Highly keratinized conical papillomas ("cutaneous horns") have been reported from the skin of the neck (Head, 1953; Moulton, 1978) and axilla (Scott, 1980), and multiple cutaneous horns, unresponsive to surgical removal, have been described on the footpads of cats infected with feline leukemia virus (Center et al., 1982).

## Sebaceous Gland Tumors

Lesions of sebaceous glands are rare in the cat (Theilen and Madewell, 1979; Scott, 1980). So-called sebaceous cysts are, in fact, epidermal inclusion cysts or, more often, hyperplastic sebaceous nodules or adenomas of the types to be described.

**NODULAR HYPERPLASIA.** Nodular hyperplasia, the most frequent lesion, was seen in 12 cats at AMAH. The only purebreds were a Himalayan and a Siamese. The cats were aged 2 to 14 years, only one being under 7. Of eight females, six were spayed; two of the four males were castrated. Two cats had more than one lesion. Seven lesions were on the head (chin, external ear canal, at the base of an auricle, above the eye, and at the margin of the upper lip). Two were on the neck and two on the proximal part of the tail. One cat had an unusual aggregation of lesions on one side of the thorax and abdomen. These first appeared when the cat was only a year old and continued to develop over a 10-year period (Fig. 11–5). At the last surgery when the cat was 11, one adenoma was removed as well as several hyperplastic lesions.

The hyperplastic nodules ranged from 0.2 to 1.4 cm (average 0.5). Most were firm, raised, and covered centrally with intact but hairless skin. On sectioning they appeared pale yellow, sharply demarcated, and finely lobulated. The larger nodules contained yellow material that oozed or could be expressed from the cut surface. In some cats the lesions were itchy and inflamed.

Microscopically, the lesions consisted of one or more hypertrophic and hyperplastic glands composed of mature lobules and ducts, some of which were cystic. These ducts and lobules were larger than those of adjacent normal glands, but their cells were of normal size. The nodules were sharply circumscribed but not encapsulated.

Both lesions that occurred in the ear canals of two cats 10 and 12 years old were wide-based, pedunculated, firm masses of identical microscopic appearance: tightly grouped, enlarged glands with dense interlobular and interglandular collagenous stroma. A clinician might well have interpreted these lesions as the more frequent growths of ceruminous glands.

**ADENOMA.** Two sebaceous gland adenomas were diagnosed in elderly cats. One, an 11-year-old, also had multiple areas of hyperplasia, described earlier. In the other cat, a 14-year-old, a 0.6 cm sessile adenoma, firm, pink, and lobulated, was situated on the tail near the base. The two adenomas were characterized microscopically by lobules with an excessive number of reserve (basal) cells and a variable number of differentiated lipid-laden epithelial cells.

**EPITHELIOMA.** A single sebaceous epithelioma was found in the AMAH group—a 0.5 cm, ulcerated, firm, dark gray nodule on an upper eyelid. Lobules of tarsal (modified sebaceous, meibomian) gland varied in the number of reserve cells and of round or fusiform basal cells. Melanin within the epithelial cells was abundant. Lymphocytes, plasma cells, and foci of lipogranulomatous inflammation surrounded many of the lobules. This sebaceous epithelioma had poorly differentiated areas resembling a pigmented basal cell tumor.

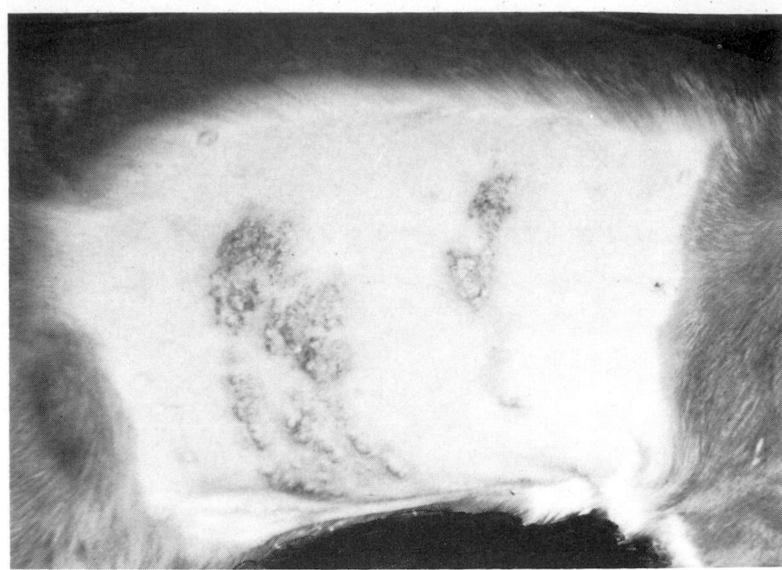

**Figure 11–5** Nodular sebaceous hyperplasia involving numerous sites on the right lateral chest and abdomen, two-year-old male red tabby. The hair has been clipped to disclose the variably sized, papular, sessile, and often confluent nodules, which were pale yellow, some with dark central debris.

**ADENOCARCINOMA.** Only two cats had malignant tumors of sebaceous glands. A six-year-old castrated male longhair had recurrent growths removed from the dorsum of the base of the tail three times during a two-year period. At the third excision, the mass elevated the overlying intact skin and on cut surface was spherical, 0.8 cm in diameter, solid, and uniformly white. It was seen on microscopic examination to displace the adjacent normally large sebaceous glands and to infiltrate the dermis, subcutis, and lymphatic vessels. It consisted of large cells with one or more pleomorphic, eccentric nuclei, some having a nucleolus almost the size of a red blood cell. The abundant, eosinophilic cytoplasm contained a globule with a basophilic, stippled periphery and a lightly eosinophilic, foamy, central region that stained light red-purple with PAS. Rare foci of squamous differentiation suggested attempts at duct formation. Foci of necrosis were present.

The other cat, an 18-year-old spayed female Siamese, had a 2.0 cm, raised, ulcerated, bleeding mass on a digit of a forepaw. It was white and lobulated on cut surface and composed of reserve cells with a vesicular nucleus and a single, large, central nucleolus. Reserve cells made up 70 to 95 per cent of the lobules and had up to 12 mitotic figures per high-dry field. Sebaceous cell differentiation, areas of atypical duct formation resembling squamous cell carcinoma, and a point of continuity with a sebaceous gland near the ulcer made identification of the cell of origin easy. The tumor had not recurred when the cat died a year later of renal failure.

## Glandular Tumors of the Anal Area

Although the cat has no glands analogous to the circumanal (perianal) glands of the dog, examination of sections (by JLC) identified clusters of glands partially in the wall and about the duct of the anal sac that have characteristics of both sebaceous and hepatoid glands. The anal sac is lined by stratified squamous epithelium and has coiled apocrine glands in its wall that empty into its lumen. Additional apocrine glands arranged in lobules lie between smooth and striated muscles of the anal sphincter and empty at the anocutaneous junction.

A few tumors of "perianal" glands or of anal glands have been reported: anal gland adenomas (Mugera, 1968), malignant "anal and perianal sac gland tumors" (Macy and Reynolds, 1981), and a "perianal gland adenoma" (Poppensiek, 1961). A "perianal gland adenocarcinoma" described by Weissman and Pulley (1974) was more likely a poorly differentiated sebaceous gland tumor arising from the sebaceous glands associated with the anus and anal sacs of the cat (Stannard and Pulley, 1978).

A 17-year-old white spayed female domestic longhair seen at AMAH had an adenocarcinoma of the apocrine glands of the anal sac. The tumor destroyed and replaced the left anal sac and metastasized to the pelvic nodes, pulmonary arteries, lungs, and liver (Fig. 11–6).

## Apocrine Sweat Gland Tumors

Sweat glands are of two types, apocrine and merocrine (eccrine). The former are numerous in the haired skin; the latter occur only in the foot pads. Ceruminous glands of the external auditory meatus are modified apocrine glands, as are mammary glands; their cysts and tumors are discussed elsewhere. Apocrine sweat glands empty into hair follicles above the point of entry of sebaceous ducts. These coiled tubular glands have two rows of cells—the inner secretory cuboidal or columnar cells and the basal smaller, usually flattened myoepithelial cells—both contained within the basement membrane.

**CYSTS OF APOCRINE SWEAT GLANDS.** Cysts of apocrine glands, common in dogs, are rare in cats. Only five were on record at AMAH, all occurring on the head—two each on the chin and near an ear, one near the medial ocular canthus. The cats were aged from 1½ to 13 years; only one was under 6. Three were males and two females.

The cysts formed elevated, round or oval, fluctuant, intradermal and subcutaneous nodules, covered by sparsely haired epidermis. From 0.2 to 2.0 cm in diameter, they contained clear, watery or viscid fluid and were lined by epithelium ranging from simple squamous to tall columnar with a basal layer of myoepithelial cells. Golden brown pigment was present in some of the epithelial cells.

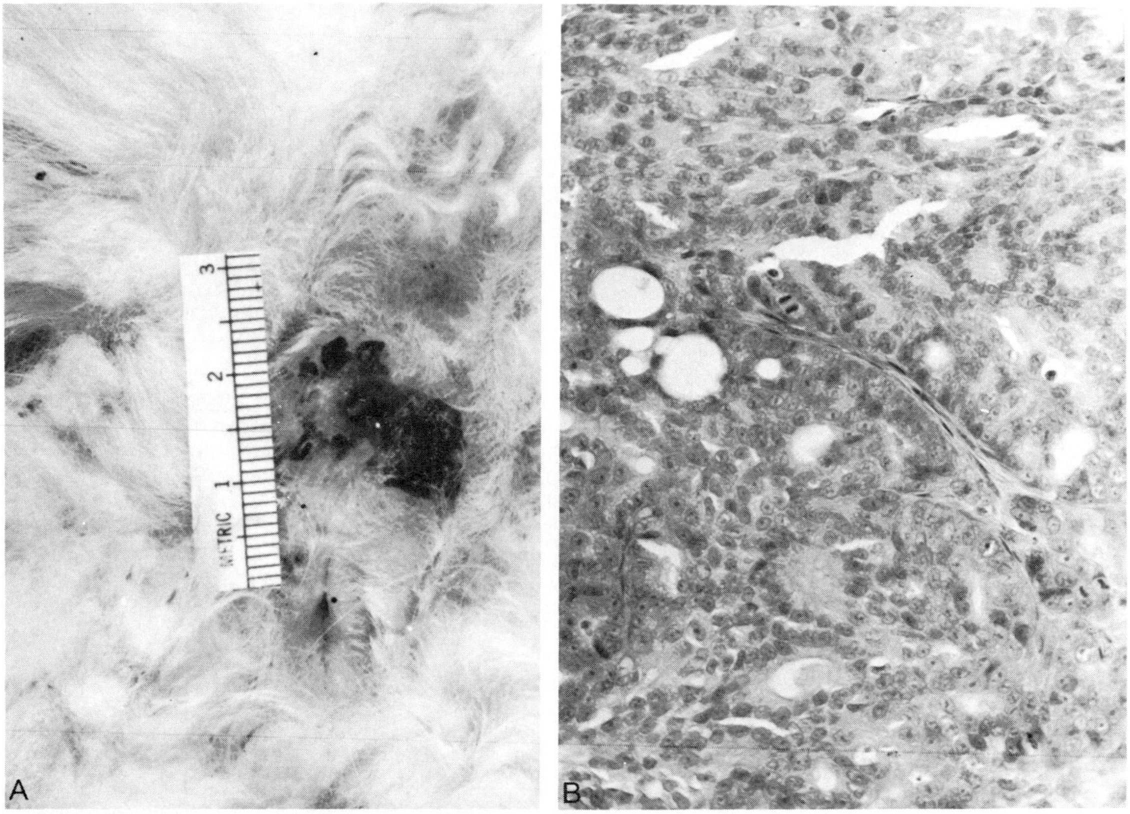

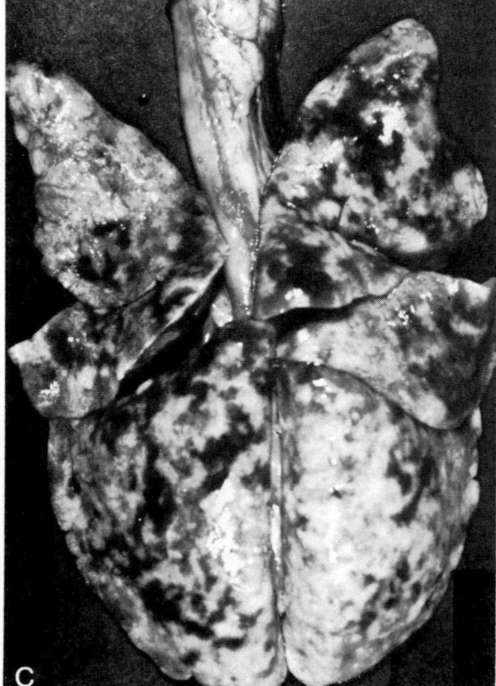

**Figure 11–6** Adenocarcinoma of apocrine glands of the right anal sac, 17-year-old spayed female white domestic longhair. Dark exudate on the hair surrounds a fistula that communicates with the neoplastic anal sac. The vulva is located below and to the right of the ruler. *B*, The predominantly solid adenocarcinoma of the apocrine glands of the anal sac also had alveolar (center) and tubular patterns (not shown). H & E, × 200. *C*, All lung lobes are mottled and irregularly consolidated owing to disseminated metastases from the adenocarcinoma of the anal sac.

**ADENOMA AND ADENOCARCINOMA.** Tumors of apocrine glands are rare in cats but yet more frequent than those of sebaceous glands. Twenty-four adenomas were on record at AMAH and 16 adenocarcinomas. Only two cats were purebreds, both Siamese with adenocarcinomas. Cats with adenomas were aged from 9 to 17 years (mean 12), those with adenocarcinomas from 6 to 24 years (mean 12.9). In the total group of 40 cats, 26 were females (20 spayed) and 14 males (8 castrated).

The head and neck were the sites of 80 per cent of the adenomas but only about a third of the adenocarcinomas. A third of the adenomas had been present from six months to three years, but only one had ruptured before excision. A majority were fluctuant and thought by the examining veterinarian to be cysts. Most caused dome-shaped elevation of the skin. A few were papillary or pedunculated. Most were white, but a few appeared blue or black owing to pigmentation of the overlying epidermis. All were sharply demarcated and ranged from 0.2 to 3.0 cm in diameter (average 1.4).

Unlike the adenomas, the adenocarcinomas were usually ulcerated and poorly circumscribed. Most were firm or hard, rather than fluctuant, and were larger than adenomas, averaging 2.4 cm in greatest dimension. On cut surface many adenomas consisted of a smooth-walled cyst, as well as papillary or lobulated white or pale yellow regions. Fluid in the cysts was usually clear and watery, occasionally rust-colored. Fixation caused the fluid in some cysts to assume a pale yellow mucoid or gelatinous character.

Microscopically, some apocrine adenomas are difficult to distinguish from cystic basal cell tumors that have foci of apocrine glandular differentiation, unless the basal cells are abundant or contain melanin granules; however, melanin granules can be observed rarely in epithelium of normal apocrine glands. Tumors of apocrine glands arise from existing glands, whereas most basal cell tumors originate from epidermal basal cells and therefore tend to be more superficial in the dermis and subcutis and more often ulcerated. Furthermore, the majority of adenomas have one or more regions in a single microsection where a double layer of cells resembles the wall of a cystic apocrine gland.

The most common histologic type of benign apocrine gland tumor is the papillary syringoadenoma (papillary cystadenoma), exemplified in 24 tumors at AMAH: a cystic mass with a glandular wall consisting of papillae composed of two double rows of cells separated by minimal intervening stroma. The irregular spaces formed by the branching papillae may be empty or may contain eosinophilic secretion. Cells edging the papillae and lining spaces have cytoplasmic apices with features suggesting the apocrine mode of secretion. Within the papillae, and especially near the edge of the cyst, the inner layer of the double row of cells is sometimes effaced by a sheet of fusiform or squamoid cells. The epithelial cells forming the cyst wall are cuboidal or low columnar and are distinct from the underlying fusiform or squamoid cells. In tumors of this pattern sections of the outer border are often composed only of a double row of cells resembling the wall of a cystic apocrine gland. The other six adenomas were of the same pattern but lacked a prominent fusiform or squamoid component. Pure cystadenomas without any papillary growth were not observed.

The adenocarcinomas were most reliably differentiated by invasion of stroma or vessels, or both. Absence of a uniform double row of cells, piling up of cells, irregular and poorly demarcated border, high mitotic index, foci of necrosis, fibroplasia, cellular pleomorphism, and ulceration also suggested malignancy. The precise site of origin of the adenocarcinomas was impossible to ascertain except for one tumor that was seen to originate from the epidermis. Some malignant tumors of apocrine glands on the ventral abdomen or near the vulva may be impossible to differentiate from disseminated mammary tumor.

To summarize, benign tumors of apocrine glands rarely ulcerate, whereas over half the malignant tumors are ulcerated. Benign tumors are seldom accompanied by inflammation, again in contrast with adenocarcinomas, which can be mistaken for injuries and infections of the skin. Benign tumors often feel cystic, whereas malignant growths are usually firm and nonfluctuant. Adenocarcinomas metastasize by lymphatics, so regional nodes should be examined. Excision should be generous, especially with firm, poorly demarcated, ulcerated growths.

Metastasis of a sweat gland adenocarcinoma to the eye has been described (Moise et al., 1982).

## Merocrine (Eccrine) Sweat Gland Tumors

Merocrine sweat glands, limited to the footpads, are composed of light and dark cuboidal cells as well as myoepithelial cells. Tumors of these glands should be differentiated from tumors of apocrine glands. According to Muller et al. (1983), no tumors of eccrine glands have been reported in the cat. One adenocarcinoma was on record at AMAH, in a seven-year-old spayed female Siamese. The tumor caused lameness and, when first seen, was very hard, ulcerated, callus-like, and located in the center of a metacarpal pad. It was first diagnosed and treated as an old wound, but continued growth prompted excision five months later, when it reached 1.0 cm in diameter (Fig. 11–7). The tumor recurred in six months and was excised again, along with most of the metacarpal pad. The recurrent mass was solid, yellow, and 0.8 cm in diameter. Two years later, a solid, nodular, whitish yellow, metastatic tumor, 2.0 × 1.5 × 1.2 cm, was removed from the subcutis cranial to the ipsilateral elbow. Four years after the neoplasm was first observed, the cat was in apparent good health but was euthanatized for personal reasons of its owner. At autopsy, a hard, white nodule of metastatic tumor, 0.5 × 0.3 cm, was found between the second and third metacarpals above the small, scarred metacarpal pad. Regional nodes and lungs were free of metastases.

## Trichoepithelioma

This benign, well-differentiated tumor of hair follicles is common in dogs, but reports of its occurrence in cats are few (Austin, 1975; Bostock, 1977; Frese, 1968; Macy and Reynolds, 1981; Nielsen, 1983; Priester and McKay, 1980; Stannard and Pulley, 1978; Theilen and Madewell, 1979). One trichoepithelioma was on file at AMAH. The tumor was cystic, 0.9 cm in diameter, and located on the shoulder of an 11-year-old female Siamese (Fig. 11–8).

## Hair-Matrix Tumor (Pilomatrixoma)

This tumor of hair follicles is less well differentiated than the trichoepithelioma and may become calcified. Also common in dogs, it is reported only rarely in cats

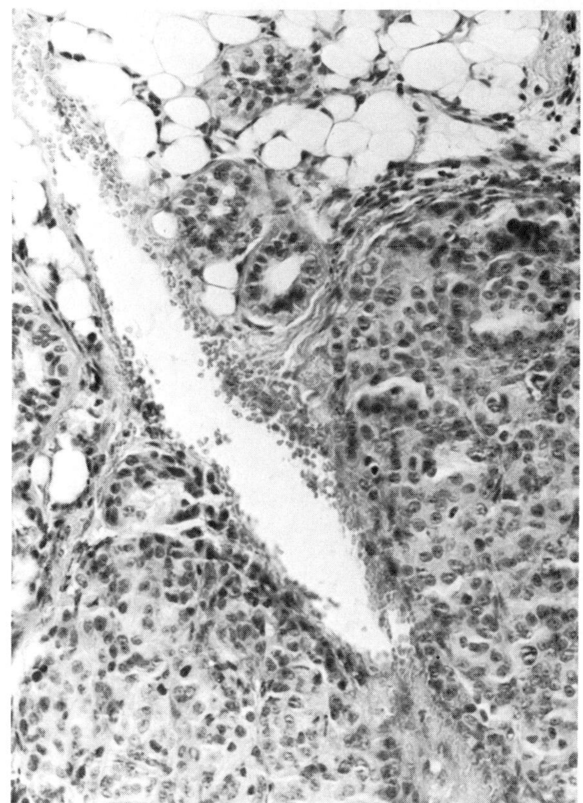

**Figure 11–7** Adenocarcinoma of eccrine sweat gland in a metacarpal pad, seven-year-old Siamese. The solid carcinoma is subdivided into poorly defined compact packets. Three sections of normal sweat glands (top center) border on the tumor and lie within fat. The tumor recurred in the pad and was again excised. It also metastasized, over a period of four years, to two sites in the same limb. H & E, × 200.

(Macy and Reynolds, 1981; Priester and McKay, 1980). Only one hair-matrix tumor was on file at AMAH. A well-circumscribed dermal and subcutaneous mass on the right shoulder of a 12-year-old spayed female Siamese, it measured 2.5 × 1.4 × 1.3 cm and on cut surface had two distinct zones, one cystic and yellow-white, the other hard with tan granular foci. Microscopically the tumor was cystic with a wall composed of several layers of viable basal cells of hair-matrix type, some in foci suggesting attempts at follicle formation. As these cells grew farther from their basement membrane and blood supply, they underwent coagulation necrosis, appearing as ghost or shadow cells.

## Intracutaneous Cornifying Epithelioma ("Keratoacanthoma")

This benign tumor, frequent in dogs, is apparently extremely uncommon in cats. The description given by Austin (1975) does not wholly correspond with the features seen in the canine tumor. None has been diagnosed at AMAH.

## Fibroma and Fibrosarcoma

**FIBROMA.** Cutaneous fibromas are, in general, infrequent in cats (Scott, 1980), although they appear in significant numbers in some surveys, e.g., 11 in a total of 45 tumors (Austin, 1975) and 16 of 125 (Cotchin, 1961).

At AMAH only five fibromas were recorded, all in domestic female cats aged 3 to 14 years, with only one being under 7. The tumors, measuring from 1.2 to 2.0 cm, involved the dermis or subcutis, or both, and were located in the external auditory meatus or on the back, hip, or toe. Solitary, firm, and white or pale gray, they were discrete but unencapsulated and were homogeneous on cut surface. The largest, over a hip, was ulcerated and secondarily infected.

Microscopically fibromas are a benign neoplastic prolif-

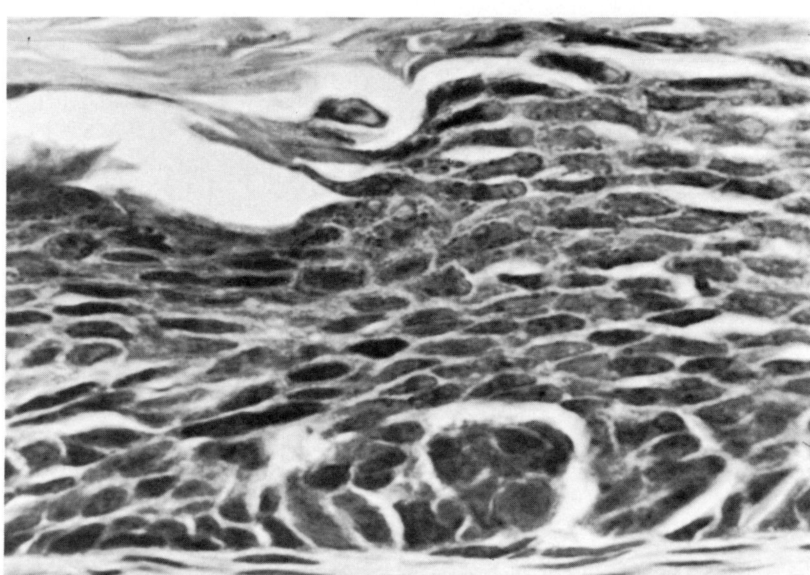

**Figure 11–8** Trichoepithelioma, shoulder, 11-year-old female Siamese. Hair matrix cells make an abortive attempt to form a follicle, and many contain cytoplasmic trichohyaline granules that appear dark here but stained brilliantly acidophilic (upper center). H & E, × 900.

eration of fusiform or, less often, stellate cells, which produce varying amounts of collagen, reticulin, and ground substance. They are of three types: durum (hard), molle (soft), and myxoma. The five at AMAH consisted of dense collagen bundles and fusiform fibroblasts. Mitotic figures were absent or rare, as were stellate cells. One tumor was less firm, owing to a small amount of fat and less dense collagen, thus qualifying as a fibroma molle.

**FIBROSARCOMA.** Aggressive tumors that sometimes metastasize widely, fibrosarcomas are the most common mesenchymal tumor of the skin and subcutis. A virus (FeSV) is the cause of the tumor in about half of cats with naturally occurring, multiple fibrosarcomas (Theilen and Madewell, 1979). Cats, both old and young, with solitary fibrosarcoma are usually uninfected. Feline sarcoma virus, unlike FeLV (of which it is probably a mutant), is not transmitted horizontally. Cats with FeSV, most often young cats with multicentric tumor, are FeLV-positive, and FeSV, a "defective" virus, requires helper FeLV for replication. Experimental inoculation of cats with FeSV has produced malignant melanoma and rhabdomyosarcoma as well as fibrosarcoma. (For detailed discussion of FeSV, its various strains, and pathogenicity, see Sarma et al. [1971a,b, 1972] and the chapter on virus diseases.)

Brown et al. (1978) reported that 13 of 23 cats with soft-tissue sarcomas were tested by the indirect fluorescent antibody test for FeLV and all were test-negative. Six of 77 cats with fibrosarcoma at AMAH were tested and found to be negative.

Fibrosarcomas account for 12 to 25 per cent of feline skin tumors (Bostock, 1977; Brodey, 1970; Cotchin, 1961). In the experience of many (see Scott, 1980) and at AMAH, fibrosarcomas are the third most frequent skin tumor of cats, but they were fourth in order after basal cell tumors, mast cell tumors, and squamous cell carcinomas in the survey of Priester and McKay (1980). It is likely that many of the spindle cell sarcomas should be regarded as fibrosarcomas. No breed or sex predisposition for fibrosarcomas has been reported. Most occur in adults, but some have been found in cats six months of age or even younger, and most are found in the subcutis (Moulton, 1978).

Since fibrosarcomas are among the most important tumors of cats, a word about diagnosis is in order. Most pathologists would agree with Moulton, who stated (1978) that "the category of fibrosarcoma probably represents a heterogeneous group consisting, not only of malignant tumors of fibroblasts, but also unclassifiable and mixed mesenchymal cell tumors capable of collagen production." To assure differentiation from neurofibrosarcomas, Frankhauser et al., writing in the WHO Bulletin (1974), would require that, in the latter, continuity with a nerve be seen. Searching an entire specimen for this feature seems to us (JLC) impractical as a routine procedure. We have accordingly eliminated from our group of fibrosarcomas any tumor in which morphologic characteristics of neurofibrosarcoma were prominent, i.e., storiform pattern, palisading, or whorls about a central core of collagen. Some of our tumors could have been called undifferentiated sarcomas.

At AMAH, among 77 fibrosarcomas of all body sites, 68 involved the skin and subcutis (other sites were oral and nasal cavities, bone, and mediastinum). No breed or sex predisposition was evident. The cats ranged in age from 1 to 20 years (mean 8.7). Lesions were situated on the head (23) (Fig. 11–9); neck (1); forelimb (12, the majority at or above the elbow) (Figs. 11–10 and 11–11); thorax (17) (Fig. 11–12); abdomen (8); lumbar region (6); hind leg (11, all but one above the tarsus); and tail (3). Twelve cats had more than one mass, sometimes in more than one anatomic region.

**Gross Features.** The tumors ranged in size from a 0.6 cm nodule on a rear digit to an 11.5 cm mass on the back. Growths raised the overlying skin, but only two were pedunculated, one on the neck and the other on a forearm. Most masses involved the dermis and subcutis, and occasionally a mass infiltrated the underlying muscles. The majority of growths were described as firm but rubbery, nodular, and on cut surface white to grayish white, lobulated, solid, unencapsulated, and poorly demarcated, with fine glistening bundles or striations. Fewer masses had cystic, fluid-filled foci and areas of hemorrhage. Ulceration of overlying skin occurred in seven cats with tumors greater than 1.8 cm in greatest dimension. Twelve of the 77 cats had multiple fibrosarcomas (3 to 15) usually close together, but one cat had masses in the lumbar, flank, and tail base regions, and another had a mass on top of the head and one under the jaw.

**Microscopic Features.** All the fibrosarcomas had the characteristic interwoven bundles of fibroblasts but otherwise varied in degree of cellularity and amounts of collagen, reticulin fiber, and ground substance (Fig. 11–13). Necrosis, hemorrhage, and edema were common in the larger masses. The cells and their nuclei were much larger than those in fibromas. The size and shape of the nuclei varied from tumor to tumor and even in the same tumor, but most were fusiform. The number of mitoses also varied. Some tumors had bizarre or multinucleated giant cells, the large number being especially characteristic of some feline fibrosarcomas. Other tumors had stellate cells, abundant ground substance, and invisible borders so that they had a myxomatous appearance. Some cells

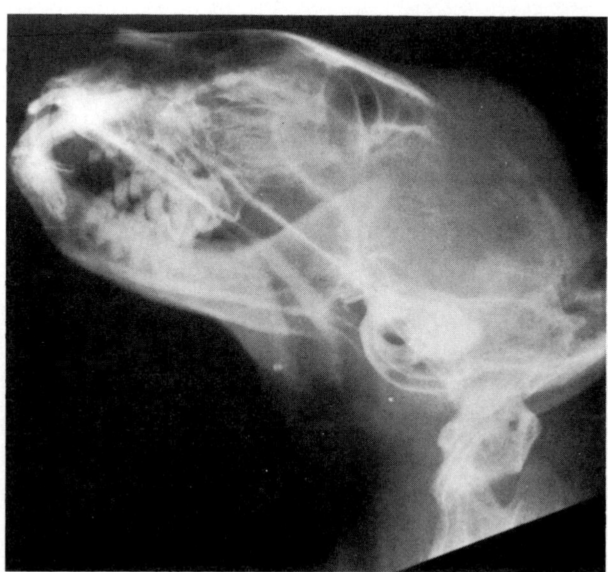

**Figure 11–9** Fibrosarcoma involving subcutis, temporalis muscles, frontal and parietal bones, and dura mater, with compression of the cerebrum, two-year-old Siamese.

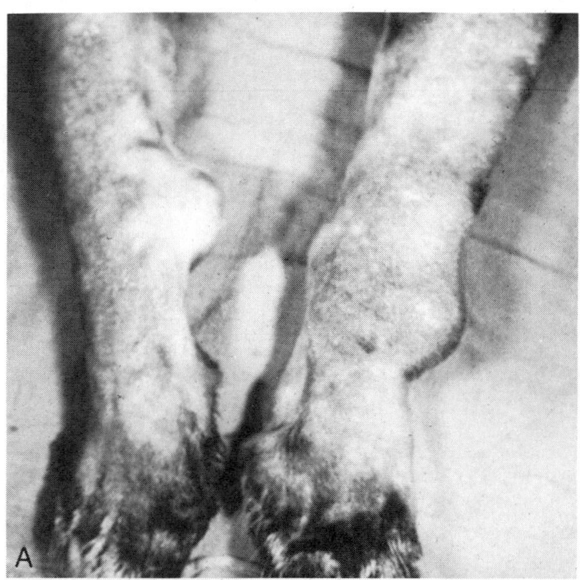


**Figure 11–10** *A*, Fibrosarcomas of both forelimbs, four-year-old castrated male tabby. Many scars (pale foci) from cat fights suggest that the numerous tumor nodules were caused by FeSV and FeLV that may have been transmitted by saliva through cat bites. Tumor nodules extended above the elbow in the left limb, but distant metastases were not found at autopsy. Tests for suspected viruses were not available in 1969 when this case occurred. *B*, Anteroposterior view, forelimbs, same cat. Soft tissue densities of fibrosarcoma extend over the medial distal right forearm and also from the left carpus to above the elbow. Exostosis of the right medial radial tuberosity and lysis of the left radial epiphysis and carpal bones are striking lesions caused by the tumor. *C*, Lateral view of left forelimb, same cat. Extensive lysis of the carpus and distal radius and diffuse soft tissue densities of the arm and forearm are unusual features of fibrosarcoma that are best explained by viral inoculation through cat bites.

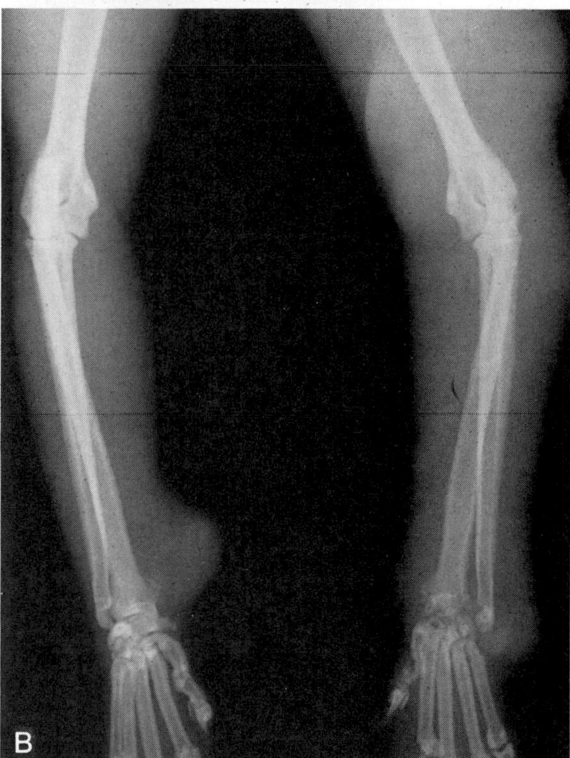


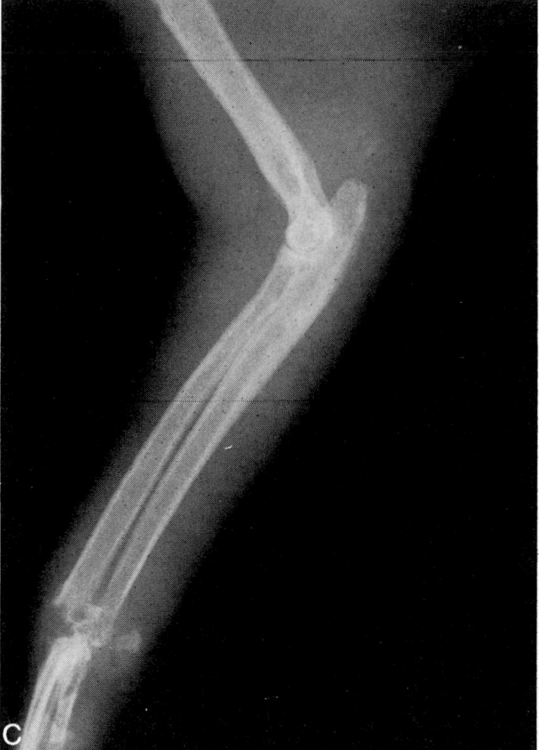

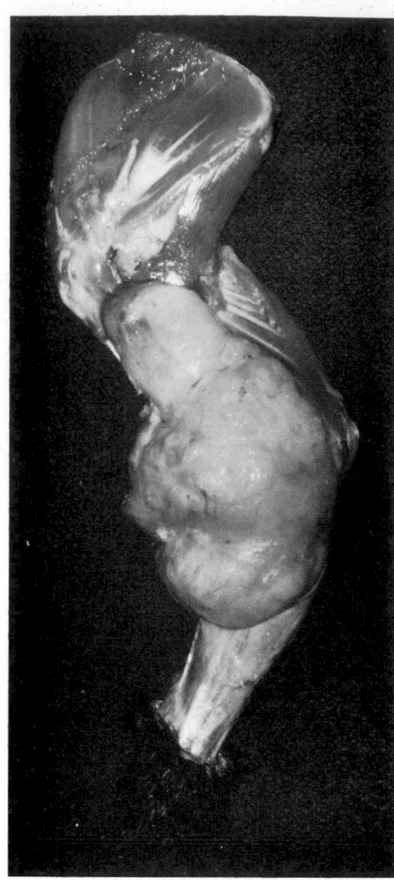

**Figure 11–11** Fibrosarcoma with a myxomatous component on the medial aspect of the right arm and forearm, 15-year-old castrated male black cat. The spongy tumor had gelatinous and cystic areas rich in mucicarmine-positive intercellular matrix and both fusiform and stellate fibroblasts. Lymphoma involving heart, lungs, and kidneys was also present at autopsy in 1955, a finding that would today suggest that the cat was infected with both FeLV and FeSV.

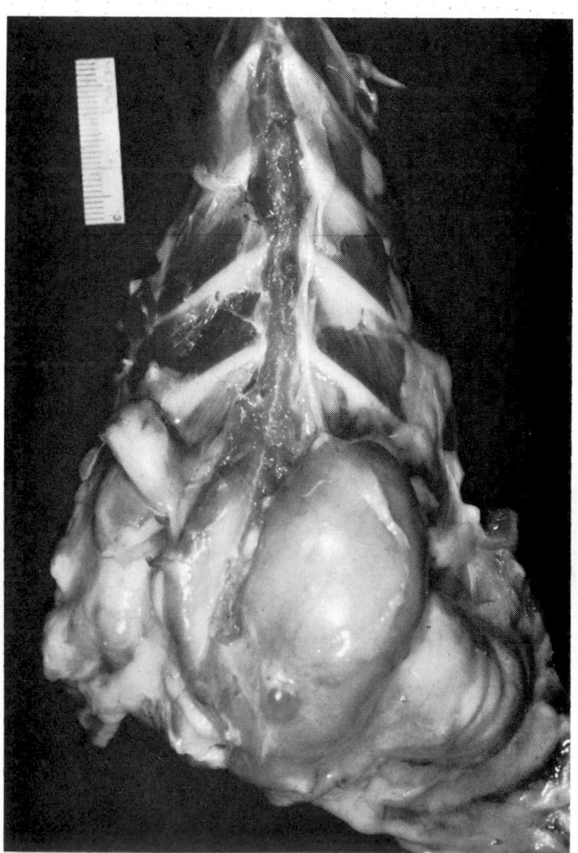

**Figure 11–12** Fibrosarcoma of the thoracic subcutis, which extended into a pleural cavity and invaded the diaphragm, two-year-old cat. A similar tumor occurred in the soft tissue around the left tarsus.

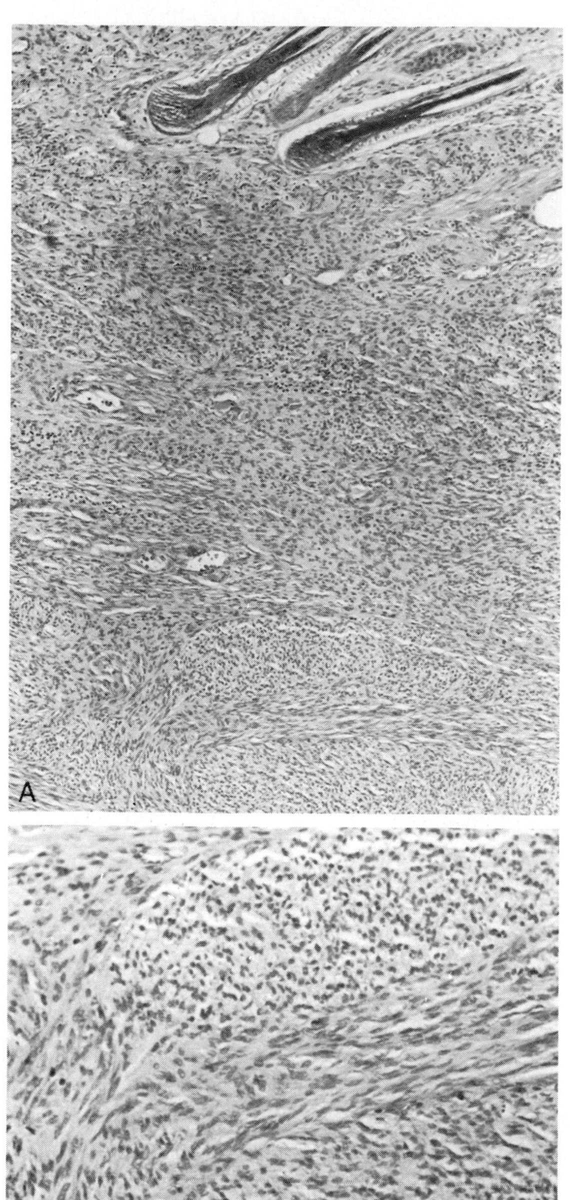


**Figure 11–13** *A,* Fibrosarcoma with interweaving bundles composed of spindle cells in the reticular dermis and subcutis of the shoulder, nine-year-old cat. H & E, × 50. *B,* Fibrosarcoma, detail from lower edge of *A.* H & E, × 175.

with cytoplasmic borders in spindle form or strap shape resembled muscle cells without striations. The tumors lacked capsules, and infiltration of dermis and muscle was common. Vascular invasion was rare but more frequent than lymphatic spread.

**Prognosis.** In a report on 44 cats with fibrosarcomas it was found that mitotic index and tumor site were of prognostic significance but that duration of growth, tumor mass, and microscopic appearance were not (Bostock and Dye, 1979). A mitotic index of six or more in 10 HPF was significant in the rapidity of recurrence but not the rate. Masses on the pinna did not recur after excision; 71 per cent of tumors in the flank recurred, but none caused death in cats followed for three years or until their death from other causes. Twenty-four of 35 cats with growths of head, back, or limbs were destroyed because of local recurrence, usually within nine months of surgery. Median survival time for cats with tumors with a mitotic index of six or more located on the head, neck, or limbs was 16 weeks after excision. Five of the 44 cats developed pulmonary metastases, and all these cats had had local recurrence.

Postoperative data on the 77 cats at AMAH were inadequate for statistical analysis, but certain observations can be made. Cats with local recurrence were returned for evaluation of a new growth between three weeks and three years. Six cats had locally recurrent tumors a year or more after surgery. Only 3 of the 68 cats were autopsied; two had metastatic tumor. A three-year-old with a midtibial tumor had metastases to popliteal and iliac nodes and lungs. A well-differentiated fibrosarcoma above the right eye of a two-year-old cat metastasized as a myxofibrosarcoma to the eye, subcutis of thorax, footpad, kidney, heart, and lung; pulmonary arterial and venous neoplastic thrombi were seen.

Cats with local tumor recurrence have a poorer prognosis owing to increased likelihood of metastases. Metastases occur more often by way of veins than by lymphatic vessels. Wide excision or amputation carries a better prognosis because fibrosarcomas are infiltrative and grow along fascial planes.

Surgery with a wide surgical margin results in a better prognosis than does cryosurgery or chemotherapy. It is reported that fibrosarcomas are composed of cells with thick membranes, making them resistant to cryosurgery (Goldstein and Hess, 1976).

## Tumors of the Melanogenic System

Melanomas constitute about 2 per cent of feline skin tumors, according to Scott (1980), who gives an extensive list of references. At AMAH cutaneous malignant melanoma occurred in ten cats and benign nevi in five. The majority of growths occurred on the head. They are discussed in detail in the section on all tumors of the melanogenic system.

## Hemangiopericytoma

Hemangiopericytoma, a common tumor of dogs, is considered to be a form of fibrosarcoma (Weiss, 1974). Its distinctive feature, present in some areas, is the onionskin arrangement of tumor cells around small vessels. Such tumors are rare in cats. An hemangiopericytoma was described from the subcutis below one eye in a 15-year-old male white cat (Dommert, 1961). The epidermis was degenerated in one area, exposing friable, light-colored tissue. The microscopic pattern was that of hemangiopericytoma with elongated cells forming whorls about the small vascular spaces. Other hemangiopericytomas in cats have been recorded (Brodey, 1970; Poppensiek, 1961) but without details.

Whether hemangiopericytoma identical with that of man occurs in other species is doubtful (Moulton, 1978). This author (JLC) agrees with Moulton that the lesion called hemangiopericytoma in dogs is not identical with hemangiopericytoma of humans, in which the cells, arranged in whorls around an excessive number of small blood vessels, have their own basement membranes as demonstrated by reticulin stains. Two tumors, one from a dog and one from a cat, classified as hemangiopericytomas by veterinary pathologists at AMAH, were examined by a medical pathologist (Hajdu, 1981), who identified the lesions as dermatofibrosarcoma protuberans (benign fibrous histiocytoma). Moulton (1978) also suggested the term canine dermatofibrosarcoma as a more appropriate designation for the hemangiopericytoma of dogs.

It is believed that the oval and spindle fibrous cells of dermatofibrosarcoma protuberans are not fibroblasts derived from fibrocytes but facultative fibroblasts derived from histiocytes; hence the synonymous term of fibrous histiocytoma (Stout and Lattes, 1966). This identification of the fibroblast-like cells as histiocytes is based on the observation that histiocytes rather than fibroblasts or Schwann cells grow out in tissue culture of such tumors.

The single feline hemangiopericytoma on file at AMAH, a tumor with fibroblast-like cells in whorls around small blood vessels and with other areas characterized by a storiform and palisading pattern (Fig. 11–14), was more likely a neurofibroma or dermatofibrosarcoma protuberans. The precise classification of such tumors remains obscure.

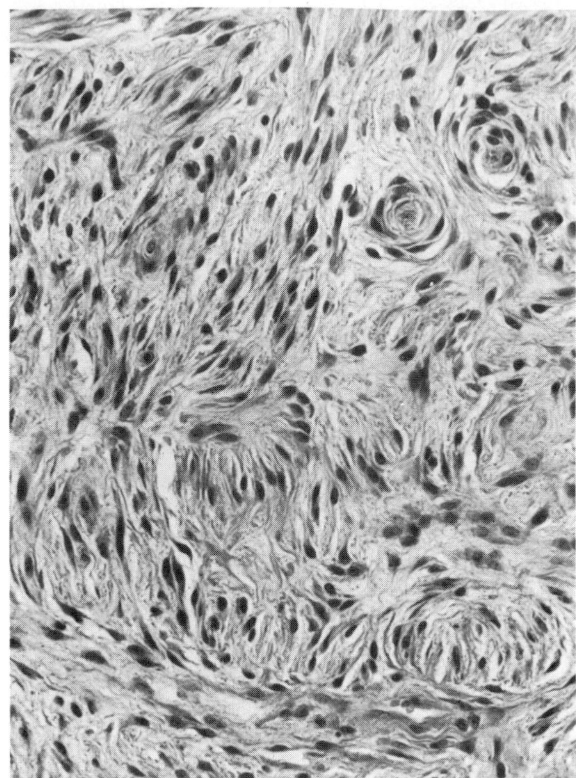

**Figure 11–14** Tumor of uncertain origin that was diagnosed as an hemangiopericytoma, subcutis, stifle of an adult male cat. Whorls of fusiform cells about capillaries (upper left), nuclear palisading (center), tissue clefts (scattered), and short, narrow, and interlacing fascicles also suggest the diagnoses of neurofibroma and dermatofibrosarcoma protuberans. H & E, × 300.

## Other Sarcomas

It is likely that many of the spindle cell sarcomas reported in the literature were fibrosarcomas (Weiss, 1974). Myxosarcomas, occasionally reported from cats, can be considered fibrosarcomas with abundant myxomatous ground substance.

Lymphomas, the most frequent of all neoplasms of cats (e.g., Priester and McKay, 1980), sometimes involve the skin and underlying soft tissue. Cutaneous lymphomas are almost always part of a generalized or multicentric neoplastic process. These cutaneous tumors are discussed in the section on neoplasms of hematopoietic tissue.

Epithelioid sarcoma, a distinctive tumor of the subcutis in humans, was described in two middle-aged spayed female domestic shorthairs (Scott, 1984). Beginning as solitary, poorly circumscribed, firm nodules in the subcutis of the shoulder region, the tumors ulcerated as they enlarged. In one cat the tumor metastasized to regional nodes and lung. A nodular arrangement of plump spindle cells and large round or polygonal epithelioid cells is characteristic, with areas of necrosis most prominent in the center of the nodules. The cell types merged imperceptibly, with frequent mitotic figures. Occasional binucleate cells and rare multinucleate giant cells were seen.

Some sarcomas defy classification and must be described simply as undifferentiated.

## Tumors of Fat Tissue

Tumors of adipose tissue are uncommon in the cat, as is apparent from numerous surveys and from records at AMAH. Twenty-three cases of lipoma, one of symmetric lipomatosis and two of liposarcoma, were recognized at AMAH. Myelolipomas are discussed with tumors of the liver and spleen.

**LIPOMA.** Among the 23 cats in which lipomas were diagnosed, obesity did not appear to be a predisposing factor, as it is in the human and the dog. Neutering, however, may be a factor, since among the cats for which sex was specified, 10 of 11 males were castrated and all 11 females were spayed. Except for two Siamese and one Persian, all were domestic shorthairs. The age range was 2 to 16 years (average 9.6); all but six were between 6 and 12.

Lipomas can occur in adipose tissue anywhere, but of those at AMAH all were found in the subcutis, except for a 2.3 cm lipoma of the omentum palpated as an incidental finding during routine examination of a nine-year-old spayed female domestic cat. Five cats had two lipomas, one had three, and an 11-year-old castrated male had many masses, of which only two were removed. None was reported from the head or distal to the elbow or stifle; there appeared to be a slight predilection for location over the thorax (five). Most lipomas grow slowly and continuously and are asymptomatic. The largest, 13.5 cm in greatest dimension, interfered with mobility owing to its weight and axillary location.

Lipomas arise from the subcutis or the reticular dermis, from which they extend into the subcutis. The overlying skin may be elevated but remains intact. Only one lipoma was pedunculated, a nipple-shaped, 2.0 × 0.7 cm mass adjacent to the vulva. The subcutaneous lipoma is soft to firm, usually discoid, well circumscribed, and unattached to the skin. The lipomas varied from 0.7 to 13.5 cm (average 2.7 cm) in greatest dimension. The cut surface, white or pale yellow and usually lobulated, has the appearance of fat with a delicate capsule.

Microscopically, a thin collagenous capsule often establishes differentiation from normal fat. Lipomas arising in the subcutis have a complete capsule, whereas those arising in the reticular dermis have a distinct capsule only on their deeper surface. Rarely a lipoma has a prominent component of mature collagen bundles; such a growth is termed a fibrolipoma (Fig. 11–15). In nearly all lipomas the lipocytes are variably larger than in adjacent normal adipose tissue. A lobular pattern may not be present in small growths. Lipocytes may be multilocular, but most are mature with a single large globule displacing and compressing the nucleus to one side.

It is of interest that three cats with lipomas had subclinical steatitis ("yellow fat" disease) that also involved the lipoma; therefore a microscopic examination of what appears to be a simple lipoma may result in more than one diagnosis.

Although benign, a suspected lipoma should be excised to confirm the diagnosis and to prevent further growth leading to possible ischemic necrosis and inflammation. Surgical removal is relatively easy with blunt dissection, unless there are fat necrosis and inflammation, as in some larger lipomas. One should remember that if a lipoma is found, there is approximately a 30 per cent chance that one or more may be present elsewhere.

**LIPOMATOSIS.** One case of lipomatosis, an entity recognized in man and dogs, has been recorded at AMAH. A four-year-old spayed black-and-white cat weighing 7 kg had symmetric lipomatosis of the thighs and chronic perineal dermatitis owing to inability to void urine normally. There had been a past episode of perineal myiasis. The growths first became noticeable when the cat was six months old and within three and a half years enlarged to masses 12 × 8 × 6 cm sagging from the caudal aspect of each thigh where the fur was constantly soaked with urine. Partial excision of the subcutaneous masses revealed nonencapsulated benign fat that infiltrated the dermis between muscles and also the muscles themselves. The fatty tissue, like fat elsewhere, was orange-brown owing to pansteatitis. Episioplasty necessitated by the lipomatosis was performed, and treatment for cystitis was administered with success.

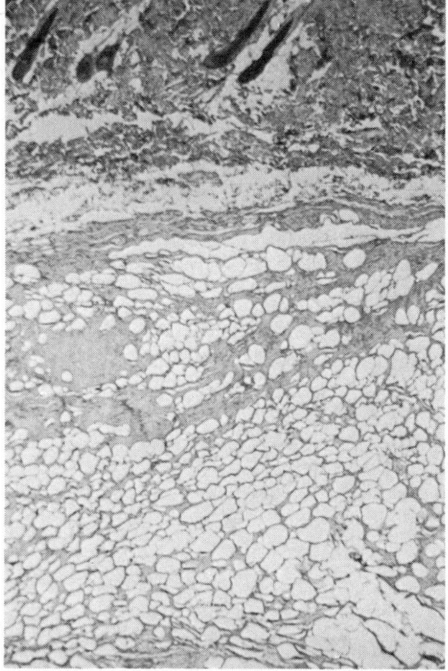

**Figure 11–15** Fibrolipoma in the subcutis of the back, seven-year-old spayed female black Persian. Abundant collagen within a benign proliferation of adipose tissue lies below the hair follicles of the dermis (left). H & E, × 30.

**LIPOSARCOMA.** Liposarcoma is exceedingly rare in cats (e.g., Priester and McKay, 1980; Scott, 1980). It has been produced experimentally by injection of the feline leukemia virus (Rickard et al., 1969) and has also occurred spontaneously in a young cat infected with feline leukemia virus (Stephens et al., 1983). Material from the latter cat failed to transmit liposarcoma when inoculated into newborn kittens, but most of the kittens did develop lymphoma (Stephens et al., 1984). Although no firm evidence was found for a causative role of either feline leukemia or sarcoma virus, the association with feline leukemia virus in both an experimental and a natural case seems more than coincidental, and an etiologic role for this virus must still be considered (Stephens et al., 1984).

Two liposarcomas were diagnosed at AMAH. One, 2 cm in diameter, was removed from the left popliteal area of a 10-year-old castrated male domestic shorthair. The collagenous capsule was wide and dense in some areas and sent trabeculae composed of fibroblasts and collagen fibers into the mass, dividing it into lobules. Many of the lipocytes were multilocular, some with bizarre nuclei and prominent nucleoli; the majority, however, appeared mature.

Another liposarcoma extended from the subcutis of the perineum into the pelvic canal of a female cat and interfered with urination. The tumor was not encapsulated, and complete excision was impossible. The biopsy specimen contained immature lipocytes, some with variably sized fat globules. Maturation from lipoblasts to mature fat cells was observed as well as numerous mitotic figures. The owner had the cat destroyed but did not permit an autopsy. Vascular invasion of venules and lymphatic vessels, which would portend metastasis, was not evident in either case.

## Tumor of Smooth Muscle

Tumors of smooth muscle are exceedingly rare in the skin (Ball, 1913; Bostock, 1977; Brodey, 1970). The one leiomyosarcoma on record at AMAH involved the skin of the lumbar region (see discussion of tumors of muscle).

## Tumors of Blood and Lymph Vessels

Tumors of blood and lymph vessels are infrequent in the cat. AT AMAH, 7 hemangiomas and 25 hemangiosarcomas of the skin were on record, as well as 9 cases of lymphangioma or lymphangiosarcoma. Reports in the literature and the cases at AMAH are discussed in the section on tumors of the cardiovascular system.

## Neurofibroma and Neurofibrosarcoma

Neurofibromas are tumors of peripheral nerves. Synonyms are schwannoma, neuroma, neurinoma, neurilemmoma, and perineural fibroblastoma. The cell of origin of this tumor category in man has been shown to be the Schwann cell (Cravioto, 1969; Waggener, 1966). However, the epineurial, perineurial, or endoneurial fibroblast cannot be excluded as a possible source of tumor arising in a peripheral or cranial neve.

For a clinician, it is important to be aware that the diagnosis of a given tumor in this group may be difficult and that pathologists may differ as to the precise classification and prognosis for some of these tumors as well as other soft tissue tumors composed of spindle cells. Whether a tumor is classified as a neurofibroma or a neurofibrosarcoma often makes little difference from a clinical viewpoint: Both are likely to recur locally, for complete removal is difficult owing to poor demarcation and lack of encapsulation. Even when appearing microscopically to be malignant, neural tumors rarely metastasize.

Neurofibromas, while common in cattle and dogs, are rare in cats (Scott, 1980). Neurofibrosarcomas are also infrequent. In a study of 23 soft-tissue sarcomas of seven cats, five males and two females ranging in age from 5 to 11 years (mean 7.5) were reported to have neurofibrosarcomas located in the perineum (two) and thoracic wall (one), and on the carpus (two), hock (one), and a rear digit (one) (Brown et al., 1978). A major survey of tumors of domestic animals (Priester and McKay, 1980) recorded three benign neuromas—two in males, one in a female—in a forelimb, in a peripheral nerve, and in an unspecified site. Two malignant neuromas, both in males, involved a forelimb and a hindlimb.

At AMAH, 28 tumors originally interpreted as arising from peripheral nerve tissue were carefully reviewed; of these, 18 could with confidence be classified as neurofibromas.* No breed predilection was apparent among affected cats. Ten were males (seven castrated), eight were females (two spayed), aged 5 to 13 years. The tumors measured 4.6 ± 2.5 cm in diameter and were similar in color, consistency, and depth to the prototypes to be discussed. The 18 neurofibromas arose from the dermis or subcutis of thoracic limb (eight) (Fig. 11–16*A*), head or neck (six), thorax (two), pelvic limb (one), and multiple sites on pelvic limbs (one). Four neurofibromas recurred at the same site within three years of excision. They did not differ in microscopic features from the nonrecurrent tumors, nor did the recurrent tumors differ histologically from their predecessors. None of the tumors metastasized.

*Diagnosis and discussion by Damon R. Averill, Jr.

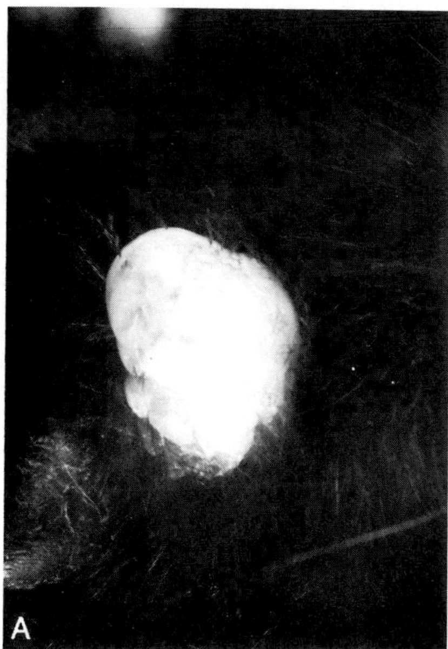


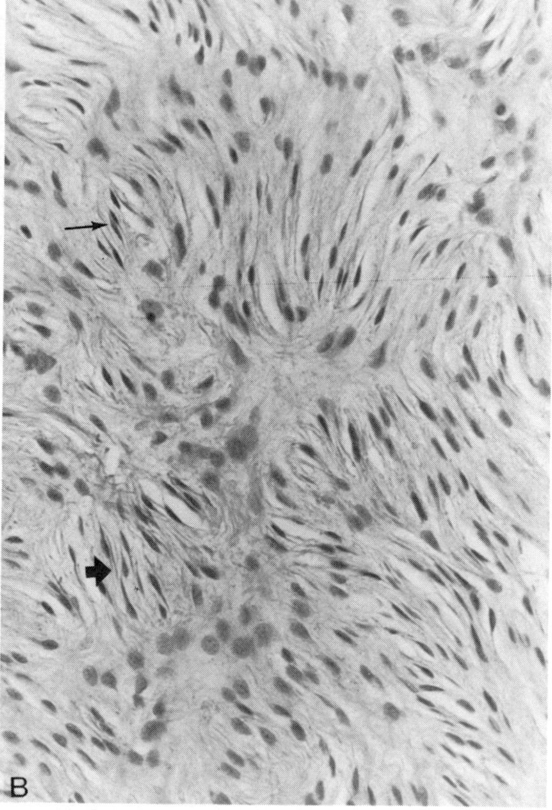


**Figure 11–16** *A*, Cutaneous neurofibroma above the pigmented accessory carpal pad (lower left corner), five-year-old Siamese. The white, nodular, sessile mass was soft and covered by nearly hairless skin. × 2.5. *B*, Neurofibroma of dermis and subcutis, carpal region, five-year-old Siamese. Conspicuous microscopic features are fusiform cells in a storiform arrangement (center), often with nuclear palisading (small arrow), and short narrow fascicles of parallel fusiform cells (large arrow), sometimes accompanied by lenticular clefts. H & E, × 300.

Criteria for the classification of neurofibroma used in this discussion are based on the features of the 3 of the 18 tumors that were observed microscopically to arise from a peripheral nerve. These three prototype tumors were 2 to 4 cm in diameter, soft or fluctuant, white or pinkish gray, dermal or subepidermal masses of weeks' or months' duration. The three tumors had a variety of microscopic features: (1) Two had Antoni type A architecture, one had Antoni types A and B (terms referring to the arrangement and concentration of cells), and one had neither; (2) two had storiform architecture (Fig. 11–16), one plexiform architecture (patterns described by Harkin and Reed, 1969); (3) the tumors were solid, of low or medium cellular density, composed of elongated cells with oval or elongated nuclei, no axons, and rare or no mitotic figures; (4) stroma mucin was present in one; (5) necrotic areas were present in one; (6) one tumor was multinodular, one had perivascular whorls, one was encapsulated, and one had hyalinized blood vessels.

The 15 other tumors were classified as neurofibromas if any of the characteristic patterns described in (1) or (2) above was present. Eleven had Antoni type A pattern, and seven Antoni Type B pattern. A storiform pattern was seen in 12 (Fig. 11–16*B*) and a plexiform pattern in four. The majority were multinodular and none was encapsulated. Mitotic figures were absent or rare except in three tumors that had a very high index of 20 or more mitoses per 10 HPF. About two thirds of the tumors had perivascular whorls, and a third stromal mucin.

The ten neoplasms excluded were reclassified as undifferentiated sarcoma (seven), fibroma (two), and melanoma (one). The sarcomas and fibromas may have originated from epineurium but exhibited no continuity with neural structures in any section examined and did not meet other criteria. One multicentric tumor previously reported as neurofibromatosis (Fankhauser and Luginbühl, 1968) was reviewed and reclassified as aggressive fibromatosis (discussed further on).

In contrast with neurofibromas, neurofibrosarcomas are distinguished by greater cellularity, pleomorphism, and anaplasia; the mitotic index is higher, and the cells are less regularly arranged. Prompt excision or amputation offers the best hope for a cure; trials of adjunctive treatment with levamisole were too limited to be evaluated (Brown et al., 1978).

## Aggressive Fibromatosis

Aggressive fibromatosis (musculoaponeurotic fibromatosis, desmoid tumor) is a lesion of humans with microscopic features common to exuberant proliferation of benign fibrous connective tissue and low-grade fibrosarcoma. Although infiltrative, it is not a malignancy that can metastasize by embolism (Robbins et al., 1984; Stout and Lattes, 1967). The mass lesions of aggressive fibromatosis are unencapsulated, gray-white, and rubbery. They arise in aponeuroses, fascia, and supportive connective tissues of skeletal muscles and infiltrate among muscles, muscle bundles, and muscle cells. Women are most often affected, incidence peaking in the third decade. Etiology is unknown; genetic factors, trauma, and estrogen stimulation are suggested.

A feline case of aggressive fibromatosis seen at AMAH in 1958 was originally reported as neurofibromatosis (Fankhauser and Luginbühl, 1968) but was later restudied. The cat, a 10-year-old spayed female domestic shorthair, had several firm subcutaneous swellings over and between the scapulae. Thick yellow fluid aspirated from the masses was sterile on aerobic cultures. Over a two-month period the masses slowly enlarged and others developed. When the cat lost weight and appetite, euthanasia was requested.

At autopsy, symmetric linear masses of the dermis and subcutis were found along each side of the spine from C3 to L1. Firm, white, and nodular, with maximum thickness of 3.5 cm over the shoulders, the masses displaced the scapulae laterally and infiltrated the cervical and intercostal muscles. A third mass, 5.3 cm thick, extended in the subcutis and muscles from the right scapula to the right elbow (Fig. 11–17), and another, measuring 6.0 × 3.5 × 1.5 cm, infiltrated the subcutis lateral to the right knee. The most extensive lesion involved the intercostal muscles near the sternum, adhered to the pleura of the left cranial lung lobe, surrounded the sternal node, infiltrated the cranial mediastinum, and encased the thymus. A growth

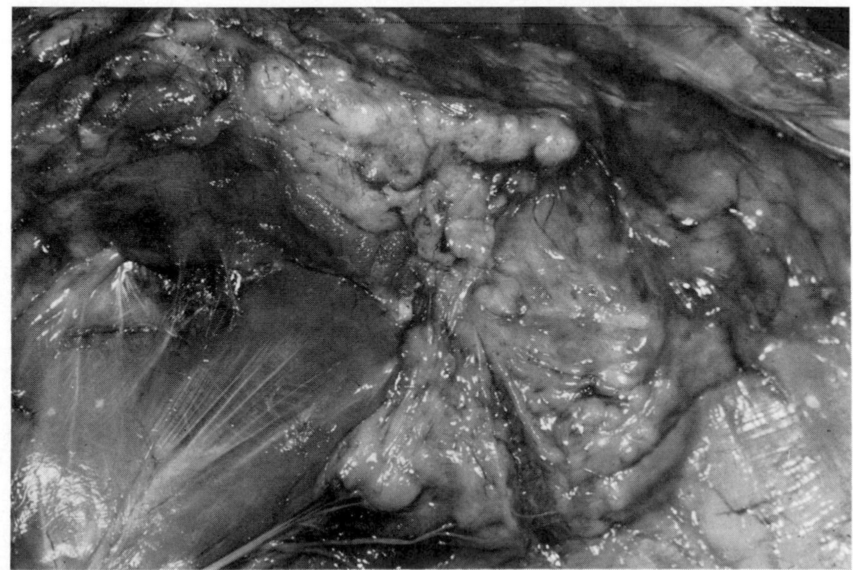

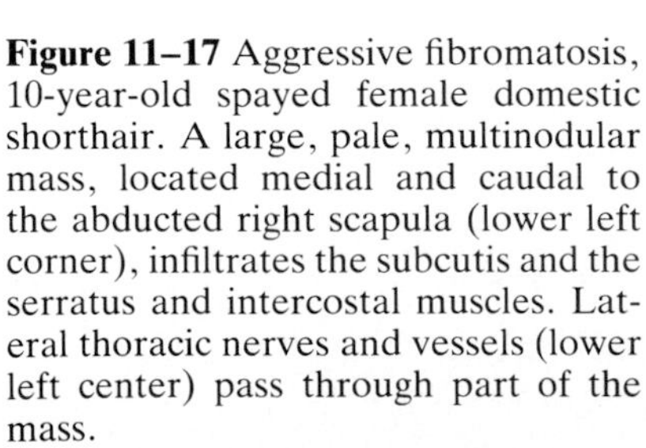

**Figure 11–17** Aggressive fibromatosis, 10-year-old spayed female domestic shorthair. A large, pale, multinodular mass, located medial and caudal to the abducted right scapula (lower left corner), infiltrates the subcutis and the serratus and intercostal muscles. Lateral thoracic nerves and vessels (lower left center) pass through part of the mass.

of similar appearance on the right caudal lung lobe measured 2.8 × 1.3 × 0.8 cm.

Microscopically, the lesions involved dermis, subcutis, fascia, epimysium, perimysium, endomysium, mediastinum, and visceral pleura. One surrounded but did not infiltrate the sternal node and thymus. The masses were unencapsulated and varied from well-differentiated fibrous connective tissue to foci with fibrosarcomatous features. Centers of the larger masses were necrotic. Although nerves passed through the masses, no origin from nerves or neural lesion could be found. Replacement or atrophy of muscle cells was not preceded by neurogenic atrophy. Masses often appeared lobulated owing to total replacement of muscle bundles by the fibrous proliferation (Fig. 11–18).

The paravertebral growths blended into the full thickness of the dermis, replaced the subcutaneous fat, and in some areas had distinct deep margins without muscle infiltration (Fig. 11–19*A*). Much of the linear masses had fibroblasts and collagen fibrils arranged parallel to the overlying skin (Fig. 11–19*B*), but significant portions had long, wide interweaving bundles resembling well-differentiated fibrosarcoma with a low mitotic index (Fig. 11–19*C*).

The pleural lesions excited curiosity, for they did not represent metastases. The right cranial lung lobe adhered to the sternal mass at a site of chronic lipid aspiration

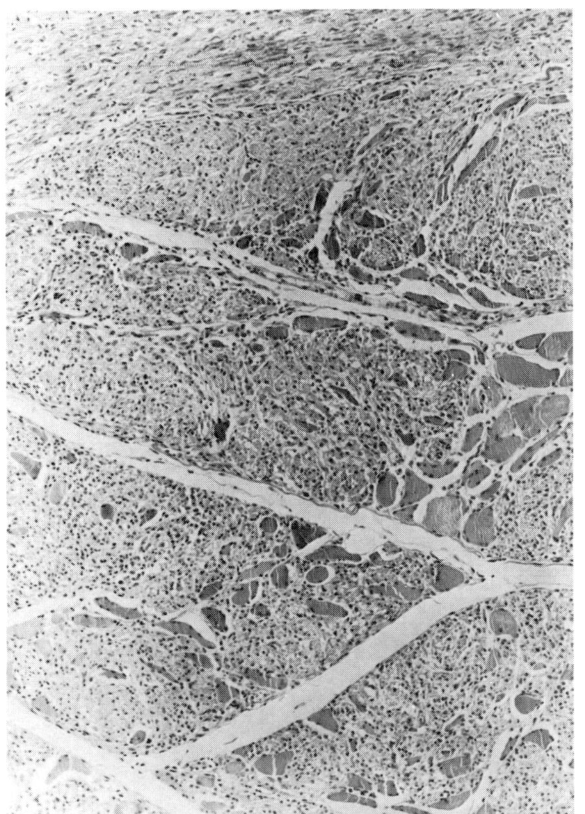

**Figure 11–18** Aggressive fibromatosis, same cat as in Figure 11–17. Fibroblasts and collagen replace most of the myocytes within the still visible individual muscle bundles. A hypercellular and widened perimysium is seen at the top. H & E, × 75.

pneumonia, but the pleural lesion of the right caudal lobe was an independent growth mostly composed of collagen and fibroblasts arranged in parallel beneath the pleural elastic lamina, while the exuberant tissue external to the lamina was in a more random pattern (Fig. 11–20).

As seen in this case, aggressive fibromatosis differs strikingly from a somewhat similar lesion of fibrodysplasia ossificans. Although both conditions may have fascial, epimysial, and pleural involvement, only aggressive fibromatosis shows muscle bundle infiltration and replacement. Even more conspicuous is the absence of foci of cartilaginous and osseous metaplasia. Finally, aggressive fibromatosis can simulate fibrosarcoma or neurofibrosarcoma, in contrast to the obviously benign fibrodysplasia ossificans.

## Mast Cell Tumors

Although splenic mast cell neoplasms of cats were reported by French pathologists in the nineteenth century, cutaneous tumors in this species were apparently rarely encountered before the 1950s. In some geographic areas (e.g., Illinois) they are now second or approximately equal in frequency to basal cell tumors (Macy and Reynolds, 1981). At AMAH they numbered 89, or 22 per cent of all the skin tumors, and were second in frequency after basal cell tumors.

They may be solitary, multiple, or part of a systemic mastocytosis involving spleen, liver, and bone marrow. Some take the form of nodules, which may be ulcerated. Others resemble the multiple flattened lesions of chronic dermatitis or eosinophilic granuloma. Mast cell tumors of skin are described in detail in the section on mast cell neoplasms.

## Histiocytoma

This benign tumor, common in young dogs, is said by some not to occur in cats; rare instances have been recorded, however (Austin, 1975; Priester and McKay, 1980; Scott, 1980). A tumor of the lower eyelid in an 8-year-old cat was reported on histologic examination to resemble a histiocytoma (Lawrence, 1965), and small, solitary tumors with microscopic features resembling those of histiocytoma were reported in four young adult cats by Macy and Reynolds (1981). No histiocytoma was recorded in a cat at AMAH.

## Malignant Fibrous Histiocytoma

A rare and poorly understood feline tumor is the malignant fibrous histiocytoma, also known as extraskeletal giant cell tumor or giant cell tumor of soft tissue. An extraskeletal giant cell tumor of the left foreleg of an eight-year-old male cat appeared to have its origin in tendon sheaths (Nielsen, 1952) and is included with synovial tumors elsewhere in this chapter.

From the following reported cases, common features of malignant fibrous histiocytoma appear to be subcutaneous origin, invasiveness, and recurrence, but failure to metastasize.

An extraskeletal giant cell tumor involving the right arm, shoulder, and axilla extended across the back and sternum of a 10-year-old spayed female domestic shorthair (Alexander et al., 1975). At the time of its partial removal

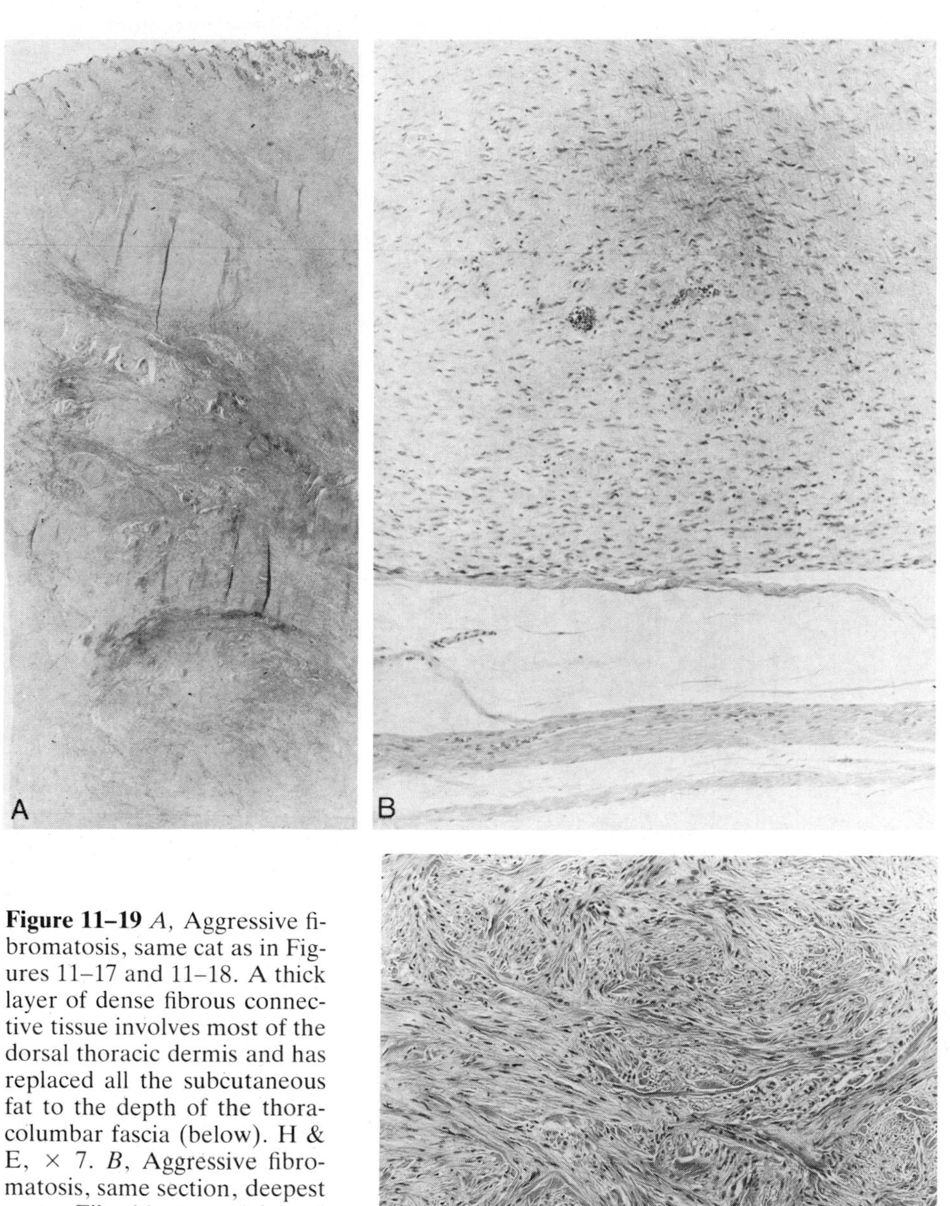

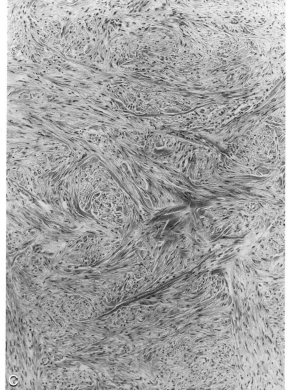

**Figure 11–19** *A*, Aggressive fibromatosis, same cat as in Figures 11–17 and 11–18. A thick layer of dense fibrous connective tissue involves most of the dorsal thoracic dermis and has replaced all the subcutaneous fat to the depth of the thoracolumbar fascia (below). H & E, × 7. *B*, Aggressive fibromatosis, same section, deepest part. Fibroblast nuclei and abundant intercellular collagen are parallel, as in benign dense regular collagenous connective tissue. The thoracolumbar fascia is below the tissue separation artifact. H & E, × 75. *C*, Aggressive fibromatosis, same section, central part. Distinct interdigitating bundles, resembling those of a fibroma or well-differentiated fibrosarcoma, are formed by fibroblasts having small hyperchromatic fusiform nuclei and prominent collagen bundles. H & E, × 75.

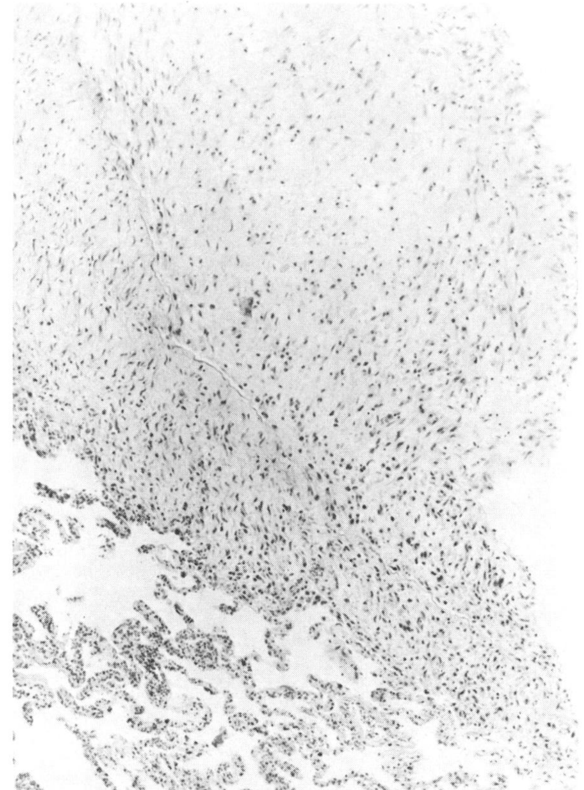

**Figure 11–20** Aggressive fibromatosis of visceral pleura, same cat as in Figures 11–17 to 11–19. The fibrous connective tissue below the pleural elastic lamina (diagonal line) is denser and more regularly arranged than that on the outer pleural surface. The pattern suggests benign primary pleural fibroplasia rather than a metastatic fibrosarcoma. H & E, × 75.

six months previously, it had been the size of a golf ball and was situated along the vertebral border of the right scapula. Muscle invasion had prevented total excision, and the extent of the recurrent tumor prohibited further surgery. Bony involvement and metastases were not seen radiographically. The cat was lost to follow-up.

A 12 × 4 × 3 cm giant cell tumor of soft tissue was incompletely removed from the femoral canal of a seven-year-old female cat (Ford et al., 1975). It deeply infiltrated fascial planes but did not involve tendons or bones. As is the case with other reported cats with malignant fibrous histiocytoma, no metastases were found at autopsy.

A giant cell variant of malignant fibrous histiocytoma was seen in three cats, 4, 9, and 12 years old (Gleiser et al., 1979). Two were males, one castrated; the other an entire female. The three tumors were located in the subcutis, but all three involved bone (radius, humerus, and tuber calcis) to a lesser degree. The tumors, in general, were firm, dense, fibrous, and unencapsulated. There was local recurrence in both cats that survived surgery.

Another malignant fibrous histiocytoma caused left rear leg lameness and atrophy in a two-year-old spayed female domestic shorthair (Seiler and Wilkinson, 1980). The rapidly growing 10 × 7 cm subcutaneous mass caused extensive lysis of the left ilium and compressed and displaced the sciatic nerve. It was not decided whether the tumor arose in the ilium or adjacent soft tissue. No metastases were found.

In a nine-year-old castrated male domestic shorthair a movable 2 cm subcutaneous mass developed between the blades of the scapulae (Confer et al., 1981). The tumor was removed surgically but recurred six times over the next 15 months. Local tumor invasion of muscle was seen in the latter surgical specimens, but no metastases were found. No viral particles were seen ultrastructurally, and blood smears were negative for FeLV by indirect immunofluorescence.

A fibrous histiocytoma involving the mandible of an 11-year-old castrated male domestic shorthair was removed by hemimandibulectomy and the cat was tumor-free 11 months later (Bradley et al., 1984).

Histologically, the tumors are described as being characterized by fibroblast-like cells, a degree of fibrogenesis, histiocyte-like cells, bizarre tumor giant cells, multinucleate giant cells, inflammatory cells (mostly lymphocytes), foam cells, anaplasia of stromal cells and mitotic figures, and a storiform pattern (Seiler and Wilkinson, 1980). In a storiform pattern, fibroblast-like or Schwann cells are arranged in short narrow fascicles that radiate from a central point having few nuclei.

This author (JLC) has reviewed some published and unpublished tumors classified as malignant fibrous histiocytomas at other institutions and has found that an extremely wide range of tumor features are included in this category. Tumors that might be classified as fibrosarcoma, osteosarcoma, and neurofibroma/sarcoma have been included in this group. Today, the classification of malignant fibrous histiocytoma of cats is a very nebulous and ill-defined entity. That group of tumors probably also includes a variety of anaplastic tumors having many multinucleate giant cells that have evoked a variable inflammatory response.

### Miscellaneous Tumors

An oddity reported by Head (1953) was a solitary subcutaneous ulcerated tumor of eosinophils on a digit.

Multiple plasmacytomas of the skin were observed in a cat at AMAH. The case is described in the section on hematopoietic neoplasms.

## TUMORS OF THE HEMATOPOIETIC SYSTEM

Hematopoietic malignancies far outnumber all others in the cat. They include lymphocytic tumors and leukemias, myeloproliferative malignancies, thymomas, and plasma cell tumors. Lymphocytic leukemia and the myeloproliferative disorders are discussed in the chapter on the hematopoietic system, and the nature and behavior of the feline leukemia virus in the chapter on viral infections.

### Lymphoma

Lymphocytic neoplasms of cats have long attracted the interest of students of animal tumors and have been described and reported with increasing frequency over more than a century, at first in Europe and then in

America and elsewhere (Holzworth, 1960). Possibly the earliest reported in the United States was that described by Bloom (1937) in a cat with orbital infiltration by atypical lymphocytes and immature lymphocytes in the blood.

Since the 1950s hematopoietic malignancies of many varieties have been recognized with increasing frequency in cats, and a vast number of studies and case reports have been published. In 1964 Jarrett and his colleagues at the University of Glasgow isolated from a cat with lymphoma a virus (FeLV) that is now believed to be responsible for most of the hematopoietic neoplasia of cats.

Lymphoma was reported to constitute about a third of all feline tumors in two California counties (Dorn et al., 1968a). In a Philadelphia survey 20 per cent of 375 feline tumors were lymphomas (Engle and Brodey, 1969). Data collected from 15 veterinary colleges in the United States and Canada indicate that of a total of 2207 neoplasms, 843 were lymphoma (795) or lymphocytic leukemia (48) (Priester and McKay, 1980). At AMAH, among a total of 3248 feline solid tumors diagnosed microscopically over a 35-year period there were 1329 lymphomas. In the total cat population it was estimated that as many as 0.05 per cent suffer from lymphoma (Dorn et al., 1968b).

Whether there is a breed predisposition for lymphocytic malignancies is difficult to determine with certainty. The proportion of purebred cats may not be the same in all geographic areas or cities, and the proportion of purebred cats in a hospital population may be greater than in a general population, because valuable cats are more likely to receive veterinary care and also to be exposed to infections endemic in catteries. The date of a survey can also be a factor in its data, since owners increasingly favor purebreds. More Siamese than expected were reported among the lymphoma cases by Dorn et al. (1968b). In a survey of 150 cases of lymphoreticular malignancies in cats in the greater New York City area, 21 per cent were pedigreed (Meincke et al., 1972). A survey of a 150-cat sample of cases of lymphoma at AMAH from 1979 to 1982 indicated that 13 per cent were Siamese, whereas Siamese constitute about 5 per cent in the AMAH hospital population generally.

Unlike all other malignancies of cats, those associated with FeLV affect cats of all ages, from as young as 4 months to as old as 19 years (e.g., Meincke et al., 1972). The peak incidence is in young adults two to three years of age; there is a second rise beginning at seven to eight years (e.g., Meincke et al., 1972; AMAH, unpublished data). Domestic pet cats tend to develop the illness later, on average, than purebreds, most of which are bred and reared, or live, in catteries in which the possibility of exposure to FeLV may be high (Meincke et al., 1972). A cat's FeLV status also affects age at onset. The average age of occurrence is three years in cats that are FeLV-positive but seven years for FeLV-negative cats (Hardy, 1981).

There is conflicting evidence as to whether there is a sex predisposition to lymphocytic malignancies. In a survey of 140 cats with lymphocytic malignancies at AMAH before 1960, males outnumbered females by about two to one, a ratio estimated to be the proportion in ill cats generally at that time (Holzworth, 1960). In a 150-cat sample of cases at AMAH in the period 1979 to 1982, the sex incidence again appeared to be the same as in the hospital population; i.e., there was a slight preponderance of males. In a California survey, however, the relative risk of male cats' developing lymphoma was more than twice that of female cats (Dorn et al., 1968b). Similarly, of the 843 cats with lymphocytic neoplasia in the survey by Priester and McKay (1980), 529 were males and 260 females, in contrast with a male:female ratio estimated to be about 8:7.5 for the reference population.

Involving so many body sites, lymphoma appears in the most varied forms of any feline neoplasm and provides endless surprises for the clinician and pathologist. Although a few tumors are truly solitary, most that appear to be so are actually associated with gross lesions or microscopic infiltration in other sites. Occasionally bone marrow presents a definitively neoplastic picture of which there is no reflection in the circulating blood. Terminally, many cases of lymphoma become leukemic. For this reason blood films should be carefully scanned for the occasional telltale primitive lymphocyte.

A negative result with the IFA or ELISA test for FeLV never definitively excludes the possibility of lymphoma, especially among older cats.

**LYMPHOID ORGANS.** Splenic or generalized lymph node enlargement due to lymphoma is far less frequent in cats than in dogs. Lymphocytic reactive hyperplasia is a more common cause of generalized lymphadenopathy in cats. Lymphoma of one or a few regional nodes is, however, fairly frequent in cats and may easily be mistaken clinically for lymphadenitis or reactive hyperplasia. Nodes with advanced neoplasia are enlarged, firm, and less movable than normal owing to capsular and perinodal infiltration, thereby resembling adenitis with capsulitis and perinodal inflammation; however, pain, heat, and redness are usually absent. On cut surface a lymphomatous node bulges and is of homogeneous appearance because of loss of cortical, medullary, and follicular features.

An imprint from an entire node is more helpful in diagnosis than a fine-needle aspirate because cellular distribution as well as cellular detail can be better evaluated. Imprints of a complete transverse cut surface, which has been cut a second time to remove the bulging tissue before the imprint is made, best assure the accurate assessment of all cellular components. A complete cross section that includes the cortical and medullary regions should also be submitted for histologic study. If a stained imprint of the fresh tissue indicates lymphadenitis rather than hyperplasia or neoplasia, some nodal tissue can be cultured before the specimen is fixed in 10 per cent formalin. Surgical removal of a normal-sized node is not likely to be of diagnostic value and is seldom justified, although an early stage of lymphoma may occasionally be detected.

Enlargement of mesenteric nodes accompanying segmental intestinal lymphoma does not in itself indicate neoplastic involvement. It may be due to hyperplasia with or without lymphadenitis secondary to mucosal erosion and ulceration, both common with intestinal lymphoma. When an intestinal mass is present, both the mass and a mesenteric node should be removed for study. With a tonsillar mass, however, a nodal biopsy is preferable because there is less chance for error in diagnosis of early lesions.

Splenic lymphoma can be diffuse, nodular, or follicular, the last being rare in cats. The diffuse form is characterized by palpable, uniform enlargement, which must be differentiated microscopically from reactive hyperplasia, extramedullary hematopoiesis, and diffuse forms of granulocytic or mast cell neoplasia. The nodular lymphoma must be differentiated from organized hematoma, nodular lymphocytic or myeloid hyperplasia, myelolipoma, granulomas of FIP, and primary and secondary tumors of the spleen, both of which are uncommon.

**MEDIASTINUM.** Lymphoma of the cranial mediastinum most often arises in the thymus but sometimes originates in mediastinal or sternal nodes. It is almost always of T-cell type. It is often a solitary lesion but may be associated with involvement elsewhere. In some geographic areas the mediastinal tumor is the most common lymphoma. While it may appear in cats of any age, it is the form that occurs in the youngest age group of cats (as young as four months). Affected kittens are usually Siamese. The mediastinal mass is usually large when detected, causing dorsal displacement of the trachea, caudal and dorsal displacement of the heart, and crowding of the lungs. The tumor may extend through the thoracic inlet (Fig. 11–21) and compress the esophagus against the left first rib, causing regurgitation even before dyspnea is evident. The mass may surround most of the pericardium and is thickest on the left side, resulting in right lateral displacement of the heart. Presence of a mass is sometimes recognized when the examiner is unable to compress the cranial rib cage. Neoplastic infiltration of thoracic muscles can occur (Fig. 11–22). The tumor is pale yellow or white, often with foci of necrosis and hemorrhage on both natural and cut surfaces. A thoracic effusion, which develops gradually, ultimately compresses the lungs and leads to severe dyspnea. The fluid is usually pale amber and cloudy but may be bloody. Rarely it is milky-looking and mistaken for chyle. The correct interpretation of such an effusion is easy, owing to the numerous lymphocytes of varying maturity, including blast forms (Fig. 11–23), but occasionally necrosis or hemorrhage in the mass or a secondary intrathoracic infection can complicate evaluation of the fluid.

For detailed discussion of differential diagnosis and treatment by chemotherapy refer to the chapter on hematopoietic disorders. Remission has also been achieved with serum containing FOCMA antibody (Hardy, 1981).

**ALIMENTARY SYSTEM.** The organ of the alimentary tract most often involved is the liver, but there is always tumor elsewhere as well. The most common form of involvement is diffuse portal infiltrate, resulting in a sometimes massively enlarged liver with a prominent pale yellow reticular pattern. Less often the tumor takes the form of nodules—dull white, soft to firm, solid, unencapsulated, and bulging only slightly on cut surface. Sharply demarcated pure white foci of necrotic tumor and red foci of hemorrhage may also be present. The liver may range from normal to massive size, and it may be friable, especially when hypoxic centrilobular fatty change has resulted from anemia. Rarely, jaundice is associated with severe hepatic involvement.

Most lymphomas localized solely in the gastrointestinal tract (stomach, intestines, and mesenteric nodes) are B-cell tumors arising from B-lymphocytes in the lamina propria. Cats with these tumors are usually older than cats with other forms of lymphoma, averaging eight years, and 90 per cent or more with tumor of the stomach or intestines are FeLV-negative (Hardy, 1981).

The jejunum and ileum are the most frequent sites of gastrointestinal lymphoma. The usual form of intestinal lymphoma is segmental with extension to the mesentery. The typical lesion is a pale annular thickening of the intestinal wall, with an enlarged lumen. The dilatation of the lumen is due to tumorous replacement of smooth muscle and intrinsic neural tissue, resulting in impaired muscle tone and peristalsis. Ulceration of the mucosa is common, but stenosis is rare. Grossly the lesion may be confused with mast cell tumor or toxoplasmal granuloma. Fibroplasia is not a feature of lymphoma, so the constriction characteristic of adenocarcinoma is absent. Enlarged mesenteric nodes may be neoplastic, but hyperplasia and lymphadenitis secondary to ulceration of the intestine may account for the increase in their size. Multiple segmental involvement of the intestine is common, and there may be gross or microscopic tumor elsewhere. The prognosis

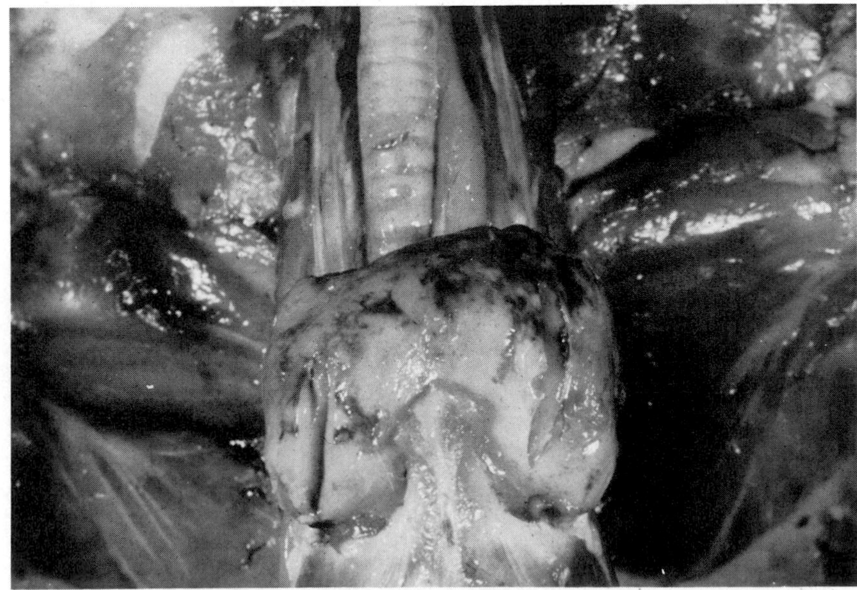

**Figure 11–21** Lymphoma of the cranial mediastinum protruding through the thoracic inlet, eight-month-old Siamese. The manubrium is at bottom center.

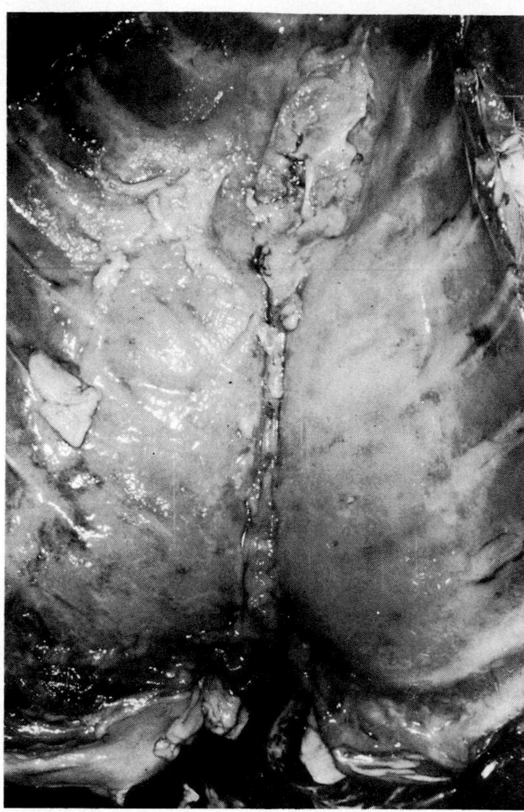

**Figure 11–22** Lymphoma of the parietal pleura, transversus thoracis and intercostal muscles in a one-year-old tricolor with a mediastinal tumor. The neoplastic lymphocytic infiltrate caused a voluminous milky pleural effusion. (From Holzworth J, Nielsen SW: J Am Vet Med Assoc 126 [1955] 26–36.)

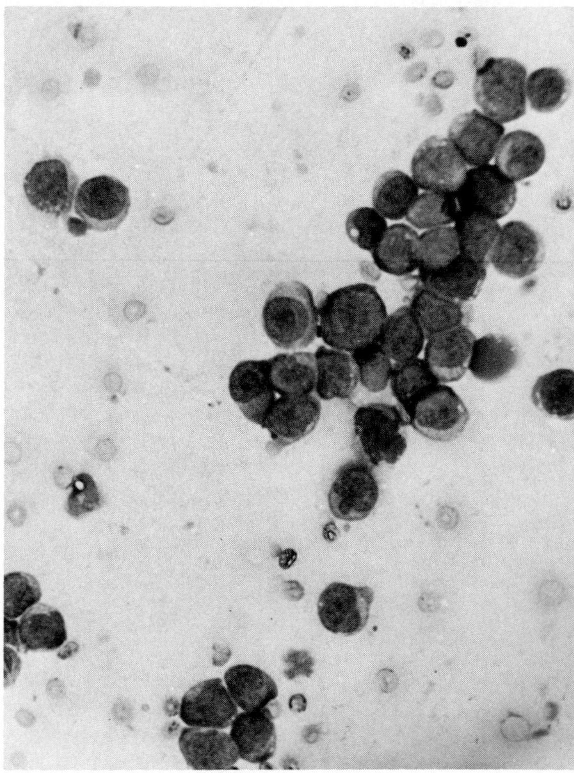

**Figure 11–23** Large, immature lymphoid cells, mostly "blasts," in a smear of clear transudate associated with a lymphoma of the mediastinum. Wright's stain, × 450. (From Holzworth J: J Am Vet Med Assoc 136 [1960] 47–69.)

for surgical resection is therefore poor. Rarely, intestinal lymphoma assumes a diffuse form that imparts a ropiness to the entire small intestine and presents as chronic enteritis, impairing digestion so that the feces resemble those in pancreatic exocrine deficiency, malabsorption, or hyperthyroidism. Lymphoma of the colon and rectum occurs much less often in cats than in dogs.

Gastric lymphoma, relatively uncommon, assumes infiltrative, nodular, and polypoid forms. The tumor may be ulcerated. Characteristic signs are inappetence, vomiting, and progressive anemia. Abnormalities of the stomach wall may be demonsrated radiographically (Fig. 11–24). Gastric lesions are usually massive when discovered, but an 11-year-old cat from which two small lesions were resected received postoperative chemotherapy and survived for two months (Weller and Hornof, 1979).

Esophageal lymphoma is very rare. It has not been accompanied by clinical signs in cats at AMAH but has been discovered incidentally at autopsy as a microscopic mural infiltration.

Oral lymphoma is relatively rare and, when present, is most often misdiagnosed as inflammation until a biopsy specimen is examined. Labial, gingival, lingual, and tonsillar lesions have been seen (Fig. 11–25). The pharyngeal as well as palatine tonsils have been involved, although rarely. A mass in the nasopharynx is most often an inflammatory polyp arising in the middle ear but occasionally proves to be a lymphoma originating in the nose or a pharyngeal tonsil (Fig. 11–26). Infrequently a salivary gland is the site of tumor.

Lymphoma of the cat's pancreas has occurred at AMAH as part of a multicentric disease but has not caused clinical signs of illness. The dull white neoplastic infiltrate thickens and obliterates the lobular pattern.

**UROGENITAL SYSTEM.** Renal lymphoma most often takes the form of bilateral enlargement and is nearly always part of a more generalized neoplastic process. Rarely, there is a solitary unilateral tumor, as in a cat that underwent nephrectomy for a single mass involving half a kidney and had no recurrence over a three-year period. (See tumors of the kidney.)

Grossly, renal lymphoma may be either nodular or diffuse. In the nodular type, masses are of varying size, dull white, soft or firm, homogeneous, unencapsulated, poorly demarcated, and located mainly in the cortex. Larger nodules elevate the capsule, causing a palpably lumpy kidney. These nodules must be distinguished from those of feline infectious peritonitis, in which there may be yellow granular foci associated with capsular inflammatory changes with a vascular distribution. Rarely, a tumor extends through the kidney capsule, extensively involving the perirenal and retroperitoneal tissue (Fig. 11–27).

The diffuse form of renal lymphoma can be overlooked by the inexperienced eye. The enlarged kidney may have a smooth capsular surface and an amazingly uniform,

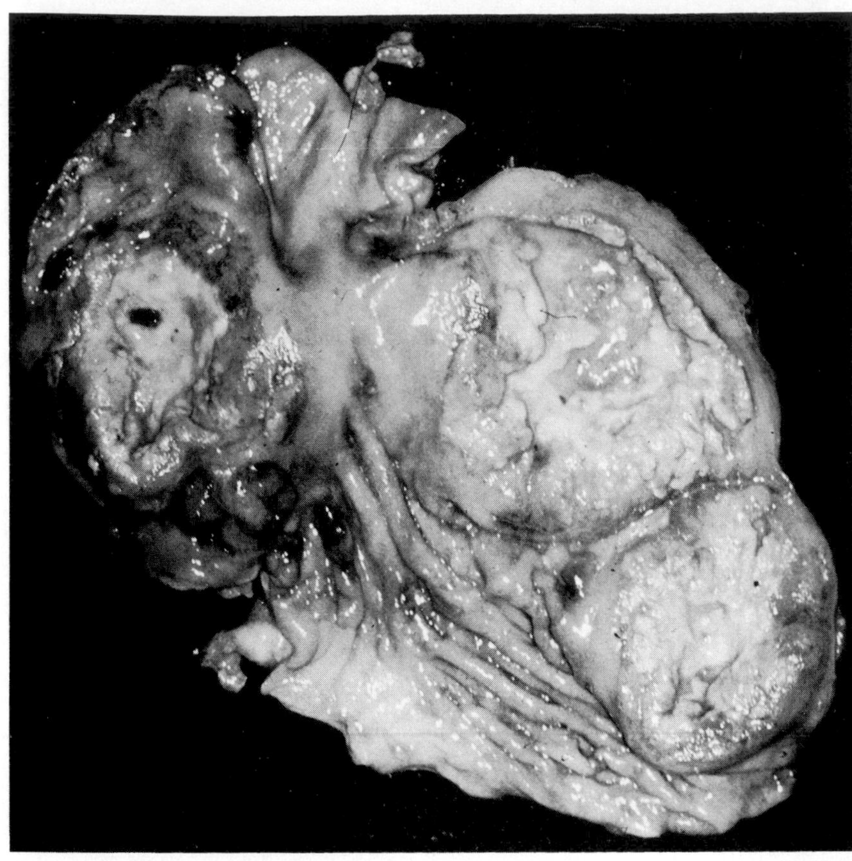

**Figure 11–24** Stomach wall with lymphoid tumors, one of which is ulcerated. (From Holzworth J: J Am Vet Med Assoc 136 [1960] 47–69.)

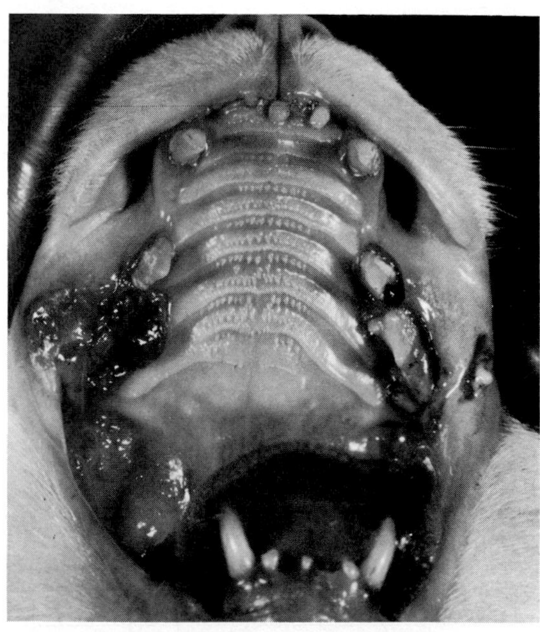

**Figure 11–25** Lymphoma of the inside of the cheeks, maxillary gingiva, and palatine margins, four-year-old white domestic longhair. Oral ulceration, hemorrhage, and gingivitis were secondary consequences.

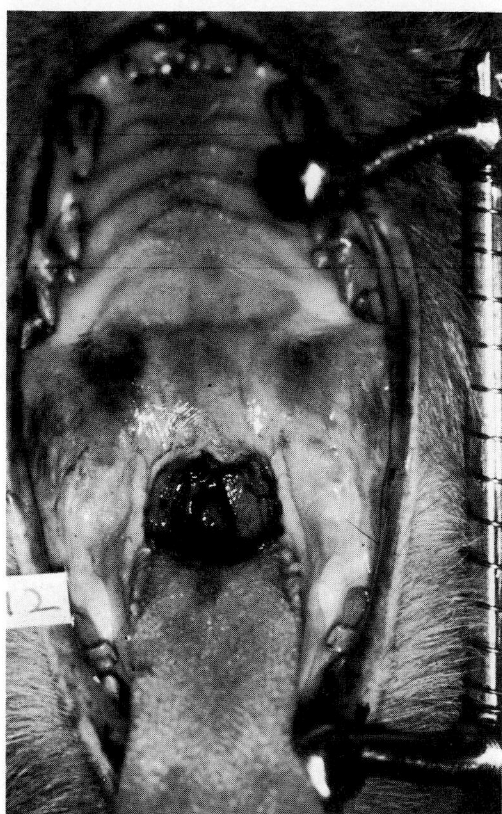

**Figure 11–26** Lymphoma of the nasopharynx. The caudal border of the soft palate, which was forced down by the growth, has been trimmed away. (From Holzworth J: J Am Vet Med Assoc 136 [1960] 47–69.)

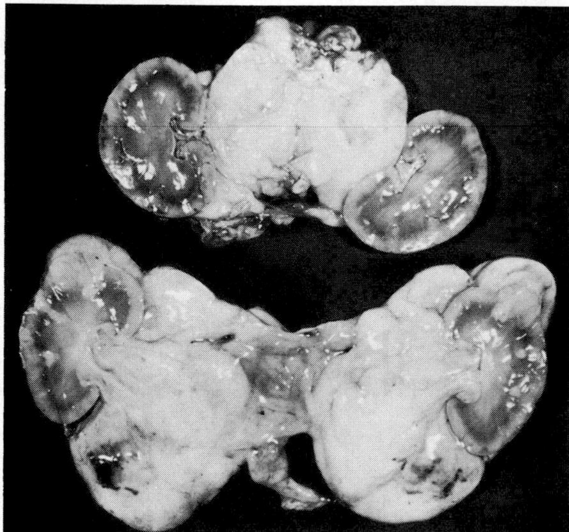

**Figure 11–27** Lymphoma involving both kidneys surrounds the arcuate vessels, infiltrates the cortex, and invades the retroperitoneal fat. Capsular and pelvic involvement are striking features in the lower kidney.

wide cortex with minor tumorous encroachment here and there on the outer medulla but with preservation of most of the corticomedullary junction. Close inspection, however, reveals variation in cortical color and width. Unless fibrosis or signs of acute inflammation suggest pyelonephritis, the diffuse infiltrative form of lymphoma should be suspected.

Examination of stained cortical imprints quickly provides the diagnosis of lymphoma when a unicellular population of lymphocytes is seen among exfoliated tubular epithelial cells. Clinical signs due solely to lymphoma are usually absent until normal tissue is largely replaced by tumor. These signs are low urinary specific gravity, rarely hematuria, and finally, increasing azotemia.

Illness related to ureteral involvement with lymphosarcoma has not been recognized at AMAH, but palpable bladder masses sometimes associated with hematuria have been diagnosed and have been observed as part of multicentric disease (e.g., Morgan and McMillan, 1981).

Also, in multicentric disease lymphoma has occasionally involved the female reproductive tract (Figs. 11–28 and 11–29) and the testes.

**NERVOUS SYSTEM.** The most common manifestation of lymphoma of the nervous system is posterior paresis, which is sometimes preceded by hyperesthesia of the skin of the corresponding somites, the result of epidural and spinal root lesions (e.g., Schappert and Geib, 1967; Swain and Shields, 1971). In fewer cats the pia-arachnoid is involved, and only one cat at AMAH in a 15-year review had a mass that invaded the spinal cord itself. The poorly demarcated, dull white epidural infiltrate may be mistaken for fat by an inexperienced prosector. An air-dried smear stained with new methylene blue allows quick and easy differentiation. A majority of cats do not have bone lesions grossly detectable by radiography or at autopsy, but marrow in the adjacent vertebrae and sometimes marrow at other body sites is involved.

Cats may be affected even under a year of age. They are usually FeLV-positive. Myelography is an important aid in diagnosis and in localizing the lesion for possible surgery. The technique is excellently described by Parker, O'Brien, and Sawchuk (1983). Chemotherapy gives good results with many extradural tumors (see chapter on the hematopoietic system).

Lymphomas of spinal nerve roots, brachial plexus, and sciatic nerve have been seen at AMAH. Horner's syndrome occurred in two cats with lymphoma of the brachial plexus (see also Fox and Gutnick, 1972), and in a cat with lesions in the mediastinum and stellate ganglion. The nerves, dull white, rounded, and enlarged, varied in diameter and had lost their cross striations.

Intracranial lymphoma usually involves the meninges, choroid plexuses, and rarely the neuropil. The dura may be several millimeters thick, forming a dull white or pale yellow mat easily lifted free of the brain (Fig. 11–30). Meningeal lesions cause compression of the brain, and impaired circulation of blood and cerebrospinal fluid results in edema, swelling, and herniation of the cerebrum and cerebellum. The choroid plexuses are gray-white and lack their usual red villous features. Lesions of the meninges and choroid plexus can lead to obstructive hydrocephalus.

Sudden blindness, nasal discharge, and, finally, circling were the signs resulting in a seven-year-old neutered male

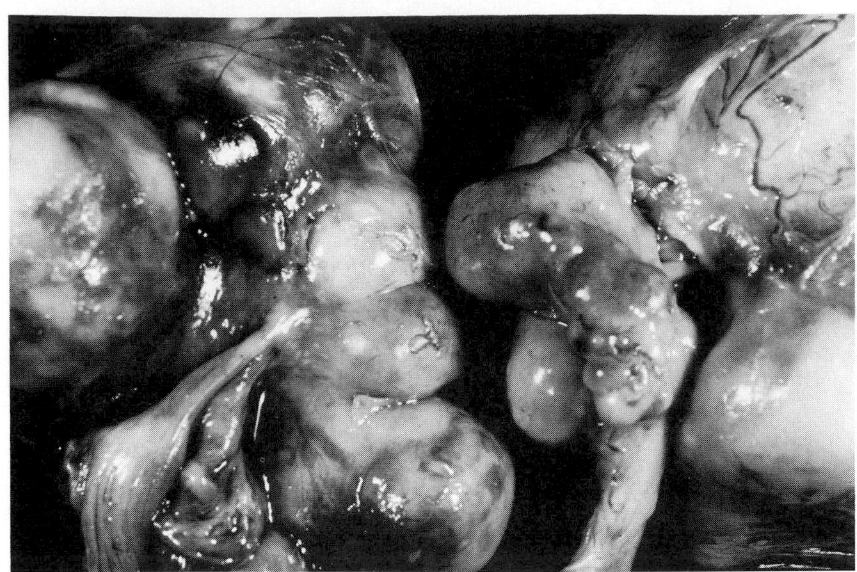

**Figure 11–28** Ovarian lymphoma, bilateral, three-year-old tricolor. Confluent tumor nodules mask all of the left and most of the right ovary and are continuous with the uterine horns (below).

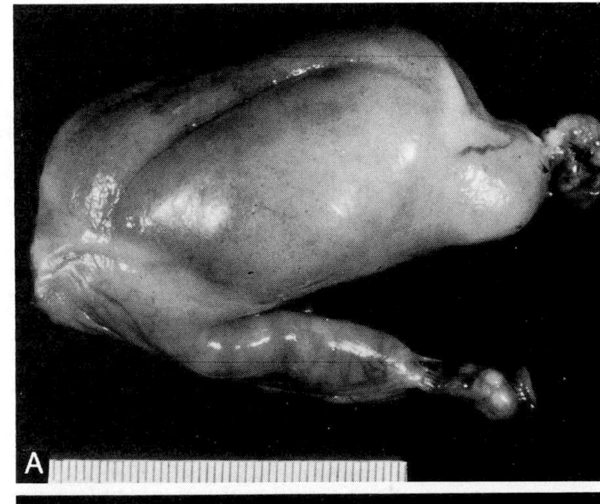


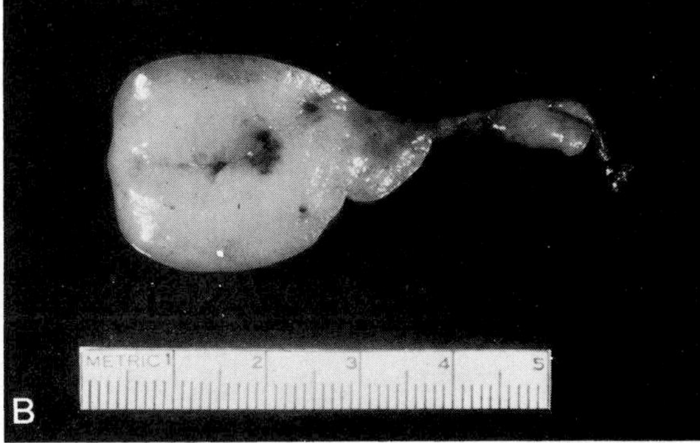


**Figure 11–29** Lymphoma of the uterus, six-year-old tabby. *B*, Lymphoma of uterine horn and broad ligament, same cat. The transverse cut surface discloses a circumferential and transmural infiltrate and foci of hemorrhage.

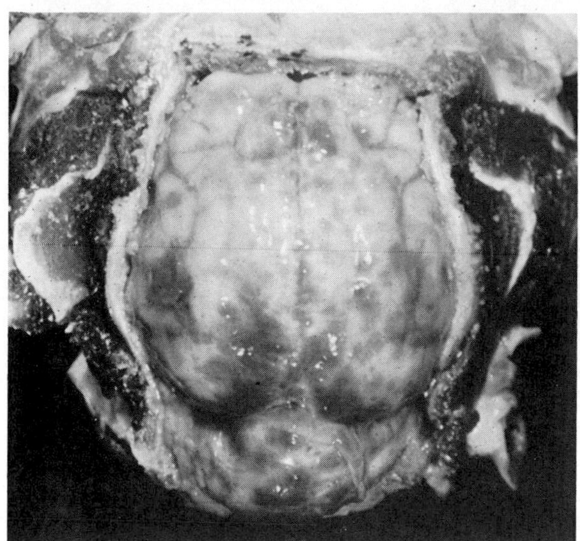

**Figure 11–30** Lymphoma of the cerebral dura mater, one-year-old tabby. The diffusely thickened and opaque dura has several dark areas of hemorrhage.

from a highly undifferentiated lymphoid tumor involving the olfactory bulbs, optic nerves, optic chiasm, and other left-sided structures (Barker and Greenwood, 1973). The tumor appeared to have arisen from the frontal sinus and nasal cavity.

**EYE.** Orbital lymphoma occasionally causes protrusion of the eyeball. The third eyelid and palpebral conjunctiva may be infiltrated and bulge through the palpebral fissure (Fig. 11–31). Tissue for examination can be obtained by needle aspiration.

Intraocular lymphoma is fairly frequent, taking the form of gross or microscopic lesions of the uvea and, less often, of the retina. The iris may appear thickened, fuzzy, and irregular (Fig. 11–32), and there may be an aqueous flare. The condition should be differentiated by needle aspirate from uveitis due to feline infectious peritonitis, toxoplasmosis, cryptococcosis, and other inflammatory disturbances.

**SKIN.** Experience at AMAH and elsewhere (e.g., Caciolo et al., 1984) indicates that lymphoma of the skin is uncommon and assumes widely different forms that may mimic other kinds of tumor or non-neoplastic lesions. Affected cats tend to be middle-aged or elderly and to test negative for FeLV. Microscopically the tumor cells are usually of primitive type.

Multiple small nodules in the dermis are firm and easily palpable and may resemble mast cell tumors, except that rubbing of the overlying skin is less likely to cause erythema and swelling. While mast cells have some predilection for the head and neck, no tendency to localization has been observed with lymphoma. On cut surface, nodules are solid, uniform, and gray-white, often poorly defined, and never encapsulated. The nodules may rarely involve underlying muscle as well as skin, as was the case in an otherwise clinically normal 12-year-old Siamese (Dallman et al., 1982). Although the cat's IFA test was negative, C-type virus was identified in tissues, and gross or microscopic tumor was present elsewhere in the body.

Another type of lymphoma is diffuse, soft, and pliable and may resemble thickened, redundant skin with varying degrees of erythema. Diffuse, aggressive histiocytic growths, such as one that involved the skin and subcutis of an entire paw in an Angell patient, may be mistaken for deep-seated infection.

In an Angell case of multiple lymphoblastic tumors the gross appearance of the lesions suggested burns, except that they came in succession, new ones appearing as earlier ones dried, sloughed, and developed scar tissue (Fig. 11–33). In this cat, as in most of the others, there proved to be tumor elsewhere.

Among nine cases of cutaneous lymphoma reported by Caciolo et al. (1984) was one of mycosis fungoides that had been previously described. Mycosis fungoides, a special form of skin lymphoma, is a T-cell tumor of humans and dogs. The early lesions, which may be single or multiple and itchy, resemble patches of eczematous dermatitis both grossly and microscopically and may regress spontaneously. In time, plaques and then tumors develop, and ultimately there is visceral involvement. Diagnostic morphologic characteristics are the presence in the dermis of "mycosis cells," atypical lymphocytes with hyperchromatic, convoluted nuclei, and clustering of these cells within intraepidermal vesicles (Pautrier's microabscesses).

A case of skin lymphoma with similarities to mycosis fungoides was reported in a five-year-old male domestic shorthair (Legendre and Becker, 1979). Multiple masses 1 to 3 cm in diameter extended into the subcutis, and a midabdominal mass was palpated. Seventy-five per cent of atypical lymphocytes in the circulating blood were considered to be neoplastic lymphocytes. The IFA test for FeLV in this cat gave negative results. Part of an excised mass was diagnosed histologically as lymphoma, and 44 per cent of the lymphoid cells in the remainder of the mass were identifed by rosette testing as T-lymphocytes, as were 48 per cent of the peripheral blood lymphocytes. Treatment was started with cyclophosphamide, vincristine, and prednisolone. The tumors regressed in 10 days but then resumed growth, and the cat died after six weeks of therapy. An autopsy was not permitted.

Mycosis fungoides was reported in a 10-year-old spayed female domestic cat with a mildly pruritic plaque on the thoracic wall (Caciolo et al., 1983, 1984; Caciolo, personal communication). This had been diagnosed clinically as an eosinophilic plaque but did not respond to treatment with corticosteroids or megestrol acetate. The IFA test for FeLV and all other hematologic and biochemical tests gave negative results. On the basis of morphologic features of the excised lesion and regional node, as well as immunologic testing of tissue, including identification of a majority of the lymphoid cells as T cells, the diagnosis of mycosis fungoides was considered to be confirmed. As chemotherapeutic agents were reported to be ineffective in humans and dogs, intravenous and intralesional treatment was given with fibronectin. For some months there was no progression of the original lesion or systemic involvement; eventually, however, patches identified as mycosis fungoides appeared on the abdomen, and the cat died of congestive cardiomyopathy after about a year of therapy. No visceral involvement was found at autopsy.

Cutaneous mycosis fungoides was also diagnosed in a 12-year-old castrated male domestic shorthair that was consistently FeLV-negative (Miller, 1981). The lesions responded well to topical treatment, but after a long course the cat died of pneumonia believed to be secondary to immunoincompetence.

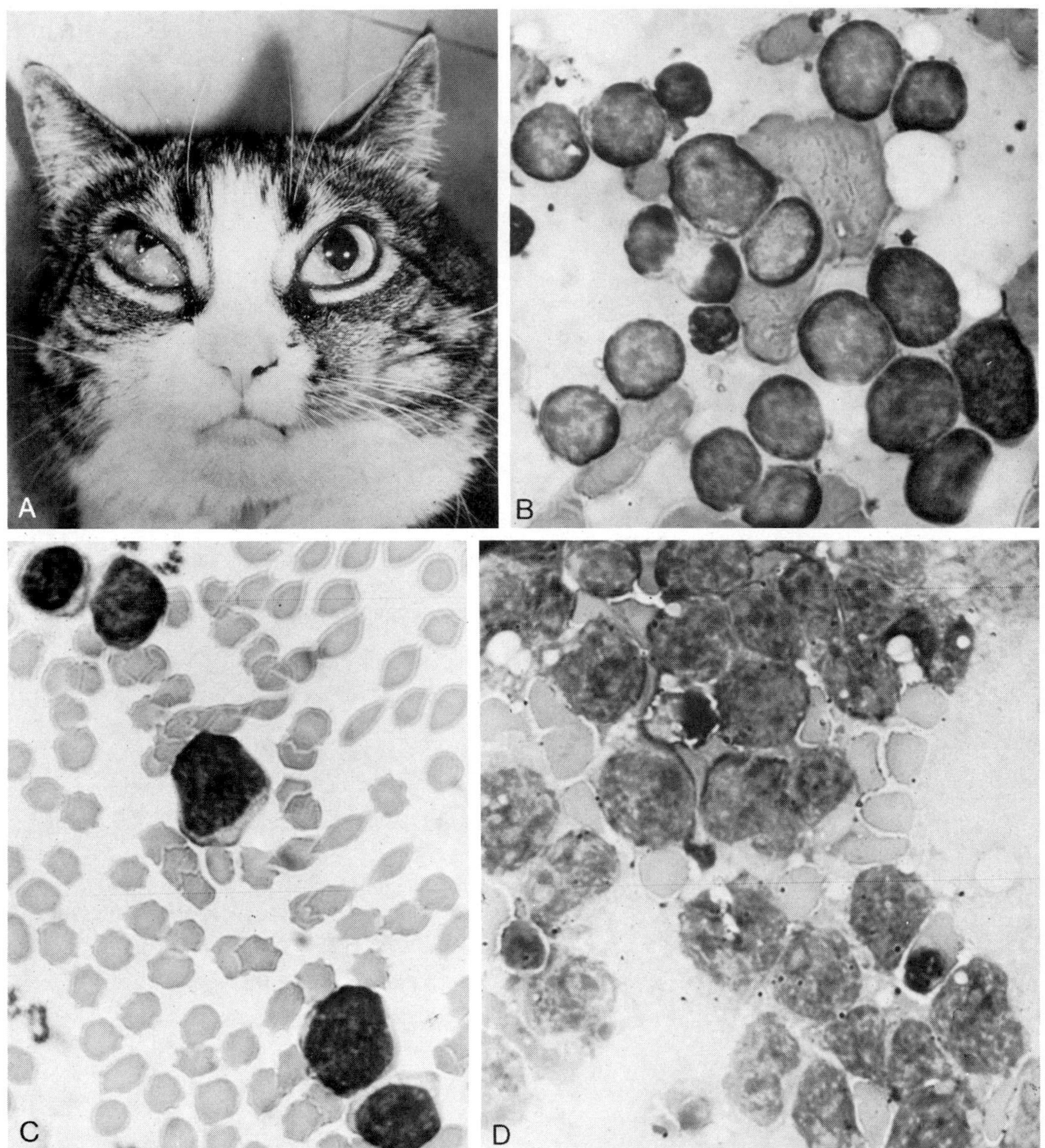


**Figure 11–31** *A*, Lymphoblastic lymphoma with retrobulbar tumor infiltration. *B*, Impression film of tumor tissue curetted from a necrotic area behind the last upper right molar. *C*, Blood, WBC 41,000/μl, lymphocytes 72 per cent (majority atypical) and 15 per cent "smudges." *D*, Marrow, numerous immature and atypical lymphoid cells. (From Holzworth J: J Am Vet Med Assoc 136 [1960] 47–69.)

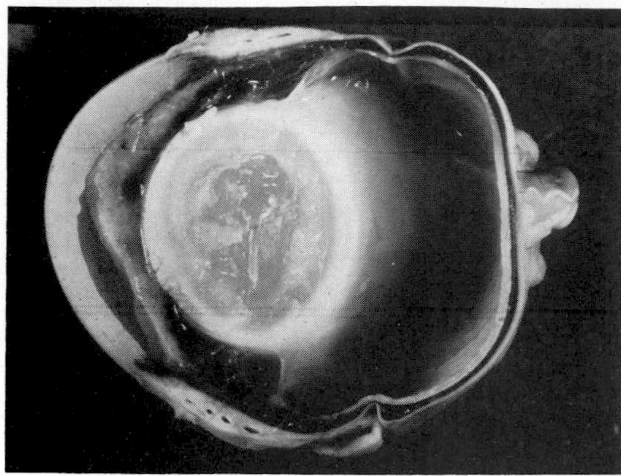

**Figure 11–32** Ocular lymphoma, eight-year-old domestic longhair, causing iridic thickening, an anterior synechia, and a closed drainage angle. A white proteinaceous exudate adheres to the caudal lens capsule.

In a dog with mycosis fungoides, treatment with a placental lysate and a low dose of prednisone achieved long-term remission (Bender, 1984).

**RESPIRATORY SYSTEM.** The respiratory tract is not a prime site for lymphoma but may occasionally be involved.

Masses in the nose are associated with sneezing, nasal discharge, and lysis of turbinate bones and may block drainage of secretion from the frontal sinuses. Eventually, facial bones may be destroyed but without the new bone formation typical of most other tumors. A polypoid mass arising in the nose may lie dorsal to the hard or soft palate and interfere with nasal breathing. Those developing from nasopharyngeal tonsils cause gagging as well. A lymphoma large enough to depress the soft palate is accessible but, when farther forward in the nose, may be suspected only from a radiograph. Differentiation among nasal masses, including cryptococcal granulomas, is by laboratory examination of material obtained by a small curette or by nasal flushing. Occasionally the frontal sinus is also involved (e.g., Legendre and Dade, 1975). Radiographs often show unilateral soft tissue density and destruction of the septum and turbinates.

In the larynx, diffuse but more often focal nodular lesions apparently arise from lymphocytic aggregates normally present in the lamina propria. Early signs are an inability to mew and tinny or rattly purring. As the laryngeal lumen is reduced, dyspnea of the expiratory type may be mistaken for asthma-like breathing. Breathing becomes progressively labored, with open mouth and cyanosis.

The trachea is frequently displaced or compressed by adjacent tumor, but lymphoma of the trachea itself is very rare and is usually recognized as a microscopic finding only at autopsy. Gross infiltration of the bifurcation occurred in a cat with a lymphoma dorsal to and surrounding the trachea (Guariglia and Rankin, 1970). A four-ring section of trachea with a large histiocytic lymphoma both outside and within the lumen was successfully removed from a seven-year-old male Siamese that was FeLV-positive (Schneider et al., 1979). For six weeks after surgery the cat was treated with cyclophosphamide, prednisone, and vincristine and at eight months was asymptomatic.

Pulmonary lesions of malignant lymphoma are most often observed as microscopic perivascular and peribronchial accumulations of immature lymphocytes or as large numbers of lymphocytes within alveolar capillaries in cases of leukemia. Masses resulting from alveolar filling by infiltrating lymphocytes may occasionally take the form of gray-white consolidated lesions large enough to be seen radiographically (>0.4 cm) and grossly, and sometimes occupy most of one or more lobes. Mucus retention within the bronchi of extensively involved lobes is to be expected. Tracheobronchial nodes are usually enlarged and neoplastic when the lung has gross lesions of lymphoma.

**CARDIOVASCULAR SYSTEM.** Cardiac lesions of lymphoma are sometimes restricted to the atria but are

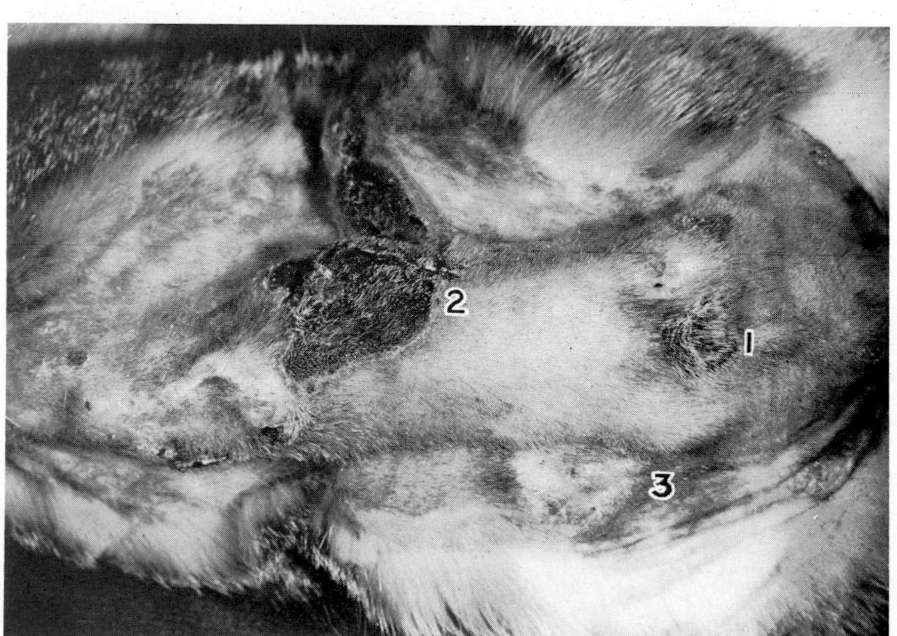


**Figure 11–33** Multiple areas of histiocytic lymphoma of the skin as they appeared after clipping. (1) Incipient lesion with thickening, loss of hair, and oozing of serum. (2) Next stage, circumscribed dry area, before sloughing. (3) Final stage, scarring. (From Holzworth J: J Am Vet Med Assoc 136 [1960] 47–69.)

more often multifocal, with the atrial lesions exceeding in severity those in the ventricles (Fig. 11–34). Atrial myocardium can be totally replaced by focal masses without tearing or perforation. Endocardial thrombi, some containing malignant cells, may be present. Cardiac function is impaired, and fluid accumulates in the chest (e.g., Wilkinson, 1967).

Arterial walls, unlike those of veins and venules, are infrequently involved.

**ENDOCRINE GLANDS.** Gross or microscopic lymphoma may occasionally involve any one of the endocrine glands but, in our experience, without recognized clinical effect (Fig. 11–35).

**BONE.** Bone is most often involved when lymphoma originating within vertebral marrow extends into the spinal epidural space and infiltrates nerve rootlets as well as compressing the cord. Only rarely is the cord itself invaded.

Ott (1983) has referred to osseous lymphoma, which may cause lameness and limb pain. Radiographs disclose lytic lesions and some evidence of new bone formation. Lymphoma involving both tarsal joints with soft tissue enlargement as well as destructive lesions affecting all the bones of the joints was described in a 13-year-old domestic cat that tested negative for FeLV (Barclay, 1979).

**MICROSCOPIC FEATURES.** Lymphoma is a neoplasm composed of lymphocytes that infiltrate and eventually replace normal tissue in a nodular or diffuse fashion without provoking fibroplasia. Traditionally the lymphomas have been characterized, according to the dominant cell, as lymphocytic, lymphoblastic, and histiocytic (reticulum cell sarcoma)—these categories also corresponding roughly to the degree of aggressiveness (modified Rappaport classification). Within the past few years, on the premise that lymphomas are neoplasms of the immune system, medical pathologists (Lukes and Collins) have proposed categorizing them on the basis of their origin from T- or B-lymphocytes or histiocytes and on classification of their cells as small or large, and nuclei as noncleaved or cleaved (indented).

Although it is recognized that the Lukes-Collins classification has advanced the understanding of the histogenesis of the lymphomas, its superiority in respect to prognostication and patient management has not been established (Robbins et al., 1984). The National Cancer Institute, together with experts elsewhere, has suggested a Working Formulation for Clinical Usage that attempts to correlate the morphologic and functional classifications (NCI, 1982; see also Robbins et al., 1984).

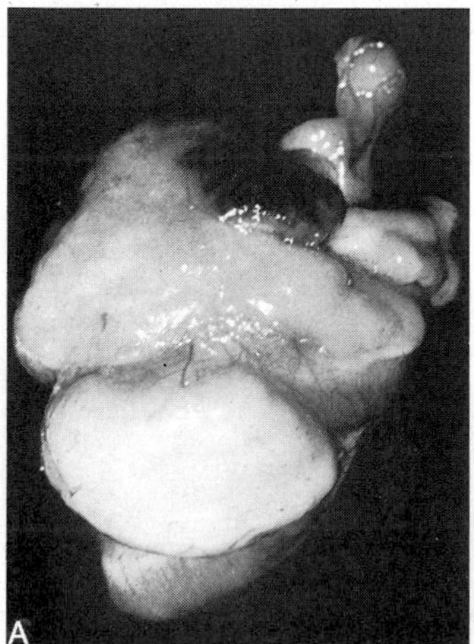


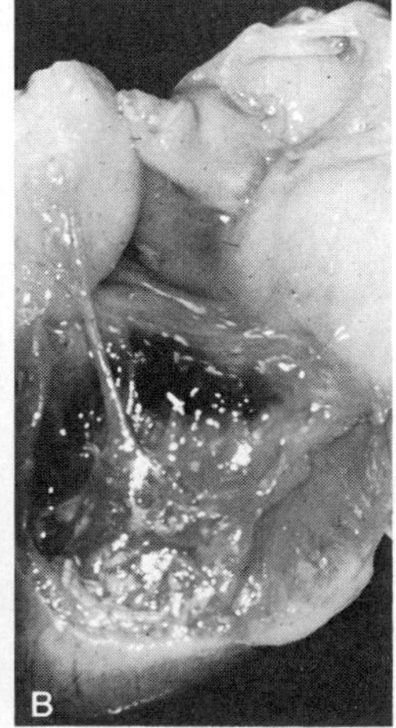


**Figure 11–34** *A* and *B*, Lymphoma of the right atrium and right ventricle, five-year-old castrated male domestic shorthair. (From Holzworth J: J Am Vet Med Assoc 136 [1960] 47–69.)

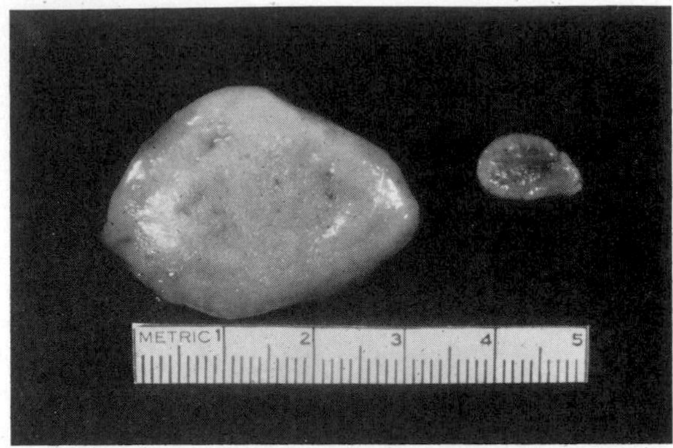


**Figure 11–35** Lymphoma of the left adrenal, six-year-old spayed female domestic shorthair. Cut surfaces of both adrenals disclose unilateral effacement.

In a study by Valli et al. (1981), feline, canine, and bovine lymphomas were characterized traditionally as nodular or diffuse and also according to the Lukes-Collins classification based on cell size and non-cleavage or cleavage of the nucleus. Seventy-nine of 81 feline tumors were duffuse, and 59 of these had non-cleaved nuclei. Only two tumors were nodular, both having non-cleaved nuclei. Over half the 81 lymphomas were of small cell type (75 per cent or more of cells with a nuclear diameter of one red cell), and none were classified as large lymphocytic type (nuclei having a diameter of three or more red cells). Many had a mixed population of cells, usually small-medium rather than medium-large.

As in man, a significant correlation was found in cats, dogs, and cows between tumor type and age at death (Valli et al., 1981). Cats with cleaved-cell lymphomas died at a mean age of 5.4 years, while those with the more common non-cleaved tumors lived a mean of 4.6 years. The two cats with tumor of nodular pattern averaged 8.3 years at death, while the 79 cats with a diffuse form averaged 4.7 years. There was no apparent relationship between cell size and age at death. Sex or neutering had no influence on tumor type.

In man, the majority of non-Hodgkin's lymphomas are of B-cell type. By contrast, the majority of feline lymphomas are of T-cell origin except for those of the gastrointestinal tract (Hardy, 1981; Holmberg et al., 1976).

Although the proponents of the immunologic classification of lymphomas maintain that B- and T-cell tumors can be distinguished by morphologic characteristics, others have not found this to be always the case (Holmberg et al., 1976; Robbins et al., 1984), and it has been advocated that markers be routinely used as an adjunct.

At AMAH over 1300 lymphomas have been diagnosed, and it is clearly impossible to carry out a retrospective morphologic review of such a vast number. Moreover, the tissues were fixed in formalin, whereas fixation in B-5, a mercuric fixative, is considered desirable for accurate identification of nuclear features. However, on the basis of almost everyday experience with feline lymphomas, we have the impression that a significant majority are of non-cleaved type. The nodular (follicular) pattern has rarely, if ever, been recognized at AMAH (JLC). With the exception of a minority of the intestinal lymphomas the feline tumors have a highly aggressive behavior. The majority are composed of lymphocytes of varying size but predominantly lymphoblasts. The behavior of any one tumor depends on its mitotic index; thus the lymphoblastic and histiocytic lymphomas are more aggressive than lymphomas in which the predominant cell is the small (mature) lymphocyte and in which mitotic figures are few. In general, histiocytic lymphoma is the most aggressive and is likely to be found not only in lymphoid organs but also in sites normally devoid of lymphoid tissue (e.g., nasal cavity, kidney, skeletal muscle).

A minority of the intestinal lymphomas are of the lymphocytic type and occur diffusely in the mucosa. A clinical course of months precedes dissemination of the tumor to other sites. It is possible that "chronic lymphocytic enteritis" may precede, or represent an early stage of, this form of lymphoma. We have learned from intestinal biopsies that there is an interval when it can be difficult to distinguish between inflammatory and neoplastic lymphocytosis.

**HODGKIN'S LYMPHOMA.** This form of lymphoma occurs rarely, if ever, in animals. A possible case of Hodgkin's disease was described in a cat by Roperto et al. (1983), and three cases of histiocytic lymphoma with multinucleated giant cells were reported, one of which was considered to resemble Hodgkin's disease (Nakayama et al., 1984).

## Thymoma

Almost all tumors of the cranial mediastinum are lymphomas. Rarely, such a tumor proves to be a mast cell tumor or—if a cat is lucky—a thymoma. An "endotheliosarcoma" and a lymphangioma have also been recorded (Mettler, 1975).

Thymomas are neoplasms of entodermal thymic epithelium and are most often benign. At least 28 feline thymomas have been reported (Carpenter and Holzworth, 1982; Cotchin, 1952; Dubielzig and Dehaney, 1980; Hardy, 1981; Hauser and Mettler, 1984; Ladds et al., 1970; Loveday, 1959; Mackey, 1975; Mettler, 1975; Parker and Casey, 1976; Priester and McKay, 1980; Richards, 1977; Willard et al., 1980). Two unpublished cases, one in a Siamese, are on record at the Armed Forces Institute of Pathology (AFIP).

Subsequent to publication of 11 cases from AMAH (Carpenter and Holzworth, 1982), six more thymomas were diagnosed at AMAH in cats 6 to 10 years old, three castrated males and three spayed females. Three were domestic shorthairs, two were Siamese, and one was an Abyssinian.

**BREED, AGE, AND SEX.** Among the 28 cats in the published reports and the later group of six at AMAH, no breed or sex predisposition was apparent. Five cats were Siamese. Fourteen of 29 cats of known gender were males, ten of them castrates. Fifteen were female, of which 11 were spayed. The age range was 1½ to 18 years (mean about 10).

**CLINICAL FEATURES.** Dyspnea is the most common sign of mediastinal thymoma and is almost always associated with a pleural effusion and a tumor large enough to be seen radiographically. Several cats coughed or vomited. A curious association with polymyositis occurred in three cats, two of which were found at autopsy also to have myocarditis (Carpenter and Holzworth, 1982). Signs were lethargy, extreme weakness, muscle-wasting, difficulty in swallowing, and decreased esophageal peristalsis (Fig. 11–36). Two cats were so weak that the head rested on the forepaws; one used its forepaws to place food in its mouth. Two other cats had a diffuse, moist dermatitis (Carpenter and Holzworth, 1982; Loveday, 1959). A remarkable feature accompanying the thymoma in a one and a half-year-old cat was severe hypertrophic osteoarthropathy involving the fore- and hindlimbs as far distally as the carpal and tarsal joints (Richards, 1977).

**RADIOGRAPHIC FEATURES.** Most cats have cra-

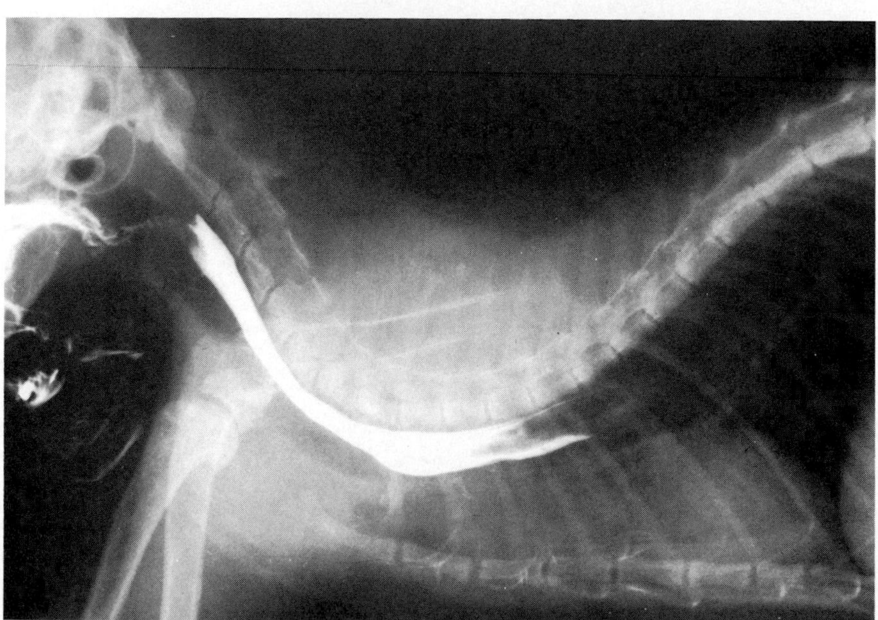

**Figure 11–36** Lateral radiographic view of a 13-year-old cat five minutes after oral administration of barium sulfate. Contrast material has been retained in the mouth, pharynx, and cranial portion of the esophagus owing to difficulty in swallowing and to greatly diminished esophageal peristalsis. The radiodensity cranial to the heart proved to be a mediastinal thymoma. (From Carpenter JL, Holzworth J: J Am Vet Med Assoc 181 [1982] 248–251.)

nial mediastinal masses accompanied by pleural effusion. Esophageal paralysis may be apparent. Tracheal elevation and caudal displacement of its bifurcation, as well as elevation of the heart to the right, are seen with the larger thymomas. Radiographically, thymoma is indistinguishable from lymphoma.

**CLINICOPATHOLOGIC FEATURES.** In none of the reported cases was a cat anemic; two had hypogammaglobulinemia. Cats suspected of having polymyositis should have serum aldolase, creatine kinase, and glutamic oxaloacetic transaminase (SGOT) determinations. Two of the cats had an absolute lymphocytosis (7430 and 12,000 per μl). The 11 cats tested for FeLV were test-negative.

Pleural effusions were pale yellow, bloody, or, in two cases, chylous; none suggested lymphoma because the lymphocytes in the effusions were mature. In several cases mast cells were also present in the fluid. They may serve as a clue to thymoma, since mast cells occur normally in the medulla of the thymus. One effusion had malignant epithelial cells, and fluid aspirated from another cat with a cystic thymoma contained atypical cells suggestive of an epithelial malignancy.

**GROSS FEATURES.** All thymomas of cats have been situated in the cranial mediastinum and have ranged from 1.2 to 11.0 cm in greatest dimension. Most were smooth, firm, and lobulated, and many were observed to be cystic, usually on cut surfaces. Most were yellow-white, others gray (Fig. 11–37). In some there were foci of necrosis or hemorrhage. Invasive growth occurred with one clear cell thymoma (Mackey, 1975). The one malignant tumor at AMAH disseminated within the mediastinum, and a neoplastic effusion was present. Another malignant tumor metastasized to the lung, and many small lung veins were occluded by tumor cell aggregates (Hauser and Mettler, 1984). Three other thymomas were listed as malignant (Priester and McKay, 1980).

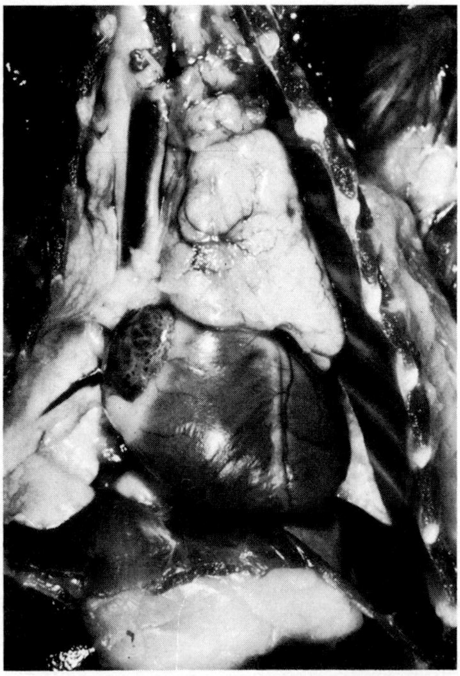

**Figure 11–37** Large thymoma in the cranial portion of the mediastinum, eight-year-old cat. (From Carpenter JL, Holzworth J: J Am Vet Med Assoc 181 [1982] 248–251.)

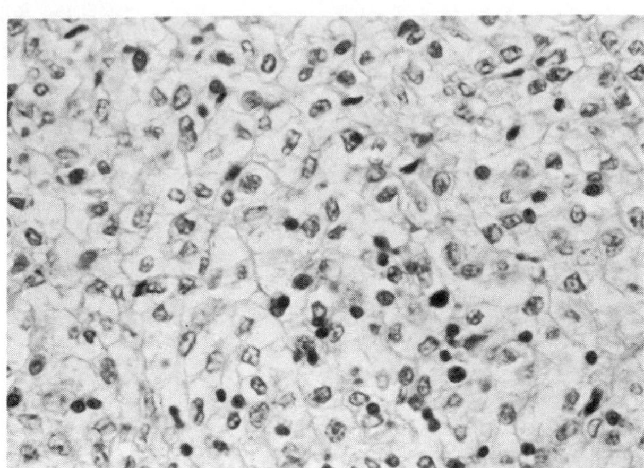

**Figure 11–38** Thymoma, 13-year-old cat. In this compact group of thymic epithelial cells the cytoplasm in some cells stains lightly, in others (clear cells) not at all. H & E, × 350. (From Carpenter JL, Holzworth J: J Am Vet Med Assoc 181 [1982] 248–251.)

Advanced muscle atrophy was prominent in two cats with polymyositis. Severe diffuse moist dermatitis was striking in two.

**MICROSCOPIC FEATURES.** The neoplastic cell in a thymoma is the thymic epithelial cell, which may have a round, oval, or fusiform nucleus. It may be arranged in rows, nests, cysts, sheets, or thymic corpuscles. Cells with clear cytoplasm have been reported (Mackey, 1975; Richards, 1977) and were seen in two tumors at AMAH (Fig. 11–38). All the thymomas described microscopically have had some areas of lymphocytes, varying in number but always of small size (Fig. 11–39*A*). Five tumors at AMAH had prominent perivascular spaces containing mainly small lymphocytes and a few macrophages, mast cells, or red cells. The outer border of the space was formed by thymic epithelial cells, which in normal thymus can be discerned only by electron microscopy as part of the blood-thymus barrier.

Ten of the 17 thymomas at AMAH had prominent cysts containing eosinophilic granular and fibrillar precipitate, a few macrophages, occasionally red blood cells, and rarely cholesterol clefts. The cysts were lined by thymic epithelial cells, most often of the fusiform type, arranged in a sheet of parallel cells. Such cysts and the prominent fibrous bands that lie within the tumor are characteristic patterns that differ strikingly from that of thymic lymphoma. Occasionally cysts lined by respiratory-type epithelium, also derived from branchial pouch, can be trapped within the tumor. Such cysts may contain mucin.

Thymic corpuscles were observed in about half of the cases, some large with abundant keratinization (Fig. 11–39*B*). In the cases at AMAH, mast cells were often more numerous and less evenly distributed than in normal feline thymuses. As noted earlier, some of the pleural effusions at AMAH reflected the mast cell component of the tumor. Eosinophils within the tumor were rare; lymphocytic follicles were not observed. In one tumor there were small areas with large plump cells containing considerable acid mucopolysaccharide (Hauser and Mettler, 1984).

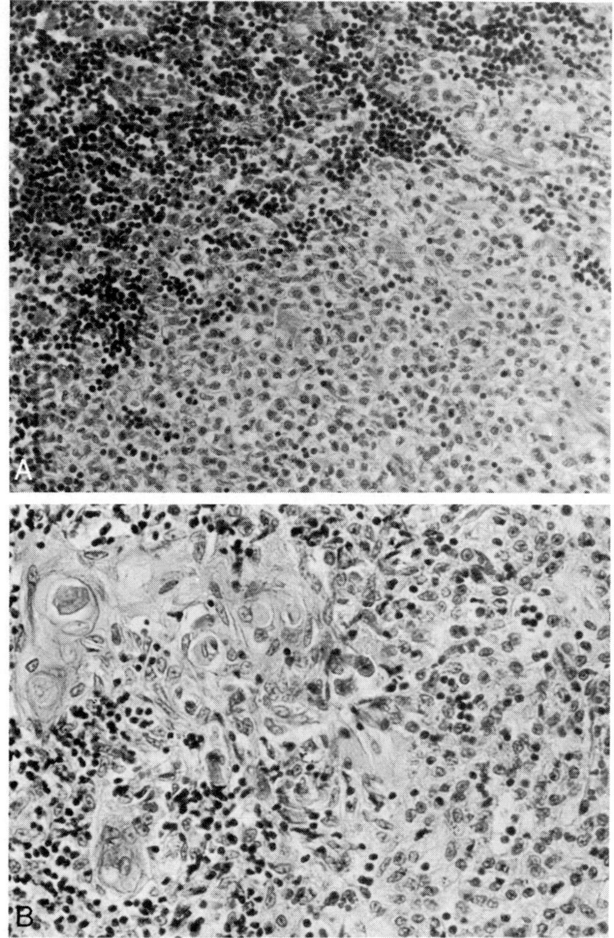


**Figure 11–39** *A*, Thymoma, same cat as in Figure 11–38. Notice solid area of polyhedral thymic epithelial cells (lower right) adjacent to a region where small lymphocytes predominate. H & E, × 350. *B*, Prominent thymic corpuscles (upper left), many lymphocytes, and larger, paler epithelial cells. H & E, × 350. (From Carpenter JL, Holzworth J: J Am Vet Med Assoc 181 [1982] 248–251.)

The reported mitotic index for benign thymomas was 0 to 1 per 10 HPF and 15 for the malignant neoplasm at AMAH. Mitotic figures and vascular invasion were common in the other malignant tumor (Hauser and Mettler, 1984). Necrosis was prominent in the malignant tumors but was also observed in the larger benign growths. Mineralization and foci of cholesterol clefts were rare.

Polymyositis was characterized by atrophy and a multifocal infiltrate, mainly of lymphocytes and macrophages, and only a few neutrophils and plasma cells. Necrosis and regeneration of myocytes were observed within the foci of inflammation, but fibrosis was minimal (Fig. 11–40).

Dermatitis, reported in two cats, was described in one as a diffuse, superficial, histiocytic and lymphocytic inflammation that often obliterated a distinct epidermal-dermal junction (Carpenter and Holzworth, 1982). The epidermis had edema, clefts, necrotic keratinocytes, intercellular neutrophils, and mononuclear cells. Foci of purulent bacterial epidermatitis were interpreted as a secondary event.

**PROGNOSIS.** Surgery may be curative or palliative for thymoma, since most lesions are benign and growth is slow. It is therefore important to differentiate thymoma from mediastinal lymphoma and the rare mast cell tumor. Small lymphocytes and the absence of lymphoblasts in a pleural effusion strongly suggest that a cranial mediastinal mass may be a thymoma. Total excision of the tumor is not necessary in order to significantly benefit the patient. The tumor growth rate in man and dogs is quite slow and may also be so in cats. A biopsy of the mass is essential for a definitive diagnosis.

In two cases resective surgery, combined with chemotherapy, appeared to be curative (Willard et al., 1980). At AMAH three cats were treated surgically by a split-sternum approach. One died three days later. In another, recurrent tumor had grown, two years later, through the previous sternotomy site and around the anterior vena cava and carotid arteries. The third cat was in apparent excellent health 15 months after surgery.

## The Spleen

**TUMOR-LIKE LESIONS.** Hematomas due to trauma or vascular disease are uncommon in cats, occurring with about a twentieth of the frequency observed in dogs at AMAH. Other tumor-like nodules may be heterotopic pancreas, pyogranulomatous inflammation, or nodular hyperplasia.

Heterotopic pancreatic tissue within the spleen occurs less often than splenic tissue within the pancreas. Pyogranulomatous inflammatory nodules are nearly always caused by feline infectious peritonitis virus and are more frequent in the noneffusive form of the disease. Certain less common infections may also cause nodular inflammation in the spleen, e.g., tuberculosis.

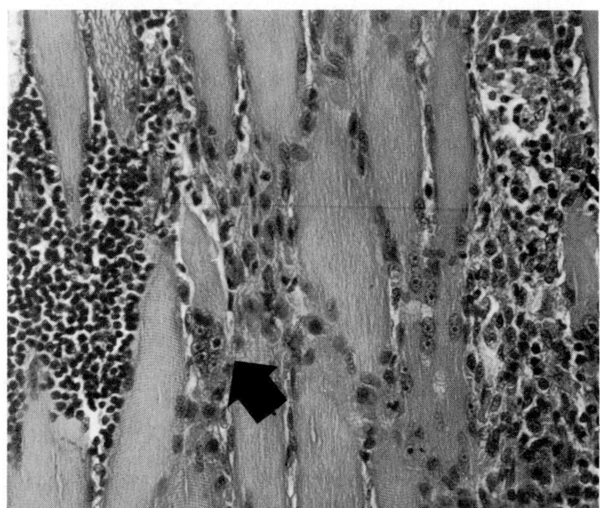

**Figure 11–40** Myositis in a section of temporalis muscle from a 13-year-old cat with thymoma and muscular impairment evidenced clinically by dysphagia and ventriflexion of the neck. Aggregates of lymphocytes (left) and histiocytes with a few neutrophils (right) are interspersed among necrotic fragmented myocytes. An attempt at regeneration is evident in one fiber (arrow). H & E, × 350. (From Carpenter JL, Holzworth J: J Am Vet Med Assoc 181 [1982] 248–251.)

Nodular hyperplasia is of several types: lymphocytic, lipocytic, lymphocytic-lipocytic, lymphocytic-reticuloendothelial, and lipocytic-hematopoietic (myelolipoma).

Nodular lymphocytic hyperplasia was observed in six cats aged 5 to 15 years. The nodules, one to three in number and 0.5 to 3.5 cm in diameter, were most often located on the ventral extremity of the spleen, forming a smooth convex mass on the parietal surface. They were red-blue or purple, and mottled white, pale gray, and red on their bulging cut surface. They were clearly demarcated but not encapsulated. Microscopically the masses were expansile, compressing and distorting adjacent trabeculae and parenchyma, and were composed of large follicles separated by red pulp.

Multiple choristomas consisting of nodules of mature fat cells were an incidental finding in a two-year-old female Siamese with a scapular osteosarcoma. A single instance of lymphocytic-lipocytic proliferation occurred in a 15-year-old spayed female tricolor, and one mass characterized by lymphocytic-reticuloendothelial hyperplasia was an incidental finding in a six-year-old cat.

Myelolipomas of the spleen and liver, usually asymptomatic, have been reported in both wild and domestic cats, as well as in some other animals and man. A splenic myelolipoma about 1.3 cm in diameter was described in a 16-year-old female domestic shorthair that was destroyed for an unrelated illness (Sander and Langham, 1972).

At AMAH splenic myelolipomas were incidental findings in four cats—three castrated male domestic shorthairs, tabby, black, and white, aged 11, 12, and 13 years. The fourth was a 13-year-old spayed female tricolor. None was anemic or had other sites of extramedullary hematopoiesis. Two cats had one nodule, one had two, and one had six. The masses, ranging from 0.7 to 4.0 cm in diameter, were smooth, convex, and soft to firm, bulging on cut surface. They were mottled yellow and brown, yellow and orange, or red and brown.

Microscopic examination revealed well-demarcated but somewhat infiltrative and nonencapsulated nodules of fat and hematopoietic cells. The ratio of the two cell types varied from one nodule to another, even within the same spleen, as did also the numbers of megakaryocytes, granulocytes, and nucleated red cells. Splenic trabeculae were spaced farther apart than in adjacent normal parenchyma. Indications of rapid expansile growth were absent, and adjacent trabeculae were less distorted than with nodular lymphocytic hyperplasia.

In none of the spleens was there extramedullary hematopoiesis. Two had only a few megakaryocytes unassociated with the nodules. One spleen was involved in mast cell neoplasia. In none of the cats were there myelolipomas in other sites.

**BENIGN TUMORS.** Although benign tumors have perhaps been observed or reported in cats, they are apparently extremely rare, and none were on record at AMAH.

**MALIGNANT TUMORS.** Lymphomas, too numerous to count, constitute by far the most common neoplasm of the cat's spleen; mast cell neoplasia is next in frequency (55 cases) at AMAH. While either can take the form of nodular growths, the usual pattern is diffuse, producing uniform enlargement. With lymphoma, the spleen is pale, whereas mast cell infiltrates are typically red-brown, becoming redder with exposure to air. Although primary splenic involvement is possible with both tumors, only a primary mast cell tumor has been documented at AMAH. There is a greater association between cutaneous and splenic growths with mast cell neoplasia (13 of 55 cats) than with malignant lymphoma.

Patnaik et al. (1975) reported four hemangiosarcomas, one neurofibrosarcoma, and one leiomyosarcoma of the spleen. Ten hemangiosarcomas were on record at AMAH and are discussed in the section on tumors of the cardiovascular system.

**SECONDARY TUMORS.** If hematopoietic malignancies and mast cell tumors are excluded, secondary tumors of the spleen are rare in cats but occur more often than primary tumors. Secondary growths seen at AMAH included tumors of mammary gland, lung, kidney, intestine, and pancreas, the last being most numerous (seven).

**BEHAVIOR AND MANAGEMENT.** Splenectomy is of no value for any of the asymptomatic tumor-like masses or for the rare benign tumor unless it is very large. Splenectomy for enlargement due to lymphoma, leukemia, or hemangiosarcoma carries a near-hopeless prognosis, since primary and solitary involvement is extremely rare. However, when the spleen is the sole, or even the principal, site of mast cell malignancy, splenectomy may sometimes prolong life significantly. (See discussion of mast cell tumors and also the chapter on the hematopoietic system.)

The most common cause of splenomegaly in the cat is extramedullary hematopoiesis in response to anemia. Therefore, considering the frequency of latent hemobartonellosis, partial splenectomy or a biopsy may be the diagnostic measure of choice when splenic abnormality is encountered at the time of abdominal surgery.

## Plasma Cell Myeloma and Plasmacytoma*

Plasma cell myeloma (multiple myeloma) is characterized by the proliferation of plasma cells or their precursors, which often produce monoclonal immunoglobulin or a subunit of immunoglobulin. Usually the bone marrow is infiltrated multifocally.

Myeloma is rarely diagnosed in the cat. Single cases have been described by Farrow and Penny (1971), Hay (1978), Holzworth and Meier (1957), Hribernik et al. (1982), Mills et al. (1982), and Saar et al. (1973). In a series study, MacEwen and Hurvitz (1977) at The Animal Medical Center examined the clinical and immunochemical findings in six cats and Drazner (1982) described five cases that were also characterized immunochemically. The 17 cats ranged in age from 6 to 13 years. Eleven were males and nine females. One cat was a Burmese, one a Persian, and one a Manx.

Other cases of myeloma recorded with no details are one of the humerus and tibia in a male cat (Engle and Brodey, 1969), one involving the eye (Peiffer, 1981), three of unspecified site and one involving vertebrae (Priester and McKay, 1980), and one of unspecified site (Theilen and Madewell, 1979).

The clinical signs of plasma cell myeloma are referable to the infiltration of organs by neoplastic plasma cells and the harmful effects of the cells' protein product, termed paraprotein or M component. Infiltration of the bone

*By Margaret L. Harbison.

marrow may result in anemia or granulocytopenia. In one reported case of feline myeloma, leukopenia, nonregenerative anemia, and thrombocytopenia were all found; a bone marrow biopsy revealed solid clusters of plasma cells replacing other marrow constituents (Hribernik et al., 1982).

Osteolytic skeletal lesions are frequent in dogs and humans with the tumor. In one study 56 per cent of dogs with the disease had these lesions (MacEwen and Hurvitz, 1977). Radiologic bone disease is an initial finding in approximately 80 per cent of people with multiple myeloma (Kyle, 1975; Woodruff, 1981). In addition to directly invading bone, neoplastic plasma cells produce osteoclast-activating factor, which plays a significant part in the bone resorption in humans (Durie et al., 1981). Skeletal lesions have been described in only five cats (Engle and Brodey, 1969; Hay, 1978; MacEwen and Hurvitz, 1977; Mills et al., 1982; Priester and McKay, 1980).

Clinical findings such as hepatomegaly or splenomegaly are attributable to infiltration of soft tissues with plasma cells. Microscopically, diffuse or multifocal plasma cell infiltrates in liver, spleen, and lymph nodes have been found at autopsy of cats with the tumor (Farrow and Penny, 1971; Hay, 1978; Holzworth and Meier, 1957; Hribernik et al., 1982).

Abnormalities associated with the production of M component by the plasma cells include bleeding disorders, renal impairment, hyperviscosity syndrome, and decreased production of normal immunoglobulins. Often the presenting sign in dogs with myeloma is a bleeding episode such as epistaxis (Morrison, 1979; Thrall, 1981), since M component can interfere with normal platelet function. Nosebleed was a prominent sign in the feline case reported by Hay (1978). Renal impairment in plasma cell myeloma has many causes, including Bence Jones proteinuria, amyloidosis, and plasma cell infiltration of the kidneys (Woodruff, 1981). Light chains of immunoglobulin in the urine (Bence Jones protein) may damage renal tubules and have been found in eight feline cases (Drazner, 1982; Farrow and Penny, 1971; MacEwen and Hurvitz, 1977); in addition, proteinaceous casts in the renal tubules have been discovered microscopically in three cats (Farrow and Penny, 1971; Hay, 1978; Hribernik et al., 1982). One cat developed a nephrotic syndrome and renal failure, and massive amyloid infiltration of the glomeruli was discovered at autopsy (Drazner, 1982).

The deleterious effects of hyperviscous blood depend on the concentration, size, and shape of M component in the blood. Some of the manifestations of the hyperviscosity syndrome are retinopathy with engorged retinal vessels and hemorrhages, bleeding diathesis, and neurologic disturbances. In The Animal Medical Center and the Drazner studies, none of the 11 cats with myeloma had signs of serum hyperviscosity. More recently reported was a nine-year-old cat with IgG myeloma and a serum viscosity of 6.2 compared with 2.5 for normal cats studied by the authors (Hribernik et al., 1982).

Serum electrophoresis allows detection of M component and is fundamental for the diagnosis of plasma cell myeloma. A monoclonal spike seen with this test can be characterized with immunoelectrophoresis. In the cases in which serum immunoelectrophoresis was done, 13 cats with myeloma had IgG monoclonal gammopathies (Drazner, 1982; Hay, 1978; Hribernik et al., 1982; MacEwen and Hurvitz, 1977; Mills et al., 1982). IgA was the immunoglobulin class in only one cat (Drazner, 1982).

In addition to the case published by Holzworth and Meier (1957), three cases of plasma cell myeloma in cats have been recognized at AMAH. The animals were all castrated males and were 11 or 12 years old. The clinical pictures were dissimilar. The neoplasm in one animal was an unexpected autopsy finding. Treated for cardiomyopathy, this cat had a recent history of behavioral change and then an abrupt onset of severe depression and ataxia that progressed to involve all limbs and the trunk. In addition to cardiac lesions, plasma cell myeloma was discovered at autopsy: an epidural mass at C1 (Fig. 11–41) and a small splenic nodule, both composed of neoplastic plasma cells. Similar to this case was the report of a cat with lumbar pain and bilateral hindleg weakness progressing to paraparesis (Mills et al., 1982). At autopsy, epidural masses at L1 and L4 were found, and microscopically, plasma cells filled the medullary cavities of these vertebrae. Lesions causing spinal cord compression are not uncommon in dogs with myeloma (Werner, 1983).

In a second case at AMAH, a cat was examined because of chronic constipation, poor appetite, and anemia. Biopsy was performed on the palpably thickened small intestine during an exploratory laparotomy. Several firm, gray regions (about 1.5 cm long) in the jejunal wall and a similar lesion (18.0 cm) in the ileum were observed. Histologically the small intestine was diffusely infiltrated with plasma cells. Electrophoresis of the cat's serum showed hypergammaglobulinemia; the urine was negative for Bence Jones protein. Unfortunately, follow-up and further evaluation of this cat were not permitted.

Another cat initially had several small (0.3 cm diameter), raised skin masses on its foreleg and thorax. When many new masses appeared during the following month, biopsies were taken and revealed cutaneous plasmacytomas. A globulin spike was then detected by serum elec-

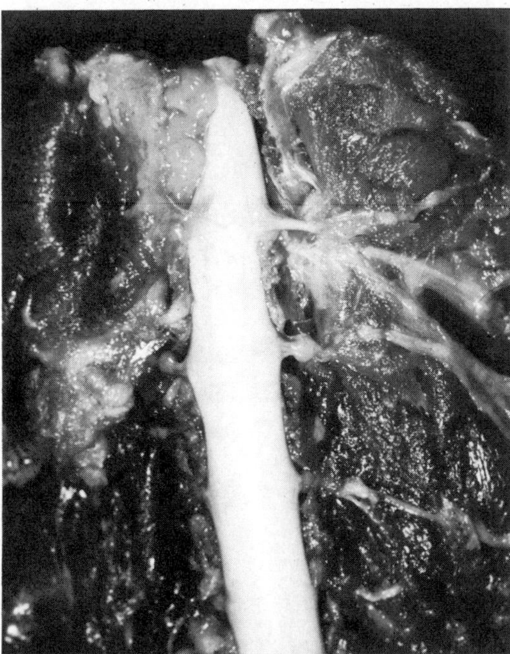

**Figure 11–41** A plasma cell myeloma of the first cervical vertebra extends into the epidural space (upper left) and compresses the spinal cord of an 11-year-old black domestic shorthair.

trophoresis; 55 per cent of the elevated total protein (10.4 gm/dl) was in the alpha globulin region. Leukopenia and anemia were present. Bence Jones proteinuria, radiologic bone disease, and increased numbers of plasma cells in the bone marrow biopsy were not found. However, at autopsy two months later, the plasma cell myeloma involved bone marrow (Fig. 11–42*A*), liver (Fig. 11–42*B*), spleen, and kidneys.

Signs common in the feline cases of myeloma were anorexia, weight loss, listlessness, and fever. Polyuria and polydipsia were sometimes present. Total white-cell counts ranged from leukopenia to leukocytosis. Anemia was usual. Total protein levels ranged as high as 13.8 gm/dl (MacEwen and Hurvitz, 1977).

Most cats died or were destroyed soon after the condition was diagnosed, but one cat's signs were relieved for two months by treatment with prednisolone (Mills et al., 1982). Drazner's five cats were treated with melphalan and prednisone, as well as supportive measures, and survived from four to nine months before being destroyed—two for chronic renal failure, two for deep skin infections (dermatomycosis with secondary bacterial infection; sporotrichosis), and one for nocardial pyothorax. The infections were thought perhaps to be due to impaired immunocompetence.

## TUMORS OF BONE, CARTILAGE, JOINTS, AND TENDON

Primary bone tumors reported in cats are, in order of decreasing frequency, osteosarcoma, osteochondroma and osteochondromatosis, fibrosarcoma, osteoma, chondrosarcoma, juxtacortical (parosteal) osteosarcoma, giant cell tumor, myeloma, and osteoblastoma (Misdorp and van der Heul, 1976; Priester and McKay, 1980; Turrel and Pool, 1982; AMAH collection). Rare tumors of other types recorded in the same four sources are a fibroma, ossifying fibromas of the mandible and digit, and angiomas of thoracic and lumbar vertebrae. Lymphoma, commonly involving marrow but only rarely bone itself, has been excluded as a primary bone tumor because of its frequent multicentric origin. Myeloma is discussed with hematopoietic neoplasia elsewhere in this chapter.

It has been reported that the incidence of bone "cancer" in cats is 4.9 per 100,000, in contrast with 7.9 in dogs (Dorn et al., 1968b). Several other striking differences exist between primary bone tumors of cats and dogs. For example, tumors of long bones are fewer in cats, although they still occur 2.4 times more often than those of the axial skeleton. Reviewing the literature, Turrel and Pool (1982) found that 80 to 90 per cent of primary bone tumors were malignant, while in their group of 15 cases, 67 per cent were malignant. At AMAH about 70 per cent of the primary tumors were malignant.

Major surveys (Misdorp and van der Heul, 1976; Moulton, 1978; Priester and McKay, 1980; Turrel and Pool, 1982) found that osteosarcomas account for 70 to 80 per cent of all primary malignant bone tumors of cats. Osteosarcomas of dogs are more aggressive than those of cats, occurring at an earlier age (7.5 vs. 10.2 years), and have a much higher percentage of metastases (60 vs. 10) (Turrel and Pool, 1982). In contrast with the canine tumors, osteosarcomas of cats occur more often in the hindlimbs than in the forelimbs; microscopically, they often have more multinucleate giant cells. Multiple osteochondromas in cats, unlike those in dogs, develop after skeletal maturity, seldom involve long bones, are rarely symmetric, and appear to be of viral rather than familial origin.

### Osteoma—Ossifying Fibroma—Fibrous Dysplasia

Osteoma, ossifying fibroma, and fibrous dysplasia are benign growths that have a certain degree of morphologic similarity but differ mainly in the amount of bony, fibrous, and vascular tissue (Pool, 1978). Osteoma is a solitary, slow-growing tumor of dense, well-differentiated bone that arises from the surface of bone, the underlying cortex remaining intact (Turrel and Pool, 1982). Ossifying fibroma, by contrast, is an expansile fibro-osseous lesion that replaces alveolar and cortical bone in the maxilla or mandible. Either growth can be asymptomatic or cause damage by pressure. Osteomas, uncommon in all species and occurring most often in the skull, have the largest proportion of bone. The bone of fibrous dysplasia arises by metaplasia of fibrous connective tissue rather than by production by osteoblasts as in osteomas. The ossifying fibroma has an intermediate architecture.

Fourteen cases of osteoma or ossifying fibroma were reviewed by Turrel and Pool (1982). The cats ranged in age from 2 to 12 years (mean 6.5). Seven tumors occurred in the skull, and one each involved the radius, humerus, pelvis, and chest wall; no site was recorded for the other three. Ten osteomas were recorded by Priester and McKay (1980), the site being specified for only one as the vertebral column. An unusual intramedullary osteoma was described as causing a pathologic fracture of the humerus in a 17-year-old female (Quigley and Leedale, 1983). An osteoma of the zygomatic arch in a six-year-old female Siamese was successfully removed (Knecht and Greene, 1977).

At AMAH an ossifying fibroma was removed, without recurrence, from the first toe of a forepaw of a 14-year-old spayed female domestic shorthair (Fig. 11–43).

Operable tumors may be managed surgically. Progression of an ossifying fibroma of the mandible was arrested for over two years by radiotherapy (Turrel and Pool, 1982).

### Osteoid Osteoma

In man this benign lesion has protean manifestations (Spjut et al., 1971). It usually involves the lower limbs of young adults but may affect any bone except sternum, clavicle, and skull. Typical signs are increasing pain, tenderness on palpation, and, if an extremity is involved, a limp. It is often confused with inflammatory conditions. The lesion may be located in cortical, cancellous, or subperiosteal bone. Radiographically, it is characterized by a central nidus, which is usually radiolucent but may have a dense core with a radiolucent periphery. The nidus is surrounded by densely sclerotic bone. Microscopically, the nidus is composed of a maze of tightly packed osteoid trabeculae, often outlined by osteoblasts. Cement lines and small calcified deposits are common, but cartilage is not present. The center of the nidus may be heavily

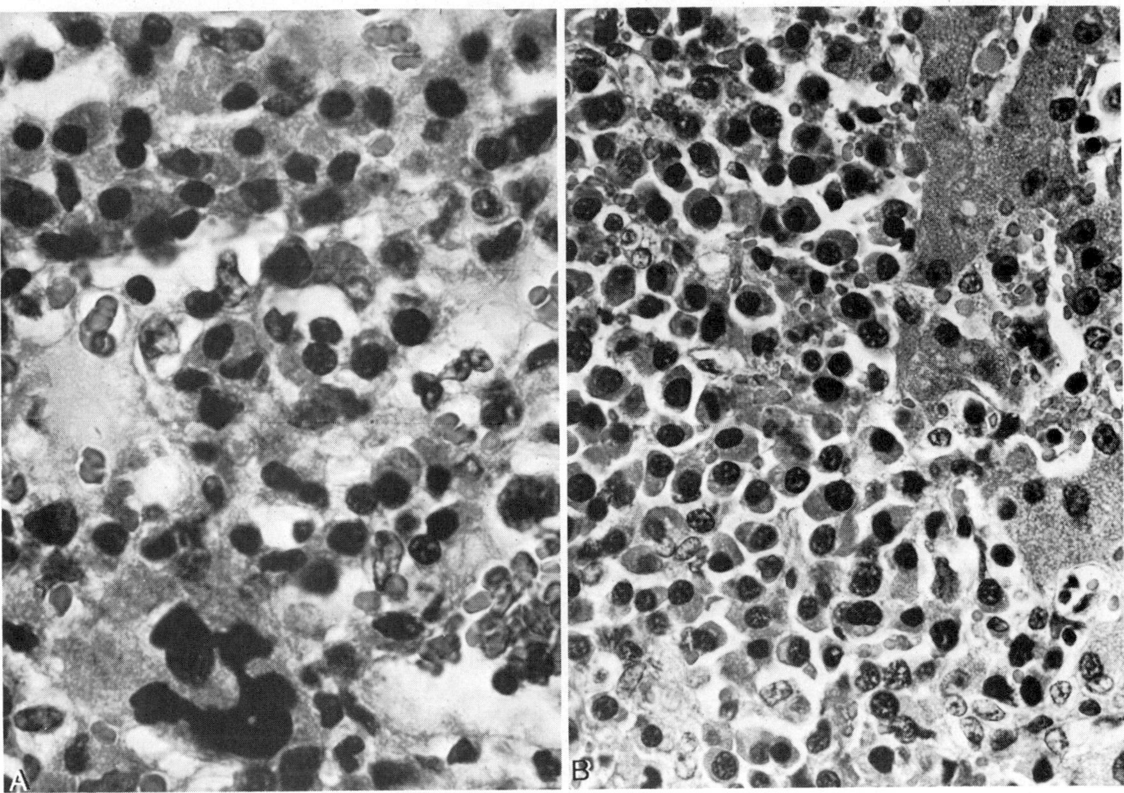

**Figure 11–42** *A*, Multiple myeloma, 11-year-old castrated male domestic longhair. Numerous plasma cells (top and center) and a megakaryocyte (below) are seen in a section of bone marrow. The PCV was 20 per cent; total serum protein was 10.4 gm/dl, of which 55 per cent was gamma globulin. H & E, × 1000. *B*, Myeloma, liver, same cat. Dense aggregates of plasma cells formed 0.1 to 0.3 cm foci throughout the liver. Cords of dissociated hepatocytes are at upper right. H & E, × 1000.

calcified with little, if any mineralization at the periphery. The intertrabecular tissue has a good blood supply provided by small, thin-walled vessels. Osteoclasts, but not fat or hematopoietic cells, are present within the fibrous connective tissue. Block excision is preferred to curettage for the human lesion.

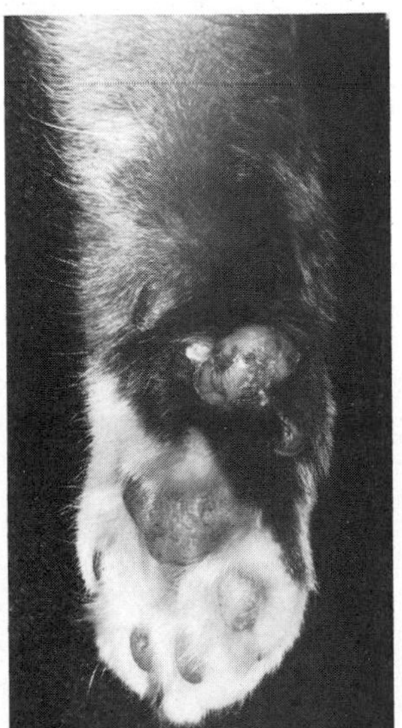

**Figure 11–43** Ossifying fibroma, first digit of left forepaw, 14-year-old spayed female blue-and-white domestic shorthair.

Osteoid osteoma, a rarity in cats, occurred in the body of the tenth thoracic vertebra of a 14-year-old domestic shorthair (Liu et al., 1974). A central rounded zone of increased radiodensity was demarcated by a thin radiolucent zone in an otherwise sclerotic vertebral body. The vertebral body was expanded and compressed the spinal cord, so that the cat ceased jumping and was unable to turn around to lick itself. Microscopically, the central dense core consisted of osteoid trabeculae, fibrous connective tissue, and multinucleated giant cells. The tumor was clearly demarcated from the surrounding sclerotic bone.

## Benign Osteoblastoma

Two vertebral lesions of cats resembling human osteoblastoma were examined by Misdorp and van der Heul (1976). Microscopically, this tumor has many similarities to osteoid osteoma.

## Osteosarcoma

**BREED, AGE, AND SEX.** No breed predisposition for osteosarcoma has been reported. The age range is 1 to 20 years (mean 10.2), and the male:female ratio is 1.7:1 (Turrel and Pool, 1982). At AMAH, 50 cats with osteosarcomas ranged in age from 15 months to 17 years

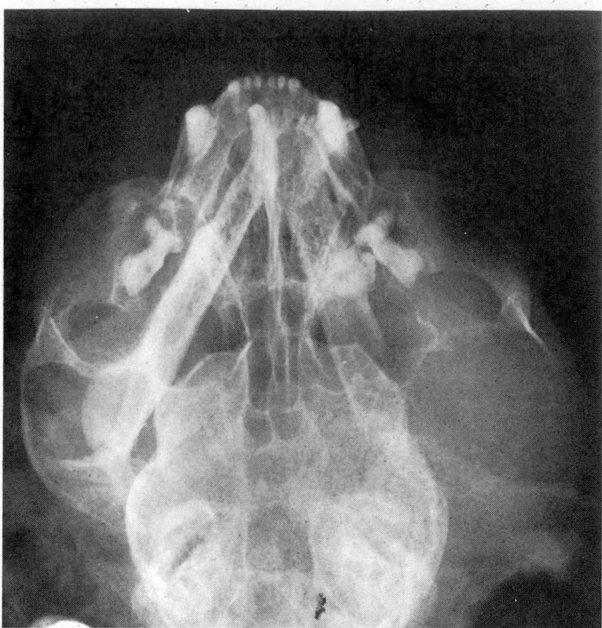

**Figure 11–44** Osteolytic osteosarcoma having numerous multinucleate giant cells involved the angle of the left mandible and zygomatic arch and displaced the left eye, 12-year-old black domestic shorthair.

(mean 10.8). The male:female ratio was 1:1.7, in contrast with that in the previously cited report. The life span of female cats, according to surveys at AMAH, tends to be longer than that of males, and this fact may partly explain why more females at AMAH had osteosarcoma, which is mainly a tumor of the aged cat.

**SITES.** Data compiled from 15 veterinary schools (Priester and McKay, 1980) listed 29 osteosarcomas of cats, eight involving the face and cranium, six the hindlimbs, four the scapula or forelimbs, two the vertebrae, one the nose, and eight in sites not specified. A literature review and a study of 15 additional cats, three of which had osteosarcoma (Turrel and Pool, 1982), revealed that feline osteosarcomas 2.4 times more often involve the appendicular skeleton than the axial skeleton and that hindlimbs are 1.6 times more frequently involved than forelimbs. The most common long bone sites are the distal femur, proximal humerus, and proximal tibia. The skull, vertebrae, scapula, and pelvis are the flat and irregular bones most often affected. Of 50 osteosarcomas at AMAH, sites of origin were frontal bone (seven), proximal tibia (six), distal femur (five), proximal humerus (four), vertebrae (three: C3, L4, and sacrum), rib (three), mandible (three) (Fig. 11–44), maxilla, pelvis (Fig. 11–45) and proximal femur (two each), scapula, distal radius, distal ulna, carpus, metacarpus, distal tibia, hock, distal rear phalanx, nasal bone, maxilla, zygomatic arch, calvaria, and temporal bone (one each). In summary, of the 50 osteosarcomas, 28 involved the appendicular skeleton, mainly tibia, femur, and humerus, and 22 the axial skeleton (skull 15), making the appendicular:axial skeletal ratio 1.4:1 in contrast to the 2.4:1 reported by Turrel and Pool (1982). The hindlimbs were affected 1.9 times more often than the forelimbs.

**CLINICAL FEATURES.** The duration of clinical signs before examination ranged from one hour to nine months (mean 2.25 months), which is close to the three months previously reported (Turrel and Pool, 1982). The cat with signs for only an hour was asymptomatic until it jumped into a snowbank and suffered a pathologic fracture of the proximal tibia. It is surprising that the two cats with signs of nine months' duration did not receive attention sooner. One had an 11 × 8 × 6 cm mass of the proximal humerus, the other a bulging tumor of the frontal bone that displaced the left cerebral hemisphere, causing compression atrophy of both hemispheres, incoordination, and poor vision.

In the group generally, the most common initial signs were deformity and lameness with limb or spinal lesions, and deformity of the skull if the head was involved. Signs were also influenced by the size and location of the tumor. A previously cantankerous 13-year-old cat with a tumor of the frontal bone compressing the cerebrum became friendly and affectionate (to the surprise of the owner), developed unilateral exophthalmos, and had periods of blank gazing (Fig. 11–46).

In man and dogs, osteosarcoma occasionally develops

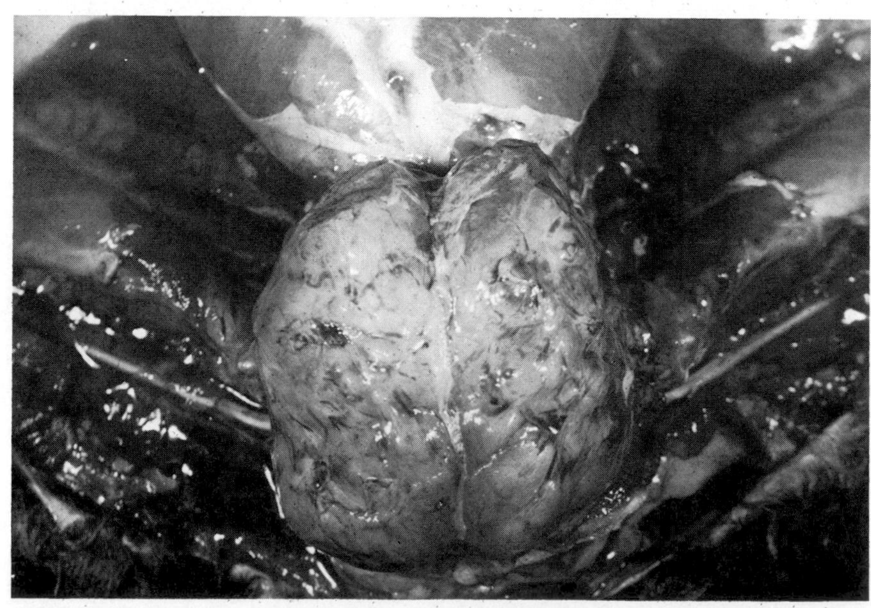

**Figure 11–45** Osteosarcoma, pubic region, 15-year-old tabby. The bilobed tumor (center) destroyed the pelvic floor, compressed the rectum, and caused obstipation with distention of the abdomen (upper center).

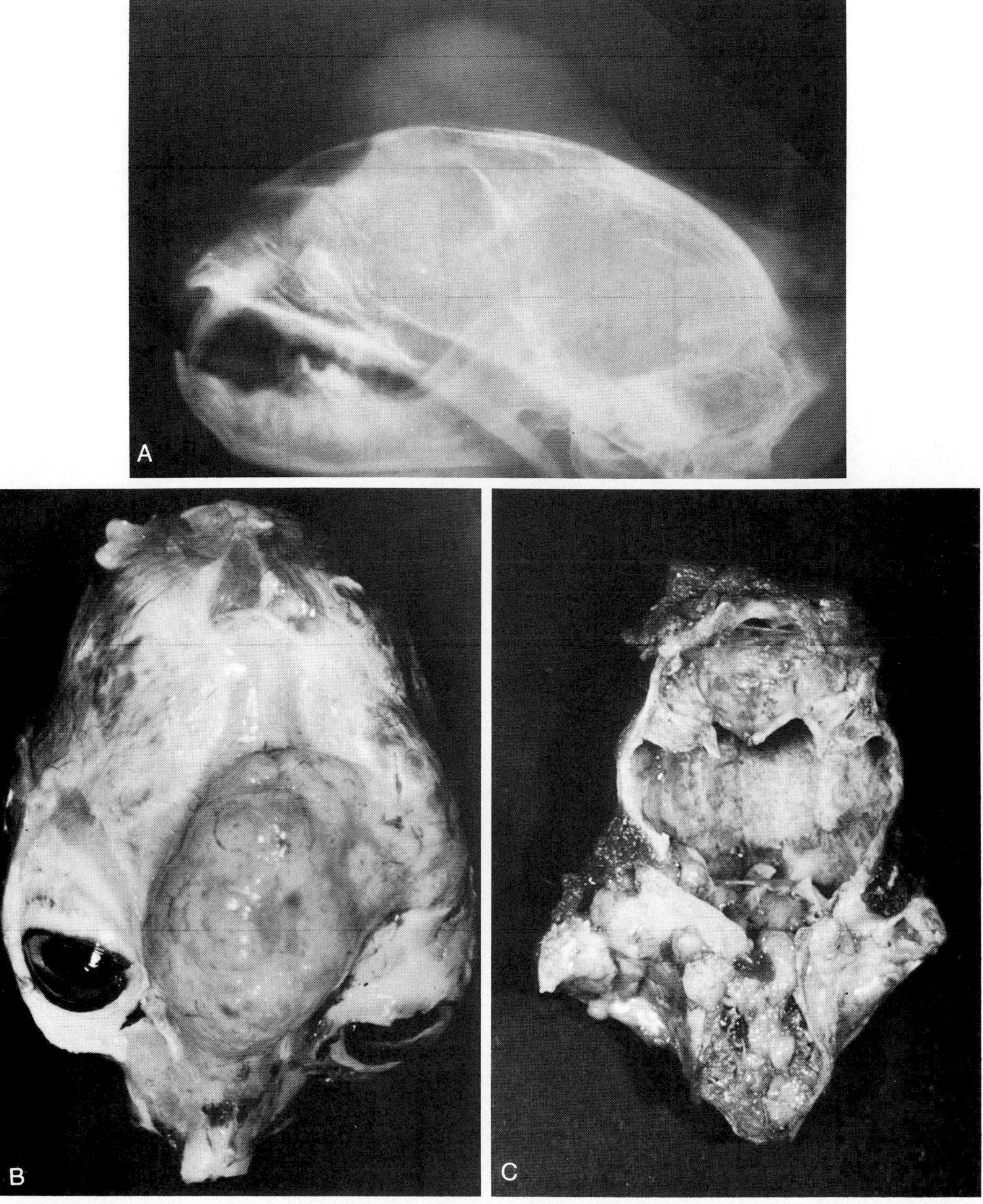

**Figure 11–46** *A*, Osteosarcoma, skull, 13-year-old black-and-white cat. The tumor involved the frontal bones, frontal sinuses, nasal cavity, left orbit, and cranial vault; compressed and displaced the cerebrum; and evoked behavioral changes. *B*, Osteosarcoma, shown in *A*. The pale, firm, elevated, and irregular-surfaced tumor covered most of the frontal bones and caused exophthalmos of the left eye. *C*, Osteosarcoma, shown in *A* and *B*. The tumor invaded the sinuses, nasal cavity, and left orbit and deformed and reduced the cranial vault.

at the site of a previous bone injury repaired by internal fixation. In a 16-year-old cat, a pathologic fracture due to a femoral tumor arose close to the site of a traumatic fracture that had occurred six months before and had been repaired with an intramedullary pin (Bennett et al., 1979). In two cats osteosarcomas were associated with severe osteodystrophies related to excessive feeding of liver (Brodey, 1970). Osteogenic sarcoma, as well as hemangiosarcoma of bone, developed in a cat that had been subjected to irradiation (Berman and Wright, 1973).

**RADIOGRAPHIC FEATURES.** Osteosarcomas can be classified radiographically as sclerosing osteogenic sarcomas when the osteoid is mineralized, or as osteolytic sarcomas when there is destruction with little or no bone formation. Telangiectatic or highly vascularized osteosarcomas also have an osteolytic appearance.

The majority of osteosarcomas of cats are osteolytic. Many appear completely so and are accompanied by an extraosseous soft tissue density (Fig. 11–47); others have minimal subperiosteal bone formation (Fig. 11–48). Osteolysis predisposes to pathologic fractures (Fig. 11–49) resulting in sudden lameness that may be the first indication of long-standing, undetected bone tumor. Not surprisingly, osteolysis is the outstanding radiographic feature of feline osteosarcomas, because the conspicuous microscopic features of the 50 at AMAH were a predominant fibrosarcomatous component (66 per cent), cartilage formation (28 per cent), and numerous multinucleate giant cells (50 per cent). All such components, as well as accumulation of malignant osteoblasts, appear radiographically as soft tissue densities.

Elevation of the cortical periosteum with formation of subperiosteal reactive woven bone adjacent to the tumor (Codman's triangle) (Fig. 11–49) is infrequent in feline osteosarcomas. Another striking difference from osteosarcomas of dogs is the lower incidence of radiographically recognizable metastatic lesions; metastases occur later and less often in cats.

**GROSS FEATURES.** Most osteosarcomas of cats at AMAH were firm or hard, and painless. They ranged in size from a 0.6 cm diameter nodule of the fourth lumbar vertebra compressing the spinal cord to a mass 38 cm in circumference that replaced the proximal femur. The majority measured from 4 to 12 cm in greatest dimension. Most were gray-white and varied from fibrous to bony on cut surface. Osteolysis, sometimes with complete loss of large segments of original bone, predominated over osteogenesis.

Metastases occur with 60 per cent of canine osteosarcomas but were reported in less than 10 per cent of cats with osteosarcoma (Turrel and Pool, 1982). In the 50 cats at AMAH, metastatic lesions were recognized at autopsy

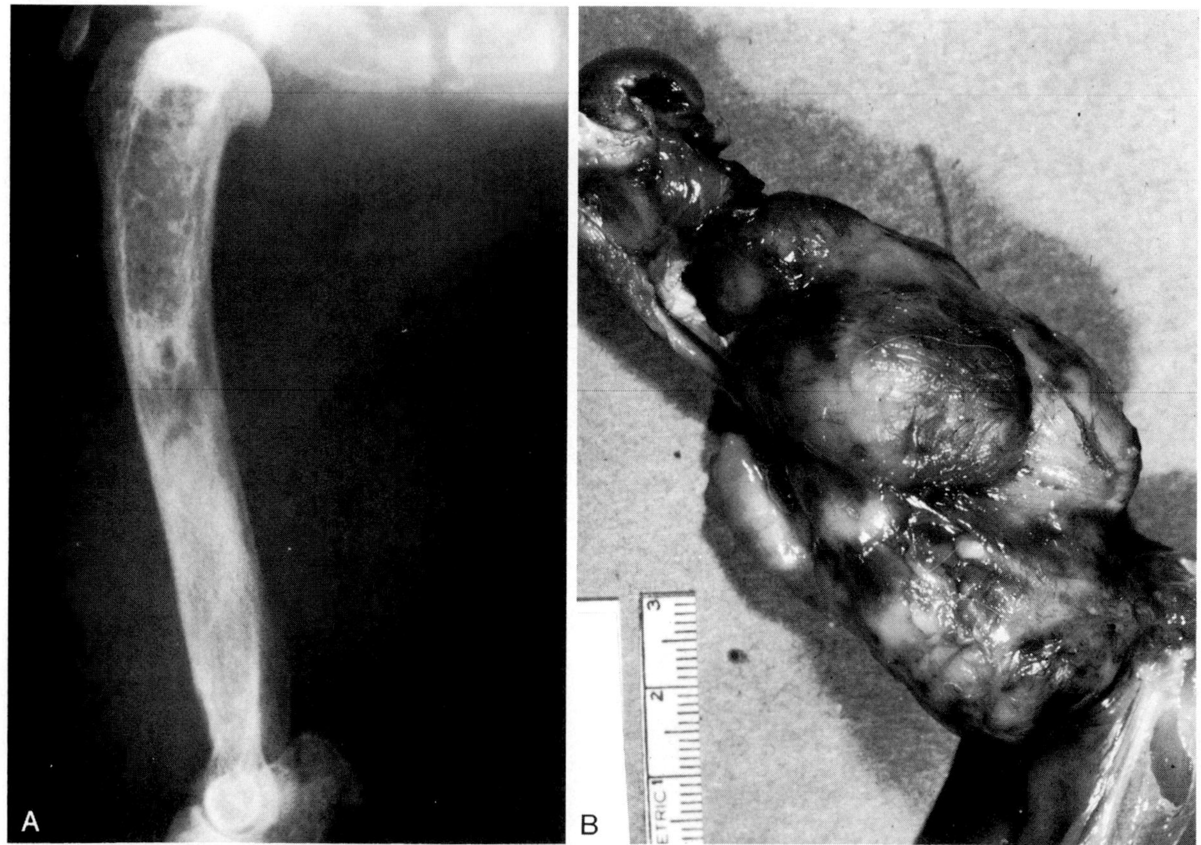


**Figure 11–47** *A*, Osteosarcoma, humerus, 14-year-old spayed female Persian. The proximal half of the bone has numerous lytic areas without bone proliferation. Excess soft-tissue density surrounds most of the humerus. *B*, Osteosarcoma, same cat. Massive multinodular tumor surrounds all but the humeral head (upper left). The neoplasm was composed of abundant fibrosarcomatous and chondrosarcomatous tissues, and only occasional small foci of malignant osseous tissue justified its classification as an osteosarcoma.

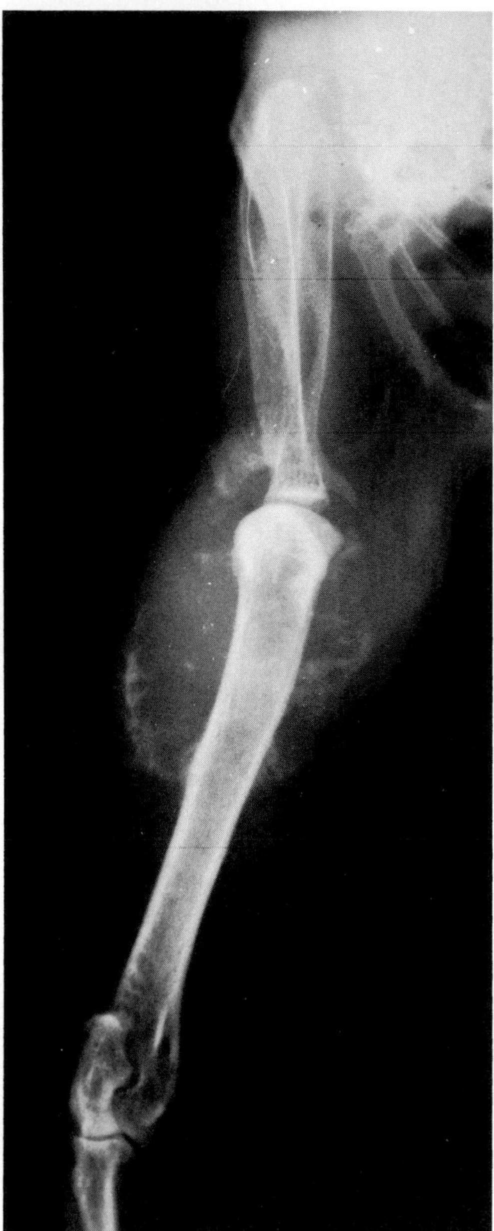

**Figure 11–48** Osteosarcoma, proximal left humerus, 12-year-old longhair tabby. The non-bony portions of the tumor were fibrosarcomatous with many multinucleate giant cells. No metastases were found at autopsy.

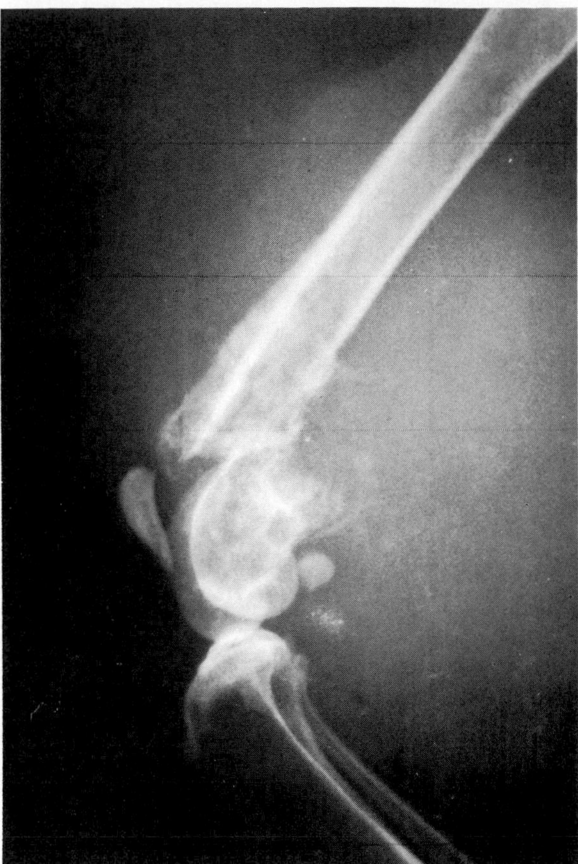

**Figure 11–49** Osteosarcoma and pathologic fracture of a distal femur in a 10-year-old cat that had pulmonary metastases. Osteolytic foci in the diaphysis, metaphysis, and epiphysis consisted of malignant nonmineralized osteoid, cartilage, and many multinucleate giant cells. Benign subperiosteal bone proliferation can be seen as Codman's triangle on the cranial surface of the proximal fragment.

in five, but only 25 of the 50 came to autopsy, many being lost to follow-up. Metastases occurred in the lungs (five), pleura (two), kidney (one), and iliac node (one). Others have reported metastases in lungs, kidneys, liver, brain, and spleen (Turrel and Pool, 1982). Hypertrophic pulmonary osteoarthropathy has apparently not been reported with osteosarcoma in the cat.

**MICROSCOPIC FEATURES.** Osteosarcomas consist of variable amounts of sarcomatous stroma, malignant osteoid, and bone. Malignant cartilaginous tissue may also be present and, in some osteosarcomas, may predominate. The sarcomatous stroma may contain so little osteoid as to resemble a fibrosarcoma (Fig. 11–50*A*), or it may contain abundant irregular islands of osteoid, permitting easy identification of the tumor (Fig. 11–50*B*). The presence of even a small amount of malignant osteoid dictates the diagnosis of osteosarcoma. Multinucleate giant cells may be so numerous in some feline osteosarcomas as to give the impression of a giant cell tumor; however, their nuclear features, in contrast to those of giant cell tumors of bone, differ from those of the rest of the cells composing the osteosarcoma (Fig. 11–50*C*). Mitotic figures can usually be found in all types of osteosarcoma. Remnants of original bone may be seen within the tumor, and the surrounding soft tissues may be compressed or infiltrated. Reactive subperiosteal cortical bone proliferation is frequent.

Of the 50 osteosarcomas in the AMAH group, 33 had one or more conspicuous fibrosarcomatous regions, 14 had areas of cartilage formation, 25 had an obvious giant cell component, and 2 had prominent cavernous blood vessels. Regional variations in pattern and cell type within the same tumor were often a striking feature that emphasized the need for examining large, or preferably multiple, sections to permit accurate identification of the tumor.

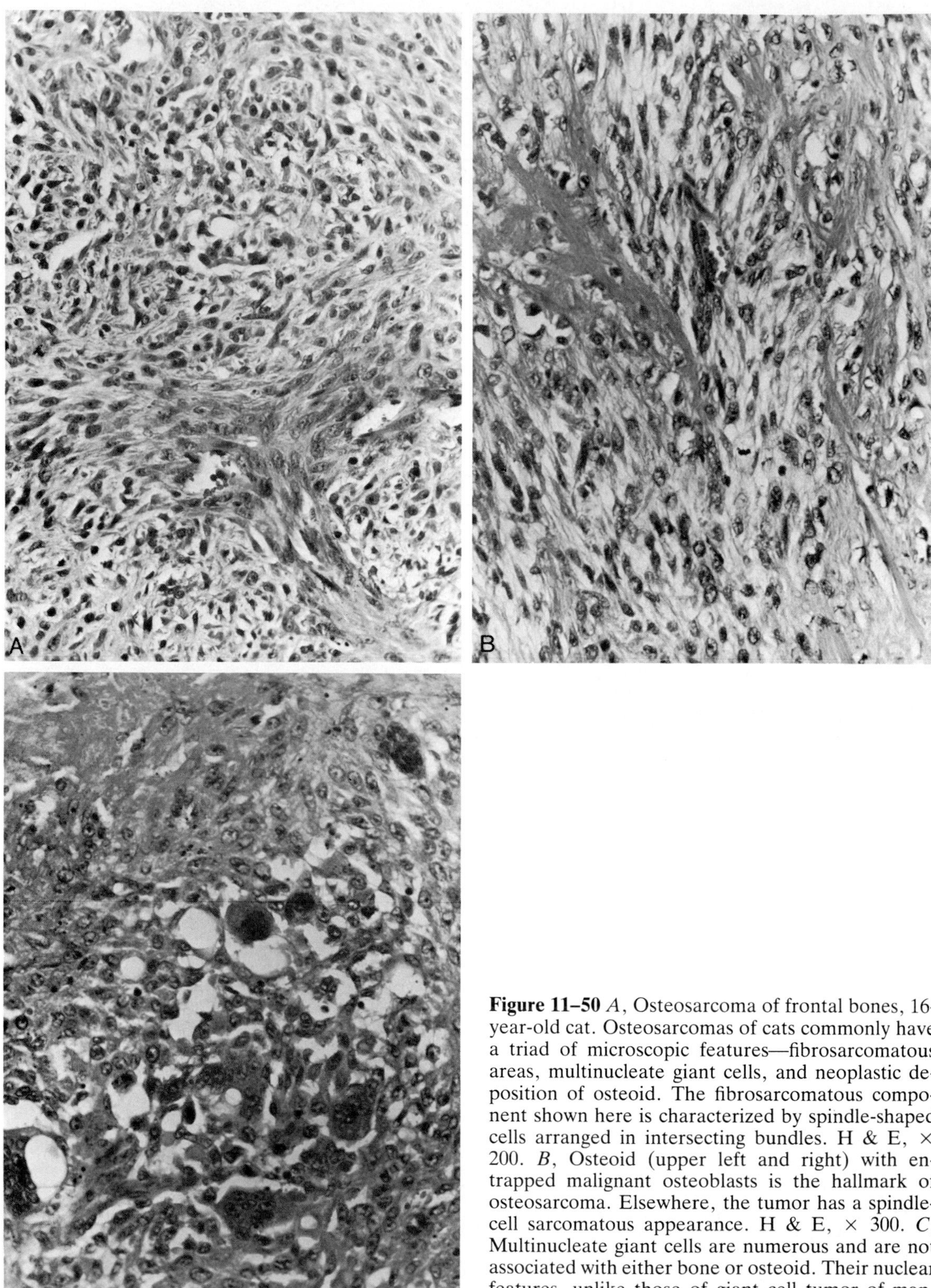


**Figure 11–50** *A*, Osteosarcoma of frontal bones, 16-year-old cat. Osteosarcomas of cats commonly have a triad of microscopic features—fibrosarcomatous areas, multinucleate giant cells, and neoplastic deposition of osteoid. The fibrosarcomatous component shown here is characterized by spindle-shaped cells arranged in intersecting bundles. H & E, × 200. *B*, Osteoid (upper left and right) with entrapped malignant osteoblasts is the hallmark of osteosarcoma. Elsewhere, the tumor has a spindle-cell sarcomatous appearance. H & E, × 300. *C*, Multinucleate giant cells are numerous and are not associated with either bone or osteoid. Their nuclear features, unlike those of giant cell tumor of man, are not identical to the nuclei of adjacent uninucleated neoplastic cells. H & E, × 300.

Variable features, in addition to sarcomatous pattern, cartilage, and giant cells, were the amount of intercellular matrix, orderliness of cellular distribution, degree of mineralization of osteoid, degree of necrosis of tumor and bone, and amount of benign reactive bone and proliferating collagen.

**DIAGNOSIS.** Radiographic features of osteosarcoma are suggestive but not pathognomonic. Radiographs of osteosarcomas at a variety of sites are shown in Figures 11–51 to 11–54. Microscopic examination of biopsy tissue, amputated specimens, or autopsy material is necessary to establish the diagnosis. Among the 40 feline bone tumors cited in the WHO Bulletin (Misdorp and van der Heul, 1976), some were reported to be particularly difficult to classify. The same was true of some tumors in the collection at AMAH. The number of sections of a tumor examined, as well as choice of sample(s) and the diagnostic prowess of the viewer, strongly influence the accuracy of diagnosis. Differentiating a fibrosarcoma from an anaplastic osteosarcoma with little osteoid can be a tremendous challenge. Errors have occurred when osteosarcomas with minimal osteoid and abundant cartilage have been classified as chondrosarcomas rather than being identified on the basis of the most differentiated component (osteoid) (Linnabary et al., 1978). Correlation of biopsy specimens with pre- and post-biopsy radiographs is a vital part of the examination. Post-biopsy radiographs are desirable to ensure that the surgeon has provided the pathologist with an appropriate sample. Many superficial or eccentric biopsy specimens from malignant bone tumors are composed only of benign reactive bony and fibrous tissue.

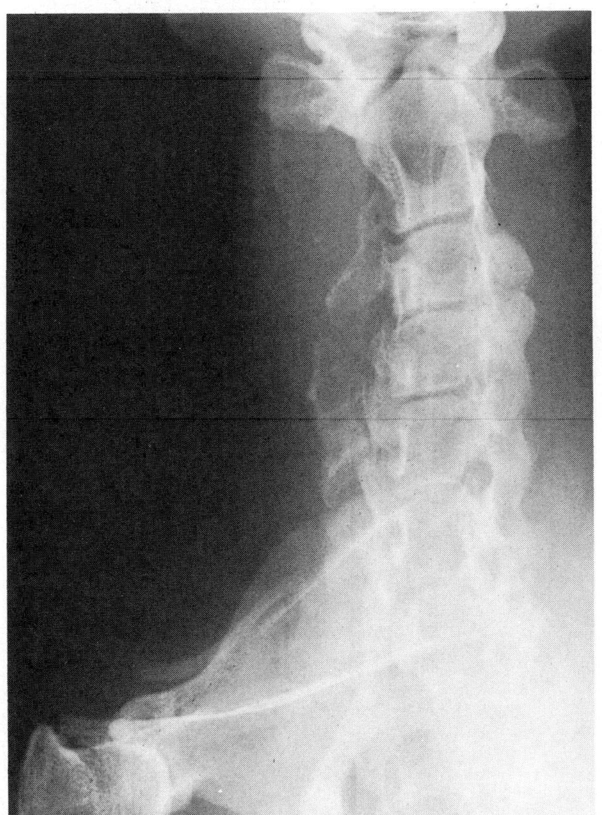

**Figure 11–51** Osteosarcoma, vertebrae C3–C5, seven-year-old cat. Lysis of the right transverse processes, most severe in C4, was associated with lysis of the body of C4, compression of the spinal cord, cervical pain, and stiff and stumbling gait of the forelegs.

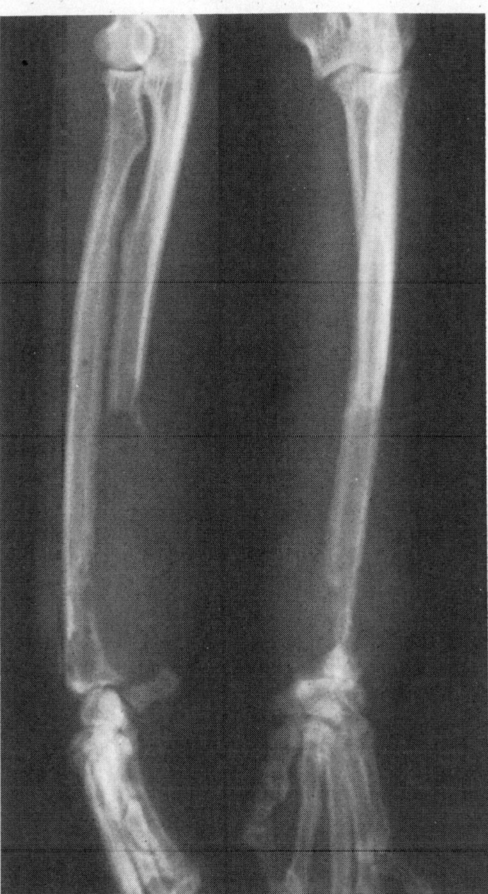

**Figure 11–52** Osteosarcoma, distal ulna and radius, in a 14-year-old domestic shorthair with a lameness of three months' duration. The bones were replaced by an osteolytic tumor having abundant fibrosarcomatous tissue and minimal mineralization of malignant osteoid.

The problem of differentiating an osteosarcoma with numerous giant cells from a giant cell tumor also needs clarification, and the latter diagnosis should be made with caution, until there is a universal understanding among veterinary pathologists about the criteria for diagnosing a giant cell tumor of bone.

Only two cats among the 50 with osteosarcoma at AMAH were tested for FeLV, and both tested negative. Osteosarcoma has not to date been associated with a virus, in contrast with osteochondromatosis of cats.

**PROGNOSIS.** As already noted, osteosarcomas of cats appear to be less aggressive and less apt to metastasize than those of dogs. If an osteosarcoma is in an operable site and there is no evidence of metastasis, amputation may be lifesaving. In one case, a tumor of the distal femur was resected and replaced with an allograft (Herron, 1983). One year later the cat was alive and showing no signs of tumor or lameness.

Limited trials with postoperative chemotherapy have been conducted in dogs and a few cats. Immunotherapy

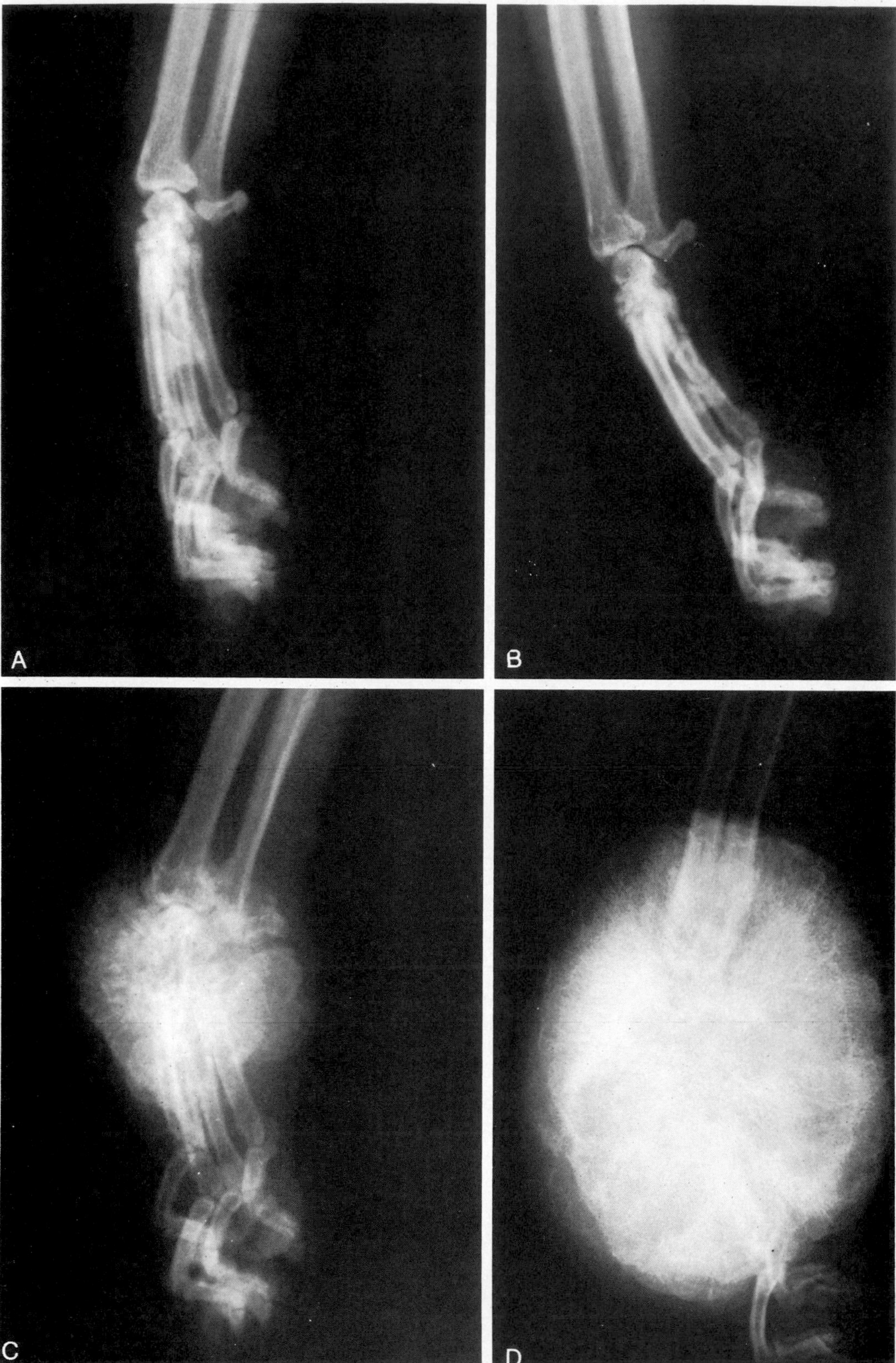


**Figure 11–53** *A*, Osteosarcoma in the left carpal bones of a lame four-year-old black domestic longhair. Minimal change with possible loss of joint spaces was the only observation recorded. *B*, Three weeks later, osteolysis and fuzzy mineralized exostoses of carpal bones were barely apparent. Biopsy at this time suggested benign bony proliferation. *C*, Seven months later, destruction of carpal bones and extensive circumferential osteogenesis prompted a second biopsy, which revealed an osteosarcoma. The owner refused amputation at this time. *D*, Eleven and a half months after the first radiograph (shown in *A*). The leg was amputated and the cat was reported to be well two and a half years after surgery.

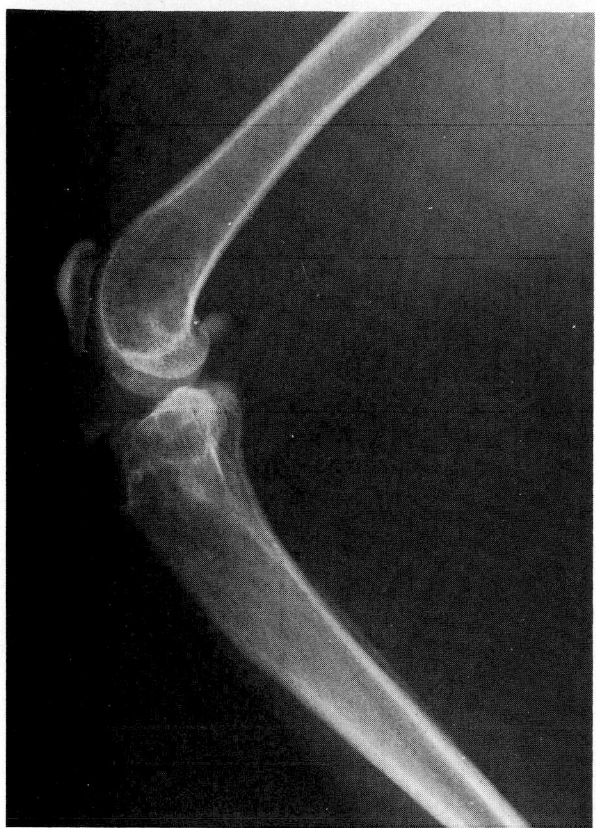

**Figure 11–54** Osteolytic osteosarcoma and avulsion of the tibial tuberosity, seven-year-old domestic longhair. The lytic foci consisted of solid masses of malignant osteoblasts with a small amount of nonmineralized osteoid. Cartilage formation and multinucleate cells were absent.

with BCG vaccine appeared to lengthen survival time in one trial with dogs. These studies are reviewed by Theilen and Madewell (1979). In a few cases treated by irradiation, results were poor, partly, it was believed, because of the stress of repeated anesthesias (Theilen and Madewell, 1979; Turrel and Pool, 1982). Successful treatment of osteogenic sarcoma of the nasal cavity with surgery followed by radiation and metronidazole has been described (Lord et al., 1982).

## Juxtacortical (Parosteal) Osteosarcoma

This malignant growth arises from periosteum. Since it is composed of well-differentiated fibrous, osseous, and in some cases cartilaginous tissues, it has also been called an ossifying perosteal sarcoma (Spjut et al., 1971).

Juxtacortical osteosarcoma of man is often a large, irregular, bosselated, firm mass intimately adherent to the periosteum and cortex (Spjut et al., 1971). It may, after prolonged growth, destroy the cortex; less often it extends into the medulla. The abundant osseous component accounts for the marked radiographic tumor density. Without radiography, parosteal osteosarcoma may be difficult to distinguish from osteochrondroma (especially an older lesion) in which the cartilaginous cap becomes attenuated or disappears, and from myositis ossificans and ossifying fibrodysplasia. Most biopsy specimens, if interpreted without radiographic findings, would be called benign because of the benign appearance of the fibrous and bony tissues (Spjut et al., 1971).

A similar warning applies to the veterinary pathologist, who must be aware of the hazard of being misled by benign-appearing core biopsies, with the result that the parosteal osteosarcoma is mistaken for osteochondroma.

Currently parosteal osteosarcoma is a poorly defined entity of domestic animals, and further study is necessary to determine whether this parosteal tumor of animals is analogous to the human parosteal osteosarcoma in clinical behavior and in radiographic and histomorphologic appearance (Pool, 1978).

Seventeen cases were reviewed by Turrel and Pool (1982), two of them cases studied by the authors. Ten cats were male and seven female, ranging in age from 1 to 14 years (mean 6.6). No breed predisposition was apparent. Both skull and long bones were involved, although in man the tumor is reported to occur most often around the distal metaphysis of long bones. In the two cats studied by Turrel and Pool (1982), the tumor involved the diaphysis of a humerus and a femur, respectively, appearing radiographically as a spiculated osteoblastic mass that had elicited no host bone involvement. In early stages a radiolucent line is described as separating the cortical bone from the tumor.

In comparison with osteosarcoma, this is a slow-growing tumor of cats with a clinical course averaging almost a year. When it involves the limb it causes lameness. In the four cats examined for metastasis, none was found.

## Giant Cell Tumor (Osteoclastoma)

A few giant cell tumors of bone have been reported for the cat, but whether they are genuinely comparable to those of man is at present open to some question.

The giant cell tumor of man occurs mainly in persons 20 to 50 years of age and is a lytic and expansile tumor of the epiphysis of long bones (Spjut et al., 1971). If a tumor arises in the metaphysis in man, it almost certainly is not a giant cell tumor. The human tumor is benign in over 90 per cent of cases and is successfully treated by curettage and bone chip implantation and sometimes also by radiation. In man, the multinucleate giant cells have been shown by histochemical technique and electron microscopy to be osteoclasts—hence the synonym osteoclastoma. Not all the foregoing criteria have been met for published feline giant cell tumors of bone. A similar caution has been voiced by Cotchin (1983) in a discussion of his group of feline bone tumors. "Some limb bone tumours showed prominent giant cell formation but did not tally in structure with the osteoclastoma of man."

Skeletal tumors of cats diagnosed as giant cell tumors have appeared in a number of surveys and reports (Cotchin, 1956b; Crocker, 1941; Howard and Kenyon, 1967; McClelland, 1941; Pool, 1978; Popp and Simpson, 1976; Thornburg, 1979; Turrel and Pool, 1982; Whitehead, 1967). At least three of the reported cases had similar radiographic features characterized by intramedullary origin, marked lysis of the cortex and trabeculae of the metaphysis, indistinct margins, little periosteal reaction, and pathologic fractures (Turrel and Pool, 1982). In one of those cases, pulmonary and renal metastases were seen (Howard and Kenyon, 1967).

In the same three reported cases, the presence of multinucleate cells, together with round or oval cells and variable numbers of spindle cells, was the principal criterion for the diagnosis of giant cell tumor. It must be cautioned, however, that multinucleate cells can occur in a wide variety of tumors as well as reparative granulomas, and designating a mass as a giant cell tumor may be more descriptive than informative as to the true tumor type. The radiographic appearance and, more importantly, the biologic behavior should determine whether a well-defined pathologic entity of giant cell tumor has been identified in cats. Many osteosarcomas and fibrosarcomas of cats have multinucleate giant cells, so that it is difficult to be confident that a given tumor warrants classification as a giant cell tumor. Many more "giant cell" tumors of cats with long-term follow-ups are needed before such classification is meaningful.

Numerous C-type viral particles were found budding from cells of a giant cell tumor occurring in the distal ulna of a young male cat (Popp and Simpson, 1976). This finding, together with the viral association in osteochondromatosis, as well as the well-documented existence of a mouse osteosarcoma virus, suggests that feline bone tumors should be studied closely for a possible viral etiology.

## Osteochondroma and Osteochondromatosis

A tumor of special interest in cats is the osteochondroma, which may occur singly or multicentrically (osteochondromatosis, multiple cartilaginous exostoses). Although the tumor occurs in man, horse, and dog, only the cat's tumor has an apparent viral etiology. Nearly all cats with the polyostotic form of osteochondroma that have been tested for FeLV have tested positive. In tumors that have been examined by electron microscopy or immunofluorescence, C-type viral particles have been found in the cartilaginous cap of the neoplasm (Pool and Carrig, 1972; Pool and Harris, 1975). In other species, osteochondromatosis is inherited, and tumors occur most often on growing long bones opposite or near areas of cartilaginous growth plates, often in a bilaterally symmetric distribution. Growth of the tumor usually ceases when skeletal growth stops. In the cat, by contrast, the tumor develops after cessation of skeletal growth and involves flat or irregular bones more often than long bones. Malignant transformation with metastases is rare in the cat and other species and is signaled by a period of sudden rapid growth and change in shape.

**BREED, AGE, AND SEX.** Inheritance does not seem to play an etiologic role in osteochondroma of cats. The cats in three reported early cases (Riddle and Leighton, 1970; Brown et al., 1972; Pool and Carrig, 1972) were Siamese, but in cases since reported there does not seem to be a breed predisposition. Three of 19 cats at AMAH were Siamese. No sex predilection was evident among the cases reviewed by Turrel and Pool (1982). In the group of 13 cats at AMAH with single osteochondromas, six were males, seven were females. Of those with osteochondromatosis, three were males and three were females.

The age range of the cats with single tumors in the published reports cited was from 4 to 12 years. Cats with osteochondromatosis were aged 1.3 to 8 years (mean 3.2). The 13 cats at AMAH with a single tumor were aged 1 to 11 years (mean 6.3), while the six with multiple tumors ranged in age from 1.5 to 6 (mean 3.2). These figures suggest that multiple tumors may be more likely to occur in younger cats, and it will be of interest in future studies to learn whether this group more often tests positive for FeLV.

**CLINICAL FEATURES.** Signs of tumor depend on the location, size, and number of osteochondromas. In reported cases generally, any bone in the body may be involved. Rather rapidly progressive bony enlargements have often developed to conspicuous disfigurement before a cat evinces mechanical disability or pain. In an unusual case described by Turrel (1979), sneezing dislodged nodules of tumor from the nasal passage.

In cats seen at AMAH, tumors of the limbs caused disfigurement and locomotor signs. A cat with a tumor of the scapula also proved to have tumors of cervical vertebrae and the nasal turbinates (Fig. 11–55). Massive involvement of cranial ribs also led to lameness. The largest scapular tumor, 14.0 × 7.3 × 6.5 cm, caused loss of balance as well as severe limb atrophy and loss of function. Tumors of the facial bones interfered with mastication and respiration (Fig. 11–56). One of four cervical vertebral tumors in a one and a half-year-old domestic shorthair compressed the spinal cord so that tetraparesis resulted.

In a five-year-old Siamese, two osteochondromas, grossly resembling meningiomas, arose in the cerebral dura mater along the longitudinal and transverse venous sinuses, giving rise to stupor, central blindness, and episodes of opisthotonos related to cerebral and cerebellar pressure atrophy and brain edema. Asymptomatic osteochondromas also involved four ribs.

Dyspnea due to chylothorax occurred in a six-year-old male domestic shorthair and was successfully relieved by ligation of the thoracic duct. Three months later the cat again became dyspneic, and radiographs disclosed intrathoracic masses with mineralization. At exploratory surgery, a bonelike cranial mediastinal mass was found, as well as three nodules on the thoracic surface of the diaphragm. Microscopic study revealed lymphoma and osteochondroma of soft tissues intermingled at both sites. The liver was extensively infiltrated with lymphoma. The cat was FeLV-positive, as were two of three others that were tested.

**SITES.** Bones involved in the AMAH group of 13 single tumors included scapula, the tumor apparently arising from the spine (four), angle of the mandible (two), distal femur (two), proximal tibia (one), rib (one), coccygeal vertebra (one), maxilla with projection into the nasal cavity (one), and humerus, medial epicondyle (one).

In the six cats with osteochondromatosis, tumor distribution was as follows: (1) maxillary turbinates, occipital bone, four cervical vertebrae, scapula; (2) cerebral dura of the longitudinal and transverse sinuses, left ribs 9 and 13, right ribs 4 and 9; (3) scapula, rib; (4) maxillary turbinate, proximal tibia; (5) turbinates, temporal bone, scapula, lumbar vertebra 7, ilium; and (6) cranial mediastinum and diaphragm without apparent bone involvement.

**RADIOGRAPHIC FEATURES.** Radiographic features in reported cases and also as exemplified in the AMAH group have been well described (Pool, 1981). Osteochondromas appear as sessile or pedunculated excrescences from the surfaces of bones, their margins blending evenly with the cortical surfaces, while their bony substance merges imperceptibly. They tend to arise toward the ends of the diaphyses or in the metaphyses of ribs and long bones. Epiphyses are rarely affected. The

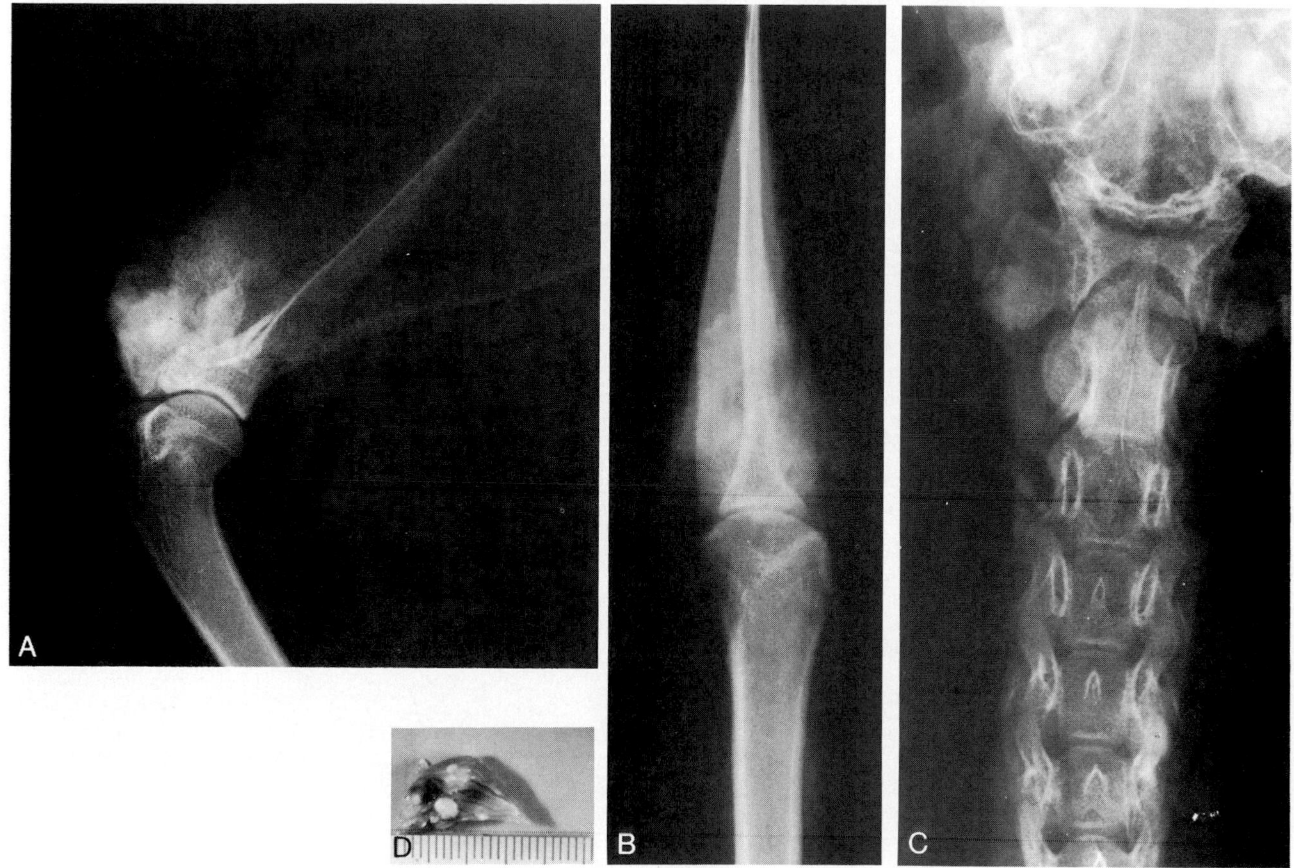


**Figure 11–55** *A*, Osteochondroma of the scapula in a one and a half-year-old FeLV-positive black cat that had a visible, hard, shoulder mass and lameness for five weeks. The lateral view shows an irregular, multinodular, radiodense mass originating at the neck of the scapula and sparing the joint. *B*, Anteroposterior view of the autopsy specimen. The osteogenic mass extends beyond both medial and lateral surfaces of the scapula. *C*, In the same cat a tumor of the axis, one of four cervical vertebral osteochondromas, caused compression of the spinal cord and ataxia. The two tumors on the wings of the atlas and the one on the left transverse process of C5 were clinically silent. *D*, Osteochondromas in a maxillary turbinate, same cat. Many discrete, glistening white, hard tumors measuring up to 0.4 cm involved both nasal passages but had not caused respiratory signs.

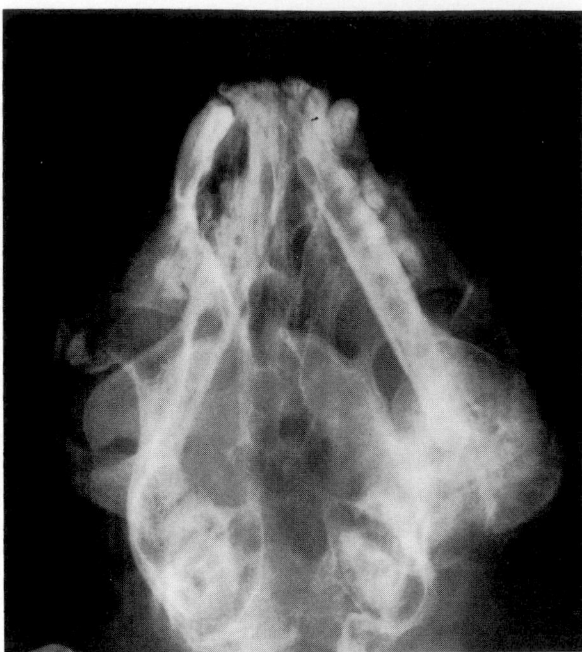

**Figure 11–56** Osteochondroma, left coronoid process of the mandible, 11-year-old tabby. The tumor had been growing for six months and interfered with prehension and mastication.

shape of affected tubular bones is typically unaltered, although the metaphyses sometimes exhibit irregular expansion.

Lesions on limbs may arise as spurs with a flat, domed, or bosselated apex. Sessile osteochrondromas, frequent on vertebral spines, ribs, scapulae, and occasionally long bones, may be smoothly contoured and cystic or cauliflower-like with intermingled radiolucencies and radiodensities. During active growth such mottling may suggest malignancy. Loss of smooth contours with bone destruction or proliferation within the mass or along its base may indicate malignant transformation or response to injury. Radiographic monitoring or bone biopsy, or both, will clarify the nature and progression of the growth.

**GROSS AND MICROSCOPIC FEATURES.** Osteochondroma is a benign, hard, and irregular cartilaginous exostosis having a fibrous and cartilaginous cap (Fig. 11–57) of variable extent and depth, from which trabecular bone arises by endochondral ossification. The mesenchymal tissue between bony trabeculae consists of variable proportions of fibrous connective tissue, osteoclasts, fat, and hematopoietic components and communicates with the medulla of the parent bone. The hyaline cartilaginous element of the cap is glistening gray-blue. The gray-white fibrous portion of the cap is more irregular and tends to blend with adjacent soft tissues, making surgical removal and cleaning of the specimen difficult. The underlying bone cannot be cut with a scalpel but, when sawed, exhibits a red, bony surface that blends at a limited area of its base with the underlying cortex and medulla of the bone from which it arose. Sections of the cartilaginous cap have features of chondroma, while those of the bony part have characteristics of osteoma. Therefore proper biopsy technique and orientation of a biopsy specimen are essential in making the correct histologic diagnosis.

**PROGNOSIS.** The prognosis for an osteochondroma is for many reasons unfavorable. The diagnosis is often delayed until a mass is so large or in such a location (e.g., cranial or vertebral) that removal is difficult or impossible. Secondly, the surgeon must be sure to remove the entire proliferative cap, leaving behind with adjacent soft tissues no remnant that could give rise to recurrence. Thirdly, the presence of one osteochondroma warns that others may be present or may develop, and a total skeletal search should be made for other tumors. Fourthly, nearly all cats with osteochondromatosis are FeLV-positive, an ominous sign for long-term health. Lastly, an osteochondroma occasionally undergoes malignant transformation and metastasizes.

## Chondroma

A few feline chondromas are mentioned in the literature (e.g., Priester and McKay, 1980). An unusual type of chondroma known as multilobular chondroma (chondroma rodens) has been reported in at least two cats (Jacobson, 1971; Morton, 1985). This tumor, far more common in the dog, arises from flat bones of the skull and is locally invasive but late to metastasize. It has a

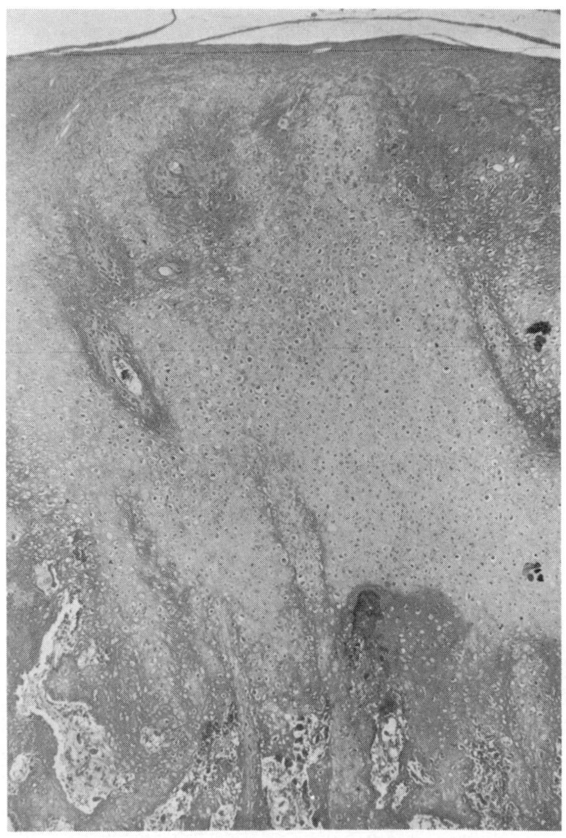

**Figure 11–57** Osteochondroma, scapula, three-year-old tabby. A narrow outer zone of dense collagen and a much broader region of hyaline cartilage (pale zone) form a cap over the trabeculae of bone (below) that forms by endochondral ossification. H & E, × 25.

distinctive lobular growth pattern with a trilaminar arrangement in which there is a central region of hyaline cartilage with varying degrees of necrosis and mineralization (rarely bone), a middle layer of plump mesenchymal cells, and an outer zone of fibrous connective tissue. One of the reported tumors underwent what was described as malignant transformation to a chondrosarcoma (Morton, 1985). The tumor arose from the parietal and occipital region of the skull of a castrated male cat of unknown age. Part of the tumor lost its benign trilaminar appearance and had cysts, foci of necrosis, and poorly differentiated cells with scattered irregular islands of cartilage. No metastases were found.

## Chondrosarcoma

Chondrosarcoma, according to a literature review and a study of four additional cases by Turrel and Pool (1982), is the third most common malignant primary bone tumor of cats, ranking after osteosarcoma and fibrosarcoma. According to the survey of these investigators, at least 25 cases had been reported previously, representing less than 10 per cent of all feline bone tumors. Two chondrosarcomas of bone, one each in a male and female, were recorded by Priester and McKay (1980), and another by Hinko et al. (1979). Myxochondrosarcoma in a 10-year-old cat was described by Herron (1975).

**BREED, AGE, AND SEX.** No breed predisposition is apparent. Of 20 cats with chondrosarcoma, 14 were males and 6 females, ranging in age from 2 to 15 years (mean 8.8) (Turrel and Pool, 1982). Of four cats with chondrosarcoma at AMAH, all were females (three spayed). Their ages were 6, 9, 12, and 14 years.

**SITES AND CLINICAL SIGNS.** Chondrosarcomas recorded in the literature involved the scapula (six), humerus (four), pelvis (three), femur (four), foot (three), skull (three), tibia (one), and other sites not specified (eight) (Hinko et al., 1979; Priester and McKay, 1980; Turrel and Pool, 1982).

Chondrosarcomas, according to Turrel and Pool (1982), are firm, fixed, rapidly developing growths that may cause lameness or pain on palpation, symptoms being present from a month to six years (median six months). A chondrosarcoma causing lameness involved the distal diaphysis of a femur of a seven-year-old male domestic shorthair (Hinko et al., 1979). Radiographically, an elevated periosteal reaction and formation of Codman's triangle, together with linear mineral densities radiating into adjacent soft tissues, suggested a proliferative osteosarcoma rather than a characteristically destructive chondrosarcoma.

An unusual tumor on the top of the skull of a castrated male of unknown age was a chondrosarcoma arising in a multilobular chondroma (Morton, 1985).

Sites of four chondrosarcomas at AMAH were femur (two), mandible (one), and nose (one). The six-year-old female tabby with the nasal tumor had a two-year history of sneezing before mouth-breathing, left-sided nasal discharge, and a nasal fistula were observed. After removal of the tumor the cat did well until hemorrhagic rhinitis occurred six months postoperatively owing to tumor recurrence.

**RADIOGRAPHIC FEATURES.** Chondrosarcomas usually appear less malignant that osteosarcomas and are almost entirely of soft-tissue density (Fig. 11–58). Areas having abundant cartilaginous matrix are, like normal cartilage, essentially radiolucent. Benign subperiosteal woven bone proliferation (Codman's triangle) can also be seen, as in osteosarcoma.

**GROSS AND MICROSCOPIC FEATURES.** Glistening gray-blue tissue is characteristic of both natural and cut surfaces of chondroid and cartilaginous matrix. Yellow foci, often present, represent mineralized necrotic matrix.

Microscopic criteria for diagnosing a chondrosarcoma are high cellularity; scant intercellular matrix; marked variation in cell size; multinucleate cells; and nuclei with irregular outline, clumps of heterochromatin, prominent nucleoli, and mitotic figures (Fig. 11–59).

**PROGNOSIS.** In man, the location of the tumor, the radiographic features, and the microscopic findings must be considered together for predicting tumor behavior. In three cases reviewed by Turrel and Pool (1982), pulmonary metastases occurred. In rare cases, surgical excision may be curative. Two years after removal of a chondromyxosarcoma by caudal hemipelvectomy, an aged cat was still alive (Herron, 1975).

## Hemangiosarcoma

Hemangiosarcomas rarely involve bone. In a two-year-old cat that had been involved in a radiation study, a hemangiosarcoma developed in the distal left femur and metastasized to the lungs; an osteosarcoma also developed in one tibia (Berman and Wright, 1973). A primary hemangiosarcoma caused a pathologic fracture in the humerus of a 12-year-old male (Witt, 1984). Hemangiosarcomas were also reported in the humerus, with metastasis, and in another cat, in a tibia (Quigley and Leedale, 1983); whether they were considered to have originated in bone was unclear.

## Fibrosarcoma

Primary fibrosarcoma of bone originates from the fibrous components of the medulla. In man, this tumor constitutes less than 4 per cent of malignant primary bone tumors (Spjut et al., 1971) and has a strong predilection for the long bones of the leg, particularly the region of the knee in the area of a neighboring metasphysis. Many other bones are sites of fibrosarcoma except those of the hand or foot (Spjut et al., 1971).

In advanced cases in both man and animals there can be difficulty in differentiating between a primary bone tumor and a tumor of adjacent tissue that has invaded bone. There is also the occasional difficulty in distinguishing a fibrosarcoma of bone from an osteosarcoma having a small amount of malignant osteoid and bone (Misdorp and van der Heul, 1976).

In a study by Liu et al. (1974), fibrosarcoma ranked second after osteosarcoma in frequency of primary bone tumors. Of 11 tumors, 6 involved bones of the skull (maxilla, four; mandible, one; frontal bone, one); three tumors involved bones of the forelimb (humerus, carpus, digit); one had invaded a hind digit, and one, the ribs. No metastasis had occurred in the 10 cats that came to autopsy. Tumor was excised from the carpal region in one cat that remained free of recurrence for at least 10 months. Another survey lists fibrosarcoma of the mandible, vertebral column, and two others of axial skeleton (Priester and McKay, 1980). Five periosteal fibrosarcomas of the

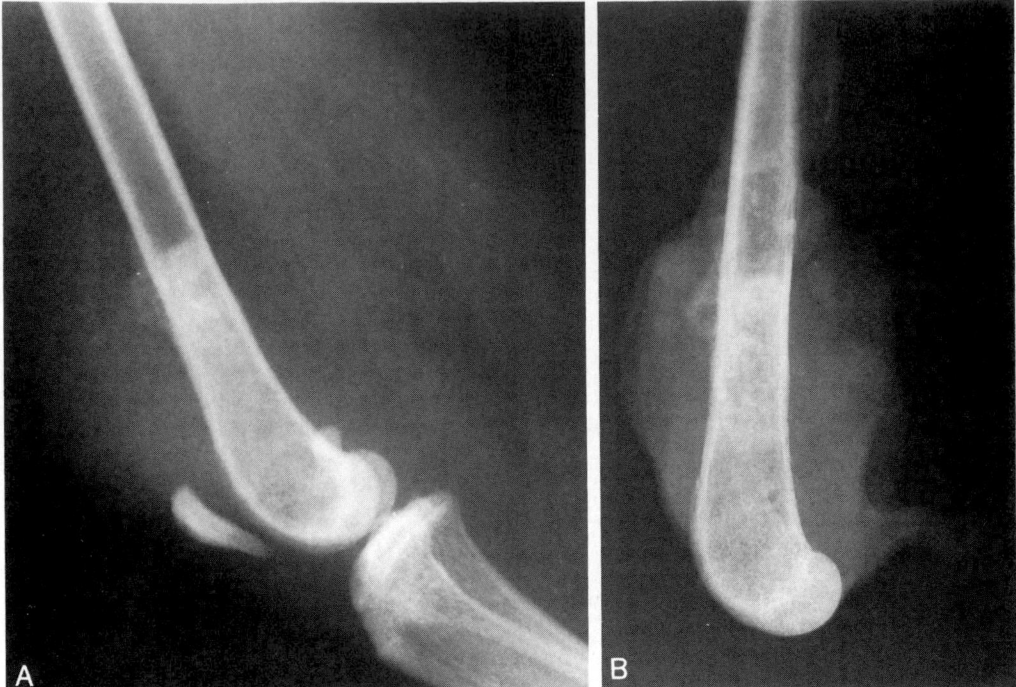


**Figure 11–58** *A*, Chondrosarcoma, distal femur, nine-year-old domestic shorthair. The extraosseous tumor, of soft-tissue density, has displaced the patella cranially. Much of the distal femoral medulla has an increased density owing to necrosis and mineralization (infarction) of the enclosed tumor. A small zone of benign subperiosteal bone proliferation is barely visible on the upper cranial surface of the cortex. *B*, The post-mortem dissection demonstrates the extent of the tumor, which is no longer covered by normal soft tissues. Medullary and cortical changes described in *A* are more clearly seen. There were no metastases.

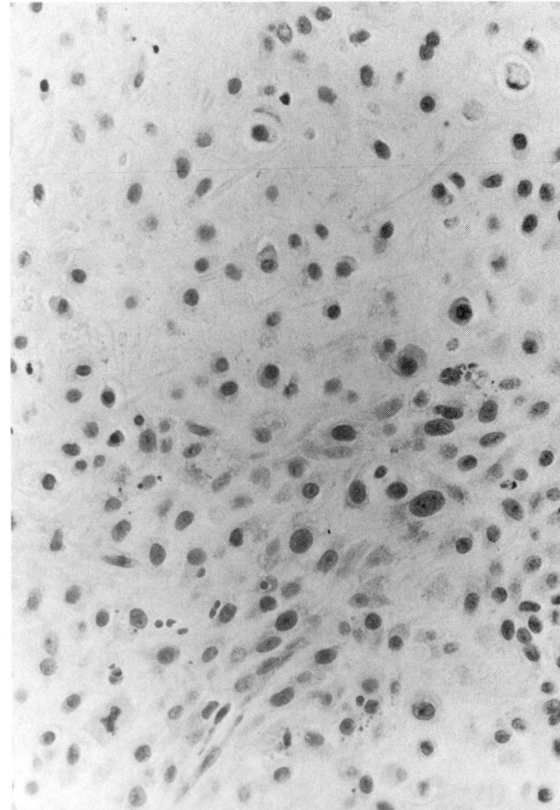

**Figure 11–59** Chondrosarcoma, mandible, 12-year-old domestic shorthair. Varying amounts of intercellular hyaline matrix separate the pleomorphic chondrocytes. Nuclei vary in size, shape, and chromatin distribution. A mitotic figure (lower left) indicates tumor growth, while pyknosis and karyorrhexis (scattered) are signs of tumor cell death. H & E, × 300.

skeleton, distinguished from osteosarcoma by the absence of osteoid, were reported by Nielsen (1964). Only one, originating on the carpus, metastasized to lymph nodes, lung, and kidney.

A fibrosarcoma believed to be assocated with use of an intramedullary splint was reported in the femur of a 13-year-old cat (Sinibaldi et al., 1982).

At AMAH no fibrosarcoma, with one possible exception, could be confidently diagnosed as having arisen within bone. That mass, 38 cm in circumference, replaced the proximal femur of a 13-year-old spayed female domestic shorthair (Fig. 11–60) and metastasized to the iliac nodes and lungs.

The radiographic feature most characteristic of fibrosarcoma is bone lysis. Periosteal response is less than with most osteosarcomas. Fibrosarcomas are much slower to metastasize than the far more frequent osteosarcomas. Radiographic differentiation of a central (medullary) fibrosarcoma from a giant cell tumor of bone, undifferentiated sarcoma, chondrosarcoma, hemangiosarcoma, or solitary lymphoma or plasmacytoma will in most cases be impossible.

Gross findings, like the radiographic features, are dominated by osteolysis. Bone is replaced by gray-white, solid, lobulated tissue that is sharply demarcated and in most cases continuous with extraosseous tumor. Usually both bone and soft tissues are involved so that the site of origin is difficult to determine. Hemorrhage and necrosis accompany tumors associated with pathologic fractures.

Microscopically, the classic fibrosarcoma is composed of interweaving bundles of spindle-shaped fibroblasts with variable amounts of collagen but without an osteoid matrix. Poorly differentiated tumors are composed of greater numbers of plump or round cells with pleomorphic nuclei, more mitotic figures, and often multinucleate giant cells. The presence of metaplastic bone or osteogenesis, representing an attempt at bone repair and remodeling, may contribute to a misleading appearance of osteosarcoma.

## Secondary Tumors of Bone

Secondary bone tumors are recognized far less often in cats than in man. The most frequent appear to be squamous cell carcinomas invading adjacent bone, with bones of the head being most often affected (14 cases, Priester and McKay, 1980). Of eight other squamous cell carcinomas, six invaded the maxilla or mandible and two involved digits (Liu et al., 1974). When such a tumor involves dental alveoli, it typically causes spontaneous loosening of the teeth (Miller et al., 1969). What appears to be an angry-looking hypertrophic gingivitis in an older cat should always arouse a clinician's suspicion of tumor if the teeth fall out and are rapidly replaced in the alveoli by proliferating reddish tissue. If the lymph nodes are not involved, radical en bloc excision combined with radiation is an aggressive approach that is sometimes attempted.

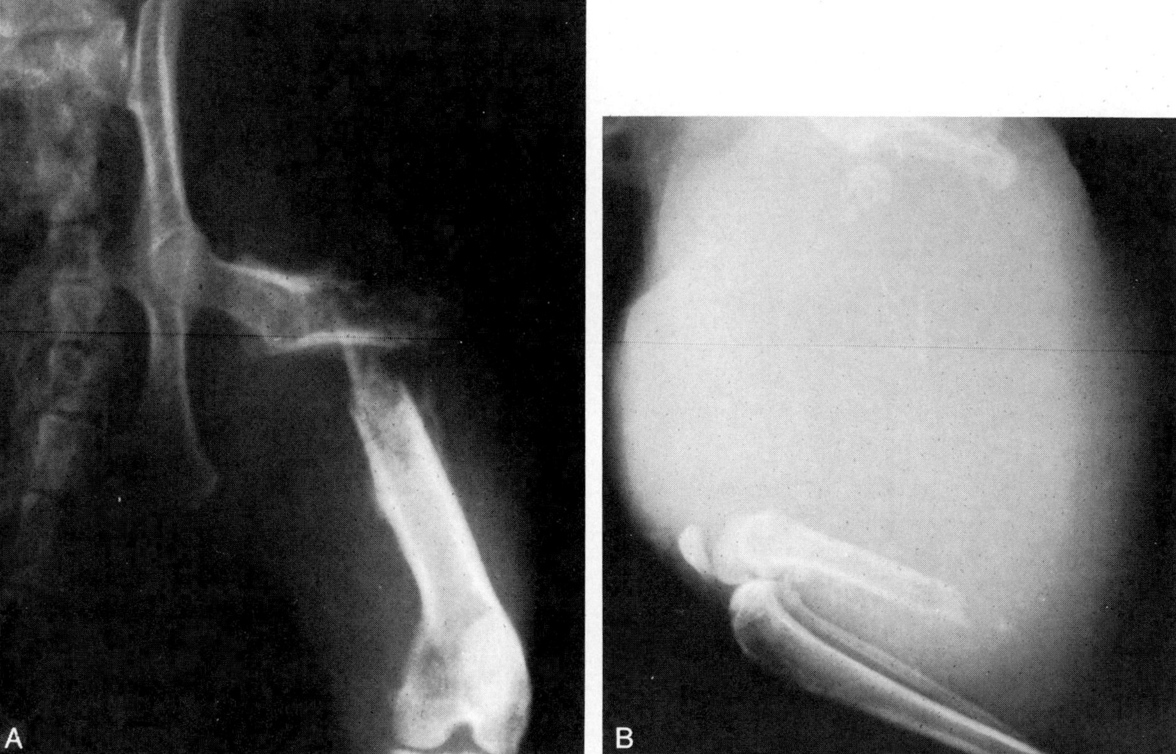


**Figure 11–60** *A*, Fibrosarcoma and a recent pathologic fracture of the left proximal femur in a 13-year-old cat. Osteolysis and subperiosteal bone formation extend beyond the site of the fracture. *B*, Same fibrosarcoma, 13 weeks later, radiographed at autopsy. The tumor had grown to 38 cm in circumference and had metastasized to the iliac nodes and all lung lobes. Pneumothorax was a complication of the pulmonary metastases. Half actual size.

Squamous cell carcinomatous invasion of bone is characterized by extreme osteoblastic reaction that has a characteristic radiographic appearance. In most cases there is more extensive bony enlargement than would be seen with osteomyelitis.

Odontogenic tumors of the mouth also invade bone.

Sarcomas of various types, originating in soft tissues, invade adjacent bone, causing lysis rather than proliferation. Wide excision or amputation is advisable even if a tumor is tiny, as sarcomas have a high recurrence rate with aggressive local invasion and also a tendency to metastasize. Some of these sarcomas present as stubbornly bleeding proliferations or ulcers on digits. In a two-year-old Angell patient, such a bleeding lesion of a toepad was removed together with the digit for diagnostic study. When a highly anaplastic sarcoma was recognized, the owner consented to amputation of the limb and the cat lived a long life, tumor-free.

Fibrosarcomas may invade or metastasize to bone, sometimes causing pathologic fracture (Alexander and Roenigk, 1977; Tepper, 1980).

Lymphoma, malignant melanoma, hemangiosarcoma, reticulum cell sarcoma, and meningioma occasionally involve bone (Liu et al., 1974).

Tumors metastatic to bone are uncommon—or at least are infrequently recognized. Characteristically they are very painful. Lung carcinomas occasionally surprise the clinician by giving rise to distant lesions (e.g., Gustaffson and Wolfe, 1968). Several cats that were presented at AMAH with a presumptive diagnosis of fungal infection of the toes proved to have digital metastases from pulmonary cancer. In one aged cat at AMAH, a minute eyelid carcinoma gave rise to massive metastases to both long and flat bones throughout the body. In another cat, lameness in a hind leg, then constriction of the pelvis by a bony mass, and finally bony tumors elsewhere in the skeleton proved to have arisen from a pancreatic adenocarcinoma—a course unusual in the cat but all too frequent in man.

Lymphoma (lymphoreticular neoplasia), the most common neoplasm of cats, occasionally affects cortical bone. The unusual coincidence of similar reticulum cell sarcomas, all apparently primary in radioulnar and radiocarpal joints of the right foreleg in four related, two- to four-year-old male domestic shorthair pet cats, was reported by Wilson (1973). Virus particles were identified in the tumor by electron microscopy, and passage into unrelated cats produced the same type of tumor.

## Giant Cell Tumors of Tendon Sheath—Synovioma

Tendon sheaths are composed of dense fibrous connective tissue and lining synovial cells. Tumors arising from tendon sheaths are rare in cats. Six cases have been described in some detail. In the four cats of known age, the range was 6 to 16 years; two were males and two females.

Two giant cell tumors of tendon sheath origin were reported by Nielsen (1952b, 1964). One, in an eight-year-old cat at AMAH, developed about the carpus and extended to the elbow joint, displacing muscles but not invading periosteum or bone. The second tumor, on the foot of a 16-year-old cat, was locally invasive. Neither of the tumors metastasized.

A benign giant cell synovioma developed on the extensor surface of the carpus of a six-year-old male tabby. Difficulty was experienced in dissecting the tumor from the extensor tendons, and it recurred locally three times before the cat was killed by a motor vehicle (Hulse, 1960).

A synovioma of the tibiotarsal joint invaded bone of a cat of unknown breed, age, and sex but did not metastasize during its 15 months of growth (Engle and Brodey, 1969).

A synovioma arising from the flexor tendon sheaths in a hind paw of an eight-year-old spayed female shorthair tabby was well described by Davies and Little (1972). The circumscribed, pear-shaped tumor encircled, and was firmly bound to, the flexor tendon sheaths of the lateral digit but did not involve the phalanges. The digit was amputated together with the distal end of the metatarsal bone. Three months later, the cat was destroyed because of a 4.5 × 3.5 × 3.0 cm recurrent tumor that was not accompanied by metastasis.

Another synovioma was described as an ulcerated, rounded, lobulated mass, 3.5 cm in diameter, attached to the common digital extensor tendon on the craniolateral aspect of the carpus of an adult female (Thoday and Evans, 1972). The surgical wound healed by secondary intention, and the tumor did not recur in a seven-month postoperative period.

Cotchin (1983) stated that in his collection of bone tumors "some fibrous tumours of the limbs, not attached to bone, appeared to be synoviomas."

Tendon sheaths rather than synovial membranes of joints gave rise to the reported synoviomas. All six arose at or below the carpus or tarsus; one extended up to the elbow. Apparently only one caused bone destruction (Engle and Brodey, 1969). Microscopically the synoviomas were characterized by nodules that were varyingly fibrous, myxomatous, or chondroid. Synovial clefts in some nodules were lined by polygonal cells. Multinucleate giant cells were scattered among the predominating spindle cells. In one tumor (Nielsen, 1952) fibroblasts predominated with development of giant cells by hyperplasia or agglomeration of the fibroblasts.

Local recurrence, but not metastasis, occurred in two cats. Too few feline synoviomas have been published to permit further comments on their biologic behavior.

## Tumor-Like Lesions of Bone

Uncommon non-neoplastic lesions that must be differentiated from tumor are aneurysmal bone cyst, myositis ossificans, and fibrodysplasia ossificans.

**ANEURYSMAL BONE CYST.** This is an expanding osteolytic lesion composed of blood-filled spaces separated by septa containing bone or osteoid and osteoclast giant cells. The lesion in man is discussed extensively by Spjut et al. (1971). The cause is unknown. Long bones, ribs, or vertebrae may be involved. The radiographic appearance often facilitates precise diagnosis. The lesion appears to destroy bone by expansion. The cortex is often thinned but usually intact. Local resection is sometimes successful. In dogs aneurysmal bone cyst occurs most often in the distal radius, ulna, and tibia.

Aneurysmal bone cysts were reported in three female cats, two of which were 2 years old, and the third, 14 (Liu et al., 1974). Sites were the sacrum, coccygeal vertebrae, and wing of an ilium.

Two aneurysmal bone cysts were diagnosed in cats at AMAH. One occurred in the left tibia of a five-year-old spayed female that became increasingly lame over a two-week period. The lesion was painful, large, and firm except for tense, fluctuant areas. After about 40 ml of dark blood was aspirated from one undulant region it was possible to palpate a deep bony enlargement in the midtibia. After aspiration, the pockets promptly filled again. Radiographs showed a small osseous excrescence on one side of the tibia and some fuzziness about the cortex at that site as well as proximal to the knee. The cat was euthanatized and an autopsy was performed.

The subcutaneous surface of the 12 × 8 × 8 cm mass was bluish, and on incision much blood drained from many cavities separated by tissue arising from the tibia. The walls of the cysts nearest the bone resisted cutting and appeared ossified. Centrally, a roughly circular hole passing through the interosseous space of the tibia and fibula appeared to originate from the proximal end of the tibia. White strands of tissue radiated from the central linear blood-filled space. No lesions were found elsewhere.

Microscopic examination revealed medullary blood-containing cysts lined by flattened cells and granulation tissue with walls formed by fibrous tissue and endosteum-derived, woven, trabecular bone (Fig. 11–61). Similar cystic spaces continued through the cortex to lie between compact cortical lamellar bone and subperiosteal trabecular woven bone.

The prominence of the blood-filled cysts raises a question as to the origin of aneurysmal bone cysts. Vascular malformation, acquired arteriovenous fistula, and hemangioma must be considered as possible precursors of this benign lesion.

The second case, diagnosed from a specimen submitted by the Chicago Cat Clinic, involved the third cervical vertebra and caused a pathologic fracture that damaged the spinal cord (Fig. 11–62).

**MYOSITIS OSSIFICANS.** This infrequent lesion may occur in muscle or near bone or it may involve the periosteum. A knowledge of its pathogenesis is essential for differentiating it from tumor. The term myositis ossificans is misleading because inflammation of muscle is absent and mineralization of osteoid may not occur, in man, during the first four months of a lesion's maturation (Spjut et al., 1971). Most cases of myositis ossificans in man follow local trauma, rarely infection. The lesion begins with muscle necrosis and a central proliferation of primitive cells suggestive of sarcoma. The clue to accurate diagnosis of the lesion is its orderly maturation, with benign features located peripherally where orderly osteoid is first recognized and where mineralization of osteoid begins. The early lesion may regress and disappear or, once matured, may persist as a hard, bony mass. In man, the lesion is painful in the early stage of development.

Lesions diagnosed as myositis ossificans occurred on the elbows of a two-year-old female cat and were associated with both mild and severe periosteal bony reaction (Liu et al., 1974). Except for the significant histologic features of more mature osseous tissue disposed peripherally, it would be difficult to distinguish the lesions from those of osteochondromatosis.

Myositis ossificans was also diagnosed microscopically in a young adult castrated male domestic longhair at Rowley Memorial Hospital of the MSPCA in Springfield, Massachusetts. The cat had been presented previously for generalized tenderness of the subcutaneous tissue, and because of its dark-tuna diet a provisional diagnosis of steatitis was made and vitamin E prescribed. A year later, small firm structures that "felt like little pieces of eggshell" could be palpated in the thigh muscles of both hind legs. The condition was otherwise asymptomatic. Radiographs disclosed multiple small irregular areas of mineralization in muscle or between muscle bellies behind the knee joints (Fig. 11–63). On biopsy the condition was diagnosed as myositis ossificans. No treatment was given, and the condition remained unchanged and asymptomatic until the cat died at 13 years of unrelated causes. An autopsy was not obtained.

Another case of myositis ossificans described as generalized in a 10-month-old female cat (Norris et al., 1980) would seem actually to have been fibrodysplasia ossificans.

**FIBRODYSPLASIA OSSIFICANS.** Fibrodysplasia ossificans, of unknown cause and rare in cats, is characterized by proliferative fascial and epimysial changes (Fig. 11–64), causing increased muscle girth, altered gait, and progressive limitation of mobility. It is a benign, disseminated hyperplasia of fascia and epimysium containing islands of mineralized bone formed by cartilaginous and osseous metaplasia (Fig. 11–65*A* and *B*) and in some older lesions by endochondral ossification (Fig. 11–65*C*). Fibrodysplasia ossificans differs from localized myositis ossificans in that it does not involve muscle itself and is multicentric, often symmetric, and unrelated to trauma. It also differs microscopically from myositis ossificans, in which a pathognomonic feature of the lesion is a peripheral zone of orderly maturation.

Fibrodysplasia in cats exhibits soft tissue changes similar to those in fibrodysplasia ossificans progressiva of man; to date, however, evidence is lacking that it is, like the human disease, inherited or strongly associated with skeletal abnormalities.

The disease was diagnosed at AMAH in three domestic shorthairs, two year-old males and a six-year-old female (Warren and Carpenter, 1984). All appeared well except for an awkward gait and impaired mobility, signs reported to have progressed over periods of weeks or months. Two of the cats had to be helped to stand. When handled, the cat in the most advanced stage of disease felt rigid, blocky, and unusually heavy for its size. Palpation and manipulation elicited pain in all three cats and revealed increased muscle mass of abnormal firmness in the limbs and severely restricted movement of most limb joints. The tissues underlying the skin and subcutis in other areas, such as shoulders, thorax, and groin, felt abnormally firm. Radiography and biopsy were done, and eventually all the cats were destroyed and came to autopsy.

Radiography disclosed linear mineralized densities up to 4 cm long in areas corresponding to muscle fascial planes (Fig. 11–65*D* and *E*).

At autopsy the essential finding was a striking abnormality of epimysium. Sites of involvement common to the three cats were the forearms, arms, shoulders, withers, thighs, and calves. Other sites affected in at least one case were neck, lateral thorax, midback, and groin. The microscopic findings have already been mentioned. In one cat an irregular weblike net of firm tissue extended over the pleural surface of all lung lobes. Microscopically, the tissue consisted of proliferative fibroblasts lying outside the elastic layer of the pleura. The immediate subjacent

*Text continued on page 468*

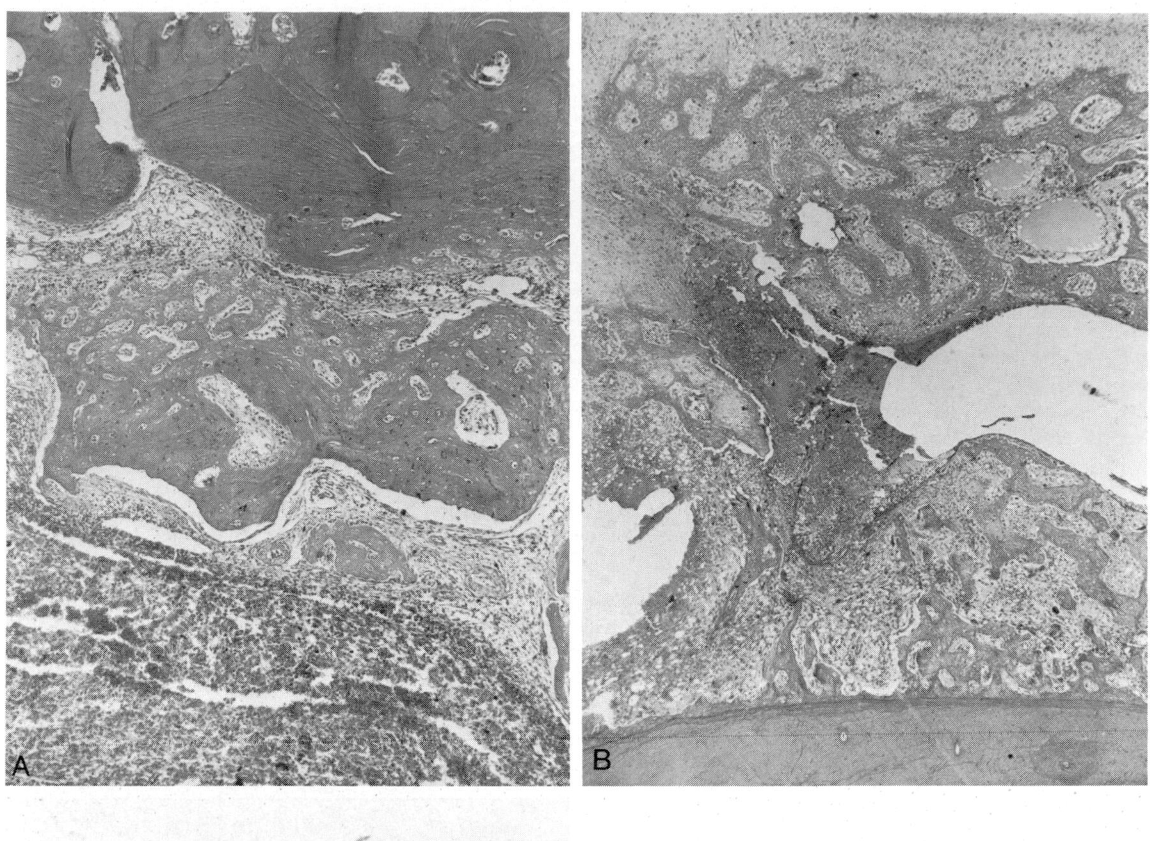


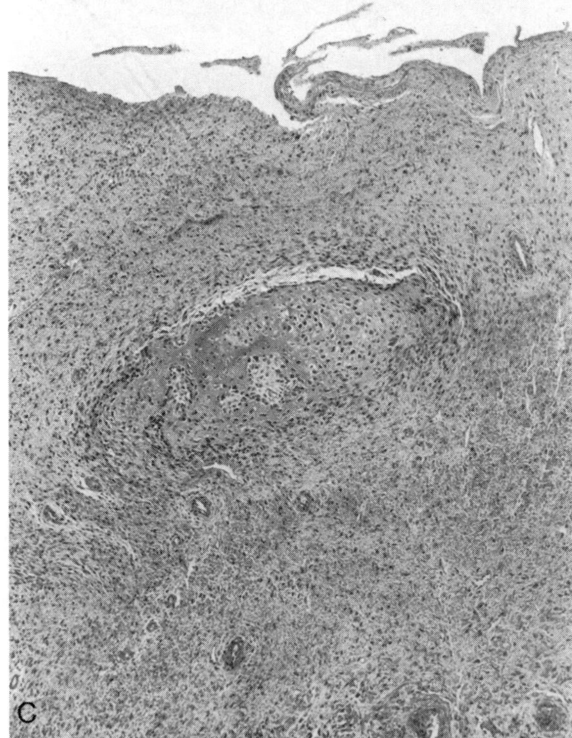


**Figure 11–61** *A*, Aneurysmal bone cyst, tibia, five-year-old black-and-white spayed female. Blood-filled spaces (bottom third) lined by granulation tissue are separated from the cortex (top) by endosteal woven bone and medullary fibrosis (center). H & E, × 50. *B*, Dilated, branching, venous-like channels (center) are within the subperiosteal woven bone. These channels were seen in other sections to pass through the cortex (below) to communicate with medullary vascular spaces seen in *A*. H & E, × 50. *C*, Blood-filled medullary space (top, now empty) is separated from other similar spaces (not shown) by trabeculae of dense fibrous tissue having cartilaginous foci undergoing endochondral ossification (center). H & E, × 100.

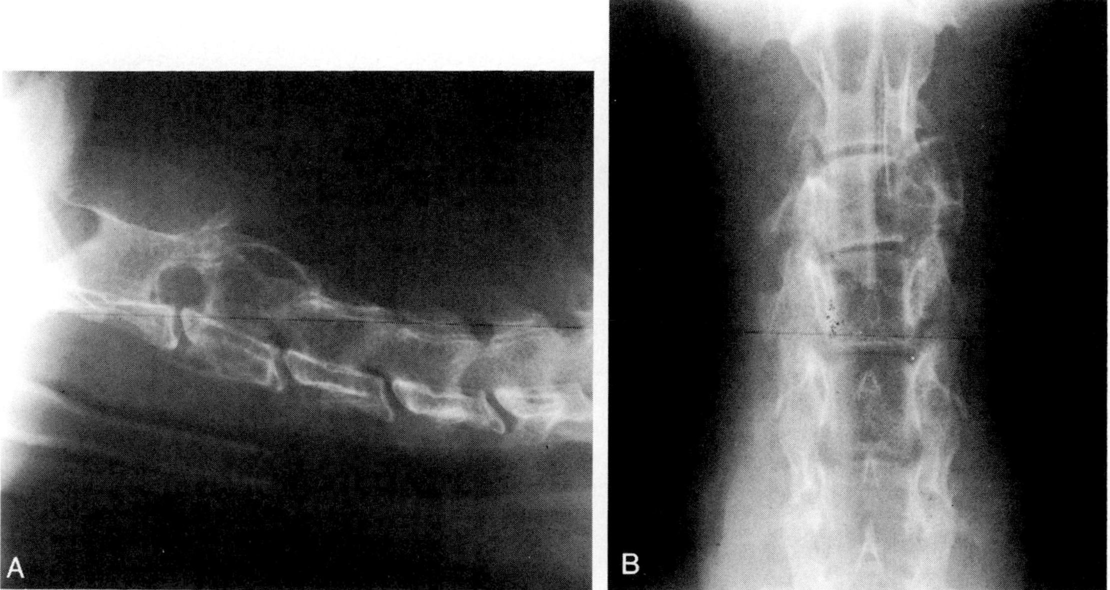


**Figure 11–62** *A*, Aneurysmal bone cyst, third cervical vertebra, in a two and a half-year-old castrated male black domestic shorthair that had a brief episode of posterior paresis six months before the sudden onset of quadriplegia. Lytic and proliferative changes are best seen in the dorsal vertebral arch. *B*, The lateral expansile growth of vertebra C3 has radiolucent cavities consisting of fibrous connective tissue and large vascular channels and a multiloculated, thin-shelled wall composed of benign bone. (Courtesy Dr. Barbara S. Stein.)

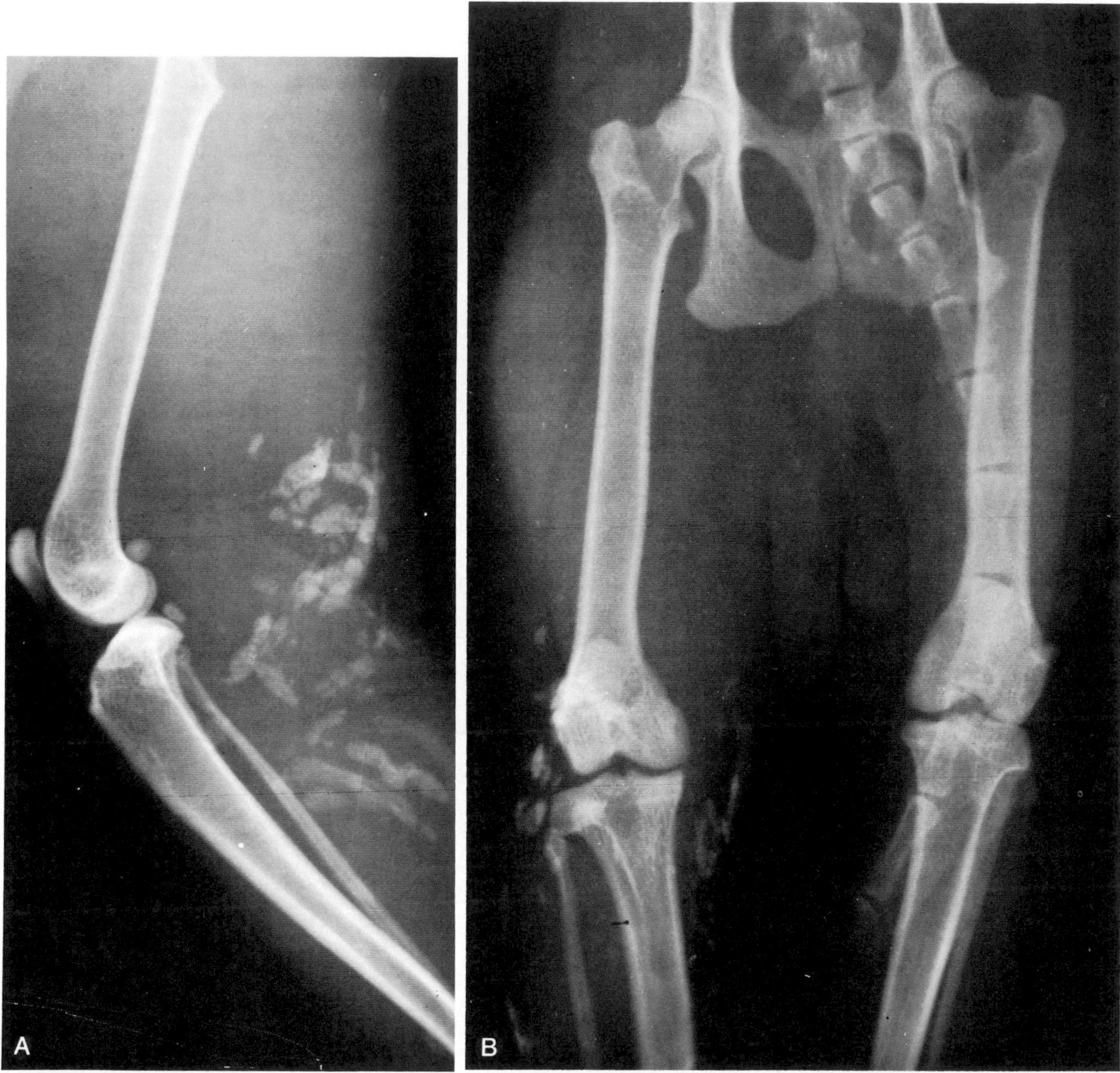


**Figure 11–63** *A* and *B*, Myositis ossificans, young adult castrated male domestic cat. The areas of mineralization in the leg muscles remained palpable throughout the cat's life but caused no significant signs of discomfort. The anteroposterior view suggests that the areas of mineralization involve fascia or epimysium rather than muscle substance—a feature more characteristic of fibrodysplasia ossificans.

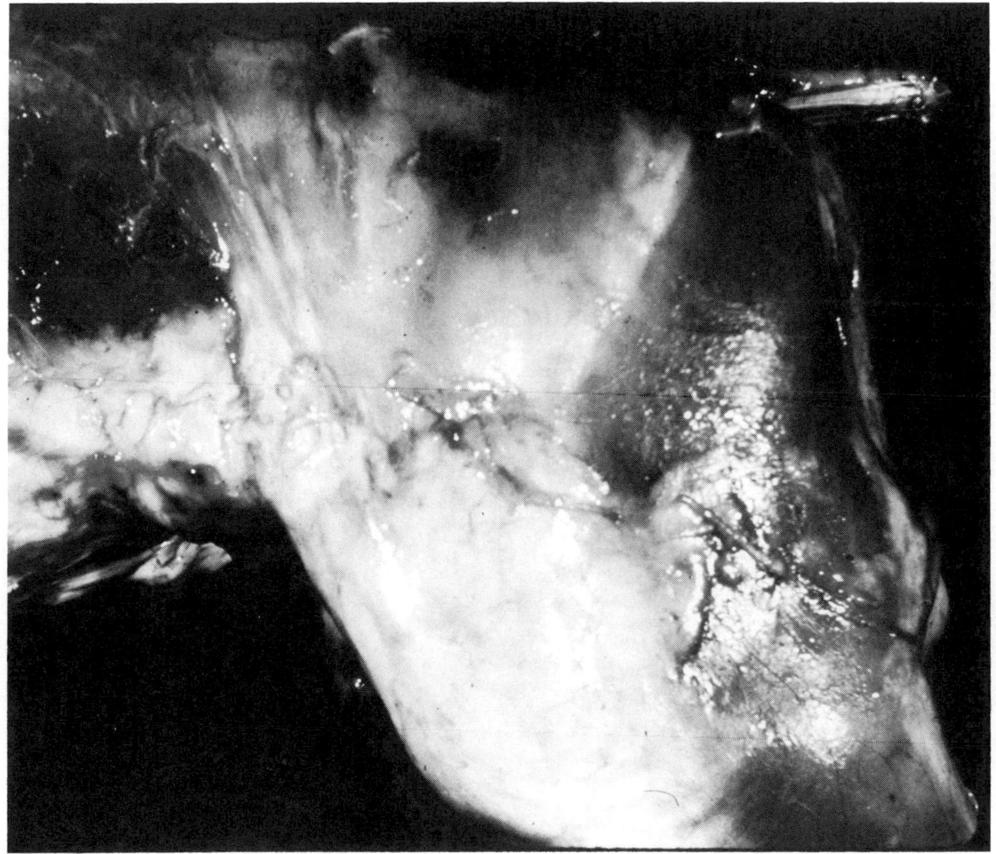

**Figure 11–64** Fibrodysplasia ossificans in a one-year-old domestic longhair. The lumbodorsal, deep gluteal, and lateral femoral fasciae are greatly thickened and opaque white.

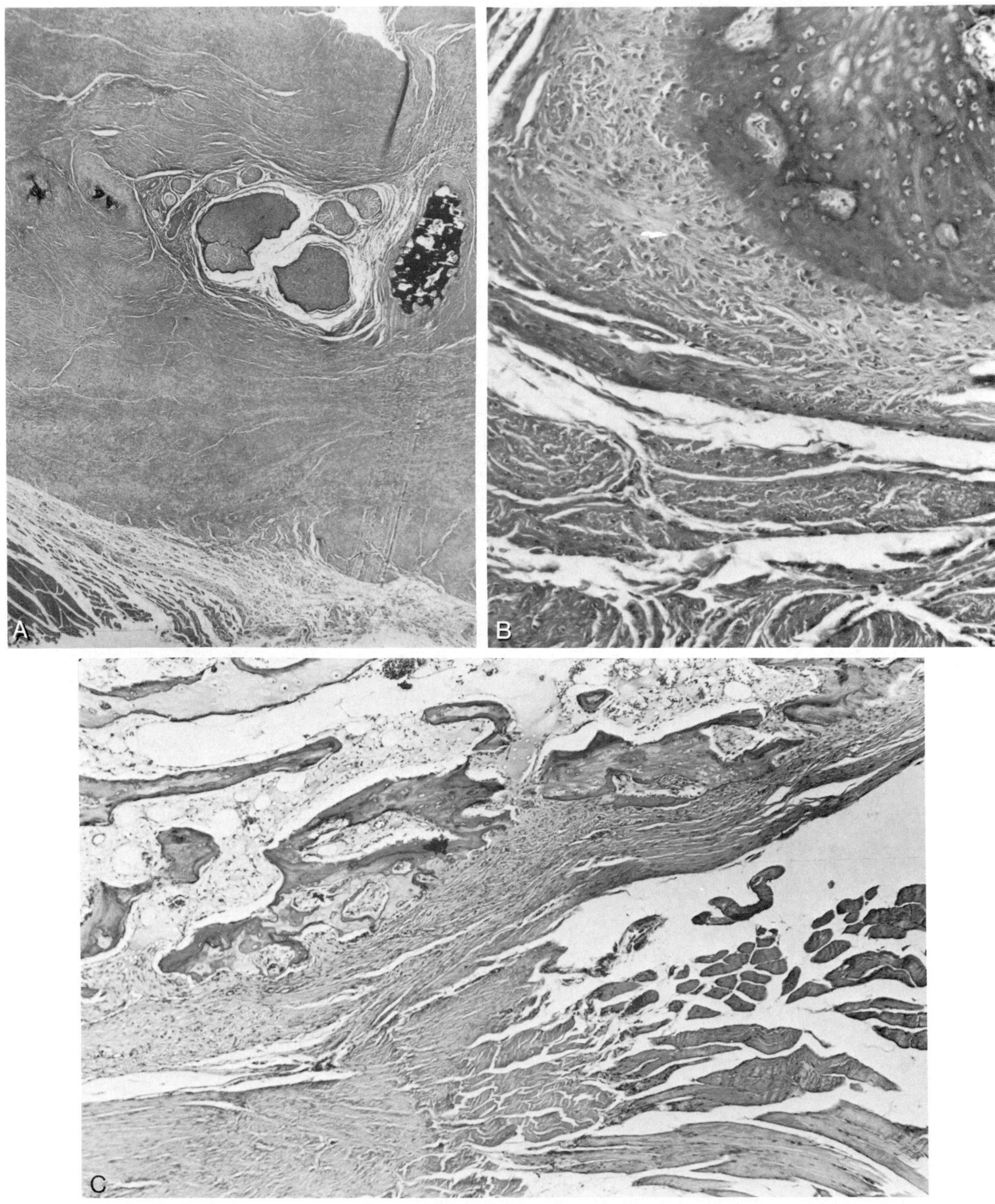


**Figure 11–65** *A*, Fibrodysplasia ossificans, thigh, six-year-old spayed female. Tremendously thickened epimysium encases branches of the sciatic nerve and vessels (center). Three dark foci of osseous metaplasia are to the right and left of the nerves. Muscle (lower left) underwent atrophy owing to compression by epimysium and to disuse. H & E, × 30. *B*, A nodule of osseous metaplasia (upper right) lies within thick, dense collagenous bundles of epimysium. H & E, × 100. *C*, Benign osseous and cartilaginous trabeculae with intertrabecular adipose and fibrous marrow (upper left) developed within the hyperplastic epimysium. H & E, × 50.

*Illustration continued on opposite page*

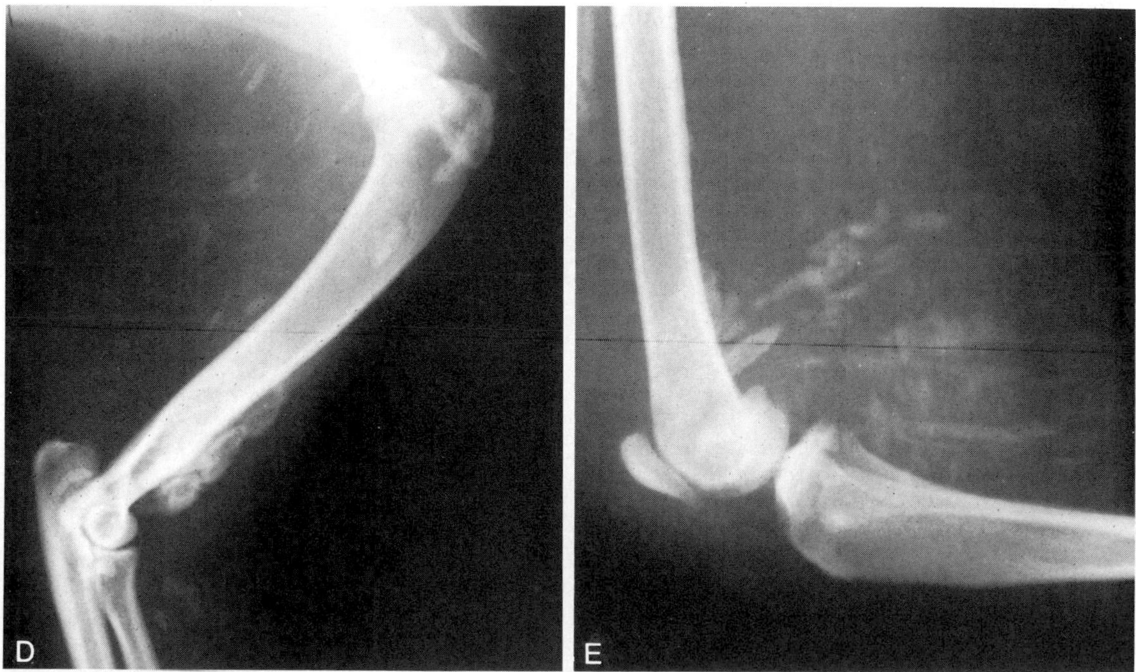


**Figure 11–65** *Continued D*, Fibrodysplasia ossificans, same cat as in Figures 11–65*A*, *B*, and *C*. Linear and oval radiographic densities proved at autopsy to be bone within epimysium of muscles of the arm. *E*, Epimysial bony densities about the knee appear to form a quilted pattern where such densities overlap.

pulmonary parenchyma was atelectatic and without inflammation. The significance of this pleural lesion in a single cat is unclear.

## TUMORS OF MUSCLE

Tumors of muscles are extremely rare in cats. In a survey of 226 neoplasms in cats, there were two leiomyomas of the uterus and no tumors of striated muscles (Cotchin, 1952). Two rhabdomyosarcomas were reported by Blähser (1961a). In a survey of 174 feline tumors, no tumor of smooth or cardiac muscle was found, and only two rhabdomyosarcomas were reported (Smith and Jones, 1966). Three rhabdomyosarcomas were listed in another survey (Schmidt and Langham, 1967). In a study of 3145 feline autopsies at The Animal Medical Center, in which 289 tumors of nonhematopoietic origin were reported, one leiomyosarcoma of the spleen, two leiomyomas of the intestine, and two rhabdomyosarcomas of skeletal muscle were listed (Patnaik et al., 1975). Through the courtesy of Dr. A. I. Hurvitz, sections of these two rhabdomyosarcomas and of four others were made available for review by us and by three other pathologists, who considered the tumors more likely to be poorly differentiated sarcomas of uncertain type.

### TUMORS OF SMOOTH MUSCLE

Ten leiomyomas (eight of uterus, two of vagina) and seven leiomyosarcomas (three of uterus, one each of vagina, urinary bladder, tongue, and skin) were on record at AMAH. For details on the smooth muscle tumors of the uterus, vagina, and bladder, the reader is referred to the discussion of tumors of the urogenital tract. The leimyosarcoma of the tongue occurred in a three-year-old spayed female Siamese. It was in the underside of the tongue and measured 1.2 cm in greatest dimension. A change in vocal sounds had attracted the owner's attention to the lingual mass for three weeks before surgery. The cutaneous leiomyosarcoma involved the lumbar region in a 13-year-old spayed female white domestic shorthair and appeared to arise from a pilomotor muscle.

### TUMORS OF STRIATED MUSCLE

Two rhabdomyomas of entire female domestic cats, aged five months and one year, were described (Syvrud, 1959). The older cat had a firm circumscribed mass, 5.5 cm in diameter, in the axilla; the other had a mass the size of a large egg in the ventral abdominal wall just caudal to the last rib, beneath the external abdominal oblique muscle. The growth extended retroperitoneally into the abdominal cavity, and one fibrous band penetrated the peritoneum and joined the tumor to the pancreas. Surgery was successful in both cases.

Sections lent for microscopic examination, through the courtesy of the Department of Pathology, Washington State College of Veterinary Medicine, revealed that both tumors had a similar microscopic appearance. Myocytes, many with obvious cross-striations, were arranged in a haphazard pattern of broad fascicles often at sharp angles to one another (Fig. 11–66).

Tumors of striated muscle are too rare in the cat to predict behavior. The prognosis should be guarded. Local recurrence due to incomplete excision is always a possibility with unencapsulated neoplasms. Wide excision, when possible, is indicated.

## TUMORS OF THE RESPIRATORY SYSTEM

Tumors of the respiratory system are uncommon. The nasal passages and frontal sinuses are most often involved, tumors in these sites representing about 1 per cent of feline tumors (Legendre et al., 1981).

### TUMORS OF THE NASAL CAVITY AND FRONTAL SINUS

#### Tumor-like Growths

Inflammatory polyps within the nasal cavity and nasopharynx of cats are more frequent than true tumors, and many have been described (Bradley, 1984). At AMAH they outnumbered primary nasal and sinal neoplasms by

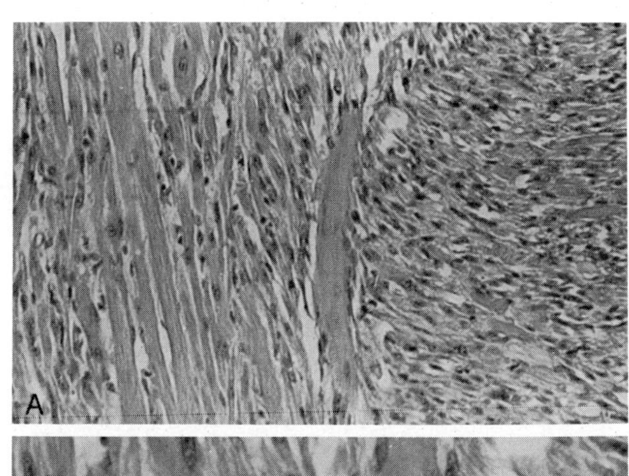


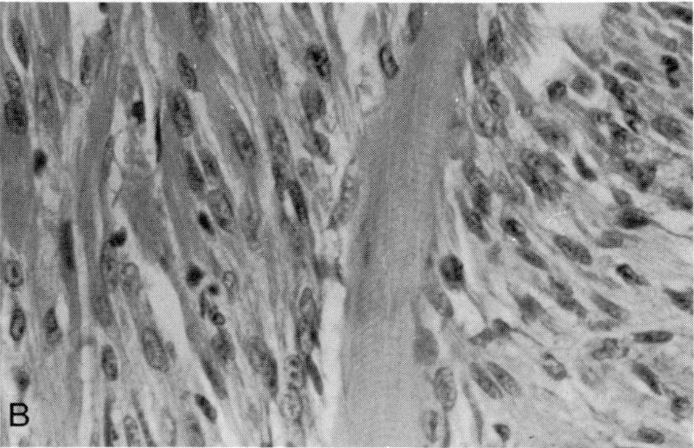


**Figure 11–66** *A*, Rhabdomyoma, ventral abdominal wall, five-month-old kitten. Bundles of striated myocytes of varying size intersect at different planes. H & E, × 200. *B*, Size, orientation, and banding of myocytes are striking cellular variations. H & E, × 500. (Sections courtesy Department of Veterinary Pathology, College of Veterinary Medicine, Washington State University, Pullman, Washington.)

3:2. They also outnumbered cases of nasal cryptococcosis by the same ratio. They occur almost exclusively in kittens and young adult cats. Varying views as to site of origin of the polyps, whether internal auditive (Eustachian) tube or bulla, have been reviewed by Bedford (1982). Over 80 per cent of inflammatory polyps in the upper respiratory tract lie within the nasopharynx, and over 75 per cent of those arise as a result of chronic proliferative infection in the middle ear, whence they pass through the internal auditive tube and then undergo expansile growth in the nasopharynx. Occasionally such a polyp passes into the nasal passage and may emerge at a nostril.

Signs of obstruction of the nasopharynx are snorting, sneezing, noisy or oral breathing, inspiratory dyspnea, gagging, seromucoid nasal discharge, and often secondary bacterial rhinitis and sinusitis. Depression of the soft palate or blockage of the pharynx can result in dysphagia.

Inflammatory polyps arising from turbinates (Fig. 11–67) are much less common than those originating from the mucosa of the middle ear and differ from them in three ways. They have a prominent vascular component characterized by cavernous blood vessels often containing organizing thrombi. Second, unlike otic polyps, they have woven bone as part of their proliferating stroma. Third, nosebleed is frequent with nasal polyps but rarely accompanies polyps of otic origin.

Inflammatory polyps of turbinate origin, most frequent in young cats weeks or months after an upper respiratory infection, have been misdiagnosed as hemangiomas and fibro-osteomas with large blood channels. Rare vascular anomalies of turbinates have been similarly misinterpreted.

In the diagnosis of nasopharyngeal masses, cryptococcal granuloma, which occasionally assumes polypoid form, and malignant tumors must be considered. Inflammatory polyps are discrete and noninvasive, whereas cryptococcosis and malignant neoplasms destroy and deform turbinates and facial bones. Malignant tumors, except for lymphoma, were not seen at AMAH in cats under three years of age. India ink preparations of moist exudate, a variety of stains, culture on blood agar, and histopathologic examination enable differentiation of polyps, granulomas, and tumor. It is well to remember that a cat with cryptococcosis may have a concurrent malignancy elsewhere, the most likely being lymphoma.

When a cat is examined under anesthesia, a polyp is often recognized as a discrete, movable mass occluding the nasopharynx. If dorsal to the soft palate, it may be palpated and can be seen and grasped when the edge of the soft palate is pulled forward. In lateral, dorsoventral, and open-mouth radiographic views it appears as soft tissue density in the nasal cavity or nasopharynx. Density in one or both of the tympanic bullae may represent inflammatory exudate or the presence of a polyp. Occasionally a polyp is present in the external ear canal as well as the nasopharynx.

Polyps are usually attached within the middle ear by a slim stalk and when removed by twisting and traction rarely recur. Sometimes it is necessary to slit the soft palate in order to grasp a polyp. If there is associated disease of the bulla, a bulla osteotomy may be indicated for curettage and drainage. Transient Horner's syndrome occasionally follows removal of a polyp or drainage of the bulla.

## Benign Tumors

Benign tumors of the nasal cavity and frontal sinus of cats are so rare that they should be regarded as nonexistent for practical clinical purposes. In a survey of tumors at 15 veterinary colleges only a half dozen adenomas, papillomas, and fibromas were reported as compared with 70 malignant neoplasms (Priester and McKay, 1980). In our experience (JLC), differentiation of such benign tumors from inflammatory polyps is not always easy.

Only one benign neoplasm, a hemangioma of the nasal passage, was on record at AMAH. It occurred in a 10-year-old spayed female Siamese and was removed nearly two years after it was first observed to cause a bump on the bridge of the nose. When episodes of nosebleed finally prompted its removal, it measured 1.5 × 0.6 cm. There was benign proliferation of the overlying bone.

Multiple osteochondromas of the turbinates (Fig. 11–55*D*) and other bones as well (calvaria, vertebrae, scapula) were seen in two cats at AMAH, a one and a half-year-old castrated male domestic shorthair and a four and a half-year-old spayed female Siamese. Both tested FeLV-positive.

## Malignant Tumors

In the survey of Madewell et al. (1976), cats were at greatest risk for malignant tumors of the nasal cavity and paranasal sinuses between 10 and 15 years of age, and

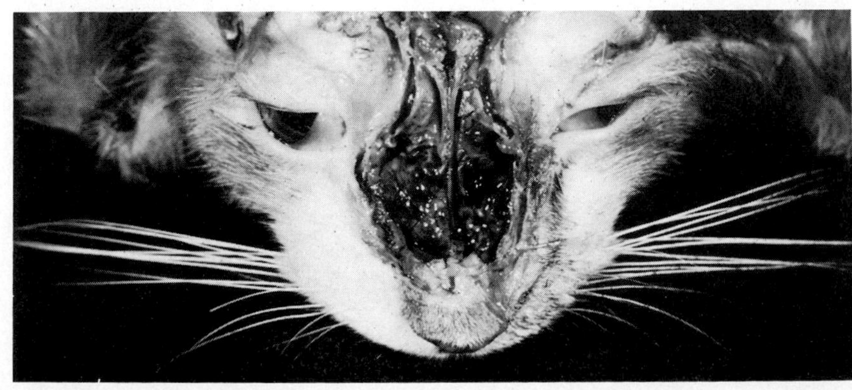

**Figure 11–67** Bilateral nasal polyps, nine-month-old tabby. The maxillary turbinates are enlarged, deformed, and discolored. The dark nodules and spots are cavernous vascular spaces within an irregular proliferation of fibrous and bony tissues. One pathologist termed the lesions osteofibromas.

males were affected twice as often as females. The frontal sinuses are involved far less often than the nasal cavity. In order of reported frequency, the malignant tumors are squamous cell carcinoma, adenocarcinoma, carcinomas of unspecified type, lymphoma, sarcomas of undetermined type, fibrosarcoma, and osteosarcoma (Cotchin, 1983; Moulton, 1978; Priester and McKay, 1980). Unusual tumors reported were a sympathicoblastoma (Madewell et al., 1976) and a tumor of myeloblasts and myelocytes (Godglück, 1950).

Twenty-seven malignant neoplasms of the nasal cavity and frontal sinus were diagnosed at AMAH. Squamous cell carcinomas arising in the oral cavity and secondarily involving the nasal cavity and lymphoma were not included in this group. Comprising the 27 tumors were three squamous cell carcinomas, seven carcinomas arising from pseudostratified epithelium, five simple tubular adenocarcinomas probably of glandular origin, two pigmented epithelioid malignant melanomas arising in the external nares, and one carcinosarcoma. Almost a third of the group were sarcomas: four osteosarcomas (Fig. 11–68), three fibrosarcomas, one chondrosarcoma (Fig. 11–69), and one hemangiosarcoma.

**BREED, AGE, AND SEX.** Six of the 27 cats (22 per cent) were Siamese, all having growths of epithelial origin, whereas Siamese represent only 5 per cent of all feline admissions at AMAH. The male:female ratio was 4:5 as compared with the male:female ratio of 3:2 in the hospital population generally and in sharp contrast with the male:female ratio of 2:1 reported by Madewell et al. (1976). Eleven of the 15 females and 8 of the 12 males were neutered. The age range for the cats was 1 to 19 years (mean 10.2) for cats with the epithelial tumors as well as for those with mesenchymal growths.

**CLINICAL FEATURES.** Four signs nearly always accompany malignant nasal tumors and usually occur in the following order: sneezing, unilateral nasal discharge, noisy breathing, and epistaxis. Noisy breathing, variously

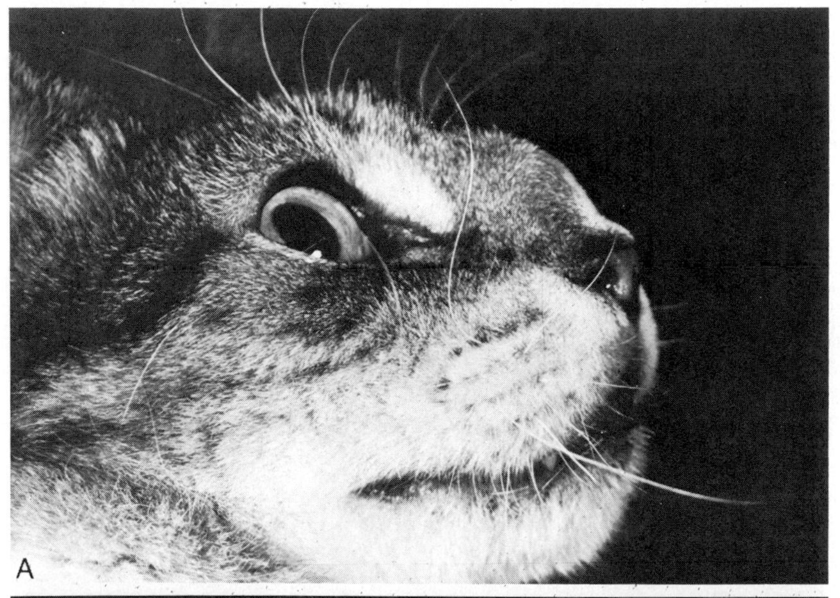


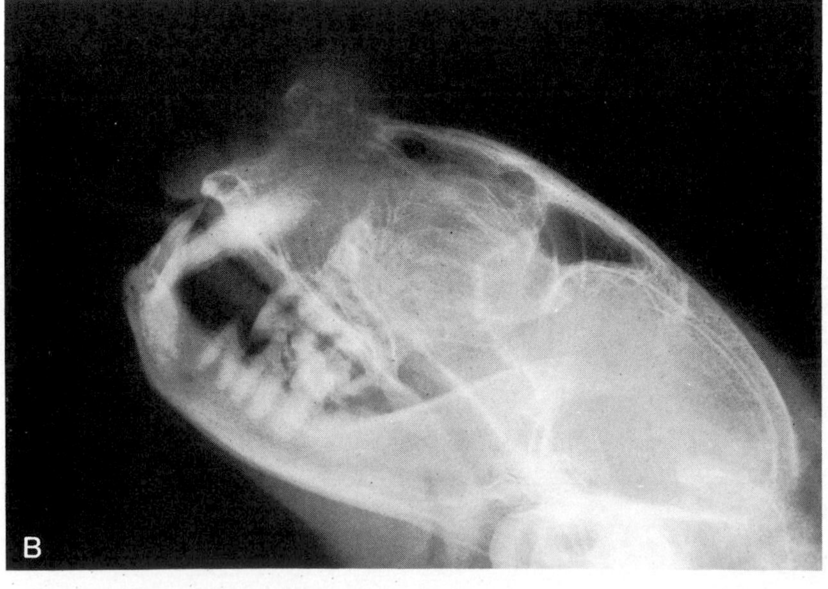


**Figure 11–68** *A*, Osteosarcoma of nasal bones and maxillae, seven-year-old tabby. The tumor caused facial swelling and a Roman nose, obstructing the nasal airways and necessitating oral breathing. *B*, Same cat, later. The tumor has partially lysed and elevated the nasal bones, infiltrated the maxilla, and caused a more prominent soft tissue swelling.

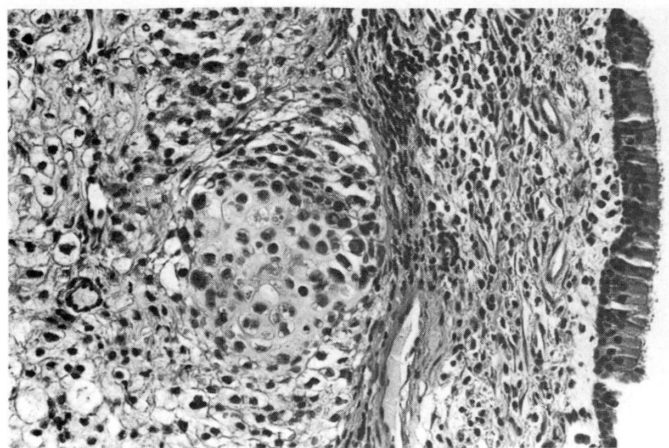

**Figure 11–69** Chondrosarcoma of the nose in a six-year-old female tabby-and-white domestic shorthair that had signs of rhinitis for two years. The tumor, which lies below the respiratory epithelium (right), consists of chondroblasts, chondrocytes, and a varying amount of intercellular matrix. H & E, × 160.

described as wheezing, snuffling, snorting, or snoring, was sometimes first noticed when cats would eat, groom, or sleep. One cat avoided its usual curled-up sleeping posture and assumed a crouched position to allow easier breathing. Some cats breathed with greater depth or with the mouth slightly opened.

Nine cats had facial disfigurement at the time of diagnosis at four weeks to two years into the clinical course: elevation of the bridge of the nose, facial swelling, fistulae, exophthalmos, ocular deviation, or a mass in the external nares. Two cats had an ocular discharge due to lacrimal duct obstruction as well as a nasal discharge on the same side as the tumor. The tumors involved one or the other side of the nose with about equal frequency.

Common radiographic findings were soft-tissue density of one side of the nasal cavity, usually with a soft-tissue or fluid density of the ipsilateral sinus. Bone changes, when present, may be purely lytic or take on a sunburst appearance caused by both lysis and bony proliferation, the latter being most characteristic of squamous cell carcinoma.

Material for diagnosis can usually be obtained by needle biopsy or with a small curette. A saline flush may provide a diagnosis if malignant cells are obtained. If these procedures are unrewarding, the nasal passage must be opened and explored.

**COURSE OF ILLNESS.** The diagnosis of nasal tumor was not made in any cat in less than four weeks after signs appeared. The longest course before detection of an adenocarcinoma was eight months, by which time destruction of the maxilla and frontal bone was advanced. The longest course was that of a sarcoma in a six-year-old female tabby with a two-year history of sneezing. At the time of surgery, mouth breathing and a left nasal discharge and fistula were observed. A chondrosarcoma was removed from the left nasal cavity, but recurrence caused hemorrhagic rhinitis six months later.

A four-year-old Siamese had nasal signs for two months before drops of blood from the right nostril prompted the owner to seek veterinary care. Exensive nasal and sinal surgery for a tubular adenocarcinoma appeared to be curative, but the cat was destroyed two months later because of recurrence.

**GROSS FEATURES.** Eight of the 28 cats came to autopsy. All had involvement of facial bones. One with a solid and tubular adenocarcinoma suffered extension to the brain through the cribriform plate. Two cats had metastases to the retropharyngeal node and lung. A one-year-old tabby with a fibrosarcoma in the right nasal passage had venous thrombi and metastases to lung, heart, and kidney. Most cats are humanely destroyed before distant metastases occur.

**MICROSCOPIC FEATURES.** Only carcinomas of the nasal cavity are described because other tumors closely resembled similar growths elsewhere in the body. Three basic types of carcinomas were obseved. The most frequent was an almost solid pattern of large, pleomorphic, polyhedral, eosinophilic cells with round nuclei of varying diameter and cytoplasm with visible margins (Fig. 11–70). The eosinophilic granules were PAS-positive and were often situated in neighboring cells so as to give the appearance of a nonpatent acinus; occasionally capillary-size lumens and larger spaces were formed. The attempt at acinar formation was better seen with the PAS stain. A fine fibrovascular stroma separated the cells into poorly

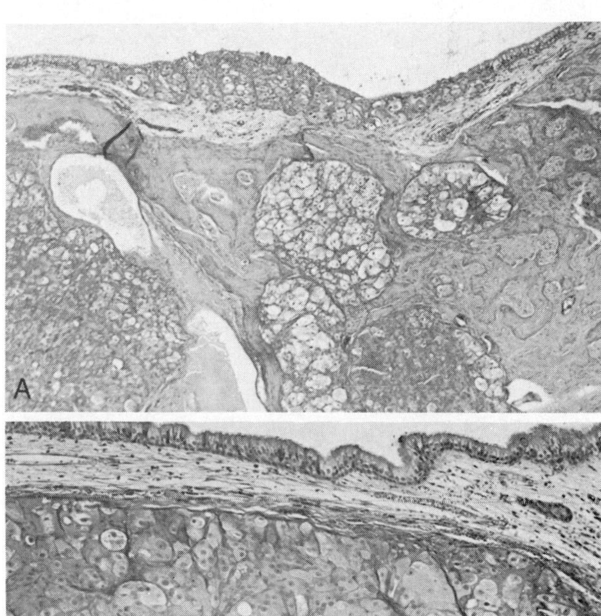


**Figure 11–70** *A*, Nasal carcinoma, 16-year-old spayed female. The tumor originates in the surface epithelium of a turbinate (upper center) and is scattered as solid-cylindrical masses deep in the turbinate. PAS, × 125. *B*, The carcinoma, in a solid pattern with thin fibrous trabeculae, lies deep in the turbinate and is unassociated, at this point, with the surface epithelium from which it arose. The neoplastic cells vary in cytoplasmic volume, some appearing globoid (top). PAS, × 312.

defined packets. Large, irregular, branching spaces were lined by cells having a brush border and, rarely, cilia.

Another variety of nearly solid pattern was a cylindroid arrangement of eosinophilic columnar cells having round basal nuclei and resting on fine, relatively straight, fibrovascular trabeculae. Between opposing rows of cells within cylinders there was sometimes a detectable central space, either empty or containing shrunken eosinophilic secretion. Some of the lining cells had a brush or ciliated border. Continuity with dysplastic and neoplastic nasal surface epithelium could be seen in both varieties of predominantly solid carcinomas.

The second basic epithelial pattern was that of simple tubular adenocarcinoma. Variable amounts of mucin were present within the cytoplasm and the lumens. The tubules were formed by cuboidal or low columnar epithelium resembling that of glandular rather than surface epithelium.

Squamous cell carcinomas, the third type of carcinoma of nasal cavity origin, resemble squamous cell carcinoma elsewhere in the body. Care must be taken to demonstrate a primary origin because secondary involvement of the nose by extension of oral neoplasms is much more common.

An unusual epithelial neoplasm in the left nasal cavity of an 11-year-old cat was characterized by squamous metaplasia of surface respiratory epithelium and regions of tubular, adenosquamous, and squamous cell carcinoma.

**MANAGEMENT.** Procedures for obtaining biopsy material and removing as much of a tumor as possible are described by Bright and Bojrab (1976). Surgical excision is often palliative and may lengthen life but is rarely curative.

**PROGNOSIS.** All malignant tumors of the nasal cavity have a poor prognosis. Recurrence after surgery is expected even when adjuvant radiation is employed (Theilen and Madewell, 1979). Intervals between nasal surgery and euthanasia ranged from two to eight months.

## Tumors of the Larynx

Tumors of the larynx are uncommon but must be considered in the differential diagnosis when a cat exhibits a gradual change in vocal character or completely "loses its voice." Other signs of laryngeal tumor are a progressive course with cough, gagging, rasping sounds of impaired air flow, and eventually life-threatening obstruction. The likeliest laryngeal tumor is lymphoma.

Primary tumors are rare. No benign tumor appears to have been reported. In man, almost all malignant tumors are squamous cell carcinomas, adenocarcinomas of mucous glands being rare. In the cat, too, squamous cell carcinomas outnumber adenocarcinomas. Whichever the type, the lesion involves the wall of the larynx and usually one or both vocal folds, proliferates into the lumen, and may also invade skeletal muscle outside the larynx.

Three cases of squamous cell carcinoma have been described, in one of which there was metastasis to a regional node (Collet, 1935; Hänichen, 1965; Wheeldon and Amis, 1985). Other squamous cell carcinomas were recorded with few or no details, three by Cotchin (1983), one by Engle and Brodey (1969), and one by Priester and McKay (1980). Two adenocarcinomas were described, in one case metastasizing to a cervical node (Vasseur and Patnaik, 1981) and in another also to lung, spleen, and adrenal (Lieberman, 1954). Another adenocarcinoma was listed without details by Engle and Brodey (1969). Of the seven cats for which age was given, one was five years old, the others from 10 to 16. Four were recorded as neutered males and two as females. Surgery was attempted in two cases but without success (Vasseur and Patnaik, 1981; Wheeldon and Amis, 1985).

At AMAH a single squamous cell carcinoma of the larynx was on record. The tumor, in an 18-year-old castrated male, occluded most of the lumen and invaded the pharynx (Fig. 11–71).

Rarely, the laryngeal orifice may be massively involved by eosinophilic granuloma that may be mistaken for tumor. A biopsy establishing the correct diagnosis would permit successful treatment.

## Tumors of the Trachea

Tracheal tumors are extremely rare in cats and, when they do occur, are usually lymphoma detected microscopically after autopsy. However, a rare symptomatic tracheal lymphoma of histiocytic type, large enough to be seen by tracheoscopy and fluoroscopy, was described in a seven-year-old intact male, FeLV-positve Siamese (Schneider et al., 1979). The mass had caused progressive dyspnea over a six-week period. A four-ring segment of the trachea was removed with its tumor, and the remaining tracheal segments were pulled and sutured together. A six-week course of treatment combining cyclophosphamide, vincristine, and prednisone was administered. The amazingly fortunate cat was apparently well eight months after surgery.

An adenoma originating in submucous glands at the bifurcation of the trachea was reported in a six-year-old cat with poor appetite, persistent retching, and dyspnea (Glock, 1960/1961).

An adenocarcinoma was described in a 10-year-old Siamese with a three-month history of stridulous breath-

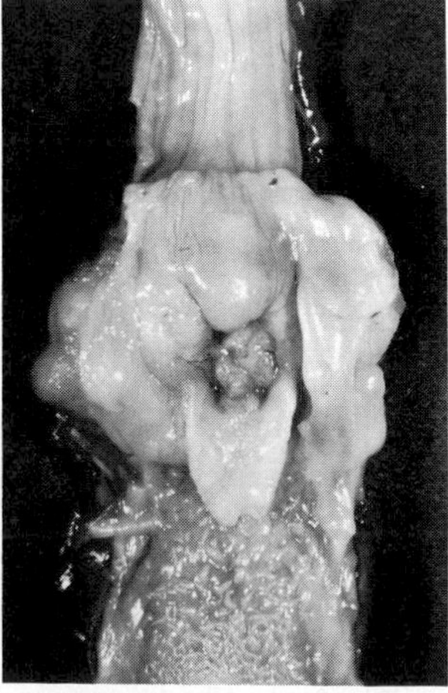

**Figure 11–71** Squamous cell carcinoma of the larynx, 18-year-old castrated male. The pale, bulky, and nodular tumor caused extreme dyspnea by occluding the laryngeal airway.

ing, coughing, periodic gagging, and marked inspiratory dyspnea (Cain and Manley, 1983). Radiography disclosed an intraluminal mass just cranial to the tracheal bifurcation. The involved segment of trachea was resected, an anastomosis was performed, and the cat recovered. The tumor, tan-white, firm, and multilobulated, obstructed over half the air passage. An adenocarcinoma of tubular and alveolar patterns, it was surmised to have arisen from glands of the tracheal submucosa.

A most interesting lesion reported as a squamous cell carcinoma in the trachea of a domestic shorthair only two years old was described as an ulcerated, well-circumscribed, granular-surfaced ridge, 8 × 4 × 3 mm, that extended transmurally through the tracheal cartilage at the level of the third intercostal space (Veith, 1974). The cat had been dyspneic for several days, was cyanotic, and died during bronchoscopy. A squamous cell carcinoma would seem most unusual in a young cat. The gross description of the lesion and of its location suggest the possibility of an injury. In a cat at AMAH a similar obstructive tracheal lesion examined at autopsy was originally interpreted as a squamous cell carcinoma but on review appeared more likely to be a tracheal tear with granulation tissue and foci of squamous metaplasia at the margins and in islands partly buried within the reactive tissue of repair. Several cats at AMAH have had partial or complete traumatic separation of the trachea at or just caudal to the thoracic inlet—the same site as in the case reported as squamous cell carcinoma.

In the only other reference to a squamous cell carcinoma of the trachea, in a 12-year-old cat, the pharynx was also involved (Schneider et al., 1979). Two carcinomas originating from the trachea were reported without details by Patnaik et al. (1975).

## Tumors of the Lung

Primary lung tumors are infrequent in cats, being found at autopsy in only about 0.4 or 0.5 per cent of cats in North America and Europe (Moulton et al., 1981; Stünzi et al., 1974). About 150 cases have been recorded in the past century, according to figures from several surveys (de Boer, 1969; Monlux, 1952; Moulton et al., 1981; Patnaik et al., 1975; Pool et al., 1974; Stünzi, 1976) and from additional reports. However, because of changing fashions in terminology over the years, the true nature of some of the tumors is uncertain; furthermore, some diagnosed as primary may actually have been metastatic.

### Benign Lesions

Benign lung tumors or tumor-like lesions are exceedingly rare in cats. The lung of the cat is notable for its abundant bronchial glands (in fact, feline lungs can be identified by this feature). These glands sometimes undergo intense adenomatous hyperplasia (Ball, 1907; de Boer, 1969; Petit, 1908; Walzl and Hunyady, 1967). Adenomas have been reported by Kronberger (1960), Patnaik et al. (1975), and Stünzi and Höfliger (1975). A "bronchial adenoma" was reported in a cat in India in association with the lung fluke *Paragonimus westermani* (Purohit and Sardeshpande, 1967).

Primary hemangioma of the lung has been recorded (Cotchin, 1966; Engle and Brodey, 1969), and a massive cholesteatoma of the left lung in a 15-year-old cat (Ball and Collet, 1932). It should be noted that a cholesteatoma is not a neoplasm but a mass consisting of granulomatous inflammation with high cholesterol and lipid content.

In cats at AMAH a few benign-appearing lesions, involving peripheral bronchioles and adjacent alveoli and resembling adenomatosis, were found. In two such cases, examination of additional sections revealed focal granulomatous foreign body inflammation within the area of columnar and cuboidal bronchioloalveolar cell proliferation. The nature of the foreign material was not determined.

### Malignant Tumors

With rare exceptions, malignant primary pulmonary tumors in the cat are of epithelial origin, most being adenocarcinoma and relatively few, epidermoid (squamous cell) and bronchial gland carcinoma. The age range in reported cases was from 2 (Nielsen, 1964) to 15 years (Jonas and Hukill, 1968; Stünzi, 1976), with the average in several studies varying from 10 to 14 years. No sex predilection has been reported, except for a markedly higher frequency in females at The Animal Medical Center (Patnaik et al., 1975). Only a few cats have been recorded as purebreds (Persians and Siamese) (Moore and Middleton, 1982; Nielsen, 1964; Slatter, 1972; Stünzi, 1958; Troy, 1955).

Hypertrophic pulmonary osteoarthropathy, which is not infrequent in dogs, is a rare complication in cats (Carr, 1971; Roberg, 1977).

Types of malignant lung tumors classified by the World Health Organization (Stünzi et al., 1974) as very rare in animals are carcinoid, mixed tumors, and sarcomas. In the cat a carcinoid was described by Schiller (Nielsen, 1970) and a mixed tumor (carcinosarcoma) by Patnaik et al., (1975). Primary sarcomas—a reticulum cell sarcoma, a spindle cell sarcoma, and a hemangiosarcoma—have been reported, respectively, by de Boer (1969), Roncaglio (cited by Monlux, 1952), and Patnaik et al. (1975).

We subscribe wholeheartedly to the important caution expressed by Stünzi et al. in the WHO Bulletin (1974), that it may be difficult to differentiate primary and secondary lung tumors, especially when the available autopsy material is incomplete. A review of 59 feline neoplasms diagnosed as primary lung tumor at AMAH in a 35-year period disclosed that only 46 were actually primary; the other 13 were metastatic from such sites as mammary gland and kidney. Incomplete autopsy material, neoplastic thrombi in major pulmonary arteries, an arterial pattern of spread, and in some cases cellular features were grounds for doubting a diagnosis of primary tumor.

**AGE, SEX, AND BREED.** The 46 cats with malignant lung tumors at AMAH ranged in age from 4 to 18 years (mean 12.5). Thirty-two were females (27 spayed) and 14 were males (13 castrated). There was thus a greater than 2:1 female:male ratio, as compared with a female:male ratio of 2:3 in the hospital population generally. Although data on breed and color were available for only 27 cats, it may possibly be of significance that 7 of the 46 (16 per cent) were tricolors, a larger proportion than in the general hospital population (7 per cent). Only four cats were noted to be purebreds (three Siamese, one Himalayan).

**SITES OF TUMOR.** It has been reported that in domestic animals the caudal lobes are most often involved and the right more often than the left (Moulton, 1978). In the AMAH group, solitary tumors occurred in 13 cats, 7 of the 13 in the caudal lobes. The right lung was involved in 8 of the 13 cats. In 13 other cats with tumor in all lobes of both lungs, sites of origin could not be determined.

The majority of papillary adenocarcinomas were intimately associated with, or could be seen arising from, large or small bronchi, while bronchioloalveolar carcinoma arose more peripherally in terminal and respiratory bronchioles and possibly in alveoli. All carcinomas of bronchial glands, epidermoid carcinomas, and the single combined tumor (adenosquamous carcinoma) were associated with the tracheal bifurcation (in two cats) or with primary bronchi.

**CLINICAL FEATURES.** Many cats have no signs or only nonspecific signs until late into the course of the neoplasm. Some tumors are asymptomatic autopsy findings incidental to other fatal conditions. In some cases the presenting complaint is unrelated to the respiratory tract and acts as a red herring to delay the correct diagnosis. Painful skeletal metastases are especially misleading.

Among the 46 cats at AMAH, disturbances that could be related to the tumor were present from three days to two months, over half the cats showing signs for only two weeks or less before the tumor was detected. Signs, in order of decreasing frequency, included rapid or difficult respiration (57 per cent), decreased appetite, weight loss, dehydration, weakness or lethargy, cyanosis, cough (13 per cent), fever, central nervous disturbance, painful lameness, and vomiting.

The respiratory difficulty may be due to extensive tumor of the lung parenchyma, to airway obstruction or compression by tumor or neoplastic nodes, to neoplastic thrombi, and to pleural effusion.

Signs limited to the nervous system in one cat were circling and falling to the left, decreased proprioception of right limbs, anisocoria, and a left visual-field deficit. Emboli of papillary adenocarcinoma from the main bronchi of the right middle and caudal lung lobes had caused left cerebral infarction due to obstruction of the left middle cerebral artery.

Locomotor difficulty was the presenting sign in one case. Episodes of hind-leg lameness and weakness over a period of a month, accompanied by muscle necrosis and atrophy, resulted from emboli of papillary adenosquamous carcinoma to both femoral arteries and their caudal femoral and popliteal branches.

Interestingly, three cats had lameness due to tumor metastases to several digits. Lameness and loss of a third phalanx when the cat clawed a carpet were the presenting complaints in a four-year-old female. Metastatic adenocarcinoma of bronchial gland origin was responsible for destruction of the bone and also for lesions resembling paronychia in other digits of both right paws. Several digits fell off during autopsy, which disclosed other metastases to eyes, skeletal muscles, duodenum, colon, and tracheobronchial, retropharyngeal, prescapular, colic, iliac, and popliteal nodes. In another cat, a seven-year-old castrated male gray Persian cross, painful metastases of a papillary bronchial adenocarcinoma to all four feet had been previously interpreted by a referring veterinarian as a deep fungal infection. Several toes were 2 cm in diameter (Fig. 11–72*A*) owing to destructive and proliferative bone changes in the second and third phalanges as seen in radiographs (Fig. 11–72*B*). Lytic and proliferative changes were evident radiographically in the dorsal spinous process of T6 (Fig. 11–72*C*). Autopsy disclosed adenocarcinoma of the right middle lung lobe and neoplastic thrombi to the toes (Fig. 11–72*D*) and to vertebra T6. The third cat, a 10-year-old spayed female white domestic shorthair, had painful metastases to all four paws. It too had been treated for mycotic pododermatitis by a referring practitioner. There were metastases to the heart, kidneys, and sixth thoracic vertebra.

Vomiting is rare and results when the wall of the esophagus is infiltrated by tumor or is compressed or fixed by nodal and other contiguous lesions. Such lesions were found in a cat that for a month ate less but retched with increasing frequency. During examination the cat coughed up pinkish foam and later, while being radiographed, frank blood, then became dyspneic, and died. A 3.5 cm tumor bound the adventitia of the esophagus to the diaphragm at the esophageal hiatus. Primary adenocarcinoma was present in all lung lobes, with metastases to mediastinum, tracheobronchial nodes, and adrenal glands. Evidence of previous hemorrhages was present in the

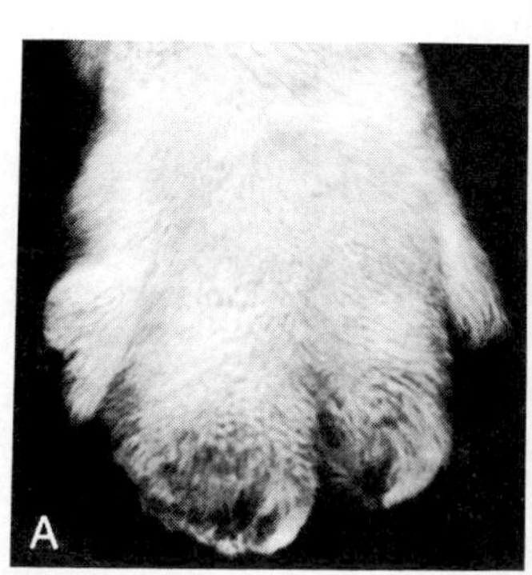


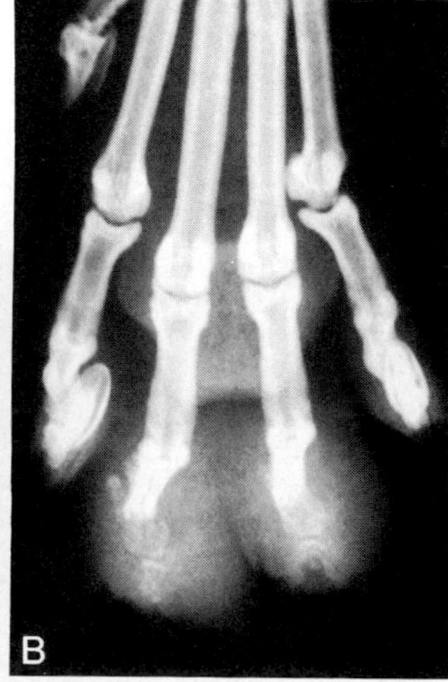


**Figure 11–72** *A*, Metastatic bronchial adenosquamous carcinoma in a forepaw of a seven-year-old castrated male gray Persian cross. The third and fourth digits are swollen, and their ends are crusted where nails have been lost. *B*, An anteroposterior view shows soft-tissue swelling and bony destruction caused by metastatic tumor to the second and third phalanges of the third and fourth digits.

*Illustration continued on opposite page*

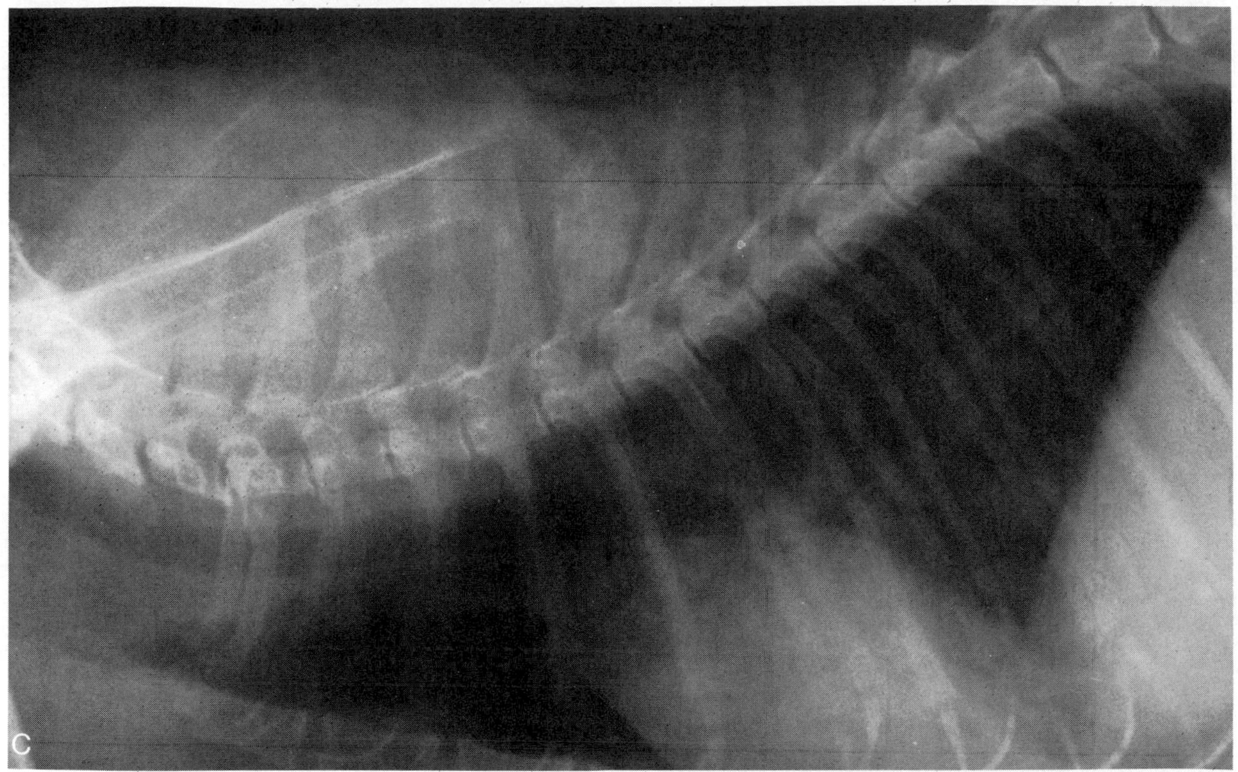


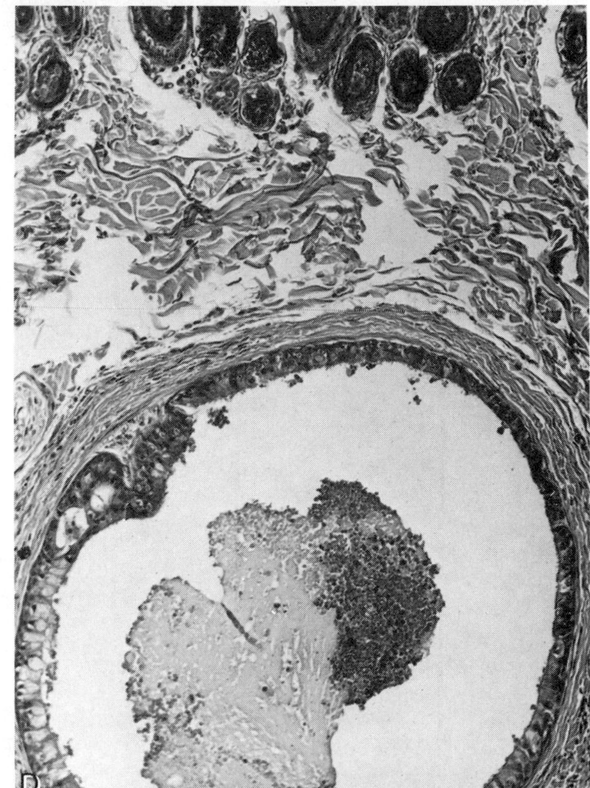


**Figure 11–72** *Continued C*, Metastasis of the carcinoma to the sixth thoracic vertebra caused osteolysis and osteogenesis of the dorsal spinous process. The primary tumor developed in the right middle lung lobe (concealed by the heart). Chronic lipid aspiration pneumonia involved the ventral portions of both caudal lung lobes. *D*, Same cat, same paw as in *A* and *B*. A dilated vessel in the subcutis is lined by metastatic pseudostratified columnar epithelium with ciliated and goblet cells. Mucus secreted by the goblet cells is mixed with blood in the lumen. H & E, × 50.

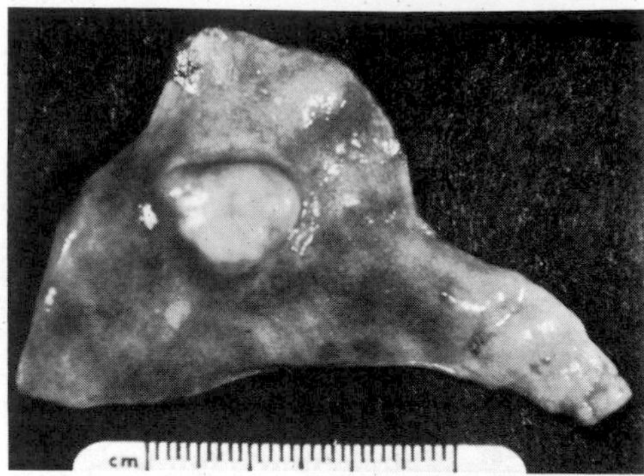


**Figure 11–73** Papillary adenocarcinoma in a cranial lung lobe, seven-year-old cat. The solitary, light yellow, spongy tumor arose from a small bronchus or a bronchiole.

tumor of the right caudal lobe, and recurrent hemorrhage was the immediate cause of death.

**LABORATORY FINDINGS.** The total white-cell count was usually in the normal range, but several were elevated, the highest to 41,250/μl. Progressive anemia was not uncommon. Pleural effusions were present in eight cats. Specific gravity ranged from 1.017 to 1.037 (mean 1.026). The white-cell count ranged from 900 to 14,520/μl (average 4300). Neutrophils predominated. Macrophages and mesothelial cells outnumbered lymphocytes in five effusions. Red cells numbered 3000 to 210,000/μl. Neoplastic cells were identified in two samples.

**RADIOGRAPHIC FEATURES.** A lateral view taken with the cat standing gives the most accurate indication of the presence and amount of fluid in the chest cavity. After aspiration of as much fluid as possible, lateral and ventrodorsal views disclose tumor involvement that varies widely from case to case. Single densities may range from a small nodule to involvement of virtually an entire lobe. Multiple or diffuse densities are more frequent. Single or multiple lesions may be predominantly hilar or peripheral. Mineralization, occasionally seen, is most likely to accompany papillary adenocarcinoma.

**PATHOLOGIC FEATURES.** Lung tumors are characterized on the basis of microscopic architecture, and the analysis of the AMAH tumors was based in general on the classificatiion of tumors of domestic animals recommended by the World Health Organization (Stünzi et al., 1974). The types of tumor in order of frequency were:

| | | |
|---|---|---|
| Adenocarcinoma | | 34 (73%) |
| Papillary | 25 (54%) | |
| Bronchioloalveolar | 9 (20%) | |
| Bronchial gland carcinoma | | 8 (18%) |

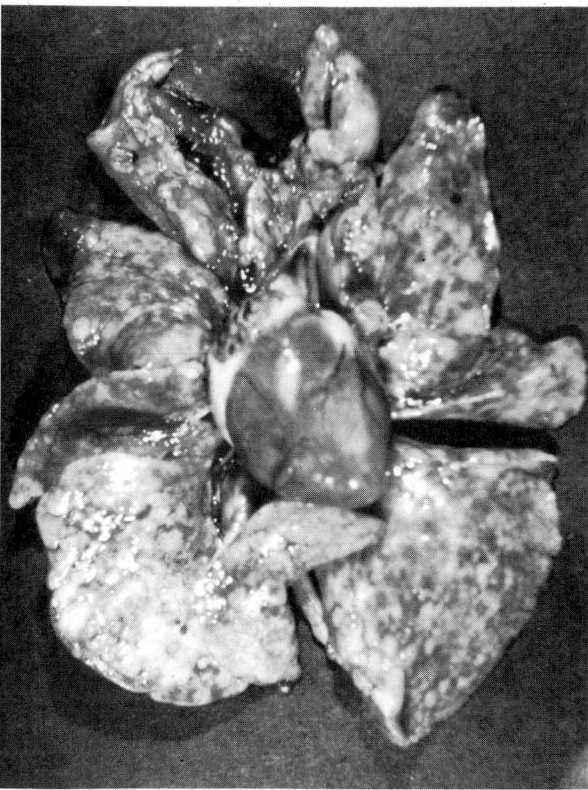

**Figure 11–74** Papillary adenocarcinoma of the lung, 13-year-old cat. The tumor apparently started in the bronchus of the right caudal lobe and extended to involve all lobes, pleura, and mediastinal nodes (top). Metastases involved the heart, thyroid, adrenals, kidneys, bladder, spleen, esophagus, and stomach.

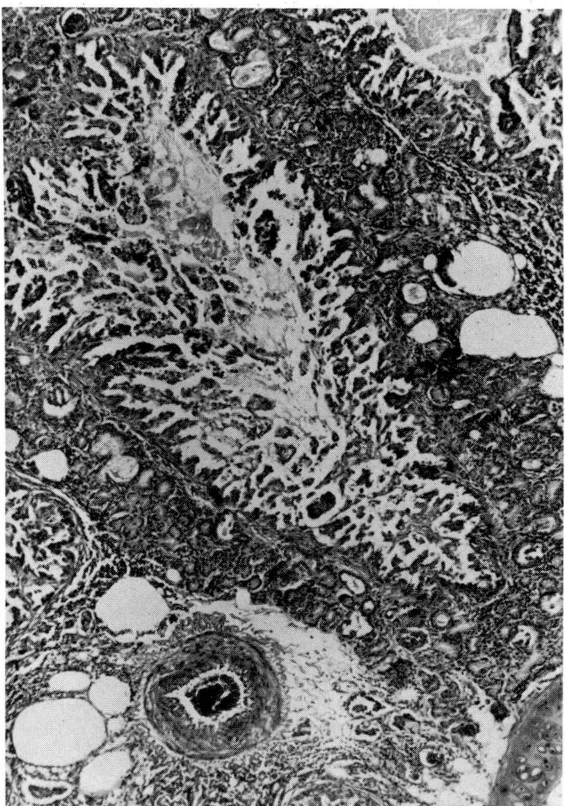

**Figure 11–75** Bronchial papillary adenocarcinoma, 11-year-old cat. Neoplastic papillary projections diffusely line the bronchus (center) and replace lung parenchyma (top right). Only a few ducts of the bronchial glands that completely surround the bronchus show neoplastic change. Also shown are a hypertrophied bronchial artery (bottom) and a cartilaginous plaque (lower right). H & E, × 50.

| | |
|---|---|
| Epidermoid (squamous cell) carcinoma | 3 (7%) |
| Combined epidermoid and adenocarcinoma (adenosquamous) | 1 (2%) |

No case of anaplastic carcinoma, carcinoid, or sarcoma was recognized in the AMAH group.

**Adenocarcinomas.** Papillary adenocarcinomas constituted 25 of the 34 adenocarcinomas. Single or multiple and ranging from minute to 8.0 cm in diameter, they were soft or firm, pale yellow or tan, and solid or cystic, sometimes with a mucoid exudate (Figs. 11–73 and 11–74). Most were poorly circumscribed, and all lacked a true capsule. Eighteen cats had metastatic lesions, most often of the pleura and tracheobronchial nodes. Five had severe mediastinal involvement, and three had metastases to the kidneys. Metastatic lesions were found only once: in brain, thyroid, esophagus, heart, stomach, liver, spleen, adrenal, and urinary bladder.

Microscopically, some papillary adenocarcinomas consisted of well-differentiated, simple columnar (cylindrical) cells or of cuboidal epithelium that formed glandular structures resembling enlarged alveoli with papillae composed of similar cells (Figs. 11–75 and 11–76). Other tumors consisted of less differentiated pleomorphic cells characterized by a larger ratio of nucleus to cytoplasm; by greater variety in shape, size, and location of nuclei; and by foci of squamous metaplasia (Fig. 11–77). As well as single rows of epithelium, some papillary tumors had well-differentiated areas of stratification and pseudostratification, occasionally with cilia and rarely with goblet cells. Vascular invasion was observed in 17 cases. Fibrosis was rare and usually associated with bronchiectasis and regions of necrosis rather than being within the papillary pattern of the tumor. Mucin accumulation was prominent in only four tumors, although mucin has been reported to be commonly demonstrable within cells by special stains. Cilia were seen on some cells in fewer than half the cases. Psammoma bodies occurred in eight tumors. Focal necrosis was a constant finding, varying only in degree.

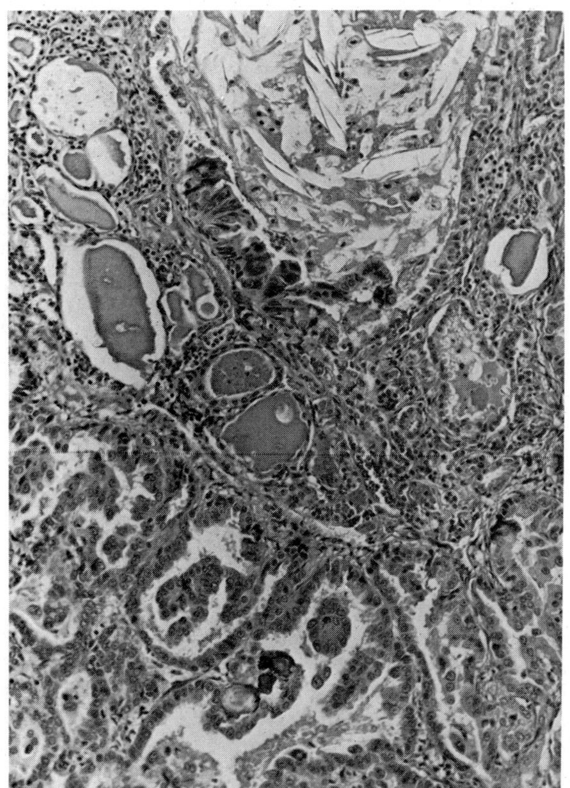

**Figure 11–76** Bronchial papillary adenocarcinoma, 18-year-old cat. The tumor, composed of cuboidal and columnar cells, surrounds the bronchial wall (bottom) and arises focally from the bronchial epithelium (top center). The bronchial lumen (top) is filled with macrophages and cholesterol clefts, and the bronchial glands are dilated and filled with secretion. Concretions (psammoma bodies) are within the tumor (bottom center). H & E, × 150.

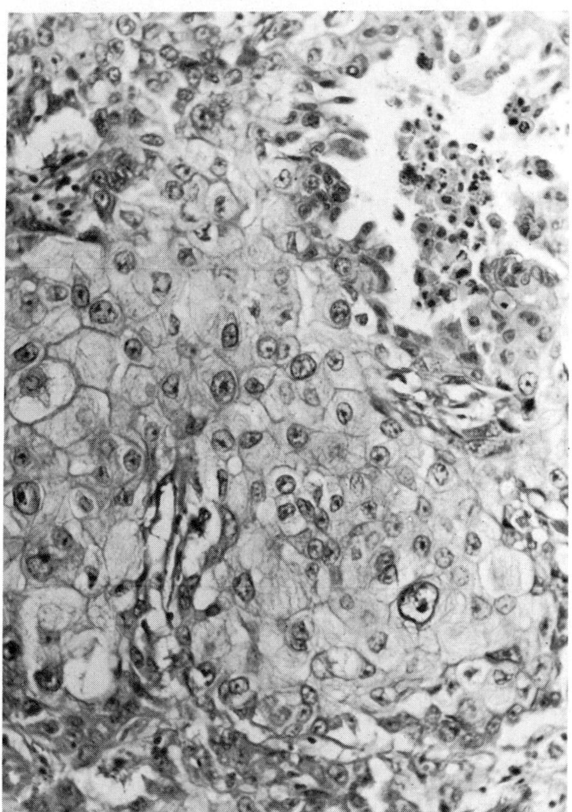

**Figure 11–77** Papillary adenocarcinoma of bronchial origin in a 10-year-old male tabby. Squamous differentiation without keratinization (left center) is a prominent feature. H & E, × 200.

The cylindrocellular and poorly differentiated tumors were more invasive and gave rise to more metastatic lesions than did those characterized by cuboidal epithelium of terminal and respiratory bronchioles.

Medial hyperplasia and hypertrophy of pulmonary arteries were present in 13 cats, and a coexisting chronic lipid aspiration pneumonia in four.

Bronchioloalveolar adenocarcinoma was represented by 9 in the group of 33 adenocarcinomas. According to criteria presented by Kress and Allen (cited by Moulton, 1978), this tumor should be solitary; however, multicentric origin appeared likely in some cats rather than spread by lymphatics or airways. Grossly, most of the tumors resembled papillary adenocarcinomas, except that they were more often solitary, more peripheral lesions, with less tendency to metastasize. Metastases, detected in only three cats, involved the pleura, tracheobronchial nodes, mediastinum, and kidneys.

Microscopically, the cuboidal or columnar cells appeared to arise from bronchioles and alveolar ducts, and lined alveolar septa without altering the architectural framework of the lung (Fig. 11–78). Some alveoli contained collections of large epithelial cells with a variable amount of cytoplasm. These intra-alveolar cells were arranged in rosettes, small irregular packets, or solid masses completely filling the alveoli.

**Bronchial Gland Carcinoma.** Bronchial gland tumors have been distinguished as an entity that may occur more often in dogs and cats than in man (Stünzi et al., 1974). Originating in the glands of the bronchial mucosa, they are in one view predominantly epidermoid (Stünzi, 1976; Stünzi et al., 1974). In the experience of others, the pattern tends to adenocarcinoma, although there are areas of squamous differentiation of carcinoma cells and of mixed adeno- and squamous carcinoma (Moulton et al., 1981).

Bronchial gland carcinomas constituted 8 of the 45 AMAH lung tumors. Seven were associated with major bronchi at, or close to, the hilus, one having tracheal lesions at the bifurcation; the eighth involved the distal 3 cm of the major bronchus of the left caudal lobe. In general, the tumors grossly resembled most papillary adenocarcinomas, except for the greater frequency of hilar involvement and the increased firmness attributable to significant fibroplasia. Bronchial sclerosis, although not recorded in these cases, is more likely with this tumor than with papillary adenocarcinoma.

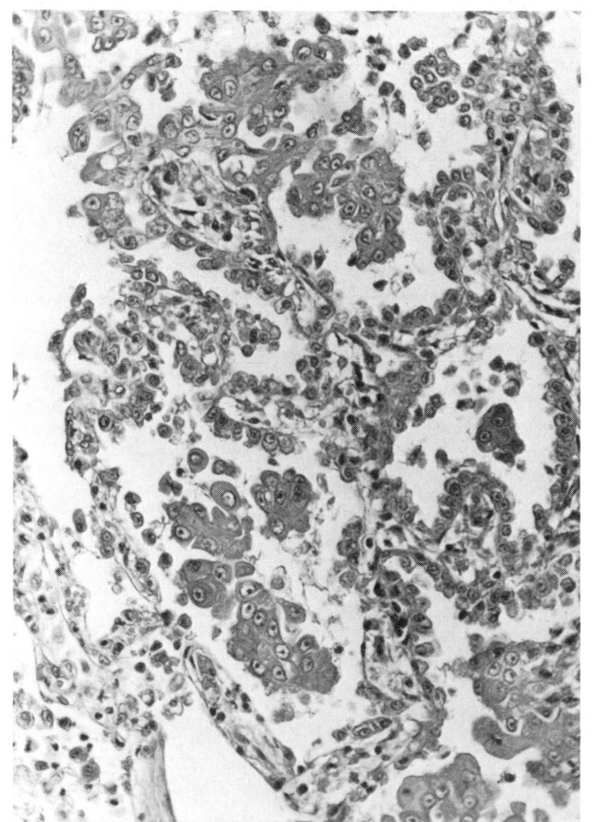

**Figure 11–78** Alveolar cell carcinoma in a 12-year-old cat that died of cardiomyopathy. The 3 mm tumor was found by chance during routine microscopic examination of lung. The tumor arises from and projects into alveoli. H & E, × 200.

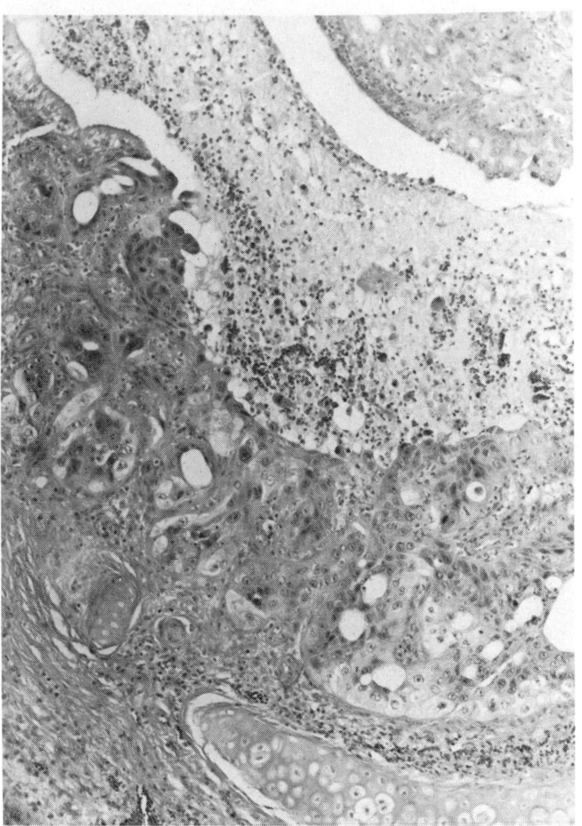

**Figure 11–79** Adenosquamous carcinoma of bronchial epithelial and glandular origin, 12-year-old domestic shorthair. The bronchus is lined by normal pseudostratified epithelium (upper left), squamous cells (upper right), and malignant cells (lower left) appearing to arise from surface and glandular epithelium. H & E, × 75.

Microscopically, no tumor appeared to arise solely from tracheal or bronchial glandular epithelium, but also had one or more sites of origin in metaplastic or neoplastic surface epithelium—a finding at variance with the published descriptions (Fig. 11–79). Pleomorphism and, often, squamous differentiation without keratinization were characteristic of this acinar (tubuloalveolar) tumor. Six cats had widespread tumor in both lungs. Seven had prominent lymphatic and venous neoplastic thrombi, and one also had a thrombus in a pulmonary artery, possibly by embolism from a distant metastatic lesion or by spread in the vasa vasorum.

Pathologists may mistake bronchial lymphatic and venous spread of another type of tumor for one arising from bronchial glands. Such spread was often observed with other malignant primary as well as secondary lung tumors.

Fibroplasia can be so severe as to mimic a primitive myxo- or fibrosarcoma. In one cat with a bronchial gland tumor (and in another with epidermoid carcinoma) there was the suggestion of sarcoma induced by the carcinoma; the accompanying fibrous tissue proliferation had tissue pattern and cellular features common to fibrosarcomas.

**Epidermoid (Squamous Cell) Carcinoma.** Only 3 of the 46 tumors were epidermoid carcinoma. All arose in the hilar region and were firm, white, and poorly demarcated. Central cavitation was prominent owing to tissue necrosis and destruction of bronchi.

Microscopically, these tumors were characterized by compact foci of large epithelial cells with sharply defined borders and occasional desmosomes. Keratinization was absent. Fibroplasia and necrosis were constant findings. None of the tumors was pure squamous cell carcinoma, since all had a small component of gland formation similar to bronchial gland carcinoma. The tumors originated from bronchial surface epithelium and very likely glandular epithelium too, because squamous metaplasia, as well as neoplasia, appeared to involve the ducts of glands. In metastatic lesions the glandular component predominated (whereas in the tumors reported by Stünzi [1976], the metastases were epidermoid).

As Stünzi (1976) observed, the presence of both epidermoid and adenocarcinomatous structures might favor the designation of "combined tumor."

Intraocular metastasis from a pulmonary squamous cell carcinoma has been described (Hamilton et al., 1984).

**Combined Epidermoid and Adenocarcinoma** This tumor, also called adenosquamous carcinoma, is composed nearly equally of epidermoid carcinoma and adenocarcinoma. It is necessary that several sections of a tumor be examined before this diagnosis is made (Stünzi et al., 1974). Only one tumor of this type was identified among the 46 in the AMAH group. Both components were evident not only in the primary tumor but also in neoplastic thrombi of both femoral arteries, in metastases to a kidney, and in several pulmonary arteries. The pulmonary arterial thrombi most likely represented the return of metastases from distant tumor sites. In one branch of the pulmonary artery the intima was covered with squamous cells and in another branch, with simple and pseudostratified columnar cells, some ciliated.

**Conclusions.** It is clear from previous reviews and case reports and from study of lung tumors in cats at AMAH that the predominant lung tumor in cats, as in dogs, is adenocarcinoma and that it occurs mostly in elderly animals. Both at The Animal Medical Center and at AMAH, females were affected with significantly greater frequency.

Although it is obviously impossible to follow the development of a given tumor chronologically, personal observation (JLC) is that multicentric origin of adenocarcinomas is not uncommon. The small number of solitary masses and the distribution of tumors support this opinion. Furthermore, many of the tumors have an overlap in patterns that complicates differentiation of bronchial papillary adenocarcinoma and bronchioloalveolar carcinoma. There is also an overlapping in morphology of adenocarcinoma and epidermoid carcinoma, since both patterns can exist in a given tumor. Squamous cell metaplasia or differentiation was present in 15 of the 42 adenocarcinomas and bronchial gland carcinomas. Keratinization did not occur in any tumor, not even in the "combined" (adenosquamous) or epidermoid tumors.

### Tumors of the Thoracic Cavity

Lymphoma of the cranial mediastinum is notoriously common. Next in frequency is thymoma. Both are discussed in the section on hematopoietic neoplasms and also in the chapter on hematopoietic disorders. Rarely, mast cell tumor and mesothelioma are found in the mediastinum (see sections on those neoplasms). Fibrosarcoma of the cranial mediastinum was diagnosed in one cat at AMAH.

## TUMORS OF THE CARDIOVASCULAR SYSTEM*

### Tumors of the Heart

The heart is occasionally the site of lymphoma in cats with multicentric tumor. Involvement may be massive or microscopic. There are rare reports of primary sarcomas of muscle (Cordy, 1978; Priester and McKay, 1980) and of primary fibrosarcomas (Nielsen, 1964; Ryan and Walder, 1980). A myxosarcoma of the pericardium weighing 350 gm and displacing the heart and lungs was reported by Mollereau (cited by Lombard, 1940), and a mesothelioma of the pericardial sac was described by Tilley et al. (1975). A malignant tumor at the base of the heart, reported by Graubmann and Sander (1965), was believed to have originated from ectopic parathyroid tissue.

The heart is the most frequent site of metastasis for hemangiosarcoma in the cat (Patnaik and Liu, 1977). Other metastatic tumors that have been observed include mammary carcinoma, salivary gland carcinoma, and oral melanoma (Tilley et al., 1981).

Although less frequent in cats than in dogs, the principal tumors of the cardiovascular system are hemangiomas and hemangiosarcomas. In many instances they may be differentiated only by microscopic study from other lesions such as hematomas, granulation tissue, vascular malformations and acquired telangiectasia, telangiectatic osteosarcoma, and cysts of apocrine and ceruminous glands containing dark fluid.

### Tumors of Vessels

#### Telangiectasia

Telangiectasia is non-neoplastic but may have the gross appearance of tumor. It is rare in cats. Instances observed at AMAH included telangiectasia of cerebellum (Fig. 11–80), ovary, and liver. The first two were congenital, but the pathogenesis of the hepatic lesion was unknown.

#### Hemangioma

Hemangiomas are benign growths of blood vascular endothelium. A survey of 395 feline tumors included two of the skin and one of the lung (Engle and Brodey, 1969). Eight "hemangiomas and lymphangiomas" were listed in another survey of 621 tumors (Dorn et al., 1968a). In a

*Laura K. Andrews, principal author, tumors of the heart and blood vessels.

nerve as it emerges from the stylomastoid foramen at the base of the skull and courses through the parotid gland may cause unilateral facial nerve palsy. Two of 13 cats examined at AMAH had moderate dyspnea owing to aspiration pneumonia. Both cats had large invasive tumors, one of the mandibular and one of the parotid gland. Both cats had been force-fed by their owners.

**GROSS FEATURES.** Most adenocarcinomas of salivary glands are firm, bosselated, white or tan masses closely adherent to the overlying subcutis. On cut section, firm, yellow, gritty areas of necrosis may be seen. Cystic and hemorrhagic foci are common. Because adenocarcinomas grow rapidly and are rarely detected early, they may be quite large at diagnosis. One adenocarcinoma of a parotid gland measured 8.0 × 8.0 × 6.0 cm.

Adenomas may resemble adenocarcinomas grossly or may be soft and pink. They are well circumscribed and do not adhere to overlying skin.

**MICROSCOPIC FEATURES.** Salivary gland tumors are classified as epithelial or mesenchymal. Benign epithelial tumors include monomorphic and pleomorphic adenomas (benign mixed tumors). The latter have not been reported in the cat. The monomorphic adenoma consists of epithelial cells in a regular glandular pattern. There is no proliferation of myoepithelial cells and no altered ground substance. Only two adenomas of a feline salivary gland were found in a review of the literature (Bastianello, 1983; Case and Simon, 1966). The tumor described by Case and Simon as an oncocytoma (oxyphilic granular adenoma), a rare benign tumor of the parotid salivary gland, was removed successfully.

One of two adenomas diagnosed at AMAH was an ovoid, soft, pink mass, 0.8 × 0.6 × 0.3 cm in the right molar salivary gland of a seven-year-old castrated male domestic shorthair. On microscopic examination, it consisted of pale-staining cuboidal to columnar epithelial cells resembling goblet cells, with basally located nuclei arranged in a papillary glandular pattern (Fig. 11–88). There were extensive multifocal, mucus-filled cystic spaces, into which papillary processes of the tumor projected. The tumor did not recur after removal of the affected gland. The other adenoma, in a nine-year-old female domestic shorthair, was an ovoid, gray-brown, firm, lobulated mass, 1.5 × 1.5 × 1.0 cm, involving the right mandibular gland and the caudal aspect of the right sublingual gland. It consisted of circumscribed foci of low cuboidal to columnar epithelial cells arranged in a pattern of small tubules. The nuclei were basal and the cytoplasm granular or vacuolated. The neoplasm had been noticed for a month and had fluctuated in size. The cat was destroyed shortly after surgical removal because of concomitant lymphoma.

The malignant epithelial tumors include adenocarcinoma, mucoepidermoid tumor, acinic cell tumor, squamous cell carcinoma, undifferentiated carcinoma, and carcinoma in pleomorphic adenoma (malignant mixed tumor). Undifferentiated carcinoma and acinic cell tumors have not been reported in the cat.

Adenocarcinomas, the most numerous salivary neoplasms in the cat, may arise from acinar or ductal epithelium. They are classified on the basis of pattern as tubular or ductular. The ductular pattern consists of low cuboidal epithelium with papillary projections. The tubular type may be subdivided into simple tubular, alveolar, trabecular, and solid patterns. Although it is common to find more than one pattern within a given tumor, one pattern usually predominates. Of 11 adenocarcinomas examined at AMAH, 4 had a simple tubular pattern, 2 a papillary (Fig. 11–89) or ductal pattern, 3 a solid pattern (Fig. 11–90), 1 a mixed tubular and papillary pattern, and 1 an alveolar pattern. Nuclei were round or oval, usually with a single prominent nucleolus. The degree of cellular atypia and number of mitotic figures varied. Necrosis, inflammation, and desmoplasia were common, as were vascular, perineural, lymphatic, and stromal invasion. Mucus secretion, cyst formation, and squamous or osseous metaplasia were less frequent. In one neoplasm, there was an inflammatory response to a ruptured cyst.

Of the 11 adenocarcinomas at AMAH, 8 had metastasized to regional lymph nodes at the time of diagnosis. All were locally invasive. In a cat with an adenocarcinoma of the minor salivary glands of the cheek, the tumor invaded the buccal mucosa and spread to regional lymph nodes, lung, heart, brain, pancreas, and adrenals. Another cat with an adenocarcinoma of the left parotid gland had metastases to the subcutaneous tissue over the head, neck, and scapula.

The mucoepidermoid tumor consists of solid masses of squamous cells with intercellular bridges and rare keratin formation surrounding mucus-secreting cells. The latter characteristically form cystic structures. The degree of differentiation of the two cell types varies. PAS, alcian green, or mucicarmine stain may be used to demonstrate mucin in the mucoepidermoid tumor (Koestner and Buer-

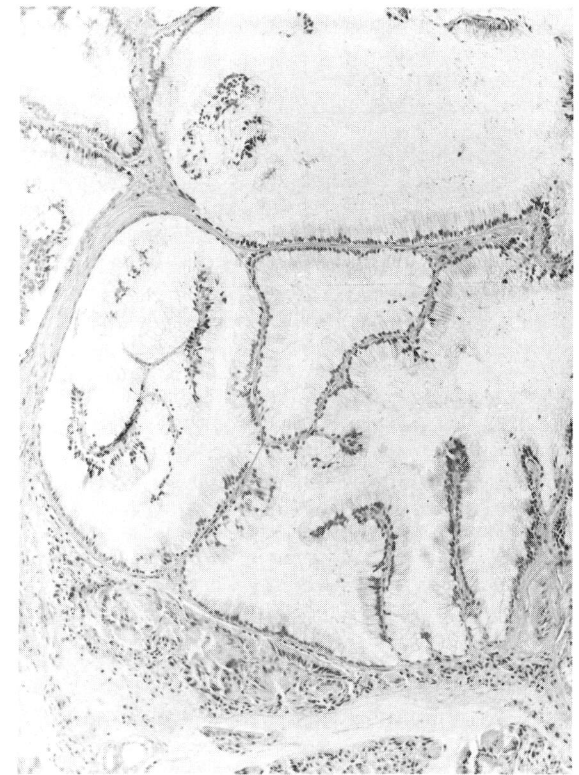

**Figure 11–88** Papillary adenoma of the molar salivary gland, six-year-old castrated male domestic shorthair. Papillae, lined by mucus-laden, tall, simple columnar epithelium, project into dilated mucus-filled glandular spaces. H & E, × 75.

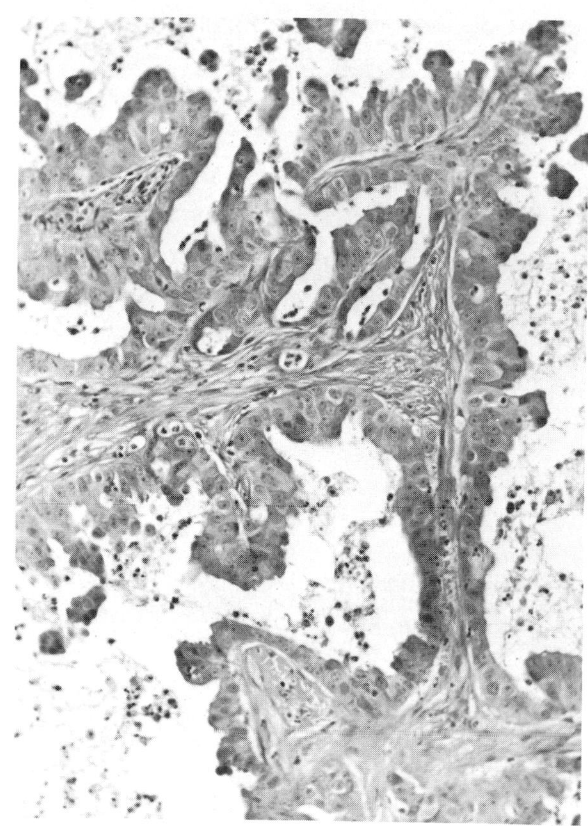

**Figure 11–89** Papillary adenocarcinoma of the parotid salivary gland, five-year-old male cat. Repetitive branching papillae form irregular spaces containing secretion, neutrophils, and macrophages. Epithelium varies from simple cuboidal to stratified columnar. H & E, × 150.

ger, 1965). A 12-year-old male Siamese cat had a 2.0 × 1.0 × 1.0 cm mucoepidermoid tumor of the parotid gland that metastasized to the lungs (Karbe and Schiefer, 1967).

One squamous cell carcinoma was reported as arising in the sublingual salivary gland (Koestner and Buerger, 1965). The morphology resembled that of squamous cell carcinomas generally, characterized by cords, islands of squamous epithelial cells with intercellular bridges, and occasional keratinization. There is some doubt as to whether primary squamous cell carcinomas of the salivary gland exist. Most squamous cell carcinomas in salivary glands are extensions of tumors arising in the oral cavity or skin.

Carcinoma in pleomorphic adenoma (malignant mixed tumor) consists of epithelial cells intermingled with a mucoid, chondroid, myxoid, or osteoid matrix. Either the epithelial or the myoepithelial component is malignant and is capable of local invasion and metastasis. Such a tumor was described in a 12-year-old spayed female domestic cat with a firm subcutaneous swelling 2.0 cm in diameter in the right submandibular area (Wells and Robinson, 1975). The mass had gradually increased in size for three weeks. On biopsy it was diagnosed as a malignant mixed tumor. Five months after surgery the cat was destroyed because of weight loss and increased tumor size. At autopsy the tumor measured 8.0 × 7.0 × 6.0 cm and extended from the base of the right ear to the commissure of the lips. It ensheathed the caudal third of the mandible and extended medially, approaching the midline of the oral cavity. It was pale gray, nodular, and ovoid, had a thin capsule, and was well circumscribed. It invaded the soft tissues of the head to the tympanic bulla and replaced part of the right sternocephalicus muscle. On cut section there were cavities 1.0 cm in diameter containing brown, viscid fluid. Culture yielded *Pasteurella septica*. Other areas of the tumor were firm and gritty. Microscopic examination revealed two kinds of tissue: sarcomatous mesenchymal cells of varied morphology forming osteoid and cartilage, and malignant cuboidal epithelial cells forming acini in a cellular mucinous stroma. The right mandibular lymph node was not found, but there was no evidence of distant spread.

Other salivary gland tumors described were a branchial epithelioma situated within the left parotid gland (Ball and Collet, 1934) and a primary melanoma also in the parotid gland (Ball, 1934). Primary mesenchymal tumors have not been reported in the cat. For correct diagnosis of a primary mesenchymal tumor in a salivary gland, it should have no other possible primary source and should infiltrate the gland diffusely rather than in circumscribed foci.

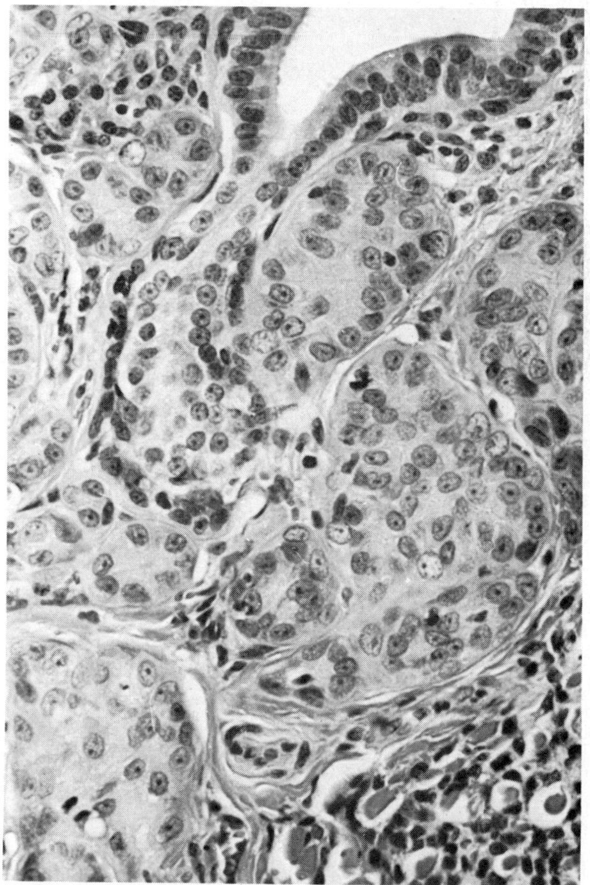

**Figure 11–90** Adenocarcinoma of the mandibular salivary gland, adult male Siamese. The tumor is arranged in solid packets and is of ductal origin. Multifocal malignant transformation involved small ducts (top) as well as the major duct (not shown). H & E, × 312.

Metastatic tumors in salivary glands are rare and are most likely to be squamous cell carcinoma or malignant lymphoma. It is important to distinguish primary neoplasms of the salivary gland from adenocarcinomas of ceruminous gland originating in the external ear.

**DIAGNOSIS.** Diagnosis of salivary gland tumors requires careful microscopic examination. Cytologic examination of fine-needle aspirates from the tumor may merely reveal clumps of malignant epithelial cells not identifiable as to origin. Thick, viscid, clear or brown fluid may be obtained if a cystic area is aspirated.

**TREATMENT.** The best treatment for salivary gland tumors is surgical removal. Except for adenomas, however, complete excision is difficult or impossible because by the time a cat is presented, most tumors are large, have ill-defined margins, and have invaded surrounding tissues to which they are firmly adherent. Attempted removal of a parotid cancer was followed by development of a fistula and recurrence of the tumor in fulminant form a month later (Bosselut et al., 1951).

## Tumors of the Esophagus

### Benign Tumors

Papillomatosis believed to be secondary to chronic esophagitis appears to be the only reported instance of a benign tumor of the esophagus (Wilkinson, 1970). The cat, a one-year-old spayed female domestic shorthair, had signs of respiratory disease, did not eat, and sat in a crouched position, gulping frequently and licking its lips. Contrast radiography revealed dilatation of the caudal esophagus, with marked irregularity of the mucosa. Autopsy disclosed diffuse, cauliflower-like growths in the intrathoracic part of the esophagus. The papillomas decreased in size from the thoracic inlet to the cardia. Lymphocytes, plasma cells, and mast cells infiltrated the tumors and the muscular tunic.

### Squamous Cell Carcinoma

This tumor is a rarity except in cats in Britain, where several cases were described in the early literature (e.g., Gray, 1935; Vincent, 1927; Wooldridge, 1913) and a total of 29 were diagnosed at the Royal Veterinary College, London (Cotchin, 1983). A few instances have been reported in France (Jonquières, 1935; Lamouroux and Lebeau, 1953) and in the United States (Patnaik et al., 1975; Poppensiek, 1961; Vernon and Roudebush, 1980). Four cases were diagnosed at AMAH.

Squamous cell carcinoma usually occurs in the middle third of the esophagus just caudal to the thoracic inlet but has been found in the cervical and terminal segments. More males than females have been affected. No breed predilection has been recognized. Except for one 3½-year-old (Lamouroux and Lebeau, 1953), the cats ranged in age from 6 to 20 years (mean 12).

The outstanding clinical sign is regurgitation shortly after swallowing of solid food. The cat often salivates, loses weight, and becomes depressed and inappetent. Some, however, manifest ravenous hunger (Joshua, 1965). If the tumor is in the cervical esophagus, palpation of the ventral neck may cause gagging and excessive swallowing. Contrast radiographs usually reveal an annular stenotic lesion or roughening of the esophageal mucosa with intramural filling defects. Cranial to the obstruction the esophagus is dilated (Fig. 11–91*A*). In one cat, examination with a fiberoptic endoscope revealed multiple small, white nodules in the mucosa of the proximal 5.0 cm of the esophagus (Vernon and Roudebush, 1980).

Grossly, most of the carcinomas are irregular, moderately firm, white stenotic growths, almost encircling the esophagus (Fig. 11–91*B* and *C*). The mucosa is nodular and frequently ulcerated. Occasionally the tumor is diffuse. One cat at AMAH had a hiatal hernia that resulted from an ulcerated stenotic tumor in the caudal esophagus. Microscopically, the tumor resembles squamous cell carcinomas found in the oral cavity.

The prognosis for this tumor is poor. The tumor most often metastasizes to the tracheobronchial or mediastinal lymph nodes.

### Other Malignant Tumors

In a cat at AMAH, a well-demarcated intramural mass in the cranial esophagus caused stenosis and regurgitation. It was surprising that the growth was an adenocarcinoma, since the cat's esophagus is devoid of glands, and a careful search discovered no primary tumor elsewhere. A sarcoma of the thoracic esophagus characterized by large round cells was described as subannular, stenosing, and ulcerated (Roy, 1938). Rarely, there may be infiltration of the esophagus by lymphoma or by tracheopulmonary or thyroid carcinoma.

## Tumors of the Stomach

Primary tumors of the stomach, rarely reported for the cat, include polyps, squamous cell and undifferentiated carcinoma, adenocarcinoma, leiomyoma, and leiomyosarcoma. Although the stomach is an infrequent site for malignant lymphomas, these constitute the majority of gastric neoplasms in the cat.

Gastric polyps were found in three elderly cats at AMAH, a Siamese, a Burmese, and an "Angora-Manx" cross. The two cats with fundic tumors had no clinical signs, but one with multiple, 0.1 to 0.2 cm, nodular growths in the pylorus vomited after eating and lost weight for a month before it was taken to a veterinarian. The polyps in the other cats, ranging in size from 0.1 to 0.6 cm, were pedunculated, cauliflower-like masses that projected from the gastric mucosa. In all three cats the polyps consisted of tubules of well-differentiated epithelium covering a narrow connective tissue stalk. Polyps are thought not to recur after surgical resection.

Adenocarcinomas are very rare in the cat. Only six appear to have been reported (Lingeman et al., 1971; Poppensiek, 1961; Turk et al., 1981). A squamous cell carcinoma (Poppensiek, 1961) and an undifferentiated carcinoma (Turk et al., 1981) have also been recorded, as well as nonfunctional argentaffinoma (carcinoid) (Jubb et al., 1985).

Mesenchymal tumors reported, other than lymphoma, are sarcoma (Cadéac, 1909; Cotchin, 1983) and leiomyosarcoma (Engle and Brodey, 1969; Priester and McKay, 1980); lymphoma is most frequent, taking the form of one or more thickened areas, sometimes ulcerated. The stom-

| | |
|---|---|
| Epidermoid (squamous cell) carcinoma | 3 (7%) |
| Combined epidermoid and adenocarcinoma (adenosquamous) | 1 (2%) |

No case of anaplastic carcinoma, carcinoid, or sarcoma was recognized in the AMAH group.

**Adenocarcinomas.** Papillary adenocarcinomas constituted 25 of the 34 adenocarcinomas. Single or multiple and ranging from minute to 8.0 cm in diameter, they were soft or firm, pale yellow or tan, and solid or cystic, sometimes with a mucoid exudate (Figs. 11–73 and 11–74). Most were poorly circumscribed, and all lacked a true capsule. Eighteen cats had metastatic lesions, most often of the pleura and tracheobronchial nodes. Five had severe mediastinal involvement, and three had metastases to the kidneys. Metastatic lesions were found only once: in brain, thyroid, esophagus, heart, stomach, liver, spleen, adrenal, and urinary bladder.

Microscopically, some papillary adenocarcinomas consisted of well-differentiated, simple columnar (cylindrical) cells or of cuboidal epithelium that formed glandular structures resembling enlarged alveoli with papillae composed of similar cells (Figs. 11–75 and 11–76). Other tumors consisted of less differentiated pleomorphic cells characterized by a larger ratio of nucleus to cytoplasm; by greater variety in shape, size, and location of nuclei; and by foci of squamous metaplasia (Fig. 11–77). As well as single rows of epithelium, some papillary tumors had well-differentiated areas of stratification and pseudostratification, occasionally with cilia and rarely with goblet cells. Vascular invasion was observed in 17 cases. Fibrosis was rare and usually associated with bronchiectasis and regions of necrosis rather than being within the papillary pattern of the tumor. Mucin accumulation was prominent in only four tumors, although mucin has been reported to be commonly demonstrable within cells by special stains. Cilia were seen on some cells in fewer than half the cases. Psammoma bodies occurred in eight tumors. Focal necrosis was a constant finding, varying only in degree.

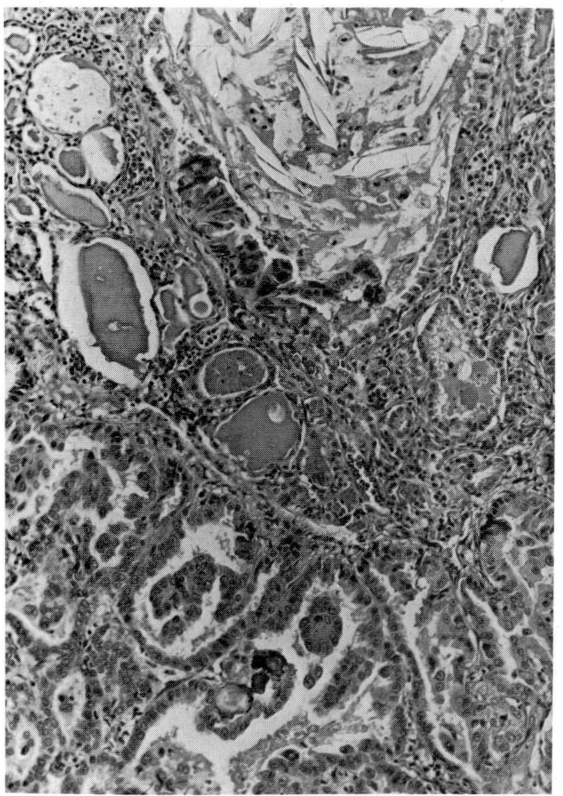

**Figure 11–76** Bronchial papillary adenocarcinoma, 18-year-old cat. The tumor, composed of cuboidal and columnar cells, surrounds the bronchial wall (bottom) and arises focally from the bronchial epithelium (top center). The bronchial lumen (top) is filled with macrophages and cholesterol clefts, and the bronchial glands are dilated and filled with secretion. Concretions (psammoma bodies) are within the tumor (bottom center). H & E, × 150.

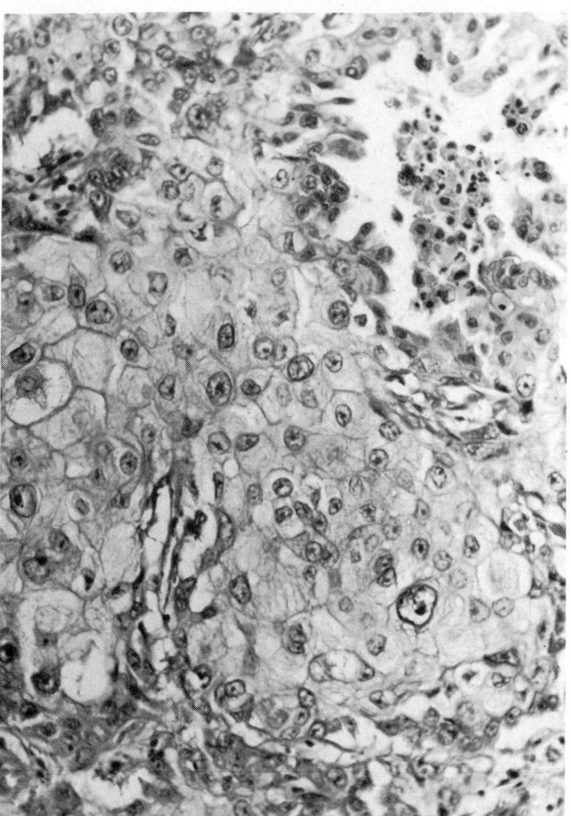

**Figure 11–77** Papillary adenocarcinoma of bronchial origin in a 10-year-old male tabby. Squamous differentiation without keratinization (left center) is a prominent feature. H & E, × 200.

The cylindrocellular and poorly differentiated tumors were more invasive and gave rise to more metastatic lesions than did those characterized by cuboidal epithelium of terminal and respiratory bronchioles.

Medial hyperplasia and hypertrophy of pulmonary arteries were present in 13 cats, and a coexisting chronic lipid aspiration pneumonia in four.

Bronchioloalveolar adenocarcinoma was represented by 9 in the group of 33 adenocarcinomas. According to criteria presented by Kress and Allen (cited by Moulton, 1978), this tumor should be solitary; however, multicentric origin appeared likely in some cats rather than spread by lymphatics or airways. Grossly, most of the tumors resembled papillary adenocarcinomas, except that they were

more often solitary, more peripheral lesions, with less tendency to metastasize. Metastases, detected in only three cats, involved the pleura, tracheobronchial nodes, mediastinum, and kidneys.

Microscopically, the cuboidal or columnar cells appeared to arise from bronchioles and alveolar ducts, and lined alveolar septa without altering the architectural framework of the lung (Fig. 11–78). Some alveoli contained collections of large epithelial cells with a variable amount of cytoplasm. These intra-alveolar cells were arranged in rosettes, small irregular packets, or solid masses completely filling the alveoli.

**Bronchial Gland Carcinoma.** Bronchial gland tumors have been distinguished as an entity that may occur more often in dogs and cats than in man (Stünzi et al., 1974). Originating in the glands of the bronchial mucosa, they are in one view predominantly epidermoid (Stünzi, 1976; Stünzi et al., 1974). In the experience of others, the pattern tends to adenocarcinoma, although there are areas of squamous differentiation of carcinoma cells and of mixed adeno- and squamous carcinoma (Moulton et al., 1981).

Bronchial gland carcinomas constituted 8 of the 45 AMAH lung tumors. Seven were associated with major bronchi at, or close to, the hilus, one having tracheal lesions at the bifurcation; the eighth involved the distal 3 cm of the major bronchus of the left caudal lobe. In general, the tumors grossly resembled most papillary adenocarcinomas, except for the greater frequency of hilar involvement and the increased firmness attributable to significant fibroplasia. Bronchial sclerosis, although not recorded in these cases, is more likely with this tumor than with papillary adenocarcinoma.

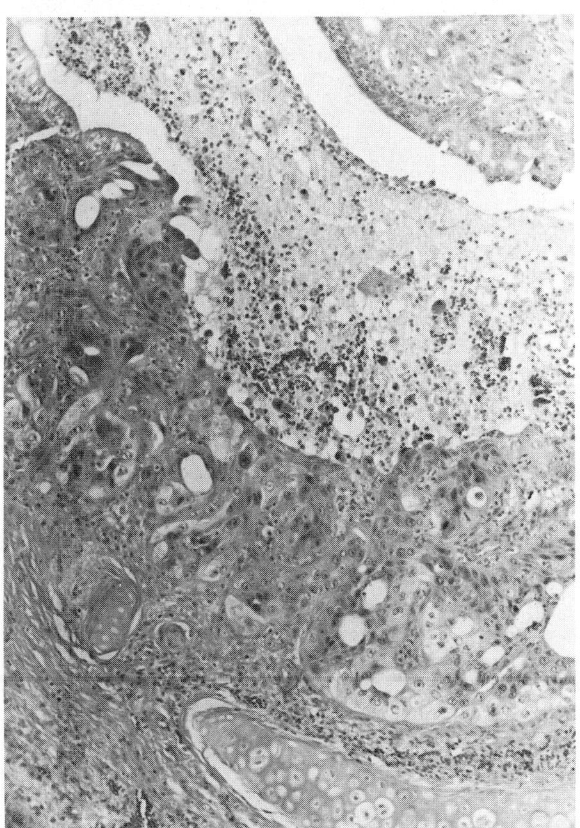

**Figure 11–79** Adenosquamous carcinoma of bronchial epithelial and glandular origin, 12-year-old domestic shorthair. The bronchus is lined by normal pseudostratified epithelium (upper left), squamous cells (upper right), and malignant cells (lower left) appearing to arise from surface and glandular epithelium. H & E, × 75.

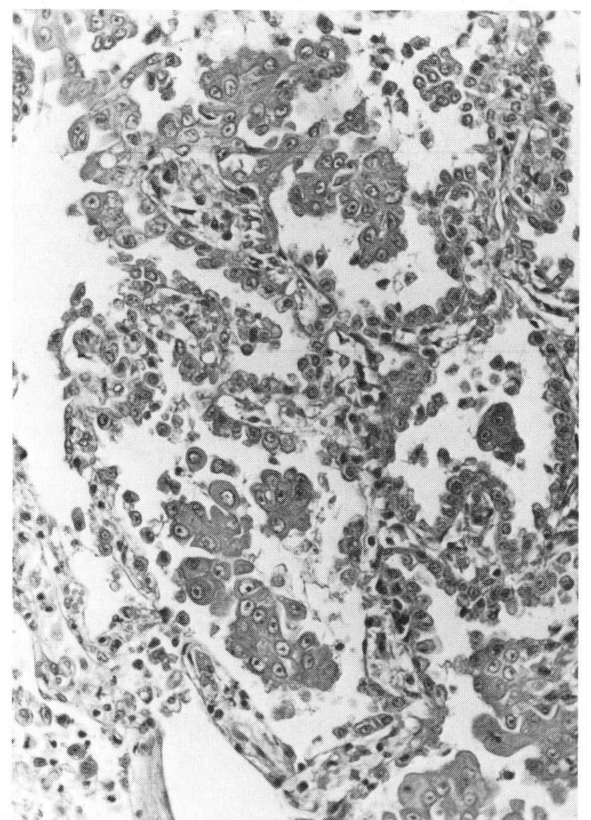

**Figure 11–78** Alveolar cell carcinoma in a 12-year-old cat that died of cardiomyopathy. The 3 mm tumor was found by chance during routine microscopic examination of lung. The tumor arises from and projects into alveoli. H & E, × 200.

Microscopically, no tumor appeared to arise solely from tracheal or bronchial glandular epithelium, but also had one or more sites of origin in metaplastic or neoplastic surface epithelium—a finding at variance with the published descriptions (Fig. 11–79). Pleomorphism and, often, squamous differentiation without keratinization were characteristic of this acinar (tubuloalveolar) tumor. Six cats had widespread tumor in both lungs. Seven had prominent lymphatic and venous neoplastic thrombi, and one also had a thrombus in a pulmonary artery, possibly by embolism from a distant metastatic lesion or by spread in the vasa vasorum.

Pathologists may mistake bronchial lymphatic and venous spread of another type of tumor for one arising from bronchial glands. Such spread was often observed with other malignant primary as well as secondary lung tumors.

Fibroplasia can be so severe as to mimic a primitive myxo- or fibrosarcoma. In one cat with a bronchial gland tumor (and in another with epidermoid carcinoma) there

was the suggestion of sarcoma induced by the carcinoma; the accompanying fibrous tissue proliferation had tissue pattern and cellular features common to fibrosarcomas.

**EPIDERMOID (SQUAMOUS CELL) CARCINOMA.** Only 3 of the 46 tumors were epidermoid carcinoma. All arose in the hilar region and were firm, white, and poorly demarcated. Central cavitation was prominent owing to tissue necrosis and destruction of bronchi.

Microscopically, these tumors were characterized by compact foci of large epithelial cells with sharply defined borders and occasional desmosomes. Keratinization was absent. Fibroplasia and necrosis were constant findings. None of the tumors was pure squamous cell carcinoma, since all had a small component of gland formation similar to bronchial gland carcinoma. The tumors originated from bronchial surface epithelium and very likely glandular epithelium too, because squamous metaplasia, as well as neoplasia, appeared to involve the ducts of glands. In metastatic lesions the glandular component predominated (whereas in the tumors reported by Stünzi [1976], the metastases were epidermoid).

As Stünzi (1976) observed, the presence of both epidermoid and adenocarcinomatous structures might favor the designation of "combined tumor."

Intraocular metastasis from a pulmonary squamous cell carcinoma has been described (Hamilton et al., 1984).

**COMBINED EPIDERMOID AND ADENOCARCINOMA** This tumor, also called adenosquamous carcinoma, is composed nearly equally of epidermoid carcinoma and adenocarcinoma. It is necessary that several sections of a tumor be examined before this diagnosis is made (Stünzi et al., 1974). Only one tumor of this type was identified among the 46 in the AMAH group. Both components were evident not only in the primary tumor but also in neoplastic thrombi of both femoral arteries, in metastases to a kidney, and in several pulmonary arteries. The pulmonary arterial thrombi most likely represented the return of metastases from distant tumor sites. In one branch of the pulmonary artery the intima was covered with squamous cells and in another branch, with simple and pseudostratified columnar cells, some ciliated.

**CONCLUSIONS.** It is clear from previous reviews and case reports and from study of lung tumors in cats at AMAH that the predominant lung tumor in cats, as in dogs, is adenocarcinoma and that it occurs mostly in elderly animals. Both at The Animal Medical Center and at AMAH, females were affected with significantly greater frequency.

Although it is obviously impossible to follow the development of a given tumor chronologically, personal observation (JLC) is that multicentric origin of adenocarcinomas is not uncommon. The small number of solitary masses and the distribution of tumors support this opinion. Furthermore, many of the tumors have an overlap in patterns that complicates differentiation of bronchial papillary adenocarcinoma and bronchioloalveolar carcinoma. There is also an overlapping in morphology of adenocarcinoma and epidermoid carcinoma, since both patterns can exist in a given tumor. Squamous cell metaplasia or differentiation was present in 15 of the 42 adenocarcinomas and bronchial gland carcinomas. Keratinization did not occur in any tumor, not even in the "combined" (adenosquamous) or epidermoid tumors.

### TUMORS OF THE THORACIC CAVITY

Lymphoma of the cranial mediastinum is notoriously common. Next in frequency is thymoma. Both are discussed in the section on hematopoietic neoplasms and also in the chapter on hematopoietic disorders. Rarely, mast cell tumor and mesothelioma are found in the mediastinum (see sections on those neoplasms). Fibrosarcoma of the cranial mediastinum was diagnosed in one cat at AMAH.

## TUMORS OF THE CARDIOVASCULAR SYSTEM*

### TUMORS OF THE HEART

The heart is occasionally the site of lymphoma in cats with multicentric tumor. Involvement may be massive or microscopic. There are rare reports of primary sarcomas of muscle (Cordy, 1978; Priester and McKay, 1980) and of primary fibrosarcomas (Nielsen, 1964; Ryan and Walder, 1980). A myxosarcoma of the pericardium weighing 350 gm and displacing the heart and lungs was reported by Mollereau (cited by Lombard, 1940), and a mesothelioma of the pericardial sac was described by Tilley et al. (1975). A malignant tumor at the base of the heart, reported by Graubmann and Sander (1965), was believed to have originated from ectopic parathyroid tissue.

The heart is the most frequent site of metastasis for hemangiosarcoma in the cat (Patnaik and Liu, 1977). Other metastatic tumors that have been observed include mammary carcinoma, salivary gland carcinoma, and oral melanoma (Tilley et al., 1981).

Although less frequent in cats than in dogs, the principal tumors of the cardiovascular system are hemangiomas and hemangiosarcomas. In many instances they may be differentiated only by microscopic study from other lesions such as hematomas, granulation tissue, vascular malformations and acquired telangiectasia, telangiectatic osteosarcoma, and cysts of apocrine and ceruminous glands containing dark fluid.

### TUMORS OF VESSELS

#### Telangiectasia

Telangiectasia is non-neoplastic but may have the gross appearance of tumor. It is rare in cats. Instances observed at AMAH included telangiectasia of cerebellum (Fig. 11–80), ovary, and liver. The first two were congenital, but the pathogenesis of the hepatic lesion was unknown.

#### Hemangioma

Hemangiomas are benign growths of blood vascular endothelium. A survey of 395 feline tumors included two of the skin and one of the lung (Engle and Brodey, 1969). Eight "hemangiomas and lymphangiomas" were listed in another survey of 621 tumors (Dorn et al., 1968a). In a

*Laura K. Andrews, principal author, tumors of the heart and blood vessels.

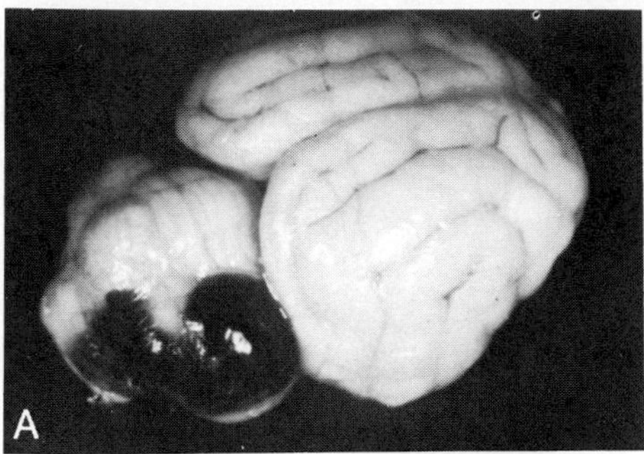


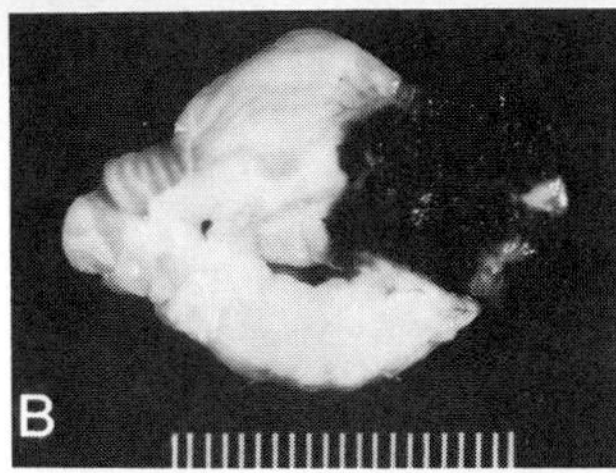


**Figure 11–80** *A*, Telangiectasia, cerebellum, two-year-old female Siamese. Ataxia and right-sided head tilt developed five weeks before sudden collapse and central nystagmus occurred at parturition. The red-black mass, 2.5 × 1.4 cm, involved most of the right cerebellar hemisphere. *B*, Telangiectasia occupies most of the right cerebellar hemisphere. Hemorrhage within and adjacent to the anomaly caused brain swelling and collapse, necessitating euthanasia.

survey of tumors at 15 veterinary colleges, five angiomas from various sites, including tongue, liver, and soft tissue, all occurred in females (Priester and McKay, 1980). Three hemangiomas, one on the thigh and two in the liver, were reported in elderly females by Nielsen (1964). A hemangioma of the lung was recorded by Cotchin (1983). A subcutaneous angioma was reported from a 10-month-old female domestic shorthair (Feldman et al., 1974) and lingual hemangiomas from a two and a half-year-old female Siamese (Crow et al., 1981). A cat with multiple hemangiomas of the tongue was treated several times by surgical excision and cryosurgery, but without success (Theilen and Madewell, 1979).

Of eight hemangiomas at AMAH, seven occurred on the skin, one in the liver; two angiomas involved vertebrae. The cats ranged in age from 7 to 21 years. No sex predisposition was evident, in contrast with the predominance of females in the reported cases in which age was given. Six cats were domestic shorthairs, two were Siamese. Breed was not specified for the others.

**CLINICAL FEATURES.** Cats with cutaneous hemangiomas are usually presented because of bleeding. One cat with lingual hemangioma had difficulty eating and developed significant anemia from recurrent bleeding (Crow et al., 1981). The hepatic hemangioma at AMAH was asymptomatic and an incidental finding at autopsy. A two-year-old cat with an angioma of the tenth thoracic vertebra had progressive paraparesis for six months and evinced pain over the dorsal midthorax (see Fig. 11–177). In a nine-month-old cat with an identical lesion of L1, use of the hindlimbs was progressively impaired.

**GROSS FEATURES.** Hemangiomas of the skin are red or blue-black raised dermal or subcutaneous nodules from pinpoint to 3.0 cm in diameter. Lobulated and soft or spongy, they contain blood in multiple spaces separated by fine trabeculae. The tumors are usually well delineated. The lingual hemangioma had multiple soft vesicular masses that bled readily (Crow et al., 1981). The hepatic hemangioma took the form of multiple, slightly elevated, spongy red masses 0.5 cm in diameter. The vertebral angiomas were firm, pink masses extending from the medullary cavity into the epidural space.

**MICROSCOPIC FEATURES.** Hemangiomas are described as capillary or cavernous, depending on the size of vascular spaces. In most, a prominent fibrous stroma separates small or large anastomosing blood-filled spaces lined by plump but uniform endothelial cells, usually in only one layer but occasionally forming sheets. Thrombosis and sclerosis are common. Necrosis is rare except in large tumors. The endothelial cells are spindle-form with minimal variation in size or shape (Fig. 11–81). Nuclei are oval and heterochromatic. Occasional vesicular (euchromatic) nuclei may be seen. Mitotic figures are rare and multinucleated cells absent.

It is sometimes difficult to distinguish hemangiomas from vascular malformations, telangiectasia, or hemangiosarcoma. In telangiectasia, tissue of the parent organ forms the intervascular stroma. The vessels of the vascular malformations usually resemble normal vessels. The endothelial cells of hemangiosarcomas are usually more pleomorphic than those of hemangiomas. Hemangiosarcomas often have multinucleated tumor cells, and the mitotic index usually exceeds 5 per 10 HPF. Necrosis is more frequent in hemangiosarcomas.

Angiomas are distinguished from hemangiomas by the presence of mural smooth muscle. The two at AMAH may have originated as congenital malformations (vascular hamartomas).

**BEHAVIOR AND MANAGEMENT.** Hemangiomas are expansile but do not metastasize. Wide excision is necessary because the growth often recurs if removal was incomplete. Hemangiomas may be difficult to treat if they are multiple or in a location subject to trauma. In one cat, multiple hemangiomas of the tongue recurred six weeks after electrosurgical resection (Crow et al., 1981). Because bleeding from the tumor was recurrent and sometimes severe and resection would be difficult, the cat was given oral cyclophosphamide, 12.5 mg four times a week, and prednisone, 5.0 mg every second day. When the tumors recurred, a 90 Sr probe was used to give a surface dose of 4100 rads directly to the tumors. This was followed by orthovoltage irradiation of the tongue with 1500 rads given in three fractions over five days. The cat did well but had occasional mild bleeding 10 months after discharge.

## Hemangiosarcoma

Hemangiosarcoma, a malignant tumor of blood vascular endothelial cells, is more frequent in the cat than its benign counterpart hemangioma. It most often arises in the skin, visceral lymph nodes, spleen, and liver, but primary tumors also occur in the nasal cavities, lung, pancreas, bone, and cranial mediastinum. Hemangio-

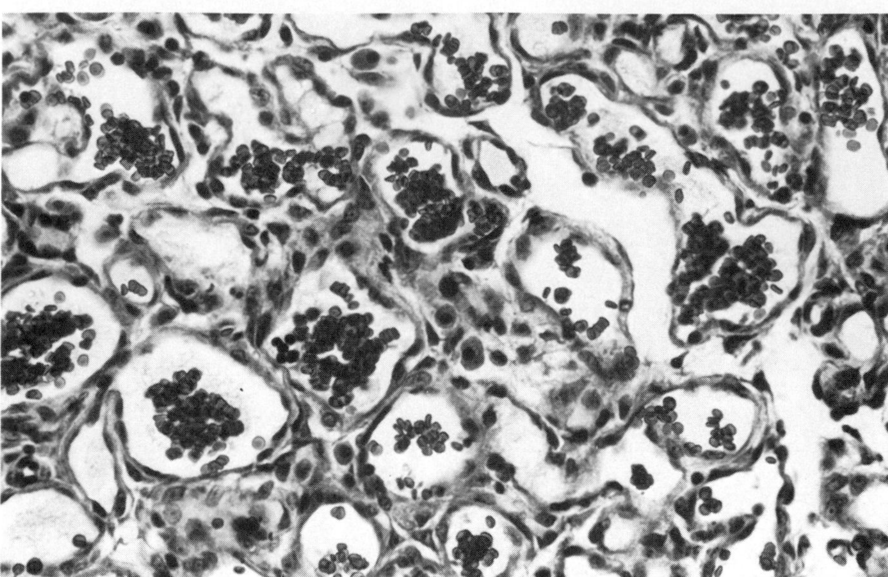

**Figure 11–81** Hemangioma, subcutis of shoulder, eight-year-old domestic longhair. The cavernous tumor, present for two years, was sharply demarcated and lobulated and measured 1.8 × 1.0 × 0.8 cm. The clearly defined, blood-filled vascular channels are lined by simple squamous endothelial cells with widely separated hyperchromatic nuclei. H & E, × 312.

sarcomas were diagnosed in 18 of 3145 cats examined at autopsy at The Animal Medical Center: six in the liver, four in the spleen, four in the mesentery, three in the mediastinum, and one in the lung (Patnaik and Liu, 1977). In a later study of 31 surgical cases from the same institution, the sites of hemangiosarcoma were abdominal cavity (15), subcutis (13), thoracic cavity (2), and nasal cavity (1) (Scavelli et al., 1985). In five surveys, 20 of 1006 tumors were hemangiosarcomas (Cotchin, 1952; Engle and Brodey, 1969, MacVean, 1978; Mulligan, 1951; Schmidt and Langham, 1967). One hemangiosarcoma of the tongue (Lombard, 1964) and two of the liver (Blähser, 1962; Carb, 1968) were described in case reports. A hemangiosarcoma in the mesentery of a nine-year-old female tricolor was reported by Nielsen (1964). An "endotheliosarcoma" of the thymus is on record (Mettler, 1975).

Fifty-six hemangiosarcomas were diagnosed at AMAH—25 in the skin, 11 in the mesentery, 10 in the spleen, 4 in the liver, 2 in the nasal cavity, 2 in the tongue, and 1 each in the hard palate and cranial mediastinum. The cats ranged in age from 5 months to 17 years (mean 10 years), a finding in accord with other reports (Cotchin, 1952; Patnaik and Liu, 1977; Scavelli et al., 1985). Males and females were equally represented. Seventy-five per cent of the tumors occurred in domestic shorthairs.

**CLINICAL FEATURES.** Signs of hemangiosarcoma depend on the location and extent of the primary and metastatic tumors. The tumors were present for three weeks to a year before diagnosis. A formerly quiescent skin tumor may enlarge rapidly owing to proliferation of tumor cells or to hemorrhage or thrombosis within the tumor. Cats with visceral tumors usually have a history of lethargy, anorexia, vomiting, dyspnea, or distended abdomen. On physical examination, pallor, pleural or peritoneal fluid, and a palpable abdominal mass are often found. Bleeding, common because vascular channels in the tumor are fragile, may be intermittent, causing episodic weakness, or acute, causing sudden collapse, sometimes in an apparently healthy cat. Bleeding usually results from trauma, such as licking or palpation. If the tumor is large or necrotic or if it invades a large vessel, bleeding may be spontaneous and severe. Cats with visceral tumors may be presented in hypovolemic shock with blood in the pleural or peritoneal cavity. The blood fails to clot readily. Bleeding is often difficult to control because of location and extent of the tumor and may be complicated by disseminated intravascular coagulation.

Most cats with visceral hemangiosarcomas are anemic. The anemia may be mild or severe and may have more than one cause. Recurrent hemorrhage may cause a regenerative anemia characterized by polychromasia, anisocytosis, hypochromasia, reticulocytosis, and nucleated red blood cells in the peripheral blood. Chronic wasting and poor nutrition in cats with widespread tumor may cause bone marrow suppression. Fragmentation of red cells, which occurs in humans and dogs with hemangiosarcoma (Rebar et al., 1980), has not been documented in cats but may well contribute to their anemia. Four causes have been proposed for this fragmentation: (1) local mechanical trauma to red cells traversing irregular vascular spaces of the tumor; (2) formation of spherocytes and destruction of older red cells with lower ATP when blood flow is sluggish and oxygen tension low; (3) increased fragility of red cells made hypochromatic by blood loss and lowered iron content; (4) altered cholesterol: phospholipid ratios in red-cell membranes due to altered hepatic lipoprotein metabolism, possibly accounting for acanthocytosis and fragmentation in dogs with hepatic hemangiosarcomas.

**DIAGNOSIS.** Diagnosis of hemangiosarcoma is most reliably made by biopsy or removal of the primary or a metastatic tumor. Cats with visceral hemangiosarcoma often have pleural or peritoneal effusions. The fluid, ranging from 50 to 400 ml, may be clear, milky-looking, or bloody. Fusiform neoplastic cells are only rarely detected in cytologic examination of such fluids.

**GROSS FEATURES.** Hemangiosarcomas are lobulated red or red-black masses of firm, fluctuant, or spongy consistency. Margins are usually ill defined. On cut section the tumors may appear solid or may have irregular spaces

formed by fragile trabeculae. The spaces may contain free or clotted blood or pink fluid that oozes from the cut surface. There are usually pale gray fibrous bands or foci and yellow-pink friable areas of necrosis.

Tumors involving the skin may be in the dermis or subcutis. The epidermis over the tumor is usually ulcerated because of trauma or ischemia, and bleeding is common. Skin tumors, varying in size from pinpoint to 10 cm in diameter, occur mainly on the head, in the axillary and inguinal areas, and on the flank and limbs.

Hemangiosarcomas occasionally arise in the mesentery (Fig. 11–82) or within or adjacent to mesenteric, duodenal, or colonic lymph nodes. They vary in size and may measure up to 7.0 cm in largest dimension. Tumors of the liver usually occur as a large, soft, lobulated, red mass in one lobe with multiple smaller discrete, slightly elevated, red or gray masses in other lobes. Hemangiosarcomas of the spleen may be single or multiple. In two cats at AMAH the tumor originated in splenic implants in the omentum. One of the cats had both diaphragmatic and umbilical hernias with the primary tumor in a splenic implant in omentum within the umbilical hernia. Tumors arising in the cranial mediastinum may be as large as 144 cmm (Patnaik and Liu, 1977) and are diffuse. One tumor arising in the lung had nodules of 6 to 8 mm in all lobes (Patnaik and Liu, 1977).

Both lingual hemangiosarcomas in the AMAH group, like the tumor described by Lombard (1964), were raised, soft, red masses on the ventrolateral surface near the frenulum. One of two cats at AMAH with tumor in the nasal cavity had a soft 3 cmm mass involving the bridge of the nose. Proliferation and lysis of nasal bone and obliteration of nasal turbinates and septum were evident in radiographs. Surgery disclosed a soft bloody mass involving both sides of the nasal cavity. Hemangiosarcomas of the gum are soft, bloody, often necrotic masses, which may invade bone and loosen nearby teeth. Like other gingival neoplasms, they may be mistaken for reactive lesions of primary dental disease.

**MICROSCOPIC FEATURES.** Hemangiosarcomas may have a variety of patterns, and more than one is usual within a single tumor. Well-differentiated tumors have blood-filled spaces of varying size lined by one or more layers of endothelial cells. These cells may pile up, forming projections into the vascular spaces. Single tumor cells or small groups forming abnormal capillaries may appear to be free within the spaces. Cells may also proliferate into and obliterate a vascular space, causing it

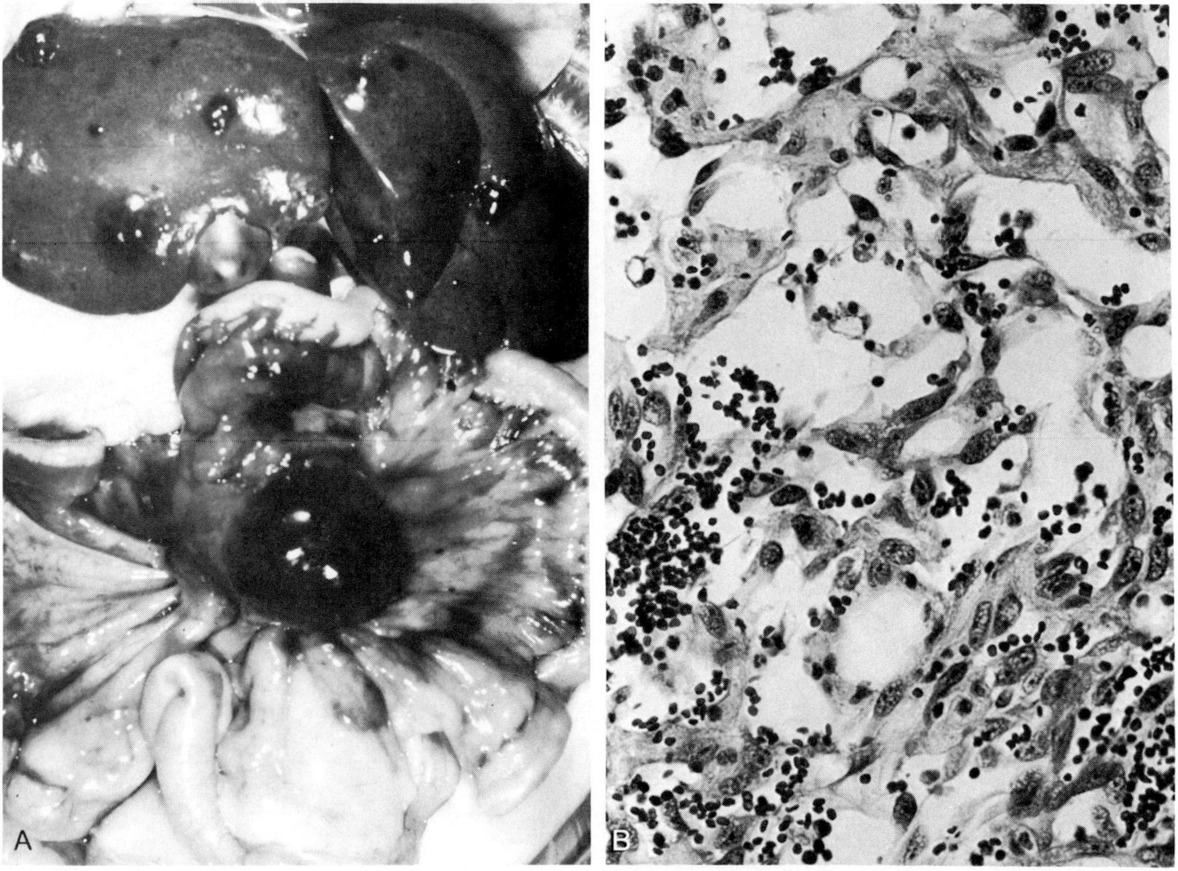

**Figure 11–82** *A*, Hemangiosarcoma originating at the root of the mesentery and metastasizing to the liver, 13-year-old domestic shorthair. The cat appeared normal except for abdominal distention with a milky orange fluid. Effusion of this sort is common when hemangiosarcoma involves the root of the mesentery and mesenteric nodes, a site of predilection in cats. *B*, The large, pleomorphic, and euchromatic endothelial cells formed branching, poorly demarcated, blood-filled vascular spaces. The tumor metastasized to mesenteric and pancreatic nodes, pancreas, and jejunal serosa, as well as liver. H & E, × 312.

to resemble a glomerulus. Other tumors have solid sheets of cells with occasional blood-filled clefts. The neoplastic endothelial cells are plump and usually fusiform. The large nucleus may be oval and vesicular with large nucleoli, or oblong and heterochromatic. Neoplastic multinucleated giant cells were seen in 39 of the 56 tumors diagnosed at AMAH. The mitotic index varied from 1 to 31 per 10 HPF.

The tumor stroma, which differs from mature connective tissue, may be hyalinized or may consist of loose myxomatous tissue containing cells resembling fibroblasts as well as varying numbers of reticulin fibers. The stroma may be inconspicuous in solid tumors. Thrombosis and necrosis are constant features. Some skin tumors contain moderate numbers of mast cells, lymphocytes, and plasma cells.

It was emphasized at the outset that blood vascular tumors may have to be distinguished microscopically from a number of lesions, but the differentiation of hemangiosarcoma from some fibrosarcomas and from telangiectatic osteosarcoma can be very difficult.

**TUMOR BEHAVIOR.** The prognosis for hemangiosarcoma is poor. At AMAH all 12 cats that had skin tumors and were followed for a year or until death had local recurrence of the primary tumor within a month to a year after surgical removal. One cat had metastasis to the lung, and one developed multiple tumors on the tail, in a mammary gland, and on the gum. Average time to recurrence was four and a half months.

Visceral hemangiosarcomas are aggressive and metastasize readily. Of 4 mesenteric hemangiosarcomas at The Animal Medical Center (Patnaik and Liu, 1977) and 11 at AMAH, 13 were found at autopsy to have metastasized. The liver was most often the site of metastasis, followed by omentum, diaphragm, pancreas, and lung.

All four cats at AMC and six of the ten at AMAH with hemangiosarcomas of the spleen had metastasis, most often to liver and regional lymph nodes. None of the four mediastinal tumors at The Animal Medical Center and AMAH had metastasized outside the thoracic cavity, but all the cats had hemothorax. The two tumors of the nasal cavity at AMAH did not metastasize, but one invaded the hard palate and the other the overlying nasal bone. None of the tumors of the oral cavity metastasized (Brodey, 1966; Lombard, 1964), but most were locally invasive and recurred. The pulmonary hemangiosarcoma spread to the spleen, skull, and brain (Patnaik and Liu, 1977).

Hemangiosarcomas of the liver may be less aggressive than those arising elsewhere in the viscera. Only one of six at The Animal Medical Center and one of three at AMAH metastasized. An eight and a half-year-old male with a single large ruptured cystic tumor of the liver had no evident metastases at laparotomy when the affected liver lobe was removed. Five months after surgery the cat was doing well (Carb, 1968).

In a study of 31 surgical cases of hemangiosarcoma at The Animal Medical Center, 9 of 15 cats with abdominal tumor had extrathoracic metastasis, but there was no evidence of metastasis from tumor in other sites (Scavelli et al., 1985).

The cause of hemangiosarcoma is not known, although the lesion has been induced experimentally in various species by chemicals and viruses. Feline sarcoma viruses may induce hemangiomas and hemangiosarcoma-like tumors and may cause hepatic and multicentric angiosarcomas in rats and mice (Hong et al., 1980; Theilen and Madewell, 1979). C-type virus particles were identified in a rapidly growing subcutaneous angioma in a 10-month-old female domestic shorthair (Feldman et al., 1974). Of 10 AMAH cats with hemangiosarcoma that were tested for feline leukemia virus, none was positive.

## Tumors of Lymphatic Vessels

Lymphangioma and lymphangiosarcoma are uncommon tumors in man and animals and must be carefully distinguished from hemangioma and hemangiosarcoma. Neoplasms of lymphatics should contain few red cells; pericytes present peripherally about blood vessel endothelial cells are not present around lymphatics. Some lymphangiomas assume a cavernous form analogous to that of the cavernous hemangioma. Lymphangiosarcoma in man arises in the skin and, sometimes after long periods, metastasizes to the thoracic wall, lungs, and occasionally other organs. Many lesions in humans originate in areas of lymphedema in the extremities, notably in the arms of women who have had radical mastectomies. Rarely, there are other types of tumor in the same patient.

Lymphangioma was described in an obese five-year-old entire female cat within a year after she had her first litter (Schindelka, 1892). A swelling first involved the inguinal nipples and eventually advanced cranially until all were swollen and the cat had difficulty in moving about. At the time of examination the tumors varied from hazelnut to hen's-egg size. The masses were transparent and yellow-red, resembling pendulous sacks half full of fluid. They felt cooler than surrounding tissue. With the cat's movement the fluid would undulate. The skin was paper thin, but bands of firmer tissue could be felt circumscribing the various pockets of fluid. Aspiration established that the tumors consisted of many small cystic spaces, and 150 ml of fluid was removed. The fluid, at first yellow-red and opaque, cleared after a red sediment settled out. It then contained a few red cells and some large white cells filled with fat droplets. The filtered fluid was pale yellow and slightly opalescent, with a specific gravity of 1.008 and much albumin. Two weeks later the cat's condition was the same as before drainage except that the skin over the sites of puncture felt like parchment. Unfortunately the cat perished in a fall from a window, so that the diagnosis of lymphangioma was not confirmed microscopically.

Other tumors of lymphatics reported without details were a lymphangioma/lymphangiosarcoma (MacVean et al., 1978), a lymphangioma of the thymus (Mettler, 1975), and two lymphangiosarcomas, one of the mediastinum and the other of the liver (Poppensieck, 1961). Three others were the subjects of case reports. One lymphangiosarcoma, in a 12-year-old domestic female, involved the skin and wall of the caudal abdomen and extended down both hind legs; the tumor was invasive, but mitoses were few and there were no metastases (Patnaik and Liu, 1977). Two cases of lymphangiosarcoma were reported from the New York State College of Veterinary Medicine (NYSCVM) (Walsh and Abbott, 1984), and one of the two was also described, with illustrations, by Walton et al. (1983). In the cat discussed in both reports, a spayed female domestic shorthair five to six years old and FeLV-negative, the initial interdigital wound of the left forepaw was unresponsive to surgical and antibiotic treatment, and when contrast radiography revealed numerous tracts in

the forearm, the limb was amputated. Nine months later, drainage from tracts on the ventrum prompted surgical exploration, and a biopsy provided the diagnosis of lymphangiosarcoma. Autopsy revealed no metastases.

In the other case at the NYSCVM there was bleeding from a cystic area on the ventrum of a two-year-old spayed female Persian. The biopsy diagnosis was lymphangiosarcoma. The cat died two weeks later at home, and an autopsy was not obtained.

At AMAH nine tumors of lymphatic vessels were diagnosed within a recent four-year period. In three cases tissues were submitted by out-of-state practitioners. Five cats were domestic shorthairs, two of these tricolors; one was a domestic longhair, and one a Persian. Breed was unspecified for the other two. Four cats were males, two castrated; the other five were spayed females. Like the cats in the reported cases they ranged in age from 2 to 12 years (mean 7.6). The tumors, situated in the dermis and subcutis, involved some portion of the ventral body wall in four cats and a limb in five: forepaw (Fig. 11–83), metacarpus, carpal pad, metatarsus, and caudal knee.

**CLINICAL AND PATHOLOGIC FEATURES.** In clinical and pathologic features the neoplasms had many similarities to those reported, but in several cases there were details of special interest.

Excessive serum-like drainage from a cutaneous sore of the left carpal pad in a two-year-old spayed female tricolor was subsequently followed by sloughing of the pad and adjacent skin (Fig. 11–84*A*). The continued drainage of much fluid and lack of healing prompted a biopsy that led to the diagnosis of lymphangiosarcoma (Fig. 11–84*B*). The limb was amputated, and tumor was found extending from the carpal area along blood vessels and nerves in the dermis and subcutis to the elbow and possibly beyond the amputation margin. These findings closely resembled those in the case described by Walton et al. (1983) and Walsh and Abbott (1984). Unfortunately the cat was lost to follow-up.

In a seven-year-old castrated male, a symmetric cystic lesion extending on the ventrum from the navel to the perineum yielded clear, pale yellow fluid with a specific gravity of 1.022, TSP 4.5 gm/dl, and mainly lymphocytes. Biopsy disclosed a cavernous lesion composed of lymphatic channels. Four months later the cat developed dyspnea associated with a pleural effusion. Autopsy revealed a chronic restrictive pleuritis, believed to represent a reaction to the effusion. There were also mucus-filled bronchi and medial hypertrophy of the pulmonary arteries. Lesions resembling those of the ventral abdominal wall were present about the thyroid lobes and retropha-

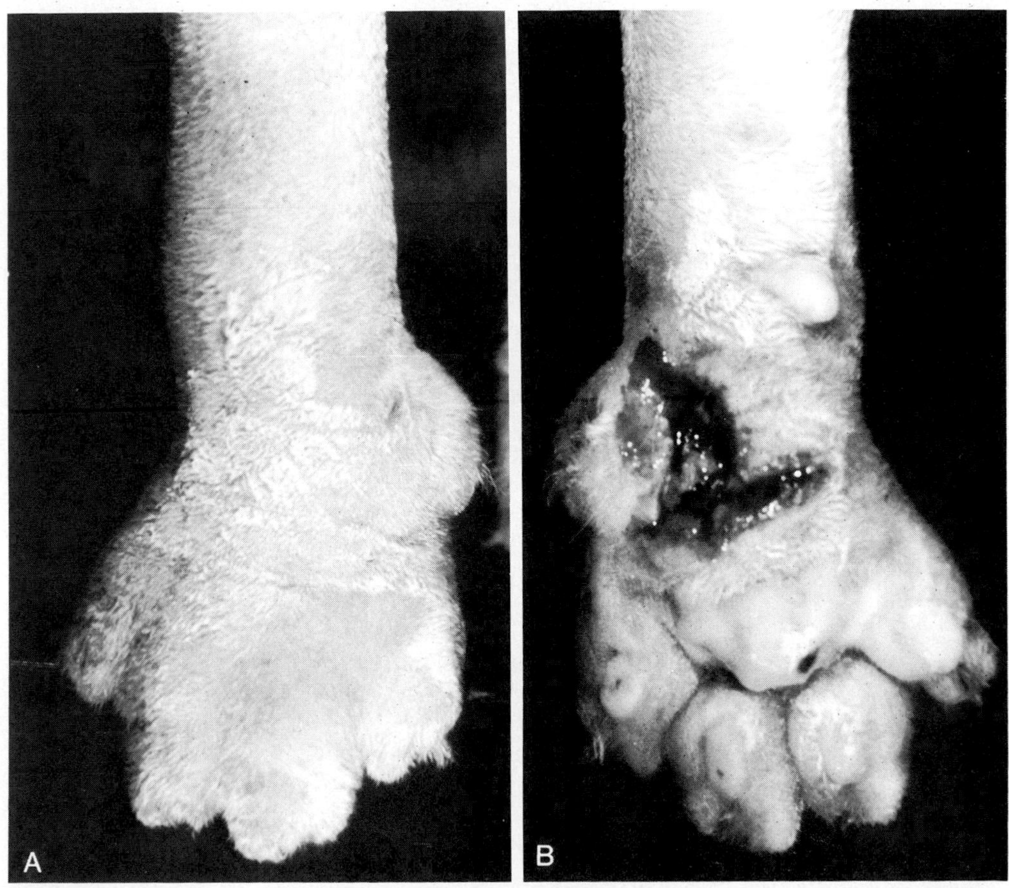


**Figure 11–83** *A* and *B*, Lymphangiosarcoma of a paw and forearm, 10-year-old male orange-and-white tabby. The forelimb is swollen and ulcerated at the biopsy site above the metacarpal pad (*B*). An unusually large volume of clear fluid continued to drain, necessitating frequent bandage changes. The tumor extended from the digits almost to the elbow. Actual size.

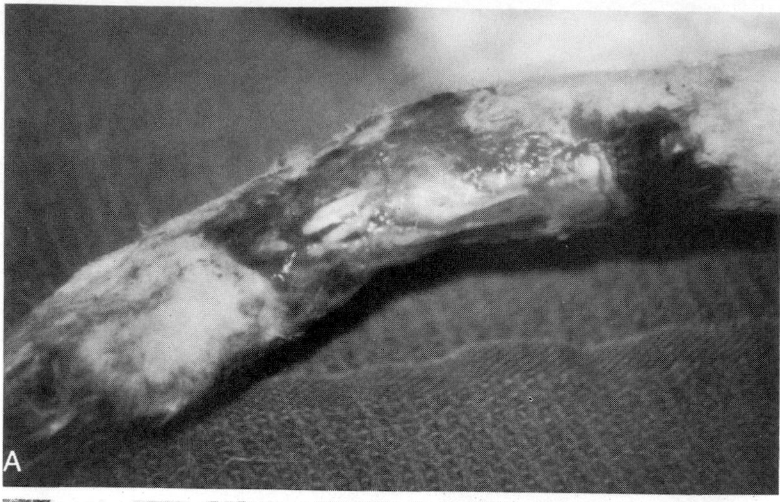


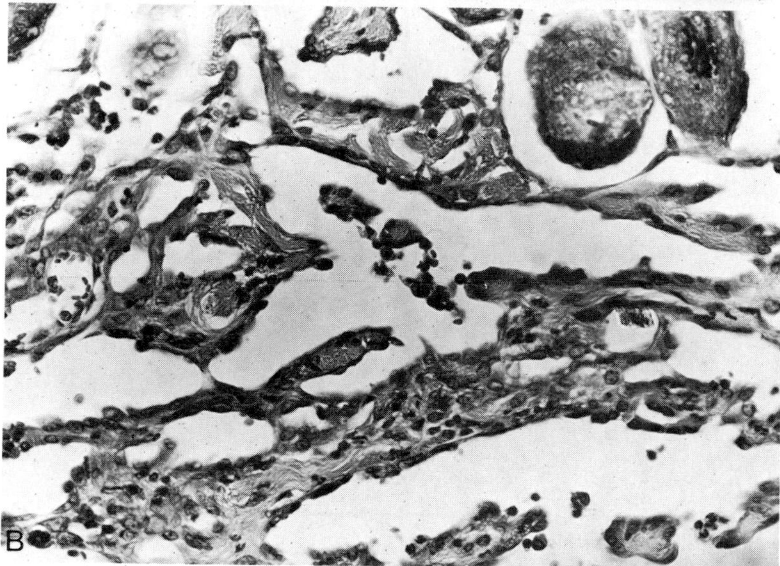


**Figure 11–84** *A*, Lymphangiosarcoma of paw and forearm, two-year-old tricolor cat. The tumor first appeared at the nailbed of the dewclaw, then became ulcerated, discharged a large volume of watery fluid, and spread up the forearm to the elbow. Granulation tissue and excessive lymph-like discharge in the area of the sloughed skin and carpal pad prompted biopsy. *B*, Irregular, open, empty, and branching neoplastic lymphatic channels lie about hair bulbs (upper right) and within the subcutis. Vascular spaces are lined by endothelial cells with oval to flattened nuclei. H & E, × 300.

ryngeal nodes, as well as retropleurally and retroperitoneally along the vertebral column. In this case, multicentric origin would best explain the distribution of lesions.

Local recurrence and pulmonary metastases developed despite amputation of the leg of a cat with a popliteal fistula and biopsy diagnosis of lymphangiosarcoma. The margin of the amputated leg was not "clean," forewarning of the recurrence.

A remarkable finding in two 12-year-old cats, a spayed female Persian and a castrated male domestic longhair, was the coexistence of other types of tumor. In the left inguinal region of the Persian, several palpable intraductal mammary papillomas measuring 0.2 to 0.3 cm were accompanied by considerable cutaneous edema and fluid accumulation in the inguinal fat deep to the inguinal mamma. Microscopic findings, beside the papillomas, included an extensive lymphangiosarcoma of the dermis, subcutis, and mammary gland and a 0.1 cm hemangiosarcoma near a nipple within the lymphatic tumor. The hemangiosarcoma had cells with nuclear features and numbers of mitoses suggesting a higher grade of malignancy than in the lymphatic vascular tumor. In the other cat with a combination of tumors, a massive subcutaneous fibrosarcoma extended from the left fifth to the twelfth rib near the dorsum, and a flat, ulcerated lymphangiosarcoma measuring 2.0 × 1.9 × 0.5 cm involved all layers of the skin on the right volar metacarpal area. As already noted, tumors of more than one type are occasionally present in humans with lymphangiosarcoma. In cats, the possibility of a common viral origin might be considered.

**PROGNOSIS.** Although follow-up reports were not available for all cats, the prognosis appears poor. Limited experience suggests that most of the tumors tend to be only locally invasive, thus raising the question as to classifying the lesion as lymphangioma or lymphangiosarcoma.

**CONCLUSIONS.** When the published cases and those at AMAH are considered together, a number of conclusions may be drawn about this unusual neoplasm. (1) No breed disposition is apparent, and the tumor may occur at any age; however, about twice as many females as males were affected. (2) The pathologic process seems to start with about equal frequency in the ventral abdominal wall and in the limbs, but the caudal abdominal wall and the forelimbs are most often involved. All but one of the cases of ventral involvement occurred in females. (3) The

neoplasm presents insidiously as draining tracts or cystic areas, and the correct diagnosis is made, often after considerable delay, only by biopsy. (4) The tumor is slowly invasive, recurs despite amputation, and only rarely metastasizes. Not one cure was achieved. (5) Microscopically, differentiation between lymphangioma and lymphangiosarcoma may be difficult and in some cases may be settled only by the behavior of a given tumor.

## TUMORS OF THE ALIMENTARY SYSTEM*

Lymphomas, because of their high incidence in the intestine, outnumber all other tumors of the digestive tract. They are discussed in the section on hematopoietic tumors and in the chapter on hematopoietic disorders. Other special features of digestive tract neoplasia in the cat are the predominance of carcinoma in the oropharynx, the strikingly high incidence of cancer of the upper alimentary tract in British cats, the rarity of stomach cancer, and the predisposition of the Siamese breed to adenocarcinoma of the small intestine.

### Tumors of the Oropharynx

The most frequent tumors arising in the oral cavity of the cat are squamous cell carcinoma and fibrosarcoma (e.g., Cotchin, 1983; Dorn and Priester, 1976; Engle and Brodey, 1969; Nielsen, 1964; Patnaik et al., 1975; Priester and McKay, 1980). Adamantinoma (ameloblastoma), epulis, papilloma, fibroma, hemangioma, hemangiosarcoma, and lymphoma are less common. Melanoma, alveolar soft-part sarcoma (granular cell myoblastoma), and adenocarcinomas of the minor salivary glands are rare.

#### Squamous Cell Carcinoma

Squamous cell carcinoma of the oral cavity was diagnosed in 80 cats at AMAH. Thirty-eight tumors involved the tongue, 21 the mandibular gingiva, 13 the maxillary gingiva, and 8 a tonsil. None arose from the cheeks. The palate was involved by extension, but carcinoma arising in the palate was not documented. Proliferation of gingival tissue and loosening of the teeth are in early stages often mistaken for dental disease. Tumor may extend from the maxillary gingiva to the palate, facial bones, turbinates, frontal sinuses, and bullae (e.g., Cucuel and Schelling, 1973). By the time gingival and palatine lesions are found, bone is almost certainly altered by destruction and reactive bone proliferation. In two cats the mandible was enlarged to six times normal size; the enlargement could have been mistaken for chronic osteomyelitis, especially actinomycosis. Such massive change in the mandible also mimics primary bone tumor (Miller et al., 1969; Quigley and Leedale, 1972).

Accurate diagnosis depends on examination of adequate biopsy tissue. Surgical excision is the treatment of choice together with removal of any involved lymph nodes; however, surgery often achieves only palliation and not a cure, since inaccessible tumor may be left behind. Cryosurgery often attains the best result, as it involves minimal risk for the animal and conserves bone (e.g., Harvey, 1980). Radiation might be effective as primary or adjunctive therapy if applied early (Theilen and Madewell, 1979). Results were disappointing, however, in a small number of feline oropharyngeal cancers that were irradiated (McClelland, 1957). Mandibular resection is an aggressive approach with a somewhat better prospect of removing all of an advanced tumor (Withrow and Holmberg, 1983). One of five cats with squamous cell carcinoma (and one with fibrous histiocytoma) were alive and tumor-free a year after hemimandibulectomy (Bradley et al., 1984).

Squamous cell carcinomas of the tongue and tonsil are described later.

#### Fibrosarcoma

This highly destructive tumor, details of which are discussed in the section on tumors of the skin and subcutis, was diagnosed in five cats at AMAH (Fig. 11–85). In three cats it involved the region of an upper molar, and in two, the mandibular gingiva.

#### Ameloblastoma (Adamantinoma)

Odontogenic tumors are uncommon, and differentiation of the types requires biopsy.

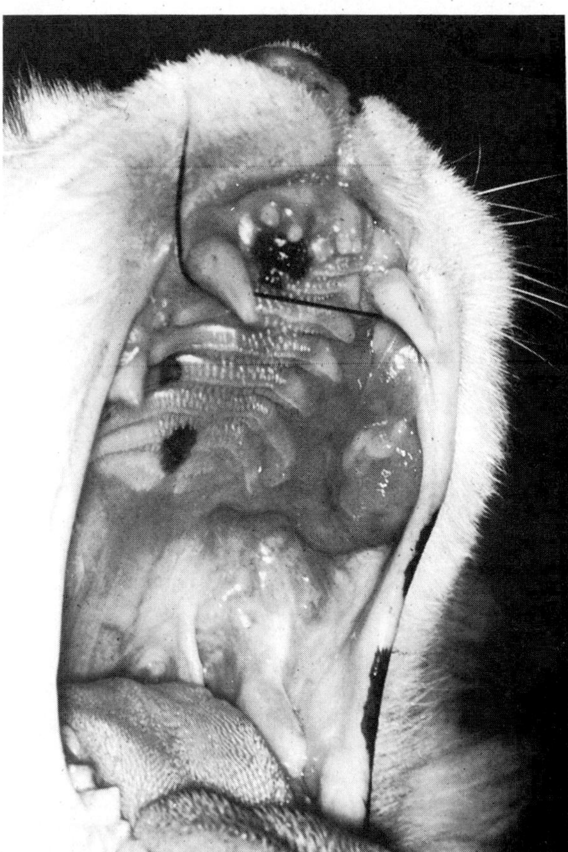

**Figure 11–85** Fibrosarcoma of left upper jaw and palate, 12-year-old cat. The nodular, proliferative tumor has caused the loss of teeth and is beginning to obscure the palatine ridges.

*Laura K. Andrews, principal author.

Adamantinomas, for which the term ameloblastoma is now preferred, have been reported in the cat by Bastianello (1983), Dorn and Priester (1976), Fölger (1913), Hoogland (1926), Liénaux (1900), Mulligan (1951), Nieberle and Cohrs (1931), Olafson (1939), Poppensiek (1961), and Whitehead (1967). These tumors are slow-growing and tend to occur in middle-aged or old cats, with no breed or sex predilection.

Two ameloblastic fibromas were reported in cats six and eight months of age (Brodey, 1966; Engle and Brodey, 1969), and "inductive" fibroameloblastomas were described in four cats aged 7 to 14 months (Dubielzig et al., 1979). Four of the cats in the two reports were domestic shorthairs and two Siamese; all five tumors for which site was given were on the maxillary gingiva.

Both ameloblastomas and ameloblastic fibromas are rounded or lobulated, firm or rubbery masses projecting from the gum of the maxilla or mandible. Cysts or spicules of bone may be present. The cat may salivate and have difficulty eating. If the tumor is large, it may ulcerate and bleed. Ameloblastomas and fibroameloblastomas commonly invade the bone of the jaw and loosen the teeth. Radiographically, ameloblastomas are characterized by multiloculated radiolucent areas and resorption of tooth roots (Fig. 11–86*A*).

Ameloblastomas arise from a dental primordium. Microscopically the tumor consists of irregular cords and islands of epithelium in a dense collagenous stroma, which may be hyalinized. Within the masses of epithelial cells there may be "star-cells" resembling embryonal connective tissue. These are sometimes replaced by cysts (Fig. 11–86*B*); sometimes they undergo squamous metaplasia and form keratin, in which case the tumor may be difficult to distinguish from squamous cell carcinoma (Head, 1976a; Moulton, 1978).

Ameloblastomas may be difficult to distinguish from certain epulides. One group of investigators considered that many tumors diagnosed as ameloblastomas are fibromatous epulides (Gorlin et al., 1959). Another view is that if both epulides and ameloblastomas arise from the enamel organ and dental lamina, they may be variations of the same tumor (Moulton, 1978).

Tumors with both ameloblastic epithelium and dental pulp–like stroma are designated fibroameloblastoma. The fibroameloblastomas reported by Dubielzig et al. (1979) occurred in the areas of the upper incisor, canine, or premolar teeth and measured 1 to 3 cm. Radiographs of three showed varying degrees of infiltration and bone destruction. One cat was destroyed because of invasion of the nasal cavity. One was free of recurrence seven months after excision, and another was tumor-free five years after the second excision. In one from which the tumor was excised twice, adjuvant radiation failed to prevent recurrence of the tumor 10 months later.

Microscopically, multiple nodules of epithelial tissue were often arranged in cords resembling dental laminar epithelium. The cords tended to form cuplike structures, in which there was frequently a tightly woven nodule of spindle cells similar to dental pulp stroma. The term inductive was applied to the unique cuplike arrangement of epithelial components seen in these four tumors. This feature has not been described in other species but has been reported in one other cat (Gorlin et al., 1963). Metastases were not reported in any of the cases.

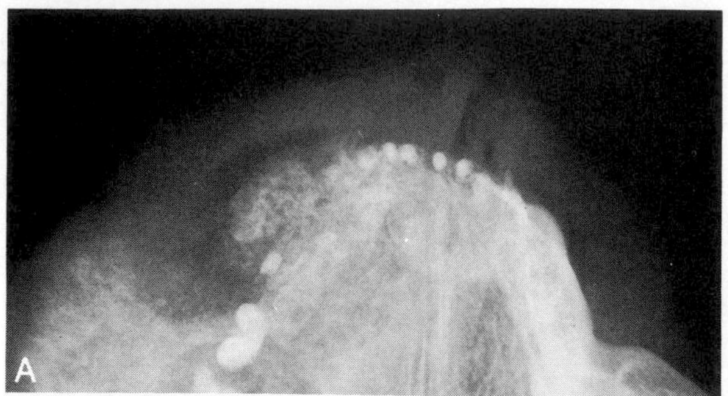


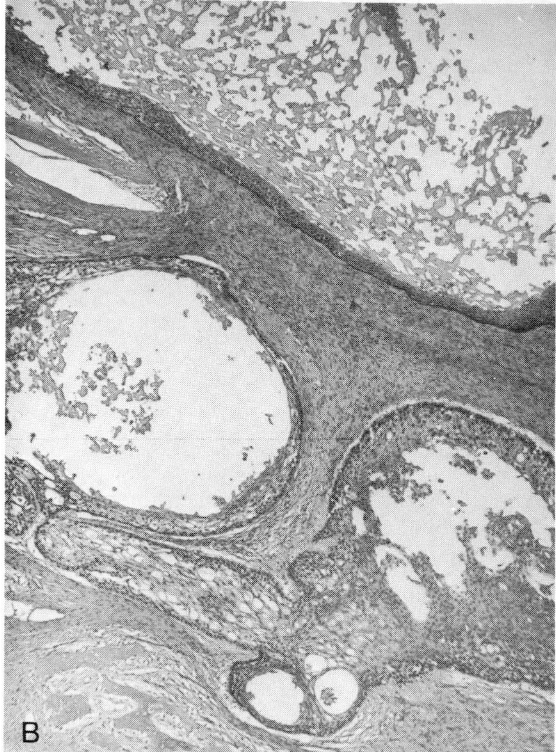


**Figure 11–86** *A*, Ameloblastoma, right maxillary and palatine bones, eight-year-old castrated male orange-and-white tabby. Lysis and proliferation of bone are features that also suggest squamous cell carcinoma as well as osteomyelitis. *B*, Dense fibrous trabeculae contain foci of new bone (upper and lower left) and separate cystic islands of epithelium. H & E, × 50.

## Epulis

Epulis is a descriptive term that has been applied confusingly to a variety of gingival excrescences, some neoplastic and some non-neoplastic. Happily, such growths are rare in cats. One was reported in a 10-year-old castrated male (Cotchin, 1956b), and two were reported without details (Bastianello, 1983; Engle and Brodey, 1969). A "giant cell epulis" was described in the lower jaw of a nine-month-old female where the root of a broken canine tooth had been removed three months before (Schneck, 1975). The growth shelled out like a pea, and the site healed uneventfully. Microscopically, many giant cells were seen in a stroma of spindle-shaped

connective tissue cells. Similar giant cell epulides develop in children when they lose deciduous teeth and could be interpreted as reparative granulomas.

Three epulides are on record at AMAH in cats aged 9, 11, and 17 years, a Persian, a Siamese, and a domestic shorthair. Two were castrated males and the third a spayed female. The tumors, which bulged from the mandibular gingiva, had been present for 5 to 10 months and were small, the largest being only 1.3 × 0.6 × 0.5 cm. They were white or pink, smooth, firm, and fibrous.

Two tumors, like that reported by Engle and Brodey (1969), were fibromatous epulides of periodontal origin. Cords of squamous epithelium resembling rete pegs branched and anastomosed in intimate contact with dense collagenous stroma similar to that of periodontal ligament. There were dentin-like foci in the stroma. The third tumor was an acanthomatous epulis consisting mainly of anastomosing sheets of cells with prominent intercellular bridges (acanthocytes). The stroma was dense, collagenous in some areas, fibrillar in others.

Epulides are benign but may recur locally if not completely excised.

## Other Oral Tumors

Two extremely rare and interesting benign oral tumors were reported in cats aged five and seven years (Levene, 1984). Both arose from gingival epithelium and were composed of basal-type and sebaceous cells, suggesting sebaceous gland differentiation (metaplasia). One of the tumors had the appearance of an oral papilloma with subsequent sebaceous metaplasia. Sebaceous differentiation has often been observed in salivary gland tumors of man, but no salivary gland tissue was seen in either of the feline growths.

A fibroxanthoma of the gum was reported by Gorlin et al. (1959) and also a possible alveolar soft-part sarcoma (malignant granular cell myoblastoma) of the upper gingiva in an eight-year-old female cat. The latter had rounded cells grouped in discrete masses separated by a delicate fibrous stroma. The nuclei were central and hyperchromatic; the cytoplasm was granular, faintly eosinophilic, and sometimes vacuolated. The tumor recurred five months after surgery, extending into the posterior nasal cavity.

Oral hemangiomas, hemangiosarcomas, melanomas, and lymphomas are discussed in the sections on those tumors.

## Tumors of the Tongue

Lingual tumors other than squamous cell carcinoma are rare. Papillomas (Engle and Brodey, 1969; Lombard, 1940; Priester and McKay, 1980) and hemangiomas have been reported (Crow et al., 1981; Priester and McKay, 1980), and one hemangioma is on record at AMAH. Uncommon malignant tumors recorded are a "vegetating hemangioendothelioma" (Lombard, 1964), a fibrosarcoma (Engle and Brodey, 1969), and a reticulum cell sarcoma (Stünzi, 1967). Hemangiosarcoma, leiomyosarcoma, and lymphoma are on record at AMAH. (See sections on those tumors.)

Squamous cell carcinoma in cats occurs predominantly in the oral cavity, most often involving the tongue. In a group of 864 tumors surveyed at the Royal Veterinary College in London, 98 were squamous cell carcinomas of the upper alimentary tract, and of these 28 were lingual, with almost equal incidence in the gum, palate, and pharynx (26) and esophagus (29); there were 15 tonsillar tumors (Cotchin, 1983). As Cotchin points out, the cat is the only species, apart from man, to suffer at all commonly from cancer of the tongue or esophagus. It has been suggested that soot from the environment is licked by cats from their coats and results in a high exposure of the upper digestive tract to carcinogens. Elsewhere lingual carcinoma is encountered only occasionally. Eight cases were reported in a group of 395 tumors from the Philadelphia area (Engle and Brodey, 1969) and 2 among 289 tumors in a New York City survey (Patnaik et al., 1975). In a total of about 2200 tumors at North American Veterinary Colleges, 24 squamous cell carcinomas of the tongue were recorded (Priester and McKay, 1980). In a survey limited to oral disease, half of 33 feline carcinomas involved the tongue (Gorlin et al., 1967). Isolated cases from the early literature were cited by Lombard (1940), and case reports appear from time to time (e.g., Bond and Dorfman, 1969; Herman, 1967). The tumor's rarity in Australia may possibly be of some epidemiologic significance (Young, 1978).

In Cotchin's (1983) group of cats with carcinoma of the upper digestive tract, of 80 cats of known sex, 68 were males (57 castrated) and 12 were females (8 spayed). In the group of lingual carcinomas reported by Priester and McKay (1980) the male:female ratio was exactly 1:1.

Of 105 feline squamous cell carcinomas diagnosed at AMAH, 80 were oral and 38 of those involved the tongue. Twenty-two of the affected cats were females (eight entire) and 16 were males (10 castrated). The age range was 6 to 19 years (mean 11.8), figures in general accord with ages given in other reports. None of the cats was a purebred.

Cats with lingual carcinoma have difficulty eating and drinking, and fetid bloody saliva may flow from the mouth. Most of the lingual squamous cell carcinomas reported by others and most of those seen at AMAH developed on the ventral surface of the tongue at or near the frenulum (Fig. 11–87*A*). Lateral growths on the body of the tongue are more common than tumors of the root; rarely a tumor arises from the dorsum. The tumors are pink or white-yellow, firm, and usually ulcerated. Early tumors, which may resemble granulation tissue, can be mistaken for eosinophilic granulomas or for injuries caused by string, needles, or other foreign bodies.

Microscopically, sheets of cells with desmosomes, autonomous cells undergoing individual keratinization, and keratin "pearls" may be seen as in squamous cell carcinoma of the skin, but keratinization is less likely when the tumor arises from a mucous membrane. Therefore the pathologist must be aware of more subtle changes indicative of carcinoma in order to distinguish tumor from benign epithelial proliferation with deep rete peg formation. Lack of normal polarity and transition of the outer layer of epithelial cells, marked variation in size of adjacent cells, occasional very large cells, many and atypical mitotic figures, and the absence of a normal transition of cells undergoing keratinization are all indicative of malignancy (Fig. 11–87*B*).

Successful surgical excision of carcinomas of the tongue is unlikely, because they tend to penetrate deeply and are

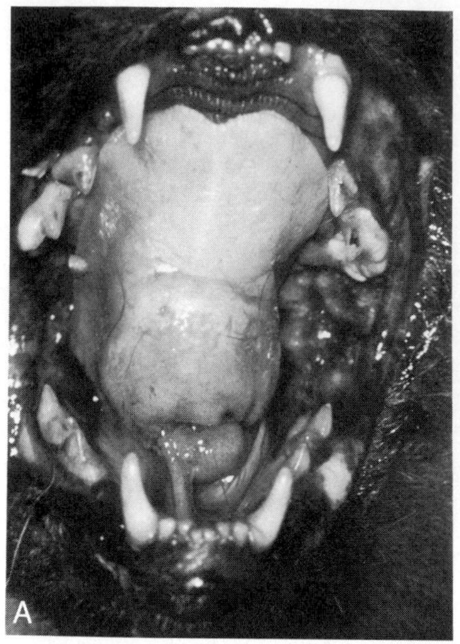


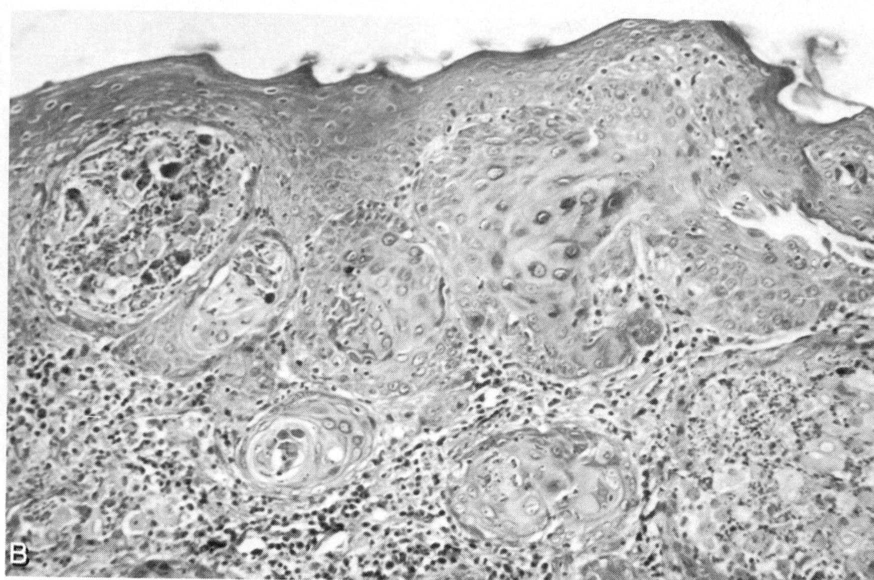


**Figure 11–87** *A*, Squamous cell carcinoma, underside of the tongue and extending back into the left side of the mouth, 12-year-old cat. The large, raised, infiltrative tumor distorts the frenulum, a common site of this neoplasm in cats. *B*, Malignant squamous cells (upper right) extend from the oral epithelium and form solid packets surrounded and infiltrated by numerous inflammatory cells. H & E, × 180.

usually well advanced by the time they are detected. The tumors metastasize very slowly, and regional nodes are rarely involved at the time most cats are euthanatized.

## Tumors of the Tonsil

Cysts and tumors of the tonsil of cats are rare. A squamous epithelium–lined cyst, 1.0 cm in diameter, containing debris, cholesterol clefts, and foci of mineralization was on record at AMAH in a 13-year-old cat.

Squamous cell carcinoma is the most frequent of feline tonsillar neoplasms recorded in the literature and seen at AMAH. Fifteen cases were reported by Cotchin (1983), four by Stünzi (1967), and one each by Engle and Brodey (1969) and Nielsen (1964). Eight cats at AMAH had carcinoma arising in or involving the tonsil by extension. In Cotchin's (1983) experience, tonsillar carcinomas appeared as firm, nodular, whitish masses causing excessive salivation and difficulty in swallowing; they tended to metastasize early to the regional lymph nodes.

In gross and microscopic appearance the tumors are similar to squamous cell carcinoma of the tongue.

A primary lymphoepithelioma of the tonsil was reported by Quarante (1938). A few cases of tonsillar lymphoma are on record at AMAH.

## Tumors of Salivary Glands

Tumors of the salivary glands are uncommon in the cat; the great majority are malignant. They may arise from the major glands (parotid, mandibular, sublingual, molar, and zygomatic), as well as from the minor glands of the lip, cheek, palate, gingiva, tongue, and floor of the mouth. Over 35 tumors have been reported: two adenomas, a mucoepidermoid tumor, at least 30 adenocarcinomas, a malignant mixed tumor, a squamous cell carcinoma, an acinar epithelioma, and a melanoma (Ball, 1934; Ball and Collet, 1934; Bastianello, 1983; Bosselut et al., 1951; Case and Simon, 1966; Engle and Brodey, 1969; Godglück, 1948; Goldberg, 1920; Gorlin et al., 1959; Head, 1976a; Karbe and Schiefer, 1967; Koestner and Buerger, 1965; Nielsen, 1964; Patnaik et al., 1975; Petit, 1902b; Priester and McKay, 1980). Of the 22 tumors for which site of origin was specified, 15 were of the parotid, 6 of the mandibular, and 1 of the sublingual gland.

Thirteen salivary gland tumors were diagnosed in cats at AMAH: 11 adenocarcinomas and 2 adenomas. Five of the adenocarcinomas were of the mandibular salivary gland, three of the parotid, and two of the minor salivary glands of the cheek; one involved both the mandibular and the sublingual glands. Most salivary gland tumors occur in aged cats. At AMAH the mean age was 11 years, with a range of 3 to 20. No breed or sex predilection was apparent. All tumors reported in the literature and those on record at AMAH were unilateral.

**CLINICAL FEATURES.** Tumorous salivary glands are enlarged, nodular, and firm or hard. The tumor may fluctuate in size if salivary ducts are compressed or obstructed. The gland may also become infected or abscessed, and occasionally the skin over a rapidly growing tumor is invaded and ulcerates. The cat often salivates profusely and, if the tumor compresses or invades the oropharynx, will have difficulty eating and swallowing. It may gag frequently, make repeated exaggerated attempts to swallow, and drop its food. The owner usually reports gradual weight loss.

Chronic otitis externa may be a complication of tumors of the parotid if the tumor obstructs the external ear canal, and meningitis and central nervous disturbances may result. Compression or invasion of the seventh cranial

nerve as it emerges from the stylomastoid foramen at the base of the skull and courses through the parotid gland may cause unilateral facial nerve palsy. Two of 13 cats examined at AMAH had moderate dyspnea owing to aspiration pneumonia. Both cats had large invasive tumors, one of the mandibular and one of the parotid gland. Both cats had been force-fed by their owners.

**GROSS FEATURES.** Most adenocarcinomas of salivary glands are firm, bosselated, white or tan masses closely adherent to the overlying subcutis. On cut section, firm, yellow, gritty areas of necrosis may be seen. Cystic and hemorrhagic foci are common. Because adenocarcinomas grow rapidly and are rarely detected early, they may be quite large at diagnosis. One adenocarcinoma of a parotid gland measured 8.0 × 8.0 × 6.0 cm.

Adenomas may resemble adenocarcinomas grossly or may be soft and pink. They are well circumscribed and do not adhere to overlying skin.

**MICROSCOPIC FEATURES.** Salivary gland tumors are classified as epithelial or mesenchymal. Benign epithelial tumors include monomorphic and pleomorphic adenomas (benign mixed tumors). The latter have not been reported in the cat. The monomorphic adenoma consists of epithelial cells in a regular glandular pattern. There is no proliferation of myoepithelial cells and no altered ground substance. Only two adenomas of a feline salivary gland were found in a review of the literature (Bastianello, 1983; Case and Simon, 1966). The tumor described by Case and Simon as an oncocytoma (oxyphilic granular adenoma), a rare benign tumor of the parotid salivary gland, was removed successfully.

One of two adenomas diagnosed at AMAH was an ovoid, soft, pink mass, 0.8 × 0.6 × 0.3 cm in the right molar salivary gland of a seven-year-old castrated male domestic shorthair. On microscopic examination, it consisted of pale-staining cuboidal to columnar epithelial cells resembling goblet cells, with basally located nuclei arranged in a papillary glandular pattern (Fig. 11–88). There were extensive multifocal, mucus-filled cystic spaces, into which papillary processes of the tumor projected. The tumor did not recur after removal of the affected gland. The other adenoma, in a nine-year-old female domestic shorthair, was an ovoid, gray-brown, firm, lobulated mass, 1.5 × 1.5 × 1.0 cm, involving the right mandibular gland and the caudal aspect of the right sublingual gland. It consisted of circumscribed foci of low cuboidal to columnar epithelial cells arranged in a pattern of small tubules. The nuclei were basal and the cytoplasm granular or vacuolated. The neoplasm had been noticed for a month and had fluctuated in size. The cat was destroyed shortly after surgical removal because of concomitant lymphoma.

The malignant epithelial tumors include adenocarcinoma, mucoepidermoid tumor, acinic cell tumor, squamous cell carcinoma, undifferentiated carcinoma, and carcinoma in pleomorphic adenoma (malignant mixed tumor). Undifferentiated carcinoma and acinic cell tumors have not been reported in the cat.

Adenocarcinomas, the most numerous salivary neoplasms in the cat, may arise from acinar or ductal epithelium. They are classified on the basis of pattern as tubular or ductular. The ductular pattern consists of low cuboidal epithelium with papillary projections. The tubular type may be subdivided into simple tubular, alveolar, trabecular, and solid patterns. Although it is common to find more than one pattern within a given tumor, one pattern usually predominates. Of 11 adenocarcinomas examined at AMAH, 4 had a simple tubular pattern, 2 a papillary (Fig. 11–89) or ductal pattern, 3 a solid pattern (Fig. 11–90), 1 a mixed tubular and papillary pattern, and 1 an alveolar pattern. Nuclei were round or oval, usually with a single prominent nucleolus. The degree of cellular atypia and number of mitotic figures varied. Necrosis, inflammation, and desmoplasia were common, as were vascular, perineural, lymphatic, and stromal invasion. Mucus secretion, cyst formation, and squamous or osseous metaplasia were less frequent. In one neoplasm, there was an inflammatory response to a ruptured cyst.

Of the 11 adenocarcinomas at AMAH, 8 had metastasized to regional lymph nodes at the time of diagnosis. All were locally invasive. In a cat with an adenocarcinoma of the minor salivary glands of the cheek, the tumor invaded the buccal mucosa and spread to regional lymph nodes, lung, heart, brain, pancreas, and adrenals. Another cat with an adenocarcinoma of the left parotid gland had metastases to the subcutaneous tissue over the head, neck, and scapula.

The mucoepidermoid tumor consists of solid masses of squamous cells with intercellular bridges and rare keratin formation surrounding mucus-secreting cells. The latter characteristically form cystic structures. The degree of differentiation of the two cell types varies. PAS, alcian green, or mucicarmine stain may be used to demonstrate mucin in the mucoepidermoid tumor (Koestner and Buer-

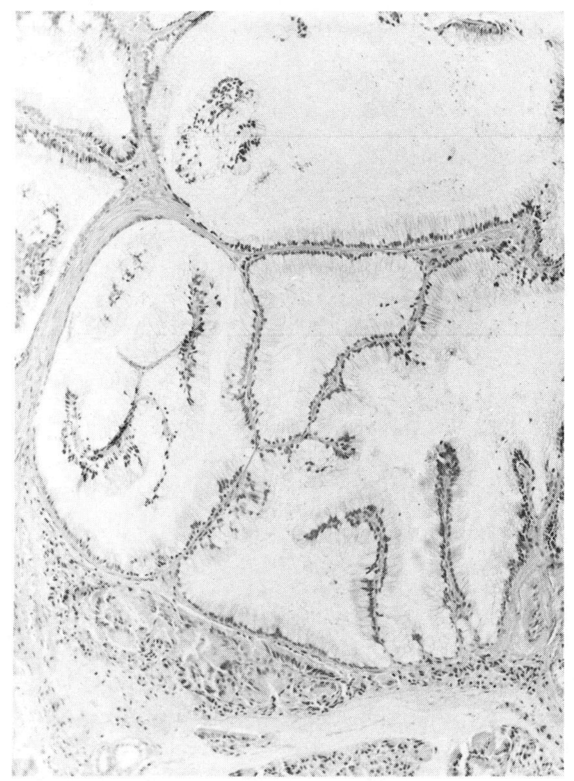

**Figure 11–88** Papillary adenoma of the molar salivary gland, six-year-old castrated male domestic shorthair. Papillae, lined by mucus-laden, tall, simple columnar epithelium, project into dilated mucus-filled glandular spaces. H & E, × 75.

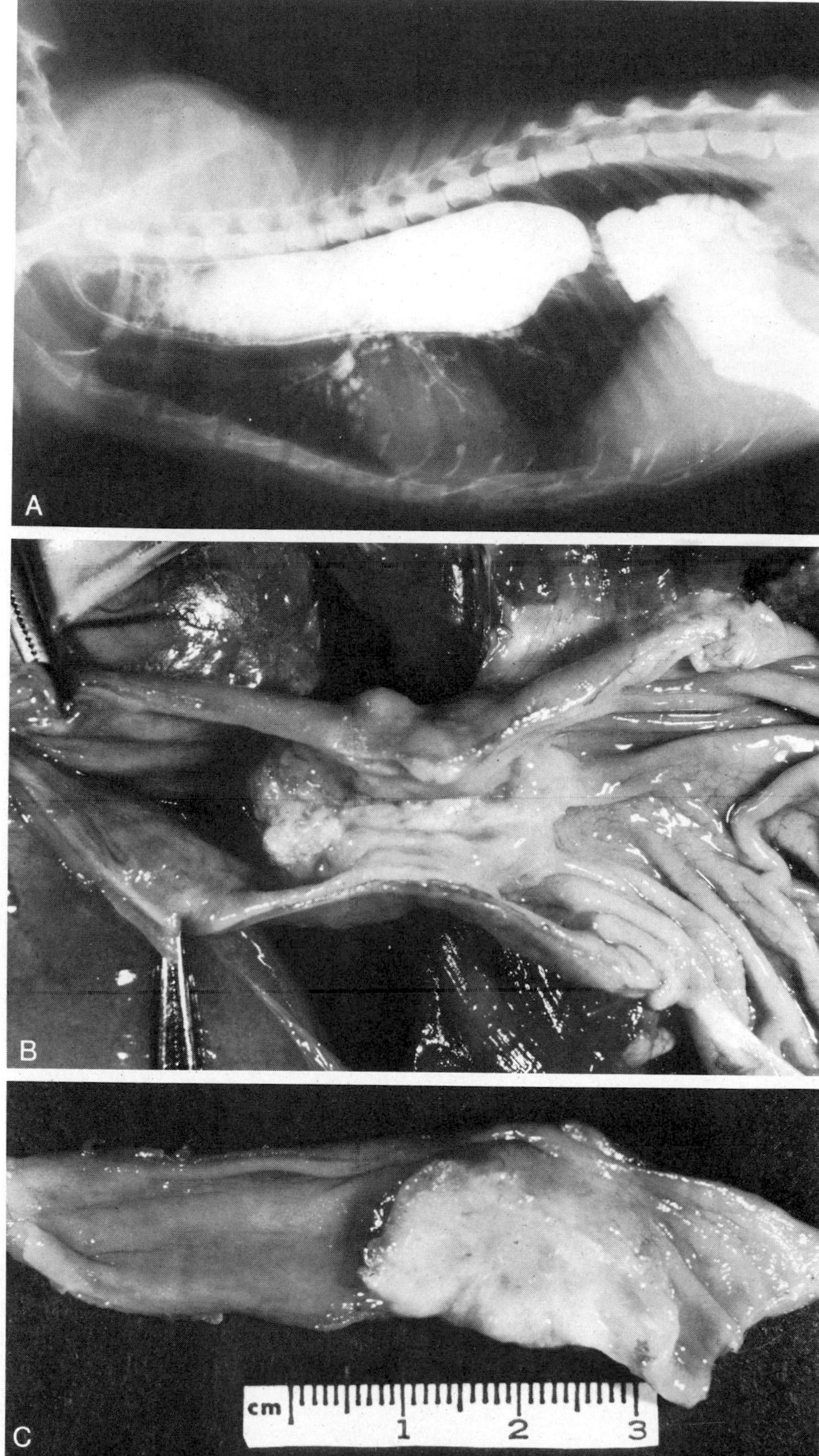


**Figure 11–91** *A*, Squamous cell carcinoma in the distal esophagus, 20-year-old white domestic shorthair. Tumor-induced fibrous stenosis caused proximal esophageal dilatation, and longitudinal contracture led to a gastric hiatal hernia. Contrast medium was administered in what would normally be a suitable amount, but reduction of the esophageal lumen to 4 mm (not shown) caused aspiration of the material. *B*, Opened distal esophagus. The proliferative tumor (center) occludes the lumen and pulls the diaphragm and stomach forward. *C*, Longitudinal section discloses that the tumor is eccentric, penetrates one area of the esophageal wall, and almost completely obstructs the lumen. Much of the tumor takes the form of white fibrous connective tissue.

ach may be so much enlarged that it is palpable behind the rib cage. Signs are vomiting, wasting, and anemia.

For gastric tumors, palpation, contrast radiography, and endoscopy can be useful in diagnosis. Prognosis is guarded.

### Tumors of the Intestine

Intestinal tumors have long been recognized as frequent in the cat, and early reports are cited by Lombard (1940). Intestinal neoplasms are most often lymphoma, adenocarcinoma, and mast cell tumor. Polyps, adenoma, leiomyoma, leiomyosarcoma, carcinoid, a ganglioneuroma, and a tumor of globule leukocytes have also been reported. A plasma cell tumor diagnosed at AMAH is described with hematopoietic neoplasms, and lymphoma and mast cell tumor are discussed in the sections on those tumors.

## Benign Tumors

Polyps are rare in the cat. A pedunculated tumor, 3.0 cm in diameter, in the rectum of a 13-year-old spayed female Siamese caused intermittent mucohemorrhagic diarrhea for 10 months. The tumor had not recurred when the cat died of other causes a year after resection. Opinion was divided as to whether the tumor was an adenoma or a polyp (Lingeman and Garner, 1972; Olin et al., 1968).

Intestinal polyps were diagnosed at AMAH in 11 cats, 3 of which had multiple polyps. One domestic shorthair with several colonic polyps passed one in the stool. Another domestic shorthair had both gastric and colonic polyps, and a Siamese had several at the anorectal junction. Sites of polyps were duodenum (one), jejunum (three), cecum (one), colon (three), and rectum (three). The cats ranged in age from 5 to 17 years. Five were intact or spayed females; six were males, five castrated.

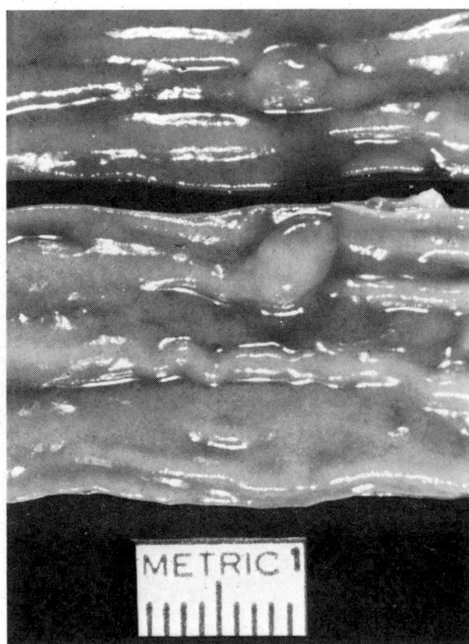


**Figure 11–92** Benign mucosal polyps, small intestine, 11-year-old tabby. The polyps were asymptomatic.

Seven were domestic shorthairs, two Siamese, one a Persian, and one a Russian Blue.

The majority of polyps were asymptomatic. One cat with a polyp in the distal jejunum had an intussusception. The cat with a cecal polyp had decreased appetite and a movable midabdominal mass. The cat with rectal polyps had blood in the stool and defecated with difficulty; the tumor was accompanied by chronic proliferative anal inflammation.

Grossly, polyps are white or pink pedunculated masses that protrude into the bowel lumen (Fig. 11–92). They may be single or multiple and range in size from minute to at least 2.0 cm in diameter. They often ulcerate and may become necrotic. They consist of fronds with well-differentiated epithelium and branching cores of lamina propria.

Intestinal adenoma is rare. A case of multiple adenomas of the small intestine was reported by Petit (1908). Multiple adenomatous tumors of the large intestine were found in a cat with *Strongyloides tumefaciens*. A cause and effect relationship was inferred but not proved (Price and Dikmans, 1941). Leiomyoma is also uncommon (Patnaik et al., 1975; Totire-Ippoliti, 1927). One seen at AMAH in a 13-year-old cat gave rise to an intussusception.

## Adenocarcinoma

Adenocarcinoma of the intestine is next in frequency after lymphoma and is one of the most important neoplasms of cats, at least 200 cases having been reported (Antoine and Brouwers, 1941; Bastianello, 1983; Burgisser, 1960; Cotchin, 1983; Engle and Brodey, 1969; Jones and Hunt, 1983; Lingeman and Garner, 1972; Mulligan, 1951; Nielsen, 1964; Palumbo and Perri, 1974; Patnaik et al., 1976, 1981; Priester and McKay, 1980; Rubarth, 1934; Stowater, 1978; Taylor and Kater, 1954; Turk et al., 1981; Whitehead, 1967). Cats with tumors of the small intestine are typically middle-aged and very often Siamese. Cats with tumors of the cecum and large intestine are older and almost always domestic cats.

Adenocarcinomas of the intestine were found in 112 cats at AMAH. About 51 per cent of the intestinal tumors were in the ileum, a predilection site noted by others (e.g., Lingeman and Garner, 1972; Patnaik et al., 1976). The next most frequent site was the jejunum (22 per cent), followed by colon (13 per cent), duodenum (9 per cent), cecum (4 per cent), and rectum (1.8 per cent). The mean age of cats with adenocarcinoma of the small intestine was 10.8 years with a range of 4 to 17. Cats with tumors of the colon averaged 16 years (range 14 to 18). The cats with rectal tumors were 9 and 12 years.

Siamese cats are predisposed to adenocarcinoma of the small intestine. One report stated that Siamese were three times more likely than domestic cats to have this tumor (Patnaik et al., 1976); in another study the incidence in Siamese was even higher (Turk et al., 1981). Seventy per cent of the cats at AMAH with this tumor were Siamese, but Siamese predominance does not hold true for adenocarcinoma located elsewhere; all cats at AMAH with tumors of the cecum (4), colon (16), and rectum (2) were domestic cats. Purebreds other than Siamese are rarely affected with intestinal adenocarcinoma (Brodey, 1966; Turk et al., 1981).

**CLINICAL FEATURES AND DIAGNOSIS.** Cats with tumors of the small intestine usually vomit intermittently and lose weight. Most become less active. Signs tend to be vague and may develop gradually for as long as a year before the cat is taken to a veterinarian. At presentation, over 25 per cent have a palpable abdominal mass. Twenty to 50 per cent have between 25 and 500 ml of clear fluid in the peritoneal cavity owing to peritoneal tumor implants (Patnaik et al., 1976). Most are dehydrated. A few have fever or diarrhea. Cats with colonic tumors are often constipated, and the stool may be streaked with blood. A cecal tumor caused an intussusception (Withrow and Greene, 1975).

Clinicopathologic findings are not usually helpful. Some cats are mildly anemic, although the anemia may be masked by dehydration. The cat that vomits frequently, has diarrhea, or does not eat may have a low serum potassium level. SGPT, SGOT, and SAP values are occasionally elevated. If a duodenal tumor invades or compresses the common bile duct, the cat may be jaundiced.

Contrast radiography with oral barium is often useful. Circumferential stenosis at the tumor site, the "napkin ring" sign, is almost pathognomonic for intestinal adenocarcinoma. The intestine proximal to the tumor is almost always dilated, and mucosal ulceration over the tumor causes irregular filling defects. Sometimes, if stenosis of the intestinal lumen is severe, functional obstruction occurs and contrast material does not pass beyond the tumor.

Cytologic examination of aspirated peritoneal fluid reveals clumps of malignant epithelial cells in about 20 per cent of cats with effusions (e.g., Jones and Hunt, 1983). The fluid is usually clear and colorless, pale yellow, or pink, but is occasionally frankly bloody. If perforation of the bowel occurs, the fluid may be septic.

Diagnosis is by biopsy or removal of the tumor. Laparotomy with excision of the tumor and at least 5 cm of intestine proximal and distal is the preferred procedure for both diagnosis and treatment. Together with this segment the surgeon should submit regional lymph nodes for examination for possible metastases. Laparoscopy may be used in a debilitated cat, but biopsies may be difficult to obtain with this technique. If the tumor is in the proximal duodenum, distal colon, or rectum, a fiberoptic endoscope or colonoscope may be used for tumor biopsy, but full-thickness biopsies cannot be obtained by this method.

**GROSS FEATURES.** Most adenocarcinomas of the small intestine are firm white masses that cause annular, segmental stenosis of the lumen of the bowel (Fig. 11–93). The tumorous intestinal wall is noticeably thickened (0.5 to 1.5 cm) compared with that of normal intestine (0.3 to 0.4 cm) for a distance of 2 to 7 cm. The intestine proximal to the tumor is usually dilated (Fig. 11–94*A*). Serosal and mesenteric metastases can occur by way of lymphatic extension as well as implantation (Fig. 11–94*B*). Tumors in the rectum may form a proliferative, cauliflower-like mass that projects into the lumen. Adenocarcinomas of the intestine are usually solitary, but occasionally multiple tumors occur, particularly in the jejunum and ileum. In advanced cases, multifocal or disseminated, firm, elevated, white tumor implants, pinpoint to 0.3 cm in diameter, are often found on the peritoneum, diaphragm, mesentery, and serosal surfaces of abdominal viscera (Fig. 11–95).

**MICROSCOPIC FEATURES.** Adenocarcinomas of the intestine originate in the epithelium and are classified on the basis of cell type and pattern as papillary, tubular, mucinous, and signet-ring (Head, 1976b). Most adenocarcinomas of the intestine have more than one pattern but are classified by the predominant cell type. The papillary tumors have well-differentiated cuboidal or columnar cells covering fingerlike projections of lamina propria. In tubular adenocarcinomas, columnar, cuboidal, or flattened epithelial cells form variably developed tubules. Solid sheets of cells may form islands within the tumor stroma. In mucinous tumors, the cuboidal or flattened epithelial cells produce excessive mucin. Often the neoplastic glands rupture, forming large lakes of mucin. Other tumor types may also produce varying amounts of mucin; therefore to be classified as mucinous, over 50 per cent of a tumor should be mucin. Signet-ring tumors are composed of poorly differentiated cells that do not form glands. Their cytoplasm usually contains mucin.

Fibrosis accompanies most adenocarcinomas, particularly if they infiltrate the tunica muscularis. Sometimes, in scirrhous carcinomas, severe fibrosis obscures individual cells or nests of epithelial cells invading the submucosa and muscular tunic. Osseous and squamous metaplasia may occur. If the tumor contains abundant bone, it is hard to cut, requiring decalcification before sectioning.

Adenocarcinomas may grow into the lumen or into the wall of the gut (Fig. 11–96). In the cat, intramural extension is more common than intraluminal growth. The tumors spread by five routes: lymphatic invasion, growth

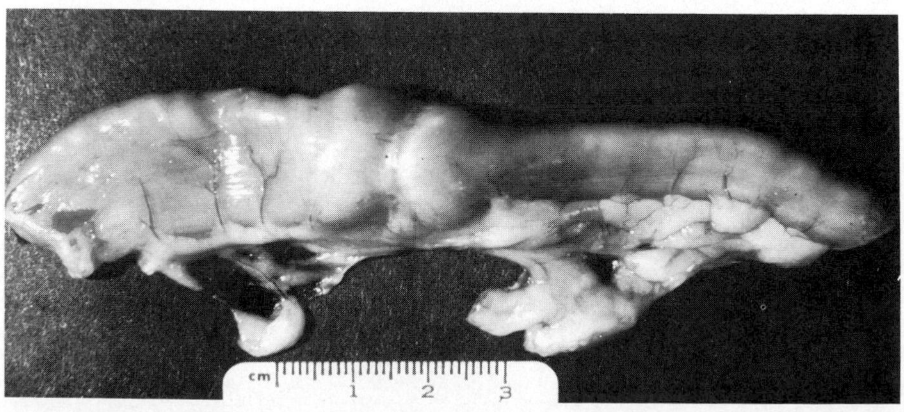


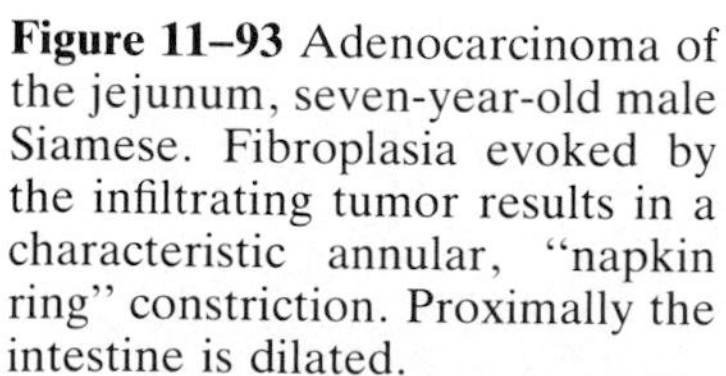

**Figure 11–93** Adenocarcinoma of the jejunum, seven-year-old male Siamese. Fibroplasia evoked by the infiltrating tumor results in a characteristic annular, "napkin ring" constriction. Proximally the intestine is dilated.

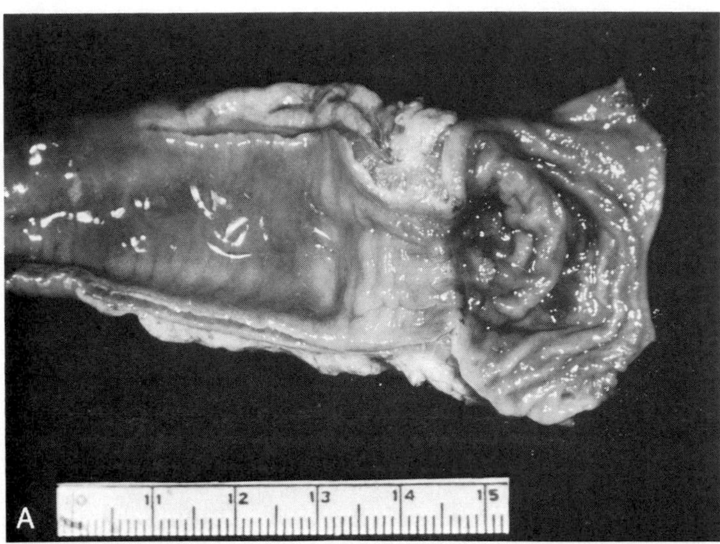

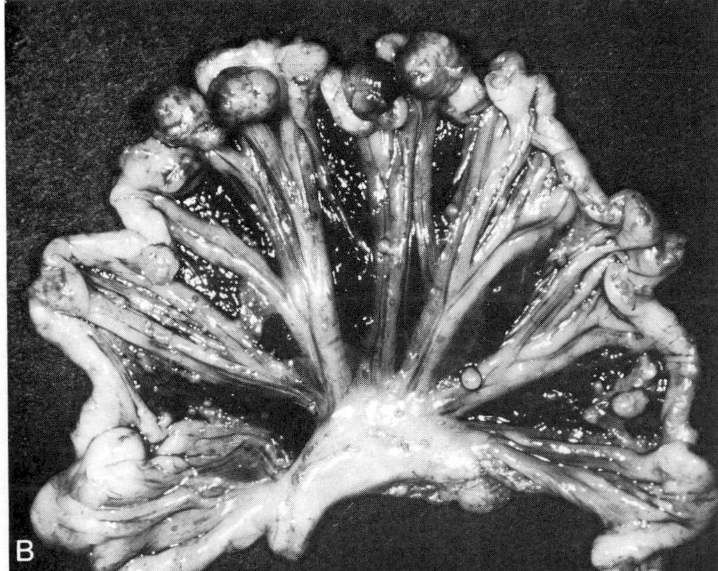

**Figure 11–94** *A*, Adenocarcinoma of the cecum, 18-year-old spayed female tricolor tabby. The cecum has been obliterated by a pale, fibrous, neoplastic mass (top center) that caused stenosis of the ileocolic junction, dilatation of the ileum (left), and seeding of the neoplasm in the abdomen. *B*, Numerous nodules, of varying size and shape, are disseminated along the bowel and mesenteric vessels. Fibrosis at the root of the mesentery (bottom) encases and hides the mesenteric nodes.

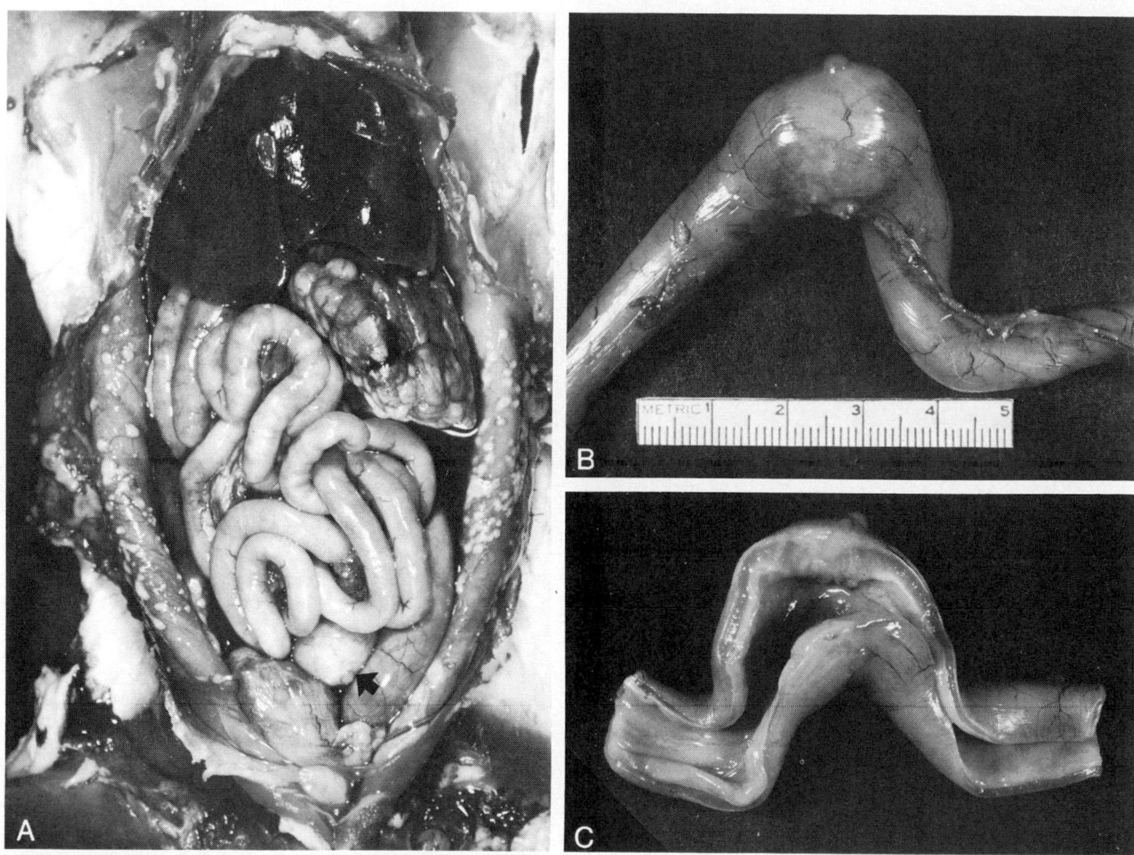


**Figure 11–95** *A*, Abdominal carcinomatosis, 13-year-old spayed female Siamese. Numerous pale nodules seed the parietal and visceral peritoneum. The liver (top) appears free of tumor, but the greater omentum, hiding the stomach, is contracted into a nodular mass by extensive neoplasia-induced fibrosis. The primary jejunal adenocarcinoma (arrow) is adjacent to the bladder. *B*, The segmental, pale enlargement with a serosal nodule is the site of the primary adenocarcinoma. The jejunum is tubularly rigid and is kinked owing to fibrosis about the tumor. *C*, The opened jejunum discloses the fibrotic distortion caused by the tumor. Stenosis of the intestine, a common feature of these adenocarciomas, is absent in this case.

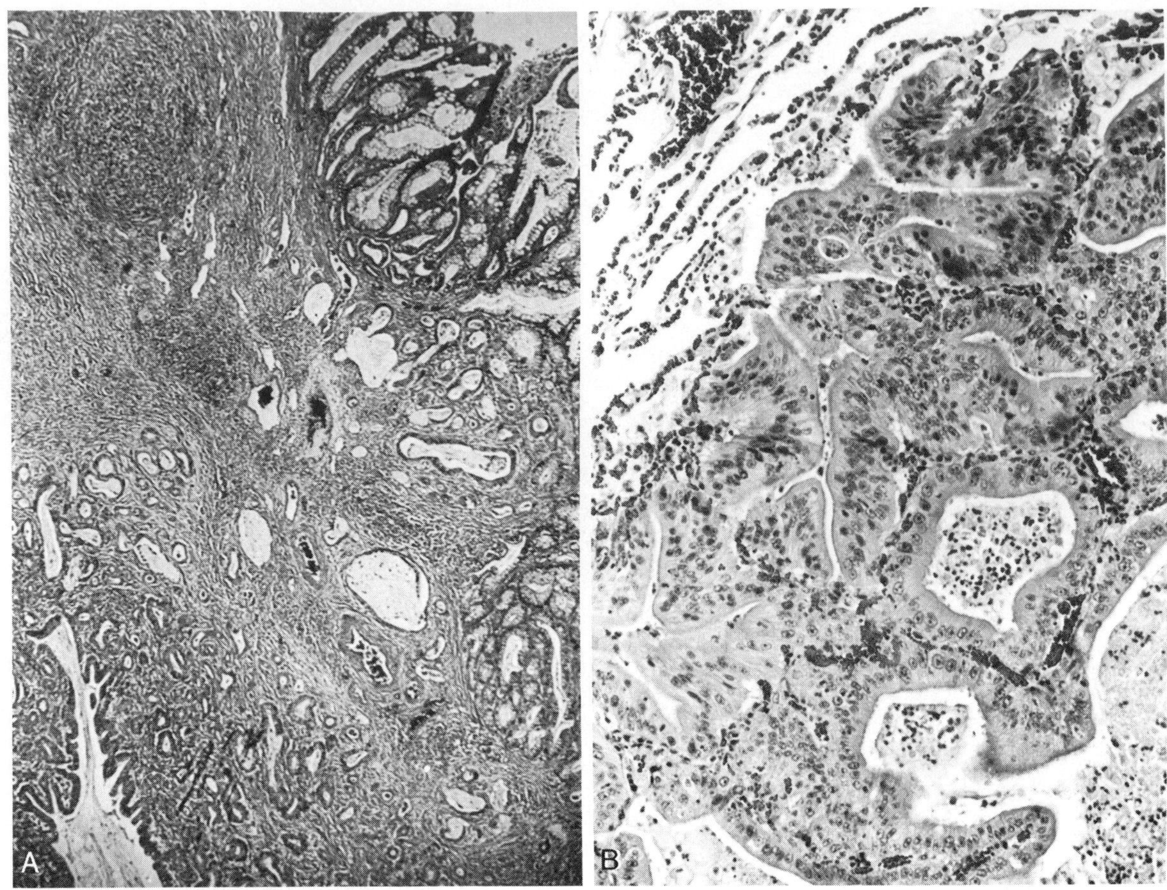


**Figure 11–96** *A*, Mucinous adenocarcinoma of the descending colon, 14-year-old castrated male blue-and-white domestic shorthair. The tumor projects into the lumen (right) and infiltrates the submucosa (center). Extension through the serosa (not shown) was accompanied by a neoplastic abdominal exudate that was yellow, opaque, sticky, and viscous. H & E, × 31. *B*, Metastatic adenocarcinoma of the colon in the lung. The neoplastic branching trabeculae are lined by simple and stratified columnar epithelium. Mucin production has elicited a histiocytic infiltrate. H & E, × 125.

into veins, direct extension to nearby structures, dissemination by way of the peritoneal cavity, and implantation (Wood, 1967). Staging, which is based on how far the tumor has spread at the time of diagnosis, may help the clinician predict its future. Stage I tumors are confined to the mucosa, Stage II tumors extend into the submucosa but not into the tunica muscularis, Stage III tumors involve the entire wall, and Stage IV tumors have spread to distant structures, such as the peritoneum and liver.

Of 65 intestinal adenocarcinomas analyzed for microscopic pattern, 58 per cent were tubular, 28 per cent mucinous, 10 per cent papillary, and 4 per cent signet-ring cell. All 112 tumors had invaded the tunica muscularis at the time of biopsy, and 40 per cent had spread to regional lymph nodes, peritoneum, mesentery, or omentum. Thirty-one per cent had metastasized to the liver, lung, spleen, stomach, urinary bladder, or uterus.

**TUMOR BEHAVIOR.** In one study the mean survival time was 20 weeks; only one cat was known to be alive two years after surgery (Turk et al., 1981). At AMAH the average survival time of cats after surgery was four to six months. However, five survived 10, 13, 14, 24 (Fig. 11–97), and 54 months, and two in published reports survived 28 and 18 months after surgical resection of their tumor (Palumbo and Perri, 1974; Patnaik et al., 1981). In all seven cats the tumors were in the small intestine, and at the time of surgery had invaded the tunica muscularis and serosa in five cats and regional lymph nodes in two.

Eventually all succumbed to recurrent or metastatic tumor, or both. However, their unexpectedly long survival times indicate that the prognosis for cats with this tumor is not always poor. Early detection, combined with wide resection of the tumor, may lengthen life significantly. Follow-up examination should include careful abdominal palpation, periodic radiographs of the thorax and abdomen, and peritoneal laparoscopy, when available. It is not known if chemotherapy or immunotherapy affects the behavior of this tumor.

## Other Intestinal Tumors

Uncommon malignant tumors include squamous cell carcinomas of the small intestine and rectum (Priester and McKay, 1980), as well as leiomyosarcoma (Engle and Brodey, 1969; Turk et al., 1981). About 20 sarcomas other than lymphoma were recorded by Cotchin (1983) and a fibrosarcoma by Turk et al. (1981).

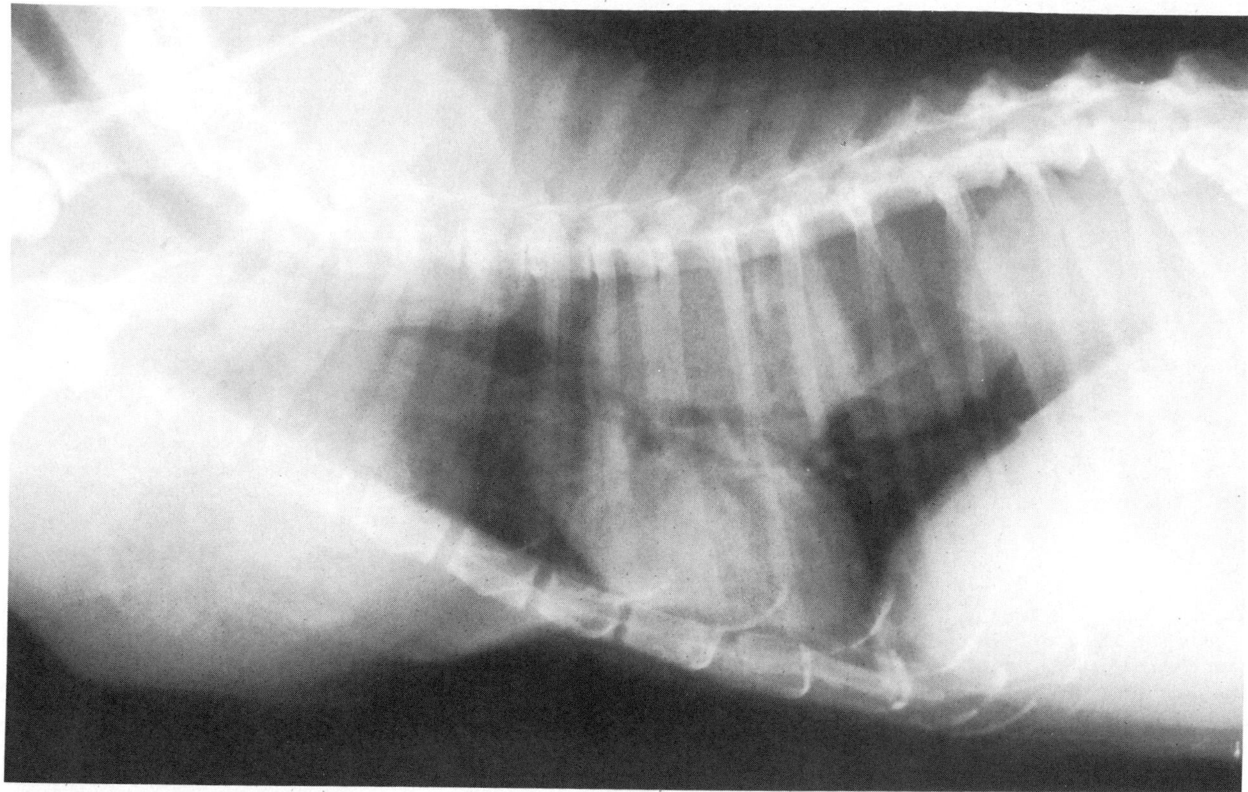

**Figure 11–97** Metastatic adenocarcinoma of the ileocolic junction in the lungs and axilla of a 12-year-old spayed female domestic shorthair. Metastases were found two years after resection of the primary tumor. The subcutaneous metastasis (left) had abundant woven bone intermingled with collagen and malignant epithelial cells.

Two carcinoids have been reported in the cat, one in the duodenum and one in the ileum (Carakostas et al., 1979; Lahellec and Joncourt, 1972). These tumors arise from enterochromaffin cells (Kulchitsky cells) of the intestine. In man, they may release 5-hydroxytryptamine (serotonin), which may cause flushing, diarrhea, and right-sided heart failure. One cat, a nine-year-old castrated male domestic shorthair, vomited frequently and lost weight for a month (Carakostas et al., 1979). A palpable nodular mass in the cranial abdomen proved to be an invasive tumor, 2.5 × 7.0 cm, involving the duodenum, pancreas, and nearby mesentery. Metastatic tumor was found in the lung and pleura at autopsy. Microscopically, the tumor consisted of a uniform population of cells having round, vesicular nuclei and arranged in solid sheets and ribbons in a delicate fibrovascular stroma. Cytoplasmic granules were argentaffin-negative, argyrophil-positive, and negative with Giemsa and PAS stains. Electron-dense granules were found in many tumor cells.

In the other cat, a 13-year-old castrated male, signs of obstruction were caused by a projecting, well-defined mass about 3 cm in diameter that completely blocked the lumen of the ileum. Because of involvement of mesenteric nodes the cat was destroyed, but a complete autopsy was not obtained. Microscopically the tumor was localized in the submucosa, but at one point it penetrated the mucosa and disrupted the muscular layer below. It consisted of anastomosing cords, sometimes broad, sometimes reduced to one layer of cells. The cells were uniformly round or polygonal with a big central nucleus and numerous eosinophilic granules. Mitoses were relatively frequent without nuclear atypia. Argentaffin-positive granules were demonstrated in many cells. Failure of the granules to stain with toluidine blue eliminated the possibility of mast cell tumor.

Carcinoids must be differentiated from intestinal mast cell tumors, which they superficially resemble. Most of the tumors diagnosed as carcinoids or argentaffinomas before 1970 have been shown to be mast cell tumors (Alroy et al., 1975).

A ganglioneuroma was reported in a six-week-old male Siamese (Patnaik et al., 1978). After several days of inappetence, vomiting, and mucoid diarrhea, the kitten was taken to a veterinarian semicomatose, dehydrated, emaciated, and hypothermic. A caudal abdominal mass was felt. A dilated, thick-walled segment of jejunum 8 cm long was resected, but the kitten died soon after surgery. Microscopically, the tumor was well circumscribed and consisted of irregularly arranged bundles of nerve fibers with spindle-form cells. Schwann cells and ganglion cells were present singly or in groups. The tumor was thought to arise from sympathetic ganglia of the submucosal plexus of Meissner.

A tumor of globule leukocytes was described in the ileum of a 12-year-old castrated male domestic shorthair (Finn and Schwartz, 1972). The cat had vomited intermittently and had a firm, painful abdominal mass. Laparotomy disclosed a thickened ileum with a nodular growth, 2.0 × 1.7 × 1.4 cm, adjacent to the mesenteric border. The tumor consisted of large cells with round, eccentric nuclei and 8 to 30 large eosinophilic globules in the cytoplasm. Chains and nests of tumor cells invaded the tunica muscularis. The cytoplasmic globules, averaging 1.15 μ in diameter, were eosinophilic with H&E stain and negative with alcian blue, PAS, and Giemsa stains. PTAH stained the granules light brown or, rarely, black.

## TUMORS OF THE LIVER AND BILIARY SYSTEM*

Primary tumors of the liver and biliary tract are uncommon in the cat, although considerable variation in prevalence is indicated by data from a number of surveys: 11 in a series of 864 tumors (Cotchin, 1966), 6 of 395 (Engle and Brodey, 1969), 20 of 289 (Patnaik et al., 1975), 23 of 2294 (Priester and McKay, 1980), 6 of 256 (Schmidt and Langham, 1967), 25 of 248 (Stünzi, 1967), 15 of 156 (Tamaschke, 1951/52), and 1 of 165 (Wlhitehead, 1967). At AMAH, among a total of 3248 feline tumors, there were 63 primary tumors of the liver and biliary tract.

The gallbladder and extrahepatic bile ducts, as will be seen, are only rarely the site of tumors.

### Hepatocellular Tumors

**ADENOMA.** This benign tumor, rare in humans, is reportedly not uncommon in some young animals (Ponomarkov and Mackey, 1976). In an extensive review of the literature on liver tumors in domestic animals, Messow (1952/53) cited what he considered to be two valid reports of liver cell adenoma in the cat, and eight liver cell adenomas were reported by Stünzi (1967). In a seven-month-old cat dying of viral rhinotracheitis an incidental finding was a 12 mm nodule diagnosed as a hepatoma (Shields and Gaskin, 1977).

Liver cell adenomas are usually solitary, well-demarcated, light tan nodules (Ponomarkov and Mackey, 1976). The cells may be arranged in a trabecular or acinar pattern, or the structure may be solid. If small, they may be difficult to differentiate from hyperplastic nodules, which, however, are usually multiple.

**CARCINOMA.** Malignant tumors of hepatocytes have been reported from the cat in several sources (e.g., Cotchin, 1966; Messow, 1952/53; Nielsen, 1964; Priester and McKay, 1980; Schmidt and Langham, 1967). Half the primary liver neoplasms (eight) in cats at The Animal Medical Center were hepatocellular carcinomas (Patnaik et al., 1975), while at AMAH these and bile duct adenomas occurred with equal frequency (18 cases each).

At AMAH the cats ranged in age from 2 to 18 years (median 11). Of 17 for which sex was recorded, 11 were males, 6 females. Sixteen were domestic shorthairs; two were Siamese.

Signs associated with hepatocellular carcinoma were nonspecific: anorexia, polydipsia, emaciation, lethargy, ascites, and a palpably or radiographically enlarged liver (Fig. 11–98). In several cats tested, SGPT was elevated. Many of the cats were destroyed owing to the poor prognosis. One died after an acute episode of "screaming," struggling, gasping for breath, and inability to rise. At autopsy, blood from a ruptured neoplastic liver nodule filled the abdominal cavity and metastatic tumor was evident in the spleen.

Grossly, hepatocellular carcinomas assume a nodular, massive, or diffuse form. In the first, there are many nodules throughout the liver (Fig. 11–99), one often larger

*By Frances M. Moore.

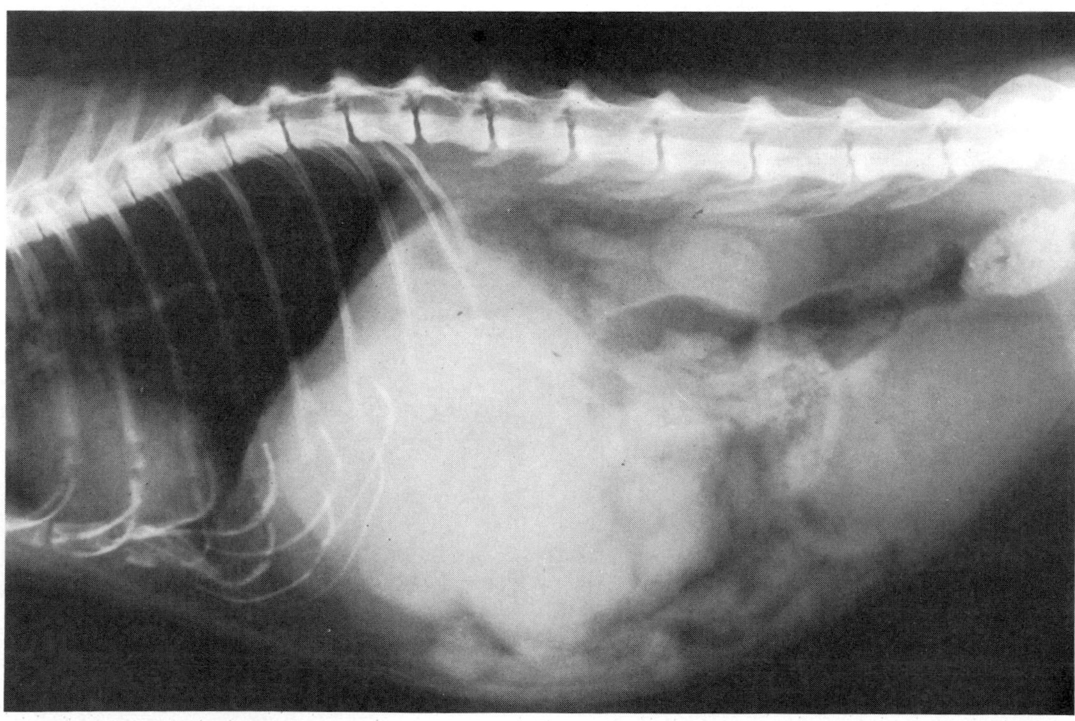

**Figure 11–98** Hepatocellular carcinoma, 16-year-old female domestic cat. The enlarged, nodular liver extends caudally far beyond the rib cage.

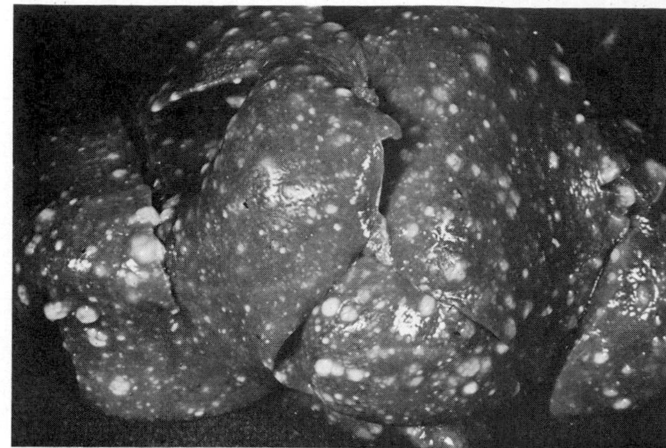

**Figure 11–99** Disseminated nodules of hepatocellular carcinoma, two-year-old castrated male domestic cat.

than the others. In the massive form, a large tumor virtually replaces a liver lobe. The diffuse form is characterized by tiny, indistinct nodules disseminated throughout the liver—lesions distinguished from regenerative nodules by disparity in size, necrosis, and variation in bile staining (Wright et al., 1979). All the hepatocellular carcinomas at AMAH were of nodular or massive type, the forms also most frequent in humans and dogs (Patnaik et al., 1980; Wright et al., 1979).

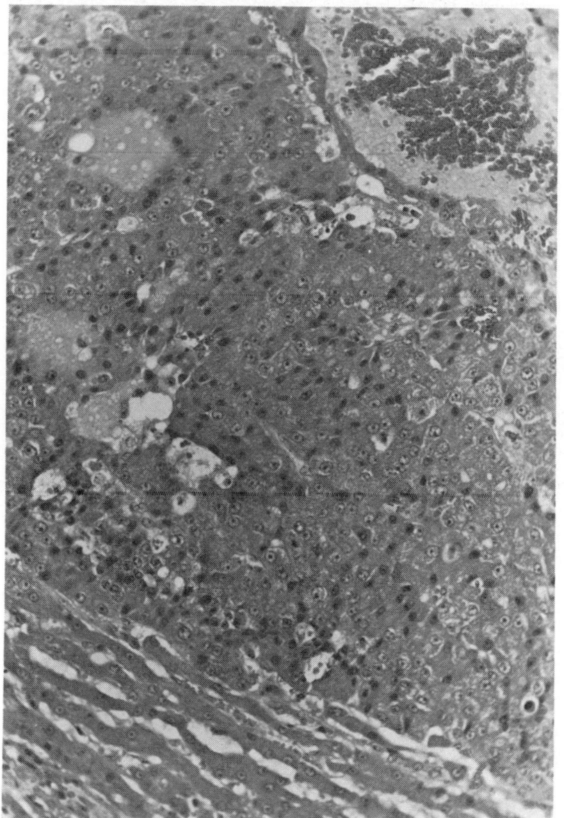

**Figure 11–100** Hepatocellular carcinoma, 12-year-old castrated male domestic cat. Broad cords of neoplastic hepatocytes form dilated sinusoid-like spaces, filled with blood and serum, and compress the adjacent, smaller, non-neoplastic hepatocellular cords. H & E, × 150.

Microscopically , the most frequent pattern was trabecular, in which cells resembling normal hepatocytes were arranged in cords or trabeculae often several cells thick. Between the cords were sinusoid-like spaces, occasionally cavernous, containing blood (Fig. 11–100). In other neoplasms the cells were arranged in tubules or acini. In several, the tumor cells compressed the surrounding non-neoplastic hepatocytes, but more often they blended almost imperceptibly with the normal liver parenchyma. Several tumors had a solid pattern. Fibroplasia was not significant.

Morphologically, the tumor cells often resembled normal hepatocytes with round or oval vesicular nuclei, abundant eosinophilic granular cytoplasm, and well-defined cell borders. Occasional cells had large, hyperchromatic nuclei and scant, slightly basophilic cytoplasm. In some tumors, multinucleated cells and cells of bizarre shapes and varying size were noted.

The distinction between benign and malignant hepatocellular tumors is not always clear. Nodular hepatocellular regeneration can also be confused with these entities. In our survey, malignancy was not well correlated with the degree of microscopic differentiation of the tumor, with one of the most well-differentiated tumors showing pulmonary metastasis. For this reason, the term "benign hepatocellular adenoma" was reserved for well-encapsulated nodules of hepatocytes. Although no tumors of this type were noted, several of the hepatocellular carcinomas were small with no evidence of metastasis at autopsy.

Five of the 18 (28 per cent) metastasized—to hepatic nodes (four), spleen (one), and lung (one). Metastasis was not consistently correlated with the degree of pleomorphism of the tumor. Coexisting liver tumors were adenoma of intrahepatic bile ducts (three), mast cell tumor (one), and myelolipoma (one).

## Tumors of Intrahepatic Bile Ducts

**ADENOMAS AND CYSTADENOMAS.** Adenomas and cystadenomas of intrahepatic bile ducts have been cited from the older literature by Messow (1952/53) and reported by Mulligan (1951) and Nunes Petisca (1956). At The Animal Medical Center, bile duct adenomas (five) were the third most frequent primary liver tumor after hepatic cell carcinoma and hemangiosarcoma (Patnaik et al., 1975).

At AMAH benign bile duct tumors (18) equaled hepatocellular carcinomas in frequency. Affected cats ranged in age from 6 to 17 years (mean 12). No sex predilection was apparent. Most were domestic shorthairs. Several had other tumors of the liver as well: hepatocellular carcinoma (3), mast cell tumor (1), and lymphoma (1). Signs in several cats were abdominal distention or a palpably enlarged liver, but most of the tumors were discovered incidentally at autopsy. One large cystadenoma (9 × 6 × 4 cm) was removed surgically from the left lateral liver lobe.

Grossly, intrahepatic bile duct adenomas in animals have been described as well circumscribed, small, solitary nodules or multilocular cystic tumors (Ponomarkov and Mackey, 1976). All the tumors at AMAH were of the latter type, varying from multiple, yellow-white, cystic foci up to 0.4 cm in diameter to multiloculated cystic and spongy structures replacing part or all of a lobe (Fig. 11–101). Microscopically, the cysts were lined by cuboidal or flattened epithelium with a scant or moderate amount of fibrous connective tissue stroma. Areas of hepatic parenchyma were often interspersed among cystic foci. Edmondson's (1958) comment on human bile duct adenomas may apply to the feline tumor:

> There is some question whether adenomas of the intrahepatic bile ducts ever occur.... The problem of distinguishing a true bile duct adenoma from the great variety of congenital cysts which may arise from bile ducts is difficult.

**ADENOCARCINOMAS.** Intrahepatic cholangiocellular carcinoma is the most frequently reported liver tumor of cats (e.g., Cotchin, 1966; Engle and Brodey, 1969; Feldman et al., 1976; Jubb and Kennedy, 1970; Jungreis, 1968; Patnaik et al., 1975; Root and Lord, 1971; Schmidt and Langham, 1967; Stünzi, 1967; Weege, 1971; Whitehead, 1967).

At AMAH 14 intrahepatic bile duct adenocarcinomas were diagnosed. The ages of the cats were from 9 to 21 years. A striking female:male (11:3) predominance was noted, similar to that in dogs (Patnaik et al., 1980). Two cats were Siamese, the rest domestic. Signs, as with hepatocellular carcinomas, were nonspecific: anorexia, lethargy, emaciation, ascites, and hepatomegaly; however, polyuria, polydipsia, and jaundice were often noted. In cats tested, SGOT and SGPT values were elevated. Most of the cats were destroyed because of clinical findings or after surgical exploration.

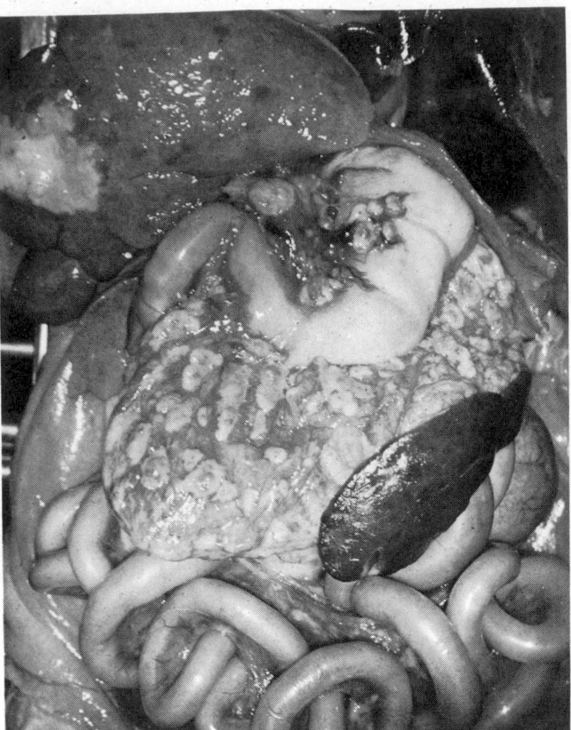

**Figure 11–102** Intrahepatic bile duct carcinoma (top left) in a 10-year-old female domestic cat with disseminated metastases to the hepatic node and to greater and lesser omentum. The walls of the stomach and duodenum and the surface of the pancreas were infiltrated.

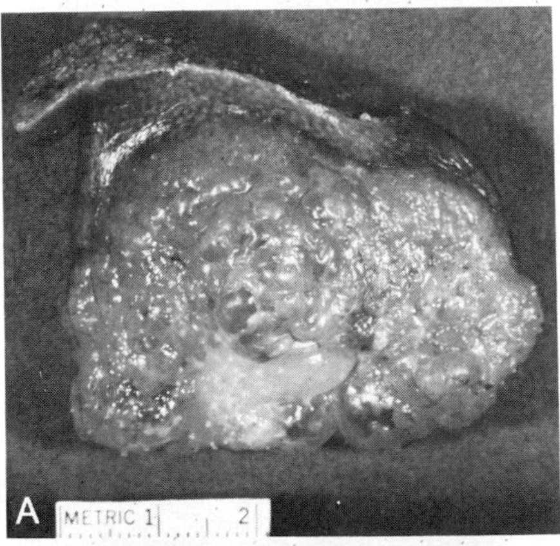


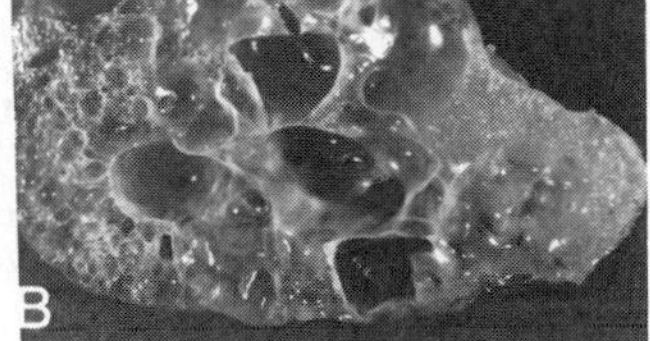


**Figure 11–101** Cystadenoma of intrahepatic bile ducts, 17-year-old castrated male domestic cat. The lobectomy specimen shows capsular (*A*) and cut (*B*) surfaces with multiple, occasionally confluent, thin-walled cysts.

Grossly, these tumors were firm, white or pale yellow, nodular masses (Fig. 11–102), sometimes replacing part or all of a liver lobe. Frequently, smaller masses were disseminated throughout all lobes. Sectioning often revealed cystic regions containing clear fluid. Metastases may be widespread.

Microscopically, the tumors usually had a tubular or papillary-tubular pattern, occasionally with amorphous, basophilic, intraluminal material. The neoplastic cells, varying from cuboidal to columnar, had round or oval vesicular nuclei, prominent nucleoli, and light-staining cytoplasm (Fig. 11–103). Sometimes pleomorphic cells with large nuclei, prominent nucleoli, and eosinophilic cytoplasm were noted either singly or in clusters. All the adenocarcinomas of intrahepatic bile ducts, in contrast to the hepatocellular carcinomas, were characterized by prominent fibroplasia.

Metastasis was evident in 11 of the 14 cats (78 per cent)—to lungs (seven), hepatic lymph nodes (five), serosa of gastrointestinal tract (four), mesenteric lymph nodes

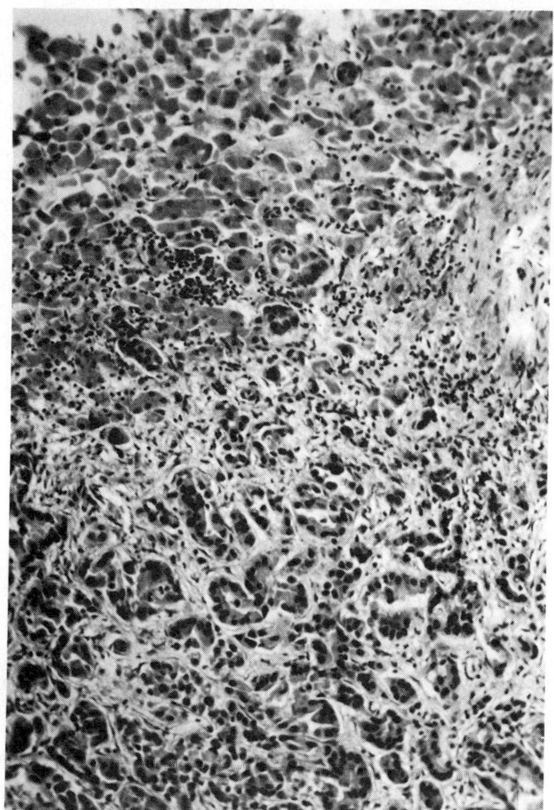

**Figure 11–103** Intrahepatic bile duct adenocarcinoma, nine-year-old male domestic cat. The neoplastic bile ducts form tubules associated with a moderate amount of connective tissue stroma that contrast with the broken cords of non-neoplastic hepatocytes. Mononuclear inflammatory cells are scattered throughout both areas but are concentrated at the tumor margin (upper left). H & E, × 180.

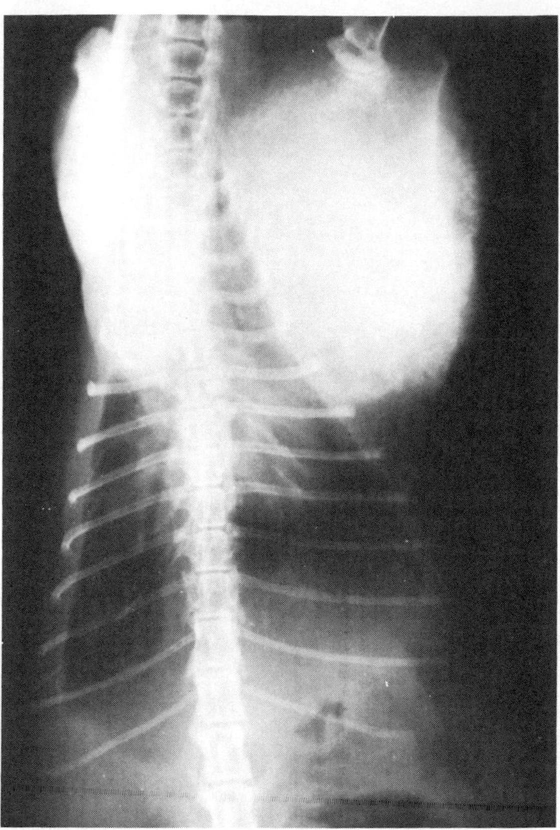

**Figure 11–104** Metastatic intrahepatic bile duct carcinoma, left scapula of an 18-year-old male tabby. Reactive bone proliferation created a hard, 6 cm mass.

(four), diaphragm (two), sternal node (two), tracheobronchial nodes (two), and in single cases to spleen, bladder serosa, mediastinal node, aortic node, adrenal, and scapula. In the cat with the scapular metastasis, the bone lesion, a firm, 6 cm mass, had been evident on the left scapula for three weeks (Fig. 11–104) and was the first sign of illness.

Two cats also had mast cell tumor in the liver.

Additional cases of bile duct carcinoma have been reported in association with liver fluke parasitism (Hoogland, 1928, 1929; Hou, 1964; Pelagatti, 1929; Santos et al., 1981). In one of Hoogland's cases, there was a tumor in the gallbladder as well as the liver, and in another case a tumor in the extrahepatic bile duct.

## Tumors of the Extrahepatic Bile Ducts

Tumors of the extrahepatic bile ducts are rare in the cat. An intra- and extrahepatic bile duct carcinoma was described in an 11-month-old female Burmese (Feldman et al., 1976) and an extrahepatic bile duct carcinoma in an 11-year-old female Siamese (Barsanti et al., 1976).

Four cats at AMAH had similar tumors. Three were female and one male. Two were Siamese, and two were domestic shorthairs. Signs common to the cases were vomiting, anorexia, and jaundice. In two cats tested, serum bilirubin, alkaline phosphatase, SGPT, and SGOT values were elevated, findings consistent with those in the reported cases. In two cats, a firm mass was palpable in the common bile duct, extending to involve adjacent pancreas and duodenum. The extrahepatic bile ducts were dilated and mucus-filled. The tumor was not recognized grossly in the other two cases, but firm hepatic lymph nodes and multiple firm, white foci, 0.1 to 0.3 cm in diameter, were present in the liver, diaphragm, and intercostal muscles. In one case the duodenum was perforated distal to the papilla of the common bile duct.

Microscopically, extrahepatic ductal carcinomas are typically characterized by a tubular pattern, although one of the AMAH cases showed both papillary and tubular patterns. The epithelial cells usually had round or oval vesicular nuclei with scant eosinophilic cytoplasm. Intramucosal tumor was often seen in adjacent bile ducts. Fibroplasia was a constant feature of those tumors, accounting for their palpable firmness. Vascular invasion caused duodenal infarction in one cat. Chronic mononuclear cholangitis was also present in two tumors. Metastases to the diaphragm and hepatic node were observed in one cat and extension to the duodenal serosa in another.

## Tumors of the Gallbladder

Neoplasms of the gallbladder are rare. One of the biliary tumors reported by Hoogland (1928, 1929) in

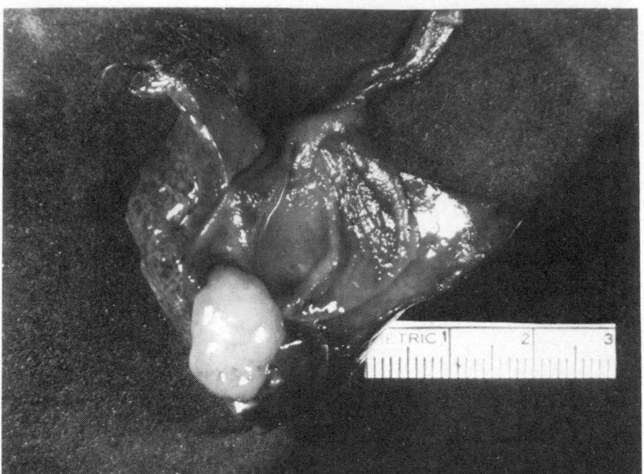

**Figure 11–105** Gallbladder adenoma, 12-year-old spayed female tabby. The gallbladder has been opened to reveal the pedunculated mass arising from the fundic mucosa.

association with fluke infestation was a papillary adenoma or incipient adenocarcinoma involving part of the gallbladder and the common bile duct. Two adenocarcinomas were recorded by Patnaik et al. (1975).

At AMAH an adenoma was found in a 12-year-old female domestic longhair and adenocarcinomas in two Siamese, a 10-year-old male and a 16-year-old female. Nonspecific signs were weakness, anorexia, and abdominal distention.

Grossly, the adenoma was a firm, yellow-orange, pedunculated mass, 2.0 × 0.5 × 0.5 cm, attached to the fundic mucosa of the gallbladder (Fig. 11–105). The carcinomas took the form of firm, white thickenings of the gallbladder wall, with extension into adjacent liver parenchyma (Fig. 11–106). Microscopically, the adenoma had a tubular pattern of columnar cells with small, round or oval, basally located, vesicular nuclei and abundant eosinophilic cytoplasm. Associated features were adenomatous mucosal hyperplasia, mast cell tumor involving both gallbladder and liver, and chronic mononuclear cholangitis with hepatocellular regeneration. The adenocarcinomas were characterized by cuboidal or columnar cells in a papillary-tubular pattern. Their nuclei were round or oval and vesicular, occasionally with prominent nucleoli. The cytoplasm was scant and eosinophilic. Both carcinomas were associated with cystic and mucinous hyperplasia of the gallbladder. Both carcinomas metastasized to mesentery, omentum, peritoneum, and lung.

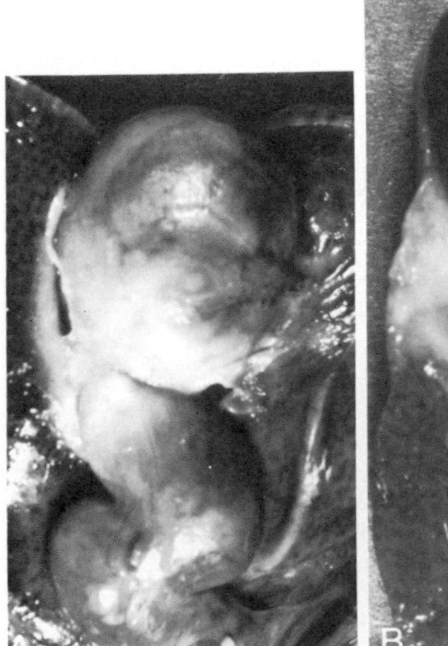

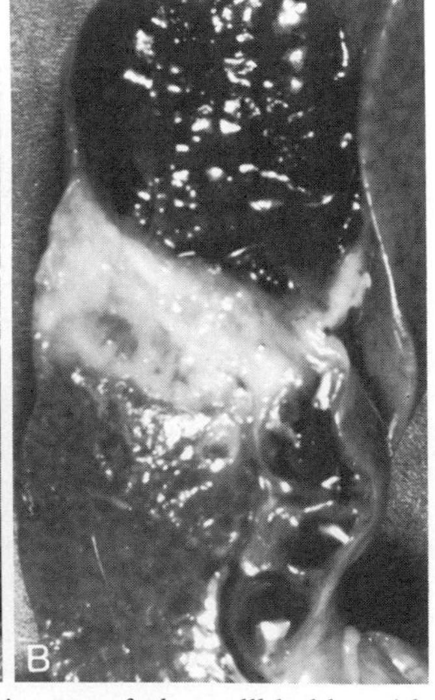

**Figure 11–106** Adenocarcinoma of the gallbladder, 16-year-old spayed female Siamese. Firm, white tissue constricts the neck of the gallbladder (*A*) and is seen on section (*B*) to extend 2.5 cm into the adjacent liver parenchyma.

## Other Epithelial Neoplasms

Of other possible epithelial neoplasms of the liver, an anaplastic carcinoma (Cotchin, 1966) and a squamous cell carcinoma (Priester and McKay, 1980) have been reported.

## Tumors of Vascular Endothelium

After tumors of liver cells and biliary epithelium, hemangiomas and hemangiosarcomas are next in frequency as primary liver tumors of cats (e.g., Blähser, 1962; Carb, 1968; Cotchin, 1966; Messow, 1952/53; Patnaik et al., 1975; Patnaik and Liu, 1977; Priester and McKay, 1980; Tamaschke, 1951/1952).

Both hemangiomas and hemangiosarcomas are characterized by blood-filled spaces that may rupture and lead to severe or fatal hemorrhage. Hemangiomas, some of which are described as cavernous, may perhaps be congenital malformations rather than true tumors. The neoplastic, malignant nature of hemangiosarcomas is all too evident from their tendency to spread widely in the abdomen and to many other sites.

One hemangioma and four hemangiosarcomas of the liver were found among cats at AMAH and are discussed among the vascular tumors. A lymphangioma was reported by Engle and Brodey (1969).

## Other Mesodermal Tumors

Fibrosarcomas and sarcomas of unspecified or undetermined type are occasionally reported as primary in the liver of cats (e.g., Joshua, 1965; Messow, 1952/53; Priester and McKay, 1980). Lymphoma and mast cell tumors may rarely be primary in the liver but are usually part of a multicentric or systemic disorder. Mesothelioma has been reported (Moulton, 1978), and one diagnosed at AMAH is described in the section on mesothelioma.

Myelolipomas are uncommon benign tumors of mature adipose tissue and bone marrow, in which primitive hematopoietic cells of all series may be found. Two instances of multiple myelolipomas have been reported in the liver of cats, one of which recovered after surgery for repair of a diaphragmatic-pericardial hernia and removal of the two tumorous liver lobes incarcerated in the pericardium (Gourley et al., 1971; Ikede and Downey, 1972).

Hepatic myelolipoma was diagnosed in two domestic shorthairs at AMAH. In a seven-year-old spayed female, masses on the liver had been palpable for at least three months. At surgery a well-defined, greasy mass 4 cm in diameter was found attached to the right lateral liver lobe and a similar mass enveloped the left lateral lobe. In the other cat, a wasted 16-year-old castrated male, a mass was palpated on the liver and the cat was destroyed with a tentative diagnosis of malignant tumor.

Microscopically, the tumor in the first case, which was unencapsulated, consisted mostly of adipose tissue. Mild fatty change was evident in the unaffected liver tissue. In the second case the palpable tumor proved to be a hepatocellular carcinoma with a microscopic focus of myelolipoma composed primarily of bone marrow stem cells mixed with fewer fat cells. The lesion spanned several lobules. Numerous foci of extramedullary hematopoiesis and hepatocellular fatty change were evident in the unaffected tissue of the liver.

## Secondary Tumors

The liver is far oftener involved with secondary tumor than with primary tumor of liver tissue or biliary tract. In cats, secondary neoplasia is most often associated with lymphocytic, myeloproliferative, and mast cell malignancies. Among a wide variety of other metastatic tumors, cancers of mammary gland, pancreas, and intestine are most frequent.

## Diagnosis and Management of Primary Liver Tumors

When a liver tumor is suspected, chest radiographs should be taken and peritoneoscopy or exploratory surgery should be performed promptly. It is important that multiple cysts or bile duct adenomas not be mistaken for malignant lesions. Provided that a tumor is confined to a single site, surgical excision or lobectomy is possible.

## Tumor-like Lesions

**TELANGIECTASIA.** Telangiectasia, a dilatation of pre-existing sinusoid capillaries, is a benign lesion occasionally seen in aging cats (Messow, 1952/1953).

**HEPATIC CYSTS.** Hepatic cysts are encountered from time to time in cats of all ages and are thought in many cases to originate in congenital malformations of the bile ducts. When they take the form of cystic dilatations that are embedded in the liver, they may be mistaken for tumor. If very large or pedunculated, the cysts may cause palpable enlargement or deformity of the liver or distention of the abdomen in an otherwise healthy cat. In these cases, surgical removal of the cyst or of the liver lobe from which it arises may be carried out (Babcock et al., 1977; Greene and Johnson, 1971; Mendham et al., 1969; Reid and Frank, 1973). Many cysts are asymptomatic and are discovered only at autopsy. If hepatic cysts are associated with polycystic renal disease or other urinary abnormalities, the predominant signs may be those of urinary disorder (Crowell et al., 1979; Lettow and Dämmrich, 1967; Scherzo, 1967).

Eight cats in the AMAH group had hepatic cysts of undetermined origin. All were domestic shorthairs and ranged from 1½ to 17 years of age. Four were male and four female. The presenting signs varied, the most consistent being an enlarged abdomen or palpable abdominal mass. In six cats other signs were polydipsia, anorexia, and vomiting associated with concurrent serious illness that resulted in death or euthanasia. In two young cats, surgical excision was successful (Fig. 11–107).

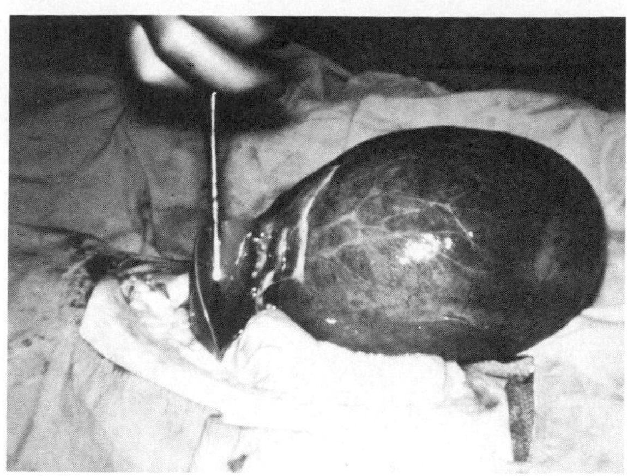

**Figure 11–107** Pedunculated hepatic cyst in an otherwise normal two-year-old spayed female domestic cat. The abdomen had become progressively distended over a period of several months. The cyst, containing about 250 ml of blood-tinged fluid, involved at its origin the gallbladder and all liver lobes except the left lateral and the caudate process of the caudal lobe. The cyst was successfully excised together with the gallbladder. The cat recovered without complications and was still in good health 11 years later. (Courtesy Dr. J. E. Easley.)

The cysts ranged from 0.4 to 20 cm in diameter and were often multiple. Thin, clear or turbid, blood-tinged fluid filled the cysts. Microscopically, the cysts were lined by epithelium that varied from squamous to columnar. Occasionally, fibrous connective tissue and inflammatory cells formed a portion of the cyst wall. These cysts were not associated with cysts of other organs.

# TUMORS OF THE EXOCRINE PANCREAS*

## Nodular Hyperplasia

Nodular hyperplasia is the most frequent pancreatic lesion of cats and is found to some degree in almost every aged animal. It is characterized by multiple unencapsulated nodules rarely larger than normal pancreatic lobules (0.1 to 0.4 cm). White or pale tan and slightly elevated, they do not compress surrounding tissue. The cells, in an acinar pattern or in solid sheets, may be large, with bright acidophilic cytoplasm or, more often, small and cuboidal with pale scant eosinophilic cytoplasm. Ducts within a hyperplastic nodule may be normal or proliferative. Inflammatory cells are absent, and there is no increase in fibrous connective tissue to suggest past or ongoing pancreatitis.

Nodular hyperplasia was present in 16 (28 per cent) of 58 cats at AMAH with exocrine carcinoma. The relationship to neoplastic disease is unknown.

## Adenomas

Adenomas are rare in the cat. In contrast with adenomatous hyperplasia, they are solitary, firm, pale masses that are partly or completely encapsulated and compress

*Laura K. Andrews, principal author.

adjacent tissue. Two described by Kircher and Nielsen (1976) were larger than normal lobules, as was the single one on record at AMAH, an incidental autopsy finding in a seven-year-old spayed female domestic shorthair. Two other adenomas were reported by Schmidt and Langham (1967), two by Owens et al. (1975), nine by Patnaik et al. (1975), and eleven by Priester and McKay (1980).

Adenomas are not likely to cause clinical signs unless they are large, such as one reported by Hjärre (1927) that was believed to have caused diabetes mellitus by encroachment on normal islet tissue. Microscopically, adenomas are of tubular or acinar pattern. Nuclei are round and vesicular with prominent nucleoli but rare mitoses. The cytoplasm is granular and stains red. Cystic spaces containing mucin are common.

## Carcinomas

Carcinomas are moderately frequent. Among 1804 tumors in four surveys there were 24 (Cotchin, 1983; Engle and Brodey, 1969; Patnaik et al., 1975; Schmidt and Langham, 1967). In a total of 2234 feline tumors at 15 veterinary colleges in North America, 16 were pancreatic carcinomas (Priester and McKay, 1980). A review of epithelial tumors of the pancreas reported before 1960 included 38 carcinomas (Rowlatt, 1967). Fifty exocrine adenocarcinomas were reviewed for the WHO Bulletin (Kircher and Nielsen, 1976). Available data for age indicated that these are tumors of older cats.

At AMAH 58 exocrine carcinomas were on record. The mean age of the cats was 12 years, with a range of 2½ to 22. Males and females were equally affected. Fifty-two cats were domestic shorthairs, four Siamese, one Himalayan, and one domestic longhair.

**CLINICAL FEATURES.** Diagnosis of pancreatic carcinoma rarely precedes laparotomy. Clinical signs appear late in the course of the disease and, like laboratory findings, are nonspecific. At the time of diagnosis, 47 of the cats at AMAH had metastatic lesions.

Signs were reported to vary in duration from a few days to more than a year before diagnosis. Those most often noted were anorexia (26 cats, 46 per cent) and weight loss (21 cats, 37 per cent). Sixteen cats (28 per cent) were depressed, weak, or lethargic, and 13 (23 per cent) vomited intermittently. Seventeen (30 per cent) had effusions due to hepatic cirrhosis, tumor implants on the peritoneum, or tumorous compression of the postcava or portal vein and its tributaries. Peritoneal fluid varied from a few milliliters to more than 2.0 liters. It was clear and colorless, pale yellow, or serosanguineous. Eight cats (14 per cent) with diffuse involvement of the pancreas or duodenum were jaundiced owing to extrahepatic bile duct obstruction. Diabetes mellitus was found in five cats before tumor was suspected. Five cats (9 per cent) were constipated, and two had diarrhea. Steatorrhea has been reported (Ball and Roquet, 1911) but was not noted in cats at AMAH.

A cranioventral abdominal mass was palpated or seen radiographically in most cats. In contrast with tumors of the small intestine or spleen, pancreatic carcinomas were usually fixed in position. Tumors of the right lobe usually displaced the duodenum to the right; tumors of the left lobe displaced the spleen and intestines caudally.

Signs of carcinoma of the pancreas may mimic those of acute pancreatitis. Tumor necrosis occurred in 40 of 58 tumors (70 per cent), and necrosis of peripancreatic fat was common. Infiltrates of inflammatory cells were prominent in 24 of 58 tumors (42 per cent). Neoplastic acinar cells may release lipase, causing necrosis of tumor and peripancreatic fat, and even of fat in distant parts of the body. In large or rapidly growing tumors, inadequate blood supply contributes to necrosis. Despite the high incidence of necrosis and inflammation, abdominal pain was recognized in only one cat.

Other clinical signs may be due to metastatic disease. One cat with a 10-month history of bone pain, lameness, and difficult bowel movements had metastases to the pelvis, ribs, humerus, and lumbar and thoracic vertebrae. Two cats with pleural effusions due to pleural and pulmonary metastases were dyspneic. Two with metastases to the quadriceps muscles had rear leg weakness and muscle pain.

Laboratory tests may be helpful but are not diagnostic. There may be mild neutrophilia, hypokalemia, bilirubinemia, hyperglycemia, and elevations in SGPT, SGOT, and SAP values. Serum amylase and lipase levels are rarely increased. Dehydration may mask mild anemia. Cytologic examination of abdominal fluid disclosed malignant epithelial cells in 25 per cent of the cats.

Surgical resection is rarely attempted. In one cat that underwent laparotomy for an asymptomatic abdominal mass, an adenocarcinoma of the left lobe of the pancreas was removed. However, vomiting, listlessness, and a peritoneal effusion developed seven months later, and autopsy disclosed widespread metastases.

**GROSS FEATURES.** Carcinoma of the exocrine pancreas may take the form of an isolated, well-circumscribed mass measuring from 0.5 to 10.0 cm in one lobe or multiple nodules of varying size involving one or both lobes. Among 41 cats for which location was specified, the tumor involved the right lobe (head) (Fig. 11–108) in 15, the left lobe (tail) in 16, and the angle (body) in one. In nine cats, tumor was disseminated throughout all lobes. Pancreatic carcinomas are usually firmer than adjacent normal pancreas and are elevated, with an irregular surface. They are usually white but may be pale yellow, tan, or brown. Soft gray or brown foci of necrosis are common, as are gritty yellow areas of mineralization. Hemorrhagic foci may be seen. Fluctuant cystic areas are rare. The carcinomas usually elicit a marked desmoplastic response. This proliferation of fibrous connective tissue tends to coat the tumor with dense, white, fibrous tissue. Adhesions to surrounding tissues are common.

**MICROSCOPIC FEATURES.** The exocrine adenocarcinomas may arise from the acini or ductules of the pancreas. Most have been assigned a ductal origin on the basis of light microscopic findings. An acinar cell carcinoma examined by both light and electron microscopy was characterized by acinus formation, colloid production, and sheets of neoplastic cells and was assigned an acinar origin on the basis of ultrastructure (Banner et al., 1979). Zymogen granules, some of which contained a tightly packed microfibrillar material, was present in many tumor cells.

Adenocarcinomas of the pancreas may be classified into three distinct morphologic types based on pattern rather than histogenesis (Kircher and Nielsen, 1976): small tu-

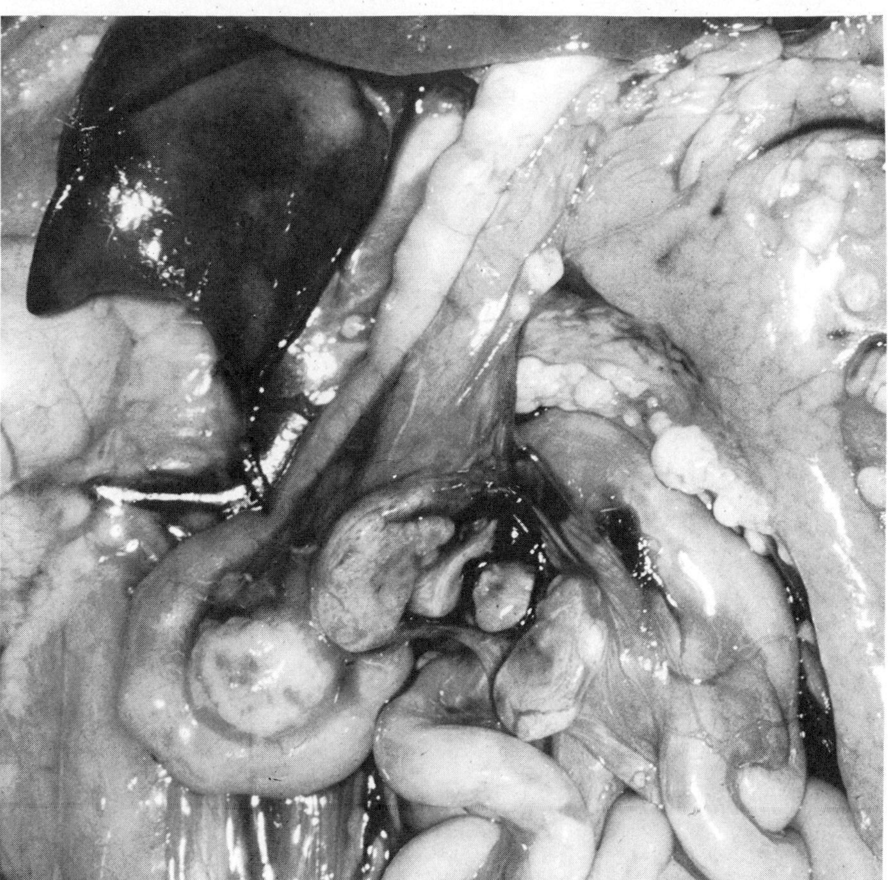

**Figure 11–108** Disseminated adenocarcinoma of the pancreas in the mesentery and omentum of a nine-year-old castrated male tabby. A solitary tumor at the free edge of the right pancreatic lobe metastasized, as firm white nodules, to the peritoneum throughout the abdomen.

bular or ductal, large tubular (ductal), and acinar. These patterns are described in detail by Kircher and Nielsen (1976).

The undifferentiated carcinomas consist of loose or solid masses of small pleomorphic cells with slightly acidophilic cytoplasm. They do not form recognizable tubules or acini. Nuclei vary from medium-sized to large and are round or oval with moderate dense chromatin and occasional nucleoli. There may be large bizarre cells with irregular nuclei. Mitoses are more numerous than in adenocarcinomas. Histiocytes are frequent. Stroma is prominent, as are central necrosis and hemorrhage.

Of the 58 pancreatic carcinomas at AMAH, 21 had a small tubular pattern (Fig. 11–109), 3 a ductal (large tubular) pattern, and 8 an acinar pattern. Sixteen had a mixed tubular and acinar pattern (Fig. 11–110), four a ductal and acinar pattern, and one a trabecular and solid pattern. Three were undifferentiated carcinomas. Tumor pattern was unrelated to tumor behavior: At the time of diagnosis all but 11 of 58 tumors had metastasized. Thirty-one cats had metastases to regional nodes, 19 to omentum or mesentery, 13 to lungs, 9 to diaphragm, 8 to peritoneum, and 7 to spleen. Occasional or rare sites of metastasis were distant lymph nodes (six), kidney (five), duodenum (five), urinary bladder (three), adrenals (three), intestine (three), quadriceps muscle (three), heart (two), bone (one), thyroid (one), esophagus (one), and ovary (one).

**PROGNOSIS.** The prognosis for carcinoma of the pancreas is poor, chiefly because the tumor is almost never diagnosed at an early, localized stage. Techniques used in man, such as upper gastrointestinal tract endoscopy with retrograde cholangiopancreatography, percutaneous transhepatic cholangiography, ultrasonography, CAT scanning, serum antigen levels, and angiography, have not been evaluated in the cat. Biopsy and resection of the tumor are currently the only known methods of diagnosis and treatment.

### Sarcoma

Multiple spindle-cell sarcoma in the tail of the pancreas with metastases to the mesenteric nodes and liver was described by Lombard (1936), but it was suggested (Cotchin, 1956a) that the site of origin might have been the mesenteric nodes.

## TUMORS OF THE URINARY SYSTEM

### Tumors of Kidney, Renal Pelvis, and Ureter

Lymphoma of the kidneys, usually bilateral and often part of a generalized process, is one of the most frequent tumors of cats. In most cases it takes the form of pale nodules originating in the cortex, lesions that must be differentiated from the granulomas of feline infectious peritonitis. If the tumorous infiltration is diffuse (so-called large white kidney), it must be distinguished from the enlargement that sometimes occurs with chronic intersti-

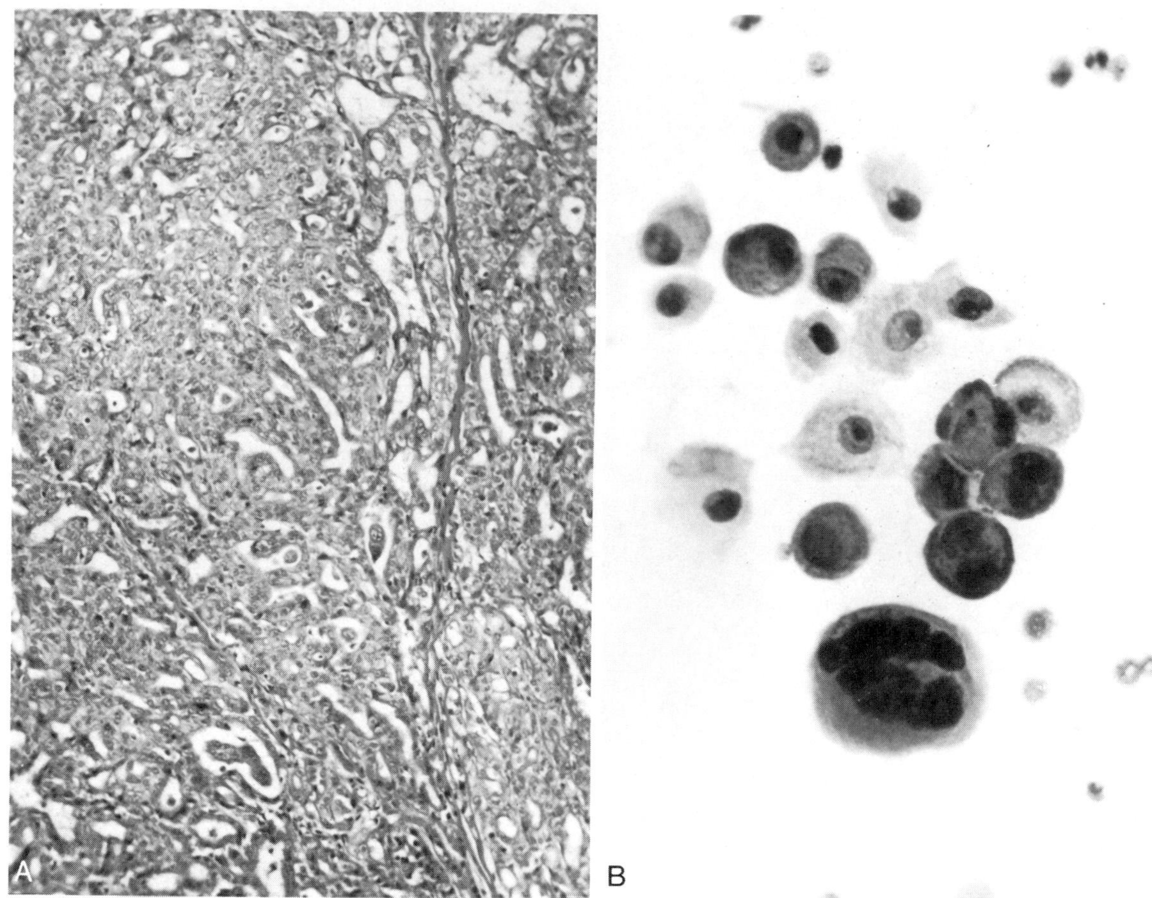

**Figure 11–109** *A*, Adenocarcinoma of exocrine pancreas. The small, irregular, branching tubular pattern is the most frequent in the cat. H & E, × 180. *B*, Abdominal effusion, same cat. The film of the neoplastic exudate shows many large cells (a few binucleate) and a multinucleate cell, the last suggesting acinar formation. Wright-Giemsa, × 760.

tial nephritis. In rare instances, a single lymphomatous kidney has been successfully removed (Fig. 11–111). (See section on lymphoma for detailed discussion.)

Primary tumors of kidney tissue are uncommon, accounting for only about 2.5 per cent of feline tumors according to Flir (1952/53) and 1.5 per cent in the survey of Priester and McKay (1980). At least 40 have been reported. Benign tumors (adenoma, leiomyoma) are rare. Malignant tumors include renal cell carcinoma of various types, nephroblastoma, squamous cell carcinoma, and transitional cell carcinoma as well as several types of sarcoma.

At AMAH 19 primary kidney tumors were diagnosed in cats, one benign and 18 malignant.

## Benign Tumors

A few renal adenomas have been reported in the cat (Flir, 1952/53; Poppensiek, 1961; Priester and McKay, 1980), and one was seen at AMAH (Fig. 11–112). In man a clear distinction between adenoma and renal cell carcinoma is often lacking, and pathologists now avoid the diagnosis of adenoma, since there are no morphologic criteria to distinguish it from a small renal cell carcinoma that has not yet metastasized. Our feline tumor was diagnosed as benign on the basis of expansile growth and the absence of mitotic figures.

A renal leiomyoma was reported by Priester and McKay (1980).

## Malignant Tumors

In the experience of Bloom (1954), renal carcinoma (also called clear-cell carcinoma, hypernephroma, and adenocarcinoma) was the most common epithelial tumor in dogs and cats, the majority of which were males and over five years of age. Renal carcinomas also constitute the largest group reported by others (Collet et al., 1952; Cotchin, 1983; Douville and Collet, 1934; Drinker et al., 1927; Engle and Brodey, 1969; Flir, 1952/53; Montoro and Botija, 1935; Plummer, 1956; Poppensiek, 1961; Priester and McKay, 1980; Purohit et al., 1964; Whitehead, 1967). The carcinoma reported by Kiesel (1950) proved on re-examination to be lymphoma. From the incomplete data on age and sex it appeared that affected cats were middle-aged or elderly; there was no clear sex predisposition.

Transitional cell carcinoma may occasionally occur in the renal pelvis and has been next in frequency (Nielsen and Howard, 1971; Osborne et al., 1971; Priester and McKay, 1980; Wimberley and Lewis, 1979).

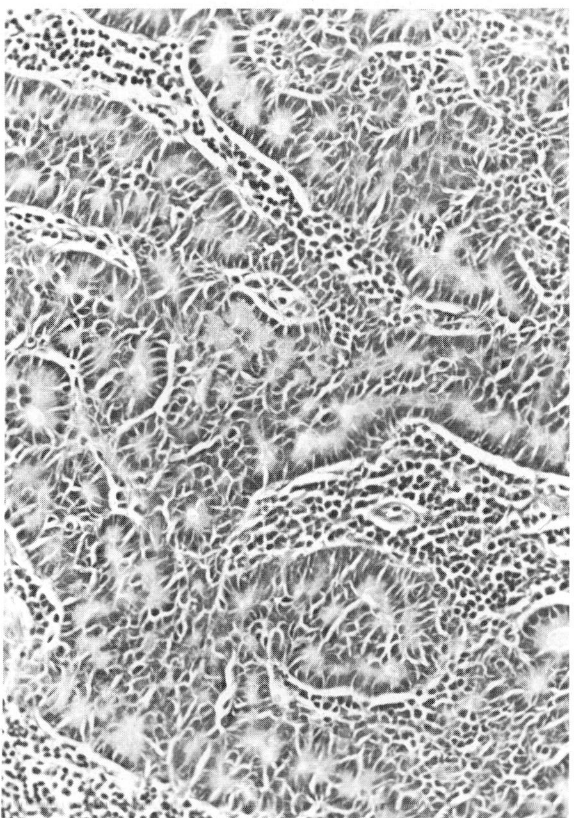

**Figure 11–110** Adenocarcinoma of the pancreas that metastasized to the mesentery and omentum, 12-year-old female domestic shorthair. The branching tubules and acini are contained within a stroma rich in lymphocytes and plasma cells. H & E, × 200.

Nephroblastoma (embryonal carcinoma) arises from vestiges of embryonic renal tissue, often in the young. Two were reported by Cotchin (1952) and two by Poppensiek (1961), and a nephroblastoma in a two-year-old cat was described by Potkay and Garman (1969). A bilateral embryonal sarcoma was diagnosed in an eight-year-old castrated male domestic cat (Fitts, 1960). Instances of squamous cell carcinoma (Priester and McKay, 1980) and of carcinosarcoma (Whitehead, 1967) have been listed, without details, in surveys.

Early reports of sarcomas such as myxosarcomas and spindle-cell sarcomas were reviewed by Lombard (1940); such tumors have also been reported by Cotchin (1983) and Priester and McKay (1980). Leiomyosarcomas were diagnosed in cats 11 (Cotchin, 1983) and 22 years old (Nielsen, 1964).

Secondary tumors of many types metastasize to the kidneys by the blood stream, taking the form of single or multiple growths localized in the cortex.

The discussion of malignant neoplasms that follows is based on 18 kidney tumors diagnosed at AMAH: eight transitional cell carcinomas, six renal cell carcinomas, one nephroblastoma, one squamous cell carcinoma, and two poorly differentiated sarcomas. The preponderance of transitional cell carcinomas contrasted surprisingly with the previous reports of tumors of cats and also with findings in humans, in whom this tumor, both of the renal pelvis and of the ureter, is only a fourth or fifth as frequent as malignant tumors of the renal parenchyma. The feline tumors strongly resembled the infiltrating tran-

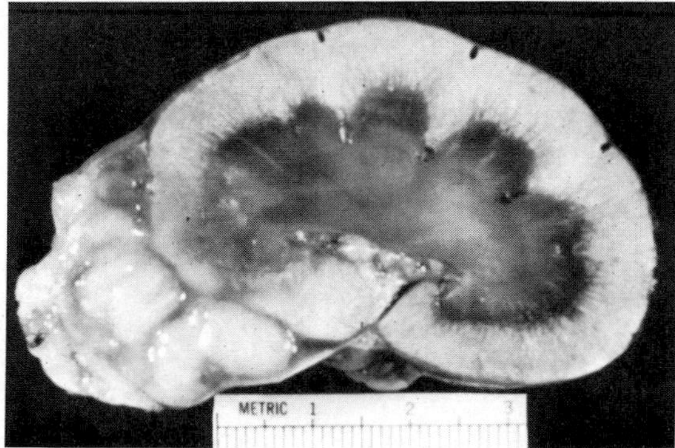


**Figure 11–111** Solitary renal lymphoma, histiocytic type, in a subcapsular and polar location, four-year-old cat. Several years after nephrectomy and without chemotherapy, this remarkably lucky cat had had no recurrence of tumor.

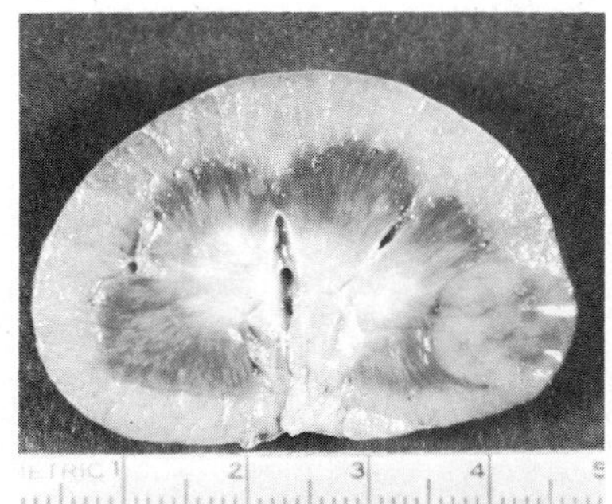

**Figure 11–112** Renal cortical adenoma, 15-year-old spayed female tricolor. The well-demarcated circular solid tumor spans the cortex and extends into the medulla.

sitional cell carcinomas with glandular and squamoid differentiation that are seen in the urinary bladder.

Only one tumor of the ureter other than lymphoma was seen—a transitional cell carcinoma that also involved the kidney.

**BREED, AGE, AND SEX.** There was only one purebred cat in the group at AMAH, a Siamese with a transitional cell carcinoma. Whatever the significance, 4 of the 18 cats (22 per cent) were tricolors, in contrast with the incidence of this phenotype in the AMAH hospital population generally (7 per cent).

The 18 cats ranged in age from 1½ to 16 years. The youngest had a nephroblastoma, the next youngest, a two-year-old, a poorly differentiated sarcoma. Cats with transitional cell carcinoma ranged from 4 to 15 years of age (mean 9.3). Renal cell carcinomas occurred in cats 4 to 16 years old (mean 9 years). Ten of the 18 cats were females, eight spayed. Seven of the eight males were castrated. Among dogs, males are predisposed to renal tumors, but no sex predisposition was apparent in cats in this or other reported studies.

**CLINICAL FEATURES.** The triad of signs frequent with human renal tumors (15 to 70 per cent)—flank mass, pain, and hematuria—was not recognized in any of the 18 cases. Abdominal enlargement and hematuria occurred in three cats. Pain was evidenced by only one, which cried after urinating. The majority of the cats had had vague signs of illness not directly related to the urinary system: decreased appetite, weight loss, and lethargy. Two cats vomited. Ten of the 18 (56 per cent) had metastatic lesions, so it was not surprising to find nonspecific signs frequent with malignancies. In this group of cats the diagnosis of renal neoplasm was made in a later stage of the disease than in humans, one third of whom had metastases. Two cats, one with metastases and one without, were asymptomatic. In both, an enlarged kidney was palpated during routine examination. One cat presented with rear leg lameness associated with metastatic lesions in the gastrocnemius and quadriceps femoris.

**LABORATORY FINDINGS.** Polycythemia, occasionally occurring in humans and dogs, was not evident in this group of cats. Anemia, frequently associated with renal neoplasia in man, was severe in two cats, both with extensive metastases. Hypercalcemia, occasionally present in man, was not detected, but serum calcium was evaluated in only a few cats. Azotemia was present only when the other kidney had severe chronic inflammation.

**DIAGNOSIS.** A renal tumor cannot always be diagnosed with certainty simply on the basis of enlargement or irregularity of the organ; benign hypertrophy, granuloma due to feline infectious peritonitis, hydronephrosis, cystic kidney, and hygroma renis (decapsulation) must be considered in the differential diagnosis. An intravenous pyelogram, renal arteriogram, or ultrasonography can aid in distinguishing among these possibilities, but exploratory laparotomy and biopsy give the most information about the nature and extent of the lesions.

**GROSS FEATURES.** All except one of the tumors were unilateral, the right kidney being involved in 10 of the 18 cats. One cat with transitional cell carcinoma of the left kidney had metastasis to the right kidney as well as to other sites.

Renal cell carcinomas ranged in size from 1.5 to 6.0 cm. The smaller tumors appeared to arise in the cortex and to grow mainly by expansion, producing a fairly well demarcated mass that distorted and compressed the adjacent parenchyma (Fig. 11–113). They were soft to firm, bulged on cut surface, and had a poorly lobulated pattern. Most were shades of yellow and brown and had red foci. One contained a blood clot 4 cm wide. The three papillary

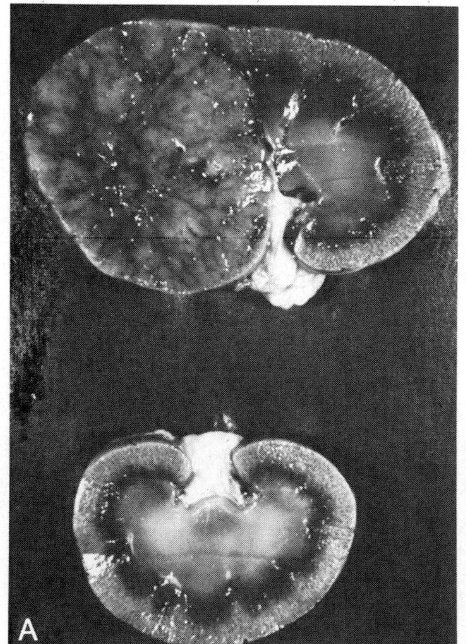


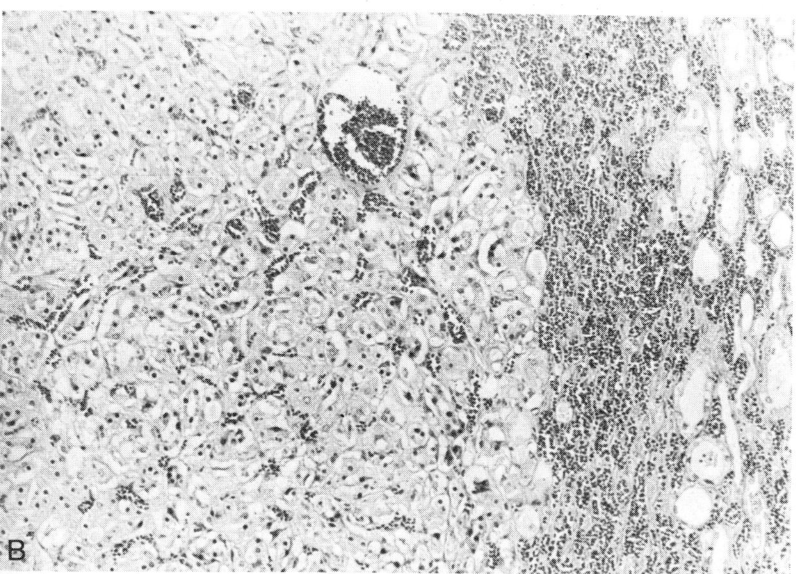


**Figure 11–113** *A*, Renal cell carcinoma was an incidental finding in one kidney (top) of a 12-year-old spayed female tricolor cat with seizures. The tumor replaced and expanded the cranial pole. The mass is sharply demarcated and lobulated. Actual size. *B*, The tumor (left) has a compact cellular and tubular pattern and very little stroma, which is in contrast to renal transitional cell carcinoma. Its expansile growth has caused adjacent congestion, tubular atrophy, and necrosis (right). H & E, × 200.

carcinomas had cysts containing yellow-brown tenacious fluid (Fig. 11–114).

The transitional cell tumors and the single squamous cell carcinoma resembled one another but differed greatly from the renal cell carcinomas. Kidneys with transitional cell tumor were hard but not greatly enlarged or deformed. The tumor itself was white or pale yellow and firm to hard, involving part or all of the pelvis (Fig. 11–115*A* and *B*). Several involved the entire kidney as well as infiltrating the capsule and surrounding tissues. A large, irregular, central cyst was usually present, with bands in its wall giving the appearance of a hydronephrotic kidney. The pelvis was also dilated in kidneys only partially involved. All the transitional cell carcinomas had an infiltrative appearance rather than a papillary growth pattern into the pelvis (Fig. 11–115*C*).

The six renal cell carcinomas were without metastases, whereas all eight transitional cell carcinomas metastasized to sites including perirenal soft tissues, adrenal, omentum, ureter, opposite kidney, sublumbar nodes, spleen, lungs, pleura, tracheobronchial nodes, heart, meninges, eye, and skeletal muscle. Neoplastic thrombi were seen in renal veins, arteries, and posterior vena cava. The cat with squamous cell carcinoma had metastases to perirenal fat; adjacent muscles; second, third, and fourth lumbar vertebrae; omentum; adrenals; sublumbar nodes; diaphragm; and pulmonary arteries.

The nephroblastoma occurred in the right kidney of a one and a half-year-old spayed female tricolor. The kidney was irregularly enlarged (8.5 × 8.0 × 7.0 cm). The cut surface bulged with white, lobulated tumor, which compressed the remaining recognizable renal parenchyma (Fig. 11–116). The tumor appeared fibrous but ranged from soft to firm. No metastases were found, and the cat made a good recovery from surgery.

The cats with poorly differentiated sarcomas were two and nine years old. Both had right kidneys measuring 10 cm in greatest dimension. Both tumors were firm, white, and lobulated; one was cystic. Metastases were not found.

**MICROSCOPIC FEATURES.** The renal cell carcinomas exhibited solid, tubular, or papillary patterns. The three with a papillary pattern (Fig. 11–114) had cysts, some grossly visible. Necrosis was extensive in two. One had a 5 cm hematoma. Fibrosis was slight or absent. The renal cell carcinomas were unencapsulated, and compression of adjacent parenchyma was a common feature.

By contrast, the transitional cell carcinomas were infiltrative and characterized by extensive fibroplasia resulting in a firm or hard white growth. Epithelial cells piled up into islands and cores, the latter often having a tubular lumen (Fig. 11–115*C* ). Squamous metaplasia without keratinization was common, foci of keratinization including "pearl" formation occurring in only one tumor. That tumor had infiltrated the capsule, the perirenal fat and muscles, and the left adrenal.

The single squamous cell carcinoma arose from pelvic transitional epithelium. Features of transitional cell and squamous cell carcinoma occurred together, the squamous component predominating in both primary tumor and metastases. Desmosomes, autonomous cellular keratinization, and keratin pearls were abundant in the metastatic lesions.

Of the two sarcomas, that in a two-year-old spayed female was composed of fasciculi of pleomorphic spindle cells, many with "racket" and "strap" shapes. Some had two or more nuclei in linear arrangement. These features

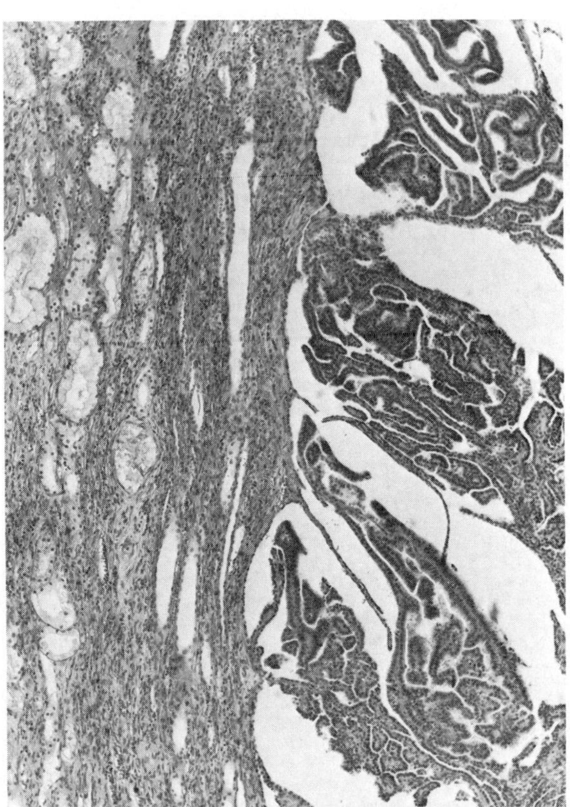

**Figure 11–114** Papillary carcinoma of a kidney weighing 174 gm, one and a half-year-old castrated male cat. Fibrous tissue and atrophic tubules (left) are compressed by the expansile growth. H & E, × 50.

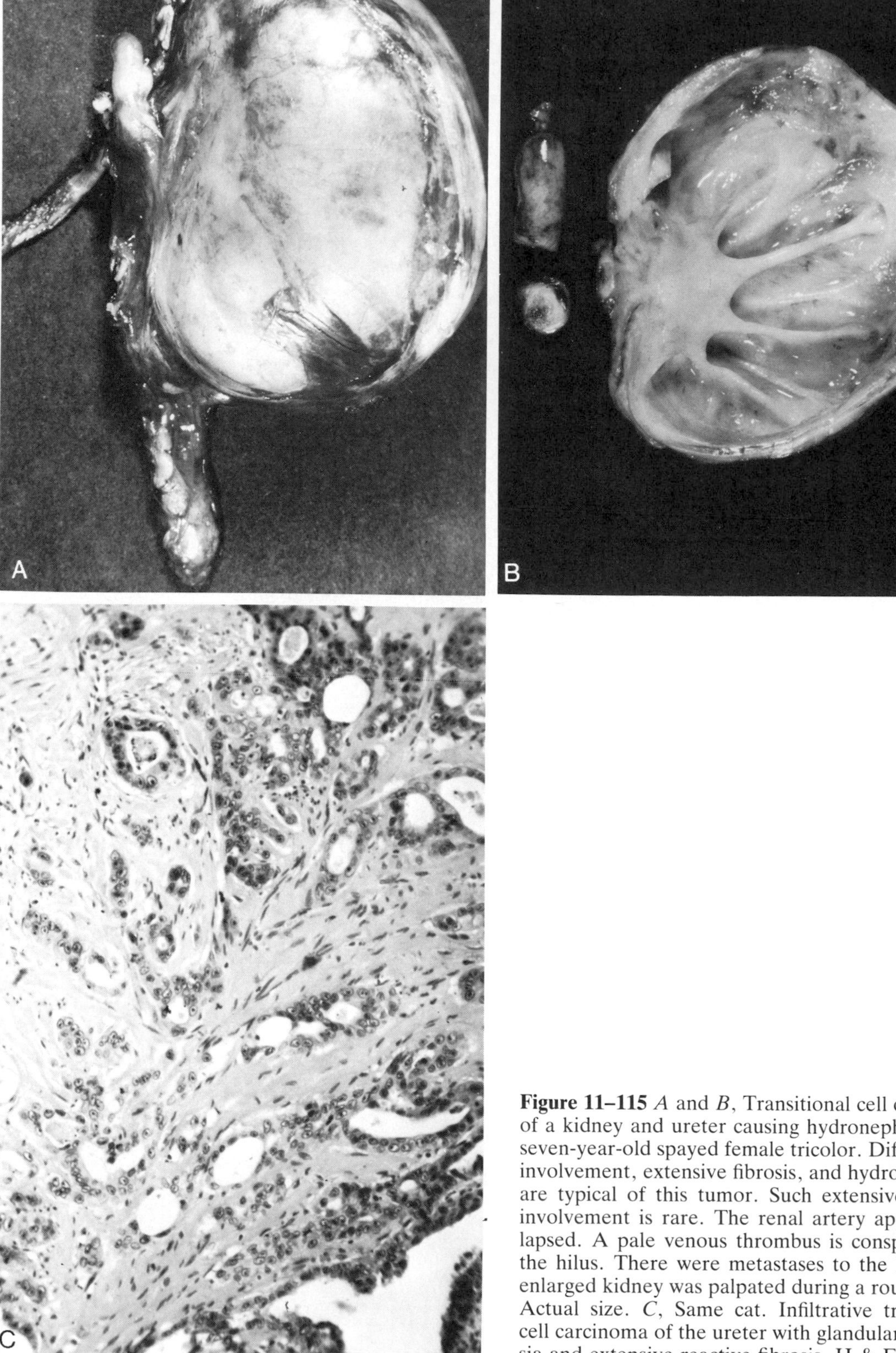


**Figure 11–115** *A* and *B*, Transitional cell carcinoma of a kidney and ureter causing hydronephrosis in a seven-year-old spayed female tricolor. Diffuse renal involvement, extensive fibrosis, and hydronephrosis are typical of this tumor. Such extensive ureteral involvement is rare. The renal artery appears collapsed. A pale venous thrombus is conspicuous at the hilus. There were metastases to the lung. The enlarged kidney was palpated during a routine visit. Actual size. *C*, Same cat. Infiltrative transitional cell carcinoma of the ureter with glandular metaplasia and extensive reactive fibrosis. H & E, × 100.

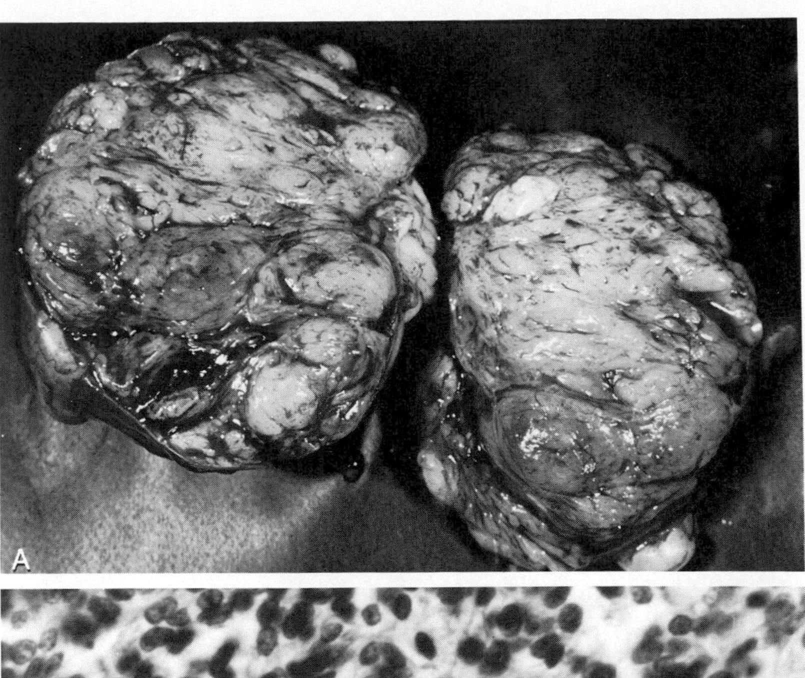

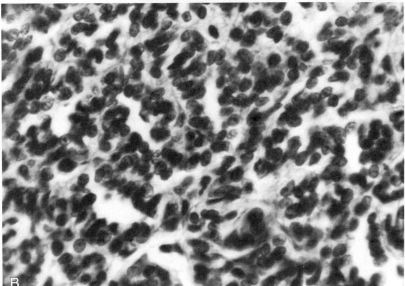

**Figure 11–116** *A*, Nephroblastoma (embryonal nephroma) successfully removed from a one and a half-year-old spayed tricolor that had periods of pain for three months and a noticeable abdominal mass for one month. The 6 cm tumor is demarcated from the compressed remnant of kidney. The bulging cut surface is glistening white and lobulated. Actual size. *B*, Ill-defined tubules are lined by cells with hyperchromatic nuclei and fewer cells with euchromatic nuclei containing a single small nucleolus. The tubules lie within a fine fibrovascular stroma. H & E, × 760.

suggested rhabdomyosarcoma, but striations could not be positively identified with special stains and electron microscopy was not done. Fat cells were also present, as were collagen fibers. The possibility of a nephroblastoma composed only of mesenchymal components (embryonal sarcoma) must be considered in this young cat. A similar tumor, a bilateral embryonal sarcoma, was reported in an eight-year-old male (Fitts, 1960). The other sarcoma in this group of cats, also poorly differentiated, would have required electron microscopy for more specific identification. It is of interest to note that fibrosarcomas and fibromas, once frequently diagnosed in humans, are now almost always shown by electron-microscopic technique to be of smooth muscle origin.

The nephroblastoma had abundant mature collagen, often arranged in a herringbone pattern, and a scattering of smooth muscle cells. A smaller component consisted of islands of small basophilic epithelial cells arranged in solid, tubular, and cystic papillary patterns (Fig. 11–116*B*). Skeletal muscle, cartilage, fat, and bone, reported in some nephroblastomas, were not seen. Growth was by expansion, which is characteristic of this tumor.

**MANAGEMENT OF KIDNEY TUMORS.** Almost all kidney tumors are malignant, and many are inoperable or have metastasized by the time they are diagnosed. A two-year-old cat with a nephroblastoma involving the posterior vena cava survived for over a year after radical surgery (Potkay and Garman, 1969), and a unilateral nephroblastoma was removed successfully from another young cat at AMAH.

If surgical resection is contemplated, it is mandatory to make certain that the other kidney is present and normal or near-normal in structure and function. Careful palpation, urinalysis, blood creatinine determination, and intravenous pyelogram as well as radiographs of the lungs, lest there are already visible metastases, should always precede nephrectomy.

Nephrectomy can be carried out by a ventral abdominal incision. The renal vessels are ligated, the organ carefully freed by blunt dissection, and the ureter isolated, ligated, and transected. Care should be taken to observe for vascular thrombi distending renal veins and lymphatics, since they are routes for metastasis. If possible, the peritoneum is brought together over the defect in the body wall.

## TUMORS OF THE URINARY BLADDER

In the dog, primary tumors of the bladder outnumber those of the kidney; in the cat the reverse is true. While papillomas and urothelial carcinomas are not infrequent in dogs, cattle, and man, they are very rare in cats. The cat's low susceptibility to such neoplasms is believed to be related to its ability to metabolize tryptophan without producing large quantities of orthoaminophenol metabolites, some of which have been implicated in the formation of human and canine bladder tumors (Leklem et al., 1971; Price et al., 1960).

Twenty-four bladder tumors of cats at the University of Minnesota were surveyed by Caywood et al. (1980) in an article that superseded an earlier study from that institution (Osborne et al., 1968b). Twenty-seven cases diagnosed at The Animal Medical Center from January 1974, to June 1983 (including one previously described by Patnaik and Greene [1979]) were studied by Schwarz et al. (1985)—a striking increase in incidence over the two cases reported for the period January 1962 to December 1972 (Patnaik et al., 1975). Isolated instances totaling about 20 have been recorded in case reports and general surveys.

Twenty-five cases of bladder tumor were diagnosed at AMAH in a 35-year period, representing a frequency less than a third that at The Animal Medical Center.

### Benign Tumors

A few benign tumors are on record: papillomas in two young cats, one a Persian (Osborne et al., 1968b); leiomyomas in a 12-year-old female (Osborne et al., 1968b), in a 5-year-old castrated male Siamese (Patnaik and Greene, 1979), and in a five-year-old Siamese, a 9-year-old Burmese, and a 14-year-old domestic shorthair, all castrated males (Schwarz et al., 1985); a cystadenoma in a 12-year-old female (Caywood et al., 1980); and a fibroma in an 8-year-old spayed female and an hemangioma in a 15-year-old castrated male (Schwarz et al., 1985).

No benign neoplasms were diagnosed at AMAH; however, six cats had inflammatory polyps, lesions that in gross appearance could be mistaken for papillomas. Three of these cats also had vesical calculi and one a persistent urachal remnant.

### Malignant Tumors

The great majority of malignant tumors reported were transitional cell carcinomas (over 30), the cats ranging in age from 3 to 16 years, and females outnumbering males (Caywood et al., 1980; Cotchin, 1983; Dill et al., 1972; Nielsen, 1964; Priester and McKay, 1980; Schwarz et al., 1985; Wimberly and Lewis, 1979). Other types of carcinoma reported were four adenocarcinomas, three in males (Caywood et al., 1980; Schwarz et al., 1985), and seven squamous cell carcinomas, four cats known to be males and two, females (Caywood et al., 1980; Dorn et al., 1978; Priester and McKay, 1980; Schwarz et al., 1985). Other tumors reported were a papillary carcinoma in a 14-year-old male (Thoonen and Hoorens, 1960), an anaplastic carcinoma (Whitehead, 1967), and five carcinomas of unspecified type (Caywood et al., 1980; Patnaik et al., 1975).

Leiomyosarcomas occurred in four neutered cats aged 5 to 11 years (mean 7 years), two males and two females (Burk et al., 1975; Nielsen, 1964; Schwarz et al., 1985). Rare sarcomas were a myxosarcoma in a six-year-old male (Caywood et al., 1980) and two hemangiosarcomas, an embryonal rhabdosarcoma, and a primary lymphoma, all in castrated males (Schwarz et al., 1985). No breed predisposition was apparent in reported cases.

Lymphoma occasionally involves the bladder as part of a multicentric neoplasia, and malignant abdominal tumors may invade the bladder by extension or implantation.

Of the 25 malignant bladder tumors diagnosed at AMAH, 23 were carcinomas. No breed predisposition was apparent, all cats but three Siamese being domestic short- or longhairs. The cats ranged in age from 9 to 18 years (mean 13). Twelve were females (10 spayed) and 11 were males (9 castrated). Leiomyosarcomas occurred in a 10-year-old male and an 8-year-old spayed female.

**CLINICAL FEATURES.** The most frequent manifestation of the bladder tumors was constant or intermittent voiding of blood and blood clots, sometimes with mucus. Some cats strained and evinced discomfort during or after urination. Signs considered to be due to cystitis were present for two weeks to as long as six months before some cats were presented for veterinary care—the presumptive diagnosis of cystitis sometimes delaying recognition of the primary neoplasm. Some cats seemed otherwise healthy. Others appeared ill and had either advanced tumor or partial urinary tract obstruction causing hydroureter and hydronephrosis; coexisting chronic nephritis was common. In a 12-year-old cat that died of cardiomyopathy and chronic renal failure, the bladder carcinoma was an asymptomatic incidental finding at autopsy.

Two spayed females and one male had histories of previous episodes of cystitis. Four spayed females and one castrated male had coexisting bladder stones; one of these females also had a persistent urachal remnant.

The bladder was sometimes palpably thickened or hardened, and in one cat an enlarging fundic mass was recognized on successive examinations. In two cats, masses palpated in and around the bladder proved to be infiltrative carcinoma extending to involve the uterine stump, omentum, and abdominal wall. Rectal examination may be helpful in confirming the presence of a tumor involving the neck of the bladder and urethra and in detecting involvement of sublumbar nodes.

**DIAGNOSTIC PROCEDURES.** Urinalyses consistently disclosed pus cells, packed fields of red cells, and proteinuria (2 to 4 plus, 100 to >1000 mg/dl). Urine culture rarely yielded significant bacterial growth. Tumor cells were occasionally identified in sediment, but these must be carefully distinguished from non-neoplastic urinary epithelium. An obstructing blood clot from the vagina of an 18-year-old cat was examined by paraffin section technique and found to contain neoplastic epithelial cells, as did the urine sediment. *Staphylococcus aureus* was cultured from the urine. Exploration revealed multiple papillary carcinomatous masses in the bladder and also diffuse infiltrating carcinoma extending 2.5 cm into the urethra.

Radiographic examination with positive, negative, and double contrast techniques frequently demonstrated abnormalities in shape, thickness, and motility of the bladder (Fig. 11–117). In most cases, however, these changes could not be definitively distinguished from those of chronic cystitis, and exploratory surgery and biopsy were necessary. Hydronephrosis and hydroureter, present in some cases, were demonstrated by intravenous pyelography.

**GROSS FINDINGS.** Precise location of the carcinomas was recorded for 17 of the 23 cats: fundus in 10, dorsal wall wholly or in part in 4, ventrolateral wall in 1, trigone in 1, and, as already described, diffuse papillary vesical masses as well as tumor of the urethra in 1. At The Animal Medical Center, by contrast, no tumor was re-

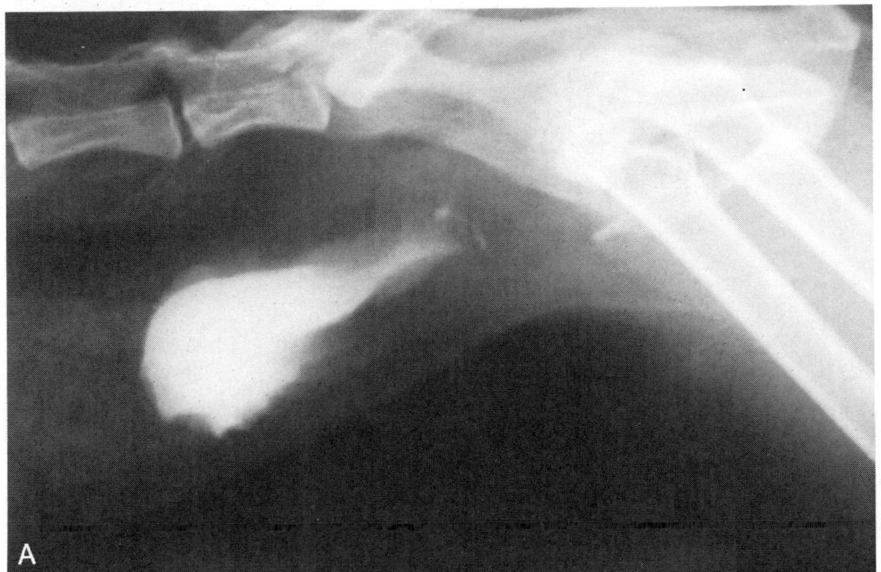


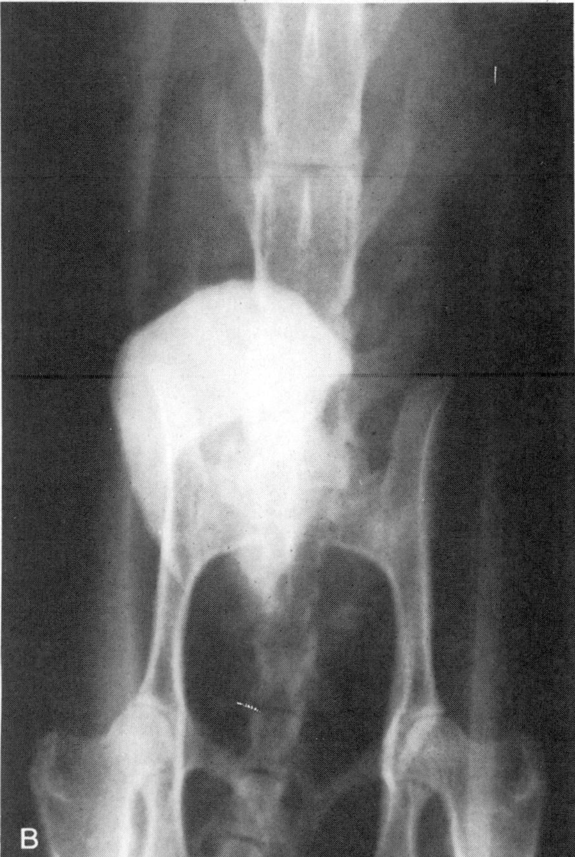


**Figure 11–117** *A*, Transitional cell carcinoma of urinary bladder, 11-year-old female domestic shorthair. Double-contrast study reveals a thickened, irregular bladder wall. The largest of the filling defects occupies the caudoventral wall. Terminal portions of the ureters are filled with positive contrast material and appear normal. *B*, A large filling defect involves the left caudal wall and trigone.

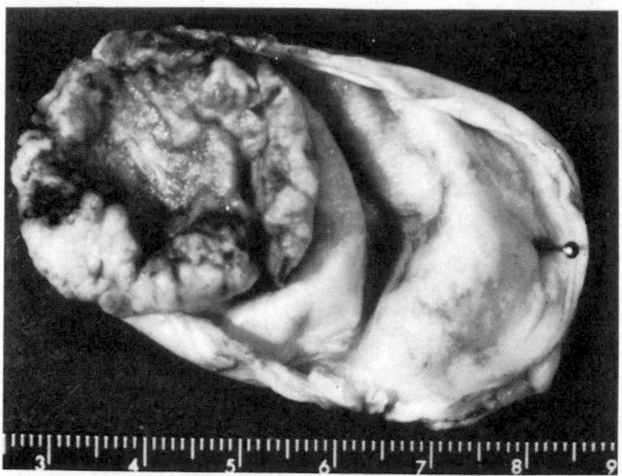

**Figure 11–118** Transitional cell carcinoma of the urinary bladder, 13-year-old spayed female Siamese. The 3 cm, nodular, umbilicated growth was of polypoid form with a wide base.

ported as originating in the dorsal wall (Schwarz et al., 1985).

The carcinomas varied in size from 1.0 cm to involvement of the entire dorsal wall. Blood clots were often found in the bladder lumen, sometimes adhering to the surface of the tumor. The mucosal aspect of the tumors was usually white, pale yellow, or pale gray, with red foci. Some of the masses were polypoid, crateriform, or both (Fig. 11–118), but most were irregularly thickened and rigid transmural lesions. One tumor appeared as a poorly demarcated, raised, rough region of the mucosa.

Two cats had secondary hydroureter and hydronephrosis, and five others had perivesical neoplastic infiltration, one with its abdomen distended by an effusion containing tumor cells. Six of the 23 carcinomas metastasized to sites including iliac nodes, uterine stump, omentum, and abdominal wall.

One leiomyosarcoma involved the cranial half of the bladder, the other the ventral wall. They were uniform, firm, rubbery, and mildly vascular. One cat was asymptomatic four months after resection, the other was euthanatized but an autopsy was not obtained.

Only one cat of the 25 with primary bladder tumors was known to have coexisting tumor of another type—a single cutaneous mast cell tumor removed at the time of resection of the bladder cacinoma. Six months later the cat was destroyed because of widely disseminated mast cell neoplasia. Recurrent carcinoma of the bladder was also found at autopsy.

**MICROSCOPIC FINDINGS.** Bladder carcinoma may be single or multiple, confined to the mucosal surface (carcinoma in situ), papillary, or invasive. Microscopically, the three basic types are transitional cell carcinoma, squamous cell carcinoma, and adenocarcinoma. The transitional epithelial cell is descended from primitive cells of the embryonic cloaca that have the potential to differentiate not only into lining cells of the bladder but also into glands of the rectum and squamous cells of the anus and terminal urethra. The mature transitional cell remains pluripotential and may thus give rise to squamous cell carcinoma and adenocarcinoma.

Many transitional cell carcinomas have squamous cell or glandular components, and it is understandable that microscopic interpretation of mixed lesions may yield varying data on the frequency of the several histologic forms (Robbins et al., 1984). The most frequent transitional cell carcinoma of cats has both squamous and glandular differentiation, but in the group at AMAH we observed no tumor that we could classify as squamous cell carcinoma or adenocarcinoma.

The 23 transitional cell carcinomas assumed a variety of forms: 15 papillary and infiltrative with glandlike and squamous metaplasia, four infiltrative with glandlike and squamous metaplasia (Fig. 11–119), two papillary and solid, one papillary, and one papillary and infiltrative with glandlike metaplasia. In the 19 carcinomas with squamous metaplasia, keratinization was seen in only two, the others being characterized by larger cells having more eosinophilic cytoplasm, visible cytoplasmic borders, and desmosomes. Foci of squamous metaplasia without keratinization were found in non-neoplastic epithelium adjacent to the tumors in several cats. The glandlike spaces observed in 20 of the carcinomas were not lined by cuboidal or columnar cells but often contained PAS-positive material that was not seen in H&E–stained sections. Similar PAS-positive substance was demonstrated in vacuoles and signet-ring cells within the tumor. All grades of malignancy were represented among the tumors. Thirteen of the 23 carcinomas had infiltrated to the serosa or extended beyond.

**DIFFERENTIAL DIAGNOSIS.** Beside chronic proliferative cystitis, lesions that may be mistaken for bladder tumors include remnants of the urachus, congenital uro-

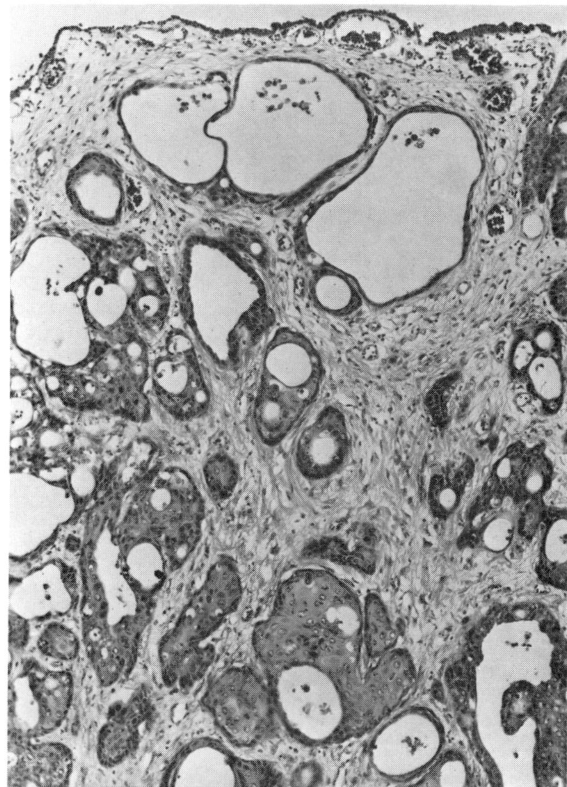

**Figure 11–119** Transitional cell carcinoma of the urinary bladder, 11-year-old female domestic shorthair. The tumor was of infiltrative type with glandular (spaces) and squamous metaplasia (lower center). H & E, × 50.

thelial cysts, Brunn's epithelial nests, and focal squamous metaplasia. Remnants of the urachus can appear as solid or cystic, tortuous or branching masses of benign transitional epithelium extending to varying depths in the ventral cranial fundus and rarely into the ventral ligament of the bladder. If they reach the umbilicus, urine may leak from that site. Urine stasis rather often occurs within a communicating remnant, predisposing the bladder to cystitis.

Cysts may sometimes have the gross appearance of tumor. A 14-year-old castrated male had a 1.5 × 1.0 × 0.8 cm mass in the ventral fundus and body of the bladder that was composed of many variably sized cysts lined by one or two layers of flat or low cuboidal epithelium (Fig. 11–120). The cysts contained PAS-positive material and macrophages with PAS-positive cytoplasm. The combination of this condition with cystitis, also present in this case, is known as cystitis cystica.

Brunn's nests are compact aggregates of benign transitional epithelium that develop in the lamina propria in association with proliferative cystitis. The nests prove to be connected with surface epithelium when examined by serial sectioning. Such nests were seen adjacent to points of origin of several of the transitional cell carcinomas. Focal squamous metaplasia is now and then seen in surface epithelium or in Brunn's nests. Keratinization has not been observed. Such metaplasia could conceivably be misinterpreted as carcinoma in situ.

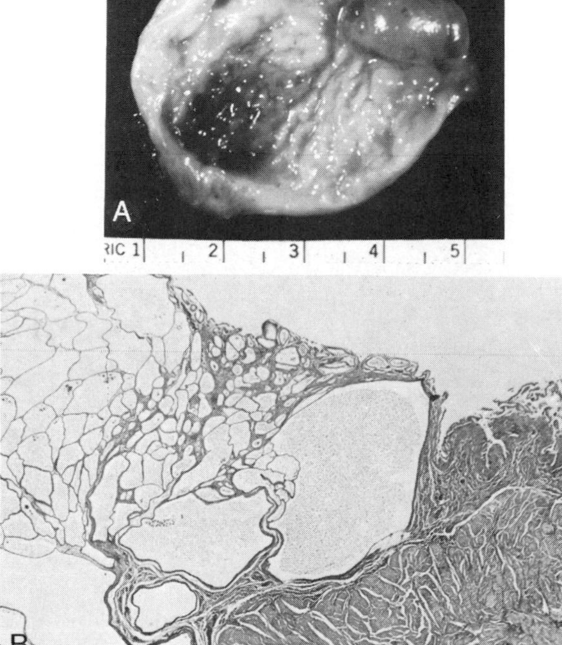


**Figure 11–120** *A*, Cystitis cystica, 14-year-old castrated male domestic cat. In addition to a congenital cystic mass (upper right), the bladder exhibits a thickened wall with an area of hemorrhagic cystitis and also pale raised areas of lymphoma. Actual size. *B*, Section of the protruding mass revealed multiple fluid-filled compartments within the thickened mucosa. PAS, × 12.5.

**MANAGEMENT OF BLADDER TUMORS.** Diagnosis and management of bladder tumors are well discussed by Osborne et al. (1968a) and by Schwarz et al. (1985). Early diagnosis and generous resection offer the best prospect for a cure. A few benign tumors have been removed successfully, but many tumors, by the time they are diagnosed, have already metastasized or are so situated or so extensive that complete resection is impossible. The majority of cats are euthanatized at once. Those undergoing surgery usually succumb within a few weeks or months as a result of progression or metastasis of the tumor. Total cystectomy with ureteral anastomosis to the skin or digestive tract is resorted to in humans but is not practical for animals. Irradiation and chemotherapy are possibilities that have not yet been sufficiently investigated in animals.

### Tumors of the Urethra

Tumors of the urethra are exceedingly rare. A transitional cell carcinoma (3.0 cm × 2.0 cm) of the proximal pelvic and prostatic urethra was reported in a six-year-old entire male cat with hematuria (Barrett and Nobel, 1976). A soft tissue mass narrowed the pelvic canal, causing a fecal impaction of the colon. Pelvic symphysectomy and a prepubic urethrostomy were undertaken, but the cat died during surgery.

## TUMORS OF THE MALE REPRODUCTIVE SYSTEM

Neoplasms of the male reproductive organs are a rarity in cats. One reason may be that most pet cats are neutered early in life and few toms survive the hazards of their life style to reach old age.

### Tumors of the Testis

Few tumors of the feline testis have been reported, and those mostly without details: a metastasizing carcinoma of unknown origin (Zettler, 1916), a cancer (Thirot, 1937), an embryonal carcinoma in a 13-year-old cat (Joshua, 1965), an adenoma of the caudal pole of the right testis (Bourgeois, 1933), and two interstitial cell tumors in old cats (Cotchin, 1983). An interstitial cell tumor has also been reported by Priester and McKay (1980) and four tumors of unspecified type by Kovacs and Somogyvari (1968). Tumor-like developmental anomalies have been described in young cats: a wolffian (mesonephric duct) "tumor" in a nine-month-old cat (Peyron and Cocu, 1938) and cysts of the rete testis and of the testis itself (Gelberg and McEntee, 1983).

A malignant seminoma occurred in a two-year-old male black domestic shorthair with bilateral retained abdominal testes. The cat ate less and was listless for three weeks before a palpable abdominal mass was detected. The testes, one with a 6 cm tumor, were removed. The tumor was diagnosed at Tufts University School of Veterinary Medicine as a seminoma. One year later the cat became obstipated, sublumbar masses were palpated, and the cat was destroyed. Diffuse metastatic tumor was found in the

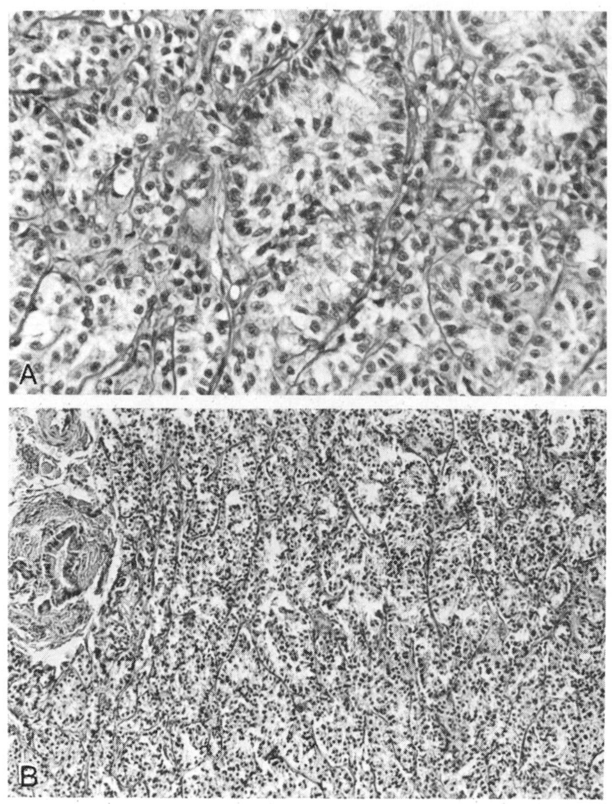


**Figure 11–121** *A*, Malignant Sertoli cell tumor, 15-year-old cat, composed of solid tubules of palisading cells with abundant clear to foamy cytoplasm. H & E, × 312. *B*, Metastatic tumor in the liver consists of tightly grouped packets of malignant cells that have replaced all but a portal triad (upper left). H & E, × 125.

nodes and soft tissues of the sublumbar region (Williams et al., 1982).

Two cases of Sertoli cell tumor were published from AMAH in 1956 (Meier) and have been restudied by us. In one cat, a 15-year-old bilateral cryptorchid with an ulcerated basal cell skin tumor, the enlarged left testis contained a Sertoli cell tumor with metastases to the liver (Fig. 11–121). The reported metastases to the spleen proved on re-examination to be primary mast cell tumor. In the other cat, of unknown age, the 43 gm right testis was composed entirely of tumor. The left testis looked grossly normal, but microscopic examination revealed a small invasive Sertoli cell tumor; it was not possible to identify the seminoma in situ mentioned in the earlier report (Meier, 1956b). Neither cat exhibited signs suggesting that these Sertoli cell tumors were hormonally functional.

Secondary tumors are rare. At AMAH lymphoma of the testis has been seen in a few cats, but it has always been a part of a more generalized disease. Disseminated metastatic carcinoma of uncertain origin involved both testes in one cat.

## Tumors of the Prostate*

The cat, in strong contrast with man and dog, very rarely suffers from prostatic tumors. A fibroadenoma was reported in a 13-year-old castrated male by Cotchin (1983).

Three carcinomas were diagnosed at AMAH in castrated males aged 15, 17, and 22 years. Two were domestic shorthairs, the third a domestic longhair. Two had hematuria and dysuria for two weeks, one also dribbled urine constantly. All were presented because of acute urethral obstruction. A urinary catheter was passed with difficulty in two cats and with ease in the third. None of the cats urinated freely, nor could the bladder be expressed after the catheterization. A hard mass at the pelvic brim was felt in two cats by rectal palpation. All three were destroyed.

In all the cats the prostates were firm, gray-white, and smooth, ranging from 0.8 to 2.0 cm in diameter (Figs. 11–122 and 11–123*A*). The cut surfaces were white or tan and appeared fibrous. Changes in the urinary bladder included muscle hypertrophy, mucosal fibrosis, and erosions, congestion, and hemorrhage in the bladder wall.

All three tumors were adenocarcinomas. In one, pleomorphic cuboidal cells with scanty granular or vacuolated eosinophilic cytoplasm and round nuclei formed irregular tubules (Fig. 11–123*B*). Many tumor cells had vesicular nuclei and a single prominent nucleolus with coarse chromatin at the nuclear margin. There were many signet-ring cells in the stroma. In the other two tumors, cells varying from columnar to squamous were arranged in acini and irregular solid sheets. Cytoplasm was eosinophilic and granular or vacuolated. Some nuclei were round or oval, some larger and irregular with prominent nucleoli. Chromatin was evenly dispersed in some cells, marginated in others. All three tumors had fibromuscular proliferation and multifocal infiltrates of mononuclear cells. The tumor invaded lymphatics and venules of the prostate in all three cats but did not extend beyond the capsule, spread to regional lymph nodes, or metastasize.

The origin of these tumors was most likely acinar or ductal prostatic epithelium. The tumor invaded the pros-

*Laura K. Andrews, principal author.

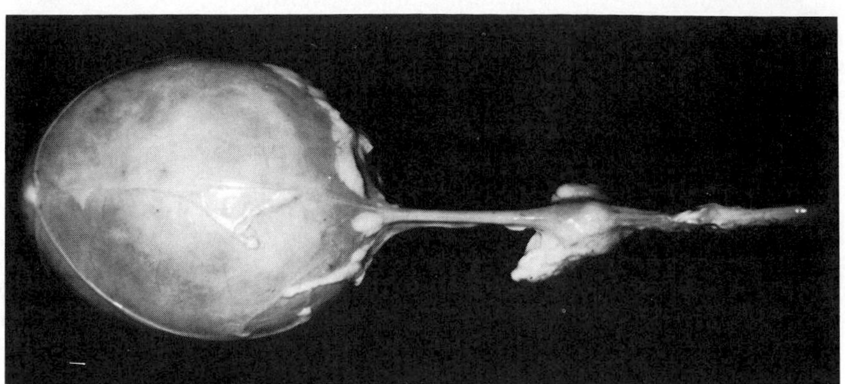

**Figure 11–122** Bladder, urethra, and adenocarcinoma of the prostate (right of center), 22-year-old castrated male red tabby. A catheter could easily be passed and urine withdrawn, but the moment the catheter was removed the cat could not urinate. The bladder was thickened and rigid, probably owing to muscle hypertrophy, and had foci of serosal hemorrhage. Actual size.

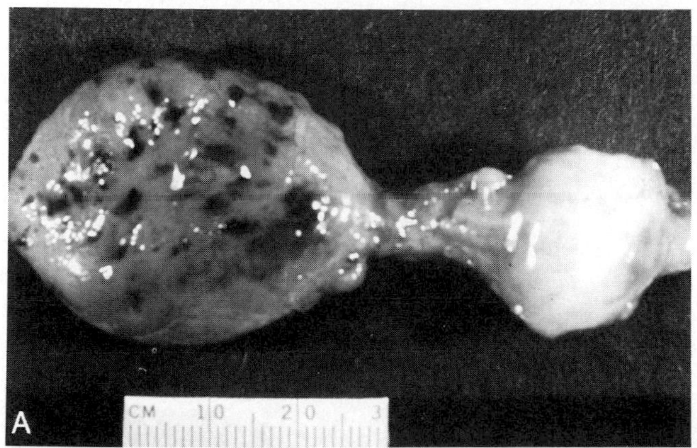


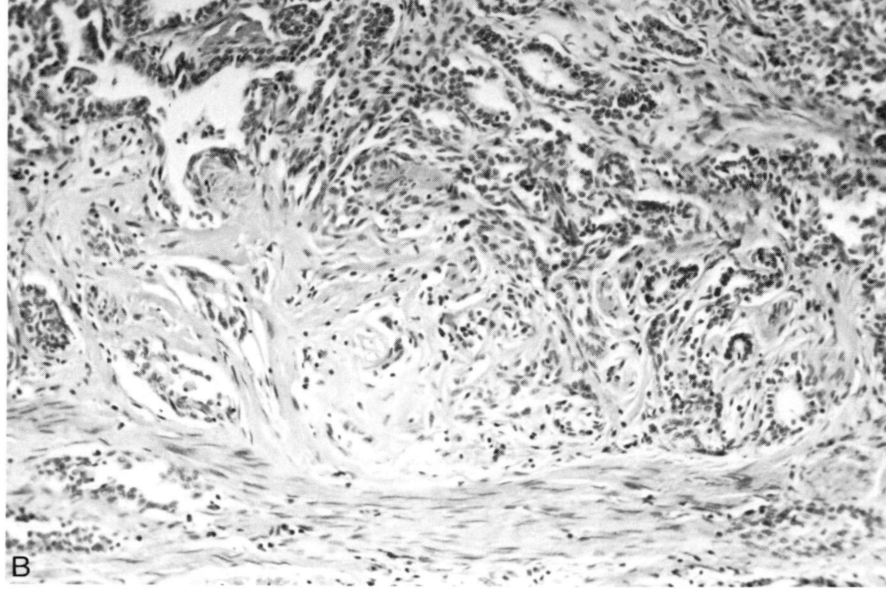


**Figure 11–123** *A*, Adenocarcinoma of the prostate, 17-year-old castrated male. The white, nodular tumor infiltrates the area surrounding the urethra. Because of chronic obstruction to urine outflow the urinary bladder has become distended, thickened, and opaque. *B*, Same cat. Irregular branching tubules are embedded in a dense fibromuscular stroma. H & E, × 180.

tatic urethra in one cat, but the pelvic urethra proximal and distal to the prostate was normal.

The prognosis for cats with this tumor is unknown. Surgical removal of the tumor and regional lymph nodes should be attempted.

### Other Tumors

Benign tumors of the scrotum have been reported—a fibroma (Milks, 1939) and a papilloma (Priester and McKay, 1980). An incipient "epithelioma" was described as originating from the scrotum of a five-month-old cat three weeks after it was castrated (Lombard, 1961).

The penis was reported as the site of a carcinoma (Sticker, 1901) and of a sarcoma (Hübner, 1920).

## TUMORS OF THE FEMALE REPRODUCTIVE SYSTEM*

### Tumors of the Ovary

The most frequent lesions in the feline ovary are follicular cysts. Because cats ovulate only after copulation, multiple estrogen-containing cysts develop in cats that come into heat repeatedly with no opportunity to mate. Such cysts sometimes give rise to nymphomania and vicious or antisocial behavior such as breaking of litter-box training.

Luteal cysts, by contrast, are rare in the cat.

Cysts of the rete ovarii, probably assumed by veterinary practitioners and pathologists to be follicular cysts, are distinct microscopically and vary in character depending on where in the rete they arise (Gelbert et al., 1984). They are grossly visible and are most often unilateral, displacing or compressing ovarian parenchyma. Among 20 cats studied, those of known age ranged from 2 to 13 years. All but one (a Siamese) were domestic shorthairs. The functional significance of the cysts is unknown.

Small, glassy-looking parovarian cysts are occasionally found in the mesovarium at spaying.

"Wolffian tumors" of the ovary have been described (Winiwarter, cited by Lombard, 1940). The wolffian (mesonephric) duct is a vestigial structure that in the male gives rise to the epididymis and vas deferens. Remnants may persist as epithelial inclusions anywhere along the course of the reproductive tract.

The subgerminal epithelial inclusion cysts common in aged dogs are seldom if ever seen in cats.

#### Sex-Cord Tumors

This group includes granulosa cell tumors, thecomas, and luteomas. Some produce estrogen or progesterone that may have nymphomanic or virilizing effects (Nielsen et al., 1976).

**GRANULOSA CELL TUMORS.** These neoplasms constitute about half of the ovarian tumors of cats (Norris et al., 1969); about half of them metastasize (Nielsen et al., 1976). Around 20 have been reported (Aliakbrai and Ivoghli, 1979; Arnbjerg, 1980; Baker, 1956; Cotchin, 1983; Di Domizio, 1947, cited by Norris et al., 1969; Engle and Brodey, 1969; Gilmore, 1965; Kitt, 1900, Norris et al., 1969; Patnaik et al., 1975; Priester and McKay, 1980). For the cats whose age was reported, the range was 3 to 16 years (mean 11). Of eight cats with available clinical histories, seven had a palpable ovarian mass; in one (Arnbjerg, 1980), both ovaries were normal and the tumor arose from the upper end of the left uterine horn. Six had signs of a functional tumor, and nine had metastases variously involving abdominal and pelvic peritoneum, lungs, liver, spleen, and kidney. Endometrial hyperplasia and partial hair loss were other effects of granulosa cell tumors.

Three granulosa cell tumors were diagnosed at AMAH, two in cats that despite spaying resumed estrous behavior. One, a three-year-old black domestic shorthair, 23 months after surgery had four episodes resembling estrus, each lasting a week and recurring at three-week intervals. At exploratory laparotomy the surgeon found and removed a piece of right ovary with a 0.4 cm solid, yellow tumor composed of vacuolated granulosa cells that partially infiltrated one of two corpora lutea. He also removed a segment of oviduct with a multiloculated cyst of the fimbria (Fig. 11–124).

The second cat, an 11-year-old tabby-and-white domestic shorthair, had been spayed eight years before experiencing two periods of abnormal behavior four months apart. During these episodes the cat "roared like a lion and screamed like a Siamese." It developed a nasty disposition and ate more without a noticeable gain in weight. Exploratory surgery revealed a firm, yellow, 0.8 × 0.5 cm tumor and two mucinous cysts involving the remnant of the right ovary. The tumor consisted in part of granulosa cells that formed follicles containing eosinophilic secretion, but its major portion was composed of sheets and packets of cells resembling luteinized and interstitial cells. The mucinous cysts, lined partly by ciliated pseudostratified, columnar epithelium, partly by

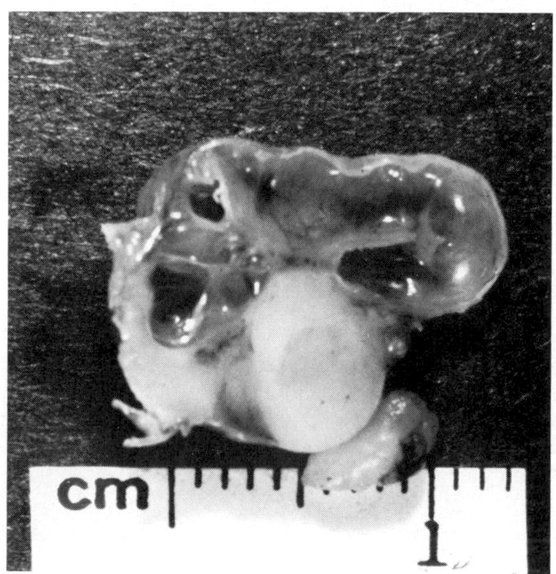


**Figure 11–124** Granulosa cell tumor removed from a three-year-old cat two years after incomplete oophorohysterectomy. Multiloculated parovarian cysts partially surround the tumor.

*A number of the AMAH tumors discussed in this section were previously reported by Gilmore (1965).

simple cuboidal epithelium, were probably remnants of the mesonephric duct. All abnormal behavioral signs disappeared by the eighth postoperative day.

The third granulosa cell tumor, functional as well as palpable, was removed from a 13-year-old Siamese that had continuous signs of estrus over a five-month period. The tumor, 3.5 cm in diameter, pale yellow, and nodular, was composed of granulosa cells arranged in sheets and small packets separated by a fine fibrovascular stroma and by round as well as irregular spaces filled with PAS-positive secretion. Other features were a very high mitotic index, extensive necrosis, and a peritheliomatous pattern of viable neoplastic cells. The uterus had undergone cystic endometrial hyperplasia. The cat recovered from surgery but was euthanatized five months later for suspected malignancy; an autopsy was not obtained.

**LUTEOMA AND THECOMA.** These sex-cord tumors are uncommon in the cat. A lipid-cell tumor believed to be derived from luteinized theca cells was found in a nine-year-old cat that had possible signs of masculinization (an enlarged head and neck and a lowered voice), as well as prolonged estrus, an ovarian cyst, and cystic endometrial hyperplasia (Norris et al., 1969).

A "so-called androblastoma with Sertoli-Leydig cell pattern" was described in a surgically removed right ovary of a six-year-old domestic cat (Hofmann et al., 1980). Measuring 7.5 × 5.4 × 3.6 cm, the ovary had a slightly bosselated surface and on section showed solid, whitish areas and also cysts up to 3 cm that contained mucinous or hemorrhagic material. No metastases were seen. The uterus was slightly enlarged, with a moderately thickened endometrium. Although no clinical evidence of hormonal activity was noted before or after surgery, the adenomatous hyperplasia of the endometrium was considered evidence of an estrogenic effect.

**INTERSTITIAL CELL TUMOR.** Interstitial cells of the ovary are often seen at sites of ovulation and atretic follicles in cats but not, in our experience (JLC), in the bitch. They arise chiefly from the epithelioid theca interna cells or from hypertrophied granulosa cells (Dellman and Brown, 1976). An ovarian tumor described as arising from interstitial cells was reported by Petit et al. (1926). It was the size of a large nut and bosselated. Microscopically the tumor was polymorphic, resembling variously fibrosarcoma, sarcoma, and myxolipoma. These features suggest that the tumor was probably a nonfunctional pleomorphic sarcoma (Norris et al., 1969).

## Germ Cell Tumors

Dysgerminoma and teratoma are ovarian germ cell tumors that may be benign or malignant, and both tumors have been reported in cats. The cells of the dysgerminoma are uniform and undergo no further differentiation, while the cells of the teratoma may differentiate into skin, muscle, fat, bone, hair, and other tissues.

**DYSGERMINOMA.** Dysgerminomas are estimated to constitute about 15 per cent of feline ovarian tumors (Barrett and Theilen, 1977). They are solid, often large masses with areas of hemorrhage and necrosis. The dysgerminoma resembles the testicular seminoma and is usually benign. An exception occurred in a seven-year-old Siamese cat with a dysgerminoma, masculine behavior, and a metastatic lesion in the omentum (Dehner et al., 1970). A dysgerminoma the size of a small apple was removed from a seven-year-old domestic cat (Sbernardori and Nava, 1968), and bilateral spherical tumors each weighing 40 gm were found in routine spaying of a one-year-old domestic shorthair (Andrews et al., 1974).

A mixed dysgerminoma-teratoma weighing 1000 gm caused sudden death from hemorrhage in a six-year-old domestic cat (Dehner et al., 1970).

A dysgerminoma reported from AMAH (Gilmore, 1965) proved on re-examination to be a metastatic carcinoma.

**TERATOMA.** Teratomas may be found in very young animals. A dermoid cyst filled with hair was found in the left ovary of a six-month-old kitten ( Cotchin, 1983) and a massive teratoma of the left ovary in a two-year-old domestic cat (McClelland, 1942). Two benign teratomas of the ovary were reported by Norris et al. (1969), one associated with hemorrhage that caused the death of a two-year-old cat that had queened three weeks before.

## Epithelial Tumors

Epithelial tumors are thought to arise from the surface (coelomic) epithelium of the ovary. They are often cystic and papillary and rarely have endocrine manifestations. Differentiation between benign and malignant tumors on morphologic grounds is sometimes arbitrary.

Benign cystomas are said to occur in cats, although less often than in dogs (Bloom, 1954). A palpable cystadenoma was reported in a cat with virilization, persistent estrus, and cystic endometrial hyperplasia (Norris et al., 1969).

At least eight adenocarcinomas have been reported, two with metastatic lesions at the time of diagnosis (Boucek, 1906; Cotchin, 1983; Nielsen, 1964; Norris et al., 1969; Priester and McKay, 1980; Schlegel, cited by Lombard, 1940; Verardini, 1935), as well as cystadenocarcinoma (Barrett and Theilen, 1977) and a mucinous carcinoma (Priester and McKay, 1980). One carcinoma of unspecified type was reported by Feldman (1932) and three by Patnaik et al. (1975).

It is generally stated that epithelial tumors, like the dysgerminoma, have no endocrine manifestations. They are often cystic and papillary. Metastases may be widespread. Implantation of exfoliated cells is the most common form of metastasis, and a careful search for secondary lesions is always indicated during surgery for ovarian masses. Both ovaries should always be examined because bilateral tumors, although rare, can occur in the cat.

## Mesenchymal Tumors

Ovarian polyps and leiomyomas are said to have been reported in the cat (Barrett and Theilen, 1977). A walnut-sized fibrosarcoma was described by Boucek (1906), and a myxochondroma was found in an aged cat by Cotchin (1983).

## Metastatic Tumor

The ovary may occasionally be the site of secondary tumor, e.g., squamous cell carcinoma of the vagina and uterine and pancreatic adenocarcinoma. It is also sometimes involved in lymphoma (Fig. 11–125).

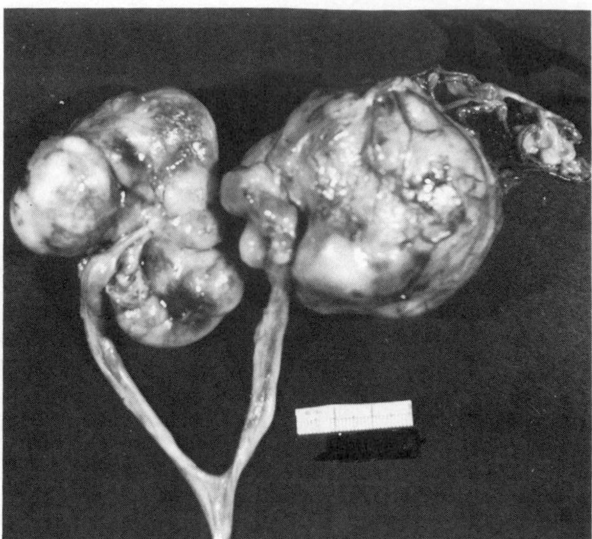

**Figure 11–125** Lymphoma involving the ovaries, three-year-old tricolor. Both masses, measuring 7 cm in greatest dimension, were pale, firm, and irregularly nodular. Half actual size.

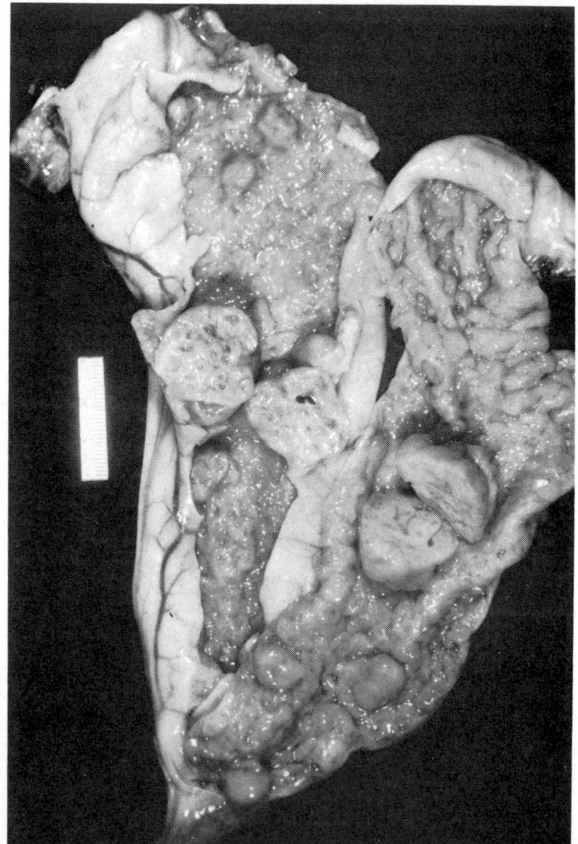

**Figure 11–126** Endometrial polyps, numerous and varying in size and shape, are scattered throughout both horns and the uterine body of a 15-year-old cat. Two large polyps have been incised to reveal their pedunculated and cystic features. The endometrial wall is diffusely hyperplastic.

## Tumors of the Uterus

### Tumor-like Lesions

Endometrial polyps, which are not neoplasms in the strict sense, are the most commonly encountered uterine masses, occurring in older cats with endometrial hyperplasia, mucometra, and pyometra. Polyps, often cystic, are the result of focal proliferation of endometrial, stromal, and epithelial components. They may be single or multiple (e.g., Thoonen and Hoorens, 1961) (Fig. 11–126). They are not considered to represent a preneoplastic change (Gelberg and McEntee, 1984).

Adenomyosis is another rather common lesion, most often seen microscopically but sometimes large enough to be visible grossly and mistaken for tumor. It consists of ectopic endometrium located in the myometrium. Massive, diffuse, symmetric enlargement of both uterine body and horns was described in a nine-year-old Siamese with adenomyosis and associated pyometra (Pack, 1980). The largest such mass seen at AMAH was also in a nine-year-old Siamese. The cat felt well but had three episodes of abdominal enlargement and uterine discharge over a nine-month period. Signs persisted after the third attack, and a uterine mass was palpated. This proved at surgery to involve the body of the uterus and measured 8.0 × 8.0 × 4.0 cm (Fig. 11–127*A*). The microscopic appearance was suggestive at first glance of adenocarcinoma, but the presence of benign-appearing glands in the same progesterone phase as the endometrium, together with benign endometrial stroma, established the true nature of the lesion (Fig. 11–127*B*).

### Benign Tumors

Benign uterine tumors greatly outnumber malignant ones in the cat. Adenomas are rare. One was recorded in a four-year-old cat (Schmidt and Langham, 1967). A fibroadenoma was reported by Zietzschmann (1901), and a large movable cystadenoma in the cavity of a uterine horn was described by Collet (1933).

The principal benign growth is the leiomyoma, a proliferation of smooth muscle that most often bulges outwardly but may occasionally occlude the lumen of the uterus or block the cervix or vagina, predisposing to dystocia and uterine infection. Many tumors of this type have been reported, some multiple (e.g., Cotchin, 1983; Feldman, 1932; Mulligan, 1951; Nava and Sbernardori, 1967; Patnaik et al., 1975; Petit, 1902a; Whitehead, 1967). A cystic fibromyoma associated with pyometra was described by Richard (1910).

Eight leiomyomas were diagnosed at AMAH. No breed predisposition was apparent. Age of the cats ranged from 3 to 15 years (mean 9). The growths varied in greatest dimension from 0.3 to 8.0 cm. The majority occurred in the body of the uterus. Four cats had more than one lesion. Of these, one 3-year-old had five and the 15-year-old had three (Fig. 11–128) as well as a leiomyoma of the vagina. Five cats had ovarian follicular cysts, and three had cystic endometrial hyperplasia. A cat with dystocia had retained dead fetuses owing to obstruction by two leiomyomas in the body of the uterus near the cervix.

It is reported that for women and dogs the leiomyoma is estrogen-dependent and the tumor decreases in size if the source of estrogen is removed. It is of interest to note

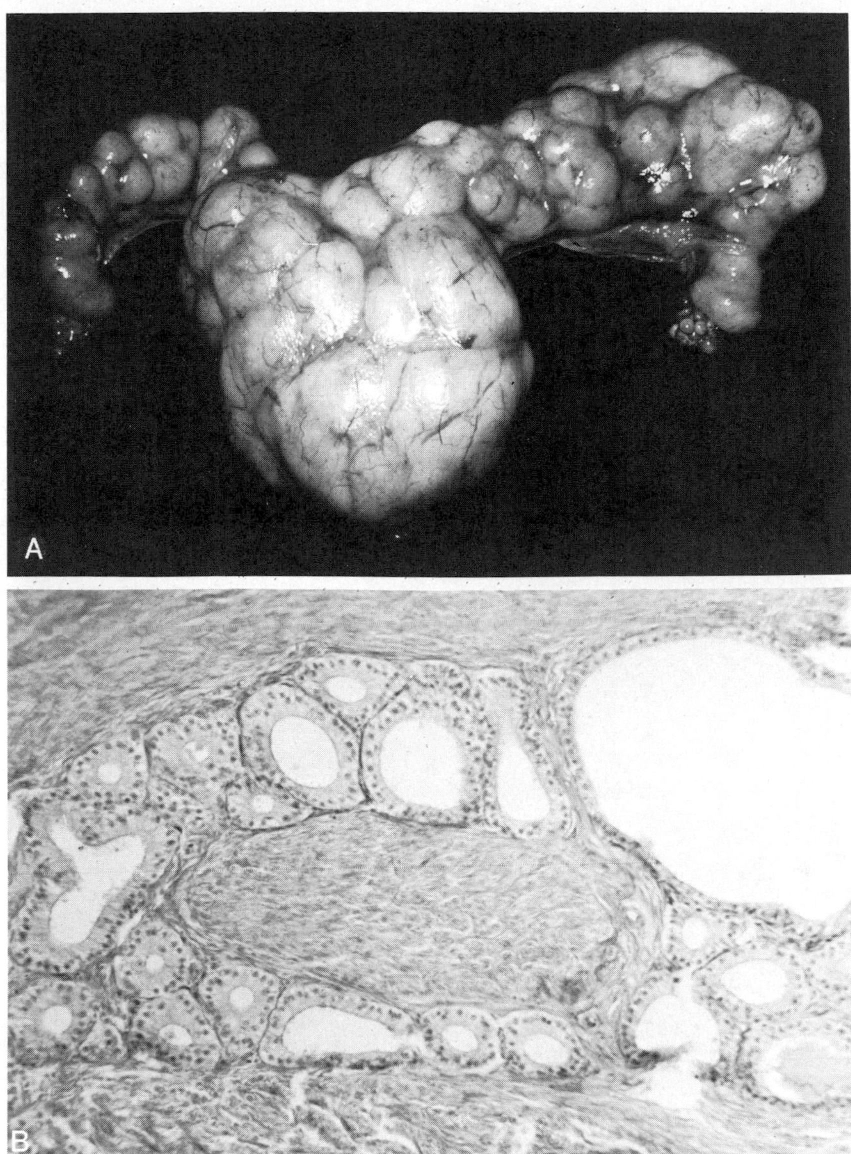


**Figure 11–127** *A*, Diffuse adenomyosis of a 330 gm uterus, nine-year-old Siamese. The bosselation of the perimetrial surface is caused by ectopic and often cystic endometrium situated within the myometrium. *B*, Benign, deeply displaced, coiled endometrial glands within scant endometrial stroma are surrounded by uterine muscle. H & E, × 180.

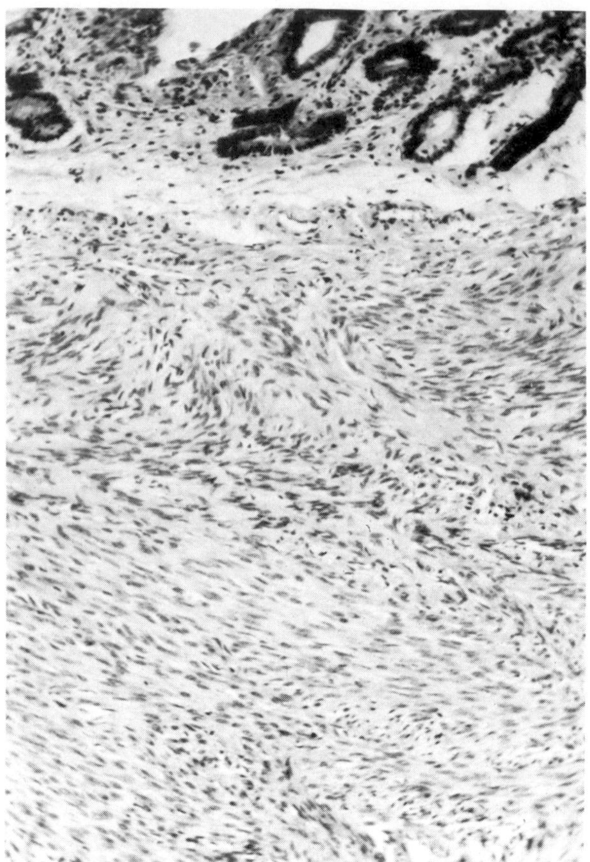

**Figure 11–128** Leiomyoma of the uterus, one of several in the uterus and vagina of a 15-year-old cat. Broad, long bundles of mature, spindle-shaped, smooth muscle cells underlie the endometrium. H & E, × 180.

the frequent association of this tumor with the ovarian and endometrial changes found in the eight cats.

Fibromas of the feline uterus have been reported (Ball and Lombard, 1925; Feldman, 1932; Lombard, 1940), as well as fibroleiomyomas (Moulton, 1978). The designation fibroleiomyoma is arbitrary and should be used only when both fibrous and smooth muscle components are prominent. Moulton (1978) reports that fibroleiomyoma is by far the most frequent tubular genital tract tumor in the dog and cat. This contrasts with the findings in cats at AMAH, because while a fibrous component was present to varying degree in our leiomyomas it was an insignificant feature.

Both leiomyomas and fibroleiomyomas are firmer and lighter-colored (white or dull pink) than the adjacent muscle. Sectioning reveals a discrete but unencapsulated mass, which may be pseudolobulated and usually has an uneven, bulging surface and barely visible swirling bundles. Cysts may be present, and if there is necrosis with mineralization, yellow caseous foci may be seen. The more abundant the fibrous component, the firmer and lighter-colored the mass will be. Leiomyomas of the uterus and vagina of cats resemble benign smooth muscle tumors found elsewhere and in other species, except that the fibrous component may be more plentiful.

## Malignant Tumors

Occurring almost without exception in old cats, primary malignant tumors are uncommon. Metastases may be widespread. Associated genital lesions include cysts of the ovary, endometrial hyperplasia, pyometra, leiomyomas of the uterus or vagina, and mammary cancer.

**CARCINOMA.** About a dozen cases have been reported, mostly adenocarcinomas (Belter et al., 1968; Cotchin, 1983; Engle and Brodey, 1969; Joest, cited by Ball, 1932; Kermen, 1935; Meier, 1956a; Norris et al., 1969; O'Rourke and Geib, 1970; Preiser, 1964; Priester and McKay, 1980; Schmidt and Langham, 1967; Whitehead, 1967). Except for one 4-year-old cat (Schmidt and Langham, 1967), all for which age was noted were at least 10 years old. A cervical adenocarcinoma was reported by Montpellier et al. (1952) and squamous cell carcinomas of the cervix by Boucek (1906) and Collignon (1936).

Of the four cats at AMAH with carcinoma of the uterus, three were 11 years old and the fourth 16. Three were tricolors. In one cat, a spayed female, constipation was caused by the pressure of tumor. Cystic masses ranging up to 5.0 cm were present at the stump of one uterine horn and in the retroperitoneum, iliac nodes, omentum, mesocolon, and diaphragm. Microscopically the tumor was a papillary and tubular cystadenocarcinoma. This case was previously described and pictured by Meier (1956a).

In a 16-year-old cat with an adenosquamous carcinoma the signs were anorexia, diarrhea, and vaginal discharge. The abdomen was distended with fluid that contained malignant epithelial cells. The uterus was enlarged, with horns up to 5 cm in diameter. A scirrhous stenotic segment in one horn proved to be a tumor composed microscopically of malignant glandular and squamous epithelium with transmural infiltration and extensive vascular invasion (Fig. 11–129). There were metastases to the ovaries, broad ligament, omentum, and peritoneal wall. As well as the malignant tumor there were 15 endometrial polyps. Ovarian follicular and parovarian cysts were also present.

The third tricolor had mucometra and in the uterine body a firm 3.5 cm adenocarcinoma with squamous metaplasia. Microscopically the tumor was composed of malignant glandular and squamous epithelium with transmural infiltration and extensive vascular invasion.

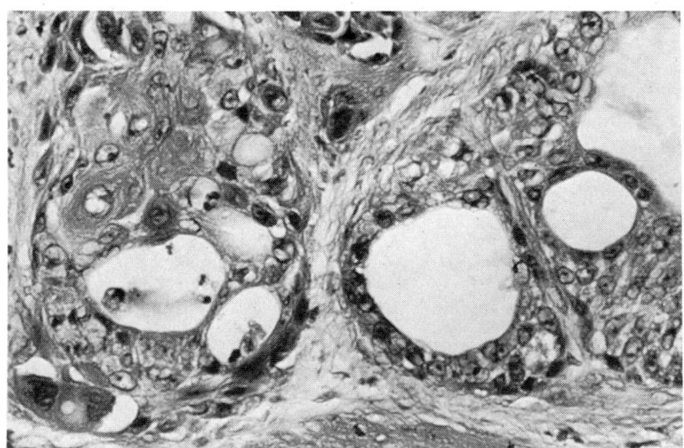

**Figure 11–129** Adenosquamous carcinoma of the uterus, 16-year-old tricolor. A tubuloalveolar glandular pattern (lower right) blends with solid nests of squamous cells (upper left) undergoing keratinization. H & E, × 312.

The fourth cat had a solid adenocarcinoma arising in the oviduct and metastasizing to the omentum and mesentery.

**LEIOMYOSARCOMA.** By comparison with their benign counterparts, uterine leiomyosarcomas are uncommon in the cat, two being recorded by Priester and McKay (1980) and one by Whitehead (1967).

Three were diagnosed at AMAH in cats 10, 11, and 17 years old. Two cats with signs of poor appetite and weight loss had pyometra and tumors of 9 and 10 cm in greatest dimension, with metastatic lesions in the mesentery and omentum. One also had metastases to the diaphragm, sternal nodes, and lungs. The third cat was asymptomatic, and the tumor was found during routine spaying, a 2 cm specimen from a larger mass being submitted for diagnosis.

Grossly, uterine leiomyosarcomas resemble leiomyomas unless metastatic lesions are present (Figs. 11–130 and 11–131*A*). Microscopically, bundles of smooth muscle cells are the prominent feature (Fig. 11–131*B* and *C*). Pleomorphism and a high mitotic index distinguished the malignant tumors from the leiomyomas. It is emphasized in medical pathology that a mitotic index of 5 or more per 10 HPF, rather than the degree of pleomorphism, is the most reliable criterion for malignant behavior of smooth muscle tumors. Our three leiomyosarcomas had mitotic indices of 7, 10, and 25, while the benign growths had no mitotic figures or two at most per 10 HPF. Necrosis, cysts, and mineralization were seen in the larger of the benign tumors but necrosis was more extensive in the malignant growths. In two of the leiomyosarcomas, strap- and racket-shaped cells and a few multinucleated cells were seen. The metastatic lesions in the diaphragm in one case could easily have been confused with rhabdomyosarcoma.

**OTHER MALIGNANT TUMORS.** Rare uterine tumors reported were a large fibrosarcoma associated with pyometra in an 11-year-old cat (Alexander, 1911), a mixed mesodermal endometrial tumor with both carcinomatous and sarcomatous components (Evans and Grant, 1977), and an hydatidiform mole (Drieux and Thiéry, 1948).

**SECONDARY TUMORS.** Secondary lymphoma has been recorded (e.g., Cotchin, 1983; Feldman, 1932), and several cats with multicentric lymphoma seen at AMAH had uterine or utero-ovarian involvement (Fig. 11–132).

## Tumors of the Vagina

Tumors of the vagina are even less frequent than uterine neoplasms. They may cause the perineum to bulge, or they may protrude from the vulva. Constipation, dystocia, interference with urination, and a chronic discharge have been due to intrapelvic vaginal tumors. Other complications or associated conditions include endometritis, oophoritis, ovarian cysts, and tumors of uterine smooth muscle. Interference with coition could lead to sterility.

Most vaginal tumors are benign. A papilloma, 4 to 5 cm long and causing urinary difficulty, was excised from a 10-year-old Siamese (Marusi, 1967). Two leiomyomas were recorded by Whitehead (1967), and two described by Wolke (1963) caused chronic constipation in 8- and 14-year-old domestic shorthairs. A fibroma was recorded by Cotchin (1983), and a myxoma at the vulvovaginal junction in a two-year-old cat by Nielsen (1964). Two tumors at AMAH previously reported as a leiomyoma and a fibroma (Gilmore, 1965) seemed on review to be best described as fibroleiomyomas (JLC). They occurred in 12- and 15-year-old cats. The older cat had, in addition, leiomyomas of the uterus, endometrial polyps, and ovarian follicular cysts.

Two malignant growths were diagnosed at AMAH. In a 12-year-old pregnant cat, a leiomyosarcoma measuring 6 × 4 × 4 cm was attached to the roof and side of the vagina, occluded the lumen, and protruded from the vulva. A satellite lesion, 2 × 1 cm, was also present. The other malignancy of the vagina, a poorly differentiated carcinoma, arose near the cervix in a five-year-old cat and metastasized to the uterus, an ovary, sublumbar nodes, diaphragm, liver, and lungs (Fig. 11–133). There had been a genital discharge for one year. Chronic endometritis and oophoritis were considered to be complications of the vaginal neoplasia. This tumor was originally interpreted as arising in the uterus (Meier, 1956a).

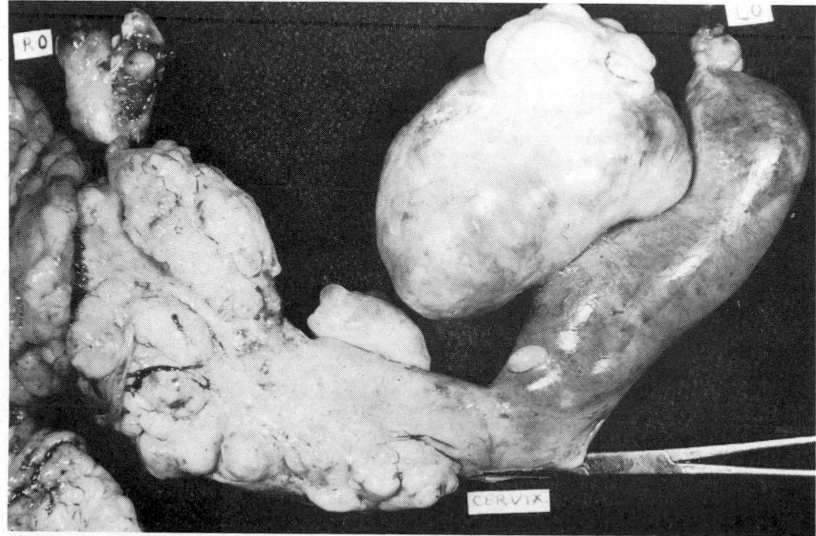


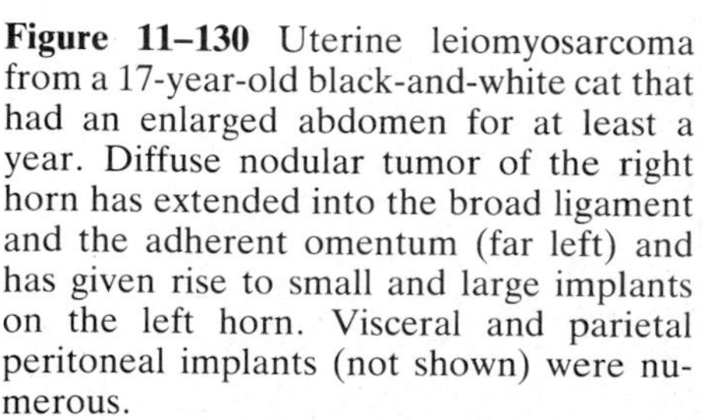
**Figure 11–130** Uterine leiomyosarcoma from a 17-year-old black-and-white cat that had an enlarged abdomen for at least a year. Diffuse nodular tumor of the right horn has extended into the broad ligament and the adherent omentum (far left) and has given rise to small and large implants on the left horn. Visceral and parietal peritoneal implants (not shown) were numerous.

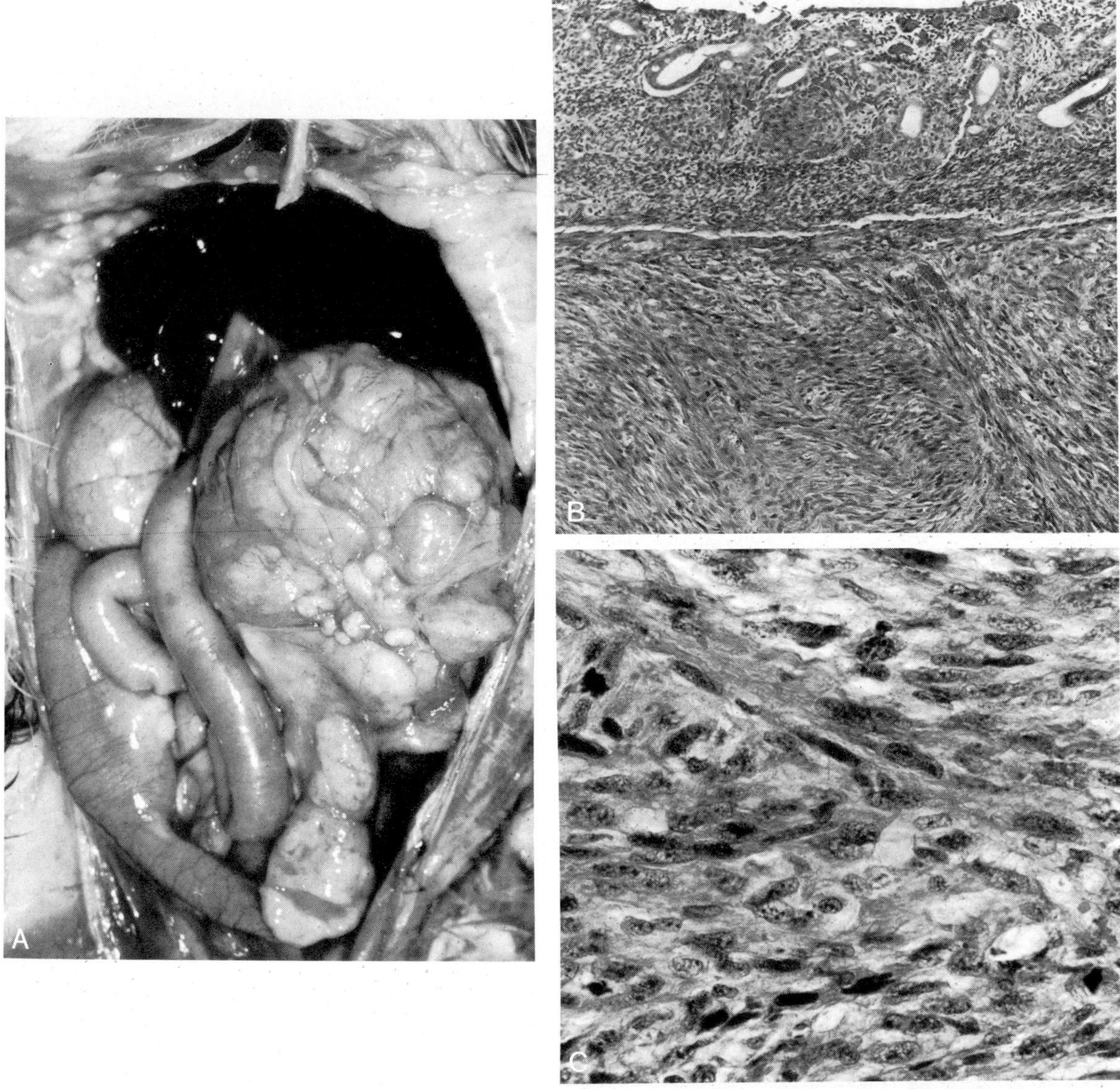


**Figure 11–131** *A*, Leiomyosarcoma of the uterus, 10-year-old cat. The tumor, which occupies most of the left side of the abdominal cavity, involves the left horn and is wrapped cranially in omentum. There are small, pale implants on visceral and parietal peritoneum. *B*, Leiomyosarcoma, same cat. Prominent interlacing fascicles of smooth muscle cells underlie attenuated endometrium. H & E, × 75. *C*, The leiomyosarcoma is characterized by dark-staining mitotic figures (upper left and lower right corners) and by spindle cells forming fascicles. H & E, × 800.

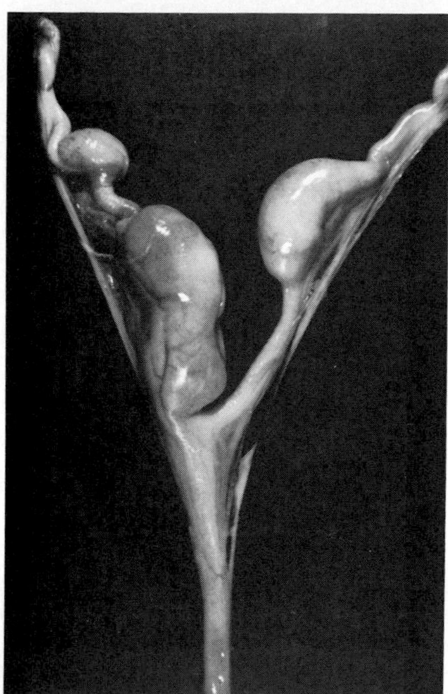

**Figure 11–132** Lymphoma involving segments of the uterine horns in a two-year-old cat with lesions elsewhere. Actual size.

Other malignant tumors reported were a squamous cell carcinoma (Bastianello, 1983) and a sarcoma of unspecified type (Priester and McKay, 1980).

### Tumors of the Vulva

Primary tumors of the vulva are rare. A leiomyoma (Patnaik et al., 1975) and a sarcoma (Petit, 1903) have been reported. Rarely, a mammary carcinoma involving a caudal mammary gland may extend to involve the vulva, infiltrating and deforming the lips (Petit, 1914–15).

## TUMORS OF THE MAMMARY GLANDS

As many surveys and case reports attest, mammary tumors are third in frequency in the cat after hematopoietic malignancies and tumors of the skin. Only in the dog is the incidence of mammary tumors higher. For over a century feline mammary tumors, as well as a variety of dysplastic lesions, have attracted the interest of pathologists and have occasioned the proliferation of a substantial and often confusing literature. The malignant tumors, especially, are of importance because of their relative frequency, their similarity to human tumors, and their lethal potential. Also of great clinical significance is fibroepithelial hyperplasia, a massive lesion unique to the cat and sometimes mistaken for a neoplasm.

An outstanding literature review and study is that of Hayden and Nielsen (1971). The most comprehensive recent work on mammary lesions of the cat is that of Weijer (1979), who brought together as a thesis, in one volume, a number of previously published studies in which he participated, supplemented them with additional material, and suggested modifications of the WHO classification for benign tumors and dysplasias of the cat. Large groups of mammary cancers diagnosed at The Animal Medical Center and at 15 veterinary teaching hospitals in North America have also been studied (Hayes and Mooney, 1985; Hayes et al., 1981; MacEwen et al., 1984a; Priester and McKay, 1980).

The majority of cats with mammary tumors are intact females, and one study indicates that they are at sevenfold greater risk than spayed females (Dorn et al., 1968b). Many of the neutered female cats were spayed within the first year of life; however, data have not been reported as to whether spaying *before* the first heat would have a further sparing effect, as it does in dogs (Fanton and Withrow, 1981). In rare instances intact and neutered male cats are affected (Hayes and Mooney, 1985). The vast majority of tumors of the breast in cats are highly malignant, spreading by both the lymphatic and the hematogenous routes. They may be well established in one or more glands and even ulcerated before they are detected beneath the cat's thick fur. Although reported in cats from 2 to 23 years old, the average age is from 10 to 12 years.

The majority of the malignant tumors are carcinomas (predominantly adenocarcinomas). Rare forms of carcinoma described from the cat are comedocarcinoma, in which areas of necrosis may become calcified (Bloom, 1954; Schönbauer, 1983), and myoepitheliomas (Gimbo, 1961; Überreiter, 1968). For definitive identification of the latter, examination by electron microscopy would be desirable to demonstrate contractile filaments. Spindle cell sarcomas, fibrosarcomas, myxosarcomas, and sarcomas of unspecified type have appeared in small numbers in various surveys.

In the small group of benign tumors are adenomas, papillomas, lipomas, cystadenomas, fibromas, and fibroadenomas (some of the latter, to judge from the descriptions, actually being non-neoplastic fibroepithelial hyperplasia).

"Mixed" mammary tumors are generally considered to be the exclusive specialty of dogs, but a few are on record in the cat (four, Kronberger, 1960; one, Schmidt and Langham, 1977; two specified as benign, Bastianello, 1983, and Überreiter, 1968; and eight as malignant, Hayes et al., 1981). An 18-year-old Siamese had a malignant mixed tumor in one gland and adenocarcinoma in another (Britt et al., 1979).

Because of the high incidence and pathogenicity of the carcinomas, excisional biopsy is the safest course with any cystic or nodular lesion in a feline mammary gland. Fibroepithelial hyperplasia in a young cat, to be described in detail, is the only exception to this rule.

In general, our discussion follows the classification of mammary lesions proposed by the World Health Organization (Hampe and Misdorp, 1974), but there will be a few divergencies or modifications based on detailed study of the large group of cases available at AMAH. Benign and malignant mammary lesions exclusive of simple cysts were diagnosed in a total of 284 cats at AMAH over a 35-year period. Several different lesions were often present in a single animal.

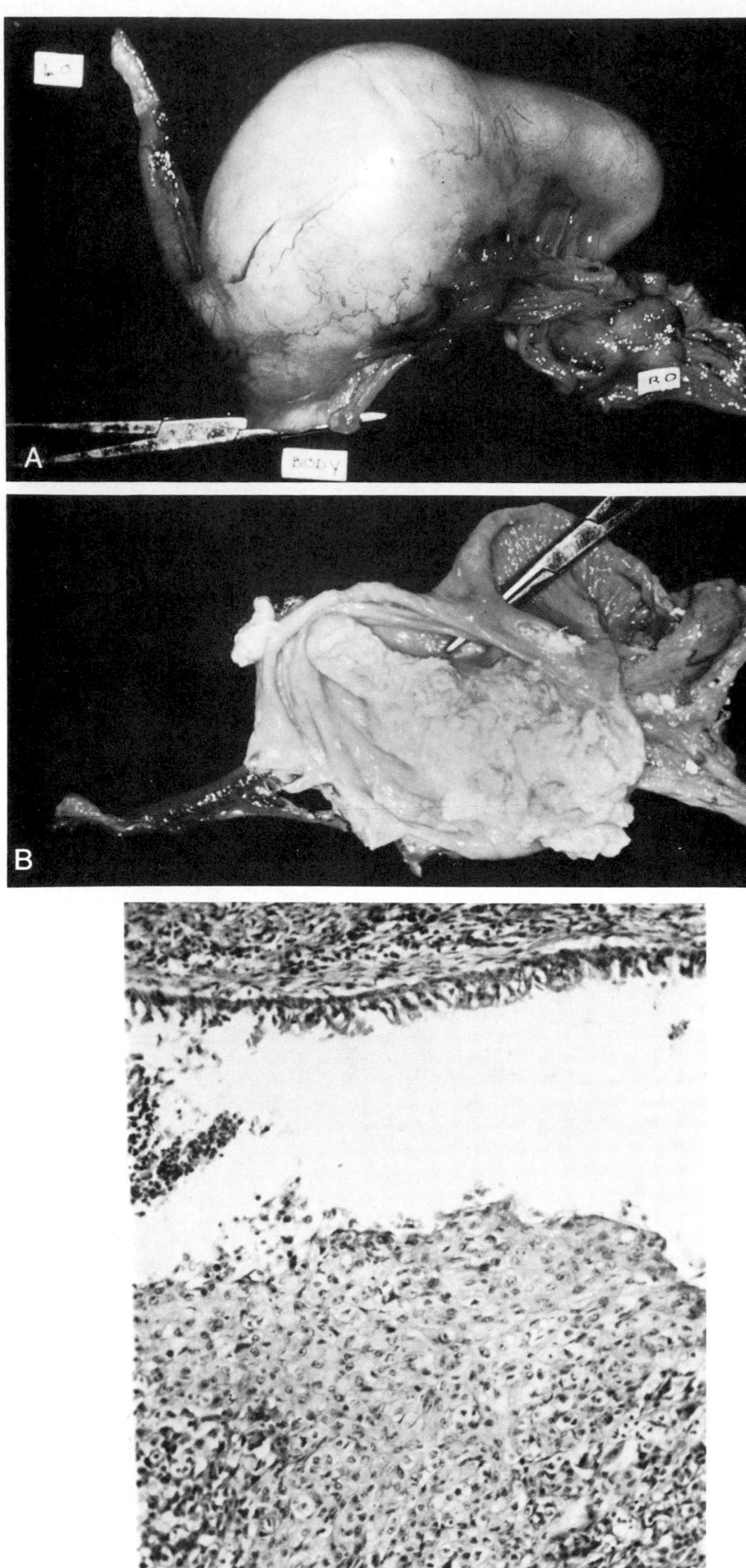


**Figure 11–133** *A*, Carcinoma of the uterus, cervix, and vagina, five-year-old cat. Enlargement of the right horn results from tumor infiltration and accumulated exudate. *B*, Opened uterine horn. Pale, raised, irregular endometrial lesions (center), which also infiltrated the cervix and vagina, were accompanied by endometritis and widespread metastases. *C*, The upper vaginal mucosal surface is inflamed, and the vaginal canal contains necrotic cells. Below, the tumor, composed of a sheet of epithelial cells with foci of necrosis, bulges into the lumen. H & E, × 180.

## Benign Dysplasias

**CYSTS AND DUCT ECTASIA.** Cysts of non-neoplastic mammary tissue are rare in cats. They may be felt in one or more glands as finely beaded or nodular areas. Grossly, they cannot be distinguished from early tumor. Microscopically the cysts appear as greatly dilated lactiferous and interlobular ducts with varying degrees of ectasia of the intralobular ducts. Hyperplasia of the cyst wall, if present, may be either an epithelial or a papillary proliferation. Varying degrees of mastitis, hyperplasia, and squamous metaplasia may accompany cystic ducts.

In mammary neoplasms, cysts varying in number and size are common and may be partly or wholly lined by neoplastic epithelium that is most often malignant.

**ADENOSIS.** Adenosis, a proliferation of ductal epithelium recognized microscopically, is said to occur rarely in the cat (Hampe and Misdorp, 1974) but was not recognized among the cases at AMAH.

**GYNECOMASTIA.** This uncommon condition, an abnormal enlargement of mammary glands in males, occurs occasionally in cats treated with progestogens for undesirable behavior or for certain skin disorders. (See discussion of fibroepithelial hyperplasia.)

**MAMMARY HYPERPLASIA.** There are two basic types of noninflammatory hyperplasia of the feline mammary gland—lobular hyperplasia and fibroepithelial hyperplasia (designated by the WHO [Hampe and Misdorp, 1974] as total fibroadenomatous change). The latter will be discussed later.

Lobular hypertrophy and hyperplasia are palpable lesions that may involve one or several glands, only a part of a lobule, or one or more entire lobules within a single gland. Enlargement is due predominantly to hyperplasia rather than to hypertrophy of cells. Lobular hyperplasia unassociated with neoplasia was recognized at AMAH in 13 cats from 1 to 14 years old (mean, 8). Only one was under four. Eight of the 12 females were entire. The thirteenth cat was an eight-year-old castrated male Siamese that had received megestrol acetate for personality changes (spraying and viciousness) that started during the owner's absence for a three-week period. The drug had been administerd at varying doses and intervals but usually at 2.5 mg daily for two to three months. The right inguinal gland was enlarged, and fluid could be expressed from the nipple. The other three caudal glands felt granular. The excised inguinal gland was uniformly hyperplastic and in an active secretory phase.

Lobular hyperplasia occurred in one to four glands simultaneously and most often in the two caudal pairs in the 13 cats. Three of the cats also had one or more malignant neoplasms, one cat had focal malignant change within the hyperplasia, another cat a focus of adenomatous change within a hyperplastic lobule. In two cats significant mastitis accompanied the hyperplasia.

The most common type of lobular hyperplasia involves one or more enlarged lobules with preservation of lobular organization, dense stroma, secretion in alveoli, and a cystic or dilated ductal component. Within some lobules one or more intralobular ducts may be lined by intensely basophilic cells. Multifocal ductal epithelial hyperplasia ("epitheliosis") is a variable component of lobular hyperplasia.

Adenomatous or malignant change might have been recognized more often elsewhere in a gland with a hyperplastic nodule if additional adjacent, normal-appearing tissue had been sectioned and examined as well as the nodule itself.

**FIBROEPITHELIAL HYPERPLASIA.** Unlike most benign mammary lesions, fibroepithelial hyperplasia is a striking entity recognizable grossly and of urgent clinical significance and apparently increasing incidence. A variety of terms have been used to describe these massive lesions. Total fibroadenomatous change (Hampe and Misdorp, 1974) is inaccurate, since not all glands and not all lobules within a single gland may be involved. Mammary hypertrophy, favored by several studies, is inaccurate, because the mechanism for enlargement of the breast is not hypertrophy but hyperplasia of both glandular epithelium and fibrous stroma. Fibroadenomatous hyperplasia (Nimmo and Plummer, 1981) is acceptable, but the designations adenoma, adenofibroma, and fibroadenoma, sometimes employed, are mistaken, since the lesion, unlike most neoplasms, regresses and disappears after estrus or spaying. In our opinion, fibroepithelial hyperplasia, suggested by Dorn et al. (1983), best describes the lesions that we have studied at AMAH.

This startling benign disorder, unique to cats, appears to have been known to two early French students of feline pathology, Petit and Germain (1912), and to have been observed in Italy by Roncati (1947), who described a case of "iperplasia mammaria di tipo virginale" in a 10-month-old female cat. In the United States, Bloom (1954) noted briefly that he had observed a "tremendous firm enlargement of unknown cause of all the mammary glands, without milk secretion, in unbred cats." He later (1974) suggested the term fibroadenomatosis as best describing the histologic characteristics.

Since the early 1970s the condition has received increasing notice. Published reports are most extensively reviewed by Nimmo and Plummer (1981) and by Mandelli and Finazzi (1983). Over 100 instances have been reported, the largest groups being the 11 cases of Allen (1973), the 9 of Hinton and Gaskell (1977), the 26 of Hayden et al. (1981), and the 27 of Hampe and Weijer (1979).

The disorder occurs predominantly in young, cycling or pregnant female cats and has even been seen in kittens believed never to have been in heat. Older unspayed females (up to 10 years) have been affected, as well as neutered cats, both males and females, treated with progestogens (megestrol acetate, medroxyprogesterone acetate) for such reasons as suppression of estrus, objectionable spraying, and skin disorders. One, several, or all glands may be affected, the most rapid development and extensive involvement occurring in young, cycling or pregnant females. One remarkable young tricolored cat went through two pregnancies in rapid succession, lactating normally despite tremendous enlargement of all glands and development of mastitis (Center and Randolph, 1985) (Fig. 11–134). Spaying terminated the process.

Thirty cases of fibroepithelial hyperplasia are on record at AMAH. The earliest was diagnosed in 1951. Three cats underwent biopsy in 1953, but no more than two cases were diagnosed in any one year until 1979 and 1980, with three and five cases, respectively.

Among the 30 cats were seven tricolors, representing three times the expected incidence at AMAH. It is of interest that none of the cats in the AMAH group was Siamese and that in other studies of this lesion they

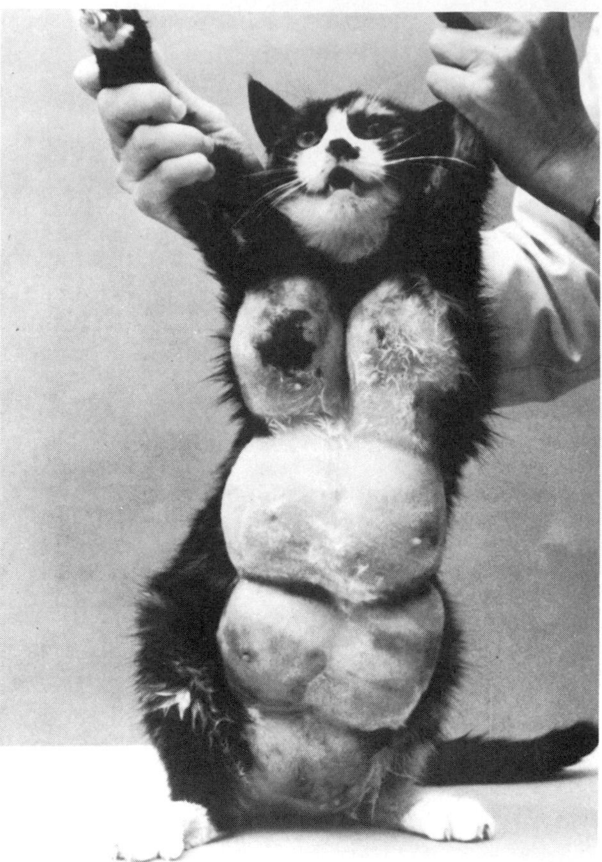

**Figure 11–134** Fibroepithelial mammary hyperplasia in a 10-month-old tricolor shorthair in late pregnancy. All breasts are tremendously hypertrophied. The sudden rapid enlargement has stretched the overlying skin, leading to focal ulceration. Although the glands are severely enlarged, they retain some identity from adjacent glands, unlike glands in most cases of acute mastitis. (From Center SA, Randolph JF: J Am Anim Hosp Assoc 21 [1985] 56–58.)

appear only rarely (Hayden et al., 1981). Whatever the significance, all but three of the 30 cats at AMAH were shorthairs.

Of 29 cats for which ages were known, the two youngest were 10 weeks and 4 months. Sixteen were aged 7 to 12 months, the age range in which most cats first come into heat. Four were aged three to five years, and five were aged eight to ten years. One of the 10-year-olds had both inguinal glands removed, and then at 13 suffered a recurrence for which the second left gland was removed.

All 30 cats were females; only one, an eight-year-old, was listed as spayed but there was some doubt about its status. The cats in the published reports were all entire females except for the neutered animals that had received progestogen therapy. Only one of the group at AMAH, a nine-year-old, had received hormone therapy (megestrol acetate), so that exogenous hormones were not a major factor. In contrast, five cats in Hinton and Gaskell's (1977) group and four in the group studied by Hayden et al. (1981) had received progestogens.

In 11 cats of the AMAH group all glands were involved, but in most of the older cats only one or two. In cats with only partial involvement the inguinal glands were affected twice as often as any of the others. There was no predilection for right or left side.

**Clinical Features.** Most affected cats exhibit mammary hyperplasia one or two weeks after their first estrus and are presented for veterinary care two or three weeks later. In the AMAH group, in contrast with cases in published reports, none of the cats was known to be pregnant when the condition was diagnosed. Affected cats usually appear to feel well, except that they may have difficulty in walking owing to enlargement of the glands, or they may be restless or show discomfort when handled. Discoloration of the overlying skin, edema, rapid increase in mammary size, and, occasionally, pain have led more than one veterinarian, unfamiliar with the condition, to diagnose mastitis.

With multiple involvement the glands vary in size even in the same pair. In one autopsy case of generalized breast enlargement, the glands weighed from 1 to 433 gm, constituting 27 per cent of the cat's body weight. The largest gland in the AMAH group of cats weighed 522 gm. The tremendously enlarged glands may be covered by pink, red, blue, or dark necrotic skin. The nipples are sometimes surrounded by a blue circular zone but may be difficult to locate because they have been stretched and flattened. Edema of the skin and subcutis of the ventrum and of one or both rear legs is common. At surgery or autopsy, the glands may adhere tightly to the skin but are easily removed, as they are sharply circumscribed and do not invade the body wall. Even the largest gland can, with patience, be separated by blunt dissection from its neighbors. One or more smaller nodules attached to the main mass were in two cases mistaken for lymph nodes.

**Gross Features.** The glands bulge on cut surface, are rubbery, and have white or bluish fibrous septa forming a reticular pattern. They contain pale yellow or pale gray foci, which may be round, linear, branching, or beaded, representing the epithelial component of the fibroepithelial hyperplasia. Edema, hemorrhage, and necrosis are variable but are most frequent and severe in the largest glands. Regional nodes are edematous and have blood-filled sinuses. Venous thrombi may be present.

**Microscopic Features.** Microscopically there are three basic patterns of fibroepithelial hyperplasia, but 83 per cent of the 30 cats studied at AMAH had only the diffuse lobular pattern, in which the degree of lobular involvement varied among the glands and within a single gland. The duration and the degree of glandular enlargement determine its microscopic appearance. The second pattern is intraductal fibroepithelial hyperplasia, and the third pattern, observed in only two cats, is a combination of the two patterns within the same gland.

The epithelial component of fibroepithelial hyperplasia accounts for only 5 to 50 per cent of the total mass, with an average of 20 per cent, the rest being stroma (Fig. 11–135). Proliferating epithelium forms repeatedly branching and often tortuous ducts lined by two to four layers of cells. This lining usually consists of an inner row of epithelial cells having round vesicular nuclei with a single prominent nucleolus, as well as a basal row of myoepithelial cells having an ovoid and less vesicular nucleus. The myoepithelial cells of the larger intra- and interlobular ducts have an oval or spindle-shaped hyperchromatic nucleus.

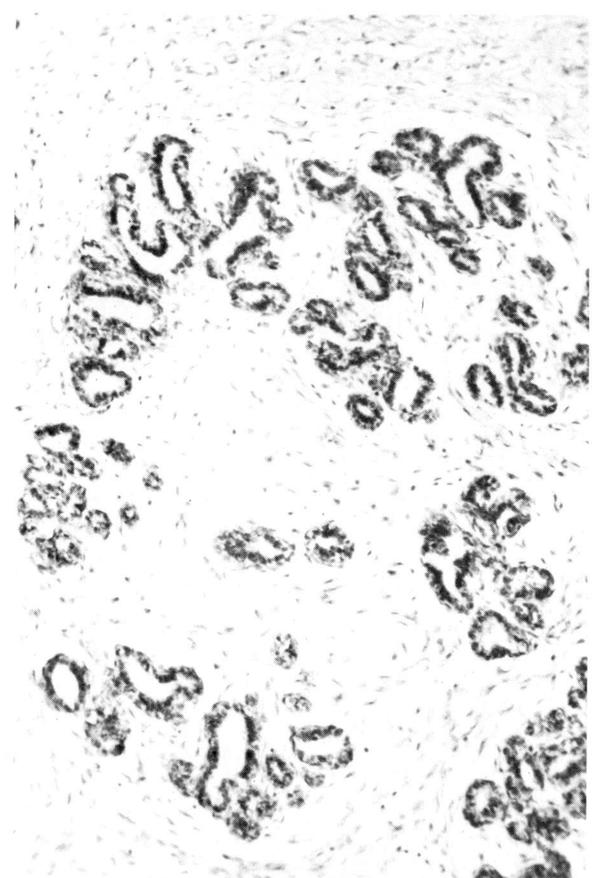

**Figure 11–135** Fibroepithelial mammary hyperplasia. Ductal and stromal proliferation, congestion, and edema account for rapid enlargement of the glands. H & E, × 180.

Alveoli with minimal secretion were observed in only 6 of the 30 specimens; the others were composed of empty ducts. Secreting alveoli had a double layer of cells, the basal myoepithelial cells being small and containing a densely basophilic nucleus variably oval, fusiform, or triangular. Intralobular ducts greatly outnumbered interlobular ducts.

The interlobular stroma contains more collagen fibers and fewer but larger fibroblasts than the paler-staining intralobular connective tissue. Arteries, large venules, and strikingly dilated lymphatics are restricted to the more eosinophilic interlobular tissue. Small venules and capillaries are not easily seen within the stroma formed by the smaller and hyperchromatic fibroblasts within the abundant intercellular matrix adjacent to the glandular epithelium. This intralobular stroma is sparse in collagen bundles but richer in acid mucopolysaccharide than the interlobular matrix. Mitotic figures are frequent in stromal and epithelial cells.

Ultrastructural studies (Hayden et al., 1983; Nimmo and Plummer, 1981) confirmed that myoepithelial cells do not participate in the formation of the intralobular stroma. Myoepithelial cells, as expected, were seen to contain cytoplasmic myofibrils.

The rapidly proliferating tissue is not encapsulated but invades the dermis, often reaching the superficial corium. The adnexa are displaced and the dermal vessels compressed, predisposing to congestion, ischemia, and, later, necrosis, ulceration, and infection. The lesion commonly extended through bundles of the panniculus carnosus but never infiltrated the deeper muscles.

The uterus and ovaries of 6 of the 30 cats were examined microscopically. Findings in five of the six cats were similar and characteristic of normal ovaries and uterus at metestrus. Large corpora lutea and follicles of expected types and size, including large secondary follicles as well as atretic follicles, were present in all the ovaries. All uteri were in the progesterone phase, characterized by numerous coiled glands having tall columnar epithelium with basally located nuclei and eosinophilic secretion in their lumina. These ovarian and uterine findings are compatible with the evidence that progesterone is implicated in the pathogenesis of this lesion and that progesterone receptors are present (Hayden et al., 1981).

The sixth cat, a four-year-old female, had parovarian cysts, a leiomyoma of the uterus, simple tubular adenocarcinoma of one mammary gland, and fibroepithelial hyperplasia of another gland that had more alveolar development and secretion than in any of the other cats.

**Autopsy Findings.** Autopsies were performed on five of the 30 cats. Three of the five had been destroyed and only mammary tissue was examined, but one had been noted to have pale mucous membranes and extensive hemorrhage in the two involved glands, which measured 12 × 9 × 5 and 8 × 7 × 4 cm. Two of the five cats had died after surgery. Both were anemic and had pulmonary arterial thrombi. One of the two, a nine-month-old female, had mammary and cutaneous venous thrombi, bacterial cellulitis, and bacteremia as well as pancreatitis and pulmonary arterial thrombi associated with severe intimal hyperplasia and infiltration by eosinophils. Causes of the eosinophilic arteritis and the pancreatitis were not determined. The other cat, a one-year-old, died with pulmonary emboli, myxomatosis of the left A-V valve, and fibroelastosis of the left ventricle. Large fibroblasts and abundant intercellular matrix indicated that the endocardial change was recent. Mild endocardial hemorrhage and macrophages, some with phagocytized red cells and hemosiderin, were also present, findings not characteristic of neonatal fibroelastosis. It was of great interest that the portal vein also had undergone intimal hyperplasia. Could it be that some types of collagen other than that of mammary gland—for example, collagen of intima and endocardium—also undergo hyperplasia in cats with this condition? More autopsy studies are needed to answer this question.

Both cats with pulmonary thrombi not only were anemic but also had pulmonary and subcutaneous edema, hydrothorax, and ascites. One had retroperitoneal and retropleural lymph accumulations, most severe about the cisterna chyli, as well as greatly dilated sublumbar lymphatics. Lymph production in the mammary glands was voluminous.

**Management.** Opinion varies as to management. Diuretics, corticosteroids, and testosterone have been suggested to reduce mammary engorgement until spaying, which is the ultimate solution (Stein, 1975). Unnecessary trauma and handling of mammary tissue should be avoided, to reduce the likelihood of venous thrombosis. Spaying should be avoided while the hyperplasia is present, but if for any reason it is considered necessary, a flank approach is indicated. In the classic case the diagnosis should be obvious, and mastectomy or biopsy is contraindicated; however, in older cats, in which neoplasia is possible, mastectomy is advisable as well as spaying to prevent recurrence. Histologic examination of mammary tissue should be performed to establish a definitive diagnosis.

The rapid, massive hyperplasia is a dramatic and severe local anabolic and general catabolic event. While development is swift, regression is slow, requiring up to five months after spaying for complete glandular atrophy.

Complications, both of the condition itself and of spaying, are common and may be lethal. Mastitis and ulceration may require hot packs and systemic antibiotic treatment. Severe cutaneous ulceration and mammary and cutaneous venous thrombi leading to emboli and pulmonary arterial thrombosis are not unusual. Intramammary and cutaneous congestion, edema, thrombosis, necrosis, and hemorrhage can result in blood loss, anemia, and hypovolemic shock. Sepsis accompanying cutaneous ischemia and necrosis caused death in one cat. The growth of mammary glands within a four-week period may reach 25 per cent of the body weight, subjecting the cat to nutritional and cardiac stress. According to experience at AMAH, the prognosis is guarded if surgery is done when the condition is full-blown. The mortality rate was 11 per cent (3 of 27) in the AMAH series of 30 cats, with the three cats dying within three days of surgery. Three others were euthanatized at the owner's wish. Owners should be reassured that the condition will usually regress naturally, at which time the cat should be spayed. Recurrence is not to be expected after spaying unless an exogenous progestogen is administered.

Male cats may develop mammary hyperplasia after progestogen therapy, but in the only affected male seen at AMAH after treatment with megestrol acetate the hyperplasia had a secretory pattern closely resembling that of normal lactating mammary gland, rather than that of fibrous and ductal epithelial hyperplasia.

## Benign Mammary Tumors

Few mammary tumors of cats are benign.

**ADENOMAS.** A relatively small number of adenomas have been reported (e.g., Bastianello, 1983; Hayden and Nielsen, 1971; Hayes et al., 1981; Schmidt and Langham, 1967; Weijer, 1979; Whitehead, 1967). Only 13 mammary adenomas were diagnosed at AMAH. All the cats were domestic, eight unspayed. They ranged in age from 6 to 16 years. Some had one growth, some several; four also had malignant mammary tumors.

Microscopically, the adenomas were of simple epithelial type. Complex adenomas, frequent in dogs, were not found. The simple adenomas were of three histologic patterns—tubular, tubular cystadenoma, and cystic intraductal adenoma. The most frequent, the tubular type, had either a lobular or a lobar pattern. The cystadenomas resembled the tubular type but had one or more cysts lined by a double layer of cells, giving the appearance of cystic ducts. One cystadenoma had foci of squamous metaplasia with abundant keratinization.

Cystic intraductal adenomas often resembled the common cystic adenoid basal cell tumors of skin and arose from papillary, lobar, or interlobular ducts. The intraductal, proliferating, pleomorphic "basal cells" formed glands, rarely with secretion, and ranged from fusiform to squamoid, the latter often lining the cyst. Keratinization was absent. Several growths were papillary and could have been termed intraductal papilloma. Similarly, Hampe and Weijer preferred to regard some of their benign tumors as papilloma rather than adenoma (Weijer, 1979).

**BENIGN MIXED MAMMARY TUMOR.** Only one of five mixed mammary tumors seen at AMAH was benign. This tumor, in a seven-year-old female, was an intraductal papillary growth consisting of epithelium, myxomatous myoepithelial tissue, hyaline cartilage, and dense, vascularized collagenous stroma. The same cat had a simple intraductal epithelial adenoma as well.

**BENIGN SOFT TISSUE TUMORS.** Hemangiomas, lipomas, and mast cell tumors may arise within or near mammary glands (Hampe and Misdorp, 1974) and may be mistaken clinically for tumors of mammary tissue. Osteochondroma and cavernous hemangioma have been reported in the mammary gland of the cat (Lasserre et al., 1938).

## Malignant Mammary Tumors

Malignant mammary tumors are an important cause of mortality in middle-aged and elderly female cats. Because they are hidden by the cats' thick fur they are often well advanced and have frequently metastasized before they are discovered.

**BREED.** Fifty-one (22 per cent) of the 227 cats at AMAH with malignant tumors were Siamese; 12 per cent were domestic tricolors. In contrast, Siamese cats represent 5 per cent of the total male and female hospital feline population at AMAH; tricolors, almost invariably female, represent 7 per cent. The relative frequency of malignant breast tumors in Siamese is generally recognized (Hayes, 1977); in a survey of 113 mammary cancers, 52 occurred in Siamese (Hayes et al., 1981).

**AGE.** The cats at AMAH ranged from 2 to 23 years of age (mean 11.1). Only four were less than five years old. Similarly, the ages of 170 cats in the Netherlands with malignant mammary tumors ranged from 2½ to 19 years (mean 10.8) (Weijer et al., 1972). An English group of 77 cats with carcinoma ranged from two to 20 years (mean 11.5) (Cotchin, 1983). Siamese are affected within a younger age range than other cats (Hayes et al., 1981).

**SEX.** Of the 227 cats at AMAH, 122 (54 per cent) were entire females, 102 (45 per cent) spayed females, and 3 (1 per cent) castrated males. Data as to age at spaying are incomplete; the majority were probably spayed before one year of age. Unfortunately, information was not available as to how many cats were spayed before the first heat. Spaying would appear to have some sparing effect, since in the general hospital population, only 27 per cent of females five years of age and over are entire. Dorn et al. (1968b), analyzing canine and feline neoplasms in California, found that intact cats had an approximately sevenfold higher relative risk of mammary cancer than cats spayed at about puberty. In the group of Netherlands cats, although data on a control population were lacking, of 154 females, 114 (74 per cent) were unspayed. Of the 50 females with malignant mammary tumors reported by Hayden and Nielsen (1971), 62 per cent were unspayed. In Cotchin's (1983) experience, mammary tumors usually occurred in entire females. The ratio of intact to spayed females was 58:52 in the study by Hayes et al. (1981).

Development of mammary cancer appears occasionally to be associated with prolonged use of a progestogen (e.g., Hayes et al., 1981; Hernandez et al., 1975; AMAH).

**CLINICAL SIGNS AND GROSS FEATURES.** Most cats with mammary cancer appear to be in good general health when first seen. In advanced cases with metastases, there may be weight loss and dyspnea.

The majority of malignant tumors of mammary gland are firm, flat, and nodular, and unless advanced are usually concealed by fur. Fluctuant cystic areas are occasionally recognizable on palpation. Often a tumor is not noticed by the owner until it is an ulcerated, foul-smelling mass plastered with soiled and matted fur. One owner mistook an ulcerated tumor for a slice of tomato stuck to the fur! About a quarter of the cats had at least one ulcerated tumor. Rarely, fistulae develop from a necrotic tumor or necrotic neoplastic node. A single ulcerated or draining tumor has occasionally been erroneously treated as a mammary abscess. Overlying skin is often tied down to a tumor even when ulceration is absent, but only rarely is a tumor fixed to the thoracic or abdominal wall. Occasionally a reddened, swollen nipple discharges bloody, yellow, or tan fluid. Sometimes a nipple is retracted and when squeezed exudes abnormal fluid, which may contain malignant cells (Engle, 1973; Hernandez et al., 1975).

Beadlike chains of tiny nodules suggesting venous or lymphatic invasion are occasionally palpated, as well as enlarged axillary or inguinal nodes. Extensive lymphatic and venous thrombi and emboli may cause diffuse swelling, edema, redness, increased local temperature, and pain, all of which can simulate mastitis.

Rarely, a tumor of great size or one characterized by severe fibrosis (desmoplasia) and contracture can prevent normal mobility and positioning of a limb. Only very rarely does a primary tumor remain small or undiscovered while giving rise to extensive metastatic lesions.

Among the 227 cats at AMAH with mammary cancer, a single gland was involved in 127 and two or more in the rest. Of 298 glands for which location was specified, 69 glands were of the cranial pair, 66 of the second pair, 71 of the third pair, and 88 of the inguinal pair. These findings contrasted with data reported by others. Cotchin (1983), Hayden and Nielsen (1971), and Moulton (1978) stated that the two cranial glands were most often involved. There was no significant difference between right- and left-sided involvement (147 and 151 glands, respectively) among the AMAH cats, although Weijer et al. (1972) reported that malignant tumors were significantly less frequent in the left second and third glands.

On cut surface mammary cancers are most often white but sometimes pale yellow, gray, or tan. They are lobulated and slightly granular and appear misleadingly as well demarcated. Foci of necrosis are common, as are cysts containing watery, milky, or puslike fluid.

In some cats variable numbers of glands may also be involved with one or more of the following lesions: chronic mastitis, hyperplasia, and adenoma.

Metastatic lesions in the cases at AMAH were most often recognized, in order of decreasing frequency, in lymphatic vessels and venules in the same gland, adjacent gland, or dermis (Fig. 11–136); regional nodes; lungs; pleural cavity; diaphragm; thoracic nodes; liver; kidney; adrenal; spleen; and bone marrow. Weijer et al. (1972) reported that in 129 autopsies, metastases were found in the regional nodes in 82.8 per cent, lung in 83.6 per cent, pleura in 42.2 per cent, and liver in 23.6 per cent. More extensive data on metastases are presented in a later study (Weijer and Hart, 1983).

**MICROSCOPIC FEATURES.** Adenocarcinoma, according to the consensus of surveys and reports, is the predominant type of mammary cancer in cats. Although we are in basic accord with the WHO classification of mammary lesions, we (JLC) have found it difficult in many cases to segregate adenocarcinomas from solid carcinomas and to further classify the adenocarcinomas into tubular, papillary, and papillary-cystic groups, because all four patterns are sometimes present within the same tumor and appear to have similar biologic behavior. In the discussion that follows, the adenocarcinomas and solid carcinomas are placed in a single category.

Of malignant tumors in 227 cats at AMAH, 180 (78

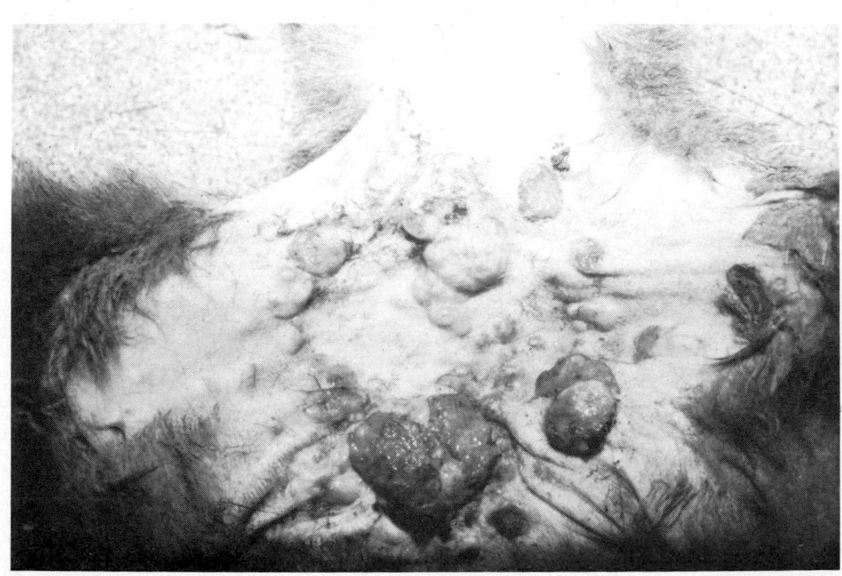

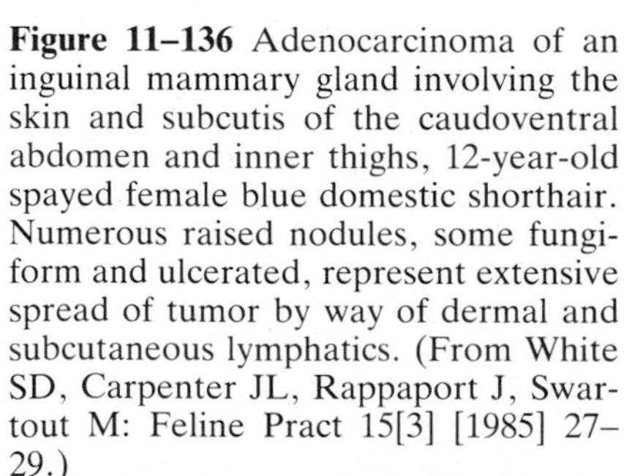

**Figure 11–136** Adenocarcinoma of an inguinal mammary gland involving the skin and subcutis of the caudoventral abdomen and inner thighs, 12-year-old spayed female blue domestic shorthair. Numerous raised nodules, some fungiform and ulcerated, represent extensive spread of tumor by way of dermal and subcutaneous lymphatics. (From White SD, Carpenter JL, Rappaport J, Swartout M: Feline Pract 15[3] [1985] 27–29.)

per cent) were adenocarcinoma–solid carcinoma; 40 (18 per cent) adenosquamous carcinoma; 4 (2 per cent) malignant mixed tumors; and 3 (2 per cent) possibly complex adenocarcinoma, although identity of the fusiform cells as myoepithelial was not clearly established. Many cats had more than one tumor and a combination of tumor types, some benign, some malignant. As noted earlier, tumors with myoepithelial cell components and tumors of mixed composition are extremely rare in cats although common in dogs.

**Adenocarcinoma–Solid Carcinoma.** The vast majority of tumors classified as adenocarcinoma–solid carcinoma had a combination of patterns, although one usually predominated: tubular in 63 per cent (Fig. 11–137), solid in 24 per cent, and papillary (Figs. 11–138 and 11–139) or papillary-cystic in 13 per cent. The tubular form most often had some tubules with epithelial proliferation resembling papillae, which, however, lacked supporting stroma and thus sometimes assumed an intratubular cribriform appearance (Fig. 11–140). Few tumors were purely solid; adenomatous differentiation could be found in over 90 per cent of the tumors with a predominantly solid pattern. Papillary and papillary-cystic growths are sometimes difficult to differentiate, since a judgment is needed as to when a space in which there is a papillary growth is to be called a cyst. In most adenocarcinoma–solid carcinomas the point of origin was impossible to ascertain, but a tubular rather than an alveolar origin was more often recognizable.

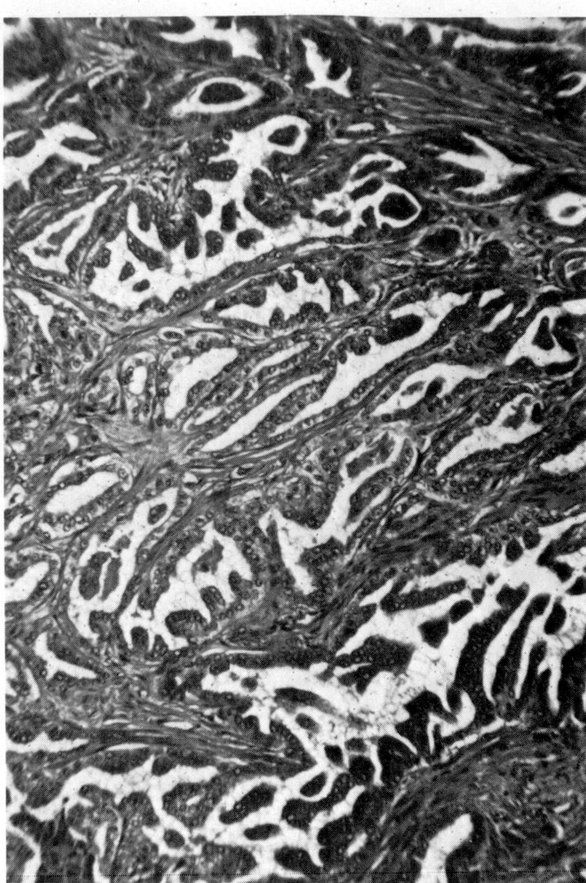

**Figure 11–138** Simple papillary adenocarcinoma, mammary gland, nine-year-old domestic cat. The pattern of branching tubules with intraluminal papillae is characteristic. H & E, × 180.

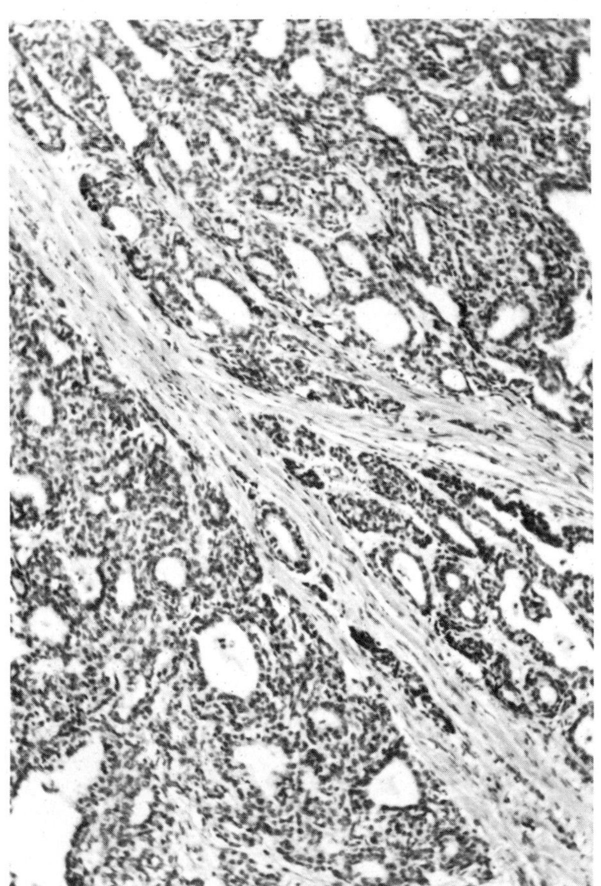

**Figure 11–137** Adenocarcinoma, mammary gland. The simple tubuloalveolar pattern with branching bands of fibrous connective tissue is the most frequent type in cats. H & E, × 180.

For the 180 cats with this type of tumor the age range was 2 to 23 years (mean 11.5).

**Adenosquamous Carcinoma.** In the adenosquamous carcinoma (adenoacanthoma), both squamous and adenoid components are malignant (Fig. 11–141). Tumors with benign squamous differentiation were not included in this category. Forty cats had this tumor type, with the squamous cells constituting from about 0.2 to 95 per cent of all neoplastic cells and always occurring in association with a glandular pattern. The squamous cells appeared in large solid regions or as individual keratinizing cells within a tubular or alveolar arrangement. Keratin "pearls" were infrequent. Fibroplasia was common in areas of the solid squamous component but not in adenoid regions. Vascular invasion was seen in 80 per cent of these tumors. Metastatic lesions usually had the same histologic appearance as the primary tumor, but a few lacked the squamous component. Sometimes an adenosquamous tumor could be clearly seen to originate from a papillary or lactiferous duct. A cystic neoplasm involving a nipple or its base often had a papillary pattern and, less often, adenosquamous differentiation. Adenosquamous carcinoma oc-

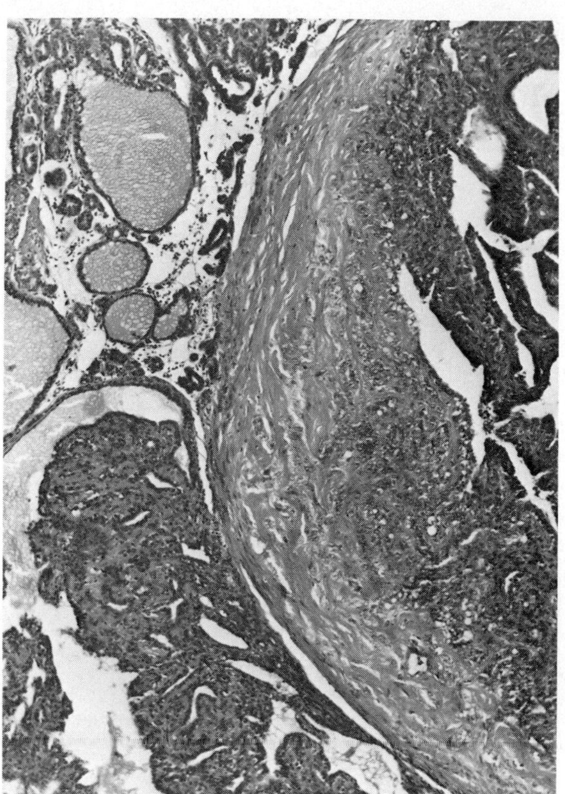

**Figure 11–139** Mammary tumor with benign and malignant elements, 12-year-old domestic cat. An invasive, sclerosing, simple adenocarcinoma (right) appeared to arise within a tubulopapillary cystadenoma (left). H & E, × 50.

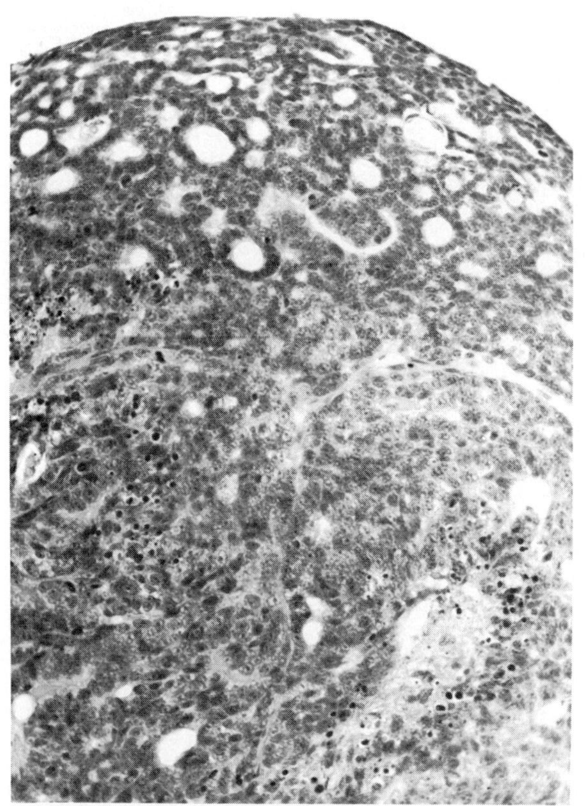

**Figure 11–140** Simple cribriform and solid adenocarcinoma, inguinal mammary gland, 10-year-old cat. The tumor, which had cribriform (top) and solid (bottom) patterns, had foci of necrosis (left center and lower right) and capsular and vascular invasion (not shown). H & E, × 180.

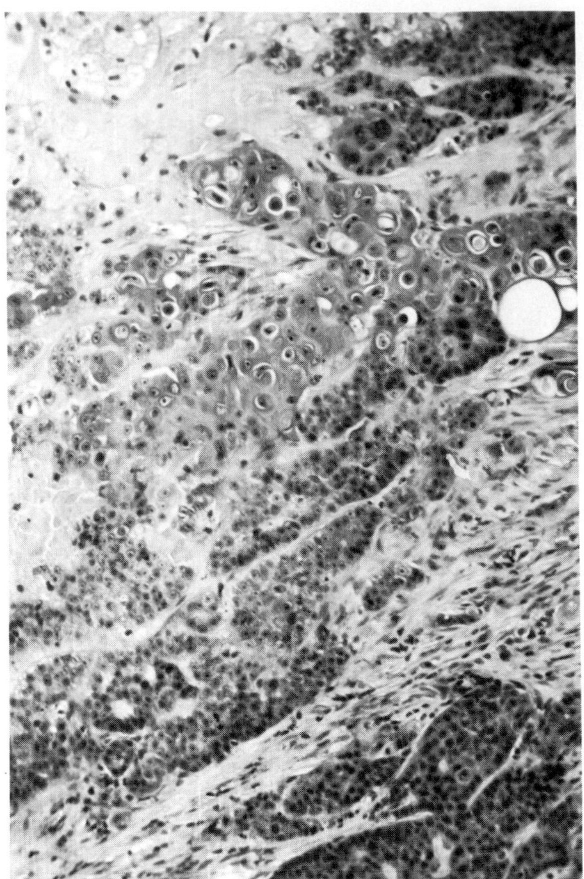

**Figure 11–141** Simple adenosquamous carcinoma (adenoacanthoma), mammary gland, 11-year-old cat. The malignant squamous cells (upper center) are accompanied by malignant glandular tissue and also by a fibrous component. H & E, × 180.

curred with about the same frequency in all glands. Ulceration was almost twice as frequent as with adenocarcinoma–solid carcinoma.

In the 40 cats with this type of tumor the age range was 2 to 23 years (mean 9.2). Eighteen of the cats were intact females.

**Malignant Mixed Mammary Tumor.** As noted earlier, mixed mammary cancer is uncommon in cats. In the AMAH group, four female cats (one unspayed), ranging in age from 9 to 12 years, had malignant mixed mammary tumors, all differing strikingly from one another. One cat had a tumor of the right second gland consisting of malignant epithelial and osseous tissue as well as an "osteosarcoma" of the skin of the perineum, which was probably a metastatic lesion. Another cat had a simple papillary-tubular adenosquamous carcinoma, with foci of hyaline cartilage within a dense fibrous stroma (Fig. 11–142). The third cat's tumor had a bizarre pattern of epithelial cells arranged predominantly in sheets but sometimes in tubules and a second population of pleomorphic cells of epithelial, spindle-shaped, and multinucleated forms. The mitotic index was high and necrosis extensive. The pleomorphic cells were associated with small foci of hyaline cartilage. Some areas of the tumor suggested a transition from neoplastic myoepithelial cells to mesenchymal cells differentiating into hyaline cartilage. The fourth mixed tumor was composed of malignant fusiform epithelial cells arranged in branching tubules in a stroma of densely packed, basophilic, spindle-shaped cells having a high mitotic index and arranged in fascicles. Within the sarcomatous areas were foci of differentiation into hyaline cartilage.

**Complex Adenocarcinomas.** Three tumors in the group at AMAH were complex adenocarcinomas or, less likely, simple adenocarcinomas. All had a prominent spindle-cell component. Electron microscopic or immunohistochemical examination would have been required to determine if the spindle cells were of epithelial or, as suspected, of myoepithelial type. The neoplasms occurred in tricolor cats aged 8, 9, and 16 years; two were entire females. Metastases were widespread in the oldest cat.

**Squamous Cell Carcinoma.** Squamous cell carcinoma of mammary gland occurs rarely in cats (Hayes et al., 1981; Kronberger, 1960; Überreiter, 1968). The records at AMAH did not note any tumors of this type. The diagnosis of a squamous cell carcinoma requires examination of several sections of a mammary tumor to be sure that no glandular component is present.

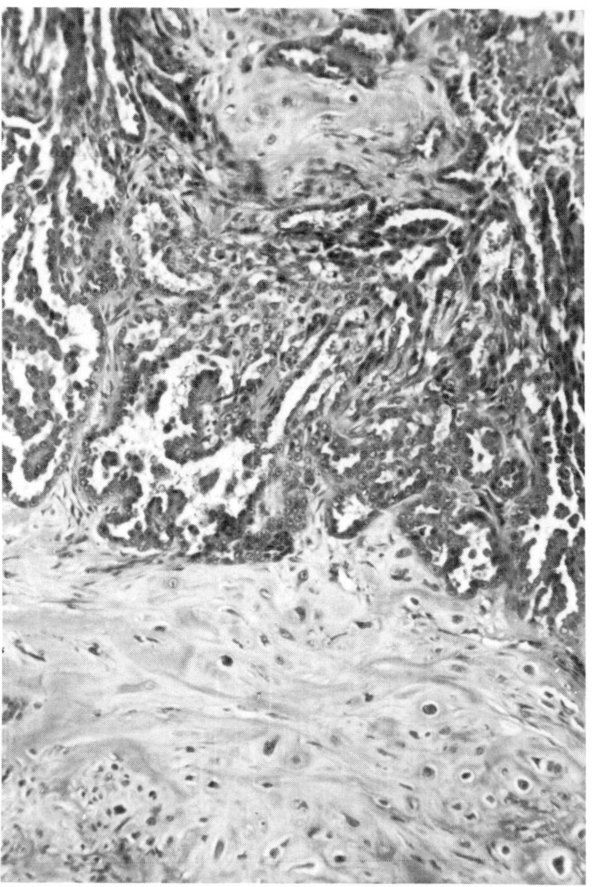

**Figure 11–142** Malignant mixed mammary tumor, nine-year-old domestic cat. This rare feline tumor consists of malignant epithelium in tubular and papillary arrangement (center) and areas of benign cartilage (top and bottom). H & E, × 180.

**PROGNOSIS FOR MALIGNANT TUMORS.** Ninety-six per cent of all mammary neoplasms of cats at AMAH were malignant. Stromal invasion was almost always seen; vascular invasion was detected in about 70 per cent of tumors studied carefully with one to three microsections, but was probably much more frequent since not all nodules present were routinely examined. These statistics dictate a poor prognosis when a mammary mass is detected, especially in a middle-aged or old cat.

Certain gross characteristics of a mammary mass are in themselves highly suggestive of malignancy: large size, poorly defined or irregular shape, discoloration and ulceration of overlying skin, fixation to the dermis or body wall, linear nodularity within the gland or adjacent skin, and enlargement of regional nodes.

Of all the factors examined for their prognostic value, tumor size is the most significant (MacEwen et al., 1984a; Weijer and Hart, 1983). Cats with a tumor measuring 8 $cm^3$ had a median survival rate of four and a half years, whereas cats with tumors of 9 to 27 $cm^3$ had a median survival time of two years; cats with still larger tumors had a median survival time of six months (MacEwen et al., 1984a). Other factors that are of prognostic value are microscopically tumor-positive lymph nodes, mitotic index, necrosis of the primary tumor, and histologic verification of completeness of surgical excision (Weijer and Hart, 1983). Older cats were found by Weijer and Hart (1983) to have worse survival rates.

Weijer et al. (1972) reported that the overall one-year survival rate was 10 per cent for cats with tumors of medium or high histologic grade and 50 per cent with low-grade malignancy. The histologic pattern or type of malignant feline mammary tumor in the AMAH group, and also in that of Weijer and Hart (1983), did not appear to be of significance in predicting length of survival. The type of surgery, conservative (segmental mastectomy) versus radical (block resection of chain and nodes) was significantly related to the disease-free interval but not to the survival time (MacEwen et al., 1984a). It is thus painfully apparent that adjuvant measures are needed in addition to surgery to prolong the life of cats afflicted with mammary cancer.

**MANAGEMENT.** With the exception of classic fibroepithelial hyperplasia, any growth in the breast of a cat two or more years of age should be promptly removed because the vast majority are malignant. Radiographs of the lungs should be taken before surgery; absence of visible lesions does not, however, guarantee that metastasis has not already occurred. The entire ventrum should be clipped and palpated to facilitate detection of small or multiple lesions. Advanced age alone is no contraindication for surgery, but a cat in poor health with concurrent disease or with evident metastatic lesions should undergo surgery only after the unfavorable prognosis is clearly discussed with the owner.

Prompt aggressive surgery offers the best hope for retarding the course of the malignancy and occasionally effects a cure or a survival period of several years. The surgical procedure is dictated by the nature of the vascular drainage of the cat's mammary glands.

The normal number of mammary glands in the cat is given by most authorities as four pairs, but in Crouch's (1969) experience, five pairs are more often present, the cranial abdominal teat sometimes being absent on one side. The two thoracic glands and the cranial abdominal gland drain into the axillary and accessory axillary nodes, the two caudal abdominal glands into the superficial inguinal node (Crouch, 1969; Nielsen, 1952a). Some of the mammary veins cross the midline (Crouch, 1969). It has been suggested that these may be a route of tumor metastasis from one chain of mammary glands to the other and also that the intercostal and intervertebral veins may serve as routes of metastasis directly through the body wall (Silver, 1966).

In view of the varied possibilities for metastasis, segmental removal of tumors with or without removal of the related nodes cannot be recommended. The protocol favored by many surgeons calls for en bloc removal of one or both affected chains and related lymph nodes if they can be located. The more severely involved chain is removed first, the other as soon as the first incision is healed. Some surgeons favor bilateral en bloc removal of glands and nodes, regardless of the numbers of mammary glands involved or the side affected. This course is justified by the finding that clinically normal glands may contain microscopic foci of tumor cells. Removal of a palpably affected node has only a slight chance of preventing further dissemination of a tumor but is of prognostic value. Although radical surgery may not affect survival time if metastases have occurred, the likelihood of recurrent tumor is reduced.

Because the majority of cats with malignant mammary tumors are not spayed, and because cystic ovaries and uterine disease of various types (cystic hyperplasia, polyps, endometritis, pyometra, and rarely tumors) often coexist with mammary cancer, it is well to spay a cat at the time the tumors are removed. In our opinion, oophorohysterectomy should precede mammary excision to decrease chances for infection and tumor transplantation. The order of surgical procedures should be reversed if an ulcerated and infected tumor lies in the surgical field of the spay incision or if the surgeon has doubt about how well the patient will tolerate prolonged surgery. A flank approach for spaying completely avoids the mammary area.

The necessity of thorough and regular follow-up examination must be stressed. The owner should be shown how to palpate the cat's ventral abdomen for early recurrence or new tumors and should be instructed to do so every two weeks and to return promptly if a nodule is detected.

Adjuvant forms of treatment (chemotherapy, immunotherapy, radiation) are still in the investigative stage (see chapter on management of feline tumors). A recent trial with levamisole gave disappointing results (MacEwen et al., 1984b). Trials with tamoxifen are in progress, but results are not yet available. Combination therapy with daunorubicin and cyclophosphamide has had some success in advanced cases (Jeglum et al., 1985).

Search for hormone receptors may someday provide a basis for other forms of treatment. In some human breast tumors the presence of estrogen and progesterone receptors is considered to enhance prognosis, since such tumors may be amenable to additive or ablative endocrine measures. In the cat, however, estrogen receptors were found in only 2 of 20 tumors (Hamilton et al., 1976), and none at all were found in other tumors studied (Johnston et al., 1984; Weijer, 1979). Progesterone receptors, however, have been demonstrated (Elling and Ungemach, 1981; Johnston et al., 1984) and may at some time provide the basis for endocrine treatment.

Virus particles (intracisternal A-particles and C-particles) as well as FeLV and RD-114 antigens have been identified in some feline mammary tumors (Calafat et al., 1977; Feldman and Gross, 1971). If a virus were shown to be involved in etiology, antiviral agents could conceivably be helpful.

## TUMORS OF THE ENDOCRINE SYSTEM*

### TUMORS OF THE PITUITARY GLAND

Tumors of the pituitary are infrequently reported in the cat. Almost all are adenomas and involve the anterior lobe (pars distalis and pars intermedia); tumors (pituicytomas) of the posterior lobe (pars nervosa) are rare. Of 289 nonhematopoietic tumors in 264 cats, four were adenomas of the pituitary (Patnaik et al., 1975). Two adenomas of the pituitary were found in a survey of 163 tumors (Whitehead, 1967) and one chromophobe adenoma in 226 tumors (Cotchin, 1983). An "epidermoid epithelioma" was reported by Diehl (1968). Five other tumors were the subject of case reports: two chromophobe adenomas, one in a 5-year-old castrated male Siamese (Nielsen, 1964) and one in an 11-year-old male domestic shorthair (Zaki and Liu, 1973); two acidophil adenomas in 6- and 12-year-old castrated males (Gembardt and Loppnow, 1976); and a pituicytoma in a 7-year-old spayed female Siamese (Zaki et al., 1975).

Eighteen pituitary adenomas were found at autopsy in cats at AMAH. Pituitaries were seldom examined before 1956 and were not always saved and examined microscopically until 1974, so the true incidence of pituitary tumors is likely to be much higher. Of the cats in which tumors were diagnosed, one was Siamese, one Persian, one a Maine Coon cat; 11 were domestic shorthairs and four were domestic longhairs. Of the 14 males, 12 were castrated; the four females were spayed. The cats ranged in age from 5 to 20 years (mean 12.7).

**CLINICAL FEATURES.** The two acidophil adenomas were associated with diabetes mellitus (Gembardt and Loppnow, 1976). One cat was destroyed because it failed to respond to insulin therapy, the other because of advanced heart disease. A space-occupying pituitary mass caused neurologic signs in three cats (Nielsen, 1964; Zaki and Liu, 1973; Zaki et al., 1975). Signs in more than one case included anorexia, behavioral changes, and altered pupillary reflexes. A chromophobe tumor that compressed the left optic nerve led to blindness (Nielsen, 1964). One cat with a chromophobe adenoma that invaded the hypothalamus and thalamus had periodic fevers and testicular atrophy and became obese (Zaki and Liu, 1973). The third cat had a large pituicytoma that compressed the ventral hypothalamus and thalamus, causing altered gait and increased patellar reflexes in both legs (Zaki et al., 1975).

Two cats at AMAH had neurologic disturbances due to compression of adjacent neural structures. One, an eight-year-old castrated male domestic shorthair, became less active and aggressive and developed a slow deliberate gait. It stopped purring, began staring into space, wandered aimlessly, and urinated and defecated outside its litter box. A CAT scan disclosed a large midline mass in the area of the pituitary (Fig. 11–143*A*). Autopsy revealed a 2.1 × 1.2 × 1.0 cm pink and gray adenoma of the pars intermedia composed of cells with lightly amphophilic granular cytoplasm and fewer cells with clear-staining cytoplasm (chromophobes). The tumor compressed and

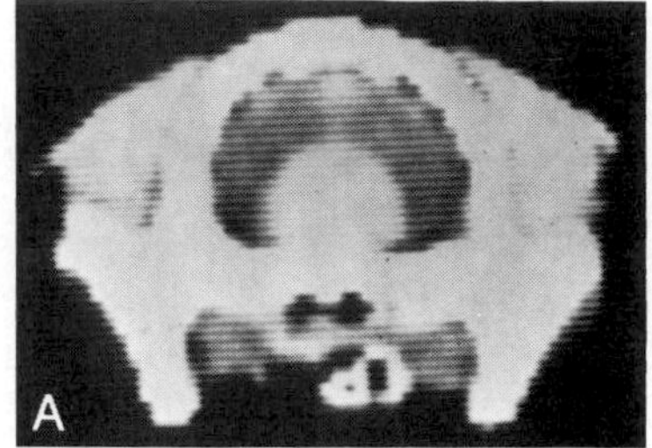


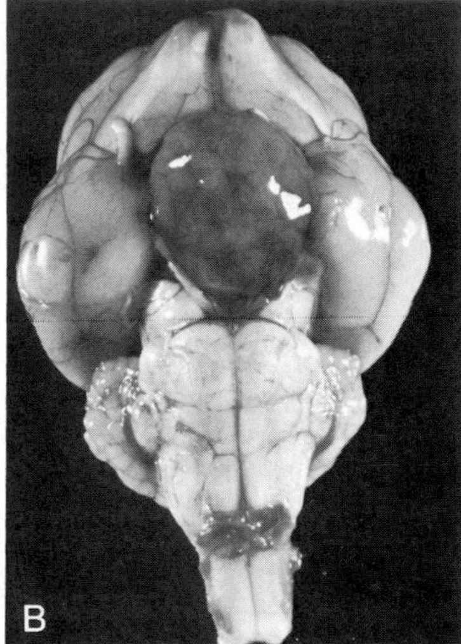


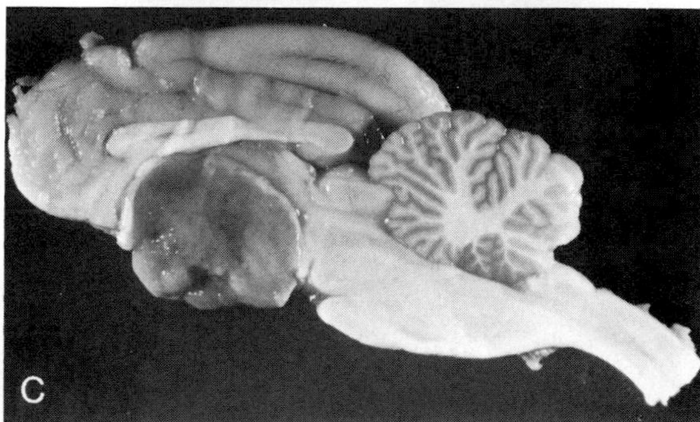


**Figure 11–143** *A*, Adenoma of the pituitary, eight-year-old castrated male domestic shorthair. CAT scan disclosed a large ventral midline mass in the region of the pituitary. There is no hydrocephalus. *B*, The smooth spherical mass arose from the pars intermedia and caused personality changes, poor vision, and slow gait. Actual size. *C*, Sagittal section shows the tumor to be discrete. It compressed and distorted the hypothalamus and thalamus and displaced the optic chiasm forward and the oculomotor nerves laterally (not shown). Actual size.

*Laura K. Andrews, principal author, except for the sections on the thyroid and parathyroid glands.

displaced the optic chiasm, optic tracts, pars distalis, and hypothalamus (Fig. 11–143*B* and *C*). Cushing's disease was diagnosed on the basis of bilateral diffuse adrenocortical hyperplasia, the cortices being 0.3 cm wide. Diffuse hepatic fatty change was believed to be related to mild obesity (4.77 kg). The second cat with neurologic signs was a seven-year-old castrated male Maine Coon cat with what appeared to be a sudden onset of blindness. Decreased locomotor activity and bumping into objects heralded the clinical course. Dilated fixed pupils, absence of menace reflex, and normal retinas, along with mental dullness, inappropriate toilet habits, decreased proprioception and hopping reflex in left limbs, and circling to the left pointed toward central blindness with a lesion involving the optic and the right cerebrospinal pathways. A 1.2 × 1.2 × 0.4 cm basophil adenoma, probably originating in the pars intermedia, was found at autopsy compressing and displacing the optic chiasm and tracts and extending cranially from the septal nucleus and caudally to the cerebral peduncles. The only other lesion was acute, bilateral, multifocal adrenal cortical necrosis at the junction of the zona fasciculata and zona reticularis, suggesting a vascular pathogenesis.

**GROSS FEATURES.** Both cats with acidophil adenomas had vacuolated beta cells of the pancreatic islets, and one had insular amyloid (Gembardt and Loppnow, 1976). In one cat, a chromophobe tumor in the sella turcica destroyed the pituitary, left optic nerve, and lower hypothalamus (Nielsen, 1964). In another cat a chromophobe adenoma of the pars distalis invaded the ventral thalamus and caused dilatation of the lateral ventricles (Zaki and Liu, 1973). In the cat with a tumor of the pars nervosa, the pituitary tumor compressed the pars distalis, hypothalamus, and thalamus (Zaki et al., 1975).

Most cats at AMAH had a subtly enlarged or normal-sized pituitary. Only six had tumors large enough to be easily seen. The tumors ranged from 0.1 to 2.1 cm in greatest dimension, only three being 1.0 cm or larger. A cystic component was seen in at least three (Fig. 11–144). When the smaller pituitaries were carefully sectioned into two or three pieces before processing, discrete, whitish yellow or pinkish foci, pinpoint to 0.3 cm in diameter, could be seen. The largest tumors were soft and tan or light gray. All cats had lesions in other endocrine organs. Thirteen had multinodular adenomatous hyperplasia of the thyroid follicular epithelium, five with signs of hyperthyroidism. A different group of 13 had diffuse or nodular hyperplasia of the adrenal cortex, and still another cat had a microscopic pheochromocytoma. Nodular hyperplasia of the exocrine pancreas was present in 14 of 17 examined. Five cats were diabetic. Sixteen of the 18 cats died or were destroyed because of one or more other disorders: diabetes mellitus (five), congestive heart failure (five), pulmonary bronchial adenocarcinoma (one), eosinophilic leukemia (one), plasma cell tumor (one), thymoma (one), osteosarcoma (one), plasma cell stomatitis (one), lingual candidiasis (one), and erosive esophagitis and duodenitis (one). Two cats were destroyed because of the severity of signs related to the pituitary tumor.

**MICROSCOPIC FEATURES.** The pars distalis was the site of 11 of the 12 tumors reported in the literature (Cotchin, 1952; Gembardt and Loppnow 1976; Nielsen, 1964; Patnaik et al., 1975; Whitehead, 1967; Zaki and Liu, 1973) and of 13 of 18 at AMAH. One pituicytoma of the pars nervosa was reported (Zaki et al., 1975).

Tumors of the pars distalis and pars intermedia are classified traditionally as basophil, acidophil, or chromophobe adenomas according to the affinity of their granules for H & E stain. All tumors of the pars distalis at AMAH were single, multiple, or confluent nodules, which were well delineated and compressed the pars distalis. Three were acidophil and ten were chromophobe-basophil adenomas. Some of the latter group had many cells with lightly staining basophilic, granular cytoplasm and fewer cells with clear cytoplasm. In five cats the tumors appeared to arise from the pars intermedia and in four cats were composed of polygonal cells with pale, granular, eosinophilic cytoplasm; the fifth tumor was similar except for its basophilia. The cells were arranged in perisinusoidal palisades and alveoli, some forming colloid-filled follicles, which were frequent in four tumors and infrequent in the

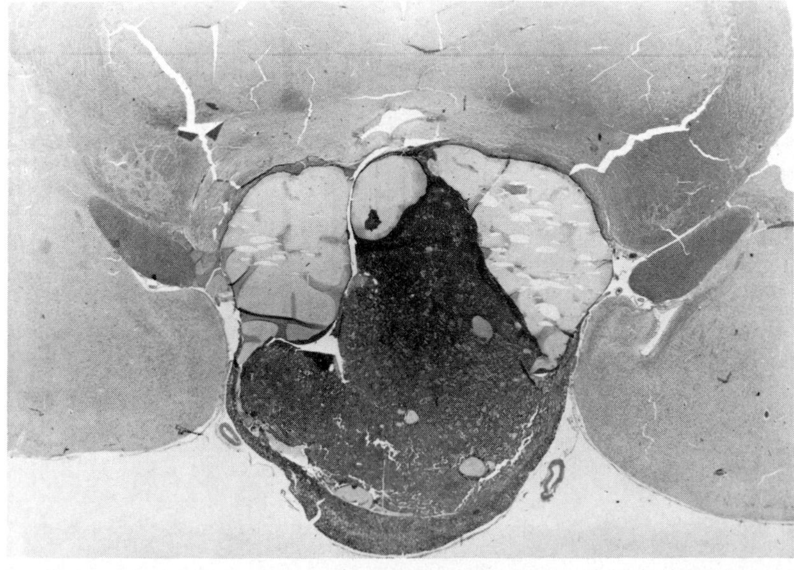

**Figure 11–144** Adenoma of the pars intermedia of the pituitary in a diabetic 11-year-old castrated male silver Persian. The tumor compressed and distorted the hypothalamus and flattened the pars distalis into a narrow crescent. Several large and small colloid-filled cysts and many follicles were formed by the basophilic cells. An additional, and possibly secondary, lesion was a striking diffuse and nodular adrenocortical hyperplasia. H & E, × 5.

fifth. Two tumors were discrete nodules; the others destroyed the pituitary, except for a small rim of pars distalis and pars intermedia, and compressed the hypothalamus.

The single tumor recognized in the pars nervosa was composed of loosely arranged, interlacing bundles of bipolar and polyhedral cells; a large cyst contained mucinous fluid (Zaki et al., 1975).

Recently, immunocytochemical techniques have enabled pathologists to identify cells of the pars distalis and pars intermedia by the content of their secretory granules. Therefore it is now possible to name tumors according to their function (El Etreby et al., 1980). Tumors of ACTH-secreting cells have been correlated with elevated serum ACTH and cortisol levels in dogs with hyperadrenocorticism, and dogs with mammary dysplasia or tumors have been found to have hypertrophy and hyperplasia of growth-hormone cells of the pituitary (El Etreby et al., 1980). Immunocytochemical staining of normal and neoplastic pituitary glands of the cat could conceivably explain the relationship between pituitary tumors and endocrine disease or lesions that appear to be common in cats—multinodular adenomatous hyperplasia of the thyroid, adrenal cortical hyperplasia, and diabetes mellitus.

It is interesting that all three cats with acidophil adenomas of the pars distalis, like the two cats reported by Gembardt and Loppnow (1976), had diabetes mellitus (Fig. 11–145). Acidophils are presumed to secrete growth hormone, and cats given growth hormone often develop diabetes (McDonald, 1980). Two cats with basophil adenomas also had diabetes (Fig. 11–146).

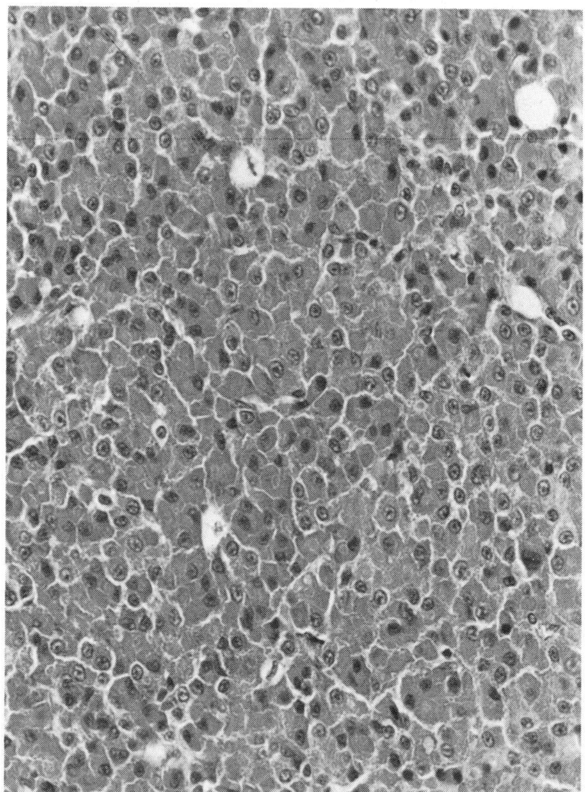

**Figure 11–145** Acidophil adenoma of the pars distalis of the pituitary in a diabetic 13-year-old castrated male tabby. The tumor consists of compact polyhedral cells with abundant granular cytoplasm and eccentric euchromatic nuclei that usually have one conspicuous central nucleolus. The cat also had diffuse adrenocortical hyperplasia. H & E, × 300.

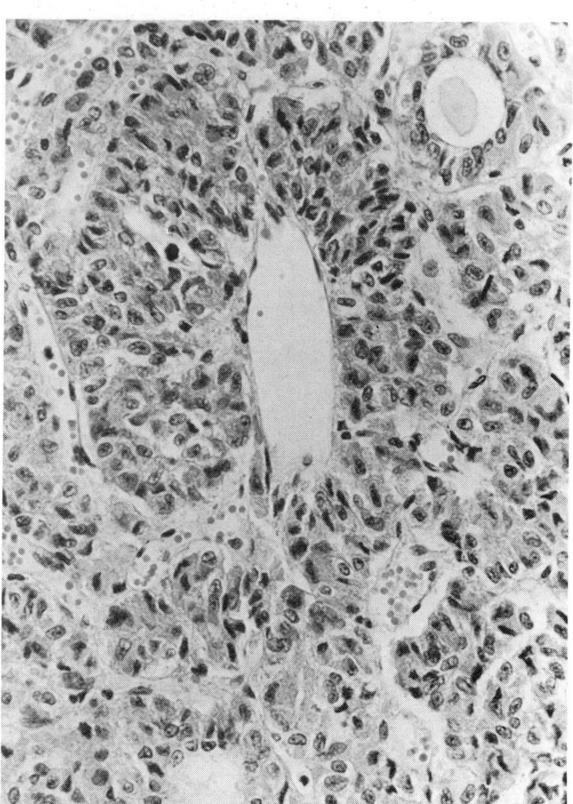

**Figure 11–146** Basophil adenoma of the pars intermedia of the pituitary in a diabetic 13-year-old castrated male tabby. The neoplastic cells are arranged in packets, cords, and follicles (upper right). Vascularity and nuclear pleomorphism are other notable features. As with the adenomas pictured in Figures 11–144 and 11–145, there was an associated finding of diffuse and nodular adrenocortical hyperplasia. H & E, × 300.

Five cats with clinical signs of hyperthyroidism had basophil-chromophobe adenomas, all of the pars distalis. Basophils are known in man to secrete TSH. Chromophobes may be degranulated cells or precursors of cells that secrete TSH. Prospective and retrospective studies of pituitary morphology and function in intact and neutered normal cats and in cats with endocrine disease are needed to clarify the relationship between pituitary tumors and endocrine disorders.

**BEHAVIOR.** Most pituitary tumors appear to be incidental findings at autopsy. Occasionally large tumors grow dorsally, compressing the hypothalamus and adjacent cranial nerves. One cat presented to a veterinarian for personality changes died seven months later from the effects of a chromophobe adenoma (Zaki and Liu, 1973).

Tumors diagnosed ante mortem have been removed successfully from dogs. The cat's pituitary, however, is surrounded by an arteriolar plexus, so that the surgical removal of a tumor would be technically more difficult (Averill, 1981).

## Hyperplasia of the Pituitary

The incidence of focal and nodular hyperplasia of the pars distalis of the pituitary of cats is unknown. This lesion is common in aged mammals (Jubb and Kennedy, 1970), but veterinarians are just beginning to recognize its importance in the dog (El Etreby et al., 1980).

In a review of 32 cats at AMAH with multinodular adenomatous hyperplasia of the thyroid, 8 for which sections of the pituitary were available had hyperplastic lesions of the pars distalis. They were neutered domestic cats ranging in age from 10 to 16 years (mean 14). Five had clinical signs of hyperthyroidism, two had diabetes mellitus, and the eighth had nutritional bone disease. The pituitary hyperplasia was a microscopic lesion consisting in six cats of focal and in two cats of diffuse, ill-defined proliferations of basophils, chromophobes, or acidophils. The pituitary was not compressed, and the cells of the hyperplastic foci were arranged in a pattern similar to that of normal pituitary.

Immunocytochemical stains and the study of additional sections would probably have increased the number of hyperplastic foci found in the 32 cats studied; however, it is difficult in a retrospective study of autopsy tissue to correlate morphologic changes of the pituitary with morphologic or functional changes in other organs. For confirmation of the apparent cause and effect relationship between adenomas or hyperplastic foci of the pars distalis and hyperplastic changes in thyroids, normal intact and neutered cats of the same age must be studied.

## Tumors of the Adrenal Gland

**TUMORS OF THE ADRENAL CORTEX.** Adrenal cortical tumors are rare in the cat. Four adenomas have been recorded in surveys (Patnaik et al., 1975; Priester and McKay, 1980; Whitehead, 1967), and a unilateral adenoma was described as the cause of hyperadrenocorticism (Meijer et al., 1978). Adrenocortical adenocarcinomas have been recorded in two surveys (Bastianello, 1983; Poppensieck, 1961).

At AMAH a 10-year-old spayed female domestic shorthair had a soft yellow-tan adenoma 1.0 cm in greatest dimension extending deep into the medulla of the left adrenal (Fig. 11–147). The tumor was composed of well-differentiated polygonal, cuboidal, and columnar cells with round or oval nuclei and granular eosinophilic cytoplasm. The cells were arranged in lobules, ribbons, and nests separated by a fine fibrovascular stroma. Nuclei were round with one or more nucleoli and had a thin rim of dense chromatin at the nuclear margin. The tumor, which was partially encapsulated, compressed adjacent cortex and medulla. Clinical signs were fever, inappetence, and painful abdomen, and autopsy disclosed chronic active pancreatitis. There were no signs of hyperadrenocorticism to prompt performance of tests that would have determined the functional status of the tumor.

Another cat, a seven-year-old castrated male, had a large adrenal cortical adenoma (Fig. 11–148*A*) that was probably functional in light of the clinical signs and pathologic findings. Increased appetite and thirst, thin soft skin, and an abscess of the neck that failed to respond to therapy could all be manifestations of hyperadrenocorticism. The character of the tumor (Fig. 11–148*B* and *C*), the atrophy of the opposite gland (Fig. 11–148*D*), and the atrophy of the skin (Fig. 11–148*E*) support the impression of a functional tumor.

Adenomas of cortical cells must be distinguished from nodular hyperplasias, which are common in the adrenals of aged cats. Hyperplasias are small, usually multiple, pale, yellow-tan nodules in the cortex or medulla that are often slightly firmer than surrounding tissue and may appear to extend beyond the capsule. These benign growths are unencapsulated but may compress adjacent tissue (Fig. 11–149). The functional significance of hyperplasia is unknown.

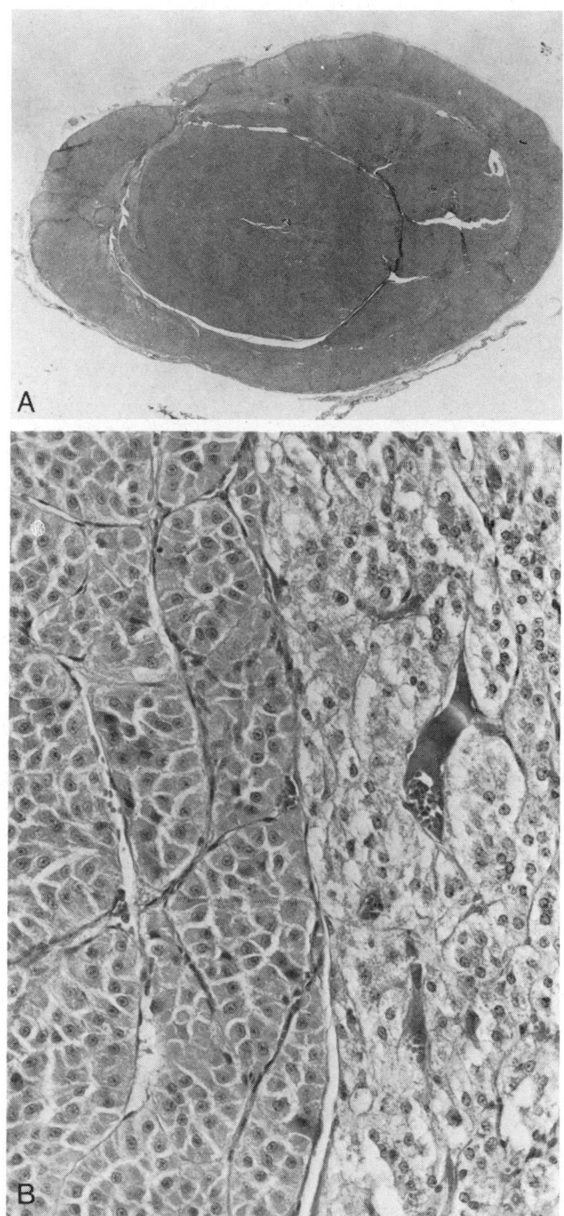


**Figure 11–147** *A*, Adrenocortical adenoma extending deep into the medulla, 10-year-old cat. The dark lobulated tumor occupies most of the gland. *B*, The adenoma (left), composed of polyhedral cells, has an insular pattern—compact packets of cells separated by a fine fibrovascular stroma. Compressed medullary cells are on the right. H & E, × 200.

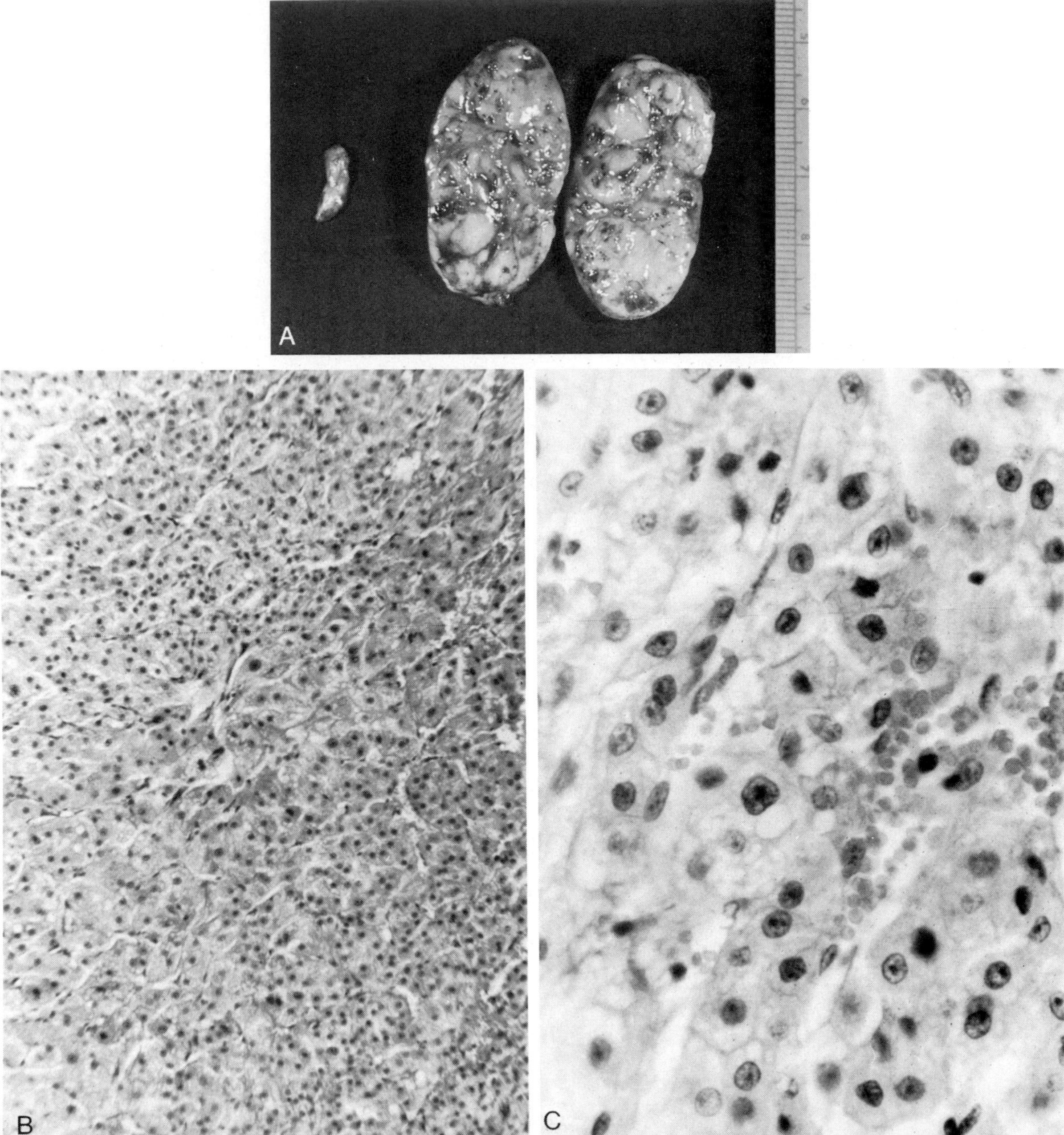


**Figure 11–148** *A*, Adrenocortical adenoma, seven-year-old castrated male. The size of the tumorous right adrenal (sectioned) and the atrophy of the left adrenal suggest that the tumor was functional. *B*, Pleomorphic cortical epithelial cells, with small cytoplasmic vacuoles and without orderly arrangement, form small packets and cords within minimal stroma. H & E, × 180. *C*, Same tumor, higher magnification. H & E, × 760.

*Illustration continued on opposite page*

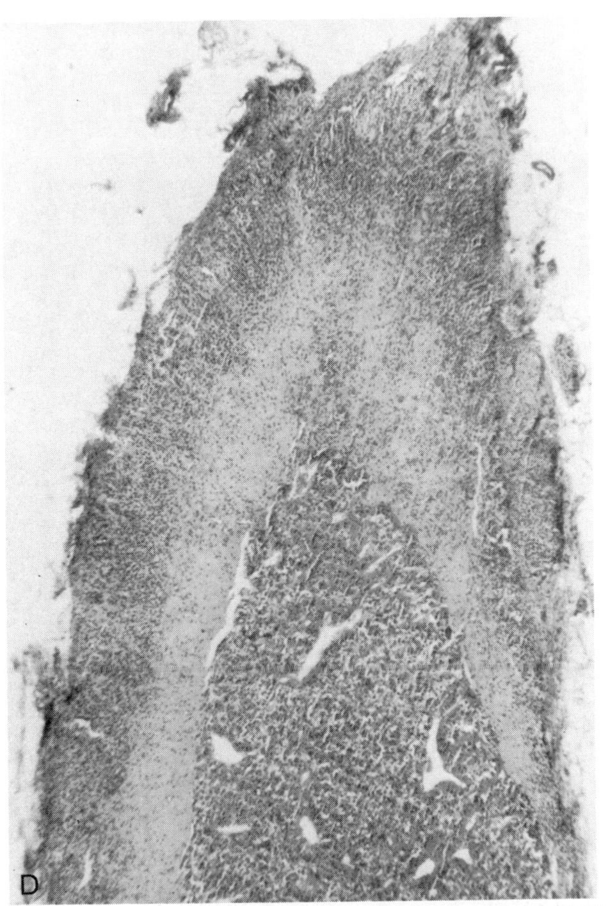


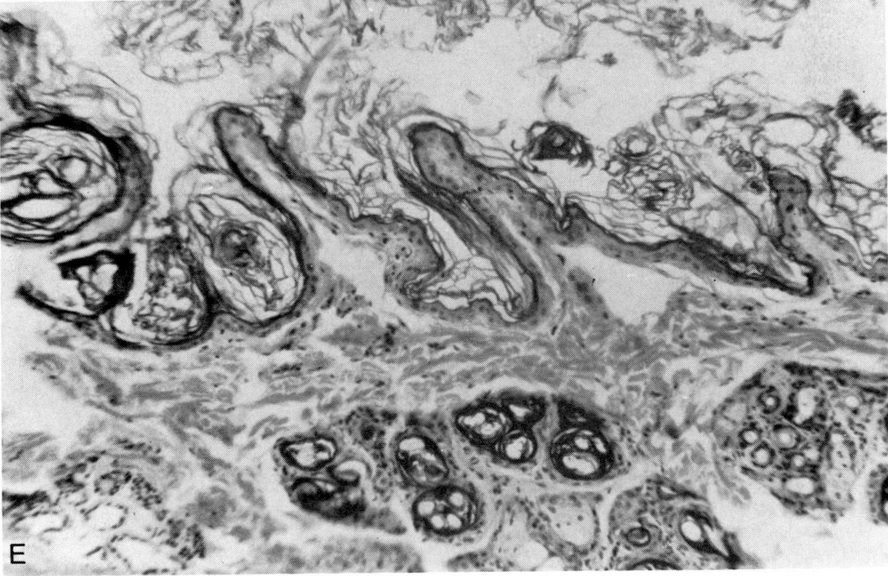


**Figure 11–148** *Continued D*, Atrophic left adrenal. A pale, broad band of collagen, largely replacing the zona reticularis and inner zona fasciculata, separates the remaining atrophic cortex from the medulla. H & E, × 64. *E*, Skin, same cat. Hyperkeratosis and epidermal and adnexal atrophy strongly suggest an endocrine dermatopathy compatible with hyperadrenocorticism. H & E, × 180.

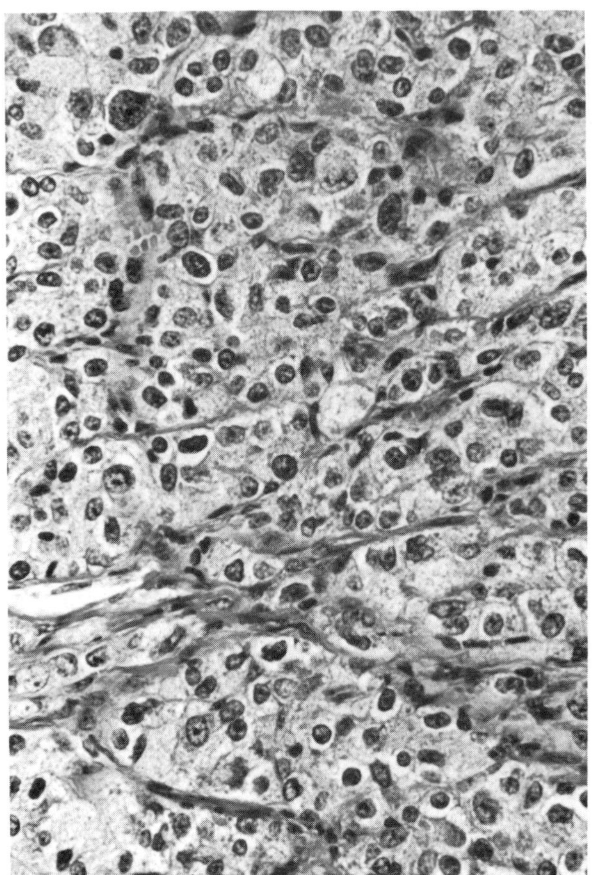

**Figure 11–160** Carotid body tumor, 15-year-old black-and-white spayed female domestic shorthair. Cells with small heterochromatic nuclei and others with larger euchromatic nuclei are in clusters separated by a fine fibrovascular stroma. Anisonucleosis, insular pattern, and argyrophilic granules are prominent features. H & E, × 312.

cussed in the section on tumors of the adrenal. Extra-adrenal chromaffin paragangliomas are rare in cats, as are the nonchromaffin paragangliomas.

Retroperitoneal paragangliomas were diagnosed in two spayed female domestic shorthairs at AMAH. The benign tumor, in a 15-year-old, was asymptomatic. The malignant tumor occurred in a 14-year-old that had many "spells" over a four-week period. The episodes began with salivation, then rapid abdominal breathing, followed by panting and twitching of the tail. The eyes dilated and the hair stood up. The pulse rate was 120 before an attack that occurred during a physical examination; it rose to over 240 during the episode and subsided to normal in two to three minutes. A palpable abdominal mass (Fig. 11–161) proved at surgery to be a 4.0 × 3.5 × 2.0 cm firm, nodular growth in the region of the celiac plexus ventral to the caudal vena cava at the base of the mesentery near the descending colon. The spells did not recur during the remaining four years of life, but at autopsy metastatic paraganglioma to the spleen was found, as well as a papillary adenocarcinoma of the lung and adenocarcinoma of the nasal cavity.

The paragangliomas in both cats were firm, nodular, and mottled gray, tan, and brown. There was a thin, well-vascularized capsule, and sectioning revealed soft, red-brown foci of hemorrhage and faint lobulation. Microscopically, the tumors were composed of irregular islands of cells separated by a fine fibrovascular stroma with prominent vascular lumina. Nuclei were round or oval and vesicular. Cytoplasm, which was distinct on hematoxylin and eosin stains, was clear or granular. The granules varied from pale pink to pale brown and were argyrophilic with the Grimelius technique. The malignancy of the second tumor was apparent only from the metastasis.

## TUMORS OF THE NERVOUS SYSTEM*

A wide variety of tumors of the nervous system have been reported in cats, but the total number is small, and in some cases an incomplete description leaves the diagnosis in doubt. For good reason greatest attention has been given to meningiomas, which are more frequent in the cat than in any other species except the dog. Lymphoma, the other neoplasm commonly involving the feline nervous system, is usually part of a generalized process and is discussed with secondary tumors.

### PRIMARY TUMORS OF THE NERVOUS SYSTEM

#### Meningiomas

Meningiomas, the most frequent intracranial tumors in cats, are variously estimated to constitute 0.9 per cent of all feline nonhematopoietic neoplasms (Patnaik et al., 1975), and 1.6 per cent of all tumors of cats (Hayes et al., 1975). A number of case series have been published (Banovcănin, 1971; Engle and Brodey, 1969; Hayes et al., 1975; Hayes and Schiefer, 1969; Lawson et al., 1984; Luginbühl, 1961; McGrath, 1962; Nafe, 1979; Zaki and Hurvitz, 1976). These tumors occur in older cats, 75 per cent being over nine years of age. Meningiomas are rare in cats less than five years old. Exceptions were a microscopic meningioma in a two-year-old cat (Luginbühl, 1961) and third ventricle meningiomas in four cats, all under three years of age, with mucopolysaccharidosis I (Haskins and McGrath, 1983). The relationship between the genetic defects of MPS I and the meningiomas is not known. There is no breed predominance for meningiomas, but in two groups a greater number of males were affected (Lawson et al., 1984; Nafe, 1979).

Tiny meningiomas (also known as meningeal whorls) are common incidental findings during careful autopsies, and those producing no clinical signs represent about 30 per cent of the reported cases. These very small meningiomas (0.1 to 0.3 cm) are located in the tela choroidea of the pineal recess of the third ventricle, in the transverse fissure, or over the cerebral convexities. The location of symptomatic meningiomas in these same regions suggests that they arise from these tiny meningiomas (Fig. 11–162).

Signs of meningiomas are related to their location. The most common site is over a cerebral hemisphere. The

*Damon R. Averill, Jr., principal author.

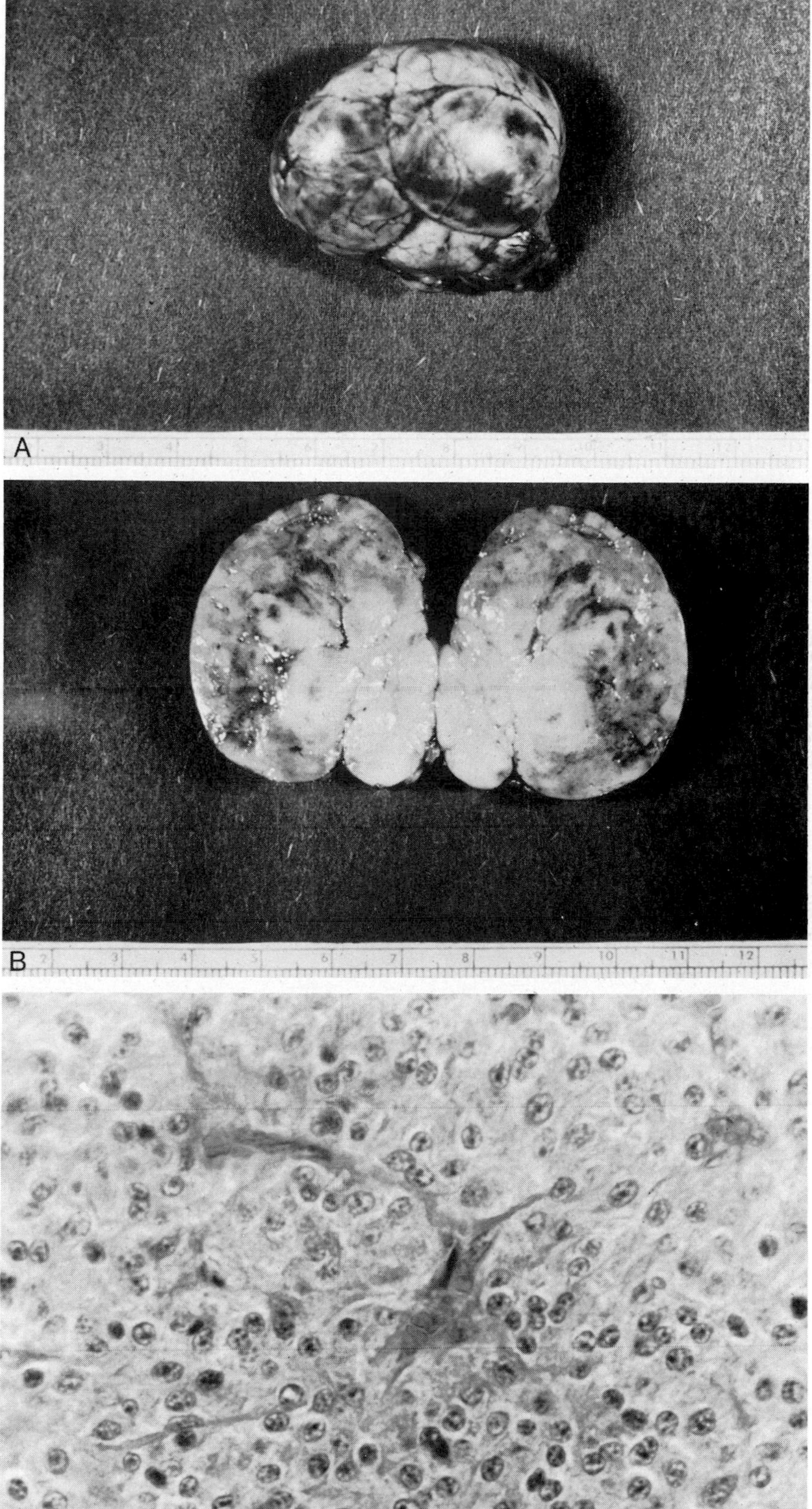


**Figure 11–161** *A*, Functional malignant paraganglioma from the dorsal retroperitoneum of a 14-year-old tricolor. The smooth but slightly nodular mass has a vascular capsule. Clinical signs presumably due to excess catecholamines ceased after its removal. Actual size. *B*, Cut surfaces reveal a mottled and partially lobulated solid growth with a smooth capsule except at one margin (lower center). A splenic metastasis was found four years later, when the cat died of an unrelated cause. *C*, Cells having euchromatic nuclei with chromatin clumps and indistinct cell borders form solid nests partially separated by fine stroma. Cytoplasmic granules were silver-positive with the Grimelius technique. H & E, × 765.

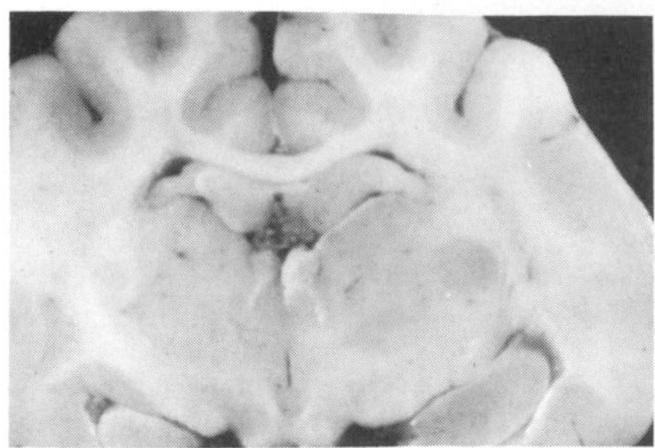

**Figure 11–162** Small meningioma attached to the meningeal surface of the pineal recess of the third ventricle, 11-year-old female cat. The hippocampal commissure is just above the tumor. As such tumors increase in size they protrude into the third ventricle and cause obstructive hydrocephalus.

earliest and most frequent sign with cerebral meningiomas is altered behavior—lethargy, dullness, inactivity, and anorexia (Lawson et al., 1984). Some cats become aggressive; rarely, an independent cat becomes affectionate. One cat at AMAH ceased to know its owners or its home; others have stopped using the litter box. Other signs of cerebral meningiomas may be circling, hemiparesis, and, occasionally, generalized seizures (Fig. 11–163). Vision on one side is sometimes lost, and there may be nystagmus. Third ventricular meningiomas may result in diffuse cerebral signs or no signs at all. Caudal fossa (e.g., Nafe, 1979) and spinal cord tumors (e.g., Engle and Brodey, 1969; Jones, 1974; McGrath, 1962) are extremely rare (Fig. 11–164).

The AMAH group does not differ significantly from reported series. Twenty-four of 64 meningiomas were symptomatic. They occurred in 16 males (12 castrated) and 8 females (five spayed) with a mean age of 11.6 years (range 3 to 17; 17 cats were 7 to 10 years old). Twelve tumors were located parasagittally over a cerebral hemisphere, with frontal, parietal, and occipital sites about equally represented. Three cats had multiple tumors over 0.4 cm in diameter (Fig. 11–165). One had large bilateral parietal lobe meningiomas (Fig. 11–166). Three tumors were found compressing the cerebellum; four were large, midline third ventricular masses, and two were in the spinal cord (one at C3, one at T12) (Fig. 11–164).

Meningiomas are considered to be benign neoplasms, but in one case metastasis to the lung was reported (Dahme, 1957).

A meningioma should be suspected when neurologic signs in an aged cat are focal and slowly progressive. Ancillary studies short of a CAT scan (Fig. 11–167) are usually not corroborative. The cerebrospinal fluid (CSF) may have elevated pressure and protein; however, the removal of CSF is considered by some to be contraindicated, since it may result in tentorial or foramen magnum herniation (Lawson et al., 1984). Some meningiomas erode the overlying neurocranium (one of the AMAH cases; also Hague and Burridge, 1969; Lawson et al., 1984; Zaki and Hurvitz, 1976) or produce overlying exostosis (Lawson et al., 1984; McGrath, 1962; Zaki and Hurvitz, 1976), which may allow palpation, radiographic demonstration, or biopsy diagnosis. Tumor calcification, although subtle, was evident radiographically in all cats in a group of 10 (Lawson et al., 1984). Abnormalities are sometimes evident in an EEG. The location of a lesion is sometimes identified by scintigraphy (Kallfelz et al., 1978) and most successfully by CAT scan (e.g., Shell et al., 1985). Nuclear magnetic imaging also gives promise (Buonanno et al., 1982).

Some meningiomas may be removed surgically (Lawson et al., 1984; Monteagudo and Purpura, 1959; Shell et al., 1985). In most cats the symptoms regressed rapidly. In one cat the tumor recurred two and a half years after removal; the recurrent meningioma was removed successfully (Lawson et al., 1984). One frontal lobe meningioma successfully removed at AMAH recurred at the same site 12 months later.

Meningiomas in the cat are meningothelial, fibrous, or transitional in histologic type; but their behavior does not vary with the histologic type.

## Ependymoma

Ependymomas arise from the ependymal cells lining the ventricular system, are composed of sheets and cords of cells, and form small rosettes around a central lumen, large tubular structures, and perivascular pseudorosettes. Ependymomas occurring in the ventricles of young adult

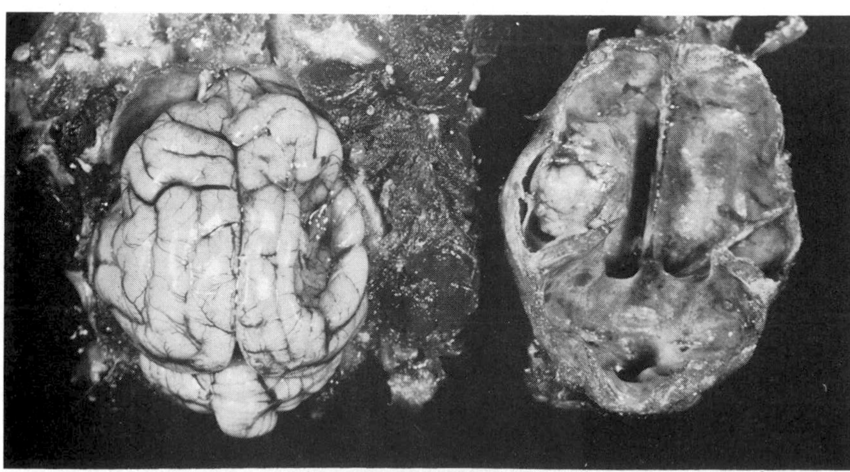

**Figure 11–163** Solitary meningioma of the right cerebral dura mater causing a linear depression in the right parietal cortex, 10-year-old tabby. The noninvasive expansile growth produced compression, ischemia, atrophy, necrosis, and gliosis of the adjacent cerebrum. Seizures with tonic-clonic spasms affecting mainly the left side of the body preceded coma and death.

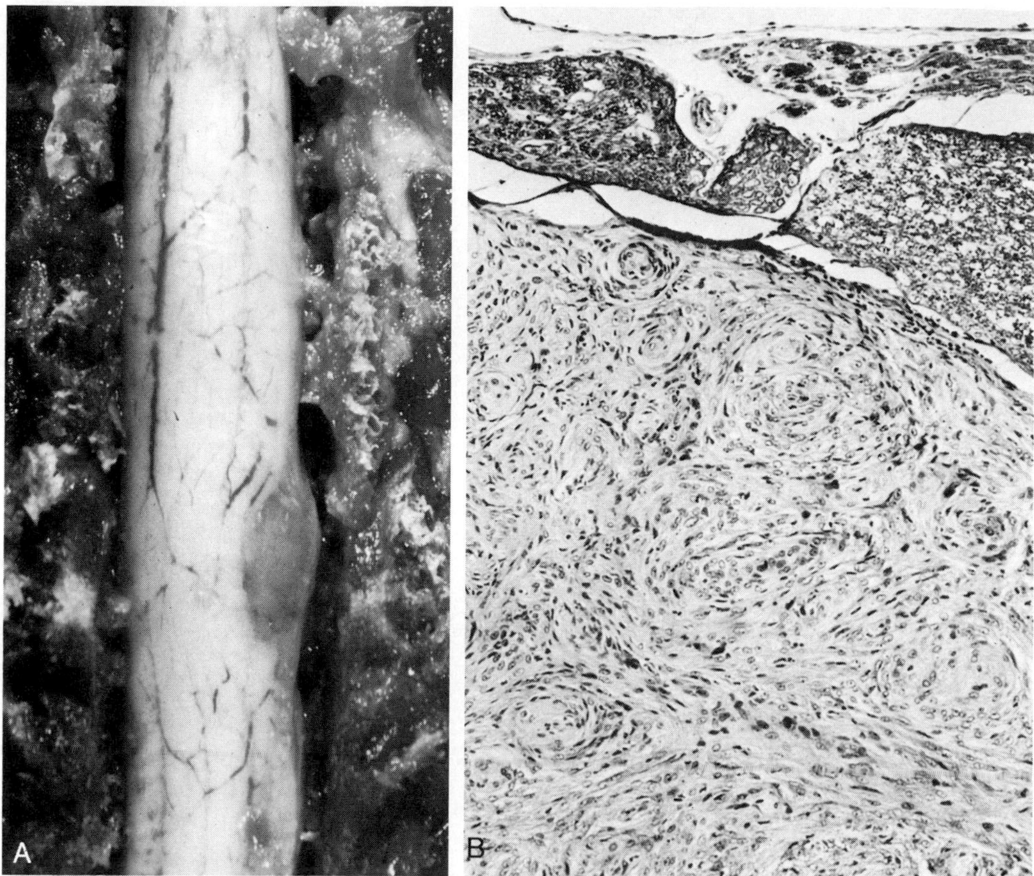


**Figure 11–164** *A*, Subdural meningioma that originated from the arachnoid on the right of the third cervical cord segment, 17-year-old black-and-white cat. Compression and displacement of the cord and spinal nerve rootlets caused progressive ipsilateral hemiparesis. × 3. *B*, The tumor, composed of cells with round, oval, and fusiform nuclei, formed whorls and bundles and compressed the cord (upper right) and spinal nerve rootlets (upper left). Luxol fast blue, × 125.

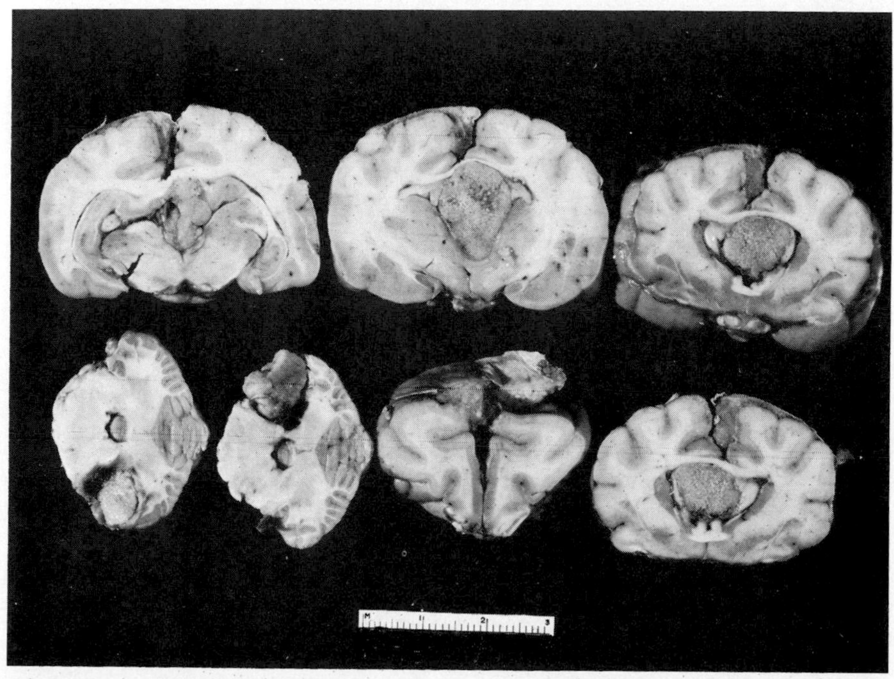

**Figure 11–165** Multiple meningiomas. Three large meningiomas are seen in transverse brain slabs as granular expansile growths that involve the dorsal meninges of the frontal and parietal lobes, the third ventricle, and the cerebellum. Hemorrhage and necrosis are conspicuous in and about the meningiomas of the cerebellum and frontal lobes. The growth within the third ventricle arose from the meninges of the pineal recess.

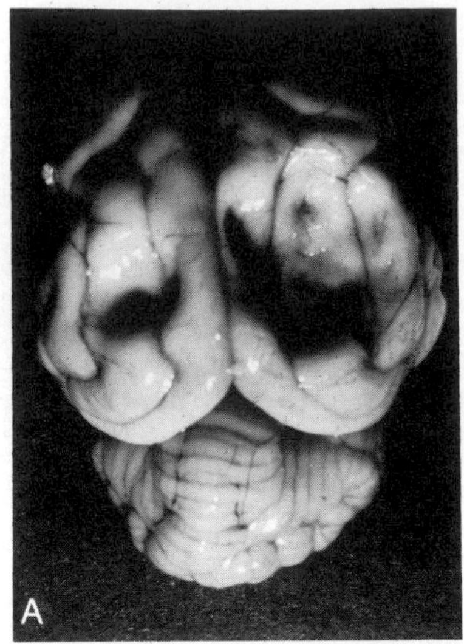


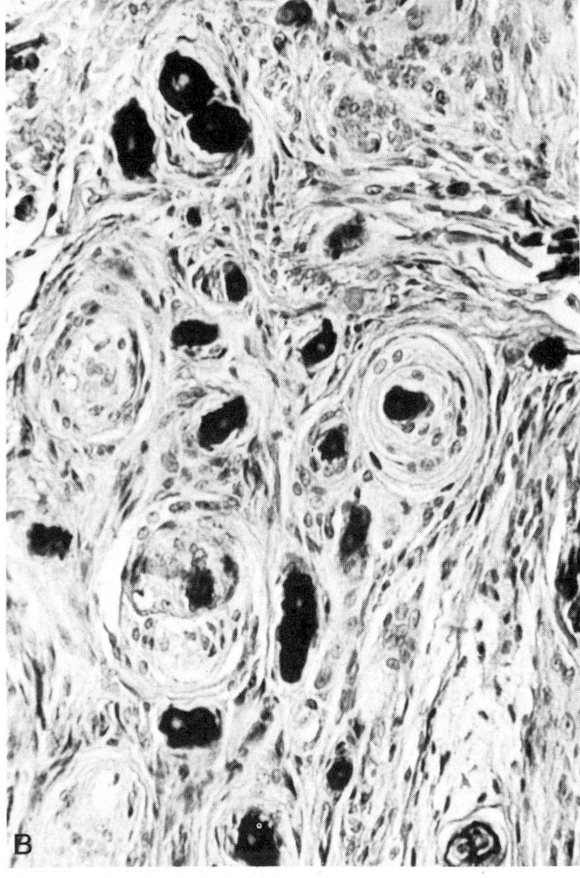


**Figure 11–166** *A*, Bilateral deep depressions in the parietal lobes caused by two meningiomas originating from the overlying dura mater (not shown). Surprisingly, the only related neurologic signs in this obese, 7.7 kg, 17-year-old domestic shorthair were urinary incontinence and great difficulty in walking. *B*, Psammoma (calcareous) bodies are numerous, appear black, and are often located in the center of fibrous whorls. Such meningiomas might, because of their high mineral content, be seen on radiographs. H & E, × 250.

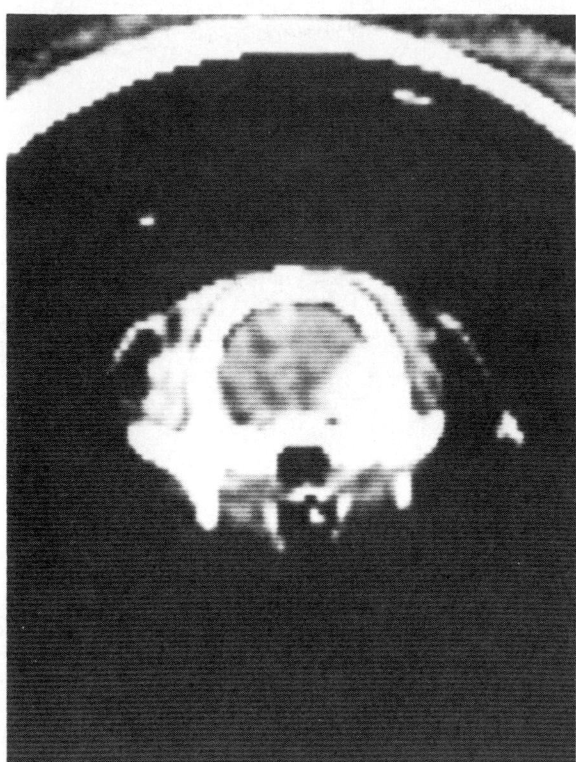

**Figure 11–167** CAT scan of meningioma arising from the dura mater over the left parietal and temporal lobes, 11-year-old castrated male blue domestic longhair. Constant pacing, circling to the left, partial loss of vision in the right eye, and dyspnea prompted a neurologic examination. The contrast CAT scan reveals homogeneous uptake of the dye by the meningioma, as well as hydrocephalus of the right lateral ventricle (dark regions). The 3 × 1 × 1 cm fibrous meningioma was successfully removed through a 4 × 3 cm rectangular craniotomy opening. Twenty months after surgery the cat was well.

and middle-aged cats have been reported by Cordy (1978), Fox et al. (1973), Luginbühl (1963), Luginbühl et al. (1968), Schiefer and Dahme (1962), Steensland (1906), and Zaki and Hurvitz (1976).

Six ependymomas were diagnosed at AMAH, two involving a lateral ventricle (Fig. 11–168) and two, the third ventricle (Fig. 11–169) in cats aged 7 (two), 8, and 12 years old; one the fourth ventricle in a 1½-year-old cat; and one the L6–L7 spinal cord segment in a 4-year-old. The principal signs of the ventricular tumors were failure to groom, stupor, and intermittent semicoma. The spinal cord tumor, which caused progressive flaccid paraparesis and responded briefly to corticosteroid administration, was found at autopsy to have produced enlargement of the vertebral canal of L6. Histologically this tumor was a myxopapillary ependymoma as described by Russell and Rubinstein (1971).

A brain tumor with distant metastasis is a rarity. One of the ependymomas at AMAH, in a seven-year-old spayed female Siamese, caused a slowly progressive two-week illness characterized by lethargy and decreased appetite. Physical examination disclosed clear bubbly nasal fluid, coughing, weakness, ataxia, and a slight head tilt to the right. Neurologic examination revealed decreased proprioception in all limbs, with greatest loss in the left forelimb. Both optic and tactile placing reflexes were slower in the left than in the right forelimb. The hopping reflex was diminished more in the forelimbs than in the hindlimbs, and again the left forelimb was most

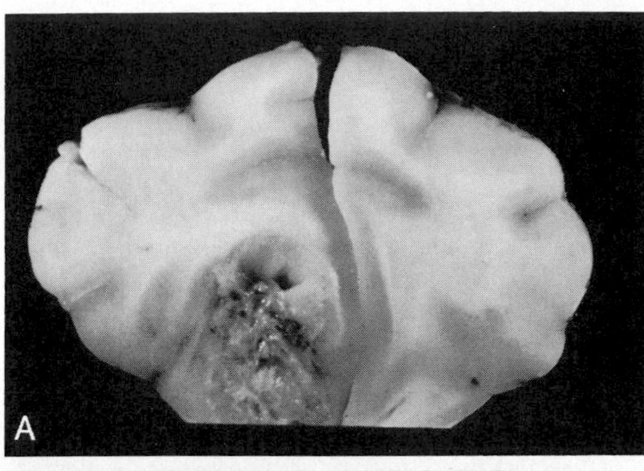



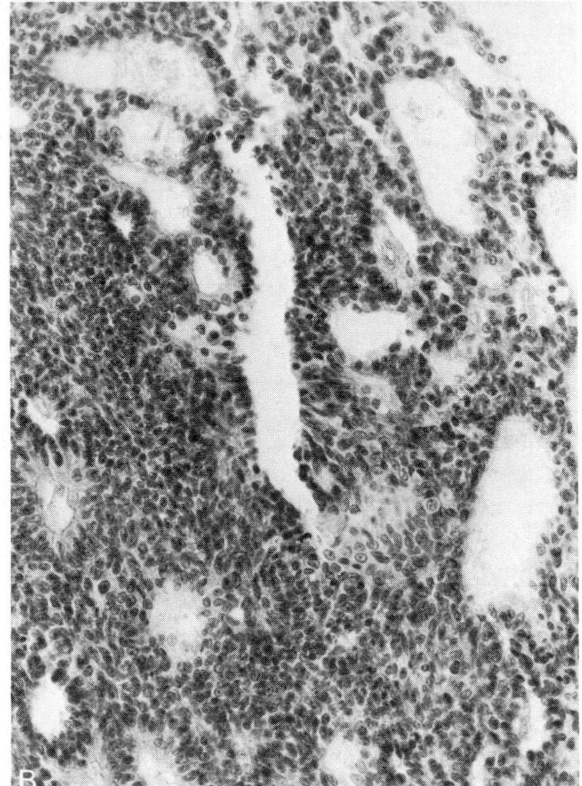



**Figure 11–166** *A*, Bilateral deep depressions in the parietal lobes caused by two meningiomas originating from the overlying dura mater (not shown). Surprisingly, the only related neurologic signs in this obese, 7.7 kg, 17-year-old domestic shorthair were urinary incontinence and great difficulty in walking. *B*, Psammoma (calcareous) bodies are numerous, appear black, and are often located in the center of fibrous whorls. Such meningiomas might, because of their high mineral content, be seen on radiographs. H & E, × 250.

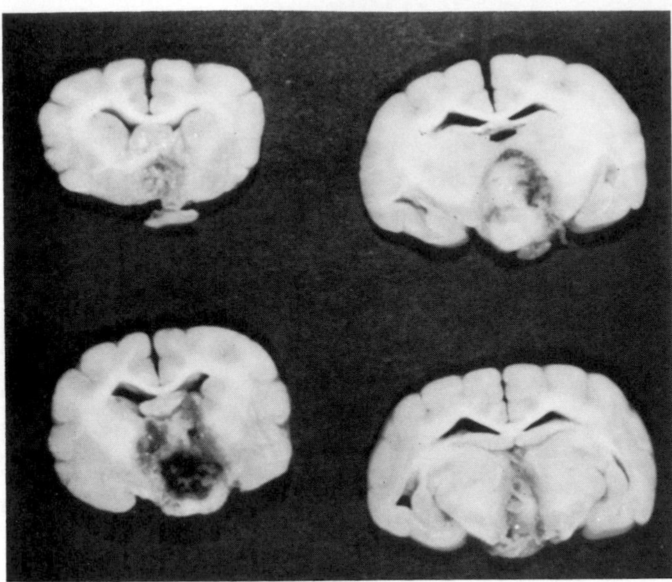

**Figure 11–169** Ependymoma in a 12-year-old spayed female Persian that was inappetent and inattentive to personal hygiene. The tumor extends from the anterior to the posterior commissure, fills the third ventricle, replaces the hypothalamus and ventral thalamus, compresses the pituitary, and displaces the optic chiasm rostrally. Cysts, hemorrhage, and necrosis are prominent gross features of this papillary ependymoma. Remarkably, the lateral ventricles are nearly normal.

affected. Autopsy disclosed that the tumor involved mainly the anterior right cerebral hemisphere and replaced much of the frontal and olfactory lobes (Fig. 11–170). It invaded vessels, extended into both ethmoid turbinates, and metastasized to regional nodes.

Two cats at AMAH had neoplasms indistinguishable histologically from ependymomas, but they arose in the olfactory epithelium, eroded the cribriform plate, and invaded the adjacent olfactory bulb and frontal lobe. These tumors (probably so-called esthesioneuroblastomas) are composed of pseudorosettes of epithelial cells. Neurologic signs were as in other frontal lobe lesions. Tumors of the olfactory epithelium have also been reported in cats aged three and six years by Pospischil and Dahme (1981).

## Other Glial Tumors

Astrocytomas have been reported in the cerebrum (Cooper and Howarth, 1956; Engle and Brodey, 1969; Luginbühl et al., 1968; McGrath, 1960; Perlstein, 1956; Zaki and Hurvitz, 1976), in the brainstem (Cusick and Parker, 1975; Jubb and Kennedy, 1970; Parker, 1981), and in the spinal cord (Luginbühl et al., 1968; Milks and Olafson, 1936). The tumor pictured by Jubb and Kennedy (1970) was reported to have metastasized to the kidney, where the lesions grossly resembled those of lymphoma.

Oligodendrogliomas are rare. Two were reported by LeCouteur et al. (1983) and Small (1964); oligoastrocytomas were described by Cooper and Howarth (1956) and Cusick and Parker (1975); and an unclassified glioma with some resemblance to a gangliocytoma was reported by Luginbühl et al. (1968).

Medulloblastoma is an undifferentiated malignant tumor that usually occurs in the cerebellum and is found in the young of various species, including humans. A feline medulloblastoma is pictured by Fankhauser et al. (1974) and another by Jubb et al. (1985).

Tumors on record at AMAH were three astrocytomas of the frontal and parietal lobes in cats aged two, six, and nine years (Fig. 11–171) and three of the spinal cord in cats aged 4 (two) and 10 years (Fig. 11–172). A cerebellar medulloblastoma was found in a three-month-old kitten.

## Other Primary Tumors of the Nervous System

Plexus papilloma, fairly common in dogs and some other species, has apparently been described only once in the cat, a young animal with hydrocephalus (Verlinde and Ojemann, 1946).

Single cases of neoplastic reticulosis, angioblastoma, and sarcoma were recorded by Luginbühl et al. (1968). Primary tumors described in the spinal cord were a sarcoma in a 5-year-old cat (Luttgen et al., 1980) and a neurofibrosarcoma in a 19-year-old (Ruben, 1983).

Capillary telangiectasia of the cerebellum is pictured in the section on the cardiovascular system.

## Peripheral Nerve Tumors

Peripheral nerve neoplasms of the cat other than malignant lymphoma are extremely rare. A thoracic neurilemmoma has been reported (Zaki and Hurvitz, 1976). Solitary neurofibromas have been found in the skin (Jubb and Kennedy, 1970) and in vertebrae (Zaki and Hurvitz, 1976). Neurofibromas of the skin and subcutis are discussed in detail among skin tumors.

An unusual disseminated tumor of the subcutis that surrounded nerves caudal to one scapula, extended along a brachial plexus, and entered the thorax, was seen at AMAH in a 10-year-old spayed female domestic cat and was pictured by Fankhauser and Luginbühl (1968). In gross features it was suggestive of neurofibromatosis, but on microscopic review it could not be demonstrated to arise from, or even to infiltrate, nerves and was reclassified as aggressive fibromatosis (see section on tumors of skin and subcutis).

## Secondary Tumors of the Nervous System

## Lymphoma

Lymphoma in its varied histologic forms is clinically the most important neoplastic disease of the feline nervous

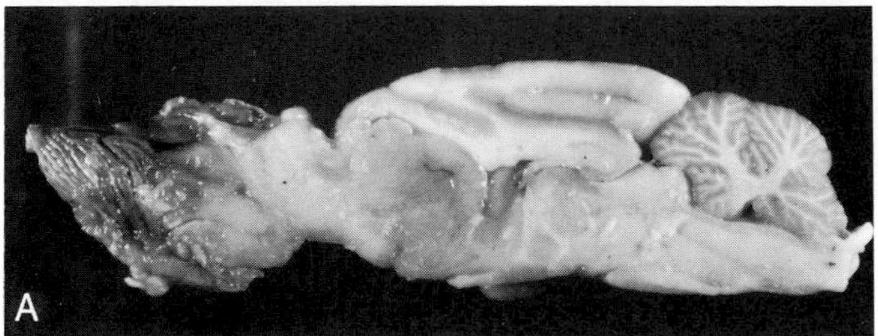


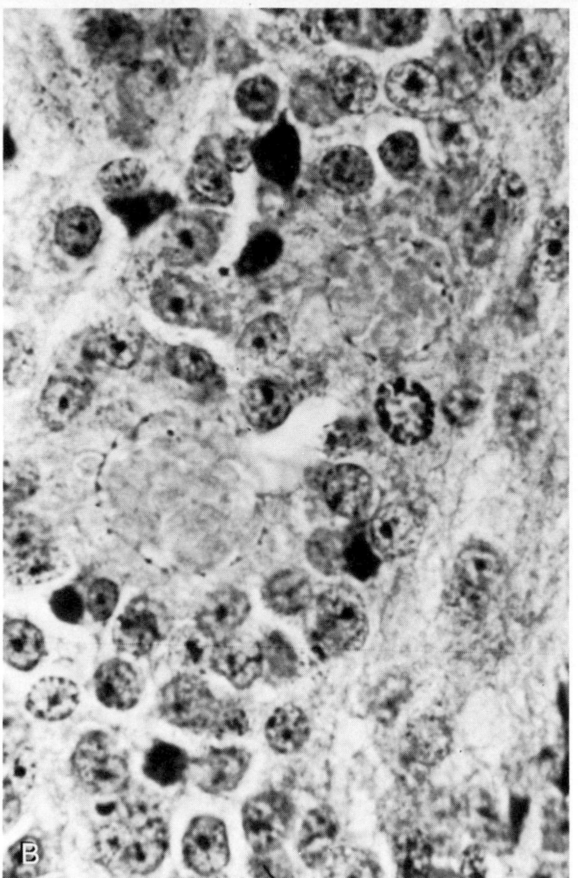


**Figure 11–170** *A*, Malignant ependymoma, seven-year-old spayed female chocolate point Siamese. The neoplasm involved the anterior right cerebral hemisphere more than the left. Its dimensions were 3.8 × 1.5 × 1.4 cm. It extended forward from above the optic chiasm adjacent to the third ventricle, compressing the lateral ventricles and elevating the corpus callosum. It replaced much of the frontal and olfactory lobes and both olfactory bulbs. Both ethmoid turbinates contained neoplastic thrombi. The tumor caused focal lysis and lateral displacement of the orbital process of the right frontal bone. Metastases were found in the right mandibular and both retropharyngeal nodes. *B*, Two rosettes (near center) are formed by ependymal cells having round euchromatic nuclei with peripheral clumped chromatin and a single centrally located nucleolus. Minute blepharoplasts appearing as dark dots in a circle within the rosettes establish the correct diagnosis of this tumor. Bielschowsky's silver technique, × 1200.

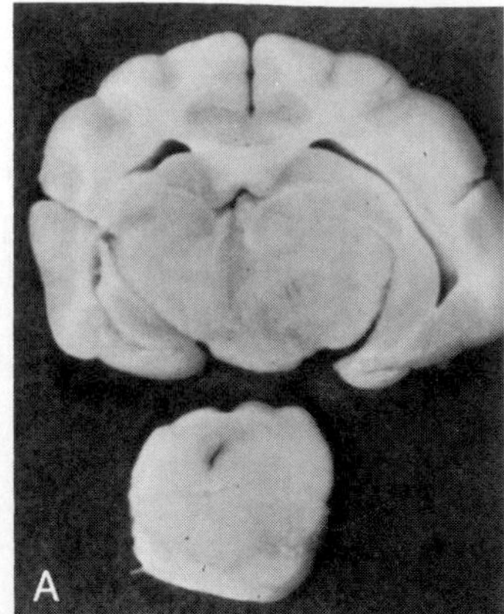


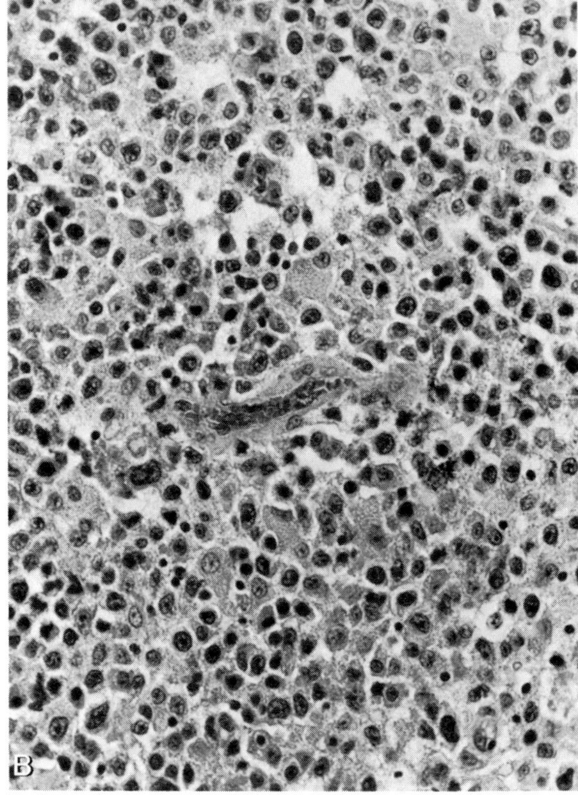


**Figure 11–171** *A*, Astrocytoma, right thalamus and right midbrain, five-year-old spayed female tricolor domestic shorthair. The tumor extended from the right caudate nucleus through the internal capsule, geniculate bodies, thalamus, and midbrain into the pons. Neurologic signs included left hemiparesis, left visual deficit, rotatory nystagmus, left head tilt, and tight circling to the left. The white, poorly demarcated tumor has enlarged and distorted the right thalamus and right midbrain. Diffuse cerebral edema is manifested by decreased contrast between gray and white matter. Actual size. *B*, Astrocytes, in a solid pattern, show conspicuous anisocytosis and anisokaryosis. H & E, × 300.

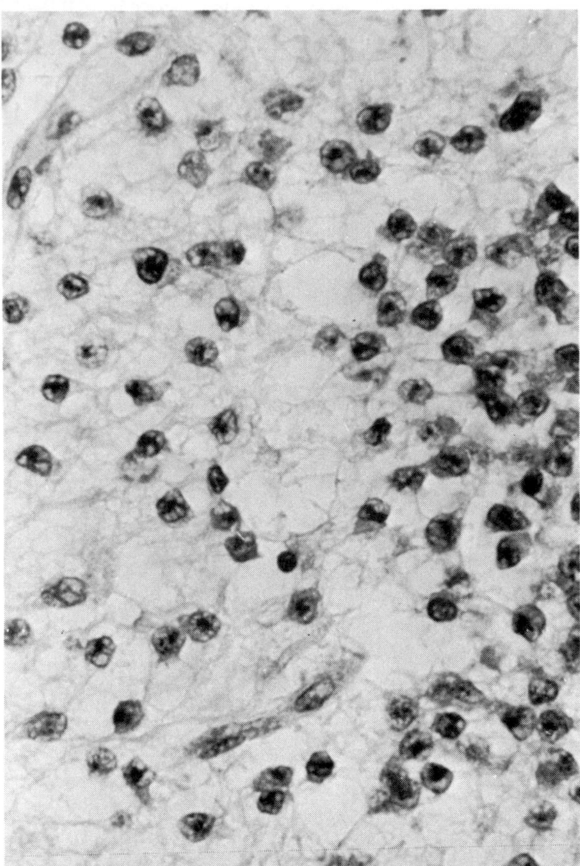

**Figure 11–172** Astrocytoma, lumbar spinal cord, four-year-old castrated male domestic shorthair. The astrocytes have many fibrillar cytoplasmic processes, a vesicular nucleus, a prominent nucleolus, and sometimes clear-staining cytoplasm. The clinical course of one year began with left rear leg weakness that completely regressed for six months after corticosteroid therapy. Weakness then recurred and progressed to involve the right rear leg about four months later. Steroid therapy was this time ineffective for the asymmetrical paraparesis. Reflexes indicated a lower motor neuron lesion in segments L6–S1. Myelography revealed widening of the spinal canal at L5 and an intramedullary lesion that was verified at laminectomy. H & E, × 500.

system. In order of decreasing prevalence, lymphoma may affect the spinal cord, lumbosacral plexus, brachial plexus, multiple cranial nerves, or the brain. In most cases, gross or microscopic tumor is also present in other sites as well as the nervous system.

**SPINAL CORD.** Spinal cord involvement may occur at any age but is rare in cats under six months. The signs may evolve over a few days or several weeks; one cat developed paraplegia over a six-month period (Heavner, 1978). Symmetric progressive paraparesis results from thoracolumbar lesions. Cases of cervical vertebral canal involvement usually begin with weakness of one thoracic limb and devolve into spastic quadriparesis. While position sense may be reduced, loss of deep pain perception or sphincter weakness is unusual.

Among eight cats that came to autopsy at AMAH with signs of a spinal cord lesion between segments T2 and L4, five had spinal column discomfort on palpation, four had atypical lymphocytes in peripheral blood, four had palpable kidney or liver lesions, and all of five tested were positive for FeLV antigen. Three of the eight had no clinical evidence of lymphoma other than the positive

FeLV test. Five cats reported in the literature were also FeLV-positive but without physical evidence of disseminated malignant lymphoma (Parker and Park, 1974; Heavner, 1978); myelograms demonstrated filling defects. In the four AMAH cases studied the CSF had elevated protein, but only one cat had abnormal cells, similar to the experience of Kornegay (1981). Kornegay found FeLV antigen in the CSF of three of five cats tested. At autopsy, all AMAH cats had either disseminated lymphoma or single-organ (e.g., mesenteric lymph node) involvement, consistent with the experience of Zaki and Hurvitz (1976).

The neoplastic lymphoid cells accumulate in the extradural space, presumably arising in extramedullary hematopoietic sites often found in epidural fat. A lesion arising in the vertebral body adjacent to the site of cord compression was present in one cat, as has been found by others (Kornegay, 1981; Zaki and Hurvitz, 1976). In four other cases, vertebral, meningeal, or muscular involvement resulted in compression of the cord, but the cord itself was not invaded (Schappert and Geib, 1967). In two cats the cells traversed the dura mater and invaded the spinal cord, as in other reported cases (Heavner, 1978; Kornegay, 1981; Parker and Park, 1974; Zaki and Hurvitz, 1976). At surgery or autopsy, extradural lymphoma may easily be confused with epidural fat owing to its gelatinous gray-white translucency (Fig. 11–173); hence the diagnosis should always be confirmed histologically. The cell type may be lymphocytic, lymphoblastic, or histiocytic without apparent difference in biologic behavior.

Treatment of vertebral canal lymphoma should be carried out with the knowledge that other focal or disseminated lesions are likely to be present. It is my experience (DRA) and that of others (Parker and Park, 1974) that the signs of spinal canal lymphoma are at first exquisitely responsive to systemic corticosteroid administration (prednisone 0.5 mg/kg t.i.d.) but become refractory after one or two courses of treatment or when systemic signs of visceral involvement prevail. We have managed six cats with biopsy-proven vertebral canal lymphoma by means of medical or surgical and medical treatment, and they survived as viable house pets for one to two years. (See also the chapter on disorders of the hematopoietic system.)

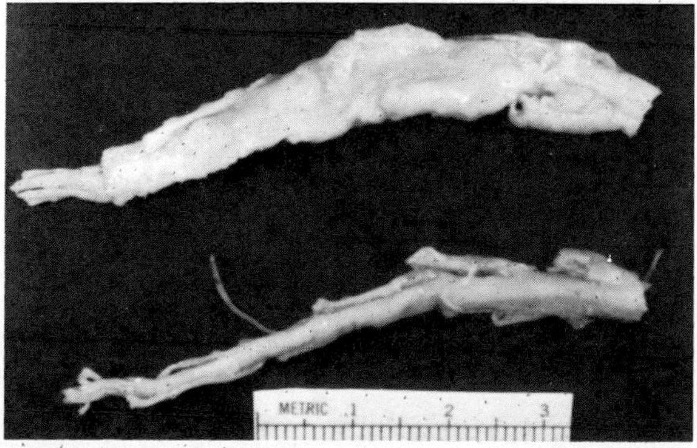


**Figure 11–173** Malignant lymphoma, lumbosacral spinal cord, 17-year-old tabby (upper specimen). These are fixed segments of two spinal cords extending from approximately the fifth lumbar segment to the end, including the cauda equina. The lower specimen is normal. The upper is ensheathed by lymphoma, which obscures the spinal roots and dura mater. This is a common location for lymphoma.

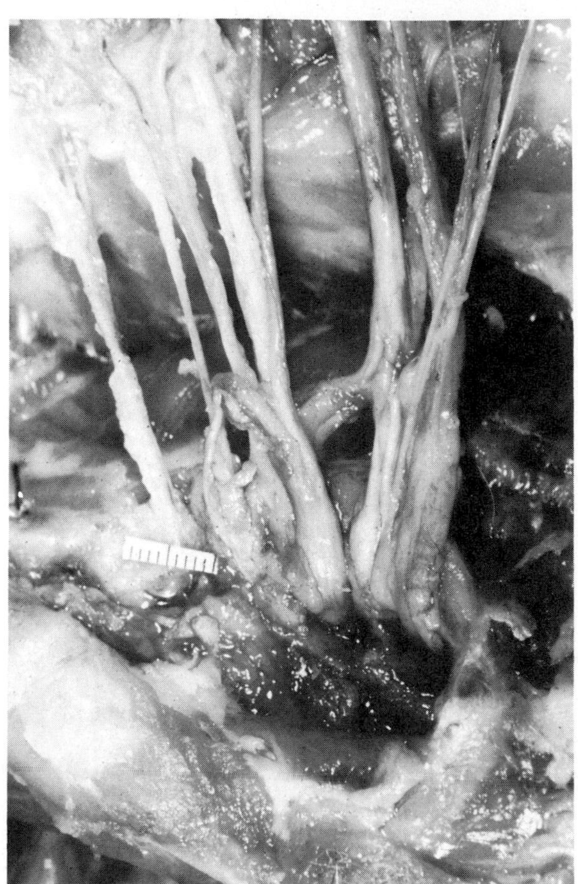

**Figure 11–174** Malignant lymphoma of most of the nerves of the left brachial plexus, seven-year-old domestic shorthair. Muscles cover the sternum and the first rib (lower edge). The left forelimb had weak and atrophic muscles and markedly decreased reflexes. Elbow drop and left-sided Horner's syndrome were evident. Lymphoma was less severe in the right brachial plexus and was not found at other sites.

**LUMBOSACRAL PLEXUS.** Lumbosacral plexus lymphoma usually begins with asymmetric weakness of muscles supplied by the sciatic nerve. The disability progresses over days or weeks to flaccid paraparesis and flaccid weakness of anal and urinary bladder sphincters with perineal anesthesia. The lumbosacral roots are enlarged with malignant lymphocytes, although the spinal fluid is normal. These cats rarely improve with medical therapy. A consideration in differential diagnosis is paralytic rabies, but usually visceral involvement with lymphoma can be demonstrated.

**BRACHIAL PLEXUS.** Unilateral lymphoma of the brachial plexus has been reported by others (Fox and Gutnick, 1972; Luginbühl et al., 1968; Zaki and Hurvitz, 1976) and is not rare. Slowly progressive flaccid monoplegia with sensory loss is usually accompanied by Horner's syndrome, if the vagosympathetic trunk or cranial thoracic roots are involved (Fig. 11–174). Treatment in three AMAH cases was unsuccessful. Trauma, which must be considered in the differential diagnosis, is associated with signs that remain static rather than worsening after hospital admission. One case of bilateral brachial plexus neuropathy has been described (Bright et al., 1978). Such signs could easily be confused with those of lymphoma.

**CRANIAL NERVES.** Involvement of multiple cranial nerves may take the form of dural or subarachnoid growth in the ventral neurocranium. Invasion of optic nerve (Barker and Greenwood, 1973), oculomotor and trigeminal nerve (Allen and Amis, 1975), and vagus nerve (Schaer et al., 1971) has been reported. Similar cases at AMAH have involved respectively cranial nerves II, V, VI and VII, IX, X, and XII; nerves II, III, VI, and VIII; and nerves II through XII. Another disease that may produce signs of involvement of multiple cranial nerves is cryptococcal meningitis. Cats with lymphoma of cranial nerves have lymphoblasts in their meninges and CSF.

Occasionally lymphoma is first manifested by a sign of involvement of a single peripheral nerve, e.g., femoral or radial paralysis.

**CEREBRUM.** Although infiltration of the cerebral meninges is not uncommon with lymphoma, invasion of the brain itself is rare. A histiocytic lymphoma arising in the parietal bone of a five-year-old male cat invaded the underlying cerebral hemisphere (Fig. 11–175).

## Primitive Lymphoreticular Tumor

Four cats were seen with local but large cerebral neoplasms of uncertain but distinctive type. All mature cats, they were presented for seizures, hemiparesis, and ipsilateral hemianopia. They had elevated CSF pressures and were destroyed or died within two weeks after the onset of signs. The affected hemispheres were swollen, and cerebellar herniation resulted in ante-mortem vestibular-brainstem signs. In each case large confluent regions of a cerebral hemisphere and thalamus were replaced by sheets of large mononuclear cells (Fig. 11–176*A*) with distinct cytoplasmic margins, clear to hazy blue cytoplasm, and large, oval, slightly eccentric nuclei with large eosinophilic nucleoli. A significant number of the cells had only a few brightly eosinophilic cytoplasmic granules (Fig. 11–176*B*). Numerous small regions of necrosis were present, individual necrotic cells were abundant, and mitoses exceeded 2 per HPF.

Special stains failed to differentiate the cells as plasma cells or malignant mast cells. Reticulin was present in small amounts. I (DRA) currently consider this a primitive lymphoreticular neoplasm akin to the poorly understood human reticulum cell sarcoma-microglioma, although the cells do not resemble microglia. Circumstantial evidence, including a previously removed popliteal lymph node containing reticulum cell sarcoma and circulating atypical lymphocytes in one cat, similar neoplastic cells in adrenal and Peyer's patches in another cat, and invasion of the dorsal neurocranium in a third cat, seems to support this tentative diagnosis. Of the four cats tested, two were FeLV-positive.

In two cases of neoplasms of similar cell type, one grew in the midline of the caudal medulla, causing ataxia, nystagmus, disorientation, and weakness. Another was disseminated throughout virtually every part of the brain, causing signs of weakness, lethargy, asymmetric quadriparesis, cerebellar ataxia, and central nystagmus. These two cats were anemic (PCV 23), and the CSF had large

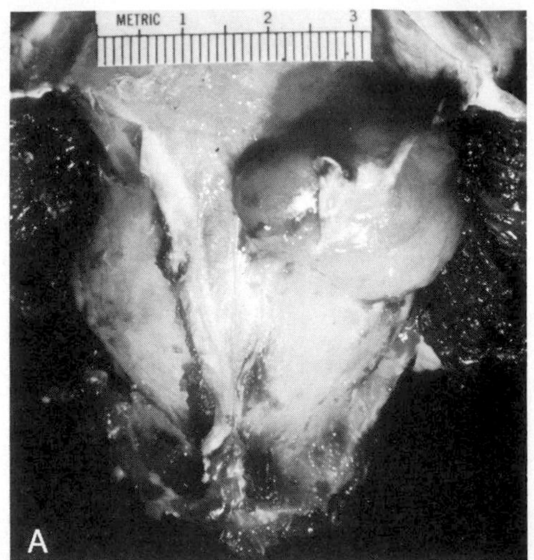


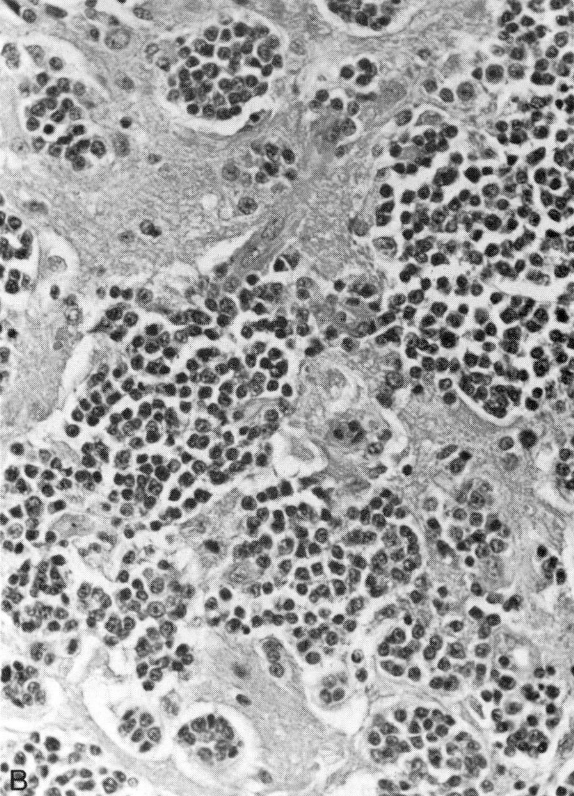


**Figure 11–175** *A*, A solitary histiocytic lymphoma, originating in the right parietal bone, formed a 3.0 × 2.5 cm nodular mass in the temporalis muscle, destroyed bone, and penetrated the meninges deep into the right cerebral hemisphere. The five-year-old male cat had lost its pleasant personality, became withdrawn, and stopped eating. It developed an ataxic gait with wandering to the left and increased weight-bearing on the right limbs. Proprioception and hopping reflexes were diminished in both left limbs. A CBC and examination of femoral marrow gave no evidence of leukemia. *B*, Aggregates of malignant histiocytic lymphocytes form compact packets located deep within the cerebrum. H & E, × 300.

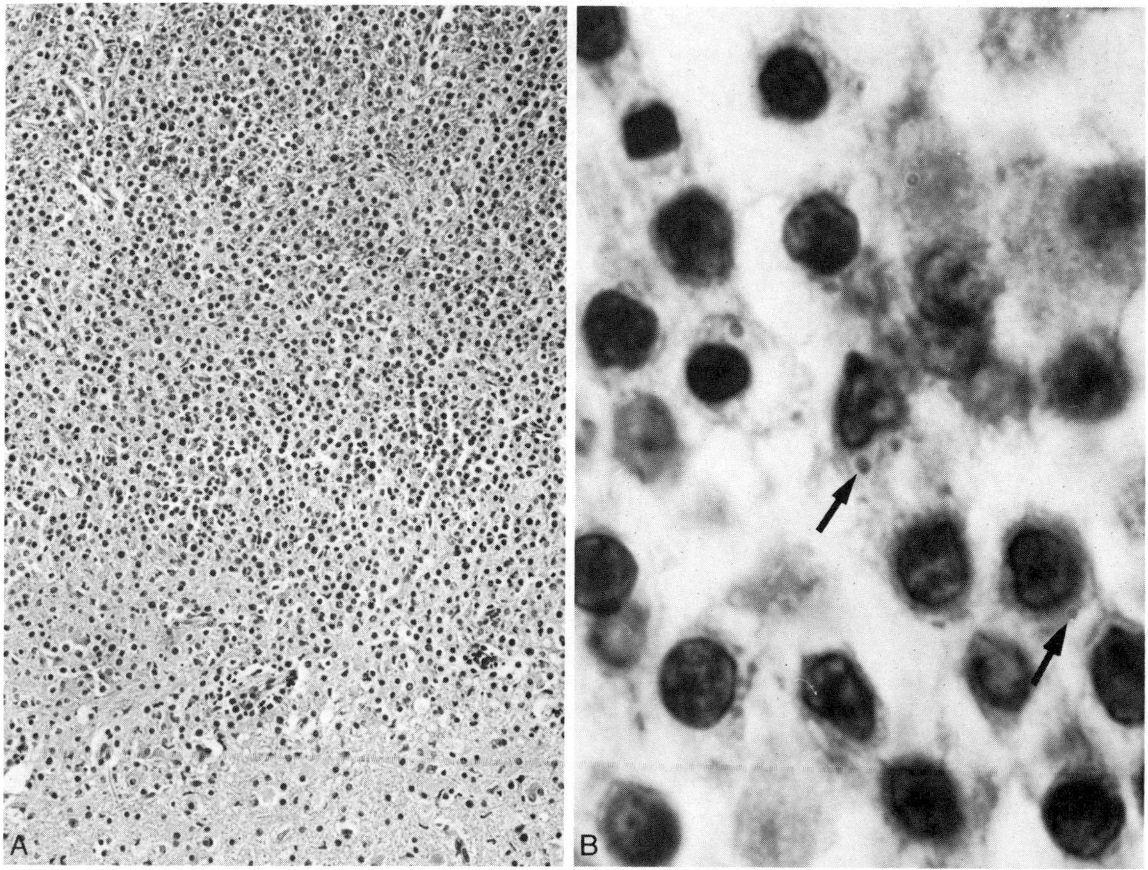


**Figure 11–176** *A*, Primitive lymphoreticular tumor at the junction of the corpus callosum (above) and the caudate nucleus (below), six-year-old castrated male domestic shorthair. The tumor caused asymmetric tetraparesis, dullness, intermittent tremor of head and trunk, and eventually inability to walk. The tumor, restricted to the nervous tissue, was found throughout most of the brain, meninges, and spinal nerve rootlets. H & E, × 125. *B*, Several of the lymphoid cells have cytoplasmic granules (arrows) that stained brightly eosinophilic. H & E, × 2000.

numbers of neoplastic cells. Similar cases have been described (Cordy, 1978; Skelley et al., 1953; Zaki and Hurvitz, 1976).

### Other Secondary Tumors

Except for lymphoma, neoplasms metastatic to the cat's central nervous system are rare. Metastatic mammary gland adenocarcinoma was reported by Luginbühl et al. (1968), and metastatic mammary and bronchial gland carcinomas were seen at AMAH. Nasal carcinomas may invade the brain through the cribriform plate, and tumors of the cranium and middle ear may compress the brain, giving rise to abnormal nervous signs.

In two young cats at AMAH, vertebral angiomas (which may have been congenital anomalies) invaded the spinal canal (Fig. 11–177).

## TUMORS OF THE EYE

Tumors of the eye are discussed in detail in the chapter on the eye. Ocular tumors diagnosed in the Department of Pathology, AMAH, are listed in Table 11–1, and the melanogenic ocular tumors are described in the section on tumors of the melanogenic system in this chapter.

## TUMORS OF THE EAR

## TUMORS OF THE EXTERNAL EAR

### Tumor-like Lesions

**INFLAMMATORY POLYP.** This is the most frequent growth of the ear of cats and may occur in cats of any age. Over 100 are on record at AMAH, and kittens as young as three months have been affected. The polyps appear to be a response to upper respiratory infection with otitis media and arise in the auditive (Eustachian) tube or middle ear (bulla) (e.g., Bedford, 1982; Harvey and Goldschmidt, 1978; Lane et al., 1981; Pearson and Hart, 1980; Stanton et al., 1985). Many push through the tympanum into the external meatus, but some remain confined to the bulla. Masses in the ear give rise to head-shaking and purulent discharge and if drainage is blocked may ultimately cause meningitis. Radiographs reveal abnormal density of the bulla.

Over 75 per cent of polyps found in the nasopharynx originate similarly, passing inward from the auditive tube (Fig. 11–178). Rarely, such polyps grow forward along the floor of the nasal cavity and emerge at the nostril. Occasionally a cat has polyps in both the external meatus and the auditive tube or pharynx (e.g., Stanton et al., 1985).

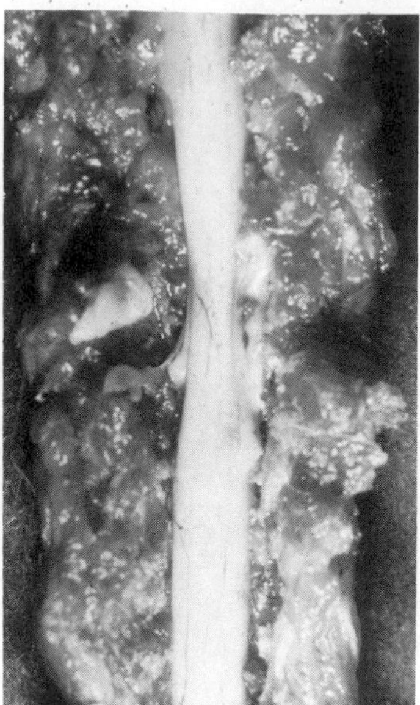

**Figure 11–177** Angioma of the tenth thoracic vertebra and spinal canal that compressed the spinal cord in a two-year-old male domestic shorthair. The angioma was composed of a proliferation of thin-walled muscular arteries arising from the vertebra. Concentric growth about the cord caused posterior paraparesis with upper motor neuron signs. Corticosteroid therapy was repeatedly shown to decrease the weakness in the rear limbs but failed to halt the progression of a paralysis occurring over a six-month period.

The polyps, usually pedunculated, are composed of proliferative inflammatory tissue, sometimes containing mucous glands. They are covered by pseudostratified columnar ciliated respiratory epithelium (near the point of origin) with a transition to stratified squamous epithelium.

Much less often polyps arise from the lining of the external meatus and are covered with stratified squamous epithelium. They are composed of proliferative inflammatory tissue, cystic and hyperplastic ceruminous glands, and hypertrophied sebaceous glands. In a rare case of recurrent cryptococcosis, that yeast gave rise to a granulomatous otic polyp. In another cat an unidentified hyphal fungus was found in a similar polyp. Demodectic mites have also been found in polyps.

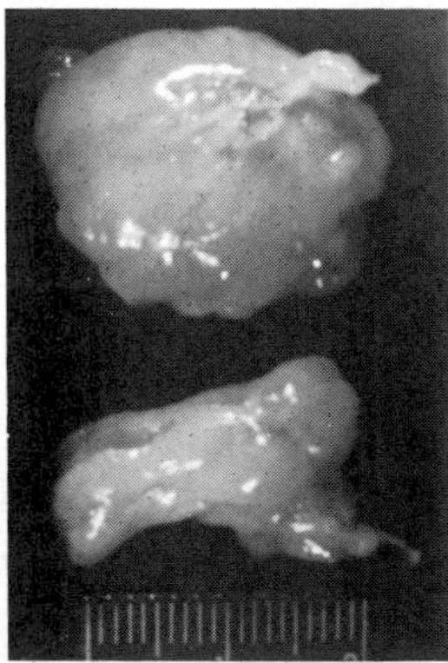

**Figure 11–178** Polyps secondary to chronic proliferative inflammation of the left middle ear in an adult cat. The nasopharyngeal polyp (upper) traversed the auditive (Eustachian) tube to lie above the soft palate; the lower polyp penetrated the tympanic membrane and occluded the external auditory canal. Bilateral nasal discharge, gagging, and a discharge from the left ear occurred over several months before successful diagnosis and treatment.

Polyps that can be grasped firmly with an Allis forceps are easily twisted free by gentle traction and rarely recur. Occasionally a lateral resection of the external meatus is required to give access to a polyp. Removal is sometimes followed by transient signs of Horner's syndrome. Bulla osteotomy is indicated if follow-up radiographs suggest persistent infection or a possible mass in the bulla.

Removal of a nasopharyngeal polyp sometimes requires an incision in the soft palate. Traction on the polyp is preferable to excision, since it is more likely to remove the pedicle.

**CYSTS.** Cyst of ceruminous glands (Fig. 11–179) is another non-neoplastic mass with a predilection for the cat. In 16 cases diagnosed at AMAH, the cats ranged from 2 to 15 years of age (mean 8). The cysts were usually multiple and in five cats involved both ears. Some cysts were present for over a year before excision. A four-year-old cat had multiple cysts, as well as hypertrophy of one pinna and external canal, from such an early age that a congenital origin was considered.

The cysts typically take the form of sessile masses, 0.1 to 0.5 cm wide, and are usually bluish or black, but occasionally pink or tan. Some look cystic or blister-like, while others appear solid until incised. An excess of brown, waxy secretion is often present in the canal, and sometimes otitis associated with otodectic mites, bacteria, or yeasts. Occasionally, multiple cysts merge into a lobulated dark mass that can be mistaken for a melanoma, hemangioma, or neoplasm of ceruminous glands. Most cysts occur in the canal, but some develop on the lower concave surface of the pinna. They are rare above the level of the ridges of the pinna.

**NODULAR HYPERPLASIA OF SEBACEOUS GLANDS.** Three middle-aged cats, two females and a male, had lesions of nodular sebaceous gland hyperplasia involving the canal (two cats) and the base of a pinna (one cat).

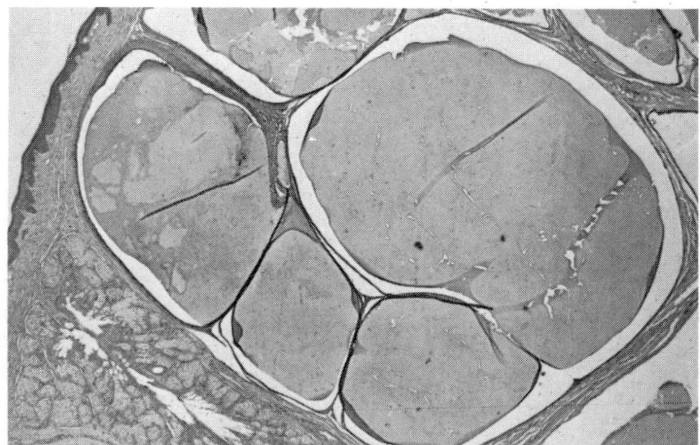

**Figure 11–179** Multiple cysts of ceruminous glands. The cystic glands, containing ceruminous secretion and occasionally blood, are seen as dark blister-like nodules in the ear canal. Adjacent sebaceous glands are often hypertrophied (lower left). H & E, × 31.

## Benign Tumors

**ADENOMA OF CERUMINOUS GLANDS.** Adenoma (adenomatous hyperplasia) of the ceruminous glands of the external meatus is the most frequent benign neoplasm of the cat's ear. The only other species in which it has been reported are man and dog, in which it is rare.

Twenty-two adenomas were diagnosed at AMAH in cats aged from 3 to 15 years (average 8.8, median 8). Only two were less than six years of age. Sixteen were males, 13 castrated. Five of the six females were spayed. Ten cats were black or white, or black and white. None were purebreds.

All the adenomas arose from the wall of the meatus except one that was located on the inner surface of the lower portion of the pinna. The lesion may be asymptomatic, but occasionally an odor, discharge, or rubbing or scratching at the ear results from an accompanying external otitis. Whether there is a relationship between otitis and the development of the tumor is not known, but at least some degree of inflammation was present in all 22 cats. Several tumors were present for from three months to a year before the owners sought advice.

Eight growths were pedunculated with either a narrow or a wide stalk, and they ranged in size from 0.2 to 1.2 cm. Shapes were described as irregular, cauliflower-like, multinodular, or grapelike, and color as dark, blue, red-black, or purple. Their consistency was variably friable, rubbery, or firm.

Although seldom seen grossly, focal or multifocal ulceration was visible microscopically in almost half the adenomas. Inflammation within and about the growth was consistent and varied from slight to severe. In the majority of tumors, purulent and mononuclear inflammation occurred between and also within the glandular proliferations. Glands and cysts often contained a purulent or histiocytic exudate, or both.

Sixteen growths had a prominent branching tubular pattern with some coiling or tortuosity. Infolding of the walls was common, as in hyperplasia. Normally oriented myoepithelial cells were seen in all adenomas. A few had glands with vacuolated cytoplasm immediately below the nuclei of the epithelial cells, making it difficult to determine if the vacuoles were subnuclear or in the myoepithelial cells (Fig. 11–180). All adenomas were simple; none was complex or of a mixed type. Four had a prominent papillary pattern as well as branching tubules. Two others with branching tubules had prominent epithelial hyperplasia simulating glandlike formation within lumens. The myoepithelial cells, although present, did not participate in intraluminal proliferation. The remaining two adenomas had proliferation of large cystic glands with mild infolding of their walls and closely resembled multiple cystic hyperplasia.

The mitotic indices of the adenomas were low, ranging from 0 to 4 per 10 HPF, with a median of 1.

All adenomas had at least some epithelial cells with granular, greenish yellow, supranuclear pigment characteristic of ceruminous glands. It varied in amount and in shades of green from tumor to tumor and within the same tumor. The columnar epithelial cells had a Golgi apparatus just above the nucleus, often with pigment granules.

Acanthosis of surface epithelium and squamous metaplasia of ducts of ceruminous glands as they approached the epidermis were frequent. Ducts of ceruminous glands of the cat usually open in common with ducts of sebaceous glands (which may or may not empty into a small hair follicle), or they may open directly to the surface as do many sebaceous glands.

**OTHER BENIGN TUMORS.** Uncommon benign tumors of the external ear are papilloma, histiocytoma, and fibroma (Priester and McKay, 1980). Extensive bilateral papillomatosis, described by Austin (1975), was treated with electrocautery. A case of sebaceous gland adenoma was reported (McAfee et al., 1979), but in gross appearance the lesions were typical of ceruminous gland adenomas, and the presence of tall columnar cells would identify the glands as ceruminous.

At AMAH there were few benign tumors other than ceruminous adenomas. The only cutaneous papilloma diagnosed microscopically in a cat was a tiny pink mass on an ear tip of a 10-year-old castrated male. One of 13 basal cell tumors on the head occurred at the base of a pinna in an eight-year-old female.

## Malignant Tumors

**ADENOCARCINOMA OF CERUMINOUS GLANDS.** Adenocarcinoma of ceruminous glands was long ago described by French pathologists in cats (Ball et al., 1938) and is among their important malignancies (Cotchin, 1983; Davenport and Eisenberg, 1984; Patnaik et al., 1975; Scott, 1980; Stookey et al., 1971). It is the most frequent of all neoplasms of the cat's ear recorded at AMAH. Specimens from 30 cats were examined. Only 15 cats were described as other than domestic short- or longhair. Of those, eight were black, blue, or black- or blue-and-white; four were tricolors, and two orange. There was only one purebred, a Siamese. The cats were slightly older than those with adenomas, ranging in age from 5 to 17 years (mean, 10.5). The median was 10 compared with 8 for cats with adenomas.

Sixteen cats were females, 11 spayed. Nine of the 14 males were castrated. These findings contrasted with the sex ratio of cats with adenomas, in which 73 per cent of the cats were males. When cats with benign and malignant ceruminous tumors are considered together, there is no sex predisposition for this tumor in a population in which male cats constitute nearly 60 per cent of hospital admissions.

**CLINICAL SIGNS.** Six cats were treated for some time for presumed chronic external otitis before the neoplasm was detected. In three cats, masses that had been previously treated as abscesses proved to be extensions of adenocarcinoma on the side of the face below an ear or at the angle of the jaw. The Siamese cat, after a three-year history of otitis, was found to have what was considered an inoperable mass in the horizontal canal. The mass enlarged in a papillary manner, finally obstructing the canal. Infection and walled-in exudate gave rise to a fistula at the junction of the cartilaginous and osseous external canal. The growth proved at autopsy to be a pedunculated papillary adenocarcinoma.

Hemorrhage from the ear occurred in two cats with bleeding neoplasms. Metastatic ulcerated tumors in the skin behind the ear, on the ventral neck, and over the shoulder occurred in one cat with a polypoid adenocarcinoma. A swelling just behind the ear of another cat was due to enlargement of the deep parotid node by a meta-

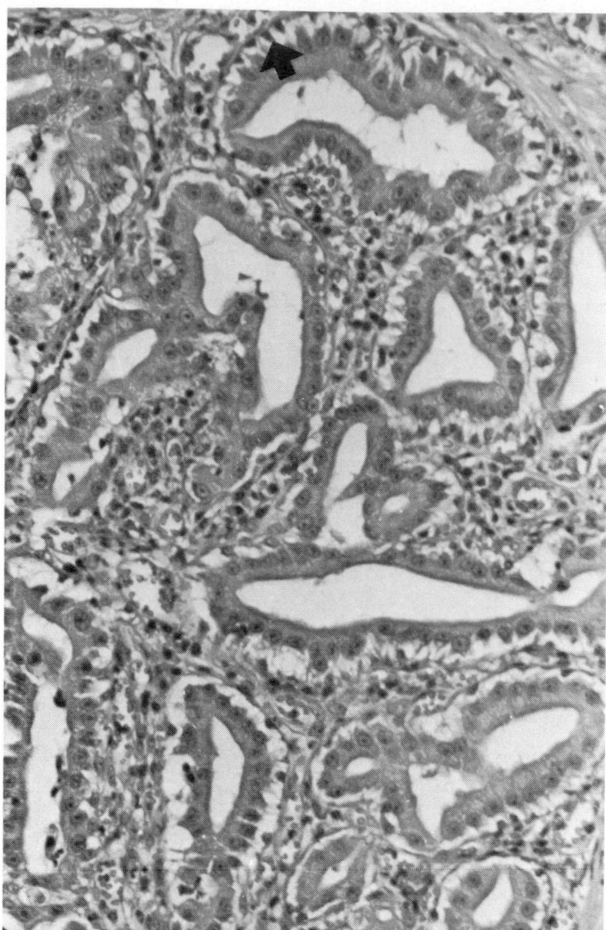

**Figure 11–180** Adenoma of ceruminous glands, eight-year-old tabby. The tumor, appearing grossly as an ulcerated polyp of the vertical ear canal, is composed of coiled tubules having normal polarity of both the outer myoepithelial (arrow) and the inner lining epithelial cells. H & E, × 200.

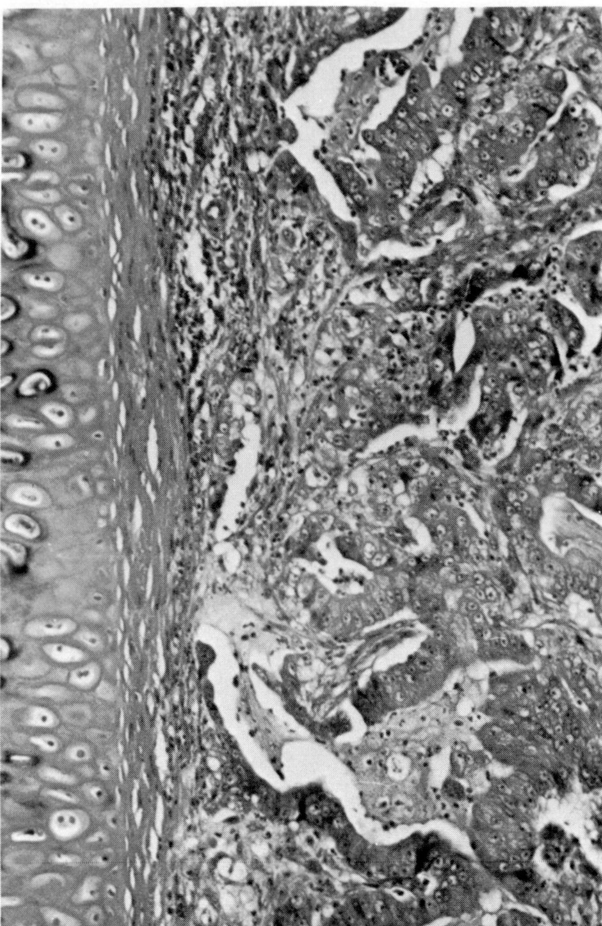

**Figure 11–181** Adenocarcinoma of ceruminous glands, eight-year-old cat, with metastases to regional nodes, lungs, and pleura. Tumor invasion approaches the cartilage (left) of the canal. It is composed of malignant epithelial cells in rows that often form incomplete glands (bottom). Inflammatory cells are within and about the imperfect tubules. H & E, × 200.

static tumor that was larger than the primary growth in the canal.

**Gross Features.** Adenocarcinomas of ceruminous glands often have features in common with adenomas but tend to be larger and more extensive. Two arose within much larger adenomas. Necrosis, ulceration, friability, and tendency to bleed are characteristics more likely to be associated with the malignant lesion. Deep infiltration of the canal, enlarged hard regional nodes, adjacent subcutaneous masses, and ulcerated lesions in the adjacent skin indicate malignancy. Deep tumors may even penetrate the eardrum and invade the middle ear.

**Microscopic Features.** Proliferation of epithelial cells in the absence of myoepithelial cells is diagnostic of malignancy; however, myoepithelial cells may be at the periphery of a group of malignant epithelial cells that form tubular, papillary, solid, or cribriform patterns.

The most common pattern of adenocarcinoma of ceruminous glands is the solid trabecular, sometimes with a tubular element. The second most common pattern is the tubular (Fig. 11–181), often with a prominent intraluminal papillary epithelial component. A papillary pattern predominated in five adenocarcinomas, and a cribriform arrangement in three. Tumors with a variety of patterns, however, were most frequent, and it is misleading to try to assign them to a single category. No complex or mixed tumors occurred among the 30 malignant or 22 benign tumors of ceruminous glands.

At the cellular level, intracytoplasmic pigment granules may be present. The mitotic indices of the malignant tumors were higher than in adenomas and ranged from 5 to 40 per 10 HPF, with a mean of 16 in those sections large enough for counting 10 fields. Malignant epithelial cells tended to be more basophilic than benign cells and often lacked the tall columnar shape and round, basally located nucleus of adenomas.

Vascular invasion was observed in 17 of the 30 adenocarcinomas. Only two cats were examined at autopsy, so knowledge of tumor behavior is limited, but five were known to have metastatic lesions involving deep parotid, retropharyngeal, and prescapular nodes; skin of head, neck, and shoulder; parotid salivary gland; skeletal muscle; and lungs and pleura.

**SQUAMOUS CELL CARCINOMA.** Auricular carcinoma of white-eared cats is an important tumor, especially in sunny climates. Carcinoma of the margin of one or both ears of five white-eared or partially white-eared cats was seen at AMAH. Two other cats had carcinoma of the external meatus. The seven cats ranged from 8 to 15 years of age. Actinic carcinoma begins insidiously over months or years as a precancerous eczematoid lesion, which eventually becomes malignant, with invasiveness and ulceration being prominent features. Regional nodes are sometimes involved and rarely there are distant metastases. Clinical features, pathologic findings, and management are discussed in the chapter on the ear.

**MAST CELL TUMOR.** The head and the neck of the cat are the most frequent sites of cutaneous mast cell tumors. Of 44 such tumors diagnosed at AMAH, 5 occurred on the pinna, 1 in a meatus, and 5 in the skin just behind the ear. A cat with disseminated cutaneous mast cell tumors also had tumors on the pinnae. (See the discussion of mast cell tumors and also the chapter on the ear.)

**FIBROSARCOMA.** The head is the most common site for fibrosarcoma of cats, according to records at AMAH. Of 23 fibrosarcomas of the head, 4 involved the pinna. (See section on skin tumors.)

### Tumors of the Middle Ear

The only growth commonly arising in the middle ear is the polyp, which is not a neoplasm but a form of proliferative inflammation. It has been discussed earlier among tumor-like lesions of the ear. Squamous cell carcinomas and a fibrosarcoma of the middle ear have been the cause of vestibular disturbances and facial paralysis (Indrieri and Taylor, 1984; Pentlarge, 1984; Rendano et al., 1980).

The only true neoplasm on record at AMAH that appeared to originate in, fill, and destroy most of the left bulla was an adenosquamous carcinoma in a five-year-old castrated male domestic shorthair. The tumor, which probably arose in the seromucous glands along the auditive (Eustachian) tube, destroyed much of the temporal bone and impinged on the pons and medulla, causing compression of cranial nerves VII through XI. It spread by lymphatics to the retropharyngeal node and lungs. Horner's syndrome of the left eye, ataxia, head tilt and falling to the left, atrophy of the left side of the tongue, flaccid paralysis of the left side of the pharynx, and occasional right rotary nystagmus were the neurologic abnormalities.

Lymphoma of the middle ear is a rarity but was found in a cat that also had lymphoma of the trachea and cervical nodes.

### Tumors of the Inner Ear

A secondary tumor occurred in a 14-year-old Siamese. The cat suddenly began to circle to the left, later developed pharyngeal paralysis, and would stand restlessly with its head against a wall or sleep with its left eye open. The left eyelid was paralyzed and the left corneal reflex was absent. The optic disks were pale gray, the pupillary responses sluggish, and the eyesight apparently impaired. The extensor thrust and righting reflexes were also affected. The tumor, a carcinoma of nasopharyngeal origin, involved the petrous temporal bone, acoustic nerve, tympanic bulla, and the dura, compressing the lower aspect of the left piriform lobe of the cerebrum and the left trigeminal, trochlear, abducent, and oculomotor nerves. It had passed through the roof of the nasopharynx and extended extradurally as far forward as the optic chiasm.

## MAST CELL TUMORS*

Mast cell tumors are the third most common tumor in cats at AMAH after lymphoma and adenocarcinoma of the mammary gland. Although Antoine reported a tumor in the spleen of a 13-year-old male cat in 1907, the incidence of feline mast cell tumors appears to have increased strikingly since about 1950.

The mast cell is a connective tissue cell thought to arise from perivascular mesenchymal cells, basophils, or lymphocytes (Ginsburg, 1963; Higginbotham, 1963; Selye, 1965). Widely distributed in the body, mast cells are most abundant in the submucosa of the respiratory and intestinal tracts, lymphoreticular tissues, bone marrow, serous membranes, skin, and the adventitia of small capillaries and venules. In normal cats, these cells are most easily identified adjacent to or surrounding small capillaries of the papillary dermis, adnexa, and subcutis. Mast cell tumors arise from tissues that normally have many mast cells: the skin, lymphoreticular organs, and the small intestine. Tumors may be single or multiple. Although a single site of origin can usually be found, some tumors appear to arise multicentrically.

### The Mast Cell—Morphology and Function

The morphology and behavior of the neoplastic mast cell parallel those of the normal mast cell. The normal mast cell is 7.0 to 10.0 $\mu$ in diameter and polygonal, fusiform, or stellate. The nucleus is oval and central; chromatin is uniformly dispersed, varies in density, and may form a thin basophilic rim at the nuclear margin. Nucleoli are rare. The cytoplasm contains granules that stain brightly eosinophilic with hematoxylin and eosin, in contrast to that of the dog, in which the granules stain more basophilic.

The ultrastructure of the cat's mast cells resembles that of other species (Alroy et al., 1975; Ward and Hurvitz, 1972). Moderate numbers of microvilli are on the cell surface. Intracytoplasmic fibrils are rare. The cytoplasm contains up to eight mitochondria and more than 70 heterogeneous granules. The diameter of the granules averages 0.6 $\mu$ but may reach 0.9 $\mu$. The granules appear to arise from the Golgi zone and have three major features: a parallel arrangement of moderately dense, fine filaments, which often contain crystalloid structures; very dense, finely granular material; and thick, curved, parallel lamellae in a fingerprint pattern. A trilaminar membrane surrounds each granule.

Neoplastic mast cells in well-differentiated tumors of cats may closely resemble normal mast cells. Light and electron microscopic studies (Alroy et al., 1975; Ward and Hurvitz, 1972) have shown that some neoplastic mast cells tend to be larger, up to 20 $\mu$ in diameter. The nucleus

*Laura K. Andrews, principal author.

is immature: larger, oval or indented, hyperchromatic or vesicular, and either central or eccentric. It may have a nucleolus. Cytoplasm is eosinophilic and finely granular or vacuolated. Cell organelles are more numerous. The cytoplasm contains up to 21 mitochondria, and there are intracytoplasmic fibrils. Granules are smaller, averaging 0.5 μ in diameter, with an upper limit of 0.7 μ; are fewer, less than 50 per cell; and are more uniform than normal granules. Metachromasia is variable. Other features of neoplastic feline mast cells have been described by Madewell et al. (1984).

Neoplastic mast cells with cytoplasmic extensions containing virus-like particles were reportedly seen by electron microscopy (Saar et al., 1969). The mast cells failed to grow in tissue culture and could not be transmitted to cats, mice, or hamsters.

Mast cell granules contain preformed or primary mediators, newly formed or secondary mediators, and substances in the granular matrix that compose up to a quarter of the granule's weight (Benditt and Lagunoff, 1964; Kaliner, 1979). Histamine and heparin are preformed mediators in the mast cells of cats and other mammals (Chiu and Lagunoff, 1972). The sulfated mucopolysaccharides permit distinctive staining of the granules with metachromatic dyes (Chiu and Lagunoff, 1972; Padawer, 1974). The granules of normal and of many neoplastic mast cells stain red with periodic acid–Schiff (PAS); magenta, purple, or blue with Giemsa; and purple with toluidine blue. The cat's mast cells probably contain other mediators, some of which have been identified in mast cells of other species. These include dopamine, serotonin and its precursors, eosinophil chemotactic factor (ECF), platelet activating factor (PAF), leukotrienes such as slow-reacting substance of anaphylaxis (SRS-A), prostaglandins, chondroitins, and other peptides (Kaliner, 1979). The concentration of these substances in the mast cell may be $10^5$ to $10^6$ times their concentration in extracellular fluid and blood (Jaques et al., 1977).

The functions of mast cells are poorly understood. Researchers have shown that mast cells function in inflammatory and allergic responses and help to defend the host from parasites having a tissue phase (Kaliner, 1979). In most mammals, the external surface of mast cells has 100,000 to 500,000 glycoprotein receptor sites for the Fc fragment of IgE (Kaliner, 1979). When allergens react with IgE on the mast cell surface, granules release biologically active mediators that cause signs of immediate hypersensitivity: increased vascular permeability, smooth muscle spasm, mucus secretion, eosinophil and neutrophil chemotaxis, pruritus, vasodilation, increased adenylate and guanylate cyclase, superoxide production, anticoagulation, and tissue destruction (Burgoon et al., 1968; Kaliner, 1979).

Commonly found within and around tumors, the mast cell may help to regulate growth (Baroni, 1964; Higginbotham and Murillo, 1965; Howard and Kenyon, 1967; Parmley et al., 1975; Takakura et al., 1966). It is not known if the mast cell's association with tumors benefits or harms the host. Histamine release by mast cells is thought to decrease cytolysis by T-lymphocytes and to decrease the delayed hypersensitivity response by suppressing macrophage inhibitory factor (MIF) (Parmley et al., 1975; Rocklin, 1976). These actions could favor tumor growth. Histamine may also induce antibody production by B-lymphocytes, a function that could inhibit tumor growth (Parmley et al., 1975).

A recently proposed theory of mast cell function, based on the study of polyelectrolytes such as heparin, suggests that mast cell granules act as ion exchangers, permitting mast cells to remove metals, amines, proteins, and other substances from tissue fluids (Melander et al., 1975; Padawer, 1974).

## Mast Cell Tumors of the Skin

If mammary tumors are excluded, mast cell tumors are the second most common skin tumor of cats at AMAH. A comprehensive review of 58 mast cell tumors reported before 1970 and of 16 RCP-AFIP cases (Garner and Lingeman, 1970) included 28 primary mast cell tumors of the skin. Holzinger (1973) reported 65 cutaneous mast cell tumors among 718 cat tumors and granulomas gathered during a five-year period at the New York State Veterinary Diagnostic Laboratory. Six of 83 cutaneous neoplasms reported by Engle and Brodey (1969) were mast cell tumors.

At AMAH, mast cell tumors were first diagnosed in cats in 1955 (Meier, 1957). Of the total of 176 mast cell tumors of all sites recorded at AMAH between 1955 and 1981, 89 (51 per cent) were primary skin tumors. The cats were aged 6 months to 21 years (mean 9 years). The tumors occurred equally in males and females. Sixty-five per cent of the cats were domestic shorthairs, 9 per cent domestic longhairs, and 15 per cent Siamese; breed was not specified for the rest. The incidence in Siamese was three times that in the hospital population generally.

**GROSS FEATURES.** A compact dermal form and a diffuse, infiltrative dermal and subcutaneous form were described by Holzinger (1973). Four types were distinguished by Scott (1980):

1. Multiple, often symmetrically shaped, raised, soft, round, poorly demarcated, edematous, pinkish masses (0.5 to 5.0 cm in diameter) fixed to overlying skin (Fig. 11–182).
2. Multiple, often symmetrically shaped, raised, firm, round, well-demarcated, white to yellow, 0.2 to 1.0 cm papules and nodules fixed to overlying skin (Fig. 11–183).
3. Single or multiple raised, firm, erythematous, well-circumscribed, 1.0 to 7.0 cm cutaneous plaques often ulcerated and pruritic (Fig. 11–184).
4. Solitary, firm, round, well-circumscribed 0.5 to 3.0 cm masses that are dermoepidermal or subcutaneous (Fig. 11–185).

Most (70 per cent) of the cutaneous mast cell tumors diagnosed at AMAH were single, firm, circumscribed, round, dermal nodules that were white or yellow on cut section (Scott's fourth type). The second type was next (20 per cent) in frequency, while the first and third (plaque type) were seen less often.

Of the 84 tumors for which site was specified, 44 (52 per cent) were on the head or neck; 15 (18 per cent) on the feet or legs; 14 (17 per cent) on the trunk, abdomen, or flank; and 11 (13 per cent) multifocal or disseminated. These findings accord with the slight predilection for the head and neck (58 per cent) reported by Garner and Lingeman (1970). On the head, the most common sites were the temples, pinnae, and periorbital area. Oral mast cell tumor, a rare finding in dogs, was diagnosed in a single cat that previously had a lip lesion with characteristics of both eosinophilic granuloma and mast cell tumor (Fig. 11–186). Sixty-five tumors (73 per cent) in cats at

*Text continued on page 575*

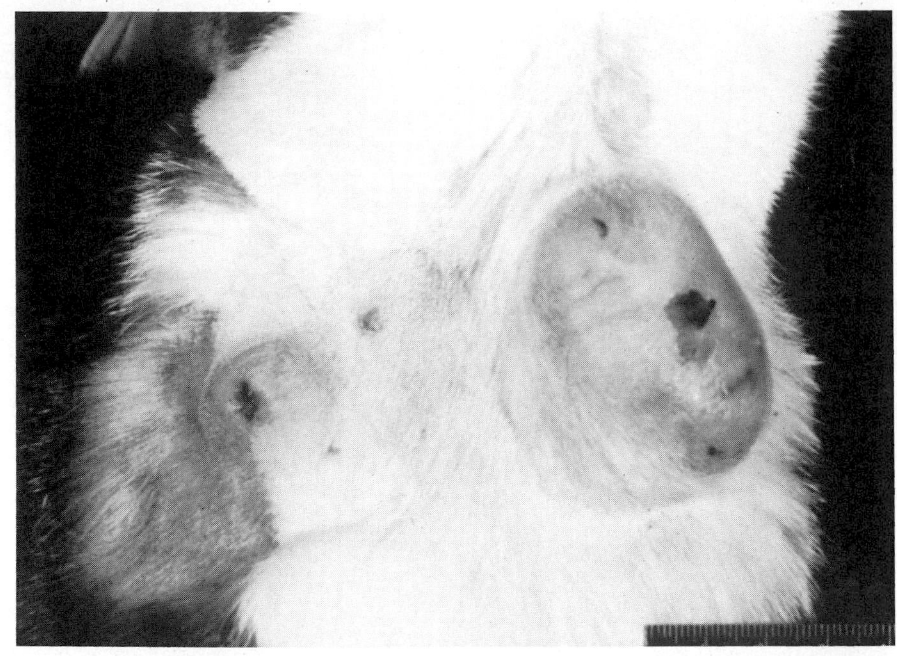

**Figure 11–182** Multiple dermal and subcutaneous mast cell tumors on the ventral thorax, 14-year-old castrated male blue-and-white domestic shorthair. Hair has been clipped around the tumors, which are covered by discolored and ulcerated skin. Several small, soft lesions appearing on the head and neck five years before were diagnosed clinically elsewhere as "wens" or "cysts"; they had increased in size and number when the cat was hospitalized at AMAH for resection of a transitional cell bladder carcinoma. At that time the skin lesions were diagnosed by needle aspirates as mast cell tumors. During the following six months the cat was treated with prednisone and the tumor remained unchanged, but the cat was euthanatized for kidney failure. Autopsy disclosed recurrent bladder tumor and malignant lymphoma of both kidneys, stomach, small intestine, pancreas, adrenal, and tracheobronchial lymph nodes.

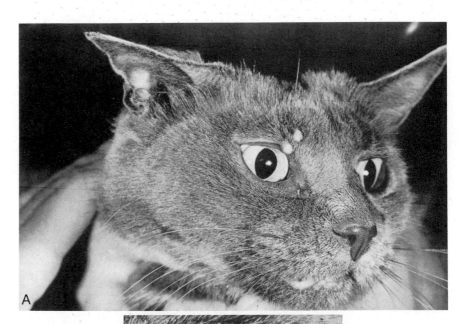


**Figure 11–183** *A*, Cutaneous mast cell tumors of ear, eyelid, and eyebrow in an eight-year-old blue domestic shorthair. Mast cells constituted 4 per cent of the nucleated cells of the blood. Autopsy revealed mast cell tumors of the skin, peripheral nodes, spleen, liver, and marrow. *B*, Two elevated circular mast cell tumors are at the mucocutaneous margin of the left upper lip.

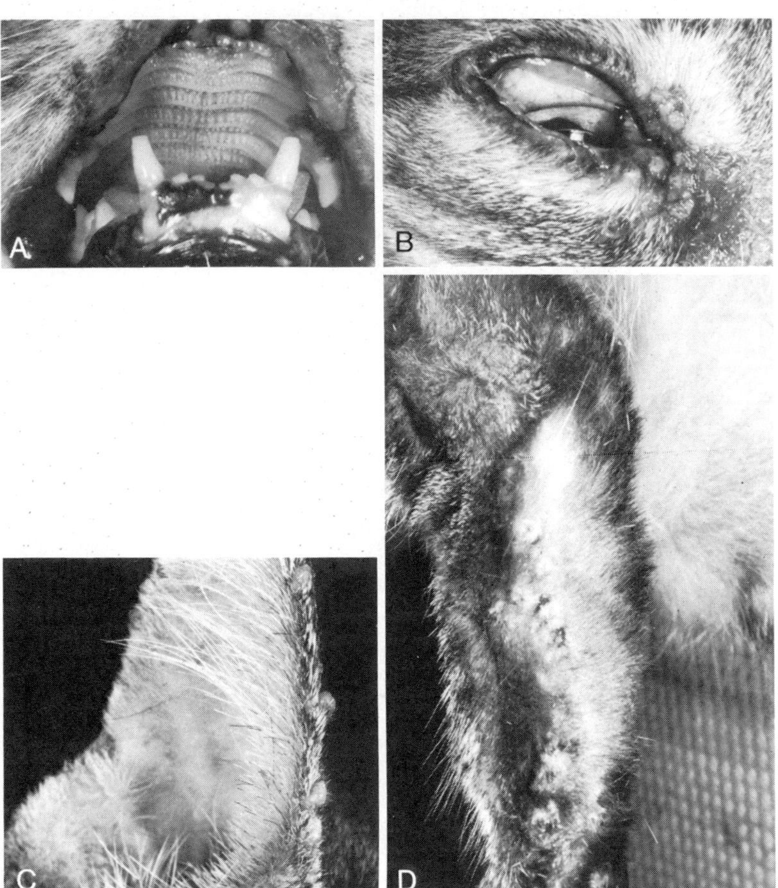


**Figure 11–184** Cutaneous and visceral mast cell neoplasia, 12-year-old spayed female tabby domestic shorthair. *A*, Bilateral ulcerated mast cell tumors of upper lip are grossly indistinguishable from eosinophilic granulomas. Several papules composed of mast cells lie within the skin adjacent to the right ulcer. *B*, Mast cell tumors forming papules within the eyelids and skin of the nose. Nasal alopecia and exudative dermatitis were sequelae of a diffuse mast cell infiltrate in the skin. *C*, Bead-like mast cell tumors and cystic apocrine glands along ear margin. *D*, Disseminated cutaneous mast cell tumors on lateral left forearm. Papular and crateriform tumors in linear array suggest tumor metastasis by lymphatics; regional lymph nodes had metastases. In gross appearance these lesions are strikingly similar to linear granuloma.

*Illustration continued on opposite page*

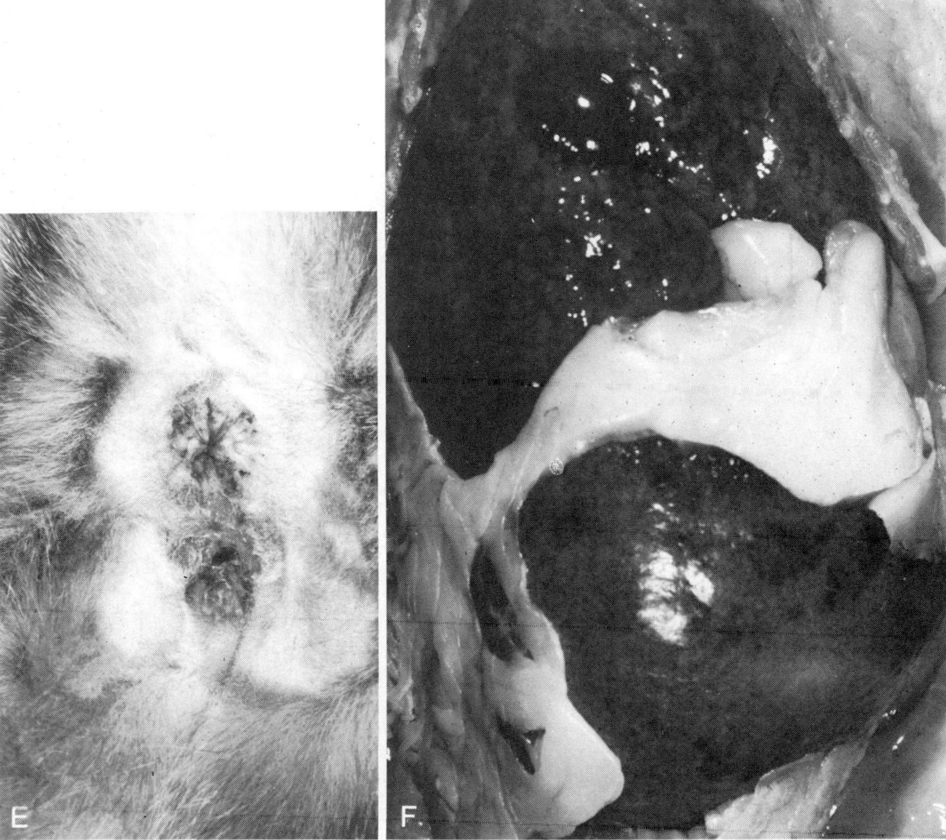


**Figure 11–184** *Continued E*, Mast cell tumors of the anus and vulva. Reddish watery fluid oozed from the lesions. *F*, Visceral mast cell neoplasia causing extraordinary hepatosplenomegaly. Both organs were diffusely infiltrated by mast cells, but much of the nodularity of the liver resulted from foci of hepatocytic hyperplasia. The cause of the splenomegaly was determined ante mortem by percutaneous fine-needle aspiration to be mast cell neoplasia. Mast cells were seen in neither blood films nor marrow sections.

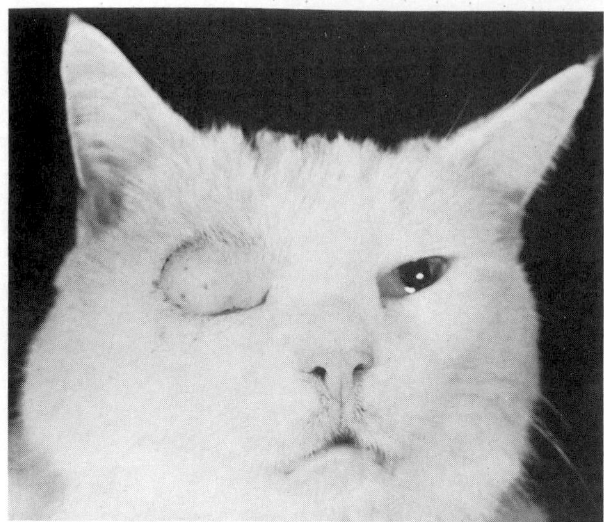

**Figure 11–185** Mast cell tumor, upper eyelid, 12-year-old white domestic shorthair. The tumor, which felt soft and almost fluctuant, was described by the owner as an inflammatory swelling that recurred and subsided over many months. The affected eyelid was removed, together with the eye, and the cat suffered no recurrence. Seen in 1958, this was only the fourth mast cell tumor diagnosed in a cat at AMAH during the 12 years from 1946. Mast cell tumor has since become the second most frequent skin tumor of cats at AMAH.

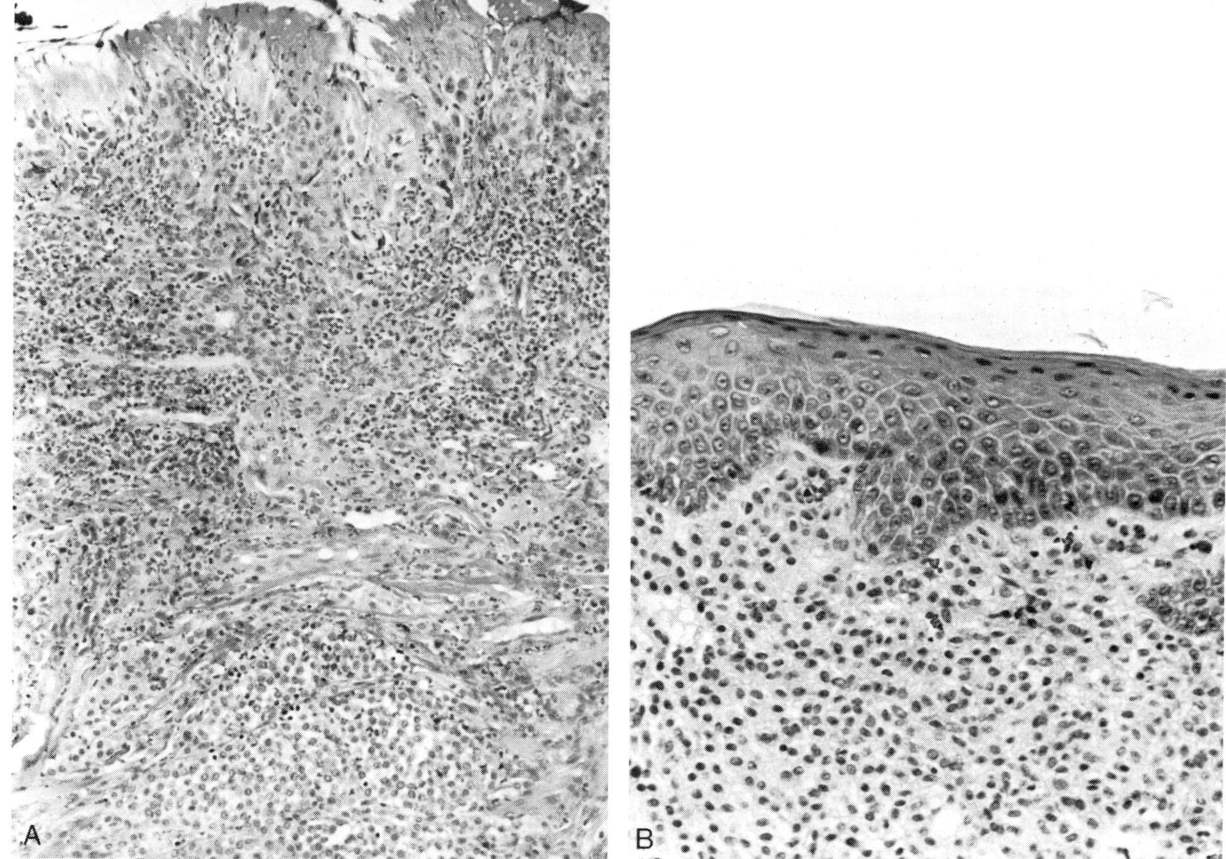


**Figure 11–186** *A*, Mast cell tumor and ulcerative cheilitis with strong microscopic resemblances to eosinophilic granuloma, upper lip, nine-year-old spayed female domestic shorthair. A solid aggregate of mast cells (below) underlies an ulcer with eosinophilic, neutrophilic, and necrotizing inflammation. The lesion was not responsive to corticosteroid therapy but did not recur after excision. H & E, × 125. *B*, Mast cell tumor of the hard palate, same cat 14 months later. Numerous white palatine plaques, 2 to 3 mm wide, were composed of compact groups of mast cells, with an occasional eosinophil, lying adjacent to the mucosal epithelium. Oral mast cell tumors are exceedingly rare in the cat. H & E, × 200.

AMAH were solitary, and 24 were multiple or disseminated.

A solitary cutaneous mast cell tumor may resemble a granuloma, cutaneous tag, unpigmented basal cell tumor, fibroma, epidermal inclusion cyst, hyperplasia or adenoma of sebaceous gland, or lymphosarcoma. Of these lesions, only basal cell tumors are common in the cat. Multiple or disseminated mast cell tumors are most often confused with lymphosarcomas or fibrosarcomas, which are rare, or with non-neoplastic allergic dermatitides, which are fairly common. Plaque-like mast cell tumors may be difficult to distinguish, both grossly and microscopically, from eosinophilic plaques. Edematous tumors may be mistaken for cellulitis or abscesses, insect bites, or infected tumors. Any tumor-like mass present for more than a week should undergo biopsy or excision, or, at the very least, be monitored vigilantly for increase in size.

**MICROSCOPIC FEATURES.** Of the 89 primary cutaneous tumors examined at AMAH, most (70 per cent) consisted of a single compact nodule of well-differentiated mast cells confined to the dermis and superficial subcutis. This type corresponds to the compact type described by Holzinger (1973) and type 4 of Scott (1980). The cells were discrete and polygonal with oval or ellipsoid central nuclei that occupied less than half the cell. Cytoplasm was granular and stained brightly eosinophilic, and cytoplasmic granules were consistently metachromatic. Cells were arranged in solid sheets or ribbons. Aggregates of plasma cells and lymphocytes were common in the deep dermis and subcutis. Numbers of eosinophils varied. Forty-one per cent of the tumors had few or no eosinophils; if present, they were mostly intra- or perivascular. Eosinophils were more numerous in tumors that were more diffuse or had greater numbers of poorly differentiated mast cells.

A second type of tumor seen was a less discrete dermal mass that infiltrated the subcutis. Cells were polygonal or fusiform. Nuclei were oval, indented, and large, constituting 50 to 70 per cent of cell volume. Cytoplasm was vacuolated, finely granular, and eosinophilic. Metachromatic staining was variable. Multinucleated cells and mitotic figures were sometimes seen. Necrosis was common, and fibrosis occurred in some tumors. This type corresponds roughly to the diffuse tumors described by Holzinger (1973), 70 per cent of which he considered malignant. Of the 20 tumors at AMAH that recurred or metastasized, six were of diffuse type.

**DIAGNOSIS.** Cutaneous mast cell tumors can be diagnosed by microscopic examination of fine-needle aspirates, imprints, or biopsy specimens. Recent excoriation, excessive handling, and injection of local anesthetic into or too close to a lesion may cause degranulation of mast cells. These factors should be considered when biopsy is performed. Mast cell granules are usually better preserved and easier to identify in fine-needle aspirates or imprints than in formalin-fixed and paraffin-processed specimens. Mast cell tumors with large numbers of eosinophils are most often confused with allergic dermatitis, eosinophilic granulomas or plaques, or chronic inflammation. Ill-differentiated or degranulated tumors, especially if poorly fixed, or in a cat that has received cortisone, may be confused with lymphoma or solid infiltrates of myeloid leukemia.

**BEHAVIOR.** An accurate estimation of the malignancy of primary cutaneous tumors is difficult. Holzinger (1973) classified 56 per cent as malignant on the basis of recurrence after surgery or cutaneous or visceral (one cat) dissemination. Garner and Lingeman (1970) diagnosed 44 per cent of 18 as malignant by the criterion of visceral involvement.

At AMAH, presence of the tumor before diagnosis had been noted by owners for periods from a few days to six and a half years. Intermittent itching and redness were common. Self-inflicted trauma or vascular compromise frequently caused ulceration. Follow-up data were available for only 34 cats. During periods of from seven months to six and a half years, 41 per cent had no recurrence or metastases after removal. Twenty-four per cent (eight) had local invasion or recurrence or developed mast cell tumors elsewhere on the skin. Time to recurrence or development of second tumors ranged from three weeks to two years but was usually within seven months. Six cats (18 per cent) later developed splenic mast cell tumor, two (four per cent) had metastases to regional lymph nodes, one had concomitant tumor in the jejunum, one had a cranial mediastinal tumor, and two had mast cells in circulating blood.

## Mast Cell Tumors of the Intestine

After lymphoma and adenocarcinoma, mast cell tumors are the third most common primary intestinal tumor in the cat. In one report, 2 of 16 cats with mast cell tumors had tumors in the intestinal tract—one in the small intestine and one in the cecum (Garner and Lingeman, 1970). At AMAH, 46 intestinal mast cell tumors were recorded. Alroy et al. (1975) described 24 diagnosed at AMAH between 1955 and 1974. Many had been formerly diagnosed as argentaffinomas. Of the 28 tumors for which complete material was available for review, 24 were in the small intestine, with approximately equal numbers in the duodenum, jejunum, and ileum. Four were in the colon. The cats ranged in age from seven to 21 years (mean 13). All were either domestic short- or longhairs. There was no sex predilection.

**CLINICAL SIGNS.** Clinical signs were most often intermittent vomiting, diarrhea, weight loss, anorexia, and depression. Stools were bloody in one cat and contained mucus in two. Most cats had a palpable or radiographically visible abdominal mass. Some had a peritoneal effusion, fever, or mild anemia. In none of the cases studied by Alroy et al. (1975) were there mast cells in the circulating blood. Most of the cats had been ill for over three months and either died or were destroyed because of the tumor.

**GROSS FEATURES.** Most of the tumors were single or multiple firm, segmental thickenings of the intestinal wall, from 1.0 to 7.0 cm in diameter (Fig. 11–187*A*). The tumor was usually confined to the submucosa and tunica muscularis. The mucosa bulged over the tumor but, in contrast with adenocarcinoma and lymphoma, was rarely ulcerated. On cut section, the tumors were poorly demarcated, smooth, and yellow.

**MICROSCOPIC FEATURES.** The mast cells of intestinal tumors are less well differentiated than those of cutaneous tumors. The cells have an eccentric, oval or indented, hyperchromatic nucleus. Chromatin may be marginated, and the nucleolus may be prominent. Cytoplasm is vacuolated or granular and pale pink or clear.

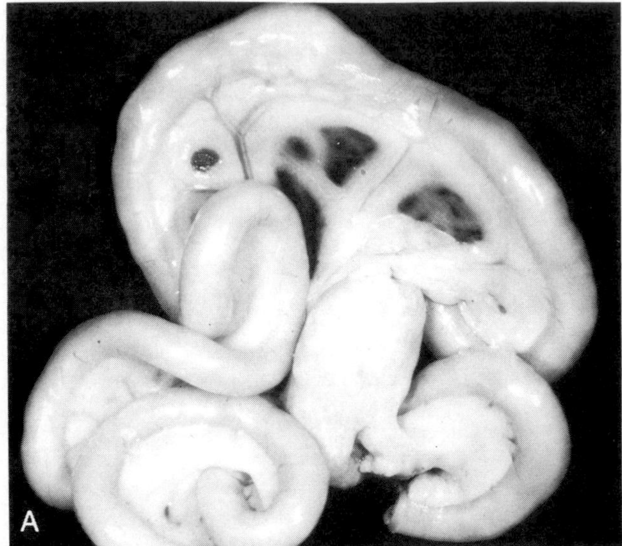


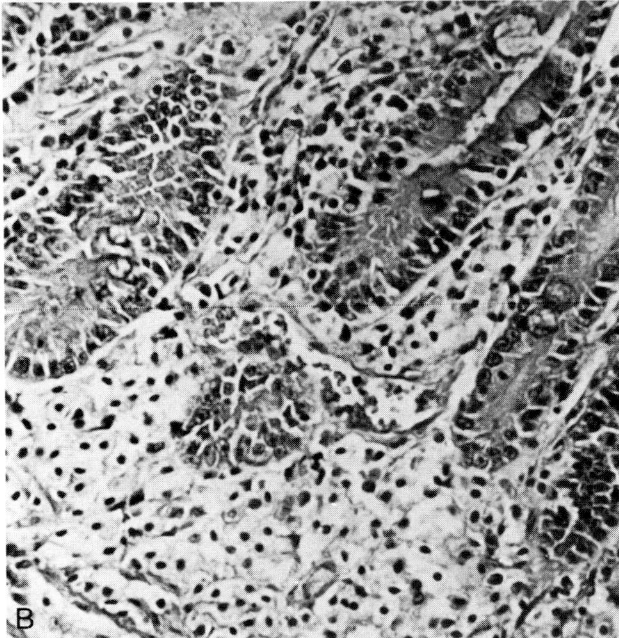


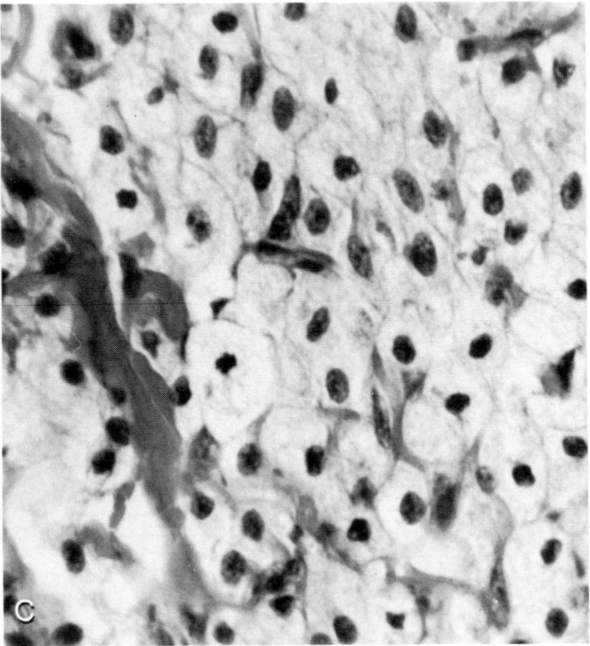


**Figure 11–187** *A*, Mast cell tumor of the jejunum (top) with metastasis to the mesenteric nodes (bottom center), six-year-old female blue-and-white domestic shorthair. In gross appearance the tumors resembled malignant lymphoma except for their color. These, like many intestinal mast cell tumors, were light yellow, whereas lymphomas tend to be white. The spleen (not shown) also had excessive mast cell neoplasia. *B*, Same cat. Mast cells diffusely infiltrate between and below crypts of the intestinal glands. H & E, × 200. *C*, Same tumor. The tightly packed, polyhedral mast cells have abundant, faintly granular, pale cytoplasm. Such cells usually do not stain metachromatically. H & E, × 760. (*B* from Alroy J, Leav I, DeLellis RA, et al.: Lab Invest 33 [1975] 159–167.)

Mast cell granules may be difficult to identify in many areas of formalin-fixed and paraffin-embedded sections, even with metachromatic stains. Electron microscopic studies showed that the granules were smaller than in normal cells and were situated at the periphery of the cell (Alroy et al., 1975). It was thought that many of the tumor cells were undergoing degranulation.

The mast cells tend to be arranged in two patterns: whorls of fusiform cells with indistinct cytoplasmic borders, and compact nests of uniformly polygonal cells 10 to 20 μ in diameter with indistinct cytoplasmic borders (Fig. 11–187*B* and *C*). Either or both patterns may occur in a given tumor (Alroy et al., 1975). The tumor cells infiltrate among smooth muscle cells of the tunica muscularis. Gut-associated lymphoid tissue may be surrounded by tumor but is rarely effaced. Tumor sometimes extends into the lamina propria, but mucosal ulceration does not occur. Fibrosis is common, and there may be a few eosinophils. Ultrastructural findings suggest that degranulated mast cells predominate (Alroy et al., 1975). None of the tumors examined had electron-dense or crystalline granules seen in normal and neoplastic mast cells in other locations. Many granules were empty vesicles surrounded by a unit membrane and containing loose, finely fibrillar material. Fused vesicles were common.

There is morphologic and histochemical evidence that mast cells in the intestinal tract differ from those in other locations (Alroy et al., 1975; Enerbäck and Lundin, 1974). Mast cells in the duodenal mucosa of the cat have fewer granules that vary in size and shape, lack microvilli, and often have indented nuclei. Degranulation does not follow administration of compound 48/80, as with other mast cells (Enerbäck and Lundin, 1974).

**DIAGNOSIS.** Excisional biopsy is the most effective way to diagnose and treat intestinal mast cell tumors. Because the tumor cells usually extend beyond the apparent margin of the tumor, 5 to 10 cm of normal intestine proximal and distal to the growth should be removed. Adjacent lymph nodes, liver, and spleen should be inspected for metastatic tumor. Touch imprints of fresh tumor tissue should always be made.

**BEHAVIOR.** All intestinal mast cell tumors should be considered malignant. Of the 28 cats at AMAH for which material was complete, 18 were found at laparotomy or autopsy to have involvement elsewhere. Mesenteric lymph nodes and liver were the most common sites, followed by spleen, lung, hepatic and cecal lymph nodes, and bone marrow. Most cats with tumors in the intestine had been ill for over three months before diagnosis. A 13-year-old female with an eight-month history of intermittent vomiting and diarrhea had a tumor 4.0 cm in diameter removed from the terminal jejunum. The mesenteric lymph node, also removed at surgery, had metastases. The cat did well for four months after surgery but then lost its appetite, became weak, and vomited. It had massive tumorous enlargement of the liver and remaining mesenteric nodes; a peritoneal effusion contained many eosinophils. The cat died five months after surgery.

## Mast Cell Tumors of Lymphoreticular Tissues

The most commonly reported visceral form of mast cell tumor arises in the spleen or other lymphoreticular tissues. More than 50 tumors have been reported, many of "leukemic" type (Allard, 1979; Confer et al., 1978; Garner and Lingeman, 1970; Guerre et al., 1979; Hauser, 1965; Kammerman-Lüscher, 1966; Labie and Fontaine, 1960; Lillie, 1931; Liska et al., 1979; Nielsen et al., 1970; Ohshima and Miura, 1965; Park, 1972; Saar et al., 1969; Schmidt and Langham, 1967; Seawright and Grono, 1964; Stünzi, 1956; Weller, 1978). Forty-one primary mast cell tumors of lymphoreticular tissues were diagnosed in cats at AMAH: 35 in the spleen, 4 in the cranial mediastinum, and 2 in peripheral lymph nodes. The cats ranged in age from 4 to 17 years (mean 10). There was no breed or sex predilection.

**CLINICAL SIGNS.** Signs of visceral mast cell tumor depend on the location and extent of involvement. Mast cell tumors usually cause splenic enlargement ranging from mild to massive. When palpated, the spleen is firm and may be smooth, with rounded borders, or nodular. Some cats have a single smooth, well-circumscribed nodule. If tumor involves the liver, the organ is enlarged, firm, and smooth or nodular. A third of cats at AMAH with visceral mast cell tumors had peritoneal or pleural effusions. The fluid was usually bloody but occasionally clear. Eosinophils, occasionally in vast numbers, or neoplastic mast cells, or both, were often present.

The four cats with tumors of the cranial mediastinum had mild or moderate pleural effusions that caused respiratory difficulty. The cranioventral thorax could not be compressed, and a mediastinal mass could be seen in thoracic radiographs.

Depression, weight loss, intermittent vomiting, and anorexia are common clinical signs. A third of cats at AMAH were mildly or severely anemic owing to hemorrhage or neoplastic infiltration of hematopoietic tissues. Twelve of the 30 cats had neoplastic mast cells in the bone marrow and peripheral blood. Chances of detecting circulating mast cells are increased by examining films prepared from the buffy coat of a centrifuged blood sample. Numbers of mast cells counted in the peripheral blood of cats at AMAH ranged from three to 32,000/$\mu$l. In one cat with mast cell leukemia, 64 per cent of 50,000 white blood cells were neoplastic mast cells when the cat died. The number of mast cells in the cat's peripheral blood fluctuated dramatically from week to week. This cat, and a few others, had a variable mild eosinophilia.

Cats with disseminated mast cell tumors sometimes have clinical signs caused by release of substances that alter smooth muscle tone, vascular permeability, and coagulation. Many of these substances, which include histamine, heparin, PAF, SRS-A, ECF, serotonin, kinin activators, dopamine, and prostaglandins, have been identified in normal and neoplastic mast cells of man and other species (Kaliner, 1979; Selye, 1965). In man, flushing, urticaria, hypotension, tachycardia, vomiting, diarrhea, pruritus, headaches, weakness, osteoporosis, cognitive changes, dyspnea, hypoxemia, and shock are clinical signs of mast cell malignancy. These signs are episodic and are due to acute mast cell degranulation (Kaliner, 1979; Kaye and Passero, 1979). Many of these signs have been observed in cats with mast cell tumors.

Release of substances such as histamine, serotonin, SRS-A, and prostaglandins, which increase gastrointestinal motility, may cause vomiting and diarrhea. Duodenal or gastric ulceration, sometimes with perforation, has been reported (Hasler and van den Ingh, 1978; Liska et al., 1979; Park, 1972; Seawright and Grono, 1964) and occurred in three cats at AMAH (Fig. 11–188). It is thought to be due to histamine-induced hypersecretion of HCl by parietal cells of the gastric mucosa and is probably abetted by vasoconstriction (Howard et al., 1969). Localized or widespread thrombosis in major organs may occur. Fibrin thrombi are often found at autopsy. One cat at AMAH had neurologic signs due to cerebral infarction and subarachnoid hemorrhage. Another cat had an hepatic infarct. Uncontrollable hemorrhage is common in cats with disseminated mast cell tumor, particularly after palpation or surgical manipulation of a large tumor. Splenic rupture is a common cause of acute shock and death, unless animals are handled and palpated very gently.

In some cats, labored respiration in the absence of anemia or space-occupying masses may be due to release of histamine, serotonin, and SRS-A, with consequent hypoxemia, pulmonary edema, and increased vascular resistance. The feline lung is extraordinarily sensitive to serotonin and is the shock organ in the cat (McCusker and Aitken, 1966). Signs of experimentally induced anaphylaxis in cats (head scratching, labored respiration, salivation, vomiting, incoordination, and collapse) are remarkably similar to signs observed in some cats with disseminated mast cell tumors (McCusker and Aitken, 1966).

Some cats with mast cell tumors have hyperglobulinemia. Of four cats described by Saar et al. (1969) one had an elevated beta fraction, one an elevated alpha fraction, and one an elevated gamma fraction. The elevated fraction was unspecified in the fourth cat. The cause of hyperglobulinemia is unknown. Howard and Kenyon (1967) found increased alpha-2 globulin in dogs with mast cell tumor. They identified a glycoprotein, the concentra-

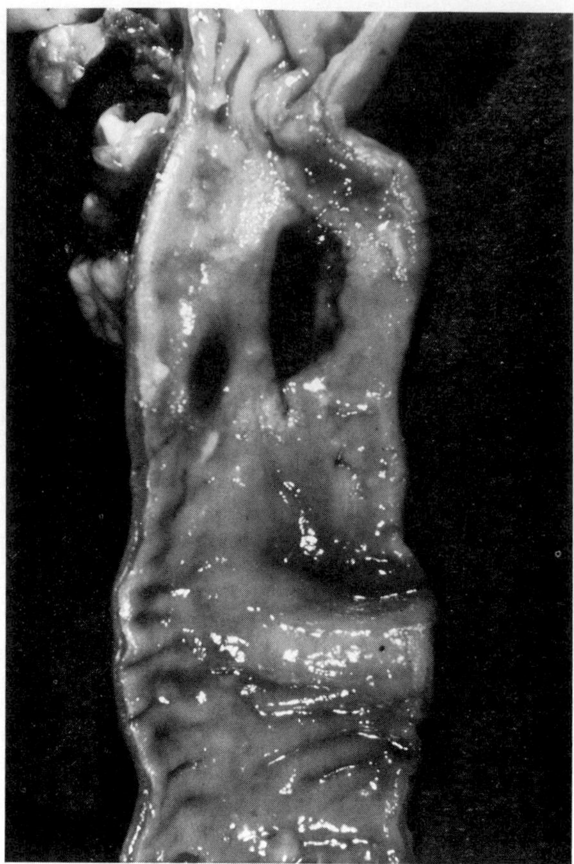

**Figure 11–188** Multiple duodenal ulcers in a four-year-old spayed female black-and-white domestic shorthair with generalized mast cell neoplasia. The largest ulcer (near pylorus, top) perforated and caused sudden death after a two-week course of vomiting.

tion of which corresponded with the size of the developing tumor. Because injection of histamine dihydrochloride causes increases in the same glycoprotein, the investigators attributed serum protein alterations to release of histamine by the tumor. Histamine may also induce B-lymphocytes to produce levels of antibody high enough to cause hyperglobulinemia. Alpha globulins are also increased by tissue destruction, a common result of mast cell tumors, and hepatic injury by metastatic mast cell tumor could elevate alpha and beta globulins.

**GROSS FEATURES.** Mast cell tumors of the spleen may be diffuse or nodular. Eight per cent of cats at AMAH with primary splenic involvement had massively enlarged, firm spleens mottled red, brown, and yellow, and weighing up to 415.0 gm. Fifteen per cent had multiple discrete, firm, elevated nodules, 0.2 to 2.5 cm in diameter, and pink or light yellow. One cat had a solitary firm, pale tan, 0.5 cm nodule on the ventral extremity of the spleen. Hemorrhage, infarction, hematomas, and capsular fibrosis may be seen.

Most cats with hepatic tumors had multiple firm, discrete, orange, pink, or pale yellow nodules in the liver. Occasionally the liver was firm, orange-brown, and diffusely enlarged. Cranial mediastinal mast cell tumors were firm and yellow-white. Hemorrhages and fibrosis were common. Three of four cats with mediastinal tumor had widespread visceral involvement. Pulmonary metastases were discrete, multifocal or disseminated, firm nodules, of pale yellow or orange color.

Most cats with peritoneal effusions had metastases to the liver, diaphragm, and peritoneum. Ulcers of the stomach or intestine, sometimes perforated, were present in a few cats.

Autopsy of 30 cats with splenic tumors revealed metastatic or multicentric tumor in the liver in 27, visceral lymph nodes in 22, bone marrow in 12, lung in 6, and intestine in 5.

**MICROSCOPIC FEATURES.** Mast cell tumors of lymphoreticular organs may be well or poorly differentiated. In the spleen, neoplastic mast cells distend the red pulp, but the lymphoid follicles are usually preserved. In 15 per cent of cases, tumor cells form indiscrete nodules in the red pulp. Hemorrhage, necrosis, and fibrosis are frequent. In the liver, the tumor cells usually distend the sinusoids. In 65 per cent of cases, discrete nodules also surround central veins or portal triads. In lymph nodes, tumor cells may distend the subcapsular and medullary sinuses. Although germinal centers are usually spared, lymph nodes are occasionally replaced by sheets of tumor cells. Fibrosis is common in severely affected nodes.

**DIAGNOSIS.** Diagnosis of mast cell tumor of lymphoreticular organs is usually easy. Sometimes mast cells are present in the circulation. Percutaneous fine-needle aspirates of spleen, liver, lymph nodes, or cranial mediastinal masses can be obtained with a 22-gauge needle. Smears of the aspirate are stained with Wright-Giemsa or methylene blue. Smears from pleural or peritoneal effusions may contain mast cells or eosinophils, or both. If examination of an aspirate or an imprint obtained at exploratory laparotomy confirms the presence of mast cell tumor, the spleen should be removed. Liver and lymph nodes should undergo biopsy and be examined for metastases. The cat should be monitored carefully, as intraoperative and postoperative death is common.

**BEHAVIOR.** Visceral mast cell tumors should be considered malignant. In cats with mast cell tumor apparently limited to the spleen, splenectomy appears to ameliorate clinical signs and increase survival time (Alroy et al., 1975; Confer et al., 1978; Guerre et al., 1979; Liska et al., 1979). Five of seven cats with splenic mast cell tumors treated at The Animal Medical Center were alive eight months after splenectomy. One survived 38 months (Liska et al., 1979). Two cats survived for 23 and 30 months after splenectomy (Confer et al., 1978). Of nine cats at AMAH that survived the immediate postoperative period, the median survival time was 12 months, with a range of two to 33 months.

**TREATMENT.** Many drugs have been used to treat cats with mast cell tumors. Oral prednisone may reduce clinical signs by inhibiting release of vasoactive substances. Intralesional injection of long-acting corticosteroids into isolated skin tumors may cause temporary regression of the tumor.

Combination chemotherapy regimens of prednisone, vincristine, cyclophosphamide, and methotrexate have been tried at AMAH and The Animal Medical Center, but these drugs do not appear to increase survival time. Vomiting, diarrhea, respiratory distress, and shock may result from rapid breakdown of tumor cells. Three drugs, i.e., cimetidine, disodium cromoglycate, and cyproheptadine, have been used to ameliorate clinical signs in cats with residual mast cell tumor. Cimetidine, an H-2 receptor antagonist that reduces HC1 production by parietal cells of the gastric mucosa, appears to reduce the incidence of gastric and duodenal ulceration in human patients with systemic mastocytosis, Zollinger-Ellison syndrome, and gastric ulceration of unknown cause. The drug has been used in dogs and cats with mast cell tumors at AMAH, The Animal Medical Center, and other institutions to prevent gastric and intestinal ulceration. The dose, empirically based on that for man, is 20 to 25 mg/kg divided into four daily doses (Liska et al., 1979). Cimetidine has not been approved for use in the cat. Although vomiting and diarrhea appear to be decreased in treated cats, the effectiveness of the drug in preventing gastric and intestinal ulceration and its role as an immunomodulator have not been assessed.

Oral disodium cromoglycate is thought to reduce histamine release from mast cells by inhibiting calcium-dependent coupled activation-secretion response of mast cells (Soter et al., 1979). The drug effectively reduced diarrhea, abdominal pain, urticaria, and flushing in three of four human patients with systemic mast cell proliferation (Soter et al., 1979). Pharmacokinetics, side effects, and effectiveness have not been evaluated, and the drug has not been approved for use in the cat.

Cyproheptadine, a serotonin antagonist, was used by the author (LKA) in a cat with visceral mast cell tumor. The drug has been shown to minimize or prevent hind leg paresis in cats with experimentally induced aortic thromboemboli when given before a clot is induced (Olmstead and Butler, 1977). The usefulness of this drug in treatment of mast cell tumors awaits clarification of the role of serotonin in producing clinical signs as well as clinical trials to measure its effectiveness.

Orthovoltage irradiation of single mast cell tumors of the skin is moderately effective in the dog but has not been adequately evaluated in the cat (McClelland, 1964). Nonspecific immunostimulators, such as mixed bacterial vaccines and *Corynebacterium parvum*, have also been tried. The use of these drugs is discussed in the chapter on management of tumors.

H-1 receptor antagonists and antihistamines, such as diphenhydramine hydrochloride and chlorpheniramine, do not appear to be effective in reducing the severity of clinical signs in cats with disseminated mast cell tumors. Drugs that cause histamine release should be avoided or used with caution in cats with mast cell tumors. These include aspirin, opiates, atropine, propranolol, dextran, decamethonium, gallamine, and d-tubocurarine (Kaye and Passero, 1979).

**ASSOCIATION WITH OTHER DISEASE.** There is no relationship between feline leukemia virus or FIP-coronavirus infections and mast cell tumors in the cat. At autopsy of 65 cats with mast cell tumors at AMAH, two also had malignant lymphoma and one had FIP. In a survey of cats at The Animal Medical Center (Hayes, 1976), none with mast cell tumors was FeLV-positive.

## TUMORS OF THE MELANOGENIC SYSTEM

Melanogenic tumors may be benign (nevi) or malignant (melanoma). They are rare in cats, most often involving the eye but occasionally other sites. Engle and Brodey (1969) in a study of 395 feline tumors described a malignant melanoma of the skin at the base of the tail of a six-year-old cat with metastases to iliac nodes, lumbar vertebrae, lungs, and liver. They also reported a malignant melanoma of the palate. Macy and Reynolds (1981) recorded 15 melanocytic tumors of the skin, 7 of which were classified as benign. Patnaik et al. (1975) found three melanomas of the skin and one of the eye among 264 cats with nonhematopoietic tumors. The primary ocular tumor had diffuse visceral metastases.

A total of 35 ocular melanomas were reported by Acland et al. (1980), Bellhorn and Henkind (1970), Blodi and Ramsey (1967), Cardy (1977), Engle and Brodey (1969), Kircher et al. (1974), Nielsen (1964), Peiffer et al. (1977), Priester and McKay (1980), and Whitehead (1967). All arose in the anterior uvea, in marked contrast with those in humans, in whom the choroid is the most common primary site.

Cutaneous melanomas are infrequent (e.g., Nielsen, 1964; Theilen and Madewell, 1979; Whitehead, 1967). They constitute about 2 per cent of feline skin tumors, according to Scott (1980), who gives a comprehensive list of references.

Feline sarcoma virus (FeSV) causes melanoma as well as fibrosarcoma in cats inoculated experimentally (Essex, 1980; Shadduck et al., 1981), but there is no evidence to date as to the role of this virus in naturally occurring melanomas.

Melanogenic tumors (melanoma or nevus) of cats were diagnosed in 39 cats at AMAH and are the basis for the following discussion of tumors of the melanogenic system. Only one cat had more than one melanoma; three cats had more than one nevus.

**BREED, AGE, AND SEX.** One of the 39 cats was a purebred red Persian. Twenty-seven were domestic shorthairs, the others domestic longhairs. Of the 19 with ocular melanomas, 2 were solid black, 5 black-and-white, 2 blue, 2 red, and 1 tricolor; color was not specified for 7. One of the 20 cats with oral or cutaneous melanomas was reported to be black; 3 were tricolors, and 2 were blue. Color was not recorded for the other 14. None of the cats with melanoma was reported to be tabby or white. These details on color are of interest because melanotic pigmentation develops naturally in the skin and oral mucosa of adult red, cream, and tricolor cats, suggesting the possibility of a predisposition to melanoma in the sex-linked color spectrum of red, black, blue, and tricolor.

The age range of the 19 cats with ocular melanomas was from 4 to 19 years (mean 11.7), and for the 20 cats with oral or cutaneous melanogenic tumors, 6 months to 18 years. The five with benign tumors (nevi) were aged 6 months, and 1, 7, 9, and 12 years. The 15 with malignant melanomas ranged from 7 to 18 years (mean 12.2).

Of the 19 cats with ocular tumors, 9 of the 12 males were castrated and five of the seven females were spayed. Among the cats with oral or cutaneous tumors, six of the nine males were castrated and 9 of 11 females were spayed.

**SITE.** It is of interest that 35 of the 39 cats had melanogenic tumors involving the head, and none had limb lesions. Of the 19 ocular tumors, 1 arose from the cornea at the limbus; 18 involved the iris. Thirteen of the latter also involved the ciliary body and five of those extended into the sclera. Metastases to lung were documented in only 1 of the 19 cats, although invasion of choroidal or scleral vessels was seen in seven. Two of the ocular tumors were incidental findings at autopsy.

The most frequent sites of tumor other than the eye were mouth (four) and skin (pinna, three; external nares, two; eyelid, four). Other cutaneous sites involved only once included skin beneath an ear, beside the nose, and in the axilla, as well as skin, subcutis, and muscle at the umbilicus, right hip, and lumbar regions in one cat. The oral melanomas involved the lip, cheek, gingiva, and pharynx. Only 1 of the 20 cats with melanoma in sites other than an eye had metastasis detected in a mandibular node two years after removal of a mandibular gingival melanoma that did not recur locally (Fig. 11–189).

Only one cat had more than one melanoma: a 1.6 cm tumor of level V at the ear tip and a 0.2 cm growth of level IV at the ear base—"level" referring to Clark's microstaging classification, which correlates increasing tumor depth (I to V) with increased potential for malignant behavior (Clark et al., 1969). It seems possible that the smaller tumor was derived by lymphatic spread from the larger.

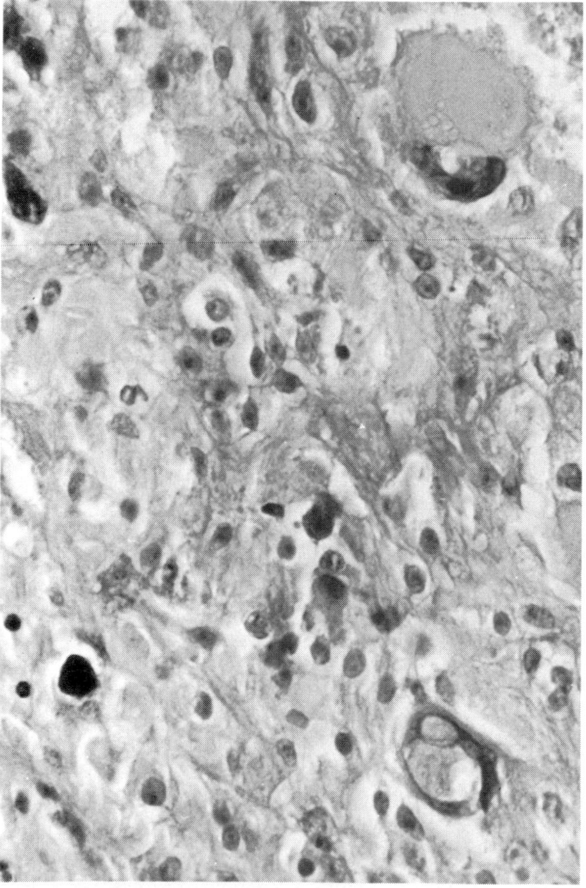

**Figure 11–189** Metastatic melanoma in a mandibular node, diagnosed two years after a gingival melanoma was excised, 18-year-old female domestic cat. An outstanding feature was astonishing nuclear and cellular pleomorphism. Melanin granules (center and upper right) and bizarre epithelioid melanocytes were numerous within the tumor, which enlarged and replaced most of one of the two left mandibular nodes. H & E, × 500.

**CLINICAL SIGNS AND GROSS FEATURES.** Unlike some melanomas in other species, all in this group were black or gray. Signs with ocular melanomas included enlarged or deviated globe, glaucoma, dilated or irregular pupil, injected scleral and conjunctival vessels, opacified cornea, hyphema, peripheral blindness, and usually a visible dark mass within the eye or, less often, involving the outer tunic and conjunctiva. One cat rubbed its diseased eye as though in pain, but pain was not apparent with any of the other melanomas.

Cutaneous melanogenic tumors, including those of the eyelids and pinnae, ranged from 0.2 to 3.5 cm in greatest dimension. Four were ulcerated; one involving the lumbar region and measuring 3.5 cm was partially covered by hairless skin and of "Jell-O-like" consistency. Another, 2.8 cm in diameter, circular, and crateriform, was located over the right hip. The third, a blue nevus located near the navel and 1.3 cm in diameter, discharged a black greasy exudate. The fourth mass, on an eyelid, was pedunculated for several years and then fell off, leaving an umbilicated, bleeding lesion.

Nonocular melanomas were variously described as papilloma-like, pedunculated, sessile, or crateriform. A botryoid, 1.6 cm mass at an ear tip burst and drained black fluid the day before surgery. Tumor consistency was usually firm.

Only 1 of the 39 cats appeared ill as a result of the neoplasm. It was a 17-year-old male red tabby that had had an enucleation five months before for an ocular melanoma (Fig. 11–190*A*) while in otherwise good health. Four months after surgery it began losing weight and sleeping more, and its abdomen enlarged. It was noticeably dyspneic and dehydrated when it was returned for examination. The cat was destroyed, and autopsy disclosed metastatic melanoma in the lungs, mediastinum, pericardium, parietal pleura, diaphragm, adrenals, peritoneum, omentum (Fig. 11–190*B*), spleen, liver, tracheobronchial and mesenteric nodes, and cerebral meninges.

**MICROSCOPIC FEATURES**

**Tumors of the Eye.** While studying intraocular melanomas of man Callender (1931) classified them as to cell type: epithelioid, spindle A, spindle B, mixed (epithelioid together with spindle cells), and necrotic (so necrotic as to prevent cell type identification).

The 19 intraocular melanomas in the cats in the AMAH group were classified by the Callender method as mixed melanomas (9), epithelioid (9), and spindle B–type melanoma (1). One tumor, in a 14-year-old black castrated male, involved the iris, ciliary body, cornea, sclera, and choroid and had characteristics of melanoma and also of fibrosarcoma and neurogenic sarcoma. Metastatic adenocarcinoma of mammary gland was found in the eye of a 19-year-old blue spayed female that had the spindle B–cell melanoma.

The single cat with distant metastases from an intraocular melanoma had a mixed-cell melanoma of the eye of epithelioid and spindle A–type cells, but only epithelioid cells in the metastases. The epithelioid cells were pleomorphic: mainly small dark cells with lymphocytoid nuclei and no or variable amounts of melanin, fewer but larger cells with a vesicular nucleus and a single central nucleolus, and also bizarre mononucleated giant cells and multinucleated giant cells.

**Tumors of the Skin and Mouth.** A melanin-pigmented macule can be benign (freckle, lentigo, nevocel-

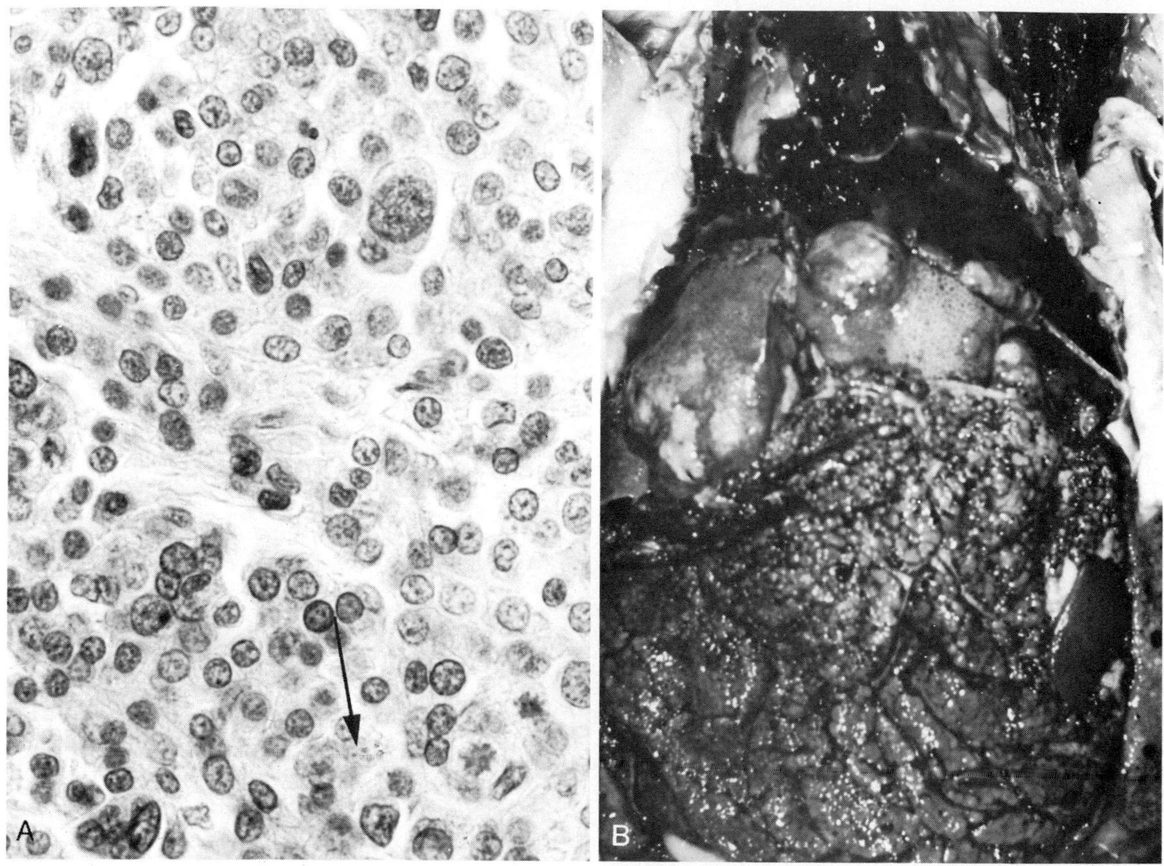


**Figure 11–190** *A*, Primary anterior uveal epithelioid melanoma that metastasized widely in a 17-year-old castrated male red tabby shorthair. Glaucoma was present for one year before the buphthalmic eye, with subtotal corneal opacification and an eccentric descemetocele, was enucleated. Anisonucleosis and mitotic figures (lower right corner) were conspicuous features. Melanin granules (arrow) were numerous, as in all of our feline melanomas. H & E, × 500. *B*, Metastatic melanoma from the anterior uvea. Within the opened thorax and abdomen, massive black pleural metastases crowd the thoracic cavity (top), less deeply pigmented metastatic nodules stud the liver (center), and diffuse black seeding thickens the omentum (below).

lular nevus) or an early stage of malignant melanoma. A freckle is a macule with increased melanin in an epidermis having a normal number of melanocytes in their normal basal location; the degree of pigmentation may vary on exposure to sunlight.

Lentigines occur on both skin and mucous membranes and are characterized by hyperplasia of melanocytes in their normal basal location. There is hyperpigmentation of the basal layer and often elongation of rete ridges. Lentigines do not darken with exposure to ultraviolet light. Lentigines are common in red, cream, and tricolor cats.

A nevus is any congenital, colored lesion. A nevocellular nevus (mole) is a benign mass located in the epithelium, the dermis (or lamina propria), or both, and composed of proliferating melanocytes or nevus cells, which can be cuboidal, epithelioid, fusiform, dendritic, multinucleate, or ballooned. A variety of nevocellular nevi have been recognized in man, such as junctional, compound, dermal, blue, congenital giant pigmented, and Spitz nevi. Moles are very frequent in man; malignant melanoma is uncommon, but its incidence has doubled every 10 years over the past few decades. In from 20 to 40 per cent of human cases of melanoma there is histologic evidence of an associated nevus (Robbins et al., 1984).

Of the 25 melanogenic tumors of the skin, oral cavity, and eyelids in 20 cats, 8 were benign (nevi). Three balloon-cell nevi in a 12-year-old spayed female were located in the cornea, scleral conjunctiva, and conjunctiva of the third eyelid of the same eye. A blue nevus and a variant of the blue nevus were seen in the umbilical area and the right nostril of nine- and seven-year-old spayed females, respectively. A six-month-old female tricolor had a dendritic and fusiform dermal nevus on each ear tip (Fig. 11–191). A dendritic and clear balloon-cell dermal nevus with junctional change occurred on the nose of a year-old castrated male domestic shorthair.

Cutaneous melanomas of man are classified by their horizontal and vertical growth patterns (Goldsmith, 1979). Superficial spreading and lentigo malignant melanomas have a centrifugal horizontal (lateral) intraepithelial growth phase and a vertical growth phase into the dermis. A nodular melanoma of man has an immediate dermal invasive phase, resulting in prominent vertical growth, and a minor lateral junctional intraepithelial spread of less than three rete ridges. Of the 16 feline nonocular

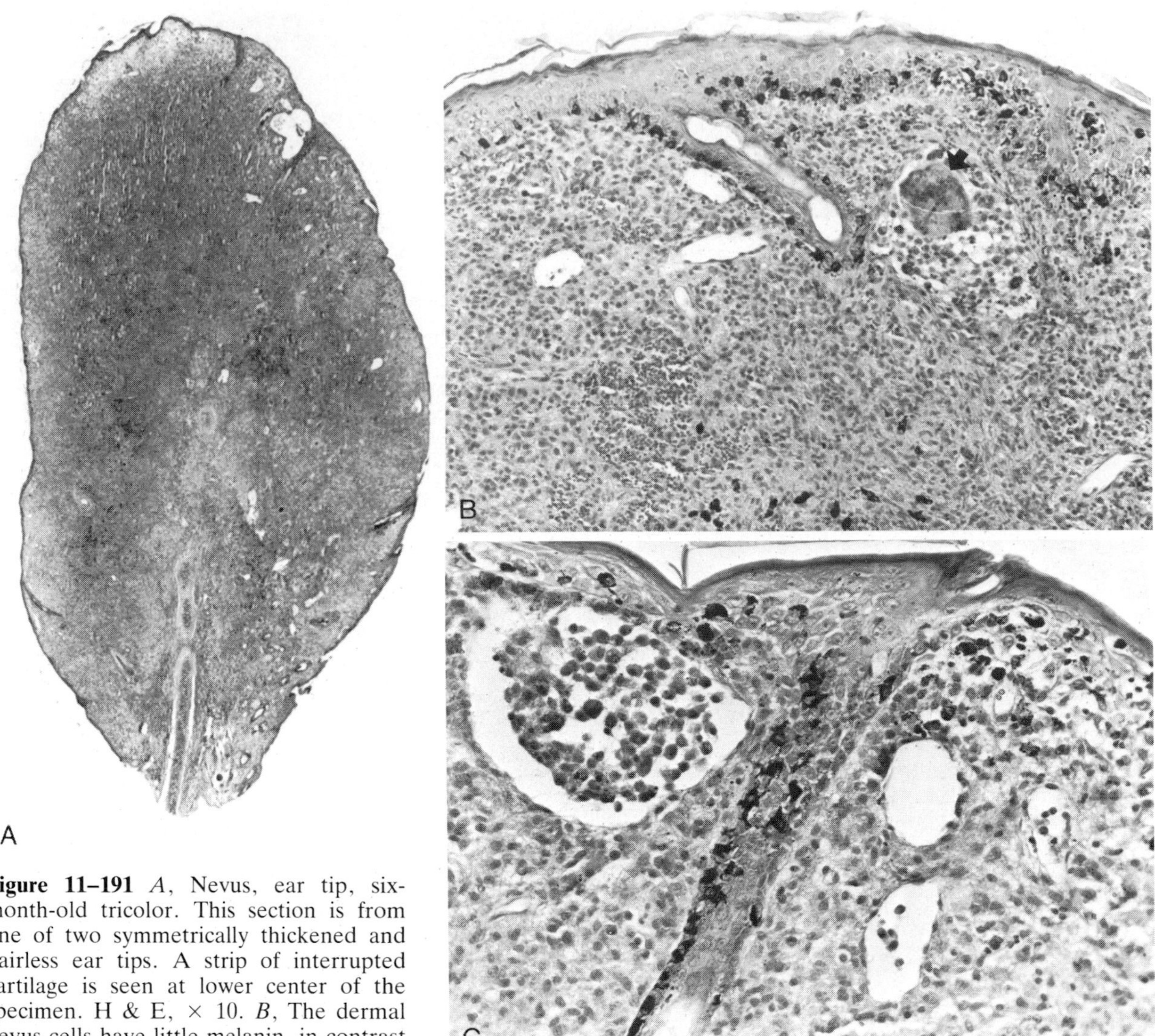


**Figure 11–191** *A*, Nevus, ear tip, six-month-old tricolor. This section is from one of two symmetrically thickened and hairless ear tips. A strip of interrupted cartilage is seen at lower center of the specimen. H & E, × 10. *B*, The dermal nevus cells have little melanin, in contrast with the denser melanosis of the epidermal cells. A collection of macrophages and a multinucleate giant cell (arrow) appear to lie in a dilated lymphatic vessel. H & E, × 100. *C*, Nevocytes with indistinct borders underlie the dermis, line the rete ridge, and surround dilated vessels, one of which contains many macrophages (upper left). H & E, × 200.

melanomas, 11 were of the nodular type, 1 was metastatic to a node so that the primary tumor could not be classified, and the 4 that were ulcerated were not sectioned in such a way as to enable the intraepithelial component to be evaluated.

Melanomas of the skin can be classified histologically by the depth of the vertical growth phase (Clark et al., 1969). Clark's level I is melanoma in situ (above the basal lamina of the epithelium); II is tumor through the basal lamina into the papillary dermis; III is tumor filling and expanding the papillary dermis; IV is tumor penetrating into the dense collagen bundles of the reticular dermis, and V is tumor invading the subcutis. The feline melanomas had all reached level IV or V. Delayed excision, lack of long-term follow-up, and insufficient number of tumors studied prevent prognostic correlation with level of invasion and probability of metastasis. In man, tumors in levels IV and V metastasize to nodes in 40 to 70 per cent of cases, respectively (Goldsmith, 1979).

Callender's cellular classification can be applied to nonocular melanomas. Of the aforementioned 16 melanomas, 10 were of epithelioid cell type (Fig. 11–192) and 6 of mixed cell type. No attempt was made to divide the spindle cells into A and B subtypes in the mixed tumors. No pure spindle cell type was seen. Sections of the primary oral melanoma removed two years earlier from a 16-year-old domestic shorthair were not available for review, but the metastasis in the mandibular node consisted of a pleomorphic population of epithelioid cells. Most of the large cells were in packets, lacked pigment, and had vesicular nuclei with a single, central, magenta-staining nucleolus. Giant cells with one or more bizarre nuclei had abundant eosinophilic cytoplasm and occasional melanin granules (Fig. 11–189).

**PROGNOSIS.** Ocular nevi (brown spots) are occasionally observed in the irides of older cats and have sometimes led to unnecessary enucleation. Ocular melanomas of cats rarely metastasize even when present for months.

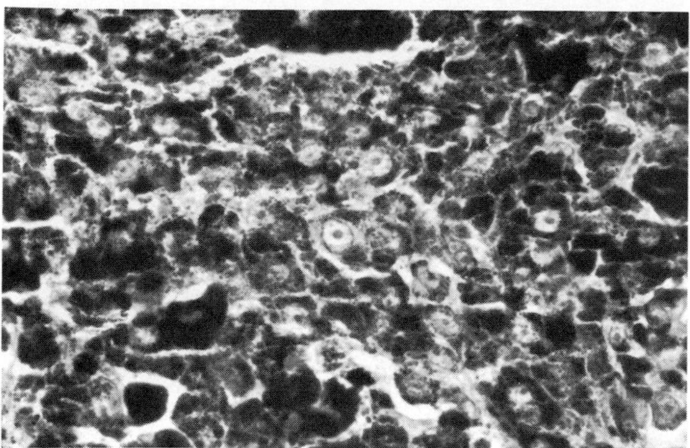

**Figure 11–192** Melanoma, eyelid, nine-year-old tricolor. This heavily pigmented malignant tumor, of epithelioid type, is composed of cells with prominently euchromatic nuclei having a single large nucleolus (center). H & E, × 500.

In the AMAH group, only one of seven that were present from one to five years metastasized. Invasion of the fibrous tunic and vortex veins, migration along the optic nerve, and infiltration of soft tissues of the orbit were observed.

Cutaneous and oral pigmented maculae of cats are recognized most often in adult red, cream, and tricolor cats, but very rarely, if ever, is biopsy done.

While only 2 of the 39 cats at AMAH were known to have had metastatic lesions, all 35 melanomas were considered on microscopic examination to be potentially malignant. Vascular invasion was observed in seven eyes and seems likely to have been present in many of the cutaneous tumors because of the amount of dermal and subcutaneous infiltration.

It is of interest that two years passed before the mandibular node became obviously involved with metastatic tumor from a lesion of the inferior gingiva. In humans, many years may pass after removal of the primary tumor before melanoma is apparent in a regional node. The speed at which melanoma cells travel within the lymphatic system is not known in any species.

Any area of pigmentation developing in the eye must be followed vigilantly. If such an area enlarges or darkens significantly or assumes the form of a mass, a malignant tumor must be suspected. The prognosis for ocular melanoma is best when enucleation is performed early, together with removal of ocular adnexa and a long piece of optic nerve. The prognosis for cutaneous melanomas is always guarded but is improved when early, wide excision includes removal of the underlying deep fascia and an incontinuity dissection is done (Goldsmith, 1979). Incontinuity dissection includes removal of the primary melanoma, regional nodes, and lymphatics connecting both areas. Unfortunately, it is not always technically and anatomically possible. In humans, the removal of a regional node with no more than 20 per cent tumor involvement carries a better prognosis than with more extensive tumor.

In summary, oral and nasal melanomas of cats appear to have a poor prognosis, ocular tumors a more favorable but somewhat guarded prognosis, and cutaneous tumors in general a guarded prognosis except for those of the pinna, which have been successfully removed, probably because wide excision can be achieved by partial amputation of the ear.

## MESOTHELIOMA

Mesotheliomas are primary tumors of lining cells of serous membranes and have been reported to arise from pleura, pericardium, and peritoneum including its extension, the tunica vaginalis. They are important neoplasms of man and have also been reported in many animal species, including cats. Asbestos is now accepted as a cause of mesothelioma in man and has also been associated with it in dogs (Harbison and Godleski, 1983). Strain MC29 avian leukosis virus has induced the tumor in chickens (Chabot et al., 1970).

Few cases of mesothelioma have been reported in Felidae, and no causal factor is known. One tumor was a pleural mesothelioma in a captive clouded leopard (Stewart, 1966). Three tumors in domestic cats have been reported (Andrews, 1973; Raflo and Nuernberger, 1978; Tilley et al., 1975). Two cases of mesothelioma were recorded without details by Bastianello (1983). Another case was diagnosed at AMAH.

Of the four mesotheliomas for which details are available, three occurred in Siamese and the fourth in a domestic shorthair. The cats' ages ranged from 1½ to 15 years. The two youngest were entire females, the others a spayed female and a castrated male. One tumor arose from the parietal pericardium, another from the pleura, and two from the peritoneum.

**CLINICAL SIGNS AND GROSS FEATURES.** The youngest cat, a domestic shorthair with a pericardial tumor, had a history of decreased appetite, nonproductive cough, and lethargy (Tilley et al., 1975). Heart sounds were muffled owing to 200 ml of serosanguineous pericardial effusion (sp gr 1.027). Multiple 0.8 to 1.2 cm masses were found on the cranioventral parietal area of the pericardial sac. The cat died shortly after exploratory surgery. Another cat, a three-year-old female Siamese presented in moribund condition, died before an examination could be performed (Andrews, 1973). Voluminous turbid white fluid occupied both pleural cavities. A noninvasive, nonmetastasizing, yellow-white friable papillomatous growth involved the parietal and visceral pleura. A third cat, a nine-year-old spayed female Siamese, had vomited, was listless, and had abdominal swelling caused by 450 ml of clear pink effusion (Raflo and Nuernberger, 1978). Widely disseminated masses ranging from 1 mm to 7.5 cm involved the peritoneum of the stomach, omentum, mesentery, splenic hilus, abdominal surface of the diaphragm, caudal mediastinum, and visceral surface of the right caudal lung lobe.

The cat at AMAH was a 15-year-old castrated male Siamese with a decreased appetite, fever of 40C (104.2F), and a greatly distended abdomen. Aspiration of 1000 ml of serosanguineous fluid (sp gr 1.026) allowed palpation of an irregular mass on or near the liver. Euthanasia was performed, and autopsy revealed a light yellow, thick, granular, plaque-like growth covering most of the visceral surfaces of the right medial and quadrate lobes (Fig. 11–193*A*). Numerous neoplastic implants took the form of glistening, pink-white, round, minute nodules up to 0.2 cm on the omentum, diaphragm, parietal peritoneum, serosa, and mesentery (Fig. 11–193*B*).

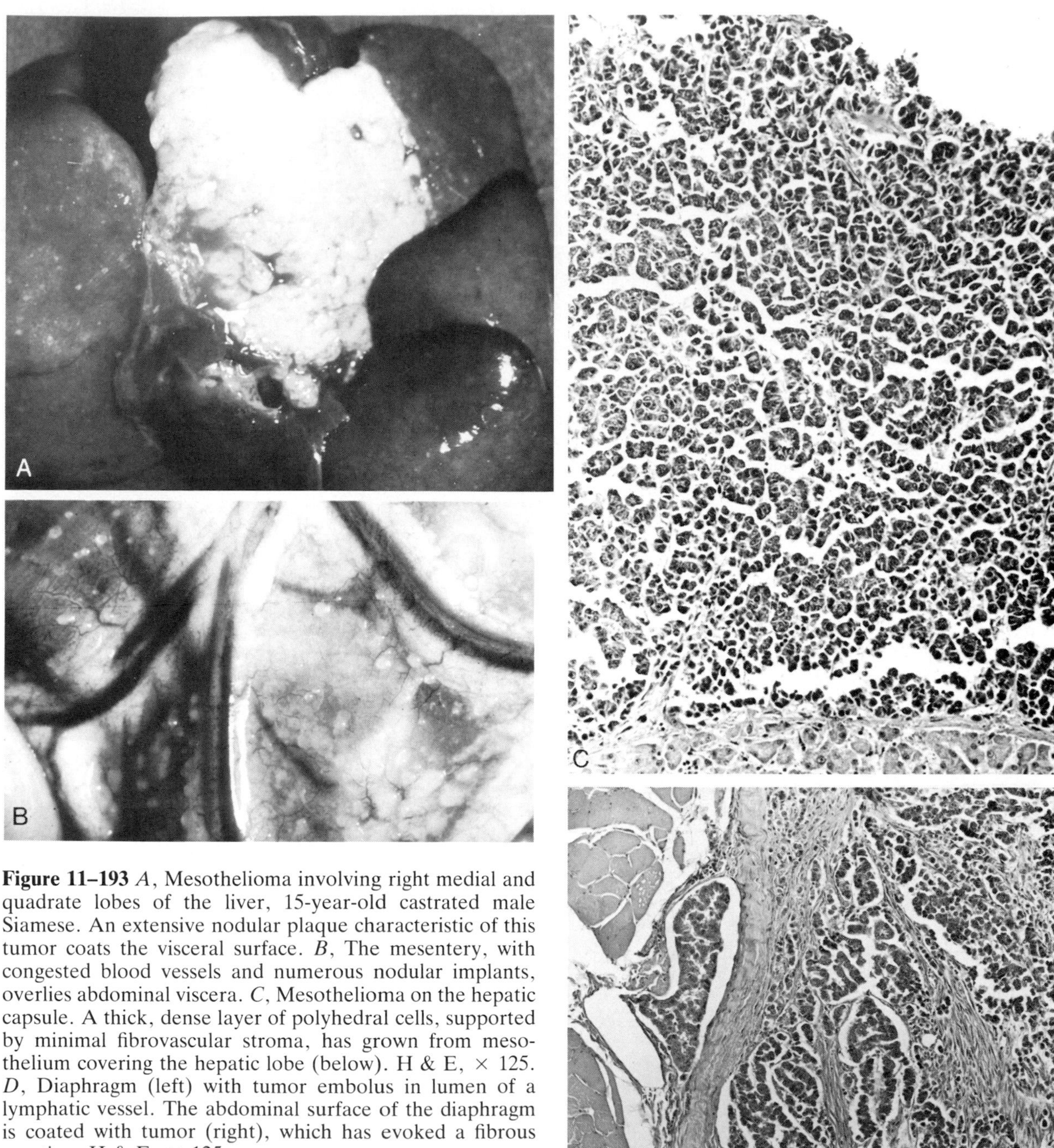

**Figure 11–193** *A*, Mesothelioma involving right medial and quadrate lobes of the liver, 15-year-old castrated male Siamese. An extensive nodular plaque characteristic of this tumor coats the visceral surface. *B*, The mesentery, with congested blood vessels and numerous nodular implants, overlies abdominal viscera. *C*, Mesothelioma on the hepatic capsule. A thick, dense layer of polyhedral cells, supported by minimal fibrovascular stroma, has grown from mesothelium covering the hepatic lobe (below). H & E, × 125. *D*, Diaphragm (left) with tumor embolus in lumen of a lymphatic vessel. The abdominal surface of the diaphragm is coated with tumor (right), which has evoked a fibrous reaction. H & E, × 125.

The clinical finding common to the four cases was a large volume of effusion associated with multiple neoplastic growths. This is also a frequent finding with mesothelioma in other species. Neoplastic cells are expected in the effusion; however, experience with a number of canine mesotheliomas indicates that some well-differentiated mesotheliomas shed many cells that could be interpreted as benign, while cells from other mesotheliomas misleadingly suggest adenocarcinoma. Cells in a neoplastic effusion associated with a mesothelioma are pictured in a study of thoracic effusions in the cat (Creighton and Wilkins, 1975).

**MICROSCOPIC FEATURES.** Mesotheliomas may resemble fibrosarcoma because mesothelial cells can act as facultative fibroblasts, or they may resemble adenocarcinoma with solid, papillary, or tubular patterns. Evidence of malignancy should be based on behavior rather than on cell type or pattern. Malignant mesothelial cells grow on the serous surface but eventually invade the underlying tissues and organs (Fig. 11–193*C* and *D*). Fluid accumulation in the affected cavity promotes exfoliation and implantation, resulting in multiple tumor growths. Most mesotheliomas can be differentiated from metastatic adenocarcinoma by special stains for mucopolysaccharides. Epithelial cells of mesothelioma are usually PAS-positive and diastase-resistant as well as Alcian blue–positive and hyaluronidase-sensitive. Electron microscopy can also assist in identification by revealing the microvilli and tonofilaments of mesothelial cells.

**PROGNOSIS.** Mesotheliomas are almost always malignant and have a grave prognosis in all species. Clinical signs appear late in the course of the disease and are often related to fluid accumulation and extensive implantation. No successful therapy is available at this time.

## REFERENCES


Acland GM, McLean IW, Aguirre GD, Trucka R: Diffuse iris melanoma in cats. J Am Vet Med Assoc 176 (1980) 52–56.

Alexander E: Neubildung im Uterus und Pyometra bei einer Katze. Berl Tierärzt Wochenschr May 11 (1911) 345–347.

Alexander JW, Riis RC, Dueland R: Extraskeletal giant cell tumor in a cat. Vet Med Small Anim Clin 70 (1975) 1161–1166.

Alexander JW, Roenigk WJ: What is your diagnosis? [Pathologic fracture of humerus due to a fibrosarcoma]. J Am Vet Med Assoc 170 (1977) 225–226.

Aliakbrai S, Ivoghli B: Granulosa cell tumor in a cat. J Am Vet Med Assoc 174 (1979) 1306–1308.

Allard AW: Splenic mastocytosis. Feline Pract 9(4) (1979) 21–22.

Allen HL: Feline mammary hypertrophy. Vet Pathol 10(1973) 501–508.

Allen JG, Amis T: Lymphosarcoma involving cranial nerves in a cat. Aust Vet J 51 (1975) 155–158.

Alroy J, Leav I, DeLellis RA, Weinstein RS: Distinctive intestinal mast cell neoplasms of domestic cats. Lab Invest 33 (1975) 159–167.

Andrews EJ: Pleural mesothelioma in a cat. J Comp Pathol 83 (1973) 259–263.

Andrews EJ, Stookey JL, Helland DR, Slaughter LJ: A histopathological study of canine and feline ovarian dysgerminomas. Can J Comp Med 38 (1974) 85–89.

Antman KH, Skarin AT, Mayer RJ, Hargreaves KH, Canellos GP: Microangiopathic hemolytic anemia and cancer: a review. Medicine 58 (1979) 377–384.

Antoine EH: Contribution à l'étude du cancer chez le chat. Medical thesis, University of Bordeaux, 1907.

Antoine G, Brouwers J: Deux cas de tumeurs primitives malignes du tube digestif chez le cheval et le chat. Ann Méd Vét 85 (1941) 293–298.

Arnbjerg J: Extra-ovarian granulosa cell tumor in a cat. Feline Pract 10(2) (1980) 26–32.

Austin VH: Common skin problems in cats. Mod Vet Pract 56 (1975) 541–545.

Austin VH: The skin. *In* Catcott EJ (ed): Feline Medicine and Surgery, 2nd ed. Santa Barbara, American Veterinary Publications, Inc, 1975.

Averill DR: Personal communication, 1981.

Babcock RE, Snodgrass CP, Bartsch RC: What is your diagnosis? [Hepatic hematocyst.] J Am Vet Med Assoc 171 (1977) 660–662.

Baker E: Malignant granulosa cell tumor in a cat. J Am Vet Med Assoc 129 (1956) 322–324.

Baker J, Greenwood AG: Intracranial lymphoid tumour in a cat. J Small Anim Pract 14 (1973) 15–22.

Ball V: Polyadénome bronchique annulaire. J Med Vét Zootech 58 (1907) 71.

Ball V: Dermatomyome chez un chat. J Med Vet Zootech 64 (1913) 409–410.

Ball V: Traité d'Anatomie Pathologique Générale. Vigot Frères, 1924 (cited by C. Lombard, 1935). [Islet-cell carcinoma.]

Ball V: Le cancer de l'utérus chez les femelles domestiques. Rev Vét 84 (1932) 72–78. [Uterine "endothelioma."]

Ball V: La pathologie comparée et la question controversée de l'existence du naevocancer parotidien chez l'homme. Bull Acad Méd Paris 111 (1934) 370–371.

Ball V, Collet P: Cholestéatome massif au poumon gauche chez une chatte brightique. Bull Soc Sci Vét Lyon 35 (1932) 19–22.

Ball V, Collet P: Le cancer des glandes salivaires chez l'homme et chez les animaux. Rev Vét 86 (1934) 545–559.

Ball V, Collet, P, Girard H: Les céruminomes. Ancien style: adénomes épithéliales des glandes cérumineuses. Rev Méd Vét 90 (1938) 390–398.

Ball V, Lombard C: Les corps fibreux de l'utérus. Rev Vét 77 (1925) 409–415.

Ball V, Roquet M: Cancer de la queue du pancréas. J Méd Vét Zootech 62 (1911) 477–483.

Banner BF, Alroy J, Kipnis RM: Acinar cell carcinoma of the pancreas in a cat. Vet Pathol 16 (1979) 543–547.

Banovcǎnin B: [Meningioma in cats.] Vet Glasnik 25 (1971) 201–205.

Barclay SM: Lymphosarcoma in tarsi of a cat. J Am Vet Med Assoc 175 (1979) 582–583.

Barker J, Greenwood AG: Intracranial lymphoid tumour in a cat. J Small Anim Pract 14 (1973) 15–22.

Baroni C: On the relationship of mast cells to various soft tissue tumours. Br J Cancer 18 (1964) 686–691.

Barrett RE, Nobel TA: Transitional cell carcinoma of the urethra in a cat. Cornell Vet 66 (1976) 14–26.

Barrett RE, Theilen GH: Neoplasms of the canine and feline reproductive tracts. *In* Kirk RW (ed): Current Veterinary Therapy VI. Philadelphia, WB Saunders Company, 1977.

Barsanti JA, Higgins RJ, Spano JS, Jones BD: Adenocarcinoma of the extrahepatic bile duct in a cat. J Small Anim Pract 17 (1976) 599–605.

Bastianello SS: A survey of neoplasia in domestic species over a 40-year period from 1935 to 1974 in the Republic of South Africa. V. Tumours occurring in the cat. Onderstepoort J Vet Res 50 (1983) 105–110.

Bedford PGC: Origin of the nasopharyngeal polyp in the cat. Vet Rec 110 (1982) 541–542.

Bellhorn RW, Henkind P: Intraocular malignant melanoma in domestic cats. J Small Anim Pract 10 (1970) 631–637.

Belter LF, Crawford EM, Bates HR: Endometrial adenocarcinoma in a cat. Pathol Vet 5 (1968) 429–431.

Bender WM: Nontraditional treatment of mycosis fungoides in a dog. J Am Vet Med Assoc 185 (1984) 900–901.

Benditt EP, Lagunoff D: The mast cell: its structure and function. Prog Allergy 8 (1964) 195–223.

Bennett D, Campbell JR, Brown P: Osteosarcoma associated with healed fractures. J Small Anim Pract 20 (1979) 13–18.

Berman E, Wright JF: What is your diagnosis? [Osteosarcoma of tibia and hemangiosarcoma of femur metastatic to lungs in an irradiated cat]. J Am Vet Med Assoc 162 (1973) 1065–1066.

Birchard SJ, Peterson ME, Jacobson A: Surgical treatment of feline hyperthyroidism: results of 85 cases. J Am Anim Hosp Assoc 20 (1984) 705–709.

Blähser S: Contribution à l'étude des tumeurs de la fibre musculaire striée chez les animaux. Thesis, Paris (Alfort), 1961 (Abstr Vet Bull 32 [1962] 841).

Blähser S: Über nichtalltägliche Todesursachen und einige plötzliche Todesfälle. Kleintierpraxis 7 (1962) 192–201.

Bloch KJ, Cygan RW, Waltin J: The IgE system and parasitism: role of mast cells, IgE, and other antibodies in host response to primary infection with *Nippostrongylus brasiliensis*. *In* Ishizaka K, Dayton DH Jr (eds): The Biological Role of the Immunoglobulin E System. Washington, DC, Government Printing Office, 1974, 119–132.

Blodi RC, Ramsey FK: Ocular tumors in domestic animals. Am J Ophthalmol 64 (1967) 627–633.

Bloom F: Unilateral exophthalmos associated with leucaemia in a cat. Vet Med 32 (1937) 29–30.

Bloom F: Pathology of the Dog and Cat. The Genitourinary System, with Clinical Considerations. Evanston, Illinois, American Veterinary Publications Inc, 1954.

Bloom F: Feline mammary hypertrophy. Vet Pathol 11(1974) 561.

Bond E, Dorfman HD: Squamous cell carcinoma of the tongue in cats. J Am Vet Med Assoc 154 (1969) 786–789.

Bosselut R, Samso A, Catanei J: Cancer des glandes salivaires chez le chat. Bull Algér Carcinol 4 (1951) 407–408.

Bostock DE: The prognosis in cats bearing squamous cell carcinoma. J Small Anim Pract 13 (1972) 119–125.

Bostock DE: Neoplasia of the skin and mammary glands in dogs and cats. *In* Kirk RW (ed): Current Veterinary Therapy VI. Philadelphia, WB Saunders Company, 1977, 493–505.

Bostock DE, Dye MT: Prognosis after surgical excision of fibrosarcomas in cats. J Am Vet Med Assoc 175 (1979) 727–728.

Bostock DE, Owen LN: Chemotherapy of canine and feline neoplasia. J Small Anim Pract 13 (1972) 359–367.

Boucek Z: Mitteilungen über 35 histologisch untersuchte Tiergeschwülste. Arch Wissensch Prakt Tierheilkd 32 (1906) 585–600.

Bourgeois E: Kropfstudien bei der Katze. Dissertation, Bern, 1933.

Bradley RL: Selected oral, pharyngeal, and upper respiratory conditions in the cat. Oral tumors, nasopharyngeal and middle ear polyps, and chronic rhinitis and sinusitis. Vet Clin North Am 14(1984) 1173–1184.

Bradley RL, MacEwen EG, Loar AS: Mandibular resection for removal of oral tumors in 30 dogs and 6 cats. J Am Vet Med Assoc 184 (1984) 460–463.

Bright RM, Bojrab MJ: Intranasal neoplasia in the dog and cat. J Am Anim Hosp Assoc 12 (1976) 806–812.

Bright RM, Crabtree BJ, Knecht CD: Brachial plexus neuropathy in the cat: a case report. J Am Anim Hosp Assoc 14 (1978) 612–615.

Britt JO, Howard EB, Ryan CP: Simultaneous mixed mammary tumor and adenocarcinoma in a cat. Feline Pract 9 (5) (1979) 41–47.

Brodey RS: Alimentary tract neoplasms in the cat: a clinicopathologic survey of 46 cases. Am J Vet Res 27 (1966) 74–80.

Brodey RS: Canine and feline neoplasia. Adv Vet Sci 14 (1970) 309–354.

Brown NO, Patnaik AK, Mooney S, Hayes A, Harvey HJ, MacEwen EG: Soft tissue sarcomas in the cat. J Am Vet Med Assoc 173 (1978) 744–749.

Brown RJ, Trevethan WP, Henny VL: Multiple osteochondroma in a Siamese cat. J Am Vet Med Assoc 160 (1972) 433–435.

Buergelt CD, Das KM: Aortic body tumor in a cat. A case report. Pathol Vet 5 (1968) 84–90.

Buhles WC Jr, Theilen GH: Preliminary evaluation of bleomycin in feline and canine squamous cell carcinoma. Am J Vet Res 34 (1973) 289–291.

Buonanno FS, Pykitt IL, Kistler JP, Vielma J, Brady TJ, Hinshaw WS, Goldman MR, Newhouse JH, Pohost GM: Cranial anatomy and detection of ischemic stroke in the cat by nuclear magnetic resonance imaging. Radiology 143 (1982) 187–193.

Burgisser E: Epithélioma ossifié de l'iléon chez le chat. Schweiz Arch Tierheilkd 102 (1960) 559–562.

Burgoon CF Jr, Graham JH, McCaffree DL: Mast cell disease. A cutaneous variant with multisystem involvement. Arch Dermatol 98 (1968) 590–605.

Burk RL, Meierhenry EF, Schaubhut CW: Leiomyosarcoma of the urinary bladder in a cat. J Am Vet Med Assoc 167 (1975) 749–785.

Caciolo PL, Hayes AA, Patnaik AK, Nesbitt GH, Pack FD: A case of mycosis fungoides in a cat and literature review. J Am Anim Hosp Assoc 19 (1983) 505–512.

Caciolo PL, Nesbitt GH, Patnaik AK, Hayes AA: Cutaneous lymphosarcoma in the cat: a report of nine cases. J Am Anim Hosp Assoc 20 (1984) 491–494.

Cadéac C: Sarcome du pylore chez une chatte atteinte de dithyridiose. J Méd Vét Lyon 60 (1909) 478–482.

Cain GR, Manley P: Tracheal adenocarcinoma in a cat. J Am Vet Med Assoc 182 (1983) 614–616.

Calafat J, Weijer K, Daams H: Feline malignant mammary tumors. III. Presence of C-particles and intracisternal A-particles and their relationship with feline leukemia virus antigens and RD-114 virus antigens. Int J Cancer 20 (1977) 759–767.

Callender GR: Malignant melanotic tumors of the eye: a study of histologic types in 111 cases. Trans Am Acad Ophthalmol Otolaryngol 36 (1931) 131–142.

Capen CC: Tumors of the endocrine glands. *In* Moulton JE (ed): Tumors in Domestic Animals, 2nd ed. Berkeley, University of California Press, 1978.

Capron M, Rousseaux J, Mazingue C, Bazin H, Capron A: Rat mast cell–eosinophil interaction in antibody-dependent eosinophil cytotoxicity to *Schistosoma mansoni schistosomula*. J Immunol 121 (1978) 2518–2525.

Carakostas MC, Kennedy GA, Kittleson MD, Cook JE: Malignant foregut carcinoid tumor in a domestic cat. Vet Pathol 16 (1979) 607–609.

Carb AV: What is your diagnosis? [Cystic hemangiosarcoma in the liver of a cat]. J Am Vet Med Assoc 153 (1968) 711–712.

Cardy RH: Primary intraocular malignant melanoma in a Siamese cat. Vet Pathol 14 (1977) 648–649.

Cardy RH, Bostrom RE: Multiple splenic myelolipomas in a cheetah (*Acinonyx jubatus*). Vet Pathol 15 (1978) 556–558.

Carlisle CH, Gould S: Response of squamous cell carcinoma of the nose of the cat to treatment with x-rays. Vet Radiol 23 (1982) 186–192.

Carpenter JL, Holzworth J: Thymoma in 11 cats. J Am Vet Med Assoc 181 (1982) 248–251.

Carr SH: Secondary hypertrophic pulmonary osteoarthropathy in a cat. Feline Pract 1(2) (1971) 25–26.

Case MT, Simon J: Oncocytoma in a cat and a dog. Vet Med 61 (1966) 41–43.

Caywood DD, Osborne CA, Johnston GR: Neoplasms of the canine and feline urinary tracts. *In* Kirk RW: Current Veterinary Therapy VII. Philadelphia, WB Saunders Company, 1980.

Center SA, Randolph JF: Lactation and spontaneous remission of feline mammary hyperplasia following pregnancy. J Am Anim Hosp Assoc 21(1985) 56–58.

Center SA, Scott DW, Scott FW: Multiple cutaneous horns on the footpads of a cat. Feline Pract 12 (4) (1982) 26–30.

Chabot JF, Beard D, Langlois AJ, Beard JW: Mesothelioma of peritoneum, epicardium, and pericardium induced by strain MC29 avian leukosis virus. Cancer Res 30 (1970) 1287–1308.

Chiu H, Lagunoff D: Histochemical comparison of vertebrate mast cells. Histochem J 4 (1972) 135–144.

Ciampi L: Su due casi di cancroide cutaneo nei gatti bianchi. Nuova Vet 15 (1949) 342–348.

Clark ST, Meier H: A clinico-pathological study of thyroid diseases in the dog and cat. Part 1. Thyroid pathology. Zentralbl Veterinärmed 5 (1958) 17–32.

Clark WH Jr, From L, Bernardino EA, Mihm MA: The histogenesis and biologic behavior of primary human malignant melanomas of the skin. Cancer Res 29 (1969) 705–727.

Collet P: Tumeur primitive de l'utérus chez une chatte. Bull Soc Sci Vét Lyon 36 (1933) 199–202.

Collet P: Cancer primitif du larynx chez une chatte. Bull Soc Sci Vét Lyon 38 (1935) 219–226.

Collet P, Lucam F, Marlier A: Métastases musculaires multiples d'un cancer rénal chez le chat. Bull Soc Sci Vét Lyon 53 (1951) 47–49.

Collignon H: Le cancer de l'utérus chez les femelles domestiques. Thesis, Lyon, 1936 (cited by Meier, 1956a).

Collins DR: Thoracic tumor in a cat. Vet Med Small Anim Clin 59 (1964) 459.

Confer AW, Enright FM, Beard GB: Ultrastructure of a feline extraskeletal giant cell tumor (malignant fibrous histiocytoma). Vet Pathol 18 (1981) 738–744.

Confer AW, Langloss JM, Cashell IG: Long-term survival of two cats with mastocytosis. J Am Vet Med Assoc 172 (1978) 160–161.

Cooper ER, Howarth I: Some pathological changes in the cat brain. J Comp Pathol 66 (1956) 35–38.

Cordy DR: Tumors of the nervous system and eye. *In* Moulton JE (ed): Tumors in Domestic Animals, 2nd ed. Berkeley, University of California Press, 1978.

Cotchin E: Neoplasms in cats. Proc R Soc Med 45 (1952) 671–674.

Cotchin E: Neoplasms of the Domesticated Mammals. Review Series No. 4 of the Commonwealth Bureau of Animal Health, Farnham Royal, England, 1956a.

Cotchin E: Further examples of spontaneous neoplasms in the domestic cat. Br Vet J 112 (1956b) 263–272.

Cotchin E: Neoplasia in the cat. Vet Rec 69 (1957) 425–434.

Cotchin E: Some tumours of dogs and cats of comparative veterinary and human interest. Vet Rec 71 (1959) 1040–1050.

Cotchin E: Skin tumors of cats. Res Vet Sci 2 (1961) 353–361.

Cotchin E: Neoplasia. *In* Wilkinson GT (ed): Diseases of the Cat. Oxford, Pergamon Press, 1966.

Cotchin E: Neoplasia. *In* Wilkinson GT (ed): Diseases of the Cat and Their Management. Melbourne, Blackwell Scientific Publications, 1983.

Cowen PN, Jackson P: Thyroid carcinoma in a cat. Vet Rec 114 (1984) 521–522.

Cravioto H: The ultrastructure of acoustic nerve tumors. Acta Neuropathol 12 (1969) 116–140.

Creighton SR, Wilkins RJ: Thoracic effusions in the cat. J Am Anim Hosp Assoc 11 (1975) 66–76.

Crocker W: Three thousand autopsies. Cornell Vet 31 (1941) 86.

Crouch JE: Text-Atlas of Cat Anatomy. Philadelphia, Lea & Febiger, 1969.

Crow SE, Pulley LT, Wittenbrock TP: Lingual hemangioma in a cat. J Am Anim Hosp Assoc 17 (1981) 71–74.

Crowell WA, Hubbell JJ, Riley JC: Polycystic renal disease in related cats. J Am Vet Med Assoc 175 (1979) 286–288.

Csaba G, Acs T, Horvath C, Mold K: Genesis and function of mast cells. Mast cell and plasmacyte reaction to induced, homologous and heterologous tumours. Br J Cancer 15 (1961) 327–335.

Cucuel J-P E, Schelling SH: What is your diagnosis? [Squamous cell carcinoma invading right maxilla.] J Am Vet Med Assoc 103 (1973) 1389–1390.

Cusick PK, Parker AJ: Brain stem gliomas in cats. Vet Pathol 12 (1975) 460–461.

Dahme E: Meningiome bei Fleischfressern. Berl Münch Tierärztl Wochenschr 70 (1957) 32–34.

Dallman MJ, Noxon JO, Stogsdell P: Feline lymphosarcoma with cutaneous and muscle lesions. J Am Vet Med Assoc 181 (1982) 166–168.

Davenport DJ, Eisenberg HM: What is your diagnosis? [Ceruminous gland adenocarcinoma]. J Am Vet Med Assoc 185 (1984) 317–318.

Davies JD, Little NRF: Synovioma in a cat. J Small Anim Pract 13 (1972) 127–133.

de Boer H: Primäre epitheliale Lungentumoren bei Hund und Katze. Eine Auswertung von 52 Fällen. Dissertation, Munich, 1969.

Dehner LP, Norris HJ, Garner FM, Taylor HB: Comparative pathology of ovarian neoplasms. III. Germ cell tumors of canine, bovine, feline, rodent, and human species. J Comp Pathol 80 (1970) 299–306.

Dellman H-D, Brown EM: Textbook of Veterinary Histology. Philadelphia, Lea & Febiger, 1976.

Diehl MP: Un cas de coexistence d'une néoplasie et de tuberculose du chat. Bull Acad Vét Fr 41 (1968) 209.

Dill GS, McElyea U, Stookey JL: Transitional cell carcinoma of the urinary bladder in a cat. J Am Vet Med Assoc 160 (1972) 743–745.

Ditchfield J, Archibald J: Carcinoma of the pancreas in small animals. A report of two cases. Small Anim Clin 1 (1961) 173–176.

Diters RW, Walsh KM: Feline basal cell tumors: a review of 124 cases. Vet Pathol 21 (1984) 51–56.

Dixon RT, Aizstrauts A: A nasopharyngeal tumour associated with oesophageal dilatation in the cat. Aust Vet J 40 (1964) 263–265.

Dommert R: Hemangiopericytoma in a cat. Southwest Vet 14 (2) (1961) 149–150.

Dorn AS, Harris SG, Olmstead ML: Squamous cell carcinoma of the urinary bladder in a cat. Feline Pract 8 (5) (1978) 14–17.

Dorn AS: Legendre AM, McGavin MD: Mammary hyperplasia in a male cat receiving progesterone. J Am Vet Med Assoc 182 (1983) 621–622.

Dorn CR: Epidemiology of canine and feline tumors. J Am Anim Hosp Assoc 12 (1976) 307–312.

Dorn CR, Priester WA: Epidemiologic analysis of oral and pharyngeal cancer in dogs, cats, horses, and cattle. J Am Vet Med Assoc 169 (1976) 1202–1206.

Dorn CR, Taylor DON, Frye FL, Hibbard HH: Survey of animal neoplasms in Alameda and Contra Costa counties, California. I. Methodology and descriptions of cases. J Natl Cancer Inst 40 (1968a) 295–305.

Dorn CR, Taylor DON, Schneider R, Hibbard HH, Klauber MR: Survey of animal neoplasms in Alameda and Contra Costa counties, California. II. Cancer morbidity in dogs and cats from Alameda county. J Natl Cancer Inst 40 (1968b) 307–318.

Douville [no init], Collet P: Le cancer du rein chez le chat. Bull Soc Sci Vét Lyon 37 (1934) 147–150.

Drazner FH: Multiple myeloma in the cat. Compend Contin Ed 4 (1982) 206–216.

Drieux H, Thiéry G: Les tumeurs du placenta chez les animaux domestiques [Hydatidiform mole]. Rev Pathol Comp 48 (1948) 445–451.

Drinker KR, Thompson PK, Marsh M: An investigation of the effect of long-continued ingestion of zinc, in the form of zinc oxide, by cats and dogs, together with observations upon the excretion and the storage of zinc. Am J Physiol 80 (1927) 31–74.

Dubielzig RR, Dehaney RG: Thymoma in a cat. Vet Med Small Anim Clin 74 (1980) 1270–1272.

Dubielzig RR, Adams WM, Brodey RS: Inductive fibroamelo-

blastoma, an unusual dental tumor of young cats. J Am Vet Med Assoc 174 (1979) 720–722.
Duffell SJ: Some aspects of pancreatic disease in the cat. J Small Anim Pract 16 (1975) 365–374.
Durie BGM, Salmon SE, Mundy GR: Relation of osteoclast activating factor production to extent of bone disease in multiple myeloma. Br J Haematol 47 (1981) 21–30.
Edmondson HA: Atlas of Tumor Pathology: Tumors of the Liver and Intrahepatic Bile Ducts. Washington, DC, Armed Forces Institute of Pathology, 1958.
El Etreby MF, Müller-Peddinghaus R, Bhargava AS, Trautwein G: Functional morphology of spontaneous hyperplastic and neoplastic lesions in the canine pituitary gland. Vet Pathol 17 (1980) 109–122.
Elling H, Ungemach FR: Progesterone receptors in feline mammary cancer cytosol. J Cancer Res Clin Oncol 100 (1981) 325–327.
Enerbäck L, Lundin PM: Ultrastructure of mucosal mast cells in normal and compound 48/80-treated rats. Cell Tissue Res 150 (1974) 95–105.
Engle GC: Mammary gland neoplasia in the cat: Prognosis and treatment. Feline Pract 3 (5) (1973) 9–12.
Engle GC, Brodey RS: A retrospective study of 395 feline neoplasms. J Am Anim Hosp Assoc 5 (1969) 21–31.
Essex M: Feline leukemia and sarcoma viruses. *In* Klein G (ed): Viral Oncology. New York, Raven Press, 1980, 205–229.
Essex M, Francis DP: The risk to humans from malignant disease of their pets: An unsettled issue. J Am Anim Hosp Assoc 12 (1976) 386–390.
Evans JG, Grant DI: A mixed mesodermal tumour in the uterus of a cat. J Comp Pathol 87 (1977) 635–638.
Eve H: An interesting growth in the fauces of a kitten [Papillomatosis]. [Br] Vet J 62 (1906) 369–370.
Fankhauser R, Luginbühl H: Das Nervensystem. *In* Dobberstein J, Pallaske G, Stünzi H (eds): Joest's Handbuch der Speziellen Pathologischen Anatomie der Haustiere, vol. 3, 3rd ed. Berlin, Paul Parey, 1968.
Fankhauser R, Luginbühl H, McGrath JT: V. Tumours of the nervous system. Bull WHO 50 (1974) 53–69.
Fanton JW, Withrow SJ: Canine mammary neoplasia: An overview. Calif Vet 35 (7) (1981) 12–16.
Farrow BRH, Penny R: Multiple myeloma in a cat. J Am Vet Med Assoc 158 (1971) 606–611.
Feldman BF: Strafuss AC, Gabbert N: Bile duct carcinoma in the cat: three case reports. Feline Pract 6(1) (1976) 33–35.
Feldman DG, Ehrenreich T, Gross L: Type-C virus particles in a feline angioma: a case report. J Natl Cancer Inst 53 (1974) 1843–1846.
Feldman DG, Gross L: Electron microscopic study of spontaneous mammary carcinoma in cats and dogs: virus-like particles in cat mammary carcinomas. Cancer Res 31 (1971) 1261–1267.
Feldman WH: Neoplasms of Domestic Animals. Philadelphia, WB Saunders Company, 1932.
Finn JP, Schwartz LW: A neoplasm of globule leucocytes in the intestine of a cat. J Comp Pathol 82 (1972) 323–326.
Fitts RH: Bilateral feline embryonal sarcoma. J Am Vet Med Assoc 136 (1960) 616.
Flir K: Die primären Nierengeschwülste der Haussäugetiere. Wissensch Z Humboldt-Univ Berlin 2(1952/53) 93–119.
Foley RH: A selection of cutaneous and related tumors of cats (A photographic essay). Vet Med Small Anim Clin 72 (1977) 43–45.
Fölger AF: Ueber Adamantinome bei den Haustieren. Monatsh Prakt Tierheilk 24 (1913) 564–575.
Ford GH, Empson RN Jr, Plopper CG, Brown PH: Giant cell tumor of soft parts. Vet Pathol 12 (1975) 428–433.
Foresti C: Su di un caso di cancro della lingua. Nuova Vet 12 (1934) 208–211.
Fox JG, Gutnick MJ: Horner's syndrome and brachial paralysis due to lymphosarcoma in a cat. J Am Vet Med Assoc 160 (1972) 977–980.
Fox JG, Snyder SB, Reed C, Campbell LH: Malignant ependymoma in a cat. J Small Anim Pract 14 (1973) 23–26.
Franc M, Guaguere E, Magnol JP, Dorchies P, Ducos de Lahitte J: Tumeurs du conduit auditif externe des carnivores. Rev Méd Vét 132 (1981) 733–739.
Frese K: Statistiche Erhebungen über die Hautgeschwülste der Haustieres. Zentralbl Veterinärmed A 15 (1968) 448–459.
Furth J: Lymphomatosis, myelomatosis, and endothelioma of chickens caused by a filterable agent. II. Morphological characteristics of the endotheliomata caused by this agent. J Exp Med 59 (1934) 501–517.
Gardner MB, Arnstein P, Rongey RW, Estes JD, Sarma PS, Rickard CF, Huebner RJ: Experimental transmission of feline fibrosarcoma to cats and dogs. Nature 226 (1970) 807–809.
Garner FM, Lingeman CH: Mast-cell neoplasms of the domestic cat. Pathol Vet 7 (1970) 517–530.
Gelberg HB, McEntee K: Cystic rete testis in a cat and a fox. Vet Pathol 20 (1983) 634–636.
Gelberg HB, McEntee K: Hyperplastic endometrial polyps in the dog and cat. Vet Pathol 21 (1984) 570–573.
Gelberg HB, McEntee K, Heath EH: Feline cystic rete ovarii. Vet Pathol 21 (1984) 304–307.
Gembardt C, Loppnow H: Zur Pathogenese des spontanen Diabetes mellitus der Katze II. Mitteilung: Azidophile Adenome des Hypophysenvorderlappens und Diabetes mellitus in zwei Fällen. Berl Münch Tieraztl Wochenschr 80 (1976) 336–340.
Gilmore CE: Tumors of the female reproductive tract. Calif Vet 19 (May–June) (1965) 12–15.
Gilmore CE: Tumors of the gastrointestinal tract of cats. *In* Kirk RW (ed): Current Veterinary Therapy V. Philadelphia, WB Saunders Company, 1974, 736–738.
Gimbo A: Su un raro caso di mioepitelioma mammario nella gatta. Rilievi istologici ed istochimici. Clin Vet (Milano) 84 (1961) 313–330.
Ginsburg H: The *in vitro* differentiation and culture of normal mast cells from the mouse thymus. Ann NY Acad Sci 103 (1963) 20–39.
Gleiser CA, Raulston GL, Jardine JH, Gray KN: Malignant fibrous histiocytoma in dogs and cats. Vet Pathol 16 (1979) 199–208.
Glock R: [Tracheal adenoma]. Iowa State Vet 23 (1960–61) 155–156.
Godglück G: Die Geschwülste der Speicheldrüse bei Hund und Katze. Monatsh Vet Med 3 (1948) 148–151.
Godglück G: Sarkome und Karzinome der Nasennöhle bei Fleischfressern. Monatsh Vet Med 5 (1950) 42–44.
Goldberg SA: The occurrence of epithelial tumors in the domesticated animals. J Am Vet Med Assoc 58 (1920) 47–63.
Goldie H, Walker M, Jones D, Lundy R: Mast cells as a factor regulating implantation of free tumor cells from the ascitic fluid into peritoneal tissues of the mouse. Fed Proc 25 (1975) 291.
Goldsmith HS: Melanoma: An overview. American Cancer Society, Inc, 1979.
Goldstein RS, Hess PW: Cryosurgery of canine and feline tumors. J Am Anim Hosp Assoc 12 (1976) 340–349.
Gorlin RJ, Barron CN, Chaudhry AP, Clark JJ: The oral and pharyngeal pathology of domestic animals: a study of 487 cases. Am J Vet Res 20 (1959) 1032–1061.
Gorlin RJ, Chaudhry AP, Pindborg JJ: Odontogenic tumors. Classification, histopathology, and clinical behavior in man and domesticated animals. Cancer 14 (1961) 73–101.
Gorlin RJ, Meskin LH, Brodey R: Odontogenic tumors in man and animals: pathologic classification and clinical behavior—a review. Ann NY Acad Sci 108 (1963) 722–771.
Gorlin RJ, Peterson WC Jr: Oral disease in man and animals (based on analysis of 1135 cases in a variety of species). Arch Dermatol 96 (1967) 390–403.
Gourley IM, Popp JA, Park RD: Myelolipomas of the liver in a domestic cat. J Am Vet Med Assoc 158 (1971) 2053–2057.

Graubmann H-D, Sander W: Herzbasistumor bei einer Katze. Kleintierpraxis 10 (1965) 13–17.

Gray H: Cancer of the esophagus in the cat. Vet Rec 47 (1935) 532–533.

Greene RW, Johnson G: What is your diagnosis? [Hepatic cyst]. J Am Vet Med Assoc 158 (1971) 381–382.

Grier GL, Brewer WG, Theilen GH: Hyperthermic treatment of superficial tumors in cats and dogs. J Am Vet Med Assoc 177 (1980) 227–233.

Guariglia CJ, Rankin JB: What is your diagnosis? [Lymphoma surrounding and infiltrating the tracheal bifurcation]. J Am Vet Med Assoc 156 (1970) 114–116.

Guerre R, Millet P, Groulade P: Systemic mastocytosis in a cat: remission after splenectomy. J Small Anim Pract 20 (1979) 769–772.

Gustaffson PeO, Wolfe D: Bone metastasizing lung carcinoma in a cat. Cornell Vet 58 (1968) 425–430.

Hague PH, Burridge MJ: A meningioma in a cat associated with erosion of the skull. Vet Rec 84 (1969) 217–219.

Hajdu, SI: Personal communication. Memorial Sloan-Kettering Cancer Center. New York, NY, 1981.

Hamilton HB, Severin GA, Nold J: Pulmonary squamous cell carcinoma with intraocular metastasis. J Am Vet Med Assoc 185 (1984) 307–309.

Hamilton JM, Else RW, Forshaw P: Oestrogen receptors in feline mammary carcinomas. Vet Rec 99 (1976) 477–479.

Hampe JF, Misdorp W: Tumours and dysplasias of the mammary gland. Bull WHO50 (1974) 111–133.

Hampe JF, Weijer K: Feline mammary benign tumours and dysplasias. *In* Weijer K (ed): Feline Mammary Tumours and Dysplasia. Oosthuizen, Drukkerij Van der Molen, 1979.

Hänichen T: Über ein Kehlkopfkarzinom bei einer Katze. Berl Münch Tierärztl Wochenschr 78 (1965) 234–235.

Hanlon GF: What is your diagnosis? [Myxomatous bladder tumor of low-grade malignancy]. J Am Vet Med Assoc 141 (1962) 263–264. [This tumor is included in Osborne et al., 1948a, 1948b, and Caywood et al., 1980.]

Harbison ML, Godleski JJ: Malignant mesothelioma in urban dogs. Vet Pathol 20 (1983) 531–540.

Hardy WD Jr: Hematopoietic tumors of cats. J Am Anim Hosp Assoc 17 (1981) 921–940.

Hardy WD Jr, Essex M, McClelland AJ: Feline Leukemia Virus. New York, Elsevier/North-Holland, Inc, 1980.

Harkin JC, Reed RJ: Atlas of Tumor Pathology: Tumors of the Peripheral Nervous System. Washington, DC, Armed Forces Institute of Pathology, 1969.

Harvey C, Goldschmidt MH: Inflammatory polypoid growths in the ear canal of cats. J Small Anim Pract 19 (1978) 669–677.

Harvey HJ: Cryosurgery of oral tumors in dogs and cats. Vet Clin North Am 10 (1980) 821–830.

Haskins ME, McGrath JT: Meningiomas in young cats with mucopolysaccharidosis I. J Neuropathol Exp Neurol 42 (1983) 664–670.

Hasler UC, van den Ingh TSGAM: Malignant mastocytosis and duodenal ulceration in a cat. Schweiz Arch Tierheilkd 120 (1978) 263–268. (Abstr Vet Bull 48 [1978] 7512.)

Hauser B, Mettler F: Malignant thymoma in a cat. J Comp Pathol 94 (1984) 311–313.

Hauser P: Ein Fall von Gewebsmastzellen-Leukämie bei einer Katze. Schweiz Arch Tierheilk 107 (1965) 487–496.

Hay LE: Multiple myeloma in a cat. Aust Vet Pract 8(1) (1978) 45–48.

Hayden DW, Johnson KH, Ghobrial HK: Ultrastructure of feline mammary hypertrophy. Vet Pathol 20 (1983) 254–264.

Hayden DW, Johnston SD, Kiang DT, Johnson HH, Barnes DM: Feline mammary hypertrophy/fibroadenoma complex: clinical and hormonal aspects. Am J Vet Res 42 (1981) 1699–1703.

Hayden DW, Nielsen SW: Feline mammary tumours. J Small Anim Pract 12 (1971) 687–697.

Hayes A: Personal communication, 1976.

Hayes A: Feline mammary gland tumors. Vet Clin North Am 7 (1977) 205–212.

Hayes AA, Hardy WD Jr, McClelland AJ: The prevention of canine and feline tumor development. J Am Anim Hosp Assoc 12 (1976) 381–385.

Hayes AA, Mooney S: Feline mammary tumors. Vet Clin North Am 15 (1985) 513–520.

Hayes HM, Milne KL, Mandell CP: Epidemiological features of feline mammary carcinoma. Vet Rec 108 (1981) 476–479.

Hayes HM, Priester WA, Pendergrass TW: Occurrence of nervous-tissue tumors in cattle, horses, cats and dogs. Int J Cancer 15 (1975) 39–47.

Hayes KC, Schiefer B: Primary tumors in the CNS of carnivores. Pathol Vet 6 (1969) 94–116.

Head KW: Neoplastic diseases. *In* Symposium on skin diseases. Vet Rec 65 (1953) 921–929.

Head KW: Cutaneous mast-cell tumours in the dog, cat and ox. Br J Dermatol 70 (1958) 399–408.

Head KW: Tumours of the upper alimentary tract. Bull WHO 53 (1976a) 145–166.

Head KW: Tumours of the lower alimentary tract. Bull WHO 53 (1976b) 167–174.

Heavner JE: Neural lymphomatosis in cats. Mod Vet Pract 59 (1978) 122–124.

Herman LH: Sublingual squamous cell carcinoma in a cat. Am J Vet Res 28 (1967) 1627–1629.

Hernandez FJ, Fernandez BB, Chertack M, Gage PA: Feline mammary carcinoma and progestogens. Feline Pract 5 (5) (1975) 45–48.

Herron ML: The musculoskeletal system. *In* Catcott EJ (ed): Feline Medicine and Surgery, 2nd ed. Santa Barbara, American Veterinary Publications, Inc, 1975.

Herron ML: The musculoskeletal system. *In* Pratt PW (ed): Feline Medicine, 1st ed. Santa Barbara, American Veterinary Publications, Inc, 1983.

Hess PW, Meierhenry EF: Management of canine and feline oral and pharyngeal tumors. Proc Am Anim Hosp Assoc 42 (vol II) (1975) 122–125.

Higginbotham RD: *In* Round table discussion on mast cells and basophils. Ann NY Acad Sci 103 (1963) 441–490.

Higginbotham RD, Murillo GJ: Influence of heparin on resistance of rabbits to infection with fibroma virus. J Immunol 94 (1965) 228–233.

Hinko PJ, Burt JK, Fetter AW: Chondrosarcoma in the femur of a cat. J Am Anim Hosp Assoc 15 (1979) 737–739.

Hinton M, Gaskell CJ: Non-neoplastic mammary hypertrophy in the cat associated either with pregnancy or with oral progestagen therapy. Vet Rec 100 (1977) 277–280.

Hjärre A: Sektionsbefund beim Diabetes mellitus des Hundes und der Katze. Arch Tierheilkd 57 (1927) 1–76.

Hoening M, Goldschmidt MH, Ferguson DC, Koch K, Eymontt MJ: Toxic nodular goitre in the cat. J Small Anim Pract 23 (1982) 1–12.

Hofmann W, Arbiter D, Scheele D: Sex cord stromal tumor of the cat: So-called androblastoma with Sertoli-Leydig cell pattern. Vet Pathol 17 (1980) 508–513.

Holmberg CA, Manning JS, Osburn BI: Feline malignant lymphomas: Comparison of morphologic and immunologic characteristics. Am J Vet Res 37 (1976) 1455–1460.

Holzinger EA: Feline cutaneous mastocytomas. Cornell Vet 63 (1973) 87–93.

Holzworth J: Leukemia and related neoplasms in the cat. I. Lymphoid malignancies. J Am Vet Med Assoc 136 (1960) 47–69.

Holzworth J, Coffin DL: Pancreatic insufficiency and diabetes mellitus in a cat. Cornell Vet 43 (1953) 502–512.

Holzworth J, Husted P, Wind A: Arterial thrombosis and thyroid carcinoma in a cat. Cornell Vet 45 (1955) 487–496.

Holzworth J, Meier H: Reticulum cell myeloma in a cat. Cornell Vet 47 (1957) 302–316.

Holzworth J, Theran P, Carpenter JL, Harpster NK, Todoroff

RJ: Hyperthyroidism in the cat: ten cases. J Am Vet Med Assoc 176 (4) (1980) 345–353.

Hong CB, Winston JM, Lee CC: Hepatic angiosarcoma. Animal model: angiosarcoma of rats and mice induced by vinyl chloride. Am J Pathol 101 (1980) 737–740.

Hoogland HJM: Ein massives Adamantinom beim Rind. Arch Wiss Prakt Tierheilkd 54 (1926) 170–183 [two cases in cats].

Hoogland HJM: Twe zeldzame carcinoomgevallen bij de kat. Ned Tijdschr Geneeskd 72 (1928) 4741–4742.

Hoogland HJM: Carcinome der Gallenwege bei Distomatose der Katze. Z Krebsforsch 29 (1929) 236–269.

Hottendorf GH, Nielsen SW, Kenyon AJ: Ribonucleic acid in canine mast cell granules and the possible interrelationship of mast cells and plasma cells. Pathol Vet 3 (1966) 178–189.

Hou PC: Primary carcinoma of bile duct of the liver of the cat (*Felis catus*) infested with *Clonorchis sinensis*. J Pathol Bacteriol 87 (1964) 239–244.

Howard EB, Kenyon AJ: Malignant osteoclastoma (giant cell tumor) in the cat with associated mast-cell response. Cornell Vet 57 (1967) 398–409.

Howard EB, Sawa TR, Nielsen SW, Kenyon AJ: Mastocytoma and gastroduodenal ulceration. Gastric and duodenal ulcers in dogs with mastocytoma. Pathol Vet 6 (1969) 146–158.

Howell J McC, Ishmael J, Tandy J, Hughes IB: A 6-year survey of tumours of dogs and cats removed surgically in private practice. J Small Anim Pract 11 (1970) 793–801.

Hribernik TN, Barta O, Gaunt SD, Boudreaux MK: Serum hyperviscosity syndrome associated with IgG myeloma in a cat. J Am Vet Med Assoc 181 (1982) 169–170.

Hübner L: Das Blutbild der Katze. Monatsh Prakt Tierheilkd 31 (1920) 499–501.

Hulse EV: A benign giant-cell synovioma in a cat. J Pathol Bacteriol 91 (1960) 269–271.

Ikede BO, Downey RS: Multiple hepatic myelolipomas in a cat. Can Vet J 13 (1972) 160–163.

Indrieri RJ, Taylor RF: Vestibular dysfunction caused by squamous cell carcinoma involving the middle and inner ear in two cats. J Am Vet Med Assoc 184 (1984) 471–473.

Jacobson SA: The Comparative Pathology of the Tumors of Bone. Springfield IL, Charles C Thomas, 1971, 102–126.

Jaques LB: The mast cells in the light of new knowledge of heparin and the sulfated mucopolysaccharides. Gen Pharmacol 6 (1975) 235–245.

Jaques LB, Sue TK, McDuffie NM, Presnell KR: Sulfated mucopolysaccharides in dog mast cell tumors. J Am Anim Hosp Assoc 13 (1977) 359–368.

Jarrett WFH, Martin WB, Crighton GW, Stewart MF: Leukaemia in the cat. Transmission experiments with leukaemia (lymphosarcoma). Nature (London) 202 (1964) 566–567.

Jeglum KA, de Guzman E, Young KM: Chemotherapy of advanced mammary adenocarcinoma in 14 cats. J Am Vet Med Assoc 187 (1985) 157–160.

Johnson KH, Osborne CA: Adenocarcinoma of the thyroid gland in a cat. J Am Vet Med Assoc 156 (1970) 906–912.

Johnston SD, Hayden DW, Kiang DT, Handschin B, Johnson KH: Progesterone receptors in feline mammary adenocarcinomas. Am J Vet Res 45 (1984) 379–382.

Jonas AM, Hukill PG: Histogenesis of a pulmonary adenocarcinoma in the cat. Arch Pathol 85 (1968) 573–579.

Jones BR: Spinal meningioma in a cat. Aust Vet J 50 (1974) 229–231.

Jones BR, Studdert VP: Horner's syndrome in the dog and cat as an aid to diagnosis. Aust Vet J 51 (1975) 329–332.

Jones TC, Hunt RD: Veterinary Pathology, 5th ed. Philadelphia, Lea & Febiger, 1983.

Jonquières [no initial]: Cancer de l'oesophage chez un chat. Bull Soc Sci Vét Lyon 38 (1935) 101–106.

Joshua JO: The Clinical Aspects of Some Diseases of Cats. London, William Heinemann Medical Books Limited, 1965.

Jubb KVF, Kennedy PC: Pathology of Domestic Animals. New York, Academic Press, 1963.

Jubb KVF, Kennedy PC: Pathology of Domestic Animals, 2nd ed. New York, Academic Press, 1970.

Jubb KVF, Kennedy PC, Palmer N: Pathology of Domestic Animals, 3rd ed. Orlando, Academic Press, 1985.

Jungreis T: [Metastasizing bile duct carcinoma]. NYC Vet 10 (5) (1968) 5–6.

Kaliner MA: The mast cell—a fascinating riddle. N Engl J Med 301 (1979) 498–499.

Kallfelz FA, de Lahunta A, Allhands RV: Scintigraphic diagnosis of brain lesions in the dog and cat. J Am Vet Med Assoc 172 (1978) 589–597.

Kammerman-Lüscher B: Blutbasophilen-Leukose beim Hund und Gewebsbasophilen-Retikulose bei der Katze. Berl Münch Tierärztl Wochenschr 79 (1966) 459–464.

Karbe E, Schiefer B: Primary salivary gland tumors in carnivores. Can Vet J 8 (1967) 212–215.

Kaye WA, Passero MA: Respiratory distress and hypoxemia in systemic mastocytosis. Chest 75 (1979) 87–88.

Kermen WR: Ovarian cyst in a cat [and adenocarcinoma of the uterus]. J Am Vet Med Assoc 86 (1935) 96–97.

Kiesel GK: Carcinoma of the kidney of a cat. Cornell Vet 40 (1950) 380.

Kircher CH, Garner FM, Robinson FR: Tumors of the eye and adnexa. Bull WHO 50 (1974) 135–142.

Kircher CH, Nielsen SW: Tumours of the pancreas. Bull WHO 53 (1976) 195–202.

Kitt T: Carcinomatose des Eierstocks mit Metastasen bei einer Katze. Monatsh Prakt Thierheilk 11 (1900) 306–311.

Knecht CD, Greene JA: Osteoma of the zygomatic arch in a cat. J Am Vet Med Assoc 171 (1977) 1077–1078.

Koestner A, Buerger L: Primary neoplasms of the salivary glands in animals compared to similar tumors in man. Pathol Vet 2 (1965) 201–226.

Kornegay JN: Feline neurology. Compend Contin Ed 3 (1981) 203–213.

Kovacs AB, Somogyvari K: Tumours of domestic animals. Acta Vet Acad Sci Hung 18 (1968) 399–408.

Kronberger H: Spontane Geschwülste bei Haussäugetieren. Nach den Sektionsprotokollen des Veterinär-Pathologischen Institutes. Monatsh Vet Med 15 (1960) 730–735.

Kyle R: Multiple myeloma—review of 869 cases. Mayo Clin Proc 50 (1975) 29–40.

Labie C, Fontaine M: Mastocytome splénique du chat. Bull Acad Vét Fr 33 (1960) 361–366.

Ladds PW, Strafuss AC, Anderson NV: A feline mediastinal tumor of probable thymic origin. J Am Anim Hosp Assoc 6 (1970) 55–58.

Lahellec M, Joncourt A: Étude clinique et histologique d'une tumeur carcinoïde du grêle chez un chat. Bull Acad Vét Fr 45 (1972) 363–365.

Lamouroux J, Lebeau C: Cancer oesophagien chez un chat. Bull Acad Vét Fr 26 (1953) 85–86.

Lane JG, Orr CM, Lucke VM, Gruffydd-Jones TJ: Nasopharyngeal polyps arising in the middle ear of the cat. J Small Anim Pract 22 (1981) 511–522.

Lasserre R, Lombard C, Labatut R: Recherches sur le cancer des animaux domestiques. Rev Méd Vét 90 (1938) 425–451.

Lawrence DE: Histocytoma [sic]. NY City Vet 7 (14) (June 1965) 16.

Lawson DC, Burk RL, Prata RG: Cerebral meningioma in the cat: Diagnosis and surgical treatment of ten cases. J Am Anim Hosp Assoc 20 (1984) 333–342.

Leav I, Schiller AL, Rijnberk A, Legg MA, der Kinderen PJ: Adenomas and carcinomas of the canine and feline thyroid. Am J Pathol 83 (1976) 61–94.

LeCouteur RA, Fike JR, Cann CE, Turrel JM, Thompson JE, Biggart JF: X-ray computed tomography of brain tumors in cats. J Am Vet Med Assoc 183 (1983) 301–305.

Legendre AM, Becker PU: Feline skin lymphoma: Characterization of tumor and identification of tumor-stimulating serum factor(s). Am J Vet Res 40 (1979) 1805–1807.

Legendre AM, Dade AW: Nasal tumor in a cat. J Am Vet Med Assoc 167 (1975) 481–483.
Legendre AM, Carrig CB, Howard DR, Dade AW: Nasal tumor in a cat [Lymphoma]. J Am Vet Med Assoc 167 (1975) 481–483.
Legendre AM, Krahwinkel DJ: Feline ear tumors. J Am Anim Hosp Assoc 17 (1981) 1035–1037.
Legendre AM, Krahwinkel DJ, Spaulding KA: Feline nasal and paranasal sinus tumors. J Am Anim Hosp Assoc 17 (1981) 1038–1039.
Leklem JE, Brown RR, Hankes LV, Schmaeler M: Tryptophan metabolism in the cat: A study with carbon-14–labelled compounds. Am J Vet Res 32 (1971) 335–344.
Lettow E, Dämmrich K: Angeborene polyzystische Leber- und Nierenveränderungen bei einer Katze. Kleintierpraxis 12 (1967) 35–43.
Levene A: Sebaceous gland differentiation in tumours of the feline oral mucosa. Vet Rec 114 (1984) 69.
Lieberman LL: Feline adenocarcinoma of the larynx with metastasis to the adrenal gland. J Am Vet Med Assoc 125 (1954) 153–154.
Liénaux E: Epulis du chat: deux cas d'épithéliomes adamantins. Ann Méd Vét 49 (1900) 19–20.
Lillie RD: Mast myelocyte leukemia in a cat. Am J Pathol 7 (1931) 713–721.
Lingeman CH: Comparative aspects of the mastocytoses. Natl Cancer Inst Monogr 32 (1969) 289–295.
Lingeman CH, Garner FM, Taylor DON: Spontaneous gastric adenocarcinomas of dogs: a review. J Natl Cancer Inst 47 (1971) 137–153.
Lingeman CH, Garner FM: Comparative study of intestinal adenocarcinomas of animals and man. J Natl Cancer Inst 48 (1972) 325–346.
Linnabary RD, Holscher MA, Page DL, Fitzpatrick D: Primitive multipotential primary sarcoma of bone in a cat. Vet Pathol 15 (1978) 432–434.
Liska WD, MacEwen EG, Zaki FA, Garvey M: Feline systemic mastocytosis: a review and results of splenectomy in seven cases. J Am Anim Hosp Assoc 15 (1979) 589–597.
Liu S-K, Dorfman HD, Patnaik AK: Primary and secondary bone tumours in the cat. J Small Anim Pract 15 (1974) 141–156.
Lombard C: Un troisième cas de épithelioma langerhansien chez les animaux. Rev Vét 87 (1935) 632–634.
Lombard C: Sarcome du pancréas chez la chatte. Rev Vét 88 (1936) 674–675.
Lombard C: Les cancers et tumeurs du chat. Recl Méd Vét 116 (1940) 193–212.
Lombard C: Contribution à l'étude des tumeurs de l'appareil génital, chez les mammifères domestiques. Rev Méd Vét 112 (1961) 509–526, 598–618.
Lombard C: Hémangio-endothéliome végétant sublingual chez la chatte. Bull Acad Vét Fr 37 (1964) 163–167.
Lombard LS, Fortna HM, Garner FM, Brynjolfsson G: Myelolipomas of the liver in captive wild felidae. Pathol Vet 5 (1968) 127–134.
Lord PF, Kapp DS, Schwartz A, Morrow DT: Osteogenic sarcoma of the nasal cavity in a cat; postoperative control with high dose-per-fraction radiation therapy and metronidazole. Vet Radiol 23 (1982) 23–26.
Loveday RK: Thymoma in a Siamese cat. J S Afr Vet Med Assoc 30 (1959) 33–34.
Lucke VM: An histological study of thyroid abnormalities in the domestic cat. J Small Anim Pract 5 (1964) 351–358.
Luginbühl H: Studies on meningiomas in cats. Am J Vet Res 22 (1961) 1030–1040.
Luginbühl H: Comparative aspects of tumors of the nervous system. Ann NY Acad Sci 108 (1963) 702–721.
Luginbühl H, Fankhauser R, McGrath JT: Spontaneous neoplasms of the nervous system in animals. Progr Neurol Surg 2 (1968) 85–164.
Luttgen PJ, Braund KG, Brawner WR, Vandevelde M: A retrospective study of twenty-nine spinal tumours in the dog and cat. J Small Anim Pract 21 (1980) 213–226.
MacEwen EG, Hayes AA, Harvey HJ, Patnaik AK, Mooney SM, Passe S: Prognostic factors for feline mammary tumors. J Am Vet Med Assoc 185 (1984a) 201–204.
MacEwen EG, Hayes AA, Mooney S, Patnaik AK, Harvey JH, Passe S: Effect of levamisole on feline mammary cancer. J Biol Resp Modif 3 (1984b) 541–546.
MacEwen EG, Hurvitz AI: Diagnosis and management of monoclonal gammopathies. Vet Clin North Am 7 (1977) 119–132.
Mackey L: Clear cell thymoma and thymic hyperplasia in a cat. J Comp Pathol 85 (1975) 367–371.
MacVean DW, Monlux AW, Anderson PS Jr, Silberg SL, Roszel JF: Frequency of canine and feline tumors in a defined population. Vet Pathol 15 (1978) 700–715.
Macy DW, Reynolds HA: The incidence, characteristics and clinical management of skin tumors of cats. J Am Anim Hosp Assoc 17 (1981) 1026–1034.
Madewell BR, Ackerman N, Sesline DH: Invasive carcinoma radiographically mimicking primary bone cancer in the mandibles of two cats. J Am Vet Radiol Soc 17 (1976) 213–215.
Madewell BR, Munn RJ, Phillips LK: Ultrastructure of canine, feline, and bovine mast cell neoplasms. Am J Vet Res 45 (1984) 2066–2073.
Madewell BR, Priester WA, Gillette EL, Snyder SP: Neoplasms of the nasal passages and paranasal sinuses in domestic animals as reported by 13 veterinary colleges. Am J Vet Res 37 (1976) 851–856.
Mandelli G, Finazzi M: Histologische Befunde bei dem Milchdrüsen-Hypertrophie-Fibroadenomkomplex der Katze. Deutsch Tierärztl Wochenschr 90 (1983) 482–485.
Mann FC, Brimhall SD: Pathologic conditions noted in laboratory animals. J Am Vet Med Assoc 52 (1917) 195–204.
Martin SL, Capen CC: The endocrine system. *In* Catcott EJ (ed): Feline Medicine and Surgery, 2nd ed. Santa Barbara, American Veterinary Publications, Inc, 1975, 454–456.
Marusi A: Papilloma della vagina di una gatta. Nuova Vet 40 (1967) 640–644.
McAfee LT, McAfee JT, Katz R: Sebaceous gland adenomas in a cat. Feline Pract 9 (2) (1979) 21–23.
McClelland RB: A giant-cell tumor of the tibia in a cat. Cornell Vet 31 (1941) 86–87.
McClelland RB: Ovarian teratoma in cat. North Am Vet 23 (1942) 172.
McClelland RB: X-ray therapy in malignant neoplastic diseases of small animals. Cornell Vet 47 (1957) 533–538.
McClelland RB: The treatment of mastocytomas in dogs. Cornell Vet 54 (1964) 517–519.
McCusker HB, Aitken ID: Anaphylaxis in the cat. J Pathol Bacteriol 91 (1966) 282–285.
McDonald LE: Veterinary Endocrinology and Reproduction, 3rd ed. Philadelphia, Lea & Febiger, 1980.
McDonough S, Larsen S, Brodey RS, Stock ND, Hardy WD Jr: A transmissible feline fibrosarcoma of viral origin. Cancer Res 31 (1971) 953–956.
McGrath JT: Neurological Examination of the Dog with Clinicopathologic Observations, 2nd ed. Philadelphia, Lea & Febiger, 1960.
McGrath JT: Meningiomas in animals. J Neuropathol Exp Neurol 21 (1962) 327–328.
McMillan FD: Insulinoma in a cat. Proc Am Coll Vet Intern Med 1983, 51.
Meier H: Carcinoma of the uterus in the cat: Two cases. Cornell Vet 46 (1956a) 188–200.
Meier H: Sertoli-cell tumor in the cat: Report of two cases. North Am Vet 37 (1956b) 979–981.
Meier H: Feline mastocytoma: Two cases. Cornell Vet 47 (1957) 220–226.
Meijer JC, Lubberink AAME, Gruys E: Cushing's syndrome due to adenocortical adenoma in a cat. Tijdschr Diergeneeskd 103 (1978) 1048–1051.
Meincke JE, Hobbie WJ, Hardy WD Jr: Lymphoreticular malig-

nancies in the cat: Clinical findings. J Am Vet Med Assoc 160 (1972) 1093–1103.

Melander A, Westgren U, Sundler F, Ericson LE: Influence of histamine- and 5-hydroxytryptamine–containing thyroid mast cells on thyroid blood flow and permeability in the rat. Endocrinology 97 (1975) 1130–1137.

Mendham JH, Roszel JF, Bovee KC: Clinico-pathologic conference [Biliary cyst in a cat]. J Am Vet Med Assoc 154 (1969) 935–944.

Messow C: Die Lebertumoren unserer Haussäugetiere. Wissensch Z Humboldt–Univ Berlin 2 (1952/53) 121–152.

Mettler F: Thymome bei Hund und Katze. Schweiz Arch Tierheilkd 117 (1975) 577–584.

Middleton DJ, Watson ADJ, Vasak E, Culvenor JE: Duodenal ulceration associated with gastrin-secreting pancreatic tumor in a cat. J Am Vet Med Assoc 183 (1983) 461–462.

Milks HJ: Some diseases of the genitourinary system. Cornell Vet 29 (1939) 105–114.

Milks HJ, Olafson P: Primary brain tumors in small animals. Cornell Vet 26 (1936) 159–170.

Miller AS, McCrea MW, Rhodes WH: Mandibular epidermoid carcinoma with reactive bone proliferation in a cat. Am J Vet Res 30 (1969) 1465–1468.

Miller WH: Personal communication, 1981.

Mills JN, Eger CE, Robinson WF, Penhale WJ, McKenna RP: A case of multiple myeloma in a cat. J Am Anim Hosp Assoc 18 (1982) 79–82.

Misdorp W, van der Heul RO: Tumors of bones and joints. Bull WHO 53 (1976) 265–282.

Moise NS, Riis RC, Allison NM: Ocular manifestations of metastatic sweat gland adenocarcinoma in a cat. J Am Vet Med Assoc 180 (1982) 1100–1103.

Monlux WS: Primary pulmonary neoplasms in domestic animals. Southwest Vet (Oct) (1952) 5–39.

Monteagudo OG, Purpura DP: Epileptogenic effects of an auditory cortex meningioma in a cat. Cornell Vet 49 (1959) 375–379.

Montoro L, Botija C Sanchez: Un caso de adenocarcinoma primario de rinon con metastasis. Rev Hig Sanid Pecuar (Madrid) 25 (1935) 504–510.

Montpellier J-M, Samso A, Catanei J: Le cancer de l'utérus en pathologie vétérinaire. Bull Algér Carcinol 5 (1952) 45–56.

Moore AS, Middleton DJ: Pulmonary adenocarcinoma in three cats with non-respiratory signs only. J Small Anim Pract 23 (1982) 501–509.

Morgan R, McMillan MC: What is your diagnosis? [Lymphoma, kidneys, bladder, ileocolic junction]. J Am Vet Med Assoc 178 (1981) 597–598.

Morozova SM, Skorodumova JV: [Tumors of pancreas in carnivores]. Veterinariia (Moscow) 49 (6) (1972) 91–93.

Morrison WB: Paraneoplastic syndromes of the dog. J Am Vet Med Assoc 175 (1979) 559–561.

Morton D: Chondrosarcoma arising in a multilobular chondroma in a cat. J Am Vet Med Assoc 186 (1985) 804–806.

Moulton JE: Tumors in Domestic Animals, 1st ed. Berkeley, University of California Press, 1961.

Moulton JE (ed): Tumors in Domestic Animals, 2nd ed. Berkeley, University of California Press, 1978.

Moulton JE, von Tscharner C, Schneider R: Classification of lung carcinomas in the dog and cat. Vet Pathol 18 (1981) 513–528.

Mugera CM: Canine and feline neoplasms in Kenya. Bull Epizoot Dis Afr 16 (1968) 367–370.

Muller GH, Kirk RW, Scott DW: Small Animal Dermatology, 3rd ed. Philadelphia, WB Saunders Company, 1983.

Mulligan RM: Spontaneous cat tumors. Cancer Res 11 (1951) 271.

Nafe LA: Meningiomas in cats: a retrospective clinical study of 36 cases. J Am Vet Med Assoc 174 (1979) 1224–1227.

Nakayama H, Nakanaga K, Ogihara S, Hayashi T, Takahashi R, Fujiwara K: Three cases of feline lymphosarcoma with formation of multinucleated giant cells. Jpn J Vet Sci 46 (1984) 225–228. (Abstr Vet Bull 54 [1984] 5815.)

Nathwani BN, Hun Kim, Rappaport H, Solomon J, Fox M: Non-Hodgkin's lymphomas. A clinicopathologic study comparing two classifications. Cancer 41 (1978) 303–325.

National Cancer Institute: Sponsored study of non-Hodgkin's lymphomas. Summary and description of a Working Formulation for Clinical Usage. Cancer 49 (1982) 2112–2135.

Nava GA, Sbernardori U: Dystocia materna nella gatta de leiomyoma del corpo dell' utero. Clin Vet (Milano) 90 (1967) 521–525.

Nieberle K, Cohrs P: Lehrbuch der Speziellen Pathologischen Anatomie der Haustiere. Jena, G Fischer, 1931.

Nielsen SW: The malignancy of mammary tumors in cats. North Am Vet 33 (1952a) 245–252.

Nielsen SW: Extraskeletal giant cell tumor in a cat. Cornell Vet 42 (1952b) 304–311.

Nielsen SW: Neoplastic diseases. *In* Catcott EJ (ed): Feline Medicine and Surgery, 1st ed. Santa Barbara, American Veterinary Publications, Inc, 1964.

Nielsen SW: Spontaneous hematopoietic neoplasms of the domestic cat. Natl Cancer Inst Monogr 32 (1969) 73–94.

Nielsen SW: Pulmonary Neoplasms in Domestic Animals. Oak Ridge, TN, US Atomic Energy Commission, Division of Technical Information, 1970, 123–145.

Nielsen SW: Classification of tumors in dogs and cats. J Am Anim Hosp Assoc 19 (1983) 13–59.

Nielsen SW, Cole CR: Canine mastocytoma—a report of one hundred cases. Am J Vet Res 19 (1958) 417–432.

Nielsen SW, Howard EB, Wolke RE: Feline mastocytosis. *In* Clarke WJ, Howard EB, Hackett PL (eds): Myeloproliferative Disorders of Animals and Man. Oak Ridge, TN, US Atomic Energy Commission, 1970, 359–370.

Nielsen SW, Howard EB: Feline neoplasia. Progr Feline Pract 2 (1971) 194–197.

Nielsen SW, Misdorp W, McEntee K: Tumours of the ovary. Bull WHO 53 (1976) 203–216.

Nimmo JS, Plummer JM: Ultrastructural studies of fibroadenomatous hyperplasia of mammary glands of 2 cats. J Comp Pathol 91 (1981) 41–50.

Norris AM, Pallett C, Wilcock B: Generalized myositis ossificans in a cat. J Am Anim Hosp Assoc 16 (1980) 659–663.

Norris HJ, Garner FM, Taylor HB: Pathology of feline ovarian neoplasms. J Pathol 97 (1969) 138–143.

Noxon JO, Thornburg LP, Dillender MJ, Jones BD: An adenoma in ectopic thyroid tissue causing hyperthyroidism in a cat. J Am Anim Hosp Assoc 19 (1983) 369–370.

Nunes Petisca JL: Cisto-adenoma solitario no fegado do gato. Rev Cienc Vet (Lisbon) 51 (1956) 86–88.

Olafson P: Oral tumors of small animals. Cornell Vet 29 (1939) 222–237.

Olin FH, Lea RB, Kim C: Colonic adenoma in a cat. J Am Vet Med Assoc 153 (1968) 53–56.

Olmstead ML, Butler HC: Five-hydroxytryptamine antagonists and feline aortic embolism. J Small Anim Pract 18 (1977) 247–259.

O'Rourke MD, Geib LW: Endometrial adenocarcinoma in a cat. Cornell Vet 60 (1970) 598–604.

Osborne CA, Low DG, Perman V: Neoplasms of the canine and feline urinary bladder: clinical findings, diagnosis, and treatment. J Am Vet Med Assoc 152 (1968a) 247–259.

Osborne CA, Low DG, Perman V, Barnes DM: Neoplasms of the canine and feline urinary bladder: incidence, etiologic factors, occurrence, and pathologic features. Am J Vet Res 29 (1968b) 2041–2055.

Osborne CA, Quast JF, Barnes DM, Fitz CR: Renal pelvic carcinoma in a cat [transitional cell carcinoma]. J Am Vet Med Assoc 159 (1971) 1238–1241.

Oshima K, Miura S: Mast-cell leukosis in cats—a report of two cases. Jpn J Vet Sci 27 (1966) 233–238 (Abstr Vet Bull 36 [1966] 3171).

Ott RL: Systemic viral diseases. *In* Pratt PW (ed): Feline Medicine, 1st ed. Santa Barbara, American Veterinary Publications, Inc, 1983.

Ottani F: Cancro cutaneo su fondo infiammatorio in un gatto. Nuova Vet 1 (6) (1923) 6–8.
Owens JM, Drazner FH, Gilbertson SR: Pancreatic disease in the cat. J Am Anim Hosp Assoc 11 (1975) 83–89.
Pack FD: Feline uterine adenomyosis. Feline Pract 10 (5) (1980) 45–47.
Padawer J: Studies on mammalian mast cells. Trans NY Acad Sci 19 (1957) 690–713.
Padawer J: The ins and outs of mast cell function (editorial). Am J Anat 141 (1974) 299–302.
Palumbo NE, Perri SF: Adenocarcinoma of the ileum in a cat. J Am Vet Med Assoc 164 (1974) 607–608.
Pamukcu AM: Tumours of the urinary bladder. Bull WHO 50 (1974) 43–52.
Park RD: Acute abdomen in the cat [Mast cell malignancy with perforated duodenal ulcer]. Feline Pract 2 (6) (1972) 51–53.
Parker AJ: Differential diagnosis of brain disease: Part 2 Lumbar ataxia, paresis, and paralysis. Mod Vet Pract 62 (1981) 839–845.
Parker AJ, O'Brien DP, Sawchuk SA: The nervous system. *In* Pratt PW (ed): Feline Medicine, 1st ed. Santa Barbara, American Veterinary Publications, Inc, 1983.
Parker AJ, Park RD: Myelographic diagnosis of a spinal cord tumor in a cat. Feline Pract 4 (3) (1974) 28–33.
Parker C, Jost RG, Bauer E, Haddad J, Garza R: Systemic mastocytosis. Am J Med 61 (1976) 671–680.
Parker GA, Casey HW: Thymomas in domestic animals. Vet Pathol 13 (1976) 353–364.
Parmley RT, Spicer SS, Wright NJ: The ultrastructural identification of tissue basophils and mast cells in Hodgkin's disease. Lab Invest 32 (1975) 469–475.
Patnaik AK, Greene RW: Intravenous leiomyoma of the bladder in a cat. J Am Vet Med Assoc 175 (1979) 381–383.
Patnaik AK, Lieberman PH: Feline anaplastic giant cell adenocarcinoma of the thyroid. Vet Pathol 16 (1979) 687–692.
Patnaik AK, Hurvitz AI, Lieberman PH: Canine hepatic neoplasms: a clinicopathologic study. Vet Pathol 17 (1980) 553–564.
Patnaik AK, Johnson GF, Greene RW, Hayes AA, MacEwen EG: Surgical resection of intestinal adenocarcinoma in a cat, with survival of 28 months. J Am Vet Med Assoc 178 (1981) 479–481.
Patnaik AK, Lieberman PH, Johnson GF: Intestinal ganglioneuroma in a kitten—a case report and review of literature. J Small Anim Pract 19 (1978) 735–742.
Patnaik AK, Liu S-K, Hurvitz AI, McClelland AJ: Nonhematopoietic neoplasms in cats. J Natl Cancer Inst 54 (1975) 855–860.
Patnaik AK, Liu S-K, Johnson GF: Feline intestinal adenocarcinoma. A clinicopathologic study of 22 cases. Vet Pathol 13 (1976) 1–10.
Patnaik AK, Liu S-K: Angiosarcoma in cats. J Small Anim Pract 18 (1977) 191–198.
Pearson GR, Hart CA: A case of otitis in a domestic cat. J Small Anim Pract 21 (1980) 333–338.
Peiffer RL: Feline ophthalmology. *In* Gelatt KN: Veterinary Ophthalmology. Philadelphia, Lea & Febiger, 1981.
Peiffer RL, Seymour WG, Williams LW: Malignant melanoma of the iris and ciliary body in a cat. Mod Vet Pract 58 (1977) 853–856.
Pelagatti V: Su di un tumore primitivo maligno del fegato nel gatto. Nuova Vet 7 (1929) 328–330.
Pentlarge VW: Peripheral vestibular disease in a cat with middle and inner ear squamous cell carcinoma. Compend Contin Ed 6 (1984) 731–733, 736.
Perlstein Z: Zur Pathologie der Gliome bei Haustieren. Dissertation, Zürich, 1956.
Peterson ME: Feline hyperthyroidism. Vet Clin North Am 14 (1984) 809–826.
Peterson ME, Becker DV: Radionuclide thyroid imaging in 135 cats with hyperthyroidism. Vet Radiol 25 (1984) 23–27.
Peterson ME, Kintzer PP, Cavanagh PG, Fox PR, Ferguson DC, Johnson GF, Becker DV: Feline hyperthyroidism: pretreatment clinical and laboratory evaluation of 131 cases. J Am Vet Med Assoc 183 (1983) 103–110.
Petit G: Myomes utérins chez une chatte. Bull Soc Anat (Paris) 77 (1902a) 390.
Petit G: Cancer parotidien du chat. Bull Soc Anat (Paris) 77 (1902b) 884–885; Bull Soc Centr Méd Vét 56 (1902b) 650.
Petit G: Sarcome de la vulve chez une chatte. Bull Soc Anat (Paris) 78 (1903) 288.
Petit G: Coexistence de plusieurs tumeurs chez le chat. [Adenomas of small intestine and bronchial adenomas]. Bull Soc Anat (Paris) 83 (1908) 86.
Petit G: Cancer de la mamelle propagé à la vulve et généralisé chez une chatte. Bull Soc Centr Méd Vét 68 (1914–15) 491–494.
Petit G, Germain R: Quelques cas intéressants de fibroadénomes, massifs ou kystiques, de la mamelle, chez les carnivores domestiques. Bull Assoc Fr Cancer 5 (1912) 104–109.
Petit G, Peyron A, Cocu J: Sur une tumeur ovarienne issue des cellules interstitielles chez une chatte. Bull Assoc Fr Cancer 15 (1926) 393–403.
Peyron A, Cocu T: Sur une petite tumeur wolfienne du testicule d'un chat de neuf mois. Bull Acad Vét Fr 91 (1938) 507–510.
Plummer PJG: A survey of six hundred and thirty six tumours from domesticated animals. Can J Comp Med 20 (1956) 239–251.
Ponomarkov V, Mackey LJ: Tumours of the liver and biliary system. Bull WHO 53 (1976) 187–194.
Pool RR: Tumors of bone and cartilage. *In* Moulton JE (ed): Tumors in Domestic Animals, 2nd ed. Berkeley, University of California Press, 1978.
Pool RR: Osteochondromatosis. *In* Bojrab MJ (ed): Pathophysiology in Small Animal Surgery. Philadelphia, Lea & Febiger, 1981, 641–649.
Pool RR, Bodle JE, Mantos JJ, Ticer JW: Primary lung carcinoma with skeletal metastases in the cat. Feline Pract 4 (4) (1974) 36–41.
Pool RR, Carrig CB: Multiple cartilaginous exostoses in a cat. Vet Pathol 9 (1972) 350–359.
Pool RR, Harris JM: Feline osteochondromatosis. Feline Pract 5 (2) (1975) 24–30.
Popp JA, Simpson CF: Feline malignant giant cell tumor of bone associated with C-type virus particles. Cornell Vet 66 (1976) 527–534.
Poppensiek GC: Neoplasms Studied in Selected Veterinary Diagnostic Laboratories. Ithaca, NY, Cornell University, 1961 (unpublished survey).
Popper H, Thomas LB, Telles NC, Falk H, Selikoff IJ: Development of hepatic angiosarcoma in man induced by vinyl chloride, thorotrast, and arsenic. Comparison with cases of unknown etiology. Am J Pathol 92 (1978) 349–376.
Pospischil A, Dahme E: Neuroepitheliale (aesthesioneurogene) Tumoren der Riechschleimhaut bei der Katze. Zentralbl Veterinärmed A28 (1981) 214–225.
Potkay S, Garman R: Nephroblastoma in a cat: The effects of nephrectomy and occlusion of the caudal vena cava. J Small Anim Pract 10 (1969) 345–349.
Preiser H: Endometrial adenocarcinoma in a cat. Pathol Vet 1 (1964) 485–490.
Price EW, Dikmans G: Adenomatous tumors in the large intestine of cats caused by *Strongyloides tumefaciens*. Proc Helminth Soc Wash 8 (1941) 41–50.
Price JM, Wear JB, Brown RR, Satter EJ, Olson C: Studies on etiology of carcinoma of urinary bladder. J Urol 83 (1960) 376–382.
Priester WA: Pancreatic islet cell tumors in domestic animals. Data from 11 colleges of veterinary medicine in the United States and Canada. J Natl Cancer Inst 53 (1974) 227–229.
Priester WA, Mantel N: Occurrence of tumors in domestic animals. Data from 12 United States and Canadian colleges

of veterinary medicine. J Natl Cancer Inst 47 (1971) 1333–1344.
Priester WA, McKay FW: The Occurrence of Tumors in Domestic Animals. Natl Cancer Inst Monogr 54, 1980.
Purohit BL, Sardeshpande PD, Joshi KV: Renal carcinoma in a cat. Indian Vet J 41 (1964) 796–798.
Purohit BL, Sardeshpande PD: Canine pulmonary neoplasms. Indian Vet J 44 (1967) 558–563.
Quarante M: Lympho-epithéliome de l'amygdale d'un chat. Bull Acad Vét Fr NS 11 (1938) 474–475.
Quigley PJ, Leedale A: Carcinoma of mandible of cat and dog simulating osteosarcoma. J Comp Pathol 82 (1972) 15–18.
Quigley PJ, Leedale AH: Tumors involving bone in the domestic cat: A review of fifty-eight cases. Vet Pathol 20 (1983) 670–686.
Raflo CP, Nuernberger SP: Abdominal mesothelioma in a cat. Vet Pathol 15 (1978) 781–783.
Rebar AH, Hahn FF, Halliwell WH, DeNicola DB, Benjamin SA: Microangiopathic hemolytic anemia associated with radiation-induced hemangiosarcomas. Vet Pathol 17 (1980) 443–454.
Reid JS, Frank RJ: Liver cyst in a cat (a case report). Vet Med Small Anim Clin 68 (1973) 1127–1130.
Rendano VT, de Lahunta A, King JM: Extracranial neoplasia with facial nerve paralysis in two cats. J Am Anim Hosp Assoc 10 (1980) 921–925.
Richard [no init]: Fibromyome kystique de la corne utérine gauche chez une chatte. Bull Soc Centr Méd Vét 64 (1910) 163.
Richards CD: Hypertrophic osteoarthropathy in a cat [with benign thymoma]. Feline Pract 7 (2) (1977) 41–43.
Rickard CG, Post JE, Noronha F, Barr LM: A transmissible virus–induced lymphocytic leukemia of the cat. J Natl Cancer Inst 42 (1969) 987–1014.
Riddle WE Jr, Leighton RL: Osteochondromatosis in a cat. J Am Vet Med Assoc 156 (1970) 1428–1430.
Robbins SL, Cotran RS: Pathologic Basis of Disease, 2nd ed. Philadelphia, WB Saunders Company, 1979.
Robbins SL, Cotran RS, Kumar V: Pathologic Basis of Disease, 3rd ed. Philadelphia, WB Saunders Company, 1984.
Roberg J: Hypertrophic pulmonary osteoarthropathy. Feline Pract 7 (6) (1977) 18, 20–22.
Roberts PL, McDonald HB, Wells RF: Systemic mast cell disease in a patient with unusual gastrointestinal and pulmonary abnormalities. Am J Med 45 (1968) 638–642.
Rocklin RE: Modulation of cellular-immune responses in vivo and in vitro by histamine receptor–bearing lymphocytes. J Clin Invest 57 (1976) 1051–1058.
Roncati G: Hyperplasia mammaria di tipo virginale in una gatta. Zooprofilassi 2 (1947) 357–362.
Root CR, Lord PF: Peritoneal carcinomatosis in the dog and cat: its radiographic appearance. J Am Vet Radiol Soc 12 (1971) 54–59.
Roperto F, Damiano S, Galati P: Hodgkin's disease in a cat. Zentralbl Veterinärmed A 30 (1983) 182–188.
Rowlatt U: Spontaneous epithelial tumours of the pancreas of mammals. Br J Cancer 21 (1967) 82–107.
Roy P: Le Cancer de l'Oesophage chez les Animaux Domestiques. Thesis, Lyon, 1938 (cited by C. Lombard, 1940, op. cit.)
Rubarth S: Några fall av primära mag- och tarmkarcinom hos husdjuren. Skand Vet Tidskr 24 (1934) 685–706.
Ruben JMS: Neurofibrosarcoma in a 19-year-old cat. Vet Rec 113 (1983) 135.
Russell DF, Rubinstein LJ: Pathology of Tumours of the Nervous System, 3rd ed. London, Edward Arnold, 1971.
Ryan CP, Walder EJ: Feline fibrosarcoma of the heart. Calif Vet 34 (8) (1980) 12–14.
Saar C, Opitz M, Lange W, Hirchert R, Burow H, Grund S, Loppnow H: Mastzellenretikulose bei Katzen. Berl Münch Tierärztl Wochenschr 82 (1969) 438–444.
Saar C, Saar U, Opitz M, Burow H, Teichert G: Paraproteinämische Retikulosen bei der Katze (Bericht über je einen Fall von Plasmazellenretikulose und Makroglobulinämie). Berl Münch Tierärzt Wochenschr 86 (1973) 11–15, 21–24.
Samso A, Catanei J: Le cancer de l'intestin chez les animaux domestiques. Bull Algér Carcinol 5 (1952) 403–414.
Sander CH, Langham RF: Myelolipoma of the spleen in a cat. J Am Vet Med Assoc 160 (1972) 1101–1103.
Santos JA dos, Lopes MA daF, Schott AC, Santos AE dos, Porfirio LC, Passos L: [Cholangiocellular carcinoma with biliary parasitism by *Platynosomum fastosum*]. Pesquisa Veterinaria Brasileira 1 (1) (1981) 31–36. (Abstr Vet Bull 51 [1981] 5123.)
Sarma PS, Baskar JF, Gilden RV, Gardner MB, Huebner RJ: "In vitro" isolation and characterization of the GA strain of feline sarcoma virus. Proc Soc Exp Biol Med 137 (1971a) 1333–1336.
Sarma PS, Log T, Theilen GH: ST feline sarcoma virus. Biological characteristics and in vitro propagation. Proc Soc Exp Biol Med 137 (1971b) 1444–1448.
Sarma PS, Sharar AL, McDonough S: The SM strain of feline sarcoma virus. Biologic and antigenic characterization of virus. Proc Soc Exp Biol Med 140 (1972) 1365–1368.
Sbernardori U, Nava A: Disgerminoma dell' ovaio nella gatta. Clin Vet 91 (1968) 733–736.
Scavelli TD, Patnaik AE, Mehlhaff CJ, Hayes AA: Hemangiosarcoma in the cat: Retrospective evaluation of 31 surgical cases. J Am Vet Med Assoc 187 (1985) 817–819.
Schaer M, Zaki F, Harvey HJ, O'Reilly WH: Laryngeal hemiplegia due to neoplasia of the vagus nerve in a cat. J Am Vet Med Assoc 174 (1971) 513–515.
Schappert HR, Geib LW: Reticuloendothelial neoplasms involving the spinal canal of cats. J Am Vet Med Assoc 150 (1967) 753–757.
Scherzo CS: Cystic liver and persistent urachus in a cat. J Am Vet Med Assoc 151 (1967) 1329–1330.
Schiefer B, Dahme E: Primäre Geschwülste des ZNS bei Tieren. Acta Neuropathol 2 (1962) 202–212.
Schiffer SP, Hitchcock P, Irwin PF: Primary cavitating pulmonary adenocarcinoma in a cat. J Am Vet Med Assoc 183 (1983) 112–114.
Schindelka H: Lymphangiome bei einer Katze. Österr Zeitschr Veterinärkd 4 (1892) 139–143.
Schlumberger HG: Comparative pathology of oral neoplasms. Oral Surg 6 (1953) 1078–1094.
Schmidt RE, Langham RF: A survey of feline neoplasms. J Am Vet Med Assoc 151 (1967) 1325–1328.
Schneck GW: A case of giant cell epulis (osteoclastoma) in a cat. Vet Rec 97 (1975) 181–182.
Schneider PR, Smith CW, Feller DL: Histiocytic lymphosarcoma of the trachea in a cat. J Am Anim Hosp Assoc 15 (1979) 485–487.
Schönbauer M: Die Bedeutung von Mikroverkalkungen im Komedokarzinom bei Hund und Katze. Zentralbl Veterinärmed A 30 (1983) 313–323.
Schwarz PD, Greene RW, Patnaik AK: Urinary bladder tumors in the cat: A review of 27 cases. J Am Anim Hosp Assoc 21 (1985) 237–245.
Scott DW: Feline dermatology 1900–1978: a monograph. J Am Anim Hosp Assoc 16 (1980) 331–459.
Scott DW: Feline dermatology 1979–1982: Introspective retrospections. J Am Anim Hosp Assoc 20 (1984) 537–563.
Scott E, Moore RA: A case of pancreatic carcinoma in a cat. J Cancer Res 11 (1927) 152–157.
Seawright AA, Grono LR: Malignant mast cell tumour in a cat with perforating duodenal ulcer. J Pathol Bacteriol 87 (1964) 107–111.
Sedlmeier H, Weiss E: Zur Beurteilung der Hauttumoren von Hund und Katze. Berl Münch Tierärztl Wochenschr 76 (1963) 181–185.
Seiler RJ, Wilkinson GT: Malignant fibrous histiocytoma involving the ilium in a cat. Vet Pathol 17 (1980) 513–517.

Sellyei M, Szonyi I: [Tumor inhibition and mast cell reaction.] Magy Onkol 8 (1964) 193–199.
Selye H: The Mast Cells. Washington, DC, Butterworth, Inc, 1965.
Shadduck JA, Albert DM, Neiderkorn JY: Feline uveal melanomas induced with feline sarcoma virus: potential model of the human counterpart. J Natl Cancer Inst 67 (1981) 619–627.
Shell L, Colter SB, Blass CE, Ingram JT: Surgical removal of a meningioma in a cat after detection by computerized axial tomography. J Am Anim Hosp Assoc 21 (1985) 439–442.
Shields RP, Gaskin JM: Fatal generalized feline viral rhinotracheitis in a young adult cat. J Am Vet Med Assoc 170 (1977) 439–441.
Silver IA: Symposium on mammary neoplasia in the dog and cat—I The anatomy of the mammary gland of the dog and cat. J Small Anim Pract 7 (1966) 689–696.
Silver IA: Use of radiotherapy for the treatment of malignant neoplasms. J Small Anim Pract 13 (1972) 351–358.
Sinibaldi KR, Pugh J, Rosen H, Liu S-K: Osteomyelitis and neoplasia associated with the use of the Jonas intramedullary splint in small animals. J Am Vet Med Assoc 181 (1982) 885–890.
Skelley JF, McGrath JT, Mark JH: Some nervous disorders in cats with clinico-pathological studies. Univ Pa Vet Ext Q 131 (1953) 84–88.
Slatter DH: Bronchogenic carcinoma in the cat. Feline Pract 2 (5) (1972) 32–34.
Small E: Diseases of the central nervous system. *In* Catcott EJ (ed): Feline Medicine and Surgery, 1st ed. Santa Barbara, American Veterinary Publications Inc, 1964, 303–314.
Smith HA, Jones TC: Veterinary Pathology, 3rd ed. Philadelphia, Lea & Febiger, 1966.
Snyder SP, Theilen GH: Transmissible feline fibrosarcoma. Nature 221 (1969) 1074–1075.
Soter NA, Austen KF, Wasserman SI: Oral disodium cromoglycate in the treatment of systemic mastocytosis. N Engl J Med 301 (1979) 465–469.
Spjut HJ, Dorfman HD, Fechner RE, Ackerman LV: Atlas of Tumor Pathology: Tumors of Bone and Cartilage. Washington, DC, Armed Forces Institute of Pathology, 1971.
Stannard AA, Pulley LT: Tumors of the skin and soft tissues. *In* Moulton JE (ed): Tumors in Domestic Animals, 2nd ed. Berkeley, University of California Press, 1978.
Stanton ME, Wheaton LG, Render JA, Blevins WE: Pharyngeal polyps in two feline siblings. J Am Vet Med Assoc 186 (1985) 1311–1313.
Steensland HS: Neuroma embryonale of the choroid plexus of the cat. J Exp Med 8 (1906) 120–126.
Stein BS: The genital system. *In* Catcott EJ (ed): Feline Medicine and Surgery, 2nd ed. Santa Barbara, American Veterinary Publications, Inc, 1975.
Stephens LC, King GK, Jardine JH: Attempted transmission of a feline virus–associated liposarcoma to newborn kittens. Vet Pathol 21 (1984) 614–616.
Stephens LC, Tsai CC, Raulston GL, Jardine JH, MacKenzie WF: Virus-associated liposarcoma and malignant lymphoma in a kitten. J Am Vet Med Assoc 183 (1983) 123–125.
Stewart HL: Pulmonary cancer and adenomatosis in captive wild mammals and birds from the Philadelphia Zoo. J Natl Cancer Inst 36 (1966) 117–138.
Sticker A: Ueber den Krebs der Tiere. Arch Klin Chir 65 (1901) 616–696; Dtsch Tierärztl Wochenschr 9 (1901) 401–423, 433–436.
Stookey JL, Dill GS Jr, Whitney GD: Ceruminal gland neoplasia in the cat. J Am Med Vet Assoc 159 (1971) 326.
Stout AP, Lattes R: Atlas of Tumor Pathology: Tumors of the Soft Tissues. Washington, DC, Armed Forces Institute of Pathology, 1967.
Stowater JL: Intestinal adenocarcinoma in a cat. Vet Med Small Anim Clin 73 (1978) 475–477.
Stünzi H: Zur pathologischen Anatomie der Mastzell-Leukämie der Katze. Monatsh Veterinärmed 11 (1956) 716–718.
Stünzi H: Zur Pathologie des Lungenkarzinoms der Katze. Zentralbl Veterinärmed 5 (1958) 665–674.
Stünzi H: The histopathology of feline lung cancer. *In* Severi L (ed): Lung Tumours in Animals. Proceedings of Third Quadrennial Conference on Cancer, Division of Cancer Research, University of Perugia, Italy, 1966, 181–188.
Stünzi H: Krebsstatistik bei Katzen. Schweiz Arch Tierheilk 109 (1967) 1–8.
Stünzi H: Das epidermoïde Karzinom der Bronchialdrüsen bei Hund und Katze. Vet Pathol 13 (1976) 277–285.
Stünzi H, Head KW, Nielsen SW: Tumours of the lung. Bull WHO 50 (1974) 9–19.
Stünzi H, Höfliger H: Das Adenom der Bronchaldrüsen beim Haustier. Schweiz Arch Tierheilk 117 (1975) 599–604.
Stünzi H, Suter P: Zur Pathologie der Pancreaskrebse bei Carnivoren. Monatsh Veterinärmed 13 (1958) 251–256.
Swaim SF, Shields RP: Paraplegia in the cat: Etiology and differential diagnosis. Vet Med Small Anim Clin 60 (1971) 787–792, 797–798.
Swift GA, Brown RH: Surgical treatment of Cushing's syndrome in the cat. Vet Rec 99 (1976) 374–375.
Syvrud R: Rhabdomyoma in the cat. Western Vet 6 (1959) 49–50.
Takakura K, Yamada H, Hollander VP: Mast cell stimulating factor in glycoprotein pituitary hormones and the inhibitory role of mast cells on plasma cell tumorigenesis. Fed Proc 25 (1966) 283.
Tamaschke C: Beiträge zur vergleichenden Onkologie der Haussäugetiere. Wissensch Z Humboldt-Univ Berlin 1 (1951/52) 37–70.
Taylor PF, Kater JC: Adenocarcinoma of the intestine of the dog and cat. Aust Vet J 30 (1954) 377–379.
Tepper JM: What is your diagnosis? [Metastatic fibrosarcoma of lumbar vertebra]. J Am Vet Med Assoc 177 (1980) 1155–1156.
Theilen GH, Madewell BR (eds): Veterinary Cancer Medicine. Philadelphia, Lea & Febiger, 1979.
Thirot T: Le cancer du testicule chez les animaux domestiques. Thesis, Lyon, 1937.
Thoday KL, Evans JG: Letter to the editor. J Small Anim Pract 13 (1972) 399–401.
Thoonen J, Hoorens J: Spontaan carcinoma in de urinblass bij een kat. Vlaams Diergeneeskd Tijdschr 29 (1960) 147–149.
Thoonen J, Hoorens J: Multiple Polypen im Endometrium einer Katze. Vlaams Diergeneeskd Tijdschr 30 (1961) 53–55.
Thornburg LP: Giant cell tumor of bone in a cat. Vet Pathol 16 (1979) 255–257.
Thrall MA: Lymphoproliferative disorders: lymphocytic leukemia and plasma cell myeloma. Vet Clin North Am 11 (1981) 321–347.
Tilley LP, Bond B, Patnaik AK, Liu S-K: Cardiovascular tumors in the cat. J Am Anim Hosp Assoc 17 (1981) 1009–1021.
Tilley LP, Owens JM, Wilkins RJ, Patnaik AK: Pericardial mesothelioma with effusion in a cat. J Am Anim Hosp Assoc 11 (1975) 60–65.
Tivollier A: Le cancer des lèvres et le cancer de la langue chez les animaux domestiques. Thesis, Lyon, 1936.
Totire-Ippoliti P: Leiomioma dell' intestino. Archivio Scienze Mediche 49 (1927) 468–471.
Troy MA: Bronchogenic carcinoma in the cat. J Am Vet Med Assoc 126 (1955) 410–411.
Turk MAM, Gallina AM, Russell TS: Nonhematopoietic gastrointestinal neoplasia in cats: a retrospective study of 44 cases. Vet Pathol 18 (1981) 614–620.
Turrel JM: Primary bone tumors in the cat. Master's thesis, Texas A & M University, 1979.
Turrel JM, Pool RR: Primary bone tumors in the cat: A retrospective study of 15 cats and a literature review. Vet Radiol 23 (1982) 152–166.

Turrel JM, Feldman EC, Hays M, Hornof WJ: Radiographic iodine therapy in cats with hyperthyroidism. J Am Vet Med Assoc 184 (1984) 554–559.

Überreiter O: Die Tumoren der Mamma bei Hund und Katze. Wien Tierärztl Monatsschr 55 (1968) 481–503.

Valli VE, McSherry BJ, Dunham BM, Jacobs RM, Lumsden JH: Histocytology of lymphoid tumors in the dog, cat, and cow. Vet Pathol 18 (1981) 495–512.

Vasseur PB, Patnaik AK: Laryngeal adenocarcinoma in a cat. J Am Anim Hosp Assoc 17 (1981) 639–641.

Veith LA: Squamous cell carcinoma of the trachea in a cat. Feline Pract 4 (1) (1974) 30–32.

Verardini G: Contributo allo studio anatomo-patologico dei tumori nel gatto [Adenocarcinoma of the ovary]. Nuova Vet 13 (1935) 225–233.

Verlinde JD, Ojemann JG: Eenige aangeboren misvormigen van het centrale zenuwstelsel. Tijdschr Diergeneeskd 7 (1946) 557–562.

Vernon FF, Roudebush P: Primary esophageal carcinoma in a cat. J Am Anim Hosp Assoc 16 (1980) 547–550.

Vincent GM: Carcinoma of the oesophagus in a cat. Vet Rec 25 (1927) 559.

Vlaovitch M: Le Cancer des Capsules Surrénales chez les Animaux. Thesis, Lyon, 1932 (cited by Lombard, 1940).

Waggener JD: Ultrastructure of benign peripheral nerve sheath tumors. Cancer 19 (1966) 699–709.

Waller T, Rubarth S: Haemangioendothelioma in domestic animals. Acta Vet Scand 8 (1967) 234–261.

Walsh KM, Abbott DP: Lymphangiosarcoma in two cats. J Comp Pathol 94 (1984) 611–614.

Walton DK, Scott DW, Berg RJ: Cutaneous lymphangiosarcoma in a cat. Feline Pract 13 (5) (1983) 21–26.

Walzl H, Hunyady G: Ein Fall von multipler adenomatöser Bronchialdrüsenhyperplasie bei der Katze. Berl Münch Tierärztl Wochenschr 80 (1967) 271–273.

Ward JM, Hurvitz AI: Ultrastructure of normal and neoplastic mast cells of the cat. Vet Pathol 9 (1972) 202–211.

Warren HB, Carpenter JL: Fibrodysplasia ossificans in three cats. Vet Pathol 21 (1984) 495–499.

Weege J: Cholangiosarcoma in a cat. Vet Med Small Anim Clin 66 (1971) 1024.

Weijer K: Feline mammary tumours and dysplasia. Thesis. Oosthuizen, Drukkerij Van der Molen, 1979.

Weijer K, Hart AAM: Prognostic factors in feline mammary carcinoma. J Natl Cancer Inst 70 (1983) 709–716.

Weijer K, Head KW, Misdorp W, Hampe JF: Feline malignant mammary tumors. I. Morphology and biology: Some comparisons with human and canine mammary carcinomas. J Natl Cancer Inst 49 (1972) 1697–1704.

Weiss E: Tumours of the soft (mesenchymal) tissues. Bull WHO 50 (1974) 101–110.

Weiss E, Frese K: Tumours of the skin. Bull WHO 50 (1974) 79–100.

Weissman S, Pulley LT: Perianal gland adenocarcinoma. Feline Pract 4 (3) (1974) 25.

Weller RE: Systemic mastocytosis and mastocytemia in a cat. Mod Vet Pract 59 (1978) 41–43.

Weller RE, Hornof WJ: Gastric malignant lymphoma in two cats. Mod Vet Pract 60 (1979) 701–704.

Wells GAH, Robinson M: Mixed tumour of salivary gland showing histological evidence of malignancy in a cat. J Comp Pathol 85 (1975) 77–85.

Werner LL: Immunologic diseases affecting internal organ systems. *In* Ettinger SJ (ed): Textbook of Veterinary Internal Medicine, 2nd ed. Philadelphia, WB Saunders Company, 1983.

Wheeldon EB, Amis TC: Laryngeal carcinoma in a cat. J Am Vet Med Assoc 186 (1985) 80–81.

White SD, Carpenter JL, Rappaport J, Swartout M: Cutaneous metastases of a mammary adenocarcinoma resembling eosinophilic plaques in a cat. Feline Pract 15 (3) (1985) 27–29.

Whitehead JE: Neoplasia in the cat. Vet Med Small Anim Clin 62 (1967) 44–45, 357–358.

Wilkinson GT: Diseases of the Cat. Oxford, Pergamon Press, 1966.

Wilkinson GT: Lymphosarcoma of the heart of a cat. Vet Rec 80 (1967) 381–382.

Wilkinson GT: Some preliminary clinical observations on the malabsorption syndrome in the cat. J Small Anim Pract 10 (1969) 87–94.

Wilkinson GT: Chronic papillomatous oesophagitis in a young cat. Vet Rec 87 (1970) 355–356.

Wilkinson GT (ed): Diseases of the Cat and Their Management. Melbourne, Blackwell Scientific Publications, 1983.

Willard MD, Tvedten H, Walshaw R, Aronson E: Thymoma in a cat. J Am Vet Med Assoc 176 (1980) 451–453.

Williams R, Veralli P, Schwarz D: Personal communication, 1982.

Wilson JW: Reticulum cell sarcoma of long bones terminating as respiratory distress. Vet Med 68 (1973) 1383–1401.

Wimberly HC, Lewis RM: Transitional cell carcinoma in the domestic cat. Vet Pathol 16 (1979) 223–228.

Withrow SJ, Greene RW: What is your diagnosis? [Intussusception of the colon associated with adenocarcinoma of the cecum]. J Am Vet Med Assoc 166 (1975) 1113–1114.

Withrow SJ, Holmberg DL: Mandibulectomy in the treatment of oral cancer. J Am Anim Hosp Assoc 19 (1983) 273–286.

Witt C: What's your diagnosis? [Primary hemangiosarcoma of the humerus]. J Am Vet Med Assoc 185 (1984) 451–452.

Wolke RE: Vaginal leiomyoma as a cause of chronic constipation in the cat. J Am Vet Med Assoc 143 (1963) 1103–1105.

Wood DA: Atlas of Tumor Pathology: Tumors of the Intestines. Washington, DC, Armed Forces Institute of Pathology, 1967.

Woodruff R: Treatment of multiple myeloma. Cancer Treat Rev 8 (1981) 225–270.

Wooldridge GH: Carcinoma of the oesophagus of a cat. Br Vet J 69 NS 20 (1913) 38–39.

Wright R, Alberti KG, Karrin S, Millward-Sadler GH: Liver and Biliary Disease. Philadelphia, WB Saunders Company, 1979.

Young PL: Squamous cell carcinoma of the tongue of the cat. Aust Vet J 54 (1978) 133–134.

Zaki F, Harris J, Budzilovich G: Cystic pituicytoma of the neurohypophysis in a Siamese cat. J Comp Pathol 85 (1975) 467–471.

Zaki FA, Hurvitz AI: Spontaneous neoplasms of the central nervous system of the cat. J Small Anim Pract 17 (1976) 773–782.

Zaki FA, Liu S-K: Pituitary chromophobe adenoma in a cat. Vet Pathol 10 (1973) 232–237.

Zettler [no init]: Inaug.-Diss. Leipzig, 1916, cited by Joest E: Handbuch der Speziellen Pathologischen Anatomie der Haustiere, vol. 3. Berlin, Richard Schoetz, 1954, 157.

Zietzschmann H: Ein Fall von Fibroadenom pericanaliculare im Euter der Katze. Bericht über das Veterinärwesen im Königreich Sachsen 46 (1901) 198–200.

# 12
CHAPTER

# MANAGEMENT OF FELINE NEOPLASMS

## SURGERY, IMMUNOTHERAPY, AND CHEMOTHERAPY

E. GREGORY MacEWEN, SAMANTHA MOONEY, NANCY O. BROWN, and AUDREY A. HAYES

Cancer is one of the most difficult diseases that veterinarians deal with. Veterinarians must be knowledgeable about the biologic behavior and prognosis of a tumor, the treatments currently available, and the effectiveness and complexities of the treatment for the particular animal being managed. Many practitioners refer their patients to oncology specialists. Because of the limited availability of veterinary oncologists, however, and because of financial or logistic reasons, practicing veterinarians must often manage the case themselves. This chapter presents current information on the most effective approach to treatment of the neoplastic diseases commonly diagnosed in the cat. Much of this information is based on studies and philosophies developed at the Donaldson-Atwood Cancer Clinic of The Animal Medical Center, New York City.

### CLINICAL EVALUATION

Before any therapeutic intervention, a thorough clinical evaluation is essential to determine the extent of disease and the presence of any concurrent medical problems or associated diseases. A complete history including the duration of clinical signs and rate of tumor growth is an important aid in establishing a prognosis and the most effective therapeutic approach.

A thorough physical examination must be performed, with particular attention to regional lymph nodes and other possible sites of metastasis. The thoracic cavity and the area affected by the tumor should be radiographed. Hematologic and biochemical profiles give further information on the cat's condition and the extent of the disease and provide guidance in the choice of therapeutic measures.

The history and physical examination are important to identify concurrent medical problems or associated paraneoplastic problems. Paraneoplastic disease syndromes are defined as disease conditions or clinical signs associated with products secreted or released from the tumor, or conditions that result secondary to the primary tumor (Creech, 1976) (Table 12–1).

**Table 12–1 Paraneoplastic Disease Syndromes**

| | |
|---|---|
| Hypoglycemia | Insulinomas<br>Liver tumors |
| Hypocalcemia | Medullary (C-cell) thyroid tumors |
| Hypercalcemia | Lymphosarcoma<br>Parathyroid tumors<br>Metastatic bone tumors<br>Myeloma |
| Hyperthyroidism (Thyrotoxicosis) | Thyroid tumors |
| Monoclonal gammopathies<br>Bleeding disorders<br>Hyperviscosity syndrome | Myeloma<br>Macroglobulinemia |
| Polycythemia | Renal adenocarcinoma |
| Anemia | Any neoplastic disease<br>Feline leukemia virus<br>Bone marrow infiltration |
| Hyperadrenocorticism | Adrenal tumors |
| Diabetes mellitus | Chondrosarcoma |
| Hyperestrogenism | Ovarian granulosa cell tumor |

## METASTASIS

The spread of tumor to distant organs involves a sequence of events. Tumor cells invade surrounding tissue and lymph vessels. Tumor cell emboli are released into the circulation and are subsequently trapped in the capillary beds of distant organs, where they penetrate capillary walls, infiltrate adjacent tissue, and multiply (Hart and Fidler, 1980). The most frequent distant sites of metastatic disease are the lungs and liver.

The host's immune response is an important factor that influences the spread of tumor cells. Inhibition of T-cell responses has been demonstrated after surgery (Bruce, 1972; Espanol et al., 1974; Lecky, 1975). Furthermore, continued depression of immune function often correlates with the appearance of metastatic foci (Brodey, 1979; Harvey, 1976). The tumor-host relationship is affected by many factors including tumor volume, concurrent disease, anesthesia, physical trauma, sex, hormone levels, genetic predisposition, cytotoxic agents, and anticoagulants.

## CLINICAL STAGING

The present system for clinically staging both solid and hematopoietic tumors was adopted by the World Health Organization and the Veterinary Cancer Society in 1978 and published in the World Health Organization TNM Classification of Tumours in Domestic Animals (Owen, 1981). The system for solid tumors is based on the TNM system currently used in human oncology. T stands for tumor and describes the tumor by size (diameter in centimeters), number (single or multiple), and invasiveness. N represents the regional lymph nodes and describes them as of normal size, enlarged, or histologically metastatic. M designates metastasis beyond the regional lymph nodes. Table 12–2 presents a representative staging system for oral tumors.

## PATHOLOGIC FINDINGS

Clinical evaluation, staging, and diagnosis depend on histologic examination of the tumor tissue. In most cases treatment is initiated on the basis of the histologic diagnosis. The reader is referred to the chapter on tumor pathology for details on particular tumors occurring in the cat.

## TREATMENT

Treatment of cancer involves a multidisciplinary approach. Although surgery remains the primary treatment for most types of cancer, the adjunctive use of immunotherapy, chemotherapy, and radiation has recently increased. In general, multi-modality therapy is the most effective approach.

## SURGERY

Surgery may be diagnostic, curative, palliative, preventive, or adjunctive (Brodey, 1979; Holland and Frei, 1973; Nealon and Russo, 1977) (Table 12–3). Surgical procedures include scalpel excision, cryosurgery, and electrosurgery. Scalpel excision is used most often. Cryosurgery is useful in areas where scalpel excision is limited (i.e., the oral and nasal cavities and the extremities). Electrosurgery combines the advantage of hemostasis with controlled dissection. The oncologic surgeon should be skilled in all these methods.

Several principles are applicable to the oncologic surgeon (Harvey, 1976; Holland and Frei, 1973; Nealon and Russo, 1977). First, perform excisional rather than incisional biopsies. Second, avoid local anesthesia, which distorts tissue planes and makes dissection difficult. Third, avoid manipulation of the tumor mass. It has been demonstrated in humans that showers of malignant cells occur in peripheral blood during manipulative procedures (Cole et al., 1961). Malignant cells have also been detected in wound washings after tumor excisions (Smith et al., 1958). The prognostic significance of this seeding is uncertain (Fisher et al., 1967). Fourth, make a wide and deep excision. Ideally there should be at least a 1 cm margin around the tumor with histologically confirmed clear margins. If necessary, allow the defect to heal as an open wound or use reconstructive surgery. Fifth, protect skin margins to prevent tumor cell seeding. Sixth, do an en-bloc dissection of regional nodes if possible. Seventh, ligate vessels early in the surgical procedure. Eighth, change gloves, drapes, and instruments frequently to avoid contaminating the surgical field with tumor cells. Ninth, examine all excised tissue histologically. If the results are doubtful, rebiopsy if possible for more definitive information.

Follow-up management involves the detection and clinical management of recurrence and metastasis. Both the tumor site and regional nodes should be examined periodically to detect and monitor the subsequent development of disease. A biopsy is indicated if tumor regrowth or metastasis is suspected. Radiography and laparoscopy are useful aids in staging disease, determining response to therapy, and planning changes in therapy (Johnson and Twedt, 1977).

Immunosuppressive effects of surgery have been much discussed (Eilber et al., 1975; Lecky, 1975; Park et al., 1971; Slade et al., 1975; Wagener et al., 1975, 1976). It is thought that tumor cell antigens elicit a specific antitumor reaction from the immune system and that this reaction may be suppressed by surgery (Old and Boyse, 1966). Some patients are started on immunotherapy preoperatively in an effort to augment the immune response and to counterbalance the immunosuppressive effect of surgery.

## IMMUNOTHERAPY

Immunotherapy or biologic response modifier therapy is an attempt to modulate or stimulate the patient's immune reactivity against the tumor. The following factors are thought to enhance the effectiveness of immunotherapy:

1. Minimal amount of tumor
2. A tumor that has specific immunogenic antigens
3. An immunologically responsive host
4. A tumor that is accessible to immune cells (lymphocytes and macrophages) or immune substances (antibodies and complement)

**Table 12–2 Clinical Stages (TNM) of Canine/Feline Tumors of the Oral Cavity (Buccal Cavity)**

Case number ................................ Name of owner ................................ Date.................
Cat/Dog .......... Age .................... Sex......... Breed......................... Body weight.......... lb
(1 kg = 2.2 lb) ....... kg

This classification applies to the anterior two thirds of the tongue, floor of mouth, buccal mucosa, the alveoli, and the hard palate.

The following are the minimum requirements for assessing the T, N, and M categories. (If these cannot be met the symbols TX, NX, and MX should be used.)

T categories: Clinical and surgical examination
N categories: Clinical and surgical examination
M categories: Clinical and surgical examination, radiography of thorax

**CIRCLE APPROPRIATE CATEGORY**

**T: Primary Tumor**

| | | |
|---|---|---|
| Tis | Preinvasive carcinoma (carcinoma in situ) | |
| T0 | No evidence of tumor | |
| T1 | Tumor $<$ 2 cm maximum diameter | |
| | T1a without bone invasion | T1b with bone invasion |
| T2 | Tumor 2 to 4 cm maximum diameter | |
| | T2a without bone invasion | T2b with bone invasion |
| T3 | Tumor $>$ 4 cm maximum diameter | |
| | T3a without bone invasion | T3b with bone invasion |

The symbol (m) added to the appropriate T category indicates multiple tumors.

**N: Regional Lymph Nodes (RLN)***

| | | |
|---|---|---|
| N0 | No evidence of RLN involvement | |
| N1 | Movable ipsilateral nodes | |
| | N1a Nodes not considered to contain growth** | N1b Nodes considered to contain growth** |
| N2 | Movable contralateral or bilateral nodes | |
| | N2a Nodes not considered to contain growth** | N2b Nodes considered to contain growth** |
| N3 | Fixed nodes | |

**M: Distant Metastasis**

| | |
|---|---|
| M0 | No evidence of distant metastasis |
| M1 | Distant metastasis (including distant nodes) detected—specify site(s).................................... |

**STAGE GROUPING**

| | T | N | M |
|---|---|---|---|
| I | T1 | N0, N1a, or N2a | M0 |
| II | T2 | N0, N1a, or N2a | M0 |
| III*** | T3 | N0, N1a, or N2a | M0 |
| | Any T | N1b | |
| IV | Any T | Any N2b or N3 | M0 |
| | Any T | Any N | M1 |

Comments: ..........................................................................................

*The RLN are the cervical, submandibular, and parotid nodes.
**(−) = histologically negative; (+) = histologically positive.
***Any bone involvement.

**Table 12–3 Oncologic Surgical Procedures**

| CATEGORY | TECHNIQUES/EXAMPLES | PURPOSE |
|---|---|---|
| Diagnostic | Biopsy, laparotomy, thoracotomy, laparoscopy, endoscopy | Determine histologic type and grade<br>Establish stage of disease |
| Curative | Local excision with clear margins, amputation, en bloc dissection (suspect tissue planes and lymphatics to regional lymph nodes) | Eliminate affected and suspicious sites of disease |
| Palliative | Reduce tumor burden | Prolong life<br>Prevent complications<br>Enhance patient immunocompetence and receptivity to other therapy |
| Preventive | Oophorohysterectomy | Remove a stimulus known to predispose to cancer development |
| Adjunctive | Perfusion, infusion, endocrine ablation, reconstruction, elimination of metastatic foci | Therapeutic |

Evidence of the importance of the immune system in cancer comes from a number of clinical and scientific observations. For example, individuals with primary immunodeficiency diseases have about 10,000 times the expected incidence of lymphoid tumors (Good et al., 1968). Furthermore, feline leukemia virus (FeLV)–infected cats have a high risk of developing lymphosarcoma (LSA) or leukemia (Hardy et al., 1976a). Persistently viremic cats are also immunosuppressed and are at a greater risk of developing various bacterial and viral infections (Cockerell et al., 1976; Cotter et al., 1975; Essex et al., 1975).

An important concept called immunologic surveillance is thought to explain the rare but well-documented spontaneous regression of certain neoplasms (Burnet, 1970). This concept is based on the fact that certain tumor cells produce tumor-specific or -associated antigens (TSA) on their surface. These antigens are not present on normal cells and can elicit immune reactivity resulting in tumor cell destruction. A tumor will develop if this surveillance system is somehow overwhelmed or if it fails because of an immunologic defect or because of a tumor escape mechanism (Hawrylko, 1978).

Studies with FeLV-inoculated cats and with cats naturally exposed to FeLV revealed that resistance to the development of lymphosarcoma was also related to an efficient humoral antibody response to the feline oncornavirus–associated cell membrane antigen (FOCMA) (Essex, 1980). The mechanism by which the immune response to FOCMA prevents the development of leukemia and lymphosarcoma appears to be complement-mediated antibody lysis (Grant et al., 1979). This is a prime example of natural immunosurveillance in the cat.

Biologic response modifiers are agents or therapeutic approaches that affect the host immune systems resulting either in a specific antitumor response or in the enhancement of a pre-existing immunologic reactivity. Biologic response modifiers can be grouped in the following categories (MacEwen, 1983):

1. Immunoaugmenting agents
2. Immunorestorative agents
3. Interferon inducers and interferon
4. Tumor-specific approaches

The immunoaugmenting agents include crude microbial adjuvants such as bacillus Calmette-Guérin (BCG), *Corynebacterium parvum*, and a Mixed Bacterial Vaccine (MBV) consisting of *Serratia marcescens* and *Streptococcus pyogenes*. These agents act by stimulating macrophage and reticuloendothelial function. Currently they must be considered experimental approaches for cancer therapy. MBV is being evaluated in our clinic for the treatment of cats with breast cancer after removal of their tumors. Other studies with BCG in cats with breast cancer are also being conducted (Jeglum, 1982).

Another important area of research regarding immunoaugmentation involves the selective removal of circulating immune complexes (blocking factors) from the blood of FeLV-infected cats with or without leukemia or LSA. Preliminary studies have yielded some interesting positive anti-tumor activity by *Staphylococcus aureus* Cowan I strain, which has protein A on its surface (Gordon et al., 1983; Jones et al., 1980; Terman et al., 1980). Protein A will selectively bind the Fc portion of the IgG immunoglobulin molecule, resulting in an absorption of IgG and a lowering of circulating immune complexes. Protein A also has mitogenic activity and is an interferon inducer in vitro. The removal of immune complexes results in enhanced immunologic reactivity and subsequent tumor necrosis (Gordon et al., 1983; Terman et al., 1980).

Immunorestorative approaches have been used in an effort to abrogate the immunosuppressive effects associated with cancer. Levamisole is one agent that has been studied in the cat. In addition to the anthelmintic properties of levamisole, studies have shown that it increases phagocytosis by polymorphonuclear cells and macrophages and normalizes T-cell function (Symoens and Rosenthal, 1977). We conducted a double-blind study using levamisole in cats with breast cancer. Sixty-four cats were clinically staged and randomized to receive levamisole or a placebo after undergoing radical mastectomy. There was no statistical difference between the two groups in recurrence rate or survival time (MacEwen et al., 1984a).

Another immunorestorative approach involves the infusion of plasma components (plasma, cryoprecipitate, and fibronectin) into cats with leukemia or LSA. Although this approach is still under investigation and not ready for clinical use, the results are encouraging (Hardy et al., 1976b; Hayes et al., 1980; Kassel et al., 1977).

Interferons are inducible secretory glycoproteins that have antiviral, immunoregulatory, and antiproliferative effects on tumor cells. Some preliminary studies using beta-type bovine interferon have shown some positive results in cats with FeLV-associated aplastic anemia (Tompkins and Cummins, 1982).

Tumor-specific treatments have centered on a fundamental concept of immunotherapy; that is, tumor cells possess associated antigens that can induce specific immune reactivity. Specific tumor cell vaccines are currently being studied as an adjuvant therapy to surgery in cats with breast cancer (Jeglum, 1982). Other studies using specific antibody therapy have shown that infusions of serum from cats with high levels of FOCMA antibody result in regression of disease in cats with leukemia or LSA (Hardy et al., 1980).

In one study of 15 cats treated with combination chemotherapy the cats were randomized to two groups. One group received no further therapy, and the other received anti-FOCMA antibody serum. Although the results were not conclusive, the anti-FOCMA–treated cats tended to maintain a longer remission (Cotter et al., 1980). Further studies are warranted using specific anti-tumor antibodies directed against distinct tumor antigens.

## CHEMOTHERAPY

Chemotherapy is the use of chemical agents that interfere with cellular proliferation or are tumoricidal by some mechanism. For the clinician the major problem with cancer chemotherapy is the lack of cellular selectivity. Many cancer cells have a high rate of proliferation, and consequently they are more susceptible to cytotoxic agents that interfere with certain critical components needed for cell growth and proliferation. Normal tissues, however, such as bone marrow and gastrointestinal epithelium, which also need the same critical components, are susceptible to the toxic effects of chemotherapy. Careful monitoring of the patient is necessary to prevent excessive toxicity to normal tissues.

The cell's response to drugs depends on the mechanism of action of the drug and the stage of cell growth in the cell's cycle. The cell cycle is divided into four phases. Mitosis (M) is the initiation of division. The postmitotic phase is termed $G_1$, and RNA and protein synthesis occur during this time, just before DNA synthesis (S). After the DNA content of the cell has doubled, the phase of DNA synthesis is complete, and the cell enters the $G_2$ phase. During this period RNA and protein synthesis proceed and the cell prepares for mitosis. Cells in the S phase are especially susceptible to drugs that prevent the formation of nucleotides or inhibit DNA repair. Anticancer drugs can be divided into six classes, according to their mechanism of action (Dowling et al., 1970):

*Alkylating agents* act by crosslinking cellular DNA, thus impeding its ability to act as a template for RNA synthesis.

*Antimetabolites* interfere with the biosynthesis of nucleic acids by substituting for normal metabolites and inhibiting normal enzymatic reactions.

*Antibiotics* are thought to bind nonspecifically to cellular DNA and inhibit transcription.

*Mitotic inhibitors* destroy the mitotic spindle of the cell and prevent further cell division.

*Hormones* are thought to act by interfering with cell membrane receptors that stimulate growth.

*Miscellaneous drugs* are those that do not act in any of the ways described above or whose mechanism or action is at present unknown.

Table 12–4 lists the chemotherapeutic agents available, recommended dosages for the cat, and major toxic side effects. The most common method of expressing drug dosages is by body weight (i.e., mg per kg). Because toxicity data are often available only for other species, however, and because the activity of most drugs depends on some physiologic process, drug doses for veterinary cancer patients are frequently expressed in terms of body surface area. A conversion table of weights to body surface area is available (Kirk, 1980).

Most chemotherapeutic drugs are toxic to all dividing cells, and the toxic side effects, if manifested, may limit the use of a single drug or combination of drugs. These side effects may be slight, such as mild alopecia, anorexia, vomiting, and diarrhea, and may necessitate only a temporary withholding of chemotherapy. Certain agents, usually given by the intravenous route, are very irritating and cause local reactions if they accidentally leak into the extravascular tissue. Severe pain, erythema, and ulceration of tissue occur. Great care should be taken, therefore, when administering vincristine, vinblastine, actinomycin D, and doxorubicin hydrochloride. If these drugs are accidentally given outside the vein, infiltration of the area with physiologic saline solution, xylocaine, and a corticosteroid will lessen the extent of tissue damage.

In general most of the anticancer drugs cause myelosuppression, but a few have unique toxic side effects. For

**Table 12–4 Specific Agents Used in Cancer**

| AGENT | PRINCIPAL ROUTE OF ADMINISTRATION | USUAL DOSE | MAJOR TOXIC EFFECTS |
|---|---|---|---|
| **Alkylating Agents** | | | |
| Cyclophosphamide (Cytoxan) | Oral<br>IV | 50 mg/m$^2$ daily<br>10 mg/kg weekly | Bone marrow depression<br>Cystitis (rare) |
| Chlorambucil (Leukeran) | Oral | 0.1–0.2 mg/kg daily | Bone marrow depression<br>Decreased appetite |
| Melphalan (Alkeran) | Oral | 0.05–0.1 mg/kg daily | Bone marrow depression |
| Busulfan (Myleran) | Oral | 0.1 mg/kg daily | Bone marrow depression |
| **Antimetabolites** | | | |
| Methotrexate | IV | 0.8 mg/kg weekly | Vomiting, diarrhea<br>Bone marrow depression |
| Cytosine arabinoside (Ara-C, Cytosar) | SQ<br>IV | 600 mg/m$^2$ or 30–50 mg/kg divided into 4 doses given every 12 hours for 2 days | Bone marrow depression |
| 5-Fluorouracil (5-FU) | | | CNS signs, death<br>*Do not use in cats* |
| **Antibiotics** | | | |
| Bleomycin (Blenoxane) | IV<br>SQ | 10 mg/m$^2$ daily × 4, then 10 mg/m$^2$ weekly to max dose 200 mg/m$^2$ | Pulmonary fibrosis |
| Doxorubicin (Adriamycin) | IV | 30 mg/m$^2$ q 3 to 5 weeks | Bone marrow depression<br>Cardiac toxicity at cumulative doses > 150 mg<br>Locally irritating |
| **Plant Alkaloids** | | | |
| Vincristine (Oncovin) | IV | 0.0125–0.025 mg/kg weekly<br>0.5–0.7 mg/m$^2$ weekly | Locally irritating |
| **Miscellaneous Agents** | | | |
| L-asparaginase | IP | 400 IU/kg weekly | Anaphylaxis |
| Hydroxyurea (Hydrea) | Oral | 40 mg/kg daily | Bone marrow depression |

example, cyclophosphamide can induce hemorrhagic cystitis. This complication is rare in cats, especially if they are receiving prednisone concurrently. Bizarre central nervous system reactions, shock, and death have resulted from the administration of 5-fluorouracil to cats (Harvey et al., 1977). In our opinion, this drug should not be given to cats. In general, however, cats tolerate most chemotherapeutic agents with minimal toxicity.

Combination chemotherapy protocols are designed to include drugs that act at different stages of the cell cycle. The design of these protocols is based on knowledge of the cell cycle and clinical observation that certain tumors are responsive to various drugs. More detailed discussions of chemotherapy in animals are available (Bostock and Owen, 1972; Hess, 1977; Hess et al., 1976; Owen, 1983; Theilen, 1975; Theilen and Madewell, 1979a,b). Specific protocols are presented when appropriate in the section on treatment of specific tumors.

**Table 12–5 Feline Lymphosarcoma Protocols**

**PROTOCOL A**

Week 1—Induction of remission:
- 0.025 mg/kg vincristine IV
- 400 IU/kg L-asparaginase IP
- 2 mg/kg prednisone daily, divided twice a day for 12 months, orally

Week 2—10 mg/kg cyclophosphamide IV
Week 3—0.025 mg/kg vincristine IV
Week 4—0.8 mg/kg methotrexate IV

**PROTOCOL B**
**(Renal Lymphosarcoma)**

Induction—2 cycles (8 weeks) Protocol A
Maintenance of remission:
1st drug —0.025 mg/kg vincristine IV
2nd drug —30 mg/kg or 600 mg/m$^2$ cytosine arabinoside SQ divided into 4 doses at 12-hour intervals over 48 hours
3rd drug —0.025 mg/kg vincristine IV
4th drug 0.8 mg/kg methotrexate IV

## RADIATION THERAPY

Radiation therapy is discussed later in this chapter.

## TREATMENT OF SPECIFIC TUMORS

From 69 per cent to 90 per cent of all neoplasms diagnosed in cats are malignant (Dorn et al., 1968; Engle and Brodey, 1969; Priester and McKay, 1980). Neoplasms originating from the hematopoietic tissues have been estimated to account for between 10 per cent (Cotchin, 1959) and 33 per cent (Dorn et al., 1968; Whitehead, 1967) of all feline tumors. Mammary gland tumors are the third most common cancer in female cats, accounting for 10 per cent of all neoplasms. Mast cell tumors and musculoskeletal tumors, although less frequent, will also be discussed.

At The Animal Medical Center in a one-year period, 455 surgical specimens from cats were submitted for histologic examination. Of these, 234 were malignant tumors.

### Lymphosarcoma

Lymphosarcoma constituted 18.5 per cent of the malignancies surgically diagnosed in a one-year period at The Animal Medical Center. The Donaldson-Atwood Cancer Clinic diagnoses and treats 35 to 50 cases of feline lymphosarcoma (excluding lymphocytic leukemias) yearly. A definitive diagnosis of lymphosarcoma in the cat is based on the following procedures:

1. A thorough physical examination
2. Radiographs of the thorax and abdomen
3. A complete blood count and differential white blood-cell count
4. A serum biochemistry profile
5. A feline leukemia virus test
6. A bone marrow aspiration

For cats suspected of having thymic lymphosarcoma, the final diagnosis is based on cytologic examination of an aspirate from the thymic mass or pleural effusion. It is important to differentiate thymic lymphosarcoma from thymomas (Carpenter and Holzworth, 1982). The diagnosis of alimentary lymphosarcoma (stomach, intestine, or mesenteric or ileocecal lymph nodes) is confirmed by laparotomy and histologic examination. Renal lymphosarcoma is diagnosed by percutaneous needle aspiration of the enlarged kidneys for cytologic evaluation.

Cats with a confirmed diagnosis of lymphosarcoma can be treated with a combination chemotherapy protocol (MacEwen et al., 1979; MacEwen et al., 1981) (Protocol A, Table 12–5) for eight weeks (two therapy cycles). After two therapy cycles, treatments are continued at 10-day intervals for two more cycles. Therapy is then continued biweekly for the next seven months. Affected cats are maintained on prednisone, 1 to 2 mg/kg daily for one year. After one year the treatment interval is extended to three weeks, and the prednisone dosage is decreased to 0.5 to 1 mg/kg daily. Therapy intervals are monthly after two years and every six weeks after three years.

The results of therapy are given in Table 12–6. Cats are judged to be in complete remission (CR) when no palpable and radiographic evidence of disease can be

**Table 12–6 Feline Lymphosarcoma: Response to Therapy**

| LYMPHOSARCOMA CLASSIFICATION | NO. CATS | % CASES FELINE LEUKEMIA (+) | (−) | % CASES RESPONDING TO THERAPY Total | CR | PR | SURVIVAL TIME RANGE |
|---|---|---|---|---|---|---|---|
| Thymic | 28 | 82 | 18 | 79 | 75 | 4 | 36 days—3½ years |
| Renal | 14 | 50 | 50 | 86 | 43 | 43 | 20 days—4 + years |
| Alimentary | 13 | 15 | 85 | 85 | 62 | 23 | 51 days—3¾ years |
| Miscellaneous | 8 | 25 | 75 | 100 | 37 | 63 | 40 days—1½ years |

found, that is, when the disease has regressed 90 to 100 per cent. Partial response (PR) indicates a >50 per cent reduction in tumor size. A complete blood count is performed at the time of treatment. Thoracic radiographs are repeated periodically to evaluate the response to therapy in cats with thymic lymphosarcoma.

Seventy-five per cent of the cats treated for thymic lymphosarcoma died of recurrence of progressive disease while receiving chemotherapy. Recurrence of the thymic tumor was accompanied, in 5 of 21 (24 per cent) of these cases, by development of lymphoblastic leukemia. The remaining 25 per cent of the cats treated died of FeLV-related disease or of other causes. Sixty to 70 per cent of the cats with alimentary lymphosarcoma died of progressive disease that became unresponsive to all chemotherapy agents. Eight cats (57 per cent) with renal lymphosarcoma died of the disease. Five cats died of FeLV-related or other causes. One cat was alive and free of disease four years after diagnosis.

Protocol B (Table 12–5) was devised to prevent central nervous system metastases in cats with renal lymphosarcoma. Three of the eight cats that died of renal lymphosarcoma had primary disease, unresponsive to therapy. The other five died of metastatic (CNS) disease diagnosed clinically and confirmed histologically at autopsy. With the incorporation of Protocol B in the treatment of renal lymphosarcoma, none of the remaining six cats developed central nervous system metastases.

The induction of remission is the same as given in Protocol A. If the patient is in remission at the end of the eight-week cycle, therapy is continued at 10-day intervals with Protocol B in the same sequence given for Protocol A.

Protocol A has also been used to treat the following forms of lymphosarcoma:

Ocular
Nasal
Peripheral nerve and spinal cord
Cutaneous
Generalized peripheral lymphadenopathy

The number of cases in each group is small, and the response to therapy varies greatly.

Protocols A and B use a mitotic inhibitor (vincristine), an alkylating agent (cyclophosphamide), an antimetabolite (methotrexate or cytosine arabinoside), an enzyme (L-asparaginase), and a corticosteroid (prednisone). The overall response rate is 92 per cent (69 per cent CR and 23 per cent PR). The median survival time for cats in remission (CR) was 210 days, whereas that for cats with a partial response (PR) was 80 days. All cats tolerated chemotherapy with minimal toxicity.

In another study of 38 cats with lymphosarcoma treated with cyclophosphamide, vincristine, and prednisone, 64 per cent achieved a complete remission, the median duration of which was five months; nine cats remained in remission for one year or longer (Cotter, 1983).

## MAMMARY TUMORS

Feline breast cancer represents about 12 per cent of all malignant tumors in the cat (Dorn et al., 1968). Eighty-five to 90 per cent of feline mammary gland tumors are malignant. Siamese cats may have a higher risk of developing mammary cancer than do other breeds and also develop mammary gland cancer at a younger age. The greater prevalence and the behavior of the malignant tumor are consistent with a genetic determinant and a familial predisposition for mammary neoplasia in the Siamese breed (Hayes et al., 1981).

The characteristics of feline mammary cancer—the rapid growth of the primary mammary tumors, the high rate of tumor recurrence (Brodey, 1970), and the poor survival statistics (Weijer et al., 1972; Weijer and Hart, 1983)—emphasize the need for the following approach:

1. Early diagnosis of the primary tumor
2. Immediate, aggressive surgical removal (radical mastectomy)
3. Frequent follow-up examinations to detect early clinical signs of recurrent disease
4. Surgical intervention for recurrence when possible

There are five ways of treating mammary cancer: (1) surgery, (2) radiation, (3) hormone therapy, (4) chemotherapy, and (5) immunotherapy. At The Animal Medical Center all cats with primary tumors with no radiographic evidence of metastatic disease and no other medical problems are treated by radical mastectomy. Radical mastectomy is defined as the removal of all four glands of the affected mammary chain together with the ipsilateral inguinal lymph nodes (unaffected axillary nodes may be difficult to locate). Surgery is the single most important treatment for breast cancer in the cat, and the oncologic surgeon should be experienced in the techniques and principles outlined previously (see section on surgery). If tumors are present in both mammary chains, two radical mastectomies are performed. The chain of glands with the larger tumor volume is usually removed first. The second mastectomy is performed 10 to 14 days after removal of the sutures from the first mastectomy (Hayes, 1977).

In a recent study of 91 cats with malignant mammary tumors, the type of surgery (radical versus conservative) was significantly ($p < 0.01$) related to the disease-free interval but was of no significance in prolonging survival time ($p = 0.12$) (MacEwen et al., 1984b). Radical surgery is still advised because of the lower recurrence rate associated with it.

There is an inverse relationship between tumor volume and survival time (i.e., the larger the tumor, the shorter the survival time). In a Donaldson-Atwood Cancer Clinic study of 91 cats with malignant mammary tumors treated by surgical excision, the single most important factor affecting prognosis after surgery was the tumor volume. Eighteen cats with a tumor size of 27 $cm^3$ (3 cm diam) or greater had a median survival time of approximately 200 days, and only 20 per cent survived longer than one year. Nineteen cats had a tumor size of 8 to 27 $cm^3$ (2 to 3 cm diam) and a median survival time of 700 days, with 20 per cent surviving two and a half years or longer. Fifty-four cats with tumor size of less than 8 $cm^3$ (2 cm diam) had a median survival of greater than three years (MacEwen et al., 1984b).

There are no published reports concerning the effectiveness of radiation therapy in feline mammary cancer.

The hormonal influence on the development of mammary neoplasia in the cat is unknown. Mammary carcinomas occur in female cats neutered during their first year of life (Weijer et al., 1972, 1983), and rare cases have occurred in both castrated and intact male cats (Lombard, 1940; Patnaik et al., 1975; Thiéry, 1946; Weijer et al., 1972; Weijer and Hart, 1983). In other studies the incidence of mammary tumors was found to be as much as sevenfold higher in intact female cats than in neutered cats (Dorn et al., 1968; Hayden and Nielsen, 1971).

There are indications that exogenous hormones may lead to the development of feline mammary tumors (Brodey, 1970; Hernandez et al., 1975). Endogenous progesterone or the administration of progestogens may influence mammary hypertrophy and the development of malignant mammary tumors (Brodey, 1970; Hernandez et al., 1975; Hinton and Gaskell, 1977). The effectiveness of hormonal therapy for the treatment of malignant mammary tumors cannot be assessed until the role of hormones in the development of mammary neoplasia is understood.

Newly developed anti-estrogen drugs are probably not applicable to the treatment of feline mammary cancer, since estrogen receptors are few or nonexistent in feline mammary tumor tissue (Hamilton et al., 1976; Weijer, 1979). Progesterone receptors and possible corticosteroid receptors, however, have been identified on the cell surfaces of hypertrophied feline mammary gland tissue (Hayden et al., 1981) and tumor tissue (Elling and Ungemach, 1981; Johnston et al., 1984).

The postoperative use of chemotherapy (cyclophosphamide) has been reported, although no results are available at this time (Theilen and Madewell, 1979a). Two chemotherapeutic protocols have been used at the Donaldson-Atwood Cancer Clinic for the treatment of metastatic or recurrent nonresectable mammary gland neoplasms or both. Low-dose chemotherapy with vincristine, cyclophosphamide, and methotrexate was found to be ineffective. Doxorubicin and cyclophosphamide in combination may limit advancing disease, but too few cases have been evaluated to substantiate this clinical indication. One cat with nonresectable tumors was able to undergo surgery after four courses of treatment. The following treatment schedule was used:

Day 1: Doxorubicin 30 mg/m$^2$ IV
Days 3, 4, 5, 6: Cyclophosphamide 50 to 100 mg/m$^2$ orally.

White blood-cell counts were performed 10 days and 21 days after treatment. An electrocardiogram was taken before each doxorubicin treatment to detect cardiac toxicity. Therapy was repeated after five weeks.

In a recent double-blind, randomized clinical study in 64 cats at the Donaldson-Atwood Cancer Clinic, 32 were treated with levamisole 5 mg/kg orally on a Monday-Wednesday-Friday schedule (MacEwen et al., 1984a). No significant difference in either survival time or recurrence rate was found between the two groups.

The use of Mixed Bacterial Vaccine (MBV) in conjunction with radical surgery is being evaluated in our clinic. Ideally MBV therapy (*Serratia marcescens* and *Streptococcus pyogenes*) is initiated before surgery in an attempt to counterbalance the immunosuppressive effects of surgery. In most cases, however, MBV therapy was started after surgery. Sixteen weekly injections are given (IM). If the cat is free of disease at the end of this four-month period, treatments are continued biweekly. In a preliminary analysis, MBV therapy has not yet been shown to increase survival time significantly beyond that of the cats undergoing radical surgery alone.

It is apparent that better methods of treating feline mammary cancer should be developed. Cooperative clinical trials in which different therapeutic regimens could be compared would hasten the development of new methods for treating this disease.

## Mast Cell Tumors

Feline mast cell tumors may involve skin, intestine, or primary hematopoietic organs. Seven and a half per cent of the malignant tumors diagnosed surgically in a one-year period at The Animal Medical Center were mast cell tumors, and 55 per cent of these were cutaneous.

Mast cell tumors may appear as multiple, raised, firm nodules or as subcutaneous soft masses, usually originating around the head and neck. Surgical excision and corticosteroids are the treatments of choice (Brodey, 1970; Slusher et al., 1967). Radiation therapy can be considered an adjunct to surgery (Banks and Morris, 1975; Bostock and Owen, 1975; Gillette, 1970). Our experience with chemotherapy (vincristine, cyclophosphamide, doxorubicin) has been unrewarding in the treatment of mast cell tumors. Other reports indicate that chemotherapy is an ineffective approach (Bostock, 1977; Bostock and Owen, 1972, 1975; Theilen, 1975).

Another form of mast cell tumor in the cat is characterized by splenomegaly, vomiting, anorexia, and sometimes mast cells in a buffy coat film and in bone marrow. Cats with primary splenic mast cell tumor may have cutaneous involvement. Therapy involves splenectomy, and these cats usually do very well after surgery, even if a positive buffy coat existed before surgery. In a report of seven cats treated with splenectomy the survival time of six ranged from 2+ to 34 months (Liska et al., 1979). One of the cats was alive and free of disease 93 months after splenectomy. Data on three more cases are given in Table 12–7 (Cases 1 to 3). Supportive therapy should include cimetidine, an H–2 receptor antihistamine. This will help to prevent gastroduodenal ulceration, a common sequela to mast cell tumors. The dose of cimetidine is 20 to 40 mg/kg orally divided q.i.d.

Solitary involvement of the small intestine is the least common presentation for mast cell tumor. A single lesion may be found with regional lymph nodes or liver as possible metastatic sites. Surgery is the treatment of choice, and no adjuvant therapy has been found to prevent recurrence. Recurrences are common and usually develop within six months of surgery. One cat with mast cell tumor involving the small intestine was followed for two years (Case 4, Table 12–7). Although gastroduodenal ulceration is reported not to occur with intestinal mast cell tumors in the cat (Alroy et al., 1975), we recommend the use of cimetidine.

## Sarcomas

Musculoskeletal tumors accounted for 5.4 per cent of the surgically treated tumors in a one-year period at The Animal Medical Center. Furthermore, feline bone tumors are more often malignant than benign (Misdorp and van

**Table 12–7 Surgically Treated Cases of Mast Cell Tumor in the Cat***

| | CASE 1 | CASE 2 | CASE 3 | CASE 4 |
|---|---|---|---|---|
| Breed | DSH | DLH | DSH | DSH |
| Sex | F/S | M/C | F/S | M/C |
| Age (years) | 16 | 9 | 9 | 16 |
| Presenting signs | Lethargy<br>Weight loss<br>Emesis | Emesis | Lethargy<br>Weight loss<br>Emesis<br>Behavior change | Emesis |
| Postoperative survival (months) | 15 | 12** | 14 | 24** |
| Cause of death | Unknown (concurrent diabetes mellitus) | Alive | Unrelated (heart) | Alive |
| Neoplastic involvement | Spleen | Spleen, liver, cutaneous lesions 13 months before surgery | Spleen | Small intestine |

*See Liska et al., 1979, for additional cases.
** = Still alive.

der Heul, 1976). Despite the high incidence of malignancy, cats with bone tumors may have a better prognosis with amputation than dogs or humans. Osteosarcomas and fibrosarcomas accounted for 31 per cent each of the malignant skeletal neoplasms diagnosed surgically in one year. The most frequent sites for osteosarcoma are distal femur, proximal humerus, and proximal tibia. Feline osteosarcomas develop in the appendicular skeleton 2.4 times more often than in the axial skeleton (Turrel and Pool, 1982).

Of five cats with osteosarcoma that were treated with amputation of the affected limb, one had pulmonary and renal metastasis five months after amputation; the other four cats were free of recurrent and metastatic disease for up to 26 months at the time of publication (Liu et al., 1974). The longest-surviving cat followed to date at the Donaldson-Atwood Cancer Clinic was still free of recurrent and metastatic disease eight years after limb amputation. Among 15 cases of primary bone tumors in cats, few had evidence of metastatic disease (Turrel and Pool, 1982).

In our experience the prognosis for osteosarcomas and fibrosarcomas is excellent if the neoplasm can be totally excised or if it occurs distally on a limb that can be amputated. Data on nonresectable or partially excised sarcomas and the use of adjunctive therapy are available from two studies at the Donaldson-Atwood Cancer Clinic (Brown et al., 1978, 1980). In a study of 11 cats with fibrosarcoma no metastases were seen in 10 *untreated* cats autopsied; one cat was reported free of disease 10 months after surgical excision (Liu et al., 1974). The Donaldson-Atwood Cancer Clinic reported on five cats with fibrosarcoma that underwent amputation (Brown et al., 1978). Only one cat died of metastatic disease. Three cats were free of the disease at the time of unrelated death. One was alive and without disease seven years after amputation. In two reported cases of chondrosarcoma with signs present from four months to six years, no metastases were found at autopsy (Liu et al., 1974). In our experience, however, chondrosarcomas recur and metastasize to the regional lymph nodes and lungs within a year after amputation (Brown et al., 1978).

Most cats with solitary fibrosarcomas are over eight years of age and test negative for the FeLV-FeSV (feline sarcoma virus) by the indirect immunofluorescent antibody (IFA) test. A small percentage of cats are presented with multicentric fibrosarcoma. These cats are usually young (<5 years) and when tested for the FeLV-FeSV by IFA or enzyme-linked immunosorbent assay (ELISA), usually test positive. It is estimated that FeSV-induced fibrosarcoma occurs only once for every 40 cats that develop solitary non-FeSV fibrosarcomas (Hardy, 1980). The solitary fibrosarcomas are usually well-differentiated, slowly invasive tumors that contain considerable amounts of collagen and reticulum. In contrast, the multicentric FeLV-FeSV–positive fibrosarcomas are less well differentiated and more invasive, contain less collagen and reticulum, and grow rapidly. Cats with multicentric fibrosarcomas have a poor prognosis, and treatment is not recommended. In addition, there appears to be a possible public health risk associated with FeSV (Hardy, 1980).

## Digestive Tract Tumors

After lymphosarcoma, carcinomas are the most common tumor in the digestive tract, pancreas, and liver (Patnaik et al., 1975). Intestinal carcinomas tend to be more frequent in males than in females. The incidence in the Siamese cat is nearly three times that in other breeds (Patnaik et al., 1975). The clinical signs typical of intestinal carcinomas are depression, anorexia, vomiting, weight loss, and abdominal effusion. The ileum is most often the site of origin and 30 to 40 per cent of the cats have peritoneal implants at the time of diagnosis. The intestinal lesions are usually annular, constrictive masses ranging from 1 to 6 cm in length. (See also the chapter on tumors.) The only possible treatment is surgical excision. On gross inspection it is very difficult to differentiate normal from abnormal tissue, as these tumors tend to infiltrate the mucosa and submucosa into areas that appear normal. Their invasiveness contributes to the extremely poor success rate with surgical excision. Our attempts to treat these tumors with postoperative chemotherapy were few, and all failed.

In a series of 264 nonhematopoietic solid tumors in the cat, 18 (6.9 per cent) were hemangiosarcomas. Most involved the liver, spleen, and mesentery (Patnaik et al.,

1975). We have successfully removed splenic hemangiosarcomas surgically, but attempts at treatment with combination chemotherapy (doxorubicin/cyclophosphamide) have yielded questionable prolongation of survival, because we lack evidence of the natural biologic behavior of this neoplasm.

The most frequent oropharyngeal neoplasm in the cat is squamous cell carcinoma (Brodey, 1970; Patnaik, 1975; Theilen and Madewell, 1979c). These tumors arise most often in the gum but also occur on the tongue and palate. They tend to be very invasive, with bone involvement; metastases to the regional lymph nodes tend to occur late in the course of the disease. Radiation can be effective for the early cases, and success depends on site, extent, and degree of bone involvement. A recent study reported on mandibulectomy for the treatment of oral squamous cell carcinoma in five cats (Bradley et al., 1984). Three died of recurrence within six months, one survived to nine months, and another had survived to 12 months at the time of publication.

# RADIATION THERAPY AND HYPERTHERMIA

JANE M. TURREL

## RADIOTHERAPY

Radiotherapy is important in the management of cancer in humans and has become increasingly important for treatment of animal neoplasms as well. There are several reasons for this. The incidence of neoplasia is increasing, as pet animals live longer and owners seek the most effective methods of treating their pets. Veterinary clinicians and surgeons are becoming more knowledgeable about radiation therapy and are more willing to refer animals with cancer to qualified veterinary radiation oncologists. Radiotherapy in cancer management has assumed a greater role, owing to increased availability of proper radiotherapy equipment and improved training for veterinary radiologists (Feeney and Johnston, 1983).

In this section, feline disorders that respond to radiotherapy and the methods of radiotherapy will be discussed. Owing to the relative newness of radiotherapy as a treatment modality in veterinary medicine, little statistical data are available about its effectiveness; most reports are anecdotal. Some data cited here are from more than 300 cats irradiated at the University of California, Veterinary Medical Teaching Hospital (UCD-VMTH). For detailed discussion on the theory and mechanics of radiotherapy, the reader is referred to other sources (Fletcher, 1980; Hall, 1978).

### Principles of Radiotherapy

The basic principle employed in radiotherapy is the cell-killing effect of ionizing radiation. Ionizing radiation penetrates cells and deposits energy within the nucleus, thus disrupting DNA synthesis and preventing continued cellular proliferation. Ionizing radiation kills proliferating normal cells to about the same extent as neoplastic cells. Therefore normal tissue response limits the total radiation dose that can be tolerated. The division of the total radiation dose into fractions enhances the killing of tumor cells and the sparing of normal cells.

Radiosensitivity is the measure of the loss of cellular reproductive integrity, or the ease with which cells are killed. As a rule, cells that divide regularly and are less differentiated (such as germinal cells of the epidermis) are more radiosensitive than those that rarely divide and are well differentiated (such as nerve and muscle cells). The radiosensitivity of neoplastic cell types usually parallels that of the normal cells from which they originate.

Radioresponsiveness refers to the gross response of tissues to radiation. This concept incorporates tumor cell radiosensitivity, tumor volume, level of oxygenation of tissues, differences in cell population kinetics, and tumor location. Because irradiated cells are killed in a logarithmic manner, large tumor volumes require large doses of radiation. Tumors with poor vascularity usually contain a large component of hypoxic cells. These cells require two and a half to three times more radiation to achieve equivalent cell killing than do well-oxygenated cells. Tumor location may prevent adequate dose administration if radiosensitive normal tissues are within the radiation field. Additional factors affecting radioresponsiveness are total duration of therapy, total radiation dose given, and the inherent characteristics of radiation. Feline tumors that appear to be relatively radioresponsive are squamous cell carcinoma, lymphosarcoma, and mast cell tumor. In general, carcinomas are more radioresponsive than sarcomas.

Radiocurability refers to the probability that curative doses of radiation can be given to a tumor without excessive damage to normal tissues. Some tumors respond quickly to radiation but have a tendency to recur within the radiation field. Therefore the rate of tumor regression is not necessarily an indication of radiocurability.

### Selection of Patients

Before radiation treatment is given, the cat must be carefully assessed for general physical condition, tumor characteristics, and presence of metastatic disease. A thorough physical examination and baseline laboratory data are essential. Concurrent diseases must be identified and treated. Cats with compensated diseases, such as renal or heart failure, must be stabilized before the start of treatment. The cat must be healthy enough to tolerate frequent but short anesthesias, as well as the stress of unfamiliar surroundings for an extended period of time if hospitalization for radiation treatment is required. Age itself is not a deterrent to radiation treatment.

The primary tumor must be evaluated to determine size, exact location, and degree of invasiveness. Histologic examination of tumor tissue is essential to establish the type of neoplasia, the degree of malignancy, and the completeness of excision. The primary tumor should be radiographed to determine the extent of tumor invasion if bone involvement is suspected.

Screening for metastatic disease must include palpation of regional lymph nodes, cytologic examination of aspirates of enlarged regional lymph nodes, and thoracic radiography. Abdominal radiographs should be made of cats with lymphosarcoma and tumors of the hindlimbs or perineal region. Alternative imaging modalities, such as computed tomography, ultrasonography, nuclear medicine, and magnetic resonance imaging, are available on a limited basis as additional screening procedures.

The decision to irradiate a cat with a tumor should be based on the condition of the animal, the likelihood of tumor control, and the expectations and wishes of the owner. Responses to irradiation are identified as probability of tumor control at a specified time after therapy, generally one to two years. For some tumors, only palliation or relief of clinical signs can be offered. The owner should be informed as to probable response, complications, and treatment cost.

## Tissue Responses to Radiation

Irradiation of tumors kills cells or destroys the ability of clonogenic cells to divide. Clinically, positive tumor response to irradiation will vary from rapid disappearance to a relatively unchanged appearance. Some carcinomas and lymphosarcomas die rapidly and undergo phagocytosis after a few radiation periods. Some sarcomas may remain for months before gradually disappearing. The rate of tumor regression has not been studied in spontaneous animal tumors; however, in some human tumors, no prognostic relationship was found between the rate of tumor regression and overall survival time (Fletcher, 1980).

Radiation reactions develop in normal tissues within the radiation field when the rate of cell killing exceeds the rate of cell repopulation. The mucous membranes of the eye and nasal and oral cavities usually develop acute radiation reactions when doses above 3000 cGy (rad)* are given in divided doses. The lesions include conjunctivitis, rhinitis, stomatitis, and glossitis. Acute radiation reactions are seen in the skin when radiation doses exceed 2500 to 3500 cGy. As the cumulative radiation dose increases, cutaneous reactions progress from erythema to dry and finally moist desquamation and epilation. Irradiated normal tissues exhibit maximal acute tissue damage 7 to 14 days after treatment. During this time, self-mutilation of pruritic irradiated sites must be prevented. Treatment for acute radiation reactions is usually unnecessary as tissues will heal after treatment has stopped. Occasionally, radiation treatments must be temporarily stopped for one or two weeks to allow healing of normal tissues before treatment is continued. Infection within the radiation field as a result of tumor or surgical intervention will severely compromise the ability of normal cells to repair radiation damage. Side effects are limited to the tissues within the radiation field. Nausea and vomiting do not occur unless a large portion of the abdomen is being irradiated.

Late radiation effects occur months or years after radiotherapy and are the dose-limiting factors. These effects include depigmentation, alopecia, thinning of skin, fibrosis, necrosis, fistula formation, and decreased resistance to infection. Damage to specific organs may severely compromise quality of life. Long-term ocular changes induced by radiation include chronic conjunctivitis and keratoconjunctivitis sicca. Chronic stomatitis, dental caries, calculus formation, and halitosis can be related in some cases to decreased saliva production from irradiation of salivary glands.

Abdominal and thoracic organs contain many radiosensitive tissues that can preclude effective therapy of tumors within these cavities. As a result, few cats with tumors overlying thoracic or abdominal organs have been irradiated. Presumably, organ sensitivities would be similar to those reported for dogs and humans, and radiation doses above the tolerance level would elicit an inflammatory reaction within a given organ (Feeney and Johnston, 1982).

## Methods of Radiotherapy

Radiation can be given either externally at a distance (teletherapy) or by applying the radiation source directly on or within the tumor (brachytherapy).

**TELETHERAPY.** Four types of teletherapy equipment currently used are: (1) orthovoltage x-ray machine, (2) cobalt-60 ($^{60}$Co) teletherapy unit, (3) cesium-137 ($^{137}$Cs) teletherapy unit, and (4) linear accelerator. Orthovoltage x-ray machines are designed for therapeutic purposes and produce relatively low-energy x-rays (100 to 300 kVp). These orthovoltage x-rays do not penetrate deeply into tissue and are absorbed differentially in bone and soft tissue. Therefore they are ideally used to treat dermal and superficial tumors less than 3 cm below the skin surface. Cobalt-60 and cesium-137 teletherapy units produce high-energy gamma rays (1.25 MeV and 0.66 MeV, respectively) that penetrate deeply and are not selectively absorbed by bone. This equipment is used to treat deep tumors or tumors involving bone. Linear accelerators produce fixed or variable-energy x-rays (2 to 35 MV) and electrons (4 to 18 MeV) that can be focused to be maximally absorbed at tumor depth. High-energy x-rays from linear accelerators have excellent depth penetration and so are used to treat deep tumors. High-energy radiation from $^{137}$Cs and $^{60}$Co units and linear accelerators have a skin-sparing effect that reduces the likelihood of superficial reactions often seen with lower-energy x-ray units. Particulate radiation (electrons) can be applied to tumors overlying radiosensitive structures, such as thoracic or abdominal wall tumors, as the range of electrons is short (2 to 6 cm of tissue).

*1 centiGray (cGy) = 0.01 Gray (Gy). 1 Gray = 100 rad.

Regardless of the teletherapy equipment used, patients are usually irradiated on alternate days two or three times a week. The sedation or anesthesia required to restrain cats for each treatment session makes more frequent radiation treatment difficult. Many treatment, time-dose fractionation schemes can be used to irradiate tumors, and all have been empirically derived. The protocol most often used is 400 to 500 cGy on a Monday–Wednesday–Friday schedule for 10 to 12 treatments. To achieve the same biologic effect when a larger dose per fraction is given, fewer treatments can be given, and each treatment must be separated by a longer interval. The total radiation dose is determined by tumor type, size, and location (Table 12–8).

**BRACHYTHERAPY.** Surface brachytherapy is used to treat small, well-delineated superficial tumors or tumors close to radiosensitive structures. Strontium-90 ($^{90}Sr$) produces a spectrum of penetrating beta particles (electrons) having a maximum energy of 2.27 MeV. Ninety per cent of the electrons are absorbed in the first 3 mm of tissue, thereby effectively limiting treatment to lesions less than 3 mm thick. Probes contain 50 to 100 mCi of $^{90}Sr$ and have an active diameter of 9 mm and an exposure rate of 2000 to 5000 cGy per minute. Eosinophilic granuloma, corneal vascularization, and superficial squamous cell carcinoma have responded well to $^{90}Sr$ beta irradiation. Total radiation doses range from 5000 to 25,000 cGy and may be repeated at two- to four-week intervals.

The direct implantation of radioactive sources into the tumor is another effective method of delivering therapeutic doses of ionizing radiation. Interstitial implants have the advantage that the radiation dose is highest in the implanted tumor, with rapid dose fall-off in surrounding normal tissues (Hilaris, 1975). Other advantages are continued low-level irradiation of the tumor, shortened hospitalization time, and a single anesthetic procedure. Disadvantages are that the implantation procedure is technically difficult, dosimetry is complex, and implants represent a radiation hazard.

Specific indications for interstitial brachytherapy are localized tumors that have a slow growth rate and low or moderate radiosensitivity. Implants are ideally suited for soft tissue tumors that have no bone involvement and are located in the oral cavity, face, perineal region, extremities, or abdominal and thoracic walls (Fig. 12–1).

Iodine-131 ($^{131}I$) treatment is another form of brachytherapy. Iodine-131 is administered orally or intravenously and is concentrated by functional thyroid tissue. Iodine-

**Table 12–8 Selected Feline Tumors and Recommended Radiation Therapy Protocols**

| TUMOR TYPE | TUMOR SITE | RECOMMENDED RADIATION SOURCE | ALTERNATIVE RADIATION SOURCES | RELATIVE TOTAL RADIATION DOSE | PROGNOSIS | COMMENTS |
|---|---|---|---|---|---|---|
| Squamous cell carcinoma | Nose, eyelids, ears | A | B, D, E | Moderate | Good | (a) Use $^{90}Sr$ only if lesion <3mm thick (b) Hyperthermia can be used alone or added |
| Squamous cell carcinoma | Oral cavity— tongue, gingiva, tonsil | A, B, C, D | F | High | Poor | |
| Fibrosarcoma | Soft tissues of extremities, head, and body wall | A, B, C, D | F | High | Fair | (a) Hyperthermia may be combined with irradiation (b) Irradiation given after surgery |
| Carcinoma and sarcoma | Nasal cavity and paranasal sinuses | B, C | A | High | Fair | Surgical debulking may worsen prognosis |
| Adenocarcinoma | Ceruminous gland | B, C | A | High | Good | |
| | Salivary gland | B, C | A | High | Poor | |
| | Mammary gland | A, D | F | High | Fair | Local control only |
| Osteosarcoma and chondrosarcoma | Axial skeleton | B, C | A | High | Fair | Tumor may be debulked before irradiation |
| Lymphosarcoma | Cranial mediastinum | B, C | A | Low | Fair | (a) Rapid control of clinical signs |
| | Nasal cavity | | | Moderate | | (b) Adjuvant chemotherapy required |
| | Any focal site | | | Low | | |
| Benign thyroid hyperplasia and adenoma | Thyroid gland | G | — | High | Excellent | Used to treat hyperfunctional thyroid tissue |
| Solitary mast cell tumor | Skin | A, D | F | Moderate | Good | Use to treat recurrent or nonresectable tumor |
| Eosinophilic or linear granuloma | Skin | A, D, E | — | Low | Fair | Used for chronic conditions |

A = Orthovoltage x-rays
B = Cobalt-60 or cesium-137 gamma rays
C = Linear accelerator x-rays
D = Linear accelerator electrons
E = Strontium-90 electrons
F = Interstitial implant ($^{192}Ir$) gamma rays
G = Iodine-131 beta and gamma radiations

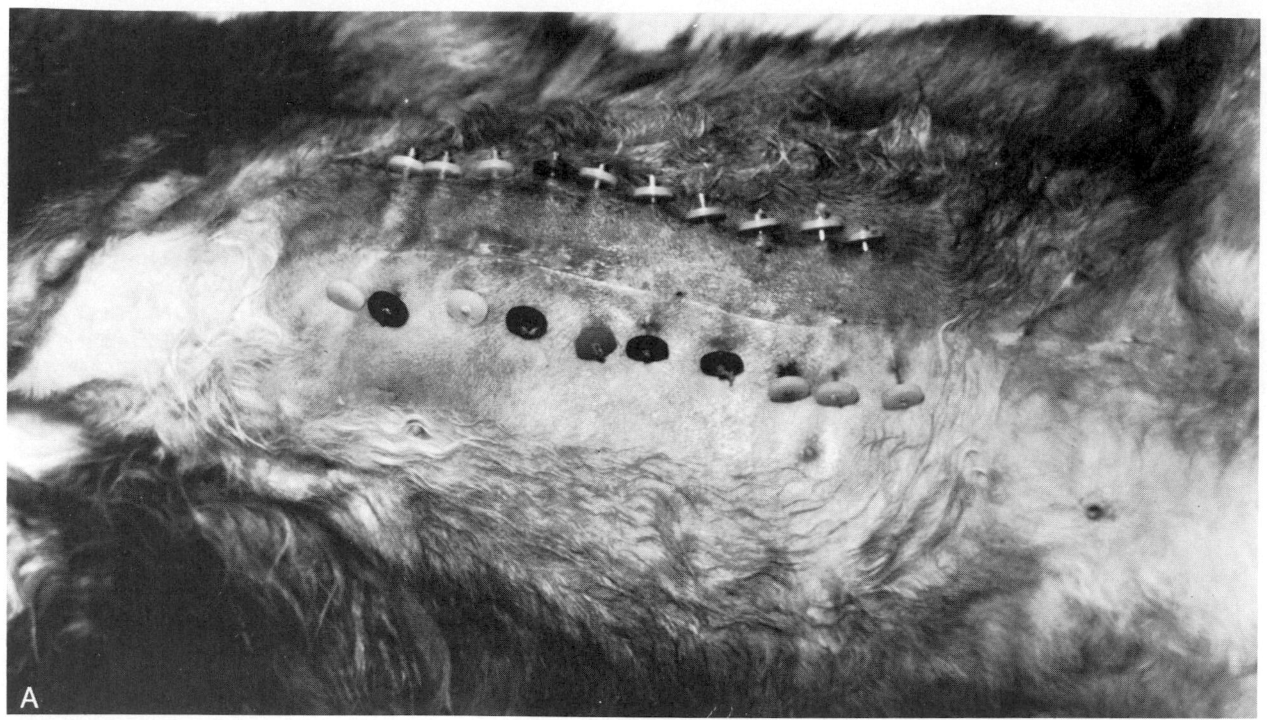

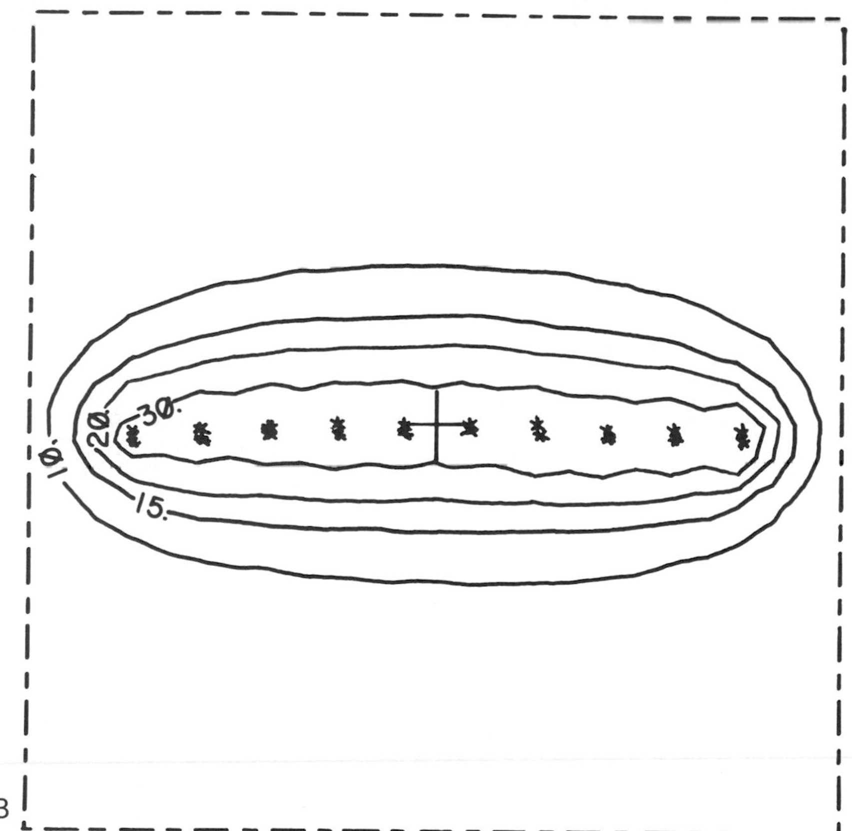


**Figure 12–1** *A*, Interstitial implant placed perpendicular to healed incision after removal of recurrent mammary gland carcinoma. Buttons at both ends of plastic tubes containing the radioisotope hold the implant in place. Tubes are spaced approximately 1 cm apart in a single plane. *B*, Lateral view of computer-generated isodose curves from the implant. The stars represent the placement of individual seeds, and the cross marks the center of the implant. The isodose curve selected (in this case, 30 cGy/hr) must encompass all tumor tissue.

131 emits gamma rays and beta particles. Eighty per cent of the radiation dose is delivered by the beta particles, which have an average penetration of 0.4 to 0.5 mm in tissue. Thus hyperfunctional thyroid tissue can be irradiated to high doses. Surrounding tissues, including atrophied thyroid follicular cells and parathyroid glands, can be relatively spared.

### RADIATION COMBINED WITH OTHER MODALITIES

Radiotherapy combined with other treatment modalities (e.g., surgery, chemotherapy, immunotherapy, and hyperthermia), can achieve more effective tumor control than radiation alone. Combined treatment not only can have an additive effect, but in some cases can also modify tumor radioresponsiveness.

**SURGERY.** Surgery and irradiation can be combined in several ways (Fletcher, 1979). Surgical salvage of recurrence of previously irradiated tumors may be effective in controlling early recurrence. Surgery and irradiation can also be useful in treating different areas for definitive control of the primary tumor, and irradiation alone can be used to treat regional lymph nodes. Surgery can also be used to allow adequate exposure and shielding of radiosensitive organs so that large radiation doses can be given to a tumor intraoperatively. Most often, however, surgery is used to eliminate gross disease. Radiation is given after surgery to eliminate microscopic disease or to treat tumor recurrence in the surgical site.

The optimum sequence of radiation and surgery is unknown. Presurgical irradiation may decrease the potential for the surgical procedure to produce distant metastases, prevent implantation of microscopic foci of tumor cells in adjacent tissues, convert inoperable lesions into operable ones by decreasing the tumor mass, and improve the blood supply to microscopic neoplasm. Increased surgical difficulty and delays in wound healing are cited as significant drawbacks to preoperative irradiation. Postoperative irradiation has been the usual sequence in veterinary medicine. The reason usually given is that radiation may not be needed if surgical resection is adequate. In most cases, radiation therapy is used in an attempt to salvage surgical failures. Advantages of postsurgical irradiation are that more accurate radiotherapy can be given because the full extent of the tumor is known, that resection of tumor and wound healing are less complicated, and that higher radiation doses can be given to already healed tissues. When irradiation is given after surgery, it should be started immediately or else postponed until wound healing is complete to avoid killing rapidly dividing cells.

Radiation has been proposed as an effective way to control surgical failures. This is not a rational approach, because irradiation is least effective against gross tumor, in which there is poorer vascularity than in microscopic tumor. Therefore, for malignancies that are likely to recur, "waiting to see if the tumor regrows" is poor tumor management. Another deterrent to effective control of surgical failures with irradiation is that viable tumor cells are often disseminated throughout the surgical field (as with mammary carcinoma and fibrosarcoma), so that very large treatment fields must often be used.

**CHEMOTHERAPY.** Treatment of tumors with combined radiation and chemotherapy is also possible. Two important drug classes relative to this discussion are radiosensitizing agents and chemotherapeutic agents (Steel and Peckham, 1979). Radiosensitizers used alone usually have no tumoricidal effect but when given with radiation can enhance the extent of tumor-cell killing. Chemotherapeutic agents, on the other hand, have significant anticancer toxicity. Many of them do not modify the radiation effect, but others have additive effects when used with radiation. Some drugs are both radiosensitizers and chemotherapeutic agents.

Chemotherapeutic agents used in combination with radiation may have minimal effect on the primary tumor; however, they are used to eradicate distant and regional metastatic disease or to treat disseminated, systemic neoplasms such as lymphosarcoma. Some drugs also enhance the effectiveness of radiotherapy by shrinking the tumor, thereby improving relative tumor vascularity. Unfortunately, the enhanced effect is also observed in normal tissues. Some agents have a synergistic effect with radiation, attributable in part to their ability to differ in activity at various stages of the cell cycle. Other chemotherapeutic agents may also inhibit repair of radiation damage to the DNA (doxorubicin) or prevent synthesis of DNA (5-fluorouracil).

## HYPERTHERMIA

Hyperthermia is the heating of tissues above 42 C (108 F) and is usually induced by radio-frequency generators and microwave and ultrasound units (Lord and Kapp, 1982). Hyperthermia can be applied locally, regionally, or to the whole body. It can be used alone or in combination with radiation. Hyperthermia does not selectively kill tumor cells; however, neoplastic cells with poor oxygenation or low pH, or in the S-phase of the cell cycle, are preferentially killed. Therefore tumors having a poor vascular supply, such as fibrosarcoma, may be susceptible to hyperthermia.

Hyperthermia is used alone when tumors are small and readily accessible (Marmor et al., 1978). Usually one treatment is given and the animal is examined two to four weeks later to determine the extent of tumor damage. If tumor regrowth or inadequate tumor kill is noted, hyperthermia can be safely repeated. Hyperthermia using 50 C (120 F) for 30 seconds has resulted in 89 per cent favorable response for feline squamous cell carcinoma of the eyelids, nose, and eartips (Grier et al., 1980). Tumor recurrence is frequent when hyperthermia is used alone, presumably because the more favorable environment of peripheral tumor cells inhibits tumor-cell death.

A complementary effect on cell killing exists when hyperthermia is combined with radiation and may be related to heat-induced inhibition of repair of cellular radiation injury (Miller et al., 1977). Although the optimum time relationship of hyperthermia and radiation is not known, radiation treatment usually precedes hyperthermia treatment. Multiple hyperthermia treatments are given after radiation at greater than 72-hour intervals. General anesthesia is required to administer each treatment.

Squamous cell carcinoma, fibrosarcoma, and eosinophilic granuloma have been treated with hyperthermia, radiation, or both (Dewhirst et al., 1982; Northway, 1982). Complete response rates were higher for hyperthermia and radiation (69 per cent) than for hyperthermia alone (25 per cent) and radiation alone (30 per cent) (Dewhirst et al., 1982). Toxemia and septicemia associated with severe tumor necrosis were observed at UCD-VMTH in cats whose tumors were heated to temperatures above 50 C (120 F). Nephrotoxicity was fatal in two cats.

## RADIOTHERAPY OF SPECIFIC TUMORS

### Dermal Squamous Cell Carcinoma

Squamous cell carcinoma is one of the common skin tumors in cats (Macy and Reynolds, 1981). Usual sites are the nasal planum, external nares, eyelids, pinnae, and preauricular area. Squamous cell carcinoma is considered to be a solar-induced lesion when it occurs in sparsely haired areas on white cats or in unpigmented areas on multicolored cats. Regardless of etiology, dermal squamous cell carcinoma is locally invasive and may be either productive or ulcerative. Solar-induced squamous cell carcinoma often has multiple primary sites where tumors have arisen simultaneously or sequentially. Cutaneous squamous cell carcinomas infrequently metastasize (10 per cent) and usually spread to the regional lymph nodes and lungs late in the disease.

Surgical excision is said to be the treatment of choice for feline squamous cell carcinoma, but this statement is unsubstantiated (Macy and Reynolds, 1981). In this author's experience, squamous cell carcinoma of the skin is often unresectable because of tumor invasiveness and location. Radiotherapy is considered to be the treatment of choice for dermal squamous cell carcinoma in cats at UCD-VMTH, because these tumors are highly radioresponsive and have a high likelihood of tumor control with irradiation, with less disfiguring results than with aggressive surgical removal (Fig. 12–2).

Superficial squamous cell carcinomas less than 3 mm deep can be treated with $^{90}$Sr applications of 10,000 to 25,000 cGy in single or divided doses. However, the majority of dermal squamous cell carcinomas are too extensive for effective treatment with $^{90}$Sr and require superficial beam teletherapy. Total radiation doses range from 3500 to 5000 cGy, given in divided doses over a three- or four-week period. Hyperthermia alone has been used successfully to treat small squamous cell carcinomas, but recurrence is common with larger tumors (Grier et al., 1980). The combination of hyperthermia and irradiation seemed to improve the therapeutic response of some highly malignant dermal squamous cell carcinomas treated at UCD-VMTH.

The prognosis for cats with dermal squamous cell carcinoma receiving radiotherapy is good; approximately 70 per cent of cats with nasal squamous cell carcinomas treated at UCD-VMTH were tumor-free at one year. Similar results were achieved with unconventional radiaton schemes of 1000 cGy per month or three times weekly for one week (Carlisle and Gould, 1982). At UCD-VMTH, the tumor-free incidence at one year was 40 per cent in cats with periocular and otic tumors. This limited success may have been due, in part, to the circumstance that cats with these tumors often had multiple tumors on the head. The prognosis was best for cats having a nasal squamous cell carcinoma less than 1 cm in diameter. When tumor did recur, approximately 50 per cent of the dermal squamous cell carcinomas were successfully reirradiated with a reduced dose (2000 to 3000 cGy).

### Oral Squamous Cell Carcinoma

Oral squamous cell carcinoma originates from the gingiva, tongue, or tonsil and is often detected late in the disease (Cotter, 1981). Extensive infiltration and tissue destruction are common, and the probability of regional lymph node metastasis is high. Tumor invasiveness may preclude treatment, as there may be a functional defi-

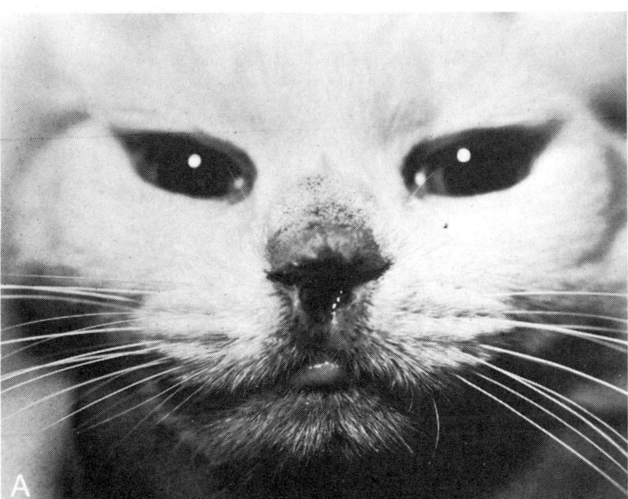


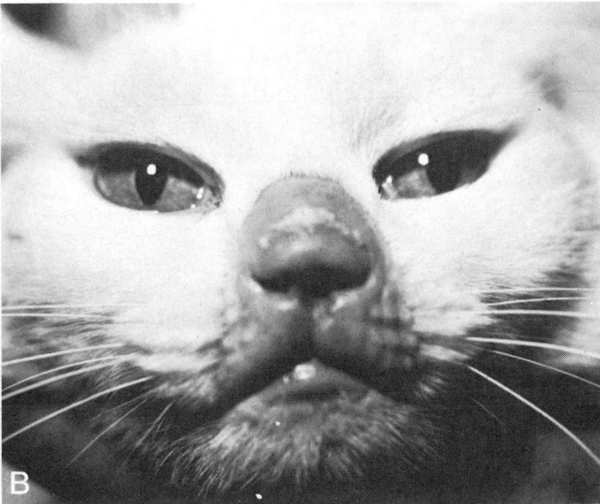


**Figure 12–2** *A*, Small squamous cell carcinoma on the nose of a cat before irradiation. The tumor was treated with 4000 cGy in 10 fractions with orthovoltage x-rays. *B*, Two months after treatment the lesion was healed, although hair loss in the surrounding irradiated area remained.

ciency or structural defect (loss of tongue) as a result of shrinking tumor mass. The cat must be carefully evaluated before treatment to determine how much functional tissue would remain.

Squamous cell carcinomas of the oral cavity respond less well to radiation than do cutaneous squamous cell carcinomas. Large radiation doses (4000 to 6000 cGy) are required with a fractionated dose schedule. The use of interstitial brachytherapy or hyperthermia or both may improve the prognosis, but the outlook is at best poor to fair and is guarded if there is secondary bone involvement. Only one of five cats with lingual squamous cell carcinoma survived to one year. The average survival time for cats with tonsillar squamous cell carcinoma was two months. Overall, the survival rate for all cats with oral squamous cell carcinomas treated at UCD-VMTH was 10 per cent at one year.

Squamous cell carcinoma invading the bones of the skull, particularly the mandible, is rare in cats (Madewell et al., 1976). This tumor stimulates a highly proliferative bony reaction and mimics osteosarcoma. No response was obtained in five cats treated with radiation doses of 4000 to 5000 cGy.

## Fibrosarcoma and Other Soft-Tissue Sarcomas

Fibrosarcomas in cats occur as two biologically different entities. Multicentric fibrosarcomas occur in young cats infected with feline sarcoma virus and will not be discussed here. Solitary fibrosarcoma typically occurs in older cats as a large, locally invasive mass that apparently arises de novo (Brown et al., 1978). The most common sites are the soft tissues of the extremities, head, and thoracic and abdominal walls. The incidence of metastatic disease is 10 to 20 per cent.

Surgical resection or amputation has been the primary method of treatment for fibrosarcoma; however, a 70 per cent recurrence rate indicates that surgery alone will not adequately control these tumors (Bostock and Dye, 1979; Brown et al., 1978). Although irradiation of fibrosarcomas and other less common soft tissue sarcomas has not been reported, radiotherapy after surgery would seem to be indicated for cats with fibrosarcoma. Superficial tumors should be given high doses with orthovoltage x-rays or linear accelerator electrons. If the tumor overlies radiosensitive structures, interstitial implants at the time of surgery can be used to give a total dose of 6000 to 8000 cGy. When the tumor mass is too large to be removed surgically, presurgical irradiation may be used to shrink the mass to an operable size.

The prognosis is fair for cats with fibrosarcomas receiving postoperative radiation. Four of nine cats at UCD-VMTH were tumor-free at one year. Unfortunately, three cats had multiple surgical procedures causing extensive seeding throughout the operative site. This required the use of large radiation fields and reduced the total radiation dose that could be tolerated. Interstitial implants and hyperthermia may improve local tumor control rates.

## Intranasal Tumors

The incidence of intranasal and paranasal sinus neoplasms in the cat is low (Legendre et al., 1981). Adenocarcinoma, squamous cell carcinoma, sarcoma, and lymphosarcoma are the most frequent tumors in those sites. All exhibit similar characteristics in that they arise in the nasal cavity, rarely involve the frontal sinuses, invade soft tissue and bony structures, often extend beyond the confines of the skull, and rarely metastasize. Most cats with nasal tumors are presented with advanced, extensive disease.

Treatment of feline intranasal tumors has rarely been reported (Legendre et al., 1975; Lord et al., 1982; Susaneck, 1982). Experience in the treatment of canine nasal tumors would indicate that radiotherapy, with or without prior surgical excision, may be the most effective treatment (Fig. 12–3). So far, only limited control or palliation of signs has been achieved by radiotherapy in cats at UCD-VMTH. Nasal tumors are irradiated to a high dose with high-energy teletherapy units. Acute radiation reactions occasionally occurring in the later stages of therapy include conjunctivitis, mucositis, loss of sense of smell, stomatitis, and superimposed infection, and may contribute to anorexia and loss of well-being. Therefore cats undergoing radiotherapy for nasal tumors must be supported and maintained in a positive nutritional status. Surgical debulking before irradiation may or may not improve treatment results.

Cats with nasal lymphosarcoma given low to moderate doses of radiation have experienced rapid remission of tumor. Chemotherapy is recommended as irradiation is considered to be adjuvant therapy.

## Adenocarcinoma

Adenocarcinomas that may be amenable to radiation therapy originate from the mammary gland, sweat gland, sebaceous gland, ceruminous gland, and salivary gland. Except for mammary gland carcinomas, they have low incidence rates and variable metastatic rates (Macy and Reynolds, 1981). Few cats with adenocarcinomas have been irradiated, but high-dose irradiation alone or with surgery may improve tumor control. Ceruminous gland carcinomas in three cats were irradiated to a total dose of 4500 cGy, and the cats were tumor-free at two years. However, two cats with salivary gland adenocarcinomas with regional lymph node metastasis had no response to 4000 cGy given after surgery.

Local tumor control of mammary gland carcinoma is a significant problem despite radical surgical procedures (Hayes, 1977). Teletherapy given after surgery or interstitial implantation at the time of surgery may significantly improve the rate of local tumor control.

## Primary Bone Tumors

Primary bone tumors are infrequent in cats (Turrel and Pool, 1982). Benign bone tumors reported in cats include osteoma, ossifying fibroma, and osteochondroma. Although feline osteochondromatosis is considered to be benign, the multicentric, progressive nature of this FeLV-related disease makes affected cats poor candidates for treatment (Pool, 1981). Two cats with osteochondromatosis were irradiated and had no response to therapy. The most frequent primary malignant bone tumors in the cat are osteosarcoma and chondrosarcoma. They are locally destructive and rarely metastasize.

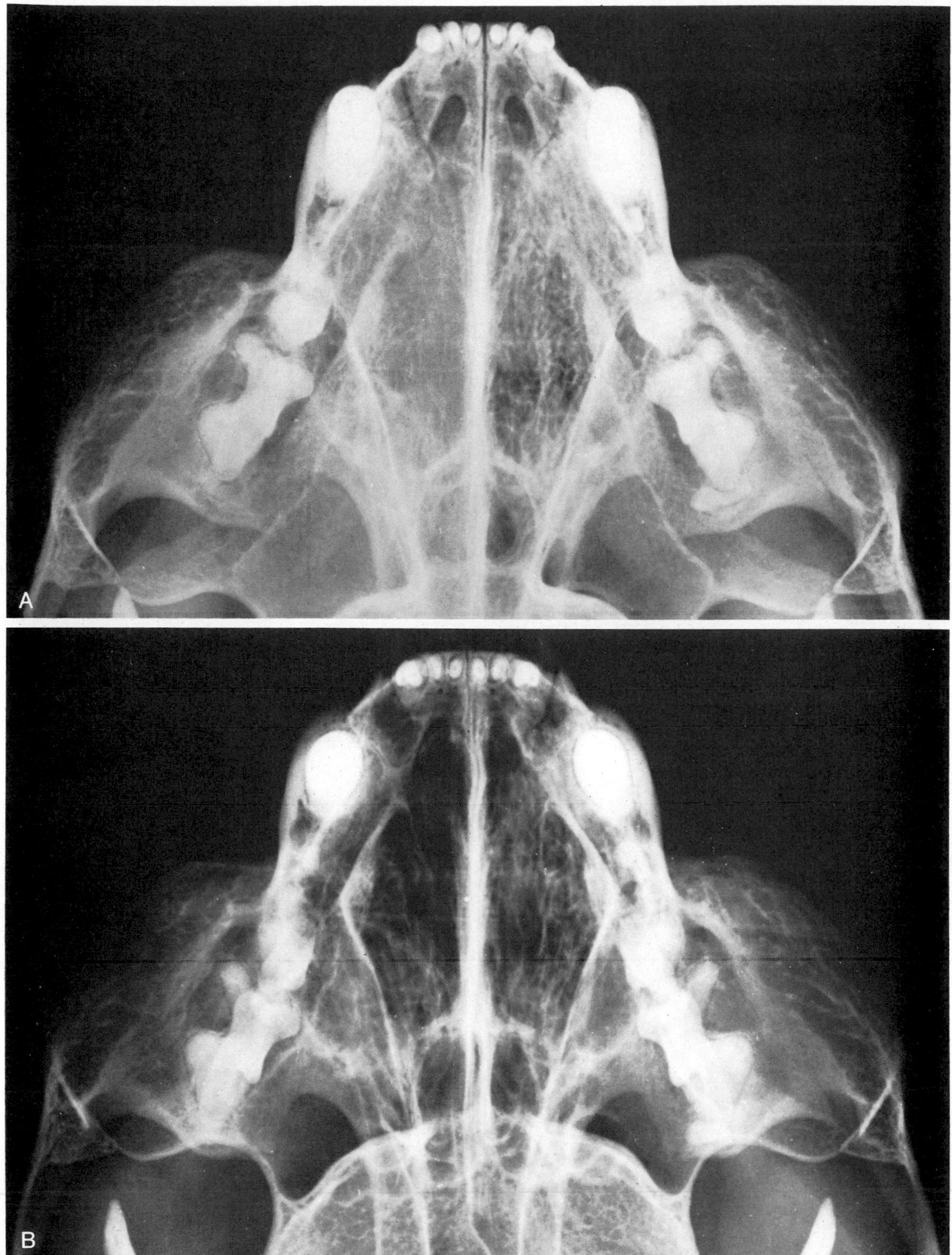


**Figure 12–3** *A*, Fibrosarcoma of the right nasal cavity. The primary finding is increased soft-tissue density. No bone destruction is evident. *B*, Same cat, six months after irradiation with 4800 cGy to the nasal cavity. There is now increased radiolucency, possibly due to erosion of nasal turbinates by tumor.

Radiotherapy should be used to treat nonresectable tumors. One cat with ossifying fibroma had regression and stabilization of tumor growth for two years after receiving 4000 cGy. The treatment of choice for malignant bone tumors of the extremities in cats is amputation. In selected cases, limb salvage procedures including radiotherapy may be an effective alternative approach. Malignant bone tumors of the skull, pelvis, and spine of cats irradiated with high doses had a fair prognosis, with 40 per cent survival at one year at UCD-VMTH.

## Lymphosarcoma

Feline lymphosarcoma is well recognized as a systemic disease. Occasionally, it may localize in a solitary site and can be controlled effectively with radiotherapy. Moderate radiation doses usually result in complete remission and tumor control. The more usual situation is the presence of a solitary mass in the cranial mediastinum, nasal cavity, or other site with concurrent systemic involvement. Chemotherapy is used with adjuvant low-dose irradiation of the mass. The mean survival time of cats treated with irradiation and chemotherapy at UCD-VMTH was 10 months compared with 6 months for cats treated with chemotherapy alone.

Lymphosarcomatous masses can compress or obstruct vital organs. A single, large dose (500 to 1000 cGy) of radiation given as emergency therapy to the tumor can achieve marked regression within 12 hours. Specific indications for prompt treatment include: (1) thymic lymphosarcoma compressing the trachea or esophagus or both (Fig. 12–4); (2) nasal, pharyngeal, or tracheal invasion causing severe dyspnea; (3) periorbital or retrobulbar lymphosarcoma causing exophthalmos and exposure keratitis; (4) involvement of brain or spinal cord, causing paralysis, seizures, or severe ataxia; and (5) abdominal lymphosarcoma (intestine, kidney, or lymph node) causing intestinal obstruction or renal failure. In these situations, radiotherapy should be considered an adjunct to

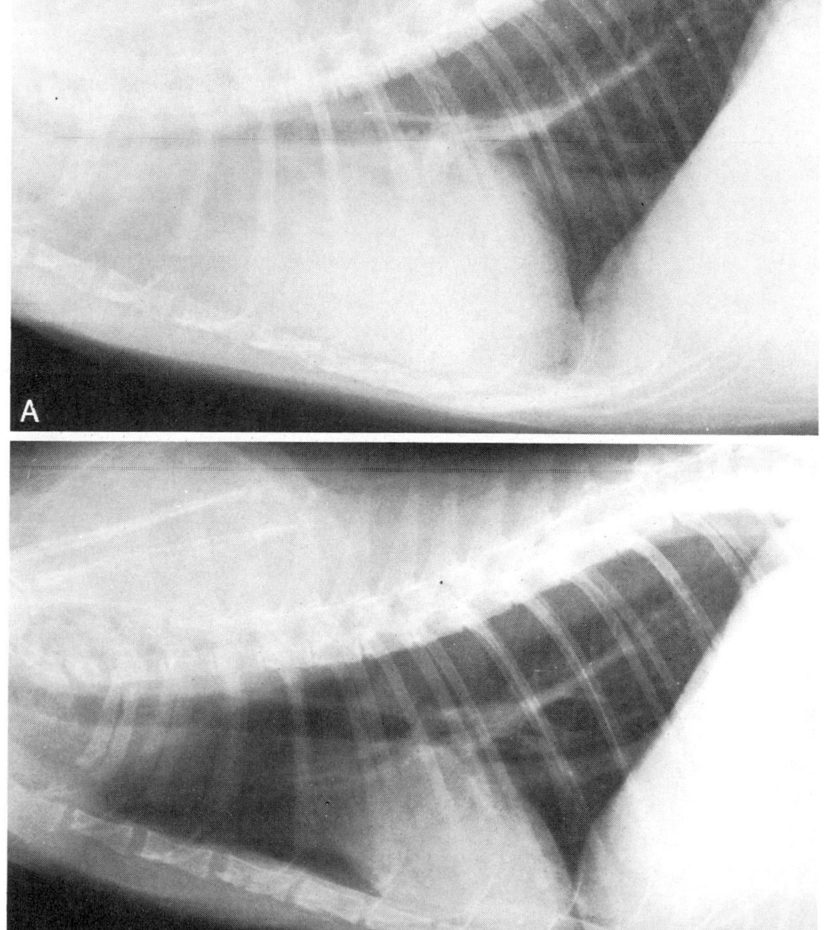


**Figure 12–4** *A*, A large cranial mediastinal mass compresses the trachea and esophagus and displaces the heart caudally, two-year-old cat. Lymphosarcoma was diagnosed by needle aspirate of the mass. *B*, Same cat three days after irradiation with 500 cGy. The dramatic reduction in tumor size typically occurs when lymphosarcomatous masses are irradiated.

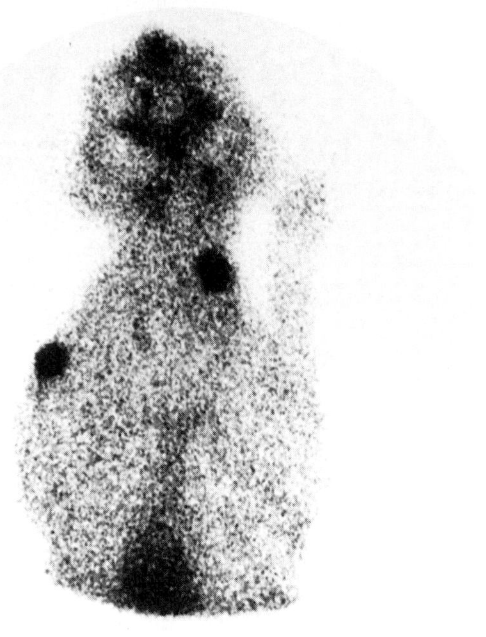

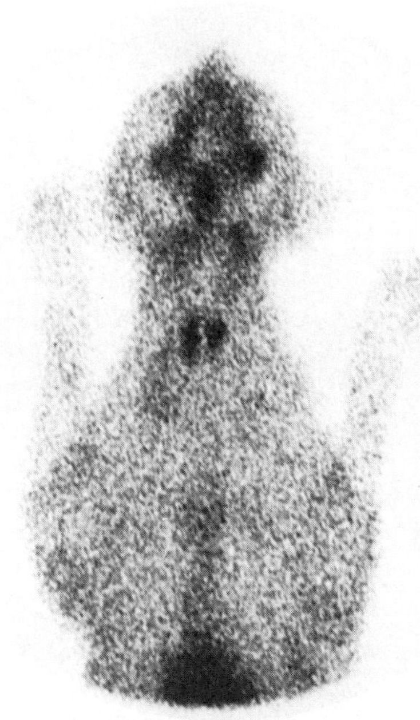

A B

**Figure 12–5** *A*, Ventral view of $^{99m}$Tc thyroid scan of a hyperthyroid cat shows unilateral left thyroid lobe enlargement. Technetium-99m is trapped in the same manner as iodine and is taken up by the thyroid gland, salivary gland, and stomach. Two areas of increased activity in the head are the salivary glands. The single area of activity on the cat's right is the site of injection. *B*, Ventral view of $^{99m}$Tc scan of same cat three months after treatment with $^{131}$I shows decrease in thyroid lobe activity and size. The contralateral lobe has regained normal function, and both thyroid lobes are of about the same intensity as salivary glands.

chemotherapy, the latter being essential for long-term survival of the cat.

Most cats with lymphosarcoma receiving irradiation and chemotherapy respond with rapid reduction in tumor size and improved hematologic values. The long-term prognosis, however, is only fair, as relapse with chemotherapeutic regimens is common. In three cats localized histiocytic lymphosarcoma treated with chemotherapy and irradiation has responded well for 8 to 12 months. Experimental treatment of cats with systemic lymphosarcoma could potentially include whole body irradiation, followed by autologous bone marrow transplantation.

## Thyroid Hyperplasia and Tumors

Thyroid diseases in cats include benign adenomatous hyperplasia, adenoma, and adenocarcinoma. The former two are usually functional and result in hyperthyroidism. Surgical excision is reported to be the treatment of choice (Theran and Holzworth, 1980). However, severe debilitation, cardiac changes, and concurrent diseases make some cats poor surgical risks. In addition, if both thyroid lobes are removed, iatrogenic hypoparathyroidism is a serious potential complication, and hypothyroidism is inevitable. Experience at UCD-VMTH indicates that radiotherapy with $^{131}$I is an effective alternative treatment for feline hyperthyroidism (Turrel, 1984). Activity of $^{131}$I administered is determined by tumor volume, percentage of iodine uptake, and biologic turnover time, and ranges from 1 to 10 mCi of $^{131}$I. Approximately 90 per cent of hyperthyroid cats given a single treatment of $^{131}$I became euthyroid within one to three months (Fig. 12–5). Cats remaining hyperthyroid usually responded to a second treatment of $^{131}$I. The only side effect associated with this therapy was the development of hypothyroidism in a small number of cats. Functional thyroid adenocarcinoma may also be treated with $^{131}$I. However, ablation (surgical or radiation) of normal thyroid tissue is necessary to increase $^{131}$I concentration in the primary and metastatic tumors. Incompletely excised nonfunctional thyroid adenocarcinomas should be given medium-dose teletherapy.

## Solitary Dermal Mast Cell Tumor and Eosinophilic Granuloma

As well as squamous cell carcinoma, other skin lesions that respond to irradiation are solitary mast cell tumor and eosinophilic granuloma. Solitary mast cell tumor is usually given moderate radiation doses. One-year tumor control was achieved in 6 of 10 cats with solitary mast cell tumors. Cats with systemic mastocytosis or miliary dermal mast cell tumors have not been irradiated, although whole body irradiation might be considered.

Eosinophilic granulomas of the lips and skin are usually treated with other therapeutic modalities, including methylprogesterone and corticosteroids. Some refractory lesions respond to irradiation. Eosinophilic granulomas less than 3 mm deep can be irradiated with strontium-90, 5000 to 10,000 cGy, for two or three treatments at biweekly intervals. Larger lesions can be treated with low-dose orthovoltage radiation.

## REFERENCES

**Surgery, Immunotherapy, and Chemotherapy**


Alroy J, Lea I, DeLellis RA, Weinstein RS: Distinctive intestinal mast cell neoplasms of domestic cats. Lab Invest 33 (1975) 159–167.

Banks WC, Morris E: Results of radiation treatment of naturally occurring animal tumors. J Am Vet Med Assoc 166 (1975) 1063–1064.

Bostock DE: Neoplasia of the skin and mammary glands in dogs and cats. *In* Kirk RW (ed): Current Veterinary Therapy VI. Philadelphia, WB Saunders Company, 1977, 493–505.

Bostock DE, Owen LN: Chemotherapy of canine and feline neoplasia. J Small Anim Pract 13 (1972) 359–367.

Bostock DE, Owen LN: Neoplasia in the cat, dog, and horse. Chicago, Yearbook Medical Publishers, Inc, 1975.

Bradley RL, MacEwen EG, Loar AS: Mandibular resection for removal of oral tumors in 30 dogs and 6 cats. J Am Vet Med Assoc 184 (1984) 460–463.

Brodey RS: Canine and feline neoplasia. Adv Vet Sci Comp Med 14 (1970) 309–354.

Brodey RS: Surgery. *In* Theilen GH, Madewell BR (eds): Veterinary Cancer Medicine. Philadelphia, Lea & Febiger, 1979, 67–78.

Brown NO, Hayes AA, Mooney S, Patnaik AK, Harvey HJ, MacEwen EG: Combined modality therapy in the treatment of solid tumors in cats. J Am Anim Hosp Assoc 16 (1980) 719–722.

Brown NO, Patnaik AK, Mooney S, Hayes AA, Harvey HJ, MacEwen EG: Soft tissue sarcomas in the cat. J Am Vet Med Assoc 173 (1978) 744–749.

Bruce DL: Halothane inhibition of phytohemagglutinin-induced transformation of lymphocytes. Anesthesiology 36 (1972) 201–205.

Burnet FM: The concept of immunological surveillance. Prog Exp Tumor Res 13 (1970) 1–27.

Carpenter JL, Holzworth J: Thymoma in 11 cats. J Am Vet Med Assoc 181 (1982) 248–251.

Cockerell GL, Hoover EA, Krakowka S, Olsen RG, Yohn DS: Lymphocyte mitogen reactivity and enumeration of circulating B- and T-cells during feline leukemia virus infection in the cat. J Natl Cancer Inst 57 (1976) 1095–1099.

Cole WH, McDonald GO, Roberts SS, Southwick HW: Dissemination of cancer. New York, Appleton-Century-Crofts Inc, 1961.

Cotchin E: Some tumours of dogs and cats of comparative veterinary and human interest. Vet Rec 71 (1959) 1040–1054.

Cotter SM: Treatment of lymphoma and leukemia with cyclophosphamide, vincristine, and prednisone: II. Treatment of cats. J Am Anim Hosp Assoc 19 (1983) 166–172.

Cotter SM, Essex M, McLane MF, Grant CK, Hardy WD Jr: Chemotherapy and passive immunotherapy in naturally occurring feline mediastinal lymphoma. *In* Hardy WD Jr, Essex M, McClelland AJ (eds): Feline Leukemia Virus. New York, Elsevier/North-Holland, 1980, 219–225.

Cotter SM, Hardy WD Jr, Essex M: Association of the feline leukemia virus with lymphosarcoma and other disorders in the cat. J Am Vet Med Assoc 166 (1975) 449–454.

Creech RH: Paraneoplastic and cancer-associated syndromes. *In* Stunick AI, Engstrom PF (eds): Oncologic Medicine. Baltimore, University Park Press, 1976, 313–331.

Dorn CR, Taylor DON, Schneider R, Hibbard HH, Klauber MR: Survey of animal neoplasms in Alameda and Contra Costa counties, California. II. Cancer morbidity in dogs and cats from Alameda County. J Natl Cancer Inst 40 (1968) 307–318.

Dowling MD Jr, Krakoff IH, Karnofsky DA: Mechanism of action of anti-cancer drugs. *In* Cole WH (ed): Chemotherapy of Cancer. Philadelphia, Lea & Febiger, 1970, 1–74.

Eilber FR, Nizze JA, Morton DL: Sequential evaluation of general immune competence in cancer patients: correlation with clinical course. Cancer 35 (1975) 660–665.

Elling H, Ungemach FR: Progesterone receptors, in feline mammary cancer cytosol. J Cancer Res Clin Oncol 100 (1981) 325–329.

Engle GC, Brodey RS: A retrospective study of 395 feline neoplasms. J Am Anim Hosp Assoc 5 (1969) 21–31.

Espanol T, Todd GB, Soothill JF: The effect of anesthesia on the lymphocyte response to phytohaemagglutinin. Clin Exp Immunol 18 (1974) 73–79.

Essex M: Feline leukemia and sarcoma viruses. *In* Klein G (ed): Viral Oncology. New York, Raven Press, 1980, 205–229.

Essex M, Hardy WD Jr, Cotter SM, Jakowski RM, Sliski A: Naturally occurring persistent feline oncornavirus infections in the absence of disease. Infect Immun 11 (1975) 470–475.

Fisher JC, Ketcham AS, Hume RB, Malmgren RA: Significance of cancer cells in operative wounds. Am J Surg 114 (1967) 514–519.

Gillette EL: Veterinary radiotherapy. J Am Vet Med Assoc 157 (1970) 1707–1712.

Good RA, Peterson RDA, Perey DY, Finstad J, Cooper MD: The immunological deficiency diseases of man. Birth Defects: Original Article Series 4(1) (1968) 17–39.

Gordon BR, Matus RE, Saal SD, MacEwen EG, Hurvitz AI, Stenzal KH, Rubin AL: Protein A–independent tumoricidal responses in dogs after extracorporeal perfusion of plasma over *Staphylococcus aureus.* J Natl Cancer Inst 70 (1983) 1127–1133.

Grant CK, Pickard DK, Ramaika C, Madewell BR, Essex M: Complement and tumor antibody levels in cats, and changes associated with natural feline leukemia virus infection and malignant disease. Cancer Res 39 (1979) 75–81.

Hamilton JM, Else RW, Forshaw P: Oestrogen receptors in feline mammary carcinoma. Vet Rec 99 (1976) 477–479.

Hardy WD Jr: The biology and virology of the feline sarcoma viruses. *In* Hardy WD Jr, Essex M, McClelland AJ (eds): Feline Leukemia Virus. New York, Elsevier/North-Holland, 1980, 79–118.

Hardy WD Jr, Hess PW, MacEwen EG, McClelland AJ, Zuckerman EE, Essex M, Cotter SM, Jarrett O: Biology of feline leukemia virus in the natural environment. Cancer Res 36 (1976a) 582–588.

Hardy WD Jr, Hess PW, MacEwen EG, Hayes AA, Kassel RL, Day NK, Old LJ: Treatment of feline lymphosarcoma with feline blood constituents. *In* Clemmesen J, Yohn DS (eds): Comparative Leukemia Research 1975. Basel, S. Karger, 1976b, 518–521.

Hardy WD Jr, MacEwen EG, Hayes AA, Zuckerman EE: FOCMA antibody as specific immunotherapy for lymphosarcoma of pet cats. *In* Hardy WD Jr, Essex M, McClelland AJ (eds): Feline Leukemia Virus. New York, Elsevier/North-Holland, 1980, 227–233.

Hart IR, Fidler IJ: Cancer invasion and metastasis. Q Rev Biol 55 (1980) 121–142.

Harvey HJ: General principles of veterinary oncologic surgery. J Am Anim Hosp Assoc 12 (1976) 335–339.

Harvey HJ, MacEwen EG, Hayes AA: Neurotoxicosis associated with use of 5-fluorouracil chemotherapy in five dogs and one cat. J Am Vet Med Assoc 171 (1977) 277–278.

Hawrylko E: Mechanisms by which tumors escape immune destruction. *In* Waters H (ed): The Handbook of Cancer Immunology. Vol 2. New York, Garland STPM Press, 1978, 1–53.

Hayden DW, Johnston SD, Kiang DT, Johnson KH, Barnes DM: Feline mammary hypertrophy/fibroadenoma complex: Clinical and hormonal aspects. Am J Vet Res 42 (1981) 1699–1703.

Hayden DW, Nielsen SW: Feline mammary tumours. J Small Anim Pract 12 (1971) 687–697.

Hayes AA: Feline mammary gland tumors. Vet Clin North Am, 7 (1977) 205–212.

Hayes AA, MacEwen EG, Matus RE, Mooney SC, Leiderman I, Old LJ: Antileukemic activity of plasma cryoprecipitate therapy in the cat. *In* Hardy WD Jr, Essex M, McClelland

AJ (eds): Feline Leukemia Virus. New York, Elsevier/North-Holland, 1980, 245–251.
Hayes HM Jr, Milne KL, Mandell CP: Epidemiological features of feline mammary carcinoma. Vet Rec 108 (1981) 476–479.
Hernandez FJ, Fernandez BB, Chertack M, Gage PA: Feline mammary carcinoma and progestogens. Feline Pract 5(5) (1975) 45–48.
Hess PW: Principles of cancer chemotherapy. Vet Clin North Am 7 (1977) 21–33.
Hess PW, MacEwen EG, McClelland AJ: Chemotherapy of canine and feline tumors. J Am Anim Hosp Assoc 12 (1976) 350–358.
Hinton M, Gaskell CJ: Non-neoplastic mammary hypertrophy in the cat associated either with pregnancy or with oral progestagen therapy. Vet Rec 100 (1977) 277–280.
Holland JF, Frei E III: Cancer Medicine. Philadelphia, Lea & Febiger, 1973.
Jeglum KA: The use of spontaneous feline neoplasms for studies of therapeutic agents. *In* Fidler IJ, White RJ (eds): Design of Models for Testing Cancer Therapeutic Agents. New York, Van Nostrand Reinhold Company, 1982, 193–205.
Johnson GF, Twedt DC: Endoscopy and laparoscopy in the diagnosis and management of neoplasia in small animals. Vet Clin North Am 7 (1977) 77–92.
Johnston SD, Hayden DW, Kiang DT, Handschin B, Johnson KH: Progesterone receptors in feline mammary adenocarcinomas. Am J Vet Res 75 (1984) 379–382.
Jones FJ, Yoshida LH, Ladiges WC, Kenny MA: Treatment of feline leukemia and reversal of FeLV by *ex vivo* removal of IgG: A preliminary report. Cancer 46 (1980) 675–684.
Kassel RL, Old LJ, Day NK, MacEwen EG, Hardy WD Jr: Plasma-mediated leukemia cell destruction: Current status. Blood Cells 3 (1977) 605–621.
Kirk RW (ed): Current Veterinary Therapy VII. Philadelphia, WB Saunders Company, 1980, 1320.
Lecky JH: Anesthesia and the immune system. Surg Clin North Am 55 (1975) 795–799.
Liska WD, MacEwen EG, Zaki FA, Garvey M: Feline systemic mastocytosis: a review and results of splenectomy in seven cases. J Am Anim Hosp Assoc 15 (1979) 589–597.
Liu S-K, Dorfman HD, Patnaik AK: Primary and secondary bone tumors in the cat. J Small Anim Pract 15 (1974) 141–156.
Lombard C: Les cancers et tumeurs du chat. Recl Méd Vét 116 (1940) 193–212.
MacEwen EG: Immunotherapy. *In* Kirk RW (ed): Current Veterinary Therapy VIII. Philadelphia, WB Saunders Company, 1983, 450–452.
MacEwen EG, Harvey HJ: Urinary tract neoplasia in dogs and cats. *In* Bojrab MJ (ed): Pathophysiology in Small Animal Surgery. Philadelphia, Lea & Febiger, 1981, 276–284.
MacEwen EG, Hayes AA, Mooney S, Patnaik AK, Harvey HJ, Passe S: Effect of levamisole on feline mammary cancer. J Biol Resp Modif 3 (1984a) 541–546.
MacEwen EG, Hayes AA, Harvey HJ, Patnaik AK, Passe S: Some prognostic factors for feline mammary tumors. J Am Vet Med Assoc 185 (1984b) 201–204.
MacEwen EG, Mooney S, Hayes AA, Patnaik AK, Harvey HJ, Hardy WD Jr: Combination chemotherapy of naturally occurring feline lymphosarcoma. Advances in Medical Oncology, Research and Education. Proc 12th Internat Cancer Cong Vol XII, Pergamon Press, 1979, 946–947.
Misdorp W, van der Heul RO: Tumors of bones and joints. Bull WHO 53 (1976) 265–282.
Nealon TF Jr, Russo EP: Surgical principles. *In* Horton J, Hill GF II (eds): Clinical Oncology. Philadelphia, WB Saunders Company, 1977, 103–125.
Old LJ, Boyse EA: Specific antigens of tumors and leukemia in experimental animals. Med Clin North Am 50 (1966) 901–912.
Owen LN (ed): T.N.M. Classification of Tumours in Domestic Animals. WHO, Geneva, 1981.
Owen LN: Cancer chemotherapy and immunotherapy. *In* Ettinger SJ (ed): Textbook of Veterinary Internal Medicine, 2nd ed. Philadelphia, WB Saunders Company, 1983, 368–392.
Park SK, Brodey JI, Wallace HA, Blakemore WS: Immunosuppressive effect of surgery. Lancet 1 (1971) 53–55.
Patnaik AK, Liu S-K, Hurvitz AI, McClelland AJ: Nonhematopoietic neoplasms in cats. J Natl Cancer Inst 54 (1975) 855–860.
Priester WA, McKay FW: The Occurrence of Tumors in Domestic Animals. Natl Cancer Inst Monogr 54, 1980.
Slade MS, Simmons RL, Yunis E, Greenberg LJ: Immunodepression after major surgery in normal patients. Surgery 78 (1975) 363–372.
Slusher R, Roenigk WJ, Wilson GP: Effects of x-irradiation on mastocytomas in dogs. J Am Vet Med Assoc 151 (1967) 1049–1054.
Smith PR, Thomas LB, Hilberg AW: Cancer cell contamination of operative wounds. Cancer 11 (1958) 53–62.
Symoens J, Rosenthal M: Levamisole in the modulation of the immune response: Current experimental and clinical state. J Reticuloendothel Soc 21 (1977) 175–221.
Terman DS, Yamamoto T, Mattioli M, Cook G, Tillquist R, Henry J, Poser R, Daskal Y: Extensive necrosis of spontaneous canine mammary adenocarcinoma after extracorporeal perfusion over Staphylococcus aureus Cowans I. J Immunol 124 (1980) 795–805.
Theilen GH: Veterinary medical oncology. *In* Ettinger SJ (ed): Textbook of Veterinary Internal Medicine. Philadelphia, WB Saunders Company, 1975, 127–149.
Theilen GH, Madewell BR: Chemotherapy. *In* Theilen GH, Madewell BR (eds): Veterinary Cancer Medicine. Philadelphia, Lea & Febiger, 1979a, 95–112.
Theilen GH, Madewell BR: Leukemia-sarcoma disease complex. *In* Theilen GH, Madewell BR (eds): Veterinary Cancer Medicine. Philadelphia, Lea & Febiger, 1979b, 204–241.
Theilen GH, Madewell Br: Tumors of the digestive tract. *In* Theilen GH, Madewell BR (eds): Veterinary Cancer Medicine. Philadelphia, Lea & Febiger, 1979c, 307–331.
Thiéry A: Épithélioma de la mamelle chez un chat castré. Recl Méd Vét 122 (1946) 258–261.
Tompkins MB, Cummins JM: Response of feline leukemia virus–induced non-regenerative anemia to oral administration of an interferon-containing preparation. Feline Pract 12 (3) (1982) 6–15.
Turrel JM, Pool RR: Primary bone tumors in the cat. A retrospective study of 15 cats and a literature review. Vet Radiol 23 (1982) 152–166.
Wagener DJT, Geestman E, Borgonjen A, Haanen C: The influence of splenectomy on cellular immunologic parameters in Hodgkin's disease. Cancer 37 (1976) 2212–2219.
Wagener DJT, Geestman E, Wessels HMC: The influence of splenectomy on the in vitro lymphocyte response to phytohemagglutinin and pokeweed mitogen in Hodgkin's disease. Cancer 36 (1975) 194–198.
Weijer K: Feline malignant mammary tumors. IV. Oestrogen receptors. *In* Weijer K (ed): Feline Mammary Tumors and Dysplasia. Oosthuizen, The Netherlands, Drukkerij Van der Molen, 1979, 51–54.
Weijer K, Hart AAM: Prognostic factors in feline mammary carcinoma. J Natl Cancer Inst 70 (1983) 709–716.
Weijer K, Head KW, Misdorp W, Hampe JF: Feline malignant mammary tumors. I. Morphology and biology: Some comparisons with human and canine mammary carcinomas. J Natl Cancer Inst 49 (1972) 1697–1704.
Whitehead JE: Neoplasia in the cat. Vet Med Small Anim Clin 62 (1967) 357–358.

**Radiation Therapy and Hyperthermia**

Bostock DE, Dye MT: Prognosis after surgical excision of fibrosarcomas in cats. J Am Vet Med Assoc 175 (1979) 727–728.

Brown NO, Patnaik AK, Mooney S, Hayes A, Harvey HJ, MacEwen EG: Soft tissue sarcomas in the cat. J Am Vet Med Assoc 173 (1978) 744–749.

Carlisle CH, Gould S: Response of squamous cell carcinoma of the nose of the cat to treatment with x-rays. Vet Radiol 23 (1982) 186–192.

Cotter SM: Oral pharyngeal neoplasms in the cat. J Am Anim Hosp Assoc 17 (1981) 917–920.

Dewhirst MW, Conner WG, Sim DA: Preliminary results of a phase III trial of spontaneous animal tumors to heat and/or radiation: Early normal tissue response and tumor volume influence on initial response. Int J Radiat Oncol Biol Phys 8 (1982) 1951–1961.

Feeney DA, Johnston GR: Abdominal radiotherapy. Vet Radiol 23 (1982) 197–202.

Feeney DA, Johnston GR: Radiation therapy: applications and availability. *In* Kirk RW (ed): Current Veterinary Therapy VIII. Philadelphia, WB Saunders Company, 1983, 428–434.

Fletcher GH: Basic principles of the combination of irradiation and surgery. Int J Radiat Oncol Biol Phys 5 (1979) 2091–2096.

Fletcher GH (ed): Textbook of Radiotherapy, 3rd ed. Philadelphia, Lea & Febiger, 1980.

Grier RL, Brewer WG, Theilen GH: Hyperthermic treatment of superficial tumors in cats and dogs. J Am Vet Med Assoc 177 (1980) 227–233.

Hall EJ: Radiobiology for the Radiologist, 2nd ed. Hagerstown, MD, Harper and Row, 1978.

Hayes A: Feline mammary gland tumors. Vet Clin North Am 7 (1977) 205–212.

Hilaris BS (ed): Handbook of Interstitial Brachytherapy. Acton, MA, Publishing Sciences Group, Inc, 1975.

Legendre AM, Carrig CB, Howard DR, Dade AW: Nasal tumor in a cat. J Am Vet Med Assoc 167 (1975) 481–483.

Legendre AM, Krahwinkel DJ, Spaulding KA: Feline nasal and paranasal sinus tumors. J Am Anim Hosp Assoc 17 (1981) 1038–1039.

Lord PF, Kapp DS: Hyperthermia and radiation therapy in cancer treatment. Vet Radiol 23 (1982) 203–210.

Lord PF, Kapp DS, Schwartz A, Morrow DT: Osteogenic sarcoma of the nasal cavity in a cat: Postoperative control with high dose-per-fraction radiation therapy and metronidazole. Vet Radiol 23 (1982) 23–26.

Macy DW, Reynolds HA: The incidence, characteristics and clinical management of skin tumors in cats. J Am Anim Hosp Assoc 17 (1981) 1026–1034.

Madewell BR, Ackerman N, Sesline DH: Invasive carcinoma radiographically mimicking primary bone cancer in the mandibles of two cats. Vet Radiol 17 (1976) 213–215.

Marmor JB, Pounds D, Hahn N, Hahn GM: Treating spontaneous tumors in dogs and cats by ultrasound-induced hyperthermia. Int J Radiat Oncol Biol Phys 4 (1978) 967–973.

Miller RC, Conner WG, Heusinkveld RS, Boone MLM: Prospects for hyperthermia in human cancer therapy. Part I. Hyperthermic effects in man and spontaneous animal tumors. Radiology 123 (1977) 489–495.

Northway RB: Hyperthermic treatment of tumors in small animals. Vet Med Small Anim Clin 77 (1982) 392–394.

Pool RR: Osteochondromatosis. *In* Bojrab MJ (ed): Pathophysiology in Small Animal Surgery. Philadelphia, Lea & Febiger, 1981, 641–649.

Steel GG, Peckham MJ: Exploitable mechanisms in combined radiotherapy-chemotherapy: The concept of additivity. Int J Radiat Oncol Biol Phys 5 (1979) 85–91.

Susaneck SJ: Nasal carcinoma in a cat. The Veterinary Cancer Society Newsletter 6 (4) (1982) 36–38.

Theran P, Holzworth J: Feline hyperthyroidism. *In* Kirk RW (ed): Current Veterinary Therapy VII. Philadelphia, WB Saunders Company, 1980, 998–999.

Turrel JM, Feldman EC, Hays M, Hornof WJ: Radioactive iodine therapy in cats with hyperthyroidism. J Am Vet Med Assoc 184 (1984) 554–559.

Turrel JM, Pool RR: Primary bone tumors in the cat: A retrospective study of 15 cats and a literature review. Vet Radiol 23 (1982) 152–166.

# 13
CHAPTER
# THE SKIN*

DANNY W. SCOTT

Although cats have undergone less evolutionary modification in basic structure and function than most animals, they have, through processes of natural selection, mutation, and human manipulation, achieved hair coats of unique variety and often striking beauty. In fact, hair coat to a great degree defines breed. Yet, with few exceptions, the skin beneath the coat is the same in all members of the species *Felis catus* and reacts similarly to harmful influences and agents of disease.

## NORMAL INTEGUMENT OF THE CAT

### GROSS ANATOMY AND PHYSIOLOGY

Important sources of information on the skin of cats are Baker (1974b), Conroy (1964), Jenkinson (1965), Jenkinson and Blackburn (1968), Kral and Schwartzman (1964), Kristensen (1975), Mann and Straile (1965), McCusker (1965), Muller et al. (1983), Ryder (1976), Scott (1980), Straile (1960), Strickland and Calhoun (1963), Swenson (1977), and Winkelmann (1957, 1960).

The cat has the thinnest skin among the domestic animals. Normal feline skin decreases in thickness from dorsal to ventral on the trunk and from proximal to distal on the limbs. It is thickest on the dorsal cervical (about 1.9 mm), lumbar, and sacral regions, and thinnest on the lateral surface of the lower hind leg (about 375 μ), thigh, and lower foreleg. Thus normal feline skin varies from about 0.4 to 2.0 mm in thickness.

Small (0.16 to 0.42 mm in diameter), hairless, knoblike enlargements are present in the haired skin. Now called tactile pads (NAV, 1983), they have been described in the literature by a variety of terms (tylotrich pad, "Haarscheibe," epidermal papilla, dermal papilla). Both dermis and epidermis contribute to the structure (see section on the microanatomy of hair).

The skin of the cat is quite pliable, especially over the neck and trunk. Skin over the dorsal cervical and lumbar areas is normally slow to return to its position when stretched and lifted. This must be kept in mind by the examiner estimating hydration by skin tone. The elasticity and loose attachment of the skin over much of the cat's body facilitate closure of large traumatic and surgical wounds.

The coat consists of stout primary (guard, outer coat) and shorter, more slender secondary (undercoat) hairs. Some breeders distinguish an intermediate (awn) hair (Robinson, 1977). Secondary hairs are far more numerous than primary hairs (10:1 dorsally, 24:1 ventrally) (Baker, 1974b). Both primary and secondary hairs are medullated. Lanugo, the fine, soft, wooly hair of fetuses and the newborn, is not medullated. Mean daily hair growth is about 295 μ for primary hairs and about 260 μ for secondary hairs.

The colors, length, and quality of the hair coat of both purebred and domestic (mixed) cats have been described in detail by Robinson (1977). The coat may be short or long. Short hair, the dominant genetic type, characterized the cat's African progenitor. The origin of the longhaired coat is uncertain. The majority of cats are nonpurebred shorthairs (domestic shorthairs, DSH); there are also a number of shorthaired purebreds (e.g., Siamese, Burmese, Abyssinian, Russian Blue, Manx, Rex, and American and British Shorthairs). Longhairs may be purebreds (e.g., Persian, Angora, Himalayan) or domestic (domestic longhairs, DLH).

The Rex breed, of which several variants have appeared in Europe and America (Robinson, 1977), has rows of curled hairs that are mostly secondary. The whiskers are crimped. It is questionable whether the Rex is hypoallergenic to people who are sensitive to cat dander, as is sometimes claimed; allergy to cats is now believed to result from feline saliva, not dander.

A dominant wirehair mutation appearing on a New York State farm gave rise to the American Wirehair

*The majority of the text and photographs in this chapter previously appeared in the *Journal of the American Animal Hospital Association*, 1980, and are appearing with the journal's gracious permission.

breed, in which the hairs are crimped and the longer hairs hooked at the end (Robinson, 1977).

Hairless mutants occur from time to time. Among recorded instances are a hairless Siamese (Letard, 1938) and a Mexican hairless (Mellen, 1939). The only hairless breed recognized by the cat fancy is the Sphinx (Canadian Hairless) (Robinson, 1973). These cats have greatly reduced hair coats with only a few guard hairs and essentially no secondary hairs.

Hospital and laboratory records often fail to describe cats accurately as to breed and color; hence statistics attempting to correlate disease incidence with breed or color must be critically evaluated.

Within the breeds and among individuals the hair coats can vary tremendously, some being thicker or softer than others. Among longhaired cats some coats mat readily, while others never mat. Whether a cat develops mats or not, daily grooming is desirable for both short- and longhairs to keep the coat sleek and to remove scurf as well as loose hair that may form hairballs in the digestive tract.

Coat color in cats is complex, but a few generalizations are possible (Muller et al., 1983; Robinson, 1977). Solid white is dominant over all colors, yet among domestic cats occurs least often, possibly because of associated lethal factors or because of owners' preferences. White spotting is governed by a separate gene. A geneticist studying gene frequencies observed that rural cats tend to be lighter colored than those in cities, New York having the largest proportion of dark cats (Todd, 1970). White is followed in order of dominance by black, tabby, and red (orange). Blue is a dilution of black, and cream a dilution of red. In the Siamese, seal point is the dominant gene, while blue point is recessive. Chocolate point is a dilution of seal point, and lilac point a dilution of blue point. Crossing Siamese with reds and tricolors has produced "color" points. Similar points are seen in Himalayans. One must read the publications of the cat fancy and attend shows to keep up with the color variations constantly developed by breeders and the new "breeds" produced by crosses or by cultivation of mutants.

Hair replacement in the cat is mosaic in pattern, unaffected by castration, and predominantly responsive to photoperiod (Baker, 1974b) and possibly ambient temperature. Normal outdoor cats in the northeast United States usually shed heavily in spring and fall. Normal indoor cats often shed noticeably all year.

Sudden excessive shedding of hair sometimes occurs when a cat is placed on a veterinarian's examination table, probably because of loss of telogen hairs when the arrectores pilorum muscles are activated by fright (Conroy, 1964).

Hair follicle activity is greatest in summer and least in winter. In summer, about 30 per cent of the primary hairs and about 50 per cent of the secondary hairs are in a resting state (telogen). In winter, these percentages increase to about 75 and 90, respectively. This must be kept in mind when one attempts to assess the ease of epilation of hairs: feline hairs are more easily epilated in the winter.

Skin surface lipids of the cat were studied by thin-layer chromatography (Lindholm et al., 1981; Nicolaides et al., 1968) and were found to contain more sterol esters, free cholesterol, and diester waxes, but fewer triglycerides, monoglycerides, free fatty acids, squalene, and monoester waxes than those of humans. It was suggested that the skin surface lipids of cats are mainly of epidermal origin, while those of humans are of sebaceous gland origin.

The pH of normal feline skin ranges from about 5.6 to 7.4 (average about 6.5) (Draize, 1942; Kral and Schwartzman, 1964; Kristensen, 1975) and is less acidic than that of man.

## Microscopic Anatomy and Physiology

Conspicuous microscopic features of feline skin generally are the thin epidermis, compound hair follicles, and dense dermis with its compacted collagen. Especially characteristic of the cat are the uniform cells of the sebaceous glands, which remind one of fried eggs. At high power, a striking feature is the appearance of the mast cells, which are oval or round with a central nucleus and cytoplasm that appears finely stippled owing to the presence of granules that stain faintly basophilic or eosinophilic. Microscopic features of the skin have been most extensively described by Baker (1974b), Calhoun (1964), and Strickland and Calhoun (1963).

### Epidermis

The epidermis consists primarily of keratinocytes, with a relatively small number of melanocytes. As many as five cellular layers may be recognized microscopically, depending on body area. The epidermis in haired skin consists of four distinct layers, the stratum lucidum usually being absent (Strickland and Calhoun, 1963). The epidermis is thin, ranging from 12 to 45 μ (average 25) and usually consists of two or three nucleated-cell layers. That of the prepuce and scrotum ranges in thickness from 70 to 60 μ. The thickest epidermis, in the footpads and planum nasale, measures up to 900 μ. The epidermis of the footpads of cats has a smooth surface, unlike that of dogs. Epidermal ridges (rete ridges, pegs) are not found at the dermo-epidermal junction in haired areas of normal cat skin but have been described in the footpads (Strickland and Calhoun, 1963).

The stratum corneum (the surface horny layer) consists of flattened, anuclear, eosinophilic keratinocytes and varies in thickness from 3 to 20 μ in haired skin. Thicker in lightly haired or glabrous skin, it is best developed in the footpads and planum nasale, where it ranges from 15 to 30 μ. The loose, "basket weave" appearance of the stratum corneum is an artifact of fixation and processing and is not seen in unprocessed sections cut by hand (Baker, 1974b). The dead keratinocytes constituting this layer form a protective surface and are continually sloughing as cells are pushed up from beneath. On the toes the stratum corneum forms a dense, hard claw surface, which is worn down by outdoor cats but needs clipping in indoor pets.

The stratum lucidum (clear layer) is a thin layer of flattened, anuclear cells containing a homogeneous hyaline material consisting of refractile droplets of eleidin, a substance related to keratin. It is usually present only in the epithelium of the footpads.

The stratum granulosum (granular layer) consists of nucleated, elliptical or spindle-shaped cells, with basophilic keratohyalin granules in their cytoplasm. This layer is usually discontinuous in haired skin where it is one cell thick, except around hair follicle openings (two to four cell layers). It is best developed in the footpads (four to eight cell layers) and the planum nasale (three to four cell layers).

The stratum spinosum (spiny layer, prickle-cell layer) consists of nucleated, lightly basophilic, polyhedral cells and is present in all skin. There are one or two cell layers in most hairy skin and up to 14 to 19 in the footpads. Intercellular bridges ("prickles") are less prominent in haired skin than in nonhaired skin.

The stratum basale (basal layer, stratum cylindricum) consists of one layer of nucleated, basophilic, slightly flattened, cuboidal or columnar cells, the flatter cells occurring in haired skin, the columnar in glabrous areas and tactile (tylotrich) pads. Mitotic figures may be present. The basement membrane zone is thin and indistinct in haired skin.

Two other terms now rarely used are stratum germinativum and stratum malpighii. They were applied in the past, with confusing inconsistency by various authors, to the deeper two or three layers alone or in combination.

Histochemical studies of normal feline epidermis have demonstrated distinct activity of oxidative enzymes in all layers except the stratum corneum (Jenkinson and Blackburn, 1968; see also other references in Scott, 1980). In addition, strong reactions for nonspecific esterases were demonstrated, especially in the stratum granulosum. Oxidative enzymes demonstrated were cytochrome oxidase, succinate dehydrogenase, malate dehydrogenase, isocitrate dehydrogenase, lactate dehydrogenase, glucose-6-phosphate-dehydrogenase, NADH, NADPH, and monoamine oxidase. Hydrolytic enzymes demonstrated were acid phosphatase, arylsulfatase, β-glucuronidase, and leucine aminopeptidase. Positive reactions for cholinesterases were not observed. Thus the enzyme pattern of normal cat epidermis shows only limited parallels to that of humans, especially in respect to esterase distribution.

## Pigment

Although melanocytes are present in haired skin in the cat, pigment tends to be concentrated in the hairs. Melanocytes (clear cells, dendritic cells) and the pigment (melanin) that they produce are most easily visualized in the epidermis of the lip, pinnae, eyelids, planum nasale, footpads, prepuce, scrotum, dorsal tail, teats, anal sac, circumanal area, umbilical skin of the fetus, and hair bulbs (Strickland and Calhoun, 1963; Baker, 1974b; Conroy, 1964). Melanophages are occasionally seen in the dermis of the scrotum (Strickland and Calhoun, 1963).

Depending on the color(s) of the coat, the eyelids, planum nasale, lips, and footpads may be unpigmented, moderately pigmented, or black. Especially striking is the mascara-like effect of the darkly pigmented eyelids of cats with chinchilla or silver coats. Tricolored and white-spotted ("piebald") cats may have bizarrely asymmetric areas of pigmentation of the eyelids, lips, and planum nasale.

As red, cream, and tricolored cats mature and age, they develop increasing numbers of freckle-like pigmented areas, starting as pinpoint dots, on the eyelids, lips, nose, ears, and footpads (Holzworth, 1983). These may first appear in cats as young as a year of age, coming and going like freckles before becoming permanently established. These dark, flat spots consist of a dense epidermal accumulation of melanin, which has been transferred to the keratinocytes from melanocytes that are heavily pigmented and present in normal numbers. Melanin in various concentrations can be seen in all layers of the epidermis, including desquamating keratinized cells as well as superficial dermal melanophages (Carpenter, 1983).

## Dermis

The dermis, many times thicker than the epidermis, is composed of collagenous, elastic, and reticular fibers, interstitial ground substance, various cells, nervous tissue, blood vessels, lymphatics, and arrector pili muscles. It is also the site of hair follicles, sweat glands, and sebaceous glands. Because the cat, like many other animals, lacks epidermal (rete) ridges formed by dermal papillae in haired skin, no clear division into papillary and reticular strata is present. The terms superficial and deep dermis will therefore be used. As described by Strickland and Calhoun (1963), the superficial dermis has fine collagenous fibers that are usually parallel to the epidermis, and a fine network of elastic fibers. The fibers of this layer interlace near the dermo-epidermal junction. The deep dermis has dense, irregularly arranged collagenous fibers about three times larger than those of the superficial dermis, as well as elastic fibers that extend in all directions and are more numerous than those of the superficial dermis. Small amounts of mucin, a blue-staining, granular- or stringy-appearing substance, are occasionally seen in the interstitial areas of the dermis, especially around appendages (Scott, 1980).

The normal feline dermis contains fibroblasts, mast cells, occasional perivascular mononuclear leukocytes, and a rare perivascular neutrophil or eosinophil (Scott, 1980). Mast cells are numerous, especially around superficial dermal blood vessels, and may range from 4 to 20 per high-power field (McCusker, 1965; Scott, 1980).

## Subcutis

The subcutis (hypodermis, panniculus adiposus) is composed of thick bands of collagenous fibers and abundant, smaller elastic fibers, which interweave and enclose the ample adipose tissue (Strickland and Calhoun, 1963).

## Hair

Hairs are dead keratin filaments. The free part of the hair, the hair shaft, consists of medulla, cortex, and cuticle. The medulla is composed of a cord of one to three longitudinal rows of flattened cells. The cells are solidly packed near the hair root but in the rest of the shaft are interspersed with air and glycogen vacuoles. The cortex consists of completely cornified, spindle-shaped cells with their long axis parallel to the hair shaft. These cells contain pigment, which gives the hair its color. Pigment may also be present in the medulla, but there it has little influence on the color of the hair. The cortex accounts for about a sixth to a quarter of the width of the hair. The hair cuticle is formed by flat, cornified, anuclear cells arranged like slates on a roof, the free edge of each cell facing the tip of the hair. Secondary hairs have a much narrower medullary cavity and a more obvious cuticle than primary hairs.

Hairs of the domestic animals, with their characteristically varied structures, are diagrammed schematically by Dellman and Brown (1976).

Hair follicles are described by Strickland and Calhoun (1963) as arranged in clusters of two, three, four, and five groups around a large, central primary (guard) hair follicle (Fig. 13–1). Clusters of two or three are more common on the back and of four to five are usual on the underside and lower limbs. Each lateral group of follicles usually contains three smaller primary hair follicles, surrounded by 6 to 12 secondary hair follicles. From 12 to 20 hairs emerge from a common opening. Dorsal oblique sections show eight or nine groups of hairs per $mm^2$, whereas sections from the underside and limbs show 12 to 16 groups per $mm^2$. All central primary hair follicles have their own sebaceous glands, apocrine sweat glands, and arrector pili muscle. Lateral primary hair follicles and secondary hair follicles, as a grouped fascicle, usually share common glands and arrector pili muscle.

The hair follicle is composed of five major parts: the dermal hair papilla, the hair matrix, the inner root sheath, the outer root sheath, and the dermal root sheath. The pluripotential cells of the hair matrix give rise to the hair and to the inner root sheath. The outer root sheath is continuous with the stratum spinosum of the epidermis. Hair follicles and the formation of hair are described in Dellman and Brown (1976) and by Trautmann and Fiebiger (1957).

Follicular folds described and pictured in the literature as involving the upper part of the inner root sheath of central primary hair follicles (e.g., Strickland and Calhoun, 1963; Dellmann and Brown, 1976) are thought to be artifacts of fixation and processing, as they are not seen in unprocessed sections cut by hand (Baker, 1974b).

Two specialized types of tactile hairs are present: sinus hairs and tylotrich hairs. Sinus hairs are present on the muzzle (whiskers), above the eyes, and as a small tuft of five or six hairs on the palmar surface of the carpus (pili carpales) associated with a tactile organ (Nilsson, 1970). These hairs are thick, stiff, and tapered distally. The cat's sinus hairs are described by Strickland and Calhoun (1963) as characterized by an endothelium-lined blood sinus interposed between the internal and external layers of the dermal root sheath. The sinus is divided into an upper nontrabecular ring or annular sinus and a lower cavernous or trabecular sinus. A cushion-like thickening of mesenchyme termed "sinus pad" ("Ringwulst") projects into the annular sinus. The large, smooth-walled sinus is about 900 μ in diameter. Above the annular sinus, a thick, circular continuation of the capsule, the conical body, encloses a sebaceous gland mass. The cavernous sinuses are traversed by trabeculae containing many nerve fibers. Skeletal muscle fibers attach to the outer layer of the follicle. Pacinian corpuscles are situated close to the sinus hair follicles. Sinus hairs are thought to function as slow-adapting mechanoreceptors.

Tylotrich hairs are scattered among ordinary hairs (Kristensen, 1975; Mann and Straile, 1965; Scott, 1980; Straile, 1960). Tylotrich hair follicles are larger than surrounding follicles and contain a single stout hair and an annular complex of neurovascular tissue that surrounds the follicle at the level of its sebaceous glands. The annular complex consists of several concentric structures. The inner component is a bilaminar arrangement of nerve fibers. This is encircled by the annulus, a connective tissue band composed of elongated cells and deeply eosinophilic fibers. Above and below the annulus are areas of randomly oriented, connective tissue–like cells. All these structures are surrounded by a thickened and highly vascularized area of the dermal root sheath. There is a large nerve at the side of each tylotrich follicle. Tylotrich hairs are thought to be rapid-adapting mechanoreceptors.

Each tylotrich follicle is associated with a tactile pad (tylotrich pad, integumentary papilla, "Haarscheibe," "touch spot," "touch corpuscle"), which is slightly raised, dome-shaped, 0.16 to 0.42 mm in diameter, and larger on the ventral than dorsal skin (Conroy, 1964; Kristensen, 1975; Mann and Straile, 1965; Scott, 1980; Straile, 1960). The tylotrich follicle opens slightly caudal, caudolateral, or, infrequently, rostral to the pad. The pads are composed of a thickened and distinctive epidermis underlain by a convex area of fine connective tissue that is highly

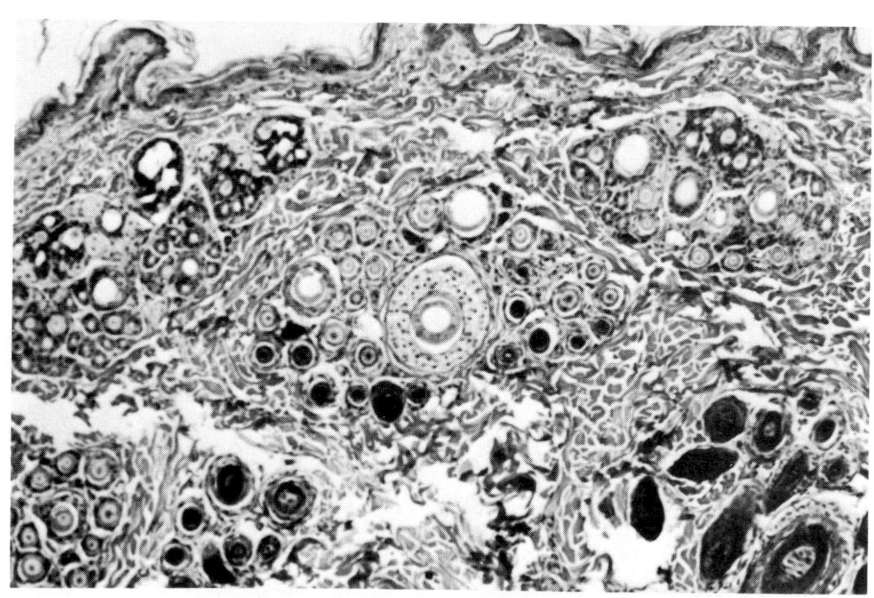

**Figure 13–1** Normal feline skin. The thin epidermis and compound follicle arrangement are characteristic. H & E.

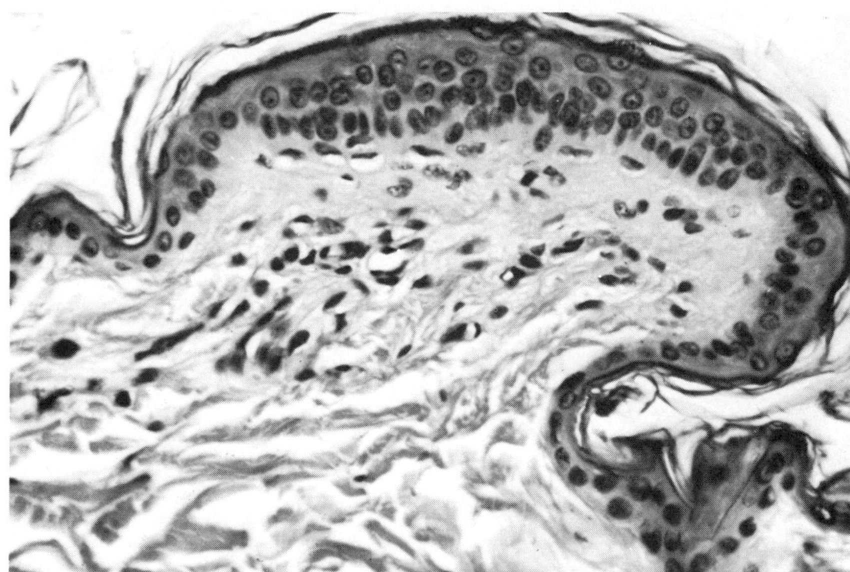

**Figure 13–2** Tactile (tylotrich) pad in normal feline skin. The epidermis is thicker over the pad, and the tactile (Merkel) cells lie below the basal cells of the epidermis (H & E). The tactile pad is occasionally mistaken for a pathologic change.

vascularized and well innervated (Fig. 13–2). The epidermis is about five cell layers thick. No adnexa are present, but there is a tuft of blood vessels, and a single myelinated nerve fiber enters the base of the pad and branches repeatedly in the dense connective tissue core. Within 10 μ of the epidermis, these nerve fibers become unmyelinated and end as tactile menisci (visible in methylene blue, silver impregnation, and electron microscopic preparations). Each meniscus is enclosed within a specialized cell in the basal cell layer of the epidermis. These cells, called tactile cells (of Merkel), serve as slow-adapting touch receptors. Histochemical investigations have revealed that feline Merkel cells are positive for neuron-specific enolase, suggesting that these cells may be of neuroendocrine origin (Gu et al., 1981).

## Sebaceous Glands

The sebaceous (holocrine) glands of the cat, as described by Strickland and Calhoun (1963), have a characteristic simple alveolar structure and are large and more numerous in certain areas. In most haired skin the glands range from 20 to 75 μ in diameter. Two or three empty by squamous epithelium-lined ducts into the upper part of the hair follicles around which they are clustered. Sebaceous glands are largest and most numerous in the lips (elongated and flask-shaped, 500 to 800 μ), chin ("submental organ", oval clusters, 800 μ) (Fig. 13–3), upper eyelids (tarsal, meibomian glands, oval clusters, 450 μ), dorsal aspect of the tail (caudal glands, oval clusters, 700 μ), prepuce (100 to 200 μ), and scrotum. Numerous large sebaceous glands are an important component of the wall of the anal sac. The circumanal glands are in part large sebaceous glands. Sebaceous glands are not found in footpads, and only rarely in other glabrous areas, where they open directly to the skin surface. Sebaceous glands do not appear to be innervated.

## Sweat Glands

Apocrine sweat glands are present in all haired skin. Saccular and coiled, 15 to 35 μ in diameter, they consist

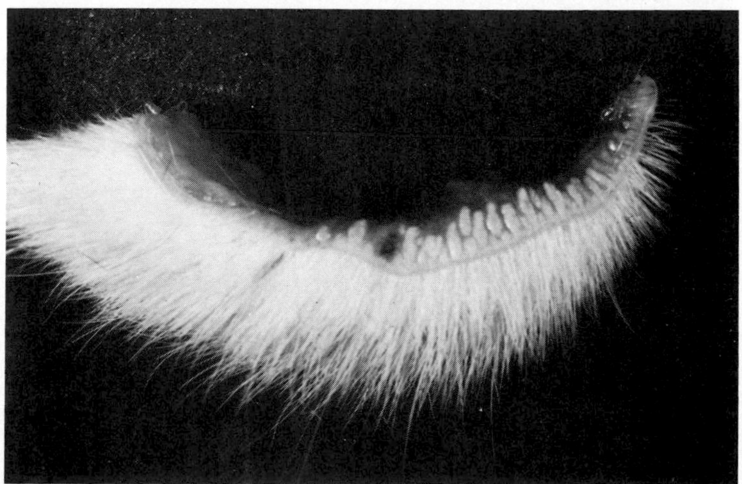

**Figure 13–3** Chin, normal skin, longitudinal section. Unstained, × 3. The pale, linear, palisading structures (upper edge of section) are sebaceous glands. They are so large that they can be seen grossly. In acne of the chin they become inflamed, and sometimes obstructing plugs of sebum and keratin lead to rupture.

of a single layer of flat or columnar epithelial (secretory) cells and a single layer of fusiform myoepithelial cells. Apocrine glands are larger (45 to 100 μ) in the lips, face, dorsal aspect of the tail, scrotum, and mucocutaneous areas. Their excretory ducts open into the upper part of the hair follicles around which they are clustered. Apocrine glands are absent from footpads and rare in other glabrous areas, where they open directly to the skin surface.

Histochemical studies of feline apocrine sweat glands (see references, Scott, 1980) demonstrated positive reactions for alkaline phosphatase and silver impregnation of the myoepithelial cells. Although apocrine glands respond to both cholinergic and adrenergic agents, histochemical preparations for cholinesterase show no nerves around most single glands in haired skin; however, glands in clusters are often surrounded by cholinesterase-reactive nerves.

Merocrine (eccrine) sweat glands occur only in the footpads. They are small (10 to 25 μ), extensively coiled, and composed of a single layer of cuboidal or columnar epithelial (secretory) cells and a single layer of fusiform myoepithelial cells. The intradermal segment of the duct consists of a double row of cuboidal epithelial cells. The duct opens directly on the footpad surface. These glands are not considered to have any temperature-regulating function (Muller et al., 1983).

Feline merocrine sweat glands and sweat have been studied by a number of workers (see references, Scott, 1980). Histochemical studies of the glands (Montagna, 1967, cited by Scott, 1980) showed positive reactions for cytochrome oxidase, succinic and other dehydrogenases, phosphorylases, and alkaline phosphatase. Secretory cells contain glycogen and some mucopolysaccharides. Merocrine glands are surrounded by nerves containing cholinesterase or pseudocholinesterase, and respond most sensitively to cholinergic agents and less so to adrenergic agents. However, when denervated, the glands retain their morphologic integrity for longer periods and continue to respond to stimulation. Nervous cats, as clinicians know, leave damp footprints on the examining table (Muller et al., 1983).

Atropine blocks merocrine gland responses to nerve stimulation. Feline merocrine sweat contains lactate, glucose, sodium, potassium, chloride, and bicarbonate. It differs from that of humans in that it is hypertonic and alkaline and contains much higher concentrations of sodium, potassium, and chloride.

## Arrector Pili Muscles

Arrector pili muscles are smooth muscle. Present in all haired skin, they are most highly developed in the lumbar, sacral, and dorsal tail regions (Strickland and Calhoun, 1963). They are about a fourth to a half the diameter of central primary hair follicles in most haired skin but of equal diameter in lumbar, sacral, and dorsal tail areas (Scott, 1980). Overall, they range in diameter from 25 to 220 μ at their attachment to the hair follicle (Strickland and Calhoun, 1963). They originate in the superficial dermis and insert on the bulge of the hair follicle. They receive cholinergic innervation, and intradermal administration of epinephrine, as well as release of adrenalin in fright or rage, evokes piloerection.

## Vessels of the Skin

Blood vessels arising from cutaneous arteries are arranged in three distinct intercommunicating plexuses of arteries and veins. The deep (subcutaneous) plexus is situated at the interface of the dermis and subcutis, with branches descending into the subcutis and ascending to supply the lower parts of the hair follicles and the apocrine sweat glands. The ascending vessels continue upward to form the middle plexus, which lies at the level of the sebaceous glands. This plexus sends branches to the arrector pili muscles, ascending and descending branches to the middle parts of the hair follicles and the sebaceous glands, and ascending branches to form the superficial plexus. Capillary loops just under the epidermis emanate from the superficial plexus, are arranged parallel to the skin surface, and supply the epidermis and upper parts of the hair follicles.

Lymphatic vessels arise from capillary networks that lie in the superficial dermis and surround the adnexa. They drain into a subcutaneous lymphatic plexus. Lymphatics are not usually visible in routine histologic preparations of normal cat skin.

## Nerves of the Skin

The innervation of the cat's skin has been extensively studied (Jenkinson and Blackburn, 1968; Kristensen, 1975; Maruhashi et al., 1952; Strickland and Calhoun, 1963; Swenson, 1977; Winkelmann, 1957, 1960; see also references, Scott, 1980). In general, nerve fibers are associated with blood vessels (providing dual autonomic innervation of arteries), various cutaneous end organs (tactile [tylotrich] pad, pacinian corpuscle, Meissner corpuscle, tactile corpuscle [of Merkel]), some apocrine sweat glands, merocrine sweat glands, arrector pili muscles, and hair follicles. They occur as a subepidermal plexus, some fine fibers of which enter the epidermis, wind through the stratum basale and stratum spinosum, and end as irregular condensations in the stratum granulosum and stratum corneum.

Cutaneous afferent nerve fibers, classified by Maruhashi et al. (1952), mediate sensations of touch, pressure, pain, scratching, cold, heat, and all kinds of mechanical stimuli. Studies on thermoreceptors and thermal nociceptors in cat skin revealed two distinct types of receptors: one for cold and one for heat (Iggo and Young, 1975; see also references, Scott, 1984). The sensitivity of cutaneous nociceptors and mechanoreceptors was shown to be increased by prior heating or by prior injections of histamine, histamine liberator 48/80, or bradykinin (Lynn, 1977; see also references, Scott, 1984).

The organization of tactile dermatomes in cat skin was described by DeBoer (1916), Kuhn (1953), and Hekmatpanah (1961).

## Histamine

Skin histamine levels in normal cats varied from 2.2 to 37.5 μg/gm and showed great regional variation (highest on the underside, lowest on the back) (McCusker, 1965; see also references, Scott, 1980). Skin histamine levels declined when cats were fed low-protein diets or daily supplements of chlortetracycline or both. It was suggested that skin histamine levels are diet-related in the cat, decarboxylation of the histidine occurring with meat diets. After administration of Compound 48/80 skin histamine was depleted for about 110 days (see references, Scott, 1980). Failure to detect histamine formation in vitro suggested that most of the histamine present in cat skin is not formed there.

### Senile Changes

After about nine years of age, normal cats often exhibit certain histologic changes in the skin (Scott, 1980). Varying degrees of hyperkeratosis and follicular keratosis are common. Occasional atrophic follicles and granular, fragmented collagen fibers may be seen. Sebaceous glands may occasionally appear atrophied and vacuolated. Occasional arrector pili muscles may appear fragmented and more vacuolated and eosinophilic than normal.

### Partial Preauricular "Alopecia"

Sparseness of the hair on the temples is normal in many cats and is unrelated to breed, sex, or age (Conroy, 1964). It is occasionally mistaken by owners for a sign of skin disease.

## DISORDERS OF THE SKIN

Data on incidence of feline skin disease are meager (Scott, 1980). At the New York State College of Veterinary Medicine the breeds of cats most frequently seen in the hospital population were domestic (mixed) (75 per cent) and Siamese (7.7 per cent). Siamese were seen less often for skin disease than would have been expected on the basis of their proportion in the hospital population. The sex ratio in the hospital cat population was equal. Neither sex exhibited a predilection for skin disease, nor did neutering appear to be a predisposing factor, except in the case of endocrine alopecia. The increasing risk of skin disease in cats over the age of six years was mostly attributable to neoplasia.

The most common feline skin disorders in order of frequency were (1) abscess or cellulitis, (2) flea infestation, (3) miliary dermatitis other than that attributable to fleas, (4) dermatophytosis, (5) eosinophilic granuloma complex, (6) seborrhea complex, (7) neoplasia, (8) psychogenic alopecia and dermatitis, (9) endocrine alopecia, and (10) acne of the chin.

### History and Physical Examination

No matter how simple a skin disorder may appear, a complete medical history, including information on a cat's life style, environment, and diet, should be taken. A thorough general examination should also be performed. In many cases these two procedures elicit clues that skin lesions alone may not provide. Scrapings, smears for staining, culturing and sensitivity testing, and biopsy are indicated far more often than many veterinarians use them. The sooner an accurate diagnosis is made, the less time and money will be wasted on ineffective, empirical measures.

These procedures are described in detail by Muller et al., 1983.

### Congenital and Hereditary Disorders

### Cutaneous Asthenia

Cutaneous asthenia embraces a number of hereditary, congenital disorders of connective tissue characterized by fragility and hyperextensibility of the skin. It resembles the Ehlers-Danlos syndrome of man, in whom at least eight forms are recognized, each with distinct clinical and pathologic features and all thought to result from defects in the metabolism of collagen. The mode of inheritance may be dominant or recessive, sometimes with sex-linkage.

In the cat, cutaneous asthenia, variously referred to as Ehlers-Danlos syndrome, "rubber kitten" syndrome, "torn skin," dermatosparaxis, hereditary fragility and hyperextensibility of the skin, is rare (Butler, 1975; Counts et al., 1979, 1980; Patterson and Minor, 1977; Scott, 1974, 1980). One form appears to be an abnormality of packing of collagen fibrils, with autosomal dominant inheritance (Patterson and Minor, 1977). Another form is associated with deficient procollagen peptidase activity (Counts et al., 1979, 1980).

Cats with cutaneous asthenia have fragile, abnormally stretchy skin that is easily and frequently torn (Fig. 13–4). Restraint, clipping, and venepuncture often result in extensive gaping tears ("fish-mouth" wounds) with minimal bleeding. The skin is often velvety, resembling chicken skin and crisscrossed with thin white scars.

The diagnosis is confirmed by histologic findings reflecting the different abnormalities characteristic of cutaneous asthenia. One study (Scott, 1974) reported epidermal atrophy, normal adnexa, dermal thinning, and disorientation, irregularity, and fragmentation of dermal collagen (Fig. 13–5). Another (Butler, 1975) described a marked deficiency of mature dermal collagen and excessive mucopolysaccharide ground substances. Collagen structure and linkage were normal on electron microscopic examination. Other workers (Patterson and Minor, 1977) reported no abnormalities on light microscopic examination, but electron microscopic examination disclosed disorganized packing of collagen fibrils, as well as collagen fibrils of different diameters (small, 56 nm, and large, 120 nm), whereas normal cats have one size of fibrils (76 ± 2 nm). The same workers demonstrated a stress modulus of 0.86 per square inch (psi) and breaking at 112.9 psi in affected cats, compared with 5.65 and 1440.1 psi, respectively, for normal cats. In the recessive form of cutaneous asthenia identified in a Himalayan cat, electron microscopic studies disclosed disorganization of collagen fiber bundles in the dermis (Holbrook et al., 1980; see also electron micrographs, Muller et al., 1983).

Affected cats, if they are to survive, must lead sheltered lives, with protection from injury. Injections should be given with small-gauge needles. Such cats may need to be surgically declawed, as even normal scratching may lacerate the skin. These cats should not be used for breeding.

### Aplasia Cutis

Aplasia cutis (epitheliogenesis imperfecta) is rare in cats (Austin, 1975a; Munday, 1970). The epidermis is congenitally absent in certain areas of skin. The hereditary aspects of this disease in cats have not been studied. Affected kittens may be presented with ulcers of the skin

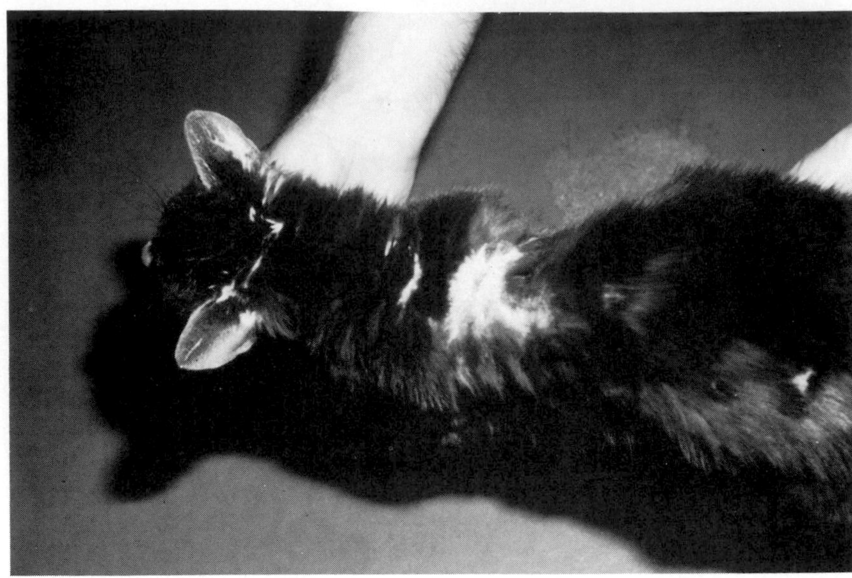

**Figure 13–4** Cutaneous asthenia. Multifocal alopecia and scarring.

or mucosae or both. The ulcers are usually secondarily infected, and kittens either die from septicemia or are eaten by the queen. Histologic examination reveals absence of the epidermis and usually of adnexa. Attempts at treatment usually fail, although small defects may be amenable to skin grafting. Breeding of surviving cats or cats that have produced affected kittens should be discouraged.

## Alopecia Universalis

Alopecia universalis is a rare hereditary disorder in cats (Austin, 1975a; Conroy, 1979; Muller et al., 1983; Robinson, 1973). It has been selectively bred for, the cats being referred to by breeders as Sphinx or Canadian Hairless. Affected cats have little or no hair except for a few short facial hairs and whiskers. The skin usually feels oily and has a rancid odor. Gray-black lipid deposits collect in the nail folds. Histologic examination reveals acanthosis and complete absence of primary hairs and follicles. Secondary follicles are few and lack well-formed bulbs. Sebaceous and apocrine glands open directly onto the surface of the skin. An antiseborrheic shampoo used once or twice weekly controls the greasiness and odor.

## Hypotrichosis

Hereditary hypotrichosis has been reported in Siamese (Letard, 1938; Scott, 1980). The condition is an autosomal recessive trait. Affected cats have thin, downy hair at

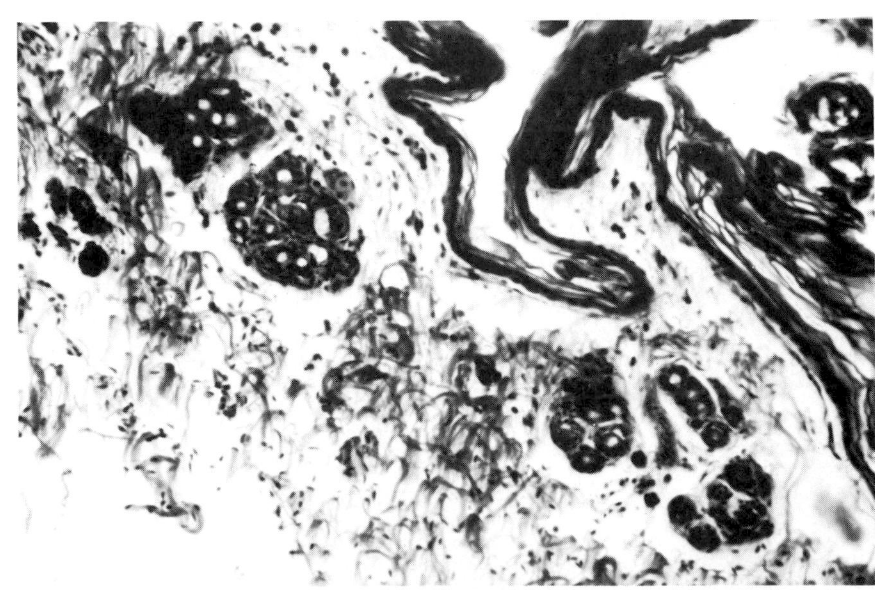

**Figure 13–5** Cutaneous asthenia. Fragmentation and disorientation of collagen. H & E.

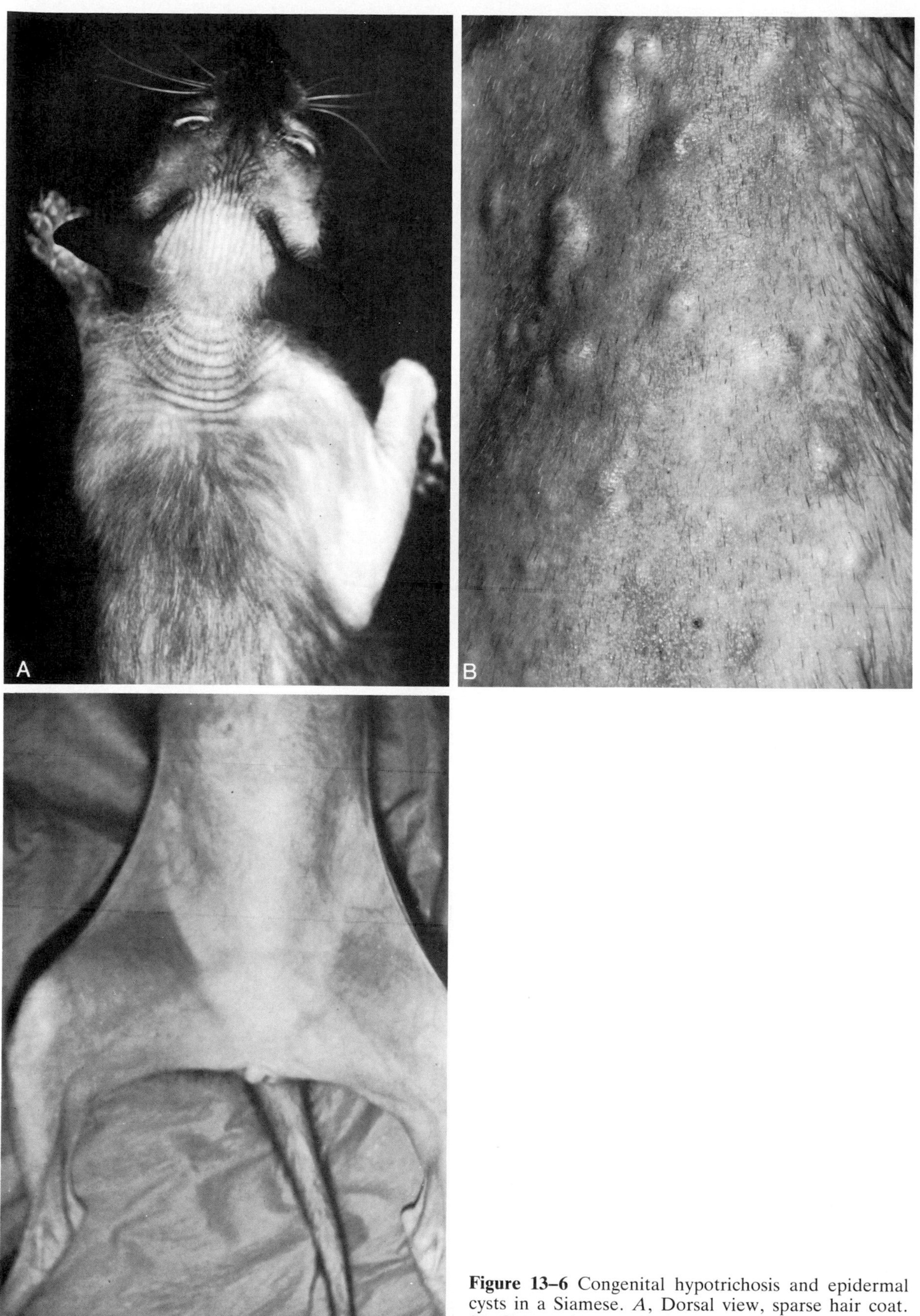


**Figure 13–6** Congenital hypotrichosis and epidermal cysts in a Siamese. *A*, Dorsal view, sparse hair coat. *B*, Closer view, multiple cysts. *C*, Alopecia of the abdomen and underside of the tail. (Courtesy Angell Memorial Animal Hospital.)

birth but are bald by 10 to 14 days of age. Some regrowth occurs by 8 to 10 weeks of age (Fig. 13–6), but total and permanent alopecia returns by about six months. A few secondary (down) hairs may remain and come and go according to season. Histologic examination reveals small, poorly developed primary hair follicles, most of which are in telogen and devoid of hair (Fig. 13–7). Secondary hair follicles are few or absent. There is no effective treatment. Affected cats and their relatives should not be bred.

Hereditary hypotrichosis has also been reported in the Devon Rex (Thoday, 1981).

## Chédiak-Higashi Syndrome

The Chédiak-Higashi syndrome (oculocutaneous albinism) is an autosomal recessive disorder reported in blue smoke Persians with light yellow or green irides and lighter than normal hair color (Kramer et al., 1977; Prieur et al., 1979). It is characterized by abnormally large melanin granules in the hair shafts, cataracts, hypopigmentation of the retina, photophobia, a bleeding tendency, an increased susceptibility to infection, and large eosinophilic granules in the cytoplasm of many neutrophils and occasional monocytes and lymphocytes. Microscopic examination of unstained hairs reveals large, elongated, irregular clumps of melanin. Melanin granules are much larger than normal but markedly decreased in number in the skin, hair follicles, and newly formed hair.

## Fetal Dermatitis

Fetal dermatitis of newborn kittens has been attributed to mycotic abortion and in-utero bacterial infections (Austin, 1975a). Details were not given.

# Disorders Caused by Physical or Chemical Agents

## Contact Dermatitis

Contact dermatitis (dermatitis venenata) is uncommon in cats (see references, Scott, 1980) and has no breed, age, or sex predilection. Most cases are caused by primary irritants such as flea collars, insecticides, kerosene, turpentine, paint, tars, phenols, cresols, various soaps, oils, and greases, highly chlorinated water, iodine compounds, quaternary ammonium compounds, naphthols, fertilizers, acids, salt, benzoyl peroxide, and various other topical medicaments.

Allergic contact dermatitis must be extremely rare in cats (see section on immunologic disorders). Cats are poorly and inconsistently responsive to experimental allergic contact dermatitis (Schultz and Adams, 1978; Scott, 1980), and naturally occurring instances have not been reported.

Signs of primary irritant contact dermatitis include varying degrees of inflammation (from mild erythema without pruritus to pigmentary changes and severe pruritic, papulovesicular eruptions, sometimes with necrosis and slough) in relatively glabrous areas such as the abdomen, medial thighs, axillae, perineum, footpads, ventral tail, chin, and pinnae. Contact dermatitis does not involve haired areas unless the contactant is in liquid or aerosol form.

Diagnosis is often by history, physical examination, and skin biopsy, but provocative exposure may be required. Microscopic characteristics are varying degrees of epidermal vesiculation, necrolysis, and ulceration with a predominantly neutrophilic response (Scott, 1980).

Measures to remove the irritant vary with the offending material. Gentle cleansing with warm water soaks or mild soap sometimes suffices. Symptomatic topical and systemic medicaments (glucocorticoids, antibiotics) may be indicated.

Exposure to road tars, asphalt, and paints deserves special comment. These substances can cause severe irritation and dermatitis if allowed to remain in contact with the skin. In addition, systemic poisoning can occur if a significant amount is swallowed owing to the cat's fastidious attempts to clean itself. If the offending material has dried, affected areas may often be clipped. Otherwise they should be soaked with vegetable oil, preferably by packing the areas in the oil for 24 hours. The oil softens tars and asphalt. The material may then be wiped off and

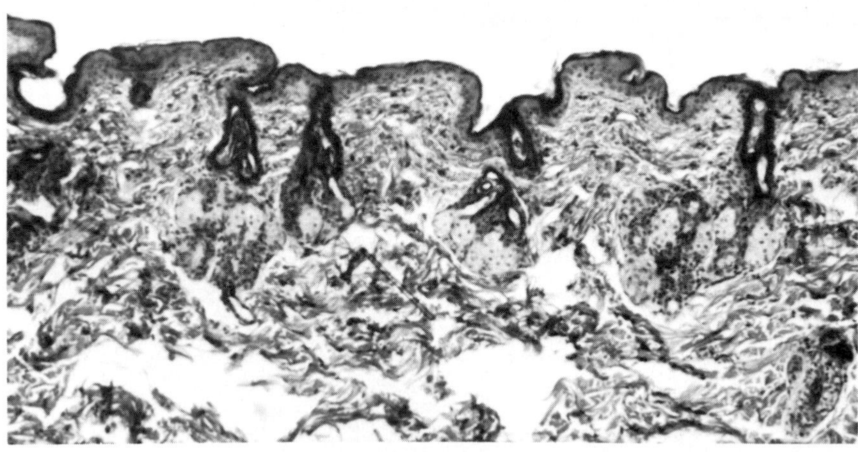

**Figure 13–7** Hypotrichosis in a Siamese. The hair follicles are poorly developed. H & E.

the cat bathed in a gentle, cleansing soap. Vegetable oil applications can be repeated if needed. Paint removers or organic solvents (e.g., kerosene, turpentine, gasoline) should never be used, for they are very irritating and may produce systemic poisoning.

Flea-collar dermatitis occurs occasionally (e.g., Bell et al., 1975; Doering, 1976; Muller, 1970, 1974b; Scott, 1980; Seawright and Costigan, 1977) and has also been reproduced in cats under experimental conditions (Bell et al., 1975). The vast majority of these cutaneous reactions represent primary irritant contact dermatitis associated with the insecticide within the collar (usually an organophosphate, especially dichlorvos; occasionally a carbamate). Flea medallions may also be offenders. It has been suggested that a small percentage of these reactions may be of allergic nature (Type IV hypersensitivity) (Muller, 1970, 1974b).

The prevalence of flea-collar dermatitis has been the subject of conflicting testimony. Most authors have stated that the incidence of skin irritations is low in proportion to the numbers of collars in use (e.g., Allen et al., 1978; Fox et al., 1969; Kodama et al., 1976; see also references, Scott, 1980). A few authors consider flea-collar dermatitis to be more common (e.g., Bell et al., 1975).

Under experimental conditions of high heat, low humidity, poor ventilation, and close confinement, cervical dermatitis, ataxia and depression, and death occurred in 74 per cent, 42 per cent, and 10 per cent, respectively, of 50 cats wearing dichlorvos flea collars (Bell et al., 1975). Other workers seriously questioned the applicability and even the validity of these findings (Allen et al., 1978; Fox et al., 1969; Kodama et al., 1976; Muller, 1970, 1974b; Scott, 1980; Seawright and Costigan, 1977). Factors thought to increase susceptibility to the flea collar–related toxicity are warm ambient temperature, low relative humidity, poor ventilation, and small body size.

Clinical signs attributable to flea collars include dermatitis under the collar varying from mild erythema and pruritus to severe papulocrustous, edematous, alopecic, ulcerated, painful eruptions. Secondary pyoderma may occur. Severely affected cats may develop generalized cutaneous eruptions, as well as constitutional signs (depression, lethargy, anorexia, fever).

Diagnosis is by history, physical examination, and response to therapy. Skin biopsy reveals varying degrees of subacute or chronic nonsuppurative dermatitis, with neutrophils predominating, and frequent epidermal vesication and necrolysis (Scott, 1980).

The collar should be removed and the hair clipped from severely affected areas, which are then treated with a wet astringent or antiseptic dressing. A topical or systemic glucocorticoid may be needed. An antibiotic is indicated for secondary infection. Healing of severe eruptions may require months. Occasionally a cat dies despite treatment.

Many suggestions for preventing flea-collar dermatitis have been offered (e.g., Doering and Jensen, 1973; Muller, 1970). The most important preventive measure would seem to be proper fit. The collar should be as loose as possible to minimize direct skin contact, but not so loose that the cat can get the collar caught on its lower jaw or on objects in its environment. It should be possible to fit two or three fingers under the collar when it is in place. Any extra length should be trimmed off. The cat should not be exposed to other agents containing organophosphates for seven days before or after a flea collar is put on or removed. The collars should not be used on sick, debilitated, convalescent, pregnant, or nursing cats, or on cats under three or four months of age.

Suggestions to "air out" collars for one to three days before applying them to cats are hard to evaluate without controlled studies. Wetting does not appear to increase the likelihood of irritation but does decrease the insecticidal power of the collar. The owner should be told to inspect the skin under the collar twice weekly and to remove the collar at the first sign of any reaction such as skin irritation, vomiting, or ataxia.

The warning not to use flea collars on Persian cats is not substantiated by published data. In fact, the long hair of the Persian should protect the neck rather than predispose it to irritation. One controlled study with both domestic shorthairs and Persians showed no increased incidence of irritation in the Persians (Fox et al., 1969).

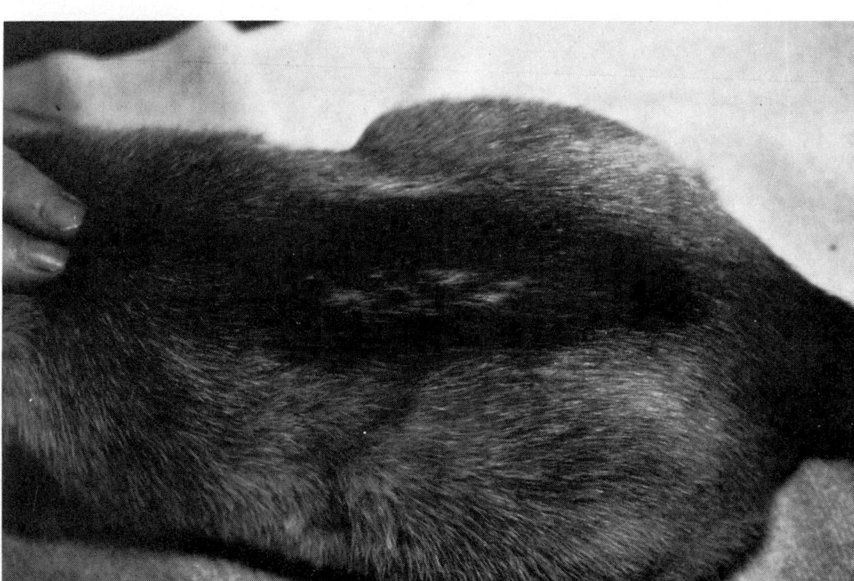

**Figure 13–8** Regrowth of darker hairs in a Siamese with psychogenic alopecia.

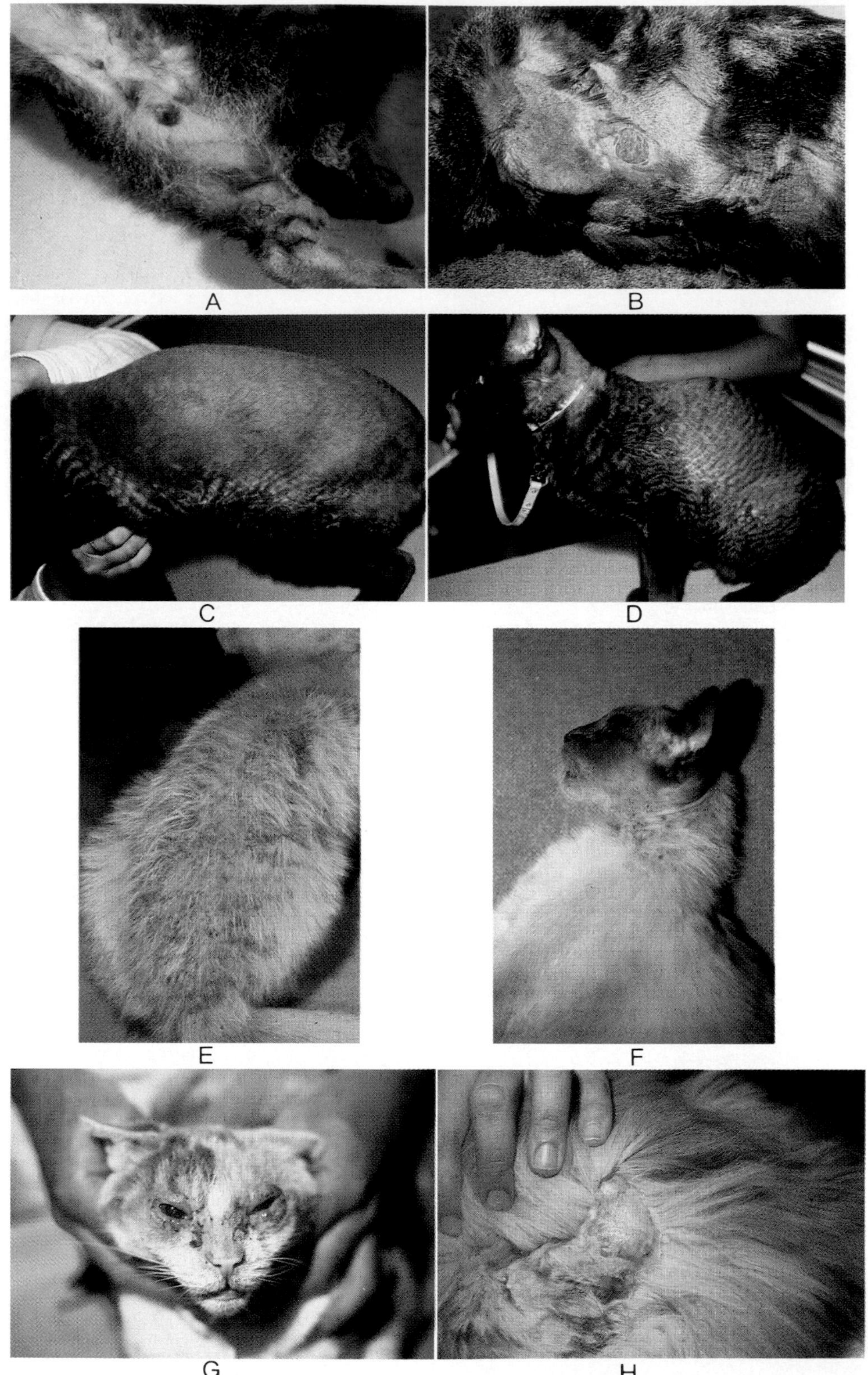


**Plate 13–1** *A*, Contact dermatitis of the perineum, underside of the tail, and hindleg associated with chronic discharge from the anal sacs. *B*, Experimentally induced hyperglucocorticoidism. The thin skin was easily bruised and torn during clipping. *C*, Hypothyroidism in a Rex cat. Alopecia of the trunk was associated with low levels of $T_4$ and $T_3$. *D*, Same cat. The hair is regrowing after 10 weeks of treatment with 0.1 mg levo-thyroxine b.i.d. *E*, Flea allergy. Severe erythema and alopecia of the back. *F*, Flea allergy. Papulocrustous dermatitis of the head and neck. *G*, Food allergy. Severe erythema, edema, and excoriation of the face are characteristic. *H*, Toxic epidermal necrolysis due to ampicillin drug eruption. An epidermal collarette surrounds the ulcer. (*A*, Courtesy Angell Memorial Animal Hospital. *C* and *D*, Courtesy Dr. Barbara S. Stein.)

Discharge from the anal sacs may cause a contact dermatitis characterized by multifocal areas of alopecia, erythema, excoriation, and hyperpigmentation on the perineum, underside of the tail, and hindlimbs (Plate 13–1*A*).

## Temperature-Dependent Changes in Hair Color

Many practitioners have noticed that the hair of a Siamese shaved for surgery or with psychogenic alopecia grows back darker (Fig. 13–8), that hair grows back lighter in the area of a previous abscess (Fig. 13–9), and that the coats of Siamese cats are darker in colder climates.

Siamese kittens are born white and develop adult "points" under the influence of external temperature. It is believed that the ability of certain parts of the coat to form pigment is hereditary (Iljin and Iljin, 1930; Innes, 1973). The same workers concluded that (1) Siamese coat color appears to be influenced by external temperature, high temperatures producing light hairs, and low temperatures producing dark hairs; (2) coat color is also influenced by physiologic factors determining heat production and loss; and (3) these phenomena appear to be associated with a temperature-dependent enzyme involved in melanin synthesis.

The coat color changes associated with various external and internal influences on heat loss and production are usually temporary. The coat usually returns to its normal color with the next hair cycle, if the temperature influences are remedied.

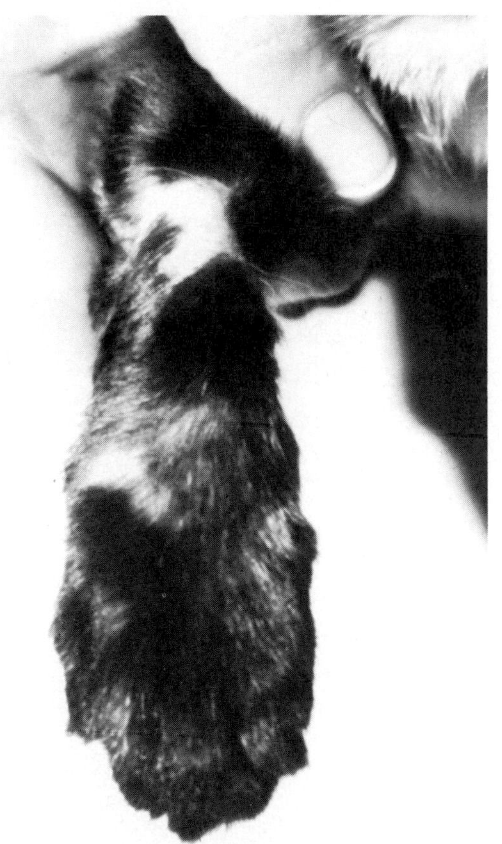

**Figure 13–9** Regrowth of lighter hairs in a Siamese with systemic lupus erythematosus.

## Burns

Burns of varying severity are occasionally caused by hot water or hot cooking oils accidentally spilled on cats (Mather, 1964; Thornton, 1963). Burned areas, characteristically on the back and extending down the sides, may for a time be concealed by the cat's thick coat. Burned feet and tails are frequent in cats that walk about on kitchen counters and stoves, and playful chewing on electric cords and wires may result in a badly burned mouth. Thanks to the protection of their thick coats, cats trapped in burning buildings sometimes survive miraculously with burns limited to the footpads, face, and ears.

A burn is treated by clipping of the fur and, if discovered within 2 hours, by cooling of the skin with ice packs or cold compresses. Silver sulfadiazine cream (Silvadene, Marion Laboratories) is an excellent antibacterial for topical application. If the area lends itself to bandaging, a light dressing may be applied, to be changed twice a day; otherwise, an Elizabethan collar should be put on the cat to prevent licking. Systemic antibiotics are ineffective for preventing local burn wound infections. Devitalized tissue must be débrided or removed by gentle bathing. Large defects in feline skin heal in remarkably by granulation and contraction, but areas of scar tissue or white fur may permanently mark the site of the burn. Extensive burns may require skin grafting.

With severe burns, treatment of shock and prevention of kidney and liver damage are of primary concern.

## Frostbite

Frostbite is rare in healthy, well-nourished cats. Well-acclimated, longhaired animals can tolerate exposure to −50 C (−58 F) for an indefinite time provided food and caloric intake are adequate (Dieterich, 1977). However, frostbite occurs occasionally in outdoor cats during the winter in the colder regions of the United States (Aronson, 1975; Dieterich, 1977; Mather, 1974b; Scott, 1980). The tips of the ears and, less often, the tip of the tail are affected. Signs of mild frostbite are scaling and alopecia of the ear tips, and the hair may be temporarily or permanently whitened. In more severe cases, the ear tips become necrotic and leathery and slough, so that after healing the margin is scarred and contracted.

Treatment is not usually needed for mild frostbite. If the cat is seen early and damage is not too severe, gentle, rapid thawing with warm water (38 to 44 C) (100 to 111 F) is indicated as soon as possible after it is known that refreezing can be prevented. Warming may be followed by application of a bland, protective ointment or cream (e.g., Vaseline or cod liver oil ointment) if needed. Severe cases with necrosis and slough are treated symptomatically with frequent water soaks and gentle cleansing with a germicide (e.g., chlorhexidine). A systemic antibiotic is indicated only for serious secondary infection. Surgical excision is postponed until a clear boundary between live and dead tissue is evident. Once frozen, tissues may have increased susceptibility to injury from cold.

## Hair Mats

Matting of hair is common in longhairs, especially behind the ears, on the underside, and on the backs of the hindlegs. Matting also occurs in obese or arthritic cats that are unable to groom themselves. If the cat is willing, small mats can usually be slit with a knife, teased apart with a comb, and combed out. If the mats are extensive or the cat cantankerous, sedation may be required. Patient and skillful grooming removes most mats. Clipping should be a last resort. Prevention of mats in longhairs requires daily combing and brushing. Shorthairs also should be brushed daily.

## Solar (Actinic) Dermatitis

Solar dermatitis occurs mainly in white cats or cats with white ears or faces (e.g., Moulton, 1961; Scott, 1980; Stannard, 1974). Porphyrin metabolism in affected cats is normal (Irving et al., 1982). The initial sign is mild erythema of the tips and margins of the pinnae and occasionally of the eyelids, nose, and lips. As dermatitis of the ear becomes more severe, alopecia, scaling, crusting, and pruritus develop along with curling of the ear margin. These lesions tend to be exacerbated during the summer and regress during the winter but worsen progressively each summer until squamous cell carcinoma develops. The most consistent indicator of malignant transformation is persistent ulceration. Although squamous cell carcinoma can develop in cats as young as three years of age, most are over seven. At an early, precancerous stage protection from sunlight and application of a sun screen preparation may bring about complete regression. Active carotenoids administered orally may also be useful in treatment (Irving et al., 1982). Well-established lesions should be generously excised. Otherwise, the tumor gradually eats away the pinna and may metastasize to regional nodes. Metastasis to distant areas occurs occasionally (see chapter on tumors).

## Thallium Poisoning

Thallium poisoning has occasionally been reported in cats (Aronson, 1975, 1977; Pile, 1956; Zook et al., 1968) but is now unlikely, as use of thallium pesticides was strictly limited in the United States in the late 1960s. Striking cutaneous signs appear to be characteristic of subacute or chronic poisoning and develop concurrently with, or several days after, constitutional signs appear (Zook et al., 1968). Usually the lips and sometimes the pinnae become progressively reddened, thickened, and crusty. The eyelids may be similarly affected. As the skin lesions evolve, a thin, dry, superficial epidermal layer cracks and loosens. This is shed or can be easily peeled away, together with the hair, leaving oozing areas of denuded skin. In cats living long enough, the same sequence of changes involves most of the body, including the footpads. Topical treatment appears to be of little value. Of 13 cats with skin lesions, the two that survived were cats that continued to eat well. In these the inflammation slowly subsided, the skin healed, and hair eventually regrew.

Microscopically, the skin lesions are characterized by severe epidermal parakeratosis and acanthosis; dilatation, parakeratosis, and plugging of hair follicles; focal purulent epidermal or perifollicular inflammation; hyperemia; and edema.

In diagnosis, the skin lesions must be differentiated from those of autoimmune dermatoses, toxic epidermal necrolysis, and drug eruption. The diagnosis is most reliably established by spectrographic demonstration of thallium in the urine.

Treatment with dithizon (diphenylthiocarbazone) is successful in dogs if given promptly. It was not tolerated by cats in the experience of Zook et al. (1968), although it has been stated elsewhere that the dose used in dogs produced no adverse effects in cats (Mather, 1974a). For subacute and chronic poisoning, ferric cyanoferrate (Prussian blue) has been recommended on the basis of experience with humans and dogs (Aronson, 1977). Supportive measures, including administration of vitamin B complex and handfeeding, are essential.

## Chlorinated Naphthalene Poisoning

About 1950, a skin disorder was recognized and experimentally reproduced in cats in Germany with exposure to wood preservatives (Wagener, 1952; Wagener and Kruger, 1953). Signs were bilateral alopecia of the trunk and encrustations on the eyelids and nostrils. The disorder in cats had many features of "X disease" ("hyperkeratosis X") of cattle, which was caused by ingestion or percutaneous absorption of chlorinated naphthalenes. The wood preservative was the same one associated with the disease in cattle.

## Warfarin Poisoning

In this uncommon poisoning of cats, hemorrhages may be found in the skin.

## Mercury Poisoning

According to Wilkinson (1983a), cats in a thermometer factory developed intensely itchy lesions on the underside of the chest and abdomen and on the medial surface of the thighs.

## Food Toxicity

Dry gangrene of the pinnae of the ears was seen in cats that ate decomposed scallops from a seafood processing plant (Holzworth, 1983).

# Nutritional Disorders

## Biotin Deficiency

First signs of experimental biotin deficiency are accumulation of dried saliva and nasal and lacrimal secretions on the face. Later, alopecia begins on the limbs and progresses over all the body. Associated changes are loss of hair pigment, drying and scaling of the skin, and finally weight loss and diarrhea (Carey and Morris, 1977) (see also chapter on nutrition and nutritional disorders).

Hepatic propionyl CoA carboxylase activity in biotin-deficient cats was found to be 4 to 24 per cent of normal (Carey and Morris, 1977). The subcutaneous injection of 0.25 mg biotin, every other day, to biotin-deficient cats resulted in clinical remission, even while the deficient diet was maintained.

Naturally occurring biotin deficiency has been suggested as a cause of miliary dermatitis in the cat (Joshua, 1965).

## Riboflavin Deficiency

Experimental dietary riboflavin deficiency in cats results in varying signs, including anorexia, weight loss, and periauricular alopecia with epidermal atrophy (Gershoff et al., 1959; Scott, 1964). Daily injections of 0.2 mg riboflavin produced clinical remission even with continued deficient diets (Gershoff et al., 1959). The daily riboflavin requirements for cats has been estimated to be 0.15 to 0.2 mg, depending on the cat's diet and metabolic demands (Scott, 1975).

## Vitamin A Deficiency

Experimental and naturally occurring dietary vitamin A deficiency has been reported in cats (Gershoff et al., 1957; Kral and Schwartzman, 1964; Scott, 1964, 1975). Chronic deficiency results in anorexia, weight loss, muscle wasting, poor coat, follicular plugging, and alopecic scaly patches of skin (Scott, 1964). These changes are followed by conjunctivitis and keratitis sicca, retinal degeneration, testicular atrophy and loss of spermatozoa in males, and anestrus or severe fetal losses in females.

Carotene is not converted by cats to vitamin A. The daily vitamin A requirement of kittens and cats has been estimated to be between 1500 and 2100 IU (500 to 700 μg) (Gershoff et al., 1957; Scott, 1975), although studies adequately defining the requirement have not been published (National Research Council, 1978). There is a serious danger of toxicity from oversupplementation, whether with liver, cod liver oil, or the vitamin itself (Muller et al., 1983). A single injection of 6000 IU aqueous vitamin A solution/kg is adequate treatment for two months for a serious deficiency. Dosage should not exceed 400 IU/kg/day orally for 10 days.

## Vitamin E Deficiency (Pansteatitis)

Pansteatitis ("yellow fat disease") has been described in cats fed largely on rations of dark-meat tuna, certain other fish diets, various canned cat foods, and excessive amounts of cod liver oil (Coffin and Holzworth, 1954; Cordy and Stillinger, 1953; Holzworth, 1971; Munson et al., 1958). The cause of this condition is deficiency of vitamin E and its antioxidant property, owing to a dietary deficit, a relative deficiency in association with highly unsaturated fatty acids, or destruction by improper processing or prolonged storage of cat food.

One study reported the course of naturally occurring untreated pansteatitis to be about 21 to 23 days from the onset of clinical signs (Cordy and Stillinger, 1953). Affected cats are usually presented with a history of anorexia, lethargy, reluctance to move, apparent lameness, and resentment of handling. Signs are fever up to 41 C (106 F) and intense generalized tenderness that may cause a cat to bite or scratch the handler when palpated. In some cases, the subcutaneous and intra-abdominal fat feels firm and lumpy. A deep yellow or mustard-colored ceroid pigment accumulates in the subcutaneous and abdominal fat and evokes an inflammatory foreign body reaction. In early cases there may be little or no discoloration of the fat, but microscopic examination of a biopsy specimen is usually diagnostic (see chapter on nutrition and nutritional disorders).

## Iodine Deficiency

Prolonged experimental iodine deficiency in kittens and cats may result in hypothyroidism, one feature of which is a sparse, short haircoat (Scott, 1964).

## Zinc Deficiency

In kittens, experimental zinc deficiency causes thinning of the hair coat, slow hair growth, scaliness of the skin, and ulceration of the buccal margins. The zinc requirement is estimated to be 15 to 50 parts per million (ppm) of the ration (Kane et al., 1981).

## Fatty Acid Deficiency

Essential fatty acid deficiency in cats fed largely on human foods or food residues has been reported (e.g., Kral and Schwartzman, 1964; Worden, 1958). The resultant clinical disorder was described as "hyperkeratotic and parakeratotic eczema," and blood levels of unsaturated fatty acids were reported to be low (Kral and Schwartzman, 1964). Less severely affected cats manifest generalized scaling, dry skin, dry hair coat, and variable alopecia. Cats apparently do not possess Δ6 desaturase and thus cannot convert linoleic and linolenic acids to arachidonic acid (Rivers et al., 1975). Therefore cats receiving only vegetable oils may develop essential fatty acid deficiency (see also chapter on nutrition and nutritional disorders). Cats recognized clinically as having "fat-responsive skin disease" (Scott, 1980) frequently are fed "complete" commercial diets, have no signs of malabsorption or liver disease, and would appear to be unlikely candidates for a fatty acid deficiency. Their excellent response to dietary supplementation of fat is mystifying.

Diagnosis is based on history, physical examination, and response to therapy. Histologic examination reveals varying degrees of hyperkeratosis, parakeratosis, and acanthosis; dermal vascular dilatation and edema; and perivascular accumulations of neutrophils, lymphocytes, and mast cells (Scott, 1980).

For supplementation of the diet a mixture of equal parts of vegetable oil and pork lard has been recommended (Scott, 1980). For the first week a quarter teaspoonful is mixed daily with the food. This amount is doubled weekly until a soft stool or diarrhea develops. The dose is then cut back to the previous week's amount and continued at that level for 12 weeks. A beneficial response should be seen by this time. Cats responding to this regimen often require maintenance therapy, at some reduced dose, for life. Commercially available fatty acid supplements have not been satisfactory. Fat-responsive skin disease may be difficult or impossible to manage in a cat that also has some sort of malabsorption disorder such as pancreatic insufficiency.

## Hormonal and Metabolic Disorders

### Feline Endocrine Alopecia

Endocrine alopecia (gonadal or castrate alopecia) is the most common hormonal skin disorder of the cat (e.g., Conroy, 1964; Doering, 1976; Joshua, 1971a; Kral and Schwartzman, 1964; Scott, 1975b; Scott, 1980). It occurs in neutered males (90 per cent of cases) and females. In Conroy's experience Siamese are most often affected. The age range is from 2 to 12 years (Conroy, 1964), with an average of 6 (Scott, 1975b).

The cause is uncertain. Sex hormone deficiencies have been hypothesized, as the disorder occurs in cats neutered before puberty (Kral and Schwartzman, 1964) and is responsive to sex hormone therapy. Why only certain cats neutered before puberty develop alopecia is unclear. It was suggested that the adrenal cortex may not produce sufficient androgens or estrogens in affected cats (Kral, 1960).

The bilaterally symmetric alopecia takes the form of diffuse thinning of hair rather than complete baldness. It starts in the groin, then involves the underside of the tail, the perineum, the caudal and medial surface of the thighs, and the abdomen (Figs. 13–10 and 13–11). In long-standing cases there may be alopecia of the lateral thorax, flanks, and forelimbs, but the back is spared. Hairs in affected areas are easily epilated and show no evidence of being bitten off. Although pruritus and skin lesions are usually absent, a rare cat manifests intense pruritus, dermatitis, and secondary seborrhea. Aside from the skin disorder, the cats are normal.

Diagnosis is based on history, physical examination, and response to therapy. Histologic examination of affected skin reveals most hair follicles to be in telogen and often devoid of hairs (Scott, 1980).

Treatment is with injections of combined androgen-estrogen or progestogens. Androgen and estrogen in combination are more effective than either hormone

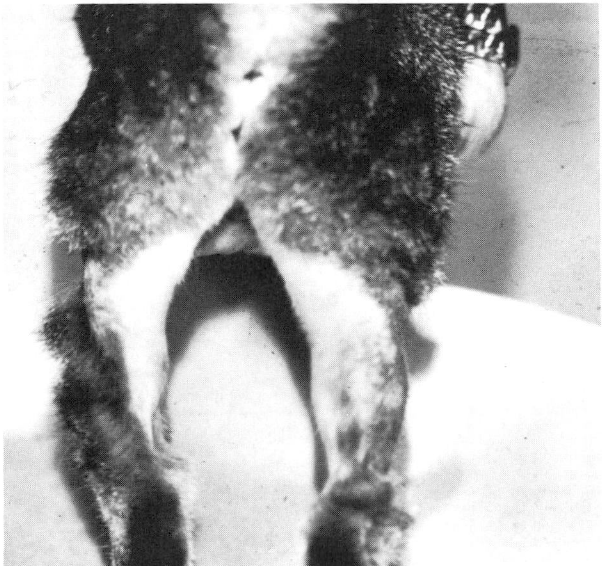

**Figure 13–10** Endocrine alopecia, caudomedial aspect of the hindlimbs.

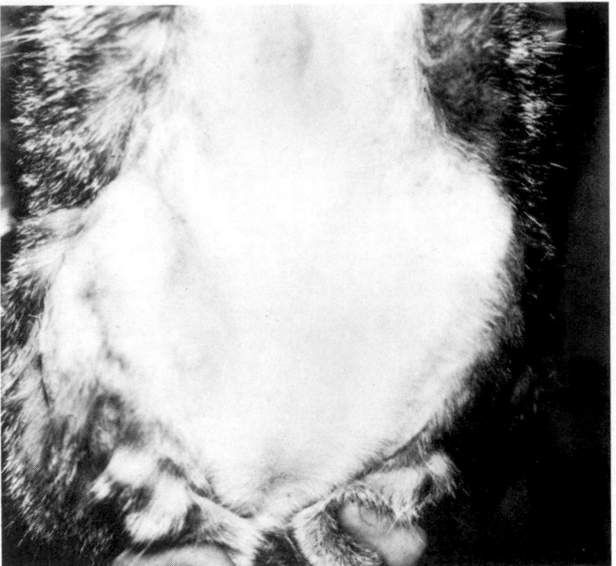

**Figure 13–11** Endocrine alopecia, abdomen.

alone. Excellent results are achieved with intramuscular injection of 0.2 ml of a repository preparation (Interstate Drug Exchange) containing 50 mg testosterone and 2 mg estradiol per ml (i.e., 10 mg testosterone and 0.4 mg estradiol). The cat is re-examined in six weeks, and if new hair growth is not evident a second injection is given. Alopecia recurs in 55 per cent of cats within six months to two years, but retreatment is effective.

Occasional transient side effects of androgen-estrogen therapy are signs of estrus in females and aggressiveness or urine spraying, or both, in males. These signs develop during the first week of therapy. If overdosed, testosterone or estrogen can cause severe liver disease (Dow, 1958; Scott, 1980; Wilkinson, 1968). Neither repository testosterone nor estradiol is licensed for use in cats.

Progestogens are also effective for the management of endocrine alopecia (McDougal, 1975; Muller et al., 1983; Pukay, 1979; Scott, 1980). Repository progesterone (2.2 to 20 mg/kg) or medroxyprogesterone acetate (50 to 175 mg, total dose) is given intramuscularly or subcutaneously. The cat is re-examined in six weeks, and a second injection is administered if hair regrowth is not evident. The relapse rate is similar to that with androgen-estrogen injections, and retreatment is similarly effective. Megestrol acetate can be given orally (2.5 to 5.0 mg) once every other day, until hair regrowth is evident. A maintenance dose of 2.5 to 5.0 mg once or twice weekly is usually required. Possible side effects of progestogens include weight gain, pyometra, diabetes mellitus, and mammary hyperplasia and carcinoma. These compounds are not licensed for use in cats.

Several workers failed to demonstrate low levels of thyroid hormone in any of their cases of endocrine alopecia (Baker, 1974a; Doering, 1976; Scott, 1975b; Scott, 1980). Muller, however, reported success with thyroid supplementation (Muller et al., 1983). Sodium levo-thyroxine (0.3 mg) is given daily for three months, then twice weekly; the maintenance dose varies from 0.1 to 0.3 mg daily. Hair usually regrows in three months, and the dose is then reduced to a level that prevents recurrence of alopecia.

Combined thyroid and gonadal hormone replacement therapy may give superior results in some cases of endocrine deficiency (Berry and Mosier, 1971). In an unusual case followed for many years at the Angell Memorial Animal Hospital, a castrated male required treatment with both testosterone (5 mg daily, Metandren, Ciba) and levo-thyroxine (0.2 mg daily) for maintenance of the coat, neither drug alone being effective (Petrak, 1983).

## Hypothyroidism

Naturally occurring hypothyroidism appears to be uncommon in cats but has in the past been diagnosed on clinical grounds and on the basis of response to empirical treatment (Austin, 1975a; Joshua, 1965, 1971a; Thornton, 1963). The first published case in which the condition was documented by determination of reduced levels of serum thyroxine ($T_4$) and triiodothyronine ($T_3$) appears to be that of Martin and Capen (1983). The cat pictured by them was obese and poorly groomed. They state that a serum $T_4$ level below 1 μg/dl and a $T_3$ level below 60 ng/dl support a clinical diagnosis of hypothyroidism and that the response of a hypothyroid cat to replacement of $T_4$ is dramatic, sodium levo-thyroxine 0.05 to 0.1 mg daily being adequate for most affected cats.

Occasional cases, unpublished but documented by low levels of thyroid hormone (usually $T_4$), have been encountered by Holzworth (1983) and Stein (1983). The thinning or loss of hair is bilaterally symmetric and often similar in distribution to that in sex hormone–responsive alopecia but may extend farther forward on the sides. The skin itself usually appears normal. Some cats are obese but others are thin and sometimes ill-tempered. Other signs may be sluggishness, slow pulse, and a tendency to seek warmth. With administration of 0.1 mg levo-thyroxine once or twice daily the hair coat and serum thyroid hormone levels return to normal.

In a congenitally hypothyroid kitten the hair coat was evenly distributed over all the body but consisted mainly of undercoat, with primary guard hair being thinly scattered throughout (Arnold et al., 1984).

In two undersized purebred Persian kittens with low levels of thyroid hormones, the hypothyroidism may have been secondary to a pituitary deficiency (Holzworth, 1983). Their fur was fine and woolly. In one the testes were abnormally small, in the other they had not descended. One kitten in particular rarely played and was abnormally sluggish and sleepy. With thyroid supplementation of 0.05 mg levo-thyroxine daily, it became much more active and grew a normal hair coat. The testes enlarged, and the cat's attempts to mate with its spayed female housemate necessitated castration. The cat still requires 0.1 mg thyroxine daily or it reverts to its former sluggishness. The other kitten succumbed to feline infectious peritonitis before thyroxine therapy could be evaluated.

Familial hypothyroidism has been diagnosed on the basis of low levels of thyroid hormone in a family of Rex cats (a brother, sister, and mother) (Stein, 1983). They first lost the curl in their hair, then the hair itself. There was a favorable response to administration of thyroid hormone (Plate 13–1*C* and *D*). It must be remembered, however, that the administration of thyroid hormone can force varying degrees of hair growth in conditions that are unrelated to hypothyroidism (e.g., feline endocrine alopecia).

Experimentally, hypothyroidism has been induced in cats and kittens by a protracted iodine deficiency that results in atrophy of the thyroid gland (Scott, 1964). The cats are stunted and have short, sparse hair coats, thickened skin, and broadening of the head owing to edema. They are slow-moving, affectionate, and gentle. Some have no sexual activity. Females that conceive may have difficult parturition and deliver deformed kittens.

Values for $T_4$ and $T_3$ may vary from laboratory to laboratory. It is important to ascertain that values at a given laboratory have been established by testing an adequate number of normal cats. Basal levels of serum $T_4$ and $T_3$ are notoriously unreliable for diagnosing hypothyroidism (Muller et al., 1983) and may be spuriously low in animals receiving various drugs (especially glucocorticoids) or having various acute or chronic illnesses (the "euthyroid sick syndrome").

At present, the most reliable method for assessing thyroid function in the cat is measurement of serum $T_4$ response to exogenous thyrotropin (TSH) (the TSH response test). Basal serum $T_4$ levels in cats, as determined by radioimmunoassay, range from 0.7 to 3.6 μg/dl (Hoenig and Ferguson, 1983; Kemppainen et al., 1984). Bovine TSH may be administered intravenously or intramuscularly at 2.5 to 5.0 IU, total dose, and causes at least a doubling of basal $T_4$ levels within 6 to 12 hours, respectively, in normal cats (Hoenig and Ferguson, 1983; Kemppainen et al., 1984; Scott, 1975b).

## Hyperadrenocorticism

Hyperadrenocorticism (Cushing's disease, Cushing's syndrome), whether naturally occurring or iatrogenic owing to steroid overdosage, is rare in the cat. Two well-studied, naturally occurring cases have been reported (Fox and Beatty, 1975; Meijer et al., 1978). The causes in these cases were, respectively, bilateral adrenocortical hyperplasia (pituitary not examined) and unilateral adrenocortical adenoma. Signs were polydipsia, polyuria, polyphagia, lethargy, pendulous abdomen, and bilaterally symmetric alopecia with thin, hypotonic, easily torn, scaly, hyperpigmented skin.

Iatrogenic hyperadrenocorticism has been observed after long-term, high-level administration of potent synthetic corticosteroids in the treatment of various corticosteroid-responsive conditions (Martin and Capen, 1983; Petrak, 1983).

Symptomatic hyperadrenocorticism was produced experimentally in two cats only after weekly intramuscular injections of repository methylprednisolone acetate, 5.5 mg/kg (five times the recommended therapeutic dose) for 15 weeks (Scott, 1980; Scott et al., 1982) (Plate 13–1*B* and Fig. 13–12).

Reported laboratory abnormalities in hyperadrenocorticism include eosinopenia, lymphopenia, elevated SALT (SGPT), hyperglycemia, and glucosuria. Histologic examination of the skin reveals hyperkeratosis, epidermal atrophy, follicular keratosis and atrophy, atrophy of sebaceous glands, dermal thinning and atrophy, and dilatation of dermal and subcuticular blood vessels (Scott, 1980).

Blood and urine corticosteroids have been studied in

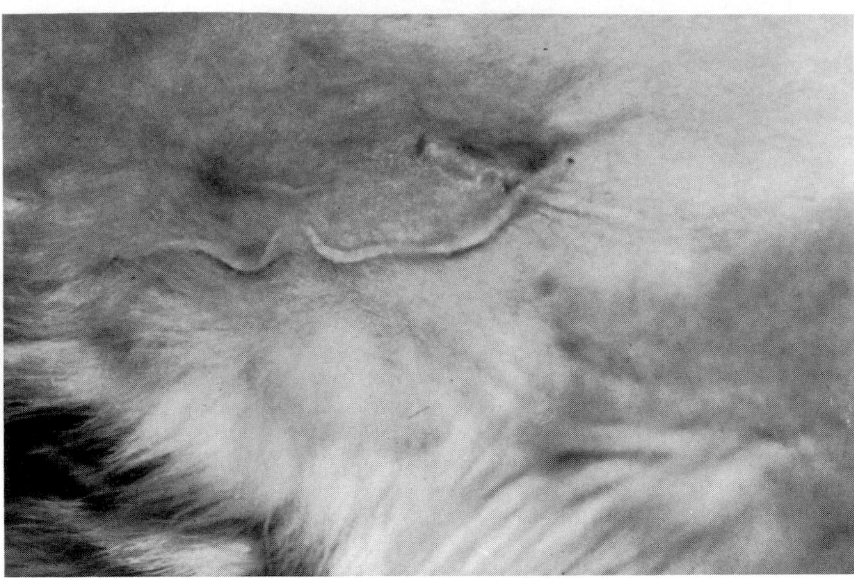

**Figure 13–12** Experimentally induced hyperglucocorticoidism. The thin hypotonic skin remains wrinkled after being lifted and released.

normal cats (see references, Scott, 1980). Virtually all corticosteroid metabolites in cats are excreted in bile (99 per cent), with only a small amount of Porter-Silber chromogens present as the free compounds in urine (1 per cent). The feline adrenal cortex secretes about five times as much cortisol as corticosterone. Plasma cortisol levels have been variously reported: 6.6 ± 0.8 μg/dl (fluorimetric method) (Garcy and Marotta, 1978; Krieger et al., 1968); 1.4 to 3.9 μg/dl (Scott et al., 1979c); 1.5 to 6.3 μg/dl (Fox and Beatty, 1975) (competitive protein binding method); and 124 to 304 nmol/l (radioimmunoassay method) (Meijer et al., 1978). Baseline cortisol levels were not of diagnostic significance in naturally occurring hyperadrenocorticism (Meijer et al., 1978).

In two studies, plasma cortisol responses to corticotropin in normal cats ranged from 11.0 to 22.4 μg/dl (Scott et al., 1979c) and from 5.0 to 12.0 μg/dl (Fox and Beatty, 1975) (two hours after 1 unit ACTH gel/pound was given intramuscularly). ACTH-response testing was diagnostic in 2 cases of feline hyperadrenocorticism: 10.8 μg/dl before and 18.7 μg/dl after administration (bilateral adrenocortical hyperplasia) (Fox and Beatty, 1975), and 166 nmol/l before and 414 nmol/l after (adrenocortical adenoma) (Meijer et al., 1978).

Plasma ACTH (radioimmunoassay method) levels in normal cats were reported to range from 151 to 503 pg/ml (Ward and Gann, 1976) and from 321 to 960 pg/ml (Ward et al., 1976).

Treatment of naturally occurring hyperadrenocorticism in the cat would probably necessitate adrenalectomy, as cats do not tolerate most chlorinated hydrocarbons (i.e., *o,p'*-DDD). The response to unilateral adrenalectomy in the cat with unilateral adrenocortical adenoma was good (Meijer et al., 1978).

## Diabetes Mellitus

Pruritus and generalized skin disease (pyoderma, seborrhea, alopecia) are associated with some cases of diabetes mellitus in cats and improve when the cat is treated for the diabetes (Conroy, 1964; Muller et al., 1983). Xanthomatosis, sometimes associated with diabetes in humans and dogs, has been described in a diabetic cat (Kwochka, 1983).

## Xanthomatosis

Xanthomatosis, a metabolic disorder, was reported in a four-year-old, castrated male Siamese (Fawcett et al., 1977). Skin lesions, first noted at one year of age, consisted of multiple, soft, well-circumscribed, smooth subcutaneous masses over the trunk and head. Hemogram, serum chemistry values, and triiodothyronine ($T_3$) were normal. The cat was destroyed.

At autopsy, the cutaneous masses were soft, brown-white, and 3.0 to 8.0 cm in diameter. Microscopically, discrete masses of densely packed cells were seen. Large histiocytes with abundant foamy cytoplasm were numerous, along with lymphoid follicles, occasional foreign body giant cells, and scattered eosinophils. Fat stains demonstrated lipid droplets within the foamy cells. The biochemical defect was not discovered.

## Excessive Shedding—Telogen Effluvium

Shedding of varying degrees is a normal event in the life of the cat (Baker, 1974b; Ryder, 1976; Scott, 1980; Thornton, 1963). As shedding is influenced by photoperiod, the process tends to be exaggerated in spring and fall in outdoor cats. Indoor cats tend to shed all year round. These patterns are not affected by neutering.

Cats are occasionally presented for excessive shedding. In most instances, physical examination reveals that the hair, predominantly of the undercoat, can be easily epilated, but areas of complete alopecia cannot be created. Treatment for these cats is limited to shortening of the abnormal photoperiod for indoor cats, if possible, and frequent, regular, thorough brushing and combing to prevent shedding on rugs, furniture, and clothing, as well as formation of hairballs in the cat's stomach.

Telogen effluvium occurs occasionally under conditions of ill health or generalized disease, stress (e.g., gestation, lactation, high fever), and drug therapy (especially with ampicillin, hetacillin, and sulfonamides) (Muller et al., 1983; Scott, 1980). The anagen phase of the hair cycle is considerably shortened, and large numbers of hair follicles are thrown into telogen at one time. Telogen hairs are more easily lost because they are less firmly anchored in the hair follicle. Frequently, upon resolution of the stressful condition, large numbers of hairs are shed simultaneously (four to eight weeks later).

Physical examination of cats with telogen effluvium reveals varying degrees of alopecia. Many hairs can be easily epilated, and areas of complete alopecia are easily produced. Therapy is not indicated. The hair coat will begin to return to normal within one to two months.

## Loss of Pigmentation

Occasionally a cat is presented for a loss of pigmentation that is hard to account for. Siamese cats are most often affected (Holzworth, 1983). For no apparent reason they sometimes lose the normal dark pigmentation of their eyelids or foot pads—an unsightly development that disqualifies them as show animals. One Siamese developed a snow-white patch on its mask during recovery from panleukopenia. Whether or not by coincidence, another lost the pigment in the planum nasale a few weeks after spaying (Fig. 13–13).

Injection of medroxyprogesterone acetate has resulted in local loss of pigment in the hair coat.

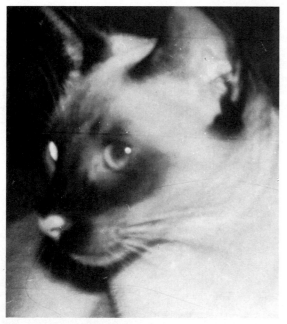

**Figure 13–13** Permanent depigmentation of the nose, cause unknown, in a nine-month-old spayed female chocolate point Siamese (courtesy Mr. and Mrs. David Kilmer). A similar loss of nasal pigment occasionally occurs in Siamese eating from a rubber or plastic dish; the pigment returns if another type of dish is provided.

# Immunologic Disorders

## Allergic (Hypersensitivity) Disorders

Allergic skin disease may be of inhalant, dietary, bacterial, fungal, parasitic, contact, hormonal, or drug origin. It is imperative to remember that a cat may manifest one or any combination of these allergies.

Allergic (hypersensitivity) reactions are classically categorized as of four basic types (Scott, 1980). In Type I (anaphylactic) reactions, complete antigens interact with IgE-coated mast cells and basophils to cause degranulation of these cells and release of numerous inflammatory mediator substances. In Type II (cytotoxic) reactions, complete antigens interact with IgG or IgM, with or without complement, with resultant destruction of the antigen. In Type III (immune complex) reactions, complete antigens, IgG, and complement interact, causing attraction of neutrophils and release of the inflammatory mediator substances. In Type IV (cellular) reactions, incomplete antigens (haptens), tissue protein, macrophages, and sensitized T-lymphocytes interact so as to cause release of inflammatory mediator substances (lymphokines) from the lymphocytes.

**FOOD ALLERGY.** Food allergy is an uncommon cause of pruritic skin disease in cats (see references, Scott, 1980), probably accounting for no more than 5 to 10 per cent of all feline "allergic" dermatitides. There are no breed or sex predilections. Such reactions are less frequent in young cats, because a period of exposure is required (Austin, 1975a). The immunologic mechanism of food allergy is not known but probably includes both immediate (Types I and III) and delayed (Type IV) hypersensitivities.

Signs vary but fall into four general categories: (1) miliary dermatitis–like eruption; (2) pruritic, ulcerative dermatitis of the head, neck, and axillae (Plate 13–1*G*); (3) pruritus without lesions; and (4) pruritic urticaria or angioedema. Varying degrees of alopecia, seborrhea, and twitching of the skin may be present. Bilateral otitis externa may accompany the dermatitis. Concurrent gastrointestinal disturbances occur in less than 10 per cent of cases.

The owner should be questioned about recent changes in the cat's diet; however, over 80 per cent of cats have been eating the offending diet for two or more years before signs of allergy appear.

Diagnosis is established by an elimination diet. Neither blood nor tissue eosinophilia is present, unless the cat has concurrent parasitism(s). Histologic findings in affected skin are varying degrees of subacute or chronic, nonsuppurative dermatitis, with neutrophils outnumbering plasma cells, lymphocytes, and mast cells (Scott, 1980).

The elimination diet is planned to avoid items that the cat is exposed to more than once weekly. Thus it can vary from case to case. A diet often used is boiled chicken, boiled brown rice, and water. Food additives (preservatives, colorings, flavorings, seasonings, other condiments) should be avoided. Never should one commercial food be substituted for another. If food allergy is present, response to the elimination diet is dramatic. Within 24 to 48 hours, pruritus and inflammatory skin changes usually regress significantly. A convincing response should certainly be evident within 14 days. Reintroduction of the offending food into the cat's diet will reproduce the clinical signs within 4 to 72 hours. Intradermal skin testing with foods has been of no benefit in cats. There is little solid information on the specific allergen(s) responsible for food allergies in cats. Many items have been faulted (cow's milk, beef, eggs, pork, fish, whole meat, chicken, rabbit, canned cat food, dry cat food, wheat, cod liver oil, benzoic acid, mutton, horse meat); however, most owners are unwilling to go through the laborious process of provocative exposure in order to identify specific allergens.

Once a cat is symptom-free, single foods are added to the elimination diet at seven-day intervals. Slowly, a variety of foods is accumulated that will not exacerbate the dermatitis. As one cannot hope to balance such diets, a daily vitamin-mineral and fatty acid supplement is provided. In addition, the cat's unique dietary requirement for taurine must be met to prevent retinal degeneration and blindness (Knopf et al., 1978). Adequate taurine may be supplied by adding half a teaspoonful of the juice from canned clams to the daily diet.

Sometimes owners are not willing to investigate "hypoallergenic" diets, or the cats refuse to eat them. In such cases, glucocorticoids are administered to suppress the signs of allergy. However, food allergy dermatitis often responds poorly to glucocorticoids (Scott, 1980). Antihistamines are of no benefit in pruritic skin diseases of the cat and may produce striking adverse reactions, varying from extreme depression and somnolence to hysteria.

**DRUG ERUPTION.** Drug eruption (drug allergy, dermatitis medicamentosa) is defined as a cutaneous or mucocutaneous reaction to the administration of a drug. The drug may have been administered orally, topically, or by injection or inhalation. Only a few cases have been reported in cats, with no apparent breed, age, or sex predilection (Aronson and Schwark, 1980; see also references, Scott, 1980). Any drug may cause an eruption, and there is no specific type of reaction for any one drug. Thus drug eruption can mimic virtually any dermatosis. Drugs that have caused eruptions in cats include sulfisoxazole (miliary dermatitis, alopecia); ampicillin and hetacillin (multifocal alopecia, pruritus, toxic epidermal necrolysis); penicillin (miliary dermatitis, urticaria, angioedema); tetracycline (urticaria, angioedema); gentamicin (pruritic erythroderma); propylthiouracil (facial edema, pruritus); neomycin, miconazole, and dichlorvos (contact dermatitis); panleukopenia vaccine (angioedema); and otic preparations containing chlorinated hydrocarbons or rotenone and derris (otitis externa).

Allergic mechanisms appear to be the most common cause of drug eruption; however, most so-called allergic drug reactions are judged as such on clinical grounds alone. The types of immunologic response thought to be involved in allergic drug reactions are Types I, II, III, and IV hypersensitivities.

In general, there are no specific or characteristic laboratory findings in drug eruption. Results of in-vitro and in-vivo immunologic tests have been disappointing. Examination of skin biopsies is often helpful, more by excluding other possibilities than by providing a specific diagnosis. Just as the eruptions vary greatly in character, so do the histologic patterns, no one change being indicative of drug eruption. Because drug eruption can mimic so many different dermatoses, it is imperative to have an accurate knowledge of the medications given to any patient with an obscure dermatosis.

At present, the only reliable test for the diagnosis of drug eruption is to withdraw the drug and observe for disappearance of the eruption (usually within 7 to 14 days); however, drug eruption may occasionally persist for weeks or months after the offending drug is discontinued. Deliberate readministration of the drug to determine if the eruption is reproduced is undesirable and dangerous.

Management of drug eruption is by (1) discontinuance of the drug; (2) evaluation of hematologic, hepatic, and renal status; (3) use of glucocorticoids; (4) use of an antihistamine (pyribenzamine, 1 mg/kg orally or IM) and epinephrine (0.25 to 0.5 ml of 1:10,000 sol IM, total dose), for urticarial or anaphylactic reactions; and (5) avoidance of chemically related drugs.

**ALLERGIC CONTACT DERMATITIS.** Allergic contact dermatitis (contact sensitivity, dermatitis venenata) is reported to be rare in cats, with no apparent breed, age, or sex predilection (Austin, 1975a; Scott, 1980; Walton, 1972, 1975). Substances reported as causes in cats include topical medication (i.e., neomycin), dichlorvos, grasses, carpeting, and cleansers. Allergic contact dermatitis is usually a Type IV hypersensitivity disorder, although Type I hypersensitivity responses can be involved. In fact, cats are poorly and inconsistently responsive to attempts to induce delayed-type (Type IV) hypersensitivity reactions under experimental conditions (Schultz and Adams, 1978; Scott, 1980). No case of allergic contact dermatitis reported in cats has been documented by patch testing. The overwhelming majority of contact dermatitides in cats result from irritants.

Signs reported are varying degress of dermatitis (mild erythema without pruritus, pigmentary changes, or severe pruritic papulovesicular eruption) in sparsely haired "contact" areas such as the chin, pinnae, axillae, abdomen, medial thighs, perineum, and ventral tail. Allergic contact dermatitis does not involve haired areas unless the allergen is in liquid or aerosol form. It may or may not be seasonal, depending on the allergen(s) involved. It is imperative to inquire about changes in a cat's environment; however, over 70 per cent of cases of allergic contact dermatitis involve items that have been in the patient's environment for over two years (Walton, 1975).

Skin biopsy should reveal a predominantly dermal reaction, with lymphocytes and histiocytes predominating. Patch testing is essential for confirming a diagnosis of allergic contact dermatitis. Patches of suspected allergens are applied to a clipped area of skin and taped in place under an occlusive dressing. Results at the test site are evaluated in 48 to 72 hours. Use of control cats is essential to rule out irritant reactions. Patch testing in cats is at present subject to procedural and interpretational pitfalls and requires study and standardization in order to yield significant results.

**URTICARIA AND ANGIOEDEMA.** Urticaria (hives) and angioedema are rare in the cat (Austin, 1975a; Parish, 1965; Scott, 1980). In humans many stimuli, both immunologic and nonimmunologic, are involved in the pathogenesis. For cats, knowledge of etiology is limited. Factors implicated include vaccine (panleukopenia), antisera, transfusions, foods, drugs (penicillin, tetracycline), and insect bites. Signs are most often acute. Urticaria is characterized by localized or disseminated wheals, and angioedema by focal or generalized large, edematous swellings. Either reaction may be accompanied by pruritus, serum leakage, or hemorrhage.

Laboratory studies may be useful in ruling out other

disorders. Skin biopsy exhibits nondiagnostic patterns varying in severity: simple vascular dilatation and edema; perivascular dermatitis with mononuclear cells, neutrophils, mast cells, and infrequently eosinophils; or leukocytoclastic vasculitis (Muller et al., 1983). A specific diagnosis can usually be made in acute cases, but a chronic condition is an extremely frustrating diagnostic challenge (over 75 per cent of human cases defy specific diagnosis).

The causative agent, when known, should be avoided. Glucocorticoids, antihistamines (pyribenzamine), and epinephrine, are used in symptomatic treatment. Acute cases (e.g., reactions to insect bites, drugs, vaccines) often regress spontaneously within 2 to 72 hours.

**ANAPHYLAXIS.** Anaphylaxis is rare in cats (Parish, 1965; Scott, 1980; Walton, 1975). I have never seen a case. A variety of heterologous proteins have been used experimentally to evoke anaphylaxis in cats, albeit with difficulty. Cutaneous anaphylaxis was produced with intradermal injections of bovine serum (McCusker and Aitken, 1967). Histologic findings in immediate cutaneous reactions were dermal edema, marked perivascular accumulations of neutrophils, and depletion and degranulation of mast cells. At 24 hours, microscopic examination of cutaneous reactions in some cats revealed massive accumulations of neutrophils that obliterated most blood vessels. Study of passive cutaneous anaphylaxis disclosed dermal edema and perivascular accumulation of neutrophils and eosinophils (Parish, 1965).

**ATOPY.** Atopy is a hypersensitivity state due to hereditary predisposition and associated with antibody of the IgE class. Although IgE has not been definitively demonstrated in the cat, possible atopy has been observed in several animals (Muller et al., 1983). These exhibited pruritus of the face, ears, and neck; miliary dermatitis; recurrent lesions of eosinophilic granuloma complex; and symmetric alopecia resembling psychogenic alopecia. Clinical signs may be seasonal or nonseasonal.

Diagnosis is confirmed by intradermal skin testing as described elsewhere (Muller et al., 1983; Reedy, 1982). Cats may be restrained in a cat bag or sedated with 30 to 50 mg ketamine given intramuscularly. Evaluation of skin test results is challenging, as feline wheals tend to be rather flat, poorly circumscribed, and nonerythematous.

Feline atopy may be managed with systemic glucocorticoids or hyposensitization. Prednisone or prednisolone may be given orally at 2 mg/kg/day until remission is achieved, and then on an alternate-day schedule. Methylprednisolone acetate may be used at a dosage of 20 mg total dose given subcutaneously as needed (*never* more often than once every two months). Reedy (1982) found that hyposensitization produced at least 75 per cent improvement in 67 per cent of the cats treated.

Results of intradermal skin testing and hyposensitization of cats with chronic skin disorders suggest that some cats with miliary dermatitis, psychogenic alopecia, or eosinophilic ulcers may have underlying atopy (Reedy, 1982).

**BACTERIAL ALLERGY.** Bacterial allergy is thought to be important in humans and dogs (Scott, 1978), but its role in cats is obscure. Suspected bacterial allergy in cats has been mentioned (Walton, 1966, 1972) but without details. Pruritic, miliary dermatitis with many small, suppurative areas was reported in a cat previously medicated with antibiotics, glucocorticoids, and topical agents (MacDonald et al., 1972). *Staphylococcus aureus* and *S. epidermidis* were consistently isolated, and histologic examination of affected skin revealed a deep-seated pustular dermatitis. An autogenous bacterin was prepared and injected twice weekly for four weeks and then weekly for four more weeks. The cat was normal within 12 weeks, relapsed in several months, but responded to "booster" injections of the bacterin. Further studies are indicated in this area.

**FUNGAL ALLERGY.** Fungal allergy (as distinct from atopic disease) is thought to be an important entity in man. Skin disorders associated with fungal hypersensitivity in the cat have been suspected (Jungerman and Schwartzman, 1972; Walton, 1966, 1972), but the classic "id" (dermatophytid) reactions have not been reported. The occasional intensely pruritic kerion and miliary dermatitis–like reactions in cats infected with *Microsporum canis* are probably examples of fungal allergy (Scott, 1980).

**ALLERGY TO INTESTINAL PARASITES.** Allergic skin reactions may occasionally be associated with intestinal parasitism with roundworms, tapeworms, or hookworms (Baker, 1968; Brownlie, 1963; Lawler, 1970; Scott, 1980; Walton, 1972). The mechanism of the "allergic" reaction is unknown, although elicitation of skin-sensitizing (IgE) antibodies (Type I hypersensitivity) is likely. Although IgE has not to date been definitively identified in cats, an association between the parasites and the dermatitis is incontestable, as elimination of the parasite(s) eliminates the dermatitis and reinfection reproduces it. The allergy may be expressed as miliary dermatitis, as pruritus with or without skin lesions, or as pruritic seborrhea sicca. Gastrointestinal signs may be present. Diagnosis is established by a fecal examination and favorable response to removal of the parasite. Symptomatic measures may also be needed.

**FLEA ALLERGY.** Flea allergy is the most common form of allergic dermatitis in the cat (see references, Scott, 1980). Flea saliva contains several antigenic substances, some of which are haptenic and require conjugation with skin collagen before they are allergenic. There is cross-reactivity among the salivas of *Ctenocephalides felis, C. canis* and *Pulex irritans* (Feingold et al., 1968). Flea allergy dermatitis may involve Type I or Type IV hypersensitivity reactions or both (Muller et al., 1983). No breed or sex predilection has been reported. Clinical signs rarely develop in animals under six months of age; as animals age, flea allergy tends to become progressively worse (Muller et al., 1983).

Signs may be seasonal or continuous, depending on geographic area and household infestation. Pruritic, papulocrustous dermatitis is typically present over the lumbosacral area (Plate 13–1*E*), caudomedial thighs, and abdomen. The head and neck are also commonly involved (Plate 13–1*F*). Occasionally, cutaneous involvement is generalized. Scratching may lead to secondary infection.

Diagnosis is primarily by demonstration of fleas, flea feces, or eggs and by response to treatment. Intradermal skin testing with various commercial flea antigens has been unrewarding in feline flea allergy (Baker, 1968; Doering, 1976; Kristensen and Kieffer, 1978; Scott, 1980). Skin biopsy reveals varying degrees of subacute or chronic nonsuppurative dermatitis with numerous eosinophils (Baker, 1968; Scott, 1980).

Owners are often reluctant to believe that their cats have fleas or that fleas could be causing such a horrid dermatitis. It is therefore essential to explain that fleas spend most of their life not on the cat but in the cat's environment, that for every flea on the cat there are many more in the house, and that the bite of a single flea is probably capable of perpetuating some degree of dermatitis and pruritus for up to four or five days.

Treatment of flea allergy is primarily a matter of flea control. The cat itself (and other cats or dogs in the household) should be thoroughly treated with a parasiticide specifically designated as nontoxic for cats. It must also be a material to which the fleas of the locality have not become resistant. Most effective are sprays in which microencapsulation of parasiticides provides slow release and therefore prolonged effect. Sprays should be applied two or three times weekly but are resented by many cats. Powders should also be applied two or three times weekly but may dry the skin and haircoat. Dips are given once a week and are especially useful for longhaired cats. Shampoos have little or no residual effect. Clipping is unnecessary. Kittens under four weeks of age should be treated only with a light dusting of rotenone or a light application of pyrethrin spray. They may be bathed in any plain pyrethrin shampoo.

Flea collars and medallions seem to control flea infestation in some cats but cannot be relied on to prevent the occasional bite that is capable of evoking allergic dermatitis. Their use should be supplemented by environmental control.

All accessible areas frequented by the cat (floors, rugs, bedding, upholstered furniture) should be vacuumed twice a week to remove fleas, eggs, and larvae. Insecticidal household sprays and "foggers" are also useful, especially for closets, garages, cellars, and crawl spaces. Some residual premise sprays act for 10 weeks or more to kill both adult fleas and larval forms. These are adversely affected by sunlight so may only be used indoors. Parasiticidal sprays are also available for the outdoor environment. As a last resort, professional exterminators may be required. (For discussion of specific agents used in flea control see later section on parasitisms.)

Glucocorticoids are a valuable adjunct in treatment of flea allergy, especially whenever total elimination of fleas is unlikely. The author prefers oral prednisolone or prednisone at 1 to 2 mg/kg b.i.d. for five to seven days, then alternate-day therapy as needed for maintenance. Alternatively, methylprednisolone acetate may be given subcutaneously, 20 mg total dose, as needed.

Hyposensitization has been reported in some uncontrolled studies to be effective (Michaeli and Goldfarb, 1968; Reedy, 1975, 1982). However, a recent double-blind trial of flea hyposensitization in cats demonstrated that hyposensitization was not only costly but also unlikely to be successful (Kunkle and Milcarsky 1985).

## Immune-Mediated Disorders

Immune-mediated disorders identified to date in the cat are toxic epidermal necrolysis, alopecia areata, erythema multiforme, sterile pyogranuloma, and possibly cutaneous vasculitis.

**TOXIC EPIDERMAL NECROLYSIS.** Toxic epidermal necrolysis (Lyell's disease) is rare in the cat (Scott et al., 1979a; Scott, 1980). It is characterized by severe mucocutaneous blistering and ulceration, moderate or marked cutaneous pain, epidermal collarette formation, a positive Nikolsky sign (i.e., the epidermis rubs off easily), and constitutional signs of fever, anorexia, and depression (Plate 13–1*H*).

In man, the disorder is associated with drug eruption (50 per cent of cases) or underlying systemic disease (25 per cent), or is idiopathic (25 per cent). Its pathogenesis is unknown, but histologic and immunopathologic studies in man and laboratory animals suggest an assault on the basal cells of the epidermis. Direct immunofluorescence studies on affected skin from humans with drug-induced toxic epidermal necrolysis have revealed immunoglobulin and complement (Ig-C) complexes in the intercellular spaces of the basal cell layer of the epidermis.

Four feline cases have been recognized: one associated with caprine anti-feline leukemia virus antiserum, one with injectable cephaloridine, and two with oral ampicillin (Scott, 1980).

Diagnosis is definitively established by skin biopsy, which reveals full-thickness coagulation necrosis of the epidermis (Fig. 13–14) and often the upper third of hair follicle epithelium, with resultant cleavage and cleft formation at the dermo-epidermal junction.

Treatment is by correction of the underlying cause; maintenance of proper fluid, electrolyte, and colloid balance; and large doses of glucocorticoids (1 to 2 mg/kg prednisolone or prednisone b.i.d.). In humans, mortality is as high as 45 per cent (mostly in "idiopathic" cases).

**ALOPECIA AREATA.** Alopecia areata has been recognized in cats (Conroy, 1979), sometimes together with hemobartonellosis (Gretillat, 1984). Thought to be an immune-mediated dermatosis with antitissue antibodies and lymphokines directed against hair follicles, it is characterized by single or multiple areas of temporary, noninflammatory alopecia. The diagnosis is established by skin biopsy revealing clusters of mononuclear cells around the bulbs of anagen hair follicles. Later the follicles atrophy and the hairs are shed. Treatment has not been reported for the cat, but in man sublesional or systemic glucocorticoids may be effective.

**ERYTHEMA MULTIFORME.** Erythema multiforme is an acute, self-limiting, frequently recurrent, inflammatory disorder of the skin and/or mucous membranes (Muller et al., 1983). It is currently considered to be an immune-mediated reaction and has been associated with infections, drugs, neoplasia, and connective tissue disorders in humans and dogs.

Erythema multiforme has been reported in a cat receiving aurothioglucose for pemphigus foliaceus (Scott, 1984). The dermatosis was characterized by the acute, asymptomatic onset of a symmetric erythematous maculopapular eruption over the trunk and proximal extremities. The lesions enlarged peripherally while healing centrally. Skin biopsy revealed hydropic degeneration of epidermal basal cells, single-cell necrosis of keratinocytes, and a superficial perivascular accumulation of mononuclear cells. The dermatosis regressed after aurothioglucose therapy was stopped.

**STERILE PYOGRANULOMA.** A condition similar to the sterile pyogranuloma of dogs (Muller et al., 1983) has been recognized in cats (Conroy, 1983; AMAH). It is characterized by a nodular dermatitis in which neither microorganisms nor foreign bodies are found. As well as surgical excision, long-term steroid therapy may be helpful.

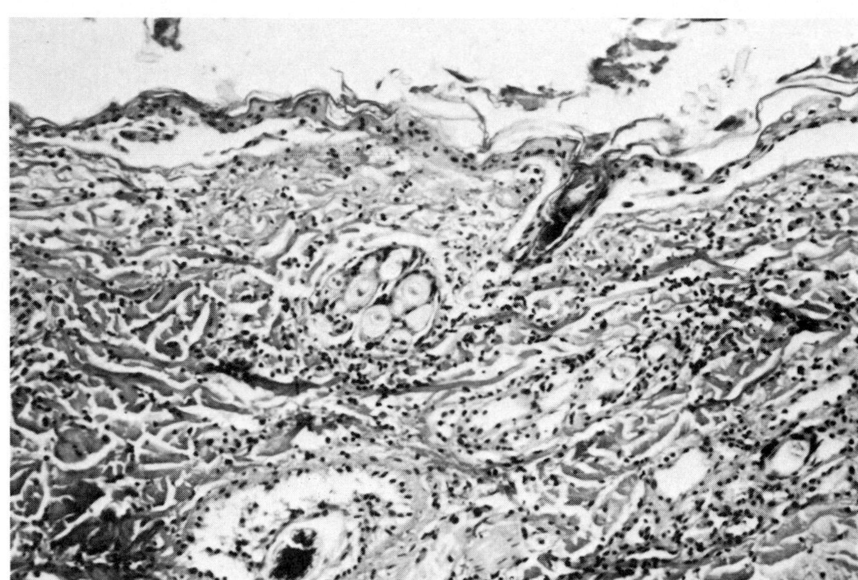

**Figure 13–14** Toxic epidermal necrolysis. Full-thickness necrosis of the epidermis. H & E.

**VASCULITIS.** Cutaneous vasculitis of the type reported in dogs (Muller et al., 1983) was suspected in a spayed female domestic cat at the Angell Memorial Animal Hospital (Holzworth, 1983). Otherwise healthy, the cat had recurrent ulcerations of the toepads, and lesions were also present on the pinna and near the lip. Sections of toepad disclosed evidence of characteristic destruction of neutrophil nuclei and also of incipient healing, although no treatment had been given. The condition was treated in a dog by oral administration of dapsone (Muller et al., 1983).

## Autoimmune Disorders

Autoimmune skin disorders are recently recognized entities in cats. Their true spectrum and impact will become more obvious as more centers become equipped to study and understand them. In general, these disorders are rare, severe, and, without proper therapy, fatal. Treatment is rigorous, with use of potentially dangerous drugs, usually for life. Thus successful management requires dedicated, well-informed veterinarians and owners.

Fundamental to diagnosis is biopsy. Proper technique, timing, and tenacity cannot be overemphasized. These lesions are usually fragile, so biopsy must be done with great care. Contiguous, normal-looking skin must be excised along with the primary or secondary lesions. The diagnostic histologic features of the bullae associated with many of the autoimmune diseases become obscured 10 to 12 hours after blister formation. Thus harvesting the earliest primary lesions is critical. Lastly, because it is often difficult to obtain tissues with diagnostic microscopic features, multiple biopsies (three to five) for serial sections should be taken whenever possible.

Direct and indirect immunofluorescence testing are the ultimate diagnostic steps and are often useful when histologic findings have been inconclusive. Direct immunofluorescence testing is preferred, as autoantibody titers in cats appear to be low or negative in most instances, making the indirect immunofluorescence testing difficult to interpret or misleading (Scott et al., 1983).

If an immunologic disorder is suspected, one set of tissues should be submitted for routine histologic studies and another reserved in Michel's fixative in case immunofluorescence studies are indicated. Pending results of routine microscopic examination, tissues may be held in the fixative at 4 C (39.2 F) up to three weeks before they are submitted for study to a qualified laboratory (for preparation of Michel's fixative see Muller et al., 1983).

**PEMPHIGUS.** Pemphigus is a group of chronic blistering diseases of skin and mucous membranes characterized microscopically by acantholysis with resultant intraepidermal bullae and immunologically by circulating and tissue-bound autoantibodies to intercellular epidermal antigen(s). It has only recently been recognized in the cat (Manning et al., 1982; Scott, 1978b; Scott, 1980; Scott et al., 1981). Owing to the thinness of the cat's epidermis, vesicles and bullae are so transient that they are often not seen. Thus one usually relies on identifying recent ulcers and erosions with epidermal collarettes, then examining the cat every three or four hours for appearance of blisters.

Pemphigus vulgaris has been recognized in several cats with no apparent age, breed, or sex predilection (Manning et al., 1982; see also references, Scott, 1984). They were presented for chronic ulceration of the oral mucosa, nasal philtrum, and mucocutaneous junctions of the lips and nostrils (Plate 13–2 *A* to *D*) and occasionally ulcers on the pinnae and footpads. Biopsies revealed suprabasilar acantholysis and cleft formation (Fig. 13–15). The basal epidermal cells remained attached to the basement membrane zone "like a row of tombstones." Direct immunofluorescence testing was positive for immunoglobulin, with or without complement, in the intercellular spaces.

In an 11-year-old castrated male treated at the Angell Memorial Animal Hospital for pemphigus vulgaris, inflammation and ulceration of the tongue, palate, and pharynx were prominent and refractory features (Holzworth, 1983). The extensive cutaneous (Plate 13–2 *E* to *H*) and mucocutaneous lesions were kept under control by prednisone and aurothioglucose administered alternately or together in the recommended dosages. The

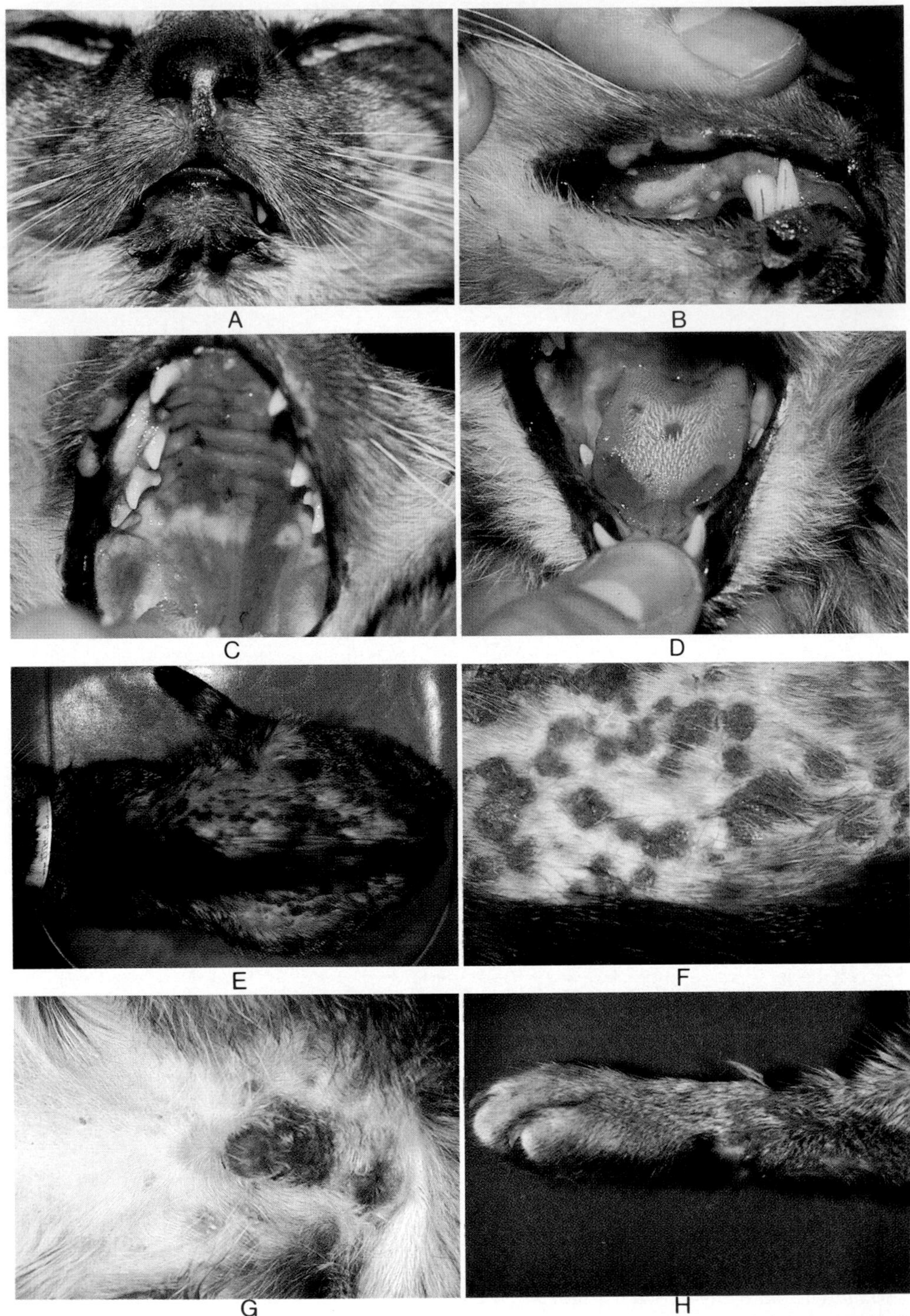


**Plate 13–2** Pemphigus vulgaris. *A*, Ulcerations of the nasal philtrum and lips. *B*, Two ulcers of the upper lip and one of the lower lip invading the skin of the chin. *C*, Multiple ulcers of the hard and soft palate. *D*, Ulcerative glossitis. *E*, Ulcerations of the back. *F*, Closer view of the back. *G*, Ulcers of the perineum. *H*, Ulcer of the metatarsus. (*E* through *H*, Courtesy Angell Memorial Animal Hospital.)

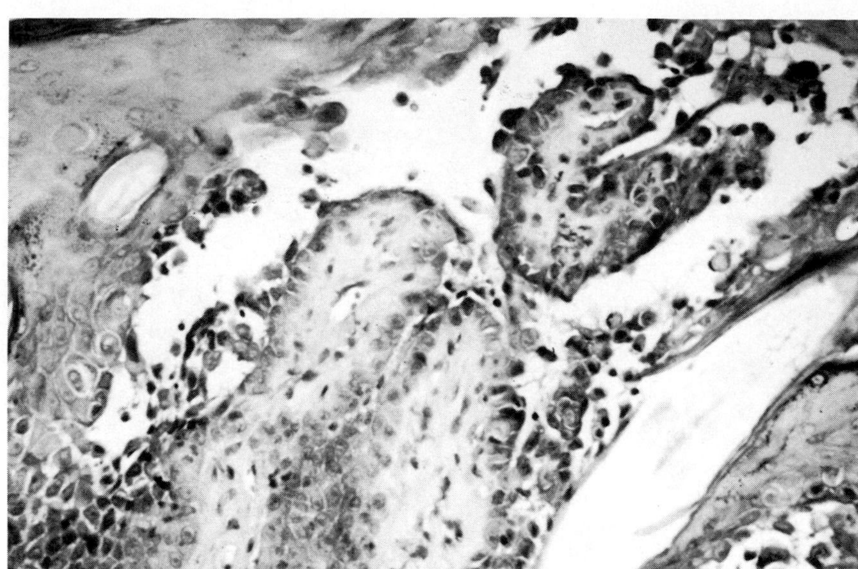

**Figure 13–15** Pemphigus vulgaris. Suprabasilar acantholysis and cleft formation are characteristic. H & E.

palatal and pharyngeal inflammation never entirely regressed, however, and the inappetence, retching, and vomiting that were present on admission recurred from time to time, although they were greatly alleviated by cimetidine. The continuing need for a high dose of steroid gradually led to extreme thinning of the skin, with frequent spontaneous tears that required suturing. After about a year and a half of treatment the cat became so weakened and emaciated that it had to be destroyed. An autopsy was not obtained.

Pemphigus foliaceus was recognized in several cats but had no age, breed, or sex predilection (Caciolo et al., 1984; Manning et al., 1982; Scott, 1978b, 1984; von Tscharner, 1984). A variably pruritic, exfoliative dermatitis, characterized by scales, crusts, erythema, alopecia, pustules, erosions, epidermal collarettes, and oozing, most often involves the face, ears, and paws. Direct smears of erosion disclose neutrophils and acantholytic keratinocytes. Biopsies reveal subcorneal to intragranular acantholysis and cleft formation. Direct immunofluorescence testing was positive for immunoglobulin in the intercellular spaces.

Pemphigus erythematosus was diagnosed in an eight-year-old intact male American Shorthair tabby (Scott, 1980; Scott et al., 1980). Signs were erythema, alopecia, erosions, epidermal collarettes, vesicopustules, oozing, crusting, and scaling affecting only the face and ears (Plate 13–3 *A* to *C*). The cat was febrile (40 C, 104.0 F) and somewhat depressed. Diagnosis was confirmed by direct smears of vesicle fluid (Plate 13–3*D*), skin biopsies characterized by subcorneal acantholysis and blister formation (Plate 13–3*E*), a positive antinuclear antibody (ANA) test (1:5), and positive direct immunofluorescence testing, which demonstrated Ig in the intercellular spaces and the basement membrane zone (Plate 13–3*F*).

All forms of feline pemphigus usually require immunosuppressive drug therapy. Prednisolone or prednisone may be given orally (3 mg/kg twice daily) until remission is attained and then administered on an alternate-day steroid schedule. However, many cases fail to respond to glucocorticoids alone (Scott, 1984).

Aurothioglucose (Solganal, Schering) may be used intramuscularly as follows: test doses of 1 mg and 2 mg a week apart, then 1 mg/kg weekly until remission (6 to 12 weeks), then once monthly (Muller et al., 1983; Scott, 1983, 1984; von Tscharner, 1984). Aurothioglucose may be used concurrently with glucocorticoids, especially during induction. Side effects, reported in man but apparently uncommon in animals, include cutaneous reactions, stomatitis, nephrotoxicity, blood dyscrasias, and anaphylactoid reactions. Careful monitoring is essential (Scott, 1983).

Recently, azathioprine (Imuran, Burroughs Wellcome) has been given orally at 1 mg/kg every 48 hours to cats with pemphigus (Caciolo et al., 1984). Leukopenia may occur, and careful monitoring is essential.

**SYSTEMIC LUPUS ERYTHEMATOSUS.** Systemic lupus erythematosus is an autoimmune disorder characterized by widespread organ involvement and the presence of a wide variety of autoantibodies in the serum. Although the etiology is unknown, most reports of human and canine disease have stressed the roles of genetic predilection, viral infection, and immunologic disorders.

Systemic lupus erythematosus with mucocutaneous lesions has been reported in five cats (Scott et al., 1979b, 1984). Four were presented for chronic dermatitis, characterized by widespread erythema, vesicles and bullae, paronychia, and pruritus (Plate 13–4 *A* to *C*). All four cats also became depressed, anorectic, and cachectic, with cyclic fever. Two had striking peripheral lymphadenopathy, and all four developed mucocutaneous ulcers of the nostrils or lip. Other complications among these cats were hemolytic anemia and glomerulonephritis. A fifth cat was presented for chronic ulcerative stomatitis and fever.

Significant laboratory findings were positive ANA tests in all the cats, histologic findings of subcorneal blister formation in three (Fig. 13–16), hydropic to lichenoid interface dermatitis in four (Fig. 13–17), and demonstration of immunoglobulin at the basement membrane of lesional skin by direct immunofluorescence testing (positive "lupus band") in three (Plate 13–4 *D*). All five cats were considered to have systemic lupus erythematosus on

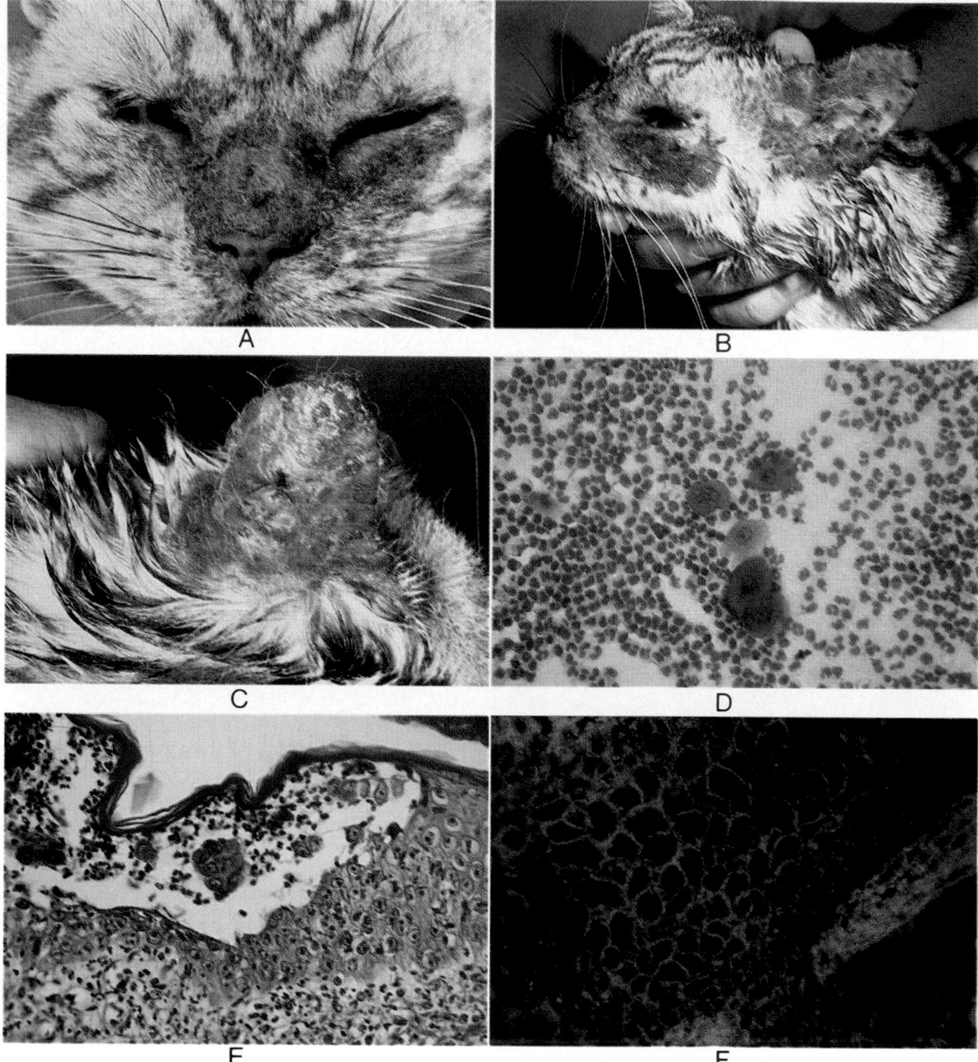


**Plate 13–3** Pemphigus erythematosus. *A*, Alopecia, erythema, oozing, and crusting of the face. *B*, Alopecia, erythema, and erosions of the face and ears. *C*, Alopecia, erythema, erosions, and epidermal collarettes on the pinna. *D*, Direct smear of vesicle fluid reveals neutrophils and acantholytic keratinocytes (new methylene blue stain). *E*, Subcorneal blister containing neutrophils and acantholytic keratinocytes. H & E. *F*, Immunofluorescence testing reveals the intercellular deposition of immunoglobulin.

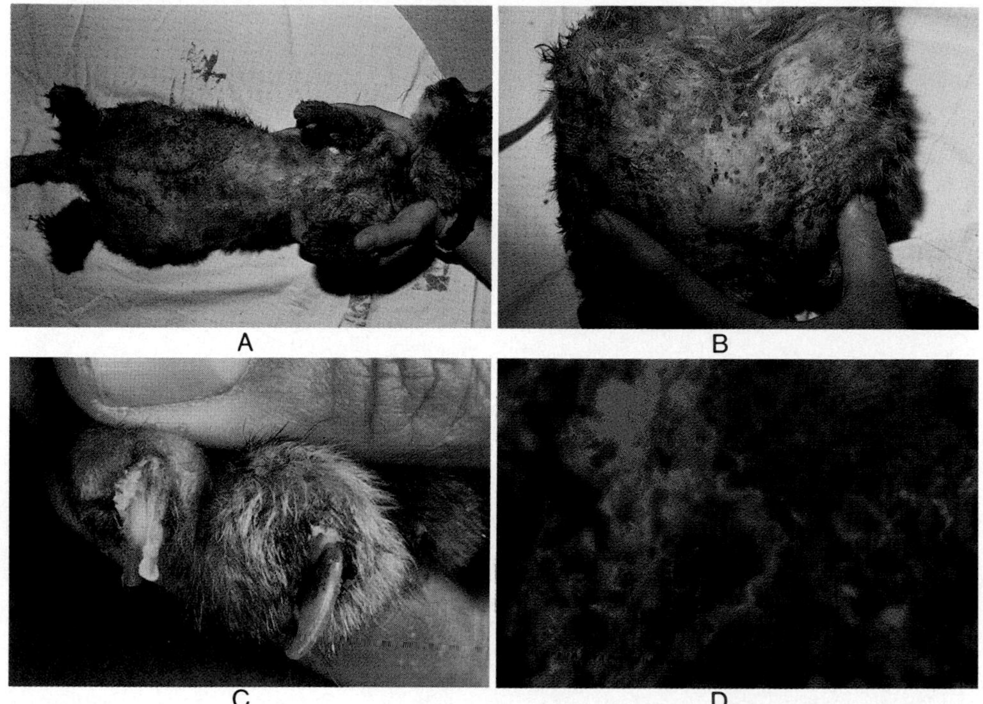


**Plate 13–4** Systemic lupus erythematosus. *A*, Patchy alopecia, erythema, and crusting. *B*, Closer view of abdominal skin, same cat. *C*, Paronychia with secondary *E. coli* and *Enterococcus* infection. *D*, Immunofluorescence testing of a skin lesion demonstrates focal deposition of immunoglobulin at the basement membrane zone.

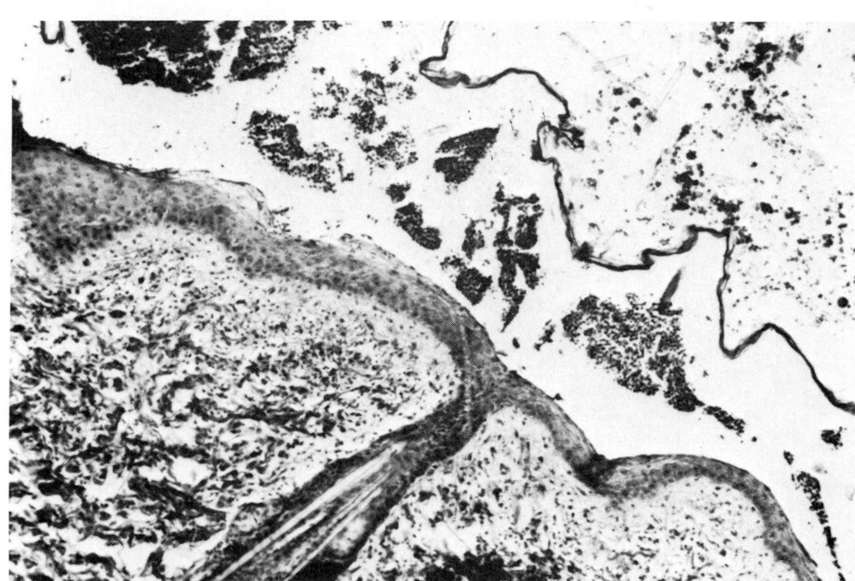

**Figure 13–16** Systemic lupus erythematosus. Subcorneal blister. H & E.

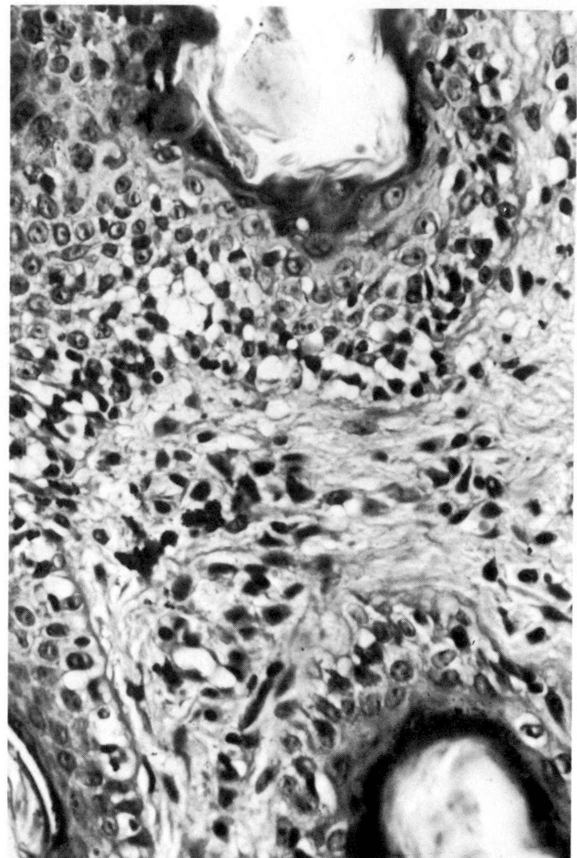

**Figure 13–17** Systemic lupus erythematosus. Hydropic degeneration of epidermal basal cells. PAS.

the basis of these findings and of other major and minor clinical criteria established by the American Rheumatism Association and others for the diagnosis of the disease in humans.

Therapy with oral prednisolone (3 mg/kg b.i.d. for induction, 2 to 4 mg/kg every other evening for maintenance) was successful in the four cats with skin disease. Residual scars and alopecia were features of the disease in these four cats. In the fifth cat the ulcerative stomatitis was controlled with methylprednisolone acetate (20 mg SC every 8 to 10 weeks).

**COLD AGGLUTININ DISEASE.** Cold agglutinin disease was diagnosed in a five-year-old spayed female Abyssinian with dry gangrene of the forepaws, ear tips, and the distal half of the tail (Schrader and Hurvitz, 1983). The spleen was moderately enlarged. The cat had been hospitalized 10 days before at another clinic for upper respiratory infection and had responded to symptomatic treatment.

The cold agglutinin titer was 1:120,000, and a direct Coombs antiglobulin test was positive.

The cat was treated for several days with prednisone. During the next six weeks the ear tips sloughed and by four months the forepaws and tail. The cat had some use of its forelimbs but supported most of its weight on the hindlimbs.

Cold agglutinin disease is associated with the IgM class of autoantibodies, which interact with red cells at temperatures below 37 C (98 F). Red cells are agglutinated in the cooler peripheral circulation, causing gangrenous necrosis. Some cases in man are associated with infection, and the disorder in this cat might have been incited by the upper respiratory infection.

## Disorders of Unknown or Multiple Origin

### Eosinophilic Granuloma Complex

The eosinophilic granuloma complex is a group of related lesions of the skin, lip, and oral cavity that constitute a common and notorious problem in domestic cats. It made its debut in the veterinary literature about a century ago with such names as "syphiloïde" and "rodent ulcer," because of gross resemblances to lesions of human syphilis and labial carcinoma, and continues to be a topic of concern to innumerable students of feline disease (e.g., Baker, 1970, 1974a; Bucci, 1966; Conroy, 1964; Doering and Jensen, 1973; Hess and MacEwen, 1977; Joshua, 1965; Muller et al., 1983; Scott, 1975a, 1980). Terms variously applied today to the common lesions of lip, mouth, and skin are eosinophilic ulcer, labial granuloma, eosinophilic granuloma, and intradermal granuloma. A curious linear lesion seen most often on the skin of the limbs and axillae and thought to belong to the complex was apparently first described in 1964 by Conroy. More recently there have been occasional reports of an eosinophilic keratitis (e.g., Brightman et al., 1979; Kipnis, 1979) that in a few instances has occurred in cats with concurrent eosinophilic granuloma (Szymanski, 1982). Whether this keratitis is indeed part of the complex is at present unknown.

Etiologies suggested for the complex have included self-inflicted trauma due to licking and grooming by the cat's spiny tongue, abrasion of the lips by the canine teeth, low-grade bacterial infection, and chronic allergy. Attempts to isolate pathogenic bacteria, fungi, and viruses from lesions have been unsuccessful (Conroy, 1964; Kral and Schwartzman, 1964; Scott, 1975a, 1980). Although lesions can be transmitted from one area to another on the same cat with autologous tissues (Hess and MacEwen, 1977; Scott, 1980), they cannot be transmitted to other cats with tissues or cell-free extracts (Kral and Schwartzman, 1964; Scott, 1980). Virus particles consistent with those of the calicivirus group were observed in fresh biopsy tissue by electron microscopy, but cross-contamination was suggested as more likely than a causal relationship (Neufeld et al., 1980). Clustering of cases has been reported, suggesting an hereditary or infectious factor (Baker, 1970, 1974a; Hess and MacEwen, 1977; Scott, 1975a, 1980). The disorder, for example, has occurred in siblings and may be contracted by suckling kittens of affected mothers (Holzworth, 1983). In my experience, there is no association with neutering. In the group of 140 cats studied by Hess and MacEwen (1977) 72 per cent of the cats were females, of which 65 per cent were spayed. Most of the cats in their group were domestic shorthairs. In a study of 19 cats with the eosinophilic granuloma complex, 13 were found to have circulating antibodies to components of normal feline epithelium—possible evidence that the condition may be an autoimmune disease (Gelberg et al., 1985).

At first sight, advanced labial and oral lesions and some of the plaques on the skin may suggest squamous cell cancer, but careful questioning may elicit a history of similar lesions in the past, and thorough examination often discloses lesions elsewhere on the body that provide a reliable presumptive diagnosis of eosinophilic granuloma complex.

This author distinguishes three separate lesions in the complex: indolent (eosinophilic) ulcer, eosinophilic plaque, and linear granuloma. Indolent ulcer occurs in cats from nine months to nine years of age (average 5.7 years), in females three times as often as in males (although females account for half the hospital population at the New York State College of Veterinary Medicine), and with no breed predilection (Scott, 1980). These lesions are well circumscribed, ulcerated, red-brown, alopecic, and glistening, with slight raised borders and a central sphacelus. They measure from 0.2 × 0.5 to 5.0 × 7.5 cm. They are usually unassociated with pain or pruritus. Indolent ulcers may occur anywhere on the skin (Plate 13–5 *A* and *B*) or in the oral cavity, but 80 per cent occur unilaterally or bilaterally on the upper lip ("rodent ulcer"). In the mouth they involve mucosa and submucosa; in the skin they are confined to the epidermis and dermis.

Diagnosis of indolent ulcer is based on history, physical examination, and sometimes skin biopsy. Usually, however, the appearance is so characteristic that biopsy is dispensed with. Blood and tissue eosinophilia are uncommon. Skin biopsy reveals chronic ulcerative dermatitis, with neutrophils, plasma cells, and mononuclear cells predominating.

Eosinophilic plaques occur in cats from two to six years of age (average 3.3 years), with no breed or sex predilection (Scott, 1980). They are well circumscribed, raised, ulcerated, exudative, fiery red, and alopecic, and range from 0.4 to 7.5 cm in diameter. Eosinophilic plaques may occur anywhere in the skin and oral cavity, but 80 per cent occur on the abdomen and medial thighs (Plate 13–5 *C*). Those of the skin are confined to the dermis and epidermis and are associated with intense pruritus, licking, and chewing.

Diagnosis of eosinophilic plaque is usually obvious from history and physical appearance. Blood and tissue eosinophilia is the rule. Skin biopsy reveals a hyperplastic or spongiotic superficial and deep perivascular dermatitis or diffuse dermatitis with epidermal vesicle formation. The dermis contains massive numbers of eosinophils and lesser numbers of mast cells in a diffuse, interstitial pattern. Lesions grossly and microscopically identical to eosinophilic plaques are occasionally seen with allergy to fleas or food. When large numbers of mast cells are present, close inspection of mast cell morphology is essential to distinguish this condition from mast cell tumor. Experienced veterinary pathologists occasionally differ on their interpretation of a given lesion, and only with the passage of time does it become clear whether the lesion was indeed an eosinophilic granuloma or a mast cell tumor.

Linear granuloma occurs in cats from six months to five years of age (average one year), in females twice as often as in males, and with no breed predilection (Scott, 1980). Both in domestic and purebred kittens it may involve littermates (Holzworth, 1983). The lesions are well circumscribed, raised, firm, yellow or yellow-pink, alopecic, and usually linear, being 0.2 to 0.4 cm wide and 5.0 to 10.0 cm long. They are confined to the dermis and are usually asymptomatic. Linear granulomas may occur anywhere in the skin but most often in linear form on the caudal aspect of the hindlimbs (Plate 13–5 *D*). On the lower lip (Plate 13–5 *E*), the paws (Plate 13–5 *F*), and within the mouth they assume a nodular form. Linear granuloma is the most frequent cause of swollen chin ("chin edema") and swollen lower lip ("pouting cat"). On the limbs and in the axillae they are often discovered only by chance when a young cat is presented for neutering. In some cases there is a moderate associated lymphadenopathy. Most linear granulomas of the skin and the related lymphadenopathy regress spontaneously.

Diagnosis of linear granuloma is usually obvious from the typical appearance. Blood and tissue eosinophilia are most often associated with the oral lesions. Biopsy of skin reveals granulomatous dermatitis with marked collagenolysis.

Constitutional signs are uncommon with the eosinophilic granuloma complex. Regional lymphadenopathy is occasionally present. In one study (Scott, 1975a), indolent ulcer occurred as the sole entity in 33 per cent of cases, eosinophilic plaque in 16.7 per cent, and linear granuloma in 28 per cent. In many a cat, however, all three lesions can be found, in any combination. Serum protein electrophoresis may reveal moderate or marked, nonspecific elevations in α2, β, and γ globulin fractions (Hess and MacEwen, 1977; Scott, 1980). Many cats with indolent ulcer tested for feline leukemia virus test positive, but the significance of this finding is unknown.

Various modes of therapy have been used for eosinophilic granuloma. Some early regimens were based on the belief that licking and irritation from contiguous canine teeth were factors in the initiation and perpetuation of the lesions. Thus some veterinarians tried the harsh expedients of removing the canine teeth or the dorsal papillae of the tongue. Topical medicaments intended to discourage licking are rapidly removed by the cat. Elizabethan collars and tranquilizers merely produce a lull in the action.

Management of the various lesions of the eosinophilic granuloma complex varies with the type and site of the lesions and their responsiveness to treatment.

Glucocorticoids are, in general, the drugs of choice (see references, Scott, 1980). It is essential that they be used in adequate dosage from the start. An oral glucocorticoid in large doses (e.g., 1 to 2 mg/kg prednisolone b.i.d.) is often successful. If a cat is difficult to medicate, an effective alternative favored by the author is methylprednisolone acetate (Depo-Medrol, Upjohn), 20 mg SC total dose for an adult cat every 2 weeks. Whatever the route of administration the glucocorticoid should be given for 30 days.

Progestogens are also effective for eosinophilic granuloma (Halliwell, 1977; Hess and MacEwen, 1977; Hutchison, 1978; Scott, 1980; Turner, 1977). Repository progesterone or medroxyprogesterone acetate may be given (2.2 to 22 mg/kg IM or SC) every two weeks. Megestrol acetate may be given orally (2.5 to 5 mg total dose or 0.5 to 1 mg/kg) every other day, until lesions are in total remission (two to six weeks). Progestogens should not be administered to intact females.

Intralesional glucocorticoid infiltration is sometimes successful with solitary lesions that have been unresponsive to systemic treatment with a glucocorticoid or progestogen. A short-acting anesthetic is required. Three mg (0.5 ml) triamcinolone (Vetalog, Squibb) is infiltrated into the lesion weekly until complete regression, usually in

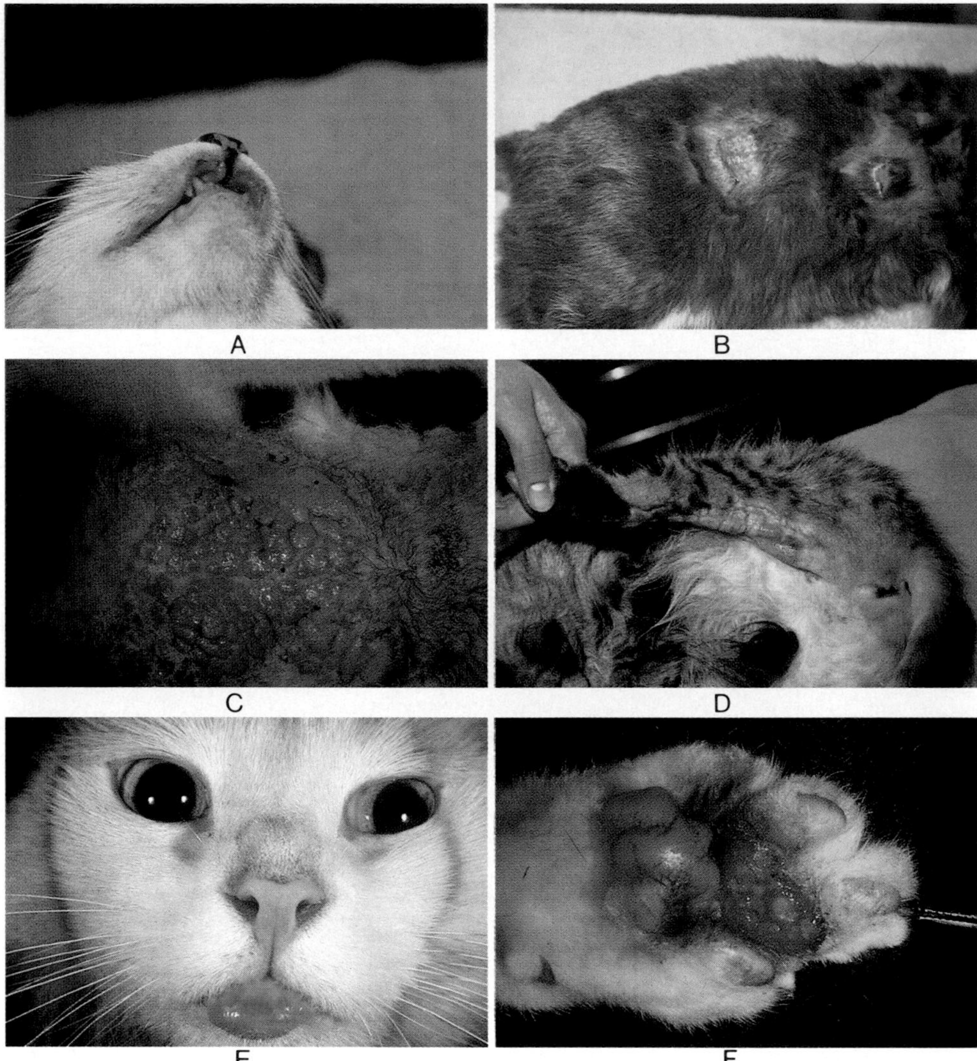


**Plate 13–5** Eosinophilic granuloma complex. *A*, Bilateral eosinophilic ulcers on the upper lip. *B*, Multiple eosinophilic ulcers on the side. *C*, Multiple eosinophilic plaques on the abdomen. *D*, Linear granuloma of the caudal aspect of the hindlimbs. *E*, This granuloma of the lower lip has the same microscopic characteristics as linear granuloma of the skin. *F*, Interdigital eosinophilic granuloma. (*E* and *F*, Courtesy Angell Memorial Animal Hospital.)

three to four weeks, after which 3 mg may be given SC for two weeks (Hess and MacEwen, 1977). Rarely, severe hemorrhage occurs with intralesional infiltration of labial lesions (Holzworth, 1983).

Owners should be alerted to observe for signs of the possible side effects of intensive and prolonged treatment with glucocorticoids or progestogens (diabetes mellitus, hyperadrenocorticism, mammary hyperplasia or neoplasia).

Two immunopotentiating imidazoles, levamisole and thiabendazole, have had limited trials for eosinophilic granuloma refractory to glucocorticoids and progestogens (Hess and MacEwen, 1977; Scott, 1980). Levamisole (5 mg/kg orally three times a week for four to six weeks, then weekly) and thiabendazole (5 to 10 mg/kg orally, on a similar schedule) have produced at least 75 per cent regression in lesion size in about half the cases treated. These agents, however, appear to be incapable of inducing a complete remission as sole treatment. They are not licensed for use in cats.

Adjunctive measures that are sometimes helpful in hastening regression of oral and labial lesions are electrocautery or cautery with silver nitrate or trichloracetic acid (Holzworth, 1983). Cryosurgery achieves varying results (Griffiths, 1977; Lane and Gruffydd-Jones, 1977; Scott, 1980), success being most likely with lip ulcers (Willemse and Lubberink, 1978).

Excision or curettage may severely deform the lips, but excision is occasionally resorted to for refractory lesions where the skin is loose enough for satisfactory suturing.

Bandaging of lesions on the neck, lower limbs, and between the toes promotes healing by protecting against the cat's licking. Bandaging over a thin film of Pellitol (Pitman-Moore), an astringent, analgesic ointment, brings about rapid regression of lesions of the toepads and interdigital skin (Holzworth, 1983), but the bandage must be well secured by tape as the material is toxic if licked off by the cat. For skin lesions where bandaging is impossible, an Elizabethan collar provides a respite from licking until a systemic drug exerts its effect.

Occasional solitary lesions, especially lip ulcers that are refractory to all other treatment, may be healed for considerable periods by irradiation (McClelland, 1954). Thirty to 50 per cent of solitary lesions not improving with medical therapy heal with 300 to 500 rads weekly for four to eight weeks (Biery, 1977). This approach, however, is costly, requiring general anesthesia and special equipment.

Rarely, an eosinophilic granuloma regresses spontaneously (Hess and MacEwen, 1977). The same workers also reported that in five cats with refractory lesions, healing occurred within 6 to 10 weeks when they were simply confined in hospital cages.

For prognosis in general, staging of lesions has been found to be more accurate than extent, location, or duration (Hess and MacEwen, 1977; Scott, 1980). Stage I lesions have received no prior treatment; Stage II lesions have responded previously to steroids but have recurred; Stage III lesions have been refractory to conventional steroid therapy. Stage I lesions, if treated aggressively with a steroid or progestogen, should respond completely with only a 10 to 25 per cent chance of recurrence. Stages II and III lesions, although responding to most regimens that are continued long enough, have a 50 per cent recurrence rate within six months.

It is therefore essential that cats with eosinophilic granuloma be treated aggressively when first presented. Incomplete response or recurrence is invited by giving inadequate doses of drugs for too short a time (less than four weeks). Although megestrol acetate is very effective for these lesions, it is infrequently used by the author, because it is not licensed for use in cats, may have serious side effects, and is no more effective than glucocorticoids properly used. Response to therapy is by no means predictable. Some granulomas respond only to glucocorticoids, some only to megestrol, and some to neither. Cats with recurrent lesions of eosinophilic granuloma complex should be checked for allergy to fleas, food, and inhalants (Kunkle, 1984; Muller et al., 1983).

## Hypereosinophilic Syndrome

A remarkable case of progressive generalized eosinophilic dermatitis that resisted all forms of therapy was accompanied by a marked eosinophilia and proved at autopsy to be associated with eosinophilic infiltration of lymph nodes, liver, spleen, and intestine (Scott et al., 1985). It was considered to be a manifestation of hypereosinophilic syndrome.

## Miliary Dermatitis (Miliary Eczema, "Scabby Cat Disease")

The veterinary literature abounds with still other terms that have been applied to this disorder and also with speculative or anecdotal testimony as to possible etiology (see references in Scott, 1980). Miliary dermatitis is now generally accepted as a descriptive term for a frequent pruritic, papulocrustous eruption of cats—a manifestation that has a number of acceptably documented causes or in occasional cases appears to be "idiopathic" (Kunkle, 1984; Muller et al., 1983).

Prominent causes are parasitic (most importantly flea allergy dermatitis, less often cheyletiellosis, pediculosis, trombiculidiasis, and intestinal parasitism), fungal (dermatophytosis), bacterial (folliculitis), and allergic (food hypersenstivity, atopy, or drug eruption) (Muller et al., 1983). Other possible causes are nutritional deficiencies (of biotin or fatty acids). These disorders are discussed elsewhere in this chapter, and when any one of them can be identified by solid clinical evidence or laboratory procedures, the specific term should be preferred to "miliary dermatitis."

Histories vary greatly depending on etiology (Muller et al., 1983). Seasonal occurrence of a dermatitis may be an important clue. If human or animal contacts are affected, contagion is suggested. Associated digestive disease may point to food hypersensitivity or internal parasitism. If response to a systemic glucocorticoid has been poor, the clinician must consider food hypersensitivity, drug eruption, fungal or bacterial infection, or an idiopathic etiology.

Signs of miliary dermatitis may occur in cats of any breed or age and in either sex irrespective of neutering. Papules and crusts associated with varying degrees of itching often begin over the back (tailhead, rump, neck, or head) but can generalize (Fig. 13–18) and result in partial alopecia. Some cats lick and rub rather than scratch; some become hyperesthetic, growl, suffer personality changes, and are subject to sudden twitching of the skin and spells of frantic running and jumping.

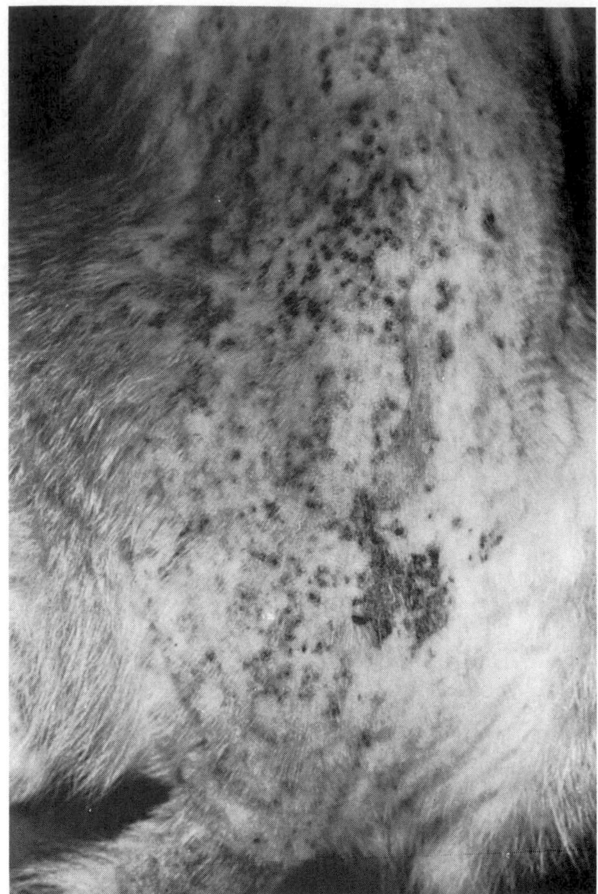

**Figure 13–18** Idiopathic miliary dermatitis. Papules, crusts, erythema, and alopecia over the back. (Courtesy Angell Memorial Animal Hospital.)

Diagnosis requires a tenacious effort to identify a specific cause, since miliary dermatitis is but a symptom (Muller et al., 1983). History alone occasionally provides an essential clue. More often a thorough physical examination, including Wood's light examination and microscopic examination of skin scrapings, identifies a fungal or parasitic cause. Laboratory procedures such as fungal or bacterial culture or fecal flotation may be required. A hemogram characterized by eosinophilia is suggestive of parasitism.

Microscopically, miliary dermatitis is characterized by subacute or chronic, nonsuppurative dermatitis with varying numbers of neutrophils, mast cells, and mononuclears (Scott, 1980). Eosinophils are prominent if the etiology is parasitic.

A diagnosis of idiopathic miliary dermatitis can only be justified if all known causes have been excluded.

In a controlled study of cats with idiopathic miliary dermatitis (McCusker, 1965) normal cats were found to have an average skin histamine level of 13.3 μg/gm of skin and an average of 7.1 mast cells/high power field, whereas cats with idiopathic miliary dermatitis had four times the skin histamine level (57.2 μg/gm) and three times the mast cell numbers (23.54/high power field).

Management of miliary dermatitis of known etiologies is discussed elsewhere in this chapter. Only treatment for the idiopathic form will be discussed here.

Idiopathic miliary dermatitis is exceedingly difficult to control with glucocorticoids (Scott, 1980). Massive doses are often needed for induction (i.e., 2 to 4 mg prednisolone/kg/day), and maintenance doses must often be given every other day. As might be imagined, steroid-induced side effects can be expected with long-term therapy at such doses.

Excellent results have been achieved with progestogens (e.g., Chesney, 1976; Halliwell, 1977; Houdeshell et al., 1977; Scott, 1980). Megestrol acetate is given orally at 2.5 to 5 mg total dose, once every other day, until lesions are gone. The cat is then given the same dose at one- to two-week intervals for maintenance. Repository progesterone (2.2 to 22 mg/kg) or medroxyprogesterone acetate (Depo-Provera, 50 to 175 mg total dose) is given intramuscularly or subcutaneously as needed (not more often than once every two to three months). Progestogen therapy will likely be needed for life, as the dermatitis tends to recur within two to six weeks after treatment is stopped. Progestogens are the most effective therapy for idiopathic miliary dermatitis. However, they should be used only as a last resort, because they are not licensed for use in cats and because serious side effects include transient or permanent diabetes mellitus, mammary hyperplasia or neoplasia (either sex), adrenocortical suppression, and pyometra in entire females.

## Seborrheic Disorders

Seborrheic skin disease is uncommon in the cat (Austin, 1975a; Carr, 1979; Conroy, 1964; Scott, 1980), and is usually generalized.

**SEBORRHEA SICCA.** Characterized by dry skin and hair coat, excessive scaling ("dandruff"), and variable pruritus, this is the most frequent form of seborrhea and may be associated with (1) ectoparasitism (especially cheyletiellosis and pediculosis), (2) endoparasitism, (3) dermatophytosis due to *Microsporum canis*, (4) malnutrition, (5) many systemic illnesses, (6) apparent fat deficiency, and (7) the "winter heat syndrome" (high indoor temperature with low humidity) (Scott, 1980, 1984). Thus the diagnostic study might include skin scrapings, fecal examination, fungal culture, a trial of dietary fat supplementation (see section on nutritional skin disorders), and appropriate laboratory tests if the cat has signs of systemic illness. Therapy should if possible correct the underlying cause(s) and may also make use of symptomatic antiseborrheic topical agents. The author prefers a nonmedicated hypoallergenic emollient shampoo (Allergroom Allerderm, Inc.). Tar preparations should be avoided, as they may be toxic to cats.

**SEBORRHEA OLEOSA AND SEBORRHEIC DERMATITIS.** These conditions, both characterized by varying degrees of scaling, greasiness, alopecia, erythema, and pruritus, are rare in the cat but have been associated with feline leukemia virus infection (with or without signs of neoplasia), chronic liver disease (usually cholangiohepatitis with cirrhosis, occasionally neoplasia), and systemic lupus erythematosus (Scott, 1980). Diagnostic study in such cases might include hemogram, serum chemistry panel, tests for feline leukemia virus infection, and an antinuclear antibody (ANA) test. Except with lupus, therapy has been disappointing.

A condition referred to as "sticky cats" has been reported (Longbottom, 1977). Affected cats (any age or breed and of either sex) were healthy in all respects, except for generalized greasiness of the hair coat. The condition apparently waxed and waned irrespective of therapy. It was suggested that it may be a form of seborrhea oleosa (Fennell, 1977).

**STUD-TAIL.** This seborrheic disorder occurs most often in sexually active purebred male cats (Persian, Siamese, Rex) (see references, Scott, 1980). The term "stud-tail" is a misnomer, however, as the condition may sometimes occur in castrated males and in females both intact and spayed. It is characterized by hyperactivity of a group of modified sebaceous glands located on the dorsal surface of the tail and corresponding to the supracaudal organ of the dog. Comedones result, and yellow-to-black, waxy material accumulates on the skin and hairs of the dorsal surface of the tail (Fig. 13–19). The condition is most apparent and objectionable in white cats. Pain and pruritus are absent, and the cats are presented for aesthetic reasons. Rarely a bacterial folliculitis develops, with draining tracts (Holzworth, 1983).

The Rex breed is especially predisposed to this form of seborrhea. Greasiness in the skin folds about the claws is also prominent in this breed (Holzworth, 1983).

Microscopically, stud-tail is characterized by pronounced hypertrophy and hyperplasia of sebaceous glands and varying degrees of hyperkeratosis (Scott, 1980).

Treatment by castration of males may be of some effect. Antiseborrheic shampoos may be needed once or twice weekly. I prefer benzoyl peroxide (Pyoben, Allerderm, Inc.). Pssssst (Clairol), a spray-on, brush-on shampoo that contains a starchy material, is reported by some owners of Persians to be effective in removing the greasy accumulation (Holzworth, 1983). Progestogen compounds (repository progesterone, medroxyprogesterone acetate, megestrol acetate) have also controlled stud-tail (Scott, 1980). It has been suggested that confinement in catteries or other limited quarters may discourage a cat from grooming properly and that an outdoor environment, fresh air, and sunshine may promote normal grooming activity (Muller et al., 1983).

## Acne

"Acne" of the chin occurs in mature cats of any breed or either sex (see references, Scott, 1980). The etiology is unclear. Feline acne is not analogous to the endocrine-related acne of adolescent dogs and humans. It involves the large sebaceous glands of the chin and the related follicles, which become plugged with sebum and keratinous debris. One suggested etiologic factor is the inability of the cat (especially one with "seborrheic" tendencies) to clean its chin thoroughly with its paws. Another is the periodic shedding cycle of the cat, acne beginning when telogen hairs are unable to push keratosebaceous plugs out of follicular openings.

Feline acne is characterized by comedo formation on the chin and lower lip (Fig. 13–20). Most cats are asymptomatic and are presented because of the unsightly appearance of the "blackheads." Occasionally, secondary bacterial infection (usually with *Pasteurella multocida*, β-hemolytic streptococci, or coagulase-positive *Staphylococcus* spp) complicates the condition, causing papules, pustules (folliculitis), edema, abscessation, and fistula formation (furunculosis) (Fig. 13–20). Folliculitis and furunculosis can be pruritic or painful and may be accompanied in severe cases by fever, depression, lethargy, difficulty in eating, and regional lymphadenopathy.

The diagnosis is apparent from physical examination, but refractory lesions should be scraped for *Demodex* mites and cultured for dermatophytes (Scott, 1980). Histologic examination, depending on the stage of the lesion, may reveal (1) follicular keratosis, plugging, and dilatation, with comedo formation; (2) development of perifolliculitis; and finally (3) folliculitis and furunculosis with pyogranulomatous dermatitis (Scott, 1980).

Treatment may not be necessary if comedones are asymptomatic, the owner being warned to observe closely for signs of secondary folliculitis or furunculosis. Many cats will live a long life, with the lesion never developing beyond this asymptomatic phase. For meticulous owners, or for cats that tend to progress into the infected stage, the condition must be held in check by constant attention: (1) gentle washing with a keratolytic shampoo (sulfur or benzoyl peroxide), and (2) the use of keratolytic or astringent topical medication or both (colloidal sulfur or benzoyl peroxide; benzoyl peroxide *gel* is often too irritating for use in cats).

Established infection usually requires treatment under sedation or anesthesia: clipping of the area, manual evac-

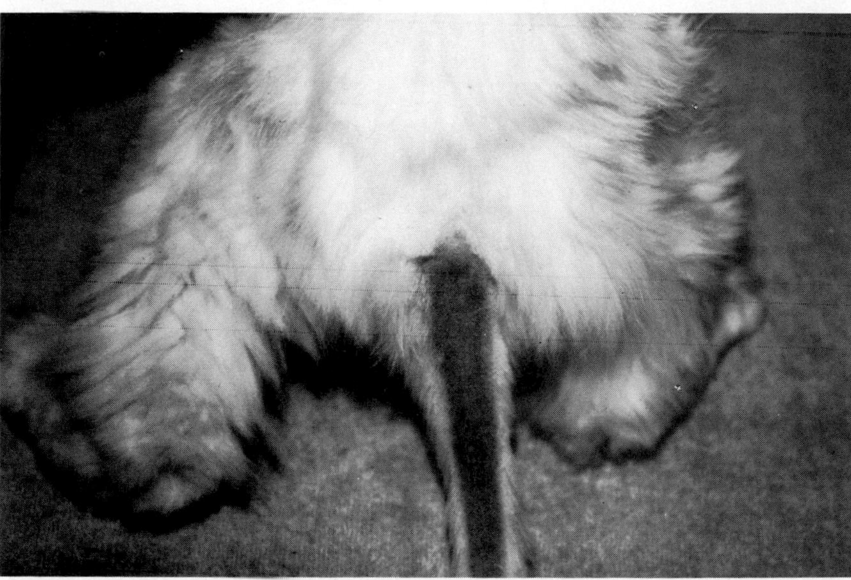

**Figure 13–19** "Stud-tail" in a male Persian.

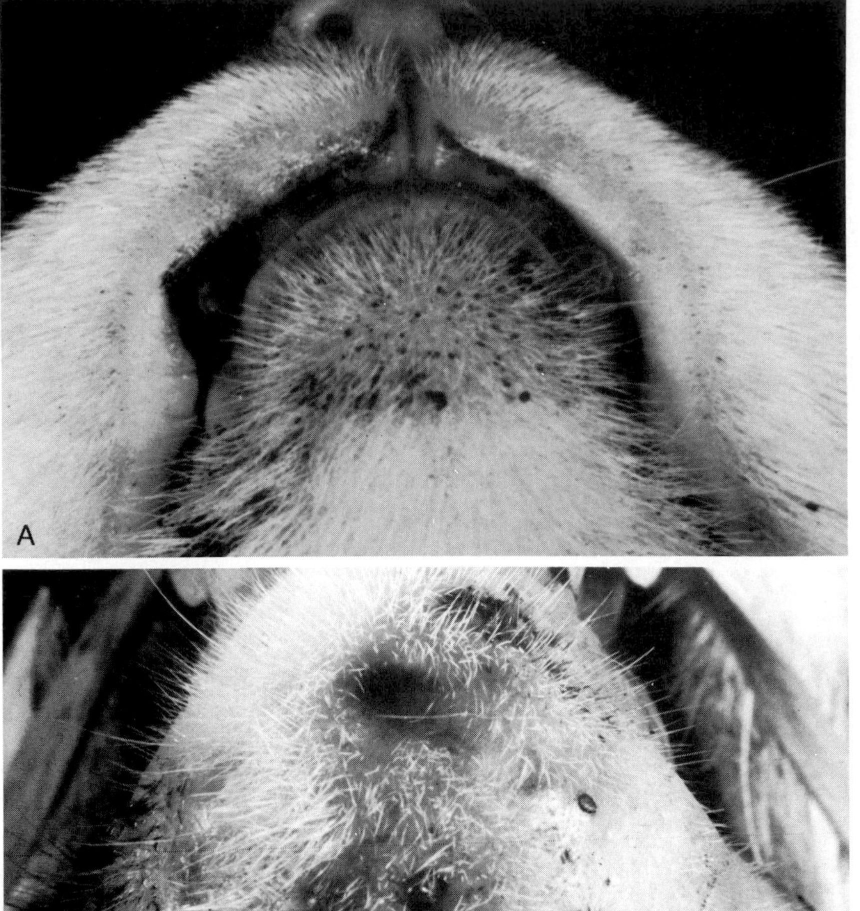


**Figure 13–20** Acne of the chin. *A*, Mild form with multiple comedones. *B*, Severe form with comedones, furunculosis, and fistulae. (Courtesy Angell Memorial Animal Hospital.)

uation of comedones, and gentle cleansing (chlorhexidine, benzoyl peroxide shampoo). Follow-up treatment includes hot packs of water, to which may be added a mild astringent (aluminum acetate) (10 minutes, t.i.d.), and a systemic antibiotic (ampicillin, hetacillin, amoxicillin, for 10 to 14 days). Fistulous tracts, which are the ultimate complication of severe infection, must be treated by surgical drainage and débridement. Flushing with chlorhexidine or benzoyl peroxide and local instillation of an antibiotic may also be indicated.

Recurrences of acne are the rule. If a cat is prone to infection or if the owner desires a clean-chinned cat, cleansing and keratolytic-astringent therapy may be required every two to seven days for life.

## Chin Edema

This rare condition, or group of conditions, affecting the chin of the cat is usually asymptomatic (Muller, 1974a; Wilkinson, 1966). Affected cats are presented for a swollen chin, which may be firm or spongy but is not tender or inflamed (Fig. 13–21). Possibly the condition is associated in some way with the large aggregation of sebaceous glands on the chin.

Another "chin lesion" characterized by acute swelling, red or brown discoloration, and alopecia has been reported (Stansbury, 1966). This condition is also asymptomatic and usually disappears spontaneously but may recur. Biopsy reveals tissue eosinophilia. Topical medications and surgical excision are not effective. Intralesional glucocorticoids hasten recovery.

It is likely that so-called chin edema is a stage of at least two feline skin disorders: acne and eosinophilic granuloma complex (Scott, 1980).

## Psychogenic Alopecia and Dermatitis

Psychogenic alopecia and dermatitis (neurodermatitis, hyperesthesia syndrome, lick dermatitis) occur in grown cats of any age or breed and of either sex, irrespective of

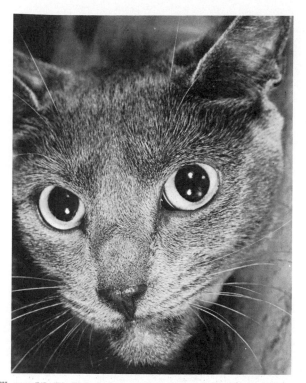

**Figure 13–21** Chin edema. This symmetric enlargement is usually asymptomatic and regresses without treatment. (Courtesy Angell Memorial Animal Hospital.)

neutering (Austin, 1975a; Brummer, 1973; Guilhon, 1962; Joshua, 1965; Muller et al., 1983; Scott, 1980). Experience at the New York State College of Veterinary Medicine indicates that Siamese, Burmese, Himalayans, and Abyssinians account for over 90 per cent of cases, although constituting only 9 per cent of the total hospital population of cats (Scott, 1980).

This psychogenic disorder takes two forms—dermatitic and alopecic. In the dermatitic form, cats are presented for excessive licking and chewing, usually concentrated on a solitary excoriated area (Fig. 13–22). Such lesions are red, alopecic, flat or raised, ulcerated, oozing, well demarcated, and of varying size (see Fig. 13–21). They are usually located on an easily accessible area (limb, abdomen, or flank). They are differentiated from eosinophilic ulcer or plaque on the basis of history (the cats *create* these lesions), clinical signs (eosinophilic ulcer is not usually pruritic), and response to therapy (glucocorticoids are of little benefit).

In the alopecic form, cats obsessively lick and groom one or more areas of the hair coat, producing partial alopecia and stubbled hairs, but leaving normal-appearing skin. These lesions often take the form of a "stripe" down the middle of the back or occur on the perineum, caudomedial thigh, or abdomen in a pattern resembling that of feline endocrine alopecia (Figs. 13–23 and 13–24). Careful inspection, however, reveals that the hairs in affected areas are broken and not easily epilated. In Siamese, hair regrowth in affected areas is much darker than normal. Normal hair color usually returns with the next hair cycle.

Diagnosis is based on a thorough history and laboratory procedures to rule out other disorders. Fungal culture should always be performed, as *Microsporum canis* can produce lesions identical to the dermatitic and alopecic forms of psychogenic alopecia (Scott, 1980). Food hypersensitivity and atopy may cause symmetric alopecia identical to that in psychogenic alopecia. Skin biopsy reveals either subacute or chronic nonsuppurative dermatitis (dermatitic form) or normal skin (alopecic form). Occasional wrinkling of the outer root sheath or intra- and perifollicular hemorrhage or both may be seen with either form (Scott, 1980).

Successful treatment depends on discovering what caused the cat to start its obsessive licking or chewing. Organic diseases should always be ruled out. Occasionally, lesions are associated with anal sac impaction or infection, taeniasis, ectoparasitism, urolithiasis, musculoskeletal disorders (arthritis, myositis), neurologic disorders (psychomotor epilepsy, "cauda equina syndrome"), foreign bodies, or prior injury.

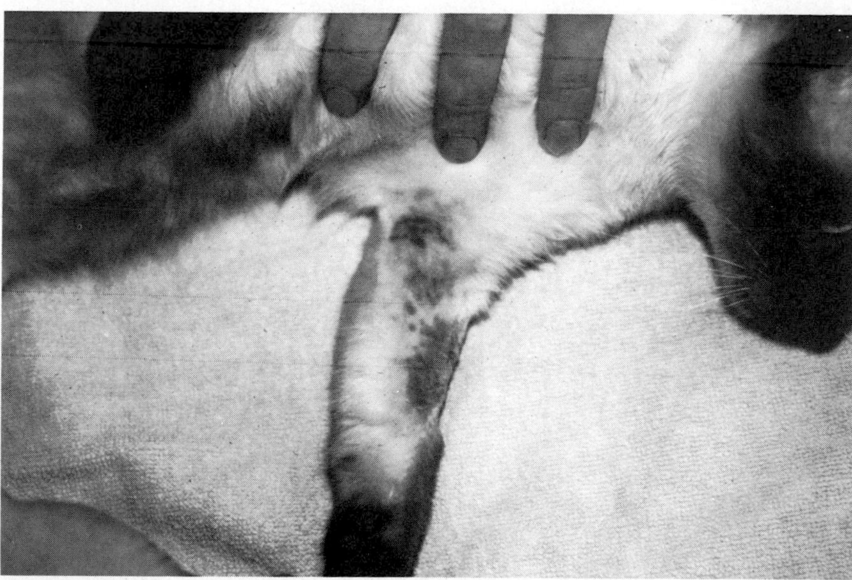

**Figure 13–22** Psychogenic alopecia and dermatitis, forelimb of a Siamese cat.

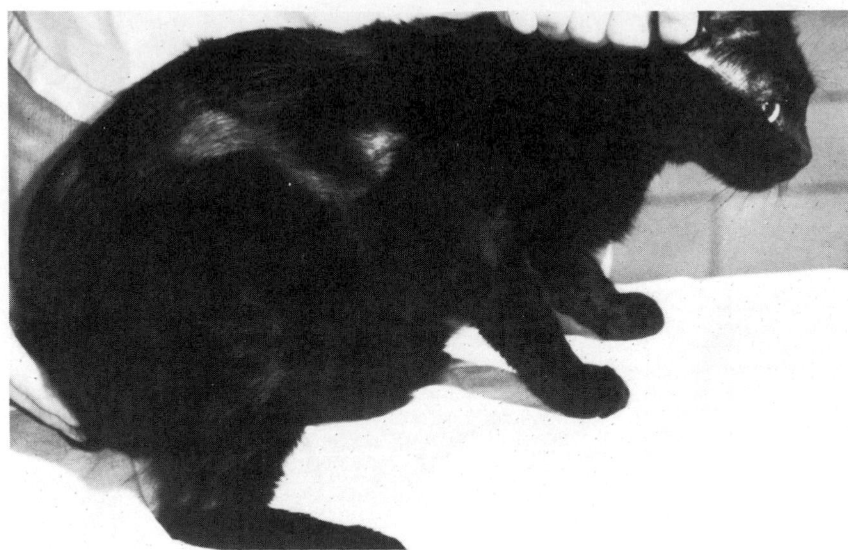

**Figure 13–23** Psychogenic alopecia, Siamese cross. Patchy alopecia on the flank.

In over 90 per cent of cases, however, the precipitating factor is some "psychic insult" (Scott, 1980). Thus it is essential to discover what change in the cat's way of life preceded the problem. Examples are endless and occasionally bizarre but are commonly change of environment (boarding, hospitalization, new home, confinement indoors), new pets or persons introduced into the household, or a new cat or dog in the neighborhood infringing on territory. Some authors have suggested that an "anxiety neurosis" is sometimes involved, since the condition is most frequently seen in breeds that tend to be high-strung and emotional.

Identification and correction of the precipitating cause often result in disappearance of the condition. Frequently, however, symptomatic treatment is the only course. Many such therapeutic approaches have been proposed, including glucocorticoids, antihistamines, vitamin-mineral supplements, radiation therapy, foul-tasting topicals, and Elizabethan collars. Such methods are usually unsuccessful. Centrally acting "anti-anxiety" drugs offer the best possibility for control and breaking of the behavior pattern. Phenobarbital (2.2 to 6.6 mg/kg orally b.i.d.) diazepam (1.25 to 2.5 mg orally b.i.d.), or both simultaneously are the drug therapy of choice. Progestogens (repository progesterone, medroxyprogesterone acetate, megestrol acetate) are a less desirable alternative. Drug treatment is usually continued for 30 days in an attempt to break the cat's "bad habit" (Scott, 1980). Some cats respond to one drug, some to another, so several may have to be tried. With megestrol acetate, some cats may need large doses initially (10 to 20 mg/dose every other day). Therapy should be stopped after a month, as some cats (especially if a precipitating factor was discovered and corrected) will be cured. Other cats will require intermittent or continuous maintenance therapy for life. Because cats with psychogenic alopecia are otherwise healthy and drug therapy may itself cause undesirable behavior, many owners choose simply to live with the condition.

## Feline Hyperesthesia Syndrome

Also referred to as "rolling skin" disease, neurodermatitis, neuritis, psychomotor epilepsy, and pruritic dermatosis of Siamese cats, this striking disorder, while discussed among practitioners since the 1960s, has received little notice in the veterinary literature (Alterman, 1977; Austin, 1975a; Mosier, 1975, 1977; Parker et al., 1983). Cases have been encountered from time to time since 1964 at Angell Memorial Animal Hospital, where

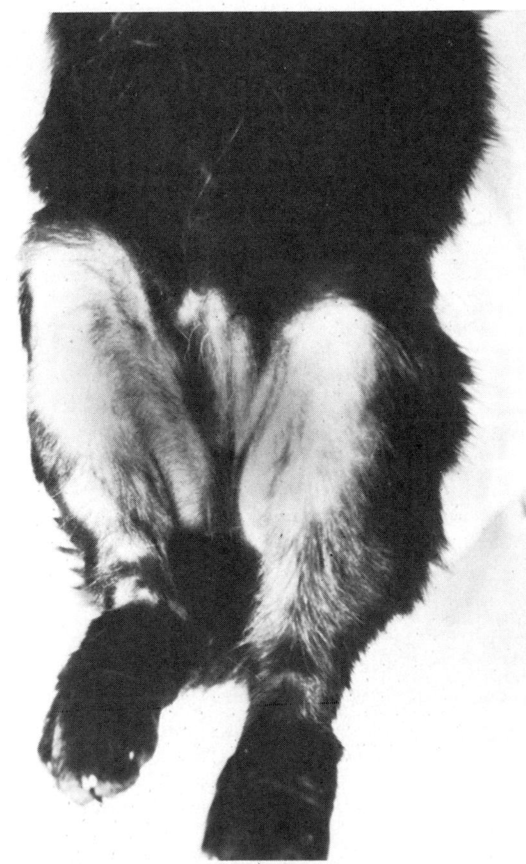

**Figure 13–24** Psychogenic alopecia of the groin and medial aspect of the hindlimbs in a Siamese cross.

the cats involved have almost always been Siamese or Siamese-crosses (Holzworth, 1983). In a large cat practice in Chicago, however, other purebreds, as well as domestic cats, have sometimes been affected (Stein, 1983).

The condition seems to be increasing in incidence, and its bizarre manifestations have been excellently described (Parker et al., 1983):

> The signs can develop at any age but usually between one and 4 years of age. Most of the signs are exhibited in moderation by many normal cats; however, in cats with the hyperesthesia syndrome the signs are carried to extremes so that normal activities are curtailed. Signs observed include rippling of the skin of the dorsum, biting or licking at the tail, flank, or pelvis, apparent hallucinations, glassy eyes with widely dilated pupils, frantic meowing, swishing of the tail, sudden violent licking when running, walking or eating, running crazily around the house, and attacking objects, including the owner, without provocation. The cats may even have generalized seizures and associated problems, such as urinating outside the litterbox. Signs may last a few seconds to a few minutes, occur at a specific time of day, vary in incidence from month to month, and occur once every few days or almost constantly all day. Between episodes the cats may be normal or slightly agitated. Once asleep, these cats seem peaceful but may wake up suddenly at night and attack their owners. Both sexes, neutered or intact, are affected.

A prodromal aura, such as may precede epileptic seizures in dogs, has been observed in some cats (Stein, 1983). Occasionally a cat gnaws compulsively on its claws. When in the throes of an attack a normally amiable cat often becomes ugly, while an habitually ill-tempered cat may become unnaturally affectionate (Holzworth, 1983).

Affected cats may have a fever but exhibit no elevation in the white-cell count (Parker et al., 1983). In severe cases the EEG may show abnormalities (slow waves, dysrhythmias, spike discharges) that disappear if treatment is successful.

No significant autopsy lesions were found by Parker et al. (1983). According to Austin (1975a), biopsy of affected skin discloses focal infiltration of the upper dermis with lymphocytes and plasma cells.

The signs, it is suggested, are manifestations of mental problems associated with an unstable personality, frustrations of various kinds, and environmental pressures, with other contributing factors such as toxins, dietary preservatives, or minimal brain damage possibly being involved as well (Parker et al., 1983).

As treatment, any kind of topical medication would be promptly licked off by the cat. Amputation of the mutilated tail has been performed in some cases, but the cat simply goes on to attack the stump or the tailhead. Tranquilizers, corticosteroids, and progestogens have been tried, but phenobarbital (4 to 10 mg/kg/day in divided doses) seems to be more effective (e.g., Austin, 1975a). Perhaps most successful of all is primidone (Mysoline, Ayerst), which in doses of 0.5 to 3.0 mg/kg (i.e., a quarter or half of a 50 mg tablet for each dose) once, twice, or three times a day, as needed, may bring relief when no other drug has had any effect (Holzworth, 1983; Mosier, 1975, 1977). Although manufacturers warn against using primidone in cats, and the drug in dosages used in dogs will very likely cause signs of toxicity (ataxia, depression, vomiting), studies at the University of Illinois indicate that in lower doses it may be given to cats without clinical signs of toxicity (Sawchuk, 1983). Within hours of receiving one or two doses a cat may become entirely asymptomatic, with return to its usual disposition (Holzworth, 1983). Other cats may require treatment for longer periods. Owners are advised to observe the cat closely and to decrease amount and frequency of drug administration to the minimum that is effective. Some cats require retreatment from time to time. Owners become very skillful in detecting early signs of recurrence (nervousness, looking at the tail, twitching of the skin) and report that brief re-administration of primidone will usually abort an attack.

In severe cases, when the cat is mutilating the tail, bandaging of the tail is helpful (Holzworth, 1983). In a young adult Siamese tom that was almost insane with discomfort and actually attempting to climb walls, the tail had to be kept bandaged for the first month of treatment with primidone. The same cat was eventually able to get along entirely without treatment, when the owner introduced a kitten to which the older cat became greatly attached. If separated from its companion, the cat would quickly show signs of agitation and twitching skin.

Study is needed to determine whether this curious disorder originates in the brain, as the response to antiepileptic drugs suggests, or whether it is a disorder of peripheral nerves or the skin itself that is relieved by the sedative effect of the drugs.

## Nodular Panniculitis

Nodular panniculitis (febrile relapsing panniculitis) is a rare disease of cats of unknown etiology (Austin, 1975a,b; Muller et al., 1983; Pandey et al., 1973; Scott, 1980). No breed or sex predilection is recognized. Affected cats are usually five to nine years of age.

The first sign is usually a premonitory period of anorexia, depression, lethargy, and fever (39.5 to 40.5 C, 103.0 to 105.0 F). Twenty-four to 48 hours later cutaneous signs appear, and the constitutional signs regress. The skin lesions are subcutaneous inflammatory nodules that are well demarcated, firm, 0.5 to 2.0 cm in diameter, and occasionally painful. As they progress they may fix the overlying skin. The nodules rapidly become fluctuant (cystlike) and rupture, giving place to ulcers and fistulae that discharge a thick, bloody exudate. Without treatment, lesions heal slowly, leaving depressed scars. The lesions are usually multiple and have a predilection for the trunk.

Diagnosis is based on history, physical examination, and laboratory studies. Nodular panniculitis is refractory to antibiotics and usual anti-inflammatory doses of glucocorticoids. On examination the disease is usually misdiagnosed as pyoderma, mycosis, cysts, or neoplasm. A hemogram usually reveals a neutrophilic leukocytosis of 25,000 to 30,000 WBC/μl. Smears of fine needle aspirates from intact lesions disclose many neutrophils and foamy macrophages but no microorganisms. Cultured exudate from intact lesions is sterile. Skin biopsy reveals panniculitis (Fig. 13–25) with varying degrees of fat necrosis, fibroplasia, neutrophilic and mononuclear cell infiltration, foamy lipid-laden macrophages, and foreign body giant cells (Scott, 1980).

Treatment with large doses of glucocorticoids (4 mg/kg prednisolone daily) usually achieves healing within 7 to 10 days. Relapses may occur and may be frequent enough to require alternate-day glucocorticoid maintenance ther-

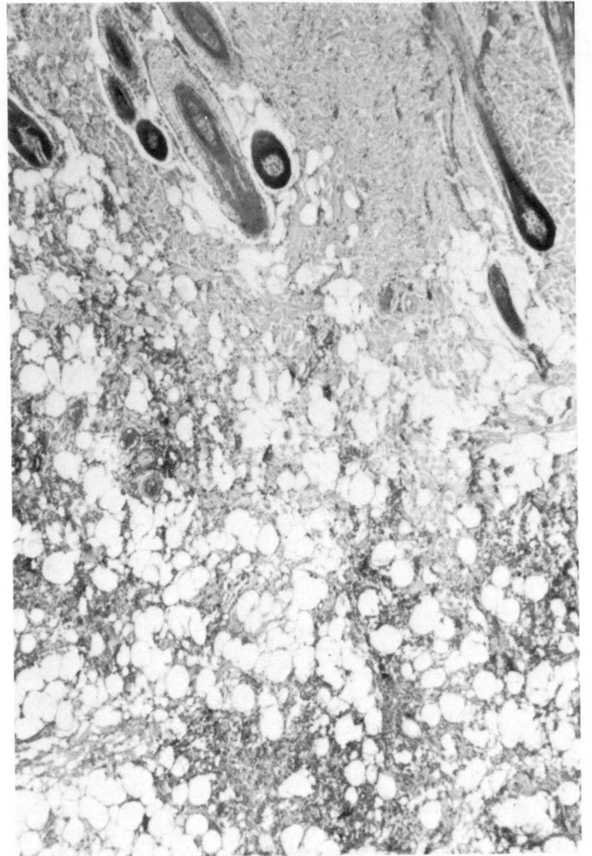

**Figure 13–25** Nodular panniculitis. Extensive fat necrosis, H & E.

apy (1 to 2 mg/kg prednisolone every other evening). The author has also had good results in two cats with oral vitamin E (dl-α-tocopherol acetate, 100 IU b.i.d.).

Nodular panniculitis has also been described as part of a systemic lipodystrophy associated with pancreatitis in a two-year-old cat (Ryan and Howard, 1981).

## Plasma Cell Pododermatitis

Plasma cell pododermatitis is a rare disorder in cats (Gruffydd-Jones et al., 1980; Kunkle, 1984; Medleau et al., 1982; Muller et al., 1983; Scott, 1980, 1984). The etiology is unknown. The condition has most often occurred in colony cats but may also affect single house pets, with no breed, age, or sex predilection noted. In colonies it can affect 15 to 33 per cent of the cats over a four-month period.

Beginning as a soft, painless swelling of the footpads, it progresses to ulceration and exuberant granulation. When ulceration occurs, pain and lameness may develop. The condition, involving one or more feet, usually affects metacarpal or metatarsal pads, less often the digital pads. In two of five cases reported by Scott (1984), the cats had concurrent bilateral proliferative ulcerated lesions in the commissures of the mouth. The microscopic features of the oral lesions were identical to those in the footpads.

Plasma cell pododermatitis must be differentiated from infection, eosinophilic granuloma, tumor, and the autoimmune dermatoses (pemphigus, pemphigoid, and lupus erythematosus).

Blood studies often reveal lymphocytosis, neutrophilia, and hyperglobulinemia. No cats tested have given evidence of feline leukemia virus infection. Cultures for viruses, bacteria, and fungi usually give negative results (Gruffydd-Jones et al., 1980; Scott, 1984).

Biopsy discloses diffuse dermatitis with the dermis and subcutis obscured in most cases by a massive infiltrate of plasma cells, many of which have prominent Russell bodies. Neutrophils vary in number with the degree of ulceration. In cats that came to autopsy, there was plasma cell infiltration of viscera and amyloidosis of liver and kidneys.

Some cases regress spontaneously; some recur seasonally. Systemic glucocorticoids are of uncertain benefit. Four cats were treated successfully with aurothioglucose (Medleau et al., 1982; Scott, 1984).

The tissue infiltration with plasma cells, the seasonal recurrence in some cases, and the response to immunomodulating therapy suggest that plasma cell pododermatitis may have an immunologic basis. Direct immunofluorescence testing has revealed immunoglobulin deposited at the basement membrane zone in two cats (Kunkle, 1984; Medleau et al., 1982) but was negative in another six cats (Kunkle, 1984; Scott, 1984). Antinuclear antibody tests were positive in two cats (Kunkle, 1984) but negative in another six (Medleau et al., 1982; Scott, 1984).

## Lymphoid Hyperplasia

A skin condition of cats (especially Siamese) characterized by elevated bluish plaques, 1.0 to 1.2 cm in diameter, beginning on the ears, then spreading to the neck, trunk, and rump, was reported (Austin, 1975b). Histologic examination revealed lymphoid hyperplasia. The condition was responsive to alternate-day glucocorticoids, although in the opinion of some pathologists the lesion was lymphoma.

# VIRAL INFECTIONS

## Feline Leukemia Virus Infection

Feline leukemia virus (FeLV) infection has been demonstrated by FeLV testing in some cats with skin disorders such as poor wound healing, chronic or recurrent pyoderma (abscess, cellulitis), chronic paronychia, generalized pruritus, eosinophilic granuloma, seborrhea, and cutaneous horns (e.g., Cotter, 1977; Muller et al., 1983; Scott, 1980). The relationship in many of these conditions is speculative, although the well-known immunosuppressive effects of FeLV infection may be involved.

It is of interest that some FeLV-associated cutaneous infections respond better to systemic antibiotics and glucocorticoids than to antibiotics alone. In addition, recurrences can be greatly reduced or eliminated with alternate-day glucocorticoid therapy.

Association of FeLV with multiple cutaneous horns of the footpads of a cat was first reported from the New York State College of Veterinary Medicine in 1982 (Center et al., 1982), and additional cases have been recognized in unrelated cats (see section on non-neoplastic tumors).

Feline leukemia virus and the closely related feline sarcoma virus are the cause of many cases of naturally occurring lymphosarcoma and fibrosarcoma and under experimental conditions may induce liposarcoma, hemangioma, and melanoma as well (see chapters on virus diseases and on tumors).

## Pox Virus Infection

Since the late 1970s, cases of infection have been reported from Great Britain and continental Europe in zoo Felidae (Baxby et al., 1979; Marennikova et al., 1977) and in domestic kittens and cats (Baxby et al., 1979; Gaskell et al., 1983; Martland et al., 1983; Thomsett et al., 1978; Schönbauer et al., 1982).

Prodromal signs may include anorexia, lethargy, and occasional vomiting. Several days later circular, well-demarcated nodules usually measuring 0.3 to 0.6 cm in diameter appear in the skin. Some eventually take the form of red glistening plaques that may be covered with scabs; others become ulcerated with purulent centers. The lesions may be itchy, and they tend to slough leaving granulating tissue and scars. They are almost always multiple and situated anywhere on the body, including lips, eyelids, and toepads.

Some cats develop dyspnea and pneumonia, sometimes with pleural fluid, and die or are destroyed. Others recover after several weeks.

In an unusual case with no systemic signs, the lesions, first on the lip and then over the body, were considered to be "lick granulomas," and the cat was treated with megestrol acetate (Martland et al., 1983). A month later the lesions were gone. However, a skin biopsy taken at the second clinic visit showed characteristic eosinophilic, intracytoplasmic inclusions in epithelial cells, and a pox virus was demonstrated by electron microscopy. Fourteen weeks after start of the disorder, the serum titer against cowpox was 1:320.

A definitive diagnosis is made by demonstration of the inclusion bodies by light and electron microscopic examination of skin scrapings or biopsy tissue, pleural fluid, or lung. Virus may be cultured from scabs, skin lesions, throat swabs, and many organs. For serologic studies samples should be taken during both acute and recovery phases. The infection can be transmitted experimentally by intravenous inoculation and scarification.

No source of infection was identified in the cases reported in domestic cats, but white rats imported as food for the zoo cats in Moscow were believed to be the source of the disease there (Marennikova et al., 1977). A zoo attendant who handled the sick animals developed skin lesions strongly resembling those of cowpox, but virus was not isolated.

## Calicivirus (Picornavirus) Infection

"Paw and mouth disease" was reported in a young cat that had been chewing at its feet (Cooper and Sabine, 1972). The feet were swollen and painful, with erosion of the pads and interdigitial webs. In addition, blisters and ulcers were present on the cat's tongue, palate, and lips. Swabs of the blisters on the tongue and of the lesions on the feet were cultured, and a calicivirus (picornavirus) was isolated from both sites. The affected tissues were not examined microscopically.

The cat was treated with a tranquilizer, corticosteroid, and topical medication, but the condition did not clear until the steroid was stopped.

## Herpesvirus (Feline Rhinotracheitis Virus) Infection

Feline rhinotracheitis virus was isolated from lesions in three cats with ulcers of the mouth and later of the skin (Johnson and Sabine, 1971). All three had been hospitalized for spaying on the same day, two developed oral ulcers within two or three days, and all three developed epidermal ulcers over most of the skin within seven days. A fourth cat, a nonsurgical patient already in the hospital when the others were spayed, developed only oral ulcers, four days after readmission of two of the spayed cats. It was suggested that one of the three females was shedding virus, which infected the others at surgery and subsequently the fourth cat as well. It is of interest that only the cats that underwent surgery developed the cutaneous lesions.

Similar skin ulcers were described in three other cats from which the virus was isolated (Flecknell et al., 1979). Secondary streptococcic and staphylococcic infections were also present. One cat died, but one of the remaining two was treated with penicillin, topical application of idoxuridine solution, and two doses of rhinotracheitis-calicivirus vaccine and made a good recovery.

## Pseudorabies (Aujeszky's Disease)

In this short and rapidly fatal infection, occasionally identified in cats, severe pruritus causes violent scratching and gnawing at the skin. Microscopic examination reveals inflammation and necrosis of the skin and subcutis. Definitive diagnosis is by isolation of virus from brain, spinal cord, or affected subcutis (see also the chapter on virus diseases).

# Bacterial Infections

Except for abscesses, the skin of the cat is not often affected by bacterial infections (Baker, 1970; Baker, 1974a; Joshua, 1965; Scott, 1980; Wilkinson, 1966). It has been suggested that the incidence of bacterial infection may be low because pathogenic bacteria are found on cat skin less often than on dog or human skin. However, evidence in support of this contention is limited. Studies on the bacterial flora of cat skin have been strictly qualitative. It is clear from studies with humans and dogs that the skin is an exceedingly effective environmental sampler, providing a temporary haven and way station for a variety of organisms. Thus only quantitative studies allow reliable distinction between resident and transient bacteria.

Baker (1970) reported a slight growth of nonhemolytic staphylococci from one of six normal adult cats (swabs taken from interscapular skin). Krogh and Kristensen (1976) swabbed the skin at seven sites (head, lumbar area, tailhead, chin, axilla, interdigital area, groin) on 10 cats (five males and five females, five breeds, aged four months to four years). *Micrococcus* sp, α-hemolytic streptococci, and *Acinetobacter* sp were consistently isolated. *Staphylococcus epidermidis* was isolated from most of the cats, although only at one or a few sites on each. *S. aureus* was isolated less often, and a *Corynebacterium* sp was isolated from one site on one cat. In general, the chin yielded the heaviest bacterial growths. Half the swabs taken were sterile. Hemolytic staphylococci are uncommonly isolated from the nasal passages of healthy cats or from septic processes of cats (Mann, 1959; Smith, 1964). Hearst (1967) swabbed 100 normal cats (several breeds) and isolated *S. aureus* from 98 per cent. It is likely that his results reflect the highly contaminated environment of the pet shop cats that he studied.

Various coagulase-negative staphylococci (*S. cohnii, S. epidermidis, S. saprophyticus, S. sciuri, S. simulans, S. warneri, S. xylosus*) and coagulase-positive staphylococci (*S. aureus, S. intermedius*) have been isolated from the skin and nares of normal cats (Devriese et al., 1984; Mardh et al., 1978). *S. aureus* is the coagulase-positive staphylococcus most often isolated from feline infections (Biberstein et al., 1984; Devriese et al., 1984).

In another study of staphylococcal species in 113 clinically healthy cats, *S. simulans, S. intermedius, S. xylosus,* and *S. aureus* were found to predominate (Cox et al., 1985).

Strains of staphylococci from feline and canine infection and their susceptibility to antibiotics have been studied by Love et al. (1981) and Biberstein et al. (1984).

## Abscesses and Cellulitis

Abscesses and cellulitis constitute the most common feline skin disorder (see references Scott, 1980). They are usually secondary to cat bites and scratches. The organisms most often involved are those of the cat's normal oral flora, namely *Pasteurella multocida,* β-hemolytic streptococci, fusiform bacilli, and *Bacteroides* spp (Joshua, 1971b; Muller et al., 1983; Oudar et al., 1972; Scott, 1980; Smith, 1964). The major pyogenic organism of the cat is *P. multocida,* which may be isolated from the mouth of 50 to 94 per cent of normal cats and is almost invariably present in fight wounds. *Corynebacterium equi,* resistant to penicillin and tetracycline, was cultured from an abscess in a cat (Higgins and Paradis, 1980).

In addition, chronic nonhealing abscesses associated with *Mycoplasma* infection were reported in three cats (Keane, 1983). Routine aerobic and anaerobic cultures for bacteria were negative. Although the lesions had been unresponsive to standard surgical and antibiotic therapy, they healed rapidly when the cats were treated with tetracycline.

Anaerobic bacteria are abundant in intestinal contents and, by fecal contamination, cause soft tissue infections. Various anaerobes have been isolated in pure or mixed culture from feline skin infections: *Actinomyces* spp; *Clostridium perfringens* and other *Clostridium* spp; *Eubacterium* sp; *Peptostreptococcus anaerobius* and other anaerobic cocci; *Propionibacterium acnes* and other *Propionibacterium* spp; *Bacteroides melaninogenicus, Bacteroides fragilis fragilis,* and other *Bacteroides* spp; and *Fusobacterium necrophorum* and other *Fusobacterium* spp (Berg et al., 1979; Biberstein et al., 1968; Love et al., 1980). The clinician's index of suspicion for anaerobic bacteria should be high (1) when dealing with abscesses, cellulitis, and draining tracts; (2) when bacteria are not isolated aerobically from wounds from which bacteria were demonstrated in direct smears; and (3) when infections respond poorly to aminoglycoside antibiotics. Unfortunately, the high cost of anaerobic culturing may preclude its use. Antibiotics of choice for anaerobic infections include ampicillin, carbenicillin, lincomycin, chloramphenicol, clindamycin, penicillin G, and cephalosporins (Muller et al., 1983).

Abscesses and cellulitis are most frequent in intact males, although intact females and neuters of either sex may be affected. The common locations for bite infections are the limbs, face, base of tail, and back, although they may occur anywhere. Clinical signs usually appear suddenly and may include pain, swelling, and regional lymphadenopathy. If a leg is involved, the cat may limp or hold it up. The initial lesions are puncture wounds and are often not at first detected.

To some extent, subsequent developments depend on the site and are related especially to the amount of subcutaneous tissue. Thus bites on a limb may result in cellulitis rather than an abscess. In areas of loose connective tissue, the course varies. Some lesions are painful from the time the bite is received; others are painful only while pus is accumulating. Still others are painless throughout, the cats being presented for a large swelling. Heat and reddening are uncommon. The skin over an abscess that is about to slough is thin and reddish purple.

The pus in abscesses varies from thin to creamy to flocculent in consistency and may be white, yellow, greenish, or red-brown. The red-brown variety is particularly foul-smelling and is often associated with fusospirochetal infection. Constitutional signs (fever, anorexia, depression, and inactivity) are usually present to some degree.

Depending on the site of primary infection, possible pyogenic sequelae to abscesses and cellulitis include pyothorax, otitis media, osteomyelitis, sinusitis, rhinitis, septic arthritis, periostitis, meningitis, and pyemia (e.g., Joshua, 1972). Recurrent or nonhealing abscesses and cellulitis should prompt consideration of possible immunodeficiency (especially associated with feline leukemia virus infection), other types of infectious agents (actinomycotic, mycobacterial, mycotic, parasitic), or neoplasia (especially lymphosarcoma and squamous cell carcinoma).

The diagnosis is usually obvious from physical examination. A hemogram often reveals leukocytosis and neutrophilia, but leukopenia and anemia are sometimes present, suggesting concurrent feline leukemia infection. Recalcitrant infections may require examination of direct smears, bacterial culture and sensitivity testing, fungal culture, skin biopsy, and testing for feline leukemia infection and immunologic competence.

"The frequency with which pyogenic infection complicates bites in cats makes prophylactic treatment with antibiotics a legitimate measure whenever it can be undertaken" (Joshua, 1965). When cats are presented within 24 hours of a bite, a single injection of procaine penicillin G will usually prevent the development of pyogenic foci (Joshua, 1971b; Scott, 1980). In fully developed abscesses, treatment includes surgical preparation, establishing ventral drainage, débriding, flushing with 3 per cent hydrogen peroxide (for its effervescent and mechanical properties), placing drains when indicated, and flushing with chlorhexidine two or three times daily until the wound is healed (5 to 10 days). Partial suturing, with placement of a drain, is occasionally indicated, but even very large defects contract and heal in rapidly once an abscess has been drained and débrided. Systemic antibiotics of choice include penicillin, amoxicillin, ampicillin, and hetacillin (Scott, 1980). Tetracycline and chloramphenicol are to be avoided in feline pyodermas—tetracycline because it is of limited efficacy and may cause vomiting, anorexia, and fever; chloramphenicol because it may cause anorexia, depression, and bone marrow toxicity.

Cellulitis should be treated with hot packs for 10 to 15 minutes three times a day and also with a systemic antibiotic until the lesion is brought to a head (abscess) or resolves. The author has occasionally used a counter-irritant poultice (Numotizine, Hobart) for a cat with cellulitis of a limb, when it was not possible to apply warm wet soaks. The poultice is bandaged in place for 24 hours. Numotizine is not, however, licensed for use in cats.

Castration of intact male cats has been shown to be an effective preventive measure (Hart, 1973). Castration results in either rapid or gradual decline in fighting and roaming in 80 to 90 per cent of cats so treated, even in adulthood (about 50 per cent stop almost immediately and about 35 per cent stop gradually). Progestogens have also been effective in modifying aggressive feline behavior so as to prevent or reduce occurrence of fight infections (Hart, 1974).

*P. multocida* is also pathogenic for humans, causing cellulitis, abscesses, tendinitis, osteomyelitis, regional lymphadenopathy, fever, and septicemia (Scott, 1980). Thus appropriate caution should be exercised when handling draining wounds and pus.

## Paronychia

Paronychia (pyogenic infection of the nail folds, understood by common usage to be bacterial) is infrequent in cats (see references, Scott, 1980) and occurs chiefly in middle-aged or older animals of either sex and any breed. Possible causes are many: trauma, dermatophytosis, demodicosis, seborrheic disease, contact dermatitis, arteriovenous fistulae secondary to trauma or declawing (Furneaux et al., 1974; Slocum et al., 1973), and states of immunodeficiency (especially with feline leukemia virus infections and systemic lupus erythematosus) (Scott, 1980). Paronychia is virtually always a secondary pyoderma. Bacteria isolated from feline paronychia are predominantly *E. coli*, with occasional concurrent isolation of β-hemolytic streptococci, *Enterococcus* spp, and *S. aureus* (Scott, 1980).

Signs are varying degrees of swelling, pain, erythema, alopecia, exudation, and crusting involving one or more digits (Fig. 13–26). A caseous, white or yellow exudate can usually be expressed from the nail beds. Claws may be brittle, split, malformed, or sloughed. The forepaws are most often affected. The cats are often lame and occasionally febrile, and they usually lick the involved paws incessantly.

Determination of etiology often requires diagnostic procedures (skin scrapings, direct smears, bacterial culture and sensitivity testing, fungal culture, radiography, antinuclear antibody test, feline leukemia virus test, biopsy). Studies of immunocompetence may be indicated.

Treatment should attempt primarily to correct the underlying cause. Other measures are removal of affected claws if indicated, warm water and chlorhexidine soaks for 10 to 15 minutes three times a day, systemic antibiotics (as determined by culture and sensitivity testing) for four to six weeks, and rarely declawing. Depending on the underlying cause, paronychia can be a chronic, relapsing, frustrating disorder.

## Acute Moist Dermatitis

Lesions comparable to the red, moist, weeping "hot spots" of dogs are almost unknown in cats but have been seen (Holzworth, 1983). Although there are many possible etiologies (Muller et al., 1983), the cause in a given case may remain unknown. Treatment includes clipping, cleansing, and application of astringent packs, and possibly systemic administration of a glucocorticoid.

## Skin Fold Dermatitis

Also called intertrigo or skin fold pyoderma, this condition is rare in the cat. In purebred Persians with excessively flattened faces, the folds of facial skin may be sites of pyoderma (Muller et al., 1983). A contributing factor is constant wetting and soiling from tears that flow down the face owing to impatency of the tear ducts.

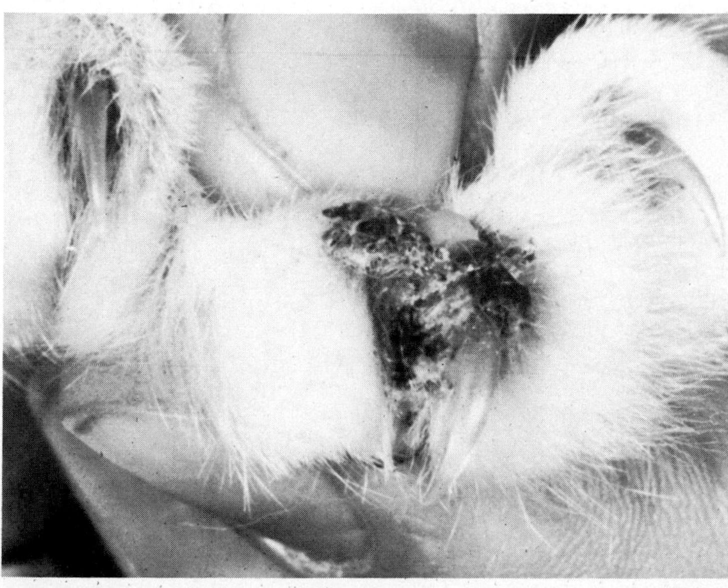

**Figure 13–26** *E. coli* paronychia in an FeLV-positive cat.

In the "rumpy" Manx, infolding of the skin in the tail dimple may lead to pyoderma (Wilkinson, 1983a). Clipping of the hair and application of antibiotic and astringent preparations are recommended. The condition is prevented by keeping the area clean.

Vulvar fold dermatitis of the type occurring in obese spayed female dogs was seen at Angell Memorial Animal Hospital in a fat spayed female cat with subcutaneous lipomatosis of the perineal area and posterior thighs (see chapter on tumors). There was associated cystitis. The condition was relieved, as in the dog, by episioplasty.

## Superficial Pustular Dermatitis

"Impetigo" was reported in young kittens by Kirk (1925). The dermatitis was preceded by anorexia and fever and was characterized by erythematous macules, evolving into vesicles, then pustules, which quickly ruptured leaving thick, yellow scabs. The eruption usually involved the neck, shoulders, and back, and was occasionally painful but never pruritic.

A similar condition has been seen in unweaned kittens (Scott, 1980). A pustular dermatitis develops on the back of the neck (Fig. 13–27) and may spread to the head, withers, chest, and abdomen. The kittens are usually otherwise healthy. One or all kittens in a litter may be affected. Cultures reveal *P. multocida,* β-hemolytic streptococci, or both. Treatment with oral penicillin, amoxicillin, or ampicillin and topical wet soaks (with aluminum acetate or chlorhexidine) is curative in seven to 10 days. The fact that the dermatitis begins on the back of the neck and yields organisms commonly found in the cat's mouth suggests an overzealous "mouthing" by the queen as she moves and carries her kittens.

## Folliculitis

Folliculitis, other than that associated with acne of the chin, is rare in cats (Scott, 1980). It is characterized by papules and pustules, from which hairs can be seen to emerge, and may progress to oozing, ulcers, crusts, and alopecia. Occasionally rupture of follicles results in furunculosis, draining tracts, and cellulitis. Lesions occur typically on the chin (secondary to acne) less often on the face and trunk, where they somewhat resemble miliary dermatitis. Pain, pruritus, and regional lymphadenopathy are variable.

Skin scrapings and fungal culture should be done to rule out demodicosis and dermatophytosis. Direct smears from papules or pustules reveal degenerate neutrophils with intracellular bacteria. Biopsy reveals varying degrees of folliculitis and furunculosis (Fig. 13–28). Bacteria isolated from feline folliculitis include β-hemolytic streptococci, *S. aureus,* and *P. multocida* (Scott, 1980).

Helpful topical measures (warm water soaks, with or without aluminum acetate or chlorhexidine, for 10 to 15 minutes three times a day, and shampoo baths with 2.5 per cent benzoyl peroxide or chlorhexidine) are combined with a systemic antibiotic (e.g., penicillin, amoxicillin, ampicillin, hetacillin, cephalexin, or lincomycin). Folliculitis of the chin (associated with acne) can be a recurrent problem, necessitating long-term prophylactic measures (previously discussed).

## Plague

Clinical infection with *Yersinia pestis* has been diagnosed in cats in areas of the western United States where plague is endemic in wild rodents. In five cats systemic signs of lethargy, inappetence, and fever were followed by development of submandibular and limb abscesses (Rollag et al., 1981). Exudate in all five cases was immunofluorescence- and culture-positive for plague. The one cat that received treatment (drainage and flushing of the abscess, penicillin) was clinically normal within six days. Plague is a potentially serious hazard for man.

## Actinomycosis and Nocardiosis

These specific bacterial infections are only occasionally recognized in cats, probably because of the difficulty of definitive diagnosis. Both are caused by coccoid, Gram-

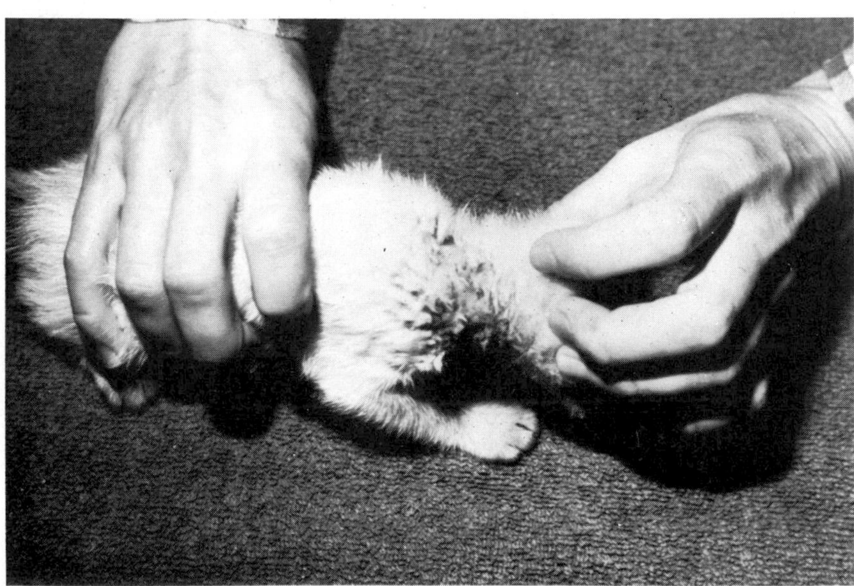

**Figure 13–27** Superficial pyoderma (*Streptococcus* sp) on the neck of a Siamese kitten.

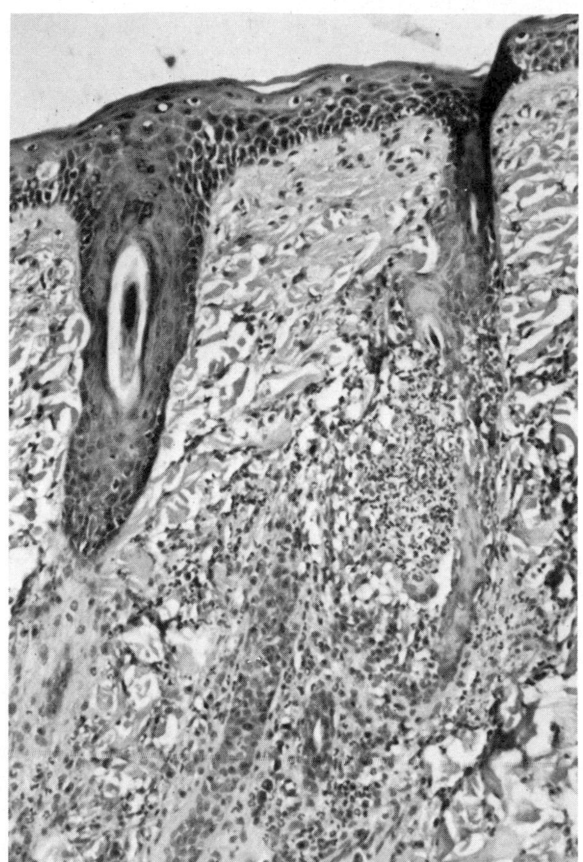

**Figure 13–28** Furunculosis, *S. aureus*. Destruction of the follicle wall by bacteria and infiltrating inflammatory cells. H & E.

positive bacteria that may also grow in branched, beaded filaments. Tangled masses of these filaments form flakes or so-called sulfur granules that may be recognizable grossly in exudate.

Staining of crushed granules may sometimes give an indication of differentiation: *Actinomyces* spp are non–acid-fast, while *Nocardia* spp may be non–acid-fast or partly or wholly acid-fast (Attleberger, 1983a,b). In exudates and tissues the granules of *Actinomyces* are seen microscopically to be surrounded by radiating clublike structures (Jones and Hunt, 1983). Culturing to confirm the diagnosis should be done at a qualified laboratory, as suitable treatment depends on reliable differentiation.

The few reports of feline actinomycosis and nocardiosis (and, in the earlier literature, of infection with *Streptothrix*, a synonym) must be evaluated with some discrimination, as not all diagnoses were made by rigorous cultural criteria.

*Actinomyces (Streptothrix)* spp (usually *A. bovis,* occasionally *A. viscosus)* appear to be normal, obligate parasites of the mouth and digestive tract and opportunistically invade wounds or are introduced by foreign bodies. Skin, subcutis, and sometimes underlying bone are most often involved, with chronic granulomas or abscesses, necrosis, and discharging tracts (Attleberger, 1983a; Bestetti et al., 1977; Jungerman and Schwartzman, 1972; McGaughey, 1951; Scott, 1977; see also references, Scott, 1980). Lesions usually occur on the limbs but occasionally on the face, ears, neck, abdomen, and tail.

Treatment is by liberal surgical drainage and débridement, flushing with iodine-containing solutions, and large daily doses of penicillin.

*Nocardia (Streptothrix)* spp *(N. asteroides, N. brasiliensis)* are mostly soil saprophytes and enter the body through skin wounds, inhalation, or ingestion. Dissemination to other parts of the body is more frequent than with actinomycosis. Cellulitis, abscesses, ulcers, and granulomas are characteristic of skin infections, often with fistulous tracts (Attleberger, 1983b; Ajello et al., 1961; Marder et al., 1973; Scott, 1977; Wilkinson, 1983b; see also references, Scott, 1980). The exudate sometimes has the consistency and appearance of tomato soup and may contain "sulfur granules." Superficial lymph nodes may be involved.

For treatment, sulfonamides are preferred (sulfamerazine, sulfadiazine, Tribrissen [Burroughs Wellcome]). A sulfonamide solution may be used to flush fistulous tracts.

Treatment for actinomycosis or nocardiosis may be required for weeks or months and should be continued for a month after regression of all clinical signs. In both infections the outlook is poor if infection generalizes.

## Actinomycetic Mycetomas (Actinomycetomas)

The term mycetoma is reserved for granulomatous swellings containing exudate characterized by granules formed by bacterial or fungal growth. Actinomycotic mycetoma refers to lesions caused by species of the bacterial genera *Actinomyces, Nocardia,* and *Streptomyces.* The granules found in tissues and exudates are composed of Gram-positive filaments that are usually 1 μ or less in diameter and do not contain chlamydospores. *Actinomyces* and *Nocardia* spp are the usual agents. In a six-year-old domestic cat, a recurrent granulomatous mass over the scapula at the site of a gunshot wound was diagnosed by culture as a mycetoma caused by a species of *Streptomyces* (Lewis et al., 1972). The prognosis for mycetomas is guarded. Surgical removal or drainage is the treatment of choice, supplemented by an appropriate microbial.

Infections with actinomycetes are discussed also in the chapter on bacterial diseases.

## Dermatophilosis (Streptothricosis)

*Dermatophilus congolensis* is a Gram-positive actinomycete characterized by filaments with parallel rows of coccoid cells that form motile zoospores. When dried, these spores may survive for long periods on carrier animals or in a contaminated environment. Infection occurs when moisture releases the zoospores and they contact sites of minor skin injuries, insect bites, or inflammation.

In horses, ruminants, dogs, and rarely man, infection takes the form of exudative dermatitis with formation of crusts, from which the causative organism can be isolated. Infection with *D. congolensis* is rarely diagnosed in the cat. Skin infections have been characterized by draining sinuses in the region of a popliteal node or on the paw (Carakostas et al., 1984; Jones, 1976; Muller et al., 1983).

Diagnostic procedures are described by Attleberger (1983a) and Muller et al. (1983). The organisms are arranged in a characteristic "railroad track" configuration in direct smears.

Superficial lesions are treated by bathing with iodine shampoos. Ampicillin and a number of other antibiotics are said to be satisfactory for systemic treatment (Muller et al., 1983). (See also chapter on bacterial diseases.)

## Botryomycosis

Botryomycosis is a chronic, suppurative granulomatous infection in which nonbranching bacteria, usually *Staphylococcus aureus,* form "grains" (compact bacterial colonies) surrounded by pyogranulomatous inflammation. It is often associated with surgery, wounds, or foreign bodies. The condition is usually a lesion of skin and subcutis; however, it is sometimes diagnosed in viscera (e.g., Habermann and Williams, 1956).

Cutaneous botryomycosis was described in an adult spayed female domestic cat with multiple bite wounds sustained five months before and still unhealed despite antibiotic treatment (Walton et al., 1983). Draining tracts on the abdomen and left flank were excised, *S. aureus* and *Streptococcus canis* were cultured from the tissues, and the cat recovered uneventfully after two weeks' treatment with amoxicillin.

Surprisingly, microscopic examination revealed a normal epidermis and dermis but almost complete replacement of the subcutis by diffuse pyogranulomatous panniculitis in which neutrophils and foamy macrophages predominated. Many of the latter contained basophilic cocci. Several round or oval basophilic "grains" showing peripheral clubbing were composed of individual cocci and homogeneous material that stained blue with acid-orcein Giemsa and Brown and Brenn stains. Special stains and cultures are mandatory in order to distinguish these grains from those of actinomycosis, nocardiosis, and mycetomas.

It has been theorized that this lesion results when an organism of rather low pathogenicity encounters a host with sufficient resistance to isolate but not eradicate the infection (Walton et al., 1983).

## Tuberculosis

Feline tuberculosis has been extensively studied and reported, especially in the European literature (e.g., Brumley, 1931; Hutyra and Marek, 1926; Kral and Novak, 1953; Oudar et al., 1965; Parodi, 1964; van Dorssen, 1960; see also other references, Scott, 1980). It is rare except in areas where bovine tuberculosis is endemic. Cutaneous tuberculosis in cats is almost always caused by *Mycobacterium bovis* and is characterized by single or multiple ulcers, abscesses, plaques, and nodules that occur most often on the head, neck, and limbs. The eyelids, lips, and nose are often the site of nonhealing ulcers. Sometimes the infection takes the form of a draining fistula under the eye or a tract from a cervical node. Often the process starts as a deformity of the forehead or bridge of the nose ("parrot's beak") and breaks through the skin over the nasal passages or frontal sinus (e.g., Foresti, 1936). Lesions usually discharge thick, yellow, or green pus with a foul odor. Regional lymphadenopathy and constitutional signs (poor appetite, lethargy, weight loss, fever) may be present. Although cutaneous tuberculosis may occasionally result from the formation of a fistula from some underlying focus of infection (e.g., a lymph node), many cases are believed to arise from bites or scratches received in fights or from licking or washing after ingestion of infected milk or meat.

Direct smears of exudate may reveal intra- and extracellular Gram-positive, acid-fast bacilli, and these may sometimes be found in biopsied tissue together with pyogranulomatous dermatitis, necrosis, caseation, and sometimes giant cells and mineralization. Serologic and tuberculin tests are unreliable for diagnosis in cats, but the lymphocyte blastogenesis test may have promise (Kramer, 1978). Definitive diagnosis can be made only by culturing or guinea pig inoculation, procedures that may require as long as eight weeks.

Attempts to treat feline tuberculosis with isoniazid would be considered inadvisable because of the public health hazard.

Tuberculosis in cats is discussed in detail in the chapter on bacterial diseases.

## Feline Leprosy and Atypical Cutaneous Mycobacteriosis

These chronic granulomatous infections are characterized by cutaneous and subcutaneous nodules, ulcers, and draining tracts associated with Gram-positive, acid-fast bacilli other than those causing skin tuberculosis.

Two recent reports include extensive surveys of the literature (Kunkle et al., 1983; White et al., 1983; see also references, Scott, 1980). First reported in the early 1960s in New Zealand and Australia and subsequently in Great Britain, the Netherlands, and western Canada, the infection was attributed to *Mycobacterium lepraemurium,* the agent of murine leprosy, and was designated "cat leprosy." Although in some cases the diagnosis was largely presumptive, since the organism could not at that time be isolated on artificial media, recent studies with animal inoculation, immunologic testing, and a suitable artificial medium support the identification. However, Schiefer and Middleton (1983) were unable to produce lesions in cats experimentally infected with *M. lepraemurium.* It is hypothesized that transmission is by the bites of infected rats.

Clinically similar infections in Australia, Great Britain, western North America, Virginia, and Florida have yielded so-called atypical mycobacteria that are environmental saprophytes: *M. xenopi* (Runyon's Group III) and *M. fortuitum, M. chelonei, M. phlei,* and *M. smegmatis* (Runyon's rapidly growing Group IV). The rapidly growing mycobacteria are frequent invaders of traumatic and surgical wounds in humans and have also been reported in dogs.

Principal features that distinguish cat leprosy from infection with the other agents are that (1) *M. lepraemurium* is cultured only with difficulty, while the other mycobacteria are easily grown on blood agar and other media; and (2) inoculation of rats and guinea pigs gives the responses typical for that organism, while for the atypical mycobacteria the mouse is the experimental animal of choice. Because of these differences it has been recommended that the designations "cat leprosy" and "atypical mycobacteriosis" not be used interchangeably (White et al., 1983).

Both cat leprosy and infection with atypical mycobacteria have been transmitted experimentally to other cats (Schiefer and Middleton, 1983; White et al., 1983).

The clinical picture is similar in both types of infection. Affected cats tend to be indoor-outdoor animals with histories of nonhealing or recurrent skin lesions, sometimes known to have developed at the site of previous wounds. The lesions start as soft, usually painless, freely movable nodules in the skin or subcutis. They may be single or multiple and anywhere on the body, with a possible predilection of the rapidly growing mycobacteria for the ventral trunk. The nodules often ulcerate and break down into fistulae and draining tracts that discharge a serosanguineous fluid. The edges of the skin defect thicken instead of healing in. Local lymphadenopathy is sometimes present.

The cats are usually otherwise healthy, and laboratory tests are noncontributory except for an occasional leukocytosis. Cats tested for feline leukemia virus gave negative results (White et al., 1983; Kunkle et al., 1983).

The differential diagnosis includes tuberculosis, actinomycetic and mycotic infections, foreign body granuloma, nodular panniculitis, chronic abscesses secondary to immunosuppression, and finally neoplasia.

The diagnosis may be suggested by direct smears of exudate or tissue if Gram-positive, acid-fast organisms can be found. These occur both extra- and intracellularly. Biopsy specimens disclose pyogranulomatous inflammation or panniculitis, sometimes with necrosis, caseation, or mineralization. Acid-fast bacilli tend to be most numerous in cat leprosy; in some biopsy specimens from atypical mycobacteriosis they may not be evident at all. The bacilli are most likely to be demonstrated in tissue processed by the rapid Ziehl-Neelsen method or by snap-freezing the formalin-fixed tissue before staining. The inflammatory reaction is characterized by infiltration with neutrophils, lymphocytes, plasma cells, and macrophages that may contain organisms.

Biopsy tissue is more useful than exudate for culturing and should be cultured in all suspect cases, not only to rule out tuberculosis but also to distinguish between cat leprosy and atypical mycobacteriosis for purposes of appropriate drug therapy. The laboratory should be alerted that mycobacteriosis is suspected because the plates may be rapidly overrun with coexisting *Staphylococcus* spp and discarded before the small mycobacterial colonies have time to grow; otherwise the laboratory may consider the mycobacterium a contaminant and not report it (Kunkle et al., 1983). In some cases, repeated culturing is necessary.

For sensitivity-testing and speciation cultures must be submitted to a qualified laboratory. Antibiotics determined by the Kirby-Bauer sensitivity test to be most effective in vitro against the rapidly growing mycobacteria are, in order of activity against *M. fortuitum* and *M. chelonei*, amikacin, kanamycin, and gentamicin. Tetracycline, chloramphenicol, and erythromycin vary greatly in effectiveness against the isolates.

Drugs that may be tried for *M. lepraemurium* infection are dapsone, 50 mg orally b.i.d. to 50 to 100 mg/kg/day (Allan and Wickham, 1976; Wilkinson, 1977), or rifampicin, 5 mg/kg daily (Wilkinson, 1977). A later report indicated that dapsone had been used successfully at a dosage of 1 mg/kg daily (Wilkinson, 1984). Dapsone must be used with caution, as it may cause hemolytic anemia and neurotoxicity in cats (Allan and Wickham, 1976, Wilkinson, 1984).

In general, effectiveness of drug therapy is difficult to evaluate, as the course of illness may also be favorably influenced by surgical excision, drainage, and débridement. Recurrences are frequent. In some cats the condition continues to resist treatment for months or years. In others, spontaneous healing eventually occurs.

Some cats are destroyed when an owner becomes discouraged by the lack of progress. Spread of the infection to internal organs is a rare finding. One of the few cats that manifested systemic symptoms (fever, depression, anorexia) recovered completely after four years of illness when an abdominal mycobacterial mass was removed (Kunkle et al., 1983).

The public health significance of nontuberculous mycobacteriosis would appear to be slight. However, since humans can be infected with the atypical mycobacteria, precautions should be observed in handling infected cats.

## Protozoan Infections

**LEISHMANIASIS.** Cutaneous leishmaniasis occurs in cats in the Near East and Mediterranean areas (Schawalder, 1977; see also chapter on protozoan diseases). Skin nodules, ulcers, and draining tracts are characteristics.

**TOXOPLASMOSIS.** *Toxoplasma gondii* may very rarely cause skin lesions in cats (see chapter on protozoan diseases).

## Fungal Infections

Fungal infections ars discussed in detail in an earlier chapter, but some general observations relating to their cutaneous forms are in order here.

Fungal infections fall into two broad groups (Muller et al., 1983; Scott, 1980). Superficial infections, such as those with the dermatophytes *Microsporum* and *Trichophyton*, invade and maintain themselves in keratinized tissues (hair, nail, and stratum corneum). These are highly contagious. Species of the yeast *Candida*, a normal inhabitant of the alimentary tract, may be involved in superficial infection of skin and mucous membrane in debilitated or immunosuppressed hosts, and *Malassezia pachydermatis (Pityrosporum canis)*, a commensal yeast in the ear canal of healthy dogs and cats, may under certain circumstances play a role in otitis externa. Saprophytic and pathogenic fungi can often be isolated from the skin and hair of normal cats (Aho, 1983; Quaife and Womar, 1982; Scott, 1980, 1984).

Dermatophytosis is both overdiagnosed and underdiagnosed. Many a lesion is labeled "grass fungus" with no supporting evidence, whereas a genuine infection often goes unrecognized because it mimics another condition, or because the clinician is inexperienced with the use of the Wood's ultraviolet light or fails to use culture media correctly or to evaluate culture growth by strict criteria.

Virtually every skin disorder of cats calls for examination with the Wood's light and fungal culture, for dermatophytes may be responsible not only for lesions of "classic ringworm" but for any of the following: (1) patchy alopecia, erythema, pruritus, and excoriations; (2) localized or generalized papulocrustous dermatitis, with or without pruritus and alopecia; (3) pigmentary changes in hair or skin, with or without other signs of skin disease; (4) large areas of papulopustular dermatitis and alopecia, with or without pruritus (especially *T. mentagrophytes*); (5) small or large areas of alopecia or broken hairs or both; (6) multifocal or generalized seborrhea sicca; (7) solitary or multiple eruptions, with hairs emerging from the centers of papules and pustules (folliculitis), with or without alopecia and pruritus; (8) plaques, granulomas, or nodules that ulcerate and develop draining tracts (*T. mentagrophytes, M. canis*); and (9) paronychia or misshapen, crumbling nails. Finally, although there may be no lesions at all, Wood's light examination or culture of brushings may detect a carrier state.

The reader is urged to become thoroughly familiar with the niceties of diagnosis of dermatophytosis as described in detail in texts on fungus infection and by Muller et al. (1983).

Another large group of fungi, members of normal plant or soil microflora, involves deeper tissues. Some are limited to the subcutis, to which they have gained access through injuries (e.g., *Drechslera, Phialophora, Prototheca,* and *Sporothrix*). Others are capable not only of skin infection but also of systemic involvement (*Aspergillus, Blastomyces, Coccidioides, Cryptococcus*, and *Histoplasma*). Compared in incidence with dermatophytosis, clinical infections with these organisms are uncommon and, except for *Sporothrix*, are believed to pose little or no threat of transmissibility to other animals or to humans.

The fungus infections that involve deeper tissues are likely to take the form of nodules, ulcers, abscesses, and draining tracts that are refractory to surgical measures and antibacterial treatment. Foreign bodies, arteriovenous shunts, and neoplasms must be considered in differential diagnosis. For example, an error that is sometimes made in the absence of diagnostic study is to mistake multiple tumor metastases to the toes for "fungus." Examination of exudate and tissue sections usually establishes a fungal etiology, but accurate identification of the agent often requires culturing.

For detailed discussion of the specific infections diagnosed in cats, the reader is referred to the chapter on mycotic diseases.

## PARASITISMS

The species of parasites to which cats play host are discussed here from the practical point of view of the clinician concerned with identifying and combating those that affect the skin and hair coat.

### Fleas

*Ctenocephalides felis* is by far the most frequent ectoparasite of cats. Other fleas that may parasitize cats are *C. canis, Pulex irritans* of man, rodent fleas, and *Echidnophaga gallinacea*, the burrowing stick-tight flea of poultry. Evidences of flea infestation include (1) flea bite dermatitis, (2) flea bite hypersensitivity (flea allergy); (3) presence of flea feces or of segments of the tapeworm *Dipylidium caninum*; (4) blood-loss anemia, especially in kittens and debilitated adults; and (5) personality changes (irritability, growling, sudden running and jumping). The cutaneous signs vary tremendously from cat to cat (see references, Scott, 1980). Many cats, literally "alive" with fleas and caked with flea feces, are totally asymptomatic. Others manifest a mild, papulocrustous, sometimes itchy dermatitis most often over the neck and lumbar regions (flea bite dermatitis), a reaction to flea saliva, which contains various proteolytic enzymes, hyaluronidases, and histamine-like substances capable of producing nonallergic skin irritation. Still other cats become hypersensitive (allergic) to flea saliva, so that a single flea is sufficient to elicit a severe, pruritic, papulocrustous dermatitis (see flea bite hypersensitivity). Flea infestation and related signs tend to peak in summer in the northern United States (unless household infestation persists) and to prevail year-round in the warmer south. All the species of fleas infesting cats will bite humans, often evoking a pruritic, papulocrustous dermatitis ("papular urticaria") of the legs and lower trunk (Hewitt et al., 1971).

Elimination or control of fleas requires treatment of all cats and dogs in a household *and* treatment of their environment as well. No single agent destroys adult fleas, larval forms, and eggs, so the best effect is achieved with more than one agent. Those that destroy by contact are more effective than ingested materials.

Pyrethrins (often combined with piperonyl butoxide) and rotenone are plant-derived contact poisons of low mammalian toxicity, although rotenone is reported to be responsible for rare instances of vomiting and liver damage (Atkins and Johnson, 1975; Clarke and Clarke, 1967; Scott, 1979a; Wilkinson 1968). These agents rapidly kill adult fleas but have little residual action. *They are the only parasiticides safe for use on kittens.*

Pyrethroids, newer synthetic contact poisons, are less costly than pyrethrins; are active againts fungi as well as ectoparasites; do not irritate eyes, nose, and throat; and break down to nontoxic compounds. Resmethrin (Dura Kyl) is available as a residual action shampoo or spray (Muller et al., 1983).

Carbamates (e.g., carbaryl, Sevin) are cholinesterase inhibitors. Varying from slow to rapid in action, they are residual contact poisons with minimal persistence in the environment. Although less toxic than the organophosphate cholinesterase inhibitors, they cannot be used on kittens.

The organophosphates, with the exception of malathion, are toxic for cats (Atkins and Johnson, 1975; Muller et al., 1983; Wilkinson, 1968). An uncommonly recognized effect of overexposure to malathion is delayed paralysis of the limbs (Georgi,1980; Holzworth, 1983).

Chlorinated hydrocarbons are notoriously toxic to cats, with the single exception of methoxychlor (Atkins and Johnson, 1975; Clarke and Clarke, 1967; Clarke, 1975; Scott, 1979b; Wilkinson, 1968).

The parasiticides listed here are available in many products for application to pets in the forms of (1) dips given every seven days; (2) powders applied every one to seven days and having good adherent property; (3) shampoos, usually of no residual activity and therefore of brief effectiveness; and (4) sprays, varying in residual effect according to the agent, and alarming to most cats. In most cases repeated powdering or spraying of cats serves as well as dips and shampoos.

Collars and medallions containing carbaryl, propoxur, dichlorvos, or stirofos give some protection to a cat for varying periods, but treatment of the environment is also required. Collars containing dichlorvos, as previously noted, may occasionally cause a severe dermatitis, especially if worn in a hot, dry enviroment (Muller et al., 1983).

In certain areas where flea infestation is severe some veterinarians have resorted to "spot" application of a twenty percent solution of the organophosphate fenthion (Spotton), although it is not approved for this use in the United States. For cats it is dropped on the *skin* of the top of the head at a dose of 0.35 ml/10 pounds once a week until remission and then as needed (every 2 to 4 weeks). The dose of 0.35 ml is not exceeded for cats over 5 kg (10 pounds), and the drug is never used on animals under 6 months or over 12 years of age (Muller et al., 1983; Scott, 1984).

Of equal or greater importance than treatment of the cat is treatment of the cat's surroundings. Floors, rugs, upholstered furniture, and the cat's bedding should be vacuumed frequently and the vacuum bag burned. Premise foggers and sprays are helpful in eliminating fleas in rugs, floor cracks, basements, garages, crawl spaces, and yards. Agents used for this purpose include carbaryl, methoxychlor, malathion, dichlorvos, and diazinon.

Microencapsulation, a relatively new form of drug delivery, "packages" liquid suspensions of insecticides (e.g., pyrethrins, diazinon) in microcapsules, some preparations of which are to be sprayed on the animal, others on furniture, floors and bedding. Here the insecticide is slowly released in small amounts for variable periods and kills the fleas by contact.

Also of great value in flea control is methoprene, a growth inhibitor that prevents larval forms from developing into adults. Of extremely low toxicity and residual effect for 75 to 90 days, it is used on floors, carpets, and furniture. As it is inactivated by sunlight, it is not effective for outdoor use. It is combined with a short-acting agent that kills adult fleas.

Pending elimination of fleas a cat that is suffering severely from flea allergy may be helped by administration of a corticosteroid.

## Pediculosis

Lice are uncommon parasites of cats and tend to be found in debilitated, anemic animals. Because *Felicola subrostratus* is a biting louse and not a red blood sucker, feline lice and the eggs ("nits") adhering to the fur look like fine dandruff and may thus escape identification. Infestations may be asymptomatic or may cause a severe pruritic dermatitis with hair loss.

Lice are easily identified by microscopic examination and are readily eliminated by the same powders, sprays, and dips that are effective against fleas (e.g., pyrethrin or carbamate shampoos and 2 per cent methoxychlor or 5 per cent carbaryl powder). Because louse-infested cats are often weak and debilitated, they will probably be least stressed by application of a powder. A second or third treatment at 10 to 14 days is recommended to ensure destruction of any remaining lice that may have hatched.

*Trichodectes canis*, the common dog louse, occasionally parasitizes kittens and aged cats in poor condition (Wilkinson, 1983a).

## Ticks

Ticks rarely parasitize cats (see references, Scott, 1980). Cats bearing ticks show little evidence of irritation and are usually presented because the owner noted "a lump on the skin" or the sudden onset of a "tumor" or "cyst." Ticks are usually found on the head and neck and in the ears of cats. Tick infestation may be seasonal (spring and summer) in the northern United States or nonseasonal in the warmer south. In Australia cats appear to be commonly parasitized by a variety of ixodid ticks and sometimes develop tick paralysis (Arundel, 1980). Clusters of larval *Ixodes cornuatus* on the feet of cats have been known to cause lesions measuring up to 0.8 cm.

Ticks should be gently pulled loose by applying a hemostat or tweezer to the head at the skin surface. The powders, sprays, and dips used to eliminate fleas are also effective against ticks.

## Otodectic Mange

*Otodectes cynotis* is by far the most frequent parasitic mite of cats (see references, Scott, 1980). Its favorite site is the external ear canal where its presence is signaled by masses of dark brown, granular material and sometimes by secondary infection. Hematomas of the pinna and excoriations of the ears, head, and neck are secondary effects. The excoriations may be indistinguishable grossly from those of notoedric mange. Treatment of otodectic ear infestation is discussed in the chapter on the ear.

"Ectopic" infestation describes the occasional cases of otodectic skin lesions on other parts of the body. These usually occur on the head, neck, rump, tail, or paws, and vary from partial alopecia to an erythematous, scaling, crusted pruritic dermatitis. It has been suggested that the cat's habit of sleeping with its head on its paws and tail is a factor in the spread of the infestation. A cat with ear mites should therefore be dusted weekly with a flea powder (Muller et al., 1983). Dusting is especially important at the time the ears are cleaned, when removal of debris may scatter large numbers of mites on the cat's coat.

Ear mites getting onto human skin may cause a transient pruritic, papular dermatitis (Herwick, 1978).

## Notoedric Mange

*Notoedres cati* is a rare parasitism of cats but is endemic and common in a few localities (Muller et al., 1983; see also references, Scott, 1980). Lesions first appear at the medial proximal edge of the pinna of the ear, then spread to the upper ear, face and eyelids, and neck. They may also extend to the feet, tail, and perineum, probably owing to the cat's habits of washing and of sleeping curled up. The female mites' burrowing into the epidermis causes minute papules. The skin soon becomes thickened and creased and is later covered with dense, adherent, yellow or gray crusts. Intense itching leads to partial alopecia and to excoriations that become secondarily infected. Notoedric mange is characteristically a disease of adult cats; rarely, however, it may present as a fulminating dermatitis in litters of kittens, in which abdomen, perineum, and limbs are most severely affected (Conroy, 1964; Holzworth, 1967; Thornton, 1963). In severe, untreated cases, death may result from secondary bacterial infection, interference with eating, anorexia, emaciation, and toxemia (Brumley, 1931; Kirk, 1925; Wilkinson, 1966).

*Notoedres cati* is much smaller than the sarcoptic mite of dogs and humans and is much more easily isolated by skin scraping. The parasitism is also more easily eliminated than scabies of humans and dogs. Since affected cats are often severely debilitated, it is wise to limit initial treatment to clipping and gentle rubbing in of a sulfur-containing lotion or cream. Several days later the cat may be given a bath to loosen crusts and a dip in 2 per cent sulfur solution, which should be allowed to dry on. Additional dips should be given at 10-day intervals until two weeks after complete cure. Malathion and carbaryl dips are effective, although less safe for debilitated animals and contraindicated for kittens. Young kittens with generalized involvement may require supportive measures if they are to survive the treatment.

Newer products may simplify treatment. A single application of amitraz (0.025 per cent, applied with a toothbrush) has been found to be successful (Wilkinson, 1980, 1983a). A single subcutaneous injection of ivermectin (1 mg/kg) was reported to cure notoedric mange in 17 cats (Bigler, 1984).

Benzyl benzoate and lindane, time-honored drugs for treatment of scabies of dogs and humans, are highly toxic to cats and should *never* be used.

*Notoedres cati* may also infest dogs, rabbits, and foxes; humans, to whom the mite is occasionally transferred by contact with cats, may experience transient irritation or dermatitis. Infestation of cats with *Sarcoptes canis* is a very rare event (Muller et al., 1983).

## Cheyletiellosis

Sometimes called colloquially "walking drandruff," this is an uncommon parasitism of cats (Fox and Hewes, 1976; McKeever and Allen, 1979; Muller et al., 1983; Scott, 1980). *Cheyletiella* spp are large mites that infest cats, dogs, and rabbits, cats usually being parasitized by *C. parasitivorax* or *C. blakei*. The adults move rapidly in epidermal debris or attach to the epidermis. Their ova, attached to hairs, are smaller than louse nits. Mites and ova can thus appear, to the naked eye, as a fine dandruff. *Cheyletiella* mites have also been seen crawling in and out of the nostrils of cats (Stein, 1982).

Cats have milder itching and skin reactions than do dogs, and cattery infestations are less severe than those in kennels. In cats the back is most often involved, but because of the cat's licking, mites may be hard to find. The white or yellow mites, eggs, and keratin scales usually give an appearance of miliary dermatitis or dandruff, but in a large cattery infestation cats had discrete dried exudate, patchy crusts, and scabs over much of their bodies (Ottenschot and Gil, 1978).

*Cheyletiella* mites moving on the skin can be identified with a high-power magnifying glass and are often easily collected by acetate tape impression, by brushing, or by a scalpel scraping; however, they may be extremely difficult to find on some cats (Scott, 1980). Mites and eggs may be found in fecal flotations even when they cannot be found in the fur (Georgi, 1980).

The mites are readily destroyed by agents effective against fleas and also by lime-sulfur dips. Three treatments should be given at weekly intervals. Premises should be sprayed with a residual insecticide (e.g., malathion).

Man may be an accidental host to mites acquired from a pet and may develop a transient dermatitis (Cohen, 1980; Fox and Reed, 1978; Hewitt et al., 1971; Thomsett, 1968). The mites do not, however, multiply on humans, and the irritation regresses spontaneously within three weeks after the source of infestation is eliminated.

## Demodicosis

Demodectic mange is rare in cats (Conroy et al., 1982; Desch and Nutting, 1979; Scott, 1980; Stogdale and Moore, 1982). It is caused by *Demodex cati* and by one or more other species as yet unnamed (Conroy et al., 1982; Muller, 1983; Wilkinson, 1983c). Infestation may be localized or generalized.

Lesions of the localized form usually occur on the eyelids and around the eyes and on the ears, neck, and skin. These lesions are characterized by alopecia, erythema, sometimes scaling, crusting, papules, and secondary pyoderma. All cats with acne of the chin should be scraped, especially if the chin and skin caudal to it are hairless, scaly, reddened, and hyperpigmented (Muller, 1983). Localized demodectic mange may be self-limiting but heals rapidly if treated with rotenone (one part Canex to four parts mineral oil). Amitraz is not recommended by the manufacturer for use in cats but was employed without ill effect for massaging into lesions of the pinnae (0.025 per cent aqueous solution twice a week for three weeks) (Wilkinson, 1983c). However, total body applications of 0.0125, 0.025, and 0.05 per cent amitraz produced various side effects in normal cats, including loose malodorous stools, anorexia, and depression (Gunaratnam et al., 1983).

Demodectic mites have also been found in cases of ceruminous external otitis. This may also be treated with Canex diluted with mineral oil.

Generalized demodicosis is very rare and not so severe as the canine form (e.g., Stogdale and Moore, 1982). It may merely take the form of a patchy thinning of the hair coat (Holzworth, 1983) or it may cause a symmetric hair loss that mimics endocrine or psychogenic alopecia (Muller et al., 1983). Other cases are characterized by multifocal or generalized alopecia, erythema, and varying degrees of scaling, papulocrustous dermatitis, and secondary pyoderma (Scott, 1980).

Mild remedies such as lime-sulfur dip or carbaryl shampoo often suffice for treatment (Muller et al., 1983).

Limited evidence suggests a possible association of generalized feline demodicosis with serious systemic disorders such as leukemia, leukopenia, and diabetes mellitus (Muller et al., 1983).

## Other Mites

***LYNXACARUS RADOVSKYI.*** The cat fur mite has been reported from Australia, Fiji, Hawaii, Puerto Rico, and most recently Florida (Greeve and Gerrish, 1981; see also references, Scott, 1984). It is easily differentiated from the cat louse by its single cylindrical, sac-like body segment and eight legs. A distinguishing feature of the adult is a pair of flap-like projections from the sternum, which wrap around the hair shaft, serving as a hold-fast. The mites, attached to the ends of the hairs, give the coat a scurfy appearance, usually along the back but occasionally all over the body. The hair is easily epilated. The skin itself is normal in some cats; in others it has lesions of miliary dermatitis. Infestation may be found on just one cat in a group.

The mites are easily obtained for identification by skin scraping or acetate tape impression. Repeated lime-sulfur dips and 5 per cent carbaryl powder have been used in treatment.

***DERMANYSSUS GALLINAE.*** *D. gallinae*, the red poultry mite, lives in cracks and nests in poultry quarters during the day and comes out at night to feed on fowl. Wild birds and rarely cats, dogs, and humans (Kral, 1960; Kral and Novak, 1953) may also be parasitized by the mites. The small gray-white mites crawling on the hair may resemble the dandruff of cheyletiellosis (Muller et al., 1983). They are red only when engorged with blood. Signs of infestation are itching and papulocrustous dermatitis, especially on the face and limbs.

The infestation is identified by skin scraping and treated by lime-sulfur or other parasiticidal dips, baths, or powders. Infested premises must be treated vigorously to prevent reinfestation of animals.

**TROMBICULID MITES.** A number of species of trombiculid larvae (chiggers, harvest mites, clover mites) may occasionally parasitize the ears, head, legs, and sometimes the back or underside of cats that roam woods and fields (Muller et al., 1983; Scott, 1980). The nymphs and adults are free-living, but the bright orange-red, six-legged larvae attach themselves tightly to the skin, where they remain for several days feeding on tissue fluid and cellular debris. They cause severe itching and dermatitis characterized by papules, pustules, and crusts. Most infestations occur in late summer or autumn.

Diagnosis is by a history of exposure and by finding the bright-colored mites on the skin. However, since they stay on the host for only 3 to 15 days, they may have dropped off by the time the cat is examined.

The parasitism is eliminated by a single lime-sulfur dip or pyrethrin or carbamate shampoo. A glucocorticoid may be given for severe pruritus. Reinfestation can be prevented only by keeping the cat indoors.

An unusually severe reaction was seen in a suburban Massachusetts cat parasitized by larvae of *Walchia americana*, a chigger of squirrels and small rodents (Lowenstine et al., 1979). A papulocrustous dermatitis involved the skin of the head, underside, perineum, and medial surfaces of the legs. The paws were swollen and the claws ragged. Skin scrapings yielded only a few damaged parasites identified as *W. americana*. An unusual feature of the case was that mites were found burrowed deep within epidermal tunnels and areas of inflammation in biopsy specimens.

Dusting with a pyrethrin-carbaryl powder and oral administration of penicillin brought about recovery within two months.

## Myiasis

Myiasis, infestation of the body by fly larvae, is caused in cats by *Cuterebra* larvae that form subcutaneous sinuses and by larvae of blowflies and fleshflies attracted to open wounds and soiled or necrotic skin.

**CUTEREBRIASIS.** *Cuterebra* larvae occasionally parasitize rural kittens and young cats in late summer. Adult flies of a number of *Cuterebra* species oviposit in the soil or on plants near rabbit and rodent burrows. Larvae may then penetrate the skin of their normal hosts or, rarely, of a cat, dog, or human and develop in subcutaneous cysts, where they remain for about a month, then leave to pupate on the ground.

Lesions take the form of firm subcutaneous swellings about 1 cm in diameter with a fistulous opening (breathing hole) through which a blood-tinged discharge exudes and the gray, spiny larva can be seen moving. These lesions usually occur in the neck or submandibular areas and are usually single and asymptomatic, but they may occasionally be multiple or may abscess. Rarely, larvae find their way to other sites in the body.

The breathing hole is enlarged, if necessary, and the "grub" (about 2.5 cm long) is gently extracted with a forceps. Care should be taken not to rupture it in situ, lest an allergic or irritant reaction occur. The infected cavity should be treated but is usually slow to heal (Muller et al., 1983).

Occasionally, the larva will have dropped out before the cat is seen, and the clinician is presented with a slowly healing wound or abscess with a telltale circular pore.

**"FLYSTRIKE."** Infestation by maggots is most likely to befall injured, debilitated, or paralyzed cats, especially those with neglected wounds, matted haircoats, or fecal or urine soiling. This form of myiasis is caused by larvae of various blowflies and fleshflies. Adult flies are attracted to the moisture and odor of feces, urine, draining wounds, and discharges. Eggs are deposited in the affected area and hatch within 12 hours. The larvae produce proteolytic enzymes and damage the skin. After three to six days of highly destructive activity, the larvae leave the host to pupate on the ground.

Most often involved is the skin around the anus, genitals, eyes, and dorsal midline, where multiple, "punched-out," round holes may coalesce to produce large defects with scalloped edges. Extensive sections of skin may become undermined and may be seen and felt to "crawl" with the large numbers of active larvae. The associated odor is pathognomonic—and the foulest known to veterinarians. Heavy flystrikes may cause death, presumably by the toxic effects of products of maggots and tissue destruction. Flystrike typically occurs in warm weather.

Treatment requires gentle clipping, and cleaning and flushing with an antiseptic such as povidone-iodine. It is essential that all larvae be removed, if necessary by a forceps, from all crevices and subcutaneous tracts. The wound should be treated with a topical antibiotic and the rest of the coat sprayed with a parasiticide. If the cat can tolerate it, parasiticidal shampoos (pyrethrins) or topical ether are extremely effective for the rapid killing and immobilization of larvae, thus facilitating flush procedures. Affected animals are often toxic, and supportive and symptomatic care may make the difference between life and death. Flystrike is a disease of neglect, and the predisposing cause must be corrected (Muller et al., 1983; Scott, 1980).

## Dracunculiasis

*Dracunculus medinensis*, the guinea worm of Africa and Asia, has been found in the cat in the USSR (Petrov and Chubabriya, 1955), but its North American relative, *D. insignis*, does not appear to have been reported in this species.

## Dirofilariasis

The cat is an unnatural host for *D. immitis*, which may find its way to sites other than the heart. A nematode found in a cutaneous granulomatous limb lesion submitted by a Massachusetts veterinarian (Dr. Howard Smith, Concord) to the Department of Pathology, Angell Memorial Animal Hospital, was identified at the Ontario Veterinary College as *D. immitis*. The locality is a notorious focus of heartworm infection, and other cases of feline dirofilariasis had been recognized there.

## Hookworm Dermatitis

Both *Ancylostoma tubaeforme* and *Uncinaria stenocephala* may cause a dermatitis similar to that in dogs (Arundel, 1980). It is seen especially in the interdigital spaces and may cause tenderness of the feet.

## Anatrichosomiasis

*Anatrichosoma* spp are nematodes known to infect humans and subhuman primates, producing a type of larva migrans lesion. Anatrichosomiasis was reported in a South African cat presented for lameness and necrosis, sloughing, and ulceration of the footpads of all four feet (Lange et al., 1980). Histologic findings included superficial perivascular dermatitis with numerous nematodes and bioperculate eggs within necrotic tracts in the epidermis.

# Non-neoplastic Tumors

## Cutaneous Horns

These are rare in cats (Scott, 1980). In man, unusual cohesiveness of keratinized material may produce a cutaneous horn on a variety of benign and malignant lesions (e.g., actinic keratosis, seborrheic keratosis, papilloma, squamous cell carcinoma). Thus the diagnosis is purely clinical, and the horn should be excised in every case and submitted for histologic diagnosis. In cats, cutaneous horns have no apparent breed, sex, or site predilection but usually occur in adult or aged animals. Hard, well-circumscribed, and fixed to surrounding skin, they may vary in length from 0.3 to 5.0 cm (Fig. 13–29). Some have arisen from basal cell tumors and papillomas (Scott, 1980).

At the New York State College of Veterinary Medicine multiple cutaneous horns were described on the footpads of a cat that tested positive for feline leukemia virus, and the virus was cultured from the lesions as well as being identified by electron microscopic examination (Center et al., 1982). Treatment was ineffective, and ultimately additional pads and the nasal planum and eyelids became involved. Subsequently, five more cases of multiple cutaneous horns of the pads were encountered, and FeLV was similarly implicated (Scott, 1984). Treatment by surgical excision, electrocautery, and cryosurgery failed to prevent recurrences.

## Cysts

Epidermal cysts (epidermoid cysts, epidermal inclusion cysts, "sebaceous" cysts, wens) are uncommon in the cat, having no apparent age, sex, or breed predilection (Conroy, 1964, 1974; Doering, 1976; Joshua, 1965; Moulton, 1961; Scott, 1980). They are usually solitary, occasionally multiple, well circumscribed, round, firm or fluctuant, bluish, fixed to the overlying skin, and filled with a caseous, greasy material ranging in color from chalk-white to brownish gray. Ulceration and secondary infection may occur. Epidermal cysts have a predilection for the neck and trunk. Conroy (1964) observed multiple epidermal cysts on the necks of cats wearing flea collars. In a Siamese

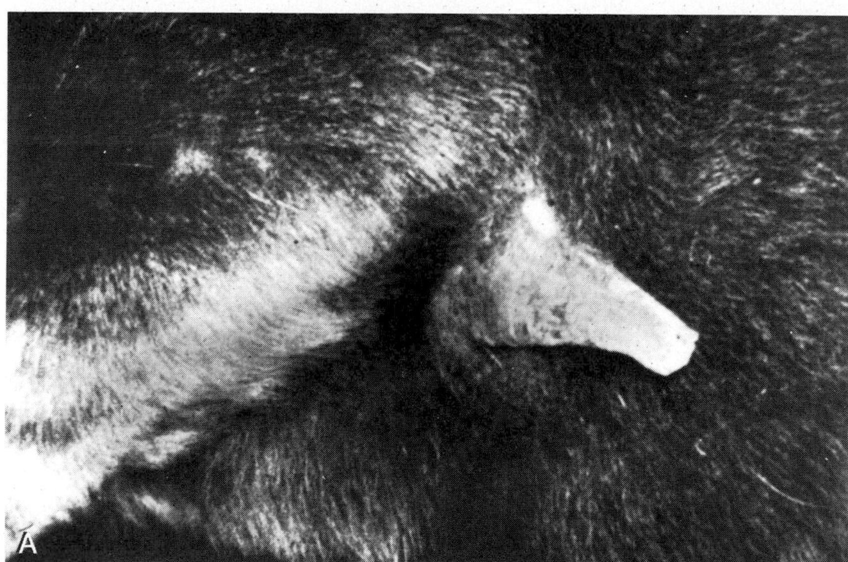


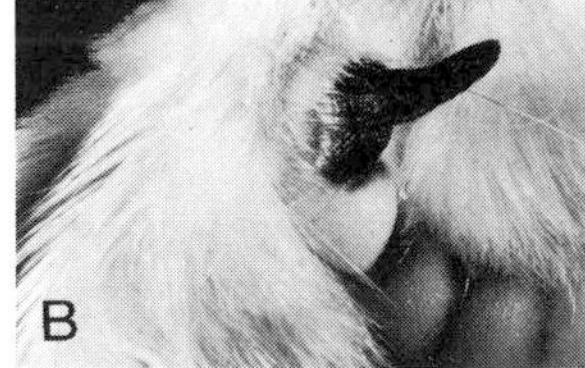


**Figure 13–29** *A*, Cutaneous horn, axilla. *B*, Pigmented cutaneous horn, digital pad. (*B*, Courtesy Angell Memorial Animal Hospital.)

cat referred to the Angell Memorial Animal Hospital, disseminated epidermal inclusion cysts were associated with congenital hypotrichosis (Holzworth, 1983) (Fig. 13–6).

True sebaceous cysts are uncommon. Multiple pedunculated apocrine cysts have been pictured by Wilkinson (1983a).

### Nevi

A nevus is a developmental malformation of the skin and may represent any combination of epithelial and mesenchymal tissues. Organoid (adnexal) nevi are of rare occurrence in the author's experience (Scott, 1980). They either have been present as long as the owner could remember or were never noticed at all. Single or multiple and measuring 0.3 to 1.0 cm in diameter, they may be firm or mushy, dome-shaped or pedunculated. They occur on the skin of the face and head, especially in the temporal area. Histologic examination reveals an overgrowth of hair follicles, sebaceous glands, and rarely apocrine sweat glands. The owner may be instructed to watch the nevi for any change in size or appearance, or they may be excised. (See also the chapter on tumors.)

### Nodular Fasciitis

This rare non-neoplastic growth of the cat (and dog) is believed to be a proliferative inflammatory process arising from the subcutaneous fascia and exhibiting a clinically aggressive behavior suggestive of a locally invasive neoplasm (Muller et al., 1983). It has been identified on the upper lip of a cat (Kemp et al., 1976) and at other sites (Scott, 1980).

Microscopically, it is characterized by a poorly circumscribed, infiltrative proliferation of pleomorphic fibroblasts growing haphazardly in a highly vascularized stroma with varying amounts of mucoid ground substance (Stannard and Pulley, 1978). Other features are mitoses, giant cells, and often a chronic inflammatory infiltrate.

Surgical excision may be successful and large doses of glucocorticoids induce striking remissions, but multiple recurrences are not uncommon (Scott, 1980).

### Dilated Pore of Winer

This rare cystic hair follicle abnormality of man has been reported in a cat (Scott and Flanders, 1984). The cat had an asymptomatic, well-circumscribed, firm, smooth, rounded mass in the skin on one side of the face. A yellowish, keratinous, conical structure protruded from the center of the lesion. Biopsy revealed a markedly dilated hair follicle filled with laminated keratin. The follicular epithelium became increasingly hyperplastic toward the base of the follicle and showed many rete ridges and irregular epithelial projections into the surrounding dermis. Surgical excision was curative.

## Neoplasms

Cutaneous neoplasms are discussed in the chapter on tumors.

## THERAPEUTICS

Therapeutic agents for skin disorders are discussed in detail in the author's monograph on feline dermatology (Scott, 1980) and by Muller et al. (1983). The appendix in the latter work gives detailed information on the constituents, actions, and uses of these products, together with the names and addresses of their makers. Agents favored by the author for cats have been specified in the foregoing chapter.

Special considerations that influence the choice and use of agents for cats merit emphasis.

Certain topical agents are contraindicated because of toxicity for cats. These include salicylic acid, tars, and other phenol derivatives (e.g., resorcinol, cresol, hexachlorophene) (Aronson, 1975; Atkins and Johnson, 1975; Clarke and Clarke, 1967; Garner, 1961; Joshua, 1965; Oehme, 1977; Scott, 1979a; Wilkinson, 1968).

Tincture of iodine and Lugol's iodine are irritating, sensitizing, and contraindicated for cats. If an iodine product is desirable, irritation is less likely with povidone-iodine (Betadine, Purdue-Frederick), which is virtually nonstinging and nonstaining, can be taped or bandaged over, and is active in the presence of blood, serum, necrotic debris, and pus.

Alcohol used as an antiseptic is disturbing to cats because of the odor and sensation of cold.

Dimethyl sulfoxide (DMSO) has been used in a wide variety of feline skin disorders, from pruritus to purulent dermatitis and abscesses (Koller, 1976; Scott, 1979a, 1980). It should be used with caution, because agents with which it is combined may be absorbed systemically and cause undesirable effects. The only commercial product licensed for use in cats is Synotic (Diamond Laboratories), in which DMSO is combined with a glucocorticoid and propylene glycol for treatment of otitis externa.

The glucocorticoids are indispensable in treatment of many feline skin disorders, but they must be used in ways appropriate to the peculiarities of cats. Topical application of glucocorticoids is limited to areas inaccessible to the cat's tongue. The author prefers betamethasone-17-valerate (Valisone, Schering), because it is available in several forms (0.1 per cent ointment, cream, and lotion, and 0.15 per cent spray) and because it is more effective in cats than the less potent glucocorticoids (hydrocortisone, prednisolone, triamcinolone). A topical glucocorticoid is applied three times daily, until the dermatosis is controlled, and can then be tapered to minimum effective frequency.

For systemic glucocorticoid therapy, cats generally require higher doses than dogs (Halliwell, 1977; Scott, 1980) and are more resistant than dogs and humans to many of the side effects of glucocorticoids (Scott et al., 1979b; Scott, 1980). Only with prolonged, excessive doses of glucocorticoid do cats develop signs of hyperglucocorticoidism. They are, however, susceptible to secondary adrenocortical insufficiency.

To minimize or avoid this suppression of the hypothalamic-pituitary-adrenocortical axis, the technique of alternate-day steroid therapy is recommended. It has been shown (Krieger et al., 1968; Scott et al., 1979b) that most cats have a daily rhythm of cortisol production opposite to that of dogs and humans, feline cortisol levels being lowest in the morning and highest from 10 PM to midnight. This finding suggests than an oral glucocorticoid should be administered to a cat every other evening (at about 10 PM).

For oral therapy, the author prefers prednisolone or prednisone at *induction* doses of 1 to 4 mg/kg b.i.d. and *maintenance* doses of 1 to 4 mg/kg every other evening. The actual dose varies with the condition and the individual cat. Rarely, one encounters steroid tachyphylaxis in the cat, when the glucocorticoid being administered appears to lose its effectiveness. I have had success in such instances by switching to another glucocorticoid, such as dexamethasone or triamcinolone, at an equipotent dose.

If a cat resists administration of tablets or if oral therapy seems ineffective, it may be necessary to resort to an injectable glucocorticoid. The author and others (e.g., Halliwell, 1977) prefer methylprednisolone acetate (Depo-Medrol, Upjohn) at a total dosage of 20 mg IM or SC every two weeks or as needed. This dosage is five times that recommended by the manufacturer but may be necessary for therapeutic effect. When administered long-term, this product should not be given more often than once every two months.

Progestogens are effective in a variety of feline skin disorders but should be used with discrimination. Available as megestrol acetate (Schering, Mead-Johnson), medroxyprogesterone acetate (Depo-Provera, Upjohn), and repository progesterone, they are not, however, licensed for use in the cat. Therefore the veterinarian should keep with the cat's medical record a drug-release form in which the owner agrees in writing to the use of an unlicensed drug for treatment of a specific skin disorder.

Among side effects of progestogens in cats are increases in appetite, weight, and water intake, personality changes for good or ill, pyometra, mammary hyperplasia and neoplasia, poor reproductive performance in males, transient or permanent diabetes mellitus, severe adrenocortical suppression, and iatrogenic Cushing's syndrome, as well as local alopecia, depigmentation, or cutaneous atrophy at injection sites (Chastain et al., 1981; Halliwell, 1977; Hart, 1974, 1976; Henik et al., 1985; Hinton and Gaskell, 1977; Houdeshell et al., 1977; Hutchison, 1978; Jones, 1975; Kunkle, 1984; Nimmo-Wilkie, 1979; Øen, 1977; Scott, 1980, 1984). Because of these drawbacks a conservative clinician will be wise to employ a progestogen only as a last resort.

## REFERENCES


Aho R: Saprophytic fungi isolated from the hair of domestic and laboratory animals with suspected dermatophytosis. Mycopathologia 83 (1983) 65–73.

Ajello L, Walker WW, Dungworth DL, Brumfield GL: Isolation of *Nocardia brasiliensis* from a cat, with a review of its prevalence and geographic distribution. J Am Vet Med Assoc 138 (1961) 370–376.

Allan GS, Wickham N: Mycobacterial granulomas in a cat diagnosed as leprosy. Feline Pract 6 (5) (1976) 34–36.

Allen LS: Eosinophilic granuloma treatment. Feline Pract 7 (5) (1977) 43–44.

Allen SD, van Kampen KR, Brooks DR: Evaluation of the feline dichlorvos (DDVP) flea collar. Feline Pract 8 (3) (1978) 9–16.

Alterman HP: [Hyperesthesia syndrome.] (Letter). Feline Pract 7 (6) (1977) 4.

Arnold U, Opitz M, Grosser I, Bader R, Eigenmann JE: Goitrous hypothyroidism and dwarfism in a kitten. J Am Anim Hosp Assoc 20 (1984) 753–758.

Aronson AL: Diseases caused by chemical and physical agents. *In* Catcott EJ (ed): Feline Medicine and Surgery, 2nd ed. Santa Barbara, American Veterinary Publications, Inc, 1975, 113–130.

Aronson AL, Schwark WS: Adverse drug reactions. *In* Kirk RW (ed): Current Veterinary Therapy VII. Philadelphia, WB Saunders Company, 1980, 155–160.

Aronson CE: Thallium intoxication. *In* Kirk RW (ed): Current Veterinary Therapy VI. Philadelphia, WB Saunders Company, 1977.

Arundel JH: Helminth and protozoan diseases of cats in Australia. University of Sydney Post-Graduate Committee in Veterinary Science. Refresher Course for Veterinarians. Proc 53 (1980) 193–200.

Atkins CE, Johnson RK: Clinical toxicities of cats. Vet Clin North Am 5 (1975) 623–652.

Attleberger MH: Actinomycosis, nocardiosis, and dermatophilosis. *In* Kirk RW (ed): Current Veterinary Therapy VIII. Philadelphia, WB Saunders Company, 1983a.

Attleberger MH: Systemic mycoses. *In* Pratt PW (ed): Feline Medicine. Santa Barbara, American Veterinary Publications, Inc, 1983b.

Austin VH: The skin. *In* Catcott EJ (ed): Feline Medicine and Surgery, 2nd ed. Santa Barbara, American Veterinary Publications, Inc, 1975a, 461–484.

Austin VH: Common skin problems in cats. Mod Vet Pract 56 (1975b) 541–545.

Baker KP: Skin allergy of the dog and cat. Ir Vet J 22 (1968) 47–50.

Baker KP: Some aspects of feline dermatoses. Vet Rec 86 (1970) 62–66.

Baker KP: The treatment of skin disease in cats. Ir Vet J 28 (1974a) 173–175.

Baker KP: Hair growth and replacement in the cat. Br Vet J 130 (1974b) 327–335.

Baxby D, Ashton DG, Denham EMH: Cowpox virus infection in unusual hosts. Vet Rec 104 (1979) 175.

Bell TG, Farrell RK, Padgett GA, Leendertsen LW: Ataxia, depression, and dermatitis associated with the use of dichlorvos-impregnated collars in the laboratory cat. J Am Vet Med Assoc 167 (1975) 579–586.

Berg JN, Fales WH, Scanlan CM: Occurrence of anaerobic bacteria in diseases of the dog and cat. Am J Vet Res 40 (1979) 876–881.

Berry JM, Mosier JE: Selected feline dermatoses. Vet Clin North Am 1 (1971) 217–224.

Bestetti G, Bühlmann V, Nicolet J, Fankhauser R: Paraplegia due to *Actinomyces viscosus* infection in a cat. Acta Neuropathol 39 (1977) 231–235.

Biberstein EL, Jang SS, Hirsh DC: Species distribution of coagulase-positive staphylococci in animals. J Clin Microbiol 19 (1984) 610–615.

Biberstein EL, Knight HD, England K: *Bacteroides melaninogenicus* in diseases of domestic animals. J Am Vet Med Assoc 153 (1968) 1045–1049.

Biery DN: Radiation therapy in dermatology. *In* Kirk RW (ed): Current Veterinary Therapy VI. Philadelphia, WB Saunders Company, 1977, 527–528.

Bigler B: Treatment of Notoedres cati with ivermectin. Proc 1st European Veterinary Dermatology Meeting, Hamburg, 1984.

Bourdin M, Destombes P, Parodi AL, Drouhet E, Segretain G: Première observation d'un mycetome à microsporum canis chez un chat. Recl Méd Vét 151 (1975) 475–480.

Brightman AH, Vestre WA, Helper LC, Godshalk CP: Chronic eosinophilic keratitis in the cat. Feline Pract 9 (3) (1979) 21–24.

Brownlie JF: Symposium: Geriatrics. Skin diseases in the aging dog and cat. J S Afr Vet Med Assoc 34 (1963) 167–174.

Brumley OV: A Textbook of the Diseases of the Small Animals, 2nd ed. Philadelphia, Lea & Febiger, 1931.

Brummer H: [Psychosomatic disorders and diseases in animals.

V. Skin, nervous system, blood, and metabolism.] Dtsch Tierärztl Wochenschr 80 (1973) 52–55.
Bucci TJ: Intradermal granuloma associated with collagen degeneration in three cats. J Am Vet Med Assoc 148 (1966) 794–800.
Butler WF: Fragility of the skin in a cat. Res Vet Sci 19 (1975) 213–216.
Caciolo PL., Nesbitt GH, Hurvitz AI: Pemphigus foliaceus in eight cats and results of induction therapy using azathioprine. J Am Anim Hosp Assoc 20 (1984) 571–577.
Carakostas MC, Miller RI, Woodward MG: Subcutaneous dermatophilosis in a cat. J Am Vet Med Assoc 185 (1984) 675–676.
Carey CJ, Morris JG: Biotin deficiency in the cat and the effect on hepatic propionyl CoA carboxylase. J Nutr 107 (1977) 330–334.
Carpenter JL: Personal communication, 1983.
Carr SH: Seborrhea in the cat. Feline Pract 9 (5) (1979) 38–39.
Center SA, Scott DW, Scott FW: Multiple cutaneous horns on the foot pads of a cat. Feline Pract 12 (4) (1982) 26–30.
Chastain CB, Graham CL, Nichols CE: Adrenocortical suppression in cats given megestrol acetate. Am J Vet Res 42 (1981) 2029–2035.
Chesney CJ: The response to progestagen treatment of some diseases of cats. J Small Anim Pract 17 (1976) 35–44.
Clarke EGC: Pets and poisons. J Small Anim Pract 16 (1975) 375–380.
Clarke EGC, Clarke ML: Garner's Veterinary Toxicology, 3rd ed. Baltimore, The Williams and Wilkins Company, 1967.
Coffin DL, Holzworth J: "Yellow fat" in two laboratory cats: acid-fast pigmentation associated with a fish-base ration. Cornell Vet 44 (1954) 63–71.
Cohen SR: *Cheyletiella* dermatitis (in rabbit, cat, dog, man). Arch Dermatol 116 (1980) 435–437.
Collier LL, Leathers CW, Counts DF: A clinical description of dermatosparaxis in a Himalayan cat. Feline Pract 10 (5) (1980) 25–36.
Comben N: Monkey glands for cats. The treatment of miliary eczema in the cat by subcutaneous implantation of testosterone. Vet Rec 65 (1953) 877–879.
Connole MD: Keratinophilic fungi on cats and dogs. Sabouraudia 4 (1965) 45–48.
Conroy JD: Diseases of the skin. *In* Catcott EJ (ed): Feline Medicine and Surgery. Wheaton, American Veterinary Publications, Inc, 1964, 321–347.
Conroy JD: Neoplasms of the skin and subcutis. *In* Kirk RW (ed): Current Veterinary Therapy V. Philadelphia, WB Saunders Company, 1974, 444–447.
Conroy JD: The etiology and pathogenesis of alopecia. Compend Contin Ed 1 (1979) 806–814.
Conroy JD: An overview of immune-mediated mucocutaneous diseases in the dog and cat. II. Other diseases based on immunologic mechanisms. Am J Dermatopathol 5 (1983) 595–599.
Conroy JD, Healey MC, Bane AG: New *Demodex* sp. infesting a cat: A case report. J Am Anim Hosp Assoc 18 (1982) 405–407.
Cooper LM, Sabine M: Paw and mouth disease in a cat (Letter). Aust Vet J 48 (1972) 644.
Cordy DR, Stillinger CJ: Steatitis ("yellow fat disease") in kittens. North Am Vet 34 (1953) 714–716.
Cotter SM: Feline leukemia virus–associated diseases. *In* Kirk RW (ed): Current Veterinary Therapy VI. Philadelphia, WB Saunders Company, 1977, 465–472.
Counts DF, Holbrook KA, Byers PH, Hegreberg GA: Dermatosparaxis in a Himalayan cat: Biochemical and ultrastructural studies of dermal collagen (Abstr). Fed Proc 38 (1979) 1339.
Counts DF, Byers PH, Holbrook KA, Hegreberg GA: Dermatosparaxis in a Himalayan cat: I. Biochemical studies of dermal collagen. J Invest Dermatol 74 (1980) 96–99.
Cox HU, Hoskins JD, Newman SS, Turnwald GH, Foil CS, Roy AF, Kearney MT: Distribution of staphylococcal species on clinically healthy cats. Am J Vet Res 46 (1985) 1824–1828.
Dall JA: A practitioner's approach to skin disease in small animals. Vet Rec 70 (1958) 1029–1039.
De Boer S: On the structure and covering of the trunk-dermatomes of the cat. Verh Akad Wet Amst 18 (1916) 1133–1146.
Dellman H-D, Brown EM: Textbook of Veterinary Histology. Philadelphia, Lea & Febiger, 1976.
Desch C, Nutting WB: *Demodex cati* Hirst, 1919: A redescription. Cornell Vet 69 (1979) 280–285.
Devriese LA, Nzuambe D, Godard C: Identification and characterization of staphylococci isolated from cats. Vet Microbiol 9 (1984) 279–285.
Dieterich RA: Cold injury (hypothermia, frostbite, freezing). *In* Kirk RW (ed): Current Veterinary Therapy VI. Philadelphia, WB Saunders Company, 1977, 205–206.
Doering GG: Feline dermatology. Vet Clin North Am 6 (1976) 463–477.
Doering GG, Jensen HE: Clinical Dermatology of Small Animals. St Louis, CV Mosby, 1973.
Dow C: The pathology of stilboestrol poisoning in the domestic cat. J Pathol Bacteriol 75 (1958) 151–161.
Draize JH: The determination of the pH of the skin of man and common laboratory animals. J Invest Dermatol 5 (1942) 77–85.
Fawcett J, Demaray SY, Altman N: Multiple xanthomatosis in a cat. Feline Pract 7 (3) (1977) 31–33.
Feingold BF, Benjamin E, Michaeli D: The allergic responses to insect bites. Ann Rev Entomol 13 (1968) 137–158.
Fennell C: "Sticky cats." Vet Rec 100 (1977) 476.
Flecknell PA, Orr CM, Wright AI, Gaskell RM, Kelly DF: Skin ulceration associated with herpesvirus infection in cats. Vet Rec 104 (1979) 313–315.
Foresti C: Su di un caso di tubercolosi del seno frontale. Nuova Vet 14 (1936) 321–324.
Fox I, Bayona IG, Armstrong JL: Cat flea control through use of dichlorvos-impregnated collars. J Am Vet Med Assoc 155 (1969) 1621–1623.
Fox JG, Beatty JO: A case report of complicated diabetes mellitus in a cat. J Am Anim Hosp Assoc 11 (1975) 129–134.
Fox JG, Hewes K: *Cheyletiella* infestation in cats. J Am Vet Med Assoc 169 (1976) 332–333.
Fox JG, Reed C: *Cheyletiella* infestation of cats and their owners. Arch Dermatol 114 (1978) 1233–1234.
Furneaux RW, Pharr JW, McManus JL: Arterio-venous fistulation following dewclaw removal in a cat. J Am Anim Hosp Assoc 10 (1974) 569–573.
Garcy AM, Marotta SF: Effects of cerebroventricular perfusion with monovalent and divalent cations on plasma cortisol of conscious cats. Neuroendocrinology 26 (1978) 32–40.
Garner RJ: Veterinary Toxicology, 2nd ed. Baltimore, The Williams and Wilkins Company, 1961.
Gaskell RM, Gaskell CJ, Evans RJ, Dennis PE, Bennett AM, Udall MD, Voyle C, Hill TJ: Natural and experimental pox virus infection in the domestic cat. Vet Rec 112 (1983) 164–170.
Gelberg HB, Lewis RM, Felsburg PJ, Smith CA: Antiepithelial autoantibodies associated with the feline eosinophilic granuloma complex. Am J Vet Res 46 (1985) 263–265.
Georgi JR: Parasitology for Veterinarians, 3rd ed. Philadelphia, WB Saunders Company, 1980.
Gershoff SN, Andrus SB, Hegsted DM, Lentini EA: Vitamin A deficiency in cats. Lab Invest 6 (1957) 227–240.
Gershoff SN, Andrus SB, Hegsted DM: The effect of the carbohydrate and fat content of the diet upon the riboflavin requirement of the cat. J Nutr 68 (1959) 75–88.
Greeve JH, Gerrish RR: Fur mites *(Lynxacarus)* from cats in Florida. Feline Pract 11 (6) (1981) 28–30.
Gretillat S: Feline hemobartonellosis. Feline Pract 14 (2) (1984) 22–27.
Griffiths BCR: The geriatric cat. J Small Anim Pract 9 (1968) 343–355.

Griffiths BCR: Eosinophilic granuloma (rodent ulcer) in the cat (Letter). Vet Rec 100 (1977) 159.

Gruffydd-Jones TJ, Orr CM, Lucke VM: Footpad swelling and ulceration in cats: A report of 5 cases. J Small Anim Pract 21 (1980) 381–389.

Gu J, Polak JM, Tapia FJ, Marangos PJ, Pearse AGE: Neuron-specific enolase in the Merkel cells of mammalian skin. The use of specific antibody as a simple and reliable marker. Am J Pathol 104 (1981) 63–68.

Guilhon J: Alopécie psycho-somatique des animaux domestiques. Recl Méd Vét 138 (1962) 839–847.

Gunaratnam P, Wilkinson GT, Seawright AA: A study of amitraz toxicity in cats. Aust Vet J 60 (1983) 278–279.

Habermann RT, Williams FP: Metastatic micrococcic infection (botryomycosis) in a cat. J Am Vet Med Assoc 129 (1956) 30–33.

Halliwell REW: Steroid therapy in skin disease. *In* Kirk RW (ed): Current Veterinary Therapy VI. Philadelphia, WB Saunders Company, 1977, 541–547.

Harari J, MacCoy DM, Johnson AL, Tranquilli WJ: Recurrent peripheral arteriovenous fistula and hyperthyroidism in a cat. J Am Anim Hosp Assoc 20 (1984) 759–764.

Hart BL: Feline behavior. Behavioral effects of long-acting progestins. Feline Pract 4 (4) (1974) 8–11.

Hart BL: Feline behavior. Quiz on feline behavior. Feline Pract 6 (3) (1976) 10–14.

Hart BL, Barrett RE: Effects of castration on fighting, roaming, and urine spraying in adult male cats. J Am Vet Med Assoc 163 (1973) 290–292.

Hearst BR: Low incidence of staphylococcal dermatitides in animals with high incidence of *Staphylococcus aureus*. Part I. Preliminary study of cats. Vet Med Small Anim Clin 62 (1967) 475–477.

Hekmatpanah J: Organization of tactile dermatomes, $C_1$ through $L_4$, in cat. J Neurophysiol 24 (1961) 129–140.

Henik RA, Olson PN, Rosychuk RA: Progestogen therapy in cats. Compend Contin Ed 7 (1985) 132–142.

Herwick RP: Lesions caused by canine ear mites. Arch Dermatol 114 (1978) 130.

Hess PW, MacEwen EG: Feline eosinophilic granuloma. *In* Kirk RW (ed): Current Veterinary Therapy VI. Philadelphia, WB Saunders Company, 1977, 534–537.

Hewitt M, Walton GS, Waterhouse M: Pet animal infestations and human skin lesions. Br J Dermatol 85 (1971) 215–225.

Higgins R, Paradis M: Abscess caused by *Corynebacterium equi* in a cat. Can Vet J 21 (1980) 63–64.

Hinton M, Gaskell CJ: Non-neoplastic mammary hypertrophy in the cat associated either with pregnancy or with oral progestagen therapy. Vet Rec 100 (1977) 277–280.

Hoenig M, Ferguson DC: Assessment of thyroid functional reserve in the cat by the thyrotropin-stimulation test. Am J Vet Res 44 (1983) 1229–1232.

Holbrook KA, Byers PH, Counts DF, Hegreberg GA: Dermatosparaxis in a Himalayan cat. II. Ultrastructural studies of dermal collagen. J Invest Dermatol 74 (1980) 100–104.

Holzworth J: Pansteatitis in cats. *In* Kirk RW (ed): Current Veterinary Therapy IV. Philadelphia, WB Saunders Company, 1971, 71–72.

Holzworth J: Personal communication, 1983.

Houdeshell JW, Hennessey PW, Bigbee HB: Treatment of feline miliary dermatitis with megestrol acetate. Vet Med Small Anim Clin 72 (1977) 573–575.

Hutchison JA: Progestogen therapy for certain skin diseases of cats (Letter). Can Vet J 19 (1978) 324.

Hutyra F, Marek J: Special Pathology and Therapeutics of the Diseases of Domestic Animals. Chicago, Alexander Eger, 1926.

Iggo A, Young DW: The Somatosensory System. Acton, Thieme Edition/Publishing Sciences Group, Inc, 1975.

Iljin NA, Iljin VN: Temperature effects on the color of the Siamese cat. J Hered 21 (1930) 309–318.

Innes DC: How temperature changes hair color in the Siamese. Feline Pract 3 (6) (1973) 27–32.

Irving RA, Day RS, Eales L: Porphyrin values and treatment of feline solar dermatitis. Am J Vet Res 43 (1982) 2067–2069.

Jenkinson DM: The skin of domestic animals. *In* Rook AJ, Walton GS (eds): Comparative Physiology and Pathology of the Skin. Philadelphia, FA Davis, 1965, 591–608.

Jenkinson DM, Blackburn PA: The distribution of nerves, monoamine oxidase and cholinesterase in the skin of the cat and dog. Res Vet Sci 9 (1968) 521–528.

Jennings S: Some aspects of veterinary dermatology. Vet Rec 65 (1953) 809–819.

Johnson RP, Sabine M: The isolation of herpesviruses from skin ulcers in domestic cats. Vet Rec 89 (1971) 360–363.

Jones RD: Pyometra in the cat (Letter). Vet Rec 97 (1975) 100.

Jones RT: Subcutaneous infection with *Dermatophilus congolensis* in a cat. J Comp Pathol 86 (1976) 415–421.

Jones TC, Hunt RD: Veterinary Pathology, 5th ed. Philadelphia, Lea & Febiger, 1983.

Joshua JO: The use of biotin in certain skin diseases of the cat. Vet Rec 71 (1959) 102.

Joshua JO: The Clinical Aspects of Some Diseases of Cats. Philadelphia, JB Lippincott Company, 1965.

Joshua JO: Some conditions seen in feline practice attributable to hormonal causes. Vet Rec 88 (1971a) 511–514.

Joshua JO: Abscesses and their sequelae in cats. Part I. Feline Pract 1 (2) (1971b) 9–12.

Joshua JO: Abscesses and their sequelae in cats. Part II. Feline Pract 2 (1) (1972) 22–23.

Jungerman PF, Schwartzman RM: Veterinary Medical Mycology. Philadelphia, Lea & Febiger, 1972.

Kane E, Morris JG, Rogers QR, Ihrke PJ, Cupps PT: Zinc deficiency in the cat. J Nutr 111 (1981) 488–495.

Keane DP: Chronic abscesses in cats associated with an organism resembling Mycoplasma. Can Vet J 24 (1983) 289–291.

Kemp WB, Abbey LM, Taylor LA: Pseudo-sarcomatous fasciitis of the upper lip of a cat. Vet Med Small Anim Clin 71 (1976) 923–925.

Kemppainen RJ, Mansfield PD, Sartin JL: Endocrine responses of normal cats to TSH and synthetic ACTH administration. J Am Anim Hosp Assoc 20 (1984) 737–740.

Kipnis RM: Corneal eosinophilic granuloma. Feline Pract 9 (6) (1979) 49–53.

Kirk H: The Diseases of the Cat and Its General Management. London, Baillière, Tindall and Cox, 1925.

Knopf K, Sturman JA, Armstrong M, Hayes KC: Taurine: An essential nutrient for the cat. J Nutr 108 (1978) 773–778.

Kodama JK, Collins JA, van Kampen KR: Toxic reactions due to flea collars (Letter). J Am Vet Med Assoc 168 (1976) 368–374.

Koller LD: Clinical application of DMSO by veterinarians in Oregon and Washington. Vet Med Small Anim Clin 71 (1976) 591–597.

Kral F: Skin manifestations of internal disorders. Vet Med 52 (1957) 437–441.

Kral F: Compendium of Veterinary Dermatology. New York, Charles Pfizer and Company, Department of Veterinary Medicine, 1960.

Kral F, Novak BJ: Veterinary Dermatology. Philadelphia, JB Lippincott Company, 1953.

Kral F, Schwartzman RM: Veterinary and Comparative Dermatology. Philadelphia, JB Lippincott Company, 1964.

Kramer JW, Davis WC, Prieur DJ: The Chediak-Higashi syndrome of cats. Lab Invest 36 (1977) 554–562.

Kramer TT: Immunity to bacterial infections. Vet Clin North Am 8 (1978) 683–695.

Krieger DT, Silverberg AI, Rizzo F, Krieger HP: Abolition of circadian periodicity of plasma 17-OHCS levels in the cat. Am J Physiol 215 (1968) 959–967.

Kristensen S: A study of skin diseases in dogs and cats. I. Histology of the hairy skin of dogs and cats. Nord Vet-Med 27 (1975) 593–603.

Kristensen S, Kieffer M: A study of skin diseases in dogs and cats. V. The intradermal test in the diagnosis of flea allergy in dogs and cats. Nord Vet-Med 30 (1978) 414–423.

Krogh HV, Kristensen S: A study of skin diseases in dogs and cats. II. Microflora of the normal skin of dogs and cats. Nord Vet-Med 28 (1976) 459–463.

Kuhn RA: Organization of tactile dermatomes in cat and monkey. J Neurophysiol 16 (1953) 169–182.

Kunkle GA: Feline dermatology. Vet Clin North Am 14 (1984) 1065–1087.

Kunkle GA, Milcarsky J: Double-blind flea hyposensitization trial in cats. J Am Vet Med Assoc 186 (1985) 677–680.

Kunkle GA, Gulbas NK, Fakok V, Halliwell RE, Connelly M: Rapidly growing mycobacteria as a cause of cutaneous granulomas: Report of five cases. J Am Anim Hosp Assoc 19 (1983) 513–521.

Kwochka KW, Short BG: Cutaneous xanthomatosis and diabetes mellitus following long-term therapy with megestrol acetate in a cat. Compend Contin Ed 6 (1984) 185–192.

Lane JG, Gruffydd-Jones TJ: Eosinophilic granulomas in cats (Letter). Vet Rec 100 (1977) 251.

Lange AL, Verster A, van Amstel Sr, de la Rey R: Anatrichosoma sp. infestation in the footpads of a cat. J S Afr Vet Assoc 51 (1980) 227–229.

Lawler DC: Allergic skin disease in the dog and cat. N Z Vet J 18 (1970) 111–114.

Letard E: Hairless Siamese cats. J Hered 29 (1938) 173–175.

Lewis GE Jr, Fidler WJ, Crumrine MH: Mycetoma in a cat. J Am Vet Med Assoc 161 (1972) 500–503.

Lindholm JS, McCormick JM, Colton SW, Downing DT: Variation of skin surface lipid composition among mammals. Comp Biochem Physiol 69B (1981) 75–78.

Longbottom GM: "Sticky cats" (Letter). Vet Rec 100 (1977) 392.

Love DN, Bailey M, Johnson RS: Antimicrobial susceptibility patterns of obligately anaerobic bacteria from subcutaneous abscesses and pyothorax in cats. Aust Vet Pract 10 (1980) 168–170.

Love DN, Lomus G, Bailey M, Jones RF, Weston I: Characterization of strains of *Staphylococci* from infections in dogs and cats. J Small Anim Pract 22 (1981) 195–199.

Lowenstine LJ, Carpenter JL, O'Connor BM: Trombiculosis in a cat. J Am Vet Med Assoc 175 (1979) 289–292.

Lynn B: Cutaneous hyperalgesia. Br Med Bull 33 (1977) 103–108.

MacDonald KR, Greenfield J, McCausland HD: Remission of staphylococcal dermatitis by autogenous bacterin therapy. Can Vet J 13 (1972) 45–48.

Mann PH: Antibiotic sensitivity testing and bacteriophage typing of staphylococci found in the nostrils of dogs and cats. J Am Vet Med Assoc 134 (1959) 469–470.

Mann SJ, Straile WE: Tylotrich (hair) follicle: Association with a slowly adapting tactile receptor in the cat. Science 147 (1965) 1043–1045.

Manning TO, Scott DW, Smith CA, Lewis RM: Pemphigus diseases in the feline: Seven case reports and discussion. J Am Anim Hosp Assoc 18 (1982) 433–443.

Marder MW, Kantrowitz MD, Davis T: Clinical pathological conference [cutaneous nocardiosis caused by *N. asteroides*]. Feline Pract 3 (5) (1973) 20–31.

Mardh PA, Hovelius B, Hovelius K, Nilsson PO: Coagulase-negative, novobiocin-resistant staphylococci on the skin of animals and man, on meat and in milk. Acta Vet Scand 19 (1978) 243–253.

Marennikova SS, Maltseva NN, Korneeva VI, Garanina NM: Outbreak of pox disease among Carnivora (Felidae) and Edentata. J Infect Dis 135 (1977) 358–366.

Martin SL, Capen CC: The endocrine system. *In* Pratt PW (ed): Feline Medicine. Santa Barbara, American Veterinary Publications, Inc, 1983, 321–362.

Martland MF, Fowler S, Poulton GJ, Baxby D: Pox virus infection of a domestic cat. Vet Rec 112 (1983) 171–172.

Maruhashi J, Mizuguchi K, Tasaki I: Action currents in single afferent nerve fibres elicited by stimulation of the skin of the toad and the cat. J Physiol 117 (1952) 129–151.

Mather GW: Diseases caused by physical and chemical agents. *In* Catcott EJ (ed): Feline Medicine and Surgery, Wheaton, American Veterinary Publications, Inc, 1964, 145–155.

Mather GW: Thallium intoxication. *In* Kirk RW (ed): Current Veterinary Therapy V. Philadelphia, WB Saunders Company, 1974a, 131–133.

Mather GW: Cold stress (hypothermia, frostbite, freezing). *In* Kirk RW (ed): Current Veterinary Therapy V. Philadelphia, WB Saunders Company, 1974b, 176–177.

McClelland RB: X-ray therapy in labial and cutaneous granulomas in cats. J Am Vet Med Assoc 125 (1954) 469–470.

McCusker HB: Histamine and mast cells in the normal and eczematous skin in the cat. *In* Rook AJ, Walton GS (eds): Comparative Physiology and Pathology of the Skin. Philadelphia, FA Davis, 1965, 427–434.

McCusker HB, Aitken ID: Immunological studies of the cat. II. Experimental induction of skin reactivity to foreign proteins. Res Vet Sci 8 (1967) 265–271.

McDougal BJ: Use of megestrol acetate for treatment of feline endocrine alopecia. Tex Vet Med J 37 (1975) 12–14.

McGaughey CA: Actinomycosis in carnivores: A review of the literature. Br Vet J 108 (1951) 89–92.

McKeever PJ, Allen SK: Dermatitis associated with *Cheyletiella* infestation in cats. J Am Vet Med Assoc 174 (1979) 718–720.

Medleau L, Kaswan RL, Lorenz MD, Dawe DL: Ulcerative pododermatitis in a cat: Immunofluorescent findings and response to chrysotherapy. J Am Anim Hosp Assoc 18 (1982) 449–451.

Meijer JC, Lubberink AAME, Gruys E: Cushing's syndrome due to adrenocortical adenoma in a cat. Tijdschr Diergeneeskd 103 (1978) 1048–1051.

Mellen IM: The origin of the Mexican hairless cat. J Hered 30 (1939) 435–436.

Michaeli D, Goldfarb S: Clinical studies on the hyposensitization of dogs and cats to flea bites. Aust Vet J 44 (1968) 161–165.

Miller RI, Ladds PW, Mudie A, Hayes DP, Trueman KF: Probable dermatophilosis in 2 cats. Aust Vet J 60 (1983) 155–156.

Moise NS, Reimers TJ: Insulin therapy in cats with diabetes mellitus. J Am Vet Med Assoc 182 (1983) 158–164.

Mosier JE: Common medical and behavioral problems in cats. Mod Vet Pract 56 (1975) 699–703.

Mosier JE: [Hyperesthesia syndrome, treatment with primidone] (Letter). Feline Pract 7 (6) (1977) 5–6.

Moulton JE: Tumors in Domestic Animals. Berkeley, University of California Press, 1961.

Muller GH: Flea collar dermatitis in animals. J Am Vet Med Assoc 157 (1970) 1616–1626.

Muller GH: Feline Skin Lesions. South Bend, IN, American Animal Hospital Association, 1974a.

Muller GH: Flea collar dermatitis. *In* Kirk RW (ed): Current Veterinary Therapy V. Philadelphia, WB Saunders Company, 1974b, 404–405.

Muller GH: Feline demodicosis. *In* Kirk RW (ed): Current Veterinary Therapy VIII. Philadelphia, WB Saunders Company, 1983, 487–488.

Muller GH, Kirk RW, Scott DW: Small Animal Dermatology, 3rd ed. Philadelphia, WB Saunders Company, 1983.

Munday BL: Epitheliogenesis imperfecta in lambs and kittens. Br Vet J 126 (1970) XLVII.

Munson TO, Holzworth J, Small E, Witzel S, Jones TC, Luginbühl H: Steatitis ("yellow fat") in cats fed canned red tuna. J Am Vet Med Assoc 133 (1958) 563–568.

National Research Council: Nutrient Requirements of Cats. Washington DC, National Academy of Sciences, 1978.

Neufeld JL, Burton L, Jeffery KR: Eosinophilic granuloma in a cat. Recovery of virus particles. Vet Pathol 17 (1980) 97–99.

Nicolaides N, Fu HC, Rice GR: The skin surface lipids of man compared with those of eighteen species of animals. J Invest Dermatol 51 (1968) 83–89.

Nilsson BY: [The tactile hair organ on the cat's foreleg. Structure and function of a group of functionally co-ordinated mechanoreceptors]. Diss Abst Int 31B, 1970, 3678.

Nimmo-Wilkie JS: Progesterone therapy for cats (Letter). Can Vet J 20 (1979) 164.

Nomina Anatomica Veterinaria, International Committee on Veterinary Gross Anatomical Nomenclature, Ithaca, NY, 1983.

Oehme FW: Poisonings from phenolic chemicals. *In* Kirk RW (ed): Current Veterinary Therapy VI. Philadelphia, WB Saunders Company, 1977, 145–147.

Øen EO: The oral administration of megestrol acetate to postpone oestrus in cats. Nord Vet-Med 29 (1977) 287–291.

Ottenschot TRF, Gil D: Cheyletiellosis in long-haired cats. Tijdschr Diergeneesk 103 (1978) 1104–1108.

Oudar J, Joubert L, Prave M, Dickelé C, Munoz Trana J-C: Le portage buccal de *'Pasteurella multocida'* chez le chat. Étude epidémiologique, biochimique et sérologique. Bull Soc Sci Vét Méd Comp Lyon 74 (1972) 353–357.

Oudar J, Viallier J, Joubert L: Tuberculose cutanée enzootique à bacille bovin chez le chien et le chat. Bull Soc Sci Vét Méd Comp Lyon 67 (1965) 321–327.

Pandey SK, Kolte GN, Singh SC: Subcutaneous lipogranuloma in a cat. Indian Vet J 50 (1973) 376–377.

Parish WE: The manifestation of anaphylactic reactions in the skin of different species. *In* Rook AJ, Walton GS (eds): Comparative Physiology and Pathology of the Skin. Philadelphia, FA Davis, 1965, 465–486.

Parker AJ, O'Brien DP, Sawchuk SA: The nervous system. *In* Pratt PW (ed): Feline Medicine. Santa Barbara, American Veterinary Publications, Inc, 1983.

Parodi A, Fontaine M, Brion A, Tisseur H, Goret P: Mycobacterioses in the domestic carnivora: Present-day epidemiology of tuberculosis in the cat and dog. J Small Anim Pract 6 (1964) 309–326.

Patterson DF, Minor RR: Hereditary fragility and hyperextensibility of the skin of cats: A defect in collagen fibrillogenesis. Lab Invest 37 (1977) 170–179.

Peterson ME: Propylthiouracil in the treatment of feline hyperthyroidism. J Am Vet Med Assoc 179 (1981) 485–487.

Peterson ME, Kintzer PP, Cavanagh PG, Fox PR, Ferguson DC, Johnson GF, Becker DV: Feline hyperthyroidism: pretreatment clinical and laboratory evaluation of 131 cases. J Am Vet Med Assoc 183 (1983) 103–110.

Peterson ME, Kintzer PP, Foodman MS, Piccolie A, Quimby FW: Adrenal function in the cat: comparison of the effects of cosyntropin (synthetic ACTH) and corticotropin gel stimulation. Res Vet Sci 37 (1984) 331–333.

Petrak M: Personal communication, 1983.

Petrov AM, Chubabriya IT: [On the discovery of *Dracunculus medinensis* L., 1758 in subcutaneous tissue of a cat in the Georgian SSR]. Trudy Gruzinskoi Nauchno-Issledovatel'sk Vet Inst 11 (1955) 231.

Pile CH: Thallium poisoning in domestic felines. Aust Vet J 32 (1956) 18–20.

Prieur DJ, Collier LL, Bryan GM, Meyers KM: The diagnosis of feline Chediak-Higashi syndrome. Feline Pract 9 (5) (1979) 26–32.

Pukay BP: A hyperglycemia-glucosuria syndrome in cats following megestrol acetate therapy (Letter). Can Vet J 20 (1979) 117.

Quaife RA, Womar SM: *Microsporum canis* isolations from show cats. Vet Rec 110 (1982) 333–334.

Reedy LM: Use of flea antigen in treatment of feline flea-allergy dermatitis. Vet Med Small Anim Clin 70 (1975) 703–704.

Reedy LM: Results of allergy testing and hyposensitization in related feline skin diseases. J Am Anim Hosp Assoc 18 (1982) 618–623.

Reinhardt R: Die Krankheiten der Katze. Hannover, M and H Schaper, 1952.

Rivers JPW, Sinclair AJ, Crawford MA: Inability of the cat to desaturate essential fatty acids. Nature 258 (1975) 171.

Robinson R: The Canadian hairless or Sphinx cat. J Hered 64 (1973) 47–49.

Robinson R: Genetics for Cat Breeders, 2nd ed. London, Pergamon Press, 1977.

Rollag OJ, Skeels MR, Nims LJ, Thilsted JP: Feline plague in New Mexico: Report of five cases. J Am Vet Med Assoc 179 (1951) 1381–1383.

Ryan CP, Howard EB: Systemic lipodystrophy associated with pancreatitis in a cat. Feline Pract 11 (6) (1981) 31–34.

Ryder ML: Seasonal changes in the coat of the cat. Res Vet Sci 21 (1976) 280–283.

Saunders EB: Hyposensitization for flea-bite hypersensitivity. Vet Med Small Anim Clin 72 (1977) 879–881.

Sawchuk SA: Personal communication to J Holzworth, 1983.

Schawalder P: Leishmaniose bei Hund und Katze. Autochthone Fälle in der Schweiz. Kleintierpraxis 32 (1977) 237–246.

Schiefer HB, Middleton DM: Experimental transmission of a feline mycobacterial skin disease (feline leprosy). Vet Pathol 20 (1983) 460–471.

Schönbauer M, Schönbauer-Längle A, Kölbl S: Pockeninfektion bei einer Hauskatze. Zentralbl Veterinärmed B29 (1982) 434–440.

Schrader LA, Hurvitz AI: Cold agglutinin disease in a cat. J Am Vet Med Assoc 183 (1983) 121–122.

Schultz KT, Maguire HC: Chemically-induced delayed hypersensitivity in the cat. Vet Immunol Immunopathol 3 (1982) 585–590.

Schultz RD, Adams LS: Immunologic methods for the detection of humoral and cellular immunity. Vet Clin North Am 8 (1978) 721–753.

Schwartzman RM: Topical dermatologic therapy. *In* Kirk RW (ed): Current Veterinary Therapy VI. Philadelphia, WB Saunders Company, 1977, 506–513.

Schwartzman RM, Kral F: Atlas of Canine and Feline Dermatoses. Philadelphia, Lea & Febiger, 1967.

Scott DW: Cutaneous asthenia in a cat, resembling Ehlers-Danlos syndrome in man. Vet Med Small Anim Clin 69 (1974) 1256–1258.

Scott DW: Observations on the eosinophilic granuloma complex in cats. J Am Anim Hosp Assoc 11 (1975a) 261–270.

Scott DW: Thyroid function in feline endocrine alopecia. J Am Anim Hosp Assoc 11 (1975b) 798–801.

Scott DW: Feline dermatology. Proc Am Anim Hosp Assoc 43 (1976a) 99–123.

Scott DW: Miliary eczema in the cat: A review. Proc Am Anim Hosp Assoc 43 (1976b) 145–152.

Scott DW: Nocardiosis and actinomycosis. *In* Kirk RW (ed): Current Veterinary Therapy VI. Philadelphia, WB Saunders Company, 1977, 1328–1330.

Scott DW: Feline skin disorders. Feline Information Bulletin 3. Ithaca, NY, Cornell Feline Research Laboratory, 1978a.

Scott DW: Immunologic skin disorders in the dog and cat. Vet Clin North Am 8 (1978b) 641–664.

Scott DW: Topical cutaneous medicine, or "Now What Should I Try?" Proc Am Anim Hosp Assoc 46 (1979a) 49–101.

Scott DW: Progestational compounds in the treatment of feline skin disorders. Small Animal Veterinary Medical Update Series 2 (1979b) 1.

Scott DW: Feline dermatology 1900–1978: a monograph. J Am Anim Hosp Assoc 16 (1980) 331–459.

Scott DW: Chrysotherapy (gold therapy). *In* Kirk RW (ed): Current Veterinary Therapy VIII. Philadelphia, WB Saunders Company, 1983, 448–449.

Scott DW: Feline dermatology 1979–1982: introspective retrospections. J Am Anim Hosp Assoc 20 (1984) 537–564.

Scott DW, Flanders JA: Dilated pore of Winer in a cat. Feline Pract 14 (6) (1984) 33–36.

Scott DW, Halliwell REW, Goldschmidt MH, DiBartola S: Toxic epidermal necrolysis in two dogs and a cat. J Am Anim Hosp Assoc 15 (1979a) 271–279.

Scott DW, Houpt KH, Knowlton BF, Lewis RM: A glucocorticoid-responsive dermatitis in cats, resembling systemic lupus erythematosus in man. J Am Anim Hosp Assoc 15 (1979b) 157–171.

Scott DW, Kirk RW, Bentinck-Smith J: Some effects of short-term methylprednisolone therapy in normal cats. Cornell Vet 69 (1979c) 104–115.

Scott DW, Manning TO, Reimers TJ: Iatrogenic Cushing's syndrome in the cat. Feline Pract 12 (2) (1982) 30–36.

Scott DW, Miller WH Jr, Lewis RM, Manning TO, Smith CA: Pemphigus erythematosus in the dog and cat. J Am Anim Hosp Assoc 16 (1980) 815–823.

Scott DW, Randolph JF, Walsh KM: Hypereosinophilic syndrome in a cat. Feline Pract 15(1) (1985) 22–30.

Scott DW, Walton DK, Lewis RM, Smith CA: Pitfalls in immunofluorescence testing in dermatology. II. Pemphigus-like antibodies in the cat, and direct immunofluorescence testing of normal dog nose and lip. Cornell Vet 73 (1983) 275–279.

Scott FW, de Lahunta A, Schultz RD, Bistner SI, Riis RC: Teratogenesis in cats associated with griseofulvin therapy. Teratology 11 (1975) 79–86.

Scott PP: Nutritional requirements and deficiencies. *In* Catcott EJ (ed): Feline Medicine and Surgery. Wheaton, American Veterinary Publications, Inc, 1964, 61–70.

Scott PP: Nutrition and disease. *In* Catcott EJ (ed): Feline Medicine and Surgery, 2nd ed., Santa Barbara, American Veterinary Publications, Inc, 1975, 131–144.

Seawright AA, Costigan P: Some toxicity aspects of dichlorvos flea collars in cats. Aust Vet J 53 (1977) 509–514.

Slocum B, Colgrove DJ, Carrig CB, Suter PF: Acquired arteriovenous fistula in two cats. J Am Vet Med Assoc 162 (1973) 271–275.

Smith JE: Symposium on diseases of cats—III. Some pathogenic bacteria of cats with special reference to their public health significance. J Small Anim Pract 5 (1964) 517–524.

Soulsby EJL: Helminths, Arthropods, and Protozoa of Domesticated Animals. Baltimore, The Williams and Wilkins Company, 1968.

Stannard AA: Actinic dermatoses (feline solar dermatitis and nasal solar dermatitis). *In* Kirk RW (ed): Current Veterinary Therapy V. Philadelphia, WB Saunders Company, 1974, 402–403.

Stannard AA, Pulley LT: Tumors of the skin and soft tissues. *In* Moulton JE (ed): Tumors in Domestic Animals, 2nd ed. Berkeley, University of California Press, 1978, 16–74.

Stansbury RL: Detecting and managing feline head lesions. Mod Vet Pract 47 (9) (1966) 45–46, 51–53.

Stein BS: Personal communication, 1982, 1983.

Stogdale L, Moore DJ: Feline demodicosis. J Am Anim Hosp Assoc 18 (1982) 427–432.

Straile WE: Sensory hair follicles in mammalian skin: The tylotrich follicle. Am J Anat 106 (1960) 133–147.

Strickland JH, Calhoun ML: The integumentary system of the cat. Am J Vet Res 24 (1963) 1018–1029.

Swenson MJ (ed): Duke's Physiology of Domestic Animals, 9th ed. Ithaca, NY, Comstock Publishing Associates, Cornell University Press, 1977.

Szymanski CM: Personal communication, 1982.

Thoday K: Skin disease of the cat. In Practice 3 (Nov) (1981) 22–35.

Thomsett LR: Reactions to food and drugs in animals. *In* Rook AJ, Walton GS (eds): Comparative Physiology and Pathology of the Skin. Philadelphia, FA Davis, 1965, 583–588.

Thomsett LR: Mite infestations of man contracted from dogs and cats. Br Med J 3 (1968) 93–95.

Thomsett LR, Baxby D, Denham EMH: Cowpox in the domestic cat (Letter). Vet Rec 103 (1978) 567.

Thornton GW: Diagnosis and treatment of common skin disorders of the cat. Cornell Vet 53 (1963) 144–157.

Todd NB: Environmental effects on cats (abstr). Vet Med Small Anim Clin 65 (1970) 444.

Trautmann A, Fiebiger J: Fundamentals of the Histology of Domestic Animals. Ithaca, NY, Comstock Publishing Company, 1957.

Turner T: Eosinophilic granuloma in cats (Letter). Vet Rec 100 (1977) 327.

Tuttle PA, Chandler FW: Deep dermatophytosis in a cat. J Am Vet Med Assoc 183 (1983) 1106–1108.

van Dorssen CA: Infectie met *Micobacterium microti* bij een kat. Tijdschr Diergeneeskd 85 (1960) 404–412.

von Tscharner C: Pemphigus in the cat. Proc 1st European Veterinary Dermatology Meeting, Hamburg, 1984.

Wagener K: Possible effects of German wood preservative on cats and dogs with special reference to hyperkeratosis. J Am Vet Med Assoc 120 (1952) 145–147.

Wagener K, Krüger A: Experimentelle Hyperkeratose ("X-disease") bei Katzen und Hunden. Dtsch Tierärztl Wochenschr 60 (1953) 312–315.

Walton DK, Scott DW, Manning TO: Cutaneous bacterial granuloma (botryomycosis) in a dog and cat. J Am Anim Hosp Assoc 19 (1983) 537–541.

Walton GS: Symposium on allergic and endocrine dermatoses in the dog and cat. I. Allergic dermatoses of the dog and cat. J Small Anim Pract 7 (1966) 749–754.

Walton GS: Allergic responses involving the skin of domestic animals. Adv Vet Sci Comp Med 15 (1971) 201–240.

Walton GS: Allergy. *In* Catcott EJ (ed): Feline Medicine and Surgery, 2nd ed. Santa Barbara, American Veterinary Publications, Inc, 1975, 145–152.

Ward DG, Gann DS: Inhibiting and facilitatory areas of the dorsal medulla mediating ACTH release in the cat. Endocrinology 99 (1976) 1213–1219.

Ward DG, Grizzle WE, Gann DS: Inhibitory and facilitatory areas of the rostral pons mediating ACTH release in the cat. Endocrinology 99 (1976) 1220–1228.

White SD, Ihrke PJ, Stannard AA, Cadmus C, Griffin C, Kruth SA, Rosser EJ, Reinke SI, Jang S: Cutaneous atypical mycobacteriosis in cats. J Am Vet Med Assoc 182 (1983) 1218–1222.

Wilkinson GT: Diseases of the Cat. London, Pergamon Press, 1966.

Wilkinson GT: A review of drug toxicity in the cat. J Small Anim Pract 9 (1968) 21–32.

Wilkinson GT: Feline leprosy. *In* Kirk RW (ed): Current Veterinary Therapy VI. Philadelphia, WB Saunders Company, 1977, 569–571.

Wilkinson GT: The University of Sydney. The Post-Graduate Committee in Veterinary Science. Refresher Course for Veterinarians. Cats. Proc 53 (1980) 443.

Wilkinson GT (ed): Diseases of the Cat and Their Management. Melbourne, Blackwell Scientific Publications, 1983a.

Wilkinson GT: Cutaneous nocardia infection in a cat. Feline Pract 13 (4) (1983b) 32–34.

Wilkinson GT: Demodicosis in a cat due to a new mite species. Feline Pract 13 (6) (1983c) 32–41.

Wilkinson GT: Diseases of Cats. Sydney, University of Sydney Post-Graduate Foundation in Veterinary Science, 1984.

Willemse A, Lubberink AAME: Cryosurgery of eosinophilic ulcers in cats. Tijdschr Diergeneeskd 103 (1978) 1052–1056.

Winkelmann RK: The sensory end-organ in the hairless skin of the cat. J Invest Dermatol 29 (1957) 347–352.

Winkelmann RK: The end-organ of feline skin: A morphologic and histochemical study. Am J Anat 107 (1960) 281–290.

Worden AN: Diet and skin disease in the dog and cat. Vet Rec 70 (1958) 189–192.

Zook BC, Holzworth J, Thornton GW: Thallium poisoning in cats. J Am Vet Med Assoc 153 (1968) 285–299.

# 14
CHAPTER
# THE EYE

CAROL SZYMANSKI

Many ocular disorders of cats are similar to those of other species, some are unique to cats, and a variety of intraocular diseases may be manifestations of systemic disease. A thorough history and physical examination are essential. Conversely, examination of the eyes, particularly the ocular fundi, should be part of every physical examination.

## EXAMINATION

The ophthalmic examination should be conducted in a systematic manner in a quiet room away from dogs. Cats object to restraint, so the examination should be done quickly and gently. An assistant who likes cats and understands cat etiquette is most helpful in providing gentle restraint and distracting the cat during the examination. Uncooperative cats may be put inside a cat bag or rolled in a large towel. Ketamine may be used to restrain unmanageable cats.

The cat should be examined first with the room lights on. Gross abnormalities such as swelling of the orbital area, abnormal ocular discharges, inversion or drooping of the eyelids, blepharospasm, or protrusion of the third eyelid (semilunar fold of the conjunctiva)* are noted.

Vision is assessed by noting eyelid closure after a threatening gesture (menace reflex). A clear plastic sheet placed between the cat's eye and the examiner's hand prevents a false-positive response due to air currents. The cat's ability to follow a moving object visually may be demonstrated by throwing a cotton ball across a cat's visual axis or dangling a roll of adhesive tape in front of the cat's eyes. The cat's short attention span requires the examiner to assess the initial responses to these tests. A simple test of vision is to place the cat on the floor in the midst of several objects and observe its ability to navigate.

Pupillary light reflexes are tested in a darkened room with a bright light source such as a Welch-Allyn focusing penlight. Before any drops are placed in the eyes, a Schirmer tear test is performed to determine tear production. Next, one drop of 1 per cent tropicamide (Mydriacyl, Alcon Laboratories) is instilled into each eye to cause pupillary dilatation for optimal examination of lens and fundus.

The ophthalmic examination is conducted from anterior to posterior. The anterior segment (eyelids, conjunctiva, cornea, anterior chamber, iris, and lens) are examined with a bright light and magnifying loupe (Donegan Optivisor, Donegan Optical Company). A biomicroscope (slit lamp) (Kowa Instrument Company) aids in detection of subtle lesions of the anterior segment. A moistened fluorescein dye-impregnated paper strip (Fluor-I-Strip, Ayerst Laboratories) touched to the dorsal bulbar conjunctiva is used to demonstrate corneal ulcers. Excess dye is rinsed from the eye with a collyrium warmed to just above room temperature. Fluorescein solution is not recommended, because it is readily contaminated with bacteria, particularly *Pseudomonas* (Havener, 1978).

After the pupil has become dilated, the lens is examined with the focusing penlight or with the direct ophthalmoscope set from +8 to 12 diopters. Lenticular opacities (cataract) or changes in lens position (luxation or subluxation) may be detected. The retina and optic disk are examined with the direct ophthalmoscope set between 0 and −3 diopters. The binocular indirect ophthalmoscope provides the advantages of depth perception and a wider field. It is relatively expensive and requires more expertise to use than the direct ophthalmoscope. The light source of the ophthalmoscope must be reduced in intensity for examination of the cat's fundus to prevent photophobia and protrusion of the third eyelid.

In some cases, material will be needed for cytologic examination or culture. Scrapings are obtained with a heat-sterilized platinum spatula after topical anesthesia. They are stained with Wright or Giemsa, as well as Gram stain. For culturing, a sterile cotton swab moistened with sterile physiologic solution is passed over the conjunctiva of the inferior fornix, and thioglycollate medium is inoculated, as well as blood agar and mannitol plates or a commercial multimedia plate.

*The common synonym "nictitating membrane" is not applicable to the cat.

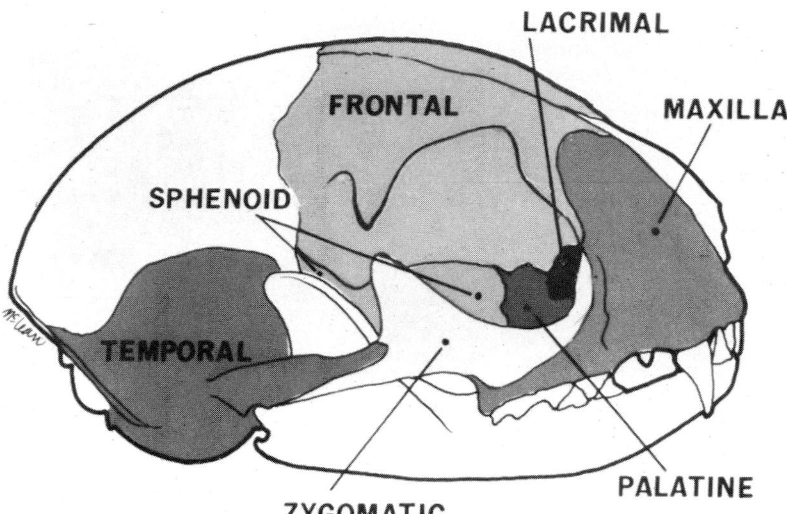


**Figure 14–1** Bone composing the cat orbit.

## THE ORBIT AND GLOBE

### Anatomy

The orbit is a cavity that is formed partly by bone, partly by periorbita. It protects the globe and provides foramina and fissures for orbital nerves and blood vessels. The orbit contains the globe, extraocular muscles, orbital fascia, fat, third eyelid, lacrimal gland, zygomatic salivary gland, and associated nerves and blood vessels. The cat's orbit is large and deep. The bony orbital wall is composed of the sphenoid, maxillary, lacrimal, zygomatic, frontal, and palatine bones as shown in Figure 14–1 (McClure et al., 1973; Walker, 1967).

The dorsal and medial walls of the orbit are formed by the frontal, sphenoid, and palatine bones. The small lacrimal bone contributes to the medial rim of the orbit and contains the lacrimal canal. The sphenoid forms the caudal extremity or apex of the orbit and contains the optic canal, orbital fissure, foramen rotundum, and foramen ovale. These and other orbital openings are listed in Table 14–1. The lateral wall of the orbit is composed of the periorbita, the zygomatic process of the frontal bone, and the frontal process of the zygomatic bone; a 5 to 6 mm gap between these two bones is bridged by the orbital ligament. The zygomatic bone also forms the lower orbital rim.

The cat's orbit lacks a bony floor except for a narrow shelf of maxillary bone above the molar teeth (Prince et al., 1960). The periorbita, a connective tissue membrane, lines the bony orbit and completes it laterally, ventrally, and caudally where there is no osseous wall. Various soft tissues—fat, pterygoid muscle, and zygomatic salivary gland—lie ventral to the orbit. Because the globe nearly fills the orbit, any space-occupying orbital mass causes exophthalmos.

In cats, in contrast with cattle, horses, and dogs, the vertical diameter of the orbit is greater than the horizontal diameter, and the orbits are relatively closer together (Martin and Anderson, 1981). The eyes of the cat are relatively larger and weigh relatively more (average 10.9 gm) than do the eyes of other domestic animals. The feline globe is spherical and notable for the large cornea. The frontal position of the globes in the cat provides the widest range of binocular vision among the domestic animals—about 45 degrees on either side of the midline, with monocular segments extending the visual field laterally to 90 degrees (Sherman and Wilson, 1975, cited by Schmidt and Coulter, 1981).

The membranous periorbita lining the bony orbit is a cone that extends from the orbital apex at the optic foramen to the orbital rim. It surrounds the globe, its vessels and nerves, and the extraocular muscles and is firmly attached to the orbital foramina and fissures and to the orbital rim. The bulbar fascia (Tenon's capsule) is a dense condensation of connective tissue that closely invests the globe, interdigitating with the sclera. It extends

**Table 14–1 Orbital Openings**

| OPENING | BONE | STRUCTURE |
|---|---|---|
| Optic canal | Sphenoid | Optic nerve<br>Ophthalmic (ciliary) artery; an internal ophthalmic artery is sometimes present |
| Orbital fissure | Sphenoid | 3rd, 4th, 6th nerves; ophthalmic division of 5th nerve<br>Branch of maxillary artery |
| Foramen rotundum | Sphenoid | Maxillary division of 5th nerve |
| Foramen ovale | Sphenoid | Mandibular division of 5th nerve<br>Branch of maxillary artery |
| Caudal palatine foramen | Palatine | Major palatine nerve and artery |
| Sphenopalatine foramen | Palatine | Sphenopalatine nerve, artery, and vein |
| Lacrimal foramen | Lacrimal | Lacrimal canal |
| Ethmoidal foramen | Frontal bone | Ethmoidal artery, vein, nerve |

Adapted from McClure et al., 1973; Prince et al., 1960; Walker, 1967; Wong and Macri, 1964; terminology modified in accord with International Committee on Veterinary Gross Anatomical Nomenclature, 1983.

from the limbus and becomes continuous with the fascia of the extraocular muscles. It is thick in cats where the rectus muscles insert near the limbus (Prince et al., 1960).

The extraocular muscles (four recti, two obliqui, and the retractor bulbi) move the globe; however, the cat relies mainly on rapid head movement to shift direction of gaze (Hyde and Eason, 1959). The rectus muscles rotate the globe in the direction of their names. The dorsal and ventral oblique muscles rotate the globe approximately on its axis. The retractor bulbi, less developed in the cat than in other species, pulls the globe back into the orbit.

The levator palpebrae superioris muscle arises above the optic canal and inserts in the upper eyelid. There are also smooth muscle fibers under sympathetic innervation among the fibers of the levator, and these aid in raising the upper eyelid.

The third cranial nerve (oculomotor) innervates the levator; the dorsal, ventral, and medial recti; and the ventral oblique. The fourth cranial nerve (trochlear) innervates the dorsal oblique. The sixth cranial nerve (abducens) innervates the lateral rectus and the retractor bulbi.

The vascular supply to the orbital structures is derived from the maxillary artery, which forms a maxillary rete covering the area from the foramen rotundum to the optic canal. This rete is a network of arteries that gives off the following branches: the ophthalmic (ciliary), two ethmoidals, the zygomatic, the lacrimal, the muscular, branches anastomosing with the arterial circle of the cerebrum (circle of Willis), and the rostral deep temporal arteries. An internal ophthalmic artery, originating from the arterial circle of the cerebrum, is present in some cats and joins the ophthalmic (ciliary) artery close to the optic nerve. The ophthalmic (ciliary) bifurcates into two long posterior ciliary arteries that supply the globe (Wong and Macri, 1964). The latter have also been found to arise directly from the rete (Prince et al., 1960).

Venous drainage of the globe is by the vortex veins and posterior ciliary veins. Other veins draining the oribt are the dorsal and ventral ophthalmic, lacrimal, ethmoidal, superficial temporal, and infraorbital (Prince et al., 1960).

The cat has a small zygomatic salivary gland in the ventral part of the orbit medial to the zygomatic arch. This gland is outside the periorbital cone and rests against the oral mucosa caudal to the upper molars (Crouch, 1969; McClure et al., 1973; Walker, 1967).

The lacrimal gland is located in the dorsolateral quadrant of the orbit within the periorbita. Its anterior edge is close to the dorsal limbus. The lacrimal gland, a tubuloalveolar gland of serous type, is the source of the aqueous portion of the tear film (Prince et al., 1960).

## Congenital Orbital Disorders

Microphthalmos (an abnormally small eye) is infrequent in the cat and may be uni- or bilateral (Fig. 14–2). Pure microphthalmos (nanophthalmos) refers to an eye that is smaller than normal but has no other gross abnormalities; functional vision in these cases is present. Microphthalmos may be associated with other ocular defects such as cataracts, persistent pupillary membranes, or colobomas; in these cases vision may be affected. Congenital microphthalmos is accompanied by enophthalmos and a small orbit. A small globe and narrow palpebral fissure are signs of microphthalmos. Microphthalmos must be differentiated from phthisis bulbi—acquired atrophy of the lobe. Phthisis bulbi is more common in cats and is an end stage of severe uveitis, endophthalmitis, or trauma. Phthisical globes have evidence of scarring and inflammation, and the size of the orbit is normal. There is no treatment for microphthalmos. Phthisical globes are not treated unless they are actively diseased or painful, in which case enucleation is recommended.

Anophthalmos (absence of the eye) has been reported (Priester, 1972), together with absence of the optic nerve and optic tract (Jones and Hunt, 1983). This rare condition should be diagnosed only when serial histologic examination of orbital tissue has excluded the possibility of microphthalmos (Yanoff and Fine, 1975).

Hydrophthalmos (infantile glaucoma) has also been reported (Priester, 1972).

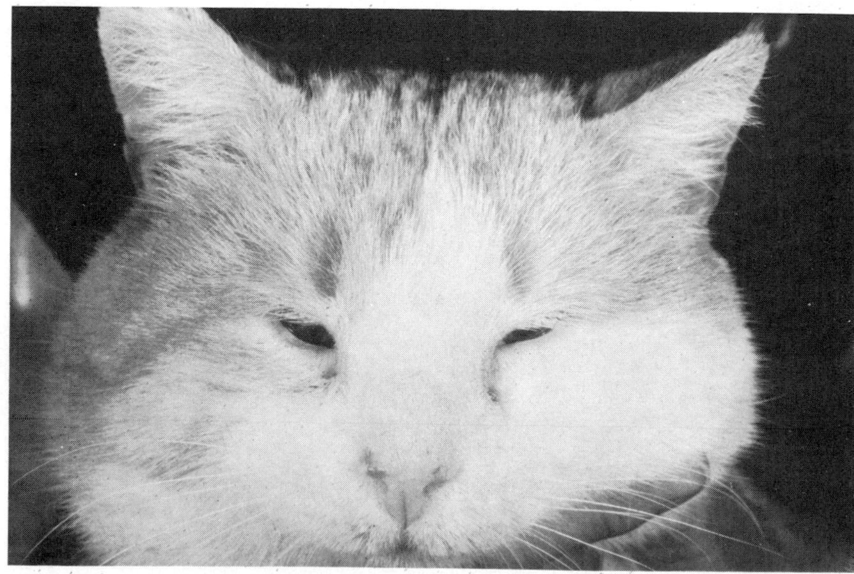

**Figure 14–2** Narrow palpebral fissures and small globe are signs of bilateral microphthalmos in a two-year-old cat.

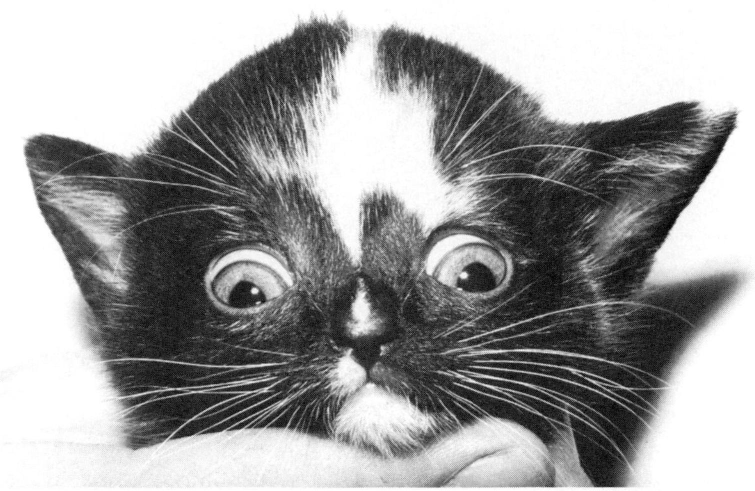

**Figure 14–3** The characteristic ventrolateral deviation of the globes is evident in a hydrocephalic kitten.

Cyclopia, a rare defect in which both orbits and their contents are fused into a single structure, was described in a stillborn kitten (Roberts and Lipton, 1975). Cyclopia is generally incompatible with life, owing to associated malformations of the brain. Cyclopia and anophthalmos, together with absence of the optic nerves and rudimentary optic tracts, were among congenital abnormalities observed in kittens of queens treated with griseofulvin (Scott et al., 1975).

Congenital hydrocephalus results in an enlargement of the calvaria and bony orbits (Fig. 14–3), with ventrolateral displacement of the globes. The appearance of this ventrolateral strabismus in hydrocephalic animals has been termed the "setting sun" phenomenon (Kay, 1981).

Strabismus (esotropia, "cross-eye") is rare in cats, except in Siamese, in which it is not related to abnormalities of the ocular muscles but to genetic defects in neural pathways (see section on the optic nerve). The trait is undesirable in show-type cats, and breeders have had some success in eliminating it. Strabismus is also a feature of mannosidosis (see chapter on inherited metabolic diseases).

Nystagmus, of a rapid lateral flickering type, occurs in some Siamese. Its cause has not been investigated. It is not associated with any apparent visual or neurologic impairment. Nystagmus also occurs in some cats with Chédiak-Higashi syndrome (see chapter on inherited metabolic diseases).

Enophthalmos, recession of the eye within the orbit, may be congenital or acquired and uni- or bilateral. Congenital enophthalmos is associated with microphthalmos. Acquired enophthalmos may result from phthisis bulbi described earlier, and in cachectic cats, from loss of retrobulbar fat. It also occurs with Horner's syndrome, owing to loss of smooth muscle tone within the fascial cone.

## Acquired Orbital Disorders

**ORBITAL TRAUMA.** Orbital trauma is common in cats and may result in orbital (retrobulbar) hemorrhage, proptosis of the globe, and fracture of the bony orbit. Retrobulbar hemorrhage due to blunt orbital trauma or bite wounds causes exophthalmos, which may be mild to severe. Subconjunctival hemorrhage may contribute to lagophthalmos (inability to close the eye), with resultant drying of the cornea and frequent ulceration (Plate 14–1*A*). Hyphema may be present.

Severe blows to the orbit may cause proptosis characterized by displacement of the globe from the orbit, with the lids posterior to the equator (Fig. 14–4). Associated trauma may include avulsion of extraocular muscles (usually the medial rectus, the ventral oblique, or both), rupture of the fibrous tunic, and avulsion of the optic nerve. Fracture of the bony orbit may occur alone or may accompany traumatic proptosis.

Treatment of orbital trauma depends on the extent and duration of damage. Lagophthalmos with resultant corneal desiccation is the main consequence of orbital and subconjunctival hemorrhage. Treatment should be directed toward protecting the cornea and reducing the orbital inflammation. Frequent instillation of artificial tears may be helpful, but a temporary tarsorrhaphy more effectively protects the cornea until the periorbital swelling has receded. A systemic corticosteroid and a broad-spectrum antibiotic are indicated. Warm compresses applied for two to four days are helpful.

A proptosed globe is an ocular emergency and must be replaced as soon as the cat's general condition allows. A general anesthetic is required. The globe should be cleansed with physiologic saline or Ringer's solution and inspected for associated damage. A soft globe indicates rupture of the fibrous tunic, and enucleation is usually indicated. Extensive avulsion of extraocular muscles with avulsion of the optic nerve also warrants enulceation. A constricted pupil carries a more favorable prognosis for vision, as efferent innervation is present. Hyphema is frequent. Blood completely filling the anterior chamber usually denotes severe damage to the iris and ciliary body, and such a globe often becomes phthisical. Replacement should be attempted, however, and prognostic statements regarding vision should be withheld until sutures are removed.

After the globe has been cleansed and inspected, strabismus hooks are used to elevate and apply traction to

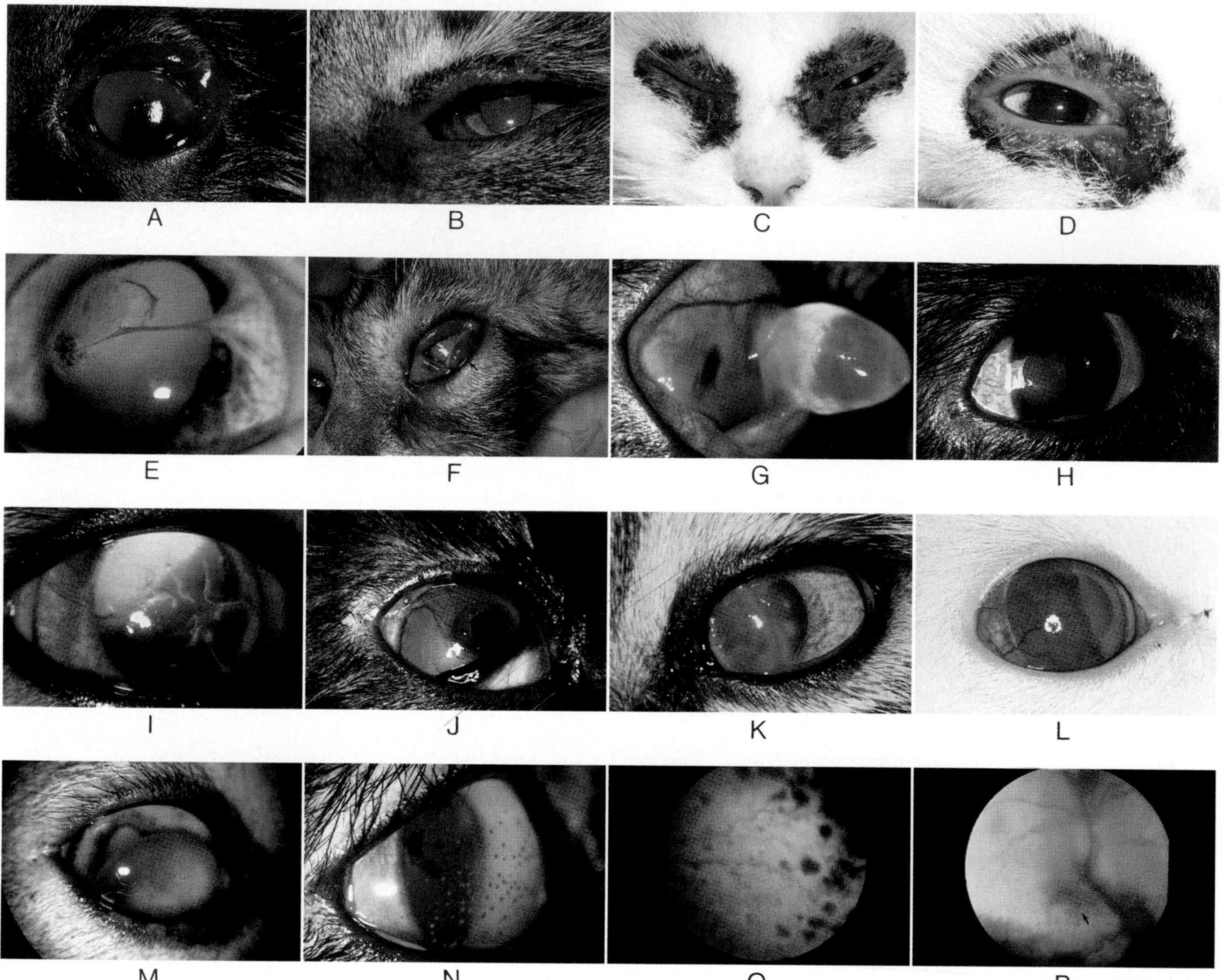

**Plate 14–1** *A*, Subconjunctival and orbital hemorrhage secondary to trauma results in lagophthalmos and corneal drying. *B*, Erythema of eyelid margin and erosion of medial canthal skin in a cat with presumed allergic blepharitis. Biopsy disclosed eosinophils and mast cells. *C* and *D*, Bilateral chronic staphylococcal blepharitis is characterized by hair loss and suppuration of eyelid margins. *E*, A persistent pupillary membrane, originating from the iris collarette, adheres to the corneal endothelium. *F*, A full-thickness laceration of the lateral aspect of the cornea with iris prolapse (arrow) was inflicted during a cat fight. *G*, A large protuberant descemetocele resulted in a cat that had been inappropriately medicated with a topical corticosteroid. The prolapsed portion of Descemet's membrane was excised and the corneal defect sutured. *H*, A descemetocele often has a crater-like appearance. Edema and superficial vascularization of the cornea are also evident. *I*, An irregular, branching corneal dendrite considered pathognomonic for feline herpesvirus (FVR) keratitis is demonstrated by fluorescein dye. *J*, A corneal sequestrum is surrounded by branching, superficial corneal vessels. (Courtesy Dr. M. Wyman.) *K*, Eosinophilic keratitis, diagnosed by cytologic examination of a scraping and by excisional biopsy, involves the nasal aspect of the cornea. *L*, Eosinophilic keratitis involves the temporal half of the cornea. Note the prominent superficial corneal vascularization. (Courtesy Dr. S. Winston.) *M*, A cataractous lens has luxated into the anterior chamber. *N*, Multiple keratic precipitates are present in a cat with feline infectious peritonitis (FIP). *O*, Well-defined choroidal lesions in a cat with feline infectious peritonitis (FIP). (From Campbell LH, Schiessl MM: Mod Vet Pract 59 [1978] 761–764.) *P*, Perivascular exudation (arrow) due to feline infectious peritonitis (FIP). Note the increase in caliber of the retinal veins. Total serum protein was 11.4 mg/dl.

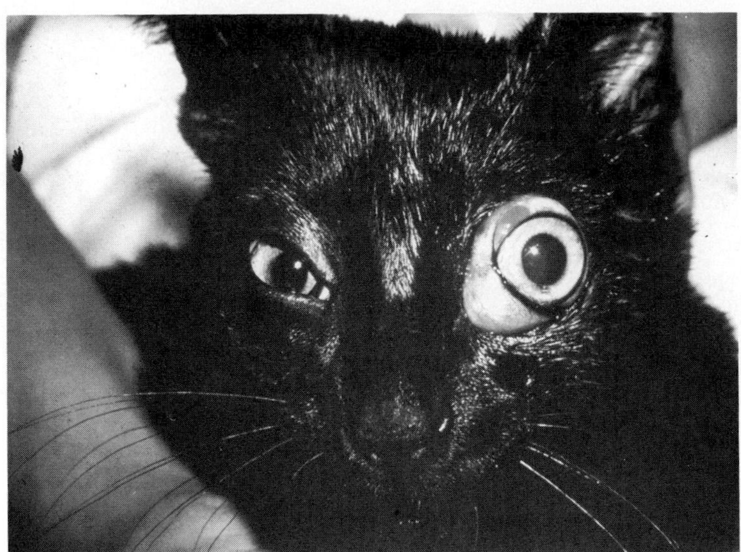

**Figure 14–4** Traumatic proptosis of the left globe was caused by an automobile injury. Replacement of the globe within the orbit and a temporary tarsorrhaphy preserved ocular function.

the eyelid margins. Simultaneously, while gentle pressure is applied to a moistened cotton ball on the cornea, the globe will "snap" back into the orbit. In difficult cases, a lateral canthotomy may be needed to enlarge the palpebral fissure so that the globe may be replaced. A temporary tarsorrhaphy is performed, with interrupted horizontal mattress sutures of 4- or 5-0 nonabsorbable material over stents of polyethylene tubing or rubber bands. Sutures should be carefully placed, entering approximately 4 to 5 mm from the eyelid margin and exiting through the tarsal (meibomian) gland openings to avoid damage to the cornea from sutures.

Oral or parenteral broad-spectrum antibiotics and a decreasing level of corticosteroid are recommended for 7 to 10 days. A retrobulbar corticosteroid seems to be contraindicated because orbital space has been compromised by hemorrhage and edema. Warm compresses are recommended for three to four days after the injury. Sutures should be left in place for about 10 to 14 days, depending on the severity of the proptosis. A common error is to remove sutures too soon.

Complications of proptosis include lateral or dorsolateral strabismus due to rupture or stretching of the medial and ventral oblique muscles. If these are stretched, the globe usually straightens out after two or three months. In the case of muscles torn loose, surgery may be needed to reappose the muscles, or, more realistically, to suture proximal muscle to orbital fascia. Blindness may result from optic nerve avulsion, damage to retinal vasculature, or retinal detachment. Keratitis sicca (usually temporary) may follow direct damage to the lacrimal gland or its nerve supply. Phthisis bulbi may occur after severe hyphema, indicating fibrosis of ciliary body and processes.

Fractures of the bony orbit sometimes accompany proptosis. The thin medial wall may be fractured. A fracture involving the nasal cavity or frontal sinus may communicate with the orbit resulting in subconjunctival emphysema (Bryan, 1977). These fractures are small and generally heal. Large factures of orbital bones occasionally require reconstructive surgery.

**ORBITAL ABSCESS—CELLULITIS.** Peri- or retroorbital cellulitis and abscessation are common in cats. Causes include foreign bodies that enter through the mouth or conjunctiva, osteomyelitis following orbital fractures or bite wounds, diseased upper molar teeth, and extension of frontal sinusitis. The orbital fat has been involved in nutritional pansteatitis in cats (Roberts and Lipton, 1975). Bilateral orbital cellulitis, sinusitis, and pulmonary granulomas due to *Penicillium* have been described (Peiffer et al., 1980).

Signs of orbital abscesses are unilateral exophthalmos, protrusion of the third eyelid, chemosis, and periorbital edema. The cat evinces pain on opening of its mouth and, with dental disease, drools fetid saliva. Anorexia, fever, and leukocytosis are usual. With retrobulbar abscess, an oral examination may disclose swelling or discoloration behind the last upper molar tooth. This area should be explored for a foreign body and lanced with a number 15 Bard-Parker blade to provide ventral drainage. The incision is enlarged with a hemostat. Periorbital abscesses may be drained over the site of maximum swelling, which is frequently at the dorsolateral rim of the orbit. Gentle blunt dissection may locate more abscess pockets or foreign body tracts. Orbital abscesses frequently communicate with the conjunctival fornix. The tract must be kept open with cotton swabs moistened with dilute povidone-iodine (Betadine) solution. Hot compresses and a systemic antibiotic are recommended. Clinical improvement is rapid once drainage has been established and maintained. Dental disease in older cats usually produces a more gradual exophthalmos than do abscesses due to bite wounds. Extraction of affected teeth and antibiotic therapy are curative.

**ORBITAL NEOPLASMS.** The incidence of orbital neoplasia is higher among cats than has been reported. It is overlooked in early stages, and affected cats are treated for secondary signs rather than for the underlying disorder.

A variety of primary tumors may originate from any of the orbital structures (muscle, connective tissue, fat, bone, lacrimal gland, zygomatic salivary gland, nerves, and vessels). Undifferentiated sarcoma, fibrosarcoma, osteosarcoma, and rhabdomyosarcoma have been reported (Peiffer, 1981). Osteosarcoma (Woog et al., 1983) and spindle cell sarcomas (Dubielzig, 1984) that may have resulted from trauma have been described. Secondary tumors may invade the orbit by direct extension from the adjacent nasal cavity, frontal sinuses, and conjunctiva. These tumors include adenocarcinoma and squamous cell carcinoma (Peiffer, 1981). Secondary involvement of the orbit by lymphosarcoma is frequent. The signs of orbital involvement may precede but usually accompany systemic disease. Exophthalmos is due to infiltration of the orbit with neoplastic lymphocytes. Orbital tumors metastatic from distant primary sites are rare.

Orbital neoplasia should be considered, especially in older cats, with gradual, painless exophthalmos. These cats are often depressed and inappetent; fever may be present with advanced neoplasia. The exceptions to old-age incidence of orbital tumors, in my experience, are lymphosarcoma and multicentric fibrosarcoma. These cats have ranged in age from eight months to two years. Involvement may be uni- or bilateral.

As with any orbital disease, early signs of orbital neoplasia include protrusion of the third eyelid, conjunctival hyperemia, lacrimation, and chemosis. Lagophthalmos produces exposure keratopathy. Exophthalmos may be detected by careful examination, and the globe cannot be pressed back into the orbit. The direction of the ocular deviation may indicate the location of the tumor. A medial mass causes lateral displacement of the globe (Fig. 14–5). Masses within the muscle cone or involving the optic nerve produce anterior displacement of the globe. Ocular motility may be decreased by lesions within the muscle cone. The mouth should be inspected for tumor extension in the area behind the last upper molar.

A localized tumor may compress or indent the sclera causing retinal striae, focal retinal detachment, or both, visible on ophthalmoscopic examination. The optic disk may be pale or edematous, and retinal vessels may be congested (Peiffer, 1981).

Skull radiographs may detect osteolytic changes compatible with neoplasia. Positive- or negative-contrast orbitography may demonstrate lesions within the muscle cone (Munger and Ackerman, 1978). As in any case of suspected orbital neoplasia, a thoracic radiograph should be obtained to exclude obvious metastases. Needle aspiration of an orbital mass for cytologic examination may be performed under general anesthesia after skull radiography. The position of the orbital mass determines the site of biopsy. Medial orbital masses may be biopsied by inserting a 20-gauge needle along the ventromedial wall of the bony orbit (Fig. 14–6). Ketamine or general anesthesia is required to obtain the specimen. Oropharyngeal masses may be biopsied directly.

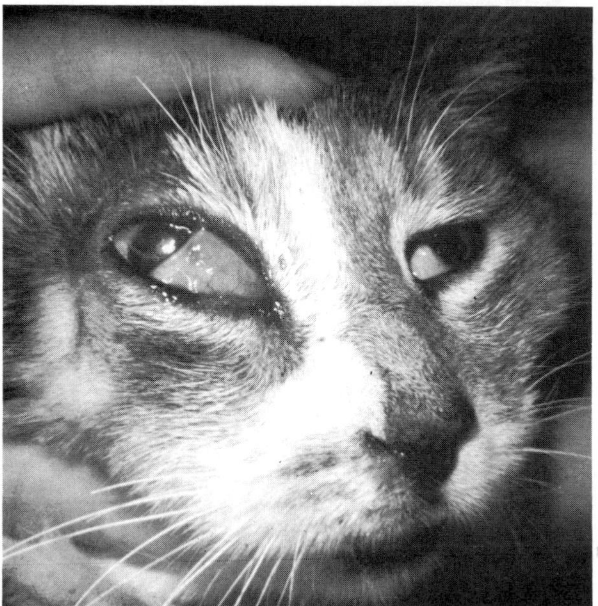

**Figure 14–5** Lateral exophthalmos and protrusion of the third eyelid are evident in a 12-year-old cat with an orbital fibrosarcoma.

Localized benign tumors may be excised via orbitotomy with resection of the zygomatic arch (Bistner et al., 1977). Exenteration (removal of the globe and all tissues within the bony orbit) is recommended for malignant tumors (Bistner et al., 1977). In my experience, most orbital tumors in the cat are malignant with involvement of adjacent sinuses. In these cases prognosis is poor, as recurrence after exenteration is common. Appropriate chemotherapy produces variable periods of remission in cats with lymphosarcoma, but long-term prognosis is poor.

**ORBITAL AND INTRAOCULAR PARASITISM.** *Cuterebra* larvae are occasionally found within the orbit. Intraocular myiasis (Brooks et al., 1984; Gwin et al., 1984) and intraocular parasitism with an unidentified metastrongylid nematode (Bussanich and Rootman, 1983) have been described.

# THE EYELIDS

## Anatomy and Function

The eyelids protect the eye and distribute the tear film across the cornea. The eyelids of the cat are in close contact with the cornea, so that little sclera is visible. Cilia are lacking from upper and lower eyelids in the cat, according to some (e.g., Schmidt and Coulter, 1981); however, Martin and Anderson (1981) state that "the leading row of hairs from the medial third of the upper lid laterally appear distinct enough in most cats to consider cilia," and a microscopic study of feline skin also reports the presence of eyelashes (Strickland and Calhoun, 1968). Cats blink infrequently, about one to five times every five minutes (Schmidt and Coulter, 1981). Kittens are born with their eyelids closed; the lids open between 3 and 15 days of age. One eye may open before the other (Blakemore and Cummings, 1975). Rarely, the lids are open at birth.

The eyelids are composed of four layers. The cutaneous layer is outermost and is covered with fine hairs. The muscular layer is next and consists of the orbicularis oculi, the levator palpebrae superioris, and smooth (Müller's) muscle fibers. The tarsus is a dense connective tissue layer between the orbicularis and the palpebral conjunctiva. Tarsal (meibomian) glands, which secrete an oily liquid, are located within the tarsus. Their excretory ducts open along the inner surface of the lid margin, and their secretion prevents overflow and evaporation of the tear film. The tarsal glands are highly developed in the cat (Martin and Anderson, 1981). The innermost layer of the eyelid is the palpebral conjunctiva, a mucous membrane that extends to the fornix, where it is continuous with the bulbar conjunctiva.

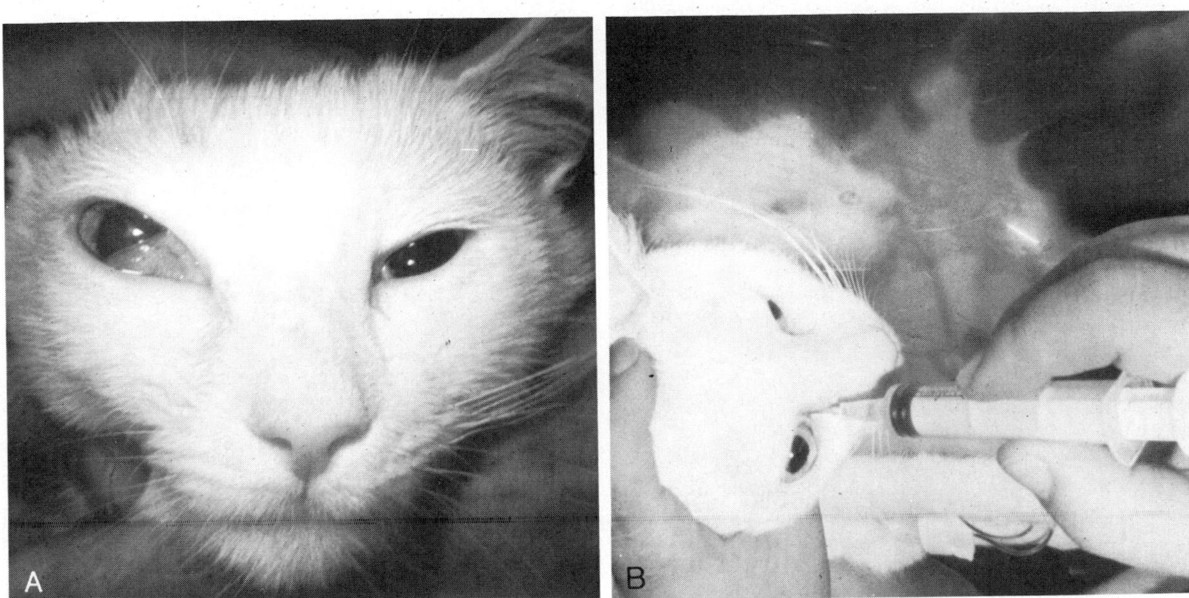

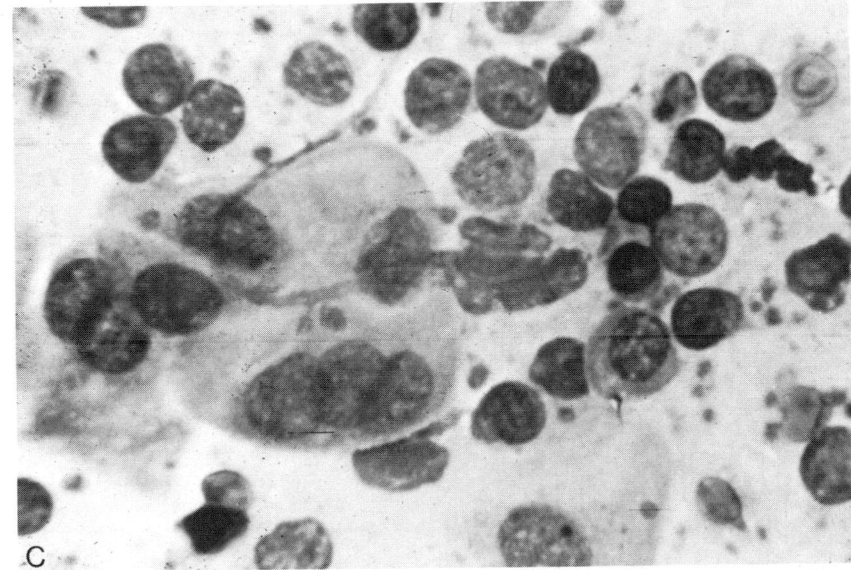

**Figure 14–6** *A*, Lateral and dorsal displacement of the right eye is due to a mass involving the medial orbit in an 11-month-old domestic shorthair. The kidneys were enlarged and the cat tested positive for feline leukemia virus. *B*, An aspiration biopsy of the medial orbital mass is obtained by careful insertion of the needle along the medial wall of the orbit. *C*, Cytologic examination of the aspirate shows numerous atypical lymphocytes compatible with a diagnosis of lymphosarcoma. Large cells with abundant cytoplasm are conjunctival epithelial cells. Wright's stain, ×1000.

Cats that are dark colored or have dark fur around the eyes, as well as purebred silvers and chinchillas, have pigmented lids that set off their eyes with a mascara-like effect. Adult red- and cream-coated cats develop small pigmented areas on the eyelids, as well as on the nose, lips, ears, and toepads. These patches become larger and darker as the cat ages.

The eyelid is raised by the levator palpebrae superioris, which is innervated by the third cranial (oculomotor) nerve. Smooth muscle fibers (M. orbitalis, Müller's muscle) also aid in widening the palpebral fissure and are under sympathetic innervation. The eyelid is closed by the orbicularis oculi, which encircles the eyelid aperture and is innervated by the seventh cranial (facial) nerve.

## Congenital Abnormalities of the Eyelids

Agenesis or congenital absence of all or part of the layers of the eyelid occurs occasionally in cats. It may be uni- or bilateral. The lateral part of the upper lid is most often affected (Roberts and Bistner, 1968). Bellhorn et al. (1971) reported three cats with upper eyelid agenesis; two also had iris colobomas. Incomplete medial or lateral canthus with dermoid formation has been observed in certain lines of Burmese (Koch, 1979).

Eyelid defects are bordered by thin, hair-covered skin lined by conjunctiva, and eyelid closure in the affected area is imperfect, as the orbicularis is lacking. If the defect is small, clinical signs are minimal. If the defect involves at least one third of the eyelid margin, signs of corneal exposure and irritation from trichiasis are present. Topical medication provides symptomatic relief in mild cases (Peiffer, 1981). If more than a third of the eyelid is involved (Fig. 14–7), a horizontal pedicle graft (Fig. 14–8) is recommended. A strip of skin and orbicularis muscle from the lower normal eyelid is transposed to a recipient bed in the affected lid corresponding to the area of agenesis (Roberts and Bistner, 1968). The hair on the transposed flap will grow downward. Vaseline may be used to direct the hair away from the eye.

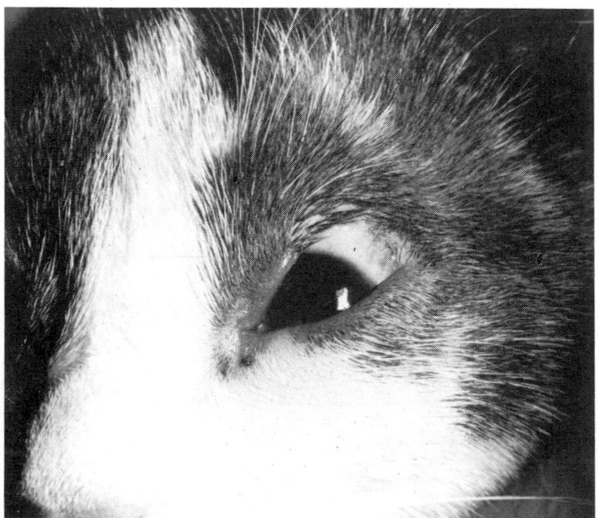

**Figure 14–7** Congenital absence or agenesis of the lateral two thirds of the upper eyelid is the most frequent congenital ocular defect in cats.

An alternative technique of repair was described by Blogg (1985).

Entropion, inversion of the eyelid margin, is usually acquired in cats, but congenital entropion has been reported (Priester, 1972). Persian cats are affected most often (Peiffer, 1981). The lower eyelid is usually involved (Fig. 14–9). Congenital entropion may also occur with microphthalmos. Signs of entropion are related to corneal irritation by the inverted lid: epiphora, blepharospasm, and corneal vascularization and ulceration. Entropion may be corrected with the modified Celsus technique (Wyman, 1979) (Fig. 14–10). Surgical results are usually excellent.

Congenital ankyloblepharon has been reported in blue Persians, in which the upper and lower lids were joined by a thick membrane (Smythe, 1958).

## Acquired Disorders of the Eyelids

**LACERATIONS.** Eyelid wounds in cats are often associated with bites or scratches. Early treatment is necessary to prevent wound contraction and permanent scarring. The laceration should be gently and minimally clipped of hair and the area cleansed with povidone-iodine soap and rinsed with sterile physiologic saline solution. Débridement should be minimal and the laceration repaired so that the tissues are anatomically realigned (Fig. 14–11). The lesion should be closed in layers, conjunctiva to conjunctiva and skin to skin. Fine absorbable suture material such as 6-0 chromic catgut is recommended for the conjunctiva and 5- to 6-0 nonabsorbable material for the skin. Skin sutures are removed in 10 days. Postoperative care consists of a systemic broad-spectrum antibiotic. Topical antibiotics are used only if corneal ulceration exists.

**ANKYLOBLEPHARON.** This refers to adhesions of the lids after the normal time for opening and may be associated with symblepharon. If it persists, gentle separation with a probe is indicated, especially if the lids are bulging owing to accumulation of exudate, as occasionally occurs in kittens with upper respiratory infection.

**ENTROPION.** Acquired entropion may be secondary to trauma but more often follows chronic conjunctivitis that has led to conjunctival scar tissue contraction (Roberts and Lipton, 1975). Both lower lids are usually affected. Signs and surgical repair are the same as for congenital entropion, discussed earlier.

Spastic entropion of upper and lower lids may be associated with corneal irritation and is alleviated by instillation of a topical anesthetic such as proparicaine. A temporary lateral tarsorrhaphy alleviates true spastic entropion by preventing inversion of the eyelids until the corneal lesion has healed. Frequently, spastic and anatomic entropion are concomitant, so careful examination and assessment must be made. For example, a topical anesthetic eliminates corneal pain so that the eyelids open; yet a mild degree of lid inversion may be detected that will require surgical correction by a modified Celsus procedure.

**ECTROPION.** Eversion of the ventral lid margin is rare in cats. It is usually secondary to unrepaired eyelid lacerations complicated by scar formation that has pulled the eyelid away from the globe (Roberts and Lipton,

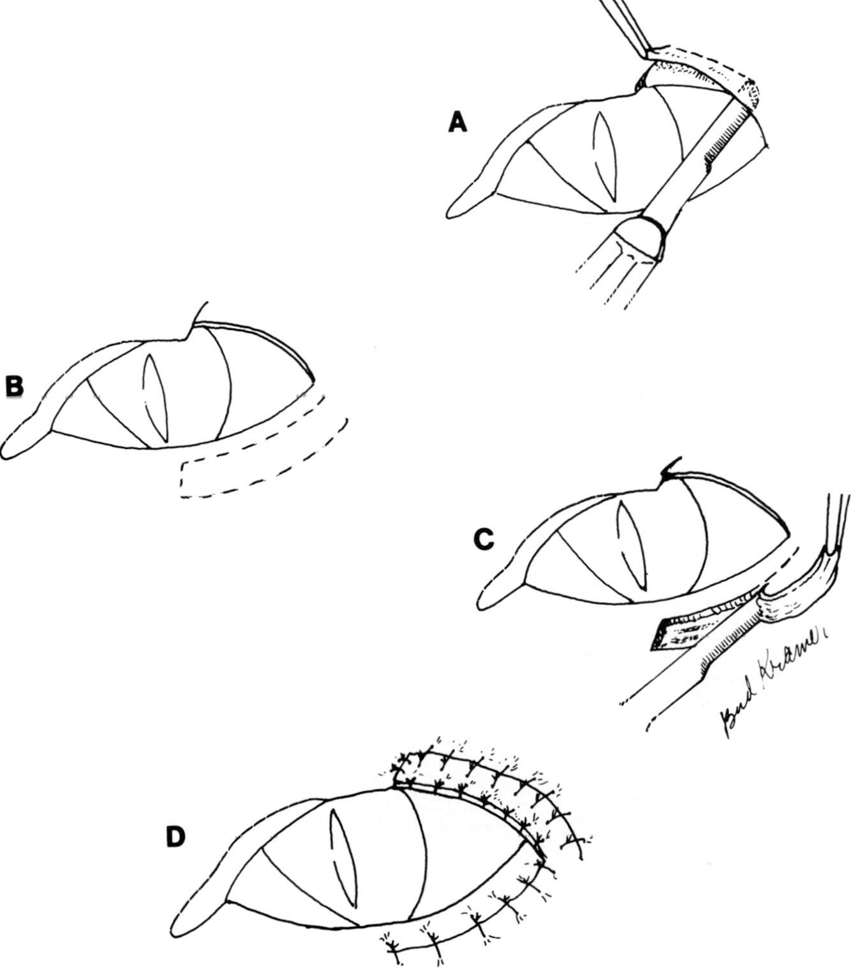


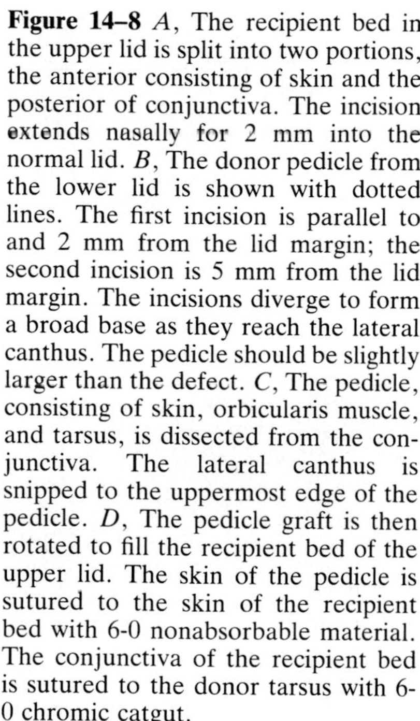
**Figure 14–8** *A*, The recipient bed in the upper lid is split into two portions, the anterior consisting of skin and the posterior of conjunctiva. The incision extends nasally for 2 mm into the normal lid. *B*, The donor pedicle from the lower lid is shown with dotted lines. The first incision is parallel to and 2 mm from the lid margin; the second incision is 5 mm from the lid margin. The incisions diverge to form a broad base as they reach the lateral canthus. The pedicle should be slightly larger than the defect. *C*, The pedicle, consisting of skin, orbicularis muscle, and tarsus, is dissected from the conjunctiva. The lateral canthus is snipped to the uppermost edge of the pedicle. *D*, The pedicle graft is then rotated to fill the recipient bed of the upper lid. The skin of the pedicle is sutured to the skin of the recipient bed with 6-0 nonabsorbable material. The conjunctiva of the recipient bed is sutured to the donor tarsus with 6-0 chromic catgut.

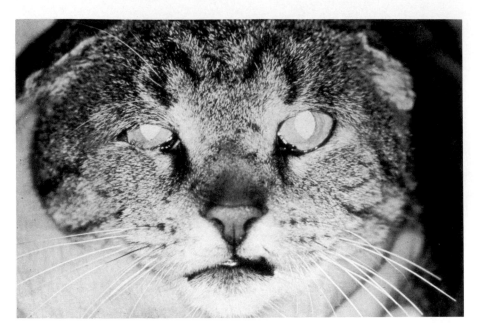

**Figure 14–9** Acquired entropion of the right lower eyelid in an aged cat. (Courtesy Dr. M. Wyman.)

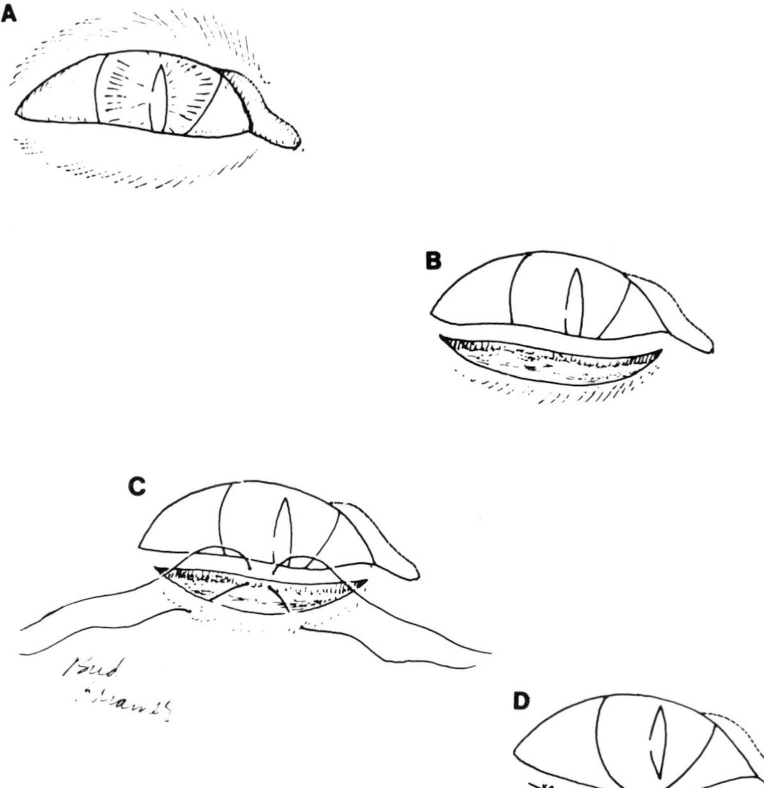


**Figure 14–10** *A*, Entropion of the lower eyelid. *B*, A crescent-shaped segment of skin corresponding to the entropic area is excised. The first incision is parallel to and 2 to 3 mm from the lid margin. The incision is extended 1 mm on either side of the inverted portion of the lid. The width of the segment of skin to be excised is determined before anesthesia. *C*, The first two sutures are placed on either side of the center, angling toward the lid. The lid is effectively everted by this method. *D*, Completed suture pattern. Five- or 6-0 nonabsorbable suture material is used.

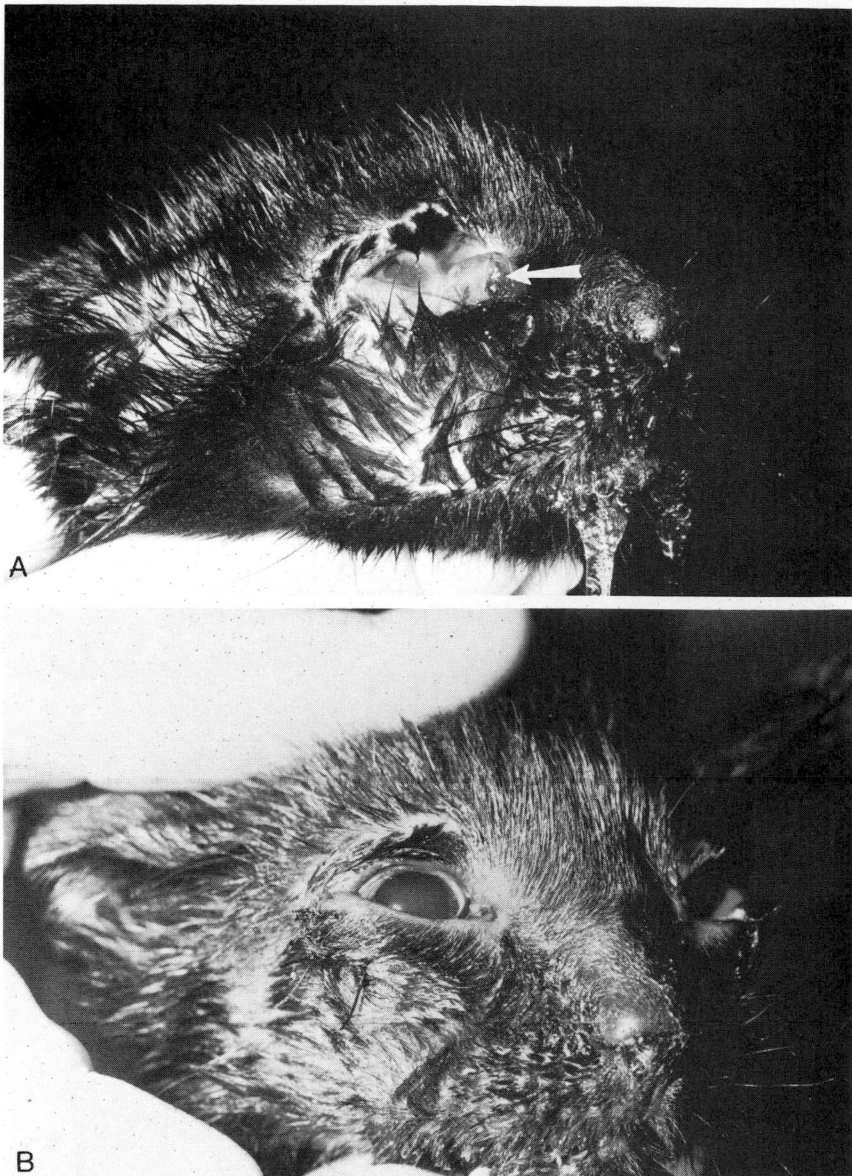


**Figure 14–11** *A*, A full-thickness laceration of the lateral lower eyelid (arrow) resulting from a dog bite. *B*, Immediate postoperative appearance after two-layer closure.

1975). Cicatricial ectropion is corrected by separating the skin from the scar and advancing the skin toward the lid margin by advancement flaps (Doherty, 1973; Roberts and Lipton, 1975).

**BLEPHARITIS.** Inflammation of the eyelid skin may accompany generalized dermatologic disorders of parasitic, mycotic, bacterial, or allergic etiology.

**Acariasis.** Feline scabies, caused by *Notoedres cati*, is rare. Typically the skin of the head and neck, including that of the eyelids and ears, is thickened and intensely pruritic. Some hair loss and adherent encrustations are characteristic (e.g., Martin, 1981). Even rarer in cats is *Demodex folliculorum*, which causes nonpruritic blepharitis (Roberts and Lipton, 1975). Diagnosis is by identification of the mite in skin scrapings. The application of rotenone ointment such as Goodwinol once daily is recommended (Roberts and Lipton, 1975). Care should be taken that the ointment does not get onto the cornea.

**Dermatomycosis.** *Microsporum canis* is the principal cause of ringworm in cats, and the eyelids may occasionally be involved (Roberts and Lipton, 1975). Signs are circular areas of alopecia with scaling and little or no pruritus. Because not all *M. canis* infections fluoresce with ultraviolet light, isolation of the organism by mycotic culture is often required. Oral griseofulvin is the recommended therapy (Roberts and Lipton, 1975). The owner should be informed that ringworm is contagious to other animals and to people.

**Allergic Blepharitis.** I have observed intensely pruritic, bilateral blepharitis characterized by severe erythema and self-mutilation of the eyelid margins (Plate 14–1*B*). Conjunctival involvement is minimal. Skin scrapings for parasites and bacterial and mycotic cultures give negative results. Eosinophils and lesser numbers of mast cells are present in biopsied skin. Systemic corticosteroids provide rapid remission of signs; most affected cats require low, alternate-day dosage of a corticosteroid to prevent recurrence. Topical medication has minimal effect. Treatment with megestrol acetate produced remission of signs in one cat.

**Bacterial Blepharitis.** *Staphylococcus* is the most frequent cause of bacterial blepharitis. The conjunctiva is usually affected as well. Erythema, exudation, ulceration of the lid margins, and variable degrees of pruritus are the signs. Involvement is usually bilateral (Plate 14–1*C* and *D*), and the condition is frequently chronic. Although a topical broad-spectrum antibiotic may be used (Peiffer, 1981), culture and sensitivity testing are helpful in choosing the most effective drug. Skin biopsy, especially in chronic cases, is highly recommended to rule out pemphigus or allergic blepharitis (Manning et al., 1982). Warm compresses three or four times daily are used to loosen and remove the exudate. As blepharitis is primarily a dermatologic problem, systemic treatment with an oral antibiotic is recommended. A systemic corticosteroid may be needed to combat the allergic exotoxins of *Staphylococcus*, especially in chronic cases with self-mutilation.

Infected bite wounds are the most common cause of suppurative blepharitis in cats. A massive abscess may involve the eyelid (Fig. 14–12) and may drain into the conjunctiva or through the cutaneous surface of the lid (Martin, 1981). The lid is swollen, warm, and painful, and the globe may not be visible. If the abscess is not draining, a needle aspiration may be performed to establish the presence of pus. Ventral drainage must be established and maintained. Antiseptic flushes or the use of a Penrose drain or an iodoform seton will keep the tract open. An oral or parenteral antibiotic and warm compresses are indicated. Prognosis is good for localized abscesses. Extensive suppuration may cause the overlying skin to slough, and blepharoplastic procedures may be needed (Doherty, 1973; Gelatt and Blogg, 1969).

**Blepharitis from Burns.** Cats exposed to fire may have severe blepharitis as well as burns of the ears and tip of the nose. Necrotic tissue must be removed. Because burned skin provides an ideal medium for bacterial growth, a topical antibiotic is indicated. The most effective is silver sulfadiazine (Silvadene Cream, Marion Laboratories).

**DISTICHIASIS.** This is uncommon in the cat but is

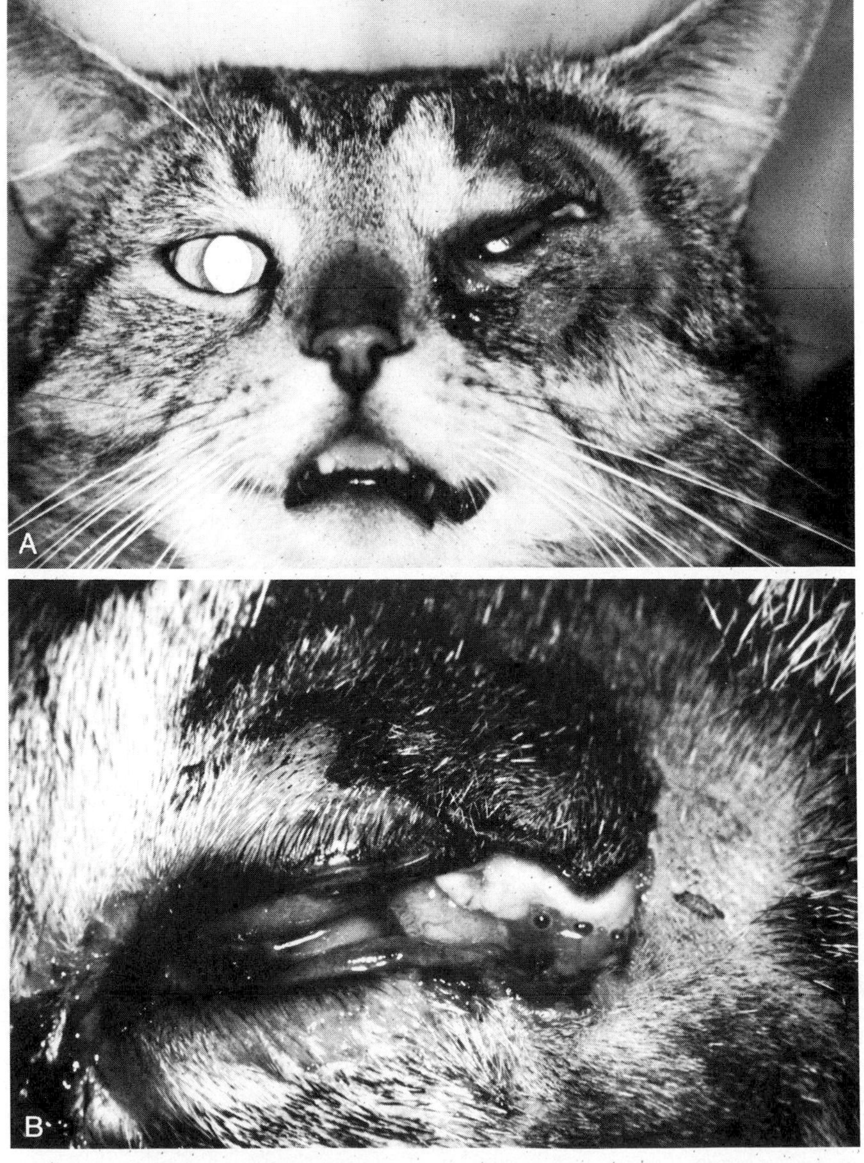

**Figure 14–12** *A*, Abscessation of the upper eyelid and periocular area was secondary to a cat fight wound. The eye was not damaged. *B*, The lateral portion of the upper eyelid is necrotic and is beginning to slough.

occasionally a complication of blepharitis. Successful epilation by cryosurgery has been described (Wheeler and Severin, 1984).

**NEOPLASMS OF THE EYELID.** Squamous cell carcinoma is the most common eyelid tumor in the cat, occurring mostly in the unpigmented lids of white or white-spotted cats. Squamous cell carcinomas originate in the epidermis and are invasive. The palpebral margin may be the site of origin; the conjunctiva, third eyelid, and cornea may also be involved primarily or secondarily (Peiffer, 1981). Squamous cell carcinomas take the form of ulcerated, proliferative masses with a red base on the eyelid or conjunctiva. Owing to the invasive growth pattern, large segments of the eyelid may be involved. Squamous cell carcinomas may metastasize to regional lymph nodes.

As wide surgical excision of squamous cell carcinoma is desirable, techniques to reconstruct the eyelid are necessary (Doherty, 1973; Gelatt and Blogg, 1969). A full-thickness bridge flap is illustrated in Figure 14–13. Squamous cell carcinomas are radiosensitive, and radiation therapy may be used in addition to surgical excision (Peiffer, 1981). Hyperthermia has also given favorable results in treatment of small superficial squamous cell carcinomas (Grier et al., 1980).

Other types of eyelid tumors are uncommon in cats, the majority being malignant (Peiffer, 1981; Roberts and Lipton, 1975). They include papilloma, adenoma, or adenocarcinoma arising from the tarsal (meibomian) glands, fibroma, fibrosarcoma, neurofibrosarcoma, hemangioma, hemangiosarcoma, and mast cell tumor (Peiffer, 1981). Histopathologic examination is indicated in all cases. If these neoplasms involve up to 25 per cent of the lid margin, a V-plasty with two-layer closure is effective (Wyman, 1979). In other cases, blepharoplastic techniques may be needed (Doherty, 1973; Gelatt and Blogg, 1969). The multicentric feline sarcoma virus (FeSV) may affect the eyelids of young cats, in which involvement is frequently extensive and bilateral. Prognosis is poor, as viral feline sarcoma is a fatal disease.

## THE LACRIMAL SYSTEM

### Anatomy and Function

The lacrimal system has secretory and excretory components. The secretory portion consists of the main lacrimal gland, the gland of the third eyelid, and the accessory conjunctival glands. The excretory portion is represented by the lacrimal puncta, canaliculi, lacrimal sac, and nasolacrimal duct. The duct passes through the lacrimal bone, along the medial surface of the maxilla, to emerge in the nasal cavity under the ventral concha.

The tear film is composed of three layers. The outer lipid layer is derived from the tarsal (meibomian) glands and prevents evaporation of tears. The aqueous middle layer is secreted by the lacrimal gland and the gland of the third eyelid. The inner mucin layer is produced by the conjunctival goblet cells. The tear film forms a continuous moist cover over the corneal and conjunctival surfaces, provides oxygen to the cornea, and forms a smooth refracting surface. Cats' tears lack the antibacterial enzyme lysozyme (Erickson et al., 1956).

The Schirmer tear test is used to measure reflex tearing. The mean one-minute value for normal cats is 16.9 mm with a standard deviation of $\pm 5.7$ (Veith et al., 1970). The tear film is spread over the cornea by the third eyelid and to a lesser extent by blinking of the eyelids.

The lacrimal puncta are circular openings near the medial angle on the mucocutaneous junction of upper and lower lids. They may be seen by slightly everting the medial margins of the lids. The lower punctum is the main route for tear drainage. Tears drain through the puncta by capillary action, and a combination of gravity and orbicularis muscle contraction during blinking propels tears from the canaliculi into the poorly developed lacrimal sac. The nasolacrimal duct empties into the vestibulum of the nasal cavity, as previously described.

The excretory portion of the lacrimal system may be evaluated for patency by irrigating the superior punctum with a 25-gauge lacrimal cannula after instillation of a topical anesthetic. As some cats object to this procedure, tranquilization may be required. Passage of fluorescein dye from the conjunctival sac through the nasolacrimal system to the nose is a test of functional patency. The dye may be seen in the nostril within 5 to 10 minutes. A negative response is not conclusive, since fluorescein fails to appear in 50 per cent of normal cats tested (Roberts and Lipton, 1975).

### Congenital Nasolacrimal Abnormalities

Congenital absence or atresia of the lacrimal puncta is rare. The primary sign is epiphora (overflow of tears onto the face). Absence of the dorsal punctum rarely causes clinical signs. Congenital occlusion caused by a thin membrane covering the lower punctum has been described (Roberts and Lipton, 1975). Correction is accomplished by cannulating the upper punctum, flushing with saline to cause the membrane covering the occluded punctum to balloon outward, and excising it, leaving a round opening. An antibiotic-corticosteroid ophthalmic solution is used every six hours for 10 to 14 days after surgery.

Congenital absence of canaliculi is another cause of epiphora and may be confirmed by dacryocystorhinography (Gelatt et al., 1973).

Congenital epiphora occurs most often in Persians. The shallow orbit, prominent globe, and constriction or occlusion of the nasolacrimal duct associated with brachycephalic conformation often combine to impair tear drainage (Peiffer, 1981; Roberts and Lipton, 1975). Among Persians, epiphora is most objectionable in white cats, in which it causes reddish staining of the face. This discoloration may be prevented by daily administration of 5 to 10 mg tetracycline (Brightman, 1983).

If epiphora is severe and results in chronic dermatitis, an alternate excretory route may be constructed by conjunctivorhinostomy, as described by Covitz et al. (1977). A Steinmann pin is used to create a fistula from the medioventral fornix to the nasal cavity. A polyethylene or silicone tube is inserted into the fistula and sutured to conjunctival mucosa for at least two months. This fistula eventually becomes lined with mucous membrane. Better results have been reported in dogs than in cats; complications include extrusion or occlusion of the tubing or occlusion of the fistula.

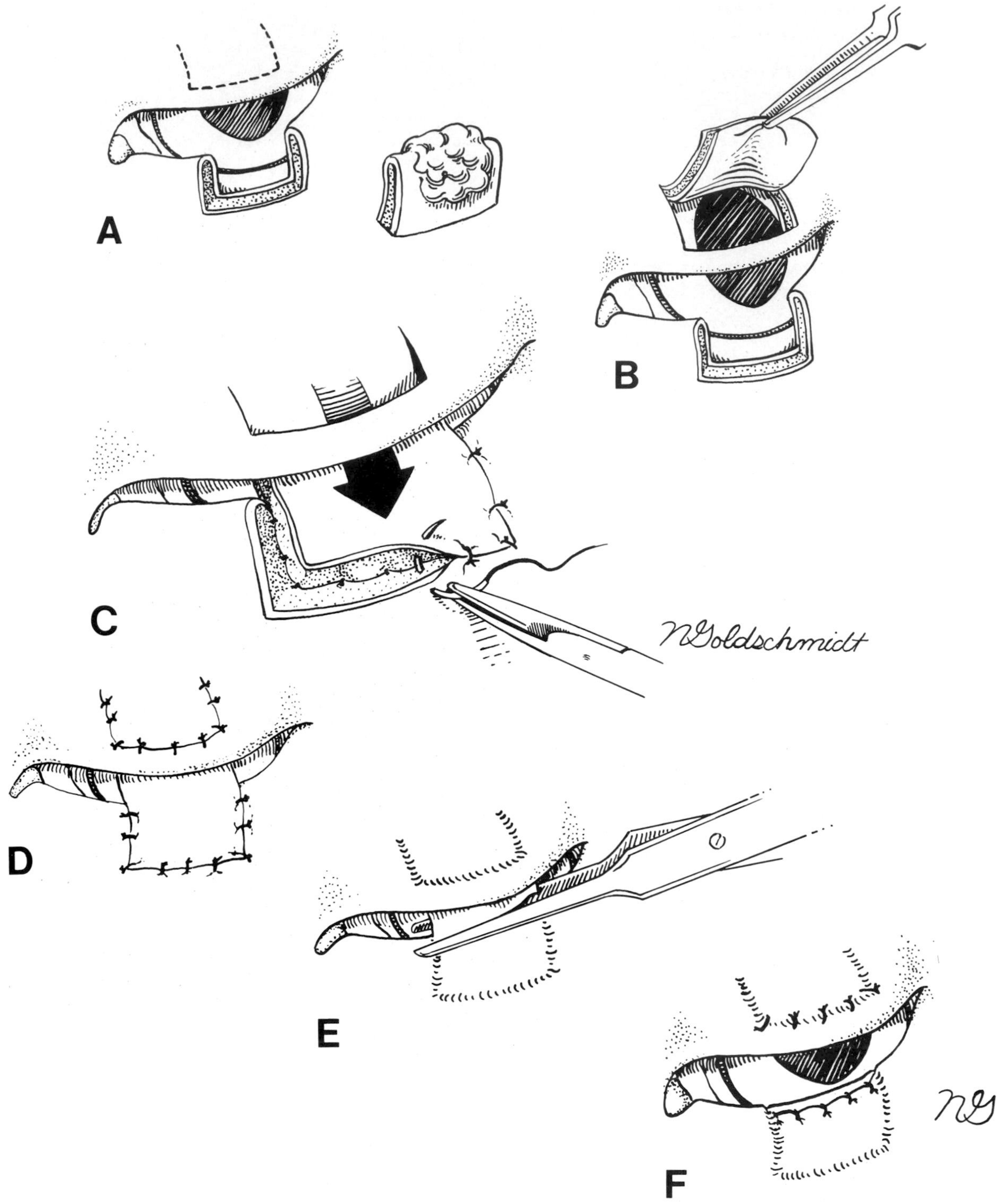


**Figure 14–13** *A*, A full-thickness defect in the lower eyelid has resulted from excision of a large tumor. The dotted lines indicate the site of a full-thickness bridge flap from the upper eyelid. *B*, The incision has been made about 4 mm from the eyelid margin and is as long as, and slightly wider than, the defect in the lower lid. *C*, The flap is pulled beneath the eyelid margin bridge and is sutured in two layers to the lower eyelid defect. The tarsal conjunctiva has been apposed with 6-0 chromic catgut. The skin is sutured with 5-0 nonabsorbable material. *D*, The bridge flap after it has been sutured in place. Skin sutures have also been placed in the upper eyelid. *E*, In three to four weeks (the second procedure) the flap is cut near the base to form the lower eyelid margin. *F*, The healed cut edge of the upper eyelid bridge was freshened and sutured in two layers to the bridge. The conjunctiva of the new lower eyelid margin has been sutured to the skin margin with 6-0 chromic catgut. (After Doherty MJ: J Am Anim Hosp Assoc 9 [1973] 238–241)

## Acquired Disorders of the Lacrimal System

**OBSTRUCTION.** Epiphora, an overflow of tears beyond the eyelid margin, is the sign common to disorders of the excretory portion of the lacrimal system.

Lacrimal duct obstruction may result from a diseased upper tooth root, from trauma to the nasal cavity in which the duct is situated, and from cryptococcal granulomas or tumors. Radiographs and nasal flushing to obtain material for culture and cytologic examination aid in diagnosis.

Punctal stenosis or occlusion may be caused by symblepharon, which frequently results from neonatal feline herpesvirus or chlamydial conjunctivitis. Surgical treatment of punctal occlusion due to symblepharon is unrewarding. A conjunctivorhinostomy procedure is not usually successful because of occlusion of the fistula with subsequent adhesions.

Dacryocystitis (inflammation of the lacrimal sac) may be an extension of bacterial conjunctivitis. Epiphora, purulent conjunctivitis, and swelling and erythema of the medial canthal skin are typical signs. Pressure on the medial canthus may express pus from one or both puncta. Treatment is by daily nasolacrimal lavage with sterile physiologic saline and broad-spectrum antibiotic solutions. Bacterial culture and sensitivity testing of the exudate flushed from the puncta, followed by specific topical antibiotic solution, are indicated in chronic cases.

Lacrimal sac abscessation is uncommon in cats but may occur during the course of dacryocystitis or result from trauma (Roberts and Lipton, 1975). Necrosis of the wall of the lacrimal sac creates a fistulous tract that drains about 1 cm below the medial canthus (Fig. 14–14). Treatment is by surgical drainage and débridement of the infected area. Culture and antibiotic sensitivity testing of exudate are recommended. Postoperative use of systemic antibiotics and warm compresses is also recommended. If the fistula re-forms a skull radiograph may reveal osteomyelitis or bone sequestration, necessitating removal of the lacrimal sac and curettage of involved bone. The resulting chronic epiphora may be treated by conjunctivorhinostomy.

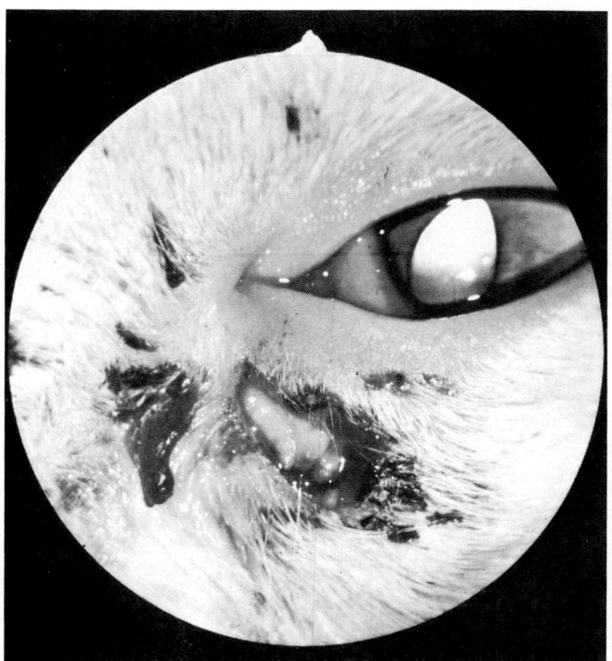

**Figure 14–14** Abscessation of the lacrimal sac resulted in a fistulous tract beneath the medial canthus in a cat with chronic dacryocystitis.

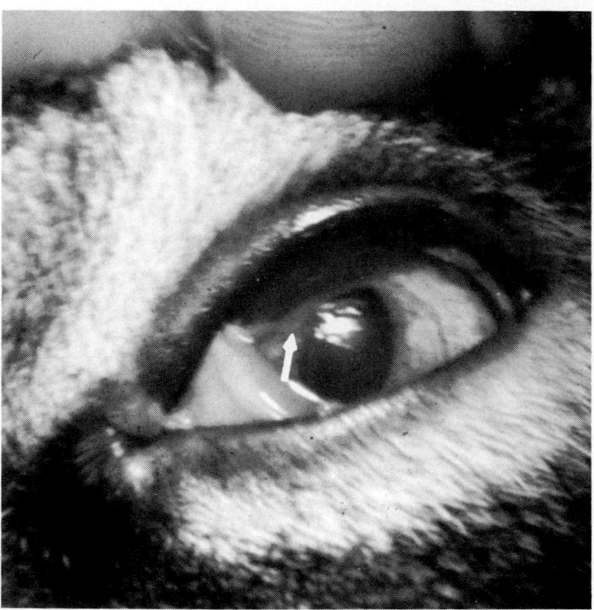

**Figure 14–15** The lusterless cornea is a sign of keratoconjunctivitis sicca. A mucin strand (arrow) adheres to the corneal surface.

Neoplasia, such as squamous cell carcinoma, may involve the medial eyelid margin or the lacrimal canaliculi or sac and obstruct tear drainage (Peiffer et al., 1978).

**DACRYOADENITIS.** Inflammation of the orbital lacrimal gland is rare in cats. Tuberculosis of the lacrimal gland and eosinophilic granuloma of the orbit involving the lacrimal gland have been described (Roberts and Lipton, 1975). Neoplasia (adenocarcinoma) of the lacrimal gland is uncommon; exophthalmos is the main clinical sign.

**KERATOCONJUNCTIVITIS SICCA (KCS).** Subnormal tear production ("dry eye") is uncommon in the cat but should be suspected in cases of uni- or bilateral chronic keratoconjunctivitis with superficial corneal vascularization and recurrent ulceration. Early signs are those of chronic conjunctivitis, but little ocular discharge is present. In addition, the cornea appears lusterless and dry (Fig. 14–15). Schirmer tear test values are below 10 mm.

Some cases of KCS may be secondary to severe conjunctivitis, particularly when associated with upper respiratory viral infections. Inflammatory KCS is often transient; however, therapy with artificial tears may be indicated, together with idoxuridine when herpes is the cause or with an antibiotic for bacterial infection.

I have observed transient drug-related KCS in cats treated for chronic cystitis with higher than therapeutic levels of sulfonamide drugs. Neurogenic KCS due to facial or orbital trauma usually responds to oral or topical 0.5 to 1.0 per cent pilocarpine solution two or three times daily. Parotid duct transposition may be performed in cases of chronic KCS that are not controllable with medical therapy (Bistner et al., 1977).

## THE CONJUNCTIVA AND THIRD EYELID

### Anatomy and Function

The conjunctiva is a thin, semitransparent mucous membrane that covers the inner surfaces of the eyelids as the palpebral conjunctiva, extends to the fornix, and continues onto the globe as the bulbar conjunctiva. The conjunctival epithelium is continuous with that of the cornea. Mucin-secreting goblet cells are present within the palpebral conjunctiva but not in the bulbar conjunctiva. The palpebral conjunctiva is the more vascular. Microscopically, the conjunctiva has two layers, the outer nonkeratinized epithelial layer and the substantia propria, which contains blood vessels, lymphatics, and accessory lacrimal glands. Conjunctival blood vessels arise from the anterior ciliary arteries (Martin and Anderson, 1981). The ophthalmic branch of the fifth cranial (trigeminal) nerve provides sensory innervation of the conjunctiva.

The third eyelid (haw) is a semilunar fold of conjunctiva supported by a T-shaped shaft of elastic cartilage curved to conform to the corneal surface (Martin and Anderson, 1981). The base of the cartilage is surrounded by the gland of the third eyelid which contributes the aqueous portion of the tear film. Lymphoid aggregates are present on the inner (bulbar) surface of the third eyelid. The edge of the third eyelid is usually pigmented.

The cat's third eyelid moves across the globe from medioventral to dorsolateral. It functions to spread the tear film and protect the cornea. By a mechanism unique to the cat, active protrusion is produced by striated muscle fibers from the lateral rectus and levator palpebrae superioris, which attach to the eyelid (Acheson, 1938; de Lahunta and Habel, 1986). The sixth cranial (abducent) nerve innervates these fibers. As in other animals, tonic retraction is maintained by smooth muscle in the periorbita and by two sheets of smooth muscle arising from the fascia of the medial and ventral recti. Postganglionic sympathetic fibers innervate the smooth muscle sheets. Passive protrusion of the third lid occurs when the retractor bulbi contracts.

### Congenital Abnormalities of the Conjunctiva and Third Eyelid

**SYMBLEPHARON.** Congenital adhesions of the bulbar and palpebral conjunctiva have been reported (Peiffer, 1981; Priester, 1972; Roberts and Lipton, 1975). The third eyelid is often involved. Repair is by incising the adhesions and allowing the conjunctiva to retract. Congenital symblepharon, unlike inflammatory symblepharon, seldom recurs after surgery.

**DERMOID.** Dermoids are congenital islands of skin and hair follicles located most often at the limbal conjunctiva. They are uncommon and are usually unilateral in cats. Familial occurrence of epibulbar dermoids has been reported in a line of British Birman cats (Hendy-Ibbs, 1985). The size of the dermoid determines the severity of the signs, which are related to corneal and conjunctival irritation. The third eyelid may be the site of a dermoid (Fig. 14–16). Dermoids are handled by surgical excision and closure of the conjunctival defect with 6- or 7-0 chromic catgut.

### Acquired Disorders of the Conjunctiva

**SYMBLEPHARON.** Inflammatory adhesions of bulbar and palpebral conjunctiva may follow caustic burns, abscesses, and most often neonatal herpetic or chlamydial infections (Roberts and Lipton, 1975). Early treatment of conjunctivitis (to be described) reduces the extent of symblepharon formation.

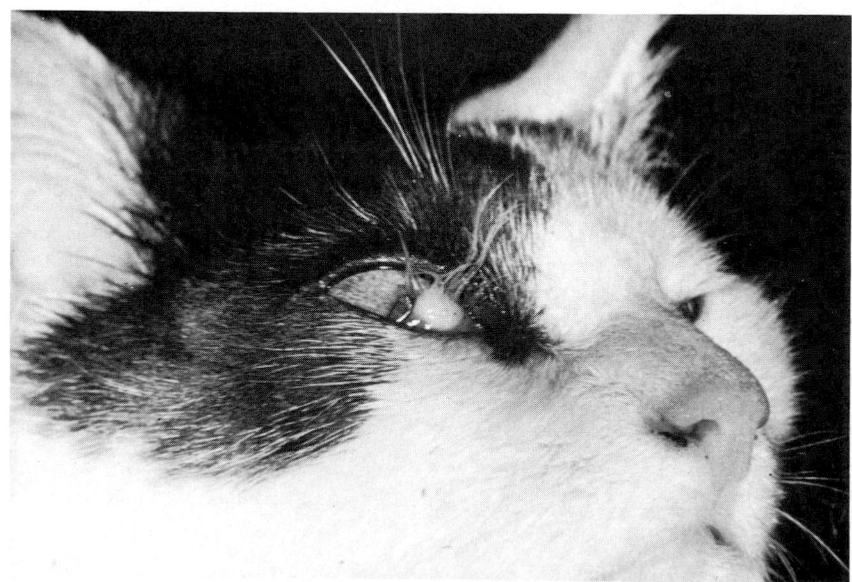

**Figure 14–16** Long hair arising from a dermoid of the third eyelid is seen at the medial canthus. (Courtesy Angell Memorial Animal Hospital.)

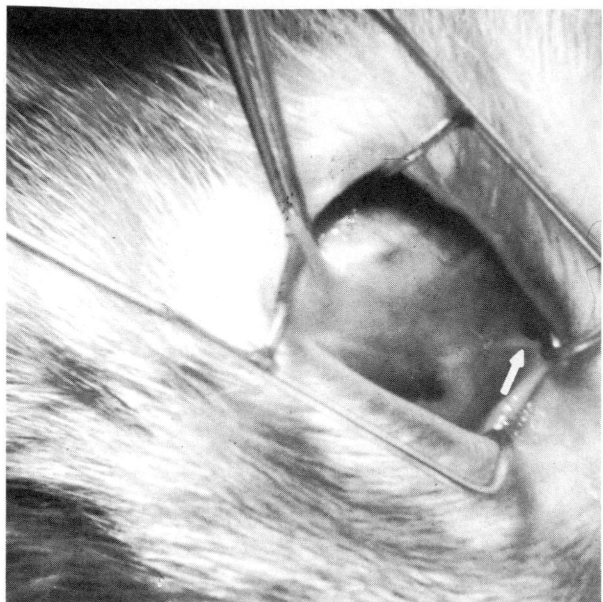

**Figure 14–17** Extensive corneal symblepharon was secondary to herpesvirus keratoconjunctivitis. The forceps grasps a portion of the symblepharon. A symblepharon also joins the third eyelid and cornea (arrow).

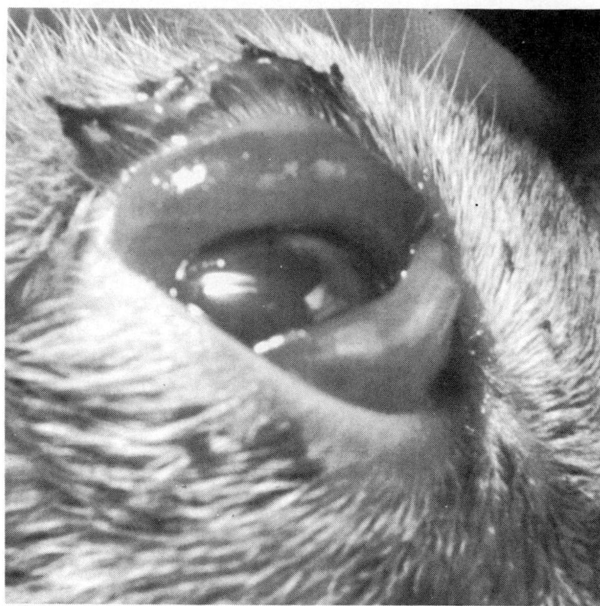

**Figure 14–18** Extensive hemorrhage of the dorsal bulbar conjunctiva and the conjunctiva of the third eyelid results in lagophthalmos.

Bands of scar tissue may bridge the bulbar and palpebral conjunctiva, and the fornices may be obliterated. The conjunctiva may adhere to the cornea (Fig. 14–17), and the third eyelid may be immobilized by cicatricial adhesions. The eyelid margins may acquire a notched appearance owing to adhesions of the palpebral conjunctiva. If scarring of the upper fornix occludes the lacrimal excretory ductules, keratitis sicca results. Occlusion of the lacrimal puncta is frequent, resulting in epiphora.

Surgery is warranted for extensive symblepharon. Superficial keratectomy frees the cornea of conjunctival adhesions. The keratectomy site is left uncovered. A topical antibiotic solution is applied after surgery until the cornea has epithelialized, then a topical antibiotic-corticosteroid solution is used for 7 to 10 days to prevent new adhesions. When large areas are involved, the conjunctival adhesions are cut, and the edges of the conjunctiva are undermined, drawn over the raw surfaces, and sutured with 6- or 7-0 absorbable material (Peiffer, 1981). Other surgical techniques for the treatment of symblepharon are described by Peiffer (1981).

**SUBCONJUNCTIVAL HEMORRHAGE.** Blunt trauma is a frequent cause of subconjunctival hemorrhage in cats. Treatment in uncomplicated cases is not necessary, as the blood is gradually resorbed in 10 to 14 days or less. Pain is absent in simple cases. If extensive subconjunctival hemorrhage causes the conjunctiva to protrude between the eyelids (Fig. 14–18), a temporary tarsorrhaphy is recommended to protect the cornea and swollen conjunctiva from exposure.

Bleeding disorders, including thrombocytopenia and autoimmune hemolytic anemia, may underlie cases of spontaneous subconjunctival hemorrhage not associated with trauma.

**CONJUNCTIVITIS.** Inflammation of the conjunctiva is common and may be uni- or bilateral. Conjunctivitis, regardless of etiology, exhibits the common signs of hyperemia, chemosis, and ocular discharge. The severity of these signs depends on etiology and duration. Pain is usually absent unless corneal disease coexists.

The diagnosis of conjunctivitis should be approached in a systematic manner. Conjunctivitis may be primary or secondary (Table 14–2). When obtaining the history, it is important to inquire whether the cat was recently hospi-

**Table 14–2 Classification of Conjunctivitis**

- **PRIMARY**
  - Microbial
    - Bacterial (including *Chlamydia*)
    - Viral
    - Mycoplasmal
    - Fungal
  - Chemical
    - Soap
    - Smoke
    - Aerosol sprays
    - Topical ophthalmic drugs
    - Chemical fumes
- **SECONDARY**
  - Mechanical Irritation
    - Entropion
    - Ectropion (cicatricial)
    - Dermoid
    - Eyelid agenesis
    - Lagophthalmos
    - Foreign body
    - Parasitic—*Thelazia*
    - Precorneal tear film deficiency
  - Periocular Extension
    - Sinusitis
    - Orbital fracture
    - Orbital abscess
    - Eyelid abscess
    - Dacryoadenitis
    - Endophthalmitis

talized, boarded, or taken to a show, and whether eye disease is present in companion cats. The owner should be asked to recall previous episodes, however mild, of upper respiratory infection. The general health of the cat should be assessed. One should inquire whether topical or systemic medication is being used. Prolonged topical medication of any kind, particularly neomycin, is capable of irritating the sensitive conjunctiva of cats. Ocular irritation subsides within 24 to 48 hours after the offending drug is discontinued.

A careful ophthalmic examination requires a good light source and magnification. The conjunctival surfaces and fornices and the bulbar aspect of the third eyelid are examined. Most helpful among diagnostic aids is conjunctival scraping for cytologic examination. A scraping to characterize the type of inflammatory response and possibly to demonstrate organisms or inclusion bodies is often more helpful than a culture. A Wright or Giemsa stain is recommended as well as a Gram stain. A bacterial culture and sensitivity test may be useful for chronic conjunctivitis or when large numbers of bacteria are seen in a conjunctival scraping. A Schirmer tear test is indicated in all cases of chronic or recurrent conjunctival disease. Nasolacrimal irrigation is also recommended, as dacryoadenitis may cause secondary conjunctivitis.

**Bacterial Conjunctivitis.** The conjuctival sac in the majority of normal cats is sterile. Among 240 samples, *Staphylococcus albus* and *Staphylococcus aureus* were cultured from 16.3 per cent and 10.4 per cent, respectively; alpha hemolytic streptococci from 2.5 per cent; *Bacillus* sp from 2.9 per cent; and *Corynebacterium* from 1.3 per cent (Campbell et al., 1973a).

Signs of acute bacterial conjunctivitis are severe conjunctival hyperemia, chemosis, purulent ocular exudate adhering to the palpebral margins, and varying degrees of blepharospasm. Acute infection may be secondary to an orbital abscess, infected eyelid wound, keratitis, or panophthalmitis, so careful examination is essential. Conjunctival scraping discloses predominantly toxic neutrophils and phagocytized bacteria.

Primary bacterial conjunctivitis, other than chlamydial, is uncommon in cats. Stress and decreased host resistance may allow opportunistic bacteria to cause infection. Unilateral conjunctivitis due to *Salmonella typhimurium* was reported in an adult cat (Fox and Galus, 1977). *Moraxella* was an uncommon organism isolated from conjunctivitis in a cattery (Withers and Davies, 1961).

Compatible clinical signs and favorable response to a topical broad-spectrum antibiotic ointment, such as neomycin-polymyxin B-bacitracin applied four to six times daily, support a diagnosis of bacterial conjunctivitis (Peiffer, 1981). Corticosteroids are not necessary in the treatment of acute bacterial conjunctivitis. If no response to therapy occurs after three to five days the condition should be reassessed. More common causes of conjunctivitis in the cat, such as herpes- or calicivirus, *Chlamydia*, or *Mycoplasma*, must be considered.

Recurrent bacterial conjunctivitis may be due to or cause dacryocystitis, for which nasolacrimal lavage is recommended. Decreased tear production, either transient or occasionally permanent, often complicates chronic conjunctivitis. A Schirmer tear test should be a routine diagnostic procedure in chronic conjunctivitis. Polyvinylpyrrolidone (Adapt*) or a petrolatum–lanolin–mineral oil ointment (Duratears†) is well tolerated by cats as a tear replacement.

**Viral Conjunctivitis.** Herpesvirus, calicivirus (picornavirus), and reovirus have been isolated from the conjunctival sac of cats. Only the herpesvirus and caliciviruses cause ocular disease of clinical importance.

Feline viral rhinotracheitis (FVR) is caused by a species-specific virus, *Herpes felis*, which is a significant ocular pathogen. Three age-related clinical types of ocular manifestations have been described (Bistner et al., 1971): (1) neonatal ophthalmia characterized by severe conjunctivitis, sometimes with corneal perforation, in kittens two to four weeks of age with systemic herpesvirus infection; (2) acute conjunctivitis in kittens one to six months of age with upper respiratory infection; and (3) keratoconjunctivitis, sometimes with upper respiratory infection, in older cats.

Signs of herpesvirus conjunctivitis are marked chemosis, serous or mucopurulent exudate, and a pseudodiphtheritic membrane. The severe conjunctivitis may result in conjunctival necrosis and symblepharon. Acute conjunctivitis is usually accompanied by signs of upper respiratory disease. Chronic herpetic conjunctivitis may be unaccompanied by obvious respiratory signs, but the owner, on questioning, may recall previous episodes of sneezing. Herpesvirus is the only respiratory virus involving the cornea. Herpetic keratitis will be discussed later in this chapter. Cytologic examination of a conjunctival scraping in herpesvirus infection discloses an initial lymphocytic response, followed by a neutrophilic response. Epithelial intranuclear inclusion bodies have not been found (Bistner et al., 1971). Definitive diagnosis may be obtained by virus isolation (from swabs in sterile skim milk or Eagle's medium), serum neutralization, hemagglutination-inhibition tests, and fluorescent antibody techniques. As these tests are seldom readily available, clinical diagnosis is based on characteristic signs and response to therapy. The keratitis associated with feline herpesvirus is effectively treated with topical idoxuridine (Stoxil, SmithKline Beckman), but whether it is helpful for herpes conjunctivitis is not known. Idoxuridine is used five or six times daily for six days. Corticosteroids are not recommended as they enhance viral growth (Peiffer, 1981). Sixty-nine per cent of cats with herpes infection may become carriers that, when stressed, develop recurrent clinical signs (Martin, 1981).

Calicivirus causes a mild conjunctivitis that may persist in chronic carriers (Ford, 1979). A topical broad-spectrum antibiotic may be used against secondary bacterial invasion.

Rarely reovirus, which produces intracytoplasmic inclusions, is identified in scrapings from naturally occurring conjunctivitis.

**Chlamydial Conjunctivitis.** Cats affected with *Chlamydia psittaci* are usually presented with a unilateral purulent conjunctivitis. Chemosis is marked (Fig. 14–19*A*). The second eye is often involved five to seven days later. Mild rhinitis is usual. Kittens born to infected or carrier queens may show severe neonatal conjunctivitis

*Burton-Parsons & Company, Washington, DC.

†Alcon Laboratories, Fort Worth, TX.

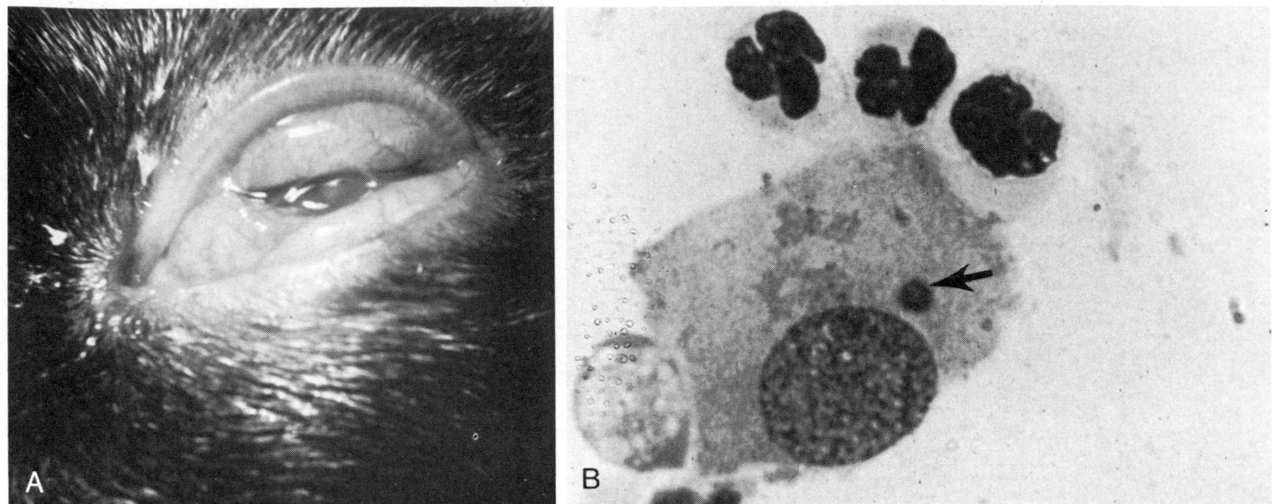

**Figure 14–19** *A*, Extensive chemosis is characteristic of acute chlamydial conjunctivitis. *B*, A chlamydial intracytoplasmic inclusion body within a conjunctival epithelial cell. Giemsa stain, ×1000.

when the eyelids open (Cello, 1967). Corneal involvement has not been reported.

Intracytoplasmic inclusion bodies (Fig. 14–19*B*) may be seen in Giemsa-stained conjunctival scrapings for as long as two weeks after infection.

Together with mild rhinitis and conjunctivitis, the demonstration of chlamydial inclusion bodies establishes the diagnosis. The organism reproduces within the cytoplasm of epithelial cells. Inclusions not recognizable with traditional stains may sometimes be demonstrated if stained with peroxidase-antiperoxidase using a monoclonal antibody for *Chlamydia** (Moore, 1985). *Chlamydia* is sensitive to topical tetracycline and chloramphenicol. Therapy should be continued for at least 28 days to cover the organisms' complete life cycle (Campbell, 1980). The untreated disease may persist for as long as 90 days (Cello, 1967).

**Mycoplasmal Conjunctivitis.** Conjunctival infection due to *Mycoplasma felis* (pleuropneumonia-like organism, PPLO) is at first characterized by epiphora, blepharospasm, and severe conjunctival hyperemia (Campbell et al., 1973). Papillary hypertrophy (minute epithelial projections surrounding a capillary core) is visible only by slit-lamp examination. Within 10 to 14 days after these initial signs, the hyperemia becomes less prominent, the papillary hypertrophy has disappeared, and the palpebral and bulbar conjunctivae have become pale, thickened, and chemotic. A pseudomembrane often forms on the conjunctival surface of the ventral cul-de-sac (Fig. 14–20*A*). Corneal involvement has not been reported.

*Ortho Diagnostic, Raritan, NJ.

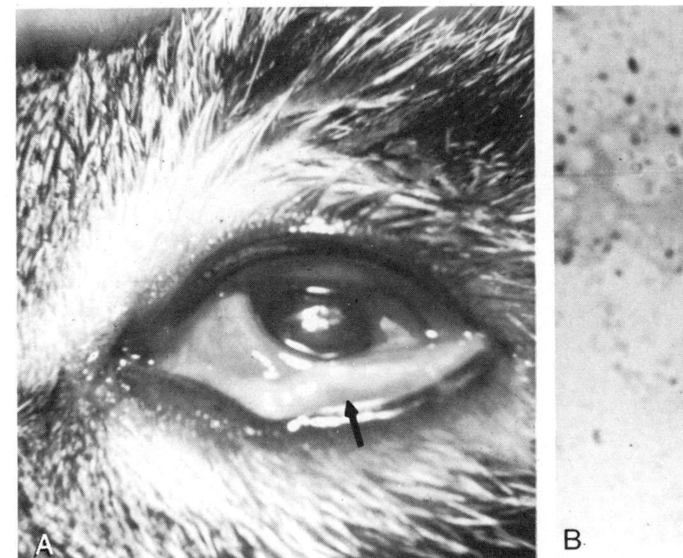

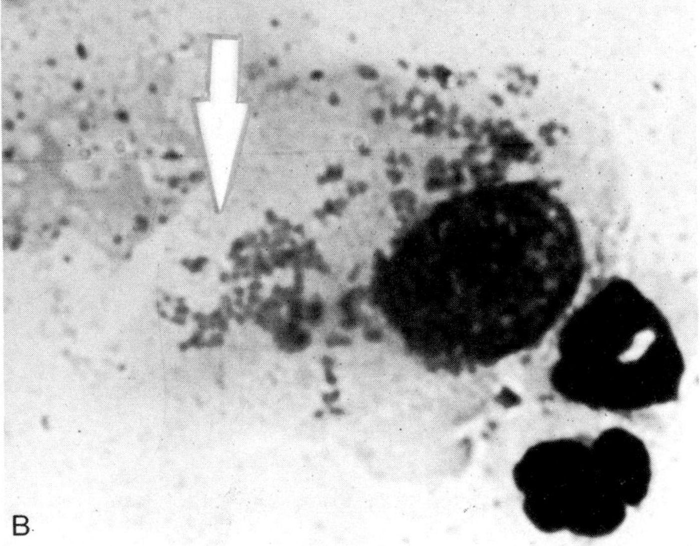

**Figure 14–20** *A*, A thick white pseudomembrane (arrow) is present in a cat with chronic *Mycoplasma*-induced conjunctivitis. Moderate chemosis is also present. *B*, *Mycoplasma* organisms (arrow) are dispersed over the surface of an epithelial cell in a conjunctival scraping. Giemsa stain, ×1000. (Courtesy Dr. L. H. Campbell.)

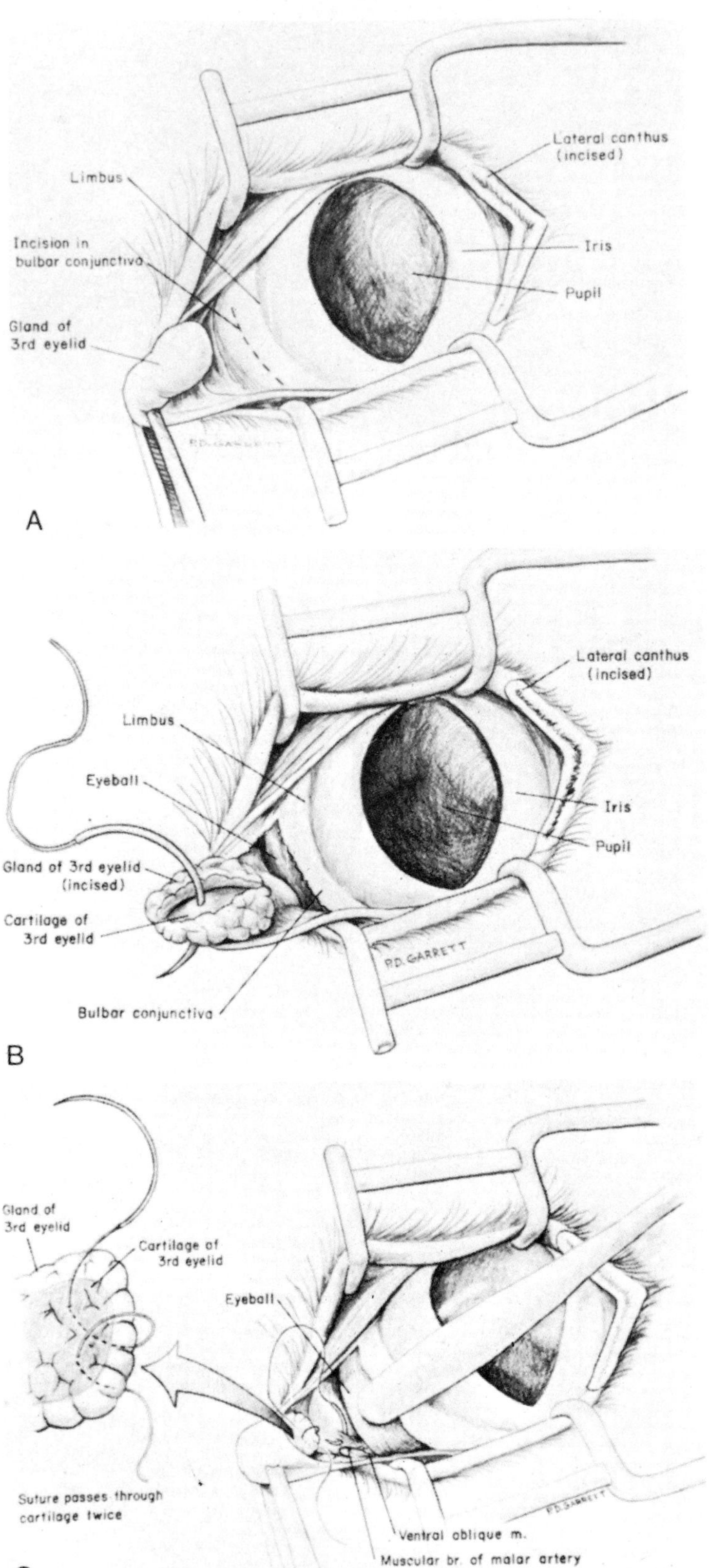


**Figure 14–21** *A*, Correction of everted cartilage of third eyelid. An initial incision through the bulbar conjunctiva is made 4 mm posterior to the limbus in the medial ventral quadrant of the globe. *B*, A second incision has been made through the inner (bulbar) aspect of the third eyelid to expose the cartilage. A 5-0 silk suture is being placed through the cartilage. *C*, The suture passes twice through the cartilage from anterior to posterior. The globe is retracted, and the initial incision is extended along the medial orbital wall to the origin of the ventral oblique muscle. The suture is passed through the muscle origin and then tied, causing the cartilage to straighten. A muscular branch of the malar artery must be avoided during suture placement.

*Illustration continued on opposite page*

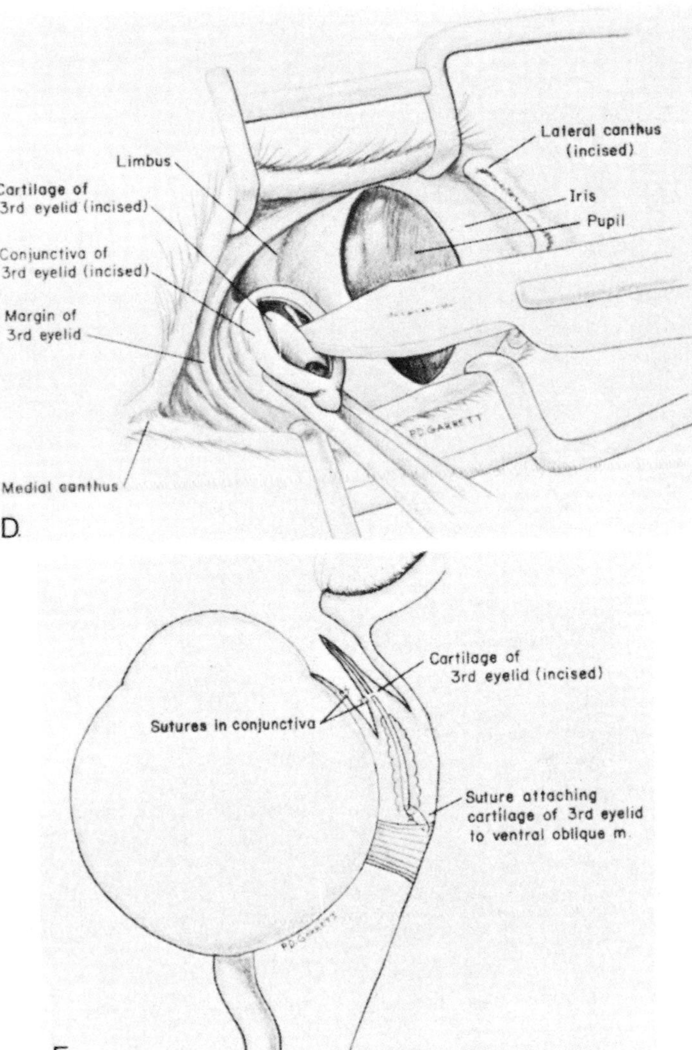


**Figure 14–21** *Continued D*, A full-thickness incision is made through the folded portion of the third eyelid. *E*, A dorsal view of the left eye shows the appearance after surgery. Compare with *A*. (From Albert RA, Garrett PD, Whitley RD, et al.: J Am Vet Med Assoc 180 [1982] 763–766.)

Giemsa-stained conjunctival scrapings may exhibit a neutrophilic response with clusters of basophilic coccoid *Mycoplasma* organisms on the surface of epithelial cells (Fig. 14–20*B*). The organism may be cultured on supplemented beef heart muscle agar (Peiffer, 1981). Mycoplasmal conjunctivitis often occurs together with other upper respiratory infections of cats.

*Mycoplasma* is sensitive to most antibiotics except penicillin and neomycin. Tetracycline is recommended, as it is also effective against *Chlamydia*, which may also be present. Dramatic improvement follows topical therapy, and clinical signs resolve in three to five days. Untreated infection may persist for up to 60 days. After regression of clinical signs, *Mycoplasma* could not be isolated from the conjunctiva of treated cats, a finding suggesting the absence of a carrier state (Campbell, 1980).

**Mycotic Conjunctivitis.** Mycotic conjunctivitis is rare in cats but has been reported in animals receiving topical antibiotics or corticosteroids for a prolonged period (Peiffer, 1981). Diagnosis is confirmed by culture of conjunctival scrapings or by biopsy.

**Parasitic Conjunctivitis.** *Thelazia californiensis* is an infrequent cause of conjunctivitis in cats living in the western United States. Signs are conjunctival hyperemia and rubbing of the eye caused by irritation from a slender worm 12 to 17 mm long behind the third eyelid. The worm is removed with a forceps after a topical anesthetic has been applied to the eye (Roberts and Lipton, 1975).

**NEOPLASMS OF THE CONJUNCTIVA.** Primary tumors of the conjunctiva are rare. A malignant melanoma has been described (Cook et al., 1985).

## Acquired Disorders of the Third Eyelid

**EVERSION OF THE CARTILAGE OF THE THIRD EYELID.** Everted cartilage of the third eyelid has been reported in two Burmese cats (Albert et al., 1982). The cartilage near the gland was folded upward and forward, displacing or prolapsing the gland. Hence the clinical appearance resembles the prolapsed gland ("cherry eye") of the canine third eyelid. The cause was stated to be deterioration of fascial attachments between the cartilage and deep orbital fascia.

Surgical correction in one cat was by repositioning the prolapsed gland of the third eyelid by passing a suture of 5-0 silk through the gland and cartilage and through the ventral oblique muscle. Tying the suture straightened the everted cartilage and returned the prolapsed gland to its normal position (Fig. 14–21*A* to *C*). In the second cat the everted cartilage was not flexible; therefore an incision was made in the everted cartilage to allow it to straighten out (Fig. 14–21*D, E*). All conjunctival incisions were closed with 6-0 chromic catgut. This technique has the advantage of preserving the gland of the third eyelid, which is a source of tears. A possible disadvantage, however, is that the third eyelid is immobilized.

**PROTRUSION OF THE THIRD EYELID.** The third eyelid may protrude (prolapse) over the corneal surface owing to corneal or conjunctival irritation, space-occupying orbital disease, or decreased orbital mass due to dehydration, loss of retrobulbar fat, microphthalmos, or phthisis bulbi. Both eyelids protrude with tetanus. Treatment and prognosis depend on the cause.

Bilateral protrusion of the third eyelid, sometimes called haw syndrome, is an entity of uncertain etiology peculiar to cats. It occurs mostly in cats under two years of age. Often they appear to be in good health, but the condition has also been observed in cats with digestive disturbances, virus infections, or heavy intestinal parasitism (Stansbury, 1966). Instillation of a sympathomimetic drug such as 1 or 2 per cent epinephrine or 10 per cent phenylephrine causes rapid retraction of the lids (Fig. 14–22). This response is suggestive of decreased sympathetic tone and postganglionic sympathetic denervation (Gelatt, 1979). The condition resolves spontaneously in several weeks or months without treatment. The sudden development and bizarre appearance of the syndrome is alarming to most cat owners, and it must be explained to them that primary lasting ocular disease is not present.

Bilateral protrusion of the third eyelid is also a conspicuous feature in autonomic polyganglionopathy (Key-Gaskell syndrome), a recently reported clinical entity among British cats. Persistent pupillary dilatation and decreased tear production are other ocular features of the condition, the gravest sign of which is a swallowing deficit due to megaesophagus. The British reports were reviewed by Barlough and Scott (1983).

Transient protrusion of the third eyelid is a common effect of certain tranquilizing drugs, and owners should be reassured that it is a phenomenon of no lasting consequence.

**HORNER'S SYNDROME.** Protrusion of the third eyelid is one of the chief components of Horner's syndrome (sympathetic denervation of the eye and adnexa). It is usually unilateral. Cats of any age may be affected. Other signs of Horner's syndrome are miosis, enophthalmos, narrowed palpebral fissure, and sometimes ptosis of the upper lid (Fig. 14–23). The syndrome is painless. The signs result from loss of smooth muscle tone in the eyeball and its adnexa (de Lahunta, 1973; Kay, 1981). All signs of Horner's syndrome are not invariably present. Lesions anywhere in the sympathetic chain may cause sympathetic denervation. The most common sites are in the T1–T3 ventral roots, cranial thoracic and cervical sympathetic trunks, and middle ear. Causes include cervical injury, surgery, mediastinal neoplasia, brachial plexus injury or neoplasia (particularly lymphosarcoma), and otitis media or removal of a middle-ear polyp. Sometimes the cause cannot be determined. Cats with Horner's syndrome should have a thorough physical examination; radiographs of the chest, neck, and middle ear; and a feline leukemia virus (FeLV) test. The condition often disappears rapidly if caused by minor injury or surgery.

**LACERATIONS.** The third eyelid is occasionally torn in a cat fight. The ragged edge will heal without treatment but should be sutured promptly if cosmetic considerations are important.

**NEOPLASMS OF THE THIRD EYELID.** Primary neoplasia of the third eyelid is rare in cats. A fibrosarcoma was reported by Morgan (1969), and another in a 15-year-old cat was successfully excised, with the affected membrane, by Buyukmihci (1975). Malignancy is the only indication for complete excision of the eyelid. Squamous cell carcinoma (Fig. 14–24) may involve the third eyelid primarily or secondarily by local invasion. Lymphosarcoma often involves the third eyelid and sometimes mast cell tumor originating in an upper or lower eyelid.

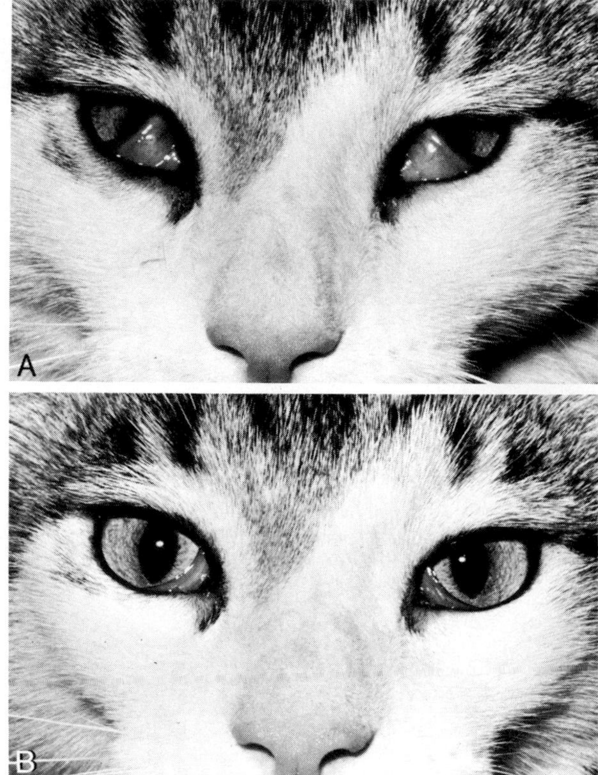


**Figure 14–22** *A*, Bilateral idiopathic protrusion of the third eyelids in a young healthy cat. *B*, Retraction of the third eyelids has occurred within five minutes after the instillation of 10 per cent phenylephrine ophthalmic solution.

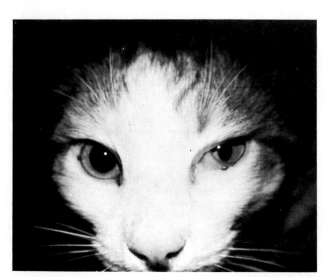

**Figure 14–23** Protrusion of the third eyelid, a miotic pupil, and ptosis (left eye) are typical of Horner's syndrome.

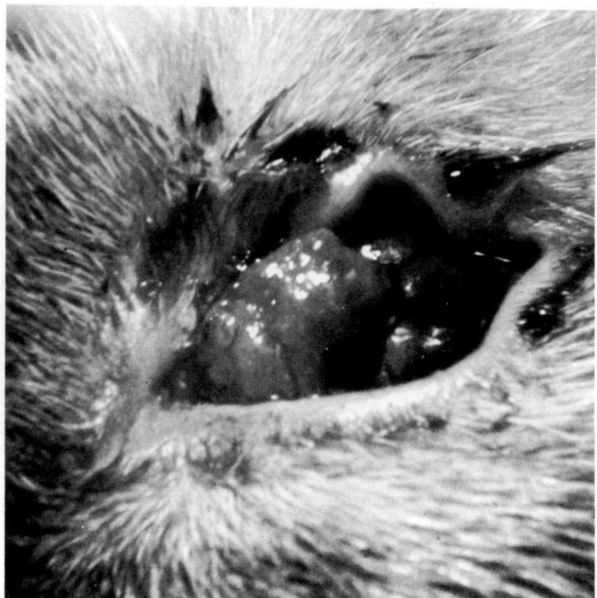

**Figure 14–24** The mass at the medial canthus is a squamous cell carcinoma of the third eyelid. Extension to the upper bulbar and palpebral conjunctiva caused lateral and ventral displacement of the globe.

# THE CORNEA

## Anatomy and Function

The cornea constitutes the transparent, avascular anterior 30 per cent of the fibrous coat of the globe. It is continuous with the sclera and together with the sclera forms the fibrous tunic that maintains the shape of the globe. The cornea is the principal refracting surface of the visual system and allows light to enter the interior of the eye.

The cat's cornea is nearly circular, with a horizontal diameter of 16.0 mm and a vertical diameter of 15.5 mm. The average corneal thickness is 0.62 to 0.68 mm (Prince et al., 1960). Its pronounced convexity increases the visual field of the cat.

The cornea is composed of four layers. From the external surface inward they are the anterior epithelium, stroma, posterior limiting (Descemet's) membrane, and the posterior epithelium (endothelium) (International Anatomical Nomenclature). The anterior epithelial cells are nonkeratinized stratified squamous cells. Although separate, the precorneal tear film is an important layer over the anterior corneal surface (Martin and Anderson, 1981). The anterior corneal epithelium regenerates rapidly after injury by sliding of adjacent cells and by mitosis. Removal of the anterior epithelium leads to stromal edema in the area of the defect. The edema disappears when the anterior epithelium regenerates.

The stroma (substantia propria) forms 90 per cent of the cornea and is composed of parallel collagen lamellae and fibroblasts (keratocytes) within a glycoprotein matrix or ground substance (Martin and Anderson, 1981).

Descemet's membrane is an acellular transparent membrane that covers the posterior surface of the stroma. It is composed of collagen fibrils, which are highly elastic in the cat. The posterior epithelium produces Descemet's membrane throughout life. Descemet's membrane does not retain fluorescein dye, an important clinical fact to remember when one is assessing corneal ulceration.

The posterior epithelium is a single layer of interdigitating polygonal cells that line the inner corneal surface. It is important in maintaining corneal deturgescence by two interrelated actions. It functions as a barrier between the aqueous and the stroma, and it is the site of the energy-dependent "metabolic pump" (Waring, 1982). Damage to the posterior epithelium allows aqueous humor to diffuse into the corneal stroma, resulting in edema that may be prolonged or permanent, as the posterior epithelium of the cat has limited regenerative ability (Van Horn et al., 1977).

The cornea is richly supplied with sensory nerves, most of which are in the anterior third of the stroma. These are derived from the ciliary nerves, which are branches of the ophthalmic division of the fifth cranial nerve. After entering the cornea the nerves are unmyelinated. In addition to the sensory cholinergic nerves, the cat has appreciable adrenergic fibers in the anterior cornea; their function is unknown (Martin and Anderson, 1981). Most of the corneal nutrients are received from the aqueous humor and the tear film. The limbal blood vessels supply nutrients to the periphery of the cornea.

## Congenital and Developmental Corneal Abnormalities

Congenital disorders of the cornea are rare in cats and may be classified as abnormalities of size or of transparency. Megalocornea is a cornea of abnormally large size, with normal intraocular pressure. Microcornea is a smaller than normal cornea, a condition not to be confused with microphthalmos. Both are rare in the cat (Roberts and Lipton, 1973).

Dermoid, not uncommon in the cat, is an elevated growth of skin and hair on the cornea, usually at the temporal limbus. Size is variable. Signs are related to corneal and conjunctival irritation by the hair. Removal is by superficial keratectomy.

Congenital opacities of the deep stroma and of Descemet's membrane may be single (Plate 14–1*E*) or multiple. Careful examination discloses remnants of fetal pupillary membranes (persistent pupillary membranes) arising from the iris collarette and attaching to Descemet's membrane. The site of attachment is opaque and white, and adjacent corneal edema may be present. Treatment is not advised. Persistent pupillary membranes must be differentiated from inflammatory adhesions (anterior synechiae) of the iris to the cornea. Anterior synechiae arise from the pupillary margin rather than from the iris collarette, which is the area between the base of the iris and the pupillary margin.

Bilateral keratoconus, an uncommon anomaly in which the cornea assumes the shape of a protruding cone, has been described (Chaillous and Robin, 1933). Keratoconus, together with anterior lenticonus, was observed in a Persian kitten (Peiffer and Belkin, 1983).

Unequal corneal curvature (astigmatism) was reported in a cat with other ocular defects (Bellhorn et al., 1971).

Corneal dystrophy, an ophthalmologic term, refers to

corneal opacification unrelated to previous ocular disease such as corneal ulceration.

A corneal dystrophy has been described in an inbred line of Manx cats (Bistner et al., 1976). Central corneal edema was noted as early as four months of age. Progression of the disease resulted in epithelial vesicles that often coalesced and ruptured, causing corneal ulceration. Histologic changes were stromal edema and intraepithelial vesicles and bullae. The endothelium appeared normal. Inheritance as an autosomal recessive trait was suggested, hence affected cats should not be bred. Prognosis is poor, and treatment is symptomatic, as topical hyperosmotic agents do not alter the course of the disease.

Suspected corneal dystrophy, characterized by central edema and recurrent ulceration has been observed in related domestic shorthairs (Peiffer, 1981).

Fine, granular, stromal opacities have been reported in cats affected with $GM_1$ gangliosidosis (Murray et al., 1977). The corneal opacities represented storage of water-soluble polysaccharide in the endothelial cells and corneal fibroblasts. Corneal clouding or stippling also occurs in $GM_2$ gangliosidosis, mucopolysaccharidosis I and VI, and mannosidosis. (See chapter on inherited metabolic diseases for the corneal and other ocular abnormalities occurring in the storage diseases.)

## Acquired Disorders of the Cornea

**CORNEAL LACERATIONS, PERFORATIONS, AND FOREIGN BODIES.** Corneal wounds are frequent in cats and are often due to claw injuries. Any area of the cornea may be involved, but the upper lateral quadrant seems especially vulnerable.

Small corneal perforations may seal with fibrin, and surgical repair may not be indicated if the anterior chamber is of normal depth. Signs of anterior uveitis, pain, miosis, aqueous flare, and possibly hyphema accompany corneal perforations. Small, sealed perforations are treated with topical and systemic antibiotics and topical atropine.

Corneal lacerations are accompanied by more severe signs. The appearance of a laceration needs little description; however, extensive chemosis is often present, and fibrin clots may adhere to the corneal surface and obscure the extent of the wound (Plate 14–1*F*). A foreign body such as a claw, splinter, or plant material may occasionally be embedded within a corneal laceration (Fig. 14–25). In these cases the eye is best examined when the cat is under general anesthesia so that its struggling will not cause prolapse of ocular contents.

Surgical repair should follow immediately. The corneal surface is gently irrigated with warmed sterile physiologic saline or Ringer's solution. Clipping of hair is not recommended, as this puts pressure on the globe. Prolapsed iris tissue may be reposited if it is viable and the wound is fresh; in most cases the iris tissue is devitalized or contaminated and should be excised. Intrastromal simple interrupted corneal sutures of chromic catgut or nylon (no larger than 6-0*) are placed to close the corneal defect. The anterior chamber is re-formed with warm sterile Ringer's solution or Balanced Salt Solution (Alcon Laboratories). If the suture line leaks, additional sutures are placed.

*Micro-point spatula GS-8 needle; Ethicon, Inc, Somerville, NJ.

Corneal lacerations that extend to the limbus should be presumed to extend into the sclera. Bulbar conjunctival dissection may be needed to determine the presence or extent of scleral laceration. These lacerations are closed with 6-0 or finer absorbable suture material.

After surgery, medication consists of topical and systemic antibiotics and topical atropine. The individual case dictates the use of topical or systemic steroids, or both; such medication is indicated if inflammation is marked. Corneal sutures may be removed in two weeks.

**SUPERFICIAL CORNEAL ULCERATION.** Superficial corneal ulceration or erosion denotes loss of the corneal epithelium. Complicating factors such as microbial infection are absent. The large and prominent cornea of the cat frequently sustains injury from mechanical irritation, scratches, smoke, thermal burns, chemical sprays, or soap. Lagophthalmos and the evaporation of tears during ketamine anesthesia may result in epithelial ulceration, unless protective ophthalmic ointment is instilled immediately after the ketamine has been given.

An acute onset of corneal pain manifested by blepharospasm and epiphora is typical of a superficial ulcer. Loss of corneal epithelium may be demonstrated by fluorescein dye–impregnated strips (Fluor-I-Strip, Ayerst Laboratories) moistened in physiologic saline solution and touched to the dorsal bulbar conjunctiva.

A superficial corneal ulcer is treated with a topical broad-spectrum antibiotic ointment or solution three or four times daily to prevent corneal infection by opportunistic bacteria. The treatment is continued until the lesion has epithelialized. Uncomplicated superficial ulcerations heal rapidly, often within 48 to 72 hours, depending on their size. Topical corticosteroids are contraindicated when the cornea is ulcerated, because they inhibit epithelial regeneration (Havener, 1978). The use of hydrophilic contact lenses is helpful in some cases of chronic superficial ulceration (Morgan et al., 1984).

**DEEP CORNEAL ULCERATION.** Deep corneal ulcerations, including descemetoceles, are regarded as complicated ulcers. Bacterial infection or corneal necrosis due to destructive enzymes such as collagenase or protease may end in corneal perforation.

Deep corneal ulcers may be secondary to any trauma but are frequently associated with cat-fight scratches. Superficial ulcers may become infected with staphylococci, streptococci, or occasionally *Pseudomonas* (Peiffer, 1981). Herpesvirus sometimes involves the deep corneal stroma. Concurrent disorders such as keratitis sicca, foreign bodies, lagophthalmos, or debilitating systemic disease may complicate corneal healing. Signs of complicated ulcers include blepharospasm, epiphora, and moderate to severe corneal edema. Corneal vascularization is evident three to five days after the onset of keratitis. Superficial vessels, derived from the bulbar conjunctiva, have a branching appearance. Deep vessels originating from the anterior ciliary vessels are straight, small, and close to the limbus. Deep vascularization indicates secondary anterior uveitis, which is frequent with complicated ulcers. Other signs of uveitis are miosis, edema of the iris, aqueous flare, and sterile hypopyon.

Deep stromal ulcers have a crater-like appearance owing to loss of corneal substance. The ulceration may extend to Descemet's membrane, causing a descemetocele. This may prolapse forward because of the cat's very elastic membrane (Plate 14–1*G*), or the descemetocele may appear as a flat, glassy membrane at the bottom of

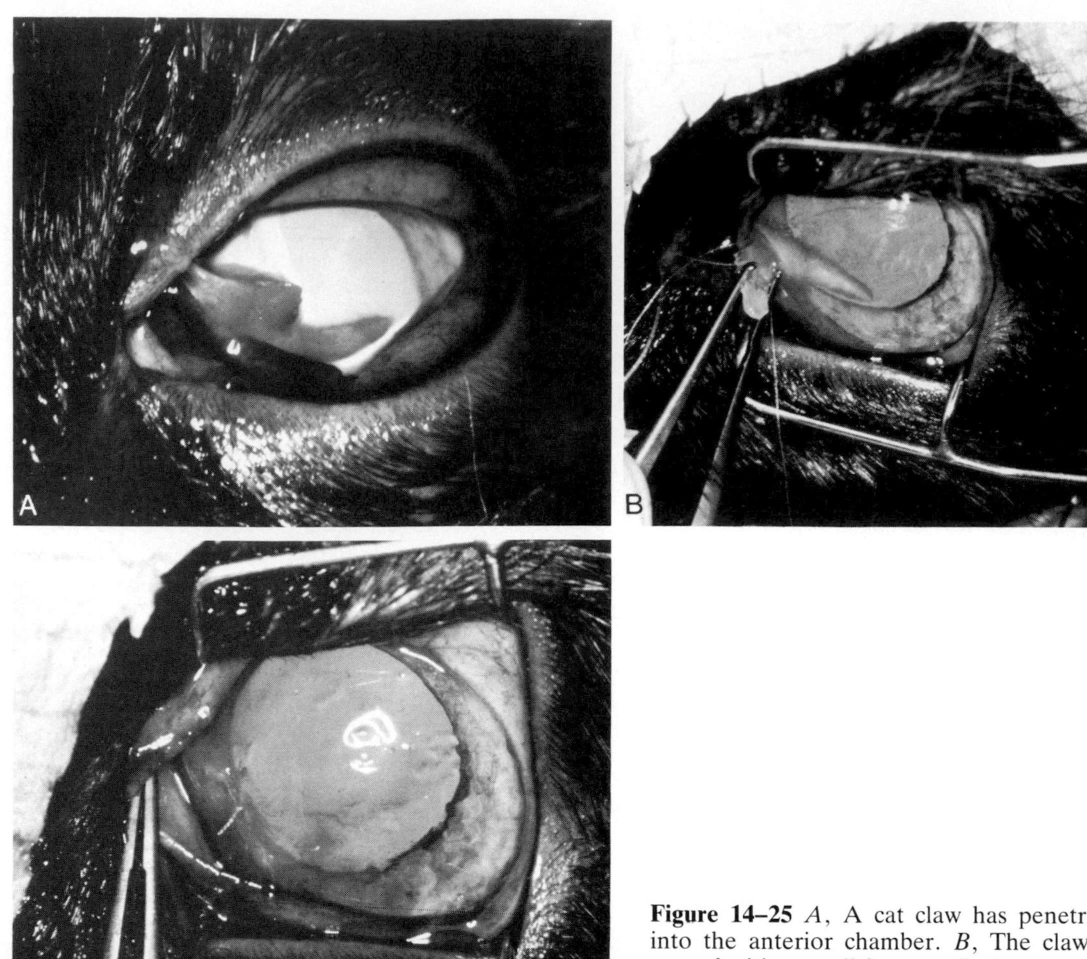


**Figure 14–25** *A*, A cat claw has penetrated the cornea into the anterior chamber. *B*, The claw is carefully removed with a small forceps. *C*, Appearance of the cornea after suturing with 7-0 chromic catgut. (Courtesy Dr. M. Wyman.)

a deep ulcer (Plate 14–1*H*). Descemet's membrane does not retain fluorescein dye. Corneal necrosis (keratomalacia) may accompany *Pseudomonas* keratitis or almost any deep ulceration.

Deep corneal ulcers or descemetoceles are urgent ocular problems. Treatment depends on etiology, although most require surgery. Bacterial culture and sensitivity testing and cytologic examination may be helpful. History may disclose inappropriate treatment with topical corticosteroids or bizarre home remedies. Failure to heal despite intensive treatment with topical broad-spectrum antibiotics is sometimes a clue to herpes keratitis.

Refractory deep corneal ulcers or descemetoceles are best managed surgically. A third eyelid flap, a thin bulbar conjunctival flap, or a corneoscleral conjunctival transposition may be used, depending on the surgeon's experience and the size of the lesion (Martin, 1981; Wyman, 1979). Postoperative medication consists of topical and systemic antibiotics and topical atropine ointment. Topical gentamicin (Schering) or tobramycin (Alcon Laboratories) is used for *Pseudomonas* keratitis. Merely suturing the eyelids together (tarsorrhaphy) is unacceptable, as observation of the eye and effective topical treatment are impossible. Proper management often results in a sighted eye, but permanent scarring of variable degree will be present.

Iris prolapse through a perforated corneal ulcer may be managed by replacing the prolapsed iris (within 12 to 24 hours) or, if the iris tissue is grossly contaminated or devitalized, by excising it flush with the wound edge. A small corneal defect may be closed with 6- or 7-0 absorbable or nonabsorbable sutures placed intrastromally. Suture placement is aided by the use of a magnifying loupe. A large corneal defect within a friable and necrotic cornea may be covered with a thin bulbar conjunctival flap. Postoperative treatment consists of a topical broad-spectrum antibiotic and atropine ointment.

**HERPETIC KERATITIS.** Keratitis due to *Herpes felis* has been described by Bistner et al. (1971). It may be uni- or bilateral and usually affects adult cats that have had recent, often mild, upper respiratory signs. Cats are presented with mild or moderate blepharospasm and serous ocular discharge. The classic corneal lesion, best demonstrated by fluorescein staining, is an irregular corneal dendrite involving the epithelium and anterior stroma (Plate 14–1*I*). The pattern of this dendritic ulcer is considered pathognomonic for feline herpes keratitis.

Not all cases are typical. Fine, linear or punctate

epithelial defects accompanied by epiphora are early lesions that may be detected only by fluorescein staining and examination with a cobalt or ultraviolet light. Some cats are presented with a chronic corneal ulcer of irregular shape and variable depth, accompanied by vascularization (Fig. 14–26). These cats are often being faithfully medicated with a topical broad-spectrum antibiotic, yet corneal healing does not progress. Corneal sensation is often diminished with herpesvirus keratitis, so that blepharospasm may not be present and hypoesthesia may be detected. Secondary anterior uveitis is frequent, as is keratoconjunctivitis sicca.

Definitive diagnosis requires special laboratory procedures (Peiffer, 1981). Clinical diagnosis is based on history, signs, and favorable response to topical idoxuridine (IDU) (Stoxil, SmithKline Beckman). IDU prevents replication of herpesvirus. To be effective, it must be given often. An empirically successful treatment regime is IDU ophthalmic ointment every four hours for five or six days. Response to treatment is evident in less than six days. Treatment should be continued every six hours for several days after healing occurs.

Adenine arabinoside (Vira-A, Parke-Davis) and trifluorothymidine (Viroptic, Burroughs Wellcome) are also effective against herpetic keratitis. Povidone-iodine (1 part to 4 parts sterile physiologic saline, 1 drop every two or three hours) has been recommended as a less costly but effective treatment (Brightman, 1983).

Two per cent aqueous iodine solution is virucidal and may be used at the start of treatment to gently débride the affected corneal epithelium. A concurrent topical broad-spectrum antibiotic is recommended to prevent secondary bacterial infection (Peiffer, 1981).

Depressed immune response as occurs with stress, corticosteroid therapy, feline leukemia virus, and feline infectious peritonitis may play a role in the recurrence of herpetic keratitis. Because herpesvirus has been isolated from the trigeminal ganglion of the cat, it has been postulated that the ganglion acts as a reservoir for latent herpesvirus, which becomes activated during periods of stress (Gaskell and Povey, 1979).

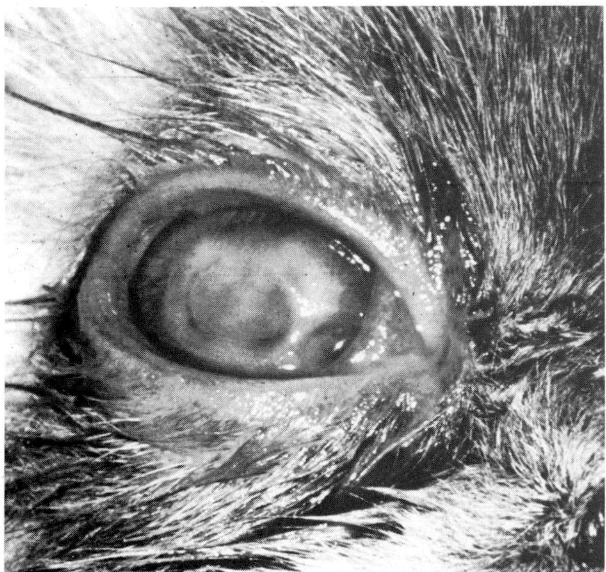

**Figure 14–26** A large midstromal corneal ulcer and corneal vascularization are present in a cat with chronic herpesvirus keratitis.

**CORNEAL SEQUESTRATION.** Corneal sequestration, a type of stromal necrosis that follows chronic ulcerative keratitis, is unique to the cat. The condition is usually unilateral. All breeds may be affected, but Persians and Siamese appear predisposed (Peiffer, 1981). The most striking sign is a flat black or brown plaque in the axial cornea (Plate 14–1*J*). The surrounding cornea may be ulcerated, edematous, or both. Superficial corneal vascularization is present. The clinical course is chronic and may be months to years in duration (Gelatt, 1979; Roberts and Lipton, 1975). The cause of feline corneal sequestation is not known, but chronic ulceration precedes most cases. Histologic examination of corneal sequestra reveals coagulation necrosis of the stroma and adjacent epithelium. The pigment has not been identified; although it is not melanin, it may be a melanin precursor (Martin, 1981).

A corneal sequestrum may occasionally slough or be extruded after a prolonged period. The most expeditious treatment is excision by superficial keratectomy. If the sequestrum extends into the deep corneal stroma it may be excised and the deep keratectomy wound repaired by a sliding lamellar, corneoscleral transposition (Fig. 14–27) (Riis, 1982). After either type of surgery, the eye should be treated with topical atropine and antibiotic ointments. A corticosteroid may be used after the keratectomy has epithelialized or after the transposition has healed.

**MYCOBACTERIAL KERATITIS.** Tuberculoma of the cornea is one of the less common ocular manifestations of this infectious disease described among European cats (Veenendaal, 1928). Dice (1977) has reported a corneal granuloma associated with a cellular infiltrate and acid-fast bacilli suggestive of feline leprosy.

**MYCOTIC KERATITIS.** Mycotic keratitis (keratomycosis) is rare in cats and may be associated with long-term topical corticosteroid therapy. *Candida albicans* and *Aspergillus* have been cited as etiologic agents (Peiffer, 1981). Involved corneas are intensely inflamed. *Drechslera spicifera* has also been recognized as a cause of mycotic keratitis (Zapater et al., 1975). Diagnosis is established by culture and demonstration of organisms in corneal scrapings.

A bilateral keratopathy presumed to be due to *Rhinosporidium* was reported in two cats by Peiffer and Jackson (1979). Signs were multiple focal corneal opacities measuring from 1 to 8 mm; a superficial corneal ulcer was present in one cat. Natamycin (Natacyn, Alcon Laboratories) is currently the only commercially available antifungal agent for topical use. Amphotericin B, clotrimazole, nystatin, and miconazole have been used topically to treat keratomycoses, but they have not been approved for ocular use. Inflammatory signs were minimal, and the condition appeared to be self-limiting. Superficial keratectomy was performed for diagnostic purposes, and spores resembling those of *Rhinosporidium* were demonstrated. Treatment was not recommended.

**PROTOZOAL KERATITIS.** A case of microsporidial infection of the cornea was reported in a three and a half-year-old domestic shorthair (Buyukmihci, 1977). Clinical signs were blepharospasm of six months' duration and

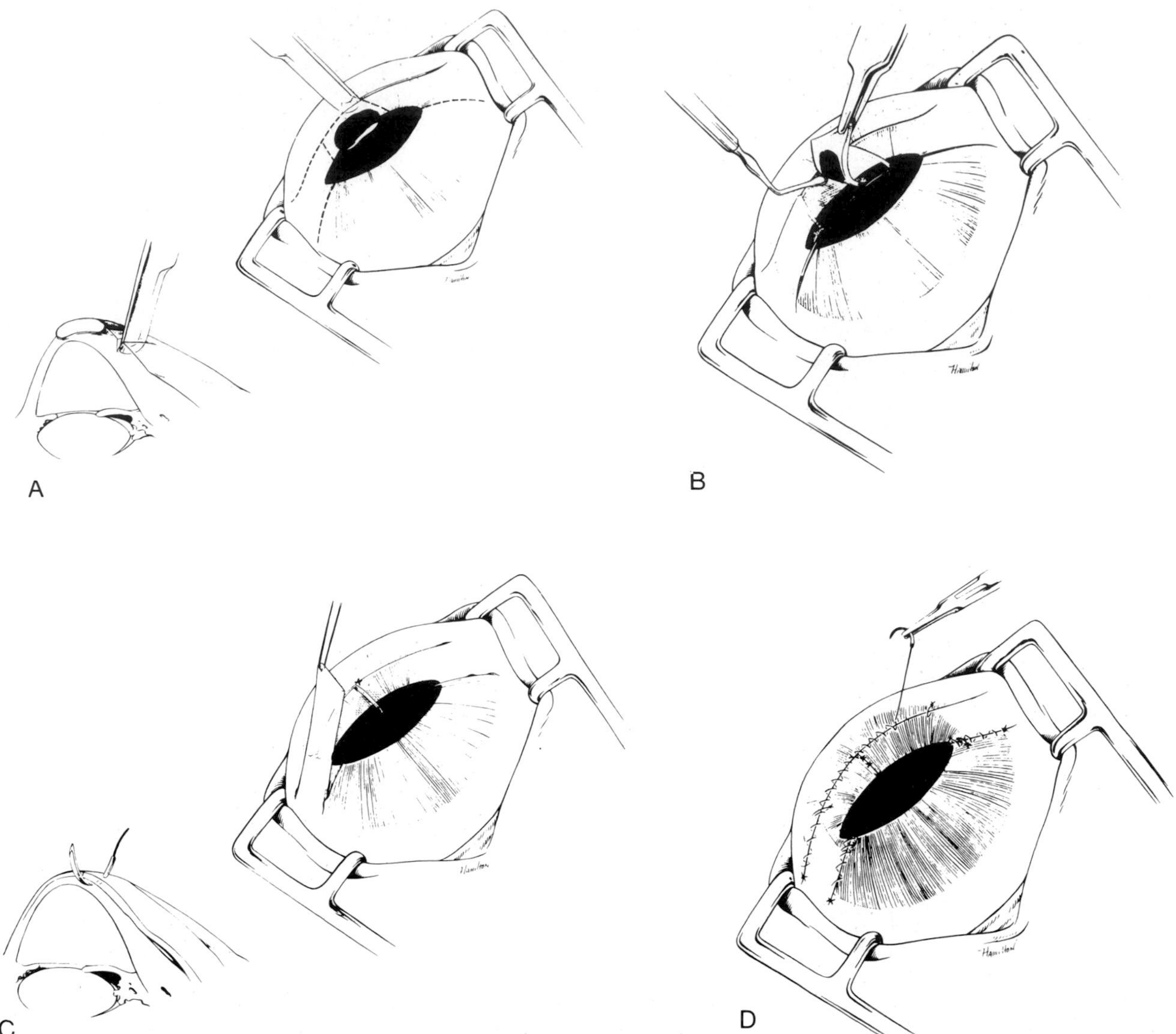


**Figure 14–27** *A*, Sliding lamellar corneal-scleral transposition was required to repair a deep keratectomy incision made for removal of a central sequestrum. A Beaver 64 blade is used to cut one-half to two-thirds the depth of the corneal thickness to excise the plaque. The incision is extended around the plaque and toward the limbus. At the limbus the incision includes conjunctival and episcleral tissue and is flared wider than the corneal incision to allow for stretching. *B*, The sequestrum is removed by grasping a corner of the incision with a fine forceps and undermining in an even plane parallel to the corneal surface. Once the plaque is removed, dissection to free the cornea is continued in the same plane and extended toward the limbus. Because the cat sclera is fairly thin, the depth of the dissection past the limbus should be conjunctival and episcleral only. *C*, The lamellar corneal graft is realigned toward the center of the cornea, and the corner is anchored with 8-0 Vicryl suture material (Ethicon). A G-S needle is used to minimize penetration into the stroma. *D*, The entire border of the transposed lamellar graft is sutured with a continuous pattern of 8-0 Vicryl sutures. Several single interrupted sutures are placed for security. These do not need to be removed. (From Riis RC: Proc Am Soc Vet Ophthalmol and Int Soc Vet Ophthalmol, Las Vegas, Nevada, 1982, 1–9).

superficial corneal opacities in a stellate pattern. Electron microscopy of the keratectomy specimen disclosed spores compatible with *Encephalitozoon* or *Nosema* of the class Microsporidia, agents once thought to be synonymous but now distinguished as separate genera. Keratectomy in this case was curative.

**EOSINOPHILIC KERATITIS.** Eosinophilic keratitis (Brightman et al., 1979) is unique to cats and is characterized by a raised, pink, proliferative lesion involving the cornea and adjacent limbus (Plate 14–1*K* and *L*). The cornea at the leading edge of the lesion may be ulcerated. Superficial corneal vascularization surrounds the mass. One or both eyes may be involved. Signs are mild blepharospasm and seromucoid discharge. The author has observed cats with eosinophilic keratitis that have had concomitant, confirmed lesions of eosinophilic granuloma of the lips. The majority of cats with eosinophilic keratitis, however, do not also have skin lesions. The etiology is at present unknown.

The mass may be excised by superficial keratectomy. Biopsy shows granulation tissue and stromal infiltration of eosinophils and fewer plasma cells and lymphocytes. Scraping of the mass and cytologic examination may provide a more rapid diagnosis. New methylene blue stain is used. Eosinophils and lesser numbers of mast cells and plasma cells are seen (Fig. 14–28). Either biopsy or cytologic examination is important, as eosinophilic keratitis must be differentiated from secondary corneal involvement of squamous cell carcinoma, lymphosarcoma, or excessive corneal granulation tissue associated with chronic keratoconjunctivitis sicca.

Megestrol acetate (Ovaban, Schering), 5 mg once daily, is given until the lesion begins to regress. The dosage is then reduced to 5 mg or less on alternate days. An effective dose is considered to be the least amount needed to keep the cornea lesion-free. Topical corticosteroids induce regression, but long-term control is best attained with megestrol acetate.

**CHRONIC PROLIFERATIVE KERATITIS.** A few cases of a curious chronic keratitis characterized by "cottage cheese"–like plaques have been described in Great Britain and the United States (Bedford and Cotchin, 1983; Pentlarge and Riis, 1984). A characteristic unidentified eosinophilic deposit is present in the corneal stroma and epithelium. It has been treated by keratectomy but is most responsive to megestrol acetate (Bedford and Cotchin, 1983).

**LIPID KERATOPATHY.** A lipid keratopathy similar to that in humans developed in a cat after a fight injury to the cornea (Carrington, 1983). A pale discoid plaque was removed but recurred in three weeks. The cat was found to have an elevated level of serum cholesterol, and the lesion was kept static by medication with liothyronine.

**NEOPLASMS OF THE CORNEA.** Primary corneal tumors are extremely rare. An infiltrative lesion resembling fibrous histiocytoma has been described (Smith et al., 1976). Secondary corneal involvement may occur when a tumor such as squamous cell carcinoma or melanoma arises from the limbus. Lymphosarcoma may involve the cornea secondarily. Diagnosis is obtained by biopsy; treatment depends on the extent of involvement.

## THE LENS

### Anatomy

The lens is an avascular, biconvex, transparent structure located behind the iris. It is relatively larger in the cat than in the dog and occupies about 10 per cent of the volume of the eye. Its transverse diameter is 12 to 13 mm and it may be up to 8 mm thick (Prince et al., 1960). It lies within the hyaloid fossa, a depression in the anterior vitreous surface. The ciliary zonule attaches the lens to the valleys between the ciliary processes (Martin and Anderson, 1981). The lens consists of about 65 per cent water and 35 per cent protein (Schmidt and Coulter, 1981). The lens capsule is the superficial layer of the lens and maintains its shape. Cats have a limited amplitude of accommodation (4 diopters) (Maguire et al., 1981). The lens epithelium, which lies under the anterior lens capsule, is the source of lens fibers, which are formed throughout life. The oldest, central portion of the lens is the embryonal nucleus. This is surrounded from within outward by the fetal and adult nuclei and finally the cortex, the region just under the capsule. The lens fibers elongate in the direction of the anterior and posterior poles of the cortex. Where the ends from the opposite sides meet, they form Y-patterned sutures. Those sutures in the anterior lens appear as an erect Y, and those in the posterior form an inverted Y. The lens derives its nutrition from the aqueous humor through the semipermeable lens capsule.

### Congenital and Developmental Anomalies of the Lens

Aphakia, total absence of the lens, is extremely rare. Bilateral aphakia associated with flat peripapillary retinal

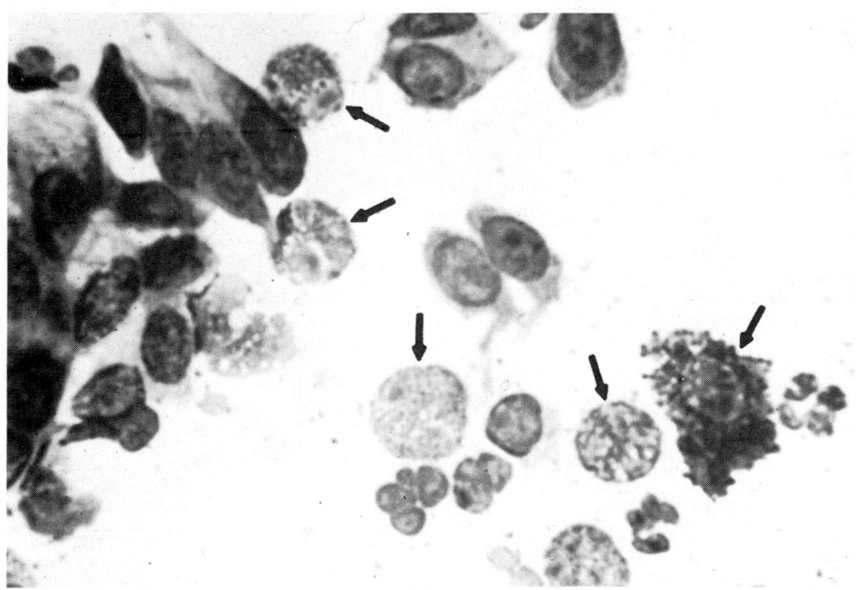

**Figure 14–28** Scraping from eosinophilic keratitis reveals characteristic mast cells and eosinophils (arrows) New methylene blue, ×1000.

detachments was reported in a three-year-old domestic shorthair (Peiffer, 1981).

Bilateral microphakia has been reported in two cats (Aguirre and Bistner, 1973). The equator of the congenitally small lens and elongated ciliary processes could be seen after pupillary dilation. Although the lenses were luxated or displaced from the hyaloid fossa, the zonular attachments were intact. In cases of anterior luxation, surgery is recommended to remove the displaced lens.

A cataract is defined as any opacity of the lens or its capsule. Congenital cataracts may be associated with persistent pupillary membrane. The anterior capsule and underlying cortex are involved. These cataracts are usually focal and nonprogressive. Congenital cataracts may involve the embryonal or fetal nucleus, or both. Prenatal inflammation or infections have been suggested as causes. Congenital cataracts were reported by Priester (1972) and by Peiffer and Gelatt (1974) and also occur in blue smoke Persian cats affected with the Chédiak-Higashi syndrome (Kramer et al., 1977; Prieur et al., 1979). Bilateral cataracts, together with cerebellar ataxia, were described in a kitten three weeks of age (Chaillous et al., 1931)—a combination suggestive of perinatal panleukopenia infection. Hereditary cataract has been reported in Himalayans (Rubin, 1986).

Congenital cataracts may occur in microphthalmic globes. Surgery is not advised, as other intraocular anomalies may be present.

Persistence of the hyaloid artery, which nourishes the lens during fetal development, has been reported (Roberts and Lipton, 1975).

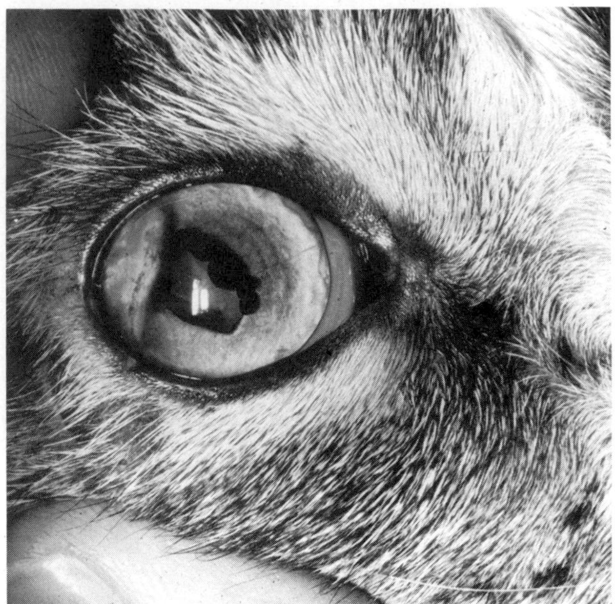

**Figure 14–29** A traumatic cataract has resulted from a corneal laceration and tearing of the lens capsule. The healed laceration is visible in the dorsolateral quadrant of the cornea. Eversion of the iris pigment epithelium (ectropion uveae) appears as black masses along the pupillary border.

## Acquired Disorders of the Lens

Nuclear sclerosis is not a disease of the lens, but rather a normal, aging change. It is seen in cats over seven years of age as a bilateral, blue-gray translucency of the lens nucleus and results from the compaction and hardening of lens fibers. It does not affect sight or impede the examiner's visualization of the fundus, characteristics that differentiate this disorder from cataract.

**CATARACTS.** Acquired cataracts are of varied etiology.

**Traumatic Cataracts.** Cataracts secondary to trauma are the type most often encountered in the cat. Corneal laceration with tearing of the anterior lens capsule is a frequent cause (Fig. 14–29). The extent and progression of a traumatic cataract is variable. Adhesions of the iris to the lens are usual with traumatic cataracts. Surgery is not advisable in most cases.

**Inflammatory Cataracts.** Inflammatory cataracts may occur with uveitis of any etiology. Posterior synechiae and alterations in the aqueous humor that disrupt the nutrition of the lens contribute to cataract formation. Cataract extraction is not successful when uveitis and synechiae are present.

**Metabolic Cataracts.** Cataracts associated with diabetes mellitus are not nearly so common in cats as in dogs. The progression of these cataracts appears to be slow (Peiffer, 1981).

**Drug-Induced Cataracts.** Systemic corticosteroids may induce cataracts that may be reversible if the drug is withdrawn. Chronic use of strong anticholinesterase agents can cause anterior cortical cataracts (Peiffer, 1981).

**Developmental Cataracts.** Developmental or primary cataracts affect young cats. They are not secondary to trauma, inflammation, or metabolic causes. Inheritance of primary cataracts has not been reported in the cat. These cataracts are usually bilateral, but the extent of involvement may differ. Spontaneous cataract resorption may occur in cats six months to three years of age. If lens-induced uveitis occurs, it should be treated with mydriatics and corticosteroids.

Cataract extraction is an elective procedure that will improve vision if the retina is normal. Techniques of cataract extraction are described (Bistner et al., 1977; Peiffer and Gelatt, 1973). If a cataract involves only the lens nucleus, a mydriatic may improve vision.

**LENS LUXATION.** Displacement of the lens from the hyaloid fossa occurs occasionally in cats. In anterior lens luxation the lens has become displaced through the pupil into the anterior chamber (Plate 14–1*M*). Secondary glaucoma may result from mechanical obstruction of the filtration angle or pupillary block. Lens extraction is the treatment of choice for anterior luxation (Bistner et al., 1977).

The lens may also luxate posteriorly into the vitreous cavity. As a result, the anterior chamber deepens and iridodonesis (quivering of the iris) is present. Surgical extraction of a posteriorly luxated lens is not recommended because of the high incidence of surgical complications, which are greater than those occurring when the lens is left in the vitreous.

# THE VASCULAR TUNIC (UVEA)

## Anatomy and Function

The vascular tunic (uvea, uveal tract) consists of the iris, ciliary body, and choroid. The iris is the anterior part of the vascular tunic and separates the anterior and posterior chambers of the eye. Its central aperture, the pupil, regulates the amount of light entering the eye. The anterior surface of the iris is green, yellow, or copper in most cats. It is dull violet-blue in young kittens. When little pigment is present, as in Siamese, Himalayans, or blue-eyed white cats, the iris appears blue. The varying types of pigment deficit in Siamese and white cats are well described by Thibos et al. (1980). Some white cats have one blue eye and one yellow or green. When pigment is absent, as in the rare complete albino, the iris appears pink (Todd, 1961).

Pupillary size is determined by the two muscles of the iris, the radially oriented dilator pupillae and the sphincter pupillae. The sphincter is parasympathetically innervated by the third cranial nerve (oculomotor); it also receives a small number of sympathetic nerve terminals (Geltzer, 1969). Contraction of the iris sphincter results in a small slit-like (miotic) pupil. The dilator in the cat is poorly developed on the vertical meridian but well developed on the horizontal (Martin and Anderson, 1981). In exotic cats, the constricted pupil is round; in the domestic cat the pupil is constricted to a vertical slit, because the sphincter pupillae includes fibers that intersect and cross at acute angles at the dorsal and ventral commissures of the iris (see figure, Trautmann and Fiebiger, 1957). McClure et al. (1973) state that the muscle fibers are thicker and longer on the medial and lateral sides of the pupil.

The anatomy of the postganglionic parasympathetic nerve supply to the iris sphincter is unique to the cat. Only two short ciliary nerves (compared with at least eight in the dog) extend from the ciliary ganglion. The medial short ciliary nerve innervates the medial half of the iris sphincter, the lateral short ciliary nerve the lateral half of the iris sphincter (Scagliotti, 1980). A lesion of the medial short ciliary nerve causes dilatation of only the medial half of the iris, while a lesion of the lateral short ciliary nerve causes dilatation of only the lateral half of the iris. This phenomenon is referred to as the D- or reverse-D effect.

Classically, the iris dilator was thought to be solely under sympathetic innervation; however, histochemical fluorescence and electron microscopic studies have identified both cholinergic and adrenergic nerve fibers in the cat's iris dilator muscle (Ehinger, 1967; Geltzer, 1969). This dual innervation may be a factor in the failure of 10 per cent phenylephrine to fully dilate the cat's iris (Gelatt, 1979).

The ciliary body lies between the iris and the choroid and is lined by two layers of epithelium. The external layer is pigmented and is continuous with the posterior iris epithelium and the retinal pigment epithelium. Aqueous humor is secreted by the two layers of the ciliary epithelium and by the core of capillaries within the ciliary processes. Aqueous humor in the cat is formed at a rate of 15 μl/min (Macri and Cevario, 1975). It flows from the posterior chamber through the pupil to the anterior chamber and exits through the iridocorneal angle.

The internal unpigmented ciliary epithelium and the endothelium of iris vessels constitute the blood-aqueous barrier (Schmidt and Coulter, 1981). Inflammation of the anterior uvea results in breakdown of the barrier, reduced aqueous production and intraocular pressure, and an increased protein content of the aqueous humor, clinically termed "flare."

The choroid (posterior uvea) is the vascular layer between the sclera and the retina and nourishes the outer two thirds of the retina. Choroidal melanocytes contribute to the brown color of the nontapetal fundus. The melanocytes are reduced or absent in blue- or pink-eyed (Siamese or albino) cats, so that the choroid appears red from the vessels within it. Tapetal cells, which reflect light, are located in a roughly triangular area within the dorsal part of the choroid.

## Congenital Anomalies of the Uvea

**PERSISTENT PUPILLARY MEMBRANES.** Remnants of the embryonal vascular tunic may remain as persistent pupillary membranes. The retained mesodermal tissue is visible as bands or fine strands that originate from the iris collarette and may bridge the pupil or attach to the cornea or to the lens. Treatment is not recommended.

**IRIS CYSTS.** Iris cysts are benign formations between the two layers of pigment epithelium of the iris. They are pigmented, spherical masses attached at the pupillary border or free within the anterior chamber. Their characteristic location, shape, and ability to transilluminate distinguish them from malignant iridic masses (Belkin, 1983; Peiffer, 1977).

**COLOBOMA.** Colobomas are rare in cats. They are cleft-like defects due to an arrest in embryologic development and may involve the iris, ciliary body, or choroid (Bellhorn et al., 1971; Roberts and Lipton, 1975).

Iris colobomas are recognized as a notch-like defect usually affecting the ventromedial pupillary border. Bilateral iris colobomas in three cats and unilateral coloboma in one cat were described by Bellhorn et al. (1971). The iris colobomas in one cat affected the lateral area of the irides and principally involved the iris sphincter muscle.

Colobomas of the choroid represent focal malformation of the choroidal blood vessels, pigment, or tapetum. They appear as pale areas within the posterior pole; the pale area is actually the underlying sclera (Martin, 1981). Choroidal colobomas may be associated with colobomas of the optic nerve (Bellhorn et al., 1971).

**HETEROCHROMIA.** Heterochromia is a difference in color between the irides ("odd-eye"). It is rare in cats with colored coats but frequent in white cats, in which blue iris color is often associated with deafness in one or both ears caused by an inherited defect in the organ of Corti. A multicolored iris is a form of heterochromia and is due to unequal pigment distribution.

**SPHINGOMYELINOSIS.** Anisocoria and abnormal color of the iris occur in this storage disorder; affected kittens may be blind by seven months of age. (See chapter on inherited metabolic diseases.)

**GLAUCOMA.** Congenital glaucoma in kittens is rare but was reported by Jakob (cited by Roberts and Lipton, 1975).

## Acquired Disorders of the Uvea

**CYSTS.** Some cysts of the iris appear to be of traumatic origin. Because of their dark color they may grossly resemble melanoma and should be carefully monitored. If cosmetic correction is desired, the cyst may be removed by an aspiration technique (Belkin, 1983).

**AGING CHANGES IN THE IRIS.** In old cats the iris may become thinned and lacy. Small pigmented areas often appear, especially in cats of orange coat color. They have the potential of becoming tumorous (Roberts and Lipton, 1975).

**GLAUCOMA.** Glaucoma is defined as elevation of intraocular pressure that damages the retina and optic nerve and causes blindness. Normal intraocular pressure in the cat varies from 15 to 30 mm Hg. The flow rate of the aqueous humor and the outflow facility are greater in cats than in other species studied. The cat's iridocorneal angle is similar to that of the dog, although pectinate ligaments are fewer and thinner, with less tendency to branch (Peiffer, 1981).

Glaucoma without antecedent ocular disease is considered primary and may be classified as open-angle, narrow-angle, or closed-angle, depending on the appearance of the drainage angle. The visualization of the angle is accomplished by gonioscopy, entailing placement of a special contact lens on the cornea. The lens bends light waves so that the angle may be observed. A bright light source and magnification are also needed. However, the deep anterior chamber of the cat's eye often allows visualization of the angle without a goniolens.

Primary open-angle glaucoma is uncommon in cats. In an open angle, the distance between the base of the iris and the cornea appears normal, and normal pectinate ligaments are seen. Precipitating causes such as anterior or posterior synechiae, red blood cells, or inflammatory exudate within the anterior chamber are absent. Usually bilateral, this type of glaucoma has been observed in Siamese, Persians, and domestic shorthairs (Peiffer, 1981). Early signs such as tearing and slight episcleral injection are subtle, and cats are often presented when glaucoma is advanced, with enlarged globes, no pupillary light reflexes, and varying degrees of corneal edema and vascularization.

Glaucoma in cats is usually secondary to intraocular disease. Uveitis due to a variety of causes such as trauma, feline infectious peritonitis, or lymphosarcoma may produce secondary glaucoma by obstruction of the iridocorneal angle by inflammatory adhesions or exudate. Iris bombé, caused by annular posterior synechiae, prevents flow of aqueous humor from the posterior to the anterior chamber. Neoplasia of the anterior uvea, whether primary (e.g., melanoma) or secondary (lymphosarcoma or metastatic tumors), may result in glaucoma by infiltration of the iridocorneal angle. Luxation of the lens into the anterior chamber may result in secondary glaucoma.

Elevated intraocular pressure is the main feature of glaucoma regardless of cause. Unless tonometry is performed, early cases are often not detected because external signs are minimal. Late signs of glaucoma include corneal edema, dilated pupil, enlarged globe, retinal atrophy, and cupping of the optic disc. Corneal vascularization and ulceration secondary to lagophthalmos are common in an enlarged globe (Fig. 14–30).

Acute glaucoma is a true emergency; however, glaucoma in most cats has an insidious onset. The initial treatment of acute glaucoma is 20 per cent mannitol, 1 to 2 gm/kg IV. Mannitol is a hyperosmotic drug that lowers intraocular pressure by reducing vitreous volume. Water must be withheld for several hours after mannitol administration. One or 2 per cent topical pilocarpine, a miotic that increases facility of aqueous outflow, is used two to four times daily. Some cats will not tolerate pilocarpine, as it is irritating. Timolol maleate, 0.25 per cent (Merck, Sharp, and Dohme), a beta-adrenergic antagonist that decreases aqueous production, may be used every 12 to 24 hours with good results in early cases. Carbonic anhydrase inhibitors such as dichlorphenamide decrease aqueous production and may be given orally at 0.5 to 1.0 mg/kg b.i.d. Long-term tolerance of dichlorphenamide is variable in cats. Inappetence, vomiting, acidosis, and lethargy are side effects that necessitate reduction in dosage (Martin, 1981). Glaucoma secondary to active anterior uveitis is treated with a topical antibiotic-corticosteroid in addition to the previously mentioned drugs.

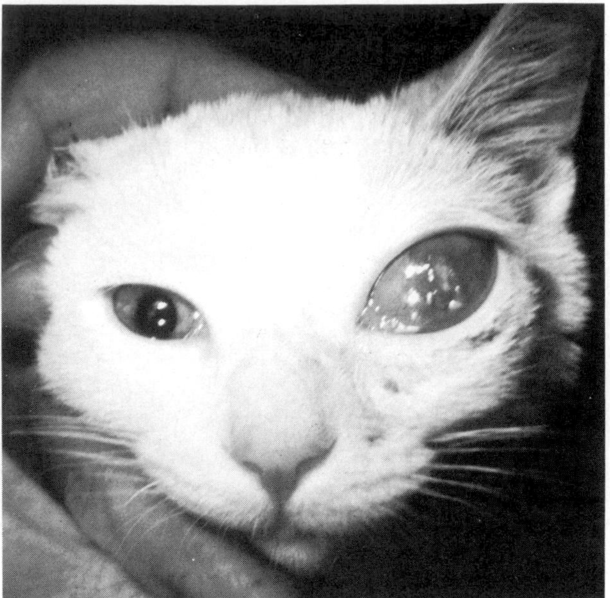

**Figure 14–30** An untreated penetrating corneal injury resulted in secondary glaucoma in a kitten. Enucleation is the treatment of choice.

If medical therapy is ineffective or if an eye is enlarged, blind, and painful owing to chronic glaucoma, surgery should be considered. Cyclocryotherapy freezes the ciliary processes and results in decreased aqueous formation. Iridectomy or iridencleisis may be performed when the pupil is immobilized by adhesions (Bistner et al., 1977); however, the long-term success rate for such procedures is limited. An anteriorly luxated lens that is causing glaucoma should be extracted. Enucleation should be performed when glaucoma is secondary to neoplasia. An evisceration with insertion of a silicone prosthesis (Jardin Plastics Research, Southfield, Michigan) into the fibrous tunic may be done in cases of glaucoma in which an intraocular tumor is not suspected and when inflammation is not active (Vestre et al., 1978). This procedure has been modified by use of a dorsal limbal incision (M. Wyman, personal communication, 1982).

**UVEITIS.** Inflammation of the uvea is common in cats. Because the iris, ciliary body, and the choroid are contiguous structures, precise clinical separation of inflammation in these tissues is seldom possible. Usually, inflammations of the iris (iritis) and of the ciliary body (cyclitis) coexist and are referred to as anterior uveitis or iridocyclitis. Choroidal inflammation is called posterior uveitis or choroiditis, and inflammation of the entire uvea is known as panuveitis.

The signs of iritis include change in color of the iris, which is often noted by the owner. It may be darkened owing to increased pigmentation. Color alterations in blue-eyed cats particularly may be detected as a dullness of color, or the iris may appear reddened (rubeosis iridis) as a result of a new formation of vessels of the iris stroma. Changes in iris texture due to edema, cellular infiltration, or both result in a thickened, velvety, or corrugated appearance. Posterior synechiae may distort the shape of the pupil. Iris neoplasia is a rare cause of alterations in color, texture, and shape.

Uveitis disrupts the blood-aqueous barrier, and protein exudes from inflamed anterior uveal vessels, producing an aqueous turbidity or flare. Exudate, which usually settles in the lower part of the anterior chamber, may take the form of fibrin, hypopyon (white blood cells), keratic precipitates (macrophages, giant cells), or hyphema (red blood cells). Disruption of the blood-aqueous barrier in hyperlipidemic cats results in a creamy white lipid flare. Other signs of uveitis are blepharospasm, photophobia, conjunctival inflammation, miosis, corneal edema, deep corneal vascularization, and ocular hypotony (reduced intraocular pressure).

Causes of uveitis may be exogenous or endogenous.

**Exogenous Uveitis.** Exogenous uveitis is usually unilateral; blunt trauma and proptosis of the globe are the common causes. Other causes are corneal ulceration, perforation, or laceration. Treatment is directed at the primary cause. In all cases of uveitis, topical atropine ointment is indicated to alleviate the pain associated with ciliary spasm, to minimize the occurrence of synechiae, and to stabilize the integrity of the iris vasculature. Atropine is used every two to four hours until the pupil is dilated, then once or twice daily.

**Endogenous Uveitis.** Not all cases of uveitis in cats are associated with systemic disease, but clinicians should be aware that uveal inflammation often occurs with feline infectious peritonitis and lymphosarcoma, less often with toxoplasmosis, histoplasmosis, blastomycosis, and cryptococcosis. Rarely, it accompanies panleukopenia. Tubercular uveitis has been described in European cats.

Feline infectious peritonitis (FIP) is perhaps the most frequent cause of uveitis in the cat. The uveitis is usually bilateral but the degree of involvement may vary. Feline infectious peritonitis is caused by a coronavirus that induces a pyogranulomatous vasculitis. Signs are chronic anterior uveitis, often with large, gray, "mutton fat" keratic precipitates adhering to the posterior corneal epithelium (Plate 14–1*N*). Choroiditis may be manifested by well-defined, red-brown lesions in the tapetum or white lesions in the nontapetal fundus (Campbell, 1978) (Plate 14–1*O*). Choroidal vasculitis may result in exudation that causes retinal detachment, and retinal hemorrhage may be present. Perivascular exudates appear as brown or gray areas adjacent to the retinal vessels (Plate 14–1*P*). If the total serum protein exceeds 9.0 gm/dl, the retinal vessels often appear dilated (Fischer, 1978). Diagnosis of FIP is based on clinical signs, a polyclonal gamma globulin elevation, and a significantly elevated coronavirus titer. Topical corticosteroids and atropine may be used as nonspecific symptomatic therapy to temporarily minimize ocular inflammation and pain.

The feline lymphosarcoma–leukemia complex (FeLLC) is the most frequent cause of intraocular neoplasia in the cat and evokes a spectrum of ocular manifestations. The orbit, third eyelid, or any part of the globe may be involved (Gelatt, 1981), but especially the richly vascular uvea. Owners frequently present their cats for ocular examination because of a change in the color or shape of the iris, which may precede systemic signs. One form of lymphosarcoma is a mass in the iris caused by infiltration of neoplastic lymphocytes. This lesion is often fleshy pink and elevated above the surface of the iris. Closer examination usually discloses flare and a fine deposit of inflammatory cells on the posterior corneal epithelium and anterior lens capsule. As the mass enlarges, the depth of the anterior chamber decreases (Plate 14–2*A*).

Chronic anterior uveitis with flare, hypopyon, hyphema, and synechiae is another frequent manifestation of FeLLC and is indistinguishable in appearance from lesions of FIP. Secondary glaucoma may result when neoplastic and inflammatory cells occlude the drainage angle or when synechiae occlude the drainage angle or block the pupil. Cats with nonregenerative anemia due to FeLLC may have uveitis accompanied by unclotted hyphema; fundic examination may disclose retinal hemorrhage, gray choroidal infiltrates, or both. Diagnosis of FeLLC is discussed in the chapter on the hematopoietic system. Cytologic examination of material obtained by aqueous or vitreous paracentesis may be diagnostic, revealing neoplastic lymphocytes. If chemotherapy is undertaken, anterior uveitis may be treated symptomatically with topical corticosteroids and atropine. A steroid alone occasionally effects prolonged remission of ocular lymphosarcoma.

Leukemia other than lymphocytic may also involve the eye.

Anterior uveitis has been produced experimentally by subcutaneous injection of feline sarcoma virus (Lubin et al., 1983).

Toxoplasmosis is primarily a disease of the retina; involvement of the adjacent choroid may occur secondarily, and anterior uveal inflammation is a late manifestation. Toxoplasmal retinitis is discussed in the chapter on protozoan diseases.

Cryptococcosis has been frequently described in the cat (e.g., Fischer, 1971; Gwin et al., 1977b; Peiffer, 1981). Ocular involvement may occur by direct extension from paranasal sinuses, by the optic meninges, or by hematogenous dissemination (Blouin and Cello, 1980) (see also the chapter on mycotic diseases). Anterior uveitis may evoke large keratic precipitates (Plate 14–2*B*). The posterior uvea is usually involved with a granulomatous reaction. Granulomas are gray-white and the overlying retina may be detached and vascularized (Plate 14–2*C*). Diagnosis is suggested by the combination of physical signs, often including pneumonia, meninigitis, and sinusitis. Centesis of the vitreous and identification of the *Cryptococcus* organism is diagnostic. Prognosis depends on the extent of involvement. Treatment with amphotericin B and with 5-fluorocytosine has had some success. Recently ketaconazole has been reported to be effective (Legendre et al., 1982).

*Histoplasma capsulatum* may involve the uvea, particularly the choroid, in cats. Bilateral uveal involvement was described in a cat with disseminated histoplasmosis

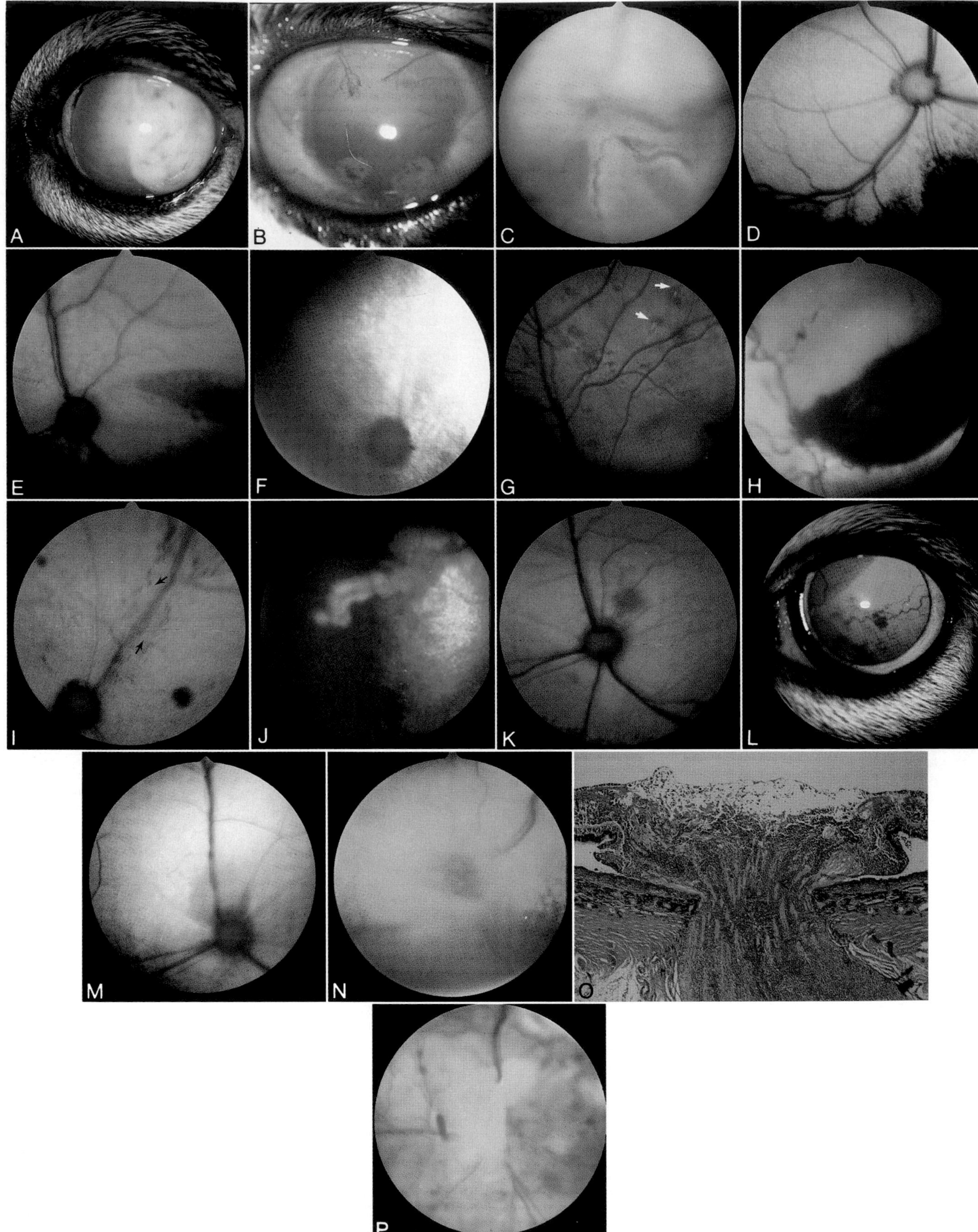


**Plate 14–2** *Legend on opposite page*

(Peiffer, 1979). The cat had hypergammaglobulinemia associated with chronic systemic infection. (See also the chapter on mycotic diseases). Bilateral focal active choroiditis (Fig. 14–31*A*) was described by Gwin et al. (1980); the anterior segments and vitreous were not involved. Causative organisms were identified by histopathologic study (Fig. 14–31*B*). Fourteen feline cases with disseminated histoplasmosis were reported by Quinn (1982). Bilateral choroidal involvement was present in all. The lesions consisted of hyperreflexia and hyperpigmentation of the tapetum, foci of decreased pigmentation, and gray exudates in the nontapetal region. All cats had nonregenerative anemia, and bone marrow aspiration resulted in identification of the organism in 13 of 14 cases. Histoplasmosis should be included in the differential diagnosis of anterior and particularly of posterior uveitis in the cat. Amphotericin B and ketaconazole have been used for treatment (Noxon et al., 1982), but the prognosis for disseminated histoplasmosis is poor.

Blastomycosis is rare in cats. In one case of ocular involvement, bilateral pyogranulomatous panuveitis was present in addition to pulmonary and central nervous involvement (Alden and Mohan, 1974). Bilateral chorioretinitis was described in another case of disseminated infection (Nasisse et al., 1985).

Immune-mediated and idiopathic are terms used to characterize numerous cases of feline uveitis, whether unilateral or bilateral, that have no demonstrable etiology. Any antigen presumably may elicit uveal inflammation. Uveal cell death triggers the infiltration of neutrophils that release lysozymes, causing further cytolysis (Fischer, 1978). Many cases resolve after treatment with a topical corticosteroid, atropine, and an antiprostaglandin such as aspirin. However, cats with uveitis should be studied in a systematic manner, beginning with a physical examination. Specific tests for the feline leukemia virus, coronavirus, and toxoplasmosis, as well as CBC and total serum protein determination and protein electrophoresis should be performed. Cytologic examination and culture of material obtained by aqueous and vitreous paracentesis are often valuable diagnostic aids.

**NEOPLASMS OF THE UVEA.** Primary intraocular tumors are rare in cats, but lymphosarcoma as a manifestation of systemic neoplasia is common (see under uveitis).

MELANOMA. This is the most frequent primary intraocular tumor in the cat and may be benign or malignant. These tumors are usually unilateral and originate from the iris and ciliary body rather than from the choroid (Bellhorn and Henkind, 1970). Older cats are affected. Reports of confirmed metastasis to distant sites or extraocular extension are infrequent (Bellhorn and Henkind, 1970; Peiffer, 1981).

Signs vary, depending on the site and extent of tumor involvement. Melanomas may appear initially as focal, slightly raised, hyperpigmented areas of the iris. Some are first noted when enlargement, distortion, or a solid mass of the iris is present. Anterior growth of the mass decreases depth of the anterior chamber; ciliary body masses often displace the lens. Malignant melanomas may cause varying degrees of iridocyclitis, hyphema, cataract, and glaucoma. These secondary changes often mask the underlying tumor. A persistent iridocyclitis, associated with iris enlargement and change in depth of the anterior chamber, suggests intraocular neoplasia. Occasionally, melanomas of cats are unpigmented (Peiffer, 1981).

A previously undescribed class of anterior uveal melanomas was reported in four cats by Acland et al. (1980). These were slowly progressive tumors characterized by diffuse neoplastic involvement of the entire iris stroma and invasion of the drainage angle that caused secondary glaucoma. Anterior uveitis was minimal. The globes were enucleated because of the glaucoma. Tumor of the iris and ciliary body was discovered by histopathologic examination. Distant metastases were not recognized.

Varying cell types of feline malignant melanoma have been reported (Bellhorn and Henkind, 1970): (1) epithelioid cells with large or small vesicular nuclei; (2) spindle cells with vesicular nuclei; (3) cells with indistinct borders and pleomorphic vesicular nuclei; and (4) plump, heavily pigmented cells with small hyperchromatic nuclei. Diffuse iris melanoma is characterized by two cell types (Acland

**Plate 14–2** *A*, A large gray-pink iridic mass is visible within the anterior chamber of a cat affected with lymphosarcoma. Consolidated fibrin is also present. *B*, Anterior uveitis due to cryptococcosis. Note the large keratic precipitates in the inferior part of the anterior chamber. *C*, Detached retina in a cat with cryptococcosis. Exudates within the vitreous contribute to the haziness of the photograph. *D*, The normal fundus of an adult domestic shorthair. *E*, An elliptical area of focal retinal atrophy temporal to the optic disk is compatible with feline central retinal degeneration (FCRD) caused by a diet deficient in taurine. *F*, Generalized retinal atrophy characterized by attenuation of retinal vessels and tapetal hyperreflexia is due to advanced FCRD. *G*, Multiple areas of active and inactive chorioretinitis are present in the tapetal fundus of a cat with feline infectious peritonitis (FIP). Inactive foci have hyperreflective centers surrounded by pigment (arrows). Active lesions appear dull gray with indistinct borders. *H*, A large preretinal hemorrhage in an aged Siamese cat with renal failure. *I*, Hemorrhages within the nerve fiber layer are flame-shaped streaks (arrows), whereas deep retinal hemorrhages appear round. *J*, Perivascular cuffing is most evident over the nontapetal fundus. Histologic examination disclosed a pyogranulomatous vasculitis due to feline infectious peritonitis (FIP). *K*, Active retinitis adjacent to the optic disk at 1 o'clock and 7 o'clock in a Siamese cat with toxoplasmosis. (Courtesy Dr. S. Vainisi.) *L*, Retinal detachment with retinal hemorrhage is visible behind the dilated pupil of a cat affected with feline infectious peritonitis (FIP). *M*, Myelinated nerve fibers are present superior to the optic disk. This is a variation of normal. *N*, Elevated optic disk with hazy margins and peripapillary infiltrate in a cat with lymphosarcoma. *O*, Photomicrograph, same cat. Note infiltration of optic nerve, disk, and peripapillary retina with neoplastic lymphocytes. H & E, ×16. *P*, Fundus of a 14-year-old female cat. The optic disk is elevated and distorted by metastatic pulmonary adenocarcinoma. Preretinal and deep retinal hemorrhages are also present.

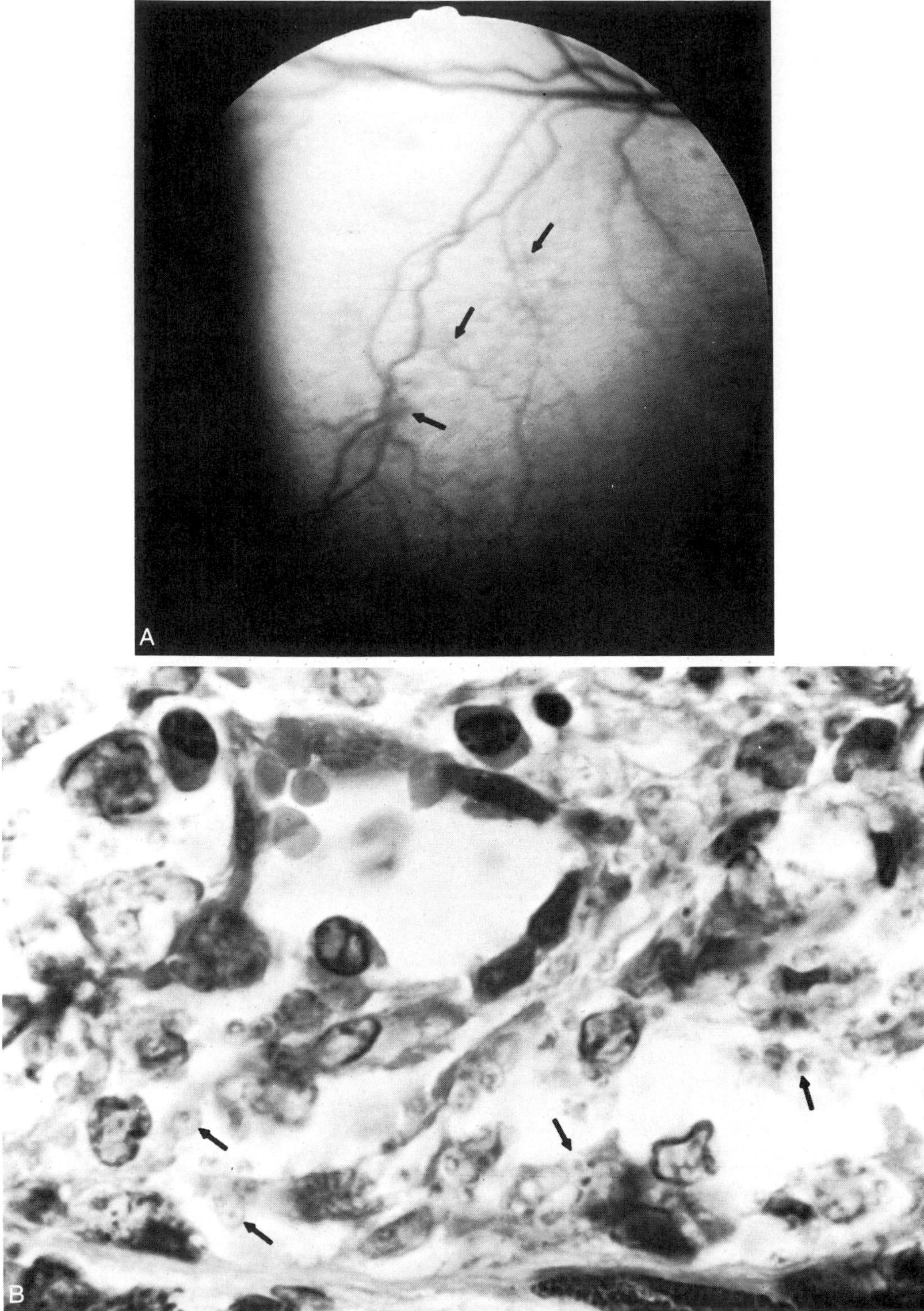

**Figure 14–31** *A*, Fundus of a two-year-old male cat with foci of active chorioretinitis caused by *Histoplasma capsulatum*. *B*, Choroid, same cat. Interspersed between the choroidal pigment and vascular channels are poorly staining extracellular and intracellular (within macrophages) *H. capsulatum* organisms (arrows). H & E, ×416. (From Gwin R, Makley TA, Wyman M, et al.: J Am Vet Med Assoc 176 [1980] 638–642.)

et al., 1980). The majority are highly anaplastic epithelioid cells with nuclei of variable size and shape (Figs. 14–32 and 14–33). The rest are balloon cells with abundant cytoplasm and round or oval nuclei.

Biopsy of intraocular masses is not recommended, lest seeding or induction of metastases occur (Peiffer, 1981). In rare cases, a small focal mass that is limited to the iris and does not invade the drainage angle may be completely excised by a wide-sector iridectomy. Examination of intraocular fluid may occasionally provide a diagnosis.

Enucleation is recommended for larger masses of the iris and ciliary body, especially if secondary signs such as uveitis or glaucoma are present. Exenteration (removal of the globe and orbital contents) is recommended when extraocular extension of the tumor is observed; however, this is uncommon. Prognosis after enucleation is good if the uveal melanoma is confined within the globe. A preoperative chest radiograph and a complete physical examination are essential and may detect the presence of metastatic disease.

Under experimental conditions the feline sarcoma virus (FeSV) induced melanomas of the iris and ciliary body in kittens (Albert et al., 1981). The sarcoma virus was injected into the anterior chamber at the inferior base of the iris. Serial histologic examinations indicated that the effect of the virus on uveal melanocytes is to induce hypertrophy, hyperplasia, and atypia, followed by development of spindle-cell, mixed-cell, and epithelioid melanomas in a focal or diffuse pattern. C-type virus particles were consistently found on melanoma cells. The role of FeLV and FeSV in the production of spontaneous feline ocular melanomas has not been studied. (Ocular melanomas are also discussed in the chapter on tumors.)

**Other Primary Tumors.** Other primary uveal tumors are adenomas and adenocarcinomas of the ciliary body epithelium. They are rare in cats (Peiffer, 1981). An hemangioma, diagnosed at the Armed Forces Institute of Pathology, was removed from a cat's iris by Magrane (1968).

**Secondary Uveal Tumors.** Feline lymphosarcoma is the most common secondary intraocular tumor. Uveal involvement predominates. Signs range from nodular iris infiltration to uveitis with hypopyon and hyphema. Choroidal involvement may result in retinal detachment.

Tumors of the uvea that are metastatic from distant primary sites have been reported. Adenocarcinomas originating in the mammary gland, lung, uterus, and sweat gland have metastasized to the choroid (Bellhorn, 1972; Hamilton et al., 1984; Moise et al., 1982; West et al., 1979), as well as a squamous cell carcinoma of undetermined primary site (Cook et al., 1984). Physical examination, history, and chest and abdomen radiographs all aid in the diagnosis of multisystemic metastatic neoplasia.

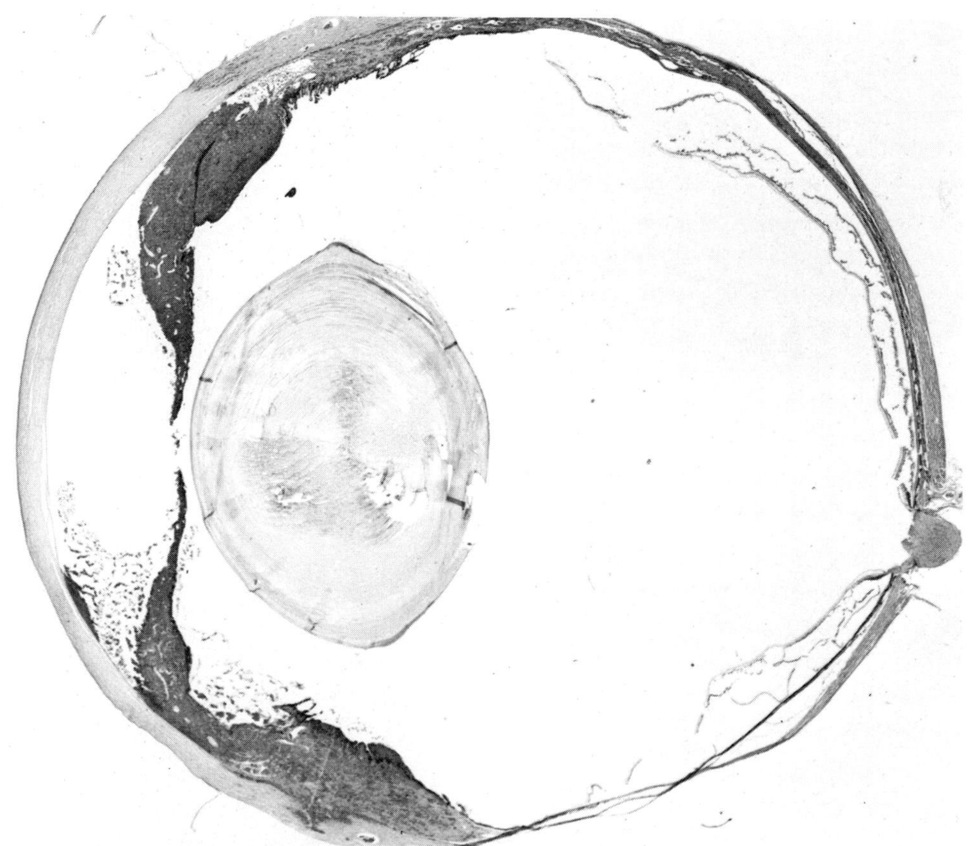

**Figure 14–32** A diffuse melanoma involves iris, ciliary body, and choroid of a 14-year-old spayed female domestic shorthair. H & E, × 7.88.

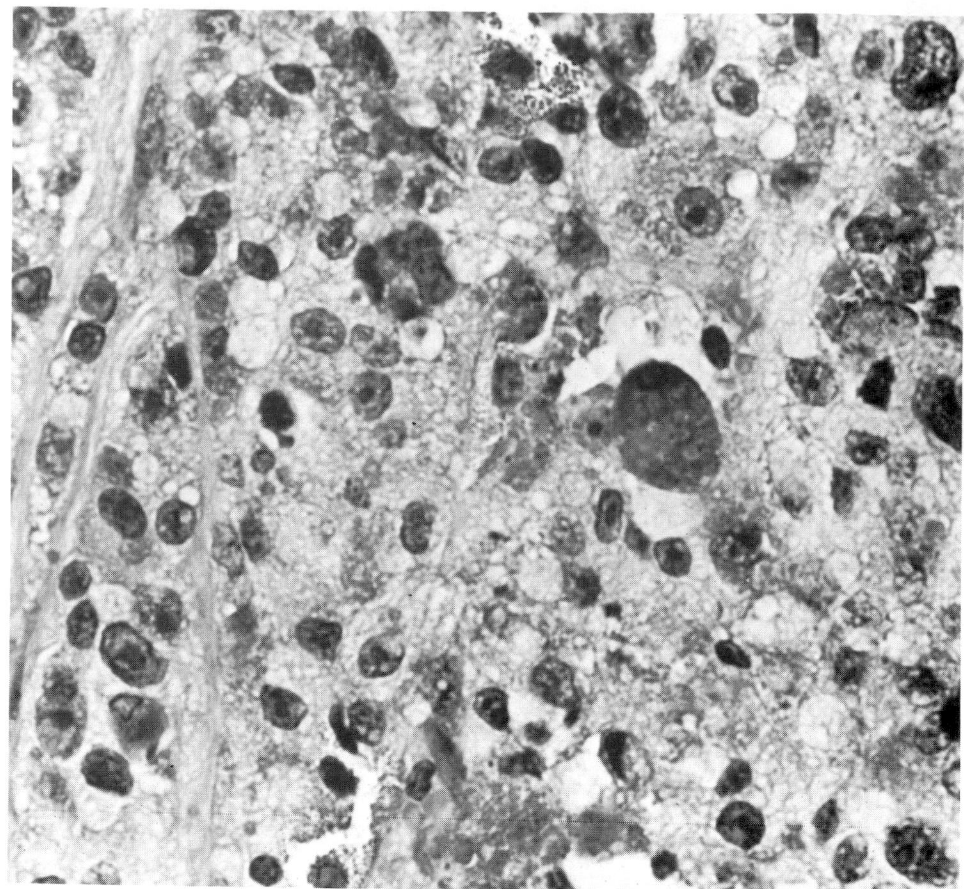

**Figure 14–33** A melanoma in which epithelioid cells predominate. Note variation in cellular and nuclear size. The large cell is a heavily pigmented melanophore. H & E, × 736.

## THE RETINA

### ANATOMY

The retina, the internal nervous tunic of the eye, is a delicate transparent membrane. It consists of 10 histologic layers; the inner neurosensory retina has nine layers, and the outer retinal pigment epithelium is the tenth layer. The retinal pigment epithelium continues over the ciliary body as the pigmented epithelial layer and onto the posterior surface of the iris. Around the optic disk (papilla) and at the ora ciliaris, the nine inner layers constituting the neurosensory part of the retina are firmly attached to the retinal pigment epithelium; elsewhere the attachment is loose. The retina consists of the following layers from without inward: (1) pigment epithelium; (2) rods and cones, the photoreceptors; (3) external limiting membrane; (4) outer nuclear layer composed of the receptor nuclei; (5) outer plexiform layer, a synaptic layer between receptor cells and bipolar cells; (6) inner nuclear layer, the bipolar cell layer; (7) inner plexiform layer, a synaptic layer between bipolar and ganglion cells; (8) ganglion cell layer; (9) nerve fiber layer made up of ganglion cell axons; and (10) internal limiting membrane.

The cat's retina has a preponderance of rods, which are most sensitive in dim light. The highest density of cones is in the central retina (area centralis), which represents the area of optimum visual acuity (Steinberg, 1973).

The fundus is the posterior portion of the globe that can be viewed with an ophthalmoscope. Familiarity with the normal feline fundus (Plate 14–2*D*) is necessary to evaluate retinal disease. Components of the fundus that are assessed by ophthalmoscopic examination are the optic disk, the tapetum lucidum, the nontapetal area, and the retinal vessels. The disk is round, unmyelinated, and gray or beige. It is usually located within the tapetum slightly lateral and inferior to the posterior pole of the eye. The disk, relatively smaller than that of the other domestic animals, measures 0.7 to 0.93 mm in diameter (Prince et al., 1960; Rubin, 1974). It may be surrounded by pigment or by a hyperreflective ring (conus). Conus is due to thinning of the peripapillary retinal layers. Three major pairs of cilioretinal arteries and veins (dorsomedial, ventromedial, and ventrolateral) radiate from the periphery of the optic disk. A central retinal artery is not usually present, although it may be vestigial, giving rise to small vessels passing from the center of the disk (Risco and Nopanitaya, 1980; Rubin, 1974). Blood vessels do not traverse the area centralis, which is located 1.5 to 2 disk diameters superior to and 3 to 4 disk diameters lateral to the optic disk. The area centralis is often slightly darker green than the surrounding tapetum.

The tapetum, triangular and usually iridescent yellow or green, is located in the dorsal half or two thirds of the fundus, extending about 40 degrees medially and 25 degrees laterally. The tapetum is within the choroid and is visible through the retina (here unpigmented). The tapetum does not develop until after 12 to 14 weeks of age; an immature tapetum is blue or violet.

The nontapetal area is brown or dark red, with irregular clumps of pigment normally present at its junction with the tapetum. Siamese and other blue-eyed cats have little pigment in the choroid and retinal pigment epithelium so that the underlying choroidal vasculature is visible. This red color should not be misinterpreted as hemorrhage. Since these albinoid cats also lack a tapetum, choroidal vessels may be seen throughout the entire fundus and are responsible for the pink "shine" when light is reflected from the eyes. In the rare "pink-eyed" (complete albino) cats, choroidal and retinal pigment are totally lacking.

On the evidence of studies to date, color perception in cats appears to be limited (Schmidt and Coulter, 1981).

## Congenital and Developmental Disorders of the Retina

**RETINAL DYSPLASIA.** This is a nonspecific response of the developing retina to various viral, chemical, or physical insults (Albert et al., 1977). The cat's retina continues to develop for six weeks after birth (Donovan, 1966). During this time, it is susceptible to the feline panleukopenia virus. Kittens exposed in utero to panleukopenia infection may exhibit retinal dysplasia characterized by irregular areas of atrophy of the tapetal fundus and mottled depigmentation of the nontapetal fundus (MacMillan, 1974; Percy et al, 1975; Rubin, 1974). This lesion is not specific but is compatible with any retinal degeneration. Histologic features are severe disorganization of retinal layers and rosette formation in the outer nuclear layer. Cerebellar hypoplasia may or may not be present. Visual function is not usually impaired since the retinal lesions are focal. Retinal dysplasia due to feline panleukopenia virus should be considered when bilateral focal areas of retinal degeneration are observed.

Retinal dysplasia was induced experimentally by feline leukemia virus (FeLV) injected intraperitoneally into fetal kittens and intravitreally into newborn kittens (Albert et al., 1977). Naturally occurring retinal dysplasia due to FeLV has not been recognized.

**$GM_1$ GANGLIOSIDOSIS.** Retinal lesions consisting of small dark spots throughout the tapetum lucidum and pale gray spots throughout the nontapetal fundi were described in kittens affected with $GM_1$ gangliosidosis, a lysosomal storage disease (Murray et al., 1977). The retinal lesions are due to glycolipid accumulation within the ganglion cells. Signs first appear at three months of age. $GM_1$ gangliosidosis has been described in mixed-breed and Siamese kittens (Baker et al., 1971; Blakemore, 1972; Farrell et al., 1973). This condition is transmitted as an autosomal recessive trait in Siamese cats (Baker et al., 1971). Progressive motor ataxia and tremor are associated signs.

Retinal abnormalities occurring in other storage disorders are discussed in the chapter on hereditary metabolic diseases.

**HEREDITARY OR CONGENITAL RETINAL DEGENERATION.** Confirmed hereditary retinal degeneration is rare in cats. Diffuse outer-segment retinal atrophy was reported in four Persian kittens in two successive litters (Rubin and Lipton, 1973). Blindness was apparent by 15 weeks of age. Ophthalmoscopic signs were tapetal hyperreflectivity and decrease in caliber of the retinal vessels. Simple autosomal inheritance was postulated.

Hereditary retinal atrophy has also been noted in Siamese (Roberts and Lipton, 1975; Severin, 1976).

Generalized advanced retinal atrophy was reported in an adult male domestic shorthair by Valle et al. (1981). Ornithine concentrations were strikingly elevated in plasma and urine owing to ornithine-delta-aminotransferase deficiency. Taurine concentration was normal. Histopathologic study disclosed absence of photoreceptors and decrease in number of small choroidal vessels. These biochemical and chorioretinal abnormalities were considered to be analogous to those in gyrate atrophy, an inherited form of human chorioretinal atrophy. Inheritance could not be studied, as this cat was infertile. Measurement of plasma or urine ornithine levels in cats with generalized retinal atrophy may detect similar cases.

Photoreceptor degeneration was reported in two generations of domestic mixed-breed cats by West-Hyde and Buyukmihci (1982a,b). Visual impairment was detected at three and a half months of age or earlier. Clinical findings were tapetal hyperreflectivity, attenuation of retinal vessels, and nearly extinguished electroretinograms. Histologic and ultrastructural changes were limited to the outer retinal layers with eventual loss of the photoreceptor layer. Plasma taurine, ornithine, and vitamin A levels were normal. Pedigree of the affected cats suggested dominant inheritance.

A high incidence of progressive retinal atrophy was reported in Sweden in Abyssinian cats (Narfström, 1983; Narfström and Nilsson, 1983). Early retinal changes of vascular thinning were first seen at one and a half to two years of age; by three to four years complete generalized retinal atrophy was present. The photoreceptor layer is primarily affected, in both the tapetal and the nontapetal areas. Simple autosomal recessive inheritance was postulated. Serum levels of vitamin A, taurine, and ornithine were not mentioned. Retinal atrophy has also been reported in British Abyssinians (Carlile, 1984). In Chédiak-Higashi syndrome of blue smoke Persians, the fundus lacks pigmentation, and there is a red light–reflection (Collier et al., 1979; Kramer et al., 1977).

## Acquired Disorders of the Retina

**NUTRITIONAL RETINAL DEGENERATION.** Feline central retinal degeneration (FCRD) refers to a nutritionally induced degeneration of the outer retinal layers related to taurine deficiency. FCRD has been produced experimentally in cats fed diets deficient in taurine (Barnett and Burger, 1980; Hayes et al., 1975) and has been observed clinically in cats fed dog food (Aguirre, 1978).

Taurine is an aminosulfonic acid present in high concentrations in the retina. Cats are unable to synthesize taurine from methionine and cysteine and must rely on exogenous dietary sources such as meat and seafood to maintain retinal function. Little or no taurine was found in commercial dog foods, and taurine content is higher in dry than in canned cat foods (Aguirre, 1978).

The earliest lesion of FCRD observable ophthalmoscopically is a granular appearance of the area centralis. This progresses to a focal round or ellipsoid area of increased reflectivity (Plate 14–2*E*) which enlarges and expands across the posterior pole from the lateral to medial quadrants. This band-shaped lesion is parallel to the junction between the tapetum and nontapetal area (Aguirre, 1978). Up to this stage, clinical impairment of vision is not detectable. Lesions are bilateral and nearly symmetric. Gradual progression results in generalized retinal degeneration (Plate 14–2*F*) with attentuation of retinal vessels and blindness. Retinal changes in experimental cats fed taurine-free diets usually required several months to develop. The shortest time was 18 weeks, but most developed after six to seven months (Barnett and Burger, 1980). The early focal stages of FCRD are reversible if adequate dietary taurine is fed (Hayes et al., 1975). Generalized retinal degeneration is irreversible.

Electroretinography disclosed reductions in rod and cone amplitudes and increased implicit time of cone a and b waves, indicating diffuse retinal involvement (Hayes et al., 1975). Electroretinograms were almost undetectable by 12 months in most cats fed taurine-deficient diets. Histologic changes are initially restricted to the photoreceptor outer segment in the area centralis. Advanced stages of degeneration result in loss of the outer nuclear layer and outer plexiform layer (Hayes et al., 1975). In addition to the photoreceptor degeneration, the tapetum of taurine-deficient cats is reduced in layers and disorganized (Wen et al., 1979).

It is noteworthy that ophthalmoscopic lesions of FCRD are often seen as incidental findings in cats being fed commercial cat foods that should contain adequate taurine levels. One may speculate that causes other than taurine deficiency, such as a deficit in protein utilization or biochemical events affecting retinal metabolism at a cellular level, are involved.

**DRUG-INDUCED RETINAL DEGENERATION.** A rapidly induced experimental retinal degeneration in adult cats that had received simultaneous injections of a neurotropic carcinogen methylnitrosourea (MNU) and ketamine hydrochloride was reported by Schaller et al. (1981). Administration of either MNU or ketamine alone failed to induce similar persistent retinal changes (Fig. 14–34*A* and *B*). Attenuation of retinal vessels, tapetal hyperreflectivity, and dullness and depigmentation of the nontapetal retina were observed five days after injection (Fig. 14–34*C*). Electroretinograms were markedly decreased. Histologic examination disclosed severe, diffuse degeneration of photoreceptor and outer nuclear layers (Fig. 14–34*D*). Except for its rapid development this retinal atrophy closely resembles the late stages of retinal degeneration resulting from dietary taurine deficiency. The authors postulated that MNU-ketamine retinal atrophy may involve reduction or failure of taurine uptake by retinal cells.

**RETINAL INFLAMMATION.** The retina may be a primary site of certain inflammations, such as toxoplasmosis; however, retinitis is most often secondary to choroiditis. Active retinal inflammation may consist of one or all of the following: cellular infiltration, edema, hemorrhage, exudation, or granulomas.

Cellular infiltrates over the tapetum appear as dull gray foci with hazy borders. Infiltrates within the nontapetal retina are white or gray with indistinct borders. Retinal edema, which has a grayish appearance, accompanies active lesions and disappears as the lesions resolve. Inactive retinitis (scars) results in retinal atrophy and appears as discrete hyperreflective areas in the tapetum and as gray or light tan areas in the nontapetal region. Active and inactive lesions may be present concomitantly (Plate 14–2*G*). Pigment clumping may be seen and is due to proliferation and migration of the retinal pigment epithelium or choroidal pigment.

A red area within the fundus usually indicates retinal hemorrhage, the character of which varies with its location. Preretinal hemorrhage originates from retinal vessels and lies between the nerve fiber layer and the internal limiting membrane (Plate 14–2*H*). The red blood cells gravitate ventrally. Hemorrhages within the nerve fiber layer also originate from the superficial retinal vessels and appear flame-shaped, because the blood is confined to the linearly aligned nerve fiber layer. Deep retinal hemorrhages are compact and round (Plate 14–2*I*), because the blood is contained in the nuclear layers and the vertically aligned plexiform layers (Fischer, 1970).

Inflammatory cellular exudates affecting the retina cause a hazy vitreous. Large vitreous exudates may cast a shadow on the retina. Exudates accumulating around blood vessels evoke perivascular cuffing (Plate 14–2*J*). Granulomas appear as solid elevated white or tan foci that may displace retinal vessels and are often accompanied by retinal edema or hemorrhage.

Toxoplasmosis primarily causes a retinitis; uveal involvement is secondary. Lymphosarcoma, feline infectious peritonitis, the systemic mycoses, and septicemia are causes of chorioretinitis. Their lesions are not specific in appearance; and diagnosis depends on history, physical signs, and laboratory data.

Treatment of active inflammation of the posterior segment depends on the cause. Topical medication does not attain therapeutic levels in the retina or choroid, so the systemic route must be used. Specific treatment for systemic diseases is covered in other chapters.

**TOXOPLASMAL RETINITIS.** Toxoplasmosis is caused by *Toxoplasma gondii*, an intracellular protozoan parasite. The ocular lesion most consistently produced in cats is retinitis or, in more advanced cases, retinochoroiditis (Campbell and Schiessl, 1978). Anterior uveal involvement sometimes develops.

Active retinal lesions are dark and slightly elevated with indistinct borders (Plate 14–2*K*). The inflamed retina is necrotic, and cellular exudation may extend into the vitreous. Retinal detachment may be caused by retinal tears or subretinal exudate (Campbell and Schiessl, 1978; Vainisi and Campbell, 1969). There may or may not be concurrent systemic involvement. Diagnosis is based on a significant (fourfold) rise in titer in serum samples drawn at two- or three-week intervals. An elevated but constant titer suggests previous infection and immunity (Jacobson, 1980; see also the chapter on protozoan diseases). The indirect fluorescent antibody and indirect hemagglutination tests are considered equally reliable (Behymer et al., 1973).

Toxoplasmosis is a zoonotic disease, and owners must be aware of this before treatment is instituted. Treatment is with pyrimethamine (Daraprim, Burroughs Wellcome) 0.5 mg/kg/day and sulfadiazine 60 mg/kg/day divided into four to six doses. These drugs act synergistically by inhibiting folic acid synthesis by the *Toxoplasma* organism. The hazard of bone marrow depression in the cat is alleviated by administration of folinic acid (leucovorin) 1 mg/kg/day. Treatment for two weeks is recommended (Jacobson, 1980).

**RETINAL DETACHMENT.** Detachment of the retina

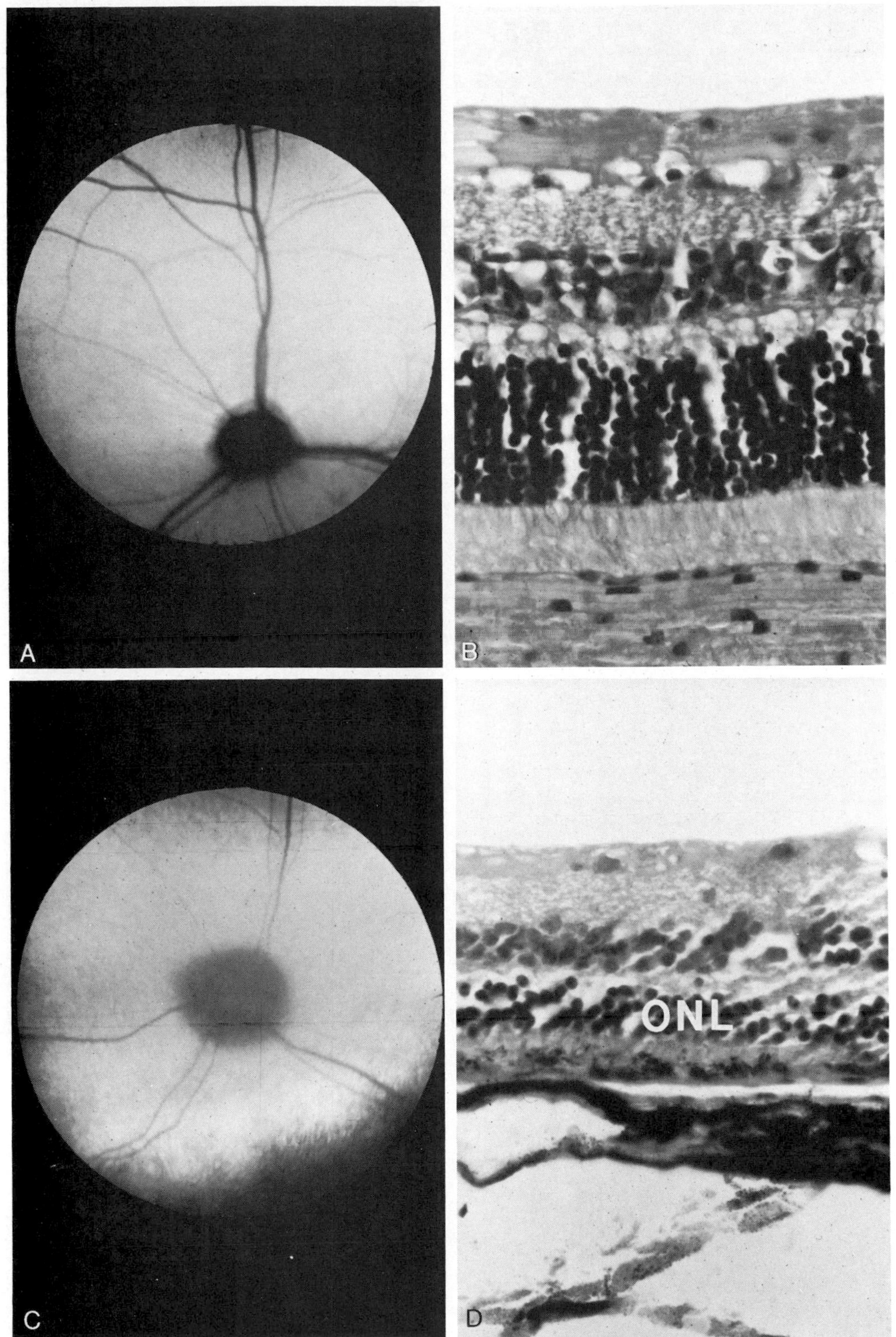


**Figure 14–34** *A*, Normal tapetal fundus of methylnitrosourea-inoculated cat shows distinct retinal vessels five days after inoculation. *B*, Normal tapetal retina from the same cat shown in *A*. H & E, ×168. *C*, Tapetal fundus of methylnitrosourea- and ketamine-inoculated cat (five days after inoculation) with markedly attenuated retinal vessels and an indistinct optic disk. *D*, Abnormal retina from same cat. Loss of rods and cones and marked reduction of outer nuclear layer (ONL) are apparent. H & E, ×168. (From Schaller JP, Wyman M, Weisbrode SE, et al.: Vet Pathol 18 [1982] 239–247.)

is a separation of the outer retinal pigment epithelium from the inner neural retina. Three causal mechanisms have been described: (1) holes or tears in the retina may permit fluid vitreous to elevate the retina, (2) contraction of inflammatory fibrous bands within the vitreous may pull the retina away from the pigment epithelium, and (3) inflammatory exudate from the choroid or the retina may elevate the neural retina (Fig. 14–35) (Roberts, 1959). In the cat, the majority of retinal detachments are secondary to inflammatory choroidal exudates due to systemic mycoses, feline infectious peritonitis, lymphosarcoma, and toxoplasmosis (Martin, 1981; Peiffer, 1981). Tuberculosis is a significant cause of retinal detachment in countries where cats are exposed to bovine tuberculosis. Other causes of retinal detachment in cats are ethylene glycol poisoning, multiple myeloma, periarteritis nodosa, and pyelonephritis (Barclay and Riis, 1979; Campbell et al., 1972; Hribernik et al., 1982; MacMillan, 1976; Roberts, 1959).

Hypertension, established by the ultrasonic Doppler method, is found in some cats with detached retina (Morgan, 1985). Renal insufficiency and hyperthyroidism are predisposing conditions in some cases; in others the cause of the hypertension may not be discovered. Typically the cat is presented for blindness or for intraocular hemorrhage. The retinal detachment may be accompanied by hemorrhage into the vitreous. As well as treatment for the underlying disorder, a low-salt diet, diuretics, and propranolol have been used with benefit. Although the retina may reattach with lowering of the blood pressure, vision is not necessarily restored to normal.

In many cases of retinal detachment no cause is discovered.

A completely detached retina may often be seen through a dilated pupil with the aid of a penlight (Plate 14–2*L*). The detachment appears as an elevated grayish veil. Focal detachments require ophthalmoscopic examination and appear as raised grayish areas. Retinal blood vessels are elevated over a detachment. Exudate and retinal hemorrhage often accompany detachment. Cats with acute, bilateral, complete retinal detachment may be presented for sudden blindness. Unilateral retinal detachment is often undetected, as cats seldom exhibit signs of monocular vision loss. If the retina remains detached for two to six weeks, the outer segments degenerate owing to lack of blood supply (Peiffer, 1981). Depending on the etiology, subretinal fluid may resorb and the retina reattach (Barclay and Riis, 1979; MacMillan, 1976). Retinal folds, which may be observed after reattachment, appear as linear dark areas overlying the tapetum and as lighter areas when in the nontapetal fundus (MacMillan, 1976).

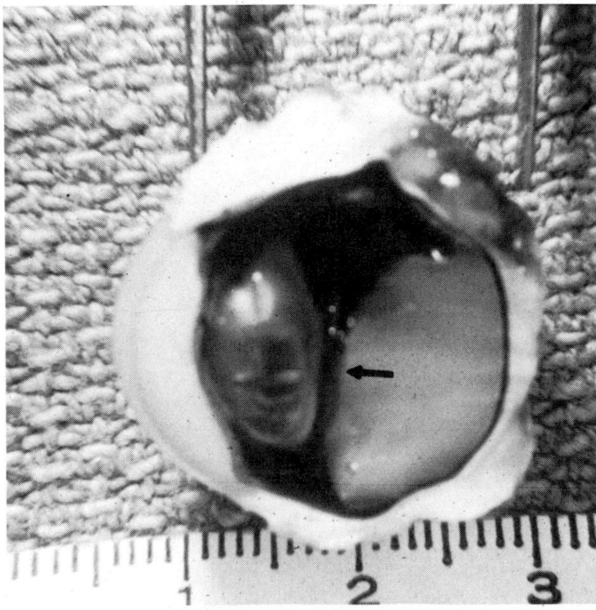

**Figure 14–35** An exudative retinal detachment was due to feline infectious peritonitis (FIP). White subretinal fluid elevates the retina (arrow).

Prognosis depends on the cause. As most exudative retinal detachments are associated with systemic disease, the need for complete history, thorough physical examination, and laboratory tests is emphasized.

**VASCULAR DISORDERS OF THE RETINA.** Abnormalities of retinal vessels may reflect systemic disorders.

**Lipemia Retinalis.** A lipemic appearance of the retinal vessels may accompany hyperlipoproteinemia or hyperchylomicronemia. The retinal vessels are pink or salmon-colored rather than red (Rubin 1974). Lipemia retinalis was reported in a cat with iatrogenic steroid-induced hyperadrenocorticism (Cushing's disease) and diabetes mellitus (Wyman et al., 1973). It may also be a sign of abnormal lipid metabolism, diabetes mellitus, or a high content of dietary fat.

**Polycythemia.** Secondary polycythemia may result from congenital or acquired cardiac anomalies in which a right-to-left shunt is present. Aguirre and Gross (1980) described the appearance of the fundus in a cat with polycythemia secondary to tetralogy of Fallot. The retinal vessels were distended, dark, and tortuous. Peripapillary retinal vascularization was present. Tortuous retinal vessels and retinal edema were observed in a cat with an atrioventricular septal defect (Rubin, 1974).

**Retinal Hemorrhage.** Retinal hemorrhages are frequent in anemic cats, when the hematocrit falls to 10 to 12 per cent (Martin, 1981). Fischer (1970) reported retinal hemorrhages in 20 to 26 cats having hemoglobin values under 5 gm/dl. Etiologies of anemic retinopathy include lymphosarcoma, reticuloendotheliosis with secondary thrombocytopenia, autoimmune hemolytic anemia, aplastic anemia, septicemia, and panleukopenia.

Hemorrhages in Fischer's series were bilateral; the severity or location of the hemorrhage, whether preretinal, superficial, or deep, could not be associated with the pathogenesis of the anemia. Focal areas of retinal atrophy may follow the subsequent resorption of retinal hemorrhage. The retinal blood vessels of anemic cats appear light red and thin.

Several mechanisms are responsible for retinal hemorrhage. The low level of red cells results in local hypoxia followed by vasodilatation and increased capillary fragility. Coagulopathies may contribute to retinal hemorrhage. The coexistence of severe anemia and thrombocytopenia predisposes to retinal hemorrhage (Fischer, 1970).

Vasculitis due to feline infectious peritonitis or secondary to chronic uremia may result in retinal hemorrhage in the cat. Retinal hemorrhage may accompany toxoplasmal retinitis depending on the intensity of the inflammatory response and the proximity of a blood vessel (Campbell and Schiessl, 1978). Nonpenetrating ocular trauma may produce retinal hemorrhage; adnexal or anterior segment injuries are generally present as well.

**Thiamine Deficiency.** Retinal hemorrhage and venous dilatation have been described in cats with thiamine deficiency. Anorexia, ataxia, mydriasis, as well as clonic convulsions and ventriflexion of the neck, are often present (Jubb et al., 1956; Rubin, 1978).

**NEOPLASMS OF THE RETINA.** Primary neoplasia of the retina is rare. A glioma was reported by Jungherr and Wolf (1939) and a neuroblastoma by Grün (1936). Lymphosarcoma of the uvea often extends to involve the retina.

**PARASITISMS OF THE RETINA.** Tracks presumably of dipterous larvae and in one cat a moving larva have been observed in the retina (Brooks et al., 1984; Gwin et al., 1984).

## THE OPTIC NERVE

### Anatomy

Axons of the cell bodies in the retinal ganglion cell layer converge at the optic disk to form the optic nerve, cranial nerve II. The optic nerve consists of intraocular, orbital, and intracranial parts. The intraocular is the disk (nerve head, optic papilla). The cat's disk is unmyelinated and acquires myelin posterior to the lamina cribrosa. Peripapillary myelinated nerve fibers may be observed occasionally as a congenital variant (Plate 14–2*M*). The orbital part of the optic nerve, which is surrounded by meninges, extends caudally in the orbit and enters the skull through the optic canal. The intracranial part is short, extending from the optic canal to the chiasm where the nerves from each eye join (Martin and Anderson, 1981). In the cat, 65 to 70 per cent of the optic nerve axons cross in the optic chiasm. In general, the axons that cross come from the nasal aspect of the retina. Axons from ganglion cells in the temporal retina do not cross and terminate ipsilaterally (de Lahunta, 1973).

The squint in Siamese is due to abnormalities in the visual pathway. Siamese cats have a greater number of axons from the temporal retina crossing over than the normal cat. This misrouting of optic nerve fibers is associated with abnormal lamination of the lateral geniculate body and abnormal input to the rostral colliculus and visual cortex (Creel, 1971; Guillery et al., 1981; Kalil et al., 1971; Levick et al., 1972). Experiments have demonstrated that Siamese cats appear to be blind for the nasal hemifield (Elekessy et al., 1973), but this defect is not observable clinically. Depth perception and binocular vision are probably impaired to some degree (Peiffer, 1981).

### Congenital Anomalies of the Optic Nerve

Aplasia or hypoplasia of the optic nerve is an uncommon congenital anomaly that may be unilateral or bilateral. Other ocular malformations such as microphthalmos may be present, or the eyes may be otherwise normal. Aplasia refers to absence of the optic nerve. Retinal vessels may also be absent. Affected animals are blind and lack pupillary light reflexes. Histologic changes are absence of the ganglion cell layer, nerve fiber layer, and retinal vasculature. Optic tracts are also absent (Barnett and Grimes, 1974). Hypoplasia of the optic nerve refers to a reduced number of ganglion cells and thinning of the nerve fiber layer. The disk is reduced in size, and retinal vessels are usually normal. Optic nerve hypoplasia has a variable effect on vision depending on the degree of involvement.

Coloboma of the optic nerve is a defect attributed to incomplete closure of the fetal fissure of the optic stalk. Optic nerve and choroidal colobomas frequently coexist. Colobomatous defects of the eyelid and iris may also be associated (Bellhorn et al., 1971). Impairment of vision is not usually detectable. A coloboma involving the entire disk has an enlarged excavated appearance that falls away from the plane of focus. A small or focal coloboma appears as a pit usually at the disk margin.

### Acquired Lesions of the Optic Nerve

Optic neuritis in the cat is usually an extension of intraocular inflammation associated with infections such as toxoplasmosis, cryptococcosis, feline infectious peritonitis, or histoplasmosis (Martin, 1981). Orbital disease such as cellulitis or proptosis may cause optic nerve inflammation. Treatment is directed at the etiology.

Optic atrophy may be the end result of optic neuritis, advanced retinal degeneration such as FCRD, or inherited retinal degeneration. Traumatic avulsion of the optic nerve due to proptosis of the globe results in optic atrophy. Glaucoma causes cupping and atrophy of the optic disk. It has been hypothesized that ischemia of the nutrient vessels to the optic nerve may be the primary event leading to glaucomatous cupping and atrophy (Henkind et al., 1977).

An atrophic optic disk appears gray and small. More of the lamina cribrosa becomes visible. The disk surface is cupped or depressed in cats with chronic glaucoma. The histologic lesions of optic nerve atrophy are loss of myelin and axons, causing shrinkage of the nerve parenchyma. Widening of the pial septa and glial proliferation occur (Yanoff and Fine, 1975).

Primary optic nerve tumors, such as meningiomas, astrocytomas, or other glial tumors, have not been reported in the cat. The intracranial optic nerve or chiasm may be compressed by an expanding brain tumor. Optic chiasmal compression by a large meningioma of the third ventricle caused bilateral blindness and pupillary areflexia in a cat (Nafe, 1979). Infiltration of the optic nerve with tumor cells may be observed in cats with lymphosarcoma (Plate 14–2*N* and *O*). The optic nerve is occasionally the site of tumor metastasis (Plate 14–2*P*) (Bellhorn, 1972).

## REFERENCES

Acheson GH: The topographical anatomy of the smooth muscle of the cat's nictitating membrane. Anat Rec 71 (1938) 297–311.

Acland GM, McLean IW, Aguirre GD, Trucksa R: Diffuse iris melanoma in cats. J Am Vet Med Assoc 176 (1980) 51–56.

Aguirre GD: Retinal degeneration associated with the feeding of dog foods to cats. J Am Vet Med Assoc 172 (1978) 791–796.

Aguirre GD, Bistner SI: Microphakia with lenticular luxation and subluxation in cats. Vet Med Small Anim Clin 68 (1973) 498–500.

Aguirre GD, Gross SL: Ocular manifestations of selected systemic disease. Compend Contin Ed 2 (1980) 144–153.

Albert DM, Lahva M, Colby ED, Shadduck JA, Sang DN: Retinal neoplasia and dysplasia. I. Induction by feline leukemia virus. Invest Ophthalmol Vis Sci 16 (1977) 325–337.

Albert DM, Shadduck JA, Craft JL, Niederkorn JY: Feline uveal melanoma model induced with feline sarcoma virus. Invest Ophthalmol Vis Sci 20 (1981) 606–624.

Albert RA, Garrett PD, Whitley RD: Surgical correction of everted third eyelid in two cats. J Am Vet Med Assoc 180 (1982) 763–766.

Alden CL, Mohan R: Ocular blastomycosis in a cat. J Am Vet Med Assoc 164 (1974) 527–528.

Baker HJ, Lindsey JR, McKhann GM, Farrell DF: Neuronal $GM_1$ gangliosidosis in a Siamese cat with β-galactosidase deficiency. Science 174 (1971) 838–839.

Barlough JE, Scott FW: Autonomic polyganglioneuropathy: A new clinical entity of cats. Cornell Feline Health Center Veterinary News, Spring 1983, 1, 8.

Barclay SM, Riis RC: Retinal detachment and reattachment associated with ethylene glycol intoxication in a cat. J Am Anim Hosp Assoc 15 (1979) 719–724.

Barnett KC: Progressive retinal atrophy in the Abyssinian cat. J Small Anim Pract 23 (1982) 763–766.

Barnett KC, Burger IH: Taurine deficiency retinopathy in the cat. J Small Anim Pract 21 (1980) 521–534.

Barnett KC, Grimes TD: Bilateral aplasia of the optic nerve in a cat. Br J Ophthalmol 58 (1974) 663–667.

Bedford PGC, Cotchin E: An unusual chronic keratoconjunctivitis in the cat. J Small Anim Pract 24 (1953) 85–102.

Behymer RD, Harlow DR, Behymer DE, Franti CE: Serologic diagnosis of toxoplasmosis and prevalence of *Toxoplasma gondii* antibodies in selected feline, canine and human populations. J Am Vet Med Assoc 162 (1973) 959–963.

Belkin PV: Iris cysts in cats. Feline Pract 13(6) (1983) 12–18.

Bellhorn RW: Secondary ocular adenocarcinoma in three dogs and a cat. J Am Vet Med Assoc 160 (1972) 302–307.

Bellhorn RW, Barnett KC, Henkind P: Ocular colobomas in domestic cats. J Am Vet Med Assoc 159 (1971) 1015–1021.

Bellhorn RW, Henkind P: Intraocular malignant melanoma in domestic cats. J Small Anim Pract 10 (1970) 631–637.

Bistner SI, Aguirre G, Batik G: Atlas of Veterinary Ophthalmic Surgery. Philadelphia, WB Saunders Company, 1977.

Bistner SI, Carlson JH, Shively JN, Scott FW: Ocular manifestations of feline herpesvirus infection. J Am Vet Med Assoc 159 (1971) 1223–1237.

Bistner SI, Aguirre G, Shively JN: Hereditary corneal dystrophy in the Manx cat; a preliminary report. Invest Ophthalmol Vis Sci 15 (1976) 15–26.

Blakemore C, Cummings RM: Eye opening in kittens. Vision Res 15 (1975) 1417–1418.

Blakemore WF: $GM_1$ gangliosidosis in a cat. J Comp Pathol 82 (1972) 179–185.

Blogg JR: Agenesis of the feline upper eyelid. Feline Pract 15(1) (1985) 31–35.

Blouin P, Cello RM: Experimental ocular cryptococcosis. Preliminary studies in cats and mice. Invest Ophthalmol Vis Sci 19 (1980) 21–30.

Brightman AH: The eye. *In* Pratt PW (ed): Feline Medicine. Santa Barbara, American Veterinary Publications, Inc, 1983.

Brightman AH, Macy DW, Gosselin Y: Pupillary abnormalities associated with the feline leukemia complex. Feline Pract 7(6) (1977) 23–27.

Brightman AH, Vestre WA, Helper LC, Godshalk CP: Chronic eosinophilic keratitis in the cat. Feline Pract 9(3) (1979) 21–24.

Brooks D, Wolf E, Merideth R: Ophthalmomyiasis interna in two cats. J Am Anim Hosp Assoc 20 (1984) 157–160.

Brown N, Hurvitz AI: A mucocutaneous disease in a cat resembling human pemphigus. J Am Anim Hosp Assoc 15 (1979) 25–28.

Bryan GM: Subconjunctival emphysema in a cat. Vet Med Small Anim Clin 72 (1977) 1087–1089.

Bussanich MN, Rootman J: Intraocular nematode in a cat. Feline Pract 13(4) (1983) 20, 24–26.

Buyukmihci N: Fibrosarcoma of the nictitating membrane in a cat. J Am Vet Med Assoc 167 (1975) 934–935.

Buyukmihci N, Bellhorn RW, Hunziker J, Clinton J: *Encephalitozoon* (*Nosema*) infection of the cornea in a cat. J Am Vet Med Assoc 171 (1977) 355–357.

Campbell FW, Maffei L, Piccolino M: The contrast sensitivity of the cat. J Physiol 229 (1973) 719–731.

Campbell LH: Toxoplasma retinitis in a cat. Feline Pract 4 (3) (1974) 36–39.

Campbell LH: Diseases of the conjunctiva. *In* Kirk RW (ed): Current Veterinary Therapy VII. Philadelphia, WB Saunders Company, 1980, 550–553.

Campbell LH, Fox JG, Drake DF: Ocular and other manifestations of periarteritis nodosa in a cat. J Am Vet Med Assoc 161 (1972) 1122–1126.

Campbell LH, Fox JG, Snyder SB: Ocular bacteria and mycoplasma of the clinically normal cat. Feline Pract 3 (6) (1973a) 10–12.

Campbell LH, Schiessl MM: Ocular manifestations of toxoplasmosis, infectious peritonitis, and lymphosarcoma in cats. Mod Vet Pract 59 (1978) 761–764.

Campbell LH, Snyder SB, Reed C, Fox JG: *Mycoplasma felis*–associated conjunctivitis in cats. J Am Vet Med Assoc 163 (1973b) 991–995.

Campbell LH, Teague HD, McCree AV: Corneal abscess in a cat: treatment by subconjunctival antibiotics. Feline Pract 8(1) (1978) 30–32.

Carlile J: Six cases of retinal atrophy in Abyssinian cats. J Small Anim Pract 25 (1984) 415–420.

Carrington SD: Lipid keratopathy in a cat. J Small Anim Pract 24 (1983) 495–505.

Cello RM: Ocular infections in animals with PLT (Bedsonia) group agents. Am J Ophthalmol 63 (1967) (Suppl) 1270–1274.

Chaillous J, Robin V: Kératocône bilateral chez un chat. Bull Soc Ophthalmol Fr 45 (1933) 153–160.

Collier LL, Bryan GM, Prieur DJ: Ocular manifestations of the Chédiak-Higashi syndrome in four species of animals. J Am Vet Med Assoc 175 (1979) 587–590.

Cook CS, Peiffer RL Jr, Stine PE: Metastatic ocular sqamous cell carcinoma in a cat. J Am Vet Med Assoc 185 (1984) 1547–1549.

Cook CS, Rosenkrantz W, Peiffer RL, MacMillan A: Malignant melanoma of the conjunctiva in a cat. J Am Vet Med Assoc 186 (1985) 505–506.

Covitz D, Hunziker J, Koch SA: Conjunctivorhinostomy: a surgical method for the control of epiphora in the dog and cat. J Am Vet Med Assoc 171 (1977) 251–254.

Creel DJ: Visual system anomaly associated with albinism in the cat. Nature 231 (1971) 465–466.

Crouch JE: Text-Atlas of Cat Anatomy. Philadelphia, Lea & Febiger, 1969.

de Lahunta A: Small animal neuro-ophthalmology. Vet Clin North Am 3 (1973) 491–501.

Dice P: Intracorneal acid-fast granuloma. Proc Am Coll Vet Ophthalmol 8 (1977) 91.

Doherty MJ: A bridge-flap blepharorrhaphy method for eyelid reconstruction in the cat. J Am Anim Hosp Assoc 9 (1973) 238–241.

Donovan A: The postnatal development of the cat retina. Exp Eye Res 5 (1966) 249–254.

Dubielzig RR: Ocular sarcoma following trauma in three cats. J Am Vet Assoc 184 (1984) 578–581.

Ehinger B: Double innervation of the feline iris dilator. Arch Ophthalmol 77 (1967) 541–545.

Elekessy EI, Campion JE, Henry GH: Differences between the

visual fields of Siamese and common cats. Vision Res 13 (1973) 2533–2543.
Erickson OF, Feeney L, McEwen WK: Filter-paper electrophoresis of tears. II. Animal tears and the presence of a "slow-moving lysozyme." Arch Ophthalmol 55 (1956) 800–806.
Farrell DF, Baker HJ, Herndon RM, Lindsey JR, McKhann GM: Feline $GM_1$ gangliosidosis: Biochemical and ultrastructural comparisons with the disease in man. J Neuropathol Exp Neurol 32 (1973) 1–18.
Fischer CA: Retinopathy in anemic cats. J Am Vet Med Assoc 156 (1970) 1415–1427.
Fischer CA: Intraocular cryptococcosis in two cats. J Am Vet Med Assoc 158 (1971) 191–199.
Fischer CA: Diseases of the uveal tract, uveitis and immunologically mediated ocular disorders. *In* Kirk RW (ed): Current Veterinary Therapy VI. Philadelphia, WB Saunders Company, 1978, 638–646.
Ford R: Feline viral respiratory disease: Current concepts. Compend Contin Ed 1 (1979) 337–341.
Fox JG, Galus CB: *Salmonella*-associated conjunctivitis in a cat. J Am Vet Med Assoc 171 (1977) 845–847.
Gaskell RM, Povey RC: Feline viral rhinotracheitis: Sites of virus replication and persistence in acutely and persistently infected cats. Res Vet Sci 27 (1979) 167–174.
Gelatt KN: Feline ophthalmology. Compend Contin Ed 1 (1979) 576–583.
Gelatt KN, Blogg JR: Blepharoplastic procedures in small animals. J Am Anim Hosp Assoc 5 (1969) 67–78.
Gelatt KN, Boggess TS II, Cure TH: Evaluation of mydriatics in the cat. J Am Anim Hosp Assoc 9 (1973) 283–287.
Geltzer AI: Autonomic innervation of the cat iris. An electron microscopic study. Arch Ophthalmol 81 (1969) 70–83.
Greene CE, Goragacz EJ, Martin CL: Hydranencephaly associated with feline panleukopenia. J Am Vet Med Assoc 180 (1982) 767–768.
Grier RL, Brewer WG Jr, Theilen GH: Hyperthermic treatment of superficial tumors in cats and dogs. J Am Vet Med Assoc 177 (1980) 227–233.
Grün K: Die Geschwülste des Zentralnervensystems und seiner Hüllen bei unseren Haustieren. Dissertation, Berlin, 1936.
Guillery RW, Hickey TL, Spear PD: Do blue-eyed, white cats have normal or abnormal retinofugal pathways? Invest Ophthalmol Vis Sci 21 (1981) 27–33.
Gwin RM, Gelatt KN, Peiffer RL Jr: Parotid duct transposition in a cat with keratoconjunctivitis sicca. J Am Anim Hosp Assoc 13 (1977a) 42–45.
Gwin RM, Gelatt KN, Hardy P, Peiffer RL, Williams LW: Ocular cryptococcosis in a cat. J Am Anim Hosp Assoc 13 (1977b) 680–684.
Gwin RM, Makley TA, Wyman M, Werling K: Multifocal ocular histoplasmosis in a dog and cat. J Am Vet Med Assoc 176 (1980) 638–642.
Gwin RM, Merideth R, Martin C, Kaswan R: Ophthalmomyiasis interna posterior in two cats and a dog. J Am Anim Hosp Assoc 20 (1984) 481–486.
Hamilton HB, Severin GA, Nold J: Pulmonary squamous cell carcinoma with intraocular metastasis. J Am Vet Med Assoc 185 (1984) 307–309.
Havener WH: Ocular Pharmacology, 4th ed. St Louis, CV Mosby Company, 1978.
Hayden DW: Squamous cell carcinoma in a cat with intraocular and orbital metastases. Vet Pathol 13 (1976) 332–336.
Hayes KC, Rabin AR, Berson EL: An ultrastructural study of nutritionally induced and reversed retinal degeneration in cats. Am J Pathol 78 (1975) 505–524.
Hendy-Ibbs PM: Familial feline epibulbar dermoids. Vet Rec 116 (1985) 13–14.
Henkind P, Bellhorn R, Rabkin M, Murphy M: Optic nerve transection in cats. Part II. Effect on vessels of optic nerve head and lamina cribrosa. Invest Ophthalmol Vis Sci 16 (1977) 442–447.
Hribernik TN, Barta O, Gaunt SD, Boudreaux MK: Serum hyperviscosity syndrome associated with IgG myeloma in a cat. J Am Vet Med Assoc 181 (1982) 169–170.
Hyde JE, Eason RG: Characteristics of ocular movements evoked by stimulation of brainstem of cat. J Neurophysiol 22 (1959) 666–678.
International Committee on Veterinary Gross Anatomical Nomenclature: Nomina Anatomica Veterinaria, 3rd ed, together with Nomina Histologica, 2nd ed. Ithaca NY, International Committee on Veterinary Gross Anatomical Nomenclature, 1983.
Jacobson RH: Toxoplasmosis—feline infections and their zoonotic potential. *In* Kirk RW (ed): Current Veterinary Therapy VII. Philadelphia, WB Saunders Company, 1980.
Jones TC, Hunt RD: Veterinary Pathology. Philadelphia, Lea & Febiger, 1983, 1689–1724.
Jubb KV, Saunders LZ, Coates HV: Thiamine deficiency encephalopathy in cats. J Comp Pathol Ther 66 (1956) 217–227.
Jungherr E, Wolf A: Gliomas in animals. Am J Cancer 37 (1939) 493–500.
Kalil RE, Jhaveri SR, Richards W: Anomalous retinal pathways in the Siamese cat: An inadequate substrate for normal binocular vision. Science 174 (1971) 302–305.
Kay WJ: Neuro-ophthalmology. *In* Gelatt KN (ed): Textbook of Veterinary Ophthalmology. Philadelphia, Lea & Febiger, 1981.
Kipnis RM: Corneal eosinophilic granuloma. Feline Pract 9(6) (1979) 49–53.
Koch SA: Congenital ophthalmic abnormalities in the Burmese cat. J Am Vet Med Assoc 174 (1979) 90–91.
Kramer JW, Davis WC, Prieur DJ: The Chediak-Higashi syndrome of cats. Lab Invest 36 (1977) 554–562.
Legendre AM, Gompf R, Bone D: Treatment of feline cryptococcosis with ketaconazole. J Am Vet Med Assoc 181 (1982) 1541–1542.
Levick WR, Cleland BG, Dubin MW: Lateral geniculate neurons of cat: Retinal inputs and physiology. Invest Ophthalmol Vis Sci 11 (1972) 302–311.
Lubin JR, Albert DM, Essex M, de Noronha F, Riis R: Experimental anterior uveitis after subcutaneous injection of feline sarcoma virus. Invest Ophthalmol Vis Sci 24 (1983) 1055–1062.
MacMillan AD: Retinal dysplasia and degeneration in the young cat: Feline panleukopenia virus as an etiological agent. PhD Thesis. University of California at Davis, 1974.
MacMillan AD: Acquired retinal folds in the cat. J Am Vet Med Assoc 168 (1976) 1015–1020.
Macri FJ, Cevario SJ: Ciliary ganglion stimulation. II. Neurogenic intraocular pathway for excitatory effects on aqueous humor production and outflow. Invest Ophthalmol Vis Sci 14 (1975) 471–475.
Magrane WG: Intraocular tumors. Proc Am Vet Med Assoc 1968. [Oral presentation.]
Maguire GW, Smith EL III, Harwerth RS, Crawford MLJ: Optically induced anisometropia in kittens. Invest Ophthalmol Vis Sci 23 (1982) 253–264.
Manning TO, Scott DW, Smith CA, Lewis RM: Pemphigus diseases in the feline: Seven case reports and discussion. J Am Anim Hosp Assoc 18 (1982) 433–443.
Martin CL: Feline ophthalmology. Proc Am Anim Hosp Assoc 48 (1981) 287–304.
Martin CL, Anderson BG: Ocular anatomy. *In* Gelatt KN (ed): Textbook of Veterinary Ophthalmology. Philadelphia, Lea & Febiger, 1981.
McClure RC, Dallman MJ, Garrett PD: Cat Anatomy. An Atlas, Text and Dissection Guide. Philadelphia, Lea & Febiger, 1973.
Moise NS, Riis RC, Allison NM: Ocular manifestations of metastatic sweat gland adenocarcinoma in a cat. J Am Vet Med Assoc 180 (1982) 1100–1103.

Moore FM: Unpublished data, 1985.

Morgan G: Ocular tumors in animals. J Small Anim Pract 10 (1969) 563–570.

Morgan RV: Chronic hypertension in four cats: ocular and medical findings. J Am Anim Hosp Assoc. In press.

Morgan RV, Bachrach A, Ogilvie GK: An evaluation of soft contact lens usage in the dog and cat. J Am Anim Hosp Assoc 20 (1984) 885–888.

Munger RJ, Ackerman N: Applications of positive contrast orbitography in small animals. Am Coll Vet Ophthalmol Ninth Ann Scientific Program (1978) 25–50.

Murray JA, Blakemore WF, Barnett KC: Ocular lesions in cats with $GM_1$-gangliosidosis with visceral involvement. J Small Anim Pract 18 (1977) 1–10.

Nafe LA: Meningiomas in cats: a retrospective clinical study of 36 cases. J Am Vet Med Assoc 174 (1979) 1224–1227.

Narfström K: Hereditary progressive retinal atrophy in the Abyssinian cat. J Hered 74 (1983) 273–276.

Narfström LK, Nilsson SEG: Progressive retinal atrophy in the Abyssinian cat: an update. Vet Rec 112 (1983) 525–526.

Nasisse MP, van Ee RT, Wright P: Ocular changes in a cat with disseminated blastomycosis. J Am Vet Med Assoc 187 (1985) 629–631.

Noxon JO, Digilio K, Schmidt DA: Disseminated histoplasmosis in a cat: Successful treatment with ketaconazole. J Am Vet Med Assoc 181 (1982) 817–820.

Olson CR, Freeman RD: Profile of the sensitive period for monocular deprivation in kittens. Exp Brain Res 39 (1980) 17–21.

Peiffer RL Jr: Iris cyst in a cat. Feline Pract 7(4) (1977) 15–17.

Peiffer RL Jr: Feline ophthalmology. *In* Gelatt KN (ed): Textbook of Veterinary Ophthalmology, Philadelphia, Lea & Febiger, 1981.

Peiffer RL: Bilateral congenital aphakia and retinal detachment in a cat. J Am Anim Hosp Assoc 18 (1982a) 128–130.

Peiffer RL Jr: Inherited ocular diseases of the dog and cat. Compend Contin Ed 4 (1982b) 152–164.

Peiffer RL Jr, Belkin PV: Ocular manifestations of disseminated histoplasmosis in a cat. Feline Pract 9(4) (1979) 24–29.

Peiffer RL Jr, Belkin PV, Janke BH: Orbital cellulitis, sinusitis, and pneumonitis caused by *Penicillium* sp in a cat. J Am Vet Med Assoc 176 (1980) 449–450.

Peiffer RL Jr, Belkin PV: Keratolenticular dysgenesis in a kitten. J Am Vet Med Assoc 182 (1983) 1242–1243.

Peiffer RL Jr, Gelatt KN: Cryoextraction of the feline cataract. Vet Med Small Anim Clin 68 (1973) 1425–1428.

Peiffer RL Jr, Gelatt KN: Cataracts in the cat. Feline Pract 4 (1) (1974) 34–38.

Peiffer RL Jr, Gelatt KN: Congenital cataracts in a Persian kitten. Vet Med Small Anim Clin 70 (1975) 1334–1335.

Peiffer RL Jr, Jackson WF: Mycotic keratopathy of the dog and cat in the Southeastern United States: A preliminary report. J Am Anim Hosp Assoc 15 (1979) 93–97.

Peiffer RL Jr, Spencer C, Popp JA: Nasal squamous cell carcinoma with periocular extension and metastasis in a cat. Feline Pract 8 (6) (1978) 43–46.

Peiffer RL Jr, Williams L, Duncan J: Keratopathy associated with smoke and thermal exposure. Feline Pract 7 (5) (1979) 23–36.

Pentlarge V, Riis RC: Proliferative keratitis in a cat: a case report. J Am Anim Hosp Assoc 20 (1984) 477–480.

Percy DH, Scott FW, Albert DM: Retinal dysplasia due to feline panleukopenia virus infection. J Am Vet Med Assoc 167 (1975) 935–937.

Priester WA: Congenital ocular defects in cattle, horses, cats, and dogs. J Am Vet Med Assoc 160 (1972) 1504–1511.

Prieur DJ, Collier LL, Bryan GM, Meyers KM: The diagnosis of feline Chediak-Higashi syndrome. Feline Pract 9 (5) (1979) 26–32.

Prince JH, Diesem CD, Eglitis I, Ruskell G: Anatomy and Histology of the Eye and Orbit in Domestic Animals. Springfield, IL, Charles C Thomas, 1960.

Quinn A: Granulomatous chorioretinitis of disseminated histoplasmosis in cats. Proc Am Soc Vet Ophthalmol Int Soc Vet Ophthalmol, Las Vegas, 1982, 159–163.

Rendano VT, de Lahunta A, King JM: Extracranial neoplasia with facial nerve paralysis in two cats. J Am Anim Hosp Assoc 16 (1980) 921–925.

Riis RC: Feline corneal sequestra. Proc Am Soc Vet Ophthalmol Int Soc Vet Ophthalmol, Las Vegas, 1982, 1–9.

Risco JM, Nopanitaya W: Ocular microcirculation. Scanning electron microscopic study. Invest Ophthalmol Vis Sci 19 (1980) 5–12.

Roberts SR: Detachment of the retina in animals. J Am Vet Med Assoc 135 (1959) 423–431.

Roberts SR, Bistner SI: Surgical correction of eyelid agenesis. Mod Vet Pract 49 (9) (1968) 40–43.

Roberts SR, Lipton DE: The eye. *In* Catcott EJ (ed): Feline Medicine and Surgery, 2nd ed. Santa Barbara, American Veterinary Publications, Inc, 1975.

Rubin LF: Atlas of Veterinary Ophthalmoscopy. Philadelphia, Lea & Febiger, 1974.

Rubin L: Hereditary cataract in Himalayan cats. Feline Pract 16 (1) (1986) 14–15.

Rubin LF, Lipton DE: Retinal degeneration in kittens. J Am Vet Med Assoc 162 (1973) 467–469.

Saperstein G, Harris S, Leipold HW: Congenital defects in domestic cats. Santa Barbara, Veterinary Practice Publishing Company, 1978. Reprinted from Feline Pract 6 (4) (1976) 18–43.

Saunders LZ: The eye and ear. *In* Jubb KYF, Kennedy PC: Pathology of Domestic Animals, vol 2. New York, Academic Press, Inc, 1963.

Saunders LZ, Barron CN: Intraocular tumours in animals. IV. Lymphosarcoma. Br Vet J 120 (1964) 25–35.

Scagliotti RH: Neuro-ophthalmology. *In* Kirk RW (ed): Current Veterinary Therapy VII. Philadelphia, WB Saunders Company, 1980.

Schaller JP, Wyman M, Weisbrode SE, Olsen RG: Induction of retinal degeneration in cats by methylnitrosourea and ketamine hydrochloride. Vet Pathol 18 (1981) 239–247.

Schmidt GM: Mycotic keratoconjunctivitis. Vet Med Small Anim Clin 69 (1974) 1177–1179.

Schmidt GM, Coulter DB: Physiology of the eye. *In* Gelatt KN (ed): Textbook of Veterinary Ophthalmology. Philadelphia, Lea & Febiger, 1981.

Scott FW, de Lahunta A, Schultz RD, Bistner SI, Riis RC: Teratogenesis in cats associated with griseofulvin therapy. Teratology 11 (1975) 79–86.

Severin GA: Veterinary Ophthalmology Notes, 2nd ed. Ft Collins, Colorado State University, 1976.

Smith J, Bistner S, Riis R: Infiltrative corneal lesions resembling fibrous histiocytoma: Clinical and pathologic findings in six dogs and one cat. J Am Vet Med Assoc 169 (1976) 722–726.

Smythe RH: Veterinary Ophthalmology, 2nd ed. Baltimore. The Williams and Wilkins Company, 1958.

Stansbury RL: Detecting and managing feline head lesions [Protrusion of membrana nictitans]. Mod Vet Pract 47 (9) (1966) 45–53.

Steinberg RH, Reid M, Lacy PL: The distribution of rods and cones in the retina of the cat (*Felis domesticus*). J Comp Neurol 148 (1973) 229–248.

Strickland JH, Calhoun ML: The integumentary system of the cat. Am J Vet Res 24 (1968) 1018–1029.

Thibos LN, Levick WR, Morstyn R: Ocular pigmentation in white and Siamese cats. Invest Ophthalmol Vis Sci 19 (1980) 475–486.

Todd NB: A pink-eyed dilution in the cat. J Hered 52 (1961) 202.

Trautmann A, Fiebiger J: Fundamentals of the Histology of Domesitc Animals. Translated and revised by Habel RE, Biberstein EL. Ithaca NY, Comstock Publishing Associates (Cornell University Press), 1957.

Vainisi SJ, Campbell LH: Ocular toxoplasmosis in cats. J Am Vet Med Assoc 154 (1969) 141–152.

Vakkur GJ, Bishop PO, Kozak W: Visual optics in the cat, including posterior nodal distance and retinal landmarks. Vision Res 3 (1963) 289–314.

Valle DL, Boison AP, Jezyk P, Aguirre G: Gyrate atrophy of the choroid and retina in a cat. Invest Ophthalmol Vis Sci 20 (1981) 251–255.

Van Alphen GW, Kern R, Robinette SL: Adrenergic receptors of the intraocular muscles: comparison to cat, rabbit, and monkey. Arch Ophthalmol 74 (1965) 253–259.

Van Horn DL, Sendele DD, Seideman S, Buco PJ: Regenerative capacity of the corneal endothelium in the rabbit and cat. Invest Ophthalmol Vis Sci 16 (1977) 597–613.

Veenendaal H: Tuberculoom op de cornea bij een kat. Tijd Diergeneeskd 55 (1928) 607–611.

Veith LA, Cure TH, Gelatt KN: The Schirmer tear test in cats. Mod Vet Pract 51 (5) (1970) 48.

Verwer MAJ: Partial mummification of the cornea in cats. Proc Am Anim Hosp Assoc 32 (1965) 112–118.

Vestre WA, Brightman AH II, Helper LC: Use of an intraocular prosthesis in the cat. Feline Pract 8 (4) (1978) 23–26.

Walker WF Jr: A Study of the Cat. Philadelphia, WB Saunders Company, 1967.

Waring GO III, Bourne WM, Edelhauser HF, Kenyon KR: The corneal endothelium. Normal and pathologic structure and function. Ophthalmology 89 (1982) 531–590.

Wen GY, Sturman JA, Wisniewski HM, Lidsky AA, Cornwell AC, Hayes KC: Tapetum disorganization in taurine-depleted cats. Invest Ophthalmol Vis Sci 18 (1979) 1200–1206.

West CS, Wolf ED, Vainisi SJ: Intraocular metastasis of mammary adenocarcinoma in the cat. J Am Anim Hosp Assoc 15 (1979) 725–728.

West-Hyde L, Buyukmihci N: Photoreceptor degeneration in a family of cats. J Am Vet Med Assoc 181 (1982a) 243–247.

West-Hyde L, Buyukmihci N: The pathology of photoreceptor degeneration in a family of cats: An update. Trans Thirteenth Ann Scientific Program Am Coll Vet Ophthalmol (1982b) 173–180.

Wheeler CA, Severin GA: Cryosurgical epilation for the treatment of distichiasis in the dog and cat. J Am Anim Hosp Assoc 20 (1984) 877–884.

Wiesel TN, Hubel DH: Effects of visual deprivation on morphology and physiology of cells in the cat's lateral geniculate body. J Neurophysiol 26 (1963) 978–993.

Withers AR, Davies ME: An outbreak of conjunctivitis in a cattery [caused by *Moraxella lacunatus*]. Vet Rec 73 (1961) 856–857.

Wong VG, Macri FJ: Vasculature of the cat eye. Arch Ophthalmol 72 (1964) 351–358.

Woog J, Albert DM, Gonder JR, Carpenter JJ: Osteosarcoma in a phthisical feline eye. Vet Pathol 20 (1983) 209–214.

Wyman M: Ophthalmic surgery for the practitioner. Vet Clin North Am 9 (1979) 311–348.

Wyman M, McKissick GE: Lipemia retinalis in a dog and cat. J Am Anim Hosp Assoc 9 (1973) 288–291.

Yanoff M, Fine BS: Ocular Pathology: A Text and Atlas. Hagerstown, Harper and Row, 1975.

Zapater RC, Albesi EJ, Garcia GH: Mycotic keratitis by *Drechslera spicifera*. Sabouraudia 13 (1975). 295–298.

# 15
CHAPTER
# THE EAR

JEAN HOLZWORTH

Whether large and pointed as in Siamese or small and rounded as in cats of Persian conformation, cats' ears are one of their handsomest features. The uniformly upright and open form of the ear is also a practical asset, sparing cats many of the ills that afflict animals with pendulous or hairy ears and hairy ear canals.

## THE NORMAL EAR

A practical familiarity with the anatomy of the normal ear is essential for effective care and treatment (Crouch, 1969; de Lahunta and Habel, 1986; McClure et al., 1973; Bourdelle and Bressou, 1953; Rose, 1976, 1978).

The auricle (pinna), erect in all breeds and facing forward and somewhat laterally, forms a roomy, well-ventilated antechamber for the deeper parts of the ear. The skin adheres tightly to the concave inner surface of the auricle, more lightly to the outer surface. The outer skin is covered with short, velvety fur. In contrast, the fur is sparse on the concave surface but varies in amount with individual cats and breeds, very little being present, for example, in the ears of Siamese, whereas Persians have long, curved "feathers." Proximally, the fur decreases steadily in amount. The fur on the temple in front of the ears is thinner than elsewhere on the face, a natural feature about which owners sometimes worry needlessly.

A little pigment is present in the skin of the auricle, as well as in the external acoustic meatus (Strickland and Calhoun, 1960).

The auricle is a thin, delicate structure, semitransparent when the covering fur is light-colored, so that the fine vascular network is often visible. The caudal auricular artery supplies medial, lateral, intermediate, and deep branches to the convex surface of the auricle, whence smaller branches penetrate the cartilage to the concave surface. Associated with the arteries of the convex surface are satellite veins. If the fur of an ear margin is flattened with a dab of Vaseline, these veins are distinguishable as fine raised cords and, with minimum discomfort to the cat, may be pricked with a stylet or curved scalpel blade when only a few drops of blood are needed for hematologic or chemical tests.

The venous drainage of the auricle differs from that of the dog in an important practical respect: the lateral auricular vein courses across the tragus, one of the processes of the auricular cartilage, and must be ligated in the operation to resect the external acoustic meatus (de Lahunta and Habel, 1986).

The auricle is constricted at its base to form the funnel-like orifice of the external auditory meatus. Directed at first ventrorostrally (forming the so-called vertical canal) and then making a medial bend at an angle of almost 90 degrees, the meatus is continued by the tube-like annular cartilage, which is attached to the bony acoustic meatus of the temporal bone and ends at the tympanic membrane. The segment of the meatus proximal to its angular bend is commonly referred to as the horizontal canal. To inspect the entire length of the meatus with an otoscope and speculum, one must draw the auricle laterally in order to straighten the meatus so that the speculum can pass the bend and get within focal distance of the tympanic membrane.

The meatus is lined with slightly pigmented, relatively hairless skin, the glandular components of which have had considerable study (Fernando, 1965a,b, 1967; Montagna, 1949; Strickland and Calhoun, 1960). Under the epidermis is a conspicuous layer of large sebaceous glands that open by ducts into hair follicles or directly to the surface. Apocrine (ceruminous) glands are situated in the deepest layer of the dermis, with ducts opening into the hair follicles just above those of the sebaceous glands. The secretions of both combine to form cerumen, which in the normal ear is neutral in reaction (Fernando, 1965a,b, 1967).

The meatus measures 3 mm in diameter, 12 mm along the length of its lower curvature, and 7 mm along the upper curvature (Benoit, 1938). It is closed at birth and opens at 10 to 14 days of age.

The skin of the deep part of the external ear canal is supplied by the auricular branch of the vagus, and irritation from ear mites or infection may provoke vomiting, because the brain interprets the afferent stimuli as originating in the stomach (Miller, 1952).

Microorganisms that may be isolated from normal feline ears include *Malassezia (Pityrosporon) pachydermatis, Staphylococcus aureus* and *epidermidis,* and nonhemolytic streptococci (Niklas, 1979).

The external acoustic meatus ends at the oval, slightly concave tympanic membrane (eardrum), which is set into the bony meatus and tilts forward and inward. The membrane is a shiny, pale gray, translucent sheet of fibrous tissue covered by a thin layer of stratified squamous epithelium. Through its upper part may be seen the manubrium (handle) of the malleus, the auditory ossicle attached to the inner surface of the membrane. In a normal membrane, vessels are visible by otoscopic examination only around the manubrium.

The middle ear (tympanic cavity) is lined with mucous membrane. It consists of two main compartments separated by a bony septum. In the tympanic (dorsal) compartment are the three auditory ossicles (malleus, incus, and stapes), which transmit sounds to the auditory components of the middle ear; two skeletal muscles, the tensor tympani and stapedius, which arise from the dorsal wall of the tympanum and regulate the vibrations of the malleus and stapes, respectively; the chorda tympani (a branch of the facial nerve); sympathetic nerve fibers; and the orifice of the auditive (Eustachian) tube. The large ventral compartment of the middle ear, commonly referred to as the bulla, is one of the cat's distinctive anatomic features. It communicates by a small opening in the bony septum with the dorsal compartment. Frequently involved in inflammatory processes and occasionally invaded by granulomas or tumors, it is easily studied by radiography (Fig. 15–1) and is also accessible to surgical drainage from the exterior.

The auditive (Eustachian) tube is short and oval, about 5 to 8 mm long and 1 mm in diameter (Carpenter, 1963; Rose, 1978b). Leaving the rostral wall of the middle ear and curving medially, it emerges by a 4-mm slit on the lateral wall of the nasopharynx dorsal to the soft palate, where it is hidden from view unless the soft palate is pulled forward. Its tympanic origin, a short bony portion, remains open. This is continued by a longer cartilaginous part that is closed in its resting state by the elasticity of the cartilage. The auditive tube, which is lined by pseudostratified columnar respiratory epithelium, opens during sneezing, swallowing, and yawning, to equalize pressure in the middle ear and to eliminate fluids. It serves as one access route for infections and granulomas of the middle ear but is most notorious as one site of origin of mucous polyps that may emerge at the external auditory meatus, the nostril, or nasopharynx.

The inner ear, separated from the tympanic cavity by a bony wall, houses the semicircular canals, utriculus, and sacculus, which regulates equilibrium, and the cochlea, which encases the organ of Corti, the receptor for hearing. One membranous opening in the wall, the vestibular (oval) window, contains the third auditory ossicle, the stapes, which transmits impulses to the perilymph circulating around the semicircular canals and cochlea. Another opening, the membranous cochlear (round) window, changes position to adjust to pressure created by fluid waves through the perilymph.

It is easy to understand that the natural opening of the auditive tube and absence or perforation of the tympanic membrane constitute serious threats to the delicate mechanisms of the middle and inner ear.

Cats have far more sensitive hearing than man. Their upper range is 50,000 to 60,000 waves or cycles (hertz, Hz) per second, while that of man is 18,000 to 20,000 (Hart, 1977). Certain very high sounds, inaudible to man, may be painful and disturbing to cats, such as those from electronic pest-repellent devices and the remote control devices used to change television channels.

## DISORDERS OF THE EAR

### Anomalies

Several congenital anomalies are reported to affect the external ear. "Four ears," in which a small extra pinna was present on either side, has been reported twice (Fasnacht, 1969; Little, 1957) and has been seen at the Angell Memorial Animal Hospital (AMAH). The mutation reported by Little was shown by breeding trials to be transmitted as a simple recessive and was associated with small eyes, undershot jaw, and sluggish temperament. The kitten seen at AMAH, a "brown mutation" female, also had small eyes.

Inward folding of the tip of the auricle appeared as a mutant in domestic shorthairs in Scotland in the 1960s. It is an autosomal dominant trait that may be associated in homozygotes with an extra upward fold of the apex of the auricle and with skeletal abnormalities such as prognathia, vertebral deformities, and incapacitating joint disease (Dyte, 1973; Todd, 1972). By breeding heterozygotes to purebred British and American shorthairs, cat fanciers developed an attractive, officially recognized breed (Fig. 15–2).

A cat with a folded ear similar to that of the Scottish Fold was also seen in Germany (Wolff, 1971). Four littermates with folded ears were born in Belgium in 1971, but at four weeks of age their ears had assumed a normal form (Robinson, 1972).

Abnormally large ears were associated in a Manx cat with a variety of skeletal defects and a cerebral malformation (Field, 1975).

Other congenital abnormalities are synotia, impatent external acoustic meatus, and absence or defect of the tympanic membrane.

Deafness in white cats, an anomaly that has fascinated laymen and scientists for about 200 years, has evoked a vast literature, which was reviewed by Bergsma and Brown (1971) and by Bosher and Hallpike (1965), and the defect has continued to be studied (e.g., Mair, 1976; Rebillard et al., 1976; Suga and Hattler, 1970; van der Velden, 1976). The degenerative changes causing this deafness are first recognizable at four to six days after birth. Inherited deafness is most often encountered in domestic (crossbred) cats but may occur in purebreds too. It is caused by an autosomal dominant gene. A single pair of alleles determines if an individual white cat will be blue-eyed, yellow-eyed, or "odd-eyed" heterochromic (Todd et al., 1968). The cat may be partly or completely deaf in one or both ears. Contrary to some reports, the deafness is not always on the same side as the blue iris. Blue-eyed cats are more often deaf than odd-eyed cats, which in turn are more often deaf than yellow-eyed cats (Bergsma and Brown, 1971). A few cats have a small gray

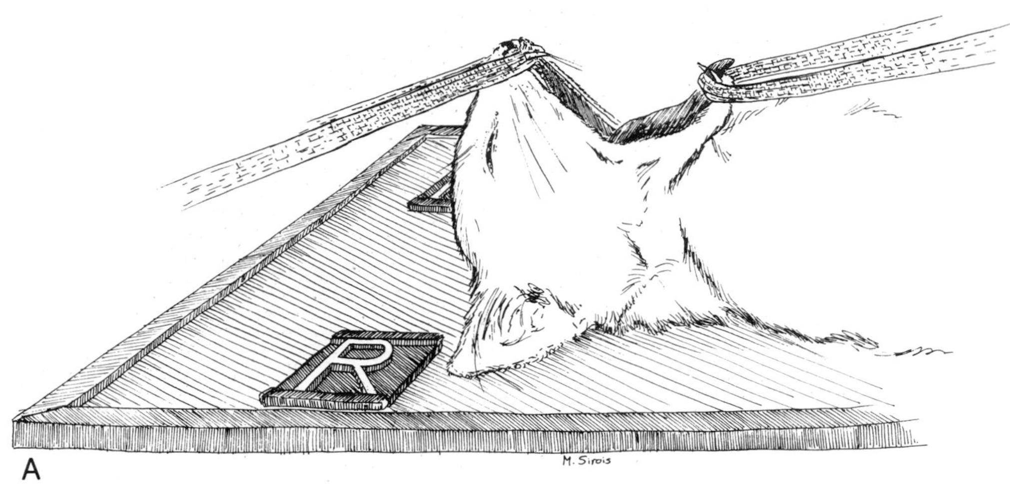


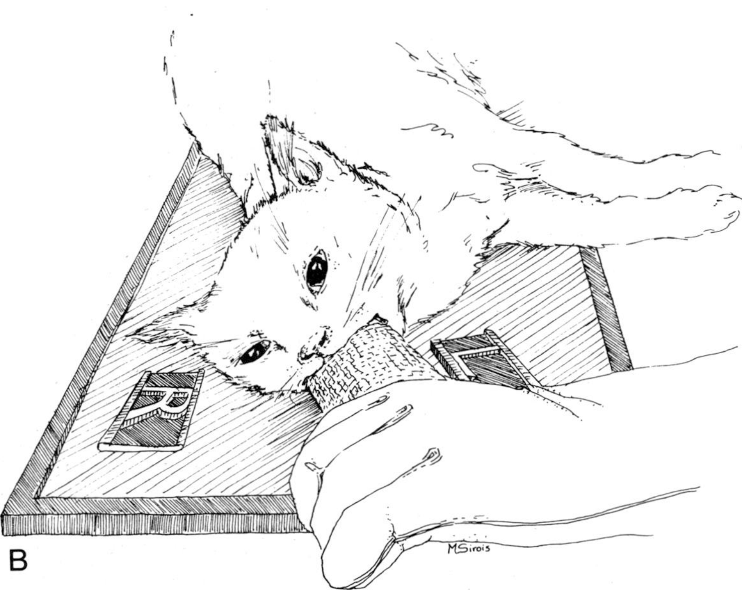


**Figure 15–1** The most informative projections for radiography of the middle ear are the frontal with open mouth and the oblique. *A*, Frontal: The anesthetized cat is immobilized squarely on its back with jaws held wide open by gauze strips hooked onto the canine teeth so that the x-ray beam is parallel to the hard palate and directed at the temporomandibular joint. The tongue is pulled forward out of the way under the gauze that secures the mandible. *B,* Oblique: With the anesthetized cat lying on its side and a roll of gauze wedged between the canine teeth, the technician rotates the roll of gauze to tilt the head downward 10 to 15 degrees so that an unobstructed exposure of the upper bulla is obtained.

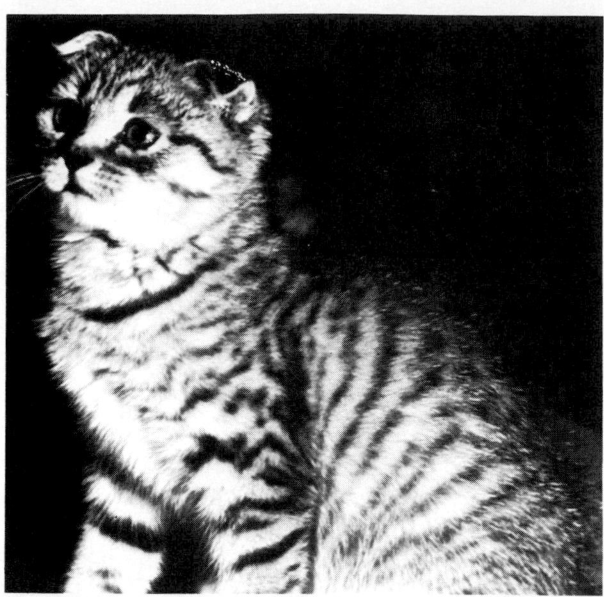

**Figure 15–2** The Scottish Fold, an officially recognized breed, was developed from a mutation in which the ear tips tilt forward. (Courtesy William Nixon.)

or black smudge on the forehead that may fade with time; others have more intense and extensive spotting that persists. Deafness tends to be less severe in the cats with transient or persistent spotting.

The defects responsible for the deafness are related to postnatal degeneration of structures derived from the embryonic neural crest. Histologic findings vary from cat to cat but include collapse of Reissner's membrane, atrophy and dysgenesis of the organ of Corti, hyaline changes of the stria vascularis, and degeneration or absence of the otoconia and collapse of the saccular macula.

Although in many respects analogous to Waardenburg's syndrome in man (Faith and Woodard, 1973), not all the associated defects occurring in man have been observed in cats. Practical problems noted in one study were that in comparison with colored cats, white cats given intravenous injections showed decreased blood vessel tone and prolonged bleeding (Bergsma and Brown, 1971). Very young deaf kittens may die of cold or malnutrition, as they cannot hear their mother's call (Jones, 1975). As a pet, a totally deaf cat is subject to serious hazards if allowed to roam outdoors.

## Acquired Disorders

The majority of aural problems of cats involve or originate in the external ear, either the auricle or the external auditory meatus.

### The Auricle (Pinna)

**INJURIES.** The auricle, because of its anatomic prominence, cutaneous covering, and delicate structure, is prone to many ills. Lucky is the cat that gets through life without a few nicks or tears inflicted by claws or teeth in play or battle. Fast-living toms run the greatest risks. Sizable lacerations should be treated to prevent infection and, if appearance is a concern, should be promptly repaired with 5-0 nonabsorbable sutures placed through the skin on each side of the auricle (Leighton, 1975).

Bites penetrating cartilage—particularly the convolutions at the base of the ear—may cause necrosis of cartilage and stubborn abscesses requiring débridement, thorough drainage, and prolonged treatment with a systemic antibiotic. One such nonhealing lesion in a cat at AMAH proved to be infected with *Nocardia,* indicating the need for culturing if a lesion is unresponsive to routine treatment. In another cat, an abscess recurring at intervals over many months was associated with a fistulous opening in the deepest part of the wall of the external auditory meatus. Resection or ablation of the meatus offered the only hope of a lasting cure but was refused by the owner.

A circumferential fracture of the cartilaginous meatus where it enters the skull is a rare but grave event and may at first go unnoticed when more conspicuous damage catches the attention. The carriage of the ears is asymmetric, the fractured auricle sliding limply sideways and failing to prick up in response to stimuli. The head may be tilted down and the eye retracted on the injured side. The entire auricle is found to be abnormally movable. As surgical reattachment is not feasible, clean-up and examination should disturb the tissues as little as possible. If the fracture is not complete, slow healing may take place; but if the cartilage is completely sheared from its attachment, the only course may be removal of the auricle.

Alterations in the tip of the auricle, other than those caused by trauma, are infrequent. Rounding and fibrous thickening of the apex in cold climates is believed to be caused by frostbite. Inward drooping of the ear tip is also rare. Owners of one cat in which both ear tips developed a permanent droop maintained that it occurred after the cat's ears were cleaned with ether.

Unilateral droop of the ear tip in a young and otherwise normal Burmese male was associated with coolness and some loss and fading of fur on the affected tip. Circulatory impairment of some sort was conjectured to be the cause. Over some months, the ear gradually returned to normal (Zagraniski, 1974, 1975).

Necrosis and sloughing of both auricles, starting at the tips, were observed in a number of cats fed scraps from fish processing on Cape Cod, Massachusetts, but the specific cause was never discovered. Several cats at AMAH with serious febrile systemic disease and hematologic abnormalities have exhibited bilateral necrosis and dry gangrene of the ear tips. Punctate necrosis of the auricle, as well as sloughing of the skin about the claws, occurred in a cat that had received a series of blood transfusions. These lesions may have resulted from disseminated intravascular coagulation.

**HEMATOMA.** Auricular hematomas have the greatest potential for spoiling a cat's looks. Rupture of blood vessels in a fight, or from headshaking or scratching, most often associated with parasitic infestation of the meatus, causes blood to accumulate between the auricular cartilage and the skin, usually on the concave surface of the auricle. The pockets of blood and serum vary in size, the largest causing the ear to puff up like a tense balloon and fall forward, obstructing the ear canal and causing the cat additional discomfort.

Surgical treatment of hematoma is discussed in the chapter on soft tissue surgery, but some comments and indication of various approaches are in order here.

Treatment should be prompt. If a hematoma is neglected, strands and sheets of fibrin form and gradually organize into fibrous tissue that eventually thickens, shrinks, and crumples the auricle into a disfiguring "cauliflower ear."

The underlying cause of the trouble must first be discovered and dealt with. The ear should be thoroughly cleaned and examined, and appropriate treatment given for ear mites if present. Both sides of the auricle must be clipped and thoroughly disinfected to prevent introduction of infection by aspiration, incision, or suturing.

Small hematomas are sometimes treated by simple aspiration, perhaps with instillation of a steroid or proteolytic enzyme, in the hope of keeping scar tissue from forming within the cavity. Large hematomas are usually opened with a straight or S-shaped incision the full length of the swelling so that blood and fibrin can be completely removed, and a narrow strip of skin is sometimes removed from one edge of the incision to prevent it from sealing and permitting the cavity to refill with fluid. In one method, the incision is made through the skin and cartilage from the convex surface (Marshall, 1959).

From here, procedures vary greatly. Many veterinarians quilt the loosened skin to the auricle by mattress sutures tied on the convex surface of the ear. The fewer the sutures and the finer the needle and suture material, the less damage there will be to cartilage and skin. In Marshall's method, the sutures are passed through small buttons on both surfaces of the auricle. Some veterinarians believe a stapler inflicts less damage than suturing, but staples may be difficult to remove. Still others neither staple nor suture but simply apply a firm dressing to prevent reaccumulation of fluid (Beard, 1954).

Dressings may either turn the ear medially, flattening it over the top of the head, or support the ear upright by bandaging it around a partly used roll of 1½-inch gauze bandage or a foam mold such as is used to keep a dog's ear upright. Another method used in the hope of restoring the ear's natural contour is to suture the edge of the ear to a wire frame molded to the inner surface of the ear (Formston, 1952; Yeats and Vaughan, 1952).

Some veterinarians do not dress the ear at all but put a protective collar on the cat or give it a tranquilizer and follow the cat carefully in the hospital or as an outpatient, to be sure that serum does not reaccumulate. Whatever the method, it is impossible to restore an ear entirely to its former undamaged state.

**INFLAMMATION.** Auricular inflammation, indicated by heat, redness, and sometimes scaliness, may evoke intense irritation, the cat shaking its head and rubbing and scratching the ears, sometimes ripping out fur and tearing the skin. Information about a cat's origin, life style, diet, and medical history is essential. The possibility of dermatophyte infection should never be overlooked, but pathogenic fungi are rarely isolated unless similar lesions are detected elsewhere on the head or body. Rarely, fungi that are generally considered harmless saprophytes are cultured (e.g., *Aspergillus* and *Hormodendrum* spp). Possibly they evoke an allergic reaction.

Questioning the owner may elicit that a cat has had outdoor exposure at a time when allergens are abundant; some cats, for instance, develop allergic reactions when hunting in new-mown hay, others by walking through a tomato patch. Still another cat may be in the habit of sitting under a hot stove. Other important causes of intense irritation of the ears are drugs, for example, unnecessarily strong parasiticidal preparations used for ear mites or simply the vehicle in topical medications. Occasional cats react badly to mineral oil, chlorinated hydrocarbons, or hexachlorophene, although these are commonly used without ill effect (Scott, 1977). That some type of allergy may be involved often seems to be confirmed by a favorable response to application of a steroid ointment or lotion.

The possibility of dietary allergy in a cat that, without apparent cause, tears at its ears and head, may be tested by a period of strict adherence to a regimen of chicken, turkey, or lamb, with rice. If this results in regression of signs, item-by-item testing of foods can be started to try to identify the offender. Meantime, the cat must receive a supplement that fulfills minimum requirements for essential dietary factors.

Irritation of the auricle may also be caused by foreign bodies, such as awns, and by various external parasites. Rabbit fleas have produced ear thickening and hair loss (Barger, 1974). The red larval forms of chigger ("harvest") mites may appear as orange patches on the head and ears (e.g., Hardison, 1977). The ears, as well as the skin of the head and occasionally other parts of the body, may undergo thickening and crusting owing to *Notoedres cati,* and rarely *Demodex cati* may be the cause of thinning fur and scaliness (Gabbert and Feldman, 1976). Chiggers are eliminated by a pyrethrin or lime-sulfur (1:40) dip, *Demodex* by rotenone (Goodwinol Ointment, Pitman-Moore), and *Notoedres* by lime-sulfur or Paramite (Vet-Kem) (½ oz/gallon). Paramite, an organophosphate agent, should be used on no more than a quarter of a cat's skin surface at one time. Ivermectin (1 mg/kg) is reported to eliminate *Notoedres* (as well as ear mites and fleas) (Bigler et al., 1984). Ticks, including nymphs of *Otobius,* are occasionally found within the auricle and should be removed by a forceps.

In pemphigus and thallium poisoning, systemic disorders, the external ears, as well as other areas of the skin, are the site of severe lesions characterized by alopecia, redness, serous oozing, and crusting (see chapter on the skin).

**NEOPLASMS.** Tumors of the auricle may be of most types that affect the skin generally, but the most distinctive is the squamous cell (actinic) carcinoma of white-eared cats that was apparently first reported in Italy (e.g., Carta, 1940; Ottani, 1923), later in California (Dorn et al., 1971; Schaffer, 1958) and that now often appears in surveys of feline tumors or animal tumors (e.g., Engle and Brodey, 1969). That an excessively sunny climate is not an invariable prerequisite was proven by two aged farm cats from the coldest corner of Connecticut and by Massachusetts cats that never went outdoors (but did bask on the sill of a plate-glass picture window). Crespeau (1974) studied a group of cases in detail and suggested that a genetic predisposition might also be involved.

Affected cats are usually middle-aged or old, but premonitory lesions on the edge of the ear were observed in a California cat less than one year old (Schaffer, 1956). Both ears, if white, are likely to be involved. Typically, the lesion develops insidiously over months or years, starting with a long, microscopically precancerous phase during which crusty eczematous lesions of the edge of the ear flare up and regress. To judge from experience with one ear of a cat of my own, the condition can be halted and reversed at the precancerous stage if a protective ointment (e.g., lanolin) is applied and the cat is kept indoors and away from sunlight. By the time proliferation and ulceration have occurred (as with the same cat's other ear), the lesion is irreversibly malignant and the edge of the ear must be trimmed back to healthy tissue. The tumor may vary greatly in microscopic appearance from area to area (Crespeau, 1974), and an accurate diagnosis may require examination of several sections.

Unless excision is ample, there may be recurrence. If the cancer is allowed to progress untreated, it eventually erodes the entire auricle and attacks the base of the ear (Fig. 15–3). Although it is slow to metastasize, it may eventually involve regional nodes and metastasize to distant sites. In one cat at AMAH, metastatic tumor appeared first as a painful enlargement in a toe of the foreleg on the same side as the affected ear, later in a hind toe on the same side, and massively involved the lungs at autopsy.

For treatment with radiotherapy, see the chapter on management of neoplasms.

Basal cell tumors, which have a predilection for the head in cats, are often found in the skin of the auricle (e.g., Foley, 1977; Rose, 1978a; AMAH).

A small mast cell tumor of the inner surface of the auricle was reported by Meier in 1957 as a rarity, but this neoplasm, varying greatly in gross appearance, has now become one of the most frequent cutaneous growths of cats, both on the ear and elsewhere, with the potentiality of becoming a fatal systemic malignancy (Fig. 15–4). (See the chapter on tumors.)

Nodular lymphomas, often indistinguishable grossly from mast cell tumors, occasionally involve the skin of the ear, also serving in some cases as the first sign of systemic disease to come.

Melanoma and fibrosarcoma may involve the pinna (see chapter on tumors). An aggressive tumor seen at AMAH was an irregularly proliferative pleomorphic spindle cell sarcoma of undetermined cell line. Starting in the skin of the base of one ear (Fig. 15–5), it recurred after excision and eventually necessitated removal of the ear.

The only cutaneous papilloma diagnosed in a cat at AMAH occurred on the auricle. An instance of histiocytoma, a rarity in cats, was reported by Priester and McKay (1980).

## External Auditory Meatus

The external auditory meatus causes far less grief in cats than in dogs, chiefly because of the upright, well-ventilated auricle and relatively hairless canal.

External ear disorders of cats—their causes, signs, and management—have been discussed by many but most fully (and forcefully) by Scott (1980, 1984). Examination with an otoscope should be a routine procedure. Depending on the condition of the ear, some form of cleaning is a prerequisite, and tranquilization or anesthesia is often required.

If an exudate is present for which culturing is desirable, the outer part of the ear should be wiped with a disinfectant and material then obtained from deeper in the meatus for Gram staining, culturing for bacteria and fungi, and sensitivity testing.

Dry or waxy masses in the meatus may have to be loosened and floated out with a softening or ceruminolytic agent. The ear is then cleaned by repeated flushing with a plastic syringe, ear bulb syringe, or, most effectively, a pulsating dental hygiene device (Water Pik, Teledyne Div., Squibb). The stream should be directed into the meatus with minimal force, lest the tympanum be ruptured. Flushing should be continued until all debris or exudate has been removed. What fluid remains should be aspirated, and the accessible parts of the ear should be dried with cotton. Cotton-tipped applicators should be

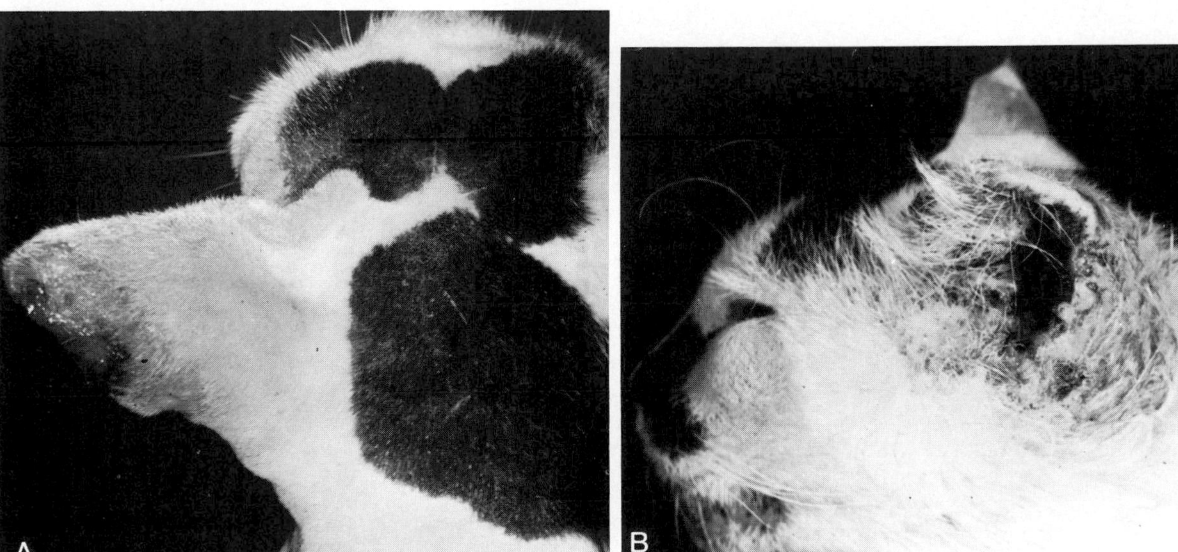


**Figure 15–3** Squamous cell carcinoma in a white-eared 12-year-old spayed domestic shorthair. *A,* In this lesion, removed after several months of oozing and crusty dermatitis, microscopic examination disclosed chronic inflammation with areas of squamous cell neoplasia. *B,* Five months after generous excision to apparently normal tissue, the cancer had recurred and destroyed most of the auricle.

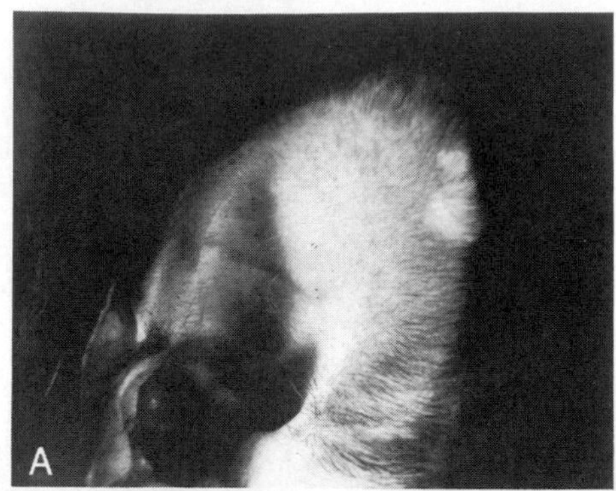


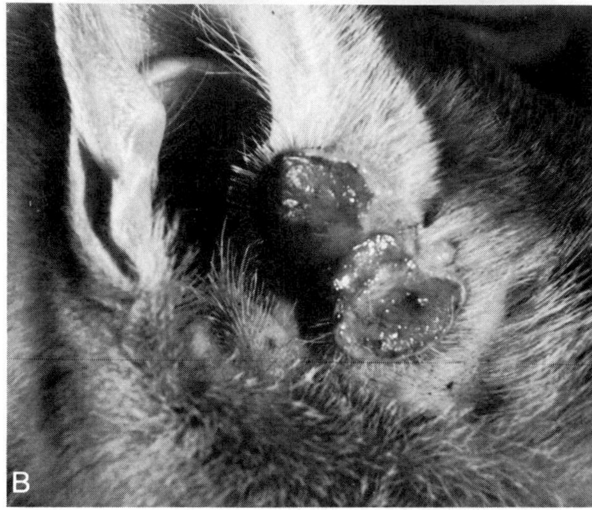


**Figure 15–4** Mast cell tumors can look deceptively innocent. *A,* "Just warts" to the owner, these nodules on the edge of the ear tip of an eight-month-old black-and-white spayed domestic longhair had already metastasized to the regional lymph nodes. *B,* Another "wart," removed four months before and not biopsied, proved to be mast cell tumor, now invading the auricle of an eight-year-old red tabby castrated domestic shorthair. The spleen was greatly enlarged, and there were 3 per cent mast cells in the blood, with PCV 24.

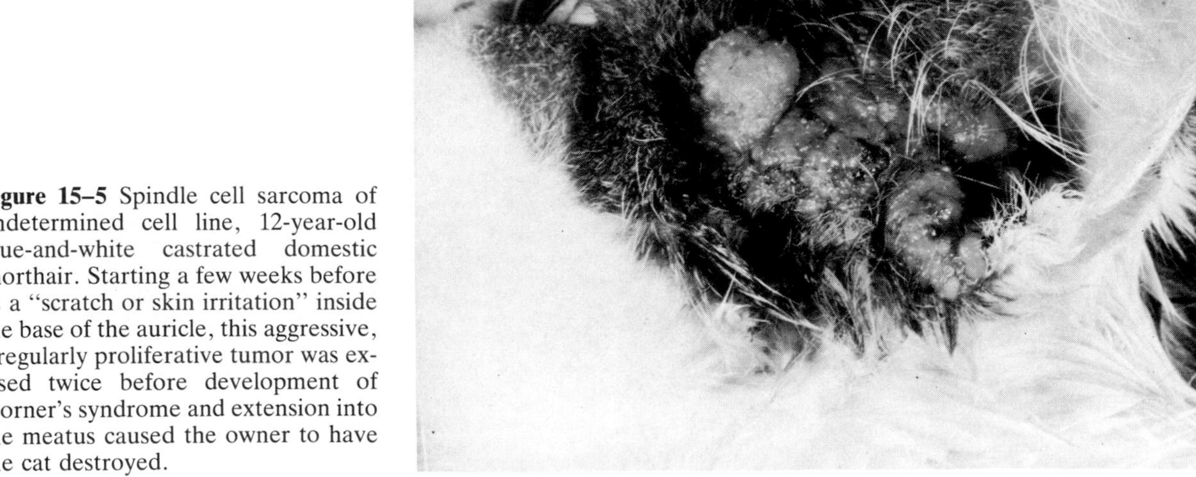

**Figure 15–5** Spindle cell sarcoma of undetermined cell line, 12-year-old blue-and-white castrated domestic shorthair. Starting a few weeks before as a "scratch or skin irritation" inside the base of the auricle, this aggressive, irregularly proliferative tumor was excised twice before development of Horner's syndrome and extension into the meatus caused the owner to have the cat destroyed.

used with caution and with additional cotton twisted over the tip, lest the meatus be traumatized. After effective cleansing it should be possible to inspect the length of the meatus and the tympanum.

A variety of solutions are used for flushing. pHisoHex, diluted 1:15 with water, has detergent and antibacterial action, but pHisoHex may be sufficiently absorbed to be toxic to some cats (Stein, 1985). A solution of povidone-iodine (Betadine) is often used but may be too irritating for some inflamed ears (Scott, 1980). Chlorhexidine solution 1:10 (Nolvasan, Fort Dodge) is active against many Gram-positive and Gram-negative bacteria but should not be used if there is any possibility of middle ear involvement (Scott, 1980). Whatever the flushing solution, it should be warmed.

Cleaning by owners should be limited to wiping of the accessible outer parts of the ear with cotton balls. Owners should be discouraged from using cotton-tipped applicators for cleaning the meatus.

**OTOACARIASIS.** The ear mite *Otodectes cynotis* is the most common cause of trouble in the cat's external auditory meatus and is readily transmitted among cats of all ages and also between cats and dogs. These parasites pass with especial virulence from queen to offspring, for kittens only a month old may have remarkably large plugs of brown debris teeming with mites in numbers rarely encountered in mature cats. Asymptomatic parasitism is common, but restlessness, headshaking, and drooping, scratched, and sometimes bleeding ears are typical signs in many cats. Occasionally, reflex vomiting and convulsions occur. If the parasitism is neglected, inflammation and secondary infection with bacteria and yeasts that normally inhabit the meatus may ensue, even leading to perforation of the tympanic membrane and involvement of the middle and inner ear and brain.

When inflamed, the skin lining the meatus thickens and its secretions are altered. The sebaceous glands, which normally produce neutral lipid, become exhausted and there is hypersecretion of acidic cerumen by the apocrine (ceruminous) glands, often with plugging of their ducts (Fernando, 1967)—hence the excessive amounts of brown wax found in many inflamed ears.

Mites should never be *assumed* to be the cause of inflammation of the meatus; they must actually be seen by the naked eye as minute, moving, whitish specks, or else they or their eggs must be demonstrated microscopically.

With simple, noninflammatory acariasis, a bland oil massaged into the meatus loosens the debris and also suffocates the mites. A solution of thiabendazole, dexamethasone, and neomycin (Tresaderm, Merck) may be used similarly. It has the additional advantages of antibacterial, antimycotic, and anti-inflammatory actions; it is thought that the thiabendazole may account for its efficacy in eliminating mites. If the material is allowed to soak in, the cat itself will shake much of the debris from the ear. Repeated treatments and massaging may be required to float the debris from the depths of the canal. Cleaning with a ceruminolytic or surfactant solution may be required so that the meatus can be inspected with an otoscope to ascertain that no deep plug of debris remains and to view the tympanic membrane. A short-acting anesthetic is required for removing deep-seated debris. For this purpose the Water Pik is most effective, used at the slowest setting, with repeated flushing and aspiration.

For eliminating ear mites, treatment should be repeated every three days for a month to break the cycle of reproduction. Many acaricidal preparations incorporate a parasiticide, but some of these, even when diluted (e.g., Canex diluted 3:1 with mineral oil), cause acute irritation of the ears in some cats, and others (benzyl benzoate, lindane) are highly toxic to cats and should never be used. Tresaderm appears to be without side effects and is the preparation of choice, as it is active against other pathogens that may be involved secondarily.

Together with treatment of the ears, the cat should be dusted with flea powder to eliminate mites that have crawled or been shaken onto other parts of the body, where they may occasionally be responsible for evoking a dermatitis (Scott, 1980, 1984).

If one cat in a group is parasitized, all others are likely to be. Dogs in contact with the cats should be checked. In catteries or laboratory colonies, treatment should be on a "herd" basis.

Excessive production of dark sebum sometimes follows treatment to eliminate ear mites. Topical medication is avoided in favor of a systemic steroid (methylprednisolone acetate, Depo-Medrol, Upjohn), one or two injections effectively drying the meatus (Stein, 1985).

The immunologic aspects of feline parasitism with *Otodectes cynotis* have been studied and are discussed in the chapter on immunology.

**MYCOTIC OTITIS.** Ear mites are not the only cause of irritation, inflammation, and infection of the external meatus. Intensely itchy inflammation characterized by a brown greasy exudate flares up from time to time in individual cats. *Malassezia (Pityrosporon)* is often isolated from such ears. Without microscopic examination or culture this condition is frequently assumed to be caused by mites, but the discharge is oily, in contrast with the dry debris typical of otoacariasis. The condition responds rapidly to cleaning with chlorhexidine solution and instillation of miconazole, thiabendazole, or nystatin. An acidifier such as aluminum acetate (Domeboro Otic, Dome) is also helpful (Scott, 1980).

*Candida* may also be cultured from feline otitis, as well as *Microsporum canis* (Dreisörner et al., 1964; Niklas, 1979).

**SUPPURATIVE OTITIS.** Frankly purulent, malodorous external otitis is not common in cats. It tends to occur if they are in poor condition, or with resistance lowered by other disease, for example, panleukopenia or leukemia. The outer part of the ear should be wiped with a disinfectant and material then obtained for culture from deeper in the meatus. Organisms commonly isolated are *Malassezia (Pityrosporon), Staphylococcus aureus* and *epidermidis,* hemolytic streptococci, less often *E. coli, Pasteurella, Proteus,* and *Pseudomonas* spp (e.g., Scott, 1980). A dark yellow or light brown purulent discharge suggests *S. aureus* or streptococci, a yellowish, thick, cheesy discharge *Pasteurella, Proteus, Pseudomonas,* and *E. coli* (Scott, 1980). Sensitivity testing should be performed to determine the most effective antimicrobial agent for treatment. A systemic antibiotic should be used if fever accompanies the otitis, and it is well to perform a CBC on the chance that there is a predisposing blood dyscrasia.

For topical treatment to be effective, the ear must be thoroughly cleaned, but it is often so painful and the meatus so eroded and necrotic that cleaning and examination must be carried out under anesthesia and perhaps postponed until the cat has been treated for several days with a systemic antibiotic. It is important to determine whether the tympanic membrane is intact, because a severe purulent otitis may be associated with otitis media. If any signs suggestive of middle ear or vestibular involvement are present, only physiologic saline solution should be used in cleaning (Venker–van Haagen, 1983). In an unanesthetized cat, excessive discomfort with frothing at the mouth when the ear is flushed is a warning that the tympanic membrane may not be intact, and introduction of cleansing solution or medication into the middle ear may speedily precipitate spectacular vestibular manifestations.

Two growths that have a predilection for cats occur in the external meatus and are often responsible for unilateral purulent discharge, otitis media, and even central nervous involvement. These are inflammatory polyps and tumors of the ceruminous glands.

**POLYPS AND TUMORS.** The polyp, sometimes referred to in the older literature as a papilloma, fibroma, or myxoma, has long been recognized as the most frequent growth in the ear of cats (see references in tumor chapter). Over 100 cases are on record at AMAH. Polyps may occur in cats of any age from as young as three months. Smooth, shiny, deep-pink, pedunculated masses, they usually arise from the respiratory epithelium of the middle ear or from the lining of the auditive tube and are believed to be a result of middle ear infection (see chapter on tumors). They may emerge at the nostril or in the nasopharynx or wedge themselves into the depths of the external meatus, rupturing the tympanic membrane. Once in a while they occur simultaneously at two different sites (Fig. 15–6). Single polyps have been found at autopsy to have expanded both into the external auditory meatus and into the nasopharynx. Occasionally a polyp arises from the lining of the external auditory meatus. Severe chronic ear mite infestation may predispose to these (Stein, 1985).

In the external meatus a polyp appears as a solid, discrete mass unattached to the wall of the canal. If it is too deep to be twisted free with an Allis forceps or tonsil snare, a lateral resection of the meatus must be performed to give access to the mass. An alternative approach is to grasp the polyp through a ventral incision in the horizontal part of the canal (Venker–van Haagen, 19083). When the polyp is pulled free, hemorrhage is sometimes profuse but can be arrested by pressure with a pledget of cotton. Transient Horner's syndrome is not unusual. Often there is no further trouble, but the growth may recur if the pedicle is not entirely removed.

Polyps may be densely fibrous or myxomatous (hence they have sometimes been called fibromas or myxomas). They are infiltrated with inflammatory cells and covered with columnar or stratified squamous epithelium. Polyps originating in the external meatus also contain ceruminous and sebaceous glands. (See also the chapter on tumors.)

Sometimes there is secondary infection of the middle ear. In one case this was suggestive of actinomycosis of the bulla (Fig. 15–7) (Bachrach and Kleine, 1974). In another case, a polyp infiltrated with *Cryptococcus* was removed from a cat in which that infection had erupted at various sites in the head but appeared to regress when treated with courses of 5-fluorocytosine. A cat with recurrent cutaneous mycetomas due to *Microsporum canis* also had a polyp containing that organism (see chapter on mycotic diseases).

Vestibular disturbance, if present, is a sign that the inner ear also is secondarily affected.

Ceruminous gland tumors occur also in man and dog (Black, 1949) but seem to be a specialty of cats (Ball et al., 1938; Courthaliac, 1938; Davenport and Eisenberg, 1984; Franc et al., 1981; Montpellier et al., 1936; Stookey et al., 1971). They appear often in surveys of feline tumors, and 52 are on record at AMAH. Unlike polyps, these growths are characteristic of middle-aged or elderly cats. Their presence or the likelihood of their future development is often indicated by small, dark, blister-like lesions at the orifice of the external meatus, usually of both ears. Microscopically, these prove to be cystic hyperplasia of the ceruminous glands, a change that precedes the development into adenomas and finally, in some cases, into adenocarcinomas. Excessive cerumen or purulent discharge may be present. The small, dark cysts are a warning to look deeper into the meatus where multiple broad-based, friable growths may be found proliferating on the skin of the wall and often obstructing the lumen (Fig. 15–8). Bits of tissue obtained for biopsy may be diagnosed as cystic hyperplasia, adenoma, or adenocarcinoma, depending on the stage of development of the

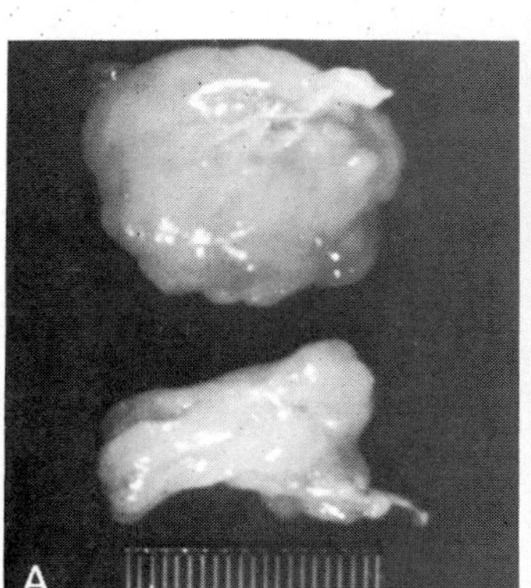


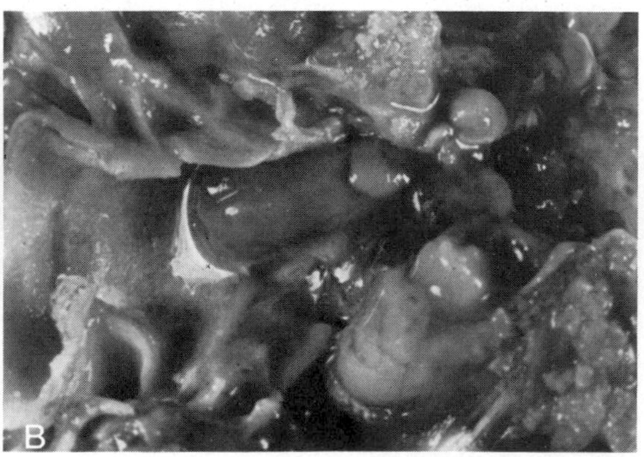


**Figure 15–6** Inflammatory polyps. *A,* The larger was removed from the nasopharynx, the smaller from the ear canal of an adult black male domestic shorthair presented for gagging and snorting as well as a purulent discharge from one ear. *B,* Ventral view of opened right external auditory meatus, bulla, and nasopharynx, six-year-old black male domestic shorthair. A polyp (center) fills the tympanic cavity and extends over 1 cm into the external meatus. Slightly above and to the right, part of the same polypoid mass occludes the orifice of the auditive tube. The thickened bulla ossea (lower right) is filled with pale semisolid exudate. The cat died after developing central nervous system signs associated with secondary meningitis involving cerebellum, pons, and medulla.

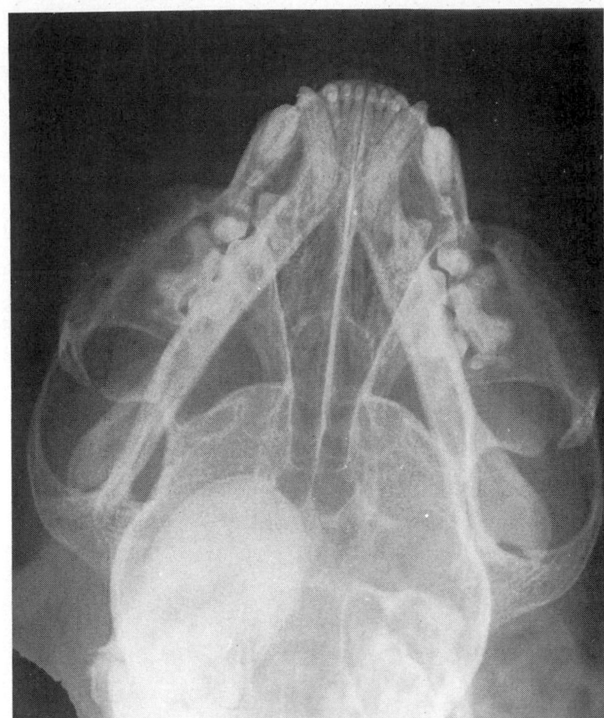

**Figure 15–7** Ventrodorsal radiographic view of tympanic bullae, two and one half-year-old tabby-and-white spayed domestic shorthair. The wall of the right bulla has undergone bony proliferation and sclerosis. A polyp originating in the right middle ear had ruptured the tympanic membrane and occluded the external meatus. The bulla was filled with thick exudate, stained smears of which showed filamentous, branching rods compatible with *Actinomyces* sp. (AMAH, in Bachrach A, Kleine W: J Am Vet Med Assoc 165 [1974] 465–466.)

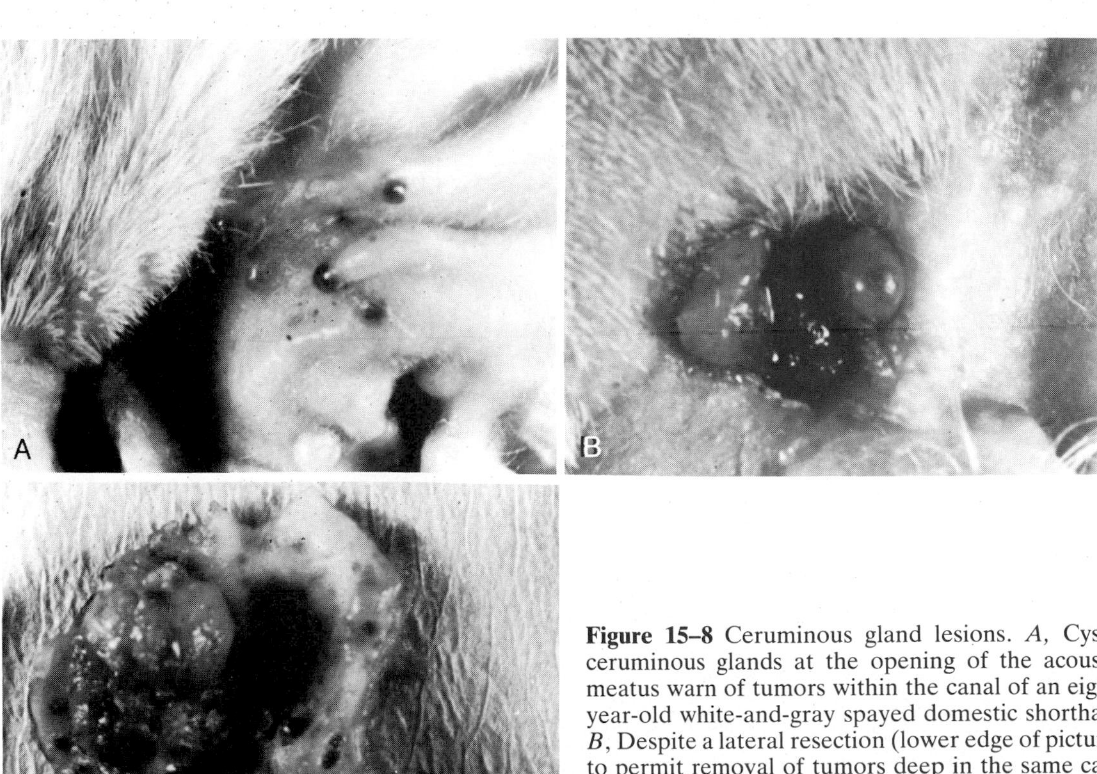


**Figure 15–8** Ceruminous gland lesions. *A,* Cystic ceruminous glands at the opening of the acoustic meatus warn of tumors within the canal of an eight-year-old white-and-gray spayed domestic shorthair. *B*, Despite a lateral resection (lower edge of picture) to permit removal of tumors deep in the same cat's vertical canal, others have now developed in the horizontal canal, necessitating ablation of the canal. *C,* In the ablated meatus, lesions range from cystic hyperplasia to adenocarcinoma.

lesions. When malignant, the tumor may penetrate the wall of the meatus or perforate the tympanic membrane and invade the middle and inner ear, as well as spread to regional nodes. Rarely the tumor spreads into the skin of the temple.

A possible familial tendency was suggested by occurrence of the tumor in a female cat at AMAH and in several of its offspring.

In one unusual case, a ceruminous gland adenoma and a squamous cell carcinoma occupied the same meatus. In another, an adenocarcinoma of the ceruminous gland penetrated the meatus and invaded the parotid salivary gland.

Although lateral resection of the meatus may relieve an obstruction and give access to deeply situated growths, such an operation is not likely to be curative. Recurrent growths, often invading the tympanic membrane and even the middle ear (Fig. 15–9), will probably require ablation of the meatus, and the most practical course is to do this at the outset. In some cats bilateral ablation is necessary. The consequent loss of hearing requires that the cat become a strictly indoor pet, but it is not otherwise handicapped. (Lateral resection and ablation of the meatus are described in the chapter on soft tissue surgery.)

Every mass from an ear canal should be submitted for microscopic diagnosis. A ceruminous gland cancer mistakenly assumed to be a polyp has killed more than one cat.

Twenty-two adenomas and 30 adenocarcinomas diagnosed at AMAH are discussed in detail in the chapter on tumors.

Other tumors reported to involve the external meatus include papillomatosis (Austin, 1975); sebaceous gland adenoma (McAfee et al., 1979); benign hibernoma (Franc et al., 1981); mucous gland adenoma, myxofibroma, a primitive lymphoreticular tumor, and an undifferentiated basosquamous carcinoma (Harvey and Goldschmidt, 1978). Squamous cell carcinoma occasionally occurs in the external ear canal (Foley, 1977; AMAH). In one cat it gave rise to difficulty in eating and swallowing and also metastasized to the orbit and eye (Hayden, 1976).

Although not an aural tumor, a neoplasm that may seriously involve the ear is adenocarcinoma of the parotid salivary gland. A firm, dense growth, it may surround and invade the external meatus, hindering normal drainage and ventilation and resulting in middle and inner ear infection that may be accompanied by signs of central nervous disturbance.

## The Middle Ear

A notable study of middle ear disease in cats is that of Lawson (1957). Although the middle ear may suffer in head injuries, disease of the middle ear almost always arises by extension from disorders elsewhere—through the external auditory meatus, by way of the auditive tube, or by the blood stream. Chronic upper respiratory infection frequently spreads to the middle ear as well as to the nasal sinuses. Parasitism, infection, and growths involving the external auditory meatus represent the other most important causes of middle ear disease. In one cat at AMAH a large, firm ball of cerumen was found in the tympanic bulla.

**OTITIS MEDIA.** As Lawson's study indicated, cats of all ages may be affected. Sometimes otitis media is asymptomatic, recognized only radiographically or at autopsy. Sometimes it simply causes a persistent purulent discharge from the external ear; sometimes it manifests itself by neurologic signs related specifically to the middle or inner ear. Disturbance of the vestibular mechanism is common. Signs of unilateral disease are head tilted sideways and down to the affected side, nystagmus with the slow phase to the affected side, and incoordinated gait with falling or rolling to the affected side. In acute bilateral involvement the head and neck are maintained in a flexed position; in

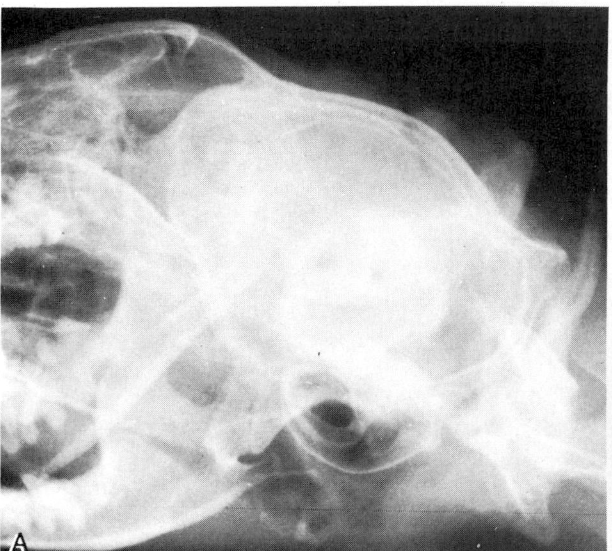


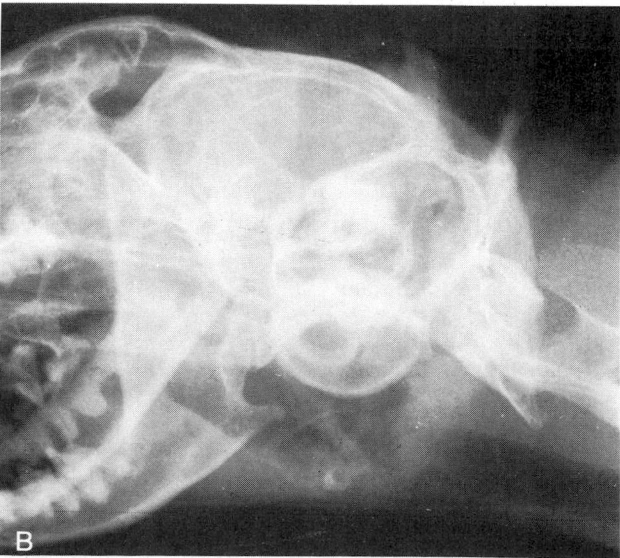


**Figure 15–9** Adenocarcinoma of ceruminous glands, 11-year-old black castrated male domestic longhair. *A,* Normal right bulla, oblique radiographic view. *B,* A growth in the left meatus, previously removed elsewhere and assumed without microscopic study to be a polyp, eventually pushed through the tympanic membrane and invaded the middle ear, producing a radiographic density in the bulla. The external meatus was ablated and the middle ear curetted. The cancer had not recurred when the cat died a year later of lymphoma.

a more chronic condition the animal may crouch with limbs spread apart or crawl in a symmetrically ataxic manner, falling to one side or the other or moving the head widely from side to side (de Lahunta, 1983; Simpson, 1983). Meningeal involvement may be the ultimate complication, with opisthotonos, rigidity of the forelimbs, and contorted attitudes.

The duration of illness and sequence of signs are important. The temperature, which may be normal in chronic cases, should be taken before the cat is disturbed by examination procedures.

The head should be examined for spasticity or paralysis of facial muscles and unequal pupillary size (decreased on the affected side). Signs of oral, pharyngeal, or nasal disease, especially the presence of polyps, should be noted; also signs of pain on opening the mouth or handling the ears, or presence of swelling or drainage below the external meatus.

A purulent exudate in the external acoustic meatus should be cultured and then removed, along with any parasitic debris or obstructing material, procedures that require anesthesia if the tympanic membrane cannot be seen in routine otoscopic examination. As already noted, only physiologic saline solution should be used for flushing.

Abnormalities of the tympanic membrane suggestive of otitis media are bulging, opacity, scarring, discoloration, vascularization, or mineralization. Perforations appear as dark spots.

If a growth occludes the terminal meatus, if the membrane is abnormal, or if signs suggest otitis media or interna, radiographs should be taken of the middle ear.

Frontal open-mouth and oblique views give the most information (Fig. 15–1). The frontal exposure is taken by placing the cat on its back with its head flexed at an angle of 80 to 90 degrees to the film, with the cat's jaws held apart by gauze strips hooked onto the upper and lower canine teeth so that the x-ray beam is centered on the temporomandibular joint. The tongue must be held firmly out of the way under the gauze that immobilizes the mandible. Lateral oblique views of each side, with the head tilted to 10 to 15 degrees and the nose appropriately supported, provide separate images of each bulla that are useful for comparison.

Serous fluid, pus, and soft tissue, such as that of granuloma or tumor, give indistinguishable densities. Chronic infection is often indicated by irregular thickening of the normally fine outline of the bulla. Long-standing infection may produce abnormal ossification.

If the tympanic membrane is abnormal or if radiographs indicate disease of the bulla, a myringotomy should be done to relieve pressure and obtain material for laboratory study. A 20-gauge, 3½ inch spinal tap needle may be used, and a 12-gauge, 3½ inch cannula to enlarge the opening if need be. The membrane should be pierced at its edge at the 6 o'clock position to avoid injury to the more dorsal structures of the middle ear. Antibiotic treatment based on a culture and sensitivity test should follow. If the cause of trouble is eliminated, the tympanum should heal in two or three weeks.

If aspiration is unproductive or if radiographs indicate severe chronic changes in the middle ear, a bulla osteotomy should be done. Earlier approaches were by way of the pharynx or through the external auditory meatus, but the technique now favored as doing least damage to internal structures is by a skin incision between the internal and external maxillary veins. After blunt dissection the ventral compartment is trephined, exudate or other abnormal material is removed, and a gauze drain is packed into the cavity to remain for several days. Aqueous antibiotic drops are instilled into the ear canal and a systemic antibiotic given for several weeks.

Bulla osteotomy is described in the chapter on soft tissue surgery.

The auditive tube may be involved in acute and chronic inflammation, allergy, and polypoid growths, but because of its small size and minimal accessibility it is not amenable to the instrumentation and treatment applicable to humans. As indicated by Rose (1978c), it may be treated only by systemic medication, indirectly by myringotomy or bulla osteotomy, and topically by otic drops and nasal sprays to reduce edema.

Insufflation of a collapsed auditive tube is a common procedure in humans and is mentioned as a possibility by both Moltzen (1962) and Rose (1978c), but this would seem to be a difficult maneuver to perform in a cat.

**NEOPLASMS.** Primary neoplasms are rare. Squamous cell carcinoma and fibrosarcoma involving the middle and inner ear have been reported to cause facial paralysis and vestibular disturbance (Indrieri and Taylor, 1984; Pentlarge, 1984; Rendano et al., 1980). As already described, most inflammatory polyps originate in the middle ear but are usually detected only when they emerge in the external meatus or nasal passages.

**PARASITISM.** Parasitism of the middle ear occurs when ear mites invade by way of a ruptured tympanic membrane. *Syngamus auris,* a nematode parasite, has been found in the middle ear of cats in China (Faust and Tang, 1934). As many as six worms, measuring from 3 to 30 mm, live in one or both chambers of the tympanic cavity. The lining of the cavity is hemorrhagic, but the tympanum is intact.

## The Inner Ear

Situated in the dorsal part of the petrous temporal bone, the inner ear houses the nervous components involved in equilibrium and hearing.

Disorders of posture and equilibrium, often referred to as vestibular disease or labyrinthitis, are frequent in cats. Etiology is varied and in many cases is never established. In some cases of labyrinthitis, 25 mg dimenhydrinate (Dramamine) twice a day for a 3- to 4-kg cat may be a helpful empirical measure (Goudy, 1970).

One important cause of vestibular disturbance, as already indicated, may be otitis media with secondary effects on the vestibular component of the inner ear. However, vestibular disturbance is produced not only when the ear itself is affected, but by a variety of lesions—neoplastic, infectious, or degenerative—that may involve the vestibular nerve (a component of the eighth cranial, or acoustic, nerve) at any point from its place of origin in the medulla along its course to the inner ear.

Certain toxic factors, for example, prolonged excessive doses of aminoglycoside drugs (streptomycin, neomycin, kanamycin, or gentamicin), damage the eighth nerve.

"Feline vestibular disease" is an acute peripheral vestibular disorder affecting cats in summer in certain areas. Slow recovery occurs over two to three weeks, although

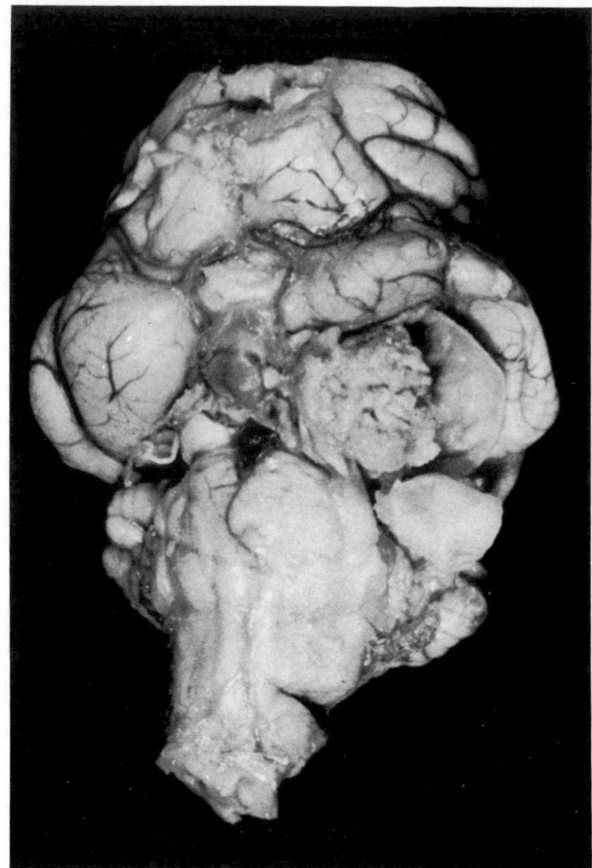

**Figure 15–10** Carcinoma of nasopharyngeal origin, inner ear, 14-year-old castrated male Siamese. On the ventral surface of the brain, left of the midline, the tumor compresses and distorts the piriform lobe. (See also the chapter on tumors).

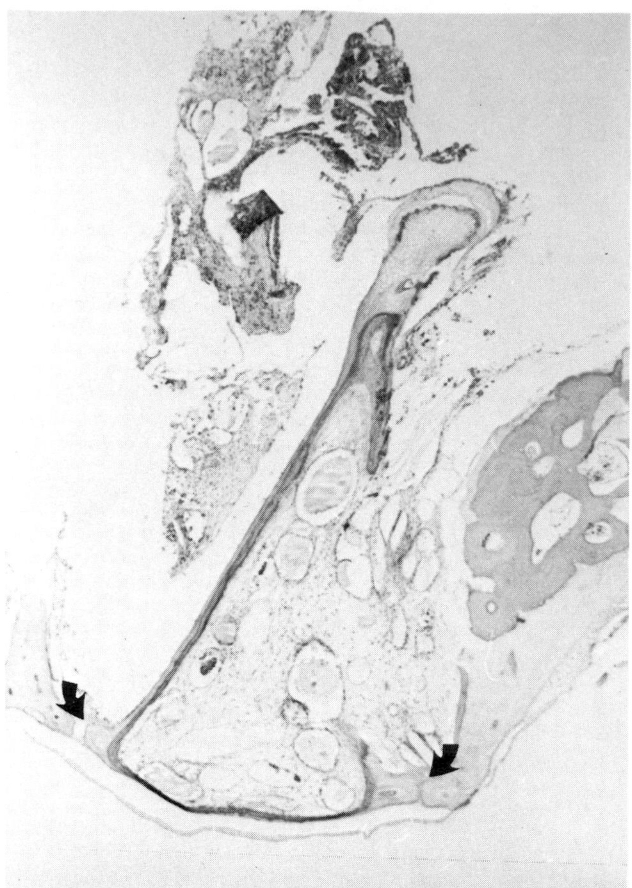

**Figure 15–11** Bilateral latent chronic otitis media causing deafness in a 17-year-old spayed female domestic smoke tabby. The stapes, located in the oval window (arrows at window margins) adheres to the petrous temporal bone (right) by fibrovascular tissue. The proliferated tissue fills the stapes, the center of which would normally be open, and replaces a part of the resorbed bony wall (right) of the ossicle. Exudate and exuberant inflammatory tissue lie within the bulla adjacent to the stapes (top center). H & E, × 400.

the cat's head tilt sometimes persists. No lesions have been found in the few cats autopsied (de Lahunta, 1983). It is suggested by some that an intoxication is caused by insecticides or by insects or other seasonal prey eaten by the cats.

Primary tumors of the inner ear have apparently not been reported. In a 14-year-old Siamese admitted to AMAH, a large secondary carcinoma of nasopharyngeal origin was found at autopsy to be the cause of signs of unilateral central nervous disturbance (Fig. 15–10). (For details see the chapter on tumors.)

Hearing, which may be affected by disturbances in conduction in the external and middle ear, is also impaired by disorders involving the receptor of the inner ear, although deafness is less easily recognized than vestibular disturbance.

The congenital deafness of white cats was previously discussed.

Acquired deafness is not often recognized in cats, even in those of venerable age, but inflammation of the inner ear doubtless affects hearing as well as the vestibular receptor. Gentamicin, kanamycin, and streptomycin administered to excess cause deafness, as well as vestibular damage.

Deafness occasionally follows periods of cerebral anoxia such as occurs in anesthetic accidents (Joshua, 1960) and has also been reported in cats poisoned with coal gas (Comben, 1949).

Hearing loss for high tones has been correlated with atrophic degenerative changes in the membranous cochlear labyrinth in some senile cats (Schuknecht, 1956). In an aged totally deaf cat autopsied at AMAH, evidence of chronic otitis media was present in both ears (Fig. 15–11), although the cat had never had an upper respiratory infection or exhibited any sign of ear disturbance. The same lesion has since been observed in other cats.

## REFERENCES

### The Normal Ear

Benoit J: Recherches sur l'Anatomie de l'Oreille Externe des Carnivores Domestiques. Toulouse, Thesis, 1938.

Bourdelle E, Bressou C: Anatomie Régionale des Animaux Domestiques. IV Carnivores Chien et Chat. Paris, J-B Baillière et Fils, 1953.

Carpenter JL: Seminar: Ear disease in cats. Unpublished, 1963.
Crouch JE: Text-Atlas of Cat Anatomy. Philadelphia, Lea & Febiger, 1969.
de Lahunta A, Habel RE: Applied Veterinary Anatomy, Philadelphia, WB Saunders Company, 1986.
Fernando SDA: The development of the glands of the external acoustic meatus of *Felis domesticus*. Am J Vet Res 26 (1965a) 734–739.
Fernando SDA: Microscopic anatomy and histochemistry of glands in the external auditory meatus of the cat (*Felis domesticus*). Am J Vet Res 26 (1965b) 1157–1162.
Hart BL: Sensory capacities and behavioral feats. Feline Pract 7 (6) (1977) 8, 10, 12.
McClure RC, Dallman MJ, Garrett PG: Cat Anatomy. Philadelphia, Lea & Febiger, 1973.
Miller ME: Guide to the Dissection of the Dog, 3rd ed. Ithaca, NY, 1952.
Montagna W: The glands of the external auditory meatus of the cat. J Morphol 85 (1949) 423–441.
Rose WR: Otitis media. Vet Med Small Anim Clin 71 (1976) 1443–1451.
Rose WR: The Eustachian tube—1: General considerations. Vet Med Small Anim Clin 73 (1978b) 882–887.
Strickland JH, Calhoun ML: The microscopic anatomy of the external ear of *Felis domesticus*. Am J Vet Res 21 (1960) 845–850.

### Disorders of the Ear

Austin VH: Common skin problems in cats. Modern Vet Pract 56 (1975) 541–545.
Bachrach A, Kleine LW: What is *your* diagnosis? [Polyp of ear canal, osteomyelitis, and possible *Actinomyces* infection]. J Am Vet Med Assoc 165 (1974) 465–466.
Ball V, Collet P, Girard H: Les céruminomes et épithéliomes des glandes cérumineuses. Rev Méd Vét 90 (NS 2) (1938) 390–393.
Barger IA: "A flea in his ear." Aust Vet J 50 (1974) 328.
Beard TG: Aural hematoma in the cat. North Am Vet 35 (1954) 855.
Bergsma DR, Brown KS: White fur, blue eyes, and deafness in the domestic cat. J Hered 62 (1971) 171–185.
Bigler B, Waber, S, Pfister K: Erste erfolgversprechende Ergebnisse in der Behandlung von *Notoedres cati* mit Ivermectin. Schweiz Arch Tierheilkd 126 (1984) 365–367.
Black MB: Adenoma of ceruminous gland in the dog. Arch Pathol 48 (1949) 85–88.
Bosher SK, Hallpike CS: Observations on the histological features, development and pathogenesis of the inner ear degeneration of the deaf white cat. Proc R Soc Lond [Biol] 162 (1965) 147–170.
Carta A: Raggi solari e cancro cutaneo dei gatti bianchi. Clin Vet (Milano) 63 (1940) 85–97.
Comben N: Deafness following coal gas poisoning in the small animals. Vet Proc 61 (1949) 128.
Courthaliac M: Contribution à l'étude des céruminomes chez le chien et le chat. Lyon, Thesis, 1938.
Crespeau F: L'épithélioma de l'oreille du chat blanc. Observations personnelles. Recl Méd Vét 150 (1974) 783–792.
Davenport DJ, Eisenberg HM: What is your diagnosis? [Ceruminous gland adenocarcinoma]. J Am Vet Med Assoc 185 (1984) 317–318.
de Lahunta A: Feline neurology. Vet Clin North Am 6 (1976) 433–452.
de Lahunta A: Veterinary Neuroanatomy and Clinical Neurology, 2nd ed. Philadelphia, WB Saunders Company, 1983.
de Lahunta A, Habel RE: Applied Veterinary Anatomy. Philadelphia, WB Saunders Company, 1986.
Dorn CR, Taylor DON, Schneider R: Sunlight exposure and risk of developing cutaneous and oral squamous cell carcinoma in white cats. J Natl Cancer Inst 46 (1971) 1073–1078.
Dreisörner H, Refai M, Rieth H: Glitis externa durch *Microsporum canis* bei Katzen. Kleintierpraxis 9 (1964) 230–234.
Dyte CE: Further data on folded-ear cats. Carnivore Genetics Newsletter 2 (5) (1973) 112.
Engle GC, Brodey RS: A retrospective study of 395 feline neoplasms. J Am Anim Hosp Assoc 5 (1969) 21–31.
Faith RE, Woodard JC: Waardenburg's syndrome. Comp Pathol Bull 5 (2) (1973) 3–4.
Fasnacht DW: Four-eared cat. J Am Vet Med Assoc 154 (1969) 1145.
Faust EC, Tang CC: A new species of Syngamus (S. auris) from the middle ear of the cat in Foochow, China. Parasitology 26 (1934) 455–459.
Fernando SDA: Certain histopathologic features of the external auditory meatus of the cat and dog with otitis externa. Am J Vet Res 28 (1967) 278–282.
Field B, Wanner RA: Cerebral malformation in a Manx cat. Vet Rec 96 (1975) 42–43.
Foley RH: A selection of cutaneous and related tumors of cats. Vet Med Small Anim Clin 72 (1977) 43–45.
Formston C: Aural hematoma in cats. Haver-Glover Messenger 32 (11–12) (1952) 33–34.
Franc M, Guaguere E, Magnol JP, Dorchies P, Ducos de Lahitte J: Tumeurs du conduit auditif externe des carnivores. Rev Méd Vét 132 (1981) 733–739.
Gabbert N, Feldman BF: A case report—feline demodex. Feline Pract 6 (6) (1976) 32–33.
Goudy J: Personal communication, 1970.
Hardison JL: *Eutrombicula alfreddugesi* (chiggers) in a cat. Vet Med Small Anim Clin 72 (1977) 47.
Harvey CE, Goldschmidt MH: Inflammatory polypoid growths in the ear canal of cats. J Small Anim Pract 19 (1978) 669–677.
Hayden DW: Squamous cell carcinoma in a cat with intraocular and orbital metastases. Vet Pathol 13 (1976) 332–336.
Indrieri RJ, Taylor RF: Vestibular dysfunction caused by squamous cell carcinoma involving the middle and inner ear in two cats. J Am Vet Med Assoc 184 (1984) 471–473.
Jones TC: Personal communication, 1975.
Joshua JO: An anaesthetic mishap. Vet Rec 72 (1960) 375–376.
Lawson DD: Otitis media in the cat. Vet Rec 69 (1957) 643–647.
Leighton RL: Surgery of the head, thorax, abdomen, genitalia, and skin. *In* Catcott EJ (ed): Feline Medicine and Surgery, 2nd ed. Santa Barbara, American Veterinary Publications, Inc, 1975.
Little CC: Four-ears, a recessive mutation in the cat. J Hered 48 (1957) 57.
Mair IW: Hereditary deafness in the white cat. Acta Otolaryngol Suppl (Stockh) 314 (1973) 1–48.
Marshall J: A new approach to the surgical treatment of haematoma in the dog and cat. Vet Rec 71 (1959) 103–105.
McAfee LT, McAfee JT, Katz R: Sebaceous gland adenomas in a cat. Feline Pract 9 (2) (1979) 21–23.
Meier H: Feline mastocytoma: two cases. Cornell Vet 47 (1957) 220–226.
Moltzen H: Otitis media in the dog and cat. Adv Small Anim Pract 3 (1962) 56–61.
Montpellier J, Dieuzeide R, Barone R: Le cancer du pavillon de l'oreille chez un chat. Épithélioma des glandes cérumineuses. Maroc Méd 16 (1936) 112–114.
Niklas W: Untersuchungen zur Keimflora in äusseren Gehörgang von Katzen. Kleintierpraxis 24 (1979) 107–111.
Ottani F: Cancro cutaneo su fondo infiammatorio in un gatto. Nuova Vet 1 (1923) 162–164.
Pentlarge VW: Peripheral vestibular disease in a cat with middle and inner ear squamous cell carcinoma. Compend Contin Ed 6 (1984) 731–733, 736.
Plummer PJG: A survey of six hundred and thirty six tumours from domesticated animals. Can J Comp Med 20 (1956) 239–251.

Priester WA, McKay FW: The Occurrence of Tumors in Domestic Animals. National Cancer Institute Monograph 54, Bethesda, 1980.

Rebillard G, Rebillard M, Carlier E, Pujol R: Histophysiological relationships in the deaf white cat auditory system. Acta Otolaryngol (Stockh) 82 (1976) 48–56.

Rendano VT, de Lahunta A, King JM: Extracranial neoplasia with facial nerve paralysis in two cats. J Am Anim Hosp Assoc 16 (1980) 921–925.

Robinson R: Folded eared kittens of Maldegem, Belgium. Carnivore Genetics Newsletter 2 (3) (1972) 68.

Rose WR: Small animal clinical otology. Tumors. Vet Med Small Anim Clin 73 (1978a) 427, 430–431.

Rose WR: The Eustachian tube—4: Therapeutics. Vet Med Small Anim Clin 73 (1978c) 1258–1262.

Schaffer MH: Personal communication, 1956.

Schaffer MH: Squamous-cell carcinomas of white-faced cats. Calif Vet 11 (Jan–Feb) (1958) 22.

Schuknecht HF: Presbycusis. Laryngoscope 65 (1956) 402–419.

Scott DW: Drug eruption in a cat due to a mitecide. Feline Pract 7 (3) (1977) 47–50.

Scott DW: Feline dermatology 1900–1978: a monograph. J Am Anim Hosp Assoc 16 (1980) 331–459.

Scott DW: Feline dermatology 1979–1982: introspective retrospections. J Am Anim Hosp Assoc 20 (1984) 537–564.

Simpson S: Diseases of the vestibular system. *In* Kirk RW (ed): Current Veterinary Therapy VIII. Philadelphia, WB Saunders Company, 1983.

Stookey JL, Dill GS Jr, Whitney GD: Ceruminal gland neoplasia in the cat. J Am Med Vet Assoc 159 (1971) 326.

Suga F, Hattler KW: Physiological and histopathological correlates of hereditary deafness in animals. Laryngoscope 80 (1970) 81–104.

Todd NB: Folded-eared cats: further observations. Carnivore Genetics Newsletter 2 (3) (1972) 64–66.

Todd NB: Jones TC, Zook BC: The inheritance of blue eyes and deafness in domestic cats. Carnivore Genetics Newsletter 1 (5) (1968) 100–104.

van der Velden NA: [Some aspects of hereditary perceptive deafness and leukism]. Tijdschr Deergeneeskd 101 (1976) 1386–1391.

Venker–van Haagen AJ: Managing diseases of the ear. *In* Kirk RW (ed): Current Veterinary Therapy VIII. Philadelphia, WB Saunders Company, 1983.

West CD, Harrison JM: Transneuronal cell atrophy in the congenitally deaf white cat. J Comp Neurol 151 (1973) 377–398.

Wolff R: Folded eared cat seen in Germany. Carnivore Genetics Newsletter 2 (2) (1971) 41.

Yeats JJ, Vaughan LC: The treatment of aural haematoma in the cat. Vet Rec 64 (1952) 531–532.

Zagraniski MJ: Drooping ear pinna. Feline Pract 4 (4) (1974) 24; 5 (1) (1975) 4.

# 16
CHAPTER

# THE HEMATOPOIETIC SYSTEM

KEITH W. PRASSE, EDWARD A. MAHAFFEY, SUSAN M. COTTER, and JEAN HOLZWORTH

## HEMATOLOGY OF NORMAL CATS AND CHARACTERISTIC RESPONSES TO DISEASE

KEITH W. PRASSE and EDWARD A. MAHAFFEY

Diseases of the hematopoietic system occupy a place of central importance in feline medicine because of their frequency and severity. Also the hematopoietic system is affected secondarily in a variety of other disease states, and hematologic manifestations are often valuable in assessing severity of disease, efficacy of treatment, and prognosis. Knowledge of the normal function of the hematopoietic system and of its response to a variety of injuries is essential to the practice of feline medicine.

### TECHNIQUES IN FELINE HEMATOLOGY

Diagnoses based on interpretation of hematologic test results are only as good as the accuracy of those results; accuracy of test results is in turn no better than the quality of the specimen from which the results are obtained. Because detailed descriptions of sampling and laboratory techniques are beyond the scope of this book, the following discussion concentrates on problems encountered in obtaining and processing of feline samples. The reader is referred to the references at the end of this chapter for additional information on these techniques.

#### Peripheral Blood

Obtaining adequate blood samples without causing artifacts is a prerequisite to evaluating the hematopoietic system of any species. Because of its size and resistance to forceful restraint, the cat presents special problems in this regard. Nevertheless, veterinarians working with cats must be able to obtain good samples if they are to evaluate the hematologic status of the animals.

Blood samples can be obtained from the jugular, cephalic, or marginal ear vein of the cat (Gilmore et al., 1964; Johnson and Perman, 1968). We prefer the jugular vein for routine use. Very small samples can be obtained by puncturing the marginal ear vein with a disposable lancet after coating the ear with petrolatum. Enough blood may be collected by this method to make films and measure the packed cell volume (PCV) and white-cell count (WBC).

With any method of collecting blood, it is important to minimize excitement of the ear. The effects of excitement on the feline hemogram have been examined and include increased PCV, hemoglobin, red-cell count (RBC), and white-cell count (Kleinsorgen et al., 1976). Such alterations can be produced by excessive or prolonged restraint.

We prefer either dipotassium or disodium ethylenediamine tetraacetate (EDTA) as an anticoagulant for routine hematology. Care must be taken to use only 1 or 2 mg of EDTA per ml of blood, because excessive EDTA causes severe cell shrinkage and artifactual lowering of the PCV (Penny et al., 1970). Heparin is used only for samples for blood gas measurement. Sodium citrate is used for coagulation studies in a ratio of one part of 3.6 per cent sodium citrate to nine parts of blood.

## Bone Marrow

Evaluation of peripheral blood is frequently inadequate to establish a diagnosis in feline hematologic disorders. In such cases examination of bone marrow often provides additional insight into the nature of the pathologic process. Specific indications for bone marrow examination include nonregenerative anemia, persistent leukopenia, thrombocytopenia, and the presence of questionable neoplastic leukocytes in the peripheral blood.

The two general techniques for examining bone marrow are histologic sections prepared from needle core biopsies and marrow aspirations. The former technique has the advantage of allowing better assessment of marrow cellularity, but it requires the preparation of histologic sections and is thus more time-consuming and expensive. Bone marrow aspiration is a more widely used technique in veterinary medicine. Because slides can be prepared and examined by the veterinarian, this technique is faster and cheaper. Cytologic detail is also much better in slides prepared from aspirates than in marrow sections.

The two common sites for bone marrow aspiration in the cat are the trochanteric fossa of the femur and the crest of the ilium (Fig. 16–1). Satisfactory specimens can usually be collected from either site. Aspiration can be performed on most cats with only local anesthetic infiltration of the subcutis and periosteum, but light sedation may be used for fractious animals. Fifteen-gauge Illinois sternal needles appropriate for dogs can be used for adult cats. An 18-gauge needle is recommended for small cats and kittens, especially if the iliac crest marrow is to be sampled. After the needle is seated in the bone, a 12-ml syringe containing one drop of 10 per cent EDTA is used to aspirate approximately two drops of marrow. A drop of the marrow sample is placed immediately on one end of a clean glass slide, which is then tilted to allow the drop to run down the length of the slide. Marrow particles adhere to the slide, reducing peripheral blood contamination. A second slide is then placed over the marrow particles at a right angle to the long axis of the first slide, and the slides are pulled apart. The second slide is then stained and examined. Detailed descriptions of the technique for sampling feline marrow are available (Gilmore et al., 1964; Penny, 1974; Schalm and Switzer, 1972; Schalm et al., 1975).

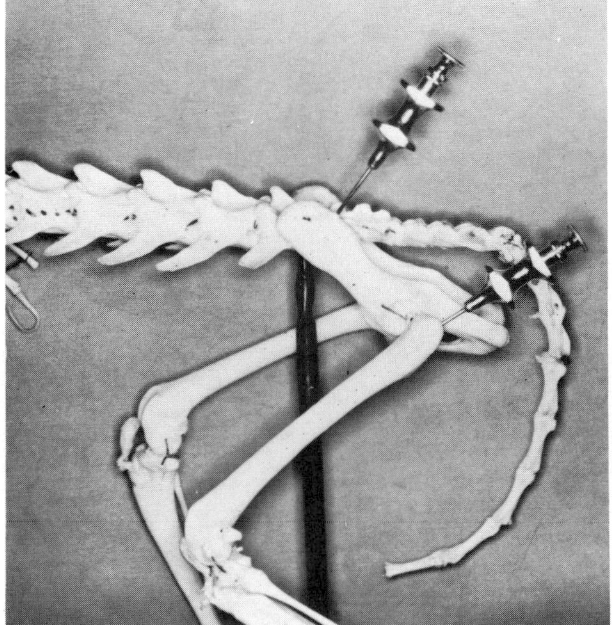

**Figure 16–1** Placement of bone marrow aspiration needles in femur and ilium. (From Switzer JW, Schalm OW: Calif Vet 22 [1968] 20.)

## Routine Hematologic Procedures

**PACKED CELL VOLUME.** The packed cell volume of the cat is routinely determined by the microhematocrit method. We are unaware of any special considerations for handling feline blood.

**HEMOGLOBIN.** Although a variety of techniques for determining the hemoglobin content of blood are available, spectrophotometric measurement of the cyanmethemoglobin derivative is by far the most popular method. One possible source of error when measuring hemoglobin spectrophotometrically is the occurrence of falsely high hemoglobin values in cats with numerous erythrocyte refractile (ER) bodies or Heinz bodies. This error is caused by interference with light transmission by the red-cell inclusions, which fail to lyse, and can be avoided by centrifuging the blood-reagent mixture before reading the absorbance in the spectrophotometer (Schalm et al., 1975).

**RED-CELL COUNT.** Because of the poor precision of the manual technique using a hematocytometer, only the automated techniques using electronic cell counters can be recommended. Two possible sources of error must be considered when interpreting feline red-cell counts from an electronic cell counter. These machines have an adjustable lower threshold setting with which one can determine the size of the smallest cells to be counted. Since normal feline red cells are smaller than either human or canine red cells, a cell counter calibrated for use with human or canine blood may not count some feline cells. For this reason, some laboratories adjust the lower threshold setting of the cell counter for each species (Schalm et al., 1975). Falsely high red-cell counts may be reported in cats with numerous large platelets or platelet clumps.

**RETICULOCYTE COUNT.** Feline reticulocytes are stained with new methylene blue by the same techniques used for other species (Schalm et al., 1975). Because of the morphologic variants of feline reticulocytes (to be described later), the reticulocyte count should be performed by someone familiar with feline hematology.

**WHITE-CELL COUNT.** White-cell counts in the cat may be performed either manually with a hematocytometer or with an electronic cell counter. Although electronically determined counts are generally considered more precise and accurate than manual counts, spuriously high values may occur with feline blood samples owing to clumping of platelets (Schalm et al., 1975).

**DIFFERENTIAL WBC.** Common problems encountered with differential white-cell counts include correct classification of band and segmented neutrophils and identification of feline basophils. Technicians in medical laboratories often overestimate the number of band neutrophils in animal blood. The criteria recommended by Schalm et al. (1975) for classifying band and segmented neutrophils are used in most veterinary laboratories (i.e., in the mature neutrophil the nucleus is irregularly lobed, and simple narrowing between lobes without filament formation is the rule; in band neutrophils the nucleus is a curved band). Also, technicians in medical laboratories often fail to recognize feline basophils, because their granules do not stain metachromatically as do granules of other species.

**COOMBS TEST.** The direct Coombs test is performed on feline blood by the same method used in other species. Feline Coombs antiserum is commercially available.*

## NORMAL VALUES IN FELINE HEMATOLOGY

### PERIPHERAL BLOOD

The veterinary literature contains numerous references to normal feline hematologic data. Many are listed in the bibliography at the end of this chapter. Examination of these references reveals significant and confusing differences in normal values, some of which can be explained by differences in methodology and criteria for identifying cells. We have chosen to list a single set of normal values that we believe to be accurate using current methodology (Table 16–1).

### BONE MARROW

Bone marrow differential counts from normal cats are listed in Table 16–2. Two schools of thought regarding the interpretation of bone marrow aspirates exist. One approach is to perform a marrow differential by counting and classifying the various cell types in a marrow preparation. This technique is time-consuming and laborious, and the information gained rarely justifies that effort. We prefer a simpler technique that provides similar diagnostic interpretative information. Under low power, the number of marrow particles and cellularity of the particles are noted. It is also convenient to evaluate the number of megakaryocytes at this magnification. Then several fields are examined closely with the high-dry or oil-immersion objective to assess the distribution of maturation stages of granulocytic (myeloid) and erythroid cells as well as the approximate ratio of granulocytic to erythroid cells. In a normal cat, approximately 80 per cent of the granulocytic cells should be metamyelocytes, bands, and segmenters, and approximately 90 per cent of the erythroid cells should be rubricytes and metarubricytes. The overall ratio of myeloid cells to erythroid cells is about 1.5:1.0 in normal cats. Hyperplasia of either the myeloid or the erythroid series is usually accompanied by an increase in the proportion of early forms of the affected series. Such shifts cannot be interpreted without knowledge of the peripheral blood findings. Asynchronous nuclear and cy-

*Miles Scientific, 30 W 475 N. Aurora Blvd, Naperville, IL 60540.

**Table 16–1 Hematologic Values of Normal Adult Cats**[a]

| | UNITS | RANGE |
|---|---|---|
| Hematocrit (PCV) | % | 30–45 (24–34)[b] |
| Hemoglobin | gm/dl | 8–15 |
| Red blood cells | n × $10^6$/μl | 5.0–10.0 |
| Reticulocytes | | |
| (aggregate) | % | 0–1.0[c] |
| (aggregate plus punctate) | % | 1.4–10.8[d] |
| Mean corpsucular volume (MCV) | fl | 39–55 |
| Mean corpuscular hemoglobin concentration (MCHC) | gm/dl | 30–36 |
| Platelets | n × $10^5$/μl | 3–7 |
| White blood cells | n/μl | 5500–19,500 |
| Segmented neutrophils | (%) n/μl | (35–75) 2500–12,500 |
| Band neutrophils | (%) n/μl | (0–3) 0–300 |
| Lymphocytes | (%) n/μl | (20–55) 1500–7000 |
| Monocytes | (%) n/μl | (1–4) 0–850 |
| Eosinophils | (%) n/μl | (2–12) 0–1500 |
| Basophils | (%) n/μl | Rare |

[a]Derived with slight modifications from Schalm et al., 1975.
[b]Lowest in kittens 4 to 6 weeks old; gradually increased to adult levels by 4 to 5 months of age.
[c]Kirk RW (ed): Current Veterinary Therapy VIII. Philadelphia, WB Saunders Company, 1983.
[d]Cramer DV, Lewis RM: J Am Vet Med Assoc 160 (1972) 61–67. (Aggregate [young] reticulocytes ranged from 0 to 0.4 per cent; the rest were punctate [mature].)

**Table 16–2 Percentage Cellular Composition of Normal Feline Bone Marrow**[a]

| | ANGELL[b] | | PENNY ET AL.[c] |
|---|---|---|---|
| | Range | Mean | Mean |
| Myeloblast | 0.0–1.8 | 0.4 | 0.74 |
| Progranulocytes | 0.6–3.8 | 1.2 | 0.88 |
| Myelocytes | 0.4–5.4 | 2.2 | 9.76 |
| Metamyelocytes | 0.6–9.6 | 4.2 | 7.32 |
| Band neutrophils | 5.0–19.4 | 11 | 25.80 |
| Neutrophils, mature | 17.8–38.6 | 27.8 | 9.24 |
| Eosinophils | 0.6–7.2 | 3.0 | 3.80 |
| Basophils | 0.0–0.4 | 0.2 | 0.002 |
| Total granulocytic cells | 39.4–64.4 | 52.0 | 58.53 |
| Rubriblast | 0.0–1.6 | 0.6 | |
| Prorubricyte and rubricyte | — | 12.4 | 12.50 |
| Metarubricyte | 15.6–32.2 | 23.6 | 11.68 |
| Total erythrocytic cells | 24.0–48.8 | 36.6 | 25.88 |
| Plasma cells | 0.0–1.2 | 0.2 | 1.61 |
| Mitotic cells | 0.0–2.0 | 1.0 | 0.61 |
| Lymphocytes | 3.2–22.6 | 11.4 | 7.63 |
| Myeloid:erythroid ratio | 0.9–2.5 | 1.5 | 2.47 |

[a]Results of other studies of normal feline marrow are tabulated by Schalm et al., 1975.
[b]Angell Memorial Animal Hospital, 1975. Study performed by Diane Ragsdale, ASCP, and Dr. James L. Carpenter.
[c]Penny et al., 1970.

toplasmic maturation is a relatively common abnormality in feline marrow and is indicated by the presence of cells with mature cytoplasmic features and immature nuclear morphology. One should also search for neoplastic cells at this magnification.

### Blood Volume

The normal blood volume of the cat has been measured by a variety of techniques including dilutional dye methods, $^{59}Fe$, and $^{51}Cr$ (Da Silva et al., 1955; Gillis and Mitchell, 1974; Reed et al., 1970; Went and Drinker, 1929). The results of these studies agree closely, and the blood volume of the cat is approximately 65 ml/kg. This figure is significantly lower than that of the dog.

## RED CELLS

### Function

The major function of the red cell is to transport oxygen from the pulmonary capillary bed to capillary beds in the rest of the body. This transport depends on the ability of hemoglobin to bind oxygen in areas of high oxygen tension and to release oxygen in areas of low oxygen concentration. The cat has two major hemoglobin types, labeled A and B, as well as three minor B components. Both type A and type B occur in the same animal in ratios varying from 1:1 to 9:1. The oxygen affinity of hemoglobin A is lowered by interaction with 2,3-diphosphoglycerate (2,3-DPG), whereas that of hemoglobin B is unaffected by 2,3-DPG or other organic phosphates (Lessard and Taketa, 1969). In experimental hemolytic anemia, the concentration of 2,3-DPG in feline red cells increases, as does the level of two minor high-oxygen affinity hemoglobins ($HbB_1$, $HbB_2$). The net effect of these changes is a slight drop in overall oxygen affinity, with an increase in oxygen binding at low oxygen tension (Mauk et al., 1974).

Feline hemoglobin is unique among hemoglobins of domestic animals in that eight free sulfhydryl groups are present on the globin beta chains (Hamilton and Edelstein, 1974). Oxidation of sulfhydryl groups is a common mechanism of protein denaturation and is thought to be important in the formation of Heinz bodies. The erythrocyte refractile (ER) bodies or Schmauch bodies that are seen commonly in the red cells of normal cats are probably Heinz bodies (Beritíc, 1965; Collins et al., 1968). Comparative studies have demonstrated that feline hemoglobin is more susceptible to oxidation than that of other species, and this susceptibility may be related to the high number of free sulfhydryl groups on feline globin (Harvey and Kaneko, 1976; Kurian and Iyer, 1977). These findings suggest that the frequent occurrence of ER bodies in feline red cells may be due to structural peculiarities of feline hemoglobin.

### Production and Destruction

Production of red cells and granulocytes in the feline embryo and fetus has been studied (Tiedemann and van Ooyen, 1978). The yolk sac is the major hematopoietic site for the first 30 days of development, and the liver is the major hematopoietic organ from day 30 until day 45. The bone marrow assumes the primary role in hematopoiesis at that time. Splenic hematopoiesis is detectable during the latter half of fetal life but is quantitatively unimportant in fetal blood-cell production. Although the distribution of active marrow in the normal adult cat has not been reported, most hematopoiesis probably occurs in the vertebrae, skull, pelvis, and ribs. Adequate samples for bone marrow evaluation can usually be obtained from the iliac crest or the proximal end of the femur.

Red-cell production is under the control of erythropoietin, a hormone produced or activated by the kidney. Although one report indicates that the feline carotid body is a source of erythropoietin, other investigators were unable to produce the results of the first study (Gillis and Mitchell, 1974; Tramezzani et al., 1971).

The life span of the feline red cell is significantly shorter than that of the other domestic animals. Estimates of mean life span vary from 66 to 79 days (Brown and Eadie, 1953; Kaneko et al., 1966; Marion and Smith, 1983; Valentine et al., 1951). This short life span is clinically significant in that it makes the cat more susceptible to depression anemias, since a relatively short period of marrow depression will result in a significant decrease in PCV. Senescent red cells are removed by fixed phagocytic cells in several organs (spleen, liver, and bone marrow). Recent ultrastructural studies of the feline spleen have revealed anatomic peculiarities that could result in poor pitting function (Weiss, 1980). Poor pitting function, the process by which the spleen removes abnormal particles from red cells, could explain in part the persistence of red cells containing Heinz bodies in the blood of normal cats.

In the last third of pregnancy a queen's PCV decreases and reticulocytosis occurs (Berman, 1974). In the first days after parturition the red-cell values return to normal. Values for red-cell numbers and hemoglobin are lower in kittens than in mature cats.

At an altitude of 7200 feet above sea level, the cat's PCV averaged 46.5 per cent and the hemoglobin 14.2 gm/dl (Velasco et al., 1971).

### Red-Cell Morphology

**MARROW PRECURSORS.** Nucleated marrow erythroid precursor cells of the cat are similar in appearance to those of other species. In general, as the cells mature, cell size decreases, the nucleus becomes smaller, and chromatin aggregates. Cytoplasmic color changes from blue to gray to orange. Nucleoli are visible only in rubriblasts. The stages of erythroid maturation are illustrated in Plate 16–1*A*.

**RETICULOCYTES.** Reticulocytes are demonstrated by supravital staining with new methylene blue, and their number is usually expressed as a percentage of the red cells. As reticulocytes mature, their cytoplasmic nucleoprotein progresses from a heavy, blue, granular network to a few faint granules. In some species the reticulocytes mature in the bone marrow and do not normally circulate; normal dogs and cats, however, may have an average of 0.5 to 1.0 per cent of the early reticulocytes in the peripheral blood (Schalm et al., 1975). A unique feature of normal feline blood is that, in addition to the classic (aggregate) reticulocytes routinely counted, there is a

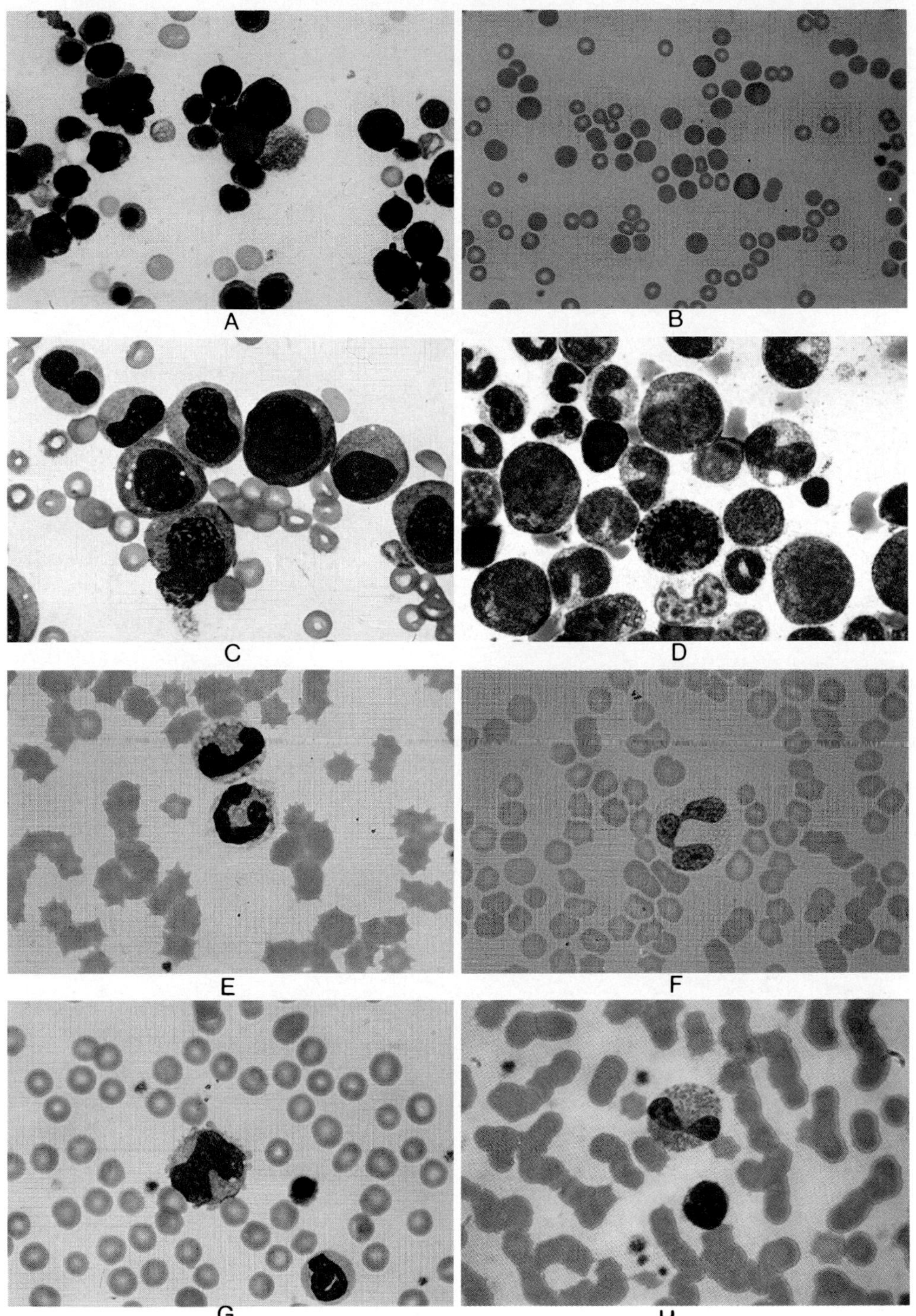

**Plate 16–1** *A*, Marrow aspirate containing rubriblasts, prorubricytes, rubricytes, and metarubricytes. Wright's, × 252. *B*, Polychromasia and anisocytosis of red cells in a cat with responding anemia. Wright-Leishman, × 252. *C*, Marrow granulocytic precursors including promyelocytes, neutrophilic myelocytes, and metamyelocytes. Wright's, × 252. *D*, Marrow granulocytic precursors, including a myeloblast (lower left), promyelocytes, a basophilic myelocyte, neutrophilic metamyelocytes, and band neutrophils. Wright's, × 252. *E*, Toxic changes in two band neutrophils including cytoplasmic vacuolation and basophilia. Wright-Leishman, × 252. *F*, Asynchronous nuclear maturation (premature segmentation) in a toxic neutrophil. Wright-Leishman, × 252. *G*, Monocyte, neutrophil, and metarubricyte. Wright-Leishman, × 252. *H*, Eosinophil and small lymphocyte. Rouleau formation is conspicuous. Wright-Leishman, × 252.

*Plate continued on following page*

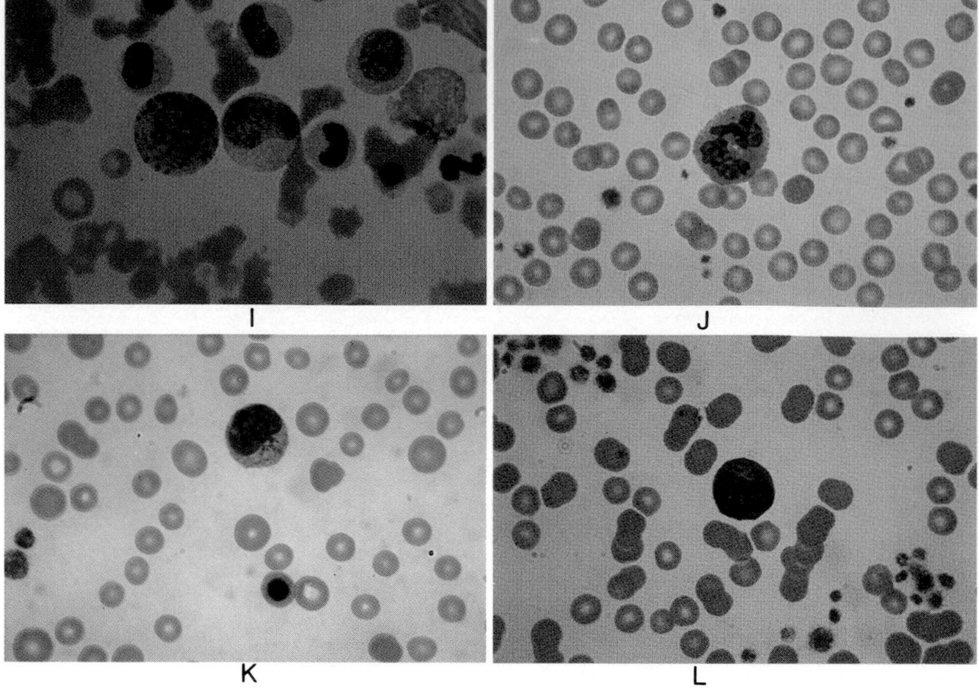


**Plate 16–1** *Continued I*, Basophilic and neutrophilic myelocytes, neutrophilic metamyelocytes, a single band neutrophil, and metarubricytes. Wright's, × 252. *J*, Mature basophil in peripheral blood. Wright-Leishman, × 252. *K*, Lymphocyte with metachromatic cytoplasmic granules and metarubricyte. Wright-Leishman, × 252. *L*, Feline immunocyte with intensely blue cytoplasm and aggregated chromatin. Wright-Leishman, × 252.

much greater number of mature (punctate) cells (Fig. 16–2). In normal cats punctate cells may raise the range of the total reticulocyte count to 1.4 to 10.8 per cent, and in responding anemias totals as high as 50 per cent may be recorded (Cramer and Lewis, 1972).

This phenomenon was studied experimentally in cats made severely anemic by bleeding (Cramer and Lewis, 1972; Fan et al., 1978). By 24 hours after severe blood loss, aggregate reticulocytes appeared. Several days later punctate forms appeared. They increased in number for about 10 to 12 days, then gradually decreased as the PCV returned to normal.

It was the conclusion of both studies that both immature and mature reticulocytes should be included in the total count and that the numbers of each should be reported. For diagnostic and prognostic purposes in naturally occurring anemia, the number of aggregate reticulocytes as an indicator of current bone marrow response was stressed by Cramer and Lewis (1972), while the punctate reticulocytes were considered by Fan et al. (1978) to be a better, although later, indicator of marrow activity.

For assessment of the regenerative response to anemia, the use of absolute reticulocyte counts (relative reticulocyte count × red cell count) avoids the potentially deceptive increase that occurs in the relative reticulocyte percentage as the number of mature red cells in circulation decreases. Absolute reticulocyte counts of greater than 60,000/μl indicate that the marrow is responding to the anemia by increasing reticulocyte output (Weiser, 1981). In severe anemia, much higher reticulocyte counts would be expected during an appropriate regenerative response.

**RED-CELL SIZE, SHAPE, AND COLOR.** The normal feline red cell is approximately 5.8 μ in diameter with slight central pallor. Rouleau formation is often prominent in blood films. Slight anisocytosis (variation in cell size) is normal in feline blood and becomes more pronounced in cats with responding anemia. Polychromasia is not observed in films from normal cats but is seen in films from cats with responding anemias (Plate 16–1*B*). The number of polychromatophilic cells in feline blood correlates well with the aggregate reticulocyte counts (Alsaker et al., 1977). Spherocytosis, a feature of autoimmune hemolytic anemias, is difficult to detect in cats, because their red cells are small and central pallor is normally slight (Schalm et al., 1975). Poikilocytosis (variation in cell shape) in the form of crenation is common in blood films from normal cats.

**RED-CELL INCLUSIONS.** Erythrocyte refractile (ER) bodies, also called Heinz bodies, Heinz-Ehrlich bodies, or Schmauch bodies, normally occur only in the blood of cats. The percentage of the red cells containing these inclusions varies widely. One investigator found ER bodies in 0.6 ± 0.24 per cent of the red cells of normal cats, but others have reported their occurrence in over 50 per cent of the red cells of individual cats with no obvious hematologic disorder (Beritíc, 1965; Jain, 1969; Penny et al., 1970). In Romanowsky-stained smears, ER bodies appear as pale, round structures usually located near the margin of the cell; however, they may be difficult to find in such preparations (Fig. 16–3). In new methylene blue-stained slides, ER bodies appear as dark blue or black inclusions that vary from 1 to 3 μ in diameter. A procedure for preparing permanent slides of feline ER bodies has been described (Jain, 1969). Similar if not identical inclusions occur in cats with oxidant-induced hemolytic anemia, discussed later in this chapter.

Howell-Jolly bodies are nuclear remnants that appear as round, dark blue inclusions within the red cell in Romanowsky-stained slides. They may be found in small numbers (less than 1 per cent of the red cells) in normal cats, and they increase in number in responding anemias.

Basophilic stippling appears as numerous fine blue dots

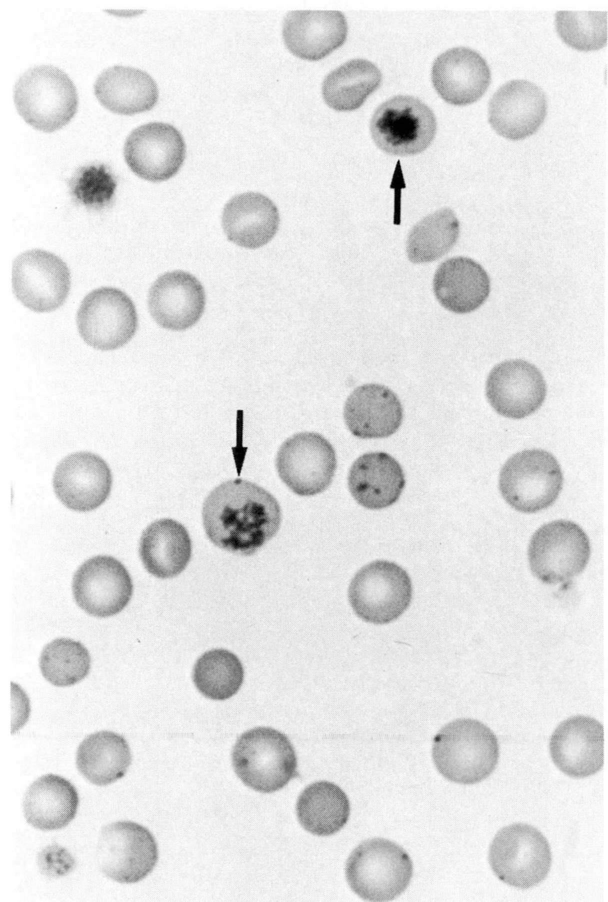

**Figure 16–2** Two aggregate reticulocytes (arrows) and numerous punctate reticulocytes. New methylene blue, × 963.

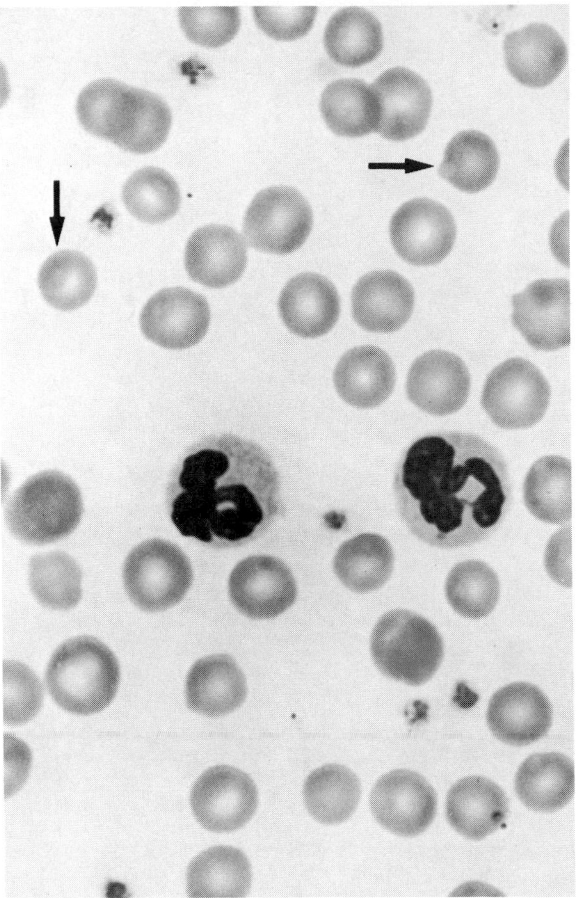

**Figure 16–3** Mature neutrophils and Heinz bodies in red cells (arrows). The Heinz bodies are barely visible as pale round structures in the red cells but are more easily recognized where they protrude from the red cell margins. Wright-Leishman, × 963.

within red cells in Romanowsky-stained slides. Although stippling may indicate lead poisoning, it often occurs in responding anemias (Schalm et al., 1975).

**ERYTHROCYTE SEDIMENTATION RATE.** The erythrocyte sedimentation rate (ESR) is a helpful procedure in humans and dogs in confirming the presence and monitoring the progress of many disease states. The strong tendency of cat blood to form rouleaux accelerates sedimentation. Furthermore, correction values for relating ESR to PCV in anemic cats have not been established. For these reasons ESR determination is at present of limited value in cats.

## CYTOLOGY OF WHITE CELLS

The morphology of feline white cells has been described and illustrated by several authors (Bentinck-Smith, 1969; Gilmore et al., 1964; Schalm et al., 1975). These descriptions, based on observations of Romanowsky-stained blood and bone marrow films, comments on feline white-cell production, distribution, and fate, and the knowledge of feline white-cell ultrastructure, histochemistry, and morphologic abnormalities are reviewed.

### Neutrophils

These cells, as well as the other granulocytes, compose a continuously renewed population that functions in defense against disease. Neutrophils phagocytize and kill bacteria or digest other foreign particles.

**MYELOBLAST, PROMYELOCYTE, AND NEUTROPHILIC MYELOCYTE.** The myeloblast, found in small numbers in bone marrow, comes from a differentiated stem cell and is committed to either the neutrophilic, eosinophilic, basophilic, or monocytic cell lines. Since it lacks specific granules, the line of commitment cannot be visually differentiated at this stage. The cell is round, measures 15 to 20 μ in diameter, and contains a round or oval nucleus (Plate 16–1*D*). The chromatin is finely granular, and one or two nucleoli or nucleolar rings are seen. The cytoplasm is deep blue but usually lighter stained than that of the erythroblast, its counterpart in the red-cell series.

In a mathematical model of feline granulopoiesis, the myeloblast was believed to divide once, with daughter cells being morphologically distinguished as promyelocytes (Prasse et al., 1973).

The promyelocyte (progranulocyte) is in low numbers in bone marrow, and it may be seen rarely in blood in disease. This cell is about the same size or slightly larger than the myeloblast, and its nucleus has slight clumping of chromatin with faintly visible nucleolar rings. The distinguishing feature is abundant cytoplasm that contains purple (often called azurophilic, a misnomer) granules (primary granules) (Plate 16–1*C* and *D*). The granules are dispersed in a deep blue cytoplasm. The cell line to which the promyelocyte is committed cannot usually be distinguished at this stage by light microscopy. The cell was thought to divide once, according to a mathematical model of granulopoiesis, with daughter cells being identified as myelocytes (Prasse et al., 1973).

Neutrophilic myelocytes are in large numbers in bone marrow but only rarely found in blood in disease. This cell is slightly smaller than the myeloblast and promyelocyte, and its nucleus is oval, developing a flattened or indented side as the cell matures, and often eccentrically positioned in a pale blue cytoplasm; nuclear chromatin is more condensed, and nucleoli are invisible. With maturation and cell division, primary granules become fewer and nearly invisible. Granules of specific cell type, however, now become visible in eosinophilic and basophilic myelocytes. The specific granules of the neutrophilic myelocyte are too small to see by light microscopy (Plate 16–1*C*). Neutrophilic myelocytes outnumber eosinophilic myelocytes, and basophilic myelocytes are few.

The neutrophilic myelocyte has about three divisions in healthy cats, with daughter cells of the third myelocyte generation being distinguished as metamyelocytes (Prasse et al., 1973). During periods of increased peripheral demand for neutrophils, more divisions occur during the myeloblast, promyelocyte, and myelocyte stages of maturation. Each additional division in the cell population doubles the output of neutrophils, and during these periods a higher proportion of these cell types is seen in bone marrow films.

Daughter cells of the promonocyte cell line are monocytes, and the term myelocyte does not apply. Monocytes, to be described, leave the bone marrow at this stage of maturation, probably without more divisions (Schmalzl and Braunsteiner, 1968). This early departure from bone marrow to blood probably explains why monocytosis sometimes precedes neutrophilia in cats recovering from granulopoietic hypoplasia.

**NEUTROPHILIC METAMYELOCYTE, BAND NEUTROPHIL, AND SEGMENTED NEUTROPHIL.** These nondividing cells constitute a storage pool of functional cells equal to about 80 per cent of the granulocyte population in feline marrow. The release of neutrophils from bone marrow to blood is ordered by cell age. In health only segmented neutrophils and rare bands are present in feline blood; the appearance of band neutrophils and perhaps neutrophilic metamyelocytes in blood (a left shift) is an indication of a depleting storage pool and an increased peripheral demand for neutrophils.

The neutrophilic metamyelocyte is variable in size but usually smaller than the myelocyte (Plate 16–1*C* and *D*). The bean-shaped nucleus, which, as maturation proceeds, becomes thinner with bulbous ends and finally elongate, distinguishes the cell. The nuclear chromatin is more clumped than that of myelocytes, and the cytoplasm is pale blue; neutrophilic specific granules cannot usually be seen. Once the nucleus is elongate with smooth, parallel nuclear edges the cell may be called a band neutrophil (Plate 16–1*D*). The band neutrophil is smaller than the metamyelocyte, and its nuclear chromatin is more clumped. Distinguishing a neutrophilic band from a metamyelocyte may be a matter of subjective judgment by the microscopist. The band neutrophil nucleus may assume a U or S shape, and the cytoplasm changes from pale blue to pale gray as the cell matures.

To achieve interlaboratory uniformity of differential white-cell counts in blood films and the assessment of severity of the left shift in diseased cats, strict attention to the morphologic differentiation between band and segmented neutrophils is required. Differentiation between band neutrophils and younger metamyelocytes is of lesser practical importance. The segmented neutrophil is numerous in bone marrow and is the most prevalent white cell in feline blood. The cell is 6 to 9 μ in diameter with pale gray cytoplasm and faint pink granulation. Any nuclear constriction classifies the cell as segmented, whereas band neutrophil nuclei lack constrictions (Plate 16–1*D*). Most feline segmented neutrophils have two or three nuclear lobes separated by constrictions, but filament formulation between nuclear lobes is less common. The nuclear female sex chromatin or drumstick lobe in feline segmented neutrophils was reported in 4.2 to 11.4 per cent of female cells, 0 to 19.0 per cent of male cells, and 1.9 to 4.0 per cent of cells in male cats with tricolor XY/XXY mosaicism (Loughman et al., 1970).

Ultrastructurally, feline neutrophils contain two types of granules (Fig. 16–4) (Ward, et al., 1972). The granules, which contain killing and digestive enzymes and reactants, fuse with phagocytosed microorganisms contained in a phagocytic vacuole. The larger primary granules contain myeloperoxidase, lysozyme, cationic proteins, and several acid hydrolases including beta-glucuronidase; smaller specific granules contain lysozyme and lactoferrin; each of these substances are in feline neutrophils in concentrations comparable to those in other species (Rausch and Moore, 1975). Feline neutrophilic granules lack alkaline phosphatase (Atwal and McFarland, 1967). The peroxidase reactivity can be used to aid neutrophil identification in leukemias (Mackey, 1977b), because myeloperoxidase is synthesized in the promyelocyte and early myelocyte stages of maturation. Another staining procedure for disease differentiation based on granule reactants is the nitroblue tetrazolium test, and the number of positive-stained neutrophils is recorded. Normal limits for cats, 0.61 to 2.33 per cent of neutrophils, were found in cats with intestinal parasites, dermatomycosis, dermatosis, or viral diseases; whereas cats with higher values had toxoplasmosis (3.5 per cent), bacterial infections (6.52 per cent), or bacterial and viral infections (7 per cent) (Poli and Faravelli, 1974).

**MORPHOLOGIC ABNORMALITIES OF NEUTROPHILS.** Many infectious and noninfectious disorders in cats cause abnormal maturation of neutrophils during granulopoiesis and abnormal appearance of the cells in blood; these abnormalities are referred to as toxic change (Schalm, 1964; Schalm and Smith, 1963a, b). The most frequent toxic change seen in feline neutrophils is the occurrence of small, angular, bluish bodies (Döhle bodies). They are aggregated endoplasmic reticulum normally disposed of during maturation, and they denote the mildest form of toxic change in cats. Another common and more severe form of toxic change is neutrophilic cyto-

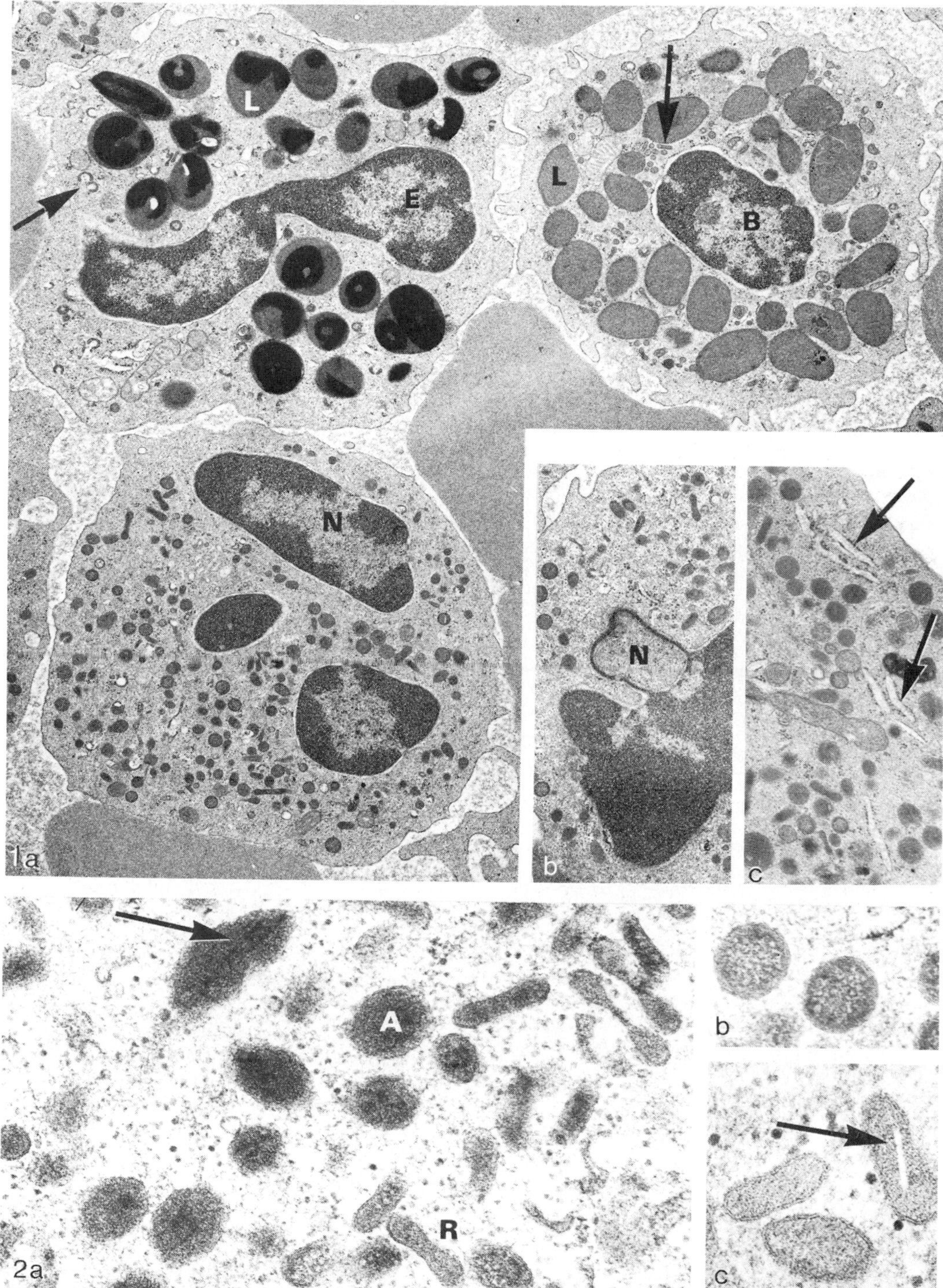


**Figure 16–4** *1a*, Buffy coat of cat with segmented neutrophil (N), eosinophil (E), and basophil (B). Large granules (L) and small granules (arrows) are seen in the eosinophil and basophil. × 8100. *1b*, A nuclear pocket (N) is seen in the neutrophil. × 10,000. *1c*, Clusters of profiles (arrows) of granular endoplasmic reticulum are observed in the neutrophil. × 15,000. *2a*, Portion of segmented neutrophil showing cytoplasmic granules. Large, dense, round primary granules (A) and smaller, dumbbell-shaped secondary granules are both limited by a unit membrane. A crystalline structure (arrow) may be present in one granule. A few reticulated, oval, dumbbell-shaped granules are seen (R). × 50,000. *2b*, Secondary granules have a reticulated internal structure. × 50,000. *2c*, A crystalline structure (arrow) is seen in the elongated granule, and the unit membrane of the granules is evident. × 86,400. (From Ward JW, Wright JF, Wharran GH: J Ultrastruct Res 39 [1972] 389–396.)

plasm that appears foamy in a basophilic (retained RNA) network; these cells are usually also enlarged (Plate 16–1*E*). Intensified staining of cytoplasmic granules is an uncommon toxic change in cats. When observed, toxic changes should signal the occurrence of significant systemic disease. Similar cytoplasmic changes have been experimentally induced with rabbit antifeline neutrophil antibody in cats (Chickering, 1980; Chickering et al., 1985). Cytoplasmic vacuoles may be seen in neutrophil precursor cells in bone marrow in chloramphenicol toxicosis (Watson, 1980).

Asynchronous maturation of neutrophil nuclei often accompanies cytoplasmic toxic change, and it usually occurs during periods of intense granulopoietic effort such as in localized suppurative disease. Asynchronous maturation is characterized by premature nuclear indentation or segmentation; cells may have nuclear filament formation coexisting with immature granular chromatin (Plate 16–1*F*).

Specific abnormalities in neutrophilic granules may be diagnostic in cats. Chédiak-Higashi syndrome in blue smoke Persian cats is characterized by autosomal recessive inheritance of partial oculocutaneous albinism, an increased susceptibility to infection, a bleeding tendency, and abnormally large eosinophilic, sudanophilic, and peroxidase-positive granules in granulocytes (Fig. 16–5) (Kramer et al., 1977; Prieur et al., 1979). In certain types of feline mucopolysaccharidosis (Haskins et al., 1980; Kramer et al., 1975), metachromatic granules, toluidine blue–positive or purple in Romanowsky-stained preparations, are seen in neutrophil cytoplasm.

## Monocytes

Monocytes are produced in the bone marrow and released to the blood at about the early myelocytic stage of maturation. The monocyte precursors, monoblast and promonocyte, are difficult to distinguish from myeloblasts and promyelocytes of the granulocytic series (Mackey, 1977b). No apparent storage pool of monocytes occurs, and this may be appreciated during recovery from granulopoietic hypoplasia in which monocytosis may precede the return of neutrophils to the blood. Monocytes transform into macrophages that constitute the monocyte-macrophage system (reticuloendothelial system), and they function in processing of antigenic information and phagocytosis of effete cells and microorganisms.

Monocytes vary from 15 to 22 μ in diameter but are usually the largest white cell, especially when vacuolated. Monocyte nuclei are round, indented, twisted, or cloverleaf-shaped, with irregular or rough nuclear membranes and lacy chromatin (Mackey, 1977b; Schalm, 1977; Schalm et al., 1975). The cytoplasm is gray-blue and always darker than neutrophilic cytoplasm, even toxic neutrophilic cytoplasm. Faintly purple granules may be seen, and cytoplasmic vacuolation is common (Plate 16–1*G*). Holding blood at room temperature for extended time before films are made enhances vacuolation of monocytes. Fine hairlike projections on the cell membrane facilitate identification of monocytes. Monocyte granules are peroxidase-positive and sudanophilic (Mackey, 1977b).

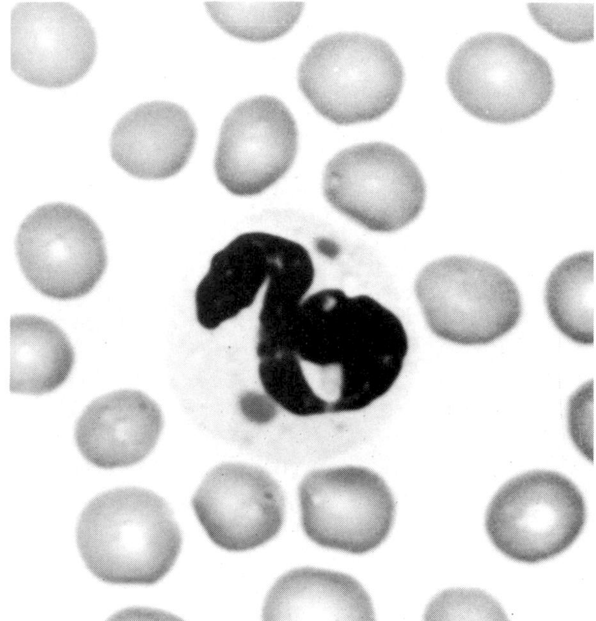

**Figure 16–5** Large cytoplasmic granules in neutrophil of cat with Chédiak-Higashi syndrome. Wright-Giemsa, × 1900. (Courtesy Dr. John W. Kramer, Washington State University, Pullman, WA.)

## Eosinophils

Eosinophils are produced in bone marrow and function in tissues at sites of specific reactions. The tissue sites are mainly beneath mucous membranes and skin, surfaces exposed to external foreign substances. Much evidence suggests that eosinophils function to contain hypersensitivity reactions and to suppress parasitic infections (Weller and Goetzl, 1980). Eosinophilopoiesis parallels neutrophil production, and the precursors are identifiable at the myelocyte stage of maturation when the specific granules become visible.

Feline eosinophil granules are elliptical and stain dull orange in Romanowsky-stained films (Plate 16–1*H*). Ultrastructurally the cell is found to contain two kinds of granules—the larger granules containing a crystalline structure and the smaller granules of varying shapes (Fig. 16–6) (Ward et al., 1972). The large specific granules of eosinophils are said to be rich in basic proteins, accounting for their staining qualities, and the other granule contents are similar to those of neutrophils. In cats, however, eosinophils are reported to lack myeloperoxidase, alkaline phosphatase, and lysozyme but to contain acid phosphatase and beta-glucuronidase (Zeya, 1978). Eosinophils have enlarged granules in cats with Chédiak-Higashi syndrome (Kramer et al., 1977).

## Basophils

Basophils are thought to function similarly to mast cells, promoting hypersensitivity reactions and as a source of the biologic anticoagulant heparin. Basophil production in bone marrow parallels neutrophil production, and the

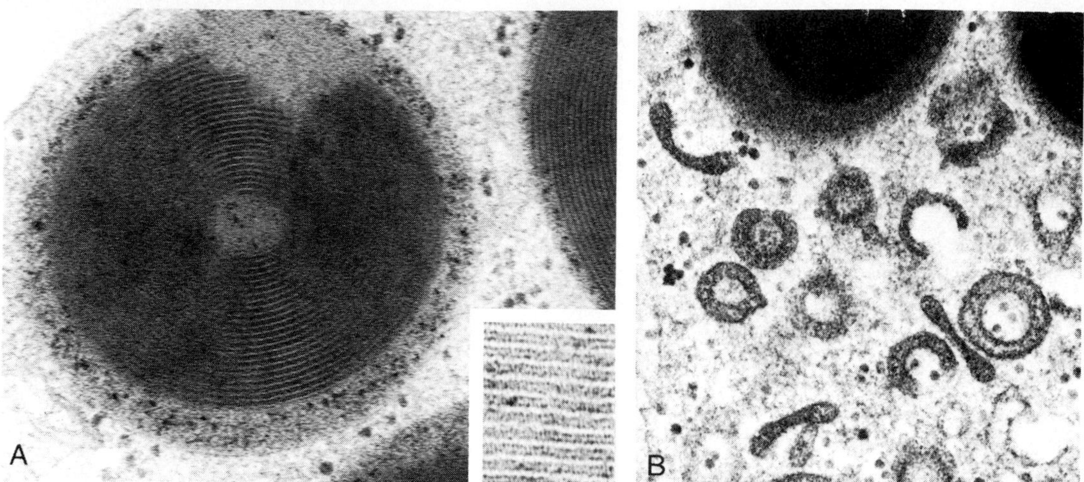


**Figure 16–6** *A*, Cross section of a typical large eosinophil granule contains ring-like structures with a repeat of approximately 10 nm. The matrix of the granule is homogeneous and contains dark granules. × 80,000. *Inset*, High magnification of rings shows triple-layered ring as well as periodicity of each ring of less than 2 nm. × 215,000. *B*, Small granules of the eosinophil are seen adjacent to the large granules. Sections appear as rings, crescents, and dumbbells. × 50,000. (From Ward JM, Wright JF, Gordon HW: J Ultrastruct Res 39 [1972] 389–396.)

precursors may be identified at the myelocyte stage of maturation when specific metachromatic granules are visible (Plate 16–1*I*). As the cell and its granules mature, the metachromatic staining quality disappears. Mature feline basophilic granules are elliptical, about the size of their counterpart in eosinophils, and numerous, 20 to 34 per cell (Ward et al., 1972). The granules stain gray in Romanowsky-stained smears (Plate 16–1*J*), and, unless a microscopist is specifically trained, the cell can be mistaken for a neutrophil or monocyte, although it is usually larger than the neutrophil. Occasionally a feline basophil retains metachromasia in a few granules, which facilitates identification (Schalm et al., 1975). Ultrastructurally the large granule has a banded or lattice pattern (Fig. 16–7), and a second smaller type of granule is also present in the cell (Ward et al., 1972).

## Lymphocytes

Lymphocyte production, distribution, and fate have been studied primarily in birds and small rodents (Greaves et al., 1973), but certain details related to these events are reported for cats. Lymphocytes are widely distributed in lymph nodes, spleen, gastrointestinal system lymphoid tissue, tonsils, thymus, bone marrow, and blood. Embryologically, stem cells from fetal liver and bone marrow populate the thymus, in which certain identifiable antigenic features are acquired, and thymic cells then populate specific anatomic sites of the lymphoid organs, designated thymic-dependent areas; this is called the T-cell population. In fetal cats, lymphoid cells appear in the thymus by 31 to 33 days of gestation and at about the same time in the primitive lymph nodes (Ackerman, 1963). A second population, also identifiable by surface markers, B cells, is hypothetically derived from bone marrow and comprises different specific anatomic regions of the lymphoid tissues.

T cells function in cell-mediated immune responses, which include delayed hypersensitivity, contact sensitivity, graft rejection, and acquired resistance to infectious organisms. B cells synthesize and secrete antibody, which is functionally manifested by immediate hypersensitivity reactions (anaphylaxis and atopy) and by antibody-mediated protection against infectious organisms. The methods of assaying immune function in cats are measuring humoral antibody levels; in-vivo manifestations of delayed hypersensitivity such as skin graft rejection; and in vitro lymphocyte blast transformation by mitogens such as concanavalin A, pokeweed, or phytohemagglutinin; cats are unusual in that they have only a minimal response to phytohemagglutinin (Cockerell et al., 1975; Taylor and Siddiqui, 1977). The proportions of T- and B-lymphocytes in the lymphoid tissues and blood of cats have been estimated: thymus, 10 to 73 per cent T and 0 to 10 per cent B; lymph node, 5 to 62 per cent T and 32 to 90 per cent B; and blood 5 to 33 per cent T and 5 to 62 per cent B (Mackey, 1977a).

Feline T and B cells are morphologically indistinguishable, although small, medium, and large lymphocytes can be seen. The size is more continuous than trimodal and relates to metabolic status and degree of flattening of the cells on films rather than any specific classification. Likewise lymphocyte life span is only arbitrarily designated as short (about two weeks) or long (several weeks, months, or years) and is defined by the time interval between two cell divisions; the interval between the last division and cell death is essentially unknown (Greaves et al., 1973). Although morphologically defined, lymphoblasts are not to be considered precursor cells or poorly differentiated cells but instead a morphologic manifestation of antigenic or mutogenic stimulation representing some stage in the life cycle of an individual lymphocyte.

Among the white cells, lymphocytes are unique because they recirculate. The majority of T cells recirculate, whereas most of the B cells found in blood are thought to be transient members of the recirculating pool; the majority of B cells do not recirculate (Greaves et al., 1973). The recirculatory route is by efferent lymph node

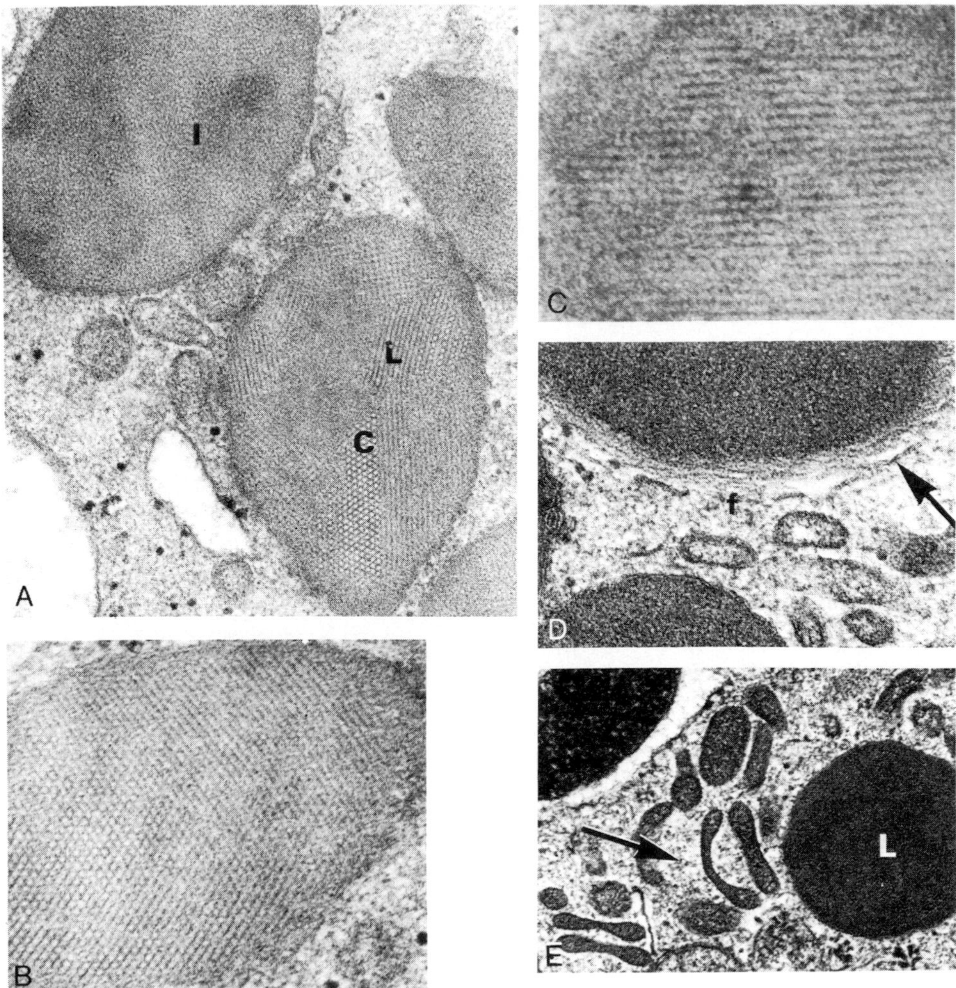


**Figure 16–7** *A*, Two large granules of the basophil. The most common granule (I) appears reticulated, while the other granule contains cross sections (C) and longitudinal sections (L) of lattice structures. × 55,000. *B*, High magnification of a granule with cross sections and longitudinal sections of lattice structures. × 86,400. *C*, A granule with only longitudinal sections of the lattice appearing as a banding pattern with a repeat of approximately 12 nm. × 120,000. *D*, On the edge of a granule, filamentous structures (f) and a unit membrane (arrow) are seen. × 50,000. *E*, The small basophil granules (arrow) appear adjacent to a large granule (L). They are round, dumbbell-shaped, and elongated. × 48,200. (From Ward JM, Wright JF, Gordon HW: J Ultrastruct Res 39 [1972] 389–396.)

ducts, thoracic duct, blood, emigration from blood through the postcapillary venule of the cortex in lymph nodes, and eventual return to efferent lymph. Knowledge of this route is essential to interpretation of blood lymphocyte counts in cats.

Feline lymphocytes are usually small, 7 to 9 μ, but range from 4 to 12 μ in diameter (Mackey, 1977b; Schalm et al., 1975; Wilkins, 1974). The nucleus nearly fills the cell, leaving visible only a narrow rim of pale blue cytoplasm (Plate 16–1*H*). The chromatin is coarsely granular, and the nucleolus is obscured from view on the light microscope. Occasionally, a few purple granules can be seen in the cytoplasm of Romanowsky-stained cells; the granules are periodic acid–Schiff–positive (Mackey, 1977b) (Plate 16–1*K*). Cells referred to as lymphoblasts (see previous discussion) are larger, stain more basophilic, and have more finely granular nuclear chromatin, and the nucleolus is usually visible. Lymphocytes and lymphoblasts stain negative in the Sudan black and peroxidase reactions (Mackey, 1977b).

Metabolically activated lymphocytes called immunocytes (Greaves et al., 1973) are seen occasionally in healthy cats and frequently with infections or other causes of antigenic challenge. Immunocytes have intensely basophilic cytoplasm on Romanowsky-stained films, and the cells vary from 7 to 15 μ in diameter; they differ from lymphoblasts in that the nuclear chromatin is densely aggregated, nucleoli are usually invisible, and the nuclear outline may be irregular (Plate 16–1*L*) (Wilkins, 1974). Plasma cells are a specific, metabolically active immunocyte; nuclear and staining characteristics are similar to those of other immunocytes, but the cell is identifiable by an eccentrically placed nucleus and a paler-staining zone of the cytoplasm caused by a well-developed Golgi apparatus (Mackey, 1977b). Plasma cells occur in lymph nodes and in small numbers in bone marrow; they are rarely encountered in feline blood.

## GENERAL WHITE-CELL RESPONSES

The total and differential white-cell counts are frequently used to aid assessment of the general health status of cats during physical examination procedures. Although seldom diagnostic, the counts and morphologic assessment of white cells provide clues to the physiopathologic status. Changes from the expected norm for cats may be called the white-cell response. The various general white-cell responses of cats will be reviewed. Sample leukograms are cited in Table 16–3.

### Physiologic Leukocytosis

Physiologic leukocytosis is a transient event produced by fear and muscular activity. Healthy cats, most often under a year of age (Schalm, 1968), are particularly prone to develop this response when force is required for handling and blood-sampling purposes; sick cats are less likely to have physiologic leukocytosis (Kleinsorgen et al., 1976; Schalm and Hughes, 1964; Schalm et al., 1975). Neutrophilia and lymphocytosis typify the response (Cases 1 through 3, Table 16–3), and lymphocytes often outnumber neutrophils.

The response is produced immediately by fear and lasts about 30 minutes, and therefore epinephrine is believed to be the mediator. Epinephrine causes a redistribution of blood neutrophils from the marginal to the circulating pools, thereby increasing the number counted (Athens et al., 1961), but the cause of lymphocytosis, unique for cats, is unknown. Delivery of thoracic duct lymphocytes may be enhanced by the muscular activity, or the return to lymph nodes of recirculating lymphocytes may be delayed. The response can be avoided if cats are not frightened or forcibly handled and if healthy cats are necessarily bled daily, they become accustomed to the routine and physiologic leukocytosis will not occur (Schalm and Hughes, 1964).

### Response to Stress and Exogenous Corticosteroids

Endogenous or exogenous corticosteroids induce leukocytosis in cats. The response occurs in cats stressed by natural disease, particularly painful disorders. It is noticeable in the leukogram within four to six hours after initiation of the stimulus, and if no further stimulation occurs, the leukogram returns to baseline values by 24 hours (Schalm et al., 1975) (Case 6, Table 16–3). The white-cell differential at the peak of the response reveals neutrophilia, monocytosis, lymphopenia, and eosinopenia (Cases 4 through 7, Table 16–3). Immature neutrophils are seldom seen unless the storage pool in bone marrow was depleted of segmented cells at the time of stimulation. The return of eosinophils and lymphocytes to normal numbers can signal the onset of convalescence (Schalm, 1968) (Case 14, Table 16–3). Monocytosis is the least consistent change in the response, but it can be observed in cats with acute and chronic stressful episodes (Prasse, 1975). Daily injections of corticosteroids cause persistence of the response, although neutrophilia may diminish. The response was inconsistently observed in cats given weekly injections of repositol corticosteroid (Scott et al., 1978), and alternate-day therapy with short-acting corticosteroids may obviate the effects.

### Neutrophil Responses

In addition to excitement and stress, a variety of feline diseases elicit certain general patterns of neutrophil responses. A normal neutrophil total (2500/μl to 12,500/μl) or neutrophilia with band or earlier neutrophils numbering 300/μl to about 1000/μl is typical in diseases in which the neutrophil is a minimal component of the inflammatory exudate, e.g., hemorrhagic cystitis, seborrheic dermatitis, tracheobronchitis, catarrhal or hemorrhagic enteritis, and certain nonsuppurative granulomatous diseases (Prasse and Duncan, 1976) (Cases 5, 7, and 16 through 20, Table 16–3).

Purulent exudative diseases may cause the blood neutrophil number to be low, normal, or high, depending on the balance between the rate of tissue utilization of neutrophils and the rate of neutrophil release from bone marrow. In any case, since the tissue utilization of neutrophils is high in purulent disease, the rate of marrow release is likewise increased, bone marrow stores of segmented neutrophils are depleted, and immature neu-

**Table 16–3 Case Examples Illustrating General White Cell Responses in Cats**[a]

**CASE EXAMPLES 1 THROUGH 5**

| | Case 1 | Case 2[b] | Case 3[c] | Case 4 | Case 5[b] |
|---|---|---|---|---|---|
| White-cell count | 23,200 | 26,200 | 22,600 | 23,600 | 21,900 |
| Segmented neutrophils | 11,368 | 14,934 | 10,396 | 23,302 | 17,850 |
| Band neutrophils | 0 | 0 | 0 | 0 | 940 |
| Earlier neutrophils | 0 | 0 | 0 | 0 | |
| Lymphocytes | 10,904 | 10,218 | 11,300 | 354 | 1,260 |
| Monocytes | 232 | 393 | 226 | 944 | 520 |
| Eosinophils | 696 | 655 | 242 | 0 | 420 |
| Basophils | 0 | 0 | 226 | 0 | 0 |
| Toxic neutrophils | – | – | ND | – | – |
| Immunocytes | – | – | ND | – | – |

Case 1. Cat, 6 months old, domestic shorthair, female. History: The healthy cat was to be neutered. Presurgical evaluation included a routine blood count. During bleeding the cat became frightened, and forced restraint was used. Interpretation: Epinephrine-mediated physiologic leukocytosis.

Case 2. Cat, 3 years old, domestic shorthair, male castrate. History: The cat had been treated for vestibular disease with chloramphenicol for 5 days. The leukogram was taken for final evaluation before release from the hospital. The cat struggled violently during sample collection. Interpretation: Epinephrine-mediated physiologic leukocytosis (normal in health). Final diagnosis: Idiopathic feline vestibular disease—recovery complete.

Case 3. Cat, 7 months old, male. History: A normal cat that lived its entire life in a cage was removed from the cage and placed in a cardboard box to await bleeding. Sample was taken from capillary blood of the ear. Interpretation: Physiologic leukocytosis resulting from fright.

Case 4. Cat, adult, castrated male. History: The cat was admitted for vomiting, abdominal distention, and abdominal pain. The urethra was obstructed, and the cat was azotemic. Interpretation: Stress-endogenous corticosteroid response with neutrophilia, lymphopenia, monocytosis, and eosinopenia. Final diagnosis: Urethral obstruction.

Case 5. Cat, 5 years old, Persian, male. History: The cat was observed by the owner to have had seizures every 8 to 12 hours for 3 days. The leukogram was obtained within 2 hours of last seizure. Interpretation: Endogenous corticosteroid–mediated neutrophilia and lymphopenia or mild inflammatory disease. Final diagnosis: Epileptiform seizures of unknown etiology.

**CASE EXAMPLES 6 THROUGH 8**

| | Case 6[d] 0 hr | Case 6[d] 8 hr | Case 6[d] 24 hr | Case 7 | Case 8 |
|---|---|---|---|---|---|
| White-cell count | 15,775 | 21,900 | 15,900 | 14,100 | 2,285 |
| Segmented neutrophils | 9,000 | 19,500 | 8,500 | 12,267 | 319 |
| Band neutrophils | 0 | 0 | 0 | 705 | 1,005 |
| Earlier neutrophils | 0 | 0 | 0 | 0 | 137 |
| Lymphocytes | 5,000 | 1,500 | 6,500 | 423 | 1,590 |
| Monocytes | 225 | 800 | 300 | 705 | 187 |
| Eosinophils | 550 | 100 | 600 | 0 | 0 |
| Basophils | 0 | 0 | 0 | 0 | 0 |
| Toxic neutrophils | ND | ND | ND | – | + |
| Immunocytes | ND | ND | ND | + | – |

Case 6. Blood white-cell changes in a cat given oral prednisolone (5 mg) at zero hour.

Case 7. Cat, adult, domestic shorthair, male. History: The cat had fever, anorexia, and depression. The fluorescent antibody test for feline leukovirus was negative. Interpretation: Neutrophilic leukocytosis and left shift consistent with mild inflammatory disease or endogenous corticosteroid–mediated neutrophilia, lymphopenia, and eosinopenia. Final diagnosis: Fever of unknown origin (possibly viral infection).

Case 8. Cat, 4 months old, domestic shorthair, male. History: The cat had fever, lethargy, and dyspnea. Opaque pleural fluid was gray-pink and contained protein, 4.7 gm/dl, red blood cells, white cells 73,400/μl, including degenerate neutrophils, and macrophages, bacteria, and yeasts. The bone marrow was hypercellular, and early granulocyte precursors predominated. Interpretation: Localized purulent disease overwhelming the granulopoietic effort, granulopoietic hyperplasia of bone marrow, and toxemia. Final diagnosis: Septic purulent pleuritis.

**CASE EXAMPLES 9 THROUGH 13**

| | Case 9 | Case 10 | Case 11 | Case 12 | Case 13 |
|---|---|---|---|---|---|
| White-cell count | 18,900 | 28,100 | 48,100 | 61,000 | 1,800 |
| Segmented neutrophils | 15,147 | 22,199 | 20,683 | 54,073 | 873 |
| Band neutrophils | 1,590 | 2,388 | 19,961 | 1,527 | 54 |
| Earlier neutrophils | 187 | 140 | 241 | 0 | 0 |
| Lymphocytes | 1,590 | 2,248 | 2,886 | 611 | 765 |
| Monocytes | 187 | 983 | 1,684 | 3,055 | 108 |
| Eosinophils | 0 | 140 | 2,404 | 1,833 | 0 |
| Basophils | 0 | 0 | 241 | 0 | 0 |
| Toxic neutrophils | + | + | + | – | – |
| Immunocytes | + | + | + | + | – |

Case 9. Cat, adult, domestic shorthair, female. History: Presenting leukogram on admission. Referred with diagnosis of pyothorax. *E. coli* isolated from blood and thoracic exudate. Interpretation: Leukogram consistent with generalized purulent inflammation and toxemia. Final diagnosis: Septicemia and septic purulent pleuritis.

Case 10. Cat, adult, domestic longhair, male. History: The cat had swelling, ulceration, and exudation around the base of the tail and perineum. *S. epidermidis* cultured. Interpretation: Localized purulent inflammatory disease. Final diagnosis: Abscess.

Case 11. Cat, 2½ years old, domestic shorthair, castrated male. History: The cat was anorectic and febrile with a distended abdomen. Fluorescent antibody test for feline leukovirus, feline infectious peritonitis titer, fecal flotation for parasites, and external parasite examinations were all negative. *S. aureus* and α and γ streptococci were isolated from peritoneal exudate composed mainly of neutrophils and macrophages with fewer eosinophils. Interpretation: Localized septic purulent inflammatory disease; unknown explanation for the eosinophils and basophils. Final diagnosis: Septic purulent peritonitis.

Case 12. Cat, 2 years old, domestic, female. History: Abdominal enlargement and fever. Radiographs indicated an enlarged uterus. Interpretation: Marked leukocytosis consistent with localized purulent inflammatory disease; neutrophilia of this magnitude with concomitant minimal left shift characterizes chronic purulent disease in which granulopoiesis has re-established bone marrow storage of neutrophils; eosinophilia often accompanies genital tract inflammatory disease; lymphopenia of stress or unknown causes. Final diagnosis: Chronic purulent metritis.

Case 13. Cat, 4 years old, domestic, male. History: Treated recently for abscesses. Currently, signs were fever, pallor, ocular discharge, and weight loss. Fluorescent antibody test positive for feline leukovirus. In addition to leukopenia, the cat had a

**Table 16–3 Case Examples Illustrating General White Cell Responses in Cats[a]** *Continued*

nonresponsive anemia, PCV 15%, and thrombocytopenia, platelets 27,000/μl. The bone marrow was hypercellular with a preponderance of early granulocyte precursors. Interpretation: Feline leukovirus–associated subleukemic granulocytic leukemia or preleukemic syndrome. Final diagnosis: Myeloproliferative disease.

**CASE EXAMPLES 14 AND 15**

| | Case 14 Days 1 through 6 | | | | Case 15 |
|---|---|---|---|---|---|
| White-cell count | 400 | 2,700 | 25,400 | 16,900 | 11,900 |
| Segmented neutrophils | (4%) | 567 | 12,573 | 11,069 | 10,591 |
| Band neutrophils | (4%) | 1,512 | 10,668 | 1,183 | 0 |
| Earlier neutrophils | 0 | 54 | 889 | 0 | 0 |
| Lymphocytes | (84%) | 513 | 889 | 3,912 | 476 |
| Monocytes | (8%) | 0 | 0 | 0 | 0 |
| Eosinophils | 0 | 54 | 381 | 676 | 833 |
| Basophils | 0 | 0 | 0 | 0 | 0 |
| Toxic neutrophils | + | + | – | – | – |
| Immunocytes | – | + | – | – | – |

Case 14. Feline infectious panleukopenia was diagnosed in a litter. One littermate was dead, and this kitten had 10% dehydration and diarrhea. On day 1, PCV was 25%, and the bone marrow was hypocellular with only scattered lymphoid cells and rare granulocytic precursors observed. The kitten was treated with fluids and antibiotics continued through day 6. On day 6 the kitten began to eat and drink, and the PCV was 18%. Interpretation: Recovery from neutropenia parallels clinical recovery from infectious panleukopenia, and often rebound neutrophilic leukocytosis with a left shift is observed; lymphopenia typifies infectious panleukopenia, and return of blood lymphocyte and eosinophil numbers signal convalescence; in this disease, the lowest point in PCV is often reached at the point of clinical recovery. Final diagnosis: Feline infectious panleukopenia.

Case 15. Cat, 2 years old, domestic shorthair, male. History: The cat had been traumatized accidentally 2 weeks earlier. The thorax contained opaque, gray-pink fluid that contained lipid and mainly lymphocytes and red blood cells. Interpretation: Lymphopenia associated with loss of thoracic duct cells into the pleural cavity. Final diagnosis: Chylothorax.

**CASE EXAMPLES 16 THROUGH 20**

| | Case 16 | Case 17 | Case 18 | Case 19 | Case 20 |
|---|---|---|---|---|---|
| White-cell count | 18,600 | 17,100 | 28,600 | 29,900 | 28,200 |
| Segmented neutrophils | 11,811 | 6,327 | 19,162 | 11,960 | 5,358 |
| Band neutrophils | 0 | 0 | 0 | 0 | 0 |
| Earlier neutrophils | 0 | 0 | 0 | 0 | 0 |
| Lymphocytes | 1,860 | 4,959 | 5,005 | 4,933 | 5,076 |
| Monocytes | 744 | 1,026 | 429 | 1,196 | 282 |
| Eosinophils | 4,185 | 4,788 | 1,144 | 11,810 | 17,000 |
| Basophils | 0 | 0 | 2,860 | 0 | 484 |
| Toxic neutrophils | – | – | – | – | – |
| Immunocytes | – | – | – | + | – |

Case 16. Cat, 8 years old, domestic shorthair, male. History: Oral and cutaneous ulcers histologically characterized by chronic granulomatous inflammation; eosinophils were among the other exudative cells. Interpretation: Eosinophilia associated with cutaneous disease. Final diagnosis: Eosinophilic granuloma complex.

Case 17. Cat, 3 years old, domestic shorthair, female. History: Coughing, sneezing, fever, and transtracheal wash containing eosinophilic exudate. Interpretation: Eosinophilia and monocytosis associated with lung disease. Final diagnosis: Eosinophilic pneumonitis.

Cat 18. Cat, 5 years old, Siamese, castrated male. History: Chronic dermatitis, which would improve upon removing the cat from its home environment for several days. Interpretation: Neutrophilic, eosinophilic, and basophilic leukocytosis associated with mild nonpurulent and possibly allergic skin disease. Final diagnosis: Atopy.

Case 19. Cat, 2 years old, domestic, castrated male. History: Flea infestation and dermatitis. Interpretation: Eosinophilic leukocytosis associated with allergic skin disease. Final diagnosis: Flea allergy dermatitis.

Case 20. Cat, 12 years old, domestic shorthair, female. Final diagnosis: Flea allergy dermatitis.

[a]All values per μl blood; – none seen on films; + seen on films; ND not done.
[b]From Prasse and Duncan, 1976.
[c]From Schalm and Hughes, 1964.
[d]From Schalm et al., 1975, values estimated from graph, p. 118.

trophils mark the differential white-cell counts in these diseases. The magnitude of left shift is some measure of the intensity of the purulent process.

Neutropenia associated with purulent exudative disease is most frequent in acute localized bacterial infections, particularly in the lung, thorax, peritoneal cavity, or uterus in cats (Case 8, Table 16–3). A similar response may occur in feline salmonellosis (Timoney et al., 1978). The majority of cats with purulent diseases have neutrophilic leukocytosis with white-cell counts from 19,500/μl to 30,000/μl; extreme counts range to 75,000/μl and on rare occasions may exceed 100,000/μl in cats (Schalm, 1962; Schalm and Smith, 1963b; Schalm et al., 1975). A wide variety of infectious and noninfectious conditions cause this response. The higher counts usually accompany localized diseases such as pyoderma, pleuritis, peritonitis, pyometra, or abscess, whereas generalized diseases such as bacterial or viral septicemias or systemic mycoses elicit a response of lesser magnitude (Cases 9 through 12, Table 16–3). The inciting agents may be pyogenic bacteria, fungi, foreign bodies (even sterile ones), and necrotic tissue. Diminishing left shifts accompany convalescence; however, such a finding in a cat with continuing localized purulent disease indicates a chronic state in which granulopoiesis has reestablished the storage pool of marrow neutrophils in spite of continued excessive tissue utilization (Case 12, Table 16–3).

Neutropenia caused by granulopoietic hypoplasia differs from neutropenia of overwhelming sepsis described previously; it is persistent and associated with disorders of insidious onset and long duration. Feline infectious panleukopenia is characterized by severe leukopenia with neutropenia and lymphopenia evident by four days after infection and persisting during the course of clinical illness

(Rohovsky and Fowler, 1971; Schalm et al., 1975). During this stage, bone marrow examination reveals a near absence of neutrophil precursors, but in cats that survive, convalescence is signaled by resurgence of granulopoiesis with granulocytic hyperplasia of bone marrow followed in a few days by neutrophilia (Case 14, Table 16–3). In a survey of 95 feline leukovirus-infected, nonleukemic cats admitted to the University of Georgia Veterinary Hospital, 50 per cent had neutropenia. Three general patterns are seen in these neutropenic cats. In the most common, neutropenia is mild and marrow granulopoiesis nearly normal. A second pattern, more severe, is characterized by granulopoietic hypoplasia, and neutropenia also accompanies the panleukopenia-like syndrome. The third pattern is characterized by severe persistent neutropenia of insidious onset accompanied by marked granulopoietic hyperplasia in the bone marrow (Case 13, Table 16–3). This syndrome has been called subleukemic granulocytic leukemia (Duncan and Prasse, 1976; Schalm, 1972), but the mechanism is not known. Affected cats may recover, die from secondary infection, or progress to overt leukemia.

### Monocytosis

Monocyte counts in excess of 850/μl were found in 27 of approximately 225 cats studied hematologically; 11 cats had acute stressful disorders, and 16 had chronic inflammatory or neoplastic diseases (Prasse, 1975). Monocytosis (Cases 4, 10 through 12, 17, and 19, Table 16–3) often accompanies neutrophilic leukocytosis in purulent inflammatory diseases in cats.

### Eosinophilia

In a survey (Prasse, 1975) of approximately 225 feline leukograms, 43 cats (19 per cent) had eosinophil counts in excess of 1000/μl at the time of admission to the University of Georgia Veterinary Hospital; all the cats were over a year of age, and eosinophilia was never seen in kittens. Usually an examination for parasites follows observation of eosinophilia; only parasitisms characterized by prolonged, intimate tissue-parasite interactions, however, seem to elicit the response. No difference in eosinophil counts was evident between 30 noninfected cats and 35 cats infected with *Taenia taeniaeformis, T. pisiformis, T. hydatigena, Hymenolepis nana, Toxocara cati, T. canis, Toxascaris leonina, Uncinaria stenocephala,* or *Ancylostoma* sp (Roth and Schneider, 1971). In contrast, aelurostrongylosis (Scott, 1973), paragonimiasis (Hoover and Dubey, 1978), trichinosis (Holzworth and Georgi, 1974), and flea infestation, particularly flea allergy dermatitis (Cases 19 and 20, Table 16–3), are parasitisms accompanied by eosinophilia in cats.

Nonparasitic causes of feline eosinophilia include the eosinophilic granuloma complex and eosinophilic pneumonitis (Cases 16 through 18, Table 16–3). One of us (KWP) has observed persistent eosinophilic leukocytosis in excess of 60,000/μl in two cats that died with gastric and mesenteric lymphosarcoma. In general, inflammatory diseases of tissues rich in mast cells, i.e., skin, lungs, genitalia (Case 11, Table 16–3), alimentary tract, and joints, frequently elicit eosinophilia (Schalm, 1977).

### Basophilia

Basophils are reported to be uncommon in the blood of cats. However, if technicians are trained to recognize the cell by its gray, nonmetachromatic granules (see earlier discussion), the cells can be found in feline diseases. Basophilia occasionally occurs concomitant with eosinophilia (Schalm, 1977) (Cases 11, 18 and 20, Table 16–3).

### Lymphopenia

Lymphopenia is one of the most common abnormalities of differential white-cell counts in sick cats. In a survey (Prasse, 1975) of 225 hospitalized cats, 66 cats (30 per cent frequency) had fewer than 1500 lymphocytes/μl; of the 66 cats, 35 died, were euthanatized or had not recovered by the time of discharge from the hospital. Lymphopenia and particularly persistent lymphopenia should be regarded as an unfavorable sign, whereas a return of lymphocyte numbers to normal limits is often evidence of convalescence (Schalm, 1968).

Lymphopenia can be easily ascribed to the effects of stress and endogenous release of corticosteroids in sick cats (see earlier discussion). Other disease mechanisms, however, cause lymphopenia, and these alternative conditions should be considered in differential diagnosis of the lymphopenic cat. Extravasation of efferent lymph rich in lymphocytes occurs in rupture of the thoracic duct (Lindsay, 1974) (Case 15, Table 16–3), chylous thoracic effusion associated with feline cardiac disease (Creighton and Wilkins, 1975), and loss of enteric lymph to the intestinal lumen in neoplastic or granulomatous intestinal diseases. Viral diseases (Cases 7, 13, and 14, Table 16–3), particularly panleukopenia (Schalm et al., 1975), cause lymphopenia, whereas febrile diseases caused by bacteria are less likely to result in lymphopenia. Congenital infection with feline leukovirus causing thymic atrophy (fading-kitten syndrome) is another mechanism for lymphopenia.

## PLATELETS

Platelets are formed by controlled cytoplasmic fragmentation of megakaryocytes, multinucleated precursor cells that are readily found in normal feline marrow.

Feline platelets are usually spherical and contain fine azurophilic granules. Size variation among feline platelets is greater than that observed in most other species; occasional platelets may be as large as red cells. Such large forms are more common in states of increased thrombopoiesis. Platelet clumping is a common artifact in feline blood and may interfere with accurate counting of platelets, white cells, and red cells.

# DISORDERS OF THE HEMATOPOIETIC SYSTEM

SUSAN M. COTTER and JEAN HOLZWORTH

Cats, of all domestic animals, suffer most often from disorders of the hematopoietic system. Anemia, granulocytopenia, and hematopoietic malignancy are the most commonly encountered conditions, and most of these are the result of infection with feline leukemia virus (FeLV). An organized approach to cats with hematopoietic disorders is essential for accurate diagnosis; it will also enable the clinician to guide an owner to a rational decision based on prognosis and, when possible, to select the most appropriate therapy.

## DISORDERS OF RED CELLS—ANEMIA

Recognition and management of the varieties of anemia constitute one of the most significant challenges to the feline practitioner. Anemia, defined as a total reduction in red cells and hemoglobin content, is a symptom rather than a diagnosis. The pathophysiology of anemia is related to reduced oxygen-carrying capacity of the blood causing tissue hypoxia. Because clinical signs are vague and the cat is able to decrease its activities in conditions of limited oxygen availability, a profound anemia may develop before signs attract an owner's attention. The most frequent presenting signs are anorexia and lethargy, sometimes with sudden collapse. Pallor, sometimes noted by owners of cats with unpigmented noses, is caused by diversion of blood to vital tissues at the expense of the periphery. Anemic cats sometimes lick soil, litter, walls, or rusty objects. A history of recent stress may be elicited, such as infection, injury, or surgery.

### Physical Findings

Pallor is evident in unpigmented skin of ears, nose, lips, and footpads and in the oral mucosa.

Decreased tissue oxygenation stimulates chemoreceptors in the aortic body causing accelerated heart rate and myocardial contractility with increased cardiac output. Systolic murmurs and gallop rhythms caused by low viscosity of the blood may develop when the packed cell volume drops to the mid-20s, and cardiac enlargement may be evident radiographically.

Splenomegaly occurs in a minority of anemic cats, primarily those with acute hemolysis, as in hemobartonellosis, or chronic anemias associated with lymphoma, myeloproliferative diseases, and mast cell tumors.

Jaundice occasionally results from severe hemolysis but is more often of hepatic origin. Protracted jaundice even with continuing hemolysis often indicates underlying liver disease, since breakdown of several grams of hemoglobin daily would be required to produce jaundice in a cat with a normal liver. Severe anemia may, in itself, cause centrilobular hepatic necrosis from anoxia.

Rarely hemoglobinuria may occur in acute hemolytic anemia. If anemia is slowly progressive and chronic, compensation occurs, and the cat may show no clinical signs even in rather severe anemia.

As anemia becomes more severe, the cat may become restless and dyspneic and may lie on its side. Fever may be present initially, but the temperature drops to normal or subnormal terminally.

Funduscopic examination in 26 cats with hemoglobin levels less than 15 gm/dl disclosed focal retinal hemorrhages in 20 (Fischer, 1970). Most often these hemorrhages were in the deep layers of the retina in cats with low platelet counts. Increased frequency of retinal hemorrhages may follow transfusion, possibly because of increased blood pressure.

When presented with an anemic cat, the clinician may be helped by information about the cat's environment—whether it is allowed outdoors, has been exposed to toxins or drugs, or has any nutritional deficiency. It is almost impossible for a cat to develop a nutritional anemia if fed a complete commercial cat food, but deficient fad diets favored by some owners may be imposed on pets as well. Questions about a cat's origin, previous illnesses, or association with other cats with similar signs might elicit a clue to exposure to feline leukemia virus.

### Diagnostic Procedures

Blood for diagnostic tests should be drawn before therapy is started, since medication or transfusions may affect the hemogram. Initial tests that are most critical are packed cell volume (PCV), total and differential white-cell counts (WBC), reticulocyte count, and examination for FeLV. Total red-cell count and hemoglobin determination are helpful for classification of an anemia, as they provide values for mean corpuscular volume (MCV) and mean corpuscular hemoglobin concentration (MCHC), but similar information can be obtained by examination of a well-made, well-stained blood film. Additional diagnostic tests can be included initially or, if the condition of the cat is critical, may be postponed until after a transfusion is given. With profoundly anemic cats, the stress of obtaining a blood sample may prove fatal, and one may have to settle initially for a blood film obtained by pricking a marginal ear vein (Fig. 16–8).

### Reticulocyte Evaluation

As reticulocytes mature, the amount of ribosomal RNA in the cells decreases, and in older reticulocytes only a few granules or threads may be found; these, as well as the younger forms, should be included in the reticulocyte count. Normal cats differ from other species in that they have significantly greater numbers of mature (punctate) reticulocytes in the circulating blood (Cramer and Lewis, 1972; Zawidzka et al., 1964). When both immature (aggregate) and mature (punctate) reticulocytes are counted, a normal cat has a total reticulocyte count of 1.4 to 10.8

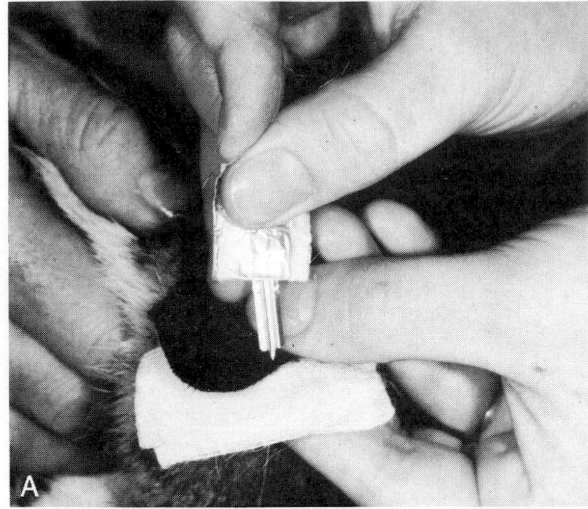

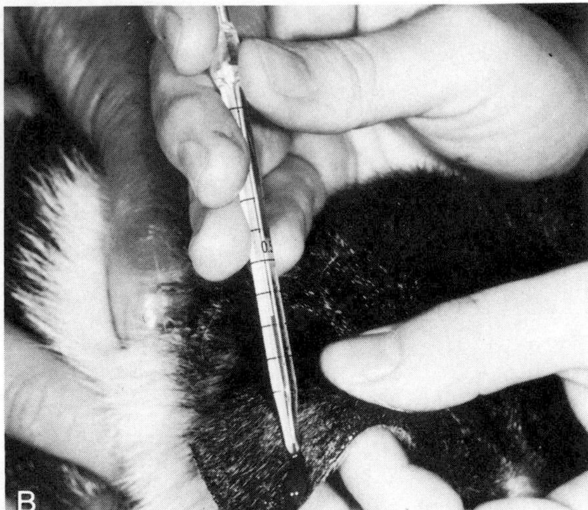

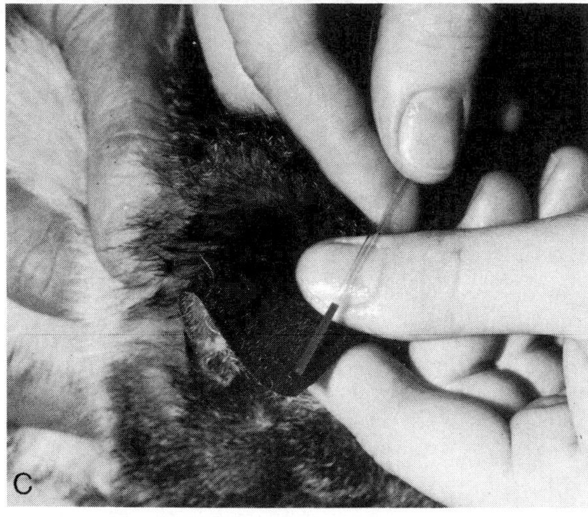

**Figure 16–8** *A* to *C*, Pricking a marginal ear vein avoids stress to a severely anemic cat and provides enough blood for films and for determining total WBC, reticulocyte count, and PCV (with Unopette vial [Becton and Dickinson] instead of the pipette pictured, and with microhematocrit tubes). No antiseptic is used. The fur is smoothed with Vaseline, which also prevents the blood from spreading out. If blood flow is poor, the tip of a curved scalpel blade should be substituted for the lancet. The collector's finger tip under the pinna must be protected by a gauze sponge.

per 100 red cells, with a mean of 4.6 per cent. Of these, 0 to 0.4 per cent are of the aggregate form (Cramer and Lewis, 1972).

An increase in aggregate reticulocytes indicates an active response to anemia (Cramer and Lewis, 1972). These peak at 3 per cent on day 4 after acute experimental blood loss and return to normal by day 11. An increase in aggregate reticulocytes correlates with polychromasia of the peripheral blood film and may represent a shift of the most immature reticulocytes from the marrow to the blood under acute stress (Alsaker et al., 1977). These cells may have undergone premature enucleation and contain more RNA and mitochondria.

After the initial response of aggregate reticulocytes, punctate reticulocytes are increased by 5 days after blood loss, reach a peak in 10 days, stay elevated for about 9 days, and return to normal by 25 days (Cramer and Lewis, 1972). The degree of response of punctate reticulocytes parallels closely the degree of blood loss (Fan et al., 1978). The response in chronic anemia is often limited to the punctate form. The prolonged presence of the punctate reticulocyte is unique to the cat, and was attributed by Cramer and Lewis to slow maturation. They stressed that the number of each form must be considered to evaluate accurately the degree of response to anemia. Adjustment of the count for the degree of anemia is discussed earlier in this chapter.

In acute blood loss, reticulocytosis is the primary response; nucleated red cells may enter the blood in a severe responsive anemia but should be accompanied by reticulocytosis. Nucleated red cells are an adverse prognostic sign in a nonregenerative anemia.

Injection of epinephrine was shown to increase reticulocyte counts of cats made anemic experimentally by blood loss (Fan et al., 1978). This finding suggests that some reticulocytes are sequestered in the spleen to be released by contraction of the spleen with excitement or stress and an adrenergic response. Splenic storage and release of blood cells may be more of a factor in a healthy cat than in a sick cat that is presumably already stressed, with a minimal storage pool remaining in the spleen.

## Classification of Anemias

Anemias can be classed as regenerative or nonregenerative, although there are occasional cases in which this distinction is not easily made. A cat with regenerative anemia may have an aplastic crisis if an infection develops. A cat with a nonregenerative anemia may at times produce red cells. Classification of feline anemias is especially difficult in the presence of concurrent illnesses (Fig. 16–9). For example, at Angell Memorial Animal Hospital (AMAH), 70 per cent of all anemic cats are carriers of

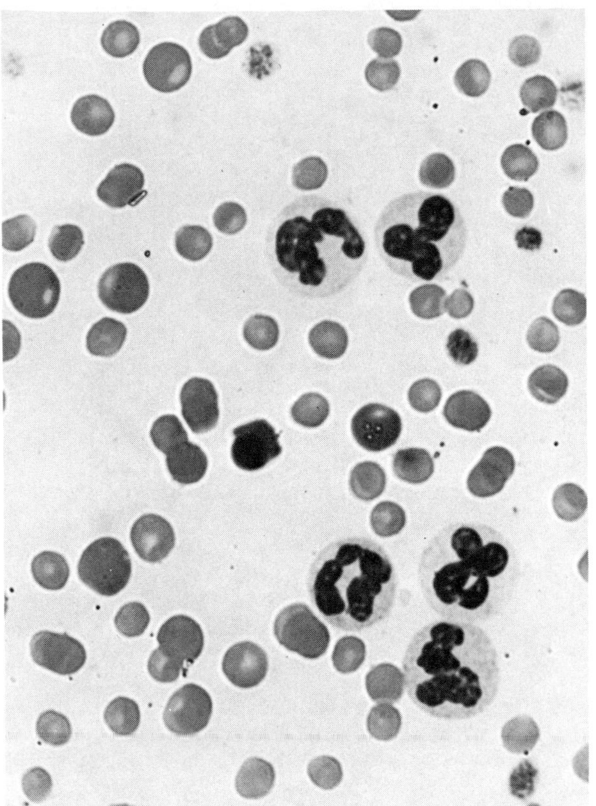

**Figure 16–9** Regenerative anemia in a cat recovering from an infection. Polychromasia and anisocytosis are pronounced, and a nucleated red cell is present. Neutrophilia often results from general marrow stimulation. Wright's, × 950. (From Holzworth J: J Am Vet Med Assoc 128 [1956] 471–478.)

feline leukemia virus (FeLV) (Cotter, 1976). *Haemobartonella felis* may be present as a latent infection in cats with nonregenerative anemias. Despite these confusing occurrences, classification is helpful in determining etiology and treatment.

## Regenerative Anemia—Blood Loss

Blood loss can be acute or chronic, external or internal. With acute blood loss, the primary concern is decreased circulating blood volume and shock rather than anemia. The PCV remains normal for about 10 to 12 hours even after severe acute blood loss, so that this test is not an accurate indicator of continuing hemorrhage. Mucous membrane color, capillary refill time, and pulse rate and strength should be monitored. An increasing pulse rate with decreasing strength is a sign of shock or continued bleeding. Fluid volume can be restored with balanced electrolyte solutions, and transfusion is required only in the most severe cases. The anemia in acute blood loss is initially normochromic and normocytic. The reticulocyte count increases after four or five days, the red cells become macrocytic and polychromatophilic, and the PCV begins to rise.

Soon after an episode of bleeding, a transient, slight decrease in platelet numbers occurs, followed within three days by an increase in their number and size. A reactive leukocytosis usually occurs within 24 hours after blood loss because of generalized stimulation of the marrow by some factor not yet well understood.

Unexpected blood loss after injury or surgery (e.g., urethrostomy) occurs occasionally and can be the first indication of a coagulation defect such as hemophilia or warfarin toxicity (Cotter et al., 1978). Severe intra-abdominal hemorrhage may occur in cats with ruptured splenic hemangiosarcoma or mast cell tumor. With bleeding into a body cavity, 80 to 90 per cent of the blood is reabsorbed if the animal survives the initial event. The history with internal hemorrhage may include episodes of collapse with apparent recovery.

Chronic blood loss occurs most often from the gastrointestinal tract, associated with ulcers, hookworms, intestinal tumors, and coagulation disorders. The anemia begins with reticulocytosis, polychromasia, and sometimes nucleated red cells but becomes hypochromic and microcytic as iron stores are depleted (Fig. 16–10). The reticulocyte count drops, and red-cell aplasia follows. Kittens have lower iron stores than adult cats and thus are more susceptible to iron deficiency anemia due to such causes as severe flea infestation. Increased iron is absorbed from the intestine soon after blood loss. In chronic iron deficiency, maturation of red cells beyond the basophilic normoblast stage is decreased because iron is needed for hemoglobinization of the developing red-cell precursors.

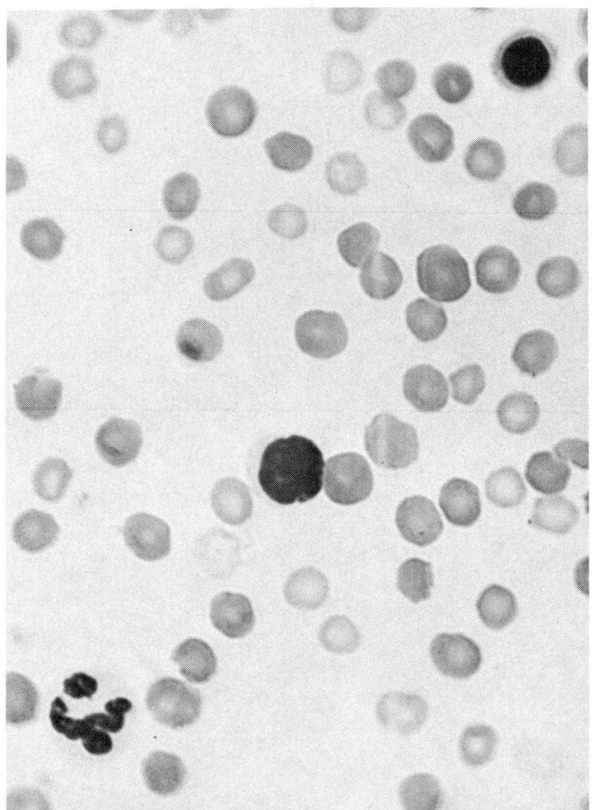

**Figure 16–10** Iron deficiency anemia in a cat with intestinal ulceration and bleeding due to a hairball. The small pale (microcytic, hypochromic) cells are typical. Numerous large basophilic red cells indicate responsive marrow activity. Wright's, × 950. (From Holzworth J: J Am Vet Med Assoc 128 [1956] 471–478.)

Fortunately, when bleeding stops and iron is administered orally, recovery is rapid. A blood transfusion supplies about 0.5 mg of iron/ml of blood, which helps replace iron stores in deficiency states. Frequent transfusions in cats with normal iron stores may lead to iron overload (Beck, 1973).

## REGENERATIVE ANEMIA—HEMOLYSIS

Hemolysis results in anemia when the rate of erythropoiesis fails to keep pace with destruction. Abnormal red cells (e.g., of rigid shape, increased fragility, or decreased life span) are predisposed to hemolysis. Because the bone marrow can expand production to 10 times the usual rate, the normal feline red-cell survival time of 70 to 80 days can be decreased to seven or eight days before anemia develops (Crosby, 1975). In compensated states of shortened red-cell life span, the only evidence of increased red-cell turnover would be reticulocytosis and perhaps hemosiderosis in tissues where hemolysis has occurred.

Hemolysis may be intravascular or extravascular. When red cells are destroyed within the circulation, they release hemoglobin, which binds irreversibly to haptoglobin, an alpha-2 globulin. This complex is then removed by the liver, as it is too large to be filtered by the glomerulus (Wintrobe et al., 1981). If the amount of free hemoglobin exceeds that of haptoglobin, excess hemoglobin circulates briefly and then dissociates into dimers that are excreted by the glomerulus. This process occurs more readily in cats than in other species (Harvey and Gaskin, 1978b). A decrease in haptoglobin has been used as an indicator of intravascular hemolysis. Harvey and Gaskin (1978b) investigated this possibility in the cat by injecting autologous hemoglobin and measuring haptoglobin levels. The levels dropped but returned to normal within 48 hours. Because of the rapid return to normal, a low value was significant but a normal value was not. In experimental hemobartonellosis, decreased haptoglobin levels were present in three cats with Coombs-positive anemias.

Haptoglobin levels increase in inflammatory disorders in the same manner as fibrinogen levels. Intravascular hemolysis can be indicated clinically by hemoglobin in serum or urine. Renal tubular cells extract iron from hemoglobin, so if these cells are sloughed into the urine, hemosiderin may be detected (Wintrobe et al., 1981). Hyperbilirubinemia of the indirect or unconjugated form is also present in some cases.

Most hemolytic anemias of the cat are characterized by extravascular hemolysis, in which red cells are removed by the reticuloendothelial system, primarily in the spleen. Hemoglobinuria is not present with extravascular hemolysis, but an increase in unconjugated bilirubin does occur because hemoglobin is degraded in situ. Bilirubin is conjugated in the liver, excreted in the bile, reabsorbed as urobilinogen, and excreted in the urine. Increased urobilinogen may appear in the urine with either intravascular or extravascular hemolysis. Intravascular and extravascular hemolysis are not mutually exclusive. For example, red cells coated by antibody may undergo direct damage resulting in intravascular lysis, but more often phagocytosis in the reticuloendothelial system leads to extravascular hemolysis.

Hemolytic anemias may also be classified according to whether the etiology is extrinsic or intrinsic to the red cell. Most hemolytic anemias of cats are due to extrinsic factors such as antibodies, toxic chemicals, and infectious organisms.

### Immune-Mediated Hemolytic Anemia

Several theories exist as to the cause of immune-mediated hemolytic anemia. The red cell itself may be altered so as to express neoantigens on the membrane. This alteration can occur by damage to the cell membrane by chemicals or microorganisms. Another theory, less likely to apply to the cat, is that of imbalance between helper and suppressor T cells, with formation of autoantibodies against normal tissues.

Presumptive cases of autoimmune hemolytic anemia were first reported by Sodikoff and Custer (1965, 1966). They concluded (1966) that a proper term for the disorder was secondary autoimmune hemolytic anemia, because affected cats often had some kind of infection (e.g., hemobartonellosis) (Plate 16–2*A*) or lymphoma.

Six of seven cats with hemolytic anemia had positive direct Coombs tests indicating antibody on red cells (Scott et al., 1973). In four cats autoagglutination of the red cells was evident when blood was drawn. In addition, four cats tested positive for FeLV by immunofluorescence. In another case, a direct Coombs test was positive in an anemic cat with hemobartonellosis (Sheriff, 1974). Autoimmune hemolytic anemia associated with systemic lupus erythematosus has been described (Heise et al., 1973; Schalm et al., 1975). The osmotic fragility of feline red cells may be increased, as in one cat with immune-mediated hemolytic anemia and in one with hemobartonellosis (Jain, 1973). Spherocytosis has been associated with autoimmune hemolytic anemia in the dog and in man, but spherocytes are difficult to detect in the cat because the normal feline red cell has very little central pallor.

Feline leukemia virus has been observed budding from the membrane of red cells, and virus structural proteins have become incorporated in the membrane of the infected cells (Oshiro et al., 1972). Hemolytic anemia has been produced experimentally in the cat by the injection of subgroup A FeLV (Mackey et al., 1975). Circulating immune complexes have also been reported in FeLV-positive cats (Jones et al., 1980). It therefore seems reasonable that FeLV antibodies attached to a red cell could alter the red-cell membrane so as to expose new host antigens or that the virus itself could be a focus of immune attack, which then destroys the red cell. A similar effect has occurred in susceptible strains of mice with murine leukemia virus–induced autoimmune hemolytic anemia (Mellors, 1969). Coombs-positive anemia occurs in lymphoproliferative malignancy in man, dog, and cat, so it is possible that tumor-related immune complexes in addition to viruses could predispose the red cell to immune-mediated destruction (Kramer and Laszlo, 1973; Madewell and Feldman, 1980).

A study evaluating 20 anemic cats by the direct antiglobulin test found that it was positive in cats with FeLV infection and also other inflammatory and neoplastic disorders (Dunn et al., 1984b). It was concluded that the test in anemic cats has diagnostic limitations and that positive reactions should be interpreted with caution in the absence of clinical or laboratory evidence of hemolytic anemia.

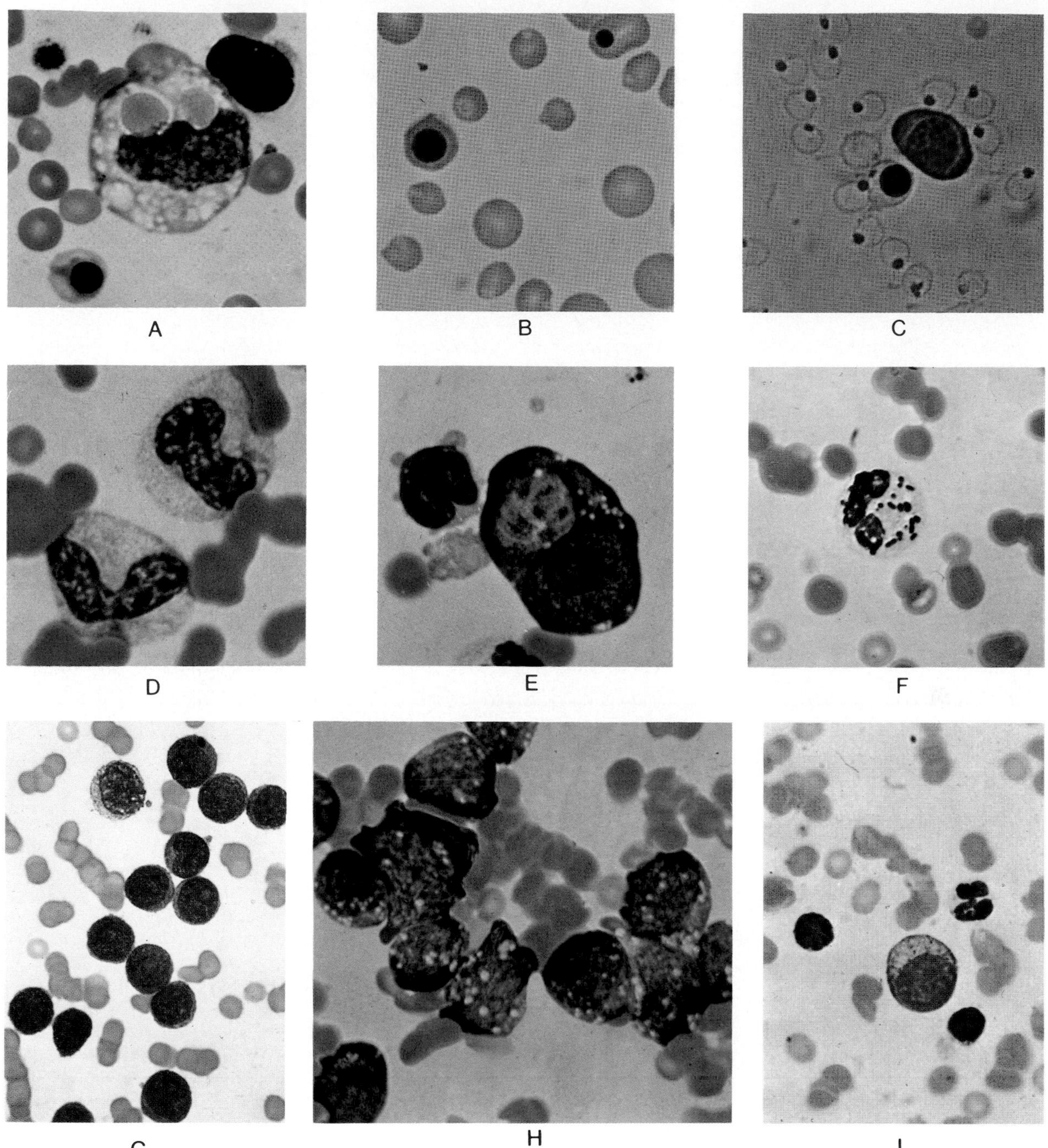


**Plate 16–2** *A*, A macrophage with two phagocytosed red cells, marrow, hemobartonellosis. Erythrophagocytosis, a feature of autoimmune hemolytic anemia, may occur in other disorders as well. A lymphocyte and a metarubricyte are also present. *B*, Heinz bodies as they appear with Romanowsky stains, such as Wright-Giemsa, in a responsive anemia characterized by nucleated red cells and large red cells, some with polychromasia. The mature red cells contain a pale, refractile structure (Heinz body) that protrudes from the edge of the cell. *C*, Heinz bodies in the same cat as they appear in a dry, unfixed blood film stained with new methylene blue. Here they stain blue and are easily seen. A metarubricyte and an unclassified cell (primitive red cell?) are present. *D*, Toxic band neutrophils, blood of a cat with pyothorax. *E*, A blast cell suggestive of a rubriblast contains a cyst of *Toxoplasma gondii*, marrow of a cat with erythroleukemia. *F*, Neutrophil containing phagocytosed staphylococci, blood, septicemia. *G*, Lymphoblastic leukemia, marrow, one-year-old cat. The uniform population of lymphoblasts is characterized by red-purple nuclei containing pale nucleoli and surrounded by a small rim of blue cytoplasm. *H*, Large, vacuolated lymphoreticular cells, marrow, histiocytic lymphoma. *I*, Reticuloendotheliosis, blood. The malignant cells are round and much larger than mature lymphocytes and neutrophils. The red-purple nucleus is eccentric and occupies much of the cell. The cytoplasm stains dull blue and contains a few azurophilic granules. Both nucleus and cytoplasm are finely stippled. (*A* to *F* and *H* from Schalm OW, Jain NC, Carroll EJ.: Veterinary Hematology. Philadelphia, Lea & Febiger, 1975. *I* from Gilmore CE, Holzworth J: J Am Vet Med Assoc 158 [1971] 1013–1225.)

Primary autoimmune hemolytic anemia has yet to be proven to exist in the cat. To demonstrate that a true anti–red cell antibody is present it would be necessary to elute the antibody from the cell and to show that it reacts with normal feline red cells.

Regardless of the cause, any Coombs-positive red cell is doomed to destruction by the immune system if complement levels are adequate, so treatment must be instituted to prevent further hemolysis. Prednisone is given at 2 mg/kg/day until the PCV increases to near normal and reticulocytosis begins to subside. Long-term corticosteroid therapy should be avoided if possible, as the immunosuppressive effect may render a cat more susceptible to infections. Blood films should be examined periodically for the emergence of latent hemobartonellosis. Transfusions should be avoided unless the anemia is life-threatening.

Most cases of immune-mediated hemolysis are caused by antibodies that are reactive at body temperature. Rarely, cold reactive antibodies cause hemolysis or agglutination of red cells at low temperatures. Cold-agglutinin disease was reported in a five-year-old Abyssinian cat presented with an upper respiratory infection that was followed by dry gangrene of the forepaws, tips of the pinnas, and tail (Schrader and Hurvitz, 1983). The serum of this cat caused autologous red cells to agglutinate when incubated overnight at refrigerator temperature. The agglutination was reversed when the blood was warmed. The sloughing of peripheral tissues occurred when red cells agglutinated in cooler tissues. Cold-agglutinin disease is associated with an IgM antibody, rarely causes significant hemolysis, and may be secondary to another disease. Treatment should include corticosteroids and a warm environment.

Isoimmune disease of newborn kittens (neonatal erythrolysis) has been reported (Cain and Suzuki, 1985; Majka, 1974, cited by Perman and Schall, 1983) (see also chapter on immunology). The study of Cain and Suzuki (1985) concerned kittens of four primiparous queens, two of which were identified as purebred Persians belonging to a breeder and one as a domestic shorthair. Typically, affected kittens seemed vigorous at birth but weakened and died within a day or two, after voiding red or brown urine and becoming jaundiced. Kittens not allowed to nurse the mother but transferred to a surrogate queen survived, with no clinical signs of illness. The offending antibodies were determined to be anti-A.

## Hemolysis Caused by Red-Cell Parasites

Hemobartonellosis is described in detail in the chapter on bacterial diseases. In a study of 121 anemic cats at AMAH, 36 had lymphoblastic leukemia, 8 myeloproliferative diseases, 64 red-cell aplasia, and 13 (11 per cent) hemobartonellosis (Cotter et al., 1975). Of the 13 with hemobartonellosis, six tested FeLV-positive, so that only seven cats (5 per cent) had a primary diagnosis of hemobartonellosis.

*Haemobartonella* is frequently an opportunist, creating a secondary problem in cats with such disorders as the immune deficiency that occurs in FeLV-infected cats. Of 374 cats with hemobartonellosis, 77 died or were destroyed during the first hospitalization (Hayes and Priester, 1973). Of those recovering, follow-up information was available on 48. Thirty-one died later, 19 of hemobartonellosis and 6 of leukemia. There was no mention of the type of anemia or FeLV status of the cats in this study.

Harvey and Gaskin (1977) induced hemobartonellosis in eight healthy cats by intravenous injection of infected blood. They found wide fluctuations in the number of parasites visible in the recipient's blood. Five of the eight cats in this study were FeLV-positive, a finding that complicates interpretation of the results. Indeed, much of the literature published before 1970 describing outbreaks of hemobartonellosis is hard to evaluate, because the role of FeLV in those outbreaks will never be known.

Parasitemia could not be induced in *Haemobartonella*-carrier cats by administration of immunosuppressive drugs such as 6-mercaptopurine and cyclophosphamide or by stress such as experimental abscess production (Harvey and Gaskin, 1978a). Splenectomy or glucocorticoid administration did, however, increase parasitemias.

In experimental hemobartonellosis the average life span of an infected red cell was 4.3 days (Maede, 1975). Infected cells were sometimes sequestered in the spleen, the organisms removed, and the red cells returned to the circulation. Survival of these previously infected cells was also shortened to 8.8 days.

Cats with hemobartonellosis may be treated with oxytetracycline, 20 mg/kg t.i.d. for about 14 days. There is no experimental evidence that arsenicals are more effective in reducing the carrier state to justify the risk of toxicity. Transfusions should be given if needed, usually if the PCV is below 10 per cent. Since some cats with hemobartonellosis are Coombs-positive, corticosteroids may be administered as well if improvement is not noted after 10 days of therapy with oxytetracycline.

Feline cytauxzoonosis, a protozoan hemolytic disorder, has been uniformly fatal (Wagner, 1976). The parasites in the red cells appear as round signet ring–shaped bodies 1 to 1.5 μ in diameter, bipolar oval safety-pin forms 1 by 2 μ, or anaplasmoid round dots measuring less than 1 μ (Kier, 1984). A single red cell usually contains only one organism, but pairs and tetrads appear occasionally. With Wright or Giemsa stain their cytoplasm is light blue and the nucleus purple or dark red. Most infections occur in rural areas of the midwestern or southern United States and are characterized by fever, jaundice, and hemolysis, with widespread dissemination of organisms throughout the body. The mode of transmission is thought to be by an arthropod vector. The bobcat (*Lynx rufus rufus*) may be a reservoir host, as asymptomatic parasitemias occur in this species (Glenn et al., 1983). (See also the chapter on protozoan diseases.)

Babesiosis, an infection causing hemolytic anemia in cats in Africa, is discussed in the chapter on protozoan diseases.

## Hemolysis Caused by Toxins or Drugs

The most significant chemically induced hemolytic anemia of the cat is that associated with Heinz bodies, which are composed of denatured hemoglobin (Plate 16–2*B* and *C*). The drugs most commonly involved are methylene blue, acetaminophen, phenazopyridine, and benzocaine, but other drugs have been implicated as well in man (Jandl, 1973). Among these are antimalarials (e.g., quinidine) and naphthalene. Deleterious effects of oxidant drugs include Heinz-body formation, hemolysis, and methemoglobin formation. Methylene blue has been used in multiagent urinary antiseptic preparations, and cats have developed hemolytic anemia with Heinz-body formation during treatment with these drugs (Harvey and Kaneko, 1974; Schalm, 1977; Schechter et al., 1973; Sodikoff, 1973).

In 1899, Schmauch described inclusion bodies of denatured hemoglobin in red cells of normal cats. These bodies, comprising a fifth to a third of the cell diameter, are usually single, round or irregular inclusions near or protruding from the periphery of the red cell and pushing the membrane outward. They do not stain with Romanowsky dyes but with supravital stains such as new methylene blue. Heinz bodies were seen in 93 of 94 normal cats in from 0.3 to 96.1 per cent of red cells examined (Berític, 1965). No variation in number was found with age or sex. Berític suggested that the term Schmauch bodies be used to describe those in normal cats, because, although indistinguishable in appearance from Heinz bodies of man, they are not always associated with anemia in the cat. The Schmauch bodies were larger in red cells of anemic cats than were Heinz bodies in human red cells. Despite Berític's valid suggestion, the term Heinz body has persisted in the veterinary literature, and the term erythrocyte-refractile body (ERB) has also been used. More red cells contain Heinz bodies in sick than in healthy cats (Schalm, 1962). Heinz bodies are most evident in lysed cells, and their rigidity makes the cell less deformable in passage through small capillaries. When the bodies are large, as in some anemic cats, attempts at removal of the bodies by the spleen ("pitting") may shorten the life span of the red cell (Jain and Keeton, 1975).

For an understanding of the predisposition of cats to form Heinz bodies, some information about red-cell metabolism and feline hemoglobin is helpful. Metabolism of glucose and glutathione in the RBC and the steps leading to formation of Heinz bodies are depicted schematically in Figure 16–11.

About 90 per cent of glucose in the mature red cell is metabolized anaerobically (Embden-Meyerhof pathway). Two products formed are adenosine triphosphate (ATP), a high-energy compound, and, farther along the pathway, reduced nicotinamide adenine dinucleotide (NADH), essential for reduction of methemoglobin. A second, aerobic pathway of glucose metabolism is the pentose phosphate pathway. This is important as the sole source of nicotinamide adenine dinucleotide phosphate (NADPH), which serves as a cofactor in the reduction of glutathione and so aids in protecting the red cell from oxidative damage (Wintrobe et al., 1981). Maintenance of glutathione in reduced form is of great importance, for it serves both as a vital link in the antioxidant function of glucose metabolism in the red cell and as a stabilizer of the sulfhydryl groups of membrane protein (Kaneko, 1980).

Heinz bodies are denatured hemoglobin formed when irreversible oxidation of hemoglobin sulfhydryl groups occurs. Whereas man has two reactive sulfhydryl groups and the dog four, the cat has at least eight (Taketa et al., 1974). Thus feline hemoglobin is especially susceptible to oxidation, and Heinz bodies are most often seen in cats.

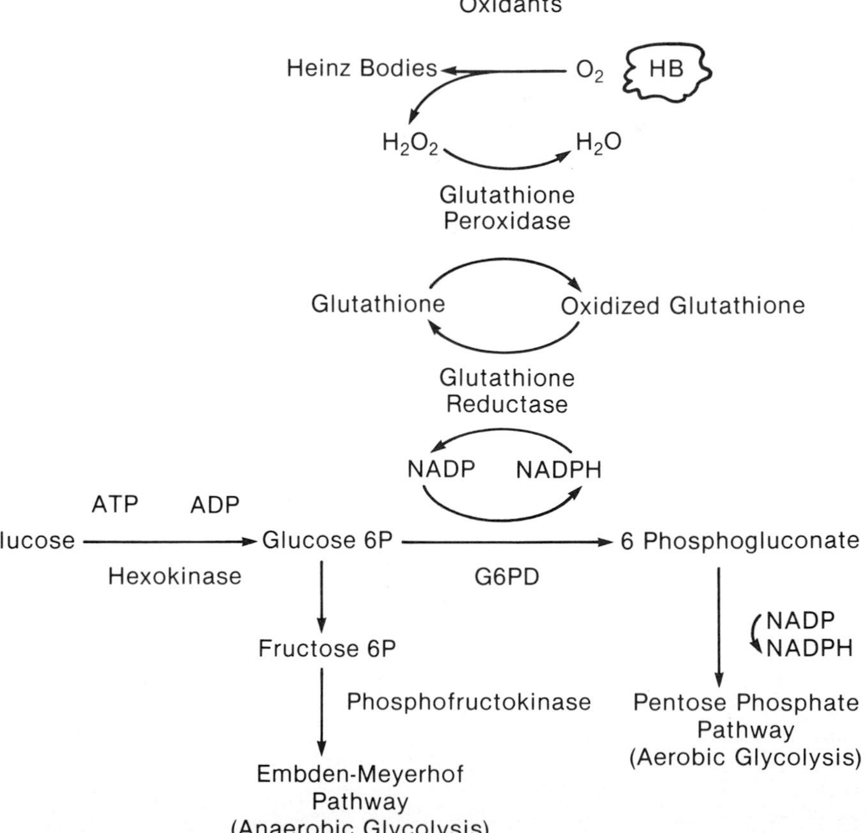


**Figure 16–11** Metabolic pathways for metabolism of glucose and glutathione in the red cell. Increased use of the pentose phosphate pathway occurs in the presence of exogenous oxidants, such as methylene blue, producing oxidized glutathione and ultimately Heinz bodies. (ATP = adenosine triphosphate, ADP = adenosine diphosphate, G6PD = glucose 6 phosphate dehydrogenase, NADP = nicotinamide adenine dinucleotide phosphate, NADPH = reduced NADP). (Adapted from Kaneko JJ: Clinical Biochemistry of the Domestic Animals. New York, Academic Press, 1980, Chapter 1, Figures 8 and 10.)

Why they are also seen in normal cats is unclear, but, as suggested earlier in this chapter in the discussion of feline red-cell physiology, recent evidence for poor pitting function of the cat's spleen might account for the persistence of red cells containing Heinz bodies.

Heinz-body hemolytic anemia as a clinical event has been most often encountered in occasional cats treated with multiagent urinary antiseptics containing methylene blue (Schalm, 1977; Schechter et al., 1973; Sodikoff, 1973). These agents were at one time used so widely, and over such long periods, without apparent ill effect that it seems likely that some individual predisposing idiosyncrasy must be present in the relatively few cats that are adversely affected. Subclinical hemolysis may have occurred in a larger number of treated cats and resolved without being detected. In some cats the anemia develops within a few days, in others only after several weeks of medication. Signs are weakness, pallor, and green-tinged urine. In white cats that become severely anemic there may be a faint greenish tinge to the mucosae, skin, and hair roots.

That the methylene blue in the preparations is the agent responsible for the anemia was demonstrated by experimental studies both with the offending drugs and with methylene blue alone. Heinz bodies were observed two hours after experimental administration and gradually enlarged over the next six hours (Harvey and Kaneko, 1974). In another study anemia developed 2 to 15 days after administration of the urinary antiseptic drug was begun (Schechter et al., 1973). As well as Heinz bodies, nucleated red cells, basophilic stippling, and reticulocytosis were sometimes present. The reticulocytes did not contain Heinz bodies. When the drug was discontinued, the Heinz bodies decreased in number and the PCV gradually returned to normal.

In many cases, discontinuance of the drug is the only treatment required, but a severely anemic cat may need supportive blood transfusion until the PCV starts to rise.

Other drugs causing hemolysis may also damage the red cell by oxidizing the iron molecule of heme from the ferrous ($Fe^{2+}$) state to the ferric ($Fe^{3+}$). With increased use of acetaminophen (paracetamol) in man, poisoning due to its uninformed use in cats is increasing (Cullison, 1984; Finco et al., 1975; Schalm, 1977; St. Omer and McKnight, 1980). Beside Heinz-body anemia, acetaminophen causes severe methemoglobinemia with cyanosis, hemoglobinuria with hemoglobin casts, and liver necrosis. At AMAH toxicity was also associated with edema of the head in four cats and also of the tail base in one of them; liver necrosis was severe in fatal cases. The cause of the edema is unclear, but the mechanism is probably similar to that of "bottle jaw," an effect of high altitude in cattle, in which edema of the head is a circulatory disturbance caused by hypoxia.

As little as half a 325-mg tablet of acetaminophen can be toxic (Cullison, 1984). The major diagnostic clue is that the blood is brown. The cyanosis changes to jaundice and pallor as hemolysis and hepatic necrosis progress. In a case reported by Schalm (1977), a cat was given six 325-mg tablets over an unspecified time. The PCV dropped from 31 to 14 per cent in two days, with appearance of ghost red cells, each containing a single large Heinz body. This cat survived with blood transfusion and supportive treatment with intravenous fluids.

A proposed mechanism for toxicity is that the cat's ability to conjugate and excrete the drug is impaired because of a decrease in glucuronyl transferase in the liver, as well as the previously described propensity of feline hemoglobin to oxidative damage.

Attempted treatment has centered on sparing stores of glutathione in the liver by giving precursors of glutathione such as cysteine (Cullison, 1984). Methionine, a similar precursor, is contraindicated, however, because it may precipitate hepatic encephalopathy.

Cats given acetaminophen experimentally were effectively treated with acetylcysteine (Mucomyst), a compound similar to glutathione (St. Omer and McKnight, 1980). The Animal Poison Control Center at the University of Illinois reported success in treating clinical cases of poisoning with administration of oxygen if cyanosis was present and with acetylcysteine orally or intravenously at a starting dose of 140 mg/kg followed every six hours for 36 hours with a dose of 70 mg/kg (Cullison, 1984). Good results were reported in cats even when treatment was begun the day after ingestion. Because many independent pharmacies do not stock acetylcysteine, veterinary practitioners should have it on hand for emergency use. Although there is some question as to the action of ascorbic acid (Mitchell et al., 1981), the Animal Poison Control Center recommends oral or parenteral administration (30 mg/kg) at the same intervals as acetylcysteine (Cullison, 1984). Fluid therapy with lactated Ringer's solution is also indicated. In poisonings characterized by life-threatening anemia, blood transfusion may be required, as in an acutely poisoned cat treated at AMAH.

Cimetidine (Tagamet) has also been proposed as a treatment because it inhibits oxidative metabolism of the p450 cytochrome oxidase system in the liver (Abernethy et al., 1982; Mitchell et al., 1981). Cimetidine has no effect on conjugation of acetaminophen but allows generation of nontoxic metabolites that are subsequently cleared from the body. Treatment must be started as soon as possible, since much of the damage occurs within the first few hours. Cimetidine may be given at an initial dosage of 10 mg/kg, followed by 5 mg/kg every six hours for the first 48 hours.

In a study comparing the antidotal effectiveness of intravenous sodium sulfate and oral or intravenous *N*-acetylcysteine it was found that the drugs were equally effective (Savides et al., 1985). The test cats were given a single oral dose of 120 mg acetaminophen/kg. Sodium sulfate 50 mg (1.6 per cent solution)/kg was given at 4½, 8½, and 12½ hours. *N*-acetylcysteine was administered in doses of 140 mg/kg at 4½ hours, then 70 mg/kg at 8½ and 12½ hours.

Phenazopyridine, an azo dye used as a urinary analgesic, has been associated in cats with fatal Heinz-body anemia (Harvey and Kornick, 1976). Methemoglobinemia and hepatic toxicity were present both in a clinically affected cat and in two of three experimentally exposed cats.

Heinz-body production and methemoglobinemia in a dog were associated with ingestion of topical benzocaine, an ester of para-aminobenzoic acid (Harvey et al., 1979). When para-aminobenzoic acid was fed to cats, Heinz-body anemia resulted (Spicer, 1949). Onion poisoning has been reported in several domestic animals including the cat (Kobayashi, 1981). Two domestic cats fed meat mixed with onion soup showed significant increases in Heinz bodies in their red cells but without development of anemia. Another cat fed a larger amount of onion soup equivalent to 28 gm/kg body weight of raw onion and one fed an extract of onion developed hemolytic anemia with hemoglobinuria. Both cats recovered after feeding of onion was stopped. Although onions are potentially toxic to cats, it is unlikely that cats would voluntarily consume enough to cause significant clinical disease.

Treatment of Heinz-body anemia and methemoglobinemia in the cat depends in many cases on restoring oxygen-carrying capacity of the blood by transfusion, perhaps even by exchange transfusion.

Other drugs have caused hemolytic anemia by other mechanisms. Propylthiouracil (PTU) is used to treat hyperthyroidism in cats; however, acute immune-mediated hemolytic anemia and thrombocytopenia occurred in 9 of 105 cats receiving PTU at a dose of 50 mg t.i.d. over periods of 19 to 37 days (Peterson et al., 1984). The cats tested Coombs-positive, with increased erythrocytic precursors and megakaryocytes in the marrow. Five of eight cats tested had a positive antinuclear antibody titer. In addition, two cats were seen at AMAH with granulocytopenia, a common side effect of PTU in man but not observed in Peterson's cats. When the drug was stopped, the hematologic and immunologic signs resolved. Prednisone was the primary therapy in Peterson's cats, along with supportive care. Because of potential hematologic toxicity, the hemogram should be monitored during PTU treatment in cats.

In addition to those mentioned, drugs containing phenyl, nitro, and hydroxy groups, naphthalene, saponin, thiazide dyes, sulfonamides, and diaminodiphenylsulfate (Dapsone) are potential causes of hemolytic anemia in the cat (Harvey and Kaneko, 1976; Holzworth, 1956; Schechter et al., 1973). Fatal hemolytic anemia from the use of dipyrone (Novin) has been observed in a cat referred to AMAH. Copper and antimony were associated with hemolytic anemia in dogs at AMAH when foreign bodies containing these materials lodged in the stomach. Presumably, either could cause similar signs in cats.

## Hemolysis Associated with Factors Intrinsic to the Red Cell

The majority of feline hemolytic anemias are caused by factors extrinsic to the red cell. These causes have been discussed earlier and include abnormal antibodies, drugs, microorganisms, and injury to red cells from abnormal endothelium or thrombosis. Less often an intrinsic defect in the red cell predisposes it to hemolysis. In this situation, the defect is not transferable, so normal transfused cells would have a normal life span.

Crystalloid bodies in red cells, similar to those in hemoglobin C disease, a hemolytic disorder of man, have been observed in a family of inbred Siamese cats (Altman, 1974). These bodies caused the affected cells to assume a rectangular or square shape, and they increased in number after splenectomy in one kitten. No apparent association with disease was noted, although one cat was anemic.

Congenital porphyria in cats is associated with overproduction of uroporphyrin I and coprophyrin I that cannot be used in heme synthesis (Giddens et al., 1975; Glenn et al., 1968). These porphyrins accumulate in developing red cells, teeth, and bones and are excreted in urine and feces. Teeth and urine may be pink-brown and fluoresce pink-red with ultraviolet light. Anemia may occur because of interruption in heme synthesis. Severe macrocytic, hypochromic anemia occurred in one cat with an enlarged liver and spleen and uremia associated with narrowing of glomerular capillaries and ischemic tubular injury (Giddens et al., 1975). Porphyria is inherited as an autosomal dominant condition and varies from an asymptomatic disorder to severe debilitating disease. Humans with porphyria have increased sensitivity to barbiturates. An asymptomatic Siamese kitten observed at AMAH had more prominent discoloration of deciduous teeth than of adult teeth, although fluorescence was detectable in both. This kitten was spayed with thiamylal-induction anesthesia and halothane maintenance, with no problems noted.

### Regenerative Anemia—Recovery from Marrow Depression

Not all nonregenerative anemias are irreversible. A regenerative marrow response often signals recovery from, or follows successful treatment for, infection, intoxication, or other stress that has depressed the marrow. An FeLV-carrier, to cite a common example, may develop what appears to be a nonregenerative anemia when suffering from a bite wound infection, but with proper drainage and antibiotic treatment the stress is overcome and red-cell production is resumed.

### Nonregenerative Anemia

Decreased marrow activity may affect either red cells only (red-cell aplasia) or red cells, myeloid cells, and megakaryocytes (pancytopenia, aplastic anemia). The majority of feline anemias are caused by decreased red-cell production. In a review at the University of Pennsylvania, 83 per cent of anemic cats had nonregenerative anemia (Maggio, 1979). This finding agrees with studies at AMAH as well as the experience of most veterinary hematologists (e.g., Cotter, 1979; Holzworth, 1956).

## Anemia Caused by Nutritional Deficiency

Nutritional deficiencies may cause anemia but are highly unlikely in cats fed "complete" commercial diets.

Megaloblastic anemia associated with folate or vitamin $B_{12}$ deficiency in man is characterized by macrocytic red cells in the absence of polychromasia or reticulocytosis. The marrow may show asynchronous maturation of nucleus and cytoplasm of red-cell precursors, with the cytoplasm more mature than the nucleus. The cell continues to enlarge but fails to divide. Folic acid deficiency was produced experimentally in cats fed a synthetic diet with sulfonamides added to decrease bacterial folate production in the intestine (Da Silva et al., 1955). Cats fed this diet for six to eight months experienced weight loss, macrocytic anemia, and leukopenia. A single dose of 2 mg folic acid produced rapid recovery. In a second trial with folate-deficient diets in cats, megaloblastic changes occurred in the marrow without changes in numbers or morphology of red or white cells in the blood (Thenen and Rasmussen, 1978). This study was terminated after five months, so anemia might have become evident had the study been continued longer.

Although folate is plentiful in most foods, it is not stored well in the body. Replacement should be considered in cats with malabsorption syndromes or debilitation from prolonged illness. Certain drugs such as methotrexate, diphenylhydantoin (phenytoin), pyrimethamine, and trimethoprim are folate antagonists and may produce signs of folate deficiency. Schalm et al. (1975) reported one case of megaloblastic anemia that may have responded to folic acid, but the most common causes of megaloblastosis in the cat are the myeloproliferative diseases (Cotter, 1979; Maggio, 1979; Schalm et al., 1975) (Plate 16–3*D*). Megaloblastic anemia was described in four cats presented with lack of reticulocytes and a mean corpuscular hemoglobin (MCV) of greater than 60 fl (femtoliter) (Hirsch and Dunn, 1983). Three of the cats tested FeLV-positive. One proved to have a red-cell malignancy in the marrow, and three tested Coombs-positive. None of the cats responded to folic acid therapy. Serum folate and vitamin $B_{12}$ levels were assayed in healthy and anemic cats, including seven infected with feline leukemia virus that had megaloblastic erythroid precursors in the marrow. No significant differences were found between the groups, indicating that the megaloblastic changes were a result of the effects of FeLV on the marrow (Dunn et al., 1984a). Experience at AMAH has been similar, in that cats with megaloblastic anemias often test FeLV-positive and many have or develop myeloproliferative disorders.

Vitamin $B_{12}$ deficiency is not known to cause anemia in cats (Keesling and Morris, 1975).

Pyridoxine deficiency, experimentally produced in cats, has caused anemia with normal marrow cellularity and elevated myeloid:erythroid (M:E) ratio (Gershoff et al., 1959). Additional effects were neurologic disturbances, oxalate nephrosis, and hemosiderosis in the spleen and liver. This deficiency is unlikely to occur naturally unless pyridoxine is inactivated during faulty processing of foods. Pyridoxine-responsive anemia has been reported in man in cases of hereditary sideroblastic anemia but does not represent a true deficiency of pyridoxine. This disease has not been described in cats.

Iron deficiency anemia has been described previously with blood-loss anemia. One case of nutritional iron deficiency anemia described in a cat resulted from a diet primarily of boiled vegetables (Holzworth, 1956).

## Anemia Caused by Toxins and Drugs

Numerous chemicals may cause nonregenerative anemia. These include heavy metals such as lead and mercury, solvents such as benzene, and drugs such as chloramphenicol, phenylbutazone, and cytotoxic antitumor drugs.

Two cases of lead poisoning in cats at AMAH were described by Holzworth in 1956, and three additional cases have been recognized since that report. The first two were characterized by normochromic, normocytic anemia and leukopenia, the latter three primarily by neurologic signs (tremors, seizures, and blindness) and by mild anemia with marked basophilic stippling of red cells and numerous circulating nucleated red cells.

One cat was studied in detail because it required treatment for lead poisoning six times in an eight-month period. This cat frequently sat licking its coat at an open window in a city area with heavy traffic, and the source of lead was presumed to be automobile fumes. The earliest sign noted by the owner on each occasion was twitching of the skin along the back. Initial laboratory data were: PCV 28 per cent, WBC 8900/μl with a normal differential white-cell count, and 28 nucleated RBC per 100 white cells. Basophilic stippling was prominent. Blood lead was 0.2 mg/dl (normal less than 0.04 mg/dl). The cat responded each time to calcium EDTA 25 mg/kg q.i.d. for five days diluted in normal physiologic saline solution and given subcutaneously. The owner's blood was found to contain a high-normal level of lead. An extensive search was made for sources of lead in the environment. The water, wall paint, and the cat's enamel bowl all tested negative. Abdominal radiographs for a lead-containing foreign body were negative. Clinical signs did not recur during a three-year follow-up period after the owner and cat moved to a new neighborhood. In two other cases the source of lead was found. One cat, owned by a worker at a smelter, habitually licked its owner's arms; another, in a house being remodeled, was exposed to paint and plaster dust.

Mercury poisoning, associated in one cat with damage to the gastrointestinal tract, liver, and kidneys, caused fatal aplastic anemia (Holzworth, 1956).

Chloramphenicol interferes with heme synthesis in dogs and cats. This effect is dose-related and reversible, in contrast with the severe, irreversible, idiosyncratic aplastic anemia that sometimes occurs in man. Chloramphenicol in cats causes depression of erythroid elements in the marrow after about two weeks (Clark, 1978). Chloramphenicol at 50 mg/kg/day caused vacuolation of both red-cell and white-cell precursors along with an increase in the M:E ratio due to erythroid hypoplasia (Penny et al., 1967a, 1970). In large doses chloramphenicol is immunosuppressive and inhibits antibody formation.

Aplastic anemia has been reported in dogs treated with estrogen or having secreting Sertoli cell tumors. In cats, however, estrogen therapy is rarely used and Sertoli cell tumors are extremely rare. It is not known whether hyperestrogenism may cause anemia in cats; however, Perman and Schall (1983) observed that cats given doses of estrogen five times greater than those causing aplastic anemia in dogs developed only mild stem-cell depression.

Some myelosuppressive chemotherapeutic drugs can cause anemia, but because of the long life span of red cells compared with that of granulocytes, granulocytopenia is generally the dose-limiting side effect of these drugs. Schalm (1978b) reported reduced cellularity in the bone marrow a few days after administration of cyclophosphamide.

## Anemia of Chronic Renal Failure

Chronic renal failure is a frequent cause of anemia in man and animals. Erythropoietin is produced in an inactive form in the kidney and is activated in the liver. Although red-cell survival may be shortened and bleeding tendencies may result from decreased platelet aggregation, the primary problem is decreased red-cell production. Only occasionally is the anemia severe enough to be a primary clinical sign of uremia. Anabolic steroids or testosterone derivatives may be of some value in treating uremic cats by stimulating erythropoietin production and increasing 2,3-DPG levels.

## Anemia Associated with Other Chronic Disease

Anemia is a frequent complication of chronic inflammatory or debilitating diseases. Although emaciation may occur, the anemia does not appear to be of nutritional origin. Because of the normally short life span of red cells in cats, these animals may be more prone to this anemia than other species. The anemia is caused by a combination of shortened red-cell life span and decreased production. Iron stores are adequate, but iron-binding capacity is often greatly decreased, leading to hemosiderin deposition in the liver, spleen, or other organs. The anemia regresses spontaneously if the underlying disorder improves.

## Anemia Associated with Infection

Anemia accompanying many infections has the hematologic characteristics of a nonregenerative anemia but often responds favorably to appropriate surgical or antibiotic treatment. In a study of feline reticulocytes at AMAH, one cat developed an upper respiratory infection after anemia was induced by phlebotomy. The reticulocyte count decreased with the onset of the infection and rose rapidly as the infection subsided; a rise in the PCV followed (Cramer and Lewis, 1972).

Reports of anemia associated with infection in cats are provided by Mahaffey and Smith (1978) and by Weiss and Krehbiel (1983). In the first study the PCV fell by day five after induction of sterile abscesses and began to rise within three to four days after drainage. In the second study the PCV began to fall three to four days after production of sterile abscesses with a mean decrease of 11.3 per cent over a one-week period. This decrease was attributed to erythrocyte destruction. Serum iron levels fell during the same period apparently because of sequestration in fixed-tissue macrophages, since iron levels and PCV returned to normal when abscesses were drained. Treatment of the cats with cobalt chloride and ferric citrate caused reticulocytosis and increases in the PCV (Weiss et al., 1983). Since these compounds may be toxic, further studies are needed in clinical settings. Any anemic cat should be examined carefully for signs of infection, since treatment of the infection often causes resolution of the anemia.

## Anemia Associated with Feline Leukemia Virus

Cats with FeLV may develop primary anemia or anemia secondary to other infections. Subgroup C FeLV has been associated experimentally with progressive, fatal, red-cell aplasia (Mackey et al., 1975). Natural isolates of this subgroup have been found only rarely and may represent a recombination of feline cellular genes with virus of subgroups A or AB.

The Kawakami-Theilen (KT) strain of FeLV induces nonregenerative anemia when injected into newborn kittens (Hoover et al., 1974). The majority of FeLV-positive cats with naturally occurring anemias have a nonregenerative anemia similar clinically to that produced experimentally by Hoover and associates.

Macrocytosis is a characteristic finding in FeLV-positive cats, both those with nonregenerative anemia and those that are not anemic (Weiser and Kociba, 1983). It was suggested that hemolysis and erythrocyte regeneration precede erythroid hypoplasia and may partly account for macrocytosis observed in the face of nonregenerative anemia. Macrocytosis in nonregenerative anemia may also be a sign of megaloblastosis (Hirsch and Dunn, 1983).

In a series of 100 FeLV-positive anemic cats at AMAH, the mean age on admission was 2.7 years, compared with 5.4 years for a group of 20 FeLV-negative anemic cats (Cotter, 1979). Among the positive cats, the ratio of males to females was 3.2:1. No clinical signs or physical findings distinguished these cats from others presented with anemia. In 22 per cent, fever or other evidence of infection suggested that erythroid hypoplasia may be secondary to infection or stress. If the infection can be managed successfully, the anemia may regress although the cat may remain FeLV-positive. Spleens were enlarged in 31 per cent of FeLV-positive cats; jaundice was present in only 10 per cent (Cotter, 1979). The median WBC was 6380/μl. Granulocytopenia and lymphopenia were frequent in cats with leukopenia. Reticulocyte counts were generally low, with a median of 3.5 per cent primarily of the punctate form.

In only 18 cats did total reticulocyte counts over 25 per cent indicate regenerative anemia. Nucleated red cells were present in the blood of 49 cats in numbers greater than one per 100 white cells, but lack of correlation between the numbers of nucleated red cells and the numbers of reticulocytes gave further evidence that nucleated red cells are not markers for responsive marrow. Platelet numbers were normal or elevated in the majority of cats and were decreased in only 18 per cent. Indeed, thrombocytopenia was present only in cats with aplastic anemia, since the mean WBC of cats with thrombocytopenia was 2294/μl. The bone marrow in FeLV-positive cats is usually normal or hypocellular with an increased M:E ratio attributable primarily to erythroid hypoplasia. Serum iron levels were measured in 13 FeLV-positive anemic cats and all were normal or elevated, with a mean level of 291 μg/dl (normal 68 to 215 μg/dl).

Anemia associated with stress from injury occurred in a one-year-old, healthy, FeLV-positive cat that suffered a fractured femur when hit by a car. The fracture was repaired surgically without complication. The PCV began to drop five days later. As the fracture healed, the anemia subsided, and two months later the cat tested FeLV-negative.

It has been questioned whether the nonregenerative anemia associated with FeLV is a primary disorder of suppression of red-cell precursors or is a preleukemic syndrome. There is evidence to support both views. Experimental anemias produced by FeLV have not progressed to leukemia (Hoover et al., 1974; Mackey et al., 1975). Follow-up examinations of anemic cats at AMAH yielded only small numbers that eventually became leukemic (Cotter et al., 1975). On the other hand, Maggio et al. (1978) reported 12 cases of preleukemic anemia. At intervals ranging from two weeks to 18 months after the onset of nonregenerative anemia, nine cats developed lymphocytic leukemia, two developed erythroleukemia, and one developed granulocytic leukemia. The majority of cats with nonregenerative anemia are destroyed if they fail to respond to treatment within a few weeks; as few cats are observed for longer, it is possible that preleukemic anemia may occur more often than we realize.

Some other hematopoietic disorders are related to preleukemic states (Madewell and Feldman, 1980). Anemia with megaloblastosis or other maturation defects may signal early leukemic change. A leukoerythroblastic reaction often indicating a malignant process in the marrow is characterized by circulating immature myeloid cells and nucleated red cells without reticulocytosis. The mechanism by which FeLV inhibits red-cell precursors is not understood. The virus is noncytopathic, so that it does not directly destroy red cells. Red-cell precursors may be destroyed by the immune response, as are mature cells in immune-mediated hemolytic anemia. In man, helper T-lymphocytes play a role in early erythroid production (Nathan et al., 1978). FeLV-positive cats have decreased numbers of T cells, as well as abnormal T-cell function (Essex et al., 1979; Perryman et al., 1972), but preliminary studies in the cat do not appear to support T-cell malfunction as the cause of FeLV-related erythroid hypoplasia (Lipton et al., 1980). Experimental infection of kittens with the KT strain of FeLV induced a rapid and selective suppression of erythroid progenitor cells (Boyce et al., 1981). This red-cell aplasia was characterized by anemia, lymphopenia, and a profound decrease in in-vitro erythroid colony-forming units ($CFU_E$). The anemia was nonregenerative with a depletion of marrow erythroid precursors. No evidence of immune-mediated red-cell destruction was found in this study. Kittens under four weeks of age were much more susceptible to this syndrome than were older cats.

With nonregenerative anemia it is important to rule out marrow infiltration by leukemic cells. Cats with such cells in the marrow may not have them in the blood. Most leukemic cats without circulating blasts have nonregenerative anemia, normal or low WBC, and normal or low platelet counts, a situation to be discussed more fully. A bone marrow aspirate is indicated in both FeLV-positive and FeLV-negative cats with nonregenerative anemia. Examination of the marrow provides information about the presence or absence of malignancy, as well as numbers and maturation of erythroid and myeloid precursors.

## Treatment of Nonregenerative Anemia

Treatment of nonleukemic cats with nonregenerative anemia is the same for both FeLV-negative and FeLV-positive cats. Blood transfusion usually produces an immediate improvement that continues for two or three weeks or longer, unless hemolysis is present. This interval allows time for further diagnostic procedures if indicated, and for other therapy.

Anabolic steroids and androgens have been advocated for treatment of nonregenerative anemias in humans (Shahidi and Diamond, 1961). Perman and Schall (1983) reported response to androgens in about a third of cats with nonregenerative anemia. Androgens may act by stimulation of erythropoietin. However, erythropoietin levels have been shown to be elevated in cats with nonregenerative anemia caused by either natural or experimental FeLV infection (Kociba et al., 1983). It thus appears that red-cell aplasia associated with FeLV is not caused by a failure in erythropoietin production and that anabolic steroids are not therefore likely to be useful in treatment of FeLV-related anemia. Oxymetholone, testosterone propionate, stanozolol, and nandrolone have been used in anemic cats at AMAH with occasional response (Cotter, 1979). Some cats respond to transfusion alone, so that apparent responses to androgens might have occurred without the drugs. In general, results of androgen therapy in anemic cats with red-cell hypoplasia have been disappointing. Side effects of androgen therapy have been minimal. One castrated male receiving androgen began spraying urine in the house. A second cat developed jaundice and cholestatic liver disease confirmed by biopsy after a month of androgen treatment. Both cats improved when androgen was stopped.

Corticosteroids may be effective in prolonging the life span of red cells by decreasing immune-mediated hemolysis and diminishing removal of older red cells by the spleen. Whether they stimulate red-cell production is not certain. Corticosteroids should be used in the FeLV-positive cat only if other causes of anemia are ruled out. These cats are already severely immunosuppressed by the virus, and further steroid-induced immunosuppression makes them more vulnerable to infection. Steroids increased the rate of conversion from FeLV-negative to FeLV-positive in exposed cats and some of these later developed lymphoma (Rojko et al., 1979). Cats that previously tested FeLV-positive and then converted to negative became positive again two or three weeks after steroid therapy (Post and Warren, 1980). Because latent FeLV may be present in previously exposed, FeLV-negative cats, it is possible that the virus may be reactivated in times of stress or immunosuppression (Rojko et al., 1982).

If an anemic cat has fever or other signs of infection, it is prudent to avoid corticosteroids and treat the infection with bactericidal drugs. Chloramphenicol, even at standard doses, should be avoided in anemic cats, as it may suppress red-cell production. Anemic cats in which fevers of unknown origin persist despite antibiotic therapy may prove to have nonbacterial diseases such as feline infectious peritonitis, toxoplasmosis, aspergillosis, cryptococcosis, or malignancies. Hematinics containing iron should be avoided in nonregenerative anemias, as they may cause iron overload and hemosiderosis.

The prognosis for recovery is less favorable for the cat with red-cell hypoplasia than for the cat with regenerative anemia. Aplastic anemia, a depression of all marrow elements, has the worst prognosis of all. Affected cats frequently succumb to infections because of granulocytopenia or hemorrhage due to thrombocytopenia. A few recover with supportive treatment. Among 25 anemic cats, 6 of 11 with regenerative anemia recovered but only 1 of 14 with nonregenerative anemia (Fischer, 1970).

In a study of 100 FeLV-positive cats at AMAH presented with PCV less than 20 per cent, 59 were destroyed within two weeks for various medical or economic reasons and 12 were lost to follow-up after that time (Cotter, 1979). Of 29 cats treated for more than two weeks, eight recovered with return to normal PCV and one converted from FeLV-positive to FeLV-negative status. The median survival time of these cats was four months, with a range of two weeks to seven years. The cats most likely to recover are those with regenerative anemia or a treatable bacterial infection.

A favorable response to FeLV-associated anemia in four cats treated with bovine fibroblast interferon has been reported (Tompkins and Cummins, 1982). The PCVs of these cats ranged from 19 to 25. Three had evidence of concurrent infection and were also treated with antibiotics. FeLV-positive cats commonly develop mild anemia in the presence of other infections, so it is possible that the response of these cats may have been related to antibiotics rather than to the interferon.

Treatment of FeLV-infected cats with BCG was reported to lessen the degree of immunosuppression but to have no effect on the incidence of illness or viremia (Guirlinger, 1983).

## Blood Transfusion Therapy

Three blood groups occur in cats, and naturally occurring isoantibodies have been described (Auer et al., 1982; Eyquem and Podliachouk, 1954; Eyquem et al., 1962; Holmes, 1953; Mulvaney and Ugenti, 1969). In a survey of 1895 Australian cats, about 73 per cent were group A and 26 per cent group B, with less than 1 per cent group AB (Auer et al., 1982). Most group B cats have some isoantibody against group A cells, whereas the group A cats usually do not have anti-B antibody. Auer and Bell (1983) reported that 16 of 29 unsensitized, anesthetized, healthy group B cats had severe, shocklike reactions when transfused with group A blood. This reaction occurred with as small a volume as 1 ml of a 50 per cent saline suspension of group A cells. The reactions were characterized by hypotension, bradycardia, and cessation of respiration. Several cats required resuscitation, and one died within five minutes. Varying degrees of AV block, including asystole for as long as 18 seconds, occurred. After this reaction cats developed hypertension, premature ventricular contractions, and tachycardia lasting from 10 to 30 minutes. PCV and WBC were transiently decreased during this time. Hemolytic reactions occurred in three group B cats. The early reaction was thought to result from release of vasoactive compounds such as histamine, serotonin, and prostaglandins stimulated by activated complement (Auer and Bell, 1983). The secondary reaction was probably stimulated by hypoxia. In view of the frequency of each blood group in cats and the fact that about half of group B cats receiving group A blood will react unfavorably, it was predicted that this reaction would occur in about one of every 11 random transfusions.

Survival time of labeled feline red cells was measured in five cats receiving autologous and allogeneic transfusions (Marion and Smith, 1983a). Autologous transfused cells had a mean survival time of 38 days. For allogeneic transfusions between cats of the same type, the mean survival time was 30 days. However, when allogeneic cells of different types were transfused, the mean survival time was only 10 to 14 days. This period was further reduced to less than five days if a second incompatible transfusion was given to a sensitized recipient. No shocklike reactions were noted in those cats even after sensitization, although only one group B cat was present

In clinical experience with large numbers of feline transfusions at AMAH and The Animal Medical Center, severe shocklike reactions have not been observed (Hayes et al., 1982). Cats receiving multiple unmatched transfusions from multiple donors appear to have progressive shortening of red-cell life span as indicated by the need for more frequent transfusions. This effect is most certainly due to sensitization to donor red cells.

The most common transfusion reaction in cats at AMAH is vomiting. This usually occurs if infusion is too rapid and can be corrected if the transfusion is stopped for a few minutes and resumed at a slower rate. The vomiting may be a reaction to the citrate anticoagulant. The citrate is metabolized in the liver within a few minutes, leaving an alkaline metabolite that is helpful in neutralizing the low pH that may be present in stored blood. When collecting blood in acid citrate dextrose solution (ACD), one must be sure that the amount of blood drawn from the donor is correct for the amount of citrate, in order to avoid hypocalcemia.

Fever beginning a few hours after transfusion is relatively frequent in cats but usually subsides in about 24 hours without treatment. It is probably a reaction to white-cell or platelet antigens. Because some anemic cats are moribund and hypothermic when presented, a post-transfusion fever could be evidence of a pre-existing disorder.

Chronically anemic cats may have cardiac enlargement indistinguishable radiographically from that of cardiomyopathy. Congestive heart failure is uncommon in anemic cats except in situations of circulatory volume overload, especially by transfusion. Acute pulmonary edema has occurred and may be treated by stopping the transfusion and giving oxygen and intravenous furosemide. The problem can be prevented by slow infusion of sedimented red cells with the plasma removed.

Hyperkalemia from transfusion of large volumes of stored blood has been reported in man. Feline red cells are high in sodium and low in potassium compared with human cells, so that in-vitro hemolysis is unlikely to cause hyperkalemia. Transmission of infections by transfusion can be minimized by using only healthy donors. Donors should have periodic hemograms, plasma protein determinations, and examinations for *Haemobartonella* and FeLV. They should be isolated from ill cats.

A large, healthy donor cat can give 50 to 70 ml of blood every two or three weeks. There is no danger to the recipient if the donor is sedated or anesthetized when blood is drawn. An equal volume of physiologic saline or lactated Ringer's solution may be given to the donor to restore circulating volume. Iron supplementation is also indicated for donor cats. Oral ferrous sulfate 250 mg twice weekly is the most effective and economic form. A 250 mg capsule of $FeSO_4$ contains 50 mg Fe, and about 20 per cent of this is absorbed from the gastrointestinal tract.

Blood is most safely collected from the jugular vein in 35 ml syringes containing 1 ml ACD/9 ml blood if the blood is to be stored; otherwise 250 units of heparin is diluted in about 2 ml normal saline/50 ml of blood if the blood is to be used within 24 hours. Blood must be collected aseptically to avoid bacterial contamination, refrigerated, and not be rewarmed unless it is to be used soon.

If many transfusions are given, as in large veterinary hospitals, donors can be anesthetized and exsanguinated aseptically by cardiac puncture, the blood being collected in ACD Vacutainer bottles. In this way 100 to 150 ml blood may be obtained from a single donor for storage up to 30 days (Marion and Smith, 1983b). Periodic mixing of the blood during storage helps to maintain contact with nutrients. This approach is limited by the supply of healthy donors but has the advantage that a larger volume of blood from a single donor can be administered to a recipient.

At AMAH the average volume of blood per transfusion is 100 ml. Sedation of the recipient is avoided in all but a few intractable cats for which the stress of a struggle would be life-threatening. Most anemic cats sit quietly once a butterfly needle or intravenous catheter has been placed in the vein. A filter is used for blood in ACD bottles, and 100 ml of blood is allowed to drip for 40 to 50 minutes. If a syringe is used, injection should be made slowly over at least 15 minutes. Stored blood may be warmed by running the tubing through a warm water bath, but care should be taken not to exceed 40 C (104 F), as hemolysis occurs at 50 C (122 F) (Tangner, 1982).

Platelets are difficult to supply in adequate numbers in whole-blood transfusions. If platelets are needed and equipment for component separation is not available, fresh blood collected in ACD in plastic bags or syringes may be given immediately after collection. A glass bottle or refrigeration causes platelet aggregation and destruction. Blood may be kept at room temperature for 24 hours and still contain viable platelets.

Because of the short life span of granulocytes these cannot be supplied by routine transfusion.

Dog blood should never be given to cats. Any short-term benefit is outweighed by a subsequent hemolytic reaction (Hessler et al., 1962).

### Bone Marrow Transplantation

Bone marrow transplantation has been used in man to treat a variety of hematologic and immunologic disorders. Marrow is removed in anticoagulant from the donor and infused intravenously into the recipient. In addition to a need for histocompatibility testing to prevent rejection, a problem with marrow transplantation not observed in other organ transplants is graft-versus-host disease. Immune-competent lymphocytes of donor origin may cause a severe immune-mediated disorder in the recipient. Because of unavailability of histocompatibility testing and difficulties in supportive care of recipients, marrow transplantation has been rarely used in cats. Several empirical transplants were done to treat apparently aplastic anemia in cats (Holzworth, unpublished data). Improvement was observed in some, although numbers were small and it was uncertain whether the improvement was a result of recovery of the patient's own marrow or of engraftment.

Recently, successful feline marrow transplantation has been accomplished (Gasper, 1984; Haskins et al., 1984). In both situations, transplantation was used to treat mucopolysaccharidosis, a metabolic disorder associated with macrophage abnormalities (Cowell et al., 1976; Jezyk et al., 1977). Because macrophages are derived from monocytes, implantation of normal marrow stem cells would be expected to supply missing enzymes.

Some anecdotal reports describe improvement of aplastic anemic in humans treated with unmatched marrow transplants. In these persons, clinical improvement occurred with recovery of the patient's own marrow. Thus the infused marrow may have acted as an immune stimulant or may possibly have supplied some missing marrow stromal elements that allowed hematopoiesis to occur. Whether some such process occurs in cats remains to be determined.

## POLYCYTHEMIA

Polycythemia is an increase in the red-cell mass of the blood. It may be relative or absolute, the latter being primary or secondary in etiology. Relative polycythemia is a common consequence of dehydration. It may also occur transiently from excitement, when the spleen contracts and releases red cells into the circulation.

Absolute polycythemia of the secondary (compensatory) type is a response to anoxia and has been described in a young Siamese cat with tetralogy of Fallot (Kirby and Gillick, 1974). The PCV was 74 per cent in the absence of dehydration, the mucosae were purple, and there was bleeding from the nose and gums.

Primary polycythemia (polycythemia vera, polycythemia rubra vera) is a myeloproliferative disorder of uncertain etiology in which abnormal proliferation of all hematopoietic marrow elements causes an absolute increase in red cell mass and often leukocytosis and thrombocythemia. A few instances have been reported in the cat (Duff et al., 1973; Reed et al., 1970; Theilen and Madewell, 1979). Polycythemia vera is discussed more fully later in this chapter.

## DISORDERS OF WHITE CELLS—NON-NEOPLASTIC

Normal white-cell production and response to various disorders are discussed earlier in this chapter. Abnormalities of granulocyte function such as failure to respond to chemotaxis or to phagocytize and kill bacteria have yet to be described in cats. Pelger-Huët anomaly of granulocytes has been reported in two cats from the same litter (Weber et al., 1981). This anomaly is characterized by failure of the cell nucleus to segment and may result in impaired granulocyte function. The cats in the Weber report were 10 years old and apparently normal, so any malfunction was not clinially important. Test-mating between another affected cat and an unaffected queen suggested autosomal dominant transmission (Latimer et al., 1985).

### Granulocytopenia

Granulocytopenia occurs with viral infections such as panleukopenia, FeLV-induced myelosuppression, and some cases of feline infectious peritonitis, toxoplasmosis, and bacterial infection. Experimental inoculation with panleukopenia virus inhibits granulopoiesis by affecting the rapidly dividing granulocyte precursors at the myelocyte stage. Because of rapid turnover and inability of more mature granulocytes to divide, granulocytopenia becomes evident three to five days after inoculation, the time required normally for maturation from myelocyte to segmented neutrophil (Ichijo et al., 1976). Erythroid and platelet precursors may also be decreased. As the cat recovers and white cells return to the blood, bizarre and atypical granulocytes and lymphocytes appear and may suggest leukemia. An important difference is that this leukemoid response is transient in convalescing panleukopenia, so that a blood count repeated in a few days shows leukocytosis with decreasing left shift.

A disorder sometimes confused with panleukopenia is the "panleukopenia-like syndrome" associated with feline leukemia virus. Here as well, a leukopenia is caused by granulocytic hypoplasia. Affected cats are often presented with fever and other signs of infection such as stomatitis. Vomiting and diarrhea may occur, as in panleukopenia. If platelets are decreased, hemorrhagic enteritis or other hemorrhage may occur. Without resort to virus isolation techniques for panleukopenia virus, it may be impossible to differentiate these disorders. Indeed, true panleukopenia may occur in an FeLV-positive cat. More typical of FeLV-related granulocytopenia than of panleukopenia are chronic illness, anemia, thrombocytopenia, and slow recovery of white-cell counts. Although the prognosis is worse in the FeLV-positive cat, treatment is the same for both: intravenous fluids, antibiotics, vitamin preparations, and possibly blood transfusion in some cases with severe anemia. (Panleukopenia and its treatment are more extensively discussed in the chapter on viral diseases.)

Granulocytopenia has been said to be a frequent response of the cat to any severe infection, but it must be realized that many such cats are also carriers of FeLV. Any cat reacting to an infection with leukopenia and a degenerative left shift should be tested for FeLV, as the FeLV-associated leukopenia may be the cause rather than the result of the infection.

Drug-induced leukopenia can be associated with numerous agents (e.g., pyrimethamine, phenylbutazone, propylthiouracil, and anticancer drugs such as cyclophosphamide, cytosine arabinoside, and doxorubicin). Vincristine is less myelosuppressive than other chemotherapeutic agents but can sometimes produce leukopenia (Todd et al., 1979). Prednisone can produce lymphopenia and eosinopenia. Many drugs have been associated with leukopenia in man, so this possibility should be a consideration if a cat will be on long-term therapy with any drug. Drugs cause neutropenia by destruction of myeloid precursors; by suppression of, or abnormalities in, neutrophilic myelopoiesis; and by idiosyncratic mechanisms (Finch, 1972).

Leukopenia can also be caused by myeloproliferative disorders (to be discussed) and by radiation. In man, immune-mediated neutropenia due to antineutrophil antibodies is well documented and may conceivably be shown to occur in cats. However, in a study of 55 clinically neutropenic cats by an indirect immunofluorescence technique, such antibodies were not demonstrated (Chickering et al., 1985).

## Inclusions in Granulocytes

**CHEDIAK-HIGASHI SYNDROME.** This hereditary systemic disorder of man, mink, mice, cattle, and killer whales also occurs in blue smoke Persian cats that have pale yellow-green irises rather than the usual copper-colored ones (Collier et al., 1979; Kramer et al., 1975; Prieur and Collier, 1978). The disorder is inherited as an autosomal recessive trait. Among its manifestations are round, eosinophilic, intracytoplasmic inclusions 1 or 2 μ in diameter, occurring principally in neutrophils but also in lymphocytes and eosinophils. The inclusions stain with peroxidase, which sometimes discloses several per cell, whereas Wright-Giemsa stain usually shows only one. Less mature myeloid cells in the marrow contain even more granules, thought to represent abnormal lysosomes. These inclusions have not been associated with increased susceptibility to infection in cats, as occurs in man.

Bleeding tendencies were suspected in affected cats because of prolonged bleeding after venepuncture but confirming tests have not been reported (Kramer et al., 1977). Cataracts are frequent and vary from opacity of posterior lenticular suture lines to generalized mature cataracts, some of which regress with age (Collier et al., 1979). Fundic pigmentation is decreased, with no difference between tapetal and nontapetal areas, and the cats are photophobic. Enlarged melanin granules are found in the hair of affected cats.

**INCLUSIONS IN GRANULOCYTES OF BIRMAN CATS.** An autosomal recessive anomaly characterized by fine acidophilic granules in neutrophils has been described in highly inbred Birman cats (Hirsch and Cunningham, 1984). Limited testing identified no functional abnormality of the affected neutrophils.

**LE CELLS.** An LE cell is a mature neutrophil containing a single, large, spherical, homogeneous inclusion representing phagocytized material from another neutrophil. It is seen in many cases of lupus erythematosus but also in other inflammatory conditions and in myeloproliferative diseases (Schalm et al., 1975).

**MUCOPOLYSACCHARIDOSES.** A group of disorders inherited in the cat and characterized by inclusions in white cells are the mucopolysaccharidoses (Cowell et al., 1976; Haskins et al., 1983; Jezyk et al., 1977). They are manifested primarily by skeletal abnormalities such as dwarfism, fusion of vertebrae, spinal cord compression, degenerative joint disease, absence of lower incisors, multiple exostoses, and central nervous deficits. Affected cats have a peculiar facial expression with a short, broad face and puffy eyelids. The mucopolysaccharidoses are lysosomal storage disorders with accumulation of coarse metachromatic granules in most of the neutrophils, in a few lymphocytes, and in some large cells resembling histiocytes (Jezyk et al., 1977). These granules, visible with Wright-Giemsa stain, are seen more easily when the blood film is stained with toluidine blue and appear to be bound to the cell membrane. The Siamese cat seems predisposed to mucopolysaccharidosis VI (Maroteaux-Lamy syndrome), which is thought to be the result of an autosomal recessive trait. Mucopolysaccharidosis I (Hurler's syndrome) has been reported in domestic shorthaired cats (Haskins et al., 1979). Although neutrophilic granules have been reported in humans with this syndrome, the granules in the affected cat were visible only with electron microscopy. Both forms of mucopolysaccharidosis may be diagnosed by a urine toluidine spot test, in which metachromasia is produced on a filter paper in the urine by reaction of the basic groups of toluidine blue dye with acid mucopolysaccharide (Cowell et al., 1976).

Large cytoplasmic granules have also been seen in neutrophils of a cat with sphingolipidosis (Prasse, 1983).

**DÖHLE BODIES.** These blue, angular granules in the cytoplasm of neutrophils indicate toxicity, often from bacterial infection. More severe toxic changes in white cells are basophilia or vacuolation of the cytoplasm, increased segmentation of nucleus, and increased cell size (Plate 16–2*D*). Blood films must be made carefully and promptly from fresh blood to demonstrate these changes. Similar changes may be produced artifactually with blood mixed with EDTA anticoagulant if several hours pass before films are made.

**MICROORGANISMS.** Microorganisms occur less often in white cells of cats than in those of dogs. Toxoplasmosis was diagnosed in a cat by the presence of tachyzoites in primitive cells in the marrow (Schalm, 1978b) (Plate 16–2*E*). Inclusions possibly related to coincidental chlamydial infection have been seen in neutrophils in cats with feline infectious peritonitis (Schalm et al., 1975). Histoplasmosis may be diagnosed occasionally by the presence of organisms in white cells. (See also the chapter on mycotic diseases.) In bacterial septicemias, neutrophils may contain organisms (Plate 16–2*F*).

## Disorders Involving Eosinophils*

In the cat some disorders associated with eosinophils, such as eosinophilic granuloma and asthma, are common; others are rare. The relationship between parasitism and eosinophilia is well documented. Eosinophilia may lead to suspicion of such conditions as intestinal parasitism, trichinosis, and dirofilariasis. Certain infrequent eosinophil-related diseases are designated as "primary" or "idiopathic," in that they arise spontaneously or from an unknown stimulus. These disorders are eosinophilic enteritis, disseminated eosinophilic disease, and eosinophilic leukemia.

The eosinophilic granuloma complex, discussed in the chapter on the skin, is a skin disease of varied clinical manifestations, characterized by infiltration of the dermis, lips, and oral mucosa with eosinophils, macrophages, lymphocytes, mast cells, and plasma cells. Eosinophilia is mild in the majority of cases but is occasionally pronounced.

Feline "asthma" is an acute respiratory disorder (Carpenter, 1974). Eosinophilic infiltrates can be seen around the bronchi and bronchioles. An absolute peripheral eosinophilia is present in most cats. The cause of feline "asthma" is not known, but it is assumed to be allergic. Two cases of dirofilariasis seen at AMAH mimicked feline "asthma," but parasites have not been found in most asthmatic cats. Chronic asthmatic bronchitis is more frequent than the acute condition and is usually accompanied by eosinophilia.

Eosinophilic enteritis is a rare disorder characterized by persistent vomiting or diarrhea with infiltration of eosinophils into the gastrointestinal wall, often with ulceration and fibrosis (Hendrick, 1981; Moore, 1983). The intestines are thick and rubbery, and the mesenteric lymph nodes may be enlarged and irregular. A moderate or marked eosinophilia has been consistently present, occasionally with immature eosinophils. The marrow is also infiltrated with eosinophils in most cats. Decreasing doses of prednisone are curative in the majority of canine cases, but cats have been more refractory to therapy. The response to corticosteroids is transient in cats, and most are destroyed or die because of progressive illness.

In some cats with eosinophilic enteritis, the infiltration of eosinophils extends beyond the intestines and mesenteric lymph nodes to other viscera including the liver, hepatic lymph nodes, spleen, pancreas, and adrenal gland. The infiltrate varies from a percolation of eosinophils along established vascular and sinusoidal channels to a frank disruption of normal architecture with replacement by eosinophils and fibrous connective tissue. The majority of invading eosinophils are mature, although occasional band cells and metamyelocytes are seen. Because of atypical infiltration patterns and the relative lack of eosinophilic immaturity, a diagnosis of eosinophilic leukemia seems inappropriate, and this disorder has been called instead disseminated eosinophilic disease (Hendrick, 1981). Some cats with eosinophilic enteritis, after a brief steroid-induced remission, go on to develop hepatosplenomegaly. When autopsied these cats have varying degrees of disseminated eosinophilic infiltration. The peripheral blood and bone marrow of these animals cannot be distinguished from those of cats with eosinophilic enteritis alone, as marked eosinophilia is present in both groups.

Eosinophilic leukemia is an extremely rare and nebulous entity. Some Scandinavian researchers go so far as to deny the existence of eosinophilic leukemia in man, at least according to the criteria for diagnosis of other leukemias (Bengtsson, 1968; Odeberg, 1965). They prefer to think of the eosinophilic proliferation as an overzealous immune response. A review of feline eosinophilic leukemias reported in the literature and of five cases at AMAH suggests that the majority would more aptly be classified as disseminated eosinophilic disease.

One case, however, was notable owing to the character of the eosinophilic proliferation (Simon and Holzworth, 1967). Although the majority of eosinophils in the peripheral blood were mature, there were significant numbers of eosinophilic bands and metamyelocytes. Rare myeloblasts and mitotic figures were also seen in the blood. Visceral infiltration by eosinophils of all stages was widespread, and in the kidneys multiple tumors were formed by the densely packed infiltrate. Another notable distinction is that in this cat steroid therapy exacerbated rather than relieved the condition.

All cases of disseminated eosinophilic disease and eosinophilic leukemia have eosinophilic infiltration of the gastrointestinal tract (i.e., eosinophilic enteritis). Vomiting and diarrhea are the usual presenting signs and eosinophilic enteritis the presumptive diagnosis, until hepatosplenomegaly or other systemic involvement develops.

The term hypereosinophilic syndrome is used in human medicine to designate a group of disorders characterized by eosinophilic infiltration and eosinophilia of the blood and bone marrow (Hardy and Anderson, 1968). Included are eosinophilic bronchitis and bronchopneumonia (Loeffler's disease), eosinophilic enteritis, disseminated eosinophilic disease, and eosinophilic leukemia. All disorders are of unknown etiology, but hypersensitivity is a possible cause. The clinical signs, response to therapy, and prognosis of the hypereosinophilic disorders in man are strikingly similar to those in the cat. Corticosteroids are the treatment of choice in the human hypereosinophilic syndrome, but some response in refractory cases has been achieved with combinations including hydroxyurea or vincristine and cytosine arabinoside (Parrillo et al., 1978; Van Slyck and Adamson, 1979).

# HEMATOPOIETIC NEOPLASIA

The domestic cat, of all animals, most nearly approaches man in the variety and complexity of its hematopoietic neoplasms. These began to be reported about a century ago, chiefly by European pathologists (see reviews of the early literature, Holzworth, 1960b; Nielsen, 1969), but have appeared to be increasing in incidence within the past 35 years—possibly because the cat population has been exploding along with that of its human owners and also because scientists are devoting more attention and diagnostic methods of increasing sophistication to a species that was traditionally the least studied of domestic animals.

*By Mattie Hendrick.

For many reasons data on the incidence of hematopoietic neoplasms in cats represent only rough approximations, and apparent differences in geographic distribution must also be taken into account. It has been estimated that from a third to a half of all feline neoplasms are hematopoietic (Dorn et al., 1968; Theilen and Madewell, 1979). A survey of data from 14 veterinary colleges in North America indicated a figure of close to 50 per cent (Priester and McKay, 1980). In two California counties it was estimated that the incidence of all types of hematopoietic neoplasms was 200/100,000 cats per year (0.2 per cent) (Theilen and Madewell, 1979).

The varieties of hematopoietic neoplasms recognized in the cat are outlined in Table 16–4. The most detailed clinical descriptions of the feline hematopoietic malignancies are those of Holzworth (1960a,b). Although predating the discovery of FeLV and recognition of its contagious nature, the observations are still valid and give clues as to the immunosuppressive nature of the virus that we recognize today.

Of the feline hematopoietic neoplasms half or more are of lymphoproliferative type (e.g., 90 per cent, Cotter et al., 1975; 90 per cent, Dorn et al., 1968; 76 per cent, Priester and McKay, 1980; 50 to 80 per cent, Theilen and Madewell, 1979). Myeloproliferative neoplasms include disorders involving marrow cell lines: reticuloendotheliosis, neoplasms of erythroid cells, and granulocytic, monocytic, and megakaryocytic leukemias. In many leukemias the cells are so undifferentiated that they cannot be classified by routine methods. Polycythemia vera (erythremia), an uncontrolled proliferation of mature red cells, is rare in the cat. Myelofibrosis and osteosclerosis are terminal events in occasional cases of myeloproliferative disorders.

Myeloma is an uncommon neoplasm of plasma cells—cells derived from B-lymphocytes. In addition "leukemic" mast cell malignancies occur from time to time in cats. These are not usually included in statistical surveys, as mast cells are of connective tissue origin.

**Table 16–4 Hematopoietic Neoplasms of the Cat**

Lymphoproliferative
- Lymphoma
- Lymphocytic and lymphoblastic leukemia

Myeloproliferative
- Reticuloendotheliosis
- Erythremic myelosis
- Erythroleukemia
- Polycythemia vera
- Granulocytic leukemia including eosinophilic and basophilic
- Monocytic leukemia
- Myelomonocytic leukemia
- Megakaryocytic myelosis and leukemia
- Myelofibrosis and osteosclerosis

Undifferentiated leukemia

Myeloma

Tumors of nonhematopoietic origin
- Mast cell neoplasia
- Thymoma

## Role of the Feline Leukemia Virus

In 1964 a virus (FeLV) isolated from naturally occurring feline lymphoma was shown to reproduce lymphoproliferative neoplasms in cats under experimental conditions Jarrett et al., 1964); in 1971 a case of granulocytic leukemia was induced by the same agent (Jarrett et al., 1971); and in 1983 a case of eosinophilic leukemia was reported in a cat inoculated with FeLV (Rickard strain) (Lewis et al., 1985; Olsen et al., 1983). Other myeloproliferative disorders have not been reproduced in cats by inoculation with FeLV, but the virus is often detected by FeLV testing or by electron microscopy in association with most forms of myeloproliferative neoplasms (Hardy, 1980; Henness and Crow, 1977; Henness et al., 1977; Herz et al., 1970; Stann, 1979). A virus strain that induces only myeloproliferative disorders is still to be found (Theilen and Madewell, 1979).

A survey of recent data (Ott, 1983) suggests that half or more of free-ranging pet cats become infected, at least transiently, with FeLV, about 1.8 per cent becoming chronically viremic. FeLV-associated disease was estimated to occur annually in about 0.2 per cent of the feline population at risk, non-neoplastic disorders outnumbering neoplastic by a ratio of 5:3 (Ott, 1983).

As well as being present in blood and marrow of infected cats, the virus is shed principally in saliva but has also been found in urine, feces, and queen's milk (Hardy et al., 1973). Thus common routes of transmission are by biting and grooming among cats and by the sharing of litter pans. Experimentally, intranasal administration of virus has resulted in viremia (Hoover et al., 1972). Infection may also be passed to offspring in utero. Outside the cat the virus survives only a short time, but clustering of cases in multi-cat households and catteries is frequent.

Blood transfusion may be a route of spread of virus. Donors should test negative and be retested at three-month intervals. They should also be segregated from other hospital patients.

The virus is more likely to replicate in malignant T-lymphocytes than in malignant B-lymphocytes, and a young cat is more likely to be viremic than an old cat (Azocar and Essex, 1979; Francis et al., 1979). About 30 per cent of cats with lymphoproliferative and myeloproliferative neoplasia test virus-negative (Cotter et al., 1975), but their neoplasms are probably caused by FeLV even though replicating virus is not present.

Aviremic latent infection in previously exposed or recovered cats, detected by culture of bone marrow, is probably more prevalent than had been realized, and in response to certain stimuli or stresses it may be reactivated. The evidence for such latent infection and its clinical implications have been well reviewed by Pedersen and associates (1984). (See also the chapter on virus diseases.)

The incubation period for FeLV-associated diseases varies from weeks to years, but one study indicated that 83 per cent of infected cats die within three and a half years (McClelland et al., 1980). Some viremic cats remain healthy for many years, and some infections are transient. These factors must be considered when the fate of an FeLV-positive cat is being contemplated. An owner may wish to retest the cat three months later, to see if it still tests positive. A positive test in a cat with signs of illness must still be followed by a thorough medical study to find the cause of the illness, as FeLV may be only a part of an otherwise treatable condition.

Because some hematopoietic malignancies are FeLV-negative and because the majority of FeLV-positive cats are not suffering from malignancy, it is important for the clinician to realize that the two available tests for FeLV, fixed-cell immunofluorescence (IFA) and the enzyme-linked immune absorbance assay (ELISA), detect viremia, not antibody or the presence of malignant disease. A diagnosis of hematopoietic neoplasia can only be made by demonstration of malignant cells in tumors, blood, marrow, or effusions.

The feline leukemia virus and the prevalence and forms of the diseases with which it is associated are discussed in more detail in the chapter on virus diseases.

## Lymphoproliferative Neoplasia

Feline lymphoproliferative neoplasms constitute the most common naturally occurring malignancy in any outbred mammalian species and are exceeded in frequency only by leukemias in inbred species of mice and chickens bred specifically for leukemia study (Nielsen, 1969).

As already noted, from 50 to 90 per cent of hematopoietic malignancies of cats have been estimated to be of lymphoproliferative type, the percentage varying according to different authorities and in different geographic areas (e.g., Hardy, 1978, 1981; Nielsen, 1969). Within the group, solid tumors (lymphoma, lymphosarcoma) are usually reported to outnumber the leukemias, in which marrow and blood are primarily involved. With some lymphomas, however, malignant cells ultimately spill over to involve blood and marrow.

Many surveys and case reports indicate that lymphoproliferative malignancies may affect all age groups, from very young kittens to cats nearing 20 years (e.g., Holzworth, 1960a). The peak age has been estimated by some authors to be from four to six years, by others as occurring bimodally at two and six years (Theilen and Madewell, 1979). In one Boston study the mean age at diagnosis was four years (Essex et al., 1975a), while in the Washington state area, the mean age was two years (Ott, 1983). Cats in the younger age range more often test FeLV-positive than do older cats (Hardy, 1981).

It is commonly said that lymphoproliferative disorders of cats occur equally in both sexes and in all breeds (e.g., Essex et al., 1975b; Meincke et al., 1972). Males, however, were found by Dorn et al. (1968) to be at a statistically greater risk for lymphoma, and a survey of records at veterinary colleges in North America disclosed that although the male:female ratio in the reference population was 8:7.5, males outnumbered females by 2:1 for all hematopoietic malignancies, including lymphoproliferative (Priester and McKay, 1980).

It has been suggested that the incidence of malignant lymphoma in purebreds, notably Siamese, may reflect a genetic susceptibility and that inbreeding may also be an adverse factor (Theilen and Madewell, 1979). Others, however, stress the intensity of exposure to which purebreds are subjected in crowded catteries (e.g., Meincke et al., 1972). In cluster households with both purebreds and domestic cats the prevalence was equal (Essex et al., 1975a).

Possibly because of differences or alterations in virus strains, forms of lymphoid malignancies may differ in prevalence in various geographic areas and possibly also change over time. Of 140 lymphomas studied at autopsy at AMAH up to 1960 the majority involved, in order of occurrence, the kidneys, intestine, mediastinum, lymph nodes, spleen, and liver, true leukemias constituting only 15 per cent (Holzworth, 1960a). However, among 184 cases studied at AMAH from 1972 to 1976 the lymphomas in order of frequency were mediastinal 27 per cent, multicentric 11 per cent, and alimentary 8 per cent, with an increase in leukemias to 42 per cent (Francis et al., 1979). In Glasgow, Scotland, alimentary lymphomas have been the most frequent (Crighton, 1968). At the University of California, among 170 cases from 1967 to 1976, alimentary and mediastinal tumors predominated, leukemias constituting only 7 per cent (Theilen and Madewell, 1979), while in New York the multicentric and thymic forms greatly outnumbered the alimentary (Hardy, 1981).

It is possible that interest at AMAH in monitoring anemic cats by frequent blood and marrow studies might account for the relatively high frequency of lymphoblastic leukemia diagnosed in Boston cats.

Most lymphocytic malignancies in the cat (i.e., virtually all mediastinal lymphomas and most multicentric lymphomas and leukemias) appear to be of T-cell origin (Cockerell et al., 1976; Hardy et al., 1977), while most alimentary tumors in older cats are of B-cell origin and are less likely to be associated with viremia or to contain virus (Essex et al., 1979).

Cytogenetic studies of leukemias and lymphomas in man give evidence that these diseases are monoclonal, and a variety of chromosomal abnormalities have been described in human tumor cells (Sandberg and Hossfeld, 1970). In one cytogenetic study of 23 cats with lymphoma, several abnormalities were noted (Jones, 1969). Aneuploidy was most often due to loss of whole chromosomes and replication of others. The modal number of chromosomes in feline tumors was 37 (normal 2n = 38). Loss usually involved a single chromosome in group D or E. Those tumors with excess chromosomes usually had trisomy in group F. Only four of the 23 cats surveyed had normal chromosomes in their tumor cells.

### Lymphoma

The term lymphoma (malignant lymphoma, lymphosarcoma) refers to a progressive malignant growth of lymphoid cells into a solid tumor. Feline lymphoma most often assumes a diffuse, poorly differentiated (lymphoblastic) form, if the Rappaport classification is used (Rappaport, 1966). Diffuse, well-differentiated (lymphocytic) lymphoma is infrequent, although mixed lymphoblastic and lymphocytic tumors are relatively common. Diffuse histiocytic lymphoma, formerly called reticulum cell sarcoma, is also frequent, especially in sites other than marrow and lymphoid tissues. The cells in histiocytic lymphoma are larger and less differentiated than lymphoblasts. The cytoplasm is more abundant and may be vacuolated. Histiocytic lymphoma has been thought to arise in man from B cells, but this possibility has not been studied in the cat (Theilen and Madewell, 1979). The follicular (or nodular) pattern often observed in human lymphomas is uncommon in the cat. Hodgkin's disease, the most frequent form of lymphoma in humans, is generally considered to have no counterpart in animals, but a possible case was recently described in a cat (Roperto et al., 1983).

Holmberg and associates (1976) attempted to classify feline lymphoma by immunologic characteristics and found that lymphoblasts failed to respond to mitogens but that cells of many tumors probably of T-cell origin formed rosettes with guinea pig red cells. They found that histiocytic lymphoma lacked both immunoglobulin of B-cell lineage and T-cell markers. They could not identify B or T cells by morphology. Morphologic classification of lymphoma in the cat has not been helpful to date in predicting response to therapy or survival times. More studies are needed to classify feline lymphomas immunologically, histochemically, and cytogenetically, as variations in prognosis probably occur in different subtypes in cats as they do in man.

Clinical signs in cats with lymphoma vary with the site of the tumor.

*Mediastinal lymphoma* occurs in cats of all ages but is the form most likely to be found in kittens and young cats (e.g., Crighton, 1968). Recently it has been the most prevalent form at AMAH, constituting 42 per cent of all lymphomas. Affected cats are usually presented in sternal recumbency with moderate or severe dyspnea of rather sudden onset. Other physical findings are incompressibility of the cranial thorax, caudodorsal displacement of apex heart beat, and muffling of heart and lung sounds by pleural effusion. Dysphagia and regurgitation may be caused by compression of the esophagus by the tumor. Sometimes the mass is palpable if it protrudes through the thoracic inlet. Rare signs are Horner's syndrome, produced by pressure on the sympathetic nerve as it ascends around the first rib, and edema of the head from pressure on the cranial vena cava. Distention of jugular veins from this pressure may be responsible for hematoma formation after jugular venepuncture.

Diagnosis of mediastinal lymphoma is by radiography and examination of aspirated thoracic fluid. The first step is to radiograph the chest. If significant fluid is present, the mass may not be discerned until the fluid is removed. A sample is saved for analysis, and as much fluid as possible is removed without stressing the cat excessively. Because cytologic examination of the fluid is diagnostic in most cases, it is not necessary to remove all the fluid, as the rest will be reabsorbed within 24 to 48 hours after chemotherapy is begun.

Typically the fluid is serosanguineous, but it may be serous or occasionally chylous from invasion of lymphatics. The nucleated cell count in the fluid is usually over 4000/μl and is composed almost entirely of lymphocytes varying in size and maturity from a few small cells through larger numbers of both large and small lymphoblasts, the larger lymphoblasts often containing vacuoles.

If the fluid analysis is not diagnostic of lymphoma, the next step is to repeat thoracic radiographs after removal of as much of the remaining fluid as possible. The cranial mediastinum may be better visualized if a horizontal beam is used with the cranial part of the cat's body elevated and both lateral and ventrodorsal views are taken. If that procedure is followed, any remaining fluid will collect in the diaphragmatic area and the presence or absence of a mediastinal mass can be determined.

Conditions that may be confused with mediastinal lymphoma are cardiomyopathy, feline infectious peritonitis (FIP) with thoracic effusion, other thoracic neoplasia such as thymoma, and diaphragmatic hernia. In cardiomyopathy, the fluid may be grossly similar to that of lymphoma but usually contains fewer lymphocytes, the majority being small mature forms. Thoracic radiography after removal of the fluid demonstrates cardiac enlargement. With FIP the fluid is usually quite different: sticky, proteinaceous, of high specific gravity, and with relatively few inflammatory cells (see chapter on viral diseases). With thymoma, as with lymphoma, a mediastinal mass is present often with pleural effusion, but the fluid usually contains predominantly small lymphocytes and occasionally neoplastic epithelial cells. Differentiation of lymphoma and thymoma may be difficult, and sometimes a needle aspirate or even a biopsy may be needed. Other tumors in the thorax may be recognized by finding malignant cells in the fluid. Diaphragmatic hernia may initially be mistaken for lymphoma, if fluid is present owing to incarceration of abdominal viscera. Once the fluid is removed, the correct diagnosis is usually evident from characteristic radiographic findings of loss of diaphragmatic line, displacement of the gastric silhouette, and the presence of intestinal loops in the thorax seen in plain radiographs or in those taken after administration of barium sulfate.

The differential diagnosis is not always easy. One cat at AMAH with mediastinal lymphoma had a superimposed pyothorax. An accurate diagnosis is essential for prognostic purposes, however, because a thymoma or diaphragmatic hernia may be managed surgically, while medical therapy offers the only hope for lymphoma, cardiomyopathy, or the rare thoracic mast cell tumor.

Mediastinal lymphomas grow quite large before pleural effusion evokes clinical signs, and they cause acute distress and death from compromised respiration within a few days of presentation if not treated by removal of fluid and chemotherapy. Figure 16–12*A* shows a normal thoracic radiograph of a cat with mediastinal lymphoma in remission after chemotherapy. The rapid recurrence of tumor only one week later gives evidence for a doubling time of the tumor cells as short as 36 hours (Fig. 16–12*B*) (Cotter et al., 1980). Mediastinal tumors may invade the pleura and occasionally the thoracic muscles. Hypercalcemia, frequent with canine lymphoma, is rarely recognized in cats but was reported with mediastinal lymphoma (e.g., McMillan, 1985; Chew et al., 1975) and has been diagnosed in two cats at AMAH. Cats with mediastinal lymphoma respond well to chemotherapy, with a 79 per cent complete remission rate at AMAH (Cotter, 1977, 1983). Occasional cats have remained in continuous complete remission for over two years after diagnosis, possibly representing cures.

Involvement of the *stomach, intestine, or mesenteric lymph nodes* is classified as alimentary lymphoma (Crighton, 1968). Clinical signs include anorexia, weight loss, vomiting, and diarrhea. Crighton reported, however, that vomiting was a presenting complaint in fewer than 50 per cent of cats with intestinal lymphoma. The progression of signs is more gradual than with mediastinal tumors. Often a large abdominal mass is palpable involving mesenteric lymph nodes. Intestinal tumors most often take the form of one or more thickened segments of lower ileum, with constriction or dilatation of the lumen. The mucosa may be ulcerated, and rarely an ulcer perforates. Occasionally, most of the small and large intestine may be diffusely thickened, a form of lymphoma less easily recognized by palpation. Biopsy is necessary to confirm the diagnosis, and if involvement is limited to a discrete intestinal tumor,

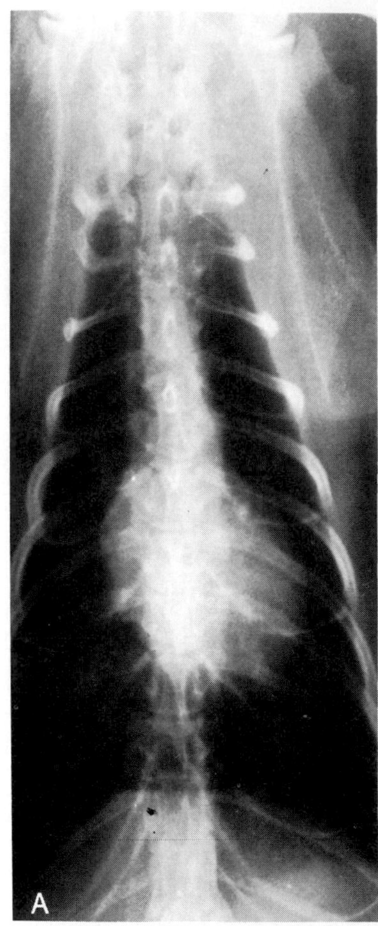


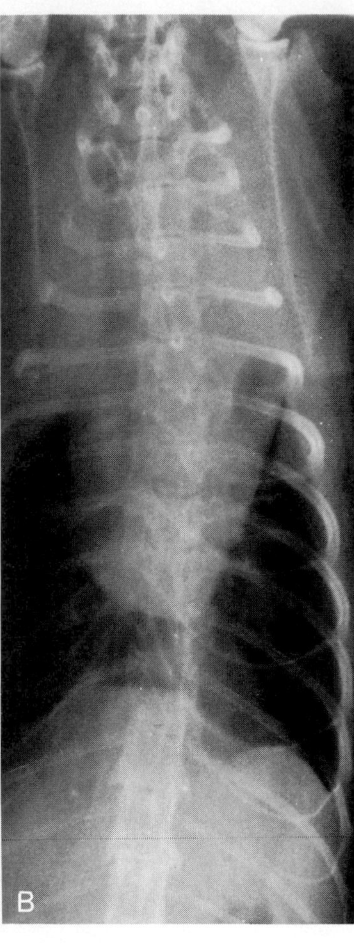


**Figure 16–12** *A*, Mediastinal lymphoma in remission. Ventrodorsal radiographic view, two-year-old spayed female Siamese. Mediastinal lymphoma was diagnosed two months earlier by radiograph and cytologic examination of fluid. Complete remission was attained with chemotherapy, as evidenced by the normal-appearing radiograph. *B*, Radiograph, same cat, seven days later, shows recurrence of a large cranial mediastinal mass. This change in such a short period gives evidence for the rapid doubling time of feline lymphoma cells.

excision may be considered (Patterson and Meier, 1955). Surgery must be followed by chemotherapy to prevent rapid recurrence of the tumor.

*Renal lymphoma* is almost always bilateral with the kidneys so large that they are easily palpated and in a thin cat may bulge visibly behind the ribs. Usually the kidney surface is studded with irregular tumor nodules, but if the tumor infiltration is diffuse, the surface may be smooth. The tumor begins in the cortex and spreads to the medulla. Wilson and Gilmore (1962) observed that 20 per cent of 98 cats with lymphoma had primary renal involvement. In a more recent survey at AMAH, the kidneys were involved in only two of 38 cats with lymphoma (Cotter et al., 1975), a more frequent cause of large, irregular kidneys being feline infectious peritonitis. The two diseases can be distinguished with certainty only by renal biopsy. With renal lymphoma, results of urinalysis and renal function tests remain normal until the tumor is far advanced. Treatment of cats in renal failure has usually been disappointing, although some improvement in renal function may occur if the tumor responds to therapy. Two cats surviving for over two years had significant involvement of only one kidney. Both were treated with nephrectomy followed by a year of chemotherapy (Cotter, 1977, 1983). One cat relapsed after two years; the other was lost to follow-up after three years.

*Lymphoma of peripheral lymph nodes and spleen* is less common in cats than in dogs. Except in some cases of multicentric lymphoma and lymphoblastic leukemia, splenomegaly in the cat is more often caused by myeloproliferative disorders, mast cell tumors, or extramedullary hematopoiesis. Slight or moderate lymph node enlargement is due more often to reactive hyperplasia than to lymphoma; but when single or multiple nodes are enlarged to three times normal size or more, one should suspect lymphoma and consider a biopsy. Complete excision of the node is desirable, as the difference between severe lymphocytic hyperplasia and lymphoma may be subtle. Loss of normal architecture of the follicles and invasion of the capsule are important criteria of malignancy that are not evident in a needle aspirate.

The *liver* is frequently affected in multicentric lymphoma, but primary involvement is uncommon. The tumor may vary from nodular to diffuse and may cause hepatomegaly and jaundice. Biopsy is necessary to confirm the diagnosis. Liver function test results become progressively more abnormal as the disease progresses, but severe elevations in liver enzymes are unusual.

Invasion of the *spinal canal* by lymphoma may compress the spinal cord, causing gradual or sudden onset of posterior paralysis. Although the majority of tumors arise in the extradural space, rare intradural lymphomas may occur (Rowe et al., 1977). In one report of 150 cats with lymphoma, eight had spinal canal involvement (Meincke et al., 1972). Conditions from which lymphoma must be distinguished include aortic embolism, spinal trauma, diskospondylitis, degenerative disk or vertebral disease, and other tumors or granulomatous infections such as feline infectious peritonitis. If treatment is contemplated, the diagnosis must be confirmed quickly because damage to the spinal cord may be irreversible after a few days. As well as a CBC, a bone marrow aspirate should be done, because the marrow is often involved in this form of lymphoma. Examination of cerebrospinal fluid (CSF) may reveal tumor cells only if the tumor is intradural. If the marrow and CSF are normal, a myelogram and laminectomy with biopsy become necessary. If a diagnosis can be confirmed and if paralysis has not been prolonged, chemotherapy is indicated. If the tumor is extradural, the response will be equally rapid with or without laminectomy. If the tumor is intradural, the chances of response are not good, because of poor penetration of chemotherapeutic agents into the CSF.

*Lymphoma of the skin* is rare in cats and varies in its presentation. Five cases were reported by Holzworth (1960a): two took the form of multiple nodules in the skin or in the subcutis and muscles; another, large areas of thickened, inflamed skin; another, a solitary thickness over one elbow; and the fifth, a diffuse growth involving the skin and subcutis of an entire forepaw. In four cases the tumors were of histiocytic type, and in all, tumor was present elsewhere in the body at the time of diagnosis or at the time of death.

Caciolo (1984) reported on nine cats with cutaneous lymphoma. The mean age was 11 years. The eight cats tested for FeLV tested negative. Five cats had single masses that recurred rapidly after excision, evidence that even solitary lymphoma must be treated as a systemic disease with chemotherapy. One cat had mycosis fungoides, a T-cell tumor characterized by the formation of lymphocytic epidermal microabscesses (Pautrier's abscesses) and often grossly resembling an inflammatory skin disease.

The *larynx* is occasionally the site of lymphoma. In three cases reported by Holzworth (1960a) early signs were inability to mew and a rattly purr; later, stridor developed and finally cyanosis and open-mouth breathing. Indirect laryngeal involvement was described in a cat in which inspiratory dyspnea developed over five months and progressed to stridor, together with dysphagia (Schaer et al., 1979). Autopsy disclosed lymphoma involving the right vagus nerve, leading to laryngeal hemiplegia, and impairing the swallowing process.

*Lymphoma of nasal passages and sinuses* may be diagnosed when treatment for presumed respiratory infection has been futile or when tumor deforms the nose by invasion and destruction of the nasal bones. To make an early diagnosis, one must obtain material with a small curet or nasal wash or perform an open biopsy of the nasal cavity. Differential diagnoses in addition to bacterial and viral rhinitis include cryptococcosis, nasopharyngeal inflammatory polyp, and other tumors.

*Retrobulbar lymphomas* (Fig. 16–13), sometimes associated with nasal tumors, are usually unilateral. The differential considerations include retrobulbar abscess and glaucoma. In a case reported by Holzworth (1960a) infiltration of both orbits was associated with lymphoblastic leukemia.

*Ocular lymphoma* most often takes the form of tumorous infiltration of the uvea and must be differentiated from the uveitis of toxoplasmosis and feline infectious peritonitis by serologic testing or by keratocentesis and demonstration of lymphoblasts. Two cases in Siamese cats were characterized by discrete white lesions in the anterior uvea (Carlton, 1976). Glaucoma may occur secondary to blockage of the drainage angle by intraocular lymphoma.

*Osseous lymphoma* is rare but has been described by Ott (1983) as causing lytic lesions and new bone formation associated with clinical signs of pain and lameness. Lymphoma involving the tarsi was diagnosed by impression smears and biopsy in a cat with a history of chronic polyarthritis (Barclay, 1979). Both joints were enlarged, with radiologic evidence of lytic bone lesions as well as soft tissue swelling.

In addition to the sites discussed, lymphoma can invade almost any organ. Others in which lymphoma has been

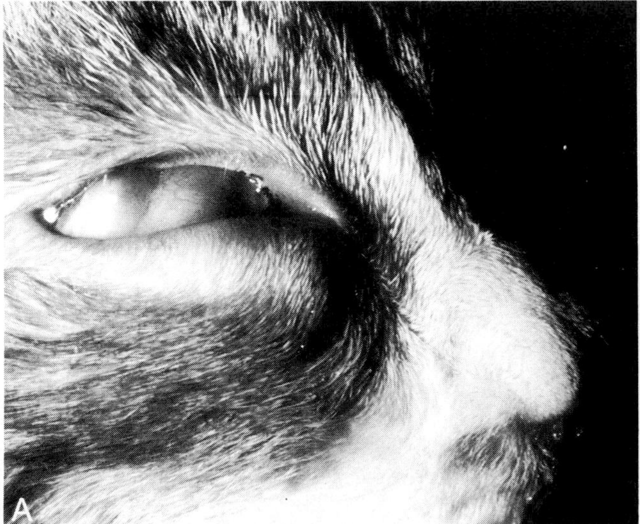


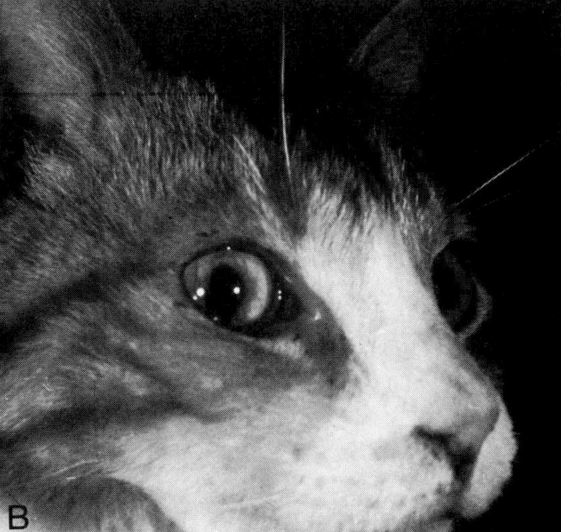


**Figure 16–13** *A*, Retrobulbar lymphoma in a five-year-old domestic castrated male cat with invasion of the right frontal sinus and nasal cavity. The right eye bulges, the third eyelid is prolapsed, and there is discharge from the right nostril. The diagnosis was established by biopsy below the right eye. *B*, The same cat in complete remission after four months of chemotherapy.

observed are the brain, lip, gum, tongue, tonsils, salivary glands, esophagus, heart, trachea, lung, ovary, uterus, urinary bladder, gallbladder, pancreas, adrenals, and thyroid (Holzworth, 1960a; Holzworth, personal comment).

Solid lymphoid tumors are also discussed in the chapter on tumors.

Hematologic findings associated with solid lymphoid tumors are most thoroughly discussed by Hardy (1981). With some tumors, especially solitary ones, the blood picture may be normal. Total white-cell counts may be elevated, normal, or decreased. Anemia, if present, is usually nonregenerative. In some cases anemia or leukopenia may result from myelosuppression in FeLV-positive cats or from infiltration of the marrow by neoplastic cells. Rarely anemia may result from blood loss from an intestinal tumor, from thrombocytopenia, or from hemolysis.

In some cats neoplastic lymphocytes from the solid tumor enter the blood and marrow. In Hardy's experience (1981) this occurred in 27 per cent of cats, while at the University of California it was observed in 62 per cent (Theilen and Madewell, 1979). The neoplastic cells may be so few that they are found only on careful inspection of blood and marrow films, or they may be so numerous as to create a frankly leukemic blood picture.

One must guard against overinterpretation of circulating atypical and immature lymphocytes in cats. Many sick cats with no evidence of neoplasia have atypical or reactive lymphocytes produced in response to some infection or other antigenic stimulus. As recovery occurs these cells disappear from the circulation. For this reason, the presence of atypical or immature lymphocytes in the circulation should simply be monitored if other signs of neoplasia are not present. A bone marrow aspirate should be done in the presence of nonregenerative anemia or any other signs suggestive of hematopoietic neoplasia.

## Lymphocytic Leukemia

Leukemia may be defined as a malignant proliferation of hematopoietic cells and their precursors in the bone marrow and blood. Manifestations in the blood vary tremendously from large numbers of blasts to severe leukopenia. Anemia is the most consistent clinical sign. Anemia, infections, and bleeding tendencies reflect the loss of normal erythroid, granulocytic, or megakaryocytic precursors rather than the presence of the leukemic cells.

Lymphocytic leukemias have been variously reported to constitute from less than 3 per cent to over 40 per cent of the lymphoproliferative malignancies of cats (Essex et al., 1975b; Francis et al., 1979; Holzworth, 1960a; Priester and McKay, 1980; Schalm et al., 1975; Theilen and Madewell, 1979).

Seventy-seven (42 per cent) of 184 cases of spontaneous feline lymphocytic malignancies recorded at AMAH from 1972 to 1976 were characterized as lymphoblastic (poorly differentiated lymphocytic) leukemia with primary involvement of the bone marrow and blood and no clinically detectable solid tumors (Francis et al., 1979). Similarities between feline lymphoblastic leukemia and childhood acute lymphoblastic leukemia are encountered in clinical findings, laboratory data, and response to treatment (Cotter and Essex, 1977). The T-cell form of human lymphoblastic leukemia represents about 20 per cent of all cases and is the most resistant to therapy (Sallan et al., 1980). In the cat the great majority of cases are of T-cell origin—a circumstance that may account for the generally poor prognosis for treatment. Thrombocytopenia is less frequent in feline than in human leukemia.

Presenting clinical signs in leukemic cats are often identical to those in cats with nonregenerative anemias: lethargy and anorexia, sometimes with weight loss and fever. Physical findings are often limited to pallor, sometimes with splenomegaly and hepatomegaly (Fig. 16–14). Confusion may arise when a cat is presented for fever and infections such as stomatitis, infected wounds, or upper respiratory infection. A diagnosis of leukemia may be made only after the cat fails to respond to antibiotic therapy.

Because of the high prevalence of FeLV-related diseases, an FeLV determination along with a CBC is indicated in any cat with severe, atypical, or chronic infection or fever of unknown origin. Although such infections are frequent in nonleukemic, FeLV-positive cats because of the immunosuppressive nature of the virus, they are even more likely in the leukemic cat because the blast cells cannot function as normal lymphocytes in the immune response, and granulocytopenia, secondary to marrow infiltration, further compromises the cat's ability to resist infection. The possibility of leukemia must also be considered in every cat with nonregenerative anemia, and a bone marrow aspirate is often necessary to establish the diagnosis.

The majority of cats with lymphocytic leukemia have normal or low white-cell counts, but extreme leukocytosis may occur, with large numbers of blast cells (Cotter and Essex, 1977). In cats with leukopenia a relative lymphocytosis may be present with or without blast cells. One cannot make a diagnosis of leukemia from blood alone in this situation, because transient neutropenia with atypical lymphocytes may occur in some infections, as in the recovery phase of panleukopenia. A bone marrow aspirate is the only way to ascertain which of these conditions is present.

Neoplastic infiltration of the marrow is characterized in some cats by solid fields of lymphoblasts and in others by cells of varying size ranging from mature lymphocytes to blasts. These blast cells, 15 to 20 $\mu$ in size, are larger than mature lymphocytes and contain a round or slightly indented nucleus with a high nucleus-to-cytoplasm ratio (Plate 16–2*G* and *H*). The nucleus is usually eccentric with a finely stippled chromatin pattern. One or more faint nucleoli are usually present.

Terminal deoxynucleotidyl transferase (TdT), an intracellular protein characteristic of some primitive lymphocytes (Bollum, 1979), is present in most cases of human lymphoblastic malignancies and absent in most cases of granulocytic leukemia. Testing for this protein was done in two dogs and three cats at AMAH. The protein was present in both dogs and two cats with lymphoproliferative malignancy and absent in one cat with granulocytic leukemia (McCaffrey et al., 1980). The differentiation of granulocytic and lymphocytic leukemia can be important, as the prognosis is better for lymphocytic leukemia.

Untreated leukemia in cats usually causes death within a month of diagnosis, because of infection or complications of anemia. The onset may be insidious, with a bone marrow aspirate showing only a slight increase in lymphocytes with a few blast cells. By contrast, cats with aplastic anemia but not leukemia may have a hypocellular marrow with the small lymphocyte as the predominant cell. In

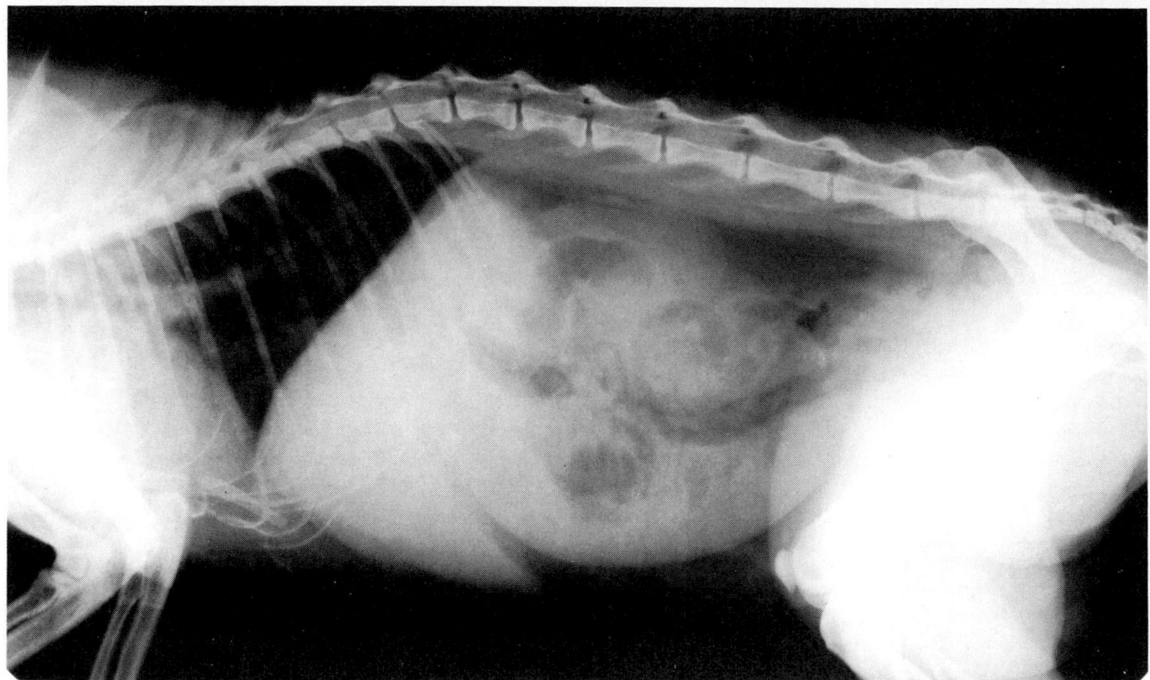

**Figure 16–14** Lymphoblastic leukemia. Lateral radiograph of a four-year-old castrated male cat. The enlarged liver is visible caudal to the rib cage, and the spleen occupies the floor of the abdomen.

these cats, lymphocytes remain normal, while depression of erythroid and myeloid lines results in a relative but not absolute lymphocytosis. With equivocal leukemia or hypocellular marrow, supportive treatment should be given and blood and marrow examinations repeated in two or three weeks. If leukemia is developing, the number of blast cells and degree of abnormality of the lymphocytes would be expected to increase. There is evidence in man that leukemic cells may suppress normal granulocytic stem cells by some factor in addition to mechanical crowding, so that normal hematopoiesis may be depressed before malignant infiltration of the marrow occurs (Broxmeyer et al., 1978). Although this phenomenon is not documented in cats, such a mechanism could account for some hypocellular marrow aspirates in cats with lymphoblastic leukemia. Leukemia is more difficult to treat than lymphoma, because aggressive use of myelosuppressive drugs may be impossible owing to coexisting granulocytopenia and thrombocytopenia.

Rare cases of chronic (well-differentiated) lymphocytic leukemia have been observed in the cat (Fig. 16–15). One case reported by Holzworth (1960a) and two additional cases, also at AMAH in elderly castrated male cats, were characterized by lymphocytosis consisting entirely of small mature lymphocytes. The white-cell counts ranged from 52,000/μl to 257,000/μl. Packed-cell volumes ranged from 12 to 30 per cent. One cat, treated with prednisone alone, achieved a remission of several months. The second, treated with vincristine and prednisone, failed to respond and was destroyed three weeks later. The third, treated with chlorambucil and prednisone, survived in partial remission for 11 months after diagnosis. Chronic lymphocytic leukemia was also described in an 11-year-old spayed female treated with prednisone and still alive after six months, when it was lost to follow-up (Thrall, 1981). In man, the dog, and probably the cat, the prognosis for long-term survival is better in lymphocytic than in lymphoblastic leukemia.

## Treatment of Lymphoproliferative Malignancy

When a diagnosis of lymphoma or leukemia is established, the decision to treat a cat depends on the owner's wishes and factors governing prognosis. Favorable indicators are normal bone marrow with adequate red cells, granulocytes, and platelets, good general physical condition, localized disease, and the absence of fever or other signs of infection. Feline lymphoproliferative malignancies are quite responsive to chemotherapy. A brief outline of treatment is given here, but more detailed recommendations are available in the chapter on management of neoplasms and in other sources (Cotter, 1977, 1983; Pedersen and Madewell, 1980; Theilen and Madewell, 1979). The most detailed discussion is that of Loar (1984).

Cats selected for treatment should be those in which the disease has not progressed to severe debility. Combinations of agents acting differently on the malignant cell are more effective than single agents. Maximum tolerable doses are most likely to produce complete and sustained remissions. Prednisone (2 mg/kg/day) as a single agent achieved only one complete remission in six cats at AMAH. The protocol of cyclophosphamide, vincristine, and prednisone (COP), shown in Figure 16–16, will produce, in lymphomas, approximately a 70 per cent complete remission rate, with a median duration of five to six months. Twenty per cent of cats are still in remission at one year, and a few surviving over two years may actually be cured. Cats with lymphoblastic leukemia have a lower remission rate (27 per cent) than those with lymphoma.

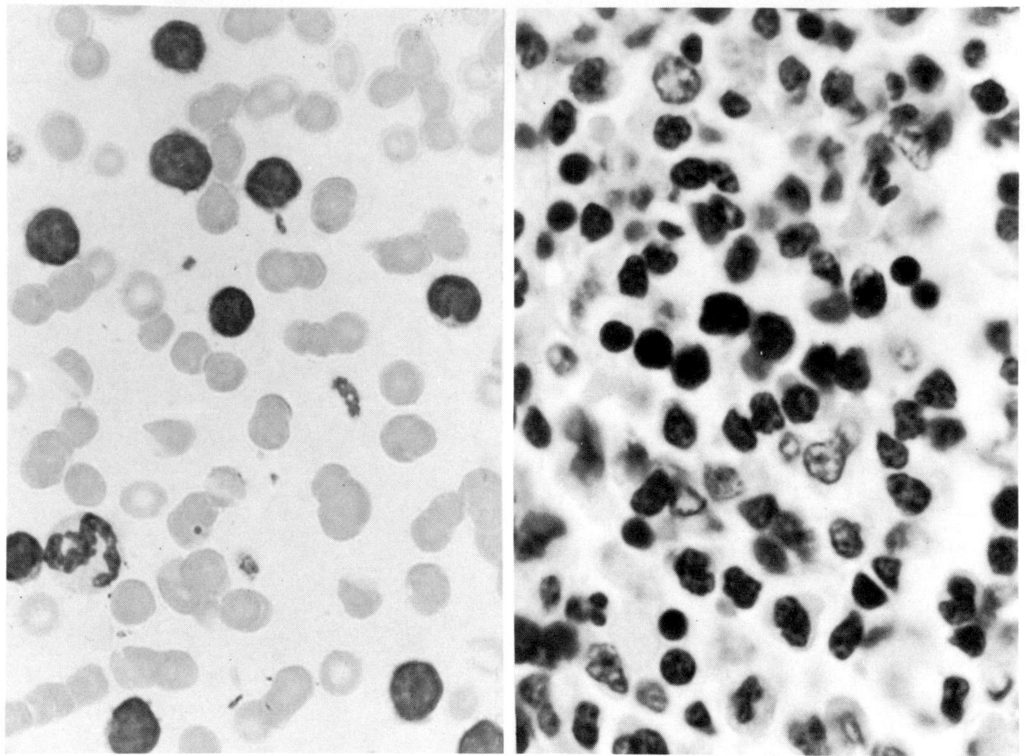

**Figure 16–15** *Left*, Chronic lymphocytic leukemia in the blood of a 12-year-old castrated male. The WBC was 257,000/μl with 86 per cent mature lymphocytes. Wright's, × 950. *Right*, A marrow section from the same cat shows a predominance of small and intermediate lymphocytes. H & E, × 950. (From Holzworth J: J Am Vet Med Assoc 136 [1960] 47–69.)

Once remission is attained, maintenance therapy is necessary to prevent rapid relapse. In seven cats in which treatment was stopped after day 22, the median duration of complete remission was only 43 days after cessation of treatment (Cotter et al., 1980).

Before chemotherapy is started, the diagnosis of lymphoproliferative neoplasm must be confirmed by biopsy of a tumor, cytologic study of malignant effusion, or, in a leukemia, by blood and usually bone marrow examination. A pretreatment CBC, urinalysis, and chemistry profile should also be done. Any coexisting infection must be treated intensively, before chemotherapy if possible, or at least concurrently. Chemotherapy should not be delayed more than a few days to treat infection. Prophylactic antibiotics do not seem to be of value in preventing infections.

Vincristine is minimally myelosuppressive and is given on days 1, 8, 15, and 22, regardless of the granulocyte count. Daily prednisone is started on day 1 as well. Cyclophosphamide regularly causes leukopenia and should not be given if the granulocyte count on day 1 is less than 3000/μl. The granulocyte count must be considered rather than the total white-cell count, because cats with lymphocytosis and leukemic cells may have a high total white-cell count, but if granulocyte counts are low before treatment severe neutropenia may follow.

Thrombocytopenia is not common, but cyclophosphamide should be withheld if the platelet count is less than

Treatment of Feline Leukemia with COP

| Drug | Week 1 | 2 | 3 | 4 | 7 | 10 | 13 | 1yr |
|---|---|---|---|---|---|---|---|---|
| Cytoxan 300 mg/m$^2$ P.O. | X | | | X | X | X | X | |
| Oncovin .75 mg/m$^2$ IV | X | X | X | X | X | X | X | |
| Prednisone 1 mg/lb P.O. | ——Daily—— | | | | | | | |

**Figure 16–16** Protocol for treatment of feline lymphoma with cyclophosphamide (Cytoxan, Mead Johnson), vincristine (Oncovin, Lilly), and prednisone. Doses for the first two drugs are given in mg/m$^2$ of body surface. Treatment is continued every three weeks for a year or until relapse.

100,000/μl. After cyclophosphamide is given, the WBC drops to a low point five to seven days later, so the CBC should be repeated on day 7 and the granulocyte count should be at least 1000/μl. If it drops below 1000/μl at any time, the dose of cyclophosphamide should be decreased by 25 per cent when the next dose is due on day 22. The white-cell count begins to rise on day 8 and usually returns to normal by day 14. After day 22, prednisone is continued daily, and vincristine and cyclophosphamide are given every three weeks for a year or until relapse. A CBC is also repeated every three weeks to ensure that the granulocyte count is adequate for treatment with cyclophosphamide.

The major danger of treatment is immunosuppression, so owners must be instructed to watch for signs of infection. Cats seem to be less prone to bacterial sepsis than dogs receiving the same treatment. Cystitis from cyclophosphamide, fairly common in man and the dog, is rare in the cat. It is not unusual for cats to lose weight in the first month of treatment, but they usually regain weight after that. Gastrointestinal side effects are rare. Extravasation of vincristine during injection can cause sloughing of skin, but peripheral neuropathies, common in man, are rare in cats. Hair loss is usually limited to loss of whiskers and thinning of hair on the head (Fig. 16–17). Rarely some of the outer hair coat is lost, exposing the soft undercoat.

Cats with lymphoblastic leukemia are more difficult to treat than those with lymphoma, bcause leukemic cats are usually anemic, often neutropenic, and occasionally thrombocytopenic. These cats often require transfusion support, as the marrow must be cleared of blasts before normal hematopoietic cells can repopulate. For this reason granulocyte and red-cell numbers may not begin to rise for two or three weeks after the start of treatment. Because of minimal granulocyte reserves, infection is a constant danger. Treatment of leukemia is the same as for lymphoma, except that cyclophosphamide may have to be omitted initially because of granulocytopenia. If granulocyte numbers increase, cyclophosphamide may then be given on day 22. Because of these difficulties, remission is difficult to achieve, and some cats may remain anemic and neutropenic and require transfusions periodically. If they do achieve complete remission, the duration of remission seems to be comparable to that of cats with lymphoma.

## Vaccination for FeLV

In 1985 vaccine to protect against FeLV became commercially available (Leukocell, Norden). It is produced from the supernatant of a malignant lymphoblast cell line that expresses all three subtypes of FeLV. The virus is inactivated, and the vaccine consists of soluble viral and cellular antigens including gp70, virus core proteins, p15e, and FOCMA. The immune response to the vaccine is protective in some cats, but the protection is not absolute.

Efficacy studies were performed with 25 vaccinated cats and 10 control (unvaccinated) cats that were immunosuppressed and exposed intranasally to purified virus. Both vaccinates and controls became viremic (FeLV-positive) after challenge, five of the vaccinates remaining so and eventually dying. Seven of the 10 unvaccinated cats also died. The vaccine thus appeared to be about 80 per cent effective.

It is claimed that the vaccine does not interfere with simultaneous vaccinations against panleukopenia, upper respiratory viral infections, and rabies, and also that it does not affect hematologic values or weight gain in kittens vaccinated at as young as six weeks of age.

The vaccine is of no value when administered to cats already FeLV-positive, but neither does it harm them. Preliminary testing would identify viremic cats for which vaccination would serve no useful purpose.

Clinical trials with about 1000 cats indicated the likely incidence of unfavorable reactions (9.0 per cent, local pain from the IM injection; 3.6 per cent, fever, lethargy, inappetence for about a day; 0.4 per cent, hypersensitivity reactions such as vomiting, diarrhea, swelling of the face or feet, erythema; and 0.2 per cent, miscellaneous reactions such as diarrhea or seizure later than 24 hours after vaccination and abortion in one queen). Most reactions occurred with the first vaccination, and some cats were revaccinated without ill effect. Because a few severe

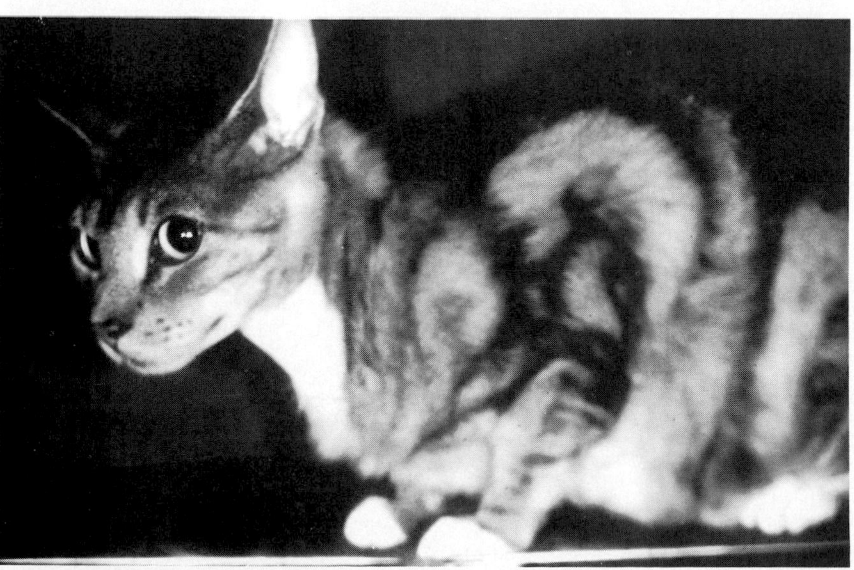

**Figure 16–17** Lymphoma of peripheral lymph nodes. A three-year-old castrated male cat in remission after a year of chemotherapy (cyclophosphamide, vincristine, prednisone). Hair loss is not significant, but the whiskers are lost and hair on head and feet is thinned.

reactions have occurred immediately after administration of the vaccine (e.g., at AMAH), it is advisable to detain vaccinated animals in the clinic waiting room for about half an hour in case emergency treatment is required.

Treatment found highly effective at AMAH for acute postvaccinal reactions is epinephrine 0.5 ml (total dose) of a 1:10,000 solution by IV or deep IM injection, together with diphenhydramine HCl (Benadryl) 0.5 ml/lb IM. The epinephrine solution *must* be made up fresh. This treatment may be followed by intravenous administration of lactated Ringer's or saline-dextrose solution to combat shock.

No information is available about efficacy of the vaccination for previously exposed cats that are FeLV-negative but may harbor latent focal infection. Vaccination should not replace testing of new cats to be introduced into catteries and multiple-cat households, and previous vaccination does not ensure that a cat is not infected.

It is recommended, although not required, that cats be tested for FeLV and vaccinated only if negative. A second vaccine is given three weeks later and a third two to four months later, with one annual booster. Vaccination would appear to be indicated principally for cats with risk of exposure (i.e., outdoor cats and those in catteries and multiple-cat households).

Neither the IFA nor the ELISA test is affected by vaccination; however, as when other vaccines are given to cats, there may for a time be a false positive coronavirus test result.

Independent studies evaluating the vaccine for immunogenicity and efficacy have raised some question as to the degree of its effectiveness (Pedersen et al., 1985). Few of the cats vaccinated, whether with two or three doses, developed virus-neutralizing antibody, and immunity to challenge with virulent virus, in cats given three vaccinations, was less than the 80 per cent protection claimed for the product.

## Myeloproliferative Neoplasia

The term myeloproliferative has been applied to abnormal proliferations of the various cell lines of the bone marrow. These disorders are less prevalent in the cat than are lymphoma and lymphocytic leukemia. Reticuloendotheliosis, as described by Gilmore and associates in 1964, is characterized by the most primitive cell type of the group. Abnormal proliferation of the red-cell series takes the form of erythremic myelosis, erythroleukemia, and polycythemia vera. The white-cell lines are involved in granulocytic, monocytic, and myelomonocytic leukemia. Platelet precursors are involved in megakaryocytic leukemia. Occasionally the myeloproliferative disorders terminate in myelofibrosis or rarely in osteosclerosis. Some myeloproliferative disorders are impossible to categorize as to cell of origin by routine means, and indeed constituted the largest proportion within the group as a whole according to tabulations from New York City (Hardy, 1981) and the University of California (Theilen and Madewell, 1979).

About 70 to 90 per cent of cats with myeloproliferative diseases test positive for FeLV (Cotter et al., 1975; Theilen and Madewell, 1979). A more recent study by Hardy (1981) found all of 50 cats positive except for four with eosinophilic leukemia. In addition, feline oncornavirus–associated cell–membrane antigen (FOCMA), an antigen found on tumor cells transformed by FeLV (Essex et al., 1977; Hardy et al., 1977), has been observed on the surface of cells from cats with erythrocytic, granulocytic, and megakaryocytic leukemia, as well as lymphoblastic leukemia and lymphoma (Hardy et al., 1977).

It is of interest, however, that only two cases of myeloproliferative neoplasia have been induced experimentally by FeLV: a myeloid leukemia (Jarrett et al., 1971) and an eosinophilic leukemia induced by the Rickard strain (Lewis et al., 1985; Olsen et al., 1983). It has therefore been questioned whether all types of myeloproliferative disease are caused by the feline leukemia virus (Prasse, 1983), and it has been suggested that a strain of virus that induces only myeloproliferative disease is still to be sought (Theilen and Madewell, 1979).

The FeLV status of the four cases of polycythemia vera at the University of California was not recorded (Theilen and Madewell, 1979); perhaps, like that of Reed et al. (1970), these cases antedated the availability of FeLV-testing.

Although some cases of feline lymphoblastic leukemia appear to evolve into leukemia of another cell type, this phenomenon is more frequent in the myeloproliferative malignancies, probably because of involvement of a stem cell that gives rise to myeloblasts, rubriblasts, or megakaryoblasts after lymphoid stem cells have evolved along a separate pathway. Thus progression from erythroleukemia to granulocytic leukemia was reported by Schalm (1978a) (Plate 16–3*D* and *E*), and a malignancy involving only the erythrocytic cell line changed to a regenerative anemia and terminated 65 days later as reticuloendotheliosis (Harvey et al., 1978).

Feline myeloproliferative disorders may also be characterized by concurrent abnormalities in more than one cell series. For example, megaloblastic dysplasia of erythrocytic precursors is frequent in cats with granulocytic leukemia. Although, at this time, there does not seem to be a prognostic or therapeutic advantage in differentiating the individual disorders, eventually there may prove to be some value in defining them as exactly as possible.

As with most cases of lymphocytic malignancy, the time of onset of myeloproliferative neoplasms may be uncertain. They are even more likely to be associated with preleukemic abnormalities such as anemias, cytopenias, atypical granulocytes and lymphocytes, large bizarre platelets sometimes with vacuoles, and leuko-erythroblastic reactions characterized by circulating immature granulocytes and nucleated red cells in the absence of reticulocytosis.

Clinical signs in a number of myeloproliferative disorders were described by Holzworth (1960b). Weakness, inappetence, pallor, and cardiac murmurs are present as with anemias of other causes. Other signs are fever, frequent infections, and sometimes bleeding due to thrombocytopenia. Splenomegaly is perhaps more frequent in myeloproliferative disorders than in lymphocytic leukemia owing partly to greater infiltration with malignant cells, but even more to severe myeloid metaplasia (extramedullary hematopoiesis), which may be so severe as to infiltrate the spleen and liver at the expense of normal cells. The lymph nodes are sometimes moderately enlarged. Solid tumors are uncommon in myeloproliferative disorders. Increased stainable iron has been reported in the marrow probably from ineffective erythropoiesis (Harvey, 1981).

In addition to difficulties in making the diagnosis, the natural history of the disorder may be confusing (Madewell et al., 1979). Schalm (1973) reported on a cat with myeloproliferative disease that underwent a spontaneous remission for two years before relapse. Cats responding to anemia or leukopenia may produce bizarre cells of both erythrocytic and granulocytic cell lines that may resemble those of myeloproliferative disorders. If a question exists as to the presence of a malignancy at the time of marrow examination, another aspirate should be examined in two or three weeks. The hematologic features of the myeloproliferative disorders are discussed in detail in *Veterinary Hematology* (Schalm et al., 1975), and the numerous excellent illustrations are an invaluable aid in diagnosis.

## Reticuloendotheliosis

The term reticuloendotheliosis was proposed by Gilmore et al (1964) to designate a disorder characterized by proliferation of undifferentiated cells appearing in the blood but, unlike those of other hematopoietic neoplasms, limited in distribution elsewhere to organs of the reticuloendothelial system. Because the abnormal cells lacked features identifying them as specific hematopoietic cells, they were classified as reticulum or reticuloendothelial cells. Since the first report from AMAH, many more cases have been diagnosed there, and this disorder has been recognized in significant numbers elsewhere in the United States (see references in Prasse, 1983; Schalm et al., 1975; Theilen and Madewell, 1979).

In the 10 cases reported by Gilmore et al. (1964), the cats, eight males and two females, were aged from one to nine years, all but two being from one to three years old. Signs of illness were inappetence, listlessness, weight loss, fever, pallor, and splenomegaly. Liver and lymph nodes were mildly enlarged in some cats. All treatment, including blood transfusion, was ineffective, and the cats deteriorated progressively, most dying or being destroyed within two weeks.

Anemia was severe. Nucleated red cells (rubricytes and metarubricytes) were present in the blood of all but two cats. Total WBC ranged from 6000 to 53,000/μl. The abnormal cells constituted up to 55 per cent (average 23) of the circulating white cells, and 16 to 77 per cent (average 50) of the same cells were found in the marrow.

The abnormal cells were round and ranged from 12 to 16 μ in diameter. The nuclei, large, round, and sometimes eccentric, occupied most of the cell and usually stained medium red-purple. The chromatin took the form of a five woven mesh and was rarely clumped. A large, pale blue nucleolus was usually visible. The cytoplasm was finely stippled and stained medium blue. Variable numbers of fine azurophilic granules were usually clumped or scattered in the cytoplasm, and a pale Golgi body was often present next to the nucleus (Plate 16–2*I*). The authors concluded that there was no evidence of progressive maturation along any cell line.

Other observers have described round or oval cells as large as 20 μ (Nielsen, 1969). Sometimes the cytoplasm is elongated into pseudopodium-like projections that may be pinched off into irregular structures resembling platelets (Schalm et al., 1975).

In spleen, liver, and lymph nodes the abnormal cells were described by Gilmore et al. (1964) as infiltrating vascular spaces, appearing as discrete round cells of nearly uniform size and staining character, never forming solid masses or invading surrounding tissues—behavior considered by some pathologists to be characteristic of this disorder. Extramedullary hematopoiesis evidenced by megakaryocytes and immature erythrocytes and granulocytes was present in those organs.

Very rarely lymphoma may occur concurrently with reticuloendotheliosis. A cat at AMAH also had lymphoma of the kidneys, and a small lymphoma of the cranial mediastinum was found in a case reported by Ward et al. (1969).

A consensus is lacking as to the nature of the primitive cell of reticuloendotheliosis. Like Gilmore et al. (1964), some observers have seen no evidence of differentiation to mature hematopoietic cells of any type (Blue, 1983; Carpenter, 1984; Nielsen, 1969). Loeb (1975) suggested that the cell was probably pluripotential, with differentiation in some cases toward monocytic, plasmacytic, lymphocytic, or erythropoietic forms, while Schalm et al. (1975) noted features of erythroid and granulocytic precursors.

That the cell is a precursor of the erythroid line was suggested by Ward et al. (1969), and Hurvitz (1970) reported that electron-microscopic examination of blood and marrow from two cats revealed surface features and chromatin patterns characteristic of erythroid cells. In humans, chromosomal abnormalities are often associated with hematopoietic neoplasia, but in examination of cells from the same two cats no cytogenetic abnormalities were found (Ripps and Hurwitz, 1971).

Harvey et al. (1978) reported on a cat with a myeloproliferative disorder in which the malignant cell appeared terminally to be that of reticuloendotheliosis. The cat initially had nonregenerative anemia (PCV 17) with many nucleated red cells from rubriblasts to metarubricytes, and a diagnosis of erythremic myelosis was considered. Two weeks later the peripheral blood picture was that of regenerative anemia, but the PCV was only 9.5; the marrow contained all maturation stages of both erythroid and myeloid series, and atypical rubriblasts suggested continued myeloproliferative disease. Without treatment the cat improved clinically and the PCV reached 30, but two months after initial examination it relapsed with anemia characterized by many circulating nucleated red cells (mostly metarubricytes, some binucleated) but with no polychromasia. One fourth of the nucleated cells in the circulation contained single or double nucleoli and fitted the description of those of reticuloendotheliosis. Similar blast cells were abundant in the marrow. Asynchronous maturation of cytoplasm and nucleus was evident in some. Abnormal binucleated rubricytes varied in size. All cell stages of the myeloid series were present but constituted only a small percentage of the total nucleated cells. At autopsy microscopic findings were similar to those reported by Gilmore et al. (1964). In addition, erythrophagocytosis was present in lymph nodes. It was concluded that the progression of disease in this case supported the hypothesis that most of the undifferentiated cells of feline reticuloendotheliosis are primitive erythroid precursors.

Until the nature of the cells is definitively established this author (SMC) also will classify feline reticuloendotheliosis with erythroid malignancies for clinical and prognostic purposes.

Because this feline disorder is not the same as human reticuloendotheliosis ("hairy cell" leukemia), other terms have been suggested such as "leukemia of undetermined cell type" (Blue, 1983), "acute erythroleukemia" or "acute erythremic myelosis" (Harvey, 1981), and "blast form of erythremic myelosis" (Prasse, 1983).

## Erythroid Malignancies

Erythremic myelosis and erythroleukemia, counterparts of DiGuglielmo's syndrome first described in man about 60 years ago, appear to have been reported in cats as early as 1940 (Bianchi and Migone) and are apparently being recognized with increasing frequency (e.g., Falconer et al., 1980; Giles, 1974; Gilmore and Holzworth, 1971; Groulade and Guilhon, 1966; Holzworth, 1960b; Maede and Murata, 1980; Saar, 1968; Schalm et al., 1975; Watson et al., 1974; Zawidzka et al., 1964). In recent years they have been the most frequent myeloproliferative neoplasms in cats at AMAH, and a similar predominance was evident in a sampling of New York cats (Hardy, 1981). Clinical signs are similar to those of reticuloendotheliosis.

The characteristic hematologic feature of erythremic myelosis is a neoplastic proliferation of red-cell precursors, which predominate in the bone marrow and appear in varying numbers in the blood (Plate 16–3*A* to *C*; Fig. 16–18). There is anemia without reticulocytosis but usually with circulating nucleated red cells. The malignant cells vary from rubriblasts to metarubricytes, although the less mature erythroid cells usually predominate in the marrow. Blood and marrow findings are described in detail by Schalm et al. (1975). Saar (1968) reported one case in which the erythroid cells were relatively mature. In such cases it can sometimes be difficult to determine whether those cells represent an impending regenerative response to anemia or are evidence of a neoplastic condition. If the nucleated red cells remain without a rise in the reticulocyte count over several days, malignancy is likely.

In erythroleukemia, immature neoplastic cells of the granulocytic series are also present (Plate 16–3*D* and *E*). Both disorders may terminate in granulocytic leukemia or myelofibrosis (Schalm et al., 1975). The distinction between erythremic myelosis and erythroleukemia is sometimes uncertain and not clinically important, as overlapping between the two is frequent. Both are associated with abnormalities in red-cell maturation. Asynchronous nuclear and cytoplasmic maturation and other megaloblastic changes are often present. In the author's (SMC) experience, megaloblastic anemia in the cat is most likely to be associated with hematopoietic malignancy, usually of erythroid origin.

## Polycythemia Vera (Erythremia)

This disorder has in common with erythroid malignancies a proliferation of red cells without the normal control by erythropoietin levels, but it differs in that the proliferating cell appears and functions like a normal mature red cell and there is a high PCV rather than anemia as occurs with all other erythroid malignancies. Although these red cells appear normal, polycythemia vera is a malignancy by definition, as there is an overproduction of a cell line that is not controlled by normal feedback inhibition.

Four cases were recorded in a survey of feline myeloproliferative disorders at the California veterinary school (Theilen and Madewell, 1979). In one case described in detail, a 15-year-old castrated male cat was presented for anorexia and vomiting of pink fluid (Reed et al., 1979). The mucosae were dark red-purple, and the PCV was 73 per cent. The WBC was 33,000/μl and the platelet count 216,000/μl. The plasma volume, oxygen saturation, and red-cell survival time were normal, but increased red-cell mass was demonstrated by a chromium-labeling technique. The cat was not treated, so response could not be evaluated. This appeared to be a case of autonomous overproduction of red cells, since other possible causes of polycythemia, such as dehydration, hypoxia, and renal lesions, were excluded.

## Treatment of Reticuloendotheliosis and Red-Cell Malignancies

Response to treatment of these disorders is at present disappointing. Four cats with reticuloendotheliosis were treated with combinations of cytosine arabinoside and prednisone; one received cyclophosphamide and 6-thioguanine as well (Crow et al., 1977). Although there was some transient improvement, no complete remissions were attained, and the mean survival time was five weeks. In another cat, treatment with cyclophosphamide and prednisone was also unsuccessful (Giles et al., 1974). Response to treatment may be poor, because transformation of malignant stem cells robs the marrow of the ability to repopulate with normal cells of any series.

The experience at AMAH with treatment has also been poor. A conservative approach has given the best results. Transfusions are given when the PCV drops to 10 per cent. Corticosteroids are used with questionable benefit. Three cats with erythroleukemia treated with blood and steroids survived for two, five, and six months, respectively. One was destroyed because of increasing need for transfusion; another developed myelofibrosis. The third cat died acutely of splenic rupture after two months of therapy.

**Plate 16–3** *A*, Erythremic myelosis, marrow. All stages of immature red cells are represented, with erythrophagocytosis by one primitive cell. *B*, Erythremic myelosis, marrow. Polyploidy involving a polychromatophilic rubricyte. *C*, Erythremic myelosis, blood. Variation in size of fully hemoglobinized red cells. *D*, Erythroleukemia, marrow, at a time when megaloblastoid rubricytes were prominent. Asynchronism between cytoplasm and nucleus of one rubricyte is marked. *E*, Erythroleukemia, marrow, same cat 10 days later. A giant rubricyte is at the right border, but granulocytic precursors now predominate, suggesting a shift toward granulocytic leukemia. *F*, Granulocytic leukemia, blood, with a total white-cell count of 369,000/μl. The neoplastic cells are myeloblasts, promyelocytes, and myelocytes. *G*, Granulocytic leukemia, marrow, same cat. Cytoplasmic primary (azurophilic) granules identify many of these cells as promyelocytes. (From Schalm OW, Jain NC, Carroll EJ: Veterinary Hematology. Philadelphia, Lea & Febiger, 1975.)

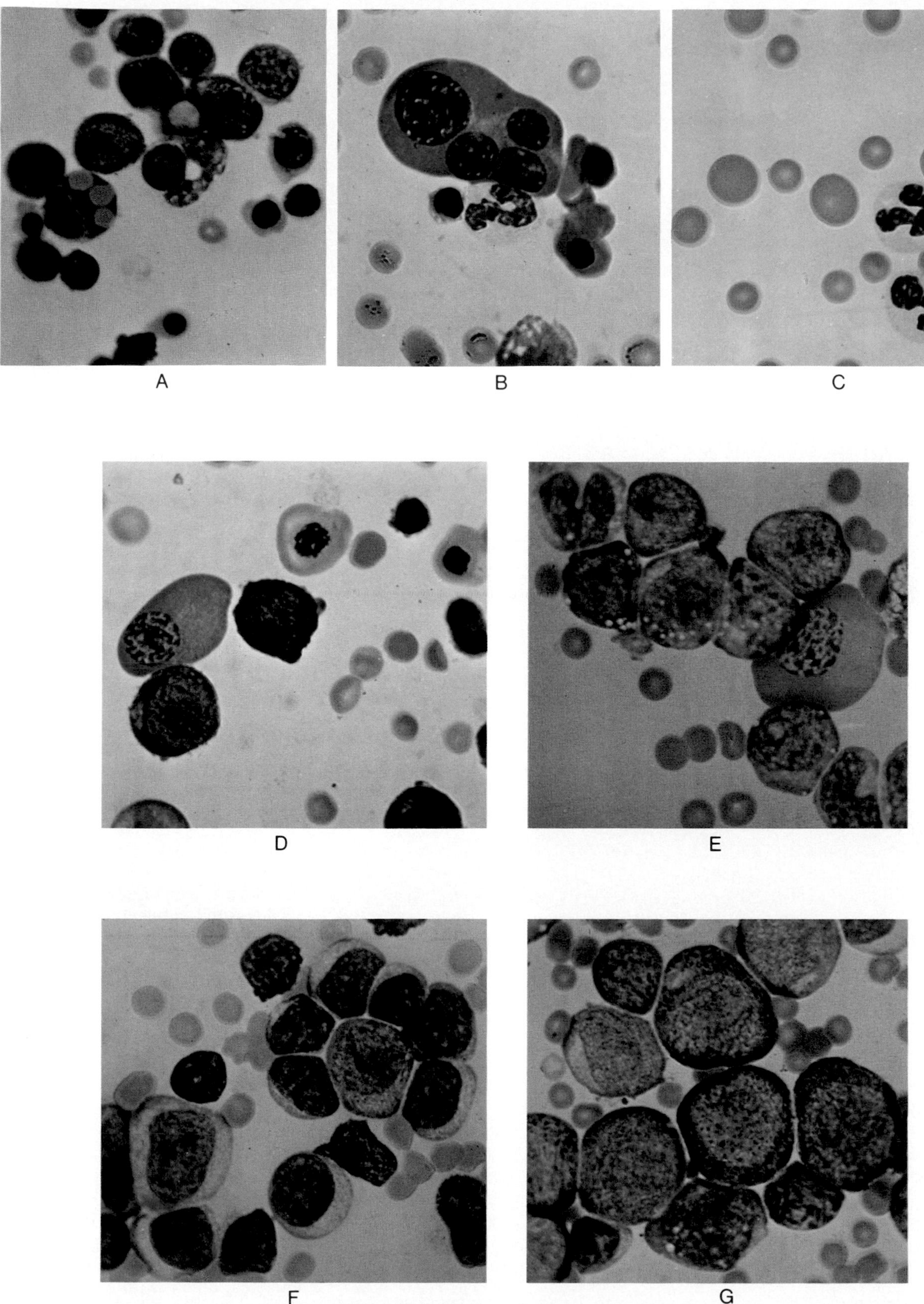


**Plate 16–3** *See legend on opposite page*

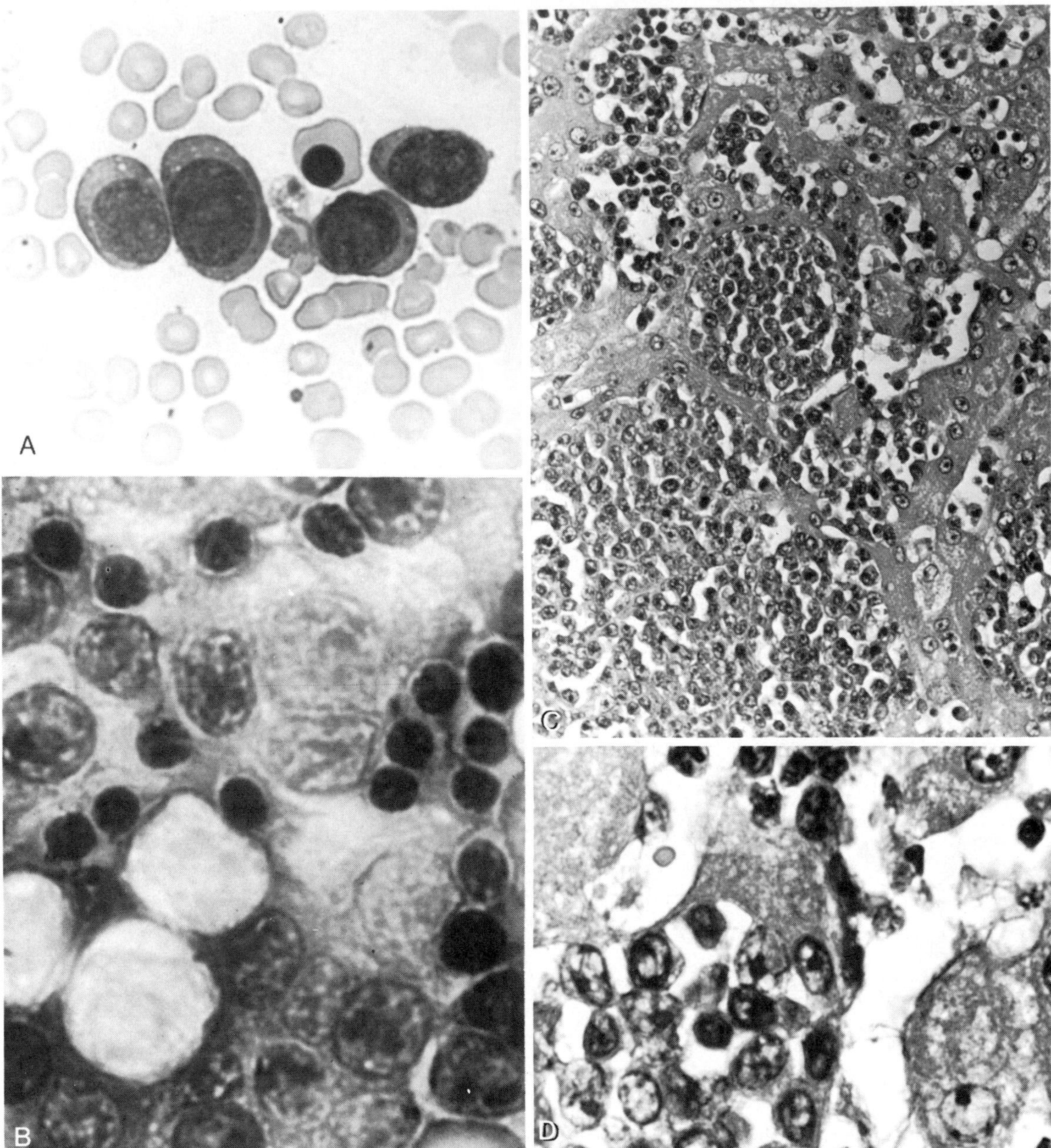

**Figure 16–18** *A*, Erythremic myelosis, blood. Red-cell precursors are represented by the three largest cells—rubriblasts with barely perceptible nucleoli. The slightly smaller cell is a prorubricyte. Above it is a metarubricyte. This cat exhibited no reticulocyte response. Wright-Giemsa, × 1000. *B*, Erythremic myelosis, impression film of marrow from the same cat taken at autopsy. The M:E ratio was 0.2:1. All nucleated cells except the three large pale ones are red-cell precursors. Wright-Giemsa, × 1200. *C*, Liver, same cat. Intrasinusoidal aggregates of primitive red cells are evident at the top of the picture. Larger aggregates (center and lower left) have virtually obliterated the hepatic cords. By contrast, in lymphoma the neoplastic cells characteristically infiltrate portal areas. H & E, × 300. *D*, Liver, same cat. All the dark-staining cells located between the large, pale hepatocytes are primitive red cells. The absence of leukocytic and megakaryocytic forms, as well as absence of red-cell maturation, distinguishes this neoplastic lesion from myeloid metaplasia. H & E, × 900.

Transfusion of cats with erythrocytic malignancy sometimes appears to decrease the number of nucleated red cells in the blood a few days later. It is possible that these malignant red-cell precursors are sensitive to oxygen tension or erythropoietin levels, so that a rise in PCV has some inhibiting effect on their proliferation. Another possibility is that some antibody or antileukemic factor is supplied with the plasma, as remissions in some lymphocytic malignancies have been produced with plasma (Hardy et al., 1976). Folate and $B_{12}$ therapy has been tried because of megaloblastic changes, but no responses were obtained (Hirsch and Dunn, 1983; Ward et al., 1969).

## Granulocytic Leukemia

In total cases recorded at AMAH over many years, granulocytic (myelogenous, myeloid) leukemia has been second in numbers to the lymphoproliferative neoplasms, but in recent years it has been diagnosed relatively less often than reticuloendotheliosis and erythroid malignancies.

Granulocytic leukemia is usually characterized by a predominance of myeloblasts and less often of promyelocytes or myelocytes (Plate 16–3*F* and *G*). The myeloblast can be difficult to distinguish from the lymphoblast but has a finer chromatin pattern, a smaller nucleus-to-cytoplasm ratio, more prominent or multiple nucleoli, and sometimes cytoplasmic granules. Histochemical stains may help to distinguish these granules from the azurophilic granules occasionally found in lymphoblasts. Myeloblast granules often stain with peroxidase, whereas those of lymphoblasts do not. The absence of granules in some cases makes histochemistry less helpful. Auer rods, metachromatic red-purple cytoplasmic inclusions often present in human granulocytic leukemia, are not known to occur in cats.

The age range in reported cases has been from under a year to advanced middle age.

Holzworth (1960b) reported on nine cases of granulocytic leukemia at AMAH. The majority of cats were males. Three were presented with leukopenia, the rest with elevated white-cell counts, the highest 65,000/μl. Anemia was severe in all. The predominant cell in the blood in most cases was the myelocyte rather than the myeloblast. In several cats, circulating nucleated red cells were abundant and sometimes of primitive form. The spleen was consistently enlarged and deep purple, with little or no trace of the lymphoid follicles often seen in lymphoblastic leukemia. Ruptured spleen was the cause of death in one cat. The liver was enlarged in most of the cats but the lymph nodes less so than in lymphocytic leukemia. The marrow was hypercellular, with myeloblasts and myelocytes predominating. Platelets were greatly increased in some cases and decreased in others. One cat bled from the nose and gums and at sites of venepuncture. In another there was hemorrhage in the brain and digestive tract (Fig. 16–19). The liver and lymph nodes were infiltrated to varying degree by neoplastic cells, and foci of neoplastic cells were sometimes observed in kidney, heart, and lung. Rarely, solid tumor formation occurs with granulocytic leukemia. In cats at AMAH masses have been seen in the subcutis and muscles, mouth, epicardium, myocardium, and kidney cortices (Fig. 16–20).

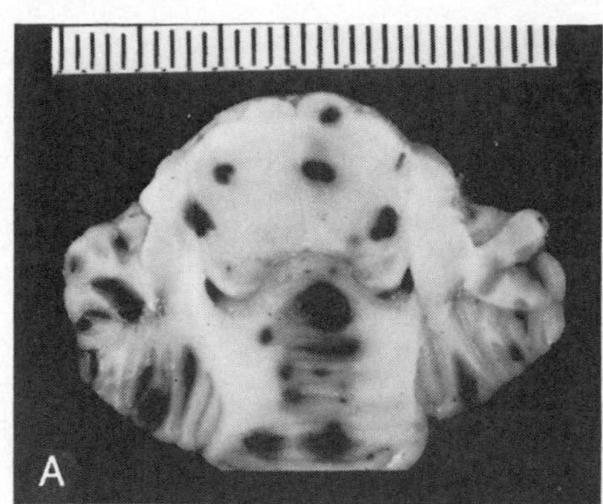


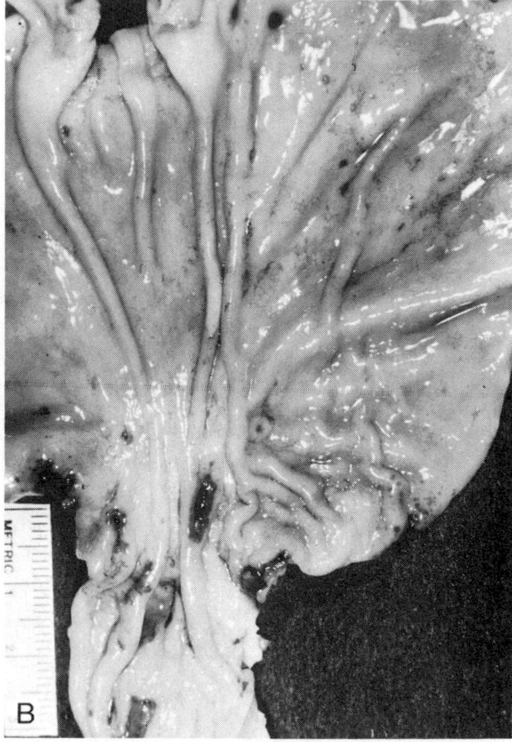


**Figure 16–19** Granulocytic leukemia, nine-year-old castrated male blue-and-white domestic cat. *A*, Small hemorrhages are scattered throughout the brain. *B*, Bleeding ulcers in the stomach and duodenum vary from pinpoint size to almost 1 cm.

Schalm et al. (1975) described 14 cases of granulocytic leukemia. Presentation was similar to that described by Holzworth (1960b). All the cats were anemic, and eight of 14 had elevated white-cell counts with primitive granulocytes in the blood and marrow, one cat having a total WBC of 389,000/μl, of which 90 per cent were myeloblasts, promyelocytes, and myelocytes.

Asynchronous maturation of nucleus and cytoplasm of myeloid cells, with gaps in maturation sequence, is sometimes seen in the marrow. Pelger-Huët cells, characterized by mature granulocytic cytoplasm without lobulation of the nucleus, may occur as well. Leukemic granulocytes are more fragile than normal cells, so that vacuolation or "smudging" may occur with rough handling or storage of blood in EDTA before preparation of blood films (Schalm et al., 1975)—characteristics that may contribute to difficulties in classification of these leukemias.

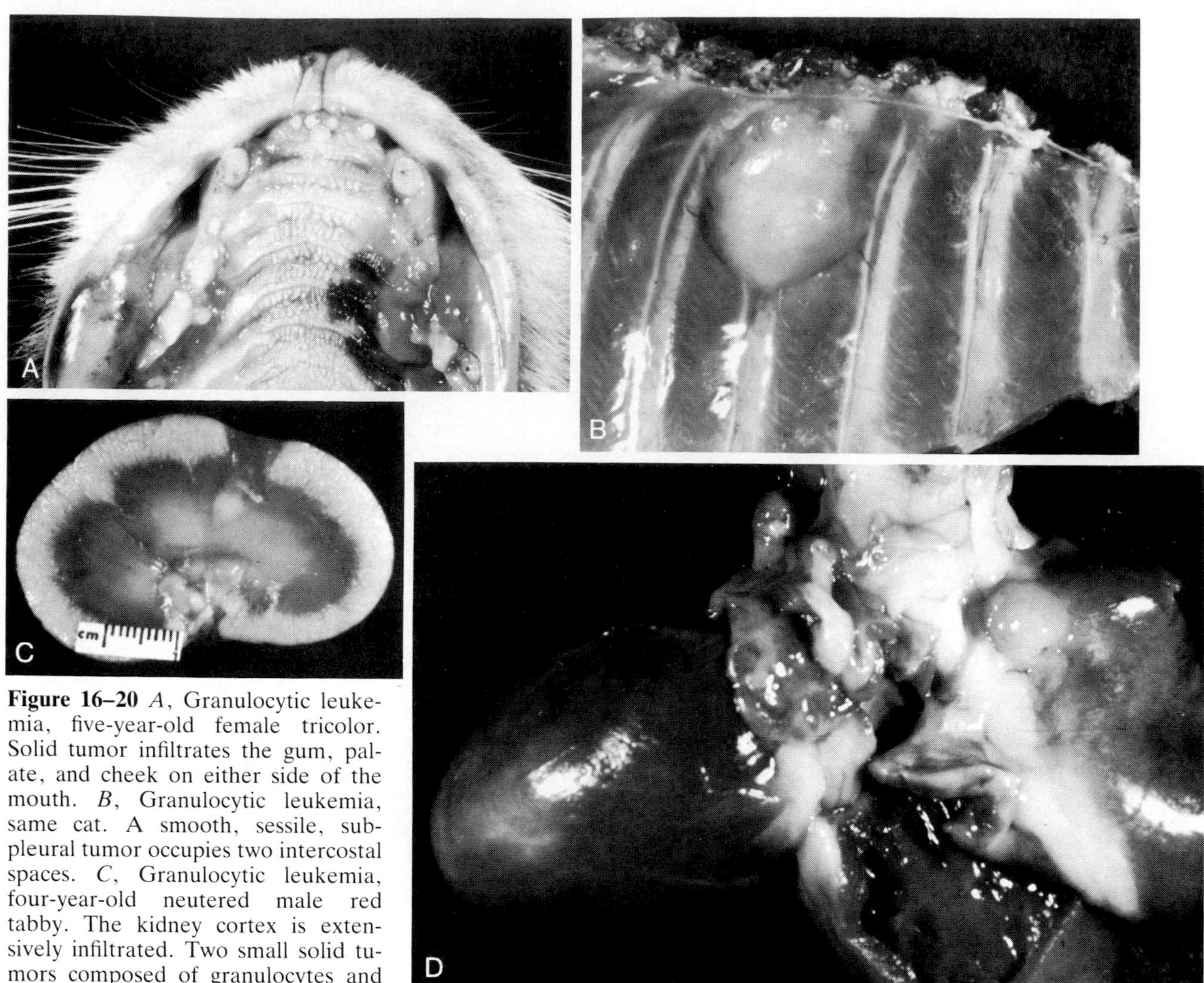


**Figure 16–20** *A*, Granulocytic leukemia, five-year-old female tricolor. Solid tumor infiltrates the gum, palate, and cheek on either side of the mouth. *B*, Granulocytic leukemia, same cat. A smooth, sessile, subpleural tumor occupies two intercostal spaces. *C*, Granulocytic leukemia, four-year-old neutered male red tabby. The kidney cortex is extensively infiltrated. Two small solid tumors composed of granulocytes and megakaryocytes extend into the medulla. One has interfered with circulation, causing an infarct. Similar small tumors in the subcutis and underlying superficial muscle were numerous over the entire body. *D*, Granulocytic leukemia, same cat. A small neoplastic nodule lies below the coronary groove on the right ventricular free wall (upper right). An irregular pale area at the apex of the left ventricle proved to be tumorous infiltration of the epicardial fat and myocardium. Budding viruses (FeLV type) were demonstrated by electron microscopy.

---

**Figure 16–21** Eosinophilic leukemia, four-year-old spayed female domestic shorthair. *A*, Blood. Segmented, band, and metamyelocytic eosinophils are present. Total white-cell count was 89,000/μl, with 83 per cent eosinophils. Wright-Giemsa, × 450. *B*, Marrow. Sixty-seven per cent of the myeloid cells are eosinophils of all stages. The myeloid:erythroid ratio is 14.6. Wright-Giemsa, × 450. *C*, Small intestine. The mucosa and submucosa are infiltrated with eosinophils. The tunica muscularis is greatly hypertrophied, accounting for the ropey thickening noted clinically—a feature also of eosinophilic enteritis. *D*, Kidney. Pale nodules composed of eosinophils bulge above the surface and crowd the cortex. (*A*, *B*, and *D* from Simon N, Holzworth J: Cornell Vet 57 [1967] 579–597.)

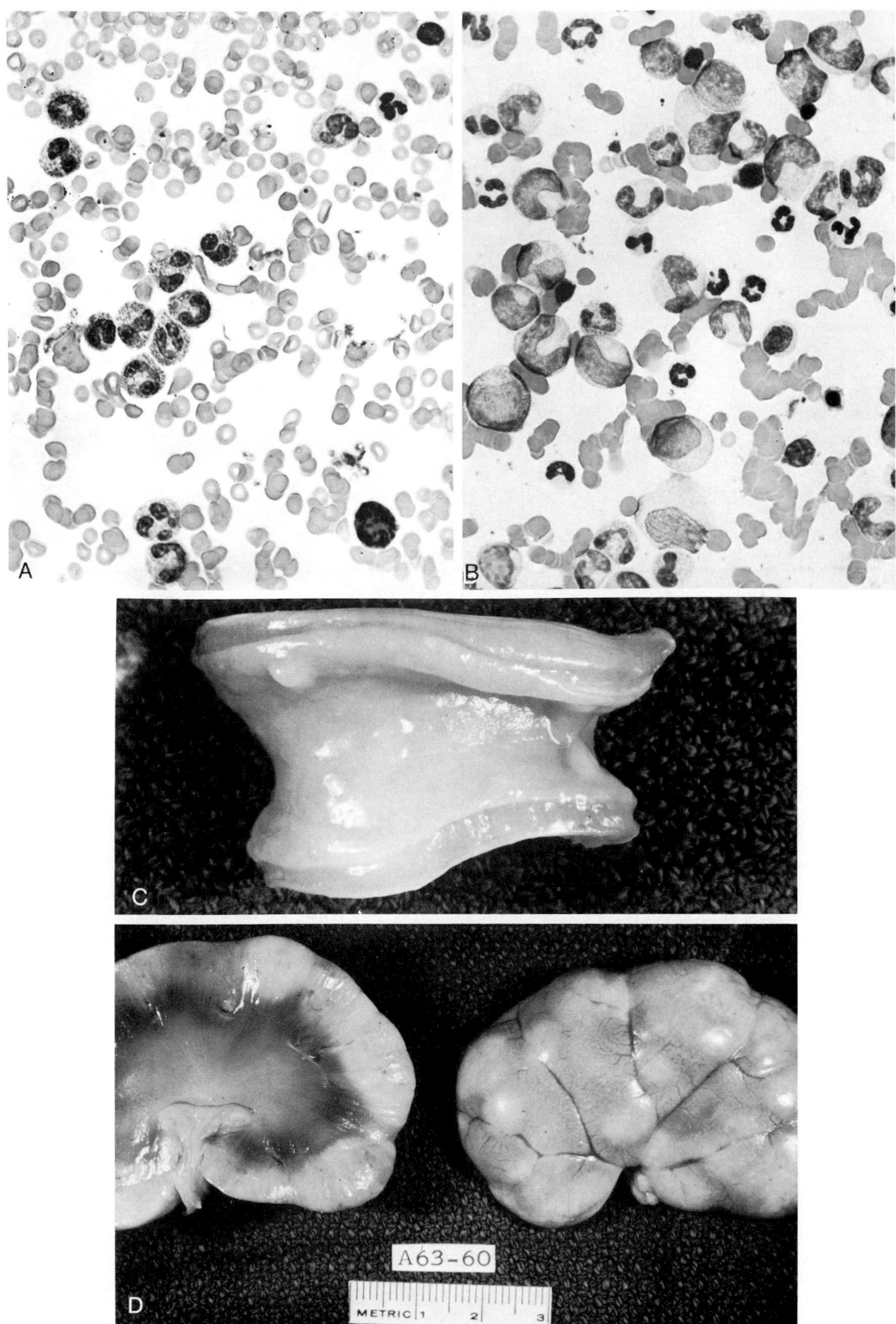


**Figure 16–21** *See legend on opposite page*

In a survey of veterinary colleges of North America, 45 cases of granulocytic leukemia were recorded, 29 in males and 16 in females (Priester and McKay, 1980). Other descriptions of granulocytic leukemia are limited to case reports (e.g., Case, 1979; Eyestone, 1951; Fraser et al., 1974; Gilbride, 1964; Henness and Crow, 1977; Meier and Patterson, 1956; Reid and Marcus, 1966). A case in which granulocytic leukemia was associated with pronounced megakaryocytic proliferation was reported by Sutton et al. (1978).

Chronic granulocytic leukemia as described in man probably occurs rarely if ever in cats. This form is characterized by large numbers of circulating granulocytic cells, most more mature than myelocytes. One cat at AMAH had severe leukocytosis with predominantly mature neutrophils for several months before a diagnosis of granulocytic leukemia was confirmed by increased immature granulocytes in the marrow. Chronic granulocytic leukemia may be difficult to distinguish from a leukemoid reaction to an infection. The latter is characterized by leukocytosis with a shift to immature granulocytes in the blood and marrow. In contrast to leukemia, however, granulocyte maturation remains orderly and the leukemoid reaction is transient. Differentiation between chronic granulocytic leukemia and leukemoid reaction in man is made easier by the presence in leukemic patients of a chromosomal marker (Philadelphia chromosome) and decreased levels of leukocyte alkaline phosphatase, whereas persons with leukemoid reactions have increased leukocyte alkaline phosphatase. The cat, however, lacks the chromosomal marker, and measurable alkaline phosphatase is absent from feline white cells (Atwal and McFarland, 1967).

## Eosinophilic Leukemia

Feline cases of this rare leukemia have been described by Holzworth (1960b), Schalm et al (1975), Silverman (1971), and Simon and Holzworth (1967). Four additional cases were encountered by Hardy (1981) and one by Henness (1984). In none of the spontaneous cases recorded since development of FeLV-testing did the cats test positive. However, in a specific pathogen–free cat inoculated with FeLV (Rickard strain), eosinophilic leukemia developed after a two-year incubation period (Lewis et al., 1985; Olsen et al., 1983). As well as eosinophilic infiltrates in the lung, heart, and intestine, there was an eosinophilic tumor in the cranial mediastinum.

In the easlier discussion of disorders of eosinophils, it was pointed out that in man some cases suggestive of eosinophilic leukemia may not represent true malignancy but rather disseminated eosinophilic disease or hypereosinophilic syndrome, possibly resulting from an overzealous immune response. Such a possibility must be considered in evaluating severe eosinophilias of cats.

In a case of true leukemia one would look for immature forms of the eosinophilic series in blood and marrow, as in the case of Simon and Holzworth (1967), in which myeloblasts and mitotic figures were present, as well as frank tumor formation in the kidneys (Fig. 16–21).

In the case reported by Schalm the initial total white-cell count was 244,000/μl, of which 84 per cent were eosinophils, some of band and metamyelocyte stages. In the marrow over 80 per cent of the white cells were eosinophils, including myelocytes and metamyelocytes.

In a number of non-neoplastic feline disorders characterized by eosinophilia the response to steroid administration is usually favorable, but in the few cases of eosinophilic leukemia treated with steroids there was only a transient response or none at all. Busulfan and vincristine, also tried in a case at AMAH, were likewise ineffective. Hydroxyurea and vincristine are the drugs of choice in humans but have not been evaluated in cats with this disorder.

## Basophilic Leukemia

This variant of granulocytic leukemia is exceedingly rare in the cat and must be distinguished by cellular morphology and staining properties from the more frequent mast cell leukemia (see section on mast cell neoplasms later in this chapter). One case was described by Henness and Crow (1977) (Plate 16–4*A* and *B*), and another was recorded without details by Hardy (1981). A third case was described by Saar and Reichel (1983) in a wasted three and a half-year-old neutered male with pale yellowish mucosae and enlarged lymph nodes and liver. The PCV was 15 and the WBC 6400, with 37 per cent leukemic cells, predominantly myelocytes and metamyelocytes with fine basophilic granules. Toluidine blue stain demonstrated metachromasia. The highly cellular marrow was infiltrated with basophils, the majority immature (promyelocytes, myelocytes, and metamyelocytes). The liver and lymph nodes were massively infiltrated with similar cells.

All three cats tested FeLV-positive.

## Monocytic Leukemia

Monocytic leukemia is uncommon in the cat. Two cases were described by Holzworth (1960b) (Fig. 16–22), one by Schalm et al. (1975), three by Henness et al. (1977), and one by Saar and Reichel (1983). One was pictured by Blue (1983), and 11 were recorded without details by Priester and McKay (1980).

---

**Plate 16–4** *A*, Basophilic leukemia. A myeloblast, with nucleolus faintly visible, is in contact with a late progranulocyte with a few specific basophilic granules. To the left is a segmented basophil. *B*, Basophilic leukemia, same cat. Two basophilic myelocytes, the larger having a nucleolus. The cell with deep blue cytoplasm and fewer specific basophilic granules (top) is a late progranulocyte. *C*, Mast cell leukemia, blood. The mast cells are large and round with round nuclei and abundant, uniform, metachromatic cytoplasmic granules. The granules may obscure the nucleus. *D*, Mast cell leukemia. The brown-red spleen is massively enlarged and partly folded to fit the confines of the abdominal cavity. The caudal border of the liver is visible (top), and the left kidney can be seen in the angle of the folded spleen (right). (*A* and *B* courtesy Dr. Anita Henness. *C* and *D* from Gilmore CE, Holzworth J: J Am Vet Med Assoc 158 [1971] 1013–1225.)

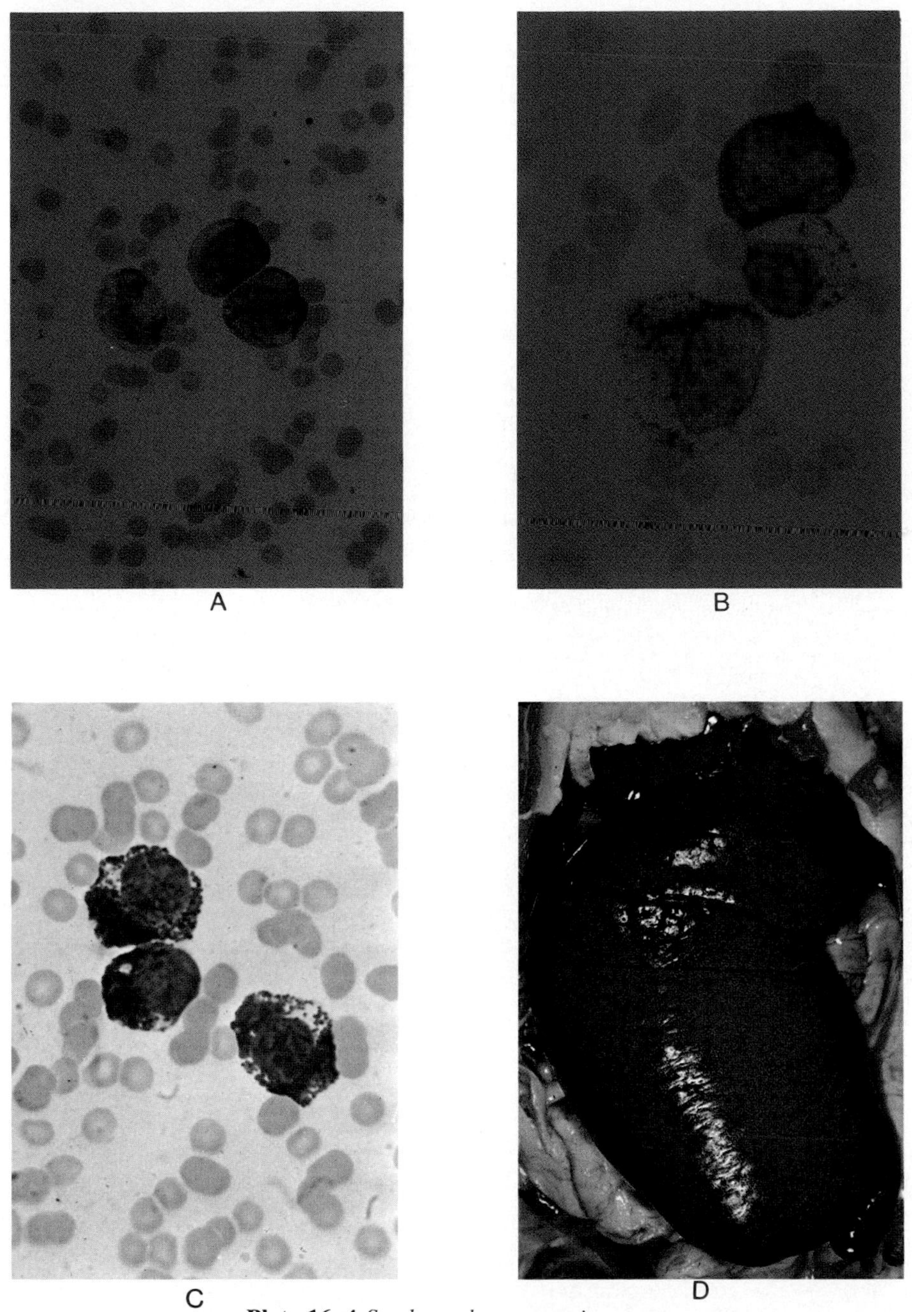


**Plate 16–4** *See legend on opposite page*

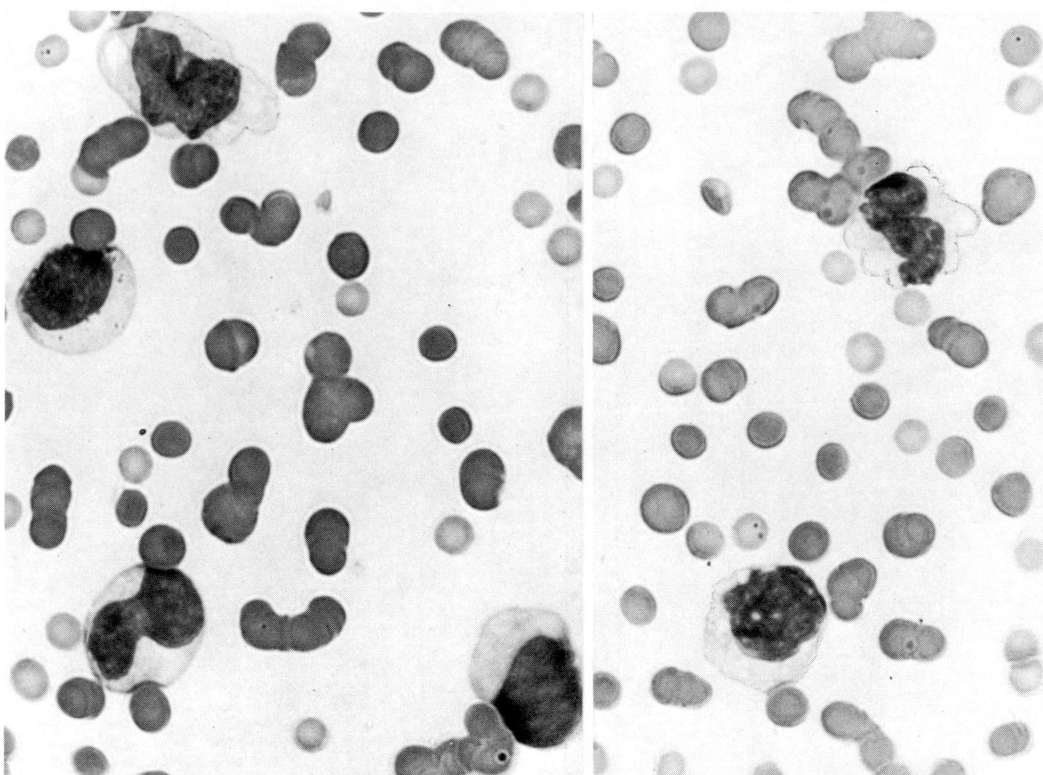

**Figure 16–22** Monocytic leukemia in a six-year-old male, with WBC 8000/μl and 29 per cent monocytes. The five monocytes have variably shaped nuclei and irregular cytoplasmic outlines. At the left is a large lymphocyte. Wright's, × 950. (From Holzworth J: J Am Vet Med Assoc 136 [1960] 107–121.)

Immature monocytes in blood and marrow in leukemia measure 15 to 25 μ and have a high nuclear:cytoplasmic ratio. The nucleus may be folded, indented, or elongated with chromatin variably described as fine or coarse. One or more nucleoli may be present, and mitotic figures may be prominent. The cytoplasm is light blue-gray and may contain a few azurophilic granules or vacuoles. An ameboid cell outline was noted in the case described by Schalm et al. (1975). In Holzworth's cases, supravital staining aided diagnosis, and a limited peroxidase reaction typical of monocytes was reported by Schalm et al. (1975). The granules in monocytes may also be tested for nonspecific esterase, a monocyte marker (Blue, 1983).

Seven of the cats, four males and three females, were aged three to six years. Common signs were inappetence, lethargy, fever, and anemia as in other forms of leukemia. The WBC in three cats was in the normal range, and one cat in time became leukopenic; in the other three cats, the WBC's were as high as 52,700, 118,200, 183,000, and 342,000/μl. The percentages of mature and immature monocytes ranged from about 25 to 96 per cent. In the cases reported by Henness et al. (1977) and by Saar and Reichel (1983), the cats tested FeLV-positive.

Multiple nodules in the kidneys and epicardium were a notable finding in one cat (Schalm et al., 1975). Hemorrhagic infarcts in the brains of two cats with high WBCs (Henness et al., 1977) may have been analogous to those caused by leukostasis, a catastrophic event in humans with granulocytic or monocytic leukemia in which large numbers of blasts aggregate and become trapped in the cerebral vessels, causing hemorrhage and infarction.

## Myelomonocytic Leukemia

Granulocytes and monocytes arise from a common precursor, and both cell lines are occasionally represented in leukemias termed myelomonocytic. Myelomonocytic leukemia has been diagnosed in several cats at AMAH and in six at the University of California (Theilen and Madewell, 1979). Other cases were described by Loeb et al. (1975), by Stann (1979), and by Raskin and Krehbiel (1985), and one was pictured by Blue (1983).

Loeb's case was characterized by anemia and splenomegaly. At autopsy the disease was widely disseminated, with chloromatous neoplastic plaques on the pleura. Examination of tissues by electron microscopy disclosed C-type virus particles. In Stann's case also, the cat tested positive for FeLV. The morphologic diagnosis was supported by cytochemical staining of blood films, marrow, and spleen for nonspecific esterase activity, which revealed positive-staining granules in granulocytes, while monocytic cells stained negatively. When stained for lipase activity, monocytes and their precursors were heavily stained, while granulocytes were unstained. In the cat reported by Raskin and Krehbiel (1985), also FeLV-positive, notable hematologic features were giant hypersegmented neutrophils, micromegakaryocytes, and erythrophagocytosis by neutrophils.

## Treatment of Granulocytic and Monocytic Leukemia

These disorders in cats have not responded well to treatment. In four cats with granulocytic leukemia (including one basophilic leukemia), partial remission was achieved with combinations of cytosine arabinoside, cyclophosphamide, vinblastine, and prednisone only in the two that were less seriously ill (Henness and Crow, 1977). Two cats with monocytic leukemia were treated with cytosine arabinoside, and one achieved a partial remission lasting over two months (Henness et al., 1977). In human granulocytic leukemia, which has been stubbornly resistant to therapy, advances are being made with aggressive therapy combining massive doses of myelosuppressive agents with supportive measures such as leukocyte and platelet transfusions. Unless veterinary oncologists are able to provide this support, they are limited in the use of chemotherapeutic agents.

### Megakaryocytic Myelosis and Leukemia (Essential Thrombocythemia)

Proliferation of megakaryocytes resulting in thrombocythemia has been reported in four cats (Hardy, 1980; Holscher et al., 1983; Michel et al., 1976; Theilen and Madewell, 1979) and observed in two at AMAH. In the case of Michel et al. (1976), in which a diagnosis of acute undifferentiated leukemia was made, blast cells with some resemblance to early erythrocytic cells were present. A platelet count exceeded 1 million/μl, and many were large and bizarre. Cells in the blood in this cat and in one at AMAH resembled megakaryocyte fragments, and increased numbers of immature megakaryocytes were present in the marrow. Megakaryocytes of a cat with a similar disorder contained the FeLV tumor-specific antigen (FOCMA) (Hardy, 1980). None of these three cats was treated. In the case of Holscher et al. (1983), factor VIII was demonstrated in the neoplastic cells in the marrow by an immunoperoxidase technique, which confirmed their origin as megakaryocytes, as factor VIII is synthesized by endothelial cells and megakaryocytes, not by other hematopoietic cells. One cat at AMAH, a six-year-old castrated male Persian, was one of a cluster household previously described in detail (Cotter et al., 1973; 1974). This cat was FeLV-positive and presented with anemia, leukopenia, and a platelet count of 1.5 million/μl (Fig. 16–23*A*). Increased numbers of immature megakaryocytes were present in the marrow (Fig. 16–23*B*). The cat lived for 13 months with no specific treatment except three transfusions and was clinically almost normal despite continuing anemia and leukopenia. Polyarthritis and endocarditis caused by *Corynebacterium* sp developed but responded well to antibiotics. Terminally, the cat developed undifferentiated leukemia with increasing numbers of blasts in the marrow and later in the blood (Fig. 16–23*C*). It is unclear whether the thrombocythemia was a preleukemic or leukemic phenomenon. No abnormality of platelet function was ever noted. Massive hepatosplenomegaly was present at autopsy.

A case characterized by proliferation of both megakaryocytes and red-cell precursors was described by Saar (1970).

### Myelofibrosis and Medullary Osteosclerosis

Myelofibrosis has been classified as a myeloproliferative disease on the basis of proliferation of fibroblasts. It occurs most often as a terminal event in cats treated for chronic aplastic anemia often associated with hepatosplenomegaly due to myeloid metaplasia (Fig. 16–24). A leukoerythroblastic reaction may be present with abnormal red-cell morphology such as teardrop–shaped cells and ovalocytes (Harvey, 1981). It may be difficult or impossible to aspirate marrow from any of several sites in cats with myelofibrosis, so that a core biopsy is necessary for confirmation of the diagnosis. One cat with myelofibrosis had radiographic evidence of thickening of the cortices of the femur and humerus and decreased size of medullary canals (Flecknell et al., 1978). At autopsy, myelofibrosis and osteosclerosis were found, with infarcts, hemosiderosis, and extramedullary hematopoiesis in the spleen.

Hoover and Kociba (1974) described bone lesions in 12 of 13 FeLV-positive cats with anemia. In most severely affected cats, dense cancellous bone filled the medullary cavity. One of the cats had focal lymphoma in the marrow. In affected cats, osteoblasts were atypical and decreased in number, and virus particles were seen by electron microscopy. The anemia in these cats was not secondary to reduced marrow space, as the anemia often preceded severe bone lesions.

A similar bone lesion was observed in an FeLV-positive anemic, leukopenic cat with hypercalcemia (serum calcium 16 mg/dl) (Zenoble and Rowland, 1979). The marrow showed maturation arrest of the granulocytic series indicative of myelogenous leukemia with myelosclerosis. T cells infected with FeLV subgroup C have been shown to produce osteoclast-activating factor, which may initiate bone changes (Onions, 1980). This syndrome has not been associated with hypercalcemia.

## Plasma Cell Neoplasms

Myeloma (multiple myeloma) is a plasma cell tumor of bone marrow that is typically multicentric. Less often, plasma cells form solitary tumors in bone or extramedullary tissue (plasmacytoma). Occasionally plasma cells spill over into the blood. Although myeloma is rare in cats, a number of cases have been reported. These as well as additional instances of myeloma and plasmacytoma on record at AMAH are discussed in the chapter on neoplasms.

Plasma cells are not ordinarily seen in the blood of normal cats and have been variously reported to constitute only 0.3 to 1.61 per cent of cells in bone marrow of normal cats (Schalm et al., 1975).

Normal plasma cells are oval or round, about the same size as lymphocytes, with a small, round, eccentric nucleus in which coarse chromatin is clumped in a wheel-spoke arrangement. The cytoplasm is dark blue, and a clear perinuclear area is usually noticeable. Plasma cells, derived from B-lymphocytes, do not divide and have a life span of about 12 hours although they may remain as memory cells for longer. Malignant plasma cells secrete an abundance of nonfunctional monoclonal immunoglobulin (M component). The monoclonal nature of the globulin suggests a single cell of origin for tumors of plasma cells. Malignant plasma cells may differ little from normal cells or they may exhibit varying degrees of pleomorphism. Plasma cells even in the malignant state can usually be distinguished from lymphocytes (Fig. 16–25). The term plasmoid lymphocyte has been used to describe cells in an occasional disorder in which differentiation has been difficult.

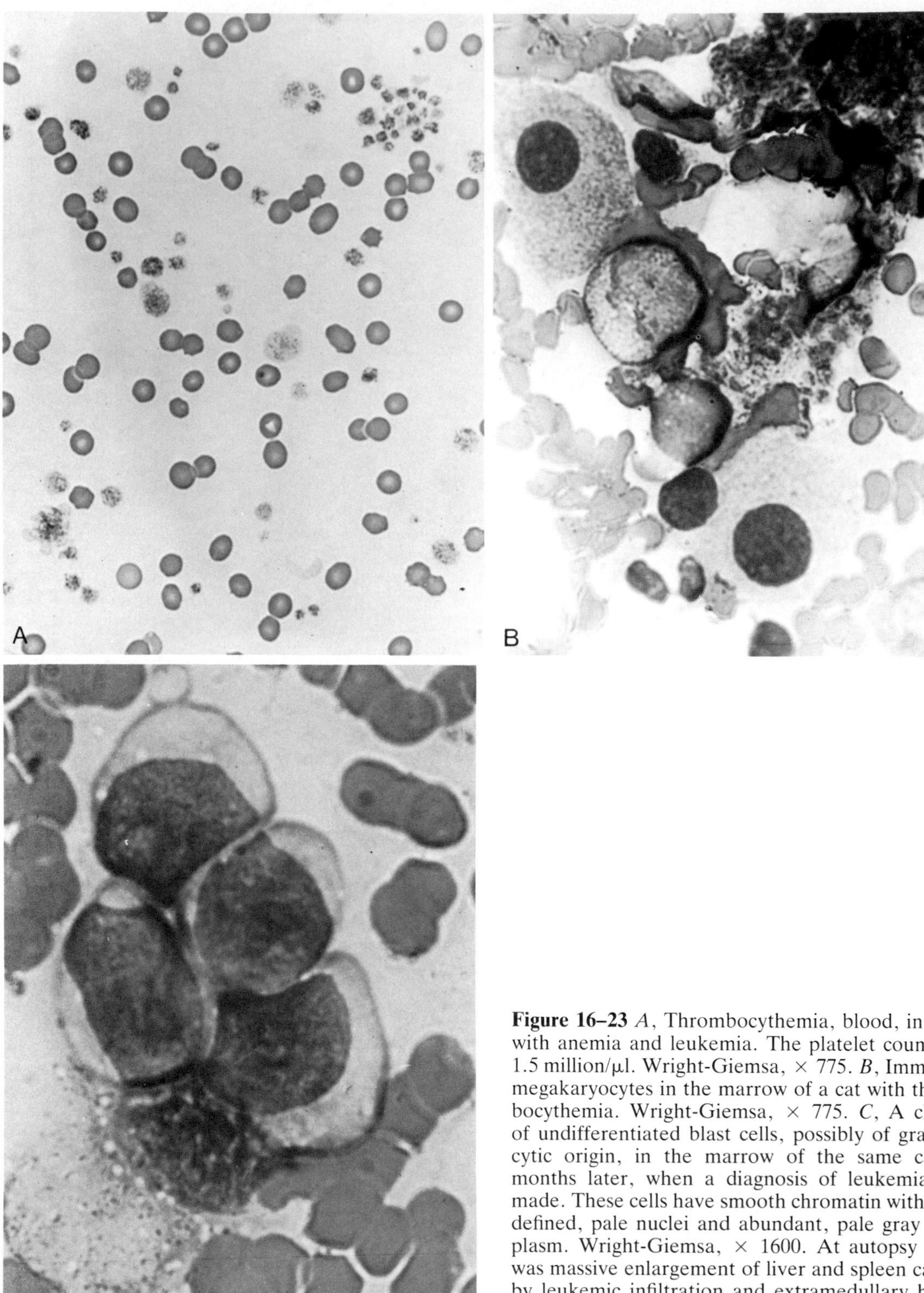


**Figure 16–23** *A*, Thrombocythemia, blood, in a cat with anemia and leukemia. The platelet count was 1.5 million/μl. Wright-Giemsa, × 775. *B*, Immature megakaryocytes in the marrow of a cat with thrombocythemia. Wright-Giemsa, × 775. *C*, A cluster of undifferentiated blast cells, possibly of granulocytic origin, in the marrow of the same cat 13 months later, when a diagnosis of leukemia was made. These cells have smooth chromatin with well-defined, pale nuclei and abundant, pale gray cytoplasm. Wright-Giemsa, × 1600. At autopsy there was massive enlargement of liver and spleen caused by leukemic infiltration and extramedullary hematopoiesis.

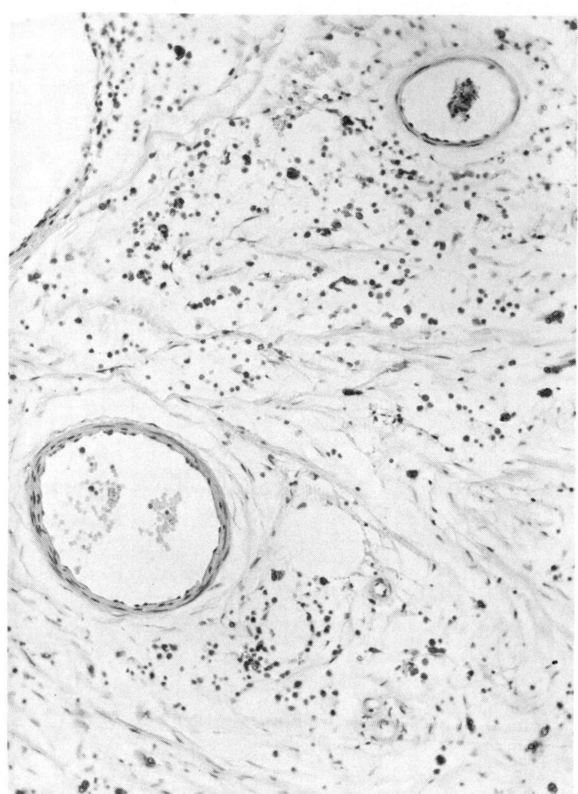

**Figure 16–24** Myelofibrosis, marrow, three-year-old spayed female with chronic, nonregenerative anemia. Only a sparse population of hematopoietic cells and rare lymphocytes survive among the proliferating fibrils of connective tissue. H & E, × 175.

Myeloma produces clinical signs in several ways. Malignant cells often infiltrate the marrow, causing a decrease in normal hematopoietic cells, so that anemia, granulocytopenia, and thrombocytopenia result. Rouleau formation of red cells is common as in other hyperproteinemic states. The combination of granlocytopenia and decreased functional immunoglobulin entails a high risk of infection. Bleeding tendencies may result from thrombocytopenia, from interference with platelet aggregation by coating of platelets with globulin, and from interaction of the M component with factors II, V, VII, and VIII (Drazner, 1982).

Hyperglobulinemia may damage renal glomeruli and form harmful protein precipitates in renal tubules. Light chains of immunoglobulin may be passed in the urine (Bence Jones protein). This protein is not detectable on "dip sticks" for urinary protein since these detect albumin only; it is best detected by electrophoresis of the urine. Albuminuria is often present as a result of glomerular damage, whether or not Bence Jones protein is present.

Hyperviscosity may occur, most often with IgM myeloma (macroglobulinemia) but also with polymerized IgA or aggregated IgG myeloma. Affected cats may develop neurologic signs and congestive heart failure with vascular changes visible on retinal examination.

Lytic bone lesions may occur in myeloma causing pain and sometimes fractures. Appearing characteristically as multiple, small, "punched-out" areas of decreased density, they are well circumscribed, without a sclerotic border, and usually develop first in the axial skeleton but may occur in long bones as well. Bone lesions have been uncommon in feline myeloma.

The criteria for diagnosis of myeloma in man, as outlined by Wintrobe et al. (1981), are, first and foremost, 10 per cent or more of plasma cells per 1000 marrow cells, together with a positive biopsy of bone or soft tissue. If only one of these findings is present, then the M component must be demonstrated electrophoretically in plasma or urine, osteolytic lesions must be radiographically evident, or myeloma cells must be seen in at least two peripheral blood films.

A remarkable case of an undifferentiated hematopoietic malignancy with clinical resemblance to myeloma was described by Saar and Scherpe (1973) in a year-old cat with hindlimb weakness, inability to urinate and defecate, and hepatosplenomegaly. Radiographs disclosed millet-sized osteolytic areas in many long bones, in the vertebrae, and in the skull. The blood picture was unremarkable except for a PCV of 28 per cent, but the marrow was overwhelmingly dominated by blast cells with no recognizable relationship to myeloid, erythroid, lymphoid, or plasma cell lines.

It must be remembered that the monoclonal gammopathies characteristic of myeloma may occur in some other disorders as well. Lymphoma of B-cell origin may cause a monoclonal gammopathy indistinguishable from that of myeloma. Two of three cats with gamma-region M spikes reported by Kehoe et al. (1972) had lymphoma; the third

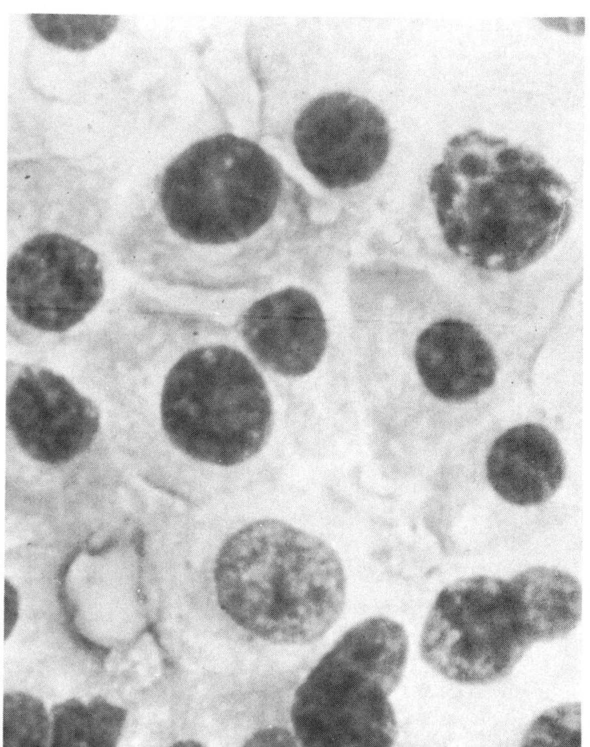

**Figure 16–25** Plasma cell myeloma, impression film of spleen, 11-year-old castrated male. The cells have abundant cytoplasm and a round, eccentric nucleus with dense chromatin. Wright-Giemsa, × 1000.

had myeloma. In the AMC series of nine cats with malignancies associated with monoclonal gammopathy, six had myeloma, one macroglobulinemia, and two lymphoma (MacEwen and Hurvitz, 1977). In an aged Siamese cat, cutaneous lymphoma was associated with hyperviscosity, hypercalemia, peripheral edema, ascites, and sepsis (Dust et al., 1982). The paraprotein in this cat was identified as IgG. In spite of the hypercalcemia, bone lesions were not evident, but the marrow was infiltrated with malignant cells. A cat at AMAH with anemia, leukopenia, and monoclonal gammopathy was found to have well-differentiated lymphocytic lymphoma involving a single enlarged prescapular lymph node. IgM macroglobulinemia was described in an elderly cat with a skin tumor and marrow infiltration characterized by highly malignant cells with some features of plasma cells but such extreme atypia that definite identification was impossible (Saar et al., 1973).

## Mast Cell Neoplasms

Mast cells are not true hematopoietic cells but connective tissue cells of uncertain origin. Mast cell malignancies are discussed in detail in the chapter on neoplasms, but also merit inclusion here, for they may assume forms that involve the hematopoietic system and sometimes behave like hematopoietic neoplasms.

The feline leukemia virus is not believed to play a causal role in mast cell tumors. In a survey at The Animal Medical Center, no cat with mast cell tumor tested FeLV-positive (Hayes, 1976); however, others have found that an occasional cat may test positive. Cell-free transmission of mast cell tumor in dogs suggested a viral etiology (Bowles et al., 1972), but in cats transmission studies with tumor extracts have not so far induced neoplasms (Muller et al., 1983).

In the past 35 years mast cell neoplasia has been encountered in cats with increasing frequency. In an early review of reports of feline mast cell malignancies, these tumors were estimated to constitute only about 1 to 6 per cent of total feline neoplasms (Garner and Lingeman, 1970). Later surveys from several institutions indicated a prevalence as high as 10 per cent (Carpenter, 1975; Engle and Brodey, 1969; Goto et al., 1974; Holzinger, 1973). By 1981, they were the third most frequent feline tumor at AMAH after lymphoid malignancies and mammary cancer. Although reported first in Europe, they appear to be described most often from the United States.

Although some early reports of mast cell neoplasia involving the blood mistakenly termed the condition basophilic leukemia (see reviews of the literature, Nielsen, 1969; Schalm et al., 1975), the mast cells and basophils of the cat are easily differentiated with Romanowsky stains (Gilmore and Holzworth, 1971; Nielsen, 1969; Nielsen et al., 1971; Schalm et al., 1975). The basophil has a multilobed nucleus and a regular, round cytoplasmic outline; the cytoplasm is grayish and contains small, round, metachromatic granules that stain pinkish or light orange in contrast to the reddish violet staining in other species; in addition, a few dark-staining granules may also be present (Schalm et al., 1975). The mast cell, by contrast, is larger and has a round or oval nucleus and variable cytoplasmic outline; the metachromatic cytoplasmic granules are larger and more numerous than those of the basophil and stain magenta, purple, or blue with Romanowsky stains or toluidine blue.

Immature mast cells may measure up to 20 μ, with a larger indented nucleus and sometimes a nucleolus. The cytoplasmic granules are smaller, fewer, and more uniform than normal granules (see chapter on neoplasms). Mast cell granules are soluble in water, so that they are sometimes lysed in improperly fixed tissue, or they may be difficult to detect in an undifferentiated tumor. Unless such a tumor is examined with a special stain such as Giemsa or toluidine blue, it could be misdiagnosed as lymphoma or reticuloendotheliosis (Nielsen, 1969).

The age range for feline mast cell tumor at AMAH has been from 6 months to 21 years (see chapter on neoplasms), but the majority of cats are adult or elderly. No sex predilection has been reported except by Garner and Lingeman (1970), who noted an apparent higher risk (2:1) in males. It is commonly said that there is no breed predisposition, but a greater prevalence in Siamese has been found at AMAH (see chapter on neoplasms).

Feline mast cells are most numerous in skin, intestine, and reticuloendothelial tissues, and feline neoplasms tend to present in three corresponding forms: skin tumors, solitary or multiple; intestinal tumors; and tumors with disseminated visceral involvement. There may be overlapping among the categories, especially as individual cases evolve.

The majority of feline mast cell neoplasms are cutaneous, or at least appear first in the skin. They take the form of nodules or of plaques resembling eosinophilic granuloma and sometimes are accompanied by a blood eosinophilia. Solitary and even several tumors, especially if widely excised, have been removed without recurrence. Multiple tumors, however, are sometimes already associated with, or later give rise to, visceral lesions that are ultimately fatal. Examination of the feathered edge of a blood film or of the buffy coat from a centrifuged blood sample may reveal a few mast cells that suggest the likelihood of systemic involvement. In one case of multiple skin lesions and visceral involvement, the WBC was 52,500/μl with 60 per cent mast cells (Hauser, 1965).

With skin mast cell tumors, a diagnosis can be made by needle aspirate, touch preparations of ulcerated lesions, or excisional biopsy. An aspirate may be done before excision and, if mast cells are identified, a wide excision can be planned. Some mast cells are present normally in chronic dermatitis and eosinophilic granuloma, but large numbers in aspirates confirm a diagnosis of mast cell tumor.

Single skin tumors should be widely excised and examined histopathologically to determine the degree of differentiation and whether the margin of the excised tissue contains tumor cells. If a well-differentiated tumor is completely excised, further treatment is not required. If tumor cells are present at the margin, wider excision should be done if feasible. With multiple tumors of undifferentiated morphology, radiation or corticosteroid therapy should be considered.

Mast cell malignancy manifested as an intestinal tumor is less frequent than cutaneous or disseminated mast cell tumor. An unusual form of intestinal mast cell tumor was studied in 24 cats at AMAH by Alroy et al. (1975). The cats were older than those with the more typical skin or visceral mast cell neoplasia. Unlike other mast cell tumors, none of these tumors was accompanied by circulating mast cells; however, tumor was present elsewhere in 16 cases, most often in mesenteric lymph nodes, liver, and spleen.

Disseminated mast cell tumor may sometimes manifest itself primarily as massive splenomegaly in an apparently healthy cat, and sudden death from ruptured spleen is not uncommon. In other cats inappetence, weight loss, gastrointestinal signs, and anemia are frequent, the anemia being less severe than with other leukemias. A devastating terminal event in cats with mast cell tumor is perforation of a gastric or duodenal ulcer resulting in peritonitis. The ulcer forms because secretion of hydrochloric acid (HCl) is increased in response to histamine release by the mast cell granules. Perforation may be preceded by vomiting or diarrhea with melena, or it may occur suddenly in a reportedly asymptomatic cat. Hemorrhagic tendencies caused by heparin or possibly by disseminated intravascular coagulation have occurred in cats with mast cell tumors.

As well as the spleen, the liver, lymph nodes, and bone marrow may become involved; rarely there is tumor in the cranial mediastinum. Varying numbers of mast cells often appear in the circulation (Plate 16–4*C*), presenting a picture sometimes referred to as mast cell leukemia. Among 30 cats with disseminated mast cell tumor at AMAH, 12 had neoplastic mast cells in the blood and bone marrow. In a case reported by Schalm et al. (1975), the total WBC was 30,000/μl, with 35 per cent mast cells in the blood and 6.3 per cent mast cells in the marrow. In other cases the percentage of mast cells is lower and often they are found only by searching the feathered edge of a blood film. Rarely a pure mast cell leukemia may occur (Theilen and Madewell, 1979).

Analysis of abdominal or thoracic fluid if present often provides a diagnosis in systemic mast cell tumor, as mast cells (and occasionally eosinophils) may be present in large numbers. Needle aspirates of spleen or liver may be done cautiously with a fine needle and good restraint of the cat. Because these organs are friable and blood coagulation may be impaired, a laceration could prove fatal.

If splenomegaly is present, splenectomy is indicated. The spleen is usually a striking cinnamon or mahogany color (Plate 16–4*D*), sometimes with a fibrin coating. For some unexplained reason, splenectomy is beneficial even in the presence of known residual disease in liver, skin, or blood. Reports of long-term survival after splenectomy are accumulating in the veterinary literature (e.g., Allard, 1979; Confer et al., 1978; Guerre et al., 1979; Liska et al., 1979). The median survival time in eight reported cases and six additional ones at AMAH was about a year, with some cats living over three years. The majority of these cats were known to have tumor elsewhere at the time of splenectomy. Additional treatment with corticosteroids (prednisone 2 mg/kg daily) after splenectomy did not seem to lengthen survival times. Splenectomy may be beneficial simply because tumor cells are removed in bulk. The spleen may also be a source of suppressor T cells, which inhibit an immune response to the tumor cells, so that splenectomy may allow the immune system to control growth of residual tumor cells for a time.

Erythrophagocytosis by cutaneous and splenic mast cells was observed in an anemic cat with cutaneous and systemic mast cell neoplasia (Madewell et al., 1983). The RBC count returned to normal after splenectomy, but progression of the skin lesions necessitated euthanasia.

Some response to steroids in cats with cutaneous mast cell tumor has been observed. Tumors resistant to prednisone appear to be resistant to other chemotherapeutic agents as well.

Three of the long-term survivors at AMAH died of intestinal ulceration. Ulceration may be prevented by prophylactic administration of cimetidine, a drug that blocks histamine ($H_2$) receptors in the stomach and thus blocks HCl production. Antihistamines such as diphenhydramine hydrochloride, which block $H_1$ receptors, are not effective. Cimetidine (5 mg/kg/day) has been used at AMAH in dogs and cats with known residual mast cell tumor. Although intestinal ulceration has not been observed in the treated animals, a controlled study of the drug's effectiveness has not been done.

## COAGULATION DISORDERS

The normal coagulation system and tests for evaluation are described elsewhere (e.g., Dodds, 1975; Green, 1983). Bleeding disorders result from platelet abnormalities or from disturbances of the intrinsic or extrinsic coagulation systems.

### Disorders of Platelets

Platelets normally aggregate to form a plug that acts as a matrix for fibrin accumulation. Platelet disorders result from a decrease in number or from abnormal function and are manifested by petechiae, ecchymoses, and bleeding from the mucosa of nose, mouth, or gastrointestinal tract (Davenport et al., 1982).

For accurate platelet counts, blood should be obtained with as little stress to the patient and as little tissue damage as possible. It is collected in EDTA, and the count should be done within four hours. The blood tube should not be refrigerated after collection, as refrigeration causes clumping of the platelets. A blood film made at the time of collection should be examined when the count is done. The platelet number estimated from the film should correlate with the count. A count of under 100,000/μl is considered significantly reduced (Dodds, 1975).

**THROMBOCYTOPENIA.** Thrombocytopenia is the most frequent clotting disorder encountered by veterinarians (Green, 1983). It is commonly classified as of three etiologic mechanisms. (1) Reduced production may be induced by infections, drugs, or radiation, or result from neoplastic replacement of the marrow (myelophthisis). Marrow aspirates show decreased numbers of megakaryocytes. (2) Accelerated destruction results from immunologic injury or disseminated intravascular coagulation (DIC) and is characterized by normal or increased numbers of megakaryocytes in the marrow. (3) Abnormal distribution or sequestration of platelets, occurring notably with hypersplenism, is characterized by normal production of platelets.

Decreased production in the cat is most often due to aplastic anemia secondary to FeLV infection and to leukemic myelophthisis. The platelets are small, and bleeding may occur when the count drops below 50,000 to 75,000/μl. Myelosuppressive chemotherapeutic drugs usually produce leukopenia before thrombocytopenia, because the eight- or nine-day life span of platelets is longer than that of granulocytes. Very few drugs selectively suppress megakaryocyte formation; a much larger group may produce generalized marrow suppression (e.g., chloramphenicol, phenylbutazone, gold compounds) (Wintrobe et al., 1981).

In immune-mediated thrombocytopenia (ITP), platelets are destroyed by action of an antiplatelet antibody. The platelets are often large and function better than normal platelets, so platelet counts may drop very low, even to less than 10,000/μl, before bleeding occurs. Immune-mediated thrombocytopenia may be primary or secondary to a variety of disorders such as hematopoietic neoplasia and systemic lupus erythematosus. In man it has been attributed to treatment with certain drugs. Not only must the diagnosis be established by demonstration of antiplatelet antibody, but a number of tests are also performed to determine possible secondary causes (e.g., urinalysis, fecal examination, coagulation studies, and testing for other immune-mediated diseases) (Jain and Switzer, 1981).

Two tests specifically detect antiplatelet antibody. The platelet factor 3 (PF-3) release test measures shortened clotting time in vitro by release of factor 3 from normal allogeneic platelets in response to antiplatelet antibodies in the patient's serum (Green, 1983). The direct immunofluorescence (DIF) test demonstrates antiplatelet antibody on megakaryocytes, if megakaryocytes can be found in the marrow. This test is considered more sensitive than the PF-3 test, but its use is limited, as few laboratories are equipped to do the test. There is no risk of significant hemorrhage in aspiration of marrow even from a severely thrombocytopenic cat.

Immune-mediated thrombocytopenia has been well characterized in man and in the dog but has rarely been reported in cats. A presumptive case of "idiopathic" thrombocytopenia was described in a kitten with severe anemia and gastrointestinal hemorrhage (Harvey and Gaskin, 1980).

Antiplatelet antibodies were demonstrated in three cats by positive PF-3 and DIF tests (Jain and Switzer, 1981; Joshi et al., 1979). The two cats tested FeLV-negative. One cat, despite treatment with corticosteroids, eventually developed an ANA titer of 1:100 and proteinuria, and a diagnosis of systemic lupus erythematosus with glomerulonephritis was made (Jain and Switzer, 1981).

Recommendations for treatment are based on experience with dogs (Jain and Switzer, 1981; Johnessee and Hurvitz, 1983). Occasional cases of primary ITP are self-limiting. If bleeding is severe, transfusion of fresh whole blood or platelets from fresh blood suspended in the donor's plasma may be given. Corticosteroids are the drugs of choice, and the dosage is adjusted according to the response as monitored by frequent platelet counts. If there is no response to corticosteroids within four or five days, vincristine may be added at low dosage. Vincristine acts both by suppressing the immune system and by stimulating megakaryocytes to divide. Platelet counts should be repeated for six months after therapy is stopped, lest there be a sudden, life-threatening relapse.

Provided all nonimmunologic causes of thrombocytopenia have been definitely excluded, splenectomy may be considered for cases unresponsive to medical treatment, since it eliminates the principal site of antibody production and of platelet removal (Johnessee and Hurvitz, 1983).

Transient ITP following viral infection or vaccination with live virus has been reported in children and puppies (Dodds, 1975). A kitten at AMAH developed transient petechiae and ecchymoses with thrombocytopenia shortly after vaccination with a modified–live-virus vaccine against panleukopenia and two respiratory viruses. The condition may resolve without treatment, but if bleeding is severe, corticosteroids hasten recovery.

Feline leukemia virus is known to replicate efficiently in megakaryocytes and could alter the antigenic structure of the membrane as it probably does with red cells in the FeLV-positive, Coombs-positive anemias of cats. Two FeLV-positive kittens at AMAH developed transient thrombocytopenia evidenced by petechiae, gingival bleeding, and epistaxis.

Two FeLV-negative cats at AMAH had thrombocytopenia, most likely primary ITP, characterized by increased megakaryocytes in the marrow indicating increased production and destruction of platelets.

Certain drugs have been associated with thrombocytopenia or abnormal platelet aggregation. Thrombocytopenia developed in a group of cats infected with feline calicivirus and treated with ribavirin, an antiviral drug (Povey, 1978). It was not determined whether the low platelet counts were caused by the virus or the drug.

Among other drugs that interfere with platelet function, sometimes by more than one mechanism, are aspirin, phenylbutazone, promazine tranquilizers, local anesthetics, nitrofurans, and sulfonamides (Wintrobe, 1981). Fatal hemorrhagic toxicity from 130 mg (2 grains) of aspirin/kg/day for nine days was reported in a group of five experimental cats (Penny et al., 1967b). Signs that developed within six days were salivation, vomiting, ataxia, hyperesthesia, and gastrointestinal bleeding. Heinz bodies were seen in small numbers in red cells, but it was not reported whether their number exceeded that before treatment. Moderate erythroid hypoplasia was evident in the marrow. At autopsy, ecchymoses were found in the lungs and mesentery and superficial bleeding ulcers in the stomach and intestine. Platelet function was not evaluated, but small doses of aspirin cause marked interference with platelet aggregation in other species (Dodds, 1975).

Platelet aggregation is decreased in uremia as well.

Disseminated intravascular coagulation, the other condition in which platelets are destroyed, is discussed with clotting disorders later in this chapter.

## Inherited Clotting Factor Deficiencies

**FACTOR VIII DEFICIENCY—HEMOPHILIA A.** A factor VIII deficiency characteristic of hemophilia A was reported first by Osbaldiston (cited by Loeb, 1975) and later by Cotter et al. (1978) in three unrelated cats with severe protracted hemorrhage after castration or declawing. Each of the three cats had a prolonged clotting and activated partial thromboplastin time (APTT), a normal prothrombin time (PT), and severe factor VIII deficiency. With intrinsic factor deficiencies, characteristic signs are hematomas and bleeding into body cavities. Bleeding after injury or surgery may be delayed in onset but protracted. Petechiae are not seen, and bleeding does not immediately follow surgery, as platelet numbers and function are normal and a platelet plug is formed to prevent capillary bleeding. With damage to larger vessels, the absence of a fibrin clot allows the plug to dissipate after a time.

Von Willebrand's disease, not yet reported in cats, was ruled out in these cats by the finding of increased levels of factor VIII–related antigen. Von Willebrand's disease is common in certain breeds of dogs and is inherited in most breeds as an autosomal, incompletely dominant trait (Dodds, 1975). It is characterized by a prolonged bleeding time, decreased platelet adhesiveness, and low factor VIII levels secondary to a low factor VIII–related antigen.

Although severe bleeding followed surgery in the three cats with hemophilia A, they did not have spontaneous hemorrhage at home as hemophiliac dogs and people commonly do. Perhaps because the cat is a light and agile animal it may be able to avoid these complications. The defect is transmitted as an X-linked genetic trait, so that the heterozygous female is an asymptomatic carrier and the disorder is evident in the male offspring. If inbreeding were to occur between a carrier female and an affected male, half the female offspring would have hemophilia and half would be carriers, while half the male offspring would have hemophilia and the other half would be normal. A heterozygous female can be identified by decreased factor VIII levels in the plasma, even though coagulation is normal.

Treatment of hemophilia requires frequent transfusion with fresh blood or plasma until bleeding stops, since factor VIII has a half-life of only 10 to 18 hours.

**FACTOR IX DEFICIENCY—HEMOPHILIA B (CHRISTMAS DISEASE).** An hereditary deficiency of factor IX has been reported in British shorthaired cats (Green, 1983). Like hemophilia A, this disorder is transmitted as an X chromosome–linked condition with identical clinical presentation. Abnormalities in the coagulation profile are also similar to those of hemophilia A. The two conditions can be differentiated by individual factor analysis. The defect in factor IX deficiency is corrected by both normal plasma and serum, because factor IX is stable in serum, whereas factor VIII is not (Dodds, 1975). The half-life of factor IX is 12 to 24 hours, so bleeding episodes should be treated by transfusion of fresh blood or plasma twice daily until bleeding stops. Both hemophilia A and hemophilia B can be eliminated from breeding stock by testing potential breeding animals for levels of factors VIII and IX.

**FACTOR XII DEFICIENCY.** The only other hereditary disorder of intrinsic coagulation so far reported for the cat is a deficiency of factor XII (Hageman factor) (Green and White, 1977; Kier et al., 1980). This defect is characterized by low levels of factor XII and prolonged activated partial thromboplastin and clotting times. It is not, however, associated with abnormal bleeding. Its significance is that the abnormal APTT may confuse testing for other diseases or experimental coagulation studies. Diagnosis must be confirmed by individual factor analysis.

## Acquired Clotting Factor Deficiencies

**WARFARIN (DICUMAROL, COUMARIN) POISONING.** The most frequent acquired abnormality in pets is caused by warfarin poisoning, but perhaps because cats are more fastidious about eating than dogs they are less often poisoned. Signs are similar to those of hemophilia: protracted bleeding from wounds and bleeding into body cavities. Petechiae are not likely. Of two cats at AMAH with warfarin poisoning, one suffered severe intra-abdominal and subcutaneous bleeding. The second was presented when blood oozed for 48 hours from a small bite wound on the nose.

Warfarin and other vitamin K–deficient states interfere with activity of the prothrombin-complex clotting factors (II, VII, IX, and X). Abnormal laboratory findings suggestive of warfarin poisoning are increased PT and APTT, as factor VII and common-pathway factors II and X are involved. The diagnosis is confirmed by specific analysis demonstrating warfarin in the plasma or liver tissue. Vitamin K therapy, with blood transfusion if needed, rapidly reverses the abnormality. The PT should return to normal by the next day. Recent introduction of new, more potent dicumarol compounds such as brodifacoum has caused severe toxicosis in dogs and cats (Beasley and Buck, 1983). These compounds also have a longer half-life, so that bleeding may recur as late as three weeks after ingestion of the material. Vitamin K should be given in the form of vitamin $K_1$ (Aquamephyton, 2 to 5 mg b.i.d.). The first dose may be given intravenously if bleeding is severe and subsequent doses subcutaneously for two days, followed by oral vitamin $K_1$ for one to three weeks depending on the compound ingested. Intravenous vitamin K must be given cautiously, as anaphylaxis may occur. Heinz-body anemia has been described in dogs treated with vitamin K, especially vitamin $K_3$ (menadione). This reaction has not been reported in cats, but since they are prone to Heinz-body formation, blood counts should be monitored during vitamin K therapy and only vitamin $K_1$ should be used (Fernandez et al., 1984).

**FACTOR VII DEFICIENCY.** A vitamin K–responsive decrease in factor VII was produced in cats by experimental administration of large doses of phenobarbital (Solomon et al., 1974). Factor VII levels fell 50 per cent in cats receiving 10 mg/kg/day. Bleeding tendencies have not been reported in cats receiving phenobarbital in clinical treatment.

**FACTOR XI DEFICIENCY.** A factor XI deficiency, presumably acquired, was described in a five-year-old cat without previous hemorrhagic problems (Feldman et al., 1983). The cat had repeated episodes of bleeding associated with a prolonged APTT and with low levels of factor XI. Although no underlying cause was found, a factor inhibitor was suspected.

**LIVER DISEASE.** Bleeding tendencies develop in some cases of severe liver disease because of decreased production of factors II, VII, IX, and X, which have short half-lives (Dodds, 1975). Although coagulation tests show the same abnormalities as those caused by warfarin, concurrent signs of liver disease and abnormal liver function tests usually make the diagnosis obvious. The coagulation abnormalities of liver disease are often unresponsive to vitamin K. Infusion of fresh plasma may temporarily restore coagulation factors.

## Disseminated Intravascular Coagulation

This severe hemorrhagic disorder is a paradox in that the clinical sign of hemorrhage is in fact an effect of the primary problem of excessive coagulation in the microcirculation. Disseminated intravascular coagulation (DIC) can occur secondarily to almost any serious disorder that affects blood flow or acid-base balance. Documented cases of DIC in animals have been associated with obstetrical complications, heat stroke, malignancy, sepsis, trauma, and mechanical injury to red cells such as might occur with vascular tumors, endocarditis, or dirofilariasis.

Cats dying of panleukopenia have been shown to have microthrombi most often in the renal cortex and medulla, glomerular capillaries usually being spared (Hoffman, 1973). Other organs affected are liver, heart, and lungs. The cause is presumed to be intestinal epithelial necrosis and sepsis due to Gram-negative bacteria. DIC has also been observed in cats with various FeLV-related infectious diseases and with vasculitis caused by FIP.

Disseminated intravascular coagulation has been produced experimentally by intraperitoneal inoculation of FIP virus into antibody-positive cats (Weiss et al., 1980). Tissue ischemia produced in cats by clamping of the abdominal aorta resulted in DIC in the lungs (Hossman and Hossman, 1977). Similar changes may occur spontaneously in some cats with cardiomyopathy. Liver disease followed by DIC occurred in a kennel of dogs fed food contaminated with aflatoxin (Greene et al., 1977).

The initial phase of DIC is capillary thrombosis, followed by consumption of platelets and clotting factors and finally by hemorrhage. The hemorrhage may be severe, with petechiae, ecchymoses, mucosal bleeding, and bleeding from injection sites. Occasionally the first sign may be hemorrhage, but more often bleeding tendencies develop in a cat already seriously ill with some underlying disease.

Diagnosis is by demonstration of multiple abnormalities in clotting tests: thrombocytopenia, prolonged PT and APTT, and decreased fibrinogen. Because fibrinolysis is accelerated, the level of fibrin split products is increased. Because DIC is the final stage of a hypercoagulable state, abnormalities in coagulation tests vary with the stage of the syndrome, and not all abnormalities described occur in each case.

Treatment of DIC has been controversial. Obviously the underlying disease should be treated vigorously with restoration of blood volume, correction of electrolyte and acid-base imbalances, and appropriate antibiotic agents. Replacement of platelets and clotting factors is also indicated. Fresh frozen plasma and platelets are given if available. Anticoagulant therapy is of value before hemorrhage becomes severe. Treatment with heparin without replacement of coagulation factors may increase the risk of hemorrhage in advanced DIC. Heparin given early to cats with DIC caused by panleukopenia produced improvement at a dose of 100 units/kg IV every 90 minutes until the status of coagulation improved (Gerbig et al., 1977; Kraft, 1980). Measurement of APTT or activated coagulation time (ACT) may be used to monitor treatment (Greene and Meriwether, 1982). Heparin accelerates the effect of antithrombin III, a coagulation inhibitor (Gerbig et al., 1977). The dose of heparin used in cats was 250 to 375 units/kg t.i.d. Changes in the ACT correlated well with changes in the APTT. The normal ACT in the cat was up to 65 seconds, less than the normal ACT in the dog of up to 120 seconds.

Others have advocated heparin in tiny doses of 5 to 10 units/kg SC b.i.d. or t.i.d. (Ruehl et al., 1982). The fact remains that heparin is likely to be of value only if used before levels of coagulation factors are severely depleted. If DIC is mild or is suspected early, aspirin may be used in cats at a dose of 100 mg (1½ grains) every three days to inhibit platelet aggregation and thrombotic tendencies.

## DISORDERS OF THE LYMPH NODES, THYMUS, AND SPLEEN

### Lymph Nodes

The normal structure and function of the lymph nodes are described in the chapter on immunology.

**LYMPHADENOPATHY.** Because the lymph nodes filter particulate matter from afferent lymphatics, they may become inflamed in response to local infection or inflammation. Some systemic infections cause generalized lymphadenopathy or lymphadenopathy in nodes draining areas of localization. A cat at AMAH had suppurative lymphadenitis of a submandibular lymph node draining an area with a raised, ulcerated, cryptococcal skin lesion. Granulomatous lymphadenitis may occur in the mesenteric or peripheral lymph nodes in FIP, especially the noneffusive form.

Two groups of laboratory cats with acute lymphadenitis have been reported (Goldman and Moore, 1973; Swindle et al., 1980). These cats developed suppurative infections of the mandibular, parotid, and retropharyngeal lymph nodes caused by Lancefield group G beta hemolytic *Streptococcus*. The infection appeared to be contagious and was experimentally reproduced in two cats by oral and subcutaneous inoculation of bacteria (Swindle et al., 1980).

The response to various antigenic stimuli has been studied in the lymph nodes of cats (Anderson and McKeating, 1970). Oxazolone, a contact sensitizing agent, was painted on the footpads before examination of the regional node. The paracortical (T-cell) areas first became hyperplastic, then the germinal centers (B-cell areas) in the follicles. This change was considered evidence of a primary cell-mediated immune response. Ovalbumin with Freund's adjuvant injected into the subcutis of the foot caused hyperplasia of both B- and T-cell areas of the popliteal lymph node.

Reactive lymph node hyperplasia may be due to a variety of causes in cats, including systemic bacterial and fungal infections. Peripheral lymph node hyperplasia without apparent cause is noted in a small number of cats, primarily cats under the age of five years. Microscopically, the majority of these cats exhibit B- or T-lymphocytic hyperplasia, while fewer show an atypical form of paracortical expansion with loss of nodal architecture (Moore et al., 1985). This distinctive form of peripheral lymph node hyperplasia differs from lymphoma by virtue of its characteristic heterogeneous cell population composed of an admixture of lymphocytes, plasma cells, histiocytes, and immunoblasts. Cats with this distinctive peripheral lymph node enlargement often have signs such as transient fever, anorexia, anemia, and lymphocytosis. They frequently test FeLV-positive. The disorder often subsides spontaneously, may persist, or rarely may precede development of lymphoma. The FeLV itself may not cause the enlargement, but another agent, possibly viral, may coexist. Bacteria cannot be cultured from these nodes.

**NEOPLASIA.** Painless enlargement of a single node may indicate metastatic neoplasia. In a cat at AMAH a subcutaneous nodule behind the pinna of one ear proved to be a lymph node not usually evident. Biopsy of the node and also of a small mass in the horizontal ear canal indicated adenocarcinoma of ceruminous glands. Regional nodes should be palpated when removal of a superficial tumor is contemplated. Enlargement of a sternal lymph node seen in a lateral thoracic radiograph may give an early clue to developing lymphoma or FIP.

## Disorders of the Thymus

A prominent thymus gland is normal in kittens until involution takes place, usually at four or five months of age.

Thymic branchial cysts are a congenital anomaly taking the form of an encapsulated cystic mass in the cranial mediastinal region (Liu et al., 1983). Dyspnea results from pleural effusion, in which lymphocytes and mesothelial cells are found. This rare condition must be differentiated from thymoma, lymphoma, and other possible mediastinal masses.

Acute thymic atrophy occurs in kittens infected with panleukopenia or FeLV (Larsen et al., 1976). This atrophy may be associated with deaths in newborn FeLV-infected kittens (Anderson et al., 1971). The depletion of T cells may be transient in panleukopenia or permanent in the cat chronically viremic with FeLV.

Thymomas occur occasionally in the cranial mediastinum in older cats. At least 28 thymomas have been reported, including 11 from AMAH (see chapter on neoplasia). Although they cannot be distinguished from lymphoma without microscopic examination, the two tumors behave differently. Lymphomas grow rapidly, whereas thymomas are usually benign, grow slowly, and may remain unchanged for weeks or months. Pleural effusion may occur with thymomas, but the fluid does not contain the large numbers of blast cells found with lymphoma. One 18-year-old cat presented at AMAH had chylothorax that was treated conservatively for six months by periodic drainage (Carpenter and Holzworth, 1982). A cystic thymoma was found at autopsy. Subsequent to publication of the 1982 report, another cat with chylothorax secondary to a thymoma was seen at AMAH. Erythroid hypoplasia in man and myasthenia gravis in man and in the dog have been reported secondary to thymoma, but neither has been observed in cats, although three cats at AMAH had clinical and histologic evidence of polymyositis (Carpenter and Holzworth, 1982). A thymoma should be removed surgically if possible, as this tumor has not been responsive to chemotherapy or radiation.

## Disorders of the Spleen

The cat's spleen varies in length from 11.4 to 18.5 cm, in width from 1.4 to 3.1 cm, and in weight from 5.5 to 32 gm (Nickel et al., 1979). When greatly enlarged, as in hemobartonellosis or hematopoietic or mast cell neoplasia, it occupies the ventral abdomen from the liver to the pubis.

Ectopic splenic tissue may occur in various organs or sites in the abdomen either as congenital "rests" or implants following traumatic fragmentation. Linear fibrous scars represent sites of healed rupture.

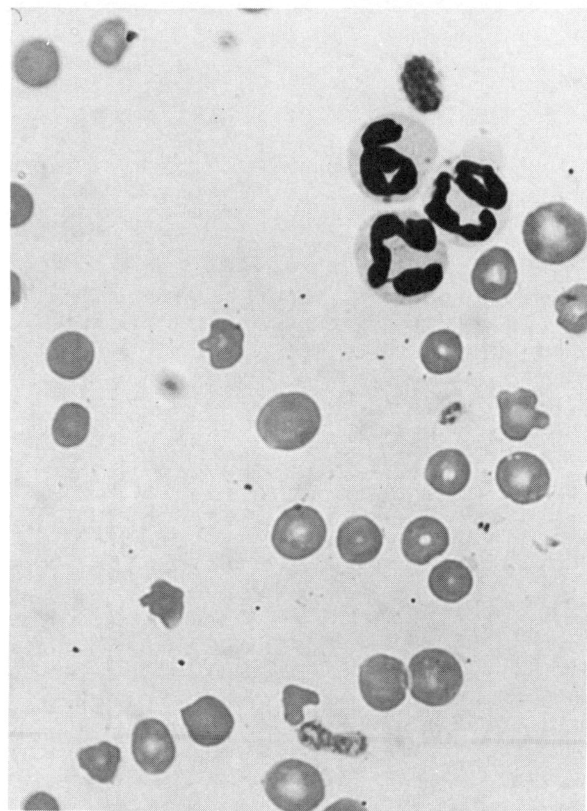

**Figure 16–26** Regenerative anemia, blood, 13-year-old male cat with abdominal hemorrhage from hemangiosarcoma of the liver. Neutrophilia, giant platelets, and large basophilic red cells indicate increased marrow activity. Distortion of several red cells suggests trauma to cells. This neoplasm can predispose to microangiopathic hemolysis and disseminated intravascular coagulation. Wright's, × 950. (From Holzworth J: J Am Vet Med Assoc 128 [1956] 471–478.)

Infarcts of unknown cause may occur, particularly when the spleen is enlarged. A 4-cm midabdominal mass was felt on routine palpation of an asymptomatic 14-year-old cat. Splenectomy was performed with histologic diagnosis of a splenic infarct. Large infarcts are relatively common in older dogs presented with palpable abdominal masses but are rare in cats.

Extramedullary hematopoiesis in the spleen and liver is a frequent compensatory mechanism in anemic cats but probably makes no significant contribution to effective hematopoiesis. In fact, the reaction may be harmful because of infiltration of hematopoietic elements at the expense of normal hepatic or splenic tissue.

Hypersplenism has been suspected as a contributing cause of cytopenias in some cats with splenomegaly (e.g., Holzworth, 1960a). The spleen has some suppressive effect in *Haemobartonella* infection, as parasitemias have occurred after splenectomy (Harvey and Gaskin, 1977).

Primary neoplasia of the spleen of the cat other than hematopoietic or mast cell malignancy is not common.

The most massive enlargement occurs with mast cell infiltration. Hemangiomas and hemangiosarcomas occur less often than in the dog. These tumors as well as mast cell tumors are fragile and may rupture, causing severe or fatal intra-abdominal hemorrhage that may sometimes be associated with DIC. They may also predispose red cells to hemolysis by trauma from abnormal endothelial surfaces in the tumor mass (Fig. 16–26). For a detailed discussion of tumor-like lesions and neoplasms of the spleen, see the chapter on neoplasms.

## REFERENCES

### The Normal Cat and Characteristic Responses to Disease


Ackerman GA: Developmental relationship between the appearance of lymphocytes and lymphopoietic activity in the thymus and lymph nodes of the fetal cat. Anat Rec 158 (1967) 387–400.

Alsaker RD, Laber J, Stevens J, Perman V: A comparison of polychromasia and reticulocyte counts in assessing erythrocytic regenerative response in the cat. J Am Vet Med Assoc 170 (1977) 39–41.

Athens JW, Haab OP, Raab SO, Mauer AM, Ashenbrucker H, Cartwright GE, Wintrobe MM: Leukokinetic studies. IV. The total blood, circulating and marginal granulocyte pools and the granulocyte turnover rate in normal subjects. J Clin Invest 40 (1961) 989–995.

Atwal OS, McFarland LZ: Histochemical study of the distribution of alkaline phosphatase in leukocytes of the horse, cow, sheep, dog, and cat. Am J Vet Res 28 (1967) 971–974.

Bentinck-Smith J: Hematology. *In* Medway W, Prier JE, Wilkinson JS (eds): A Textbook of Veterinary Clinical Pathology. Baltimore, The Williams & Wilkins Company, 1969.

Beritíc T: Studies on Schmauch bodies. I. The incidence in normal cats (Felis domestica) and the morphologic relationship to Heinz bodies. Blood 25 (1965) 999–1008.

Berman E: Hemogram of the cat during pregnancy and lactation and after lactation. Am J Vet Res 35 (1974) 457–460.

Brown IW Jr, Eadie GS: An analytical study of the in vivo survival of limited populations of animal red blood cells tagged with radioiron. J Gen Physiol 36 (1953) 327–343.

Chickering WR: Studies of immune mediated neutropenia in the cat. Athens, University of Georgia, PhD thesis, 1980.

Chickering WR, Brown J, Prasse KW, Dawe DL: Effects of heterologous antineutrophil antibody in the cat. Am J Vet Res 46 (1985) 1815–1819.

Cockerell GL, Hoover EA, LoBuglio AF, Yohn DS: Phytomitogen- and antigen-induced blast transformation of feline lymphocytes. Am J Vet Res 36 (1975) 1489–1494.

Collins JD, Jain NC, Schalm OW, Pangborn J: Ultrastructure of erythrocyte refractile bodies in the peripheral blood of cats. Am J Vet Clin Pathol 2 (1968) 75–80.

Cowell KR, Jezyk PF, Haskins ME, Patterson DF: Mucopolysaccharidosis in a cat. J Am Vet Med Assoc 169 (1976) 334–339.

Cramer DV, Lewis RM: Reticulocyte response in the cat. J Am Vet Med Assoc 160 (1972) 61–67.

Creighton SR, Wilkins RJ: Thoracic effusions in the cat. Etiology and diagnostic features. J Am Anim Hosp Assoc 11 (1975) 66–76.

Da Silva AC, De Angelis RC, Pontes MA, Guérios MFM: The domestic cat as a laboratory animal for experimental nutrition studies. IV. Folic acid deficiency. J Nutr 56 (1955) 199–213.

Duncan JR, Prasse KW: Clinical examination of bone marrow. Vet Clin North Am 6 (1976) 597–608.

Fan LC, Dorner JL, Hoffman WE: Reticulocyte response and maturation in experimental acute blood loss anemia in the cat. J Am Anim Hosp Assoc 14 (1978) 219–224.

Gillis DB, Mitchell RA: Erythrokinetics in normal cats. Am J Vet Res 35 (1974) 31–33.

Gilmore CE, Gilmore VH, Jones TC: Bone marrow and peripheral blood of cats: technique and normal values. Pathol Vet 1 (1964) 18–40.

Greaves MF, Owen JJT, Raff MC: T and B Lymphocytes. Origins, Properties and Roles in Immune Responses. New York, American Elsevier Publishing Company, 1973.

Hamilton MN, Edelstein SJ: Cat hemoglobin—pH dependence of cooperativity and ligand binding. J Biol Chem 249 (1974) 1323–1329.

Harvey JW, Kaneko JJ: Oxidation of human and animal haemoglobins with ascorbate, acetylphenylhydrazine, nitrite, and hydrogen peroxide. Br J Haematol 32 (1976) 193–203.

Haskins ME, Aguirre GD, Jezyk PF, Patterson DF: The pathology of the feline model of mucopolysaccharidosis VI. Am J Pathol 101 (1980) 657–673.

Holzworth J, Georgi JR: Trichinosis in a cat. J Am Vet Med Assoc 165 (1974) 186–191.

Hoover EA, Dubey JP: Pathogenesis of experimental pulmonary paragonimiasis in cats. Am J Vet Res 39 (1978) 1827–1832.

Jain NC: A staining technique to demonstrate erythrocyte refractile bodies in cat blood. Br Vet J 125 (1969) 437–441.

Johnson KH, Perman V: Normal values for jugular blood in the cat. Vet Med Small Anim Clin 63 (1968) 851–854.

Kaneko JJ, Green RA, Mia AS: Erythrocyte survival in the cat as determined by glycine-2-$C^{14}$. Proc Soc Exp Biol Med 123 (1966) 783–784.

Kleinsorgen VA, Brandenburg C, Brummer H: Untersuchungen über den Einfluss von Zwangsmassnahmen auf Blutparameter bei der Hauskatze. Berl Münch Tierärztl Wochenschr 89 (1976) 358–360.

Kramer JW, Davis WC, Prieur DJ, Baxter J, Norsworthy GD: An inherited disorder of Persian cats with intracytoplasmic inclusions in neutrophils. J Am Vet Med Assoc 166 (1975) 1103–1104.

Kramer JW, Davis WC, Prieur DJ: The Chediak-Higashi syndrome of cats. Lab Invest 36 (1977) 554–562.

Kurian M, Iyer GYN: Oxidant effect of acetylphenylhydrazine: a comparative study with erythrocytes of several animal species. Can J Biochem 55 (1977) 597–601.

Lessard JL, Taketa F: Multiple hemoglobins in fetal, newborn and adult cats. Biochem Biophys Acta 175 (1969) 441–444.

Lindsay FEF: Chylothorax in the domestic cat—a review. J Small Anim Pract 15 (1974) 241–258.

Loughman WD, Frye FL, Condon TB: XY/XXY bone marrow mosaicism in three male tricolor cats. Am J Vet Res 31 (1970) 307–314.

Mackey LJ: Distribution of T and B cells in thymus, blood and lymph nodes of the cat. Res Vet Sci 22 (1977a) 225–228.

Mackey L: Haematology of the cat. *In* Archer RK, Jeffcott LB (eds): Comparative Clinical Haematology. Oxford, Blackwell Scientific Publications, 1977b.

Marion RS, Smith JE: Survival of erythrocytes after autologous and allogeneic transfusion in cats. J Am Vet Med Assoc 183 (1983) 1437–1439.

Mauk AG, Whelan HT, Putz GR, Taketa F: Anemia in domestic cats: effect on hemoglobin components and whole blood oxygenation. Science 185 (1974) 447–449.

Penny RHC: The bone marrow of the dog and cat. J Small Anim Pract 15 (1974) 553–562.

Penny RHC, Carlisle CH, Davidson HA, Gray EM: Some observations on the effect of the concentration of ethylenediamine tetraacetic acid (EDTA) on the packed cell volume of domesticated animals. Br Vet J 126 (1970) 383–389.

Poli G, Faravelli G: [Nitroblue tetrazolium test in the domestic animals: normal values]. Clin Vet 97 (1974) 248–251.

Prasse KW: Disorders of the leukocytes. *In* Ettinger SJ (ed): Textbook of Veterinary Internal Medicine. Philadelphia, WB Saunders Company, 1975.

Prasse KW, Duncan JR: Clinical interpretation of leukocyte abnormalities. Vet Clin North Am 6 (1976) 581–595.

Prasse KW, Seagrave RC, Kaeberle ML, Ramsey FK: A model of granulopoiesis in cats. Lab Invest 28 (1973) 292–299.

Prieur DJ, Collier LL, Bryan GM, Meyers KM: The diagnosis of feline Chediak-Higashi syndrome. Feline Pract 9 (5) (1979) 26–32.

Rausch PG, Moore TG: Granule enzymes of polymorphonuclear neutrophils: A phylogenetic comparison. Blood 46 (1975) 913–919.

Reed C, Ling GV, Gould D, Kaneko JJ: Polycythemia vera in a cat. J Am Vet Med Assoc 157 (1970) 85–91.

Rohovsky MW, Fowler EH: Lesions of experimental panleukopenia. J Am Vet Med Assoc 158 (1971) 872–875.

Roth B, Schneider CC: Untersuchungen zur Abhängigkeit des "weissen Blutbildes" bei Hauskatzen (Felis domestica) von Wurminfektionen des Darmes. Berl Münch Tierärztl Wochenschr 84 (1971) 436–437.

Schalm OW: Leukocyte response to disease in various domestic animals. J Am Vet Med Assoc 140 (1962) 557–563.

Schalm OW: Neutrophil morphology in the cat in toxemic disease. Calif Vet 18 (1) (1964) 29–31.

Schalm OW: Notes and comments on feline hematology. Calif Vet 22 (1) (1968) 24–27.

Schalm OW: Interpretations in feline bone marrow cytology. J Am Vet Med Assoc 161 (1972) 1418–1425.

Schalm OW: Comments on feline leukocytes. Feline Pract 7 (1) (1977) 34–77.

Schalm OW, Hughes JP: Some observations on physiologic leukocytosis in the cat and horse. Calif Vet 18 (5) (1964) 23–25.

Schalm OW, Smith R: Signs of defective neutrophil maturation in the cat. Calif Vet 17 (6) (1963a) 33–34.

Schalm OW, Smith R: Some unique aspects of feline hematology in disease. Small Anim Clinician 3 (1963b) 311–318.

Schalm OW, Switzer JA: Bone marrow aspiration in the cat. Feline Pract 2 (6) (1972) 56–62.

Schalm OW, Jain NC, Carroll EJ: Veterinary Hematology, 3rd ed. Philadelphia, Lea & Febiger, 1975.

Schmalzl F, Braunsteiner H: On the origin of monocytes. Acta Haematol (Basel) 39 (1968) 177–182.

Scott DW: Current knowledge of aelurostrongylosis in the cat. Literature review and case reports. Cornell Vet 63 (1973) 483–500.

Scott DW, Kirk RW, Bentinck-Smith J: Some effects of short-term methylprednisolone therapy in normal cats. Cornell Vet 69 (1978) 104–115.

Taylor DW, Siddiqui WA: Responses of enriched populations of feline T and B lymphocytes to mitogen stimulation. Am J Vet Res 38 (1977) 1969–1971.

Tiedemann K, van Ooyen B: Prenatal hematopoiesis and blood characteristics of the cat. Anat Embryol 153 (1978) 243–267.

Timoney JF, Neibert HC, Scott FW: Feline salmonellosis. A nosocomial outbreak and experimental studies. Cornell Vet 68 (1978) 211–219.

Tramezzani JH, Morita E, Chiocchio SR: The carotid body as a neuroendocrine organ involved in control of erythropoiesis. Proc Natl Acad Sci 68 (1971) 52–55.

Valentine WN, Pearce ML, Riley RF, Richter E, Lawrence JS: Heme synthesis and erythrocyte life span in the cat. Proc Soc Biol Med 77 (1951) 244–245.

Velasco M, Landaverde M, Lifshitz F, Parra A: Some blood constituents in normal cats. J Am Vet Med Assoc 158 (1971) 763–764.

Ward JM, Wright JF, Wharran GH: Ultrastructure of granulocytes in the peripheral blood of the cat. J Ultrastruct Res 39 (1972) 389–396.

Watson ADJ: Further observations on chloramphenicol toxicosis in cats. Am J Vet Res 41 (1980) 293–294.

Weiser MG: Hematologic techniques. Vet Clin North Am 11 (1981) 189–208.

Weiss L: Personal communication, 1980.

Weller PF, Goetzl EJ: The human eosinophil. Roles in host defense and tissue injury. Am J Pathol 100 (1980) 793–818.

Went S, Drinker CK: A micromethod for determination of the absolute blood volume, with data upon the blood volume of the guinea pig, white rat, rabbit, and cat. Am J Physiol 88 (1929) 468–478.

Wilkins RJ: Morphologic features of feline peripheral blood lymphocytes. J Am Anim Hosp Assoc 10 (1974) 363–366.

Zeya HI: Myeloperoxidase absence in cat eosinophils (abstr). Clin Res 26 (1978) 360A.

**Disorders of the Hematopoietic System**

Abernethy DR, Greenblatt DJ, Divoll M, Ameer B, Shader RI: Differential effect of cimetidine on drug oxidation (antipyrine and diazepam) vs conjugation (acetaminophen and lorazepam): prevention of acetaminophen toxicity by cimetidine. J Pharmacol Exp Ther 224 (1983) 508–513.

Allard AW: Splenic mastocytosis. Feline Pract 9 (4) (1979) 21–22.

Alroy J, Leav I, DeLellis RA, Weinstein RS: Distinctive intestinal mast cell neoplasms of domestic cats. Lab Invest 33 (1975) 159–167.

Alsaker RD, Laber J, Stevens J, Perman V: A comparison of polychromasia and reticulocyte counts in assessing erythrocytic regenerative response in the cat. J Am Vet Med Assoc 170 (1977) 39–41.

Altman NH: Intraerythrocytic crystalloid bodies in cats and their comparison with hemoglobinopathies of man. Ann NY Acad Sci 241 (1974) 589–593.

Anderson LJ, Jarrett WFH, Jarrett O, Laird HM: Feline leukemia-virus infection of kittens: mortality associated with atrophy of the thymus and lymphoid depletion. J Natl Cancer Inst 47 (1971) 807–817.

Anderson LJ, McKeating FJ: Immunological responses in lymph nodes of the cat. Immunology 19 (1970) 935–943.

Atwal OS, McFarland LZ: Histochemical study of the distribution of alkaline phosphatase in leukocytes of the horse, cow, sheep, dog, and cat. Am J Vet Res 28 (1967) 971–974.

Auer L, Bell K: Transfusion reactions in cats due to AB blood group incompatibility. Res Vet Sci 35 (1983) 145–152.

Auer L, Bell K, Coates S: Blood transfusion reactions in the cat. J Am Vet Med Assoc 180 (1982) 729–730.

Azocar J, Essex M: Interactions of feline leukemia virus with lymphoid cells. *In* Proffitt MR (ed): Virus-Lymphocyte Interactions: Implications in Disease. New York, Elsevier/North-Holland Biomedical Press, 1979, 179–189.

Barclay, SM: Lymphosarcoma in tarsi of a cat. J Am Vet Med Assoc 175 (1979) 582–583.

Beasley VR, Buck WB: Warfarin and other anticoagulant poisonings. *In* Kirk RW (ed): Current Veterinary Therapy VIII. Philadelphia, WB Saunders Company, 1983, 101–106.

Beck WS: Iron metabolism and the hypochromic anemias. *In* Beck WS (ed): Hematology. Cambridge, MIT Press, 1973, 27–50.

Bengtsson E: Eosinophilic leukemia—an immunopathological reaction? Acta Paediatr Scand 57 (1968) 245–249.

Beritíc T: Studies on Schmauch bodies. I. The incidence in normal cats (Felis domestica) and the morphologic relationship to Heinz bodies. Blood 25 (1965) 999–1008.

Bianchi C, Migone L: Sindrome eritremica in un gatto. Haematologica 22 (1940) 597–620.

Blue J: The blood and blood-forming organs. *In* Pratt PW (ed): Feline Medicine. Santa Barbara, American Veterinary Publications, Inc, 1983.

Bollum FJ: Terminal deoxynucleotidyl transferase as a hematopoietic cell marker. Blood 54 (1979) 1203–1215.

Bowles CA, Kerber WT, Rangan SRS, Kwapien R, Woods W, Jensen EM: Characterization of a transplantable, canine, immature mast cell tumor. Cancer Res 32 (1972) 1434–1441.

Boyce JT, Hoover EA, Kociba GJ, Olsen RG: Feline leukemia virus–induced erythroid aplasia: in vitro hemopoietic culture studies. Exp Hematol 9 (1981) 990–1001.

Broxmeyer HE, Jacobsen N, Kurland J, Mendelsohn N, Moore MAS: In vitro suppression of normal granulocytic stem cells

by inhibitory activity derived from human leukemia cells. J Natl Cancer Inst 60 (1978) 497–511.
Caciolo PL, Nesbitt GH, Patnaik AK, Hayes AA: Cutaneous lymphosarcoma in the cat: A report of nine cases. J Am Anim Hosp Assoc 20 (1984) 491–496.
Cain GR, Suzuki Y: Presumptive neonatal isoerythrolysis in cats. J Am Vet Med Assoc 187 (1983) 46–48.
Carlton WW: Intraocular lymphosarcoma: Two cases in Siamese cats. J Am Anim Hosp Assoc 12 (1976) 83–87.
Carpenter JL: Bronchial asthma in cats. *In* Kirk RW (ed): Current Veterinary Therapy V. Philadelphia, WB Saunders Company, 1974, 208–209.
Carpenter JL: Unpublished data, 1975.
Carpenter JL: Personal communication, 1984.
Carpenter JL, Holzworth J: Thymoma in 11 cats. J Am Vet Med Assoc 181 (1982) 248–251.
Case MT: A case of myelogenous leukemia in a cat. Zentralbl Veterinärmed A17 (1970) 273–277.
Chew DJ, Schaer M, Liu SK, Owens J: Pseudohyperparathyroidism in a cat. J Am Anim Hosp Assoc 11 (1975) 46–52.
Chickering WR, Prasse KW, Dawe DL: Development and clinical application of methods for detection of antineutrophil antibody in serum of the cat. Am J Vet Res 46 (1985) 1809–1814.
Clark CH: Metabolic effects and toxicities of chloramphenicol. Mod Vet Pract 59 (1978) 663–668.
Cockerell GL, Krakowka S, Hoover EA, Olsen RG, Yohn DS: Characterization of feline T- and B-lymphocytes and identification of an experimentally induced T-cell neoplasm in the cat. J Natl Cancer Inst 57 (1976) 907–913.
Collier LL, Bryan GM, Prieur DJ: Ocular manifestations of the Chédiak-Higashi syndrome in four species of animals. J Am Vet Med Assoc 175 (1979) 587–595.
Confer AW, Langloss JM, Cashell IG: Long-term survival of two cats with mastocytosis. J Am Vet Med Assoc 172 (1978) 160–161.
Cotter SM: Feline leukemia virus induced disorders in the cat. Vet Clin North Am 6 (1976) 367–378.
Cotter SM: Feline leukemia virus-associated diseases. *In* Kirk RW (ed): Current Veterinary Therapy VI. Philadelphia, WB Saunders Company, 1977, 465–472.
Cotter SM: Anemia associated with feline leukemia virus infection. J Am Vet Med Assoc 175 (1979) 1191–1194.
Cotter SM: Treatment of lymphoma and leukemia with cyclophosphamide, vincristine, and prednisone: II. Treatment of cats. J Am Anim Hosp Assoc 19 (1983) 166–172.
Cotter SM, Essex M: Animal model of human disease—acute lymphoblastic leukemia, aplastic anemia. Am J Pathol 87 (1977) 265–268.
Cotter SM, Brenner RM, Dodds WJ: Hemophilia A in three unrelated cats. J Am Vet Med Assoc 172 (1978) 166–168.
Cotter SM, Essex M, Hardy WD Jr: Serological studies of normal and leukemic cats in a multiple case–leukemia cluster. Cancer Res 34 (1974) 1061–1069.
Cotter SM, Essex M, McLane MF, Grant CK, Hardy WD Jr: Chemotherapy and passive immunotherapy in naturally occurring feline mediastinal lymphoma. *In* Hardy WD Jr, Essex M, McClelland AJ (eds): Feline Leukemia Virus. New York, Elsevier/North-Holland, 1980, 219–225.
Cotter SM, Gilmore CE, Rollins C: Multiple cases of feline leukemia and feline infectious peritonitis in a household. J Am Vet Med Assoc 162 (1973) 1054–1058.
Cotter SM, Hardy WD Jr, Essex M: Association of feline leukemia virus with lymphosarcoma and other disorders in the cat. J Am Vet Med Assoc 166 (1975) 449–454.
Cowell KR, Jezyk PF, Haskins ME, Patterson DF: Mucopolysaccharidosis in a cat. J Am Vet Med Assoc 169 (1976) 334–339.
Cramer DV, Lewis RM: Reticulocyte response in the cat. J Am Vet Med Assoc 160 (1972) 61–67.
Crighton GW: Clinical aspects of lymphosarcoma in the cat. Vet Rec 82 (1968) 122–126.
Crosby WH: The limits of erythropoiesis: How much can the marrow produce with total recruitment? Blood Cells 1 (1975) 497–507.
Crow SE, Madewell BR, Henness AM: Feline reticuloendotheliosis: a report of four cases. J Am Vet Med Assoc 170 (1977) 1329–1332.
Cullison RF: Acetaminophen toxicosis in small animals: clinical signs, mode of action, and treatment. Compend Contin Ed 6 (1984) 315–321.
Da Silva AC, De Angelis RC, Pontes MA, Guérios MFM: The domestic cat as a laboratory animal for experimental nutrition studies. IV. Folic acid deficiency. J Nutr 56 (1955) 199–213.
Davenport DJ, Breitschwerdt EB, Carakostas MC: Platelet disorders in the dog and cat Part I: Physiology and pathogenesis. Compend Contin Ed 4 (1982) 762–772.
Dodds WJ: Bleeding disorders. *In* Ettinger SJ (ed): Textbook of Veterinary Internal Medicine. Philadelphia, WB Saunders Company, 1975, 1679–1698.
Dorn CR, Taylor DON, Frye FL, Hibbard HH: Survey of animal neoplasms in Alameda and Contra Costa Counties, California: 1. Methodology and description of cases. J Natl Cancer Inst 40 (1968) 295–305.
Drazner FH: Multiple myeloma in the cat. Compend Contin Ed 4 (1982) 206–216.
Duff BC, Allan GS, Howlett CR: A presumptive case of polycythemia vera in a cat. Aust Vet Pract 3 (2) (1973) 78–79.
Dunn JK, Hirsch VM, Searcy GP: Serum folate and vitamin $B_{12}$ levels in anemic cats. J Am Anim Hosp Assoc 20 (1984a) 999–1002.
Dunn JK, Searcy GP, Hirsch VM: The diagnostic significance of a positive direct antiglobulin test in anemic cats. Can J Comp Med 48 (1984b) 349–353.
Dust A, Norris AM, Valli VEO: Cutaneous lymphosarcoma with IgG monoclonal gammopathy, serum hyperviscosity and hypercalcemia in a cat. Can Vet J 23 (1982) 235–239.
Engle GC, Brodey RS: A retrospective study of 395 feline neoplasms. J Am Anim Hosp Assoc 5 (1969) 21–31.
Essex M, Jakowski RM, Hardy WD Jr, Cotter SM, Hess P, Sliski A: Feline oncornavirus–associated cell membrane antigen. III. Antibody titers in cats from leukemia cluster households. J Natl Cancer Inst 54 (1975a) 637–641.
Essex M, Cotter SM, Hardy WD Jr, Hess P, Jarrett W, Jarrett O, Mackey L, Laird H, Perryman L, Olsen RG, Yohn DS: Feline oncornavirus–associated cell membrane antigen. IV. Antibody titers in cats with naturally occurring leukemia, lymphoma, and other diseases. J Natl Cancer Inst 55 (1975b) 463–467.
Essex M, Sliski A, Hardy WD Jr, deNoronha F, Cotter SM: Feline oncornavirus–associated antigen: A tumor specific cell surface marker. *In* Bentvelzen P, Hilgers J, Yohn DS (eds): Advances in Comparative Leukemia Research 1977. Amsterdam, Elsevier/North-Holland Biomedical Press, 1978, 337–340.
Essex M, Grant CK, Cotter SM, Sliski A, Hardy WD Jr: Leukemia specific antigens: FOCMA and immune surveillance. *In* Neth R, Gallo RC, Hofschneider PH, Mannweiler K (eds): Modern Trends in Human Leukemia III. New York, Springer-Verlag, 1979, 453–467.
Eyestone WH: Myelogenous leukemia in the cat. J Natl Cancer Inst 12 (1951) 599–613.
Eyquem A, Podliachouk L: Les groupes sanguins des chats. Ann Inst Pasteur 87 (1954) 91–94.
Eyquem A, Podliachouk L, Millot P: Blood groups in chimpanzees, horses, sheep, pigs, and other mammals. Ann NY Acad Sci 97 (1962) 320–328.
Falconer GJ, Irving AC, Watson PR, Ludwig J: A case of erythremic myelosis in a cat. NZ Vet J 28 (1980) 83–84.
Fan LC, Dorner JL, Hoffmann WE: Reticulocyte response and maturation in experimental acute blood loss anemia in the cat. J Am Anim Hosp Assoc 14 (1978) 219–224.

Feldman BF, Soares CJ, Kitchell BE, Brown CC, O'Neill S: Hemorrhage in a cat caused by inhibition of factor XI (plasma thromboplastin antecedent). J Am Vet Med Assoc 182 (1983) 589–591.

Fernandez FR, Davies AP, Teachout DJ, Krake A, Christopher MM, Perman V: Vitamin K–induced Heinz body formation in dogs. J Am Anim Hosp Assoc 20 (1984) 711–720.

Finch SC: Granulocytopenia. *In* Williams WJ, Beutler E, Erslev AJ, Rundles RW (eds): Hematology. New York, McGraw-Hill Book Company, 1972, 628–654.

Finco DR, Duncan JR, Schall WD, Prasse KW: Acetaminophen toxicosis in the cat. J Am Vet Med Assoc 166 (1975) 469–472.

Fischer CA: Retinopathy in anemic cats. J Am Vet Med Assoc 156 (1970) 1415–1427.

Flecknell PA, Gibbs C, Kelly DF: Myelosclerosis in a cat. J Comp Pathol 88 (1978) 627–631.

Francis DP, Cotter SM, Hardy WD Jr, Essex M: Comparison of virus-positive and virus-negative cases of feline leukemia and lymphoma. Cancer Res 39 (1979) 3866–3870.

Fraser CJ, Joiner GN, Jardine JH, Gleiser CA: Acute granulocytic leukemia in cats. J Am Vet Med Assoc 165 (1974) 355–359.

Garner FM, Lingeman CH: Mast cell neoplasms of the domestic cat. Pathol Vet 7 (1970) 517–530.

Gasper PW, Thrall MA, Wenger DA, Macy DW, Ham L, Dornsife RE, McBiles K, Quackenbush SL, Kesel ML, Gillette EL, Hoover EA: Correction of feline arylsulphatase B deficiency (mucopolysaccharidosis VI) by bone marrow transplantation. Nature 312 (1984) 467–469.

Gerbig T, Kraft W, Kraft I: [Kaolin-activated partial thromboplastin time in healthy cats and the control of heparin therapy]. Kleintierpraxis 22 (1977) 293–296.

Gershoff SN, Faragalla FF, Nelson DA, Andrus SB: Vitamin $B_6$ deficiency and oxalate nephrocalcinosis in the cat. Am J Med 27 (1959) 72–80.

Giddens WE Jr, Labbe RF, Swango LJ, Padgett GA: Feline congenital erythropoietic porphyria associated with severe anemia and renal disease. Clinical, morphologic, and biochemical studies. Am J Pathol 80 (1975) 367–386.

Gilbride AP: Myelogenous leukemia in a cat complicated by an otitis media. Can J Comp Med 28 (1964) 207–211.

Giles RC, Buhles WC, Montgomery CA: Myeloproliferative disorder in a cat. J Am Vet Med Assoc 165 (1974) 456–457.

Gilmore CE, Holzworth J: Naturally occurring feline leukemia: clinical, pathologic, and differential diagnostic features. J Am Vet Med Assoc 158 (1971) 1013–1025.

Gilmore CE, Gilmore VH, Jones TC: Reticuloendotheliosis, a myeloproliferative disorder of cats: comparison with lymphocytic leukemia. Pathol Vet 1 (1964) 161–183.

Glenn BL, Glenn HG, Omtvedt IT: Congenital porphyria in the domestic cat (*Felis catus*): Preliminary investigations on inheritance pattern. Am J Vet Res 29 (1968) 1653–1657.

Glenn BL, Kocan AA, Blouin EF: Cytauxzoonosis in bobcats. J Am Vet Med Assoc 183 (1983) 1155–1158.

Goldman PM, Moore TD: Spontaneous Lancefield group G streptococcal infection in a random source cat colony. Lab Anim Sci 23 (1973) 565–566.

Goto N, Ozasa M, Takahashi R, Ishida K, Fujiwara K: Pathological observations of feline mast cell tumor. Jpn J Vet Sci 36 (1974) 483–494.

Green RA: Bleeding disorders. *In* Ettinger SJ (ed): Textbook of Veterinary Internal Medicine, 2nd ed. Philadelphia, WB Saunders Company, 1983, 2076–2098.

Green RA, White F: Feline factor XII (Hageman) deficiency. Am J Vet Res 38 (1977) 893–895.

Greene CE, Meriwether E: Activated partial thromboplastin time and activated coagulation time in monitoring heparinized cats. Am J Vet Res 43 (1982) 1473–1480.

Greene CE, Barsanti JA, Jones BD: Disseminated intravascular coagulation complicating aflatoxicosis in dogs. Cornell Vet 67 (1977) 29–49.

Groulade P, Guilhon JC: Syndrome érythrémique chez le chat. Bull Acad Vét Fr 39 (1966) 127–131.

Guerre R. Millet P, Groulade P: Systemic mastocytosis in a cat: remission after splenectomy. J Small Anim Pract 20 (1979) 769–772.

Guirlinger P: Étude de l'immunodépression due au FeLV. Essai d'immunostimulation par le B.C.G. Thesis, Alfort (abstr Vet Bull 1985, 1020).

Hardy WD Jr: Epidemiology of primary neoplasms of lymphoid tissue in animals. *In* Twomey JJ, Good RA (eds): The Immunopathology of Lymphoreticular Neoplasms. New York, Plenum Medical Book Company, 1978, 129–180.

Hardy WD Jr: Feline leukemia virus diseases. *In* Hardy WD Jr, Essex M, McClelland AJ (eds): Feline Leukemia Virus. New York, Elsevier/North-Holland, 1980, 3–31.

Hardy WD Jr: Hematopoietic tumors of cats. J Am Anim Hosp Assoc 17 (1981) 921–940.

Hardy WD Jr, Hess PW, Essex M, Cotter S: Horizontal transmission of feline leukaemia virus. Nature 244 (1973) 266–269.

Hardy WD Jr, Hess PW, MacEwen EG, Hayes AA, Kassel RL, Day NK, Old LJ: Treatment of feline lymphosarcoma with feline blood constituents. *In* Clemmesen J, Yohn DS (eds): Comparative Leukemia Research 1975, Bibl Haemat, No 43. Basel, Karger, 1976, 518–521.

Hardy WD Jr, Zuckerman EE, MacEwen EG, Hayes AA, Essex M: A feline leukaemia virus– and sarcoma virus–induced tumour-specific antigen. Nature 270 (1977) 249–251.

Hardy WR, Anderson RE: Hypereosinophilic syndromes. Ann Intern Med 68 (1968) 1220–1229.

Harvey JW: Myeloproliferative disorders in dogs and cats. Vet Clin North Am 11 (1981) 349–381.

Harvey JW, Gaskin JM: Experimental feline haemobartonellosis. J Am Anim Hosp Assoc 13 (1977) 28–38.

Harvey JW, Gaskin JM: Feline haemobartonellosis: Attempts to induce relapses of clinical disease in chronically infected cats. J Am Anim Hosp Assoc 14 (1978a) 453–456.

Harvey JW, Gaskin JM: Feline haptoglobin. Am J Vet Res 39 (1978b) 549–553.

Harvey JW, Gaskin JM: Idiopathic thrombocytopenia and hemorrhage followed by thrombocytosis in a cat. Feline Pract 10 (1) (1980) 25–31.

Harvey JW, Kaneko JJ: Interactions between methylene blue and erythrocytes of several mammalian species, *in vitro*. Proc Soc Exp Biol Med 147 (1974) 245–249.

Harvey JW, Kaneko JJ: Oxidation of human and animal haemoglobins with ascorbate, acetylphenylhydrazine, nitrite and hydrogen peroxide. Br J Haematol 32 (1976) 193–203.

Harvey JW, Kornick HP: Phenazopyridine toxicosis in the cat. J Am Vet Med Assoc 169 (1976) 327–331.

Harvey JW, Sameck JH, Burgard FJ: Benzocaine-induced methemoglobinemia in dogs. J Am Vet Med Assoc 175 (1979) 1171–1175.

Harvey JW, Shields RP, Gaskin JM: Feline myeloproliferative diseases. Changing manifestations in the peripheral blood. Vet Pathol 15 (1978) 437–448.

Haskins ME, Bingel SA, Northington JW, Newton CD, Sande RD, Jezyk PF, Patterson DF: Spinal cord compression and hind limb paresis in cats with mucopolysaccharidosis VI. J Am Vet Med Assoc 182 (1983) 983–985.

Haskins ME, Jezyk PF, Desnick RJ, McDonough SK, Patterson DF: Mucopolysaccharidosis in a domestic short-haired cat—a disease distinct from that seen in the Siamese cat. J Am Vet Med Assoc 175 (1979) 384–387.

Haskins ME, Wortman JA, Wilson S, Wolf JH: Bone marrow transplantation in the cat. Transplantation 37 (1984) 634–636.

Hauser P: Ein Fall von Gewebsmastzellen-Leukämie bei einer Katze. Schweiz Arch Tierheilkd 107 (1965) 487–495.

Hayes AA: Personal communication to LK Andrews, 1976.

Hayes A, Mastrota F, Mooney S, Hurvitz A: Safety of transfusing blood in cats [letter]. J Am Vet Med Assoc 181 (1982) 4–5.

Hayes HM, Priester WA: Feline infectious anaemia. Risk by age, sex, and breed; prior disease; seasonal occurrence; mortality. J Small Anim Pract 14 (1973) 797–804.

Heise SC, Smith RS, Schalm OW: Lupus erythematosus with hemolytic anemia in a cat. Feline Pract 3 (3) (1973) 14–19.

Hendrick M: A spectrum of hypereosinophilic syndromes exemplified by six cats with eosinophilic enteritis. Vet Pathol 18 (1981) 188–200.

Henness AM: Personal communication, 1984.

Henness AM, Crow SE: Treatment of feline myelogenous leukemia: Four case reports. J Am Vet Med Assoc 171 (1977) 263–266.

Henness AM, Crow SE, Anderson BC: Monocytic leukemia in three cats. J Am Vet Med Assoc 170 (1977) 1325–1328.

Herz A, Theilen GH, Schalm OW, Munn RJ: C-type virus in bone marrow cells of cats with myeloproliferative disorders. J Natl Cancer Inst 44 (1970) 339–348.

Hessler J, Davis LE, Dale HE: Effect of repeated transfusions of dog blood to cats. Small Anim Clin 2 (1962) 684–687.

Hirsch VM, Cunningham TA: Hereditary anomaly of neutrophil granulation in Birman cats. Am J Vet Res 45 (1984) 2170–2174.

Hirsch VM, Dunn J: Megaloblastic anemia in the cat. J Am Anim Hosp Assoc 19 (1983) 873–880.

Hoffman R: [Consumption coagulopathy in spontaneous panleukopenia in domestic and wild cats.] Berl Münch Tierärztl Wochenschr 86 (1973) 72–74.

Holmberg CA, Manning JS, Osburn BI: Feline malignant lymphomas: comparison of morphologic and immunologic characteristics. Am J Vet Res 37 (1976) 1455–1460.

Holmes R: The occurrence of blood groups in cats. J Exp Biol 30 (1953) 350–357.

Holscher MA, Collins RD, Cousar JB, Kasselberg AG, Macherey CL: Megakaryocytic leukemia in a cat. Feline Pract 13 (4) (1983) 8–12.

Holzinger EA: Feline cutaneous mastocytomas. Cornell Vet 63 (1973) 87–93.

Holzworth J: Anemia in the cat. J Am Vet Med Assoc 128 (1956) 471–488.

Holzworth J: Leukemia and related neoplasms in the cat I. Lymphoid malignancies. J Am Vet Med Assoc 136 (1960a) 47–69.

Holzworth J: Leukemia and related neoplasms in the cat II. Malignancies other than lymphoid. J Am Vet Med Assoc 136 (1960b) 107–121.

Hoover EA, Kociba GJ: Bone lesions in cats with anemia induced by feline leukemia virus. J Natl Cancer Inst 53 (1974) 1277–1284.

Hoover EA, Kociba GJ, Hardy WD Jr, Yohn DS: Erythroid hypoplasia in cats inoculated with feline leukemia virus. J Natl Cancer Inst 53 (1974) 1271–1276.

Hoover EA, McCullough CB, Griesemer RA: Intranasal transmission of feline leukemia. J Natl Cancer Inst 48 (1972) 973–983.

Hossmann KA, Hossmann V: Coagulopathy following experimental cerebral ischemia. Stroke 8 (1977) 249–254.

Hurvitz AI: Fine structure of cells from a cat with myeloproliferative disorder. Am J Vet Res 31 (1970) 747–753.

Ichijo S, Osame S, Konishi T, Goto H: Clinical and hematological findings and myelograms of feline panleukopenia. Jpn J Vet Sci 38 (1976) 197–205.

Jain NC: Osmotic fragility of erythrocytes of dogs and cats in health and in certain hematologic disorders. Cornell Vet 63 (1973) 411–423.

Jain NC, Keeton KS: Scanning electron microscopy of Heinz bodies in feline erythrocytes. Am J Vet Res 36 (1975) 1691–1695.

Jain NC, Switzer JW: Autoimmune thrombocytopenia in dogs and cats. Vet Clin North Am 11 (1981) 421–434.

Jandl JH: Hemolytic anemias II. Membrane and metabolic disorders. *In* Beck WS (ed): Hematology. Cambridge, MIT Press, 1973, 179–198.

Jarrett WF, Anderson LJ, Jarrett O, Laird HM, Stewart MF: Myeloid leukaemia in a cat produced experimentally by feline leukemia virus. Res Vet Sci 12 (1971) 385–387.

Jarrett WFH, Crawford E, Martin WB, Davie F: Leukaemia in the cat. A virus-like particle associated with leukaemia (lymphosarcoma). Nature 202 (1964) 567–568.

Jezyk PF, Haskins ME, Patterson DF, Mellman WJ, Greenstein M: Mucopolysaccharidosis in a cat with arylsulfatase B deficiency: a model of Maroteaux-Lamy syndrome. Science 198 (1977) 834–836.

Johnessee JS, Hurvitz AI: Thrombocytopenia. *In* Kirk RW (ed): Current Veterinary Therapy VIII. Philadelphia, WB Saunders Company, 1983.

Jones FR, Toshida LH, Ladiges WC, Zeidner NS, Kenny MA, McClelland AJ: Treatment of feline lymphosarcoma by extracorporeal immunosorption. *In* Hardy WD Jr, Essex M, McClelland AJ (eds): Feline Leukemia Virus. New York, Elsevier/North-Holland, 1980, 235–243.

Jones TC: Chromosomal analyses of feline lymphomas. *In* Symposium on Comparative Morphology of Hematopoietic Neoplasms, Natl Cancer Inst Monogr 32. Bethesda, MD, National Cancer Institute, 1969, 95.

Joshi BC, Raplee RG, Powell AL, Hancock F: Autoimmune thrombocytopenia in a cat. J Am Anim Hosp Assoc 15 (1979) 585–588.

Kaneko JJ: Clinical Biochemistry of Domestic Animals, 3rd ed. New York, Academic Press, 1980.

Keesling PT, Morris JG: Vitamin $B_{12}$ deficiency in the cat (abstr). J Anim Sci 41 (1975) 317.

Kehoe JM, Hurvitz AI, Capra JD: Characterization of three feline paraproteins. J Immunol 109 (1972) 511–516.

Kier AB: Cytauxzoonosis. *In* Greene CE (ed): Clinical Microbiology and Infectious Diseases of the Dog and Cat. Philadelphia, WB Saunders Company, 1984.

Kier AB, Bresnahan JF, White FJ, Wagner JE: The inheritance pattern of Factor XII (Hageman) deficiency in domestic cats. Can J Comp Med 44 (1980) 309–314.

Kirby D, Gillick A: Case report. Polycythemia and tetralogy of Fallot in a cat. Can Vet J 15 (1974) 114–118.

Kobayashi K: Onion poisoning in the cat. Feline Pract 11 (1) (1981) 22–27.

Kociba GJ, Lange RD, Dunn CDR, Hoover EA: Serum erythropoietin changes in cats with feline leukemia virus–induced erythroid aplasia. Vet Pathol 20 (1983) 548–552.

Kraft W: [Thromboelastogram of healthy domestic cats and the treatment of consumption coagulopathy in panleukopenia]. Berl Münch Tierärztl Wochenschr 86 (1973) 394–396.

Kramer JW, Davis WC, Prieur DJ, Baxter J, Norsworthy GD: An inherited disorder of Persian cats with intracytoplasmic inclusions in neutrophils. J Am Vet Med Assoc 166 (1975) 1103–1104.

Kramer JW, Davis WC, Prieur DJ: The Chediak-Higashi syndrome of cats. Lab Invest 36 (1977) 554–562.

Kramer WB, Laszlo J: Hematologic effects of cancer. *In* Holland JF, Frei E (eds): Cancer Medicine. Philadelphia, Lea & Febiger, 1973, 1085–1099.

Larsen S, Flagstad A, Aalbaek B: Experimental feline panleucopenia in the conventional cat. Vet Pathol 13 (1976) 216–240.

Latimer KS, Rakich PM, Thompson DF: Pelger-Huët anomaly in cats. Vet Pathol 22 (1985) 370–374.

Lewis MG, Kociba GJ, Rojko JL, Stiff MI, Haberman AB, Velicer LF, Olsen RG: Retroviral-associated eosinophilic leukemia in the cat. Am J Vet Res 46 (1985) 1066–1070.

Lipton JM, Nathan DG, Cotter, SM, Kudish M: Unpublished observations, 1980.

Liska WD, MacEwen EG, Zaki FA, Garvey M: Feline systemic mastocytosis: A review and results of splenectomy in seven cats. J Am Anim Hosp Assoc 15 (1979) 589–597.

Liu S-K, Patnaik AK, Burk RL: Thymic branchial cysts in the dog and cat. J Am Vet Med Assoc 182 (1983) 1095–1098.

Loar AS: The management of feline lymphosarcoma. Vet Clin North Am 14 (1984) 1299–1330.

Loeb WF: Blood and blood forming organs. *In* Catcott EJ (ed): Feline Medicine and Surgery. Santa Barbara, American Veterinary Publications, Inc, 1975.

Loeb WF, Rininger B, Montgomery CA, Jenkins S: Myelomonocytic leukemia in a cat. Vet Pathol 12 (1975) 464–467.

MacEwen EG, Hurvitz AI: Diagnosis and management of monoclonal gammopathies. Vet Clin North Am 7 (1977) 119–132.

Mackey L, Jarrett W, Jarrett O, Laird H: Anemia associated with feline leukemia virus infection in cats. J Natl Cancer Inst 54 (1975) 209–217.

Madewell BR, Feldman BF: Characterization of anemias associated with neoplasia in small animals. J Am Vet Med Assoc 176 (1980) 419–425.

Madewell BR, Gunn C, Gribble DH: Mast cell phagocytosis of red blood cells in a cat. Vet Pathol 20 (1983) 638–640.

Madewell BR, Jain NC, Weller RE: Hematologic abnormalities preceding myeloid leukemia in three cats. Vet Pathol 16 (1979) 510–519.

Maede Y: Studies on feline haemobartonellosis. IV. Lifespan of erythrocytes of cats infected with *Haemobartonella felis*. Jpn J Vet Sci 37 (1975) 461–464.

Maede Y, Murata H: Erythroleukemia in a cat with special reference to the fine structure of primitive cells in its peripheral blood. Jpn J Vet Sci 42 (1980) 531–541.

Maggio L: Anemia in the cat. Compend Contin Ed 1 (1979) 114–122.

Maggio L, Hoffman R, Cotter SM, Dainiakn N, Mooney S, Maffei LA: Feline preleukemia: an animal model of human disease. Yale J Biol Med 51 (1978) 469–476.

Mahaffey EA, Smith JE: Depression anemia in cats. Feline Pract 8 (5) (1978) 19–22.

Marion RS, Smith JE: Survival of erythrocytes after autologous and allogeneic transfusion in cats. J Am Vet Med Assoc 183 (1983a) 1437–1439.

Marion RS, Smith JE: Posttransfusion viability of feline erythrocytes stored in acid-citrate-dextrose solution. J Am Vet Med Assoc 183 (1983b) 1459–1460.

McCaffrey R, Cotter S, McLane M: Unpublished observations, 1980.

McClelland AJ, Hardy WD Jr, Zuckerman EE: Prognosis of healthy feline leukemia virus infected cats. *In* Hardy WD Jr, Essex M, McClelland AJ (eds): Feline Leukemia Virus. New York, Elsevier/North-Holland, 1980.

McMillan FD: Hypercalcemia associated with lymphoid neoplasia in two cats. Feline Pract 15 (3) (1985) 31–35.

Meier H, Patterson DF: Myelogenous leukemia in a cat. J Am Vet Med Assoc 128 (1956) 211–214.

Meincke JE, Hobbie WV Jr, Hardy WD Jr: Lymphoreticular malignancies in the cat: clinical findings. J Am Vet Med Assoc 160 (1972) 1093–1099.

Mellors RC: Murine leukemialike virus and the immunopathological disorders of New Zealand black mice. J Infect Dis 120 (1969) 480–487.

Michel RL, O'Handley P, Dade AW: Megakaryocytic myelosis in a cat. J Am Vet Med Assoc 168 (1976) 1021–1025.

Mitchell MC, Schenker S, Avant GR, Speeg KV Jr: Cimetidine protects against acetaminophen hepatotoxicity in rats. Gastroenterology 81 (1981) 1052–1060.

Moore FM, Emerson WE, Cotter SM, DeLellis RA: Spontaneous peripheral lymph node enlargement of young cats resembling human angioimmunoblastic lymphadenopathy: a feline leukemia virus (FeLV) associated lesion (abstr). Lab Invest 52 (1985) 45A.

Moore RP: Feline eosinophilic enteritis. *In* Kirk RW (ed): Current Veterinary Therapy VIII. Philadelphia, WB Saunders Company, 1983, 791–793.

Muller GH, Kirk RW, Scott DW: Small Animal Dermatology, 3rd ed. Philadelphia, WB Saunders Company, 1983.

Mulvaney DA, Ugenti J: Blood group study in the domestic cat. Carnivore Genetics Newsletter 7 (1969) 150–153.

Nathan DG, Chess L, Hillman DG, Clarke B, Breard J, Merler E, Houseman DE: Human erythroid burst-forming unit: T cell requirement for proliferation in vitro. J Exp Med 47 (1978) 324–339.

Nickel R, Schummer A, Seiferle E: The Anatomy of the Domestic Animals. New York, Springer-Verlag, 1979.

Nielsen SW: Spontaneous hematopoietic neoplasms of the domestic cat. *In* Lingeman CH, Garner FM (eds): Symposium on Comparative Morphology of Hematopoietic Neoplasms. National Cancer Institute Monograph 32. Bethesda, MD, National Cancer Institute, 1969, 73–94.

Nielsen SW, Howard EB, Wolke RE: Feline mastocytosis. *In* Clark WJ, Howard EB, Hackett PL (eds): Myeloproliferative Disorders of Animals and Man. Oak Ridge, TN, US Atomic Energy Commission Division of Technical Information, 1971, 359–370.

Odeberg B: Eosinophilic leukemia and disseminated eosinophilic collagen disease—a disease entity? Acta Med Scand 177 (1965) 129–144.

Olsen RG, Lewis MG, Kociba GJ, Rojko JL, Velicer LF: Identification of eosinophilic leukemia in cats infected with a recombinant feline leukemia virus. Leuk Rev Int 1 (1983) 111–112.

Onions D, Testa N, Jarrett O: Growth of FeLV in haemopoietic cells *in vitro*. *In* Hardy WD Jr, Essex M, McClelland AJ (eds): Feline Leukemia Virus. New York, Elsevier/North-Holland, 1980, 507–516.

Oshiro LS, Taylor DON, Riggs JL, Lennette EH: Replication of feline C-type virus at the plasma membrane of erythrocytes. J Natl Cancer Inst 48 (1972) 1419–1424.

Ott RL: Systemic viral diseases. *In* Pratt PW (ed): Feline Medicine. Santa Barbara, American Veterinary Publications, Inc, 1983.

Parrillo JE, Fauci AS, Wolff SM: Therapy of the hypereosinophilic syndrome. Ann Intern Med 89 (1978) 167–172.

Patterson DF, Meier H: Surgical intervention in intestinal lymphosarcoma in two cats. J Am Vet Med Assoc 127 (1955) 495–498.

Pedersen NC, Madewell BR: Feline leukemia virus disease complex. *In* Kirk RW (ed): Current Veterinary Therapy VII. Philadelphia, WB Saunders Company, 1980, 404–410.

Pedersen NC, Johnson L, Ott RL: Evaluation of a commercial feline leukemia virus vaccine for immunogenicity and efficacy. Feline Pract 15 (6) (1985) 7–20.

Pederson NC, Meric SM, Johnson L, Plucker S, Theilen GH: The clinical significance of latent feline leukemia virus infection in cats. Feline Pract 14 (2) (1984) 32–48.

Pedersen NC, Theilen G, Keane MA, Fairbanks L, Mason T, Orser B, Chen CH, Allison C: Studies of naturally transmitted feline leukemia virus infection. Am J Vet Res 38 (1977) 1523–1531.

Penny RHC, Carlisle CH, Prescott CW, Davidson HA: Effects of chloramphenicol on the haemopoietic system of the cat. Br Vet J 123 (1967a) 145–153.

Penny RHC, Carlisle CH, Prescott CW, Davidson HA: Effect of aspirin (acetylsalicylic acid) on the haemopoietic system of the cat. Br Vet J 123 (1967b) 154–161.

Penny RHC, Carlisle CH, Prescott CW, Davidson HA: Further observations on the effect of chloramphenicol on the haemopoietic system of the cat. Br Vet J 126 (1970) 453–458.

Perman V, Schall WD: Diseases of the red blood cells. *In* Ettinger SJ (ed): Textbook of Veterinary Internal Medicine, 2nd ed. Philadelphia, WB Saunders Company, 1983, 1938–2000.

Perryman LE, Hoover EA, Yohn DS: Immunologic reactivity of the cat: Immunosuppression in experimental feline leukemia. J Natl Cancer Inst 49 (1972) 1357–1365.

Peterson ME, Hurvitz AI, Leib MS, Cavanagh PG, Dutton RE: Propylthiouracil-associated hemolytic anemia, thrombocytopenia, and antinuclear antibodies in cats with hyperthyroidism. J Am Vet Med Assoc 184 (1984) 806–808.

Post JE, Warren L: Reactivation of latent feline leukemia virus. *In* Hardy WD Jr, Essex M, McClelland AJ (eds): Feline Leukemia Virus. New York, Elsevier/North-Holland, 1980, 151–155.

Povey RC: Effect of orally administered ribavirin on experimental feline calicivirus infection in cats. Am J Vet Res 39 (1978) 1337–1341.

Prasse KW: White blood cell disorders. *In* Ettinger SJ (ed): Textbook of Veterinary Internal Medicine, 2nd ed. Philadelphia, WB Saunders Company, 1983, 2001–2045.

Priester WA, McKay FW: The Occurrence of Tumors in Domestic Animals. National Cancer Institute Monograph 54. Bethesda, MD, National Cancer Institute, 1980.

Prieur DJ, Collier LL: Chediak-Higashi syndrome of animals. Am J Pathol 90 (1978) 533–536.

Rappaport H: Tumors of the hematopoietic system. *In* Atlas of Tumor Pathology, Section III, Fascicle 8. Washington, DC, Armed Forces Institute of Pathology, 1966.

Raskin RE, Krehbiel JD: Myelodysplastic changes in a cat with myelomonocytic leukemia. J Am Vet Med Assoc 187 (1985) 171–174.

Reed C, Ling GV, Gould D, Kaneko JJ: Polycythemia vera in a cat. J Am Vet Med Assoc 157 (1970) 85–91.

Reid JA, Marcus LC: Granulocytic leukemia in a cat. J Small Anim Pract 7 (1966) 421–425.

Ripps CS, Hurvitz AI: Myeloproliferative disorder in two cats: cytogenetic studies. Am J Vet Res 32 (1971) 93–97.

Rojko JL, Hoover EA, Mathes LE, Krakowka S, Olsen RG: Influence of adrenal corticosteroids on the susceptibility of cats to feline leukemia virus infection. Cancer Res 39 (1979) 3789–3791.

Rojko JL, Hoover EA, Quackenbush SL, Olsen RG: Reactivation of latent feline leukaemia virus infection. Nature 298 (1982) 385–388.

Roperto F, Damiano S, Galati P: Hodgkin's disease in a cat. Zentralbl Veterinärmed A30 (1983) 182–188.

Rowe WS, Bradford TS, Martin P: Posterior paralysis due to lymphosarcoma. Feline Pract 7 (6) (1977) 34–36.

Ruehl W, Mills C, Feldman BF: Rational therapy in disseminated intravascular coagulation. J Am Vet Med Assoc 181 (1982) 76–78.

Saar C: Erythrämie und Erythroleukämie bei der Katze. Bericht über je einen Fall. Berl Münch Tierärztl Wochenschr 21 (1968) 423–426.

Saar C: Erythro-Megakaryozythämie bei einer Katze. Berl Münch Tierärztl Wochenschr 83 (1970) 70–74.

Saar C, Reichel C: Einige besondere Leukoseformen bei der Katze. Prakt Tierarzt 5 (1983) 443–450.

Saar C, Scherpe W-P: Osteolytische Knochendestruktionen bei einer Katze mit unreifzelliger Leukose. Kleintierpraxis 18 (3) (1973) 82–83.

Saar C, Saar U, Opitz M, Burow H, Teichert G: Paraproteinämische Retikulosen bei der Katze. (Bericht über je einen Fall von Plasmazellenretikulose und Makroglobulinämie.) Berl Münch Tierärztl Wochenschr 86 (1973) 11–15, 21–24.

Sallan SE, Ritz J, Pesando J, Gelber R, O'Brien C, Hitchcock S, Coral F, Schlossman SF: Cell surface antigens: prognostic implications in childhood acute lymphoblastic leukemia. Blood 55 (1980) 395–402.

Sandberg AA, Hossfeld DK: Chromosomal abnormalities in human neoplasia. Annu Rev Med 21(1970) 379–408.

Savides MC, Oehme FW, Leipold HW: Effects of various antidotal treatments on acetaminophen toxicosis and biotransformation in cats. Am J Vet Res 40 (1985) 1485–1489.

Schaer M, Zaki FA, Harvey HJ, O'Reilly WH: Laryngeal hemiplegia due to neoplasia of the vagus nerve in a cat. J Am Vet Med Assoc 174 (1979) 513–515.

Schalm OW: Inclusion bodies in the erythrocytes of the cat. Calif Vet 17 (2) (1962) 34–36.

Schalm OW: Myeloproliferative disorder in a cat with a period of remission followed by a relapse two years later. Calif Vet 27 (4) (1973) 26–29.

Schalm OW: Heinz body anemia in the cat. Feline Pract 7 (6) (1977) 30–33.

Schalm OW: Progression of a myeloproliferative disorder in the cat. Feline Pract 8 (2) (1978a) 14–17.

Schalm OW: Findings in feline bone marrow. 1. Effect of cyclophosphamide. 2. Feline infectious anemia and lymphosarcoma. 3. Toxoplasmosis and erythroleukemia. Feline Pract 8 (4) (1978b) 18–22.

Schalm OW, Jain NC, Carroll EJ: Veterinary Hematology, 3rd ed. Philadelphia, Lea & Febiger, 1975.

Schechter RD, Schalm OW, Kaneko JJ: Heinz body hemolytic anemia associated with the use of urinary antiseptics containing methylene blue in the cat. J Am Vet Med Assoc 162 (1973) 37–44.

Schmauch G: Ueber endoglobuläre Körperchen in den Erythrocyten der Katze. Virchows Arch (A) 156 (1899) 201–244.

Schrader LA, Hurvitz AI: Cold agglutinin disease in a cat. J Am Vet Med Assoc 183 (1983) 121–122.

Scott DW: Feline dermatology 1900–1978: a monograph. J Am Anim Hosp Assoc 16 (1980) 331–459.

Scott DW, Schultz RD, Post JE, Bolton GR, Baldwin CA: Autoimmune hemolytic anemia in the cat. J Am Anim Hosp Assoc 9 (1973) 530–539.

Shahidi NT, Diamond LK: Testosterone-induced remission in aplastic anemia of both acquired and congenital types. N Engl J Med 264 (1961) 953–967.

Sheriff D: Feline infectious anaemia. Vet Rec 94 (1974) 385.

Silverman J: Eosinophilic leukemia in a cat. J. Am Vet Med Assoc 158 (1971) 199.

Simon N, Holzworth J: Eosinophilic leukemia in a cat. Cornell Vet 57 (1967) 579–597.

Sodikoff CH: Heinz body anemia in a cat induced by methylene blue. Feline Pract 3 (2) (1973) 38–42.

Sodikoff CH, Custer MA: Autoimmune hemolytic anemia. Anim Hosp 1 (1965) 261–262.

Sodikoff CH, Custer MA: Secondary autoimmune hemolytic anemia in cats. Anim Hosp 2 (1966) 20–23.

Solomon GE, Hilgartner MW, Kutt H: Phenobarbital-induced coagulation defects in cats. Neurology 24 (1974) 920–924.

Spicer SS: Effect of para-aminobenzoic acid on the in vivo oxidation of hemoglobin. J Indust Hyg Toxicol 31 (1949) 204–205.

Stann SE: Myelomonocytic leukemia in a cat. J Am Vet Med Assoc 174 (1979) 722–725.

St. Omer VV, McKnight ED III: Acetylcysteine for treatment of acetaminophen toxicosis in the cat. J Am Vet Med Assoc 176 (1980) 911–913.

Sutton RH, McKellow AM, Bottrill MB: Myeloproliferative disease in the cat: a granulocytic and megakaryocytic disorder NZ Vet J 26 (1978) 273–274, 279.

Swindle MM, Narayan O, Luzarraga M, Bobbie DL: Contagious streptococcal lymphadenitis in cats. J Am Vet Med Assoc 177 (1980) 829–830.

Taketa F: Organic phosphates and hemoglobin structure-function relationships in the feline. Ann NY Acad Sci 241 (1974) 524–537.

Tangner CH: Transfusion therapy for the dog and cat. Compend Contin Ed 4 (1982) 521–527.

Theilen GH, Madewell BR: Veterinary Cancer Medicine. Philadelphia, Lea & Febiger, 1979.

Thenen SW, Rasmussen KM: Megaloblastic erythropoiesis and tissue depletion of folic acid in the cat. Am J Vet Res 39 (1978) 1205–1207.

Thrall MA: Lymphoproliferative disorders: Lymphocytic leukemia and plasma cell myeloma. Vet Clin North Am 11 (1981) 321–347.

Todd GC, Griffing WJ, Gibson WR, Morton DM: Animal models for the comparative assessment of neurotoxicity following repeated administration of vinca alkaloids. Cancer Treat Rep 63 (1979) 35–41.

Tompkins MB, Cummins JM: Response of feline leukemia virus–induced nonregenerative anemia to oral administration of an interferon-containing preparation. Feline Pract 12 (3) (1982) 6–15.

Van Slyck EJ, Adamson TC III: Acute hypereosinophilic syndrome. Successful treatment with vincristine, cytarabine, and prednisone. J Am Med Assoc 242 (1979) 175–176.

Wagner JE: A fatal cytauxzoonosis-like disease in cats. J Am Vet Med Assoc 168 (1976) 585–588.
Ward JM, Sodikoff CH, Schalm OW: Myeloproliferative disease and abnormal erythrogenesis in the cat. J Am Vet Med Assoc 155 (1969) 879–888.
Watson ADJ, Huxtable CRR, Hoskins LP: Erythremic myelosis in two cats. Aust Vet J 50 (1974) 29–33.
Weber SE, Evans DA, Feldman BF: Pelger-Huët anomaly of granulocytic leukocytes in two feline littermates. Feline Pract 11 (1) (1981) 44–47.
Weiser MG, Kociba GJ: Erythrocyte macrocytosis in feline leukemia virus associated anemia. Vet Pathol 20 (1983) 687–697.
Weiss DJ, Krehbiel JD: Studies of the pathogenesis of anemia of inflammation: erythrocyte survival. Am J Vet Res 44 (1983) 1830–1831.
Weiss DJ, Krehbiel JD, Lund JE: Studies of the pathogenesis of anemia of inflammation: mechanism of impaired erythropoiesis. Am J Vet Res 44 (1983) 1832–1835.
Weiss RC, Dodds WJ, Scott FW: Disseminated intravascular coagulation in experimentally induced feline infectious peritonitis. Am J Vet Res 41 (1980) 663–671.
Wilson JE, Gilmore CE: Malignant lymphoma in a cat with involvement of the kidneys demonstrated radiographically. J Am Vet Med Assoc 140 (1962) 1068–1072.
Wintrobe MM, Lee GR, Boggs DR, Bithell TC, Foerster J, Athens JW, Lukens JN: Clinical Hematology, 8th ed. Philadelphia, Lea & Febiger, 1981.
Zawidzka ZZ, Janzen E, Grice HC: Erythremic myelosis in a cat. A case resembling Di Guglielmo's syndrome in man. Pathol Vet 1 (1964) 530–541.
Zenoble RD, Rowland GN: Hypercalcemia and proliferative, myelosclerotic bone reaction associated with feline leukovirus infection in a cat. J Am Vet Med Assoc 175 (1979) 591–595.

**Supplemental References**

Anderson L, Wilson R, Hay D: Haematological values in normal cats from four weeks to one year of age. Res Vet Sci 12 (1971) 579–583.
Aufderheide WM, Kaneko JJ: Erythrocyte 2,3-diphosphoglycerate, diphosphoglycerate mutase and diphosphoglycerate phosphatase in man, dog, cat and sheep. Fed Proc 35 (1976) 853.
Canfield PJ: An ultrastructural study of granulocytic development of feline bone marrow. Anat Histol Embryol 13 (1984) 97–107.
Canfield PJ, Johnson RS: Morphological aspects of prenatal haematopoietic development in the cat. Anat Histol Embryol 13 (1984) 197–221.
Dhindsa DS, Metcalfe J: Post-natal changes in oxygen affinity and the concentration of 2,3-diphosphoglycerate in cat blood. Respir Physiol 21 (1974) 37–46.
George JW, Duncan JR, Mahaffey EA: Comparison of pyrimidine 5′ nucleotidase activity in erythrocytes of sheep, dogs, cats, horses, calves, and Mongolian gerbils. Am J Vet Res 44 (1983) 1968–1970.
Grindem CB, Perman V, Stevens JB: Morphological classification and clinical and pathological characteristics of spontaneous leukemia in 10 cats. J Am Anim Hosp Assoc 21 (1985) 227–236.
Harvey JW, Kaneko JJ: Mammalian erythrocyte metabolism and oxidant drugs. Toxicol Appl Pharmacol 42 (1977) 253–261.
Hubner L: Das Blutbild der Katze. Monatschr Prakt Tierheilkd 31 (1920) 499–501.
Ishmael J, Howell J McC: Observations on the pathology of the spleen of the cat. J Small Anim Pract 9 (1968) 7–13.
Jain NC, Keeton KS: Scanning electron microscopy of Heinz bodies in feline erythrocytes. Am J Vet Res 36 (1975) 1691–1695.
Jain NC, Kono CS: Erythrocyte sedimentation rate in the dog and cat: Comparison of two methods and influence of packed cell volume, temperature and storage of blood. J Small Anim Pract 16 (1975) 671–678.
Jarrett O, Golder MC, Toth S, Onions DE, Stewart MF: Interaction between feline leukaemia virus subgroups in the pathogenesis of erythroid hypoplasia. Int J Cancer 34 (1984) 283–288.
Kasten-Jolly J, Taketa F: Biosynthesis of cat hemoglobins A and B: Amino terminal acetylation of the β chain of HbB. Arch Biochem Biophys 192 (2) (1979) 336–343.
Kociba GJ, Weiser MG, Olsen RG: Enhanced susceptibility to feline leukemia virus in cats with Haemobartonella felis infection. Leuk Rev Int 1 (1983) 88–89.
Lawrence JS, Valentine WN: The blood platelets: The rate of their utilization in the cat. Blood 2 (1947) 40–49.
Lester SJ, Searcy GP: Hematologic abnormalities preceding apparent recovery from feline leukemia virus infection. J Am Vet Med Assoc 178 (1981) 471–474.
Mauk AG, Huang YP, Skogen FW, Litwin SB, Taketa F: The effect of hemoglobin phenotype on whole blood oxygen saturation and erythrocyte organic phosphate concentration in the domestic cat (*Felis catus*). Comp Biochem Physiol 51 [A] (1975) 487–489.
Madewell BR, Holmes PH, Onions DE: Ferrokinetic and erythrocyte survival studies in healthy and anemic cats. Am J Vet Res 44 (1983) 424–427.
Meyers-Wallen VN, Harkins ME, Patterson DF: Hematologic values in healthy, neonatal, weanling, and juvenile kittens. Am J Vet Res 45 (1984) 1322–1327.
Middel-Erdmann I: [Blood sedimentation reaction in the cat. Determination of fibrinogen, erythrocyte volume in blood of cats with different rates of sedimentation.] Dissertation, Fachbereich Veterinärmedizin, Freie Universität, Berlin, 1983.
Osbaldiston GW: Haematological values in healthy cats. Br Vet J 134 (1978) 524–536.
Penny RHC, Carlisle CH, Davidson HA: The blood and marrow picture of the cat. Br Vet J 126 (1970) 459–464.
Rojko JL, Cheney CM, Kociba GJ, Mathes LE, Olsen RG: Infectious leukemia virus depresses erythrogenesis in vitro. Leuk Rev Int 1 (1983) 129–130.
Rojko JL, Hoover EA, Mathes LE, Krakowka S, Olsen RG: Influence of adrenal corticosteroids on the susceptibility of cats to feline leukemia virus infection. Cancer Res 39 (1979) 3789–3791.
Sawitsky A, Meyer LM: The bone marrow of normal cats. J Lab Clin Med 32 (1947) 70–75.
Schermer S: Die Blutmorphologie der Laboratoriumstiere, 2nd ed. Leipzig, Johann Ambrosius Barth, 1958.
Schryver HF: The bone marrow of the cat. Am J Vet Res 24 (1963) 1012–1017.
Skogen WF, Mauk MR, Taketa F: Hemoglobin components in peripheral and marrow erythroid cells of normal and anemic cats. Fed Proc 34 (1975) 604.
Sutton RH: The value of a single haematological examination in the diagnosis of disease in the cat. J Small Anim Pract 21 (1980) 339–345.
Taketa F: Structure of the felidae hemoglobins and response to 2,3-diphosphoglycerate. Comp Biochem Physiol 45 [B] (1973) 813–823.
Taketa F, Chen JY, Palosaari N: Hemoglobin A and B of the cat: occurrence in the same cell. Hemoglobin 2 (1978) 371–381.
Tsujimoto H, Hasegawa A, Tomoda I: A cytochemical study on feline blood cells. Jpn J Vet Sci 45 (1983) 373–382.
Turnwald GH, Pichler ME: Blood transfusion in dogs and cats. Part II. Administration, adverse effects, and component therapy. Compend Contin Ed 115 (1985) 115–122.
Weiser MC, Kociba GJ: Sequential changes in erythrocyte volume distribution and microcytosis associated with iron deficiency in kittens. Vet Pathol 20 (1983) 1–12.
Weiser MG, Kociba GJ: Platelet concentration and platelet volume distribution in healthy cats. Am J Vet Res 45 (1984) 518–522.

# 17
CHAPTER

# INHERITED METABOLIC DISEASES

MARK E. HASKINS and DONALD F. PATTERSON

That an inborn error of metabolism could be responsible for the production of disease was first postulated by Sir Archibald Garrod (1908). According to his concept, certain lifelong diseases are due to the reduction in activity of an enzyme that mediates a single metabolic step. It is now known that the cause of the enzyme abnormality usually involves a mutation in the DNA that codes for the enzyme structure. Such defects in DNA are present in germ cells, as well as somatic cells, and are therefore the basis of the inherited nature of these diseases. Animals homozygous for the normal allele (gene) have normal levels of activity of the enzyme, whereas those homozygous for the mutant allele have little or no enzyme activity and have signs of disease. The definitive diagnosis of a specific enzyme deficiency disorder is thus based on demonstration of deficient activity of that enzyme. In the heterozygote or carrier animal, only one of the pair of genes is abnormal, and the enzyme activity is approximately 50 per cent of normal. Because this is usually sufficient for normal function, heterozygotes do not show clinical signs of disease but transmit the defective gene to half of their offspring. As most of the mutant genes for recessive disorders in the cat population are carried by heterozygotes, it is important to identify carriers and prevent them from breeding. Fortunately, heterozygotes can often be identified by enzyme assay.

Because of the usual autosomal recessive inheritance of these diseases, pedigrees may be helpful in diagnosis. Affected animals are usually born of matings between two clinically normal carriers. On average, one in four offspring of such matings is affected, and males and females are equally at risk. The affected matings are often consanguineous. For example, in a number of reported cases the affected cats resulted from brother-sister or parent-offspring matings.

It is now recognized that single-gene mutations may produce defects in a variety of nonenzymatic proteins, including receptor proteins and structural proteins such as collagen. Because the presence of half-normal receptor protein activity or abnormal structural protein may cause clinical signs, these diseases are often inherited in a dominant pattern. Heterozygotes express the disease, half of the offspring of an affected individual are affected, and the homozygous state is frequently lethal.

## LYSOSOMAL STORAGE DISORDERS

In this group of recessively inherited disorders, the basic defect is deficient activity of an individual catabolic enzyme located within cellular lysosomes. Because it cannot be degraded, the substrate on which the particular enzyme normally acts accumulates within lysosomes. The lysosomes become large, often appearing to fill the cytoplasm, and produce alterations in the size and shape of the cell (Fig. 17–1). The pathologic change and subsequent clinical signs appear to be related primarily to the cellular distortion produced, rather than to a direct toxic effect of the accumulated substrate. Storage occurs in those cell types normally responsible for the catabolism of a particular substrate and, because substrate is continuously presented to the lysosome, the diseases are progressive.

The lysosomal storage disorders known to occur in the cat are inherited as autosomal recessive traits and the names given to the diseases, all of which have been described in man, reflect the substrate that accumulates.

### MUCOPOLYSACCHARIDOSES (MPS)

Glycosaminoglycans (formerly called mucopolysaccharides) are long-chain, repeating molecules that are part of

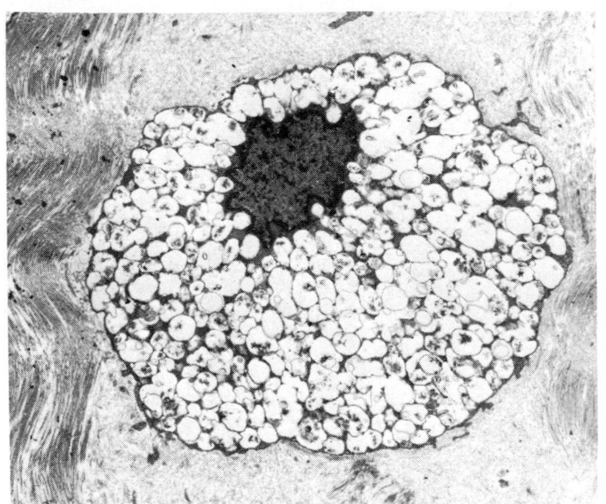

**Figure 17–1** Mucopolysaccharidosis VI, cat. This electron photomicrograph of a cell from the mitral valve illustrates the degree to which the cytoplasm of a cell can become filled with membrane-bound inclusions in a lysosomal storage disease. The accumulated substrate, in this case dermatan sulfate, has been washed out during processing, leaving empty vacuoles. Lead citrate–uranyl acetate, × 3560.

the extracellular ground substance. These compounds are continuously synthesized and degraded, and a number of lysosomal hydrolases are necessary for their sequential breakdown. In the MPS disorders, the glycosaminoglycans remain relatively uncatabolized owing to failure in one enzyme-mediated step. The glycosaminoglycans are stored within the lysosomes, appear in the serum, and are excreted by the kidney. A simple urinary screening test for these compounds can aid in the initial diagnosis of these diseases (Berry and Spinanger, 1960). This test involves placing a drop of urine on a piece of filter paper, letting it dry, staining it with toluidine blue, and washing with ethanol–acetic acid. A second order of urine evaluation involves electrophoresis to determine the individual glycosaminoglycans present in excess.

In man there are at least 10 different MPS disorders, each caused by the deficiency of an enzyme necessary for a distinct step in the catabolism of glycosaminoglycans. Each disease has a characteristic combination of clinical signs, urinary glycosaminoglycans, and enzyme deficiency. Thus far, two of these have been described in the cat.

**MUCOPOLYSACCHARIDOSIS I (MPS I).** Defective activity of alpha-L-iduronidase, resulting in the accumulation of two primary substrates, dermatan and heparan sulfates, has been described in the domestic shorthair (Haskins et al., 1979a, b, 1983a). The clinical signs of MPS I are related to the storage of these compounds in chondrocytes, keratocytes, hepatocytes, fibroblasts of the heart valves, and neurons of the central nervous system. The fully developed clinical syndrome includes a large head with small ears, pectus excavatum, and gait abnormalities referable to cervical vertebral dysplasia and bilateral coxofemoral subluxation. Corneal clouding, mild hepatomegaly, and mitral insufficiency are present. Late in the disease, after two and a half years of age, neurologic abnormalities develop, including muscular rigidity and tremors.

The earliest clinical manifestations of the disease, observed by about 10 weeks, are pectus excavatum and corneal clouding, which prevents clear observation of the fundus on ophthalmologic examination. The clouding within the cornea itself, caused by the accumulation of stored substrate within keratocytes, may not be readily apparent, requiring slit-lamp examination. An ocular discharge that stains the fur at the medial canthus may be present early or may develop later. When normal littermates are available for comparison, it can often be recognized that the affected kittens have large heads and small ears; however, the dysmorphia is not always immediately obvious (Fig. 17–2). The urine spot test for glycosaminoglycans is reliable as a screening test at six

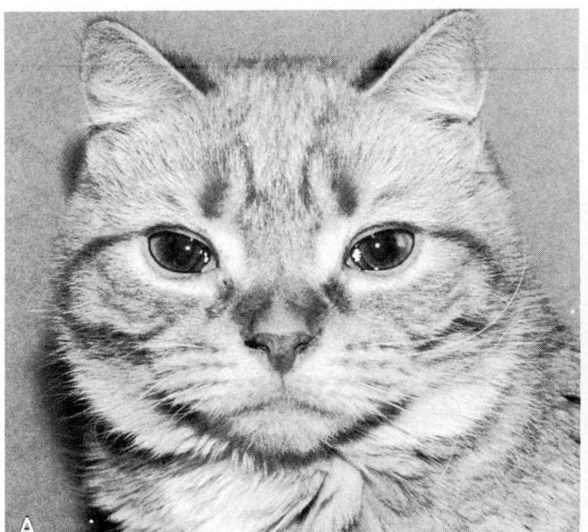


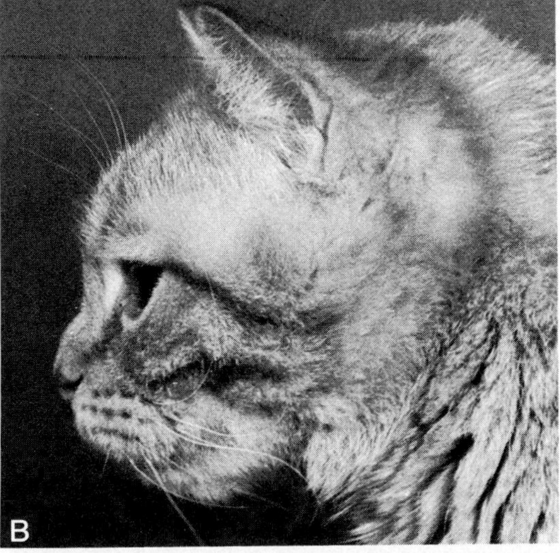


**Figure 17–2** Mucopolysaccharidosis I, one-year-old orange tabby female cat. *A*, The small ears, round head, and ocular discharge are characteristic of cats with this disease. *B*, This view of the same cat illustrates the flattened face seen in MPS I.

weeks of age. On concentration and electrophoresis, the compounds excreted in excess can be identified as heparan and dermatan sulfates. Mitral insufficiency, indicated by a holosystolic murmur best heard at the cardiac apex, is present in some cats but is not usually associated with other clinical signs of heart disease.

The most prominent outward signs of MPS I in young cats and the most likely complaint of the owner are an unsteadiness of the rear legs and some difficulty in jumping. These appear to be related primarily to the bony changes that accompany the disease. Radiographic examination reveals abnormalities of the cervical vertebrae and bilateral subluxation of the femoral heads (Fig. 17–3).

Few cats have been observed late in the course of this disease, and characterization of the neurologic signs is not precise. In those cats studied, the clinical signs of neurologic dysfunction began between two and a half and three years, lasted less than three weeks, and were progressive. Initially, clonus and extensor rigidity, primarily of the hindlimbs, were present, followed by muscle tremors and death. The neurologic signs are thought to be due primarily to lysosomal storage within neurons (Fig. 17–4), the presence of meganeurites, and axonal sprouting (Walkley and Haskins, 1982). However, hydrocephalus and meningiomas (Haskins and McGrath, 1983; Haskins et al., 1983a) have also been seen in a majority of the cats examined. Both a male and a female cat with MPS I have produced offspring. However, fertility appears to be reduced, as each animal had only a single litter.

**MUCOPOLYSACCHARIDOSIS VI (MPS VI).** In this disorder, which has been described in the Siamese cat, a deficiency of arylsulfatase B activity results in storage of the glycosaminoglycan dermatan sulfate (Cowell et al., 1976; Haskins et al., 1979c; Jezyk et al., 1977). Skeletal abnormalities, including facial dysmorphia, are the most prominent clinical signs. By 10 weeks of age, affected kittens are smaller than their littermates and have a broad, flattened face, small ears, and pectus excavatum (Fig. 17–5). The forepaws appear disproportionately large. Corneal clouding is more severe than in MPS I and is often apparent without the aid of a slit lamp.

Blood films reveal large, prominent granules in the

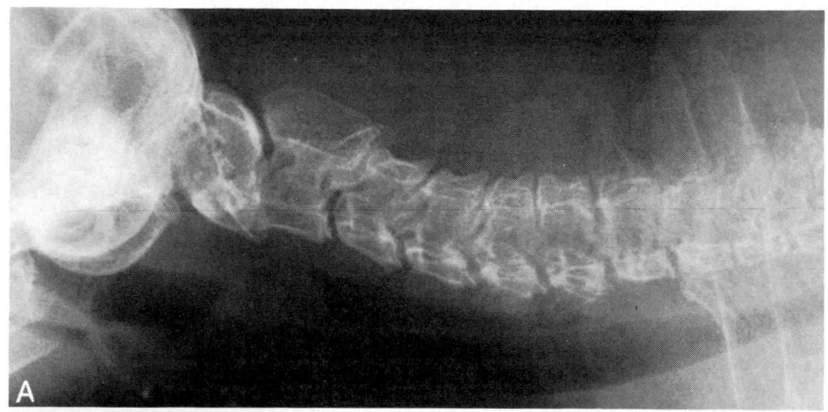


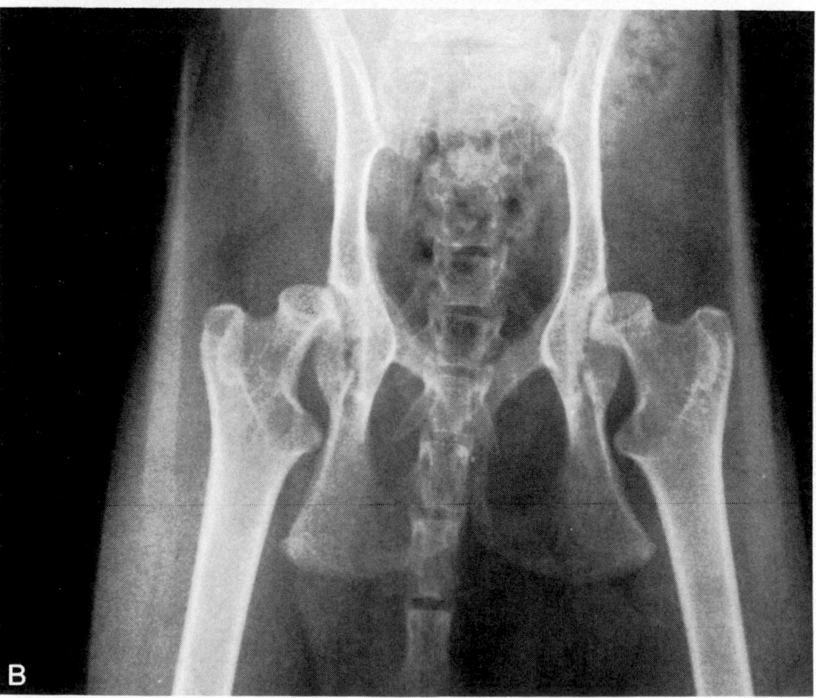


**Figure 17–3** Mucopolysaccharidosis I. *A*, A lateral radiograph of the cervical spine of a 14-month-old female cat illustrates the abnormally narrow vertebral bodies with irregular end-plates, a wide spinal canal, and a coarse trabecular pattern. *B*, A ventrodorsal radiograph demonstrates the bilaterally small femoral head and neck, shallow acetabulum, and coxofemoral subluxation occurring in cats with MPS I.

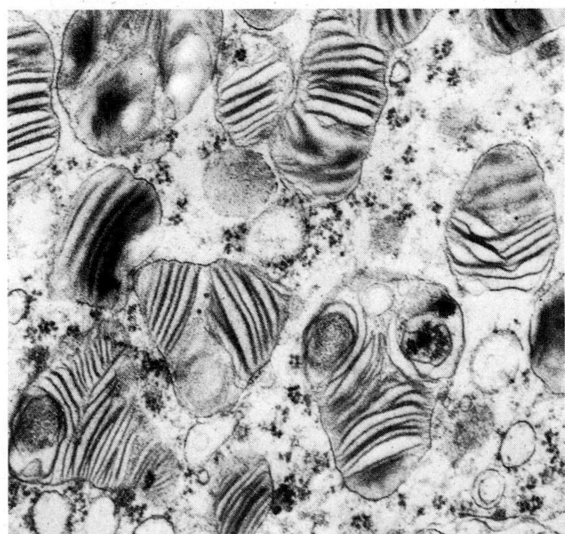

**Figure 17–4** Mucopolysaccharidosis I. Electron photomicrograph of the cytoplasm of a neuron from a one-year-old cat. Membrane-bound lysosomes contain lamellar structures ("zebra bodies") characteristic of most lysosomal storage diseases with neuronal involvement, regardless of the primary substrate that is stored. Lead citrate–uranyl acetate, × 28,500.

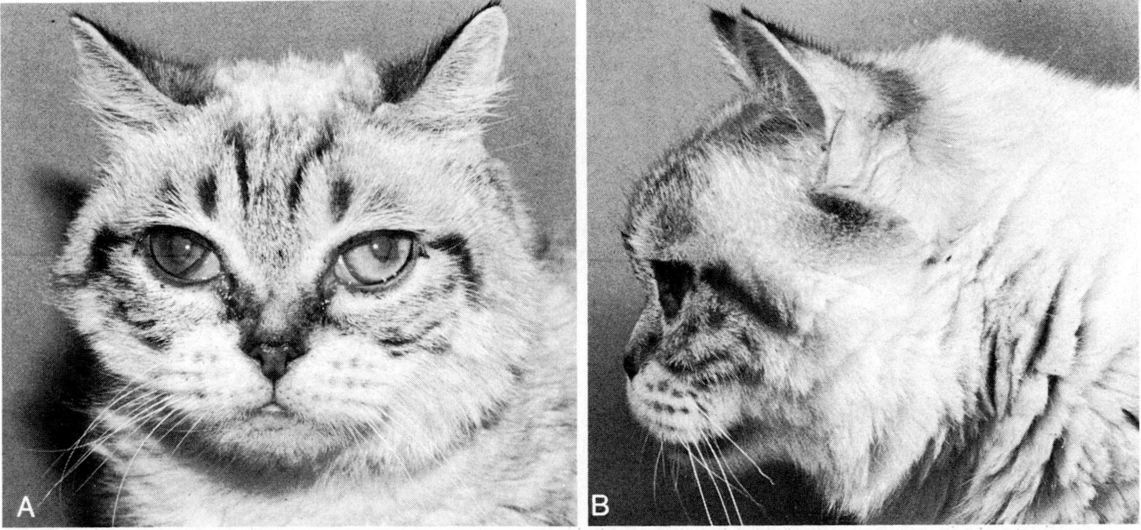


**Figure 17–5** *A*, Mucopolysaccharidosis VI. *A*, A frontal view of a two-year-old tabby point Siamese cat illustrates the hypertelorism (wide-spaced eyes), small ears, and, to some degree, the corneal clouding occurring in this disorder. The prolapsed third eyelid is frequent in these cats. *B*, Same cat as in *A*. The flattened face and frontal bossing are particularly striking in the Siamese cat, which normally has an elongated face.

polymorphonuclear leukocytes (Fig. 17–6). These granules can be seen with Wright-Giemsa stain and appear metachromatic if stained with toluidine blue. The granules have been shown by electron microscopy to be lysosomes swollen with stored material (Fig. 17–7). Vacuoles are present in mononuclear leukocytes. Spot tests of the urine indicate excessive excretion of glycosaminoglycan, which on concentration and electrophoresis is dermatan sulfate.

By five months the gait is abnormal. The cats move with short steps with the head held relatively low and extended. Usually they are incapable of jumping higher than they can reach with their forepaws. Radiographs reveal fusion of the cervical vertebrae, bilateral coxofemoral subluxation, and widespread epiphyseal dysplasia (Fig. 17–8). Approximately 25 per cent of cats with MPS VI develop posterior paresis or paralysis by 10 months, owing to bony growth into the spinal canal, impinging on the spinal cord at the thoracolumbar junction (Haskins et al., 1983b). Lysosomal storage has been demonstrated in leukocytes, hepatocytes, fibroblasts in skin and heart valves, smooth muscle, cornea, and retinal pigment epithelium (Aguirre et al., 1983; Haskins et al., 1980).

Unlike cats with all other lysosomal storage diseases, those with MPS VI have no neuronal storage and may survive to middle or old age. However, they may become increasingly disabled as a result of progressive skeletal changes. The oldest cat seen with MPS VI was a female Siamese that died at five and a half years of age. Both males and females with MPS VI have reproduced successfully, although fertility may be reduced.

Arylsulfatase B deficiency was treated in a two-year-old male Siamese with bone marrow from a normal sibling (Gasper et al., 1984). The urinary dermatan excretion returned to normal, the corneal clouding resolved, and there was improvement in facial conformation and locomotion.

## Gangliosidoses

Gangliosides are sialic acid–containing glycosphingolipids found, among other places, in the plasma membranes of nerve cells. Several syndromes, each with a deficiency of a specific enzyme required for the catabolism of gangliosides, have been described in man; two have been described in the cat. Central nervous system dysfunction is characteristic of these diseases in both man and animals.

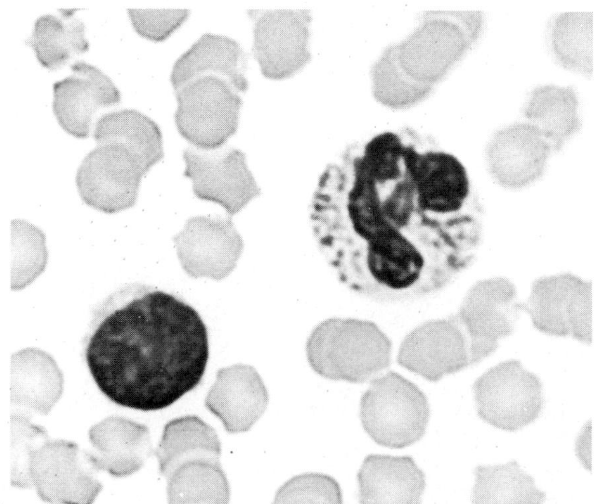

**Figure 17–6** Mucopolysaccharidosis VI. Prominent cytoplasmic granules are present in most polymorphonuclear leukocytes in routine blood films from cats with MPS VI. Wright-Giemsa, × 2000.

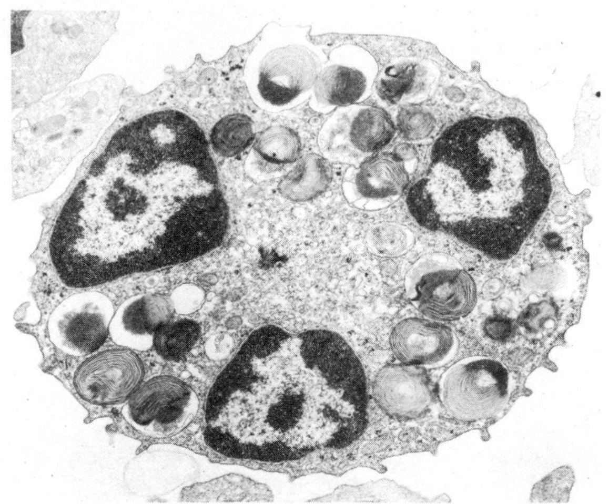

**Figure 17–7** Mucopolysaccharidosis VI. Electron photomicrograph of a polymorphonuclear leukocyte shows the membrane-bound cytoplasmic granules, containing lamellar and granular material, that are visible by light microscopy (Fig. 17–6). Lead citrate–uranyl acetate, × 8270.

**$GM_1$ GANGLIOSIDOSIS.** A deficiency of acid beta-galactosidase has been reported to produce a neurologic syndrome in Siamese, Korat, and domestic shorthairs (Baker and Lindsey, 1974; Baker et al., 1979, 1982; Blakemore, 1972). In this autosomal recessive disorder, weakness, incoordination, dysmetria, and fine muscular tremors of the head and limbs were first noted between two and three months of age. Affected kittens appeared normal at earlier ages. The neurologic abnormalities progressed to quadriplegia, somnolence, blindness, an exaggerated acoustic response, and recurring grand mal seizures by 12 months of age. One series of animals with less documentation had corneal opacities, and the retina, although difficult to examine, contained numerous pale gray and darker spots throughout the tapetum nigrum and tapetum lucidum, respectively (Murray et al., 1977). These cats also had hepatomegaly.

Unlike the cats with mucopolysaccharidoses, cats with $GM_1$ gangliosidosis have no obvious dysmorphia or bony lesions and do not excrete any urinary products detectable by simple methods. Histologic examination of the liver and nervous system reveals cytoloplasmic vacuolation of hepatocytes and neurons, which, seen by electron microscopy, are swollen lysosomes containing stored material (Farrell et al., 1973). Widespread neuronal degeneration is present. The definitive diagnosis can be made by measuring beta-galactosidase activity (pH optimum 3.8) in brain, kidney, skin, and cultured fibroblasts.

**$GM_2$ GANGLIOSIDOSIS.** A deficiency of both A and B isoenzymes of beta-D-*N*-acetyl hexosaminidase has been reported to produce in domestic shorthaired cats (Baker et al., 1982; Cork et al., 1977) and in Korat cats (Neuwelt et al., 1985) a syndrome similar to $GM_1$ gangliosidosis. However, the age at onset is earlier and the progression

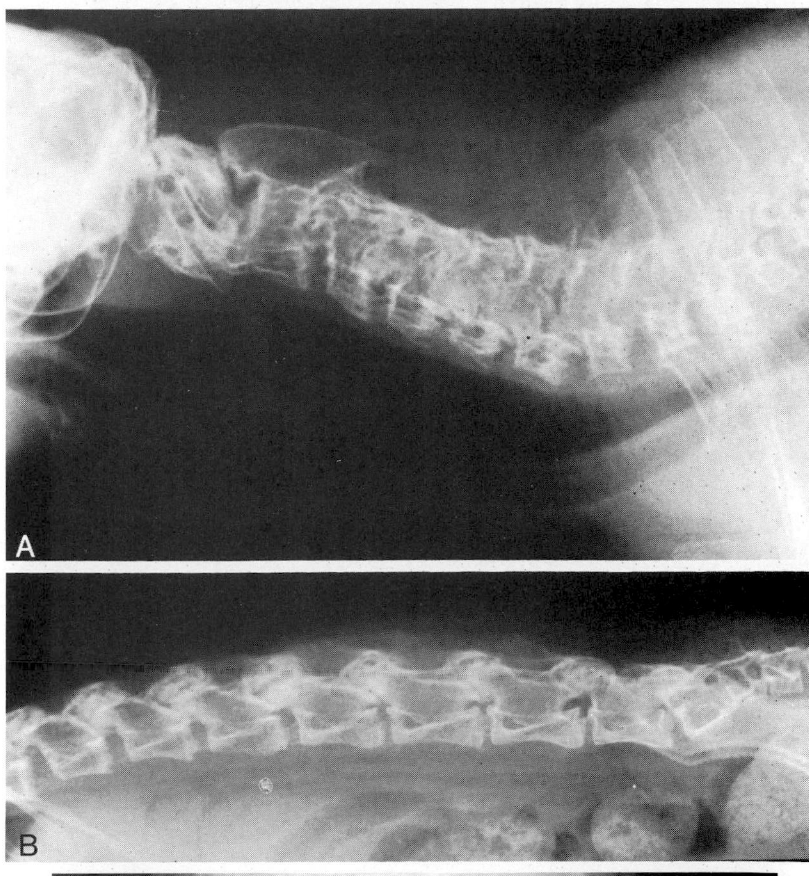


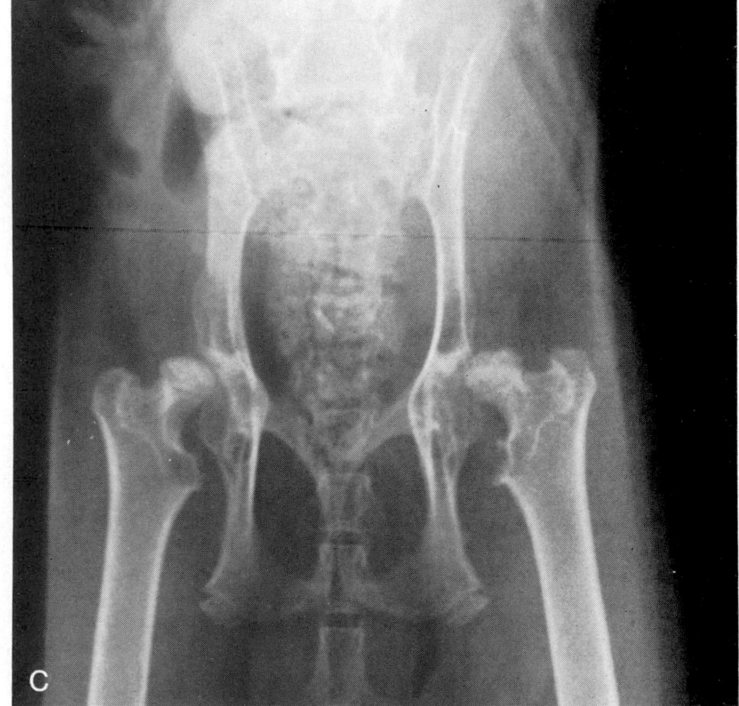


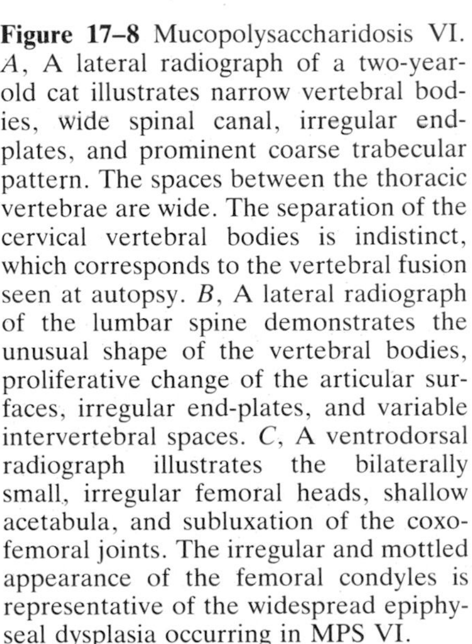
**Figure 17–8** Mucopolysaccharidosis VI. *A*, A lateral radiograph of a two-year-old cat illustrates narrow vertebral bodies, wide spinal canal, irregular end-plates, and prominent coarse trabecular pattern. The spaces between the thoracic vertebrae are wide. The separation of the cervical vertebral bodies is indistinct, which corresponds to the vertebral fusion seen at autopsy. *B*, A lateral radiograph of the lumbar spine demonstrates the unusual shape of the vertebral bodies, proliferative change of the articular surfaces, irregular end-plates, and variable intervertebral spaces. *C*, A ventrodorsal radiograph illustrates the bilaterally small, irregular femoral heads, shallow acetabula, and subluxation of the coxofemoral joints. The irregular and mottled appearance of the femoral condyles is representative of the widespread epiphyseal dysplasia occurring in MPS VI.

of signs more rapid. Ataxia, hypermetria, and head tremor occur between one and two months, and the disorder progresses to paralysis by four to five months. The cats have unusually round heads, strained facial expressions, and diffuse corneal clouding that prevents funduscopic examination. No organomegaly or bony lesions have been described, and there are no abnormal compounds in the urine to aid in diagnosis.

The histopathologic and electron microscopic findings closely resemble those of $GM_1$ gangliosidosis: neuronal degeneration and lysosomal storage (Cork et al., 1978). The specific diagnosis of $GM_2$ gangliosidosis can be made by demonstrating a combined deficiency of hexosaminidase isozymes A and B in brain, liver, or cultured fibroblasts.

## Mannosidosis

N-linked glycoproteins are a major class of glycoproteins containing dibranched alpha-mannosyl residues. They are constituents of cell membranes and also of many elements of body fluids. Deficient activity of alpha-mannosidase, which catabolizes this class of glycoproteins, has been described in man and Angus cattle and also in domestic (Burditt et al., 1980) and Persian cats (Alroy et al., 1986a; Jezyk et al., 1986; Vandevelde et al., 1982). The age at onset of clinical signs appears to be variable.

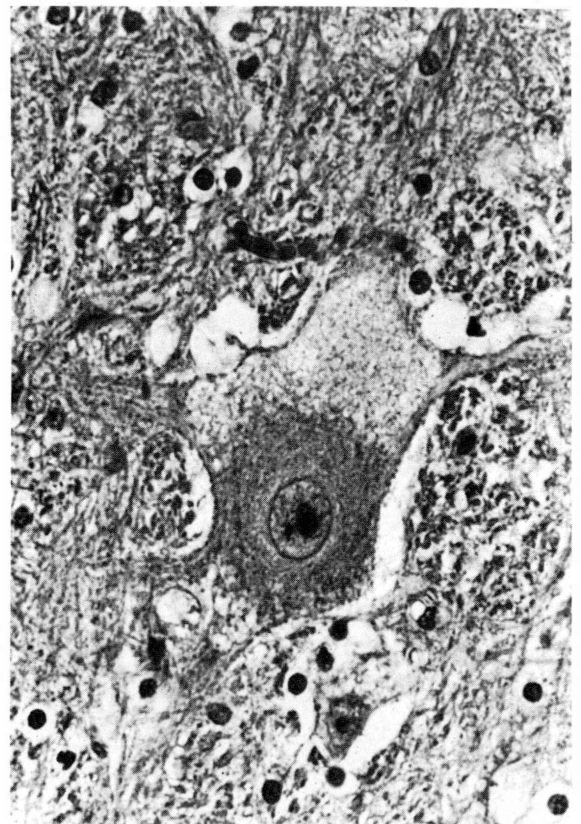

**Figure 17–9** Mannosidosis. The pale area in the cytoplasm of this neuron from the reticular formation represents lysosomal storage in a nine-month-old blue Persian cat. H & E, × 345.

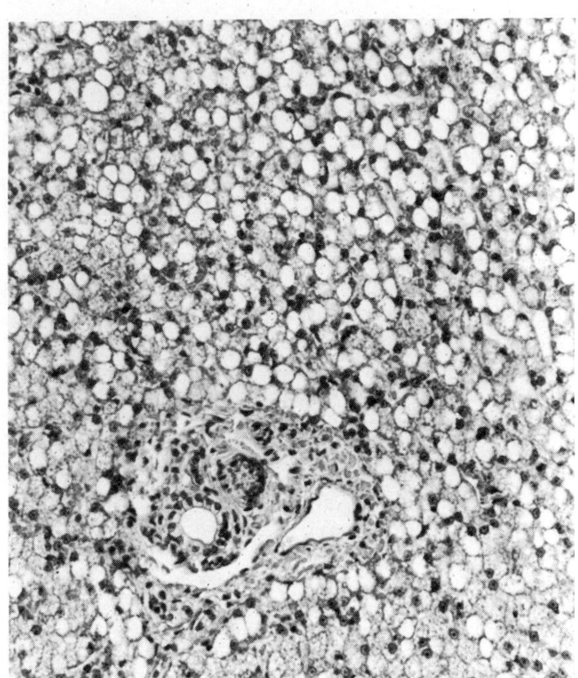

**Figure 17–10** Mannosidosis, liver. The widespread vacuolation of the hepatocytes is consistent with lysosomal storage. H & E, × 131.

Of the cats reported with this disease, some are either stillborn or die without apparent clinical signs, and some die before the age of two months with a brief clinical course of generalized weakness, apathy, and diarrhea. Other kittens may be presented with signs of central neuropathy at from three to seven months of age, although subtle signs of neurologic abnormality may be detectable in kittens at a week of age (Alroy et al., 1986a). The neurologic manifestations include severe ataxia, hypermetric gait, slow righting and flexor reflexes, intention tremor, and strabismus. These signs are progressive and ultimately necessitate euthanasia.

Non-neurologic signs are also variable. Skeletal abnormalities are probably present to some degree in all affected kittens and may include frontal "bossing." Ocular abnormalities of some sort are also present in most or all of the affected kittens. These include fine diffuse stippling of the corneas, many small vacuoles along the suture lines of the lenses, and a gray, granular lesion in the area centralis of the fundus (Aguirre et al., 1985). Cataracts also occur (Alroy et al., 1986a). Growth may be retarded, and some kittens have had enlarged livers.

Occasional autopsy findings have been thymic aplasia, polycystic kidneys, and large thyroid glands. In addition to the widespread lysosomal storage throughout the central nervous system (Fig. 17–9) and the presence of meganeurites (Walkely et al., 1981), enlargements within axons and demyelination occur consistently. Extraneural vacuolation is reported most consistently in the liver (Fig. 17–10) but also occurs in pancreatic, salivary, endocrine, renal, corneal, endothelial, and placental cells, as well as in chondrocytes (Alroy et al., 1986b).

No urinary products provide a simple screening test for the initial diagnosis of this disease. However, mannose-rich oligosaccharides can be detected by more complex methods. Blood films have been reported to contain vacuolated lymphocytes (Burditt et al., 1980), and vacuoles may also appear in other white cells. Oligosaccharides are demonstrable in the placenta of affected kittens (Warren et al., 1986).

### SPHINGOMYELINOSIS

A deficiency of lysosomal sphingomyelinase activity has been reported to produce a neurologic disease in Siamese cats (Snyder et al., 1982; Wenger et al., 1980). Sphingomyelin and, secondarily, cholesterol and gangliosides were found to have accumulated in neurons, hepatocytes, and reticuloendothelial cells. The first reported case of presumed sphingomyelinosis, with characteristic clinical and pathologic signs but without enzyme confirmation, was also in a Siamese cat (Chrisp et al., 1970).

The earliest signs of the disease include growth retardation and ataxia beginning at about four months of age. Affected kittens had anisocoria and an abnormal iridic color and were apparently blind by five months of age (Aguirre et al., 1985). The disease progressed with increasing ataxia and difficulty in eating and drinking, apparently related to a bobbing head movement. Neurologic signs became progressively more severe, and death occurred before one year of age. Blood films contained lymphocytes and monocytes with clear, cytoplasmic vacuoles.

At autopsy, the lymph nodes, livers, and spleens were enlarged. The presence of half-normal levels of sphingomyelinase activity in leukocytes from clinically normal littermates of affected cats strongly supported the hypothesis that this disease was inherited as an autosomal recessive trait (similar to its counterpart in man, Niemann-Pick disease). The definitive diagnosis can be made by demonstrating a total deficiency of sphingomyelinase activity (pH 5.0) in leukocytes, liver, and brain of affected cats.

### OTHER LYSOSOMAL STORAGE DISEASE

A suspected lysosomal storage disease has been reported in related Abyssinian kittens (Lange et al., 1977; Bland van den Berg et al., 1977). It was manifested clinically by ataxia, incoordination, and dysmetria, and microscopically by vacuolation of neurons and macrophages. Irregularly shaped membrane-bound bodies with an amorphous substance were found in the cytoplasm of affected cells. Biochemical studies did not reveal the nature of the stored material (Lange et al., 1983), and lysosomal enzyme activities were not evaluated.

## GLOBOID CELL LEUKODYSTROPHY (KRABBE'S DISEASE)

In man, a deficiency of galactocerebroside beta-galactosidase activity produces a dysmyelinating disease of the central and peripheral nervous systems (Suzuki and Suzuki, 1983). Although beta-galactosidase is a lysosomal enzyme, this disorder is not, strictly speaking, a lysosomal storage disorder, because the material that accumulates within the "globoid cells" is not contained within lysosomes. A disease with clinical and pathologic findings similar to those in man has been reported in two closely related members of an inbred family of domestic shorthaired cats (Johnson, 1970). However, enzymatic confirmation was not made in these cats (and was not confirmed in human cases until 1970).

The earliest clinical signs, occurring at five to six weeks of age in affected cats, were posterior dysmetria and incoordination. Ataxia was progressive, in one case involving the forelimbs; occasional generalized tremors were present in both cats. The cats were destroyed at six and a half and eight and a half weeks of age.

At autopsy, the white matter of the brains appeared dull white, without any abnormality in consistency. Histologically, myelin deficiency was widespread, and the characteristic PAS-positive, nonmetachromatic, and nonsudanophilic "globoid cells," thought to be macrophages, were present throughout areas of affected white matter in the central nervous system.

In human patients, galactocerebroside beta-galactosidase activity has been shown to be deficient in leukocytes, serum, cultured fibroblasts, and a variety of tissues including brain and liver (Suzuki and Suzuki, 1983). These cells, fluids, and tissues are therefore likely to exhibit the enzyme deficiency in cats.

## HYPERCHYLOMICRONEMIA

Instances of hyperlipemia in related cats have been reported (Bauer and Verlander, 1984; Jones et al., 1983). The lipemia, related to an apparent deficiency of lipoprotein lipase, was evident as a milkiness of the serum, recognized in vessels of the retina. Plasma cholesterol and triglycerides were elevated. In one young cat, numerous subcutaneous nodules palpated over bony prominences proved to be xanthomas (Jones et al., 1983). On a lower fat diet the xanthomas resolved over a six-week period. Other signs that also resolved were hindlimb lameness and right-sided Horner's syndrome. Whether these were related to the hyperlipemia was not determined. Pedigree analyses were not reported.

## CHEDIAK-HIGASHI SYNDROME

An autosomal recessive syndrome of hypopigmentation, abnormal granulation of neutrophils and melanocytes, and immune deficiency has been described in a variety of species (Lutzner et al., 1967; Padgett et al., 1964; Prieur and Collier, 1978; Sato, 1955; Taylor and Farrell, 1973). The syndrome has also been reported to occur in a family of Persian cats (Kramer et al., 1977). The pathogenesis of this syndrome, which may not be the same in different species, is not well understood. A defect in cyclic nucleotide metabolism and microtubule assembly has been postulated in the murine form of the syndrome occurring in the beige mouse (Oliver and Zurier, 1976). This explanation, however, may not apply to the cat (Meyers et al., 1982). In the beige mouse and affected humans, an immune deficiency is associated with a defect in natural killer cells (Roder, 1982).

Persian cats with Chédiak-Higashi syndrome were not reported to have severe or progressive clinical disease.

Blue smoke Persians are affected and have light yellow-green irises with an unusual "basket-weave" pattern. Ocular abnormalities include photophobia, thin irides, spontaneous nystagmus, and decreased fundic pigmentation (Collier et al., 1979, 1985). The cataracts originally described as part of this syndrome may have been the result of another inherited disorder (Aguirre et al., 1985).

Abnormally large eosinophilic, sudanophilic, peroxidase-containing granules were observed in blood and bone marrow neutrophils (Kramer et al., 1977). Eosinophils and basophils also contained abnormal granules. However, no increased susceptibility to infectious disease has been noted in the cats. Within the skin and hair, melanin granules were also abnormally large. A bleeding tendency, undocumented by clinical laboratory tests, was seen on venepuncture in affected cats. This tendency may be partly attributable to a reduction in the number of platelet-dense granules and an associated deficiency of secreted adenine nucleotides, serotonin, and reduced bivalent cations normally stored in these granules (Meyers et al., 1982). The question of whether a mild immunodeficiency is present in cats with the Chédiak-Higashi syndrome remains to be answered by further studies.

The diagnosis of Chédiak-Higashi syndrome is made on the basis of histologic and ultrastructural features, as at present no enzyme deficiency is known to be associated with this autosomal recessive disorder.

## GYRATE ATROPHY OF THE RETINA

A deficiency in activity of the mitochondrial matrix enzyme ornithine aminotransferase has been reported in a domestic shorthaired cat of undetermined ancestry (Valle et al., 1981). The animal was an adult male in good health presented for apparent blindness. Ophthalmoscopic examination revealed bilateral generalized retinal atrophy and thinning with vascular attenuation. Cataracts were not present. Plasma ornithine levels were increased 60 fold, producing an overflow ornithinuria.

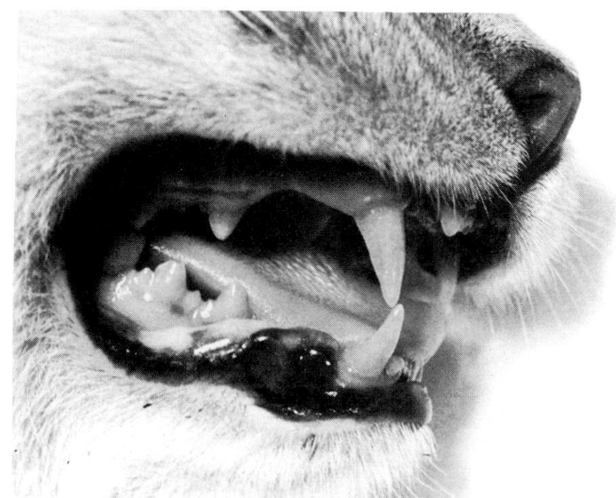

**Figure 17–11** Porphyria, adult domestic shorthair cat. The discoloration of the teeth is characteristic in cats with this disorder of heme biosynthesis.

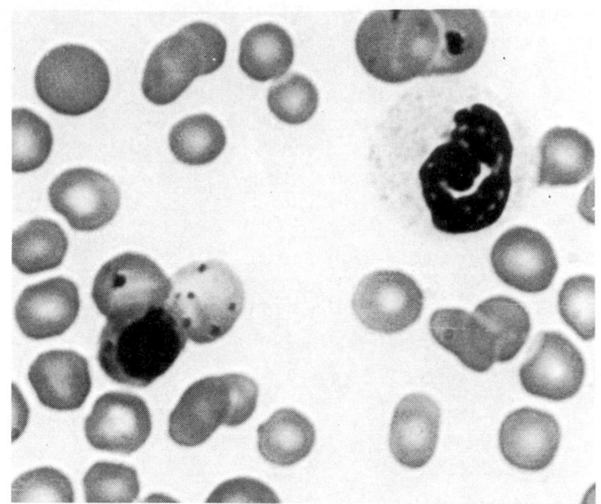

**Figure 17–12** Porphyria. Several red blood cells contain the refractile bodies common in cats with this disorder. Wright-Giemsa, × 1690.

The presence of abnormally large amounts of ornithine in the urine was detected by a paper chromatographic screening test (Jezyk et al., 1982). The definitive diagnosis of gyrate atrophy of the retina can be made by demonstrating deficient activity of ornithine aminotransferase in cultured skin fibroblasts and liver. In man, this disorder is inherited as an autosomal recessive trait (Valle and Simell, 1983).

## PORPHYRIA

Defects in the heme biosynthetic pathway result in elevations of intermediate porphyrin compounds, primarily uroporphyrin I and coproporphyrin I (Kappas et al., 1983). Two apparently distinct syndromes have been described in domestic shorthaired cats (Desnick et al., 1986; Glenn, 1970; Glenn et al., 1968; Tobias, 1964) and Siamese cats (Giddens et al., 1975). The domestic short haired cats with porphyria had a brownish discoloration of the teeth (and bones at autopsy) (Fig. 17–11) and a dark brown to red discoloration of the urine, all of which fluoresced bright pink-red under long-wave ultraviolet light. A mild variable anemia was present, and blood films revealed red blood cells that contained refractile bodies (Fig. 17–12). Photosensitization, described in other species, was not seen. No apparent systemic illness was associated with this condition.

Porphyria in the cat has been shown to be inherited as an autosomal dominant trait and has been classified as having characteristics in common with both erythropoietic and hepatic porphyrias described in man. However, a reduction of porphobilinogen deaminase activity to approximately half of normal (consistent with a dominant inheritance) has been recently demonstrated in red blood cells and liver (Desnick et al., 1985). Elevation of urinary porphobilinogen also occurred. This enzyme deficiency is similar to that described in hepatic porphyria in man (Kappas et al., 1983). The similarities to hepatic porphyria may be of importance, because a variety of drugs can induce an acute porphyric attack with neurologic signs in persons with this disorder. Whether cats with porphyria are at a similar risk has not yet been determined.

The defect in the Siamese cats produced similar pigmentation of teeth, bones, and urine. However, these animals appeared depressed and listless and had a severe macrocytic, hypochromic anemia with frequent anisocytosis, poikilocytosis, target cells, and nucleated red blood cells. Numerous Howell-Jolly bodies and red-cell refractile bodies were also observed. Blood urea nitrogen and serum creatinine were elevated in one cat, and all three cats had hepatosplenomegaly. No photosensitization was reported. Pedigree analysis of the Siamese cats with porphyria was consistent with either autosomal dominant or recessive inheritance.

## AMYLOIDOSIS

Several different pathogenic mechanisms can result in the extracellular deposition of amyloid, a substance made up of twisted beta-pleated sheet fibrils formed from various proteins (Glenner, 1984). The accumulation of amyloid, which is insoluble and resistant to proteolysis, appears to lead to pressure atrophy and cell death. Although classified into primary, secondary, and familial forms, the specific metabolic defects involved in amyloidosis are not fully understood, and the proteins that accumulate may not be the same in each subclass (Kisilevsky, 1983). The diagnosis of amyloid is made histologically by the characteristic reaction with Congo red stain and the apple-green birefringence observed under polarized light.

### Nonfamilial Amyloidosis

Generalized, primary amyloidosis (that without evidence of chronic infection or malignant disease) is rare in cats (Jakob, 1971). Three cats have been reported with generalized, primary amyloidosis (Hartigan et al., 1980). Two were dehydrated and emaciated, and the third was in very poor condition and obviously ill. All had chronic interstitial nephritis and amyloid deposition in the kidneys. The liver and adrenal glands were involved in two animals. Other cases of generalized amyloidosis without an apparent etiology have been described in cats (Crowell et al., 1972; Jakob, 1971). Six of seven cats described had chronic hypervitaminosis A, but an etiologic relationship has not been established (Clark and Seawright, 1969).

Localized, secondary amyloidosis in the cat has been reported in association with infectious peritonitis, immune-complex nephritis, and diabetes mellitus (Hauck et al., 1982; Saegusa et al., 1979; Yano et al., 1981, 1983). Insular amyloidosis, a lesion in some cats with adult-onset diabetes, was reported by one group of workers to occur in nearly 50 per cent of cats over five years of age that are not overtly diabetic (Yano et al., 1981).

### Familial Amyloidosis

Hereditary amyloidosis is a rare condition in man (Glenner et al., 1983). Renal amyloidosis has been described in related Abyssinian cats one to five years of age (Boyce et al., 1984; Chew et al., 1982; Tarr and DiBartola, 1985). Signs were weight loss, dehydration, depression, rough hair coat, gingivitis, polydipsia, and polyuria. Laboratory findings were nonregenerative anemia, hyperglobulinemia, azotemia, hyperphosphatemia, acidosis, and isosthenuria.

In some cats, amyloid deposits were also present in spleen, thyroid, parathyroid, adrenal, stomach, heart, liver, pancreas, intestine, lymph nodes, ovary, and salivary gland (DiBartola et al., 1985). In structure the renal amyloid protein strongly resembled that occurring in man and animals with spontaneous and experimentally reactive systemic amyloidosis.

In view of the familial nature of renal amyloidosis in Abyssinian cats, the condition is believed to be hereditary, but the mode of inheritance is not yet known. It is of interest to note that the generalized amyloidosis reported in association with infectious peritonitis was in an Abyssinian cat (Hauck et al., 1982).

## Acknowledgments

Supported by NIH grant AM 25759 and University of Pennsylvania Genetics Center grants GM 20138 and GM 32592. The authors would like to thank J. Hayden for photographic assistance and Dr. J. Wortman for radiographic interpretations.

## REFERENCES

Aguirre G, Stramm LE, Haskins ME: Feline mucopolysaccharidosis VI: General ocular and pigment epithelial pathology. Invest Ophthalmol Vis Sci 24 (1983) 991–1007.

Aguirre G, Stramm L, Haskins M, Jezyk P: Animal models of metabolic eye diseases. *In* Renie W (ed): Goldberg's Genetic and Metabolic Eye Diseases. Boston, Little, Brown & Company, 1986.

Alroy J, Kolodny EH, Warren LD, Schunk KL, Lamar J, Holzworth J: Mannosidosis in a family of purebred Persian cats. 1986a, in preparation.

Alroy J, Ucci A, Raghavan S, Warren CD, Kolodny EH: Feline mannosidosis: An animal model for human mannosidosis. Lab Invest 1986b, in press.

Baker HJ, Lindsey JR: Animal model of human disease: $GM_1$ gangliosidosis. Am J Pathol 74 (1974) 649–652.

Baker HJ Jr, Lindsey JR, McKhann GM, Farrell DF: Neuronal $GM_1$ gangliosidosis in a Siamese cat with β-galactosidase deficiency. Science 174 (1971) 838–839.

Baker HJ, Reynolds GD, Walkley SU, Cox NR, Baker GH: The gangliosidoses: Comparative features and research applications. Vet Pathol 16 (1979) 635–649.

Baker HJ, Walkley SU, Rattazzi MC, Singer HS, Watson HL, Wood PA: Feline gangliosidoses as models of human lysosomal storage diseases. *In* Desnick RJ, Patterson DF, Scarpelli DG (eds): Animal Models of Inherited Metabolic Diseases. New York, Alan R Liss Inc, 1982, 203–212.

Bauer JE, Verlander JW: Congenital lipoprotein lipase deficiency in hyperlipemic kitten siblings. Vet Clin Pathol 13 (1984) 7–11.

Berry HK, Spinanger J: A paper spot test useful in study of Hurler's syndrome. J Lab Clin Med 55 (1960) 136–138.

Blakemore WF: $GM_1$ gangliosidosis in a cat. J Comp Pathol 82 (1972) 179–185.

Bland van den Berg P, Baker MK, Lange AL: A suspected lysosomal storage disease in Abyssinian cats. Part I. Genetic, clinical and clinical pathological aspects. J S Afr Vet Assoc 48 (1977) 195–199.

Boyce JT, DiBartola SP, Chew DJ, Gasper PW: Familial renal amyloidosis in Abyssinian cats. Vet Pathol 21 (1984) 33–38.

Burditt LJ, Chotai K, Hirani S, Nugent PG, Winchester BG: Biochemical studies on a case of feline mannosidosis. Biochem J 189 (1980) 467–473.

Chew DJ, DiBartola SP, Boyce JT, Gasper PW: Renal amyloidosis in related Abyssinian cats. J Am Vet Med Assoc 181 (1982) 139–142.

Chrisp CE, Ringler DH, Abrams GD, Radin NS, Brenkert A: Lipid storage disease in a Siamese cat. J Am Vet Med Assoc 156 (1970) 616–622.

Clark L, Seawright AA: Generalized amyloidosis in seven cats. Pathol Vet 6 (1969) 117–134.

Collier LL, Bryan GM, Prieur DJ: Ocular manifestations of the Chédiak-Higashi syndrome in four species of animals. J Am Vet Med Assoc 175 (1979) 587–590.

Collier LC, King EJ, Prieur DJ: Tapetal degeneration in cats with Chédiak-Higashi syndrome. Curr Eye Res 4 (1985) 767–773.

Cork LC, Munnell JF, Lorenz MD, Murphy JV, Baker HJ, Rattazzi MC: $Gm_2$ ganglioside lysosomal storage disease in cats with β-hexosaminidase deficiency. Science 196 (1977) 1014–1017.

Cork LC, Munnell JF, Lorenz MD: The pathology of feline $GM_2$ gangliosidosis. Am J Pathol 90 (1978) 723–734.

Cowell KR, Jezyk PF, Haskins ME, Patterson DF: Mucopolysaccharidosis in a cat. J Am Vet Med Assoc 169 (1976) 334–339.

Crowell WA, Goldston RT, Schall WD, Finco DR: Generalized amyloidosis in a cat. J Am Vet Med Assoc 161 (1972) 1127–1133.

Desnick RJ, Tsai S-F, Bishop DF, Haskins ME: Acute intermittent porphyria: Identification and characterization of a feline analogue with deficient porphobilinogen deaminase activity. 1986, in preparation.

DiBartola SP, Benson MD, Dwulet FE, Cornacoff JB: Isolation and characterization of amyloid protein AA in the Abyssinian cat. Lab Invest 52 (1985) 485–489.

Farrell DF, Baker HJ, Herndon RM, Lindsey JR, McKhann GM: Feline $GM_1$ gangliosidosis: Biochemical and ultrastructural comparisons with the disease in man. J Neuropathol Exp Neurol 32 (1973) 1–18.

Garrod AE: Inborn errors of metabolism (Croonian Lectures). Lancet 2 (1) (1908) 73, 142, 214.

Giddens WE Jr, Labbe RF, Swango LJ, Padgett GA: Feline congenital erythropoietic porphyria associated with severe anemia and renal disease. Clinical, morphologic, and biochemical studies. Am J Pathol 80 (1975) 367–386.

Glenn BL: An animal model for human disease: Feline porphyria. Comp Pathol Bull 2 (2) (1970) 2–3.

Glenn BL, Glenn HG, Omtvedt IT: Congenital porphyria in the domestic cat (*Felis catus*): Preliminary investigations on inheritance pattern. Am J Vet Res 29 (1968) 1653–1657.

Glenner GG: Amyloid deposits and amyloidosis. The β-fibrilloses. N Engl J Med 302 (1984) 1283–1292.

Glenner GG, Ignaczak TE, Page DL: The hereditary amyloidoses. *In* Stanbury JB, Wyngaarden JB, Fredrickson DS, Goldstein JL, Brown MS (eds): The Metabolic Basis of Inherited Disease, 5th ed. New York, McGraw-Hill Book Company, 1983, 1468–1469.

Hartigan PJ, Tuite M, McAllister H: Generalized amyloidosis in the domestic cat. Irish Vet J 34 (1980) 1–6.

Haskins ME, McGrath JT: Meningiomas in young cats with mucopolysaccaridosis I. J Neuropathol Exp Neurol 42 (1983) 664–670.

Haskins ME, Aguirre GD, Jezyk PF, Patterson DF: The pathology of the feline model of mucopolysaccharidosis VI. Am J Pathol 101 (1980) 657–674.

Haskins ME, Aguirre GD, Jezyk PF, Desnick RJ, Patterson DF: The pathology of the feline model of mucopolysaccharidosis I. Am J Pathol 112 (1983a) 27–36.

Haskins ME, Bingel SA, Northington JW, Newton CD, Sande RD, Jezyk PF, Patterson DF: Spinal cord compression and hindlimb paresis in cats with mucopolysaccharidosis VI. J Am Vet Med Assoc 182 (1983b) 983–985.

Haskins ME, Jezyk PF, Desnick RJ, McDonough SK, Patterson DF: Alpha-L-iduronidase deficiency in a cat: A model of mucopolysaccharidosis I. Pediatr Res 13 (1979a) 1294–1297.

Haskins ME, Jezyk PF, Desnick RJ, McDonough SK, Patterson DF: Mucopolysaccharidosis in a domestic short-haired cat: A disease distinct from that seen in the Siamese cat. J Am Vet Med Assoc 175 (1979b) 384–387.

Haskins ME, Jezyk PF, Patterson DF: Mucopolysaccharide storage disease in three families of cats with arylsulfatase B deficiency: Leukocyte studies and carrier identification. Pediatr Res 13 (1979c) 1203–1210.

Hauck WN, Qualls CW, Hribernik TN: Concurrent generalized amyloidosis and infectious peritonitis in a cat. J Am Vet Med Assoc 180 (1982) 1349–1351.

Jakob W: Spontaneous amyloidosis of mammals. Vet Pathol 8 (1971) 292–306.

Jezyk PF, Haskins ME, Patterson DF, Mellman WJ, Greenstein M: Mucopolysaccharidosis in a cat with arylsulfatase B deficiency: A model of Maroteaux-Lamy syndrome. Science 198 (1977) 834–836.

Jezyk PF, Haskins ME, Patterson DF: Screening for inborn errors of metabolism in dogs and cats. *In* Desnick RJ, Patterson DF, Scarpelli DG (eds): Animal Models of Inherited Diseases. New York, Alan R Liss Inc, 1982, 93–116.

Jezyk PF, Newman L, Haskins ME, Patterson DF: Mannosidosis in a Persian cat. J Am Vet Med Assoc 1986, in press.

Johnson KH: Globoid leukodystrophy in the cat. J Am Vet Med Assoc 157 (1970) 2057–2064.

Jones BR, Wallace A, Harding DRK, Hancock WS, Campbell CH: Occurrence of idiopathic, familial hyperchylomicronemia in a cat. Vet Rec 112 (1983) 543–547.

Kappas A, Sassa S, Anderson KE: The porphyrias. *In* Stanbury JB, Wyngaarden JB, Fredrickson DS, Goldstein JL, Brown MS (eds): The Metabolic Basis of Inherited Disease. 5th ed. New York, McGraw-Hill Book Company, 1983, 1301–1384.

Kisilevsky R: Amyloidosis: A familiar problem in the light of current pathogenetic developments. Lab Invest 49 (1983) 381–390.

Kramer JW, Davis WC, Prieur DJ: The Chediak-Higashi syndrome of cats. Lab Invest 36 (1977) 554–562.

Lange AL, Bland van den Berg P, Baker MK: A suspected lysosomal storage disease in Abyssinian cats. Part II. Histopathological and ultrastructural aspects. J S Afr Vet Assoc 48 (1977) 201–209.

Lange AL, Brown JMM, Maree C: Biochemical studies on a lysosomal storage disease in Abyssinian cats. Onderstepoort J Vet Res 50 (1983) 149–155.

Lutzner MA, Lowrie CT, Jordan HW: Giant granules in leukocytes of the beige mouse. J Hered 58 (1967) 299–300.

Meyers KM, Hopkins G, Holmsen H, Benson K, Prieur DJ: Ultrastructure of resting and activated storage pool deficient platelets from animals with the Chédiak-Higashi syndrome. Am J Pathol 106 (1982) 364–377.

Murray JA, Blakemore WF, Barnett KC: Ocular lesions in cats with $GM_1$-gangliosidosis with visceral involvement. J Small Anim Pract 18 (1977) 1–10.

Neuwelt EA, Johnson WG, Blank NK, Pagel MA, Masien-McClure C, McClure MJ, Minwei P: Characterization of a new model of $GM_2$ gangliosidosis (Sandhoff's disease) in Korat cats. J Clin Invest 76 (1985) 482–490.

Oliver JM, Zurier RB: Correction of characteristic abnormalities of microtubule function and granule morphology in Chediak-Higashi syndrome with cholinergic agonists. Studies in vitro in man and in vivo in the beige mouse. J Clin Invest 57 (1976) 1239–1247.

Padgett GA, Leader RW, Gorham JR, O'Mary CC: The familial occurrence of the Chediak-Higashi syndrome in mink and cattle. Genetics 49 (1964) 505–512.

Prieur DJ, Collier LL: Animal model of human disease: Chediak-Higashi syndrome. Am J Pathol 90 (1978) 533–536.

Roder JC: Characterization of a murine model (beige) for a natural killer cell immunodeficiency in the Chediak-Higashi syndrome of man. *In* Desnick RJ, Patterson DF, Scarpelli DG (eds): Animal Models of Inherited Metabolic Diseases. New York, Alan R Liss Inc, 1982, 315–325.

Saegusa S, Shimizu F, Nagase M, Kasegawa A: Concurrent feline immune-complex nephritis. Arch Pathol Lab Med 103 (1979) 475–478.

Sato A: Chediak and Higashi's disease: Probable identity of a "new leukocytal anomaly (Chediak)" and "congenital gigantism of perioxidase granules (Higashi)." Tohoku J Exp Med 61 (1955) 201–210.

Snyder SP, Kingston RS, Wenger DA: Animal model of human disease: Niemann-Pick disease: Sphingomyelinosis of Siamese cats. Am J Pathol 108 (1982) 252–254.

Suzuki K, Suzuki Y: Galactosylceramide lipidosis: Globoid cell leukodystrophy (Krabbe's disease). *In* Stanbury JB, Wyngaarden JB, Fredrickson DS, Goldstein JL, Brown MS (eds): The Metabolic Basis of Inherited Disease, 5th ed. New York, McGraw-Hill Book Company, 1983, 857–880.

Tarr MJ, DiBartola SP: Familial amyloidosis in Abyssinian cats: a possible animal model for familial Mediterranean fever and pathogenesis of secondary amyloidosis. Lab Invest 52 (1985) 67A.

Taylor RF, Farrell RK: Light and electron microscopy of peripheral blood neutrophils in a killer whale affected with Chediak-Higashi syndrome. Fed Proc 32 (1973) 822.

Tobias G: Congenital porphyria in a cat. J Am Vet Med Assoc 145 (1964) 462–463.

Valle D, Simell O: The hyperornithinemias. *In* Stanbury JB, Wyngaarden JB, Fredrickson DS, Goldstein JL, Brown MS (eds): The Metabolic Basis of Inherited Disease, 5th ed. New York, McGraw-Hill Book Company, 1983, 382–401.

Valle, DL, Boison AP, Jezyk P, Aguirre G: Gyrate atrophy of the choroid and retina in a cat. Invest Ophthalmol Vis Sci 20 (1981) 251–255.

Vandevelde M, Fankhauser R, Bichsel P, Wiesmann U, Herschkowitz N: Hereditary neurovisceral mannosidosis associated with alpha-mannosidase deficiency in a family of Persian cats. Acta Neuropathol (Berl) 58 (1982) 64–68.

Walkley SU, Haskins ME: Aberrant neurite and mega-neurite development in a feline model of mucopolysaccharidosis (MPS) type I as revealed by the Golgi method. Soc Neurosci Abstr 8 (1982) 1009.

Walkley SU, Blakemore WF, Purpura DP: Alterations in neuron morphology in feline mannosidosis. A Golgi study. Acta Neuropathol (Berl) 53 (1981) 75–79.

Warren CD, Alroy J, Bugge B, Daniel PF, Raghavan SS, Kolodny EH, Lamar JL, Jeanloz RW: Oligosaccharides from placenta: Early diagnosis of feline mannosidosis. FEBS Lett 1986, in preparation.

Wenger DA, Sattler M, Kudoh T, Snyder SP, Kingston RS: Niemann-Pick disease: A genetic model in Siamese cats. Science 208 (1980) 1471–1473.

Yano BL, Hayden DW, Johnson KH: Feline insular amyloid: Incidence in adult cats with no clinicopathologic evidence of overt diabetes mellitus. Vet Pathol 18 (1981) 310–315.

Yano BL, Hayden DW, Johnson KH: Occurrence of secondary systemic amyloidosis in the pancreatic islets of a cat. Am J Vet Res 44 (1983) 338–339.

# 18
CHAPTER
# THE CARDIOVASCULAR SYSTEM

NEIL K. HARPSTER

CONTRIBUTING AUTHOR:
BERNARD C. ZOOK

## ANATOMY*

The cat's heart is pear-shaped. It is suspended between the two layers of the mediastinum, its apex directed slightly downward and to the left. Viewed from both the lateral and the dorsoventral aspects, it occupies about two and a half costal interspaces, extending from the fourth to the sixth rib or slightly beyond. The apex of the left ventricular wall may touch the diaphragm (Reighard and Jennings, 1935), although the pericardium is not directly attached to it or to the sternum (Bourdelle and Bressou, 1953). Laterally and dorsally the heart is largely covered by the lungs; the ventral and lower lateral surfaces are in contact with the chest wall.

According to one study, in the adult male the heart weighs 11 or 12 gm, in the female 9 or 10 gm (Latimer, 1942); according to another source, the average weights for the male and female heart are 18.4 and 12.7 gm, respectively (Schummer et al., 1981). The weight of the cat's heart may be compared with body length (Stünzi et al., 1959), but most prosectors compare heart weight with body weight. Percentage weights varying from 0.27 to 0.72 have been reported (Joseph, 1908; Liu, 1977; Nogalski and Szuba, 1971; Spector, 1956). Among 104 adults, the heart averaged 0.39 (females) and 0.40 (males) per cent of body weight, while the heart of 35 neonates averaged 0.76 per cent (Latimer, 1942). We have found similar values for 52 adults (mean 0.40), but 35 neonates averaged 0.93 per cent of body weight. Comparison of the mitral valve with the tricuspid valve ring circumference has been found useful to reveal dilated valve rings in dogs. The normal mitral to tricuspid valve ratio for cats is 0.66 (Zook, 1974). The ductus arteriosus, although functionally closed within hours after birth, may remain patent for several days to weeks before becoming the completely fibrotic ligamentum arteriosum. The foramen ovale normally completely seals the atrial septum, whereas in humans "probe patencies" are very common (Johnston, 1941). Lymphatic vessels draining the heart follow the major coronary vessels and then empty into a single channel that carries the lymph to a small anterior mediastinal lymph node near the thymus (Paasch, 1979).

The light microscopic or ultrastructural appearance of the cat's heart is not unique among mammals (Qayyum, 1972). Purkinje fibers are, however, more readily recognized by light microscopy than in some species, as they appear larger and lighter-staining (owing to their increased glycogen content) than regular myocardial fibers. In the left ventricle, Purkinje fibers are located just under the endocardium, whereas in the right ventricle they are located deeper, becoming superficial near the papillary muscles. The endocardium increases in thickness with age, from 1 to 5 μm in kittens to 10 μm in adults (Paasch and Zook, 1980). Cartilage may occur in the aortic anulus fibrosus and margin of the mitral valve, but less commonly than in dogs (Welsch, 1943).

Cats that are to be examined at autopsy should not be destroyed by intracardiac or intrathoracic injections. The chemicals used often damage and change the appearance of the tissues, and significant pathologic changes may be obscured. Tissues that have been exposed to a strong barbiturate solution have a rusty discoloration and may have a frosty granular surface deposit. Such tissues also have an altered microscopic appearance; affected cells may separate from one another and lose differential staining qualities.

*By Bernard C. Zook.

## PHYSIOLOGY*

For over 20 years the domestic cat has been a favored subject for the study of cardiovascular physiology and pathophysiology. The appealing aspects of this species include its small size, availability, and adaptability to confinement in small quarters for long periods of time. Yet its size is sufficient to permit extensive cardiovascular measurements by both externally and internally placed systems.

The cat heart has been found to be a useful model for the study of right ventricular hypertrophy and congestive heart failure following pulmonary artery banding (Spann et al., 1967a). Its right ventricular papillary muscle has been used extensively for in-vitro studies of myocardial performance under a variety of conditions, as its small size, cylindrical shape, and linear arrangement of muscle fibers permit easy measurements of fiber shortening and tension development. The normal parameters of this preparation for isometric tension development (Buccino et al., 1967b; Sonnenblick, 1967) and the force-velocity relationships (Parmley and Sonnenblick, 1971; Sonnenblick, 1962a) have been defined. The effects of positive inotropic interventions (Sonnenblick, 1962a, b), catecholamine depletion (Spann et al., 1967b), hyperthyroidism (Buccino et al., 1967a), and cardiac hypertrophy and failure (Spann et al., 1967b) have been reported. Although these studies have done much to further our knowledge of cardiac physiology and myocardial performance in normal and abnormal states, they do not lend themselves readily to the comparatively superficial evaluation of the feline cardiovascular system that is possible under clinical conditions.

*By Neil K. Harpster.

The heart rate in the normal unanesthetized adult cat has been variously reported. In one electrocardiographic study it ranged from 140 to 160/minute (Luisada et al., 1944), and from 160 to 240 (average 197), in another (Gompf and Tilley, 1979). The differing results can perhaps be accounted for by differences in the conditioning of the two groups of cats that were studied. It has been my experience that the heart rate in most normal cats is 120/minute or greater but not usually over 240/minute. This is indeed a wide range for normal values, but individual cats vary greatly in their acceptance of the examination and the level of sympathetic nervous system stimulation that is elicited. When the heart rate is under 120/minute or over 240/minute the presence of a cardiac arrhythmia should be considered and electrocardiography should be carried out to evaluate this possibility.

Well-defined normal values for the various cardiovascular function tests routinely performed in diagnostic studies are sparse for the cat, compared with the wealth of information available for man and the dog. Moreover, the data that have been reported are difficult to correlate owing to the differences in methods by which the values were obtained. For example, the anesthetic agents used varied from study to study, and some studies were performed without anesthetics.

In general, the normal values presented in Table 18–1 are averages based on the results obtained from small numbers of cats. When duplicate numbers for certain values are available, they do not usually differ significantly. However, some notable exceptions should be discussed further. The differences in the right ventricular mean pressure reported by Lord et al. (1974) and Reeves et al. (1963) are significant. These can be explained on the basis of environmental influences, as the latter study involved a group of cats living at 5200 feet above sea level. Similar pressure elevations have been reported in

**Table 18–1 Cardiovascular Pressures and Output Reported for the Normal Cat**

| | LORD ET AL., 1974 (SURITAL, HALOTHANE, NITROUS OXIDE) | NADEAU AND COLEBATCH, 1965 (CHLORALOSE) | WEINER ET AL., 1967 (PENTOBARBITAL) | GORDON AND GOLDBLATT, 1967 (NO ANESTHESIA) | REEVES ET AL., 1963 (SURITAL) | MIDDLETON ET AL., 1981 (NO ANESTHESIA) |
|---|---|---|---|---|---|---|
| CVP, cm $H_2O$ | | | 2.5 ± 0.4 | | 3.0 ± 1.0 | |
| RVP, mm Hg | | | | | | |
| Systolic (mean) | 15–22 (18) | | | | 36 ± 10 | |
| Diastolic (mean) | 0–8 (4) | | | | | |
| MPAP, mm Hg | | 15.1 ± 4.29 | | | | |
| MLAP, mm Hg | | 1.60 ± 1.69 | | | | |
| LVP, mm Hg | | | | | | |
| Systolic (mean) | 95–135 (106) | | | | | |
| Diastolic (mean) | 3–12 (4.5) | | | | | |
| Systemic Arterial P., mm Hg | | 148.8 ± 31.8 | 146 ± 10.0 | 149 | | |
| Mean | | | | | | |
| (Systolic/Diastolic) | | | | (177/123) | (162/118) | |
| PVR, mm Hg/100 ml/min/$m^2$ | | 0.819 ± 0.474 | | | | |
| SVR, mm Hg/100 ml/min/$m^2$ | | 7.47 ± 2.27 | | | | |
| CO, ml/min | | 439.1 ± 99.4 | 341 ± 33.0 | | | |
| Stroke Volume, ml | | 1.7 ± .526 | | | | |
| Arterial $Po_2$, mm Hg | | 91.0 ± 10.3 | | | | 102.9 ± 15.22 |
| Arterial $O_2$ Sat. % | | | | | | 95.7 ± 2.26 |
| Venous $Po_2$, mm Hg | | | | | | 38.6 ± 11.44 |
| Arterial $Pco_2$, mm Hg | | | | | | 33.6 ± 7.06 |

Abbreviations: CVP = central venous pressure; RVP = right ventricular pressure; MPAP = mean pulmonary artery pressure; MLAP = mean left arterial pressure; LVP = left ventricular pressure; PVR = pulmonary vascular resistance; SVR = systemic vascular resistance; CO = cardiac output.

man (Rotta et al., 1956) and cattle (Bisgard, 1977) living at high altitudes.

The differences in the reported values for cardiac output in Table 18–1 also are significant. These probably reflect differences in methodology, as Nadeau and Colebatch (1965) used the direct-Fick method, whereas Weiner et al. (1967) used the isotope-dilution technique. Errors in the determination of cardiac output in man by the direct-Fick method are reported to be more numerous (Selzer and Sudrann, 1958) but not to the degree seen here. The other differences in values recorded in Table 18–1 concern the arterial oxygen tensions (i.e., $Po_2$). These differences are to a great extent the result of the resting state of the animals from which they were obtained. The results reported by Nadeau and Colebatch (1965) were obtained from cats under chloralose anesthesia, while those reported by Middleton et al. (1981) were obtained from unanesthetized cats. Such observed differences are predictable from the experimental designs by which the samples were procured.

## CARDIOVASCULAR DISEASE*

### Clinical Signs

The domestic cat seems to have a great innate understanding of its physical capabilities under the limitations imposed by illness. Heart disease and anemia best exemplify this feline characteristic: the condition is frequently advanced before the owner is aware of the cat's illness and seeks veterinary attention.

In the cat, in contrast with many other species, a cough is rarely an early or common manifestation of heart disease with congestive heart failure. Far more frequently, polypnea and dyspnea due to pulmonary edema, pleural effusion, or both are the initial clinical signs following a variable period of reduced activity, lethargy, and depressed appetite. Less often, syncopal episodes resulting from marked alterations in heart rate or rhythm are the primary sign of heart disease. Lastly, the high incidence of thromboembolism in certain feline cardiovascular disorders makes this complication a significant cause of clinical signs, and it may be the only finding on presentation. Its signs can range from intermittent lameness to complete areflexic, flaccid paralysis depending on the extent and completeness of the vascular occlusion, as well as the functional status of collateral channels.

In the young kitten with significant congenital heart disease, poor weight gain and stunting may be observed. Reduced activity, exertional dyspnea, and syncope occur in kittens in which right-to-left shunting is associated with a complex congenital anomaly, such as tetralogy of Fallot and origin of both great vessels from the right ventricle (i.e., double-outlet right ventricle). Similar signs may occur with severe outflow obstruction from either the right or the left ventricle. Otherwise, the predominant clinical signs in congenital heart disease usually result from left, right, or biventricular failure. In general, the presence of clinical signs in young kittens with congenital heart disease implies a poor prognosis.

*By Neil K. Harpster.

### The Cardiovascular Examination

A complete physical examination should be considered a prerequisite for a good cardiovascular examination. The small size and body conformation of the cat aid in performance of a complete examination. A quiet, undisturbed environment is an important adjuvant in reducing stress and gaining a cat's cooperation.

During the initial history taking, it is helpful if the examiner can observe the cat for general and mental attitudes, general body condition, and the respiratory rate and effort. Such observation permits a crude assessment of the cat's stability and may supplement the history taking itself. When the history has been obtained, a complete physical examination should be carried out provided that the cat's condition is reasonably stable and emergency measures are not an immediate need. The examination should include careful abdominal palpation with the cat's forelegs elevated to facilitate cranial palpation. Special attention should be paid to size and conformation of the liver, spleen, and kidneys and the presence of any abnormal abdominal structures. The cervical area should be palpated, especially because of the increased incidence of thyroid enlargement in older cats. Also to be inspected are all visible mucous membranes and the eyes, including the retinas, the only site where arteries and veins can be seen. Attention is then turned to the cardiovascular system, which I like to separate into peripheral and central components, the latter including the heart and respiratory system.

The status of the peripheral circulation can be crudely evaluated by observing color and capillary refill of visible mucous membranes, noting skin temperature of extremities (i.e., feet, pinnae), and taking the rectal temperature. When peripheral circulation is reduced (as in congestive heart failure, volume depletion, or shock), mucous membranes tend to be pale or mildly cyanotic with slowed capillary refill, while the rectal temperature is subnormal and the skin of the extremities is cool. A more scientific and accurate method for evaluating the state of the peripheral circulatory system is to measure the circulation time by an injection of fluorescein dye or, even better, by the determination of the arteriovenous oxygen difference (normal values reported in the cat by Middleton et al. [1981] are 64.78 ± 20.22 mm Hg). The palpable characteristics of peripheral arterial pulses also serve as a crude index of cardiac performance, but they tend to be less reliable indicators of reduced peripheral circulation than the other methods discussed. When both femoral artery pulses are of equal intensity, attention should be focused on strength, rate, and rhythm characteristics.

Unequal distribution of peripheral circulation is strong clinical evidence of a localized disorder. When arterial insufficiency occurs in a single limb, lameness and some degree of discomfort are usually the initial signs. However, such signs can be transient and at times difficult to verify on examination if the vascular occlusion is distal and collateral circulation quickly reestablishes reasonable flow to the affected limb. Under these circumstances, mild lameness and cardiac abnormalities may be the only persisting evidence suggesting a vascular origin for the presenting complaints. With more severe regional arterial insufficiency, coolness and cyanosis of the affected extremity, as well as neurologic abnormalities, are found, the degree of severity depending on the extent of the ischemic process and the ability of collateral circulation to alter this process. Arterial embolism, arteriovenous fistula, and vascular disruption secondary to trauma are the common causes of arterial insufficiency in the cat. Extensive distal tissue necrosis (i.e., gangrene) results if management is inadequate or ineffective. As a rule, distal ischemia progresses much more slowly with an arteriovenous fistula than with the other conditions discussed and is invariably associated with some degree of distal subcutaneous edema (due to elevated regional venous pressure), another feature that tends to differentiate arteriovenous fistula from both arterial occlusion and disruption. A palpable thrill and a continuous murmur over the site of the shunt are other findings with peripheral arteriovenous fistula. Arterial pulses proximal to the shunt tend to be exaggerated, a result of the wide pulse pressure caused by a lowering of the arterial diastolic pressure. In contrast to these findings, proximal arterial pulses are diminished or absent when vascular occlusion or disruption is the cause of localized arterial insufficiency.

Localized obstruction or impedance to venous return may occur in the cat secondary to localized infections (e.g., cellulitis, abscesses), tissue proliferations (e.g., granulomas and neoplasia), trauma resulting in fracture or soft tissue injury, and arteriovenous fistulae. Characteristic findings are swelling and subcutaneous pitting edema distal to the obstruction. Pain and lameness are uncommon. When venous obstruction is severe, tissue fluid may exude through the intact skin. Lymphangitis and other causes of obstruction to lymphatic drainage can result in findings similar to those with venous obstruction.

Next, the central circulatory system is evaluated by examination of the thorax. By this time the examiner has had an opportunity to crudely assess respiratory function by visual observations made during the general examination. A complete physical examination of the thorax includes palpation, percussion, and auscultation.

The cat's thorax is most easily palpated with the examiner directly behind the cat, while the owner or an assistant holds the cat still in a standing position. With the finger tips of both hands on either side of the thorax a methodical examination is carried out to detect thoracic wall defects or masses, rhonchi transmitted to the chest wall, sternal abnormalities, and the position of the maximal cardiac impulse. In the majority of normal adult cats the maximal cardiac impulse (PMI) is felt in the left fifth or sixth intercostal space (ICS) at or just below the costochondral junction (CCJ). It may be difficult to define this position in some cats owing to alterations in the respiratory pattern by purring, growling, or changes in the rate and depth of respiration. Pleural and pericardial effusion, likewise, may make the heartbeat imperceptible on palpation even in the most cooperative cat. Abnormal position of the maximal cardiac impulse may be caused by right-sided or biventricular cardiac enlargement, pulmonary atelectasis, intrathoracic masses, and unilateral fluid accumulations.

Thoracic percussion is useful in detecting significant pleural effusions and large intrathoracic masses (e.g., neoplasm, localized lung consolidation with or without pleural adhesions, herniation of abdominal organs through a defect in the diaphragm) but is rarely of much benefit in distinguishing the presence of even moderate to large accumulations of free air. It is best performed with the cat standing, by gently tapping with the middle finger of one hand on the middle finger of the opposite hand, which is placed on the thorax. By percussion of various levels on the thorax, differences in resonance can be detected when pleural effusion is present, with ventral areas over the effusion being duller. Both sides of the chest should be percussed.

Thoracic auscultation is aided by patience and quiet surroundings. A cat's growling and purring interfere with successful auscultation and should be eliminated if possible. Mild digital pressure over the larynx is the most effective way to discourage purring. Both sides of the thorax should be auscultated twice, once with concentration on heart sounds and again with attention to lung sounds. Cardiac auscultation should commence with placing the stethoscope over the left cardiac apex, as determined by thoracic palpation of the PMI. From this position (i.e., mitral valve area) the examiner moves the stethoscope cranially and slightly dorsally to the left cardiac base by sliding it beneath the left scapula with the foreleg slightly abducted (i.e., to the aortic and pulmonic valve areas). When the left thorax has been examined, the right thorax is auscultated, with the stethoscope first over the cardiac apex and then over the base. As distinct sounds from the tricuspid valve cannot be discerned over the left thorax, particular attention should be focused on the right fourth ICS just above the CCJ (i.e., the tricuspid valve area), even though primary disease affecting this valve is rare in the cat.

When cardiac auscultation has been completed, attention is turned to the lung sounds. Lung auscultation is enhanced by a cooperative patient, quiet surroundings, and occlusion of one nostril to increase inspiratory effort and air volume. It should begin just behind the scapula (i.e., in a hilar position) and continue caudally over all lung fields, first over one side and then the other. In the normal cat, inspiratory sounds consist of quiet, low-pitched air-flow sounds, while expiratory sounds are absent. Next, the stethoscope is moved to various positions over the sternum, to be certain that a faint, localized murmur has not been overlooked, and then to the thoracic inlet. This latter position is particularly useful for detection of referred aortic valve murmurs (especially those resulting from congenital valvular stenosis and aortic valvular bacterial endocarditis) and for differentiation of referred upper airway sounds from primary lower respiratory noises.

In general, heart murmurs of Grade II to III/VI or greater intensity are referred from their position of greatest intensity to the opposite thorax as a less intense murmur of similar characteristics of duration and pitch. Murmurs of mitral valve incompetence usually are of greatest intensity over the left cardiac apex but occasionally are more intense over the right apex. They are typically referred to the opposite cardiac apex as a similar murmur of half to one grade less intensity. Murmurs of subvalvular aortic stenosis are most intense over the left fourth or fifth ICS at or just above the CCJ. They are usually referred to the right third and fourth ICS at the CCJ, but sometimes to a more dorsal position over the right thorax. Murmurs of aortic valve stenosis are typically referred to the thoracic inlet and up the carotid arteries, as well as to the right third and fourth ICS at the CCJ. Murmurs of both subvalvular and valvular pulmonic stenosis characteristically are referred to the right second to fourth ICS along the sternum. Although they may on occasion be heard weakly at the thoracic inlet, they are not referred up the carotids. Murmurs of tricuspid valve incompetence tend to be most intense over the right fourth ICS above the CCJ. Typically, they are referred to a wide area over the left thorax, usually from the third through the fifth ICS, and are difficult to localize well in this position. (See Table 18–2 for a summary of these and other common murmurs in the cat.)

Normally, two distinct heart sounds can be heard over the thorax, a first ($S_1$) and a second ($S_2$). The first is related to physiologic events associated with ventricular tension and muscular contraction (muscular factor), closure of the atrioventricular (AV) valves (valvular factor), and opening of the semilunar valves along with turbulence and vibrations in the great vessels at the base of the heart (vascular factor) (Burch, 1971). The second heart sound is temporally related to the onset of ventricular relaxation and is produced chiefly by closure of the semilunar valves and associated vibrations within the great vessels. As the normal positions of the heart valves in the cat are similar to those reported for the dog (Harpster, 1977c), $S_1$ is best heard over the left or right cardiac apex, while $S_2$ is most distinct over the left cardiac base.

When heart sounds in addition to $S_1$ and $S_2$ are heard, underlying heart disease should be suspected. Abnormal heart sounds may occur as systolic or diastolic murmurs, as diastolic gallop rhythms, and as abnormalities of rate and rhythm. Heart murmurs usually result from congenital or acquired shunts or valvular abnormalities but occasionally occur in cats with anemia, volume depletion, or volume overload, in which heart disease is not a contributing factor. In anemic cats, systolic murmurs are frequently heard over the left or right cardiac apex, or both, when the hematocrit is below 20 per cent. Physiologic heart murmurs also are common in kittens under four months of age. Typically, these are musical, systolic murmurs of greatest intensity over the left cardiac apex and should disappear by six months of age; otherwise congenital heart disease should be considered. Diastolic gallop rhythms result from filling abnormalities of the left ventricle due to left heart failure or to abnormal size or shape of the left ventricular chamber associated with elevated left atrial pressure. These gallop rhythms are caused by accentuation of the abnormal third and fourth heart sounds and arise within the ventricle when atrial pressure exceeds the pressure in the ventricle (Crevasse et al., 1962). Diastolic gallop rhythms may be associated with passive ventricular filling ($S_3$ or ventricular gallop), active late ventricular filling at the time of atrial contraction ($S_4$ or atrial gallop), or both passive and active ventricular filling (summation gallop). Acquired diastolic heart murmurs and other abnormal heart sounds, such as systolic clicks, venous hums, and pericardial friction rubs, are exceedingly rare in the cat.

Abnormalities of rate and rhythm heard on cardiac auscultation result from cardiac arrhythmias and in most instances point strongly to significant underlying heart disease. Arrhythmias should be suspected when the basic cardiac rhythm is regular but the heart rate is either exceedingly slow ($<$ 140/minute) or exceptionally fast ($>$ 240/minute), and also when obvious irregularities of rhythm are detected. In either circumstance, electrocardiography should be performed to confirm the examiner's clinical impression and to identify the site of origin of the arrhythmias and the possible need for therapeutic intervention.

As the final step in the cardiovascular examination the jugular veins should be inspected for evidence of elevated right-sided cardiac filling pressures (i.e., venous distention or pulsation, or both). It may be necessary, especially with longhaired cats, to moisten or clip the hair over the ventral cervical area. If other evidence from the physical

**Table 18–2 Summary of Common Heart Murmurs in the Cat and Their Typical Auscultatory Characteristics**

| VALVE ABNORMALITY | ETIOLOGIC FACTORS | MURMUR CHARACTERISTICS | SITE OF MAXIMAL INTENSITY | COMMON REFERRED POSITION(S) |
|---|---|---|---|---|
| MV incompetence | Cardiomyopathy, congenital anomaly, EF, FIP | Systolic, holosystolic, decrescendo or band-shaped | Left or right cardiac apex | Right or left cardiac apex |
| TV incompetence | Cardiomyopathy, dirofilariasis, pulmonary hypertension | Systolic, holosystolic, decrescendo or band-shaped | Right 4th ICS above CCJ | Wide area left thorax at or above CCJ. Poorly localized. |
| AS subvalvular | Congenital anomaly | Holosystolic, crescendo-decrescendo | Left 4th–5th ICS above CCJ | Right 3rd–4th ICS at CCJ. Less commonly to a more dorsal position. |
| AS valvular | Congenital anomaly, bacterial endocarditis | Holosystolic, crescendo-decrescendo | Left 3rd–4th ICS above CCJ | Thoracic inlet and up carotids. Right 3rd–4th ICS at or below CCJ. |
| PS, valvular, subvalvular | Congenital anomaly | Holosystolic | Left 2nd–3rd ICS above CCJ | Right 2nd–4th ICS along sternal border |
| AV incompetence | Bacterial endocarditis, congenital anomaly | Diastolic decrescendo | Left 4th–5th ICS at and below CCJ | Weakly to right cardiac apex |
| PDA | Congenital anomaly | Continuous | Left 3rd–4th ICS above CCJ | Right 2nd–4th ICS below CCJ |
| VSD | Congenital anomaly | Holosystolic, crescendo-decrescendo | Right 3rd–4th ICS below CCJ | Wide area left thorax 3rd–5th ICS below CCJ. Poorly localized. |

Abbreviations: AS = aortic stenosis; AV = aortic valve; CCJ = costochondral junction; EF = endocardial fibroelastosis; FIP = feline infectious peritonitis; ICS = intercostal space; MV = mitral valve; PDA = patent ductus arteriosus; PS = pulmonic stenosis; TV = tricuspid valve; VSD = ventricular septal defect.

examination suggests right-sided or biventricular heart failure (e.g., hepatomegaly, ascites, pleural effusion) and yet the jugular veins appear normal, central venous pressure should be measured to distinguish between cardiac and noncardiac causes of the other findings. This is done by means of a catheter introduced into a jugular vein and advanced into the precava.

Arterial blood pressure can be measured, if indicated, directly by percutaneous introduction of a needle into a peripheral artery and also noninvasively with the Doppler ultrasonic technique (Cowgill and Kallet, 1983; see also the chapter on sedation and anesthesia).

## Diagnostic Procedures

When cardiovascular disease is suspected from clinical signs and physical examination, further diagnostic tests will be needed to define the significance of the clinical signs and findings, establish the cause or causes of the cardiovascular disease, organize the best therapeutic approach, and establish a prognosis. The extent of the diagnostic study will be partly determined by the cat's condition and also by the nature of the disease that is present. When respiratory dysfunction is significant, because of pulmonary edema, widespread pulmonary disease of other causes, or substantial pleural effusion, extensive diagnostic procedures are potentially life-threatening. Under these circumstances it is preferable to start nonspecific therapy (e.g., oxygen, diuretics, bronchodilators, thoracocentesis) and to postpone diagnostic studies until the cat's condition has been stabilized. A CBC, SMA profile, and urinalysis are an integral part of the diagnostic study.

### Phonocardiography

Phonocardiography is the graphic recording of heart sounds. It can be considered an extension of the stethoscope but offers the added advantage of defining when the abnormal heart sound occurs as well as recording its characteristics. When recorded along with other noninvasive procedures, the phonocardiogram (PCG) has been utilized as an index for defining crude cardiac performance (Tafur et al., 1964). Finally, the PCG is a valuable teaching aid in cardiac auscultation. The phonocardiogram rarely, if ever, detects abnormal heart sounds that cannot also be detected by careful auscultation. Thus it does not replace or supersede good auscultation.

The characteristics of the normal feline phonocardiogram have been reported (Hamlin et al., 1963a; Harpster, 1977c). The first heart sound ($S_1$) usually consists of two distinct components lasting on average 74 milliseconds (range 60 to 100 milliseconds) (Pensinger, 1968). Normally four to seven vibrations are present, including the two major components. The second heart sound ($S_2$) usually consists of three to five vibrations, including a single major component, and lasts an average 41 milliseconds (range 30 to 60 milliseconds) (Pensinger, 1968). Any deviation from these phonocardiographic values in the cat can be considered abnormal (Fig. 18–1).

The main clinical uses of phonocardiography in the cat are to differentiate systolic and diastolic murmurs, particularly when the resting heart rate is rapid, and to confirm the presence of a diastolic gallop rhythm and identify its type. These objectives can be accomplished by simultaneously performing the PCG and the electrocardiogram (ECG). The ECG provides the timing sequence to which events in the PCG can be related. Systolic murmurs typically occur between the terminal portion of the QRS complex and the middle portion of the T wave (Fig. 18–2), whereas diastolic murmurs are inscribed between the termination of the T wave and initial deflection of the subsequent QRS complex (Fig. 18–3). The timing sequence of the diastolic gallop rhythms is as follows: the $S_3$ (ventricular) gallop is inscribed between the T wave and the following P wave, the $S_4$ (atrial) gallop occurs between the P wave and the initial portion of the QRS complex, and the summation gallop encompasses the intervals described for both the $S_3$ and the $S_4$ gallop (Figs. 18–4 to 18–6). In the phonocardiogram, $S_3$ and $S_4$ gallop rhythms are typically recorded as distinct deflections consisting of three or four vibrations, whereas summation gallops are prolonged deflections that may easily be mistaken for diastolic murmurs.

### Thoracic Radiography

Thoracic radiography is an essential part of the cardiovascular examination. It provides information regarding heart size and chamber enlargement. Even more important is the evidence it furnishes about other intrathoracic processes, such as pulmonary edema, pleural effusion, and intrathoracic masses—information that permits immediate decisions on the need for therapeutic interventions or additional diagnostic procedures. In addition, initial thoracic radiographs supply a baseline against which we can judge the effectiveness of therapy fairly accurately. But as with other diagnostic procedures that will be discussed, plain thoracic radiography alone does not establish a definitive diagnosis or define the status of cardiac function in cats with either congenital or acquired heart disease. More specific noninvasive (e.g., echocardiography) or invasive (e.g., nonselective angiocardiography, cardiac catheterization, cardiac nuclear imaging) procedures are required to obtain this information.

In the majority of cats, thoracic radiographs can be obtained without the administration of a sedative or anesthetic. With fractious cats, however, a low dose of a tranquilizer (acepromazine, 1.0 to 2.5 mg SC or IM) can be given safely, provided that there is cardiovascular stability, and will ensure good-quality films without excessive radiation exposure of personnel. Radiographs should always be taken in two views. I prefer them taken with the cat in right lateral recumbency and in the ventrodorsal position to maximize cardiac projection. (The dorsoventral radiographic position projects the heart in a more upright position, producing a smaller, more rounded cardiac silhouette and thus makes critical evaluation of chamber enlargement more difficult. These problems are avoided with the ventrodorsal projection, which allows the heart to be seen in a more longitudinal position.) It is sometimes useful to take both right and left lateral recumbent views to assist in differentiating the cardiac silhouette and adjacent intrathoracic masses and to more accurately define the position of intrapulmonary lesions. An attempt should be made to make exposures at the end of inspiration, but this may be difficult with unsedated cats.

Normal radiographic anatomy of the cat heart in the right lateral recumbent and dorsoventral views has been

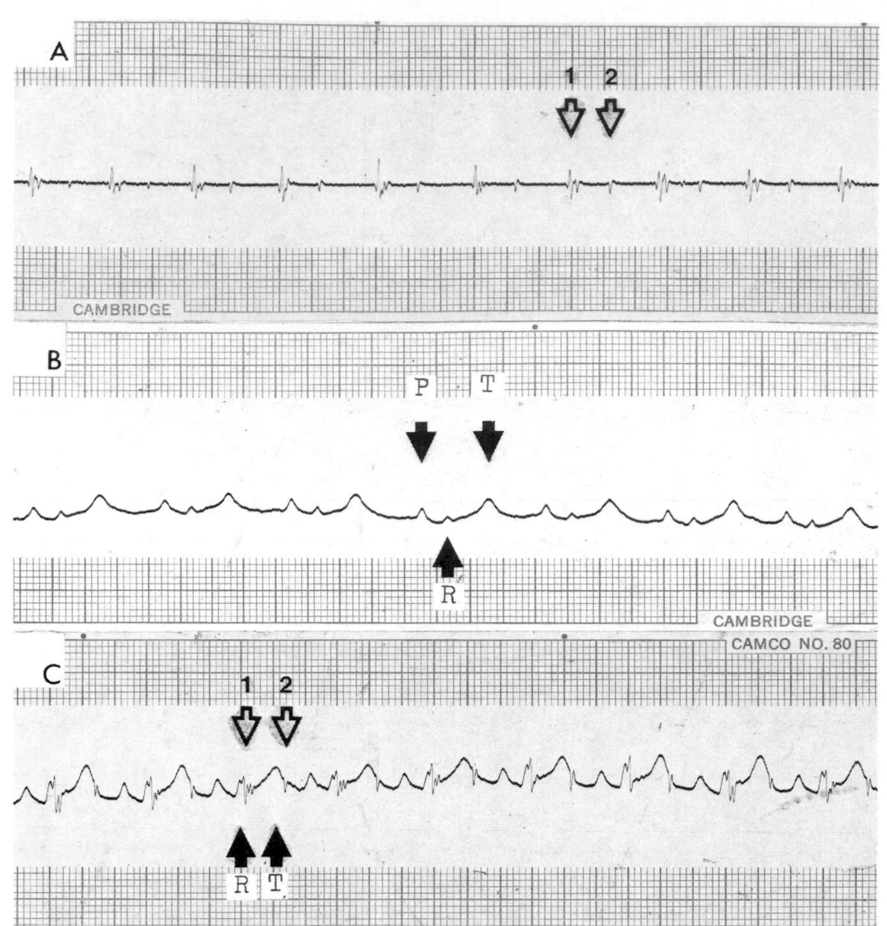


**Figure 18–1** Phonocardiogram (PCG) recorded over the mitral area of a normal one-year-old neutered male domestic shorthair. *A*, The PCG alone is presented and demonstrates two distinct and separate heart sounds. *B*, A lead II ECG strip identifies the P, QRS, and T wave complexes. *C*, The PCG and ECG recordings are superimposed. Notice the relationship of the first heart sound (1) to the QRS complex (i.e., it begins on the downstroke of the R wave), while the second heart sound (2) occurs simultaneously with terminal forces of the T wave. Normal splitting of the first heart sound can be seen but is not consistently present. 50 mm/sec. (From Harpster NK : Vet Clin North Am 7 [1977] 241–256.)

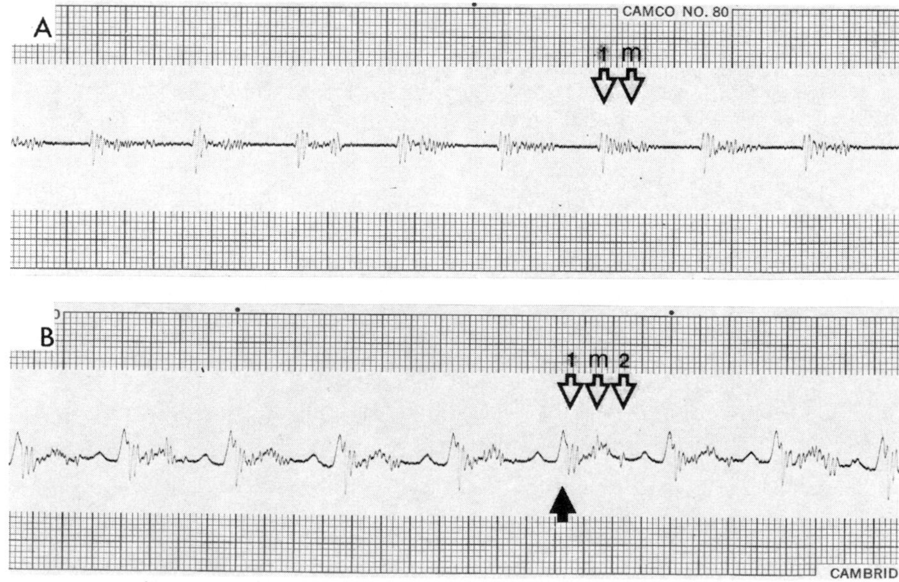


**Figure 18–2** Ventricular septal defect, phonocardiogram (PCG) recorded over the right cardiac apex of a six-month-old male domestic shorthair. *A*, The PCG, alone, demonstrates a prolonged heart sound that is not consistently separated into distinct components. The timing sequence of this sound can be appreciated in *B*, with superimposition of the PCG and ECG. Notice that the sound begins on the downstroke of the R wave (solid arrow) and continues throughout most of systole. The first heart sound (1) is responsible for the initial components of this sound, and it terminates shortly before inscription of the second heart sound (2). This is the typical phonocardiographic characteristic of a holosystolic murmur. 50 mm/sec.

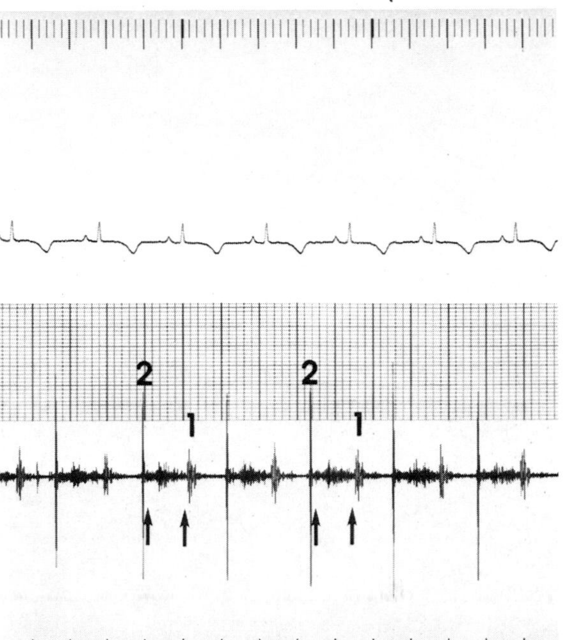


**Figure 18–3** Phonocardiogram recorded over the left cardiac apex of an 11-year-old spayed female domestic longhair presented for lethargy and anorexia of two days' duration. The murmur (arrows) encompasses the entire diastolic period (i.e., extends from the second heart sound [2] to the first heart sound [1]) and reaches a peak intensity in early diastole. These PCG features are characteristic of aortic insufficiency and what is termed a decrescendo murmur. The cause of this cat's murmur was never established.

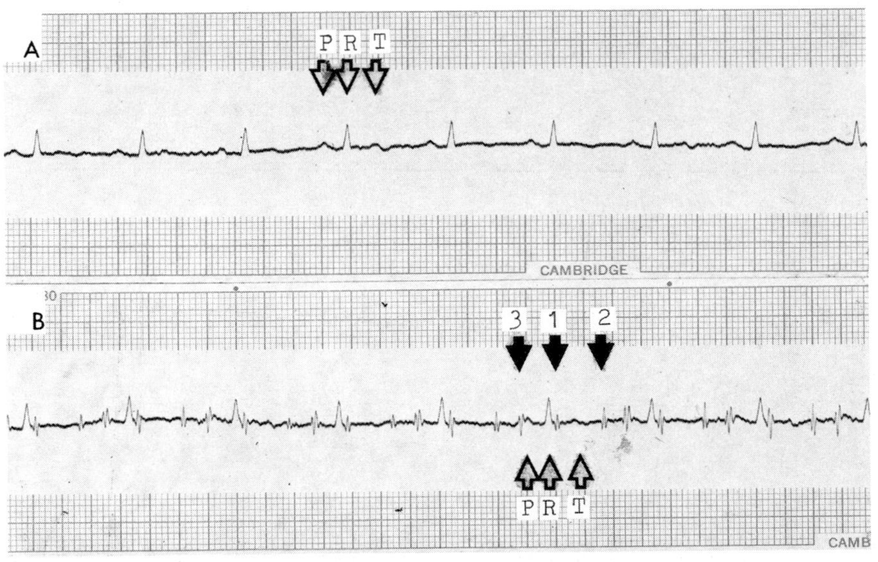


**Figure 18–4** Dilatative cardiomyopathy, phonocardiogram (PCG) recorded from a 13-year-old neutered male domestic longhair presented for acute onset of hindlimb paralysis due to an embolus at the aortic bifurcation. *A*, A lead II ECG tracing shows P, QRS (R), and T waves; the ECG and PCG are superimposed in *B*. Three distinct heart sounds can be recognized. The abnormal one (3) is inscribed during diastole (i.e., between the second [2] and first [1] normal heart sounds). Because the onset of the abnormal sound precedes the initial deflection of the P wave, it is termed a ventricular or $S_3$ gallop rhythm. Dilatative cardiomyopathy was found at autopsy. 50 mm/sec. (From Harpster NK : Vet Clin North Am 7 [1977] 241–256.)

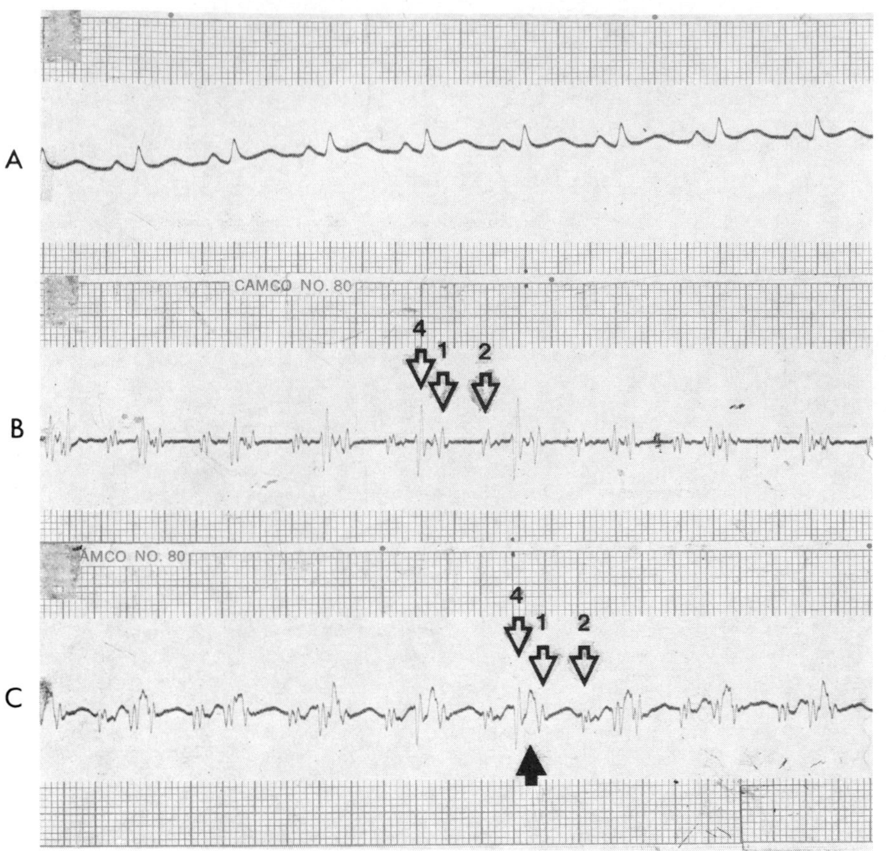


**Figure 18–5** Hypertrophic cardiomyopathy, phonocardiographic study of a five-year-old male domestic shorthair. *A*, A lead II ECG is presented for identification purposes. *B*, In the PCG three separate heart sounds can be seen. *C*, The relationship of the third, abnormal sound can be fully appreciated by superimposition of the ECG and PCG. The abnormal sound (4) occurs during the downstroke of the P wave and frequently extends to cause deformity of the initial portions of the QRS complex (solid arrow). Open arrows 1 and 2 represent the normal first and second heart sounds, respectively. The abnormal heart sound is an atrial or $S_4$ gallop rhythm. 50 mm/sec; ECG: 1.0 mV = 1.0 cm.

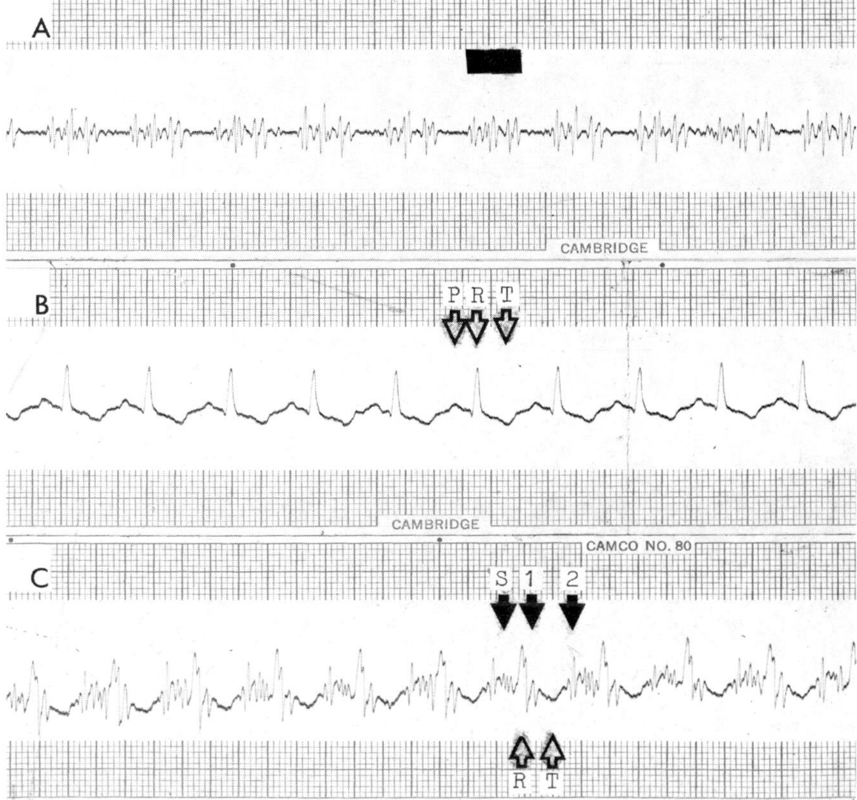


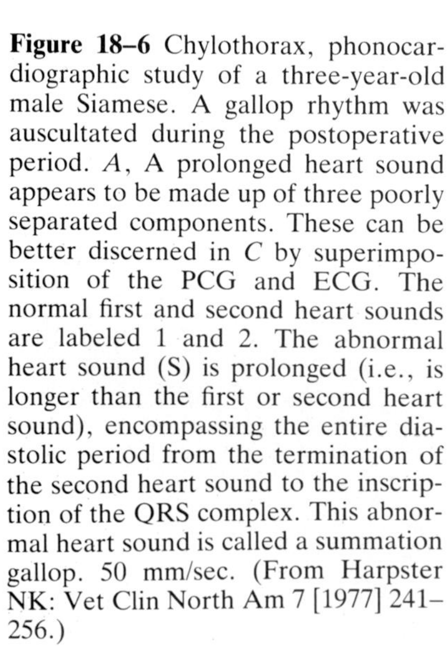

**Figure 18–6** Chylothorax, phonocardiographic study of a three-year-old male Siamese. A gallop rhythm was auscultated during the postoperative period. *A*, A prolonged heart sound appears to be made up of three poorly separated components. These can be better discerned in *C* by superimposition of the PCG and ECG. The normal first and second heart sounds are labeled 1 and 2. The abnormal heart sound (S) is prolonged (i.e., is longer than the first or second heart sound), encompassing the entire diastolic period from the termination of the second heart sound to the inscription of the QRS complex. This abnormal heart sound is called a summation gallop. 50 mm/sec. (From Harpster NK: Vet Clin North Am 7 [1977] 241–256.)

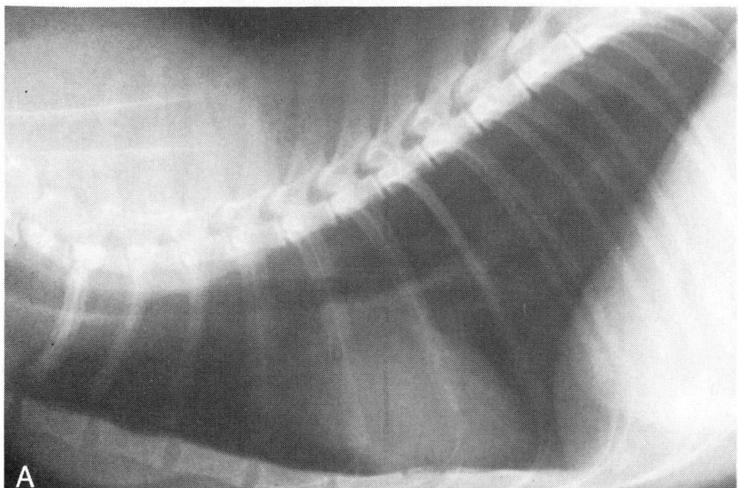


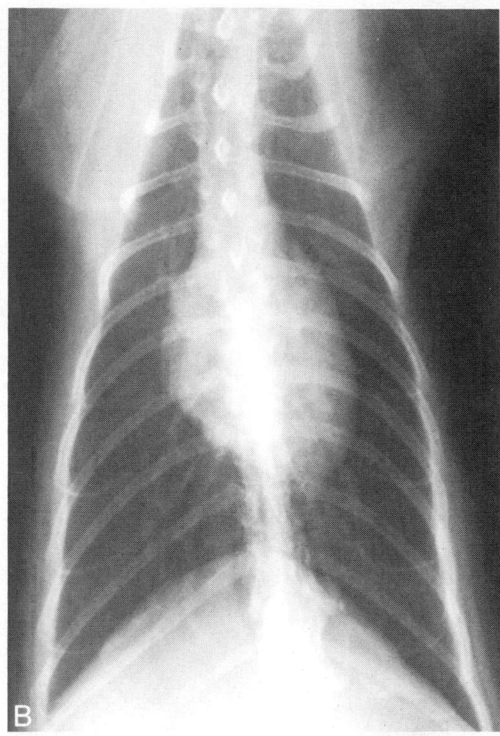


**Figure 18–7** Normal two-year-old neutered male domestic shorthair. *A*, Notice the oblique position of the cardiac silhouette in the lateral view. *B*, The silhouette is elongated in the ventrodorsal view. Cranial waist is maintained and the left cardiac border is straight. The area of cardiosternal contact is two sternebrae.

reported along with careful measurements to define its normal size and orientation (Hamlin et al., 1963b, 1964). Studies of 14 normal cats established that in the lateral projection the cardiac silhouette extends from the fourth to the sixth rib and for 70 per cent of the ventrodorsal distance between the sternum and the underside of the thoracic vertebral bodies at the level of its greatest dorsal extension. In the dorsoventral projection the apex was positioned slightly to the left of the midline in 85.7 per cent of the cats studied (Fig. 18–7). Although these studies define the normal cardiac orientation in the majority of cats, occasionally the heart sits more upright in the lateral projection, with a decreased area of sternal contact (Fig. 18–8). When this uncommon but normal variant is seen

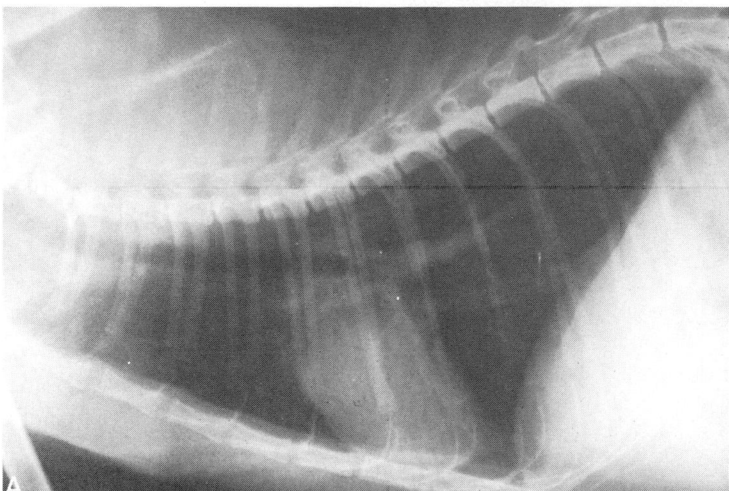


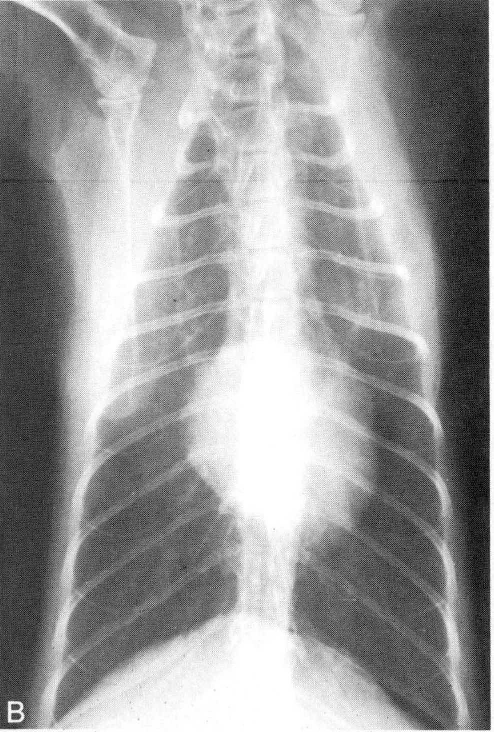


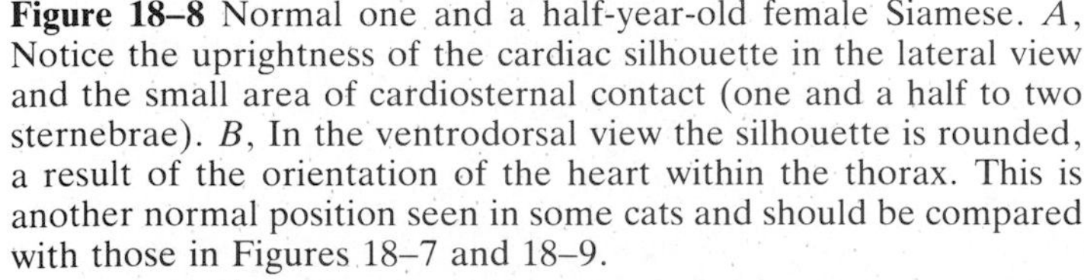

**Figure 18–8** Normal one and a half-year-old female Siamese. *A*, Notice the uprightness of the cardiac silhouette in the lateral view and the small area of cardiosternal contact (one and a half to two sternebrae). *B*, In the ventrodorsal view the silhouette is rounded, a result of the orientation of the heart within the thorax. This is another normal position seen in some cats and should be compared with those in Figures 18–7 and 18–9.

on the lateral projection, the cardiac silhouette on the ventrodorsal projection tends to be diminutive and rounded. Another normal variation, seen more often in the aged cat, is a more longitudinal orientation of the cardiac silhouette on the lateral projection, with an increased area of sternal contact and increased prominence of the aortic arch (Fig. 18–9).

In addition to these normal variations in cardiothoracic orientation, a cat's size and body weight can significantly alter the cardiac silhouette in thoracic radiographs. For example, the cardiac silhouette in young kittens tends to be more rounded in both projections, with less distinct external landmarks. In obese cats the cardiac borders are less clearly defined owing to the presence of increased amounts of mediastinal and pericardial fat (Fig. 18–10).

The normal anatomic positions of the cardiac chambers and the great vessels and their contributions to the cardiac silhouette can be identified by 70-mm rapid-sequence spot films taken after the injection of a radiopaque contrast material via a right atrial catheter (Fig. 18–11). In the lateral projection the cranial border of the cardiac silhouette, from the sternum to the thoracic vertebrae, is composed of the right ventricular outflow tract, the right auricular appendage, and the aortic arch. The ventral border consists entirely of the right ventricle. The caudal and dorsal borders of the cardiac silhouette are formed by the left ventricle and left atrium, respectively. In the ventrodorsal projection the right cardiac border is formed by the right ventricle over the caudal half, while the cranial half is supplied by the cranial and middle portions of the right atrium. The left cardiac border is formed by the main pulmonary artery cranially, the left auricular appendage at the one to three o'clock position, and the left ventricle caudally. The most caudal 1 to 1.5 cm of the cardiac apex in the ventrodorsal projection is composed entirely of the left ventricle.

Even with our detailed knowledge of normal cardiac anatomy in the cat, it is not easy to define the contribution of individual cardiac chambers to cardiac enlargement in cats with congenital or acquired heart disease. This is due to the frequent enlargement of two or more chambers in cardiac disease, to the fairly high incidence of complex and multiple anomalies in cats with congenital heart disease, and to some degree to the cardiac shifting and rotation that result from cardiac enlargement. However, even with these apparent major obstacles, considerable information can be obtained by thoracic radiography of cats with cardiac disease.

In simple right heart enlargement (Fig. 18–12) an increased area of cardiosternal contact in the lateral view may be accompanied by elevation of the apex off the sternum. In addition, there is increased prominence or fullness of the cranial border of the cardiac silhouette. In the ventrodorsal view the cardiac apex is broadened, and there is rounding of the right cardiac border, which is closer than normal to the right chest wall. There may also be some degree of tracheal elevation in the lateral view, although this is not as pronounced as with left or biventricular enlargement unless severe right ventricular enlargement is present.

In isolated left heart enlargement (Fig. 18–13) tracheal elevation and loss of caudal waist are evident in the lateral view without a significant increase in the area of cardiosternal contact. In the ventrodorsal view the apex tends to be more rounded than normal and may be shifted to the left of the pericardiophrenic ligament. A left auricular appendage bulge can frequently be seen along the left cardiac border at the one to three o'clock position.

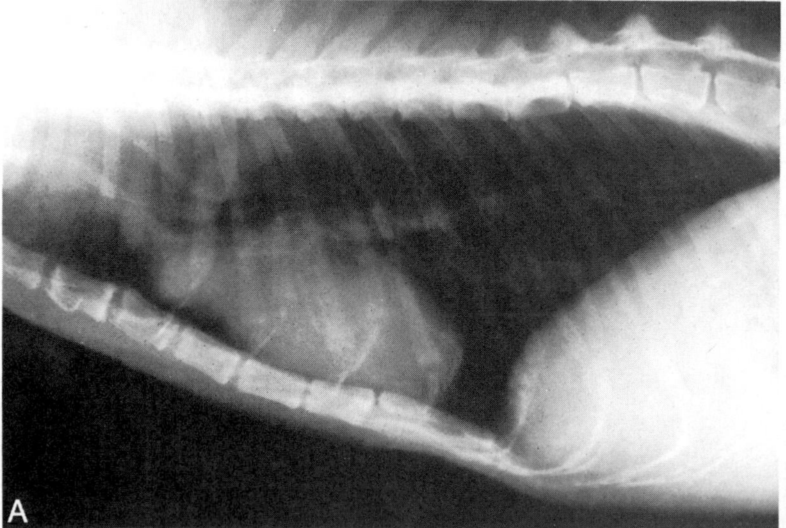


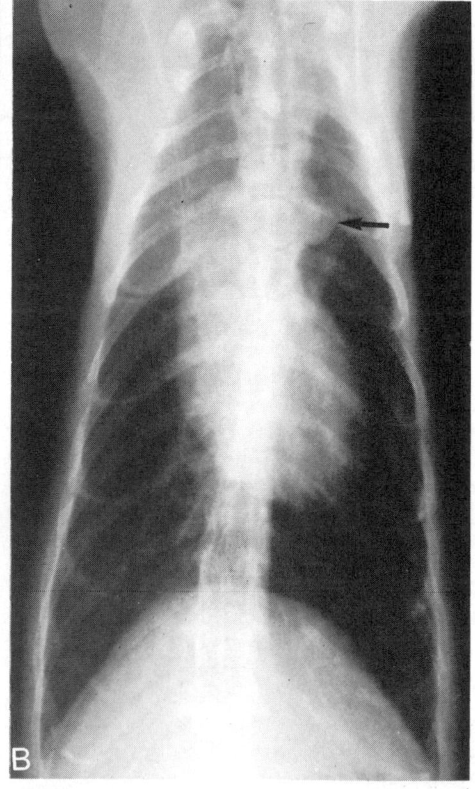


**Figure 18–9** Redundant aortic arch, 19-year-old neutered male domestic shorthair presented for a chronic urinary tract infection. *A*, Notice the horizontal position of the cardiac silhouette in the lateral view (the area of cardiosternal contact approaches four and a half sternebrae) along with the aortic prominence that results in loss of cranial waist. *B*, In the ventrodorsal view the prominence of the aortic arch is seen as widening of the cranial border of the cardiac silhouette on the right and an aortic knob on the left (arrow). This radiographic feature has been referred to as a redundant aortic arch and is common in aged cats.

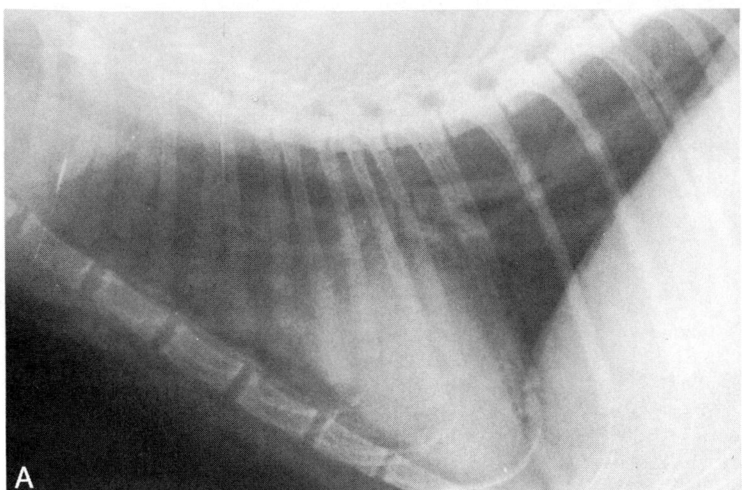


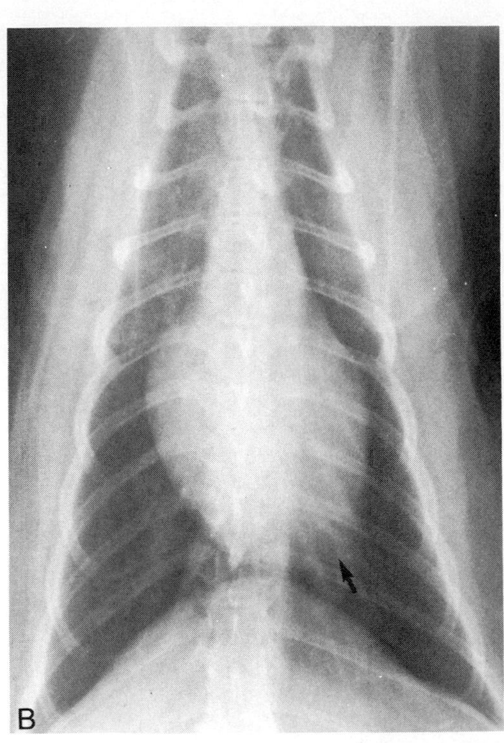


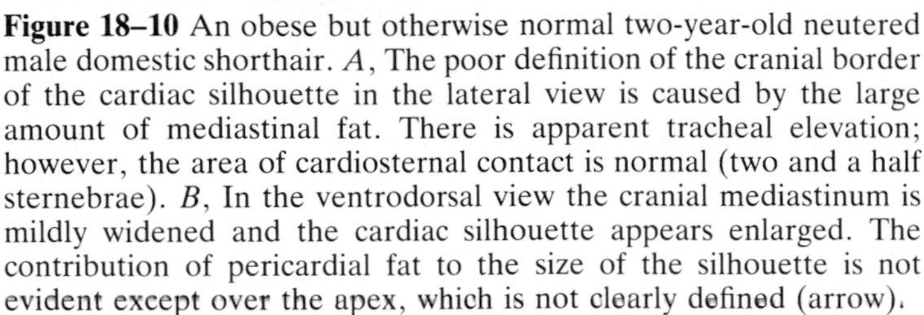

**Figure 18–10** An obese but otherwise normal two-year-old neutered male domestic shorthair. *A*, The poor definition of the cranial border of the cardiac silhouette in the lateral view is caused by the large amount of mediastinal fat. There is apparent tracheal elevation; however, the area of cardiosternal contact is normal (two and a half sternebrae). *B*, In the ventrodorsal view the cranial mediastinum is mildly widened and the cardiac silhouette appears enlarged. The contribution of pericardial fat to the size of the silhouette is not evident except over the apex, which is not clearly defined (arrow).

With biventricular cardiac enlargement, thoracic radiographs have some of the features described for both right heart and left heart enlargement (Fig. 18–14). In the lateral view there tend to be both tracheal elevation and increased cardiosternal contact. Slight fullness of the cranial border of the cardiac silhouette may also be distinguished, while caudal waist may or may not be maintained. In the ventrodorsal view the apex is frequently rounded and shifted toward the left, and the entire cardiac silhouette assumes a more rounded configuration than normal. A left auricular appendage bulge may or may not be evident.

## Electrocardiography

An ECG is an integral part of the basic cardiac study and should be performed routinely in all cats with suspected cardiac disease. The amount of information provided by the ECG will depend, in part, on the electrocardiographer's familiarity with the normal patterns seen in the cat and also on the methods used and on the time and effort spent in obtaining good tracings. An ECG is only one part of the cardiac evaluation, and, as with other species, a normal ECG does not rule out the existence of heart disease. On the other hand, the ECG can provide valuable information regarding cardiac chamber enlargement; localization and character of tachyarrhythmias, bradyarrhythmias, and conduction abnormalities; response to or toxic effects of cardioactive agents; and the existence of myocardial ischemia.

A routine, multiple-lead scalar ECG can and should be performed without tranquilization or sedation. Even the most fractious cat can be managed by a single assistant by taping the front and hind feet together. Although a sternal position for routine electrocardiography of the cat has been reported to offer certain advantages over the standard right lateral recumbent position (Gompf and Tilley, 1979), I prefer the latter position for a number of reasons. First, the cat is more easily restrained by a single assistant. Second, exact duplication of the same position is more easily obtained in subsequent ECGs, thereby eliminating artifactual errors caused by positioning. Lastly, the right lateral recumbent position permits more accurate identification of anatomic landmarks in the recording of multiple precordial leads.

**LITERATURE REVIEW.** Although the vast majority of reports dealing with feline electrocardiography have presented data only on the standard bipolar and unipolar limb leads (Blok and Boeles, 1957; Gompf and Tilley, 1979; Hamlin et al., 1963a; Massmann and Opitz, 1954; Tilley, 1985), the diagnostic value of precordial leads in man has been emphasized (Burch and Winsor, 1966) and the utilization of other leads in the domestic cat has been reported (Calvert and Coulter, 1981; Rogers and Bishop, 1971). The normal Lead II values for duration of electrocardiographic intervals, amplitudes of electrocardiographic waves, and recorded heart rates in various studies reported in the veterinary literature are presented in Table 18–3. I routinely record 12 leads: the standard bipolar limb leads (i.e., Leads I, II, and III), the standard unipolar limb leads (i.e., aVR, aVL, and aVF), and six precordial leads. The anatomic locations for the recording of these precordial leads are outlined in Table 18–4 and diagrammatically depicted in Figure 18–15. Table 18–5 identifies the normal values for these six precordial leads in 20 cats. It can be seen from these results that the cat has an intrinsicoid deflection pattern similar to that reported for man (Burch and Winsor, 1966), with a decreas-

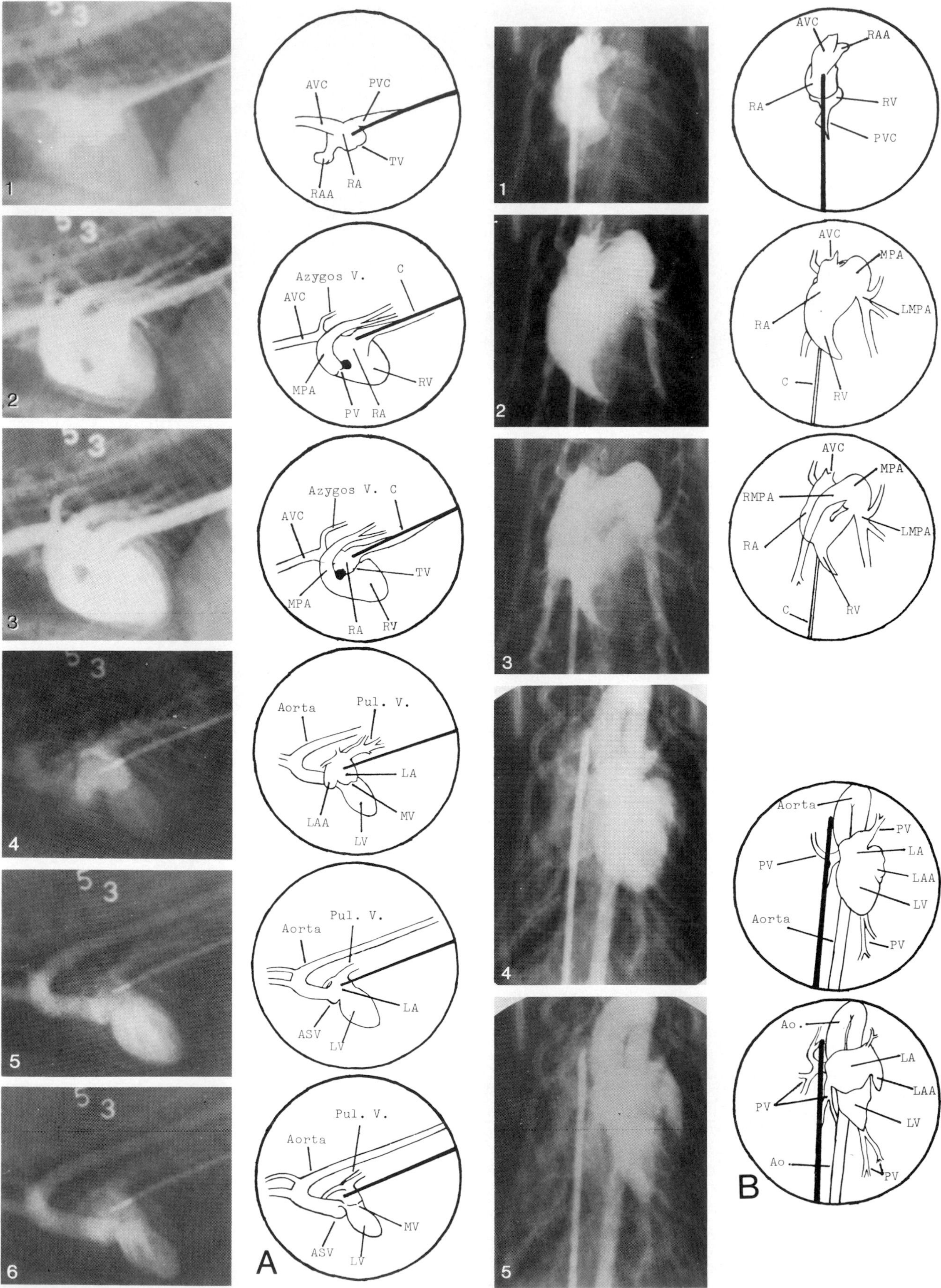


**Figure 18–11** *See legend on opposite page*

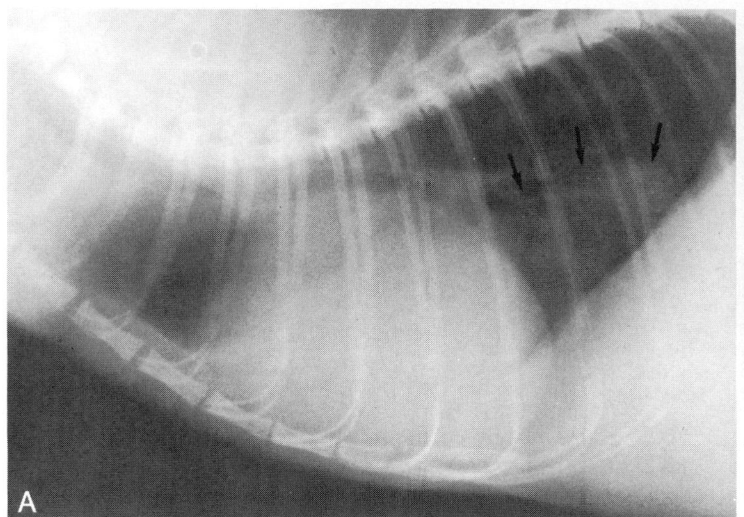


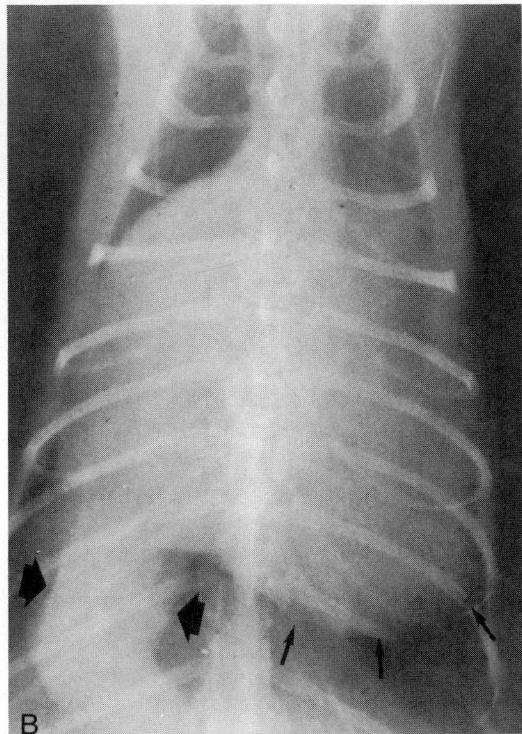


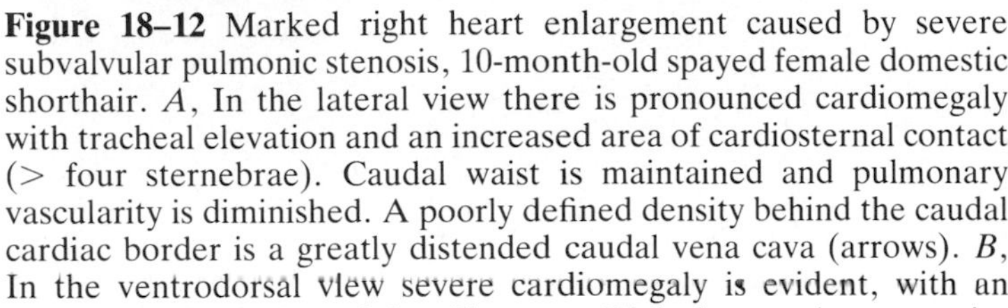
**Figure 18–12** Marked right heart enlargement caused by severe subvalvular pulmonic stenosis, 10-month-old spayed female domestic shorthair. *A*, In the lateral view there is pronounced cardiomegaly with tracheal elevation and an increased area of cardiosternal contact (> four sternebrae). Caudal waist is maintained and pulmonary vascularity is diminished. A poorly defined density behind the caudal cardiac border is a greatly distended caudal vena cava (arrows). *B*, In the ventrodorsal view severe cardiomegaly is evident, with an unusual conformation of the silhouette. Right heart enlargement is suggested by the wide area of contact between the right cardiac border and the right thoracic wall. The left caudal border of the heart is formed by the displaced left ventricle (arrows). The wide, band-like density extending caudally from the right cardiac border represents a distended caudal vena cava (between the arrowheads).

ing S-wave predominance accompanied by an increasing R-wave predominance as recordings are taken progressively from the right (i.e., r $V_2$) toward the left (i.e., $V_6$). However, the progressive increase in R-wave amplitude from right to left reported in man does not appear to occur in the cat, although R waves are of greater amplitude in the left precordial leads. It should also be noted that, with the exception of Lead $V_6$, T-wave polarity occurs in the same direction as the major QRS deflection.

In addition to the clinical uses of electrocardiography listed previously, the ECG may also aid in establishing the existence, and evaluating the response to treatment,

**Figure 18–11** Angiocardiographic anatomy in a normal cat. Nonselective angiocardiography was performed via a right atrial catheter (C), using 70 mm rapid-sequence spot films. The exposures in column A were taken with the cat in the right lateral recumbent position; those in column B are ventrodorsal views.

*Column A*: *1*, Right atrium (RA), anterior (AVC) and posterior (PVC) vena cava, right auricular appendage (RAA), and tricuspid valve (TV). The tricuspid valve is closed. *2*, The right ventricle (RV) in diastole. The pulmonic valve (PV) is closed and the tricuspid valve open (not clearly visualized). MPA = main pulmonary artery. *3*, The right ventricle (RV) in early to mid-systole. The TV is closed, and the pulmonic valve (not labeled) is not visualized. *4*, Early left-sided filling highlighting the pulmonary veins (Pul. V) and left atrium (LA). In this projection the left auricular appendage (LAA) overlies the base of the aorta, obscuring the aortic valve. This is one of the undesirable features that limit the diagnostic capabilities of nonselective angiocardiography. The mitral valve (MV) is closed, indicating left ventricular (LV) systole. *5*, The left ventricle (LV) in diastole. Notice the small size of the left atrium (LA) and the cone-shaped radiolucencies in the LV, which represent the anterior and posterior papillary muscles. ASV = aortic sinus of Valsalva. The aortic valve is not seen owing to superimposition of the left auricular appendage. *6*, The LV in systole. The papillary muscles are seen more clearly. Compare the size of the left atrium with its size in *5*. The mitral valve (MV) is closed.

*Column B*: *1*, Early study, primarily outlining the right atrium (RA). AVC = anterior vena cava, PVC = posterior vena cava, RAA = right auricular appendage, RV = right ventricle. *2*, The right ventricle (RV) in diastole. Notice its narrow, crescent-shaped outline in this view. Dye remains in the right atrium (RA) and partially obliterates the RV and its outflow tract. The main pulmonary artery (MPA) and left main lobar artery (LMPA) are clearly seen. *3*, The right ventricle (RV) in systole. Compare the size of the RV with its size in *2*; it retains a crescent-shaped form. LMPA = left main pulmonary artery; RMPA = right main pulmonary artery. *4*, The left ventricle (LV) in diastole. The papillary muscles are not well visualized in this view. LA = left atrium, LAA = left auricular appendage, PV = pulmonary vein. *5*, The left ventricle in systole. Notice the position and extent of the LA, the prominence of the LAA compared with that in *4*, and the normal course of the aorta (Ao).

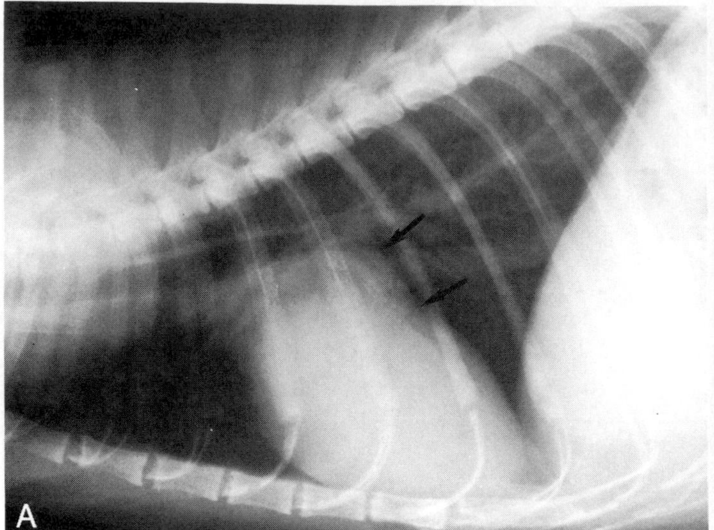


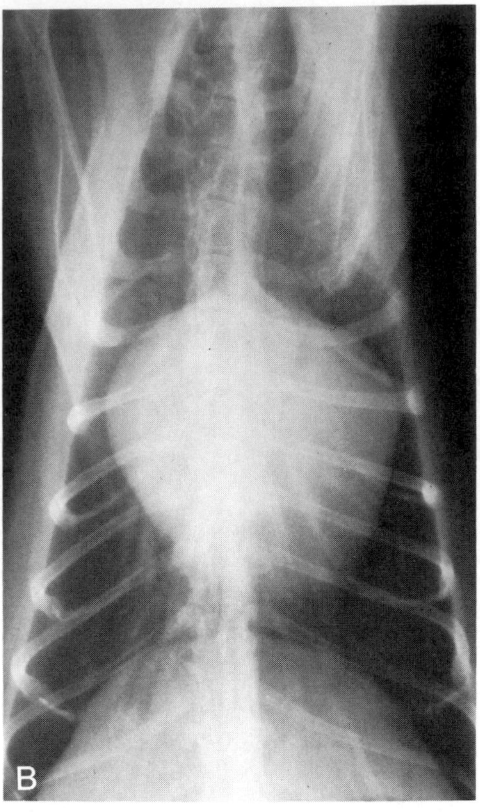


**Figure 18–13.** Nine-year-old neutered male domestic shorthair with hyperthyroidism ($T_3$ = 420 ng/dl [normal 27–220 ng/dl]; $T_4$ = 30.0 μg/dl [normal 1.0–5.0 μg//dl]). *A*, In the lateral projection there is tracheal elevation associated with prominent loss of caudal waist (arrows), although the area of cardiosternal contact is normal (two and a half sternebrae). Pulmonary vascularity is conspicuous and is accompanied by a pattern of increased interstitial density. *B*, In the ventrodorsal view also, cardiomegaly is evident, characterized by rounding of the cardiac apex and a left cranial prominence at the one o'clock to three o'clock position. The latter represents the bulge of the enlarged left auricular appendage. In an M-mode echocardiogram of this cat there was left ventricular dilatation with good preservation of septal and left ventricular free wall systolic motion, as well as left atrial dilatation. The right ventricular cavity was of normal dimensions.

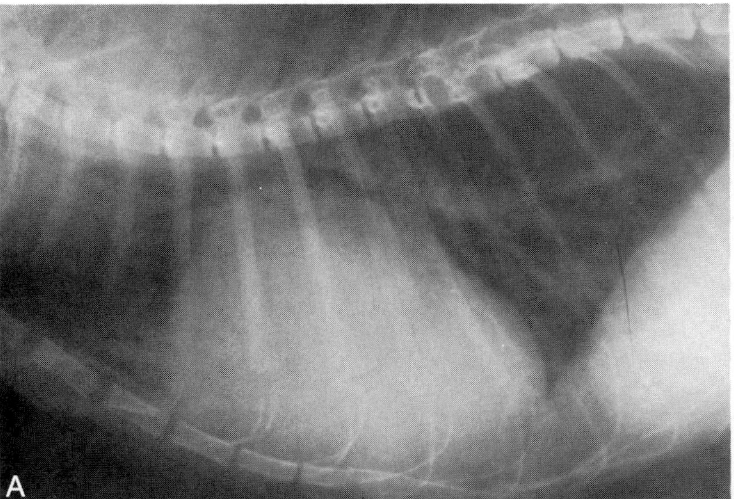


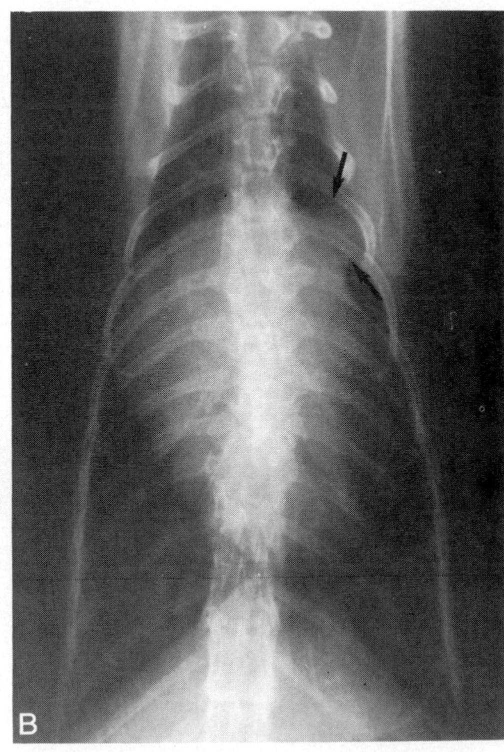


**Figure 18–14** Common atrioventricular (AV) canal, 13-month-old male Himalayan. *A,* The lateral view shows marked generalized enlargement of the cardiac silhouette, increased prominence and rounding of the cranial border of the heart, and increased cardiosternal contact. Because the caudal waist is maintained, it is likely that the prominence of the pulmonary vessels is due to increased circulation rather than congestion. *B*, In the ventrodorsal view also, generalized cardiomegaly is evident, as well as a bulging pulmonary artery segment (arrows) and increased pulmonary vascularity. A diagnosis of common AV canal was established by both nonselective angiocardiography and echocardiography.

**Table 18–3 Lead II Electrocardiographic Measurements Reported for the Normal Cat***

| INTERVAL | BLOK AND BOELES, 1957 | ROGERS AND BISHOP, 1971 | GOMPF AND TILLEY, 1979 | CALVERT AND COULTER, 1981 |
|---|---|---|---|---|
| P wave | | | | |
| Amplitude, mV | 0.15† (0.05–0.28)‡ | 0.12 [0.012]§ (0.30)[M] | 0.16±0.07‖ (0.20)[M] | 0.01 (0.03–0.28) |
| Duration, seconds | 0.03 (0.02–0.04) | NR | 0.03 (0.015–0.05) | 0.03 (0.02–0.05) |
| P-R interval, seconds | 0.07 (0.05–0.10) | 0.074 (0.055–0.10) | 0.07 (0.05–0.10) | 0.07 (0.06–0.09) |
| QRS interval, seconds | 0.02 (0.02–0.04) | 0.036 (0.02–0.045) | 0.03 (0.015–0.04) | 0.04 (0.03–0.05) |
| Q wave amplitude, mV | 0.15 (0.02–0.77) | 0.08 [0.013] (0.27) | 0.26±0.20 | 0.13±0.13 |
| R wave amplitude, mV | 0.51 (0.03–1.33) | 0.43 [0.052] (0.90) | 0.49±0.25 (0.90) | 0.46±0.33 |
| S wave amplitude, mV | 0.32 (0.03–0.70) | 0.20 [0.050] (0.50) | 0.27±0.16 | 0.08±0.06 |
| Q-T interval, seconds | 0.21 (0.18–0.26) | 0.21 (0.17–0.35) | 0.15 (0.07–0.20) | 0.16 (0.13–0.22) |
| T wave | | | | |
| Amplitude, mV | 0.16 (0.03–0.35) | 0.11 [0.015] (0.27) | 0.18±0.06 | NR |
| % Positive | 94.7 | 84.6 | 100 | 86 |
| Heart rate | NR | 159 (90–240) | 197 (160–240) | 206 (120–300) |

*Recorded in right lateral recumbent position.
†Mean value.
‡Range of values.
§Standard error of the mean [SEM] in brackets.
‖Mean ± standard deviation.
NR = Not reported.
M = Maximum value.

of hypoxemia, acid-base imbalance, and abnormal electrolyte states in cats (Coulter et al., 1975; Schaer, 1977). Although its value in identifying hypoxemia and acid-base imbalances is not well established in the clinical setting, electrocardiography is of proven benefit in identifying hyperkalemia and the associated alterations in serum calcium and metabolic acidosis that occur in cats with long-standing urethral obstruction (Schaer, 1977). The initial changes in the ECG associated with hyperkalemia are believed to develop when the serum potassium level rises to values between 7 and 8 mEq/l. T-wave peaking or spiking is the earliest recognizable change. As the serum potassium level increases further, abnormalities of impulse conduction can be identified, characterized by decreasing amplitude and prolongation of the P wave and prolongation of both the PR and the QRS intervals. At serum potassium levels approaching or exceeding 9 mEq/l, sinus arrest is frequent (i.e., absence of P waves), and the QRS complexes become more prolonged and bizarre in configuration (sinoventricular or idioventricular rhythm). How meaningful the correlations are between the serum potassium level and the observed electrocardiographic abnormalities in the cat with long-standing urethral obstruction is difficult to assess, due to coexisting hypocalcemia and metabolic acidosis.

**Table 18–4 Anatomic Locations for the Recording of Multiple Precordial Electrocardiographic Leads in the Cat**

| PRECORDIAL LEAD | ELECTRODE USED | ECG LEAD SELECTOR | ANATOMIC LOCATION |
|---|---|---|---|
| r $V_2$ ($CV_5RL$) | P or C* | V | Right 5th ICS† at sternum |
| $V_2$ ($CV_6LL$) | P or C | V | Left 6th ICS at sternum |
| $V_4$ ($CV_6LU$) | P or C | V | Left 6th ICS at CCJ‡ |
| $V_6$ | P or C | V | Left 6th ICS, midchest |
| $V_{10}$ | P or C | V | Over dorsal spine of 7th thoracic vertebra |
| Base/Apex | LA and RA | I | RA electrode attached to $V_{10}$ position; LA electrode attached to $V_4$ position |

*P or C = precordial or chest electrode.
†ICS = intercostal space.
‡CCJ = costochondral junction.

The vectorcardiogram has also been studied in the cat, as a meaningful extension of the scalar ECG, by both the Wilson and the McFee Systems (Coulter and Calvert, 1981; Rogers and Bishop, 1971). In both studies it was concluded that neither the system used for recording nor the position of the cat affected the results significantly. The McFee system for recording (i.e., X, Y, and Z leads) did result in somewhat higher amplitude QRS complexes, making the wave forms easier to study. In the majority of cats studied, the mean spatial QRS vectors were directed caudad, ventrad, and either sinistrad or dextrad, whereas mean spatial P and T vectors were usually directed caudad, ventrad, and sinistrad (Rogers and Bishop, 1971).

**ELECTROCARDIOGRAPHIC TECHNIQUE.** Like the physical examination, an electrocardiographic examination is aided by a quiet, undisturbed environment. The examination is carried out with a standard portable, properly calibrated ECG machine with copper alligator clips (teeth filed off) in place of the electrode plates or stick-on electrodes used for human patients. If the procedure is performed on a stainless steel table, a towel, light blanket, or cardboard cage mat should be placed under the cat to avoid electrical interference from contact of the copper electrodes with the stainless steel table. With the cat restrained in right lateral recumbency, the limb leads are attached to the appropriate fore- and hindlimbs (just below the elbows and just distal to the stifles), with electrical contact to the skin facilitated by

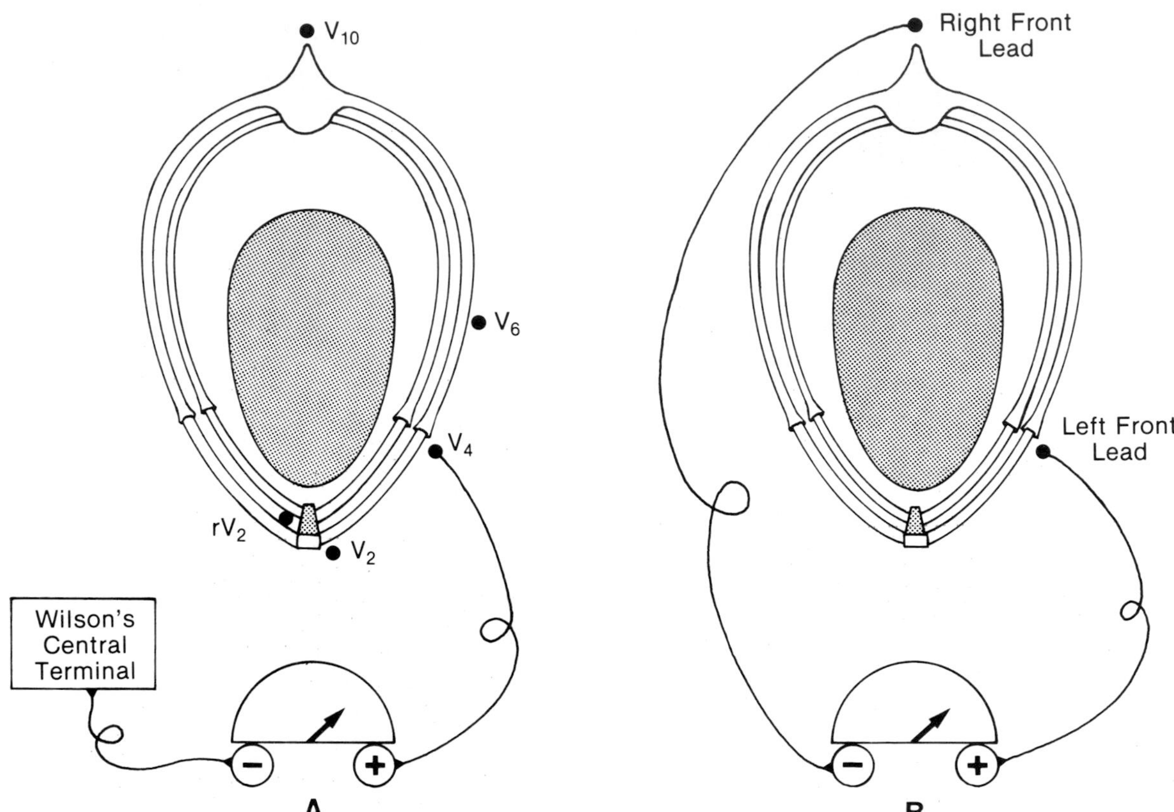


**Figure 18–15** Diagrammatic representation of the patient-electrode connections for recording the standard precordial leads (*A*) and the base/apex lead (*B*). *A*, The standard limb leads must also be attached, and they are connected to the negative terminal of the galvanometer via Wilson's central terminal. (This makes up the indifference electrode, which incorporates input from the left forelimb, right forelimb, and left hindlimb connections through a resistance of 5000 ohms, and nearly approximates zero). The exploring electrode consists of the V or P lead of the standard ECG machine, which is moved from one anatomic position to another, as marked, in order to take an accurate recording. *B*, The base/apex lead is recorded by connecting the right forelimb lead to the $V_{10}$ position and the left forelimb lead to the $V_4$ position. Lead I should be selected in the actual recording of this lead. In the interpretation of ECG recordings taken by these methods, major forces moving toward the exploring or positive electrode are recorded as positive deflections, while those moving in the opposite direction are recorded as negative deflections.

**Table 18–5 Measurements for the Precordial Leads in 20 Normal Cats***

| INTERVAL EVALUATED | PRECORDIAL LEADS rV$_2$ | V$_2$ | V$_4$ | V$_6$† | V$_{10}$ | Base/ Apex† |
|---|---|---|---|---|---|---|
| P wave amplitude (mV) | 0.029 | 0.034 | 0.060 | 0.047 | (−)0.014 | 0.059 |
| (Range) | (−0.025–+0.05) | (0.0–0.05) | (0.025–0.10) | (0.0–0.075) | (−0.025–+0.05) | (0.025–0.10) |
| %Positive | 60 | 95 | 100 | 85 | 20 | 100 |
| % Negative | 15 | 0 | 0 | 0 | 60 | 0 |
| P wave duration (sec) | 0.038 | 0.037 | 0.039 | 0.033 | 0.037 | 0.04 |
| (Range) | (0.03–0.04) | (0.02–0.045) | (0.03–0.05) | (0.025–0.040) | (0.03–0.05) | (0.03–0.05) |
| Number | 10 | 15 | 19 | 17 | 13 | 18 |
| Q wave (mV) | 0.15 | 0.025 | 0.039 | 0.094 | 0.204 | 0.031 |
| (Range) | — | — | (0.025–0.10) | (0.025–0.20) | (0.025–0.50) | (0.013–0.05) |
| Number | 1 | 2 | 9 | 16 | 20 | 2 |
| R wave (mV) | 0.310 | 0.385 | 0.371 | 0.322 | 0.128 | 0.505 |
| (Range) | (0.05–0.80) | (0.05–0.95) | (0.10–0.75) | (0.15–0.60) | (0.025–0.40) | (0.10–1.05) |
| Number | 19 | 20 | 20 | 19 | 16 | 19‡ |
| S wave (mV) | 0.275 | 0.169 | 0.113 | 0.025 | 0.0 | 0.114 |
| (Range) | (0.05–0.55) | (0.025–0.045) | (0.10–0.125) | — | — | (0.025–0.40) |
| Number | 16 | 14 | 2 | 1 | 0 | 9 |
| QRS Interval (sec) | 0.050 | 0.048 | 0.044 | 0.048 | 0.040 | 0.046 |
| (Range) | (0.03–0.065) | (0.03–0.06) | (0.03–0.06) | (0.03–0.06) | (0.03–0.05) | (0.03–0.06) |
| Number | 20 | 20 | 20 | 20 | 20 | 19‡ |
| T wave (mV) | 0.101 | 0.167 | 0.146 | 0.021 | (−)0.076 | 0.216 |
| (Range) | (0.025–0.25) | (0.025–0.50) | (−0.025–+0.30) | (−0.10–+0.20) | (−0.025–(−)0.15) | (0.05–0.35) |
| % Positive | 95 | 100 | 90 | 55 | 0 | 100 |
| % Negative | 5 | 0 | 10 | 35 | 100 | 0 |

*All performed with cats in right lateral recumbency. Average heart rate 181/minute (range 132–220/minute).
†See Table 18–3 for anatomic positioning and method of recording.
‡A base/apex recording was not taken in one cat.

applying a few drops of isopropyl alcohol or a small amount of electrode paste at the point of the electrode-skin interface. The right and left forelegs and the right and left hindlegs should be held together and the forelegs placed perpendicular to the long axis of the body. Another potential source of electrical interference can be contact between adjacent fore- or hindleg electrodes, and this must be avoided. With uncooperative cats it is extremely helpful to tape the hindlegs and the forelegs together, as well as to apply either an Elizabethan collar or a cat muzzle to eliminate the chance of injury to the assistant. For fidgety cats that are not a threat to life and limb, gentle additional restraint and soothing words by the owner or a technician may be all that are required.

Once the cat is satisfactorily restrained the electrocardiographic recording can be taken. After the sensitivity setting of the machine is registered by depressing the mV button, the bipolar limb (Leads I, II, and III) and unipolar limb (Leads aVR, aVL, and aVF) leads can be recorded in sequence by manipulation of the lead selector dial or button. If precordial leads are also to be recorded, the limb lead electrodes must remain attached while the V-lead electrode is moved from one anatomic position to another over the chest wall (Table 18–4), with recordings taken in each position.

In certain clinical situations a full-lead ECG may be unnecessary or contraindicated by the cat's condition. When a cat is presented with significant dyspnea, one should be satisfied with a standing or sternal recumbent Lead II rhythm strip to avoid stress and embarrassment to ventilation that would result from restraining the cat on its side. Additional leads can be run after the dyspnea is relieved, and without the risk that might be encountered on admission. Another situation in which a Lead II rhythm strip usually suffices is for a follow-up ECG on a cat that has recently been started on a cardioactive drug (e.g., digoxin or propranolol) or is being periodically monitored to evaluate the frequency of cardiac arrhythmias. It is unlikely that in either of these circumstances a multiple-lead ECG will be significantly altered from previously or will provide more information than the Lead II rhythm strip. My approach for the long-term cardiac patient has been to repeat full-lead ECG recordings at yearly intervals with Lead II rhythm strips run in the interim period, unless alterations in the Lead II rhythm strips suggest that the recording of additional leads will be of benefit or interest.

A few final comments should be made regarding ECG monitoring in cats. The majority are surprisingly tolerant of long-term electrode attachments and will leave them undisturbed. However, instead of the alligator clips used for routine, short-term recordings, ECG electrode plates and rubber straps are applied. It is necessary to clip hair under the electrode and to use a liberal supply of electrode paste, but only two limbs need be attached to obtain one of the bipolar limb leads. Electrocardiographic monitoring has proved useful in following the progress of cats during attempted control of aggressive cardiac arrhythmias and as a diagnostic procedure for cats presented with a history of syncopal episodes.

**INTERPRETATION OF THE ELECTROCARDIOGRAM.** In the normal cat heart the initial electrical impulse that results in total cardiac depolarization arises in specialized muscle cells (P cells) in the sinoatrial (SA) or sinus node. This is situated on the craniolateral margin of the junction between the superior vena cava and the right atrium. Other specialized muscle fibers in the sinus node, called T cells, serve to organize the distribution of impulses originating from the P cells and connect directly to three atrial internodal tracts, which preferentially and rapidly transmit the cardiac impulse from the sinus node to the atrioventricular (AV) node. Conduction in the AV node is the slowest anywhere in the heart (decremental conduction) and serves two important functions: (1) it permits time for atrial depolarization to spread from the atrial internodal tracts to atrial contractile (muscle) cells so that atrial contraction precedes ventricular contraction, thereby enhancing ventricular filling; and (2) it prevents the spread of rapid atrial tachyarrhythmias to the ventricles at the same rate, which assists in the preservation of ventricular function and maintenance of cardiac output. From the distal borders of the AV node, conduction is again very rapid, traveling first through the bundle of His and then the bundle branches. The left bundle branch divides into an anterior and posterior fascicle after a short distance. These in turn branch extensively over the left ventricular endocardium and are distributed in a manner that results in early activation of the septum and regions of the cranial and caudal papillary muscles. The right bundle branch, on the other hand, courses distally over the right side of the interventricular septum without branching. The first connections of the right bundle with the ventricular myocardium are at the apex of the right ventricle and base of the cranial papillary muscle. From the apex, the peripheral branches of the right bundle spread over the interventricular septum and free wall of the right ventricle (Bigger, 1980). The terminal Purkinje fibers ramify extensively over the endocardial surface of both ventricles and penetrate the underlying ventricular myocardium a short distance before transmitting conduction to the ventricular myocardial contractile cells (Fig. 18–16).

The science that deals with the recording and interpretation of electrical events on the surface of the body that are generated in the heart is termed scalar or surface electrocardiography. It is important to realize that not all the electrical events occurring during depolarization of the heart can be recorded from the body surface but only those that generate sufficient total electrical potential (termed electromotive force). The cell population that is undergoing simultaneous depolarization is critical in the total instantaneous electromotive force (EMF) that is generated. For example, more than 90 per cent of the total cardiac mass is composed of the contractile muscle fibers that serve its pumping function. The remainder is made up of connective tissue cells and the specialized impulse-generating and conducting cells. Thus it should not be surprising that the small population of cells in the heart responsible for impulse generation and conduction produce a small EMF that cannot be recorded from the surface of the body. The events that are recorded result from depolarization of the atrial contractile muscle fibers and both depolarization and repolarization of the ventricular contractile muscle fibers.

In examining the surface ECG, three wave forms and three intervals of importance can be identified (Fig. 18–17). The P wave is inscribed during depolarization of the atrial contractile muscle fibers. The P-R interval is the period from the onset of atrial depolarization to the beginning of ventricular depolarization. It is made up of the P wave and the P-R segment. The period from the peak of the P wave to the onset of the QRS complex is thought to represent the length of time for migration of the impulse through the AV junctional tissues and ventricular conduction pathways to the ventricular muscle (Burch and Winsor, 1966). The QRS complex is inscribed during depolarization of the ventricular contractile muscle fibers. During normal ventricular activation one, two, three, or more separate wave fronts of depolarization may be recognized. (1) The Q wave represents depolarization of the interventricular septum and limited portions of the right ventricular apex (Horan and Flowers, 1980). Major forces here are directed to the right owing to activation of the interventricular septum by the left bundle branch. (2) Inscription of the R wave is mainly the result of depolarization of the left ventricular apex and major

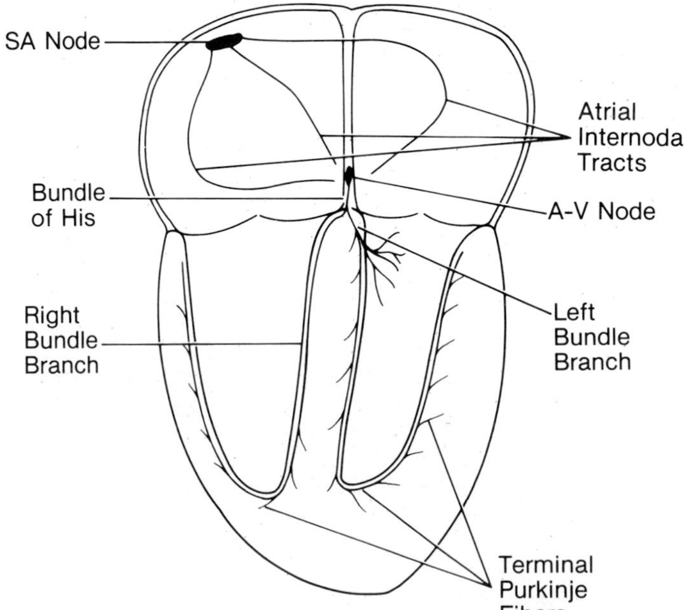


**Figure 18–16** Diagrammatic representation of the specialized conduction pathways in the heart. See text for explanation.

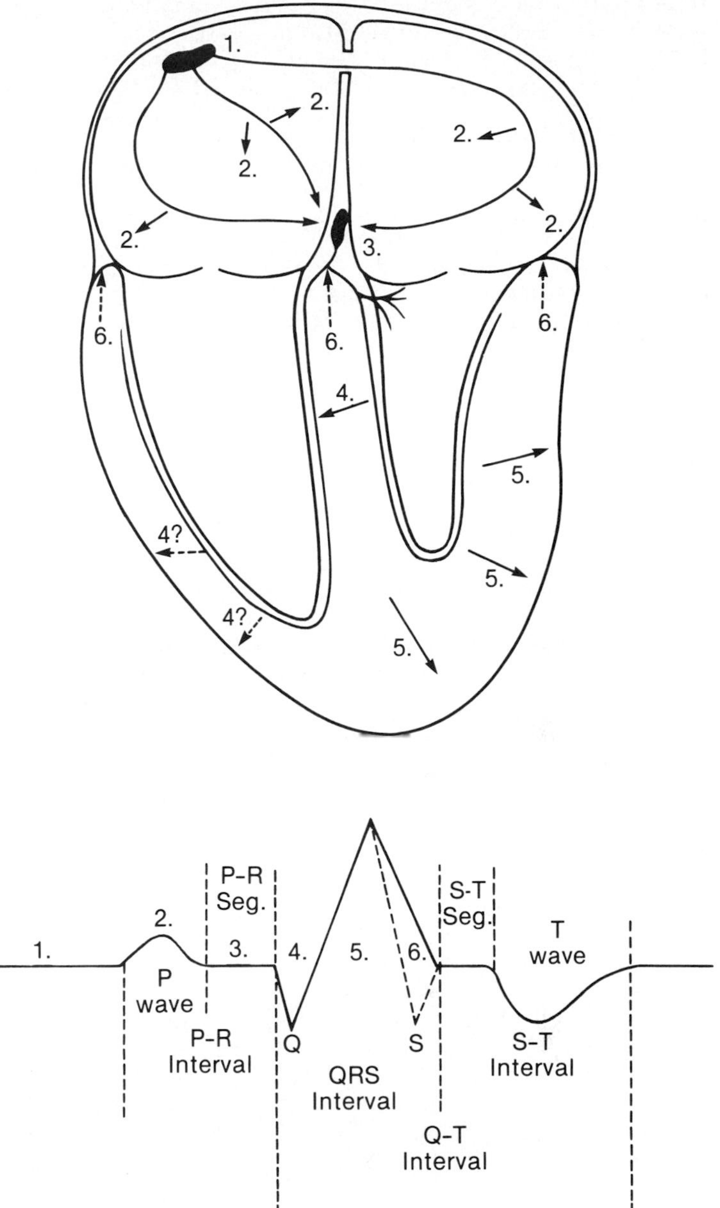


**Figure 18–17** Diagrammatic representation of the correlation between the electrical events occurring within the heart and their characteristics recorded at the external surface of the body. See text for explanation.

apical portions of the left ventricular free wall. (3) Finally, basilar portions of the left and perhaps the right ventricular free wall undergo depolarization effecting development of the S wave. It should be emphasized that during the process of ventricular depolarization there are many wave fronts of activation in a multitude of directions that are undergoing simultaneous depolarization. Many of these ongoing electrical forces are canceled by similar or greater forces occurring in the opposite direction. The final product (the inscribed QRS complex) is the result of the predominant instantaneous EMF moving in a single direction. The so-called QRS complex, therefore, may be composed of less or more than three component parts (Fig. 18–18). The Q-T interval represents the time required for depolarization and repolarization of the ventricular musculature. It is composed of the QRS interval and the S-T interval. The point of separation between the period of ventricular depolarization (QRS complex or interval) and that of ventricular repolarization (S-T interval) is termed the junction or J point. Normally the junction can be fairly easily defined on the surface ECG (Fig. 18–19). Ventricular repolarization consists of an initial period of minor reactivation (S-T segment) and the period of major reactivation (T wave). Repolarization of the ventricles occurs more slowly and diffusely than depolarization, and a cancellation of the effects of simultaneous activity in many areas results. Hence the T wave is of lesser magnitude and longer duration than the QRS complex.

Interpretations from the surface ECG must be done accurately and in a consistent fashion if meaningful values are to be obtained. Ordinarily the Lead II recording should be used for the measurement of all intervals (i.e., P-wave duration, P-R interval, QRS interval, Q-T interval). The intervals should be calculated in a manner to eliminate the width of the baseline from the measurement.

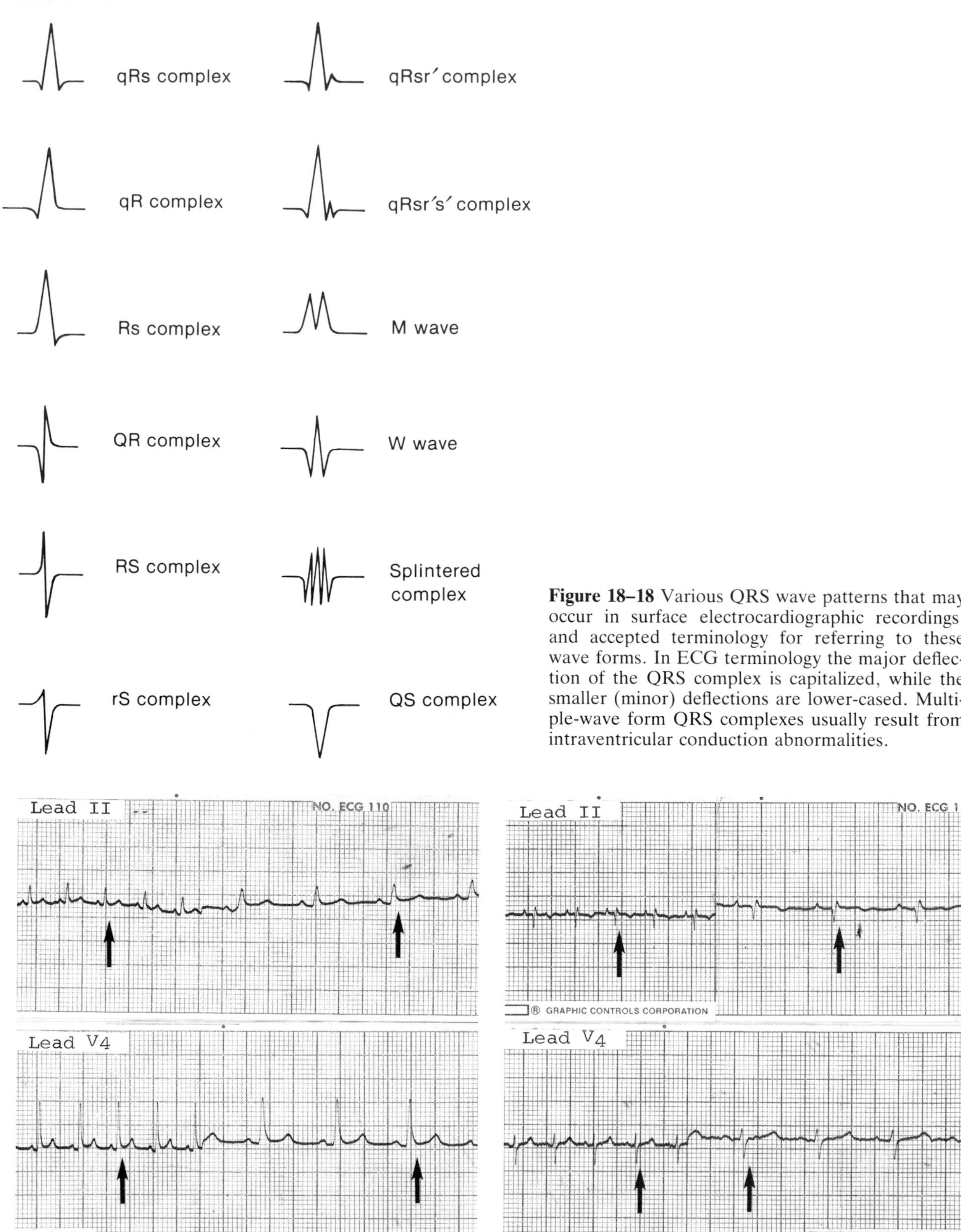


**Figure 18–18** Various QRS wave patterns that may occur in surface electrocardiographic recordings, and accepted terminology for referring to these wave forms. In ECG terminology the major deflection of the QRS complex is capitalized, while the smaller (minor) deflections are lower-cased. Multiple-wave form QRS complexes usually result from intraventricular conduction abnormalities.

**Figure 18–19** Electrocardiographic strips from two cats recorded at both 25mm/sec (*A*) and 50 mm/sec (*B*) to demonstrate the position of the junction or J point. This ECG point of importance marks the separation between the period of ventricular depolarization (i.e., QRS complex) and the onset of ventricular repolarization (i.e., S-T segment). The junction (arrows) is simply that point at which the QRS complex returns to the isoelectric baseline. It is fairly easily defined in the strips from both cats, but more easily at 25 mm/sec than at 50 mm/sec. It is far more difficult to identify exactly when S-T segment elevation or depression is present or when left ventricular strain results in S-T segment repolarization changes (compare with Figures 18–24 and 18–25). 1.0 cm = 1.0 mV.

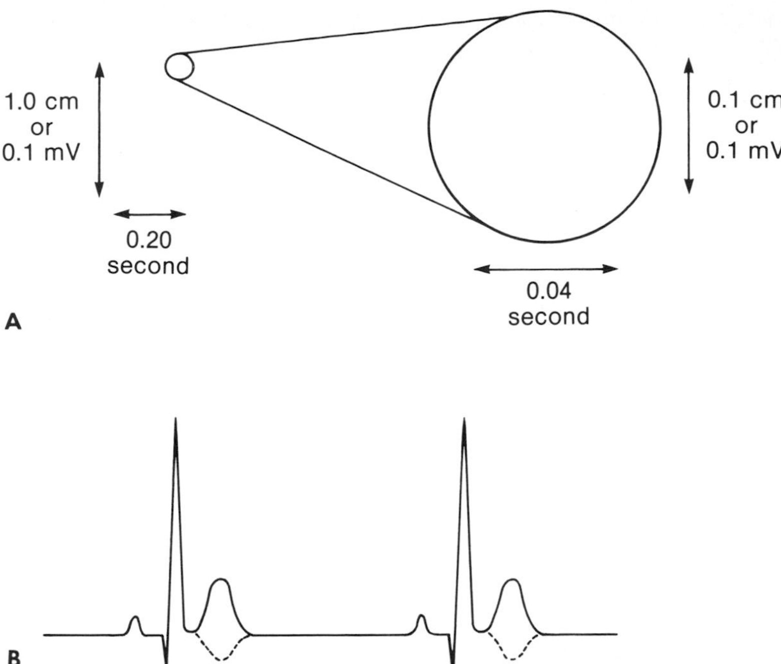


**Figure 18–20** *A*, Method for determining the duration and amplitude of the various wave forms and intervals in the standard surface electrocardiogram when recorded at a paper speed of 25 mm/sec and with the sensitivity setting at 1.0 mV = 1.0 cm. When the recording is made at a paper speed of 50 mm/sec, all calculated intervals must be halved to determine their real values by these methods. See text for further explanation and Figure 18–17 for definition of the beginning and end points for measuring the duration of these parameters. When the heart rhythm is regular (i.e., normal sinus rhythm rather than sinus arrhythmia), the heart rate can be determined by dividing 60 by the R-R interval (in the diagrammatic P-QRS-T complexes in *B*, the calculated heart rate would be 60 divided by 0.80 second, or 75 per minute).

Each is measured from the convex surface (dorsal edge of baseline on negative deflections; ventral edge of baseline on positive deflections) at its point of origin, to the convex surface (dorsal edge of baseline on negative deflection; ventral edge of baseline on positive deflection) at its point of completion. Similarly, measurements of amplitudes of inscribed waves are made to eliminate the width of the baseline. Positive deflections are made from the top of the isoelectric baseline to the convex peak of the inscribed wave, while negative deflections are made from the bottom of the isoelectric baseline to the convex tip of the inscribed wave (Fig. 18–20). Both the P-R and the Q-T intervals are inversely proportional to the heart rate; a slow resting heart rate results in lengthening, and an elevated heart rate causes some degree of shortening. Electrocardiographic values for the normal cat are presented in Tables 18–3 and 18–5.

**ELECTROCARDIOGRAPHIC DEMONSTRATION OF CARDIAC ENLARGEMENT.** An increase in cardiac chamber size is usually associated with an

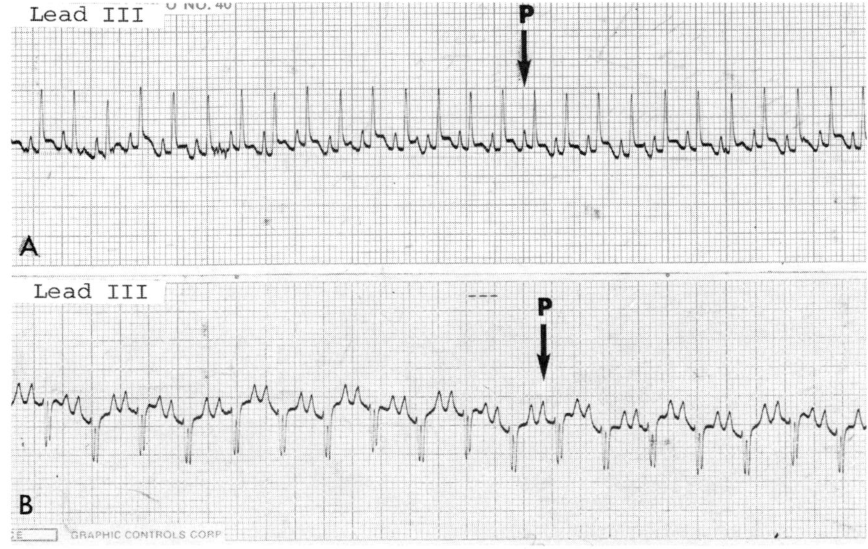


**Figure 18–21** Electrocardiographic strips from two cats to show the influence of atrial enlargement. In *A*, recorded from a five-year-old neutered male domestic shorthair with hypertrophic cardiomyopathy, the P waves are of increased amplitude (0.25 to 0.3 mV) and of normal duration (0.40 second). This pattern of atrial enlargement is fairly typical of that in hypertrophic and, less often, restrictive cardiomyopathy with predominant left atrial enlargement. Strip *B*, from a five-month-old Himalayan with common atrioventricular canal, demonstrates both increased amplitude (0.3 to 0.35 mV) and duration (0.05 second) of the P waves. This pattern of enlargement is characteristic of bilateral enlargement. 25 mm/sec; 1.0 mV = 1.0 cm.

increase in the myocardial mass of the enlarged chamber. This results in a greater EMF in one major direction, which is, as a rule, unopposed by an equal increase in forces in the opposite direction. The effect of these changes on the ECG is an increase in the amplitude of the recorded wave(s) corresponding to the enlarged chamber(s) or an increase in the duration of the influenced wave(s), or both. In general, chamber dilatation causes greater increases in amplitude than does chamber hypertrophy. The electrocardiographic amplitude of recorded waves may also be increased in circumstances unrelated to chamber hypertrophy or dilatation. Most notable of these other causes are (1) alteration in sequence of ventricular activation as seen in isolated bundle branch block, (2) a reduction in opposing forces such as occurs in myocardial infarction and underdeveloped left ventricle, and (3) alteration in cardiac position secondary to other intrathoracic pathology. All electrocardiographic examples in the following pages were recorded at 25 mm/second unless otherwise stated.

**Atrial Enlargement.** Increase in P-wave amplitude above 0.2 mV in Lead II or prolongation of its duration beyond 0.04 second, or both, are electrocardiographic findings compatible with atrial enlargement in the cat. It is far more difficult to ascribe one or the other of these changes to right or left atrial enlargement, as has been described in man and the dog, and I am not convinced that this can be done accurately. Abnormal P waves are common in young cats with congenital heart disease (e.g., common AV canal, tricuspid atresia, pulmonic stenosis) and occasionally with the hypertrophic and intermediate forms of cardiomyopathy (Fig. 18–21). P-wave abnormalities, however, are infrequent in cats with dilatative cardiomyopathy. Many cats have radiographic left atrial enlargement without electrocardiographic evidence of atrial enlargement. Abnormalities of atrial depolarization due to myocardial fibrosis and other pathologic processes may also be responsible for prolongation of $P_{II}$ (i.e., P wave in Lead II).

**Right Ventricular Enlargement.** Electrocardiographic patterns of right ventricular enlargement are not well established in the cat. This is mainly because right ventricular enlargement is infrequent except in kittens and young adults with congenital heart disease. Severe right ventricular enlargement secondary to tetralogy of Fallot, pulmonic stenosis, and double outlet right ventricle is frequently accompanied by electrocardiographic findings similar to those reported for right ventricular enlargement in man and the dog. These may include deep S waves in Leads I, II, III, and aVF, along with prominent S waves in precordial leads $V_2$, $V_4$, and base/apex (B/A) (Fig. 18–22). Other reported abnormalities of right ventricular enlargement in the cat include a clockwise mean electrical axis of the QRS complex in the frontal plane of +160° or greater, positive T waves in Lead $V_{10}$, and right atrial enlargement (Bolton and Liu, 1977; Harris and Ogburn, 1975; Tilley and Gompf, 1977). Prolongation of the QRS interval up to 0.06 second is also common.

**Left Ventricular Enlargement.** Electrocardiographic evidence of left ventricular enlargement is common in cats with either congenital or acquired heart disease. Ventricular septal defect, aortic stenosis, patent ductus arteriosus, and endocardial fibroelastosis are such congenital conditions. Left ventricular enlargement occurs with approximately the same degree of frequency in hypertrophic and dilatative cardiomyopathy, is virtually nonexistent in the intermediate form, and is prominent in hyperthyroidism secondary to adenomatous goiter. The typical ECG is characterized by an increase in R-wave amplitude to beyond 1.0 mV in Leads II and $V_4$, 0.6 mV in $V_6$, and 1.2 mV in the B/A lead. In addition there tends to be an increase in the amplitude of the R wave in Lead $V_{10}$ such that it exceeds the Q-wave amplitude (i.e., $R/Q > 1.0$), as well as a moderate prolongation of the QRS interval (0.045 to 0.060 second) (Fig. 18–23). In hyperthyroidism the increase in R-wave amplitude is often accompanied by a deep S wave, particularly in Lead II. This pattern is not seen with any of the other common causes of left ventricular enlargement. An explanation for this finding is lacking. In a few cats with hypertrophic cardiomyopathy the limb leads present a pattern of left axis deviation (mean electrical axis of the QRS complex in the frontal plane is less than 0 degrees) without prolongation of the QRS interval. It is unclear whether this latter finding is wholly related to left ventricular enlargement or is a variant of left anterior fascicular block.

**S-T SEGMENT AND JUNCTION ABNORMALITIES.** Alterations in the S-T segment and junction (J) appear electrocardiographically as elevation of the S-T segment (and junction) above the isoelectric baseline or depression of the S-T segment (and junction) below the isoelectric baseline. They are frequently accompanied by primary alterations in the T wave. S-T segment abnormalities have been shown to be the effect of the following: (1) prolongation of the period of ventricular depolarization (e.g., intraventricular conduction abnormalities, such as right and left bundle branch block; ventricular premature beats; administration of cardioactive drugs that retard ventricular depolarization, as with quinidine and procainamide in toxic doses); (2) shortening of the period of repolarization (e.g., sinus tachycardia, supraventricular tachyarrhythmias, administration of digitalis glycosides, particularly in toxic levels); (3) alterations in the resting potential of cells in adjacent areas of the ventricular myocardium. Focal abnormalities of myocardial resting potential result in what are termed currents of injury and cause a constant flow of EMF during the resting (polarized) state. These can be the consequence of myocardial infarction, myocardial trauma (surgical or accidental), pericarditis, and myocardial ischemia secondary to coronary insufficiency or cardiac hypertrophy.

In the normal cat S-T segment elevation or depression is unusual, whereas in man and the dog mild S-T segment deviations can occur without any definable cause. Thus any deviation of the S-T segment above or below the baseline in the cat can be considered an electrocardiographic abnormality, even though its presence cannot always be explained (Fig. 18–24). Abnormalities of the S-T segment in the cat have been reported in the majority of the conditions discussed earlier (Tilley, 1985), and also as a consequence of both hyperkalemia and hypokalemia (Coulter et al., 1975; Parks, 1975). In some cats with both left ventricular enlargement and congestive heart failure a different form of S-T segment depression occurs, characterized by a coving of the S-T segment along with an imperceptible or poorly defined J point (Fig. 18–25). Similar electrocardiographic changes have been reported in the dog secondary to chronic valvular disease (Edwards, 1977) and dilatative cardiomyopathy (Wood, 1983) and may occur under the influence of digitalis glycosides

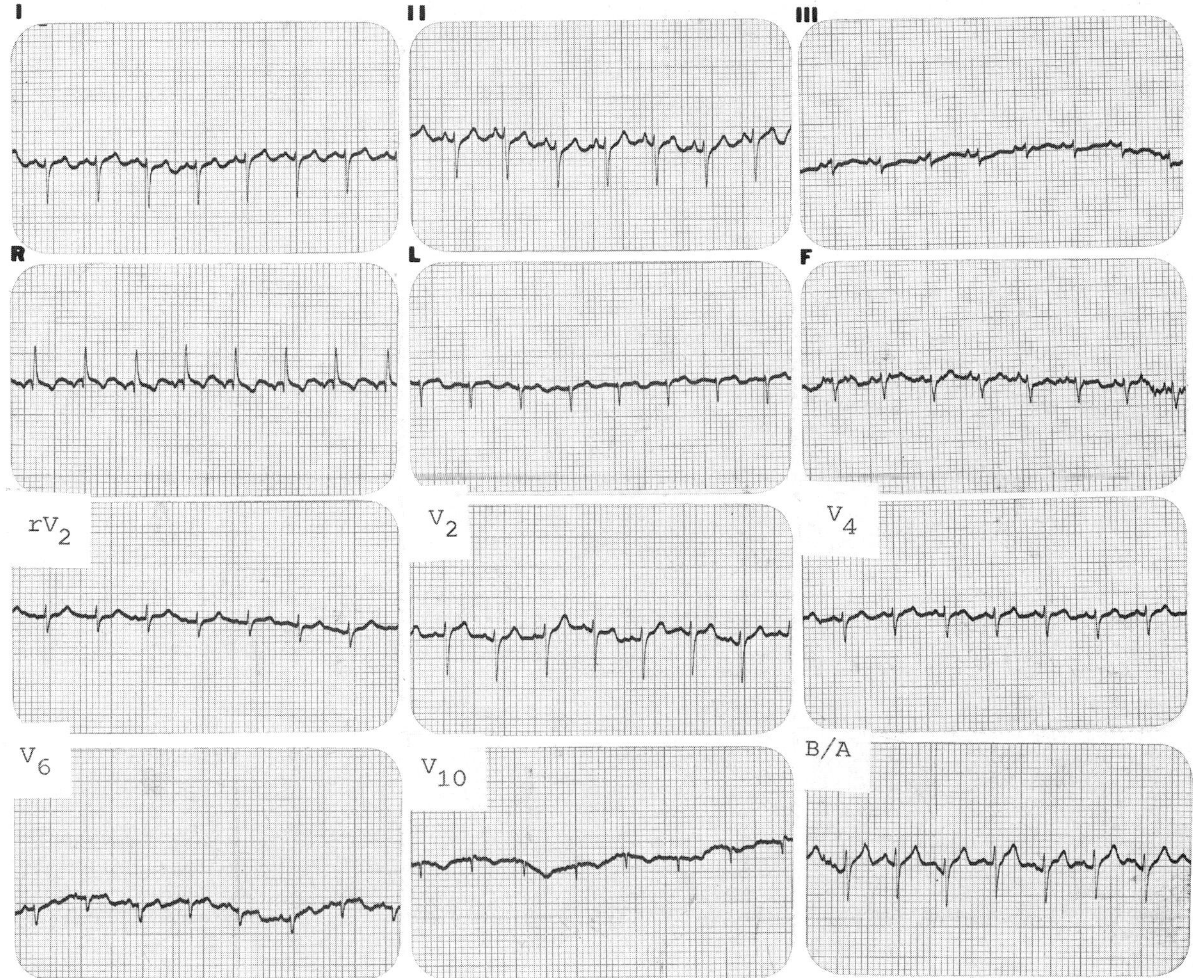


**Figure 18–22** Pulmonic stenosis, twelve-lead ECG from an 18-month-old female domestic shorthair. Deep S waves in leads I, II, and aVF and the presence of qR complexes in lead aVR are strongly indicative of major depolarization forces to the right, findings supportive of increased right ventricular mass. These changes, in conjunction with balanced QRS forces in lead III, are reminiscent of those expected in dogs with moderate to severe right ventricular enlargement (frontal plane mean electrical axis = − 160.5°). Deep S waves present in the left precordial and base/apex leads are additional evidence for right ventricular enlargement. 25 mm/sec; 1.0 mV = 1.0 cm.

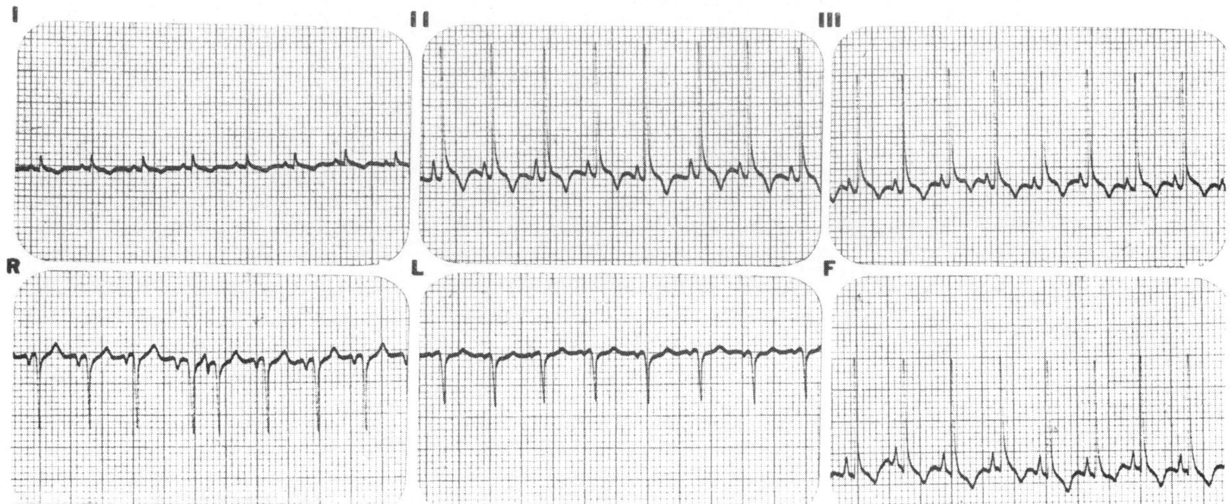


**Figure 18–23** Hypertrophic cardiomyopathy, six-lead ECG from a two-year-old neutered male domestic shorthair. Notice the high-amplitude R waves in leads II, III and aVF. Those in lead II are 2.1 mV and greatly exceed the normal limits (to 0.9 mV). P waves in lead II are increased in amplitude (0.3 mV), a finding compatible with atrial enlargement. A single atrial premature beat is recorded in aVR. This pattern of R wave amplitude is termed LVH (left ventricular hypertrophy) pattern. 25 mm/sec; 1.0 mV = 1.0 cm.

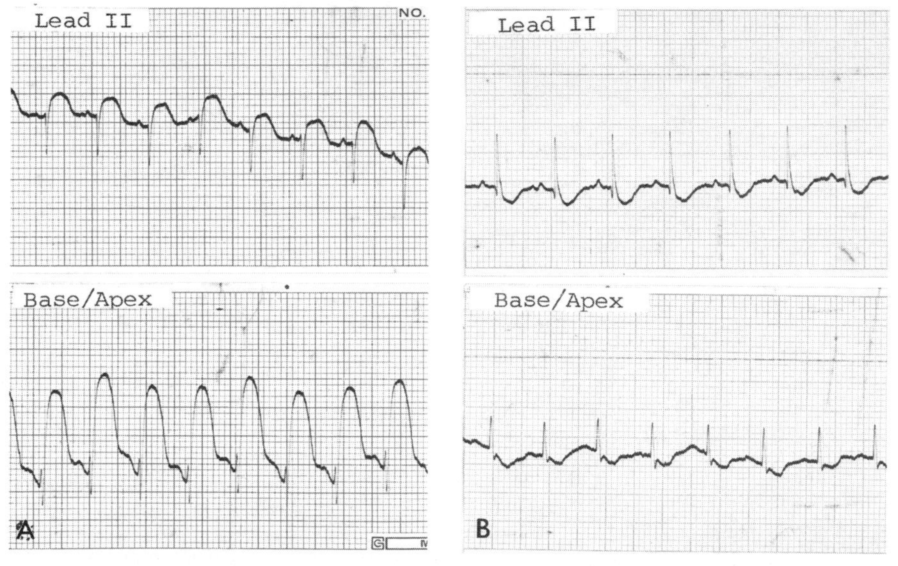


**Figure 18–24** Electrocardiographic recordings from two cats demonstrating the presence of S-T segment elevation (*A*) and depression (*B*). The five-year-old neutered male domestic longhair from which the strips in *A* were recorded developed an acute saddle embolus a few hours later. Severe myocardial ischemia, probably secondary to a coronary artery embolus, was thought to be responsible for the ECG changes. The tracings show marked elevation of the S-T segment above the isoelectric baseline (i.e., the point at which the baseline enters the QRS complex), particularly in lead B/A, where the QRS complex is virtually inseparable from the T wave. In comparison, the S-T segment depression seen in *B* is far less impressive. However, the S-T segment is squared off at the point of intersecting the T wave (in contrast with Figure 18–25, in which a more gradual blending of the two occurs). Although the cause of this finding in the two-year-old neutered male domestic longhair with hypertrophic cardiomyopathy was never established, these changes are unlike the S-T segment repolarization changes commonly seen in cats secondary to left-heart failure.

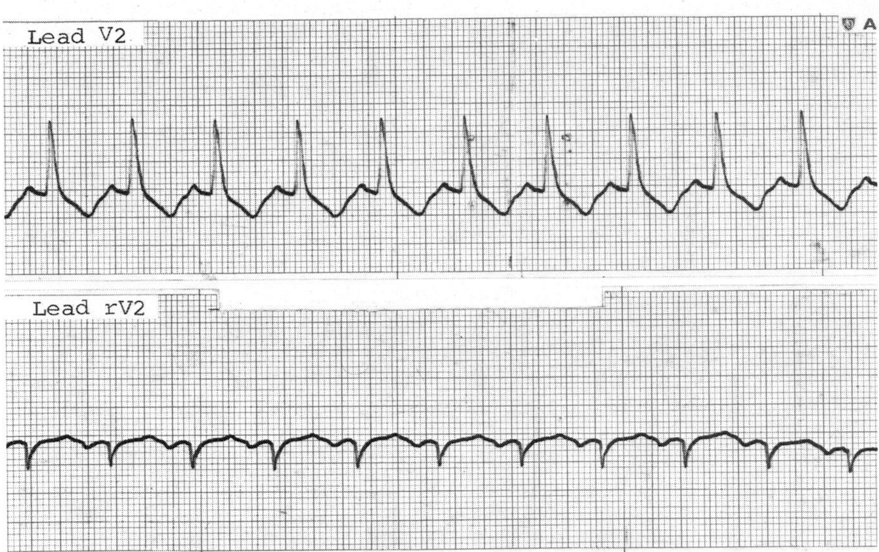


**Figure 18–25** Two precordial leads recorded from a seven-year-old female domestic shorthair presented for acute hindlimb paralysis secondary to a saddle embolus. The T wave begins at a point below the isoelectric baseline, a finding consistent with S-T segment depression. However, this is not seen to the same degree as in Figure 18–24; moreover, the J point is never clearly defined. These features represent S-T segment repolarization changes that usually result from mild left ventricular ischemia or strain, and are frequent in cats with heart failure. Hypertrophic cardiomyopathy was found at autopsy. 50 mm/sec; 1.0 mV = 1.0 cm.

(Burch and Winsor, 1966; Hahn, 1977; Tilley, 1985). Most likely these represent a combined effect of left heart enlargement and subendocardial ischemia secondary to elevated left ventricular end-diastolic pressure.

**ABNORMALITIES OF IMPULSE GENERATION AND CONDUCTION.** Cardiac rhythm in the normal cat is usually regular with considerable variation in the "resting" rate. Most reports of the normal heart rate are based on electrocardiographic studies and are probably influenced considerably by increased sympathetic tone, a result of the cat's inherent uneasiness and stressful reaction in a strange environment (Fig. 18–26). Occasionally ***sinus arrhythmia*** occurs in cats that are more relaxed or severely depressed because of illness. In these circumstances a wandering sinus pacemaker pattern may be present similar to that described for the dog (Tilley, 1985) (Fig. 18–27). On the other hand, in states of increased stress (e.g., fear, anger, pain, fever, anemia, infection, shock) ***sinus tachycardia*** is frequent. Under these conditions the ECG tends to be normal, except for the rapid sinus rate (> 240/minute) and the well-formed P waves (Fig. 18–28). In fact, P waves may exceed the upper limits of normal for amplitude (0.2 mV) but are of normal duration. The P-R interval should be constant, while the Q-T interval is frequently shortened owing to abbreviation of the period of repolarization. Similar changes may be induced by atropine, ketamine, and sympathomimetic agents. Physiologic sinus tachycardia must be differentiated from that resulting from cardiac disease and other disorders that directly affect the heart (e.g., hyperthyroidism, pheochromocytoma). The clinical approach in physiologic sinus tachycardia should be to identify and correct the cause, rather than treating the accelerated heart rate.

Primary cardiac disorders can affect the heart in a variety of ways. Arrhythmias, murmurs, and cardiac dysfunction are recognized effects. In addition, myocardial disease can affect function of impulse-generating and conduction tissues. This altered function may give rise to clinical signs or serve as an electrocardiographic signal that either myocardial disease or some extracardiac process is present. The low incidence of abnormalities of

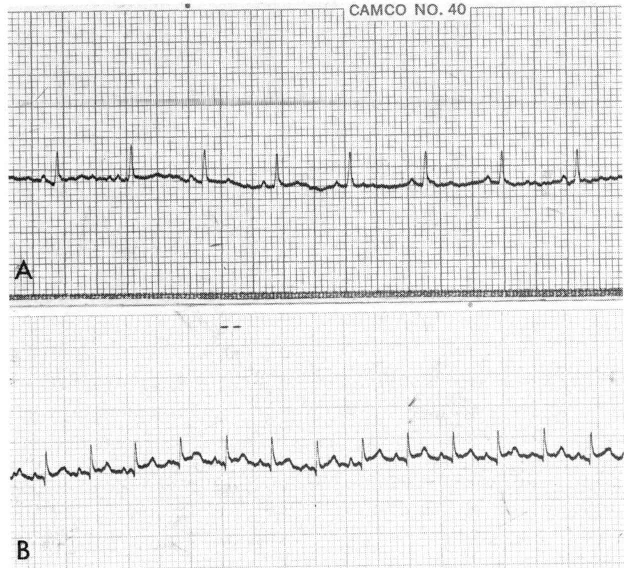


**Figure 18–26** Lead II ECG strips from two normal cats demonstrate the regular rhythm and marked variation in heart rate that are usual in this species. In *A*, recorded from a four-year-old spayed female domestic shorthair, there is normal sinus rhythm at 140/minute. The R-R intervals vary minimally, ranging from 460 to 480 milliseconds (0.46 to 0.48 second). P waves and QRS complexes are of normal duration and amplitude, and T waves are nearly isoelectric. The J point is not clearly defined on each complex. In *B*, recorded from a one-year-old female domestic shorthair, there is also normal sinus rhythm but at 210/minute. The R-R intervals range from 280 to 295 milliseconds (0.28 to 0.295 second). P waves and QRS complexes are normal in amplitude and duration, while T waves are well defined and in the same direction as the major QRS deflection—the normal pattern in most ECG leads in the cat. Variations in J point distinction are again present. 25 mm/sec; 1.0 mV = 1.0 cm.

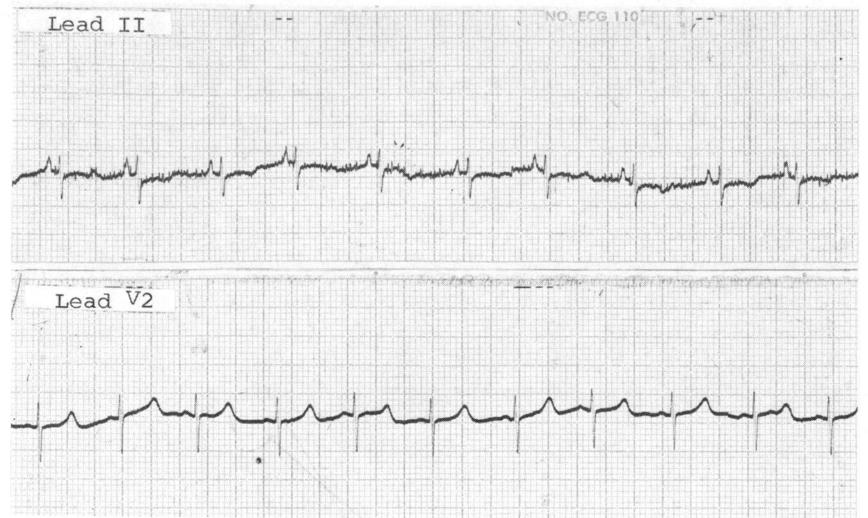


**Figure 18–27** Mild sinus arrhythmia at a rate of 108/minute in an eight-year-old neutered male presented with pleural effusion. The R-R interval ranges from 540 to 610 milliseconds during various phases of the respiratory cycle. It is longest during expiration. Notice the prominent P waves in lead II, electrocardiographic evidence of atrial enlargement. Deep S waves were present in all leads recorded from the left side, a finding suggestive of an intraventricular abnormality other than left anterior fascicular block. The QRS interval is prolonged (0.05 second). Cytologic examination of thoracic fluid provided a diagnosis of lymphoblastic lymphoma. The cause of the conduction abnormality is unclear.

impulse generation and conduction tissues in the cat is somewhat surprising in view of the prevalence of diffusely distributed myocardial disorders. A classification of these abnormalities is presented in Table 18–6.

**Abnormalities of Impulse Generation.** Because the sinus node is the primary site of cardiac electrical activation, disorders of impulse generation are usually a direct effect of its function. Alterations in function can range from mild slowing to complete cessation of sinus node activity.

***Sinus bradycardia*** can be defined in the cat as a regular sinus rhythm of less than 120/minute. This rate is taken as the lower limit of normal on the basis of a number of reports (Table 18–3), my own studies of normal cats (Table 18–5), and a telemetry study of unrestrained cats (Beglinger et al., 1977). Electrocardiographically, sinus bradycardia is characterized by a normal sinus rhythm with a fixed P-R interval. QRS complexes and T waves should be within normal limits, although the Q-T interval may be slightly prolonged (Fig. 18–29). Although sinus bradycardia may result from organic heart disease (e.g., myocarditis, myocardial fibrosis, myocardial degeneration), extracardiac factors are far more often responsible in the clinical setting. Increased vagal tone (iatrogenic, surgically induced), primary central nervous system disease, administration of anesthetics or other drugs (digoxin, propranolol, lidocaine), and hyperkalemia are common associated factors. Treatment should be directed at the underlying cause. The administration of parasympatholytic agents (atropine sulfate 0.05 mg/kg IV) or sympathomimetic agents (isoproterenol, dopamine) may be of considerable temporary benefit when indicated. Electrocardiographic monitoring should be used to evaluate and follow the response to corrective measures.

***Sinus arrest*** results from temporary, usually intermittent, failure of the sinus node to undergo spontaneous depolarization. Electrocardiographically it is distinguished by the sporadic absence of a P wave and its accompanying QRS-T complex, which may be replaced by a QRS-T complex from lower, latent pacemaker tissue (Fig. 18–30). Intermittent periods of sinus arrest may alternate with periods of normal sinus rhythm and sinus bradycardia. When long periods of sinus arrest are associated with a failure of escape of a lower latent pacemaker, syncopal episodes may occur. Although sinus arrest in man and the dog usually results from organic heart disease, the extracardiac causes and influences discussed under sinus bradycardia are more often responsible in the cat. Treatment should be directed at the cause. Experience in treating cats with sinus arrest secondary to organic heart disease has not been reported. In man and the dog, parasympatholytic and sympathomimetic drugs are rarely effective. A permanent pacemaker is usually needed for relief of syncopal episodes.

***Sinoatrial block*** is present when an impulse arising in the sinus node is delayed or blocked so that it cannot activate the atrium. In fact, sinoatrial block represents an abnormality of conduction rather than one of impulse

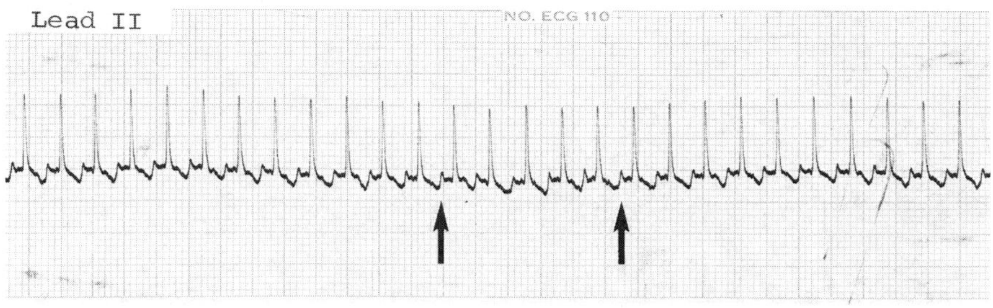


**Figure 18–28** Sinus tachycardia in a three-year-old spayed female domestic shorthair with dilatative cardiomyopathy. P waves are normal and are represented by the small positive deflections at the termination of the T waves (arrows). The R waves are 1.2 mV, a finding consistent with LVH (left ventricular hypertrophy) pattern. The rate is 270/minute. 25 mm/sec; 1.0 mV = 1.0 cm.

**Table 18–6 Abnormalities of Impulse Generation and Conduction Recognized in the Cat**

| |
|---|
| **ABNORMALITIES OF IMPULSE GENERATION** |
| Sinus bradycardia |
| Sinus arrest |
| Sinoatrial block |
| **ABNORMALITIES AFFECTING CONDUCTION PATHWAYS** |
| Isolated or peripheral |
| Right bundle branch block |
| Left bundle branch block |
| Fascicular block |
| Preexcitation syndrome |
| Complete or central |
| First-degree AV block |
| Second-degree AV block |
| Type I (Wenckebach or Mobitz type I) |
| Type II (Mobitz type II) |
| Advanced second degree |
| Third-degree AV block |

generation, but it is included here because of its similarity to, and the difficulty in differentiating it from, sinus arrest. Electrocardiographically, sinoatrial (SA) block behaves like atrioventricular (AV) block in that it may occur as first-, second-, or third-degree block. However, identification of these by surface electrocardiography is far more difficult than with AV block (Fig. 18–31). First-degree SA block, the result of a conduction delay from the SA node to the atrium without complete block, cannot be identified by surface electrocardiography but requires intracardiac electrophysiologic studies. Second-degree SA block may be of Type I, Type II, or advanced Type II. Type I second-degree SA block can be recognized electrocardiographically by the Wenckebach periodicity of the P-P intervals, which are analogous to the R-R intervals in Type I AV block. The longest P-P interval is less than twice the shortest P-P interval. After the longest P-P interval, the P-P interval shortens until block occurs. In Type II second-degree SA block there is a sudden, long P-P interval that is nearly exactly twice the duration of the usual P-P interval. More advanced second-degree SA block with fixed coupling intervals (e.g., 2:1, 3:1, 4:1 SA block) cannot be differentiated from sinus bradycardia by either surface or intracardiac electrocardiography. Third-degree SA block results in electrocardiographic changes identical to those of sinus arrest and is usually accompanied by an escape rhythm. Sinoatrial block is most commonly due to organic heart disease or an adverse drug effect (e.g., from digoxin, propranolol, or antiarrhythmic agents). Treatment is similar to that for sinus arrest.

**Abnormalities Affecting Conduction Pathways.** Alterations in the continuity of impulse transmission from the AV node to the ventricular Purkinje fibers constitute what are termed AV conduction defects or abnormalities. These may occur at various sites within the conduction pathways, causing either isolated (peripheral) abnormalities in conduction or complete (central) interference with impulse transmission (Table 18–6). Clinical signs related to these abnormalities may be totally absent or may be significant and directly related to the conduction defect.

***Right bundle branch block*** is due to the interruption of impulse conduction at some level along the course of the right bundle branch. Electrocardiographic features include prolongation of the QRS interval (> 0.06 second), prominent and late QRS forces to the right (i.e., S waves in Leads I, II, III, aVF, $V_2$, $V_4$), and a frontal plane mean electrical axis (MEA) of the QRS complex ranging from +160° clockwise to 0° (Fig. 18–32). P waves are normal unless atrial enlargement coexists, and the P-R interval is usually of normal duration. The S-T segment may be elevated owing to prolongation of ventricular depolarization. Right bundle branch block is occasionally intermittent, sometimes occurring only at faster heart rates. It can usually be differentiated from the pattern seen in right ventricular enlargement by the difference in the duration of the QRS interval. Right bundle branch block (RBBB) may occur in the absence of any definable heart disease but more often results from congenital (e.g., common AV canal; atrial septal defect, secundum type; Ebstein's anomaly [Danilowicz and Ross, 1971]) or acquired heart disease. Both dilatative and hypertrophic cardiomyopathy, bacterial endocarditis, and infiltrative neoplasms are reported acquired causes of RBBB in the

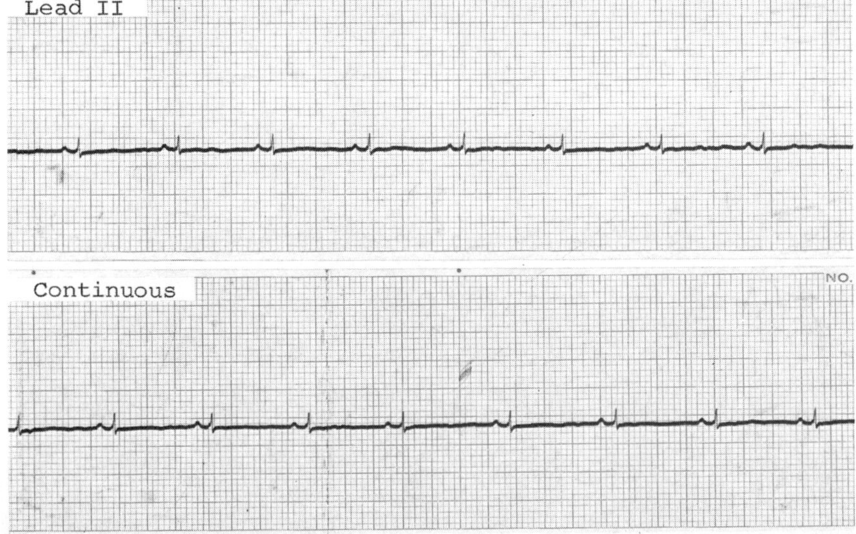


**Figure 18–29** Sinus bradycardia in a two-and-a-half year old neutered male domestic shorthair with hypertrophic cardiomyopathy. The P waves and narrow QRS complexes have a fixed relationship, occurring at a rate of 80/minute. The P-R interval is prolonged (0.12 second), and the T wave is isoelectric. This bradyarrhythmia developed under the influence of propranolol (2.5 mg b.i.d. in a 4.32 kg cat) and probably represents an unusual adverse reaction to this drug. Withdrawal of the drug and administration of atropine sulfate are indicated. See text for other potential causes. 25 mm/sec; 1.0 mV = 1.0 cm.

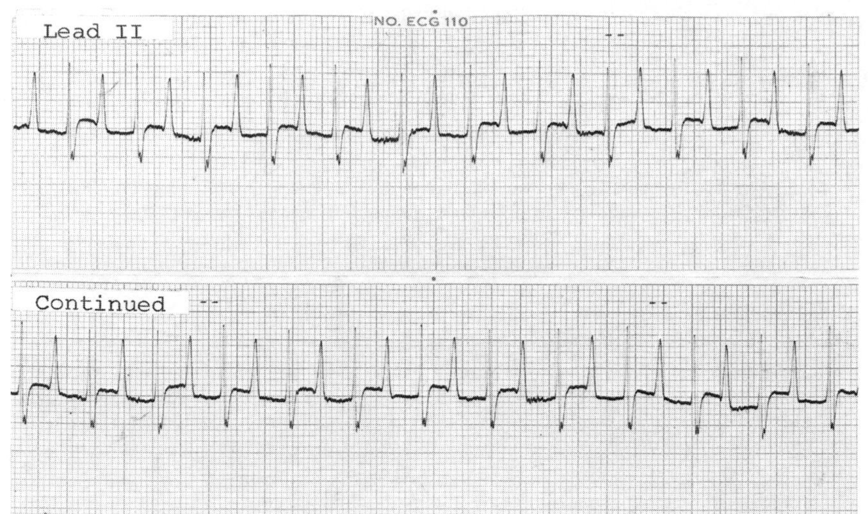


**Figure 18–30** Sinus arrest in a one-year-old female domestic shorthair with acute renal failure secondary to ethylene glycol ingestion. The absence of P waves is characteristic of this arrhythmia and may occur intermittently, but more often it is a constant finding as seen here. The origin of the escape mechanism is most likely A-V junctional tissue, with aberrant ventricular conduction accounting for the QRS widening and deformity (the pattern suggests right bundle branch block). Notice the narrow, spiked T waves and the prolonged Q-T interval (0.28 second). These latter findings are often distinguishing features of the multiple electrolyte abnormalities associated with acute renal failure. (Serum calcium 6.0 mg/dl; serum potassium 9.1 mEq/l). 25 mm/sec; 1.0 mV = 1.0 cm.

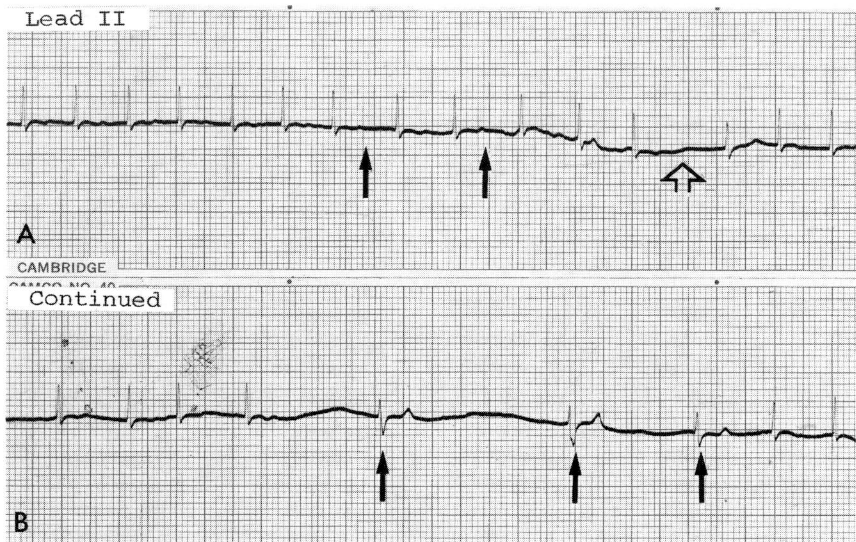


**Figure 18–31** Sinoatrial block in a five-year-old neutered male domestic longhair with acute myocardial infarction secondary to hypertrophic cardiomyopathy and thromboembolism. In *A*, the initial rhythm is normal sinus rhythm at 180/minute. This is interrupted by two brief pauses (arrows) and then by a longer pause that is terminated by an escape beat (arrowhead). Although P waves cannot be visualized, they were present in other leads during this recording, with a P-R interval of 0.12 second (prolonged). In *B*, an irregular pattern of sinus discharge continues, followed by several long pauses that are terminated by escape beats (arrows), probably from an AV junctional focus having different patterns of ventricular conduction. These strips demonstrate variable first- and second-degree sinoatrial block. The progressive prolongation of the R-R interval over a series of three beats in *B* could suggest a Wenckebach periodicity. This arrhythmia responded to atropine administration. 25 mm/sec; 1.0 mV = 1.0 cm.

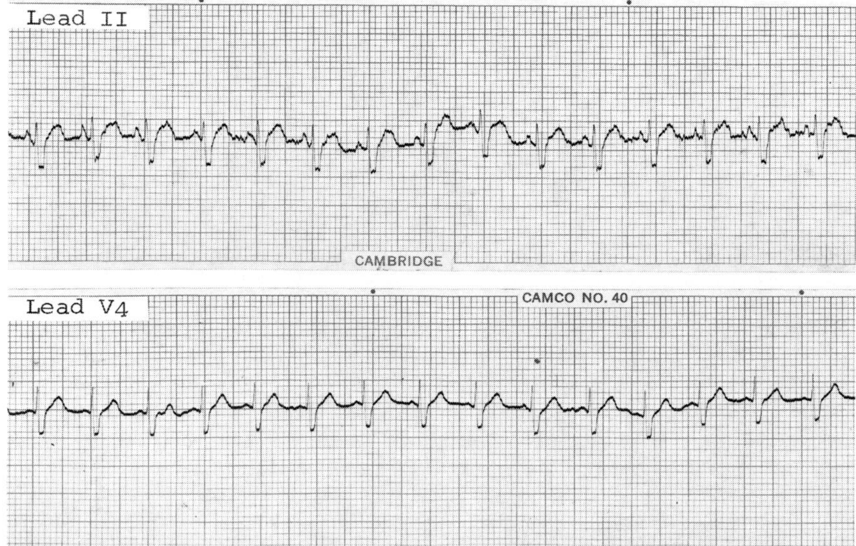


**Figure 18–32** Right bundle branch block in a seven-year-old neutered male domestic shorthair with bacterial endocarditis involving the mitral valve. Notice the narrow R waves and deep, widened S waves present in both leads. The QRS interval in lead II is 0.08 second. P waves in lead II are prolonged (0.05 second), suggesting left atrial enlargement. 25 mm/sec; 1.0 mV = 1.0 cm.

cat (Tilley, 1985; Tilley et al., 1981). Management will depend on identification of the cause, as RBBB in itself has a negligible effect on cardiac function. If the cause cannot be determined, periodic reevaluations should be carried out to detect evidence of additional conduction abnormalities.

***Complete left bundle branch block*** denotes a failure of conduction of impulses through the proximal portion of the left bundle branch. This may result from a localized lesion involving the main trunk or from a more distal, larger lesion affecting the separate fascicles. Left bundle branch block (LBBB) is characterized electrocardiographically by a prolonged QRS interval (> 0.06 second) with prominent QRS forces passing in a normal direction (R waves in Leads I, II, III, aVF, $V_2$, $V_4$, $V_6$, and B/A). Q waves are frequently missing in Leads I, II, and $V_4$ owing to alteration in the pattern of septal activation (Fig. 18–33). Complete LBBB is a strong indication of serious heart disease. Progression to third degree AV block may occur. Left bundle branch block has been reported as a sequel to hypertrophic cardiomyopathy in the cat (Tilley, 1985). Differentiation from left heart enlargement can usually be made on the basis of the QRS interval. As with RBBB, complete LBBB by itself does not result in significant functional abnormalities, and specific therapy is not indicated. The clinical approach should be directed at identifying and managing the underlying heart disease. Periodic electrocardiographic monitoring should be included in the long-term management for detection of more complex and serious conduction abnormalities.

The term ***hemiblock (fascicular block)*** refers to the interruption of conduction pathways in the separate fascicles of the left bundle branch. Such interruptions may occur as isolated conduction abnormalities or in combination with right bundle branch block. Isolated left posterior hemiblock is far less frequent than interruption of the anterior fascicle and has not been reported in the cat. In man, as well, the anterior fascicle is more vulnerable to disruption owing to its longer proximal branch and single blood supply (Horan and Flowers, 1980). The

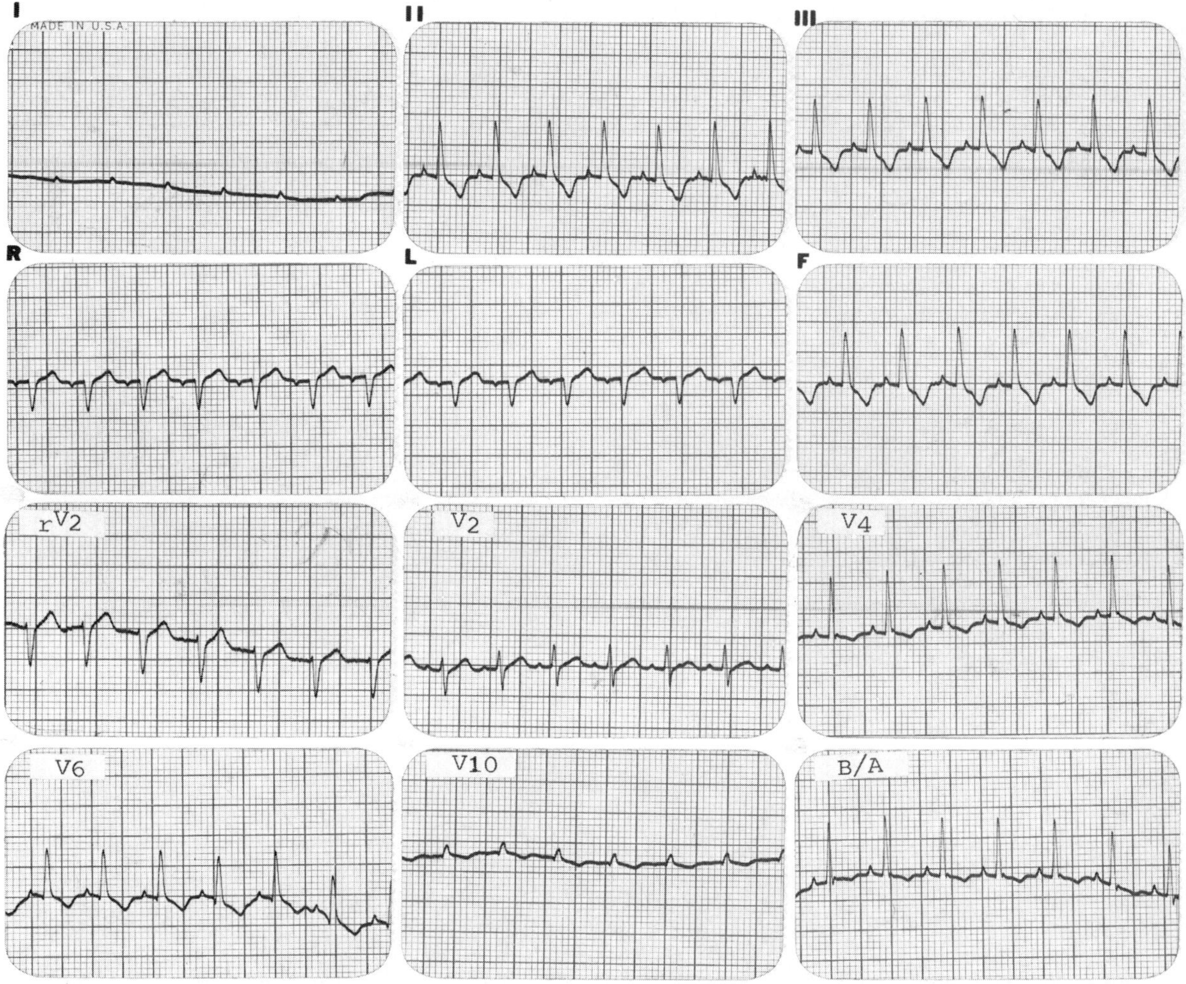


**Figure 18–33** Left bundle branch block recorded from a 13-year-old neutered male Siamese with dilatative cardiomyopathy. P waves in lead II are normal, while the P-R interval is at the upper limit of normal (0.10 second) and consistent. The QRS interval is prolonged in all leads (0.07 to 0.08 second in lead II) with deflection of the complexes in the normally expected direction. Mild S-T segment repolarization changes are most pronounced in the limb leads. 25 mm/sec; 1.0 mV = 1.0 cm.

electrocardiographic feature of isolated left anterior hemiblock (LAHB) in the cat is a normal or prolonged QRS interval (0.04 to 0.06 second) accompanied by left axis deviation in the frontal plane (ranging from −4.0° counterclockwise to −74.0° in a group of cats with HFCM confirmed by nonselective angiocardiography or postmortem examination). In the limb leads the typical findings are a small Q wave and a prominent R wave in Leads I and aVL, while deep S waves are present in Leads II, III, and aVF. Electrocardiographic findings in the precordial leads are varied and do not show any distinct, consistent pattern (Fig. 18–34). Combined RBBB and LAHB in the cat has been reported (Tilley, 1985). Left anterior hemiblock is common in cats with cardiomyopathy, particularly the hypertrophic form, and has been reported in aortic stenosis (Bolton and Liu, 1977). This conduction abnormality alone is of no real consequence to cardiac performance. Management is directed at proper identification of the underlying heart disease and appropriate treatment, if indicated.

***Preexcitation syndrome*** (Wolff-Parkinson-White syndrome, false bundle branch block, bundle of Kent syndrome) is considered by most to result from accelerated AV conduction by means of an accessory conduction pathway that bypasses the AV node (Fig. 18–35). Electrocardiographically, it is characterized by a short P-R interval and a prolonged QRS interval, which is due to the initial inscription of a delta wave (i.e., an initial slurring of the QRS complex). However, the P-J interval (period from the onset of the P wave to the termination of the QRS complex) is normal, as the shortened P-R interval compensates for the QRS prolongation (Fig. 18–36). The resulting QRS complex can vary considerably, its configuration being determined by the position of the abnormal pathway and by whether normal AV conduction is blocked or persists and contributes in any part to ventricular depolarization. A variant of the preexcitation syndrome has been reported, in which a short P-R interval is accompanied by a QRS interval of normal duration (Lown et al., 1952). This latter form is thought to be the effect of an accessory pathway within or near the normal AV conduction pathways below the AV node. Although this conduction abnormality may be tolerated without ill effect, the occurrence of supraventricular tachycardia is a well-reported complication of the preexcitation syndrome. This may result from an atrial impulse that is conducted to the ventricles by normal AV pathways. It subsequently returns to the atria over the anomalous accessory pathway to produce an atrial premature beat and, in turn, a repetitive reentry mechanism. Supraventricular tachycardia may also result from a ventricular premature beat that finds the normal AV tissue refractory to conduction and passes to the atria by the accessory pathway. It then returns to the ventricles along normal pathways, thereby initiating a supraventricular tachycardia. This complication has been reported in the cat (Ogburn, 1977). Treatment for preexcitation syndrome is not indicated unless recurring bouts of paroxysmal supraventricular tachycardia or frequent supraventricular premature beats are observed. Then an antiarrhythmic drug (e.g., propranolol, procainamide, quinidine) should be tried.

Conduction abnormalities of the central or complete type exert their effects on the AV node, proximal ventricular conduction pathways, or both. It is difficult, if not impossible, to accurately predict the exact site of obstruction without performing intracardiac electrocardiographic studies.

***First-degree AV block*** implies the presence of impeded AV conduction without complete interruption of passage.

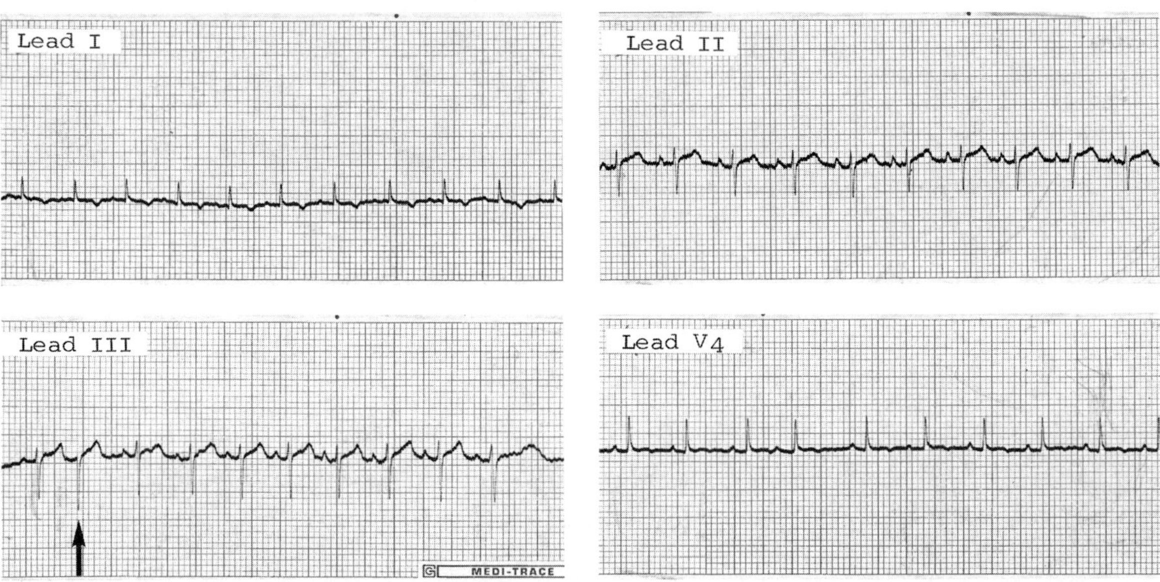


**Figure 18–34** Typical left anterior fascicular block–like conduction abnormality in an eight-year-old neutered male domestic shorthair with hypertrophic cardiomyopathy diagnosed by nonselective angiocardiography. Notice the progressive decrease in R wave amplitude and accompanying increase in S wave amplitude in leads I through III. S waves are absent in lead I. P waves in lead II are prolonged (0.05 second) and slurred, suggesting left atrial enlargement. A supraventricular premature beat with aberrant ventricular conduction can be seen in lead III (arrow). 25 mm/sec; 1.0 mV = 1.0 cm.

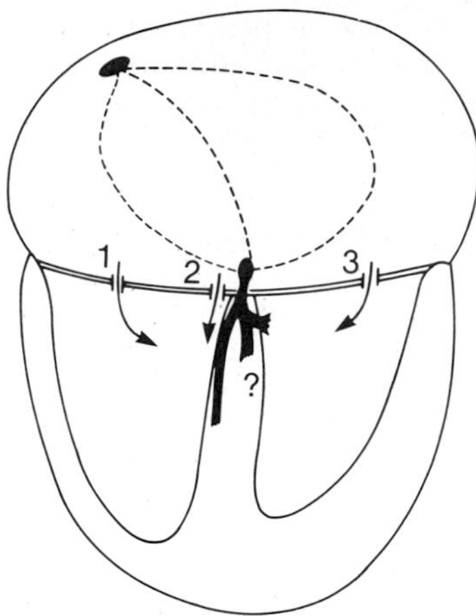


**Figure 18–35** Preexcitation (Wolff-Parkinson-White) syndrome, diagram of abnormal bypass fibers between the atria and the ventricles. Electrocardiographically, this syndrome is usually characterized by a short PR interval and a prolonged QRS interval. The morphology of the QRS complexes can vary considerably depending on the anatomic position of the bypass fibers and whether or not normal AV conduction contributes in part to ventricular depolarization. When normal AV pathways are blocked because of rapid spread of ventricular depolarization via bypass fiber conduction, QRS morphology is determined entirely by the site of the bypass fiber. For example, impulses entering the right ventricle by abnormal pathways result in QRS complexes that resemble right ventricular–originating ventricular premature beats or left bundle branch block (number 1 in the figure), while those entering the ventricle on the left are similar to left ventricular–originating ventricular premature beats or right bundle branch block (number 3 in the figure). Those impulses bypassing the AV node in an adjacent position (number 2 in the figure) may be accompanied by a normal QRS interval. When ventricular depolarization is completed by two separate impulses, one via the bypass fiber and the other along intact AV conduction tissue, QRS morphology is unpredictable. The resulting QRS complex is termed a fusion beat.

In the cat it is distinguished electrocardiographically by prolongation of the P-R interval to over 0.10 second (Fig. 18–37). Hyperkalemia, secondary to urethral obstruction or acute renal failure of other origin, drug reactions (e.g., digitalis intoxication, propranolol, general anesthesia), and increased vagal tone are common causes. Organic heart disease is another well-established association, usually the result of mild inflammation, infarction, or fibrosis of the AV conduction tissue. Treatment depends on establishing the cause. First-degree AV block is not a contraindication to the continued use of digoxin or propranolol, but when accompanied by sinus bradycardia strongly suggests an overdose. Under these circumstances and in the absence of other clinical signs, if the cat is receiving digoxin, the serum level should be measured. If it exceeds 2.0 ng/ml, the maintenance dose should be reduced by 25 per cent. When first-degree AV block occurs as a sequel to urethral obstruction, relief of the obstruction and the administration of IV fluids may be corrective. Sodium bicarbonate (1 to 2 mEq/kg over a one hour period) is also very helpful in combating the associated metabolic acidosis, as well as lowering the serum potassium level. In the presence of a very high serum potassium level accompanied by marked prolongation of the P-R interval, sinus arrest, or an idioventricular rhythm, the use of insulin and glucose (e.g., 0.5 unit of insulin to 1.0 gm glucose) may be lifesaving by effecting a rapid reduction in the serum potassium level. When first-degree AV block is of undetermined origin, a primary cardiac cause should be suspected. Periodic electrocardiographic monitoring is indicated to evaluate for evidence of change.

***Second-degree AV block*** is characterized by the occasional or periodic failure of AV conduction. Various types of second-degree AV block have been defined on the basis of their characteristic electrocardiographic features (Table 18–6). ***Type I (Mobitz Type I or Wenckebach) second-degree AV block*** is distinguished by a gradual prolongation of the P-R interval until a P wave occurs without an associated QRS complex. This is termed a dropped beat (Fig. 18–38). In some cats with Type I second-degree AV block there is not a progressive prolongation of the P-R interval, but rather the P-R interval of the first conducted beat in the cycle is always the shortest, and all subsequent P-R intervals before the dropped beat are longer. In addition, there tends to be a gradual shortening of the R-R interval between conducted beats until the dropped beat occurs. After the dropped beat the sinus node usually discharges and maintains control over the ventricular rate. However, if the pause is excessively long, owing to interference with AV conduction and perhaps also to depression of the sinus node, lower latent pacemaker tissue may fire spontaneously (i.e., an escape mechanism) and capture control of the ventricular rate for one or more beats (Fig. 18–39). Type I second-degree AV block is considered to result from impeded conduction in the proximal portion of the AV node (the A-N region). In many instances it is a temporary or transient conduction abnormality due to some extracardiac influence rather than to organic heart disease. It is a common manifestation of digitalis intoxication and has been reported as a consequence of hyperkalemia (Fisch et al., 1966). Treatment should be directed at the underlying cause.

***Second-degree AV block Type II (Mobitz Type II)*** is characterized by a periodic, sudden interruption of AV conduction for a single beat, usually following a fixed pattern (i.e., 4:3, 5:4, 8:7 conduction ratio). The P-R interval of conducted beats is fixed and may be normal or prolonged. The QRS complex is usually normal, unless additional conduction abnormalities exist in the ventricular conduction pathways (Fig. 18–40). Type II second-degree AV block may be caused by extracardiac influences (e.g., digitalis intoxication, propranolol toxicity, increased vagal tone, hyperkalemia, anesthesia) but is also common in primary organic heart disease. The anatomic site of obstruction is generally believed to be in lower portions of the AV conduction tissue (the N-H region). The clinical approach is to identify and try to correct the cause (e.g., organic heart disease such as cardiomyopathy or bacterial endocarditis). Specific management of the conduction abnormality is not indicated. Digitalis glycosides and propranolol must be used cautiously and with ECG monitoring, as they can further interfere with AV conduction.

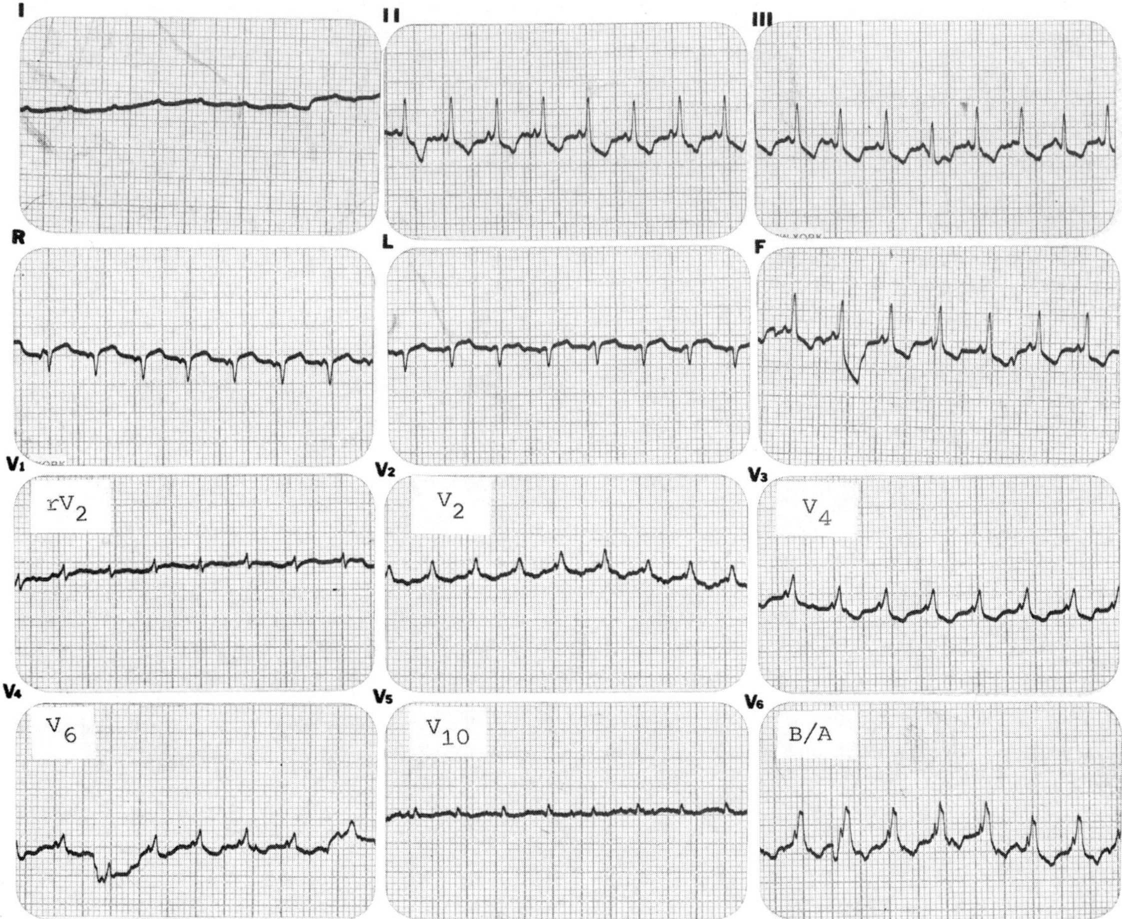


**Figure 18–36** Preexcitation syndrome, 12-lead ECG of an eight-year-old neutered male diabetic domestic shorthair. This cat was presented for coughing and wheezing of one year's duration that was partially responsive to diuretic therapy. A prominent gallop rhythm was auscultated, and generalized cardiomegaly and a mild pleural effusion were evident in thoracic radiographs. Lead I is isoelectric, while QRS complexes in the remaining 11 leads are directed in their expected patterns. However, the P-R interval is short and the QRS interval prolonged, expected findings in preexcitation syndrome. The initial gradual upstroke of the R wave, seen best in leads II and aVF, is termed the delta wave and is also expected in this syndrome. In leads $V_4$ and B/A, the P wave appears to arise within the initial part of the QRS complex. This pattern is consistent with the type B preexcitation syndrome described in man, although the validity of this classification has been questioned (Gallagher et al., 1976). M-mode echocardiography in this cat demonstrated dilatative cardiomyopathy. 25 mm/sec; 1.0 mV = 1.0 cm.

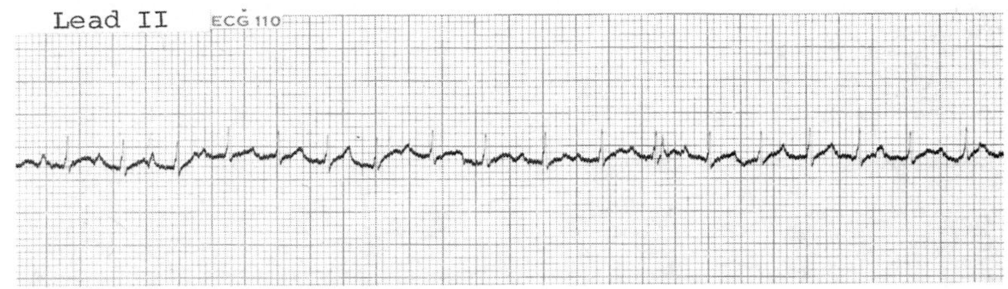


**Figure 18–37** First-degree AV block, ECG strip from a 15-year-old spayed female diabetic Persian that developed a gallop rhythm after an insulin reaction. The basic rhythm is sinus arrhythmia at 180/minute. P waves vary in configuration. The prolonged P-R interval (0.20 second) is diagnostic of first-degree AV block, as the normal P-R interval in the cat should not exceed 0.10 second. Although a specific cause of this finding was not established, fibrosis of the AV conduction pathways was suspected. M-mode echocardiographic studies were consistent with a diagnosis of intermediate feline cardiomyopathy. 25 mm/sec; 1.0 mV = 1.0 cm.

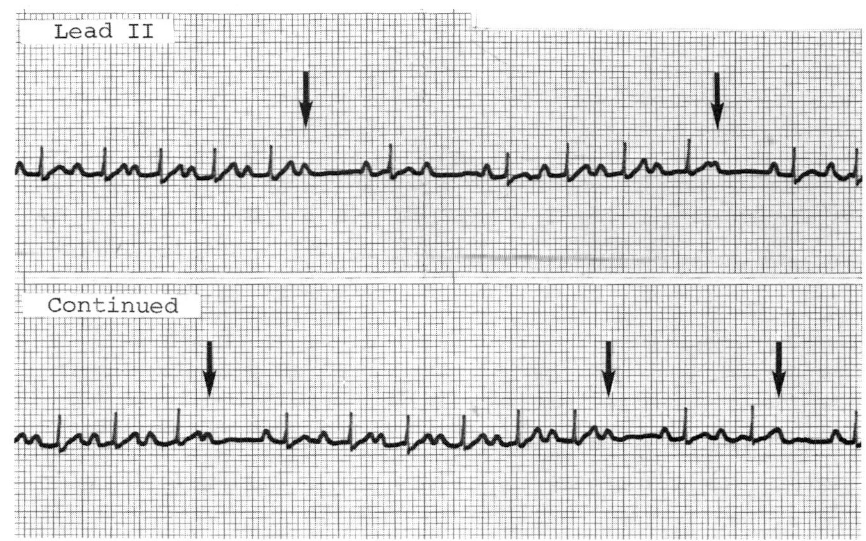


**Figure 18–38** Mobitz Type I (Wenckebach periodicity) second-degree AV block caused by digitalis overdose. The predominant pattern is a progressive prolongation of the P-R interval, accompanied by shortening of the R-R interval, until a beat is dropped (i.e., P waves unassociated with QRS complexes [arrows]). The frequency of the dropped beats is quite variable, unlike the more fixed pattern in Mobitz Type II AV block (see Figure 18–40). This rare arrhythmia results from digitalis intoxication. 25 mm/sec; 1.0 mV = 1.0 cm.

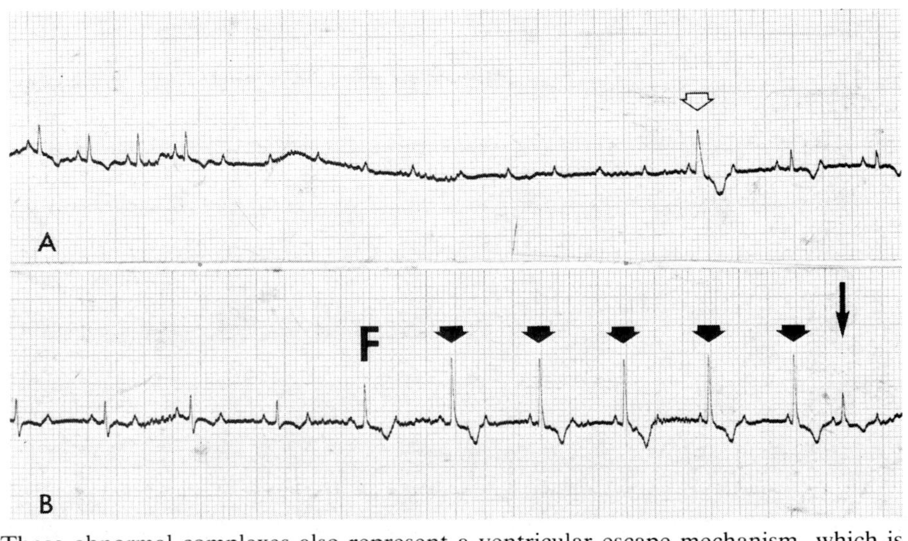


**Figure 18–39** Various patterns of escape mechanisms in advanced AV block in a 15-year-old spayed female Siamese presented for frequent collapsing spells. *A*, A normal AV conduction pattern is interrupted by a three-second period of complete AV block (i.e., P waves without QRS complexes). This period of ventricular asystole is terminated by a ventricular escape beat (open arrowhead), which is followed by a period of 2:1 AV block. In *B*, 2:1 AV block continues for a series of four conducted beats before it is interrupted by a fusion beat (F), followed by a series of five abnormal QRS complexes (arrowheads) associated with a gradual shortening of the P-R interval. These abnormal complexes also represent a ventricular escape mechanism, which is terminated by a normally conducted beat (arrow). 25 mm/sec; 1.0 mV = 1.0 cm.

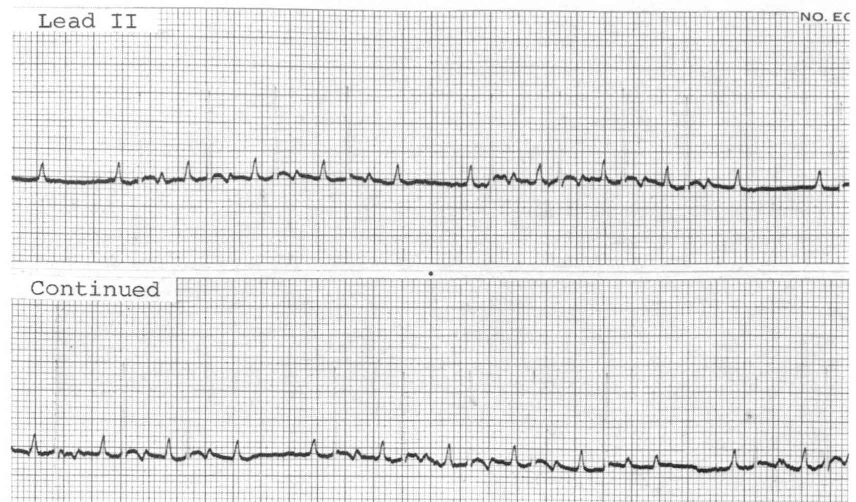


**Figure 18–40** Continuous lead II ECG strip demonstrates the features of Mobitz Type II second-degree AV block. Every fifth or sixth P wave is unaccompanied by a QRS complex (i.e., unconducted or blocked). Preceding the block or dropped beat the P-R interval of conducted beats tends to vary somewhat (from 0.16 to 0.20 second), but it does not fulfill the criteria for Wenckebach periodicity (compare with Figure 18–38). All the P-R intervals are prolonged, and the P-R interval of the first conducted beat is not shorter than the P-R intervals of the second and third conducted beats. This arrhythmia, recorded from a dog, is termed a variable 5:4 and 6:5 Mobitz Type II AV block. It suggests that the conduction abnormality lies within the N-H region of the AV node. It is most often associated with organic heart disease. 25 mm/sec; 1.0 mV = 1.0 cm.

***Advanced second-degree AV block*** implies a high degree of interference with AV conduction but with the periodic transmission of an impulse originating in the sinus node (Fig. 18–41). The pattern of nonconducted and conducted beats is usually fixed (e.g., 2:1, 3:1, or 4:1 conduction ratio) but may vary, and the P-R interval of conducted beats is usually prolonged. The QRS complex of conducted beats tends to be normal, unless ventricular conduction pathways are similarly affected (i.e., they may have right or left bundle branch block [Tilley, 1985]). Because of the slowed ventricular rate that usually accompanies advanced second-degree AV block there is an increased opportunity for spontaneous discharge of latent pacemaker tissue (i.e., escape mechanism). This advanced conduction abnormality may be a sequel of the extracardiac disorders discussed previously, although primary organic heart disease is an equally frequent cause. Granulomatous inflammation (e.g., in feline infectious peritonitis or toxoplasmosis), infection (e.g., bacterial endocarditis), and degenerative processes secondary to

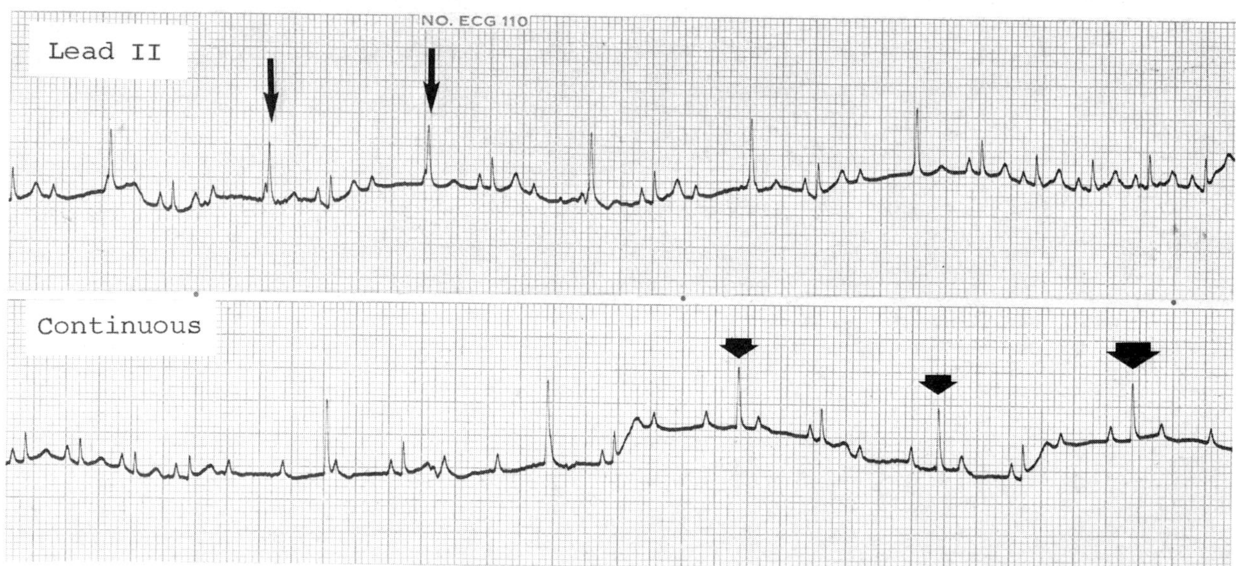


**Figure 18–41** Intermittent advanced second-degree AV block in an 11-year-old neutered male Siamese. In the upper strip, normally conducted QRS complexes (small QRS complexes with a fixed P-R interval of 0.08 to 0.09 second) occur intermittently with wide QRS complexes of increased amplitude (arrows) that follow unconducted P waves. These latter complexes represent escape beats from lower, latent pacemaker tissue (most likely from a ventricular focus), and many are deformed at their onset by the nearly simultaneous occurrence of a P wave. At the end of the upper strip and continuing at the beginning of the lower strip is a series of nine normally conducted QRS complexes. These are followed by a more advanced form of AV block characterized by normal conduction of every fourth beat. Ventricular escape beats occur similar to those in the upper strip; however, the last three are narrower and probably represent fusion beats (arrowheads). The cause of the conduction abnormality in this cat was never established. No clinical signs were present. 25 mm/sec; 1.0 mV = 1.0 cm.

ischemia, infarction, and fibrosis (e.g., vasculitis, cardiomyopathy) cause advanced second- and third-degree AV block in the cat. Cardiac and extracardiac causes can usually be differentiated by an atropine response test (Fig. 18–42). (This is performed by administering atropine sulfate, 0.04 mg/kg IV, while continuously recording a Lead II ECG for at least three minutes. A positive response is the establishment of sinus tachycardia with 1:1 AV conduction within two to three minutes. With a negative response there is an appropriate increase in the frequency of the P waves, and although there may be some increase in the number of conducted beats and the ventricular rate, consistent 1:1 AV conduction never develops. A negative response strongly suggests the presence of organic heart disease.) Treatment is directed at the underlying cause. Clinical signs are common in cats with advanced second-degree AV block secondary to primary cardiac disease and may result from either the associated slow ventricular rate (lethargy, weakness, syncope) or the combined effect of bradycardia and reduced myocardial performance (congestive heart failure, usually with ascites or pleural effusion, or both). In this latter circumstance, treatment is directed at resolution of the excess fluid state (by diuretics and low-salt diet), improvement in cardiac performance (with a vasodilator such as hydralazine or captopril), and improvement in the ventricular rate. Digitalis glycosides and propranolol are contraindicated, as they can further slow the ventricular rate by additional interference with AV conduction. One may try to increase the ventricular rate by administration of a parasympatholytic agent (but atropine or propantheline bromide is likely to be useful only if the atropine response test was positive) or a sympathomimetic drug (e.g., ephedrine sulfate or isoproterenol). In most patients, medical measures help little in accelerating the heart rate. If nonspecific methods are ineffective in eliminating clinical signs, a permanent pacemaker is indicated.

The most severe type of AV conduction abnormality is ***third-degree AV block,*** due to complete interruption of normal conduction pathways between the atria and ventricles. Electrocardiographically, third-degree AV block is characterized by complete AV dissociation, the atria (P waves) and ventricles (QRS-T complexes) beating at different, independent rates. P waves are always more frequent than QRS complexes, and the P-R interval is very variable. The atrial rate is usually normal. Both the ventricular rate and the conformation of the QRS complexes can vary considerably, depending on the anatomic site of the obstruction to conduction and the origin of the latent pacemaker tissue responsible for ventricular depolarization (Fig. 18–43). In general, the more distally in the ventricular conduction pathways the latent pacemaker arises, the slower the ventricular rate and the more bizarre the QRS complexes, while those in more proximal ventricular conduction pathways tend to discharge at a faster rate and are associated with narrower, more normal QRS complexes. Ventricular depolarization may arise from more than a single focus (i.e., competing latent pacemaker tissues). Third-degree AV block is, with few exceptions, the effect of primary organic heart disease. The site of obstruction to impulse transmission can develop at various levels within the specialized AV conduction pathways from the proximal portions of the AV node to bilateral bundle branch block distally. Causes in the cat are identical to those of advanced second-degree AV block. Medical management is rarely of benefit, but an atropine response test should be performed to identify the unusual cat that will respond. Sympathomimetic drugs occasionally effect a modest increase in the ventricular rate, but this is usually inadequate to resolve clinical signs completely and may have undesirable side effects. Diuretics and vasodilators may help to control fluid retention, although they tend to be less effective than in cats with normal ventricular rates. A permanent pacemaker is the treatment of choice.

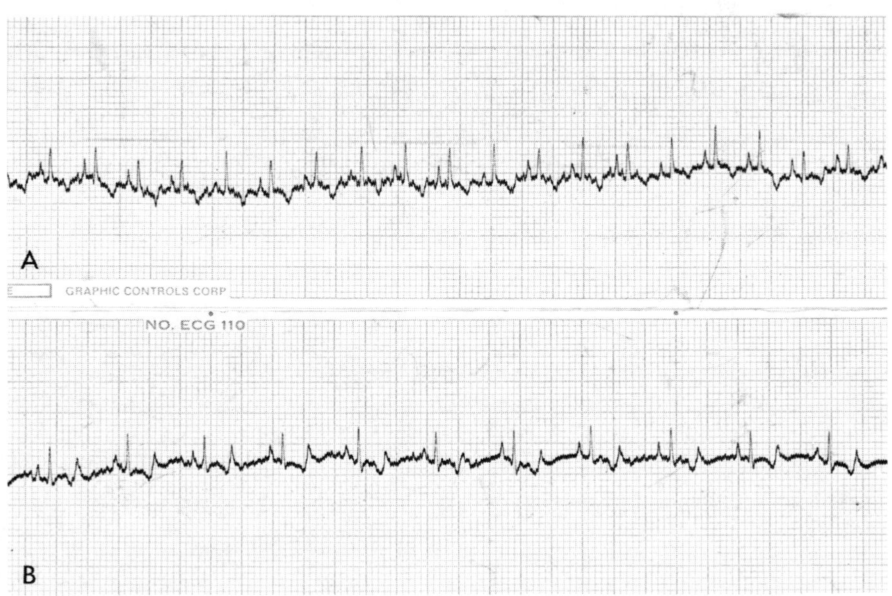


**Figure 18–42** Atropine response test in a 15-year-old spayed female Siamese presented because of daily collapsing spells. In *A*, recorded in the resting state, the rhythm is sinus tachycardia at 210/minute. P waves are prominent, suggesting atrial enlargement, but are consistently associated with the accompanying QRS–T complex by a fixed P-R interval of 0.08 second. In *B*, recorded two minutes after intravenous injection of 0.1 mg atropine sulfate, the ventricular rate has decreased to 120/minute. Notice the change in morphology of the T waves, which appear to have become biphasic. Actually, the positive deflections at the termination of the T waves represent P waves with T-P blending, and the rhythm is now 2:1 AV block. This study demonstrates the use of cardiac acceleration to uncover an A-V conduction abnormality. 25 mm/sec; 1.0 mV = 1.0 cm.

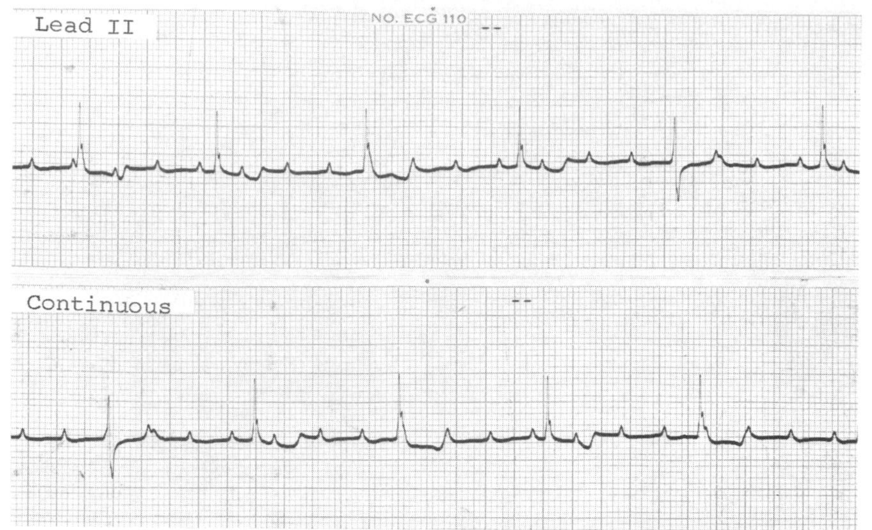


**Figure 18–43** Third-degree AV block in a 15-year-old neutered male Siamese. Notice the 3:1 ratio of P waves to QRS complexes; however, there is no fixed relationship between these two electrical events (i.e., marked variation in the P-R interval). The widened and bizarre QRS complexes suggest a ventricular origin. They assume two separate configurations, owing to competing latent ventricular pacemaker tissue. The ventricular rate is 56/minute. 25 mm/sec; 1.0 mV = 1.0 cm.

**ELECTROCARDIOGRAPHIC IDENTIFICATION OF THE CARDIAC ARRHYTHMIAS.** Having reviewed the normal variations in cardiac rhythm in the cat, as well as the bradyarrhythmias and conduction disturbances, we can consider the more commonly recognized cardiac arrhythmias. These are tachyarrhythmias, as they increase the ventricular rate (Table 18–7). They may develop by two separate electrophysiologic mechanisms: increased automaticity of latent pacemaker tissue and disturbances in impulse conductivity. In the former, the rate of spontaneous (phase 4) depolarization in latent pacemaker cells (termed automatic cells) is increased, causing them to discharge before the normal pacemaker (i.e., the sinus node). The resulting impulse spreads rapidly along normal conduction pathways, causing early ventricular depolarization. In the process, refractory conduction pathways are created that tend to partly or completely block transmission of the impulse subsequently arising from normal sinus node depolarization. The underlying electrophysiologic abnormalities leading to early diastolic depolarization of automatic cells are believed to include the rate of change of membrane potential during diastole, the absolute value of the threshold potential, and the value of the maximum diastolic potential (Hoffman, 1966). When a reduction in the resting (maximum diastolic) potential is accompanied by an increase in the threshold potential, small changes in the membrane potential are likely to decrease it to the threshold level and the development of an action potential (Fig. 18–44). On the other hand, disturbances in impulse conductivity can result in focal areas of decremental (i.e., slowed) conduction and unidirectional block, leading to the development of a reentry mechanism (Fig. 18–45). Because abnormalities in the resting state of myocardial tissue responsible for increased automaticity and those conditions necessary for a reentry mechanism are similar (i.e., reduced resting membrane potential and spontaneous phase 4 depolarization), these abnormal states can be caused by similar influences. Focal areas of myocardial ischemia, inflammation, necrosis, and fibrosis; stretching of myocardial fibers; hypoxemia; increased sympathetic tone; electrolyte disturbances; and administration of certain drugs (e.g., digitalis, procainamide, quinidine, heavy metals, anesthetics, aminophylline, and sympathomimetic amines) are recognized causes of cardiac arrhythmias. The nature of the arrhythmia is determined by its site of origin, as well as by the electrophysiologic state of the abnormal myocardial tissue.

**Atrial Arrhythmias.** Atrial tachyarrhythmias are thought to originate within specialized intra-atrial conduction tissue, since atrial myocardial contractile cells are incapable of spontaneous depolarization except under unusual circumstances. And although the electrocardiographic features of these arrhythmias are similar in certain respects, they differ considerably in their effect on ventricular rate and rhythm.

The early discharge of an atrial automatic focus, usually from an area other than the sinus node, is called an ***atrial premature beat.*** Electrocardiographically it is characterized by an earlier than expected P wave that is similar but not identical to the sinus P wave and by a P-R interval longer than those of conducted sinus beats. The refractory state of the AV junction (i.e., whether it is fully or only partially repolarized) will determine if the atrial impulse is blocked, conducted more slowly than normal (i.e.,

**Table 18–7 Classification of Cardiac Arrhythmias Recognized in the Cat**

| |
|---|
| **NORMAL VARIATIONS** |
| Normal sinus rhythm (NSR) |
| Sinus arrhythmia |
| Sinus tachycardia |
| **ATRIAL ARRHYTHMIAS** |
| Atrial premature beats (APB) |
| Paroxysmal supraventricular tachycardia (PSVT) |
| Atrial flutter |
| Atrial fibrillation (AF) |
| **ATRIOVENTRICULAR JUNCTIONAL ARRHYTHMIAS** |
| Atrioventricular junctional premature beats (AVJPB) |
| Paroxysmal atrioventricular junctional tachycardia (PAVJT) |
| **VENTRICULAR ARRHYTHMIAS** |
| Ventricular premature beats (VPB) |
| Paroxysmal ventricular tachycardia (PVT) |
| Accelerated idioventricular rhythm (AIVR) |
| Ventricular flutter and fibrillation |

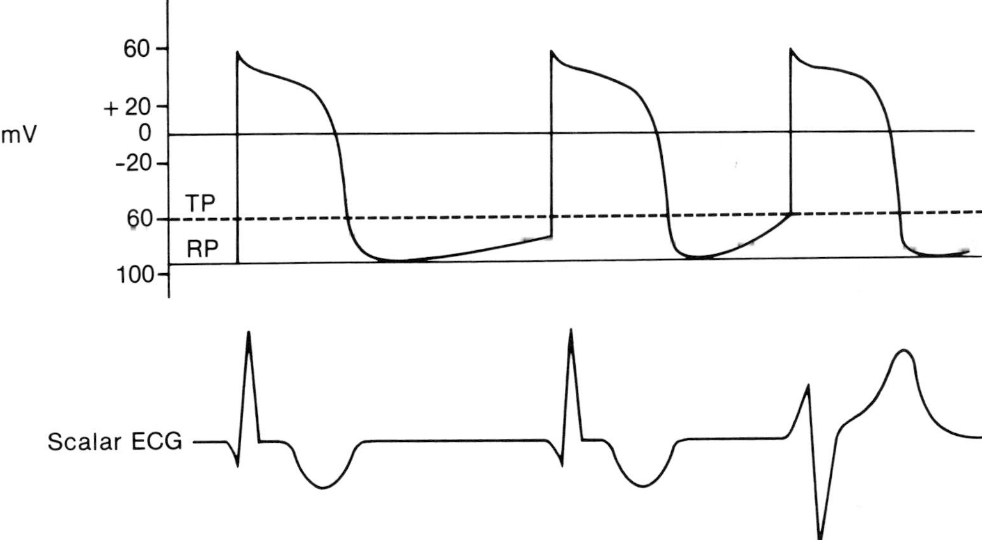


**Figure 18–44** Purkinje fiber action potential depicting progressive decrease in resting membrane potential until threshold is reached, resulting in premature development of the third action potential. Assuming that surrounding myocardial tissue was sufficiently repolarized to permit stimulation, a ventricular premature beat may occur as shown by the scalar ECG. Increase in the threshold potential can be responsible for similar effects. The normal resting membrane potential for Purkinje fibers ranges from −85 to −90 mV. TP = threshold potential. RP = resting potential.

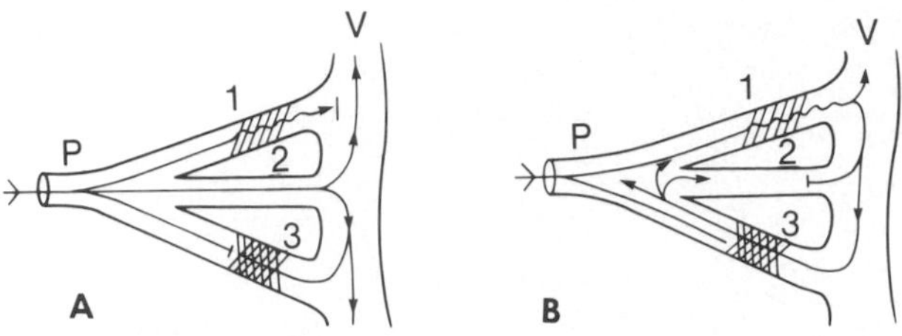


**Figure 18–45** Diagrams illustrating the mechanisms whereby delayed conduction and unidirectional block can lead to reentry and the development of ventricular premature beats and paroxysmal ventricular tachycardia. In *A*, a terminal Purkinje fiber (P) is depicted at its junction with the ventricular muscle (V). Three terminal branches are shown: fiber 1, in which there is delayed conduction; fiber 2, which conducts normally; and fiber 3, in which conduction is blocked in the antegrade direction (i.e., unidirectional block). However, arrhythmias do not develop, because the conditions for reentry mechanism are not present. In fiber 1, conduction is mildly delayed, the impulse arriving at the ventricular muscle at a time when it is depolarized by the impulse arriving from fiber 2; thus further conduction is blocked by refractory conduction pathways. Although the impulse conducted via fiber 2 is capable of being transmitted through the area of unidirectional block in fiber 3, further conduction is blocked by refractoriness created by antegrade conduction. In *B*, criteria are fulfilled for the development of a reentry circuit owing to marked delay of conduction in fiber 1. Now the impulse arrives at the ventricular muscle when the tissue is fully repolarized, and conduction can proceed in both directions. A reentry circuit is set up through fiber 3 (fiber 2 is depicted as having retrograde unidirectional block), as this fiber is now completely repolarized proximal to the site of antegrade unidirectional block (hatched area). The resulting effect may be a single ventricular premature beat by conduction proximally along the main Purkinje fiber (P) and throughout the ventricles, or a series of ventricular premature beats resulting from continued antegrade circuiting of the impulse of either fiber 1 or fiber 2, and retrograde conduction through fiber 3.

prolonged P-R interval), or conducted normally (i.e., normal P-R interval). Conduction into the ventricle and the inscribed QRS complex will depend on the resting state of the ventricular conduction pathways. When these pathways are incompletely repolarized, abnormal ventricular conduction results and the inscribed QRS differs from those arising from the normal sinus P wave (Fig. 18–46). This phenomenon of ventricular conduction along abnormal pathways is called aberrant conduction. After the fully conducted atrial premature beat there is a pause, the duration of which is determined by the effect of the atrial premature beat on sinus node function. When the sinus node is depolarized by the wave of excitation arising from the atrial premature beat (the most common finding), the timing of the sinus node is reset. This results in a shortening of the interval between the two normal sinus beats flanking the premature beat (the P-p-P interval), so that it is less than the interval between three consecutive normal sinus P waves (termed 2 P-P interval). This is called an incomplete or noncompensatory pause. Less often, atrial depolarization from the premature beat is partly blocked and the sinus node is unaffected. The sinus node, in turn, discharges at the expected time, but impulse transmission is blocked by refractory atrial conduction pathways created by the atrial premature beat. The sinus node is normally reset, and it subsequently fires at its next expected time. These conditions result in a P-p-P interval that is exactly identical to the normal 2 P-P interval. This pattern, representing the effect of a premature beat on sinus node discharge, is termed a complete or fully compensated compensatory pause and is seen more frequently with ventricular premature beats. When the atrial premature beat occurs very early, its P wave frequently falls within the T wave of the preceding QRS complex. This makes identification of P-wave morphology impossible and the differentiation of atrial and AV junctional premature beats more difficult. Under these circumstances the nonspecific term supraventricular premature beats is commonly used. Atrial premature beats may occur singly, as two in rapid succession (termed a pair or pairing), and as a series of three (called a run). Any of these patterns is strong evidence of atrial myocardial disease. In cats all forms of cardiomyopathy, congenital heart disease accompanied by heart failure or an enlarged atrium (e.g., common AV canal, Ebstein's anomaly), hyperthyroidism, bacterial endocarditis, and other infectious diseases are frequent causes. Rare or occasional (< 20/minute) atrial premature beats do not require specific treatment. Here the approach should be to define the nature of the underlying heart disease and plan its management, if indicated. Stabilization of heart failure, when present, often eliminates or markedly reduces the frequency of atrial premature beats, most likely by decreasing atrial pressure and stretch. In the presence of frequent atrial premature beats, particularly frequent pairs and runs, the electrophysiologic mechanism exists for the development of paroxysmal supraventricular (or atrial) tachycardia. Specific management of these more aggressive patterns is indicated, even in the absence of other definable heart disease. Digoxin alone, in maintenance doses, may be totally effective and should be tried first (except in cats with hypertrophic cardiomyopathy), as it offers the advantage of slowing AV conduction along with its positive inotropic effects. If this proves inadequate, propranolol or quinidine sulfate alone or in combination with digoxin may improve the response.

The regular occurrence of four or more atrial premature beats in succession constitutes ***paroxysmal atrial or supraventricular tachycardia.*** In the cat it is manifested clinically by a rapid, regular heart rhythm, usually over 240/minute, which may be brief or may persist for minutes at a time and which tends to be intermittent. It is distinguished electrocardiographically by a sudden onset, usually within a single beat, the first beat having all the features of a conducted atrial premature beat. It also tends to be terminated within a single beat and is followed by a brief pause. During the period of tachycardia the QRS complexes occur regularly with fixed R-R intervals and are usually of normal duration but may be aberrantly conducted (Fig. 18–47). With 1:1 AV conduction, P waves frequently fall within the T waves of the preceding QRS complex and cannot be discerned. Occasionally, a 2:1 or a 3:1 AV conduction ratio is found in paroxysmal atrial tachycardia, owing to extremely rapid atrial discharge or to associated inherent disease within the AV conduction pathways. P waves can then be seen to precede each QRS

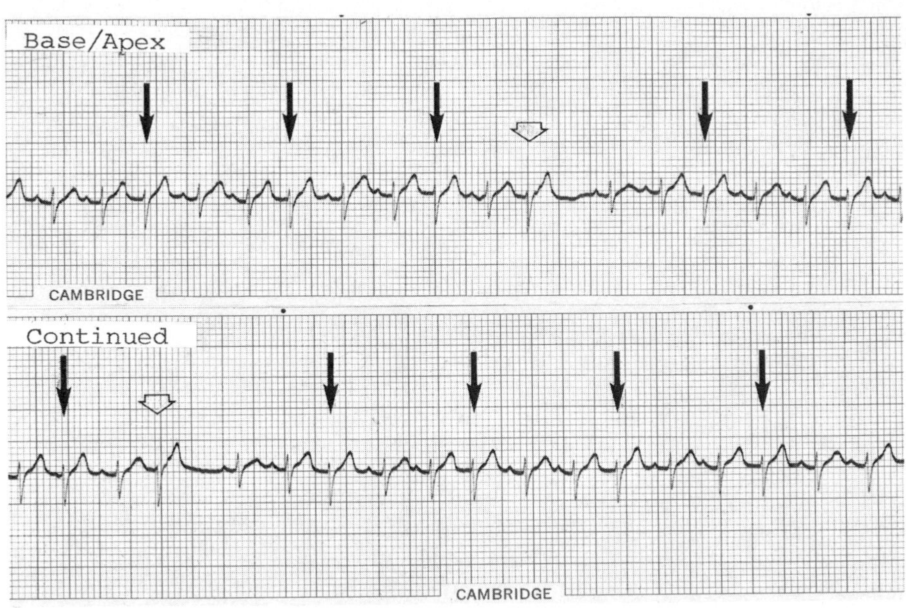


**Figure 18–46** Frequent supraventricular premature beats recorded from a 14-year-old neutered male domestic shorthair presented for a heart murmur of undefined cause. Thoracic radiographs disclosed no abnormality. Most of the premature beats (arrows) occur fairly late; are accompanied by mild deformity of the associated QRS complex, suggesting aberrant ventricular conduction; and are followed by a complete compensatory pause. However, two premature beats (open arrowheads) occur earlier than the others; are associated with greater deformity of the accompanying QRS complex, implying greater degrees of aberrant ventricular conduction; and are succeeded by a prolonged compensatory pause (i.e., reset with pause). P waves cannot be identified with any of the premature beats; thus the term supraventricular is used. These examples demonstrate the varying effect of premature beats on normal sinus node function that can result from small differences in prematurity. 25 mm/sec; 1.0 mV = 1.0 cm.

complex. However, paroxysmal atrial tachycardia with a 2:1 AV conduction ratio may be impossible to differentiate from normal sinus rhythm, especially when the nonconducted P waves fall within the preceding QRS-T complex. Vagal maneuvers or intracardiac electrocardiography will usually be required to make this distinction.

Additional diagnostic tools may be needed to differentiate paroxysmal atrial tachycardia with normal AV conduction from the other supraventricular tachyarrhythmias (atrial flutter and atrial fibrillation) and to differentiate paroxysmal atrial tachycardia with aberrant AV conduction from paroxysmal ventricular tachycardia. The use of vagal maneuvers (carotid sinus massage and eyeball pressure) and intracardiac electrocardiography (Tilley, 1985) has been most helpful in this respect. The differentiating features of the atrial tachyarrhythmias and paroxysmal ventricular tachycardia are outlined in Table 18–8.

Paroxysmal atrial tachycardia is definitive evidence of

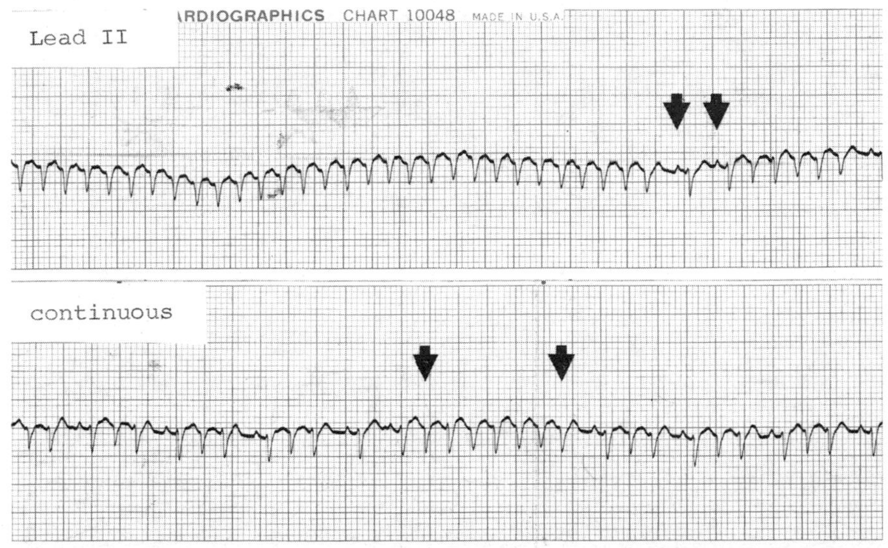


**Figure 18–47** Paroxysmal supraventricular tachycardia, continuous lead II recording from a one-year-old spayed female domestic shorthair presented for lethargy and partial anorexia of three days' duration. A single collapsing spell of five minutes' duration was observed on the day of presentation. In the upper strip a rapid, regular rhythm occurs at a rate of 400/minute. This is accompanied by prolonged QRS complexes (0.06 second) having an abnormal conformation and is terminated by two normally conducted beats (arrowheads) with a similar, abnormal QRS pattern. These normally conducted beats are followed by another burst of tachycardia (five beats) and, on the lower strip, by a repetitive pattern seen as a single normally conducted beat coupled with a pair of premature beats. This pattern is transiently broken by another short burst of tachycardia (seven beats, between the arrowheads). This example establishes the presence of paroxysmal supraventricular tachycardia. The abnormal QRS pattern is consistent with a left anterior fascicular block–like conduction abnormality. A nonselective angiocardiogram in this cat was diagnostic for hypertrophic cardiomyopathy. The arrhythmias and associated clinical signs resolved with administration of propanolol. 25 mm sec; 1.0 mV = 1.0 cm. (From Harpster NK: Vet Clin North Am 7 [1977] 355–371.)

**Table 18–8 Summary of the Electrocardiographic Features Differentiating the Supraventricular Tachyarrhythmias and Ventricular Tachycardia**

| CRITERIA | ATRIAL FIBRILLATION | ATRIAL FLUTTER | PSV TACHYCARDIA | PV TACHYCARDIA |
|---|---|---|---|---|
| Ventricular rhythm | Irregular | Regular-irregular | Regular | Regular; rarely irregular |
| P waves | Absent (f waves) | Flutter waves | Abnormal if present (frequently fall within preceding QRS complex) | Usually absent (may be seen occasionally between QRS complexes) |
| AV conduction | Variable | Usually variable | 1 : 1 | Originates in ventricles (VA conduction* may occur to interface with sinus node function) |
| Conformation of QRS complexes | Usually normal | Usually normal | Usually normal | Wide, bizarre |
| | (May be abnormal in any of the supraventricular tachyarrhythmias with aberrant ventricular conduction) | | | |
| Effect of vagal maneuvers | Slowing Remains irregular | Marked slowing Regular-irregular | Abrupt slowing or none‡ | No effect |

*Ventricular—atrial due to retrograde conduction from the ventricles to the atria; may prematurely discharge sinus node or result in exit block.

†In atrial flutter, vagal maneuvers may change the ventricular rhythm from regular to irregular or vice versa, the effect of increased vagal tone on AV conduction.

‡In some cats administration of a vagal stimulant drug, such as digitalis, may be required before response to a vagal maneuver can be elicited.

Abbreviations: PSV = paroxysmal supraventricular; PV = paroxysmal ventricular; f waves = fibrillation waves.

atrial myocardial disease. Electrophysiologic mechanisms proposed as responsible for its development include rapid discharge from an isolated atrial focus, an intra-atrial reentry mechanism, and an AV reentry mechanism similar to that discussed under preexcitation syndrome. Paroxysmal atrial tachycardia alone can be primarily responsible for precipitating congestive heart failure and is a well-recognized cause of syncopal episodes. The accompanying rapid ventricular rate markedly reduces ventricular filling, thereby depressing ventricular performance. In the cat, disease conditions associated with paroxysmal atrial tachycardia are the same as those listed for atrial premature beats. Once the underlying cause is identified, treatment is directed at its specific management. Digitalis glycosides are the initial drugs of choice for the majority of cats with paroxysmal atrial tachycardia. However, in hypertrophic cardiomyopathy, in which the use of digoxin may be contraindicated (particularly in the presence of outflow obstruction) and in hyperthyroidism, in which digoxin tends to be relatively less effective, propranolol should be tried first. If these approaches prove inadequate, other antiarrhythmic agents should be tried. In man the calcium channel–blocking agent verapamil has proved effective in the management of paroxysmal atrial tachycardia and the other supraventricular tachyarrhythmias. Diuretics should be included in the therapeutic regimen when evidence of heart failure exists.

***Atrial flutter*** is an atrial tachyarrhythmia considered to be intermediate between paroxysmal atrial tachycardia and atrial fibrillation. The electrocardiographic features include a regular or irregular ventricular rhythm, usually associated with narrow QRS complexes, and rapid, regularly occurring, saw tooth–like deflections during inscription of the isoelectric baseline (i.e., flutter waves). The variable ventricular response is the combined effect of rapid repetitive stimulation of the AV node and its inherent refractory period (Fig. 18–48). When atrial flutter is conducted with a 1:1 AV ratio, the resulting tachycardia is identical to atrial tachycardia and can be identified only by surface electrocardiography during a vagal maneuver or by intracardiac electrocardiography. S-T segment repolarization changes and aberrant ventricular conduction are more likely to be present with rapid AV conduction of atrial flutter. Electrophysiologically, atrial flutter is believed to represent a reentry mechanism within the atria.

Atrial tachyarrhythmias are rare in the cat, and, of these, atrial flutter is by far the least frequent. Tilley (1985) has demonstrated its presence in a single cat with hypertrophic cardiomyopathy and left anterior hemiblock. Its association with specific forms of heart disease is not well established. It seems reasonable to assume similar etiologic factors as for paroxysmal atrial tachycardia and atrial fibrillation. Treatment of atrial flutter is similar to that for paroxysmal atrial tachycardia. Experience in treating atrial flutter in the cat is so limited, however, that the relative benefits of drugs are unknown. Atrial flutter converts spontaneously to atrial fibrillation in a significant number of human and canine patients.

***Atrial fibrillation*** is characterized by rapid, totally chaotic atrial depolarization without contraction and by a rapid, irregular ventricular rhythm, usually with a pulse deficit. On the ECG, P waves are replaced by low-amplitude, irregularly occurring fluctuations termed f or fibrillation waves. The ventricular rhythm is rapid and irregular with marked variations in the R-R intervals, while the QRS interval tends to be narrow (Fig. 18–49). With a rapid ventricular response the QRS interval may be slightly prolonged and some variation in the QRS amplitudes is frequent, owing to aberrant ventricular conduction. Among the various electrophysiologic mechanisms proposed to explain the development of atrial fibrillation, the multiple wavelet theory of Moe (1962) is the most widely accepted.

In the cat, atrial fibrillation is infrequent, perhaps in

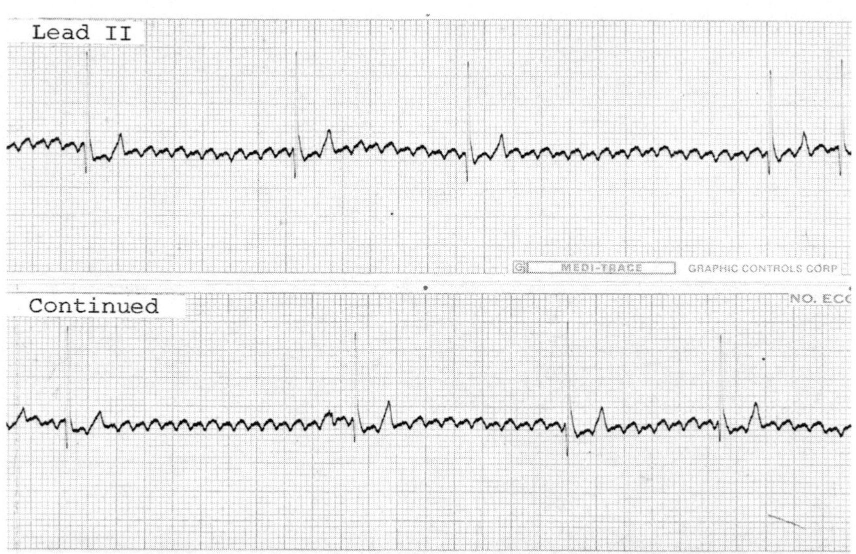


**Figure 18–48** Atrial flutter characterized by the regular occurrence of saw tooth–like deflections of the baseline (flutter waves) between the QRS complexes. The slow ventricular rate (30 to 90/minute [a dog]) suggests a high-grade AV conduction abnormality as well. (The ventricular rate in this dog was atropine-responsive, a finding consistent with high vagal tone. However, atropine administration is not recommended for this arrhythmia, because accelerated AV conduction may precipitate congestive heart failure or a fatal arrhythmia.) Atrial flutter is extremely rare in the cat, and owing to rapid A-V conduction may require vagal maneuvers to identify its presence (Tilley, 1979). 25 mm/sec; 1.0 mV = 1.0 cm.

part because of the small heart size and the inability to develop the critical atrial mass necessary to sustain this arrhythmia. Atrial fibrillation most often occurrs as a complication of cardiomyopathy, especially the hypertrophic (Tilley, 1985) and intermediate forms, in which left atrial size tends to be greater owing to imposed restrictions on left ventricular filling. As with the other atrial tachyarrhythmias, digoxin is the initial drug of choice. It is not contraindicated in atrial fibrillation secondary to hypertrophic cardiomyopathy, for the benefits gained by slowing AV conduction and the ventricular rate should improve left ventricular performance. Propranolol can be given as well if the ventricular rate is not adequately slowed (to < 180/minute) by digoxin alone. Diuretics should also be given to control excess fluid retention.

**Atrioventricular Junctional Arrhythmias.** Arrhythmias originating from latent pacemaker tissue in the AV node and most proximal ventricular conduction pathways are categorized as AV junctional arrhythmias (Table 18–7). They result from a localized disorder causing spontaneous, accelerated discharge from an ectopic focus or a reentry mechanism within this area. In many ways they resemble some of the atrial arrhythmias and can be difficult to differentiate from them by routine electrocardiographic methods.

The early discharge of an impulse arising in the AV junctional area and subsequently conducted into the ventricles, causing early ventricular depolarization, is called an ***AV junctional premature beat.*** It is distinguished electrocardiographically by a narrow, premature QRS complex, preceded or followed by a negative P wave (Fig. 18–50). Depolarization of both atria and ventricles depends on an impulse initiated at their interface and from there conducted in opposite directions. The relationship

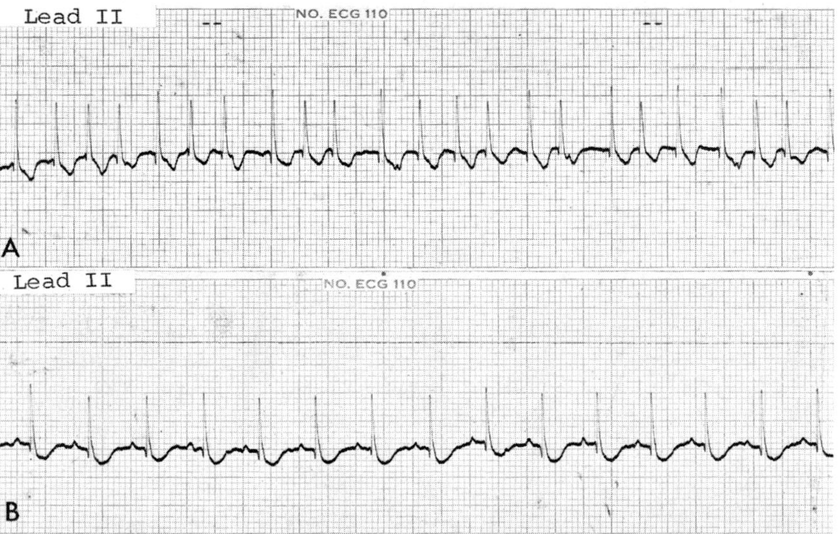


**Figure 18–49** Paroxysmal atrial fibrillation, lead II ECG strips from a two-year-old neutered male domestic longhair with hypertrophic cardiomyopathy. *A*, The basic rhythm is atrial fibrillation with a ventricular rate of 200/minute. Notice the absence of P waves, the variation in R-R intervals, and the marked differences in R-wave amplitudes. This last finding indicates aberrant ventricular conduction. R waves following long R-R intervals are of higher amplitude than those following short R-R intervals. Many R waves exceed 0.9 mV in amplitude, thereby fulfilling criteria for LVH (left ventricular hypertrophy) pattern in the cat. *B*, In a lead II strip taken 15 days later there is normal sinus rhythm at 150/minute. P waves precede each QRS complex with a constant P-R interval of 0.11 second. LVH pattern persists, and now S-T segment depression has become more pronounced, suggesting strain or ischemia. Paroxysmal atrial fibrillation has been a rare finding in my experience. 25 mm/sec; 1.0 mV = 1.0 cm.

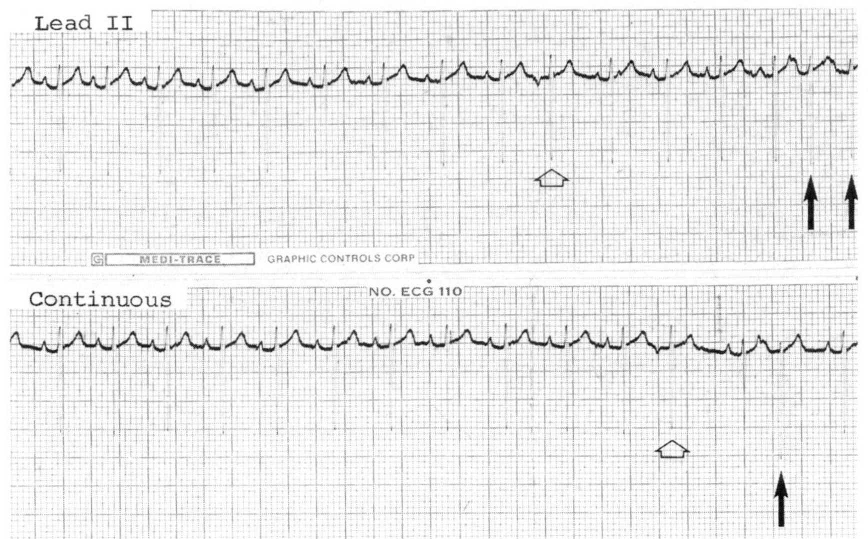


**Figure 18–50** Atrioventricular junctional premature beats, lead II ECG from a 10-year-old neutered male domestic shorthair with hypertrophic cardiomyopathy. This is the same cat as in Figure 18–34; the recording was taken 15 months later, after an episode of thromboembolism. Notice the two negative P waves (arrowheads) whose QRS complexes are followed by a complete compensatory pause. These are called A-V junctional premature beats and occur fairly late, being accompanied by QRS complexes that are similar to normal sinus QRS complexes. There are also a number of atrial premature beats (arrows) that occur early, causing T-wave deformity (due to T-P blending), and are associated with aberrantly conducted QRS complexes. 25 mm/sec; 1.0 mV = 1.0 cm.

between the inscribed P waves and QRS complex is subject to the relative rates of conduction of these separate waves of depolarization. Thus the P wave that results from retrograde atrial conduction may precede, fall within, or follow the QRS complex. The P-R interval tends to be shorter than that associated with the normal sinus beat, when the P wave comes before the QRS. If P waves are indiscernible, AV junctional premature beats cannot be clearly differentiated from atrial premature beats accompanied by T-P blending. Intracardiac electrocardiography may be helpful in making this distinction, but without this specialized study they should be termed supraventricular premature beats. Occasionally, the QRS interval may be prolonged owing to aberrant ventricular conduction.

Immediately after the AV junctional premature beat there is a pause. As with atrial premature beats its duration depends on the effect that retrograde atrial conduction has on sinus node function. Most often the sinus node is depolarized by the retrograde conduction and is reset, causing an incomplete compensatory pause (i.e., less than the 2 P-P interval). However, if retrograde atrial conduction fails to discharge the sinus node, sinus node function is unaffected and the compensatory pause is complete (i.e., 2 P-P).

The prevalence of AV junctional premature beats and the disorders responsible for their development in the cat are not clearly established. It is assumed that myocardial disorders, similar to those discussed for the more commonly found atrial premature beats, are responsible. Atrioventricular junctional premature beats do not in themselves require treatment, but their presence signals the existence of myocardial disease and the need for diagnostic studies to define its cause. Therapy is then based on the conclusions of these studies.

The regular occurrence of four or more consecutive AV junctional premature beats is called ***paroxysmal AV junctional tachycardia***. It should be suspected in a cat presented with a history of syncopal episodes or with an intermittent, rapid, regular cardiac rhythm over 240/minute. Electrocardiographically it is characterized by the sudden onset, usually within a single beat, of a series of rapidly occurring, regular QRS complexes with a narrow QRS interval (< 0.06 second). The first beat in the series has all the features of an AV junctional premature beat, being preceded by a negative P wave, and the period of tachycardia is followed by a variable pause (Fig. 18–51). Frequently the P wave cannot be identified because of failure of retrograde atrial conduction, or because atrial conduction coincides with or follows ventricular conduction. Then it may be difficult to differentiate paroxysmal AV junctional tachycardia from paroxysmal atrial tachycardia, and the term paroxysmal supraventricular tachycardia is appropriate. Vagal maneuvers may help to make this distinction by slowing or terminating the tachycardia and allowing emergence of recognizable P waves (Table 18–8).

In the cat, paroxysmal AV junctional tachycardia is strong supportive evidence of myocardial disease. Associations are similar to those for the supraventricular tachyarrhythmias already discussed: cardiomyopathy, bacterial endocarditis, hyperthyroidism, and occasionally congenital malformations. Treatment should be instituted, for the rapid ventricular response may lead to syncopal episodes and congestive heart failure. Although digoxin is the drug of choice for most disorders causing paroxysmal AV junctional tachycardia in the cat, propranolol is likely to be more effective for hyperthyroidism and hypertrophic cardiomyopathy accompanied by outflow obstruction. Other antiarrhythmic drugs may be necessary for adequate control of the tachyarrhythmia and should be tried if digoxin or propranolol alone or the two together are not effective.

**Ventricular Arrhythmias.** Those arrhythmias that arise from latent pacemaker foci within the ventricles and control ventricular depolarization for one or a number of successive beats by discharging at a rate exceeding that of normal sinus node discharge are termed ventricular arrhythmias or tachyarrhythmias (Table 18–7). These must be differentiated from ventricular escape mechanisms due to the failure of discharge of more proximal normal (i.e., sinus node) or latent pacemaker tissue or to the interruption of conduction pathways between the atria and ventricles. Ventricular arrhythmias are potentially more seri-

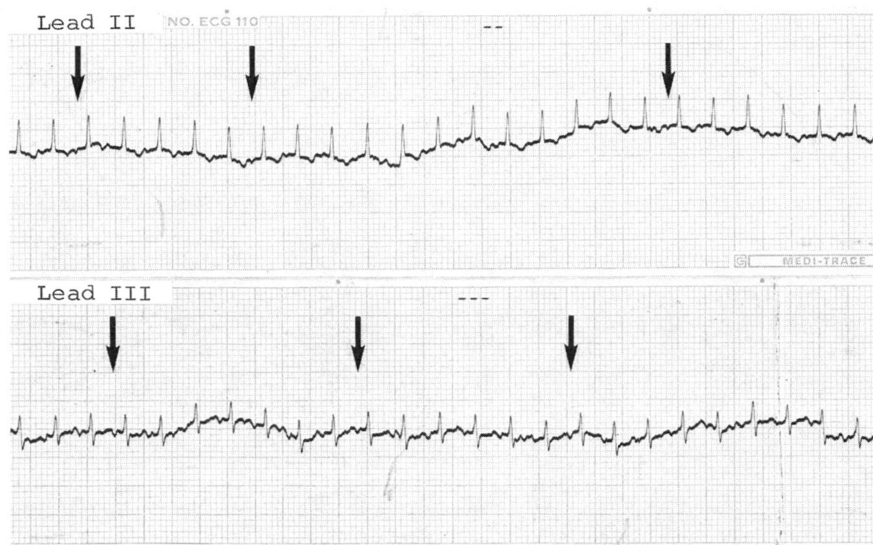


**Figure 18–51** Atrioventricular (AV) junctional tachycardia in a four-year-old neutered male domestic longhair presented for anorexia of five days' duration. A prominent gallop rhythm was auscultated, and thoracic radiographs disclosed cardiomegaly, pleural effusion, and hepatomegaly. The ECG strips show a regular rhythm at 250/minute accompanied by narrow QRS complexes. Although P waves are of low amplitude and difficult to identify consistently, when they can be distinguished they are negative in both leads II and III (arrows). Notice that they are narrow in both leads, while the P-R interval is normal (0.08 second). These findings are diagnostic for a low atrial or AV junctional tachycardia with retrograde atrial conduction. Dilatative feline cardiomyopathy was diagnosed by nonselective angiocardiography. 25 mm/sec; 1.0 mV = 1.0 cm.

ous than the supraventricular arrhythmias already discussed, because cardiac performance is impaired by the lack of atrial contribution to ventricular filling and an abnormal sequence of ventricular depolarization leading to altered contraction, and also because there is increased risk of cardiac arrest.

The early discharge of an impulse originating in the ventricles and resulting in conduction throughout the ventricles and their total depolarization constitutes a ***ventricular premature beat.*** It is characterized electrocardiographically by a wide (> 0.06 second), bizarre QRS complex that occurs earlier than expected, and is not usually preceded by a P wave. The associated T wave is usually prominent, and there is frequent significant S-T segment elevation or depression (Fig. 18–52). The electrocardiographic characteristics of the inscribed QRS complex can vary considerably, depending on its site of origin and the course followed during ventricular depolarization. (In general, ventricular premature beats arising from more peripheral positions within the ventricles have wider and more bizarre QRS complexes, while those originating more proximally, as from the major bundle branches, tend to be narrower and may clearly resemble those of normally conducted ventricular depolarization impulses.)

Occasionally, P waves precede the QRS complexes of the ventricular premature beats. When this occurs, the P-R interval is shorter than with normally conducted beats, and the accompanying QRS complex is narrower and unlike QRS complexes resulting from normal AV conduction or arising totally from ventricular foci. Under these circumstances the QRS complex is called a ***fusion beat.*** It is the effect of two separate and nearly simultaneous impulses of ventricular depolarization, one entering the ventricles by normal conduction pathways and the second originating from a ventricular focus (Fig. 18–53).

After the majority of ventricular premature beats there is a pause, as was described for both atrial and AV junctional premature beats. In most instances, conduction from the ventricular premature beat does not pass into the atria, and sinus node function is unaffected. The sinus node continues to discharge at its expected times; the impulse coinciding with the ventricular premature beat is blocked in AV conduction pathways owing to refractory tissue created by the ventricular premature beat, while the subsequent sinus node discharge is fully conducted. This results in a complete compensatory pause (2 P-P interval). Less often, retrograde conduction from the ventricular premature beat is transmitted into the atria

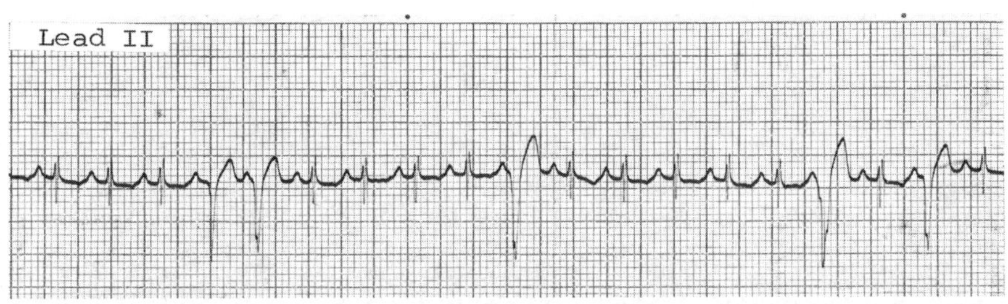


**Figure 18–52** Ventricular premature beats, lead II strip recorded from an eight-year-old neutered male domestic longhair with the intermediate form of cardiomyopathy. Frequent ventricular premature beats appear as widened, bizarre QRS complexes occurring in a downward (negative) direction, suggesting a left ventricular origin. Only the fourth premature beat is a pure one, as the others are narrower and each is preceded by a P wave with variation in the P-R interval (but always shorter than the P-R interval of normally conducted beats). All the premature beats except the fourth are fusion beats in which the ventricular ectopic focus is primarily responsible for ventricular depolarization. The QRS complexes of normally conducted beats are splintered (RSR′ complexes), suggesting an intraventricular conduction abnormality. 25 mm sec; 1.0 mV = 1.0 cm.

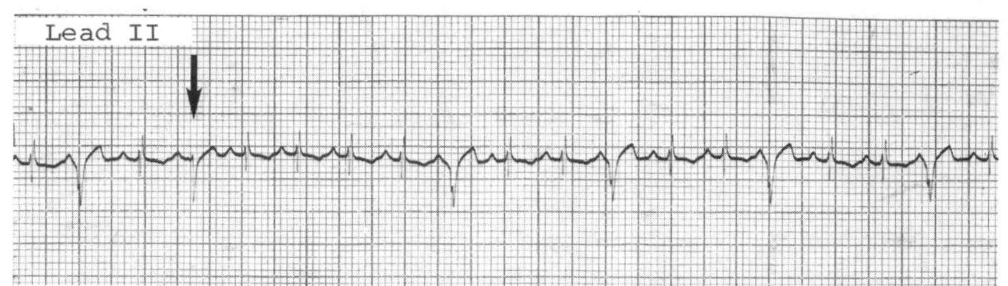


**Figure 18–53** Another lead II strip from the same cat as in Figure 18–52. The second premature beat (arrow) is much narrower than the others. It is preceded by a P wave having a normal P-R interval, and its onset is initiated by a small positive deflection. This QRS complex is a fusion beat in which normal AV conduction pathways are responsible for a greater portion of ventricular depolarization. 25 mm/sec; 1.0 mV = 1.0 cm.

(ventriculoatrial or VA conduction), causing early discharge of the sinus node. Thus the sinus node discharge pattern is reset and will not fire again until its normal refractory period is completed. The pause after the ventricular premature beat is shortened owing to resetting of the sinus node, and the interval between the two normal sinus beats flanking the premature beat is less than 2 P-P (incomplete compensatory pause). Rarely, sinus node discharge and its subsequent AV conduction is totally unaffected by the occurrence of a ventricular premature beat, so that a ventricular premature beat is sandwiched between two normal sinus beats whose relationship is exactly 1 P-P. This pattern is called an interpolated premature beat.

In the cat, ventricular premature beats are the most frequent cardiac arrhythmia (Harpster, 1977b). They have been identified in association with a variety of primary cardiac disorders, including all forms of cardiomyopathy, bacterial endocarditis (Harpster, 1977a), hyperthyroidism (Holzworth et al., 1980), myocardial infarction (Colcolough, 1974), and neoplasia (Tilley et al., 1981). They have also been reported during hypoxemia (Coulter et al., 1975) and frequently follow the administration of digitalis glycosides, catecholamines, and anesthetic agents (Tilley, 1985). The presence of ventricular premature beats is not in itself an indication for treatment. A diligent search should be made for the underlying cause and corrective measures instituted when this has been identified.

A series of four or more successive ventricular premature beats is designated ***paroxysmal ventricular tachycardia,*** although a prolonged sequence of ventricular premature beats is frequently called ***ventricular tachycardia***. These two terms can be used interchangeably; the underlying mechanism is identical for both. Electrocardiographically this arrhythmia is distinguished by a repetition of four or more rapidly occurring, widened, and bizarre QRS complexes that have no consistent relationship to P waves. When P waves can be identified, the ventricular rate always exceeds the atrial rate. Prominent T waves and S-T segment elevation or depression are other common features (Fig. 18–54). Finally, a variable pause fol-

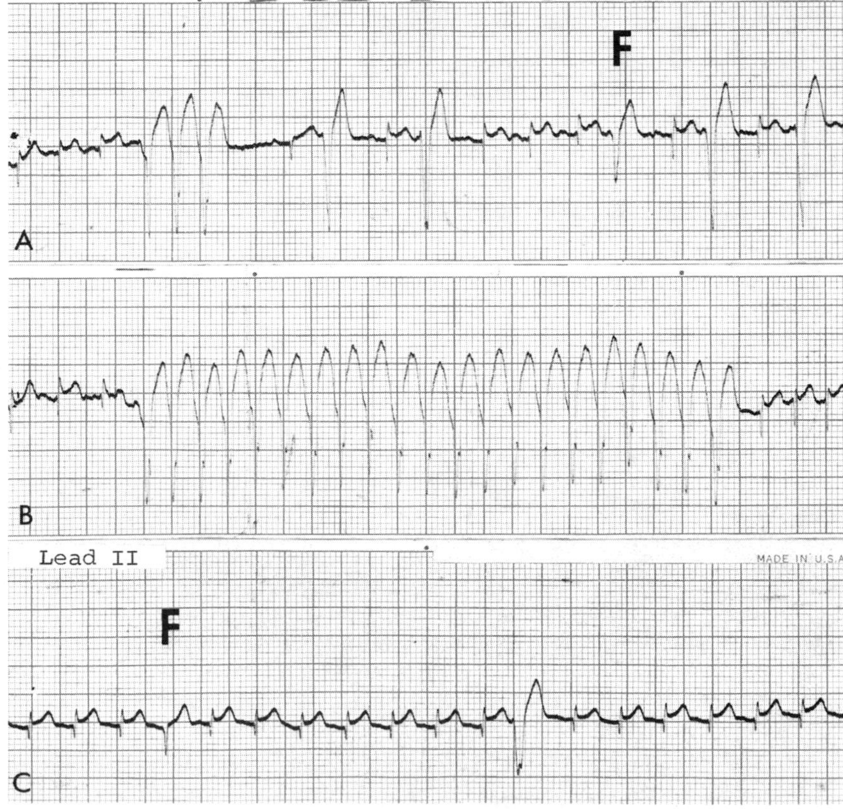


**Figure 18–54** Aggressive and potentially life-threatening ventricular arrhythmias in a 10-year-old neutered male domestic shorthair presented for partial anorexia and labored breathing of two weeks' duration. *A*, Frequent single ventricular premature beats and a run of ventricular premature beats (i.e., three ventricular premature beats occurring in succession) are evident. The ventricular premature beat that is of lower amplitude than the others probably represents a fusion beat (F). *B*, A four-second episode of paroxysmal ventricular tachycardia is characterized by a series of ventricular premature beats occurring at a rate of 300/minute. At its termination, a brief episode of apparent supraventricular tachycardia is present (a series of three rapidly occurring QRS complexes having a conformation normal for this cat). *C*, The rhythm has improved; however, a single ventricular premature beat and a fusion beat (F) remain. Notice that in each of the strips mild S-T segment elevation is present, suggesting myocardial ischemia. Although cardiomyopathy was most likely responsible for these ECG changes and the heart failure, a definitive diagnosis was never established. 25 mm/sec; 1.0 mV = 1.0 cm.

lows the series of abnormal QRS complexes, as was described for the paroxysmal supraventricular tachyarrhythmias.

For differentiating paroxysmal ventricular tachycardia from supraventricular tachycardia accompanied by aberrant ventricular conduction, vagal maneuvers (Table 18–8) or intracardiac electrocardiography may be required.

Paroxysmal ventricular tachycardia usually results from organic heart disease in the cat. Etiologic factors are similar to those discussed for ventricular premature beats. Treatment should be started as soon as possible to avoid development of a fatal arrhythmia and while diagnostic tests are in progress to establish the cause. Propranolol, quinidine, and procainamide have all been useful at times in the management of paroxysmal ventricular tachycardia in the cat, but none has been consistently effective. It is usually necessary to adopt a trial-and-error approach to determine the drug or combination of drugs that elicits the best response. Complete control of the arrhythmia is frequently difficult. Lidocaine has been reported as a potentially dangerous drug in the cat, and its use is contraindicated (Tilley and Weitz, 1977).

The independent control of the atrial and ventricular rates by discharge of two separate, unassociated pacemaker foci, in which the ventricular rate exceeds that of the atria, has been termed ***accelerated idioventricular rhythm.*** Electrocardiographically it is most often characterized by the absence of a fixed relationship between P waves and QRS complexes; P waves periodically disappear owing to merging with QRS complexes, the result of slight differences in their inherent rates of discharge (Fig. 18–55). The atrial rate is normal or increased but is slower than the accompanying ventricular rate. The QRS complexes may be normal or abnormal in conformation depending on the site of origin of the subsidiary pacemaker (normal if arising from the AV junctional focus, abnormal when originating within the ventricle). An accelerated idioventricular rhythm must be differentiated from other forms of AV dissociation, such as depressed sinus node function and the more advanced forms of AV block. In the latter abnormalities of impulse generation and conduction there is also independent control of the atrial and ventricular rates; however, the ventricular rate is the result of an escape mechanism and tends to be slower than expected.

In the cat an accelerated idioventricular rhythm is uncommon and the etiology uncertain. Frequent causes in man include anesthesia, overdose of digitalis and antiarrhythmic drugs, cardiovascular surgery, infectious diseases, and myocardial disease (Zipes and McIntosh, 1971). It is assumed that similar inciting factors are responsible in the cat. Treatment is directed at the underlying cause rather than the arrhythmia itself. If the arrhythmia develops under the influence of digitalis or antiarrhythmic agents, overdosage should be suspected, the drug should be withheld, and electrocardiographic monitoring should be carried out.

The sudden development of ineffectual cardiac func-

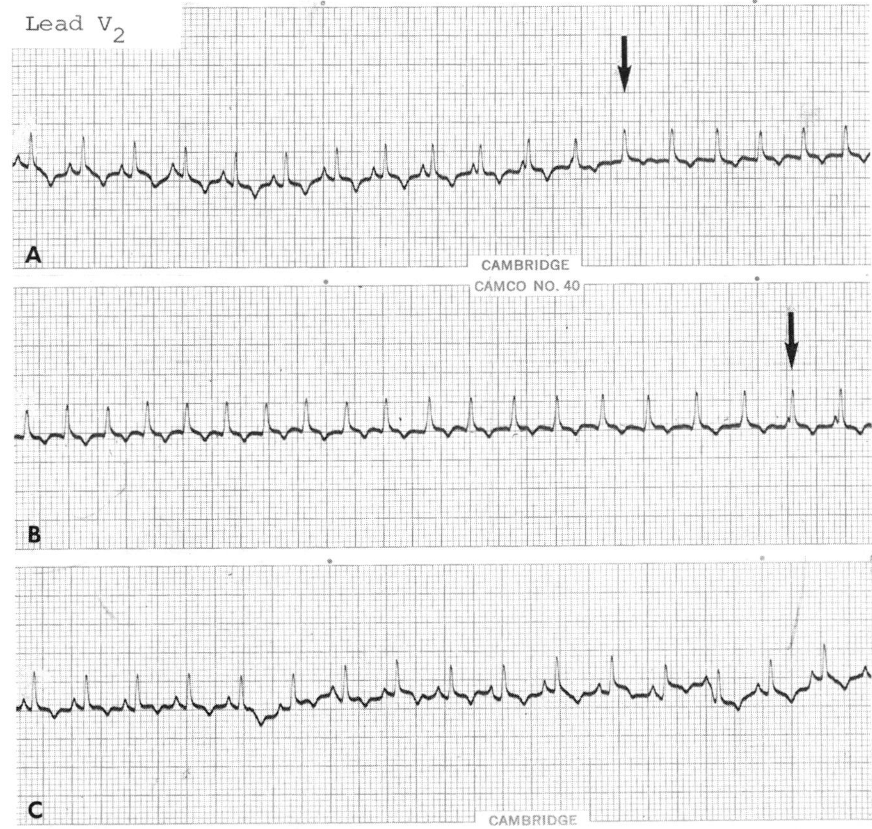


**Figure 18–55** Accelerated idioventricular rhythm (AV dissociation); continuous ECG recording from a 10-year-old spayed female domestic longhair presented for blindness of five weeks' duration. No clinical signs referable to the heart were present, and thoracic radiographs disclosed no abnormality. *A*, The P-R interval gradually shortens until the P wave disappears (arrow) without any change in the conformation of the QRS complexes but with an associated increase in the ventricular rate (from 167/minute at the beginning of the strip to 214/minute at the end). P waves then remain undetectable until the last two complexes in *B* (arrow), when P waves again emerge from the QRS complexes and continue throughout *C* with fixed P-R interval of 0.09 second. The emergence of the P waves is again associated with a gradual decrease in the ventricular rate in *B* that continues in *C*, where the rate stabilizes at 162/minute. This electrocardiographic abnormality is called accelerated idioventricular rhythm or AV dissociation. It is the result of two independent and unassociated pacemakers that occur at nearly equal rates, one controlling the rate of the atria (usually the sinus node) and the other the rate of the ventricles (usually the lower portions of the A-V node or the proximal septal tissue). This arrhythmia may occur because of drug influence (e.g., digitalis glycosides) or as a result of myocardial disorders. 25 mm/sec; 1.0 mV = 1.0 cm.

tion, usually accompanied by collapse, agonal respiration, and absence of palpable pulses, is called ***cardiac arrest.*** Electrocardiographic monitoring will demonstrate one of the following patterns: (1) ***asystole,*** the absence of any electrical activity or P waves occurring without QRS complexes; (2) ***ineffectual QRS complexes,*** also termed electromechanical dissociation and characterized by QRS complexes, usually widened and bizarre, without effectual ventricular contraction; or (3) ***ventricular flutter or fibrillation,*** characterized by rapid, continuous ventricular electrical activity in a regular or irregular pattern (Fig. 18–56). Cardiac arrest may result from progressive deterioration of intracardiac conduction, of myocardial performance, or of both, frequently as a sequel to anesthesia, hypoxemia, acid-base imbalance, electrolyte disturbance, or shock. In cardiac disease, cardiac arrest can develop suddenly without any premonitory signs, owing to the early discharge of a ventricular premature beat during the vulnerable period of the preceding QRS complex's T wave, the so-called R on T phenomenon. This event consistently results in ventricular fibrillation. Successful management of cardiac arrest demands early recognition, readily available emergency drugs and other necessary equipment, a team approach in which many staff members are familiar with the procedure, and a thorough knowledge of the management of cardiac resuscitation (Tables 18–9 and 18–10). It is extremely difficult to carry out cardiac resuscitation singlehandedly. Necessary equip-

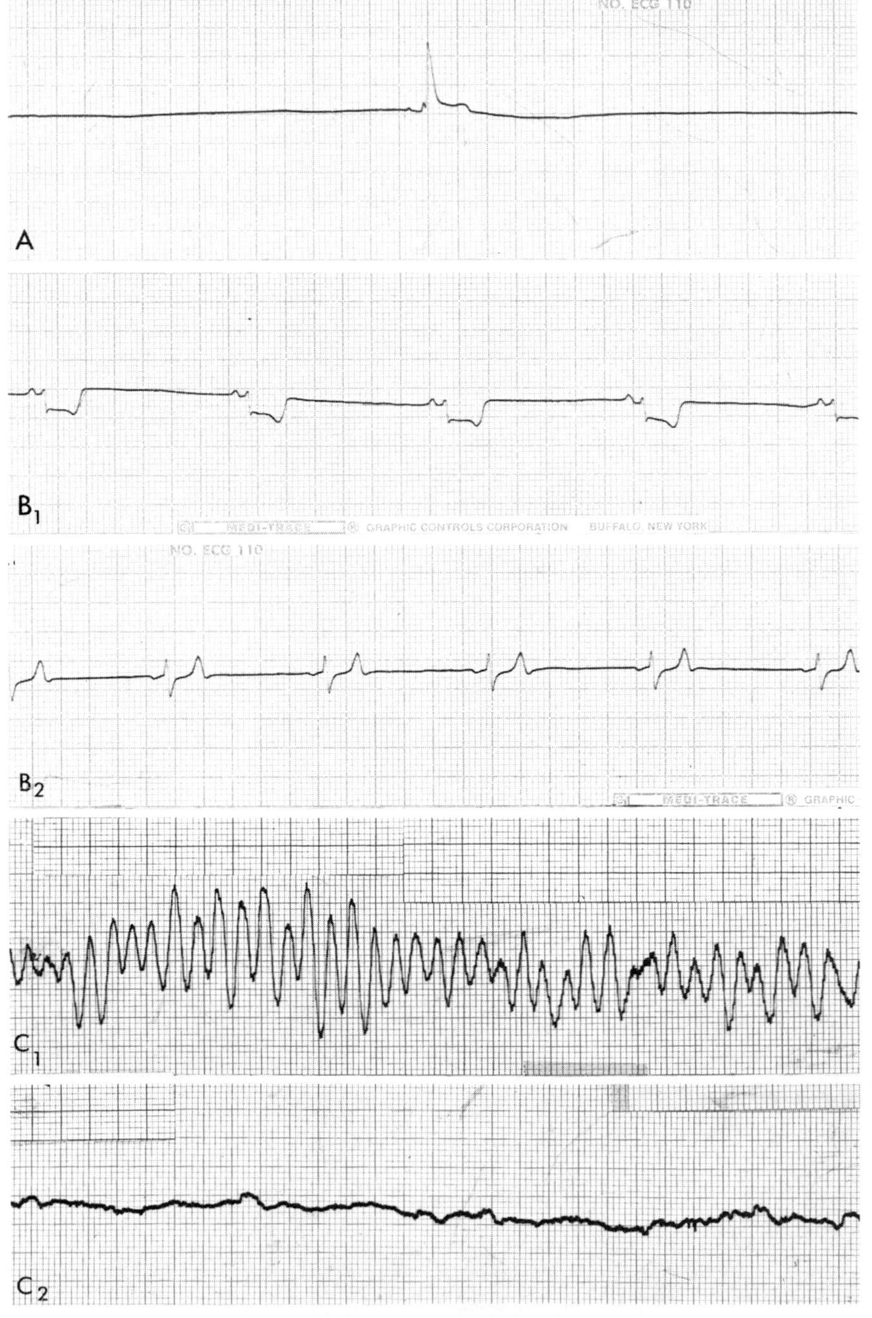


**Figure 18–56** Electrocardiographic patterns occurring in cardiac arrest. *Asystole* in *A* is characterized by a long isoelectric baseline interrupted by a widened, bizarre QRS complex preceded by a P wave. Examples of *electromechanical dissociation* are illustrated in $B_1$ and $B_2$. The recordings with this arrest pattern can vary considerably, and in an animal under anesthesia may easily be misinterpreted as sinus bradycardia if the patient is not properly monitored. In $B_1$ there is apparent sinus bradycardia at a rate of 50/minute. The low-amplitude QRS complex and especially the marked S-T segment depression usually indicate profound acidosis and the need for sodium bicarbonate administration. $B_2$, The ventricular rate is again slow at approximately 60/minute. Although the QRS complexes appear more normal than in $B_1$, they are prolonged and are preceded by a negative P wave. *Coarse ventricular fibrillation* is illustrated in $C_1$. Notice the high-amplitude, irregularly occurring fluctuations that characterize this arrest pattern. $C_1$ should be compared with $C_2$, which shows an example of *fine ventricular fibrillation*. In most instances, coarse ventricular fibrillation is more responsive to defibrillation than the fine type. 25 mm/sec; 1.0 mV = 1.0 cm.

**Table 18–9 Cardiac Resuscitation in the Cat**

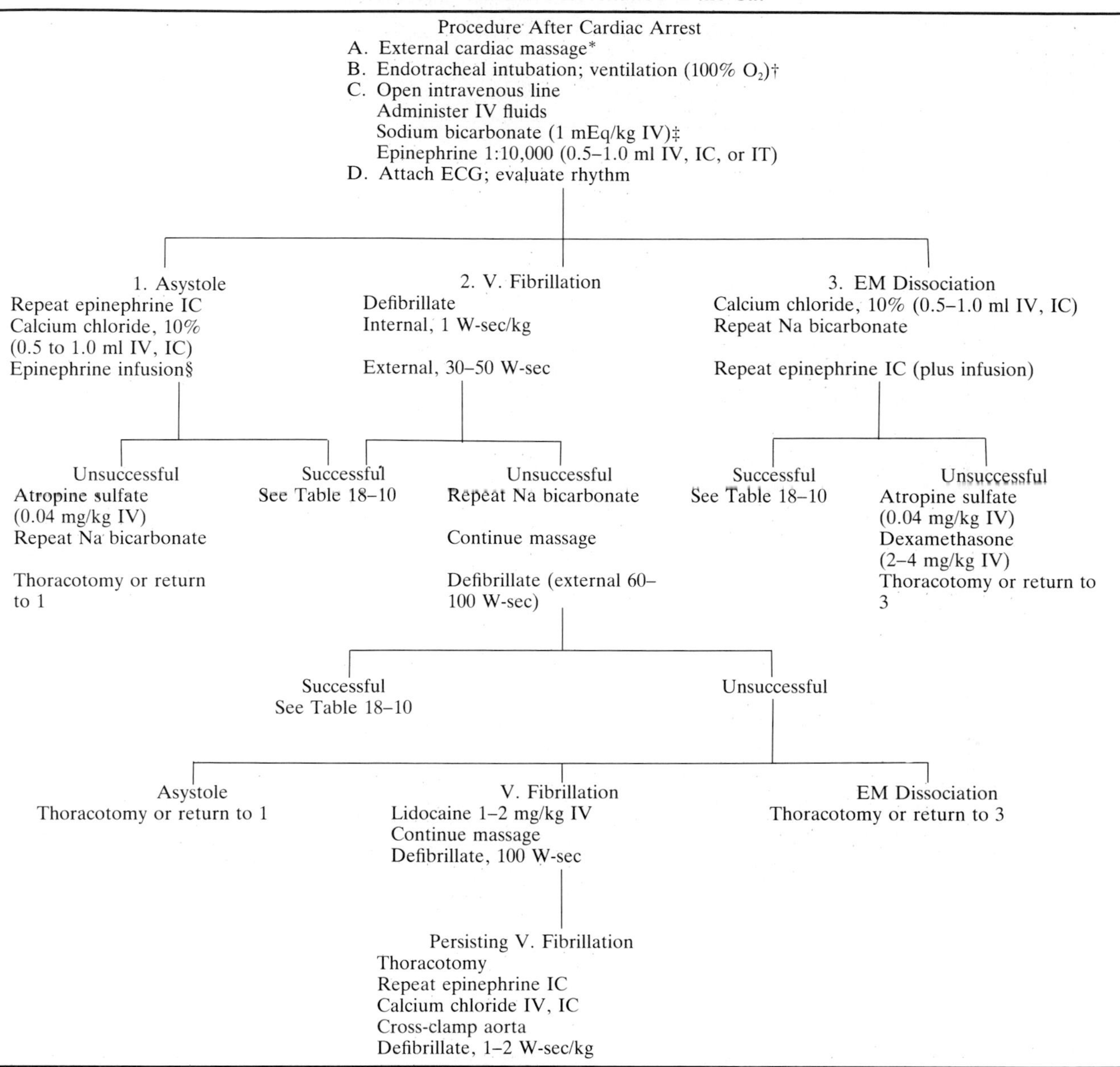
Procedure After Cardiac Arrest
A. External cardiac massage*
B. Endotracheal intubation; ventilation (100% $O_2$)†
C. Open intravenous line
Administer IV fluids
Sodium bicarbonate (1 mEq/kg IV)‡
Epinephrine 1:10,000 (0.5–1.0 ml IV, IC, or IT)
D. Attach ECG; evaluate rhythm
1. Asystole
Repeat epinephrine IC
Calcium chloride, 10%
(0.5 to 1.0 ml IV, IC)
Epinephrine infusion§
2. V. Fibrillation
Defibrillate
Internal, 1 W-sec/kg
External, 30–50 W-sec
3. EM Dissociation
Calcium chloride, 10% (0.5–1.0 ml IV, IC)
Repeat Na bicarbonate
Repeat epinephrine IC (plus infusion)
Unsuccessful
Atropine sulfate
(0.04 mg/kg IV)
Repeat Na bicarbonate
Thoracotomy or return to 1
Successful
See Table 18–10
Unsuccessful
Repeat Na bicarbonate
Continue massage
Defibrillate (external 60–100 W-sec)
Successful
See Table 18–10
Unsuccessful
Atropine sulfate
(0.04 mg/kg IV)
Dexamethasone
(2–4 mg/kg IV)
Thoracotomy or return to 3
Successful
See Table 18–10
Unsuccessful
Asystole
Thoracotomy or return to 1
V. Fibrillation
Lidocaine 1–2 mg/kg IV
Continue massage
Defibrillate, 100 W-sec
EM Dissociation
Thoracotomy or return to 3
Persisting V. Fibrillation
Thoracotomy
Repeat epinephrine IC
Calcium chloride IV, IC
Cross-clamp aorta
Defibrillate, 1–2 W-sec/kg

*Cardiac massage is continued (60–80/minute) until return of a palpable heart beat and peripheral pulse.

†Ventilation is carried out (15–20 breaths/minute) until normal, spontaneous respiration is reestablished.

‡Repeat sodium bicarbonate every 15–20 minutes during the resuscitation procedure or until normal cardiac and respiratory function return.

§An epinephrine infusion is prepared by adding 1.0 mg to 100 ml 5% dextrose in water (10 μg/ml). Administer at 0.1 μg/kg/min with a mini-drip administration set.

Abbreviations: IC = intracardiac; IT = intratracheal; V = ventricular; EM = electromechanical.

**Table 18–10 Supportive Measures After Cardiac Resuscitation**

Continue ventilation until consciousness returns.
Monitor ECG.
Evaluate pulses, blood pressure frequently. If heart slows or pulse weakens, begin infusion of dopamine* or isoproterenol.† Calcium chloride 1–2 ml IV may also be beneficial.
Administer IV fluids.
Treat CNS complications.
  Mannitol
  Corticosteroid
Take thoracic radiographs as soon as cat can be safely moved.
  Treat chest trauma by appropriate measures.
Administer broad-spectrum antibiotic.
Evaluate and monitor renal function.

*A dopamine infusion is prepared by adding 2.5 ml (40 mg/ml) to 500 ml 5% dextrose in water (200 μg/ml). Administer with mini-drip administration set at 4–10 μg/kg/min.

†An isoproterenol infusion is prepared by adding 5 ml (0.2 mg/ml) to 250 ml 5% dextrose in water (4 μg/ml). Infuse by mini-drip administration set at 0.04–0.10 μg/kg/min.

ment includes an emergency kit containing all required drugs, endotracheal tubes, IV catheters and cannulas, and IV fluids and administration sets; a readily available source of 100 per cent oxygen; a portable ECG machine or monitor; and a defibrillator. Ventricular fibrillation occurs less often in cardiac arrest in the cat than in the dog, perhaps because the cat's heart is smaller. The small size of the cat itself permits more effective external cardiac massage, a decided advantage in cardiac resuscitation. Finally, the most effective approach to cardiac arrest is prevention. This means frequent and careful monitoring of the critically ill cat in order to correct those abnormalities that could lead to cardiac arrest. Failure to do so will result in the more frequent development of cardiac arrest and less success in resuscitation procedures.

Prevention and management of cardiac arrest is also discussed in the chapter on sedation and anesthesia.

## Nonselective (Venous) Angiocardiography

Venous angiocardiography (VAC) is a valuable diagnostic procedure in the domestic cat owing to the cat's suitable size and the availability of peripheral veins of adequate diameter (Harpster, 1977b; Owens and Twedt, 1977). A bolus of radiopaque contrast medium is injected into a peripheral vein, after which one or more thoracic radiographs are taken in one or more views at a preselected time. Both Hypaque 50* and Renografin 60† provide satisfactory studies when used at 1 to 2 ml/kg. This procedure is routinely performed with chemical restraint to ensure the cat's cooperation and minimize the need for repeated studies. Ketamine hydrochloride (5 to 10 mg IV) is safe and effective but requires a well-organized and coordinated procedure, as it provides adequate restraint for no longer than 10 to 15 minutes. Although satisfactory studies can be obtained with one or two radiographic exposures in the lateral view at a preselected time, the timing of the exposure is critical although not easily calculated owing to differences in circulation time in various forms of cardiac disease. Therefore repeated studies will often be necessary with exposure time adjusted according to results of the initial study. As a rule of thumb, the first exposure should be made at eight to ten seconds after injection of contrast medium is completed to provide a satisfactory study of the left ventricle. The need for repeated studies is greatly reduced if equipment is available for multiple, rapid exposures, such as a rapid film or cassette changer or 70-mm, rapid-sequence spot films. This equipment also provides definition of the left ventricular end-diastolic and end-systolic chamber dimensions, as well as functional studies of left ventricular contractility, which are beneficial in evaluation of the cat with cardiomyopathy. The standard procedure for performing VAC in the cat is outlined in Table 18–11. Examples of VAC studies in cats with various forms of cardiomyopathy are presented as these disorders are discussed. Figure 18–11 is a normal study to be used for comparison purposes.

Complications associated with venous angiocardiography can be minimized by stabilization of the cat's cardiovascular status before the study. All pleural fluid and pulmonary edema should be eliminated by thoracocentesis, diuretic therapy, or both, and cardiac arrhythmias should be under control. In cats with reasonably normal circulation, acute vomiting is frequent, usually within one to three minutes after the injection of contrast medium. This probably results from transient stimulation of vomiting centers in the brain and is a short-lived reaction. It is sufficiently frequent to justify fasting the cat for 12 to 24 hours before the study. Far less often, and almost always in cats with dilatative cardiomyopathy, acute collapse occurs because of sudden bradycardia or cardiac arrest. Early recognition of this complication, which also tends to develop within one to three minutes after the injection of contrast medium, is essential if the cat is to survive. The majority of cats can be resuscitated by prompt cardiac massage and the IV administration of atropine sulfate or a sympathomimetic agent such as epinephrine, isoproterenol, or dopamine.

Venous angiocardiography has its greatest application in feline cardiology in differentiation of the various forms of cardiomyopathy by a properly timed study of the left ventricle. A rapid film changer or 70-mm, rapid-sequence spot film equipment provides information on left ventricular end-systolic and end-diastolic chamber characteris-

**Table 18–11 Standard Protocol for Performing Venous Angiography in the Cat**

Sedate the cat for 15 to 20 minutes before the procedure to minimize stress and improve cooperation.
  Diazepam (Valium) 1.0 mg/kg IM
  Ketamine HCl (Vetalar) 2 to 4 mg/kg IM or IV
Position a 20-gauge, 1 to 1½ inch polyethylene intravenous cannula in the left cephalic vein and bandage in place.
Restrain cat in right lateral recumbency on x-ray table.
Inject 1.5 to 2.0 ml/kg of radiopaque contrast material into the intravenous cannula as rapidly as possible (Hypaque 50 or Renografin 60).
Take 70-mm spot films, four to six per second, starting with the injection of contrast material and continuing for 10 to 12 seconds.
The procedure may be repeated twice if necessary.

*Winthrop Laboratories, New York, NY
†E. R. Squibb & Sons, Inc, Princeton, NJ

tics, size, and contractility. Venous angiocardiography is also of use in identifying pericardial disease and in differentiating pericardial effusion and intrapericardial masses. It can also be employed to identify the site of aortic occlusion in cats with thromboembolism (Fig. 18–57). A single radiographic exposure taken 10 to 15 seconds after the injection of contrast medium, with the beam centered over the abdomen, usually permits adequate definition of the obstructed site (Owens and Twedt, 1977). Finally, VAC is of use in the diagnosis of congenital cardiac anomalies, especially right-to-left shunts (Owens and Twedt, 1977). Other anomalies are more difficult to demonstrate, and angiocardiography may be misleading when more than one defect is present.

## Echocardiography (ECHO)

The use of high-frequency sound waves for noninvasive study of the heart and its internal structures is called cardiac ultrasound or echocardiography. It utilizes the principle of rapid (usually 100/second), intermittent transmission of high-frequency, inaudible (1 to 7 million cycles/second [1 to 7 megahertz]) sound waves, which upon contacting various body tissues may be absorbed,

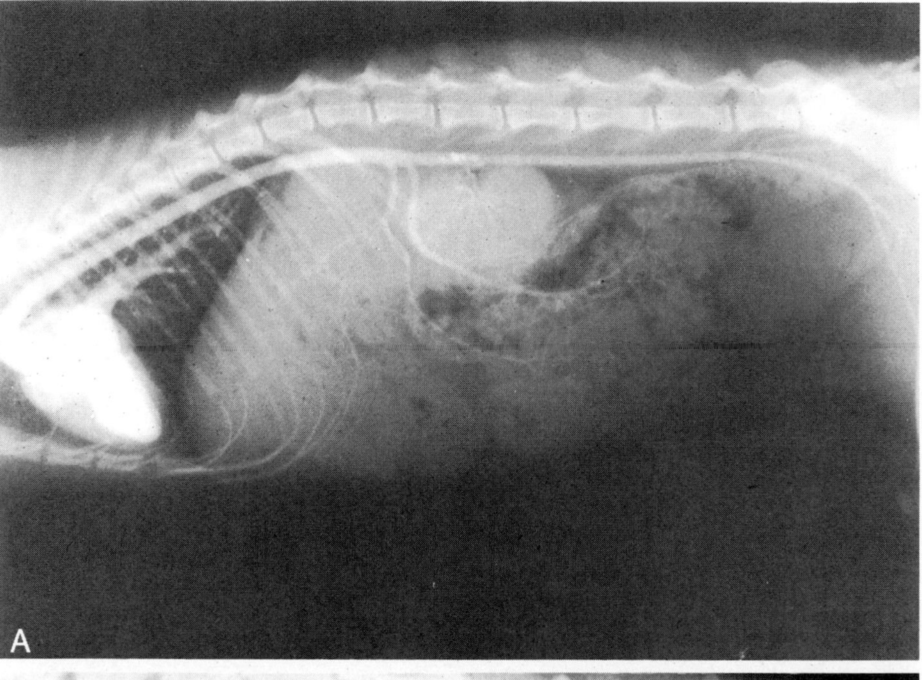


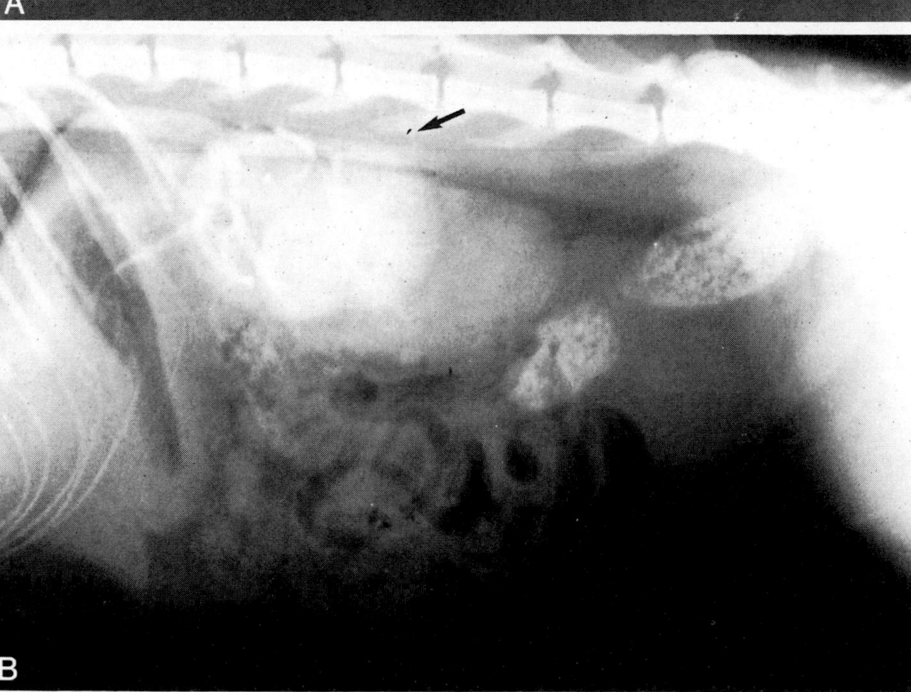


**Figure 18–57** Nonselective angiocardiography utilized to establish the patency of the descending aorta and its branches. In a normal cat (*A*) all branches of the abdominal aorta can be identified. In cranial to caudal order these include the celiac artery, the cranial mesenteric artery, the paired third lumbar arteries (the first of five pairs arising from the abdominal aorta), the right and left renal arteries, the caudal mesenteric artery, and the paired internal and external iliac arteries (the external iliac vessels are superimposed and cannot be seen as two separate vessels). *B* is a study performed in a cat with hypertrophic cardiomyopathy and presented with acute hindlimb paralysis following a thromboembolic epidode. Notice that dye in the aorta terminates just caudal to the origin of the right fourth lumbar artery (arrow). This is more cranial than the usual site of occlusion for a large embolus, which is typically at the terminal aorta where the iliac vessels originate. Occlusion at this level increases the risk of large bowel infarction.

scattered, refracted, or reflected, depending on the density and transmission characteristics of the tissue. The ideal tissue for ultrasound study is one that transmits the majority of the sound waves to deeper structures while a portion of the ultrasound energy is reflected to the sending device, called a transducer. This latter effect is the basis of imaging echocardiography. Bone and calcified costal cartilages absorb nearly all the sonic energy and block transmission to deeper tissues, thereby interfering with ultrasonic imaging; lung has a similar effect, its reflectivity of ultrasound waves approaching 100 per cent. Thus an echocardiographic study must circumvent both the ribs and the lung tissue in order to obtain useful information.

The reflected ultrasound waves picked up by the transducer may be recorded by a variety of methods. A-mode imaging produces oscilloscopic baseline deflections, whose amplitudes vary with the intensity of the signal. In B-mode display, the deflections of the A-mode images are converted into dots whose brightness represents the strength of the signal. When these dots are put into motion through a recording process, more useful information can be obtained, which is also one-dimensional and is termed M-mode echocardiography. The most recent developments in echocardiography are systems for the production of real-time, two-dimensional images of the heart. Two-dimensional (2-D) echocardiography records cardiac structure in two dimensions in real time and in various planes, equivalent to slices removed from the heart. It utilizes various systems, including an oscillating transducer (mechanical sector scanners) and the sequential activation of a variable number of crystals arranged in a linear fashion (phased-array or electronic-sector scanners; fixed-beam, linear-array systems). The interested reader should refer to echocardiographic texts to obtain more information about these systems and their advantages and disadvantages (Haft and Horowitz, 1978; Nanda and Gramiak, 1978; Talano and Gardin, 1983).

Echocardiography enables the clinician to visualize the internal structures of the heart and to obtain information about myocardial function by a noninvasive method. It has eliminated the need for cardiac catheterization in a variety of acquired cardiac conditions but at present does not provide information critical to the diagnosis and management of congenital heart disease and some acquired cardiac and valvular disorders.

Normal M-mode echocardiographic values in the awake (Pipers et al., 1979) and the sedated (Soderberg et al., 1983) domestic cat have been reported. The results of these studies are summarized in Table 18–12. They are surprisingly similar despite differences in the resting state of the two groups of cats. The major dissimilarities involve the mean values for AoED and LAES, most likely the result of differences in body size.

Satisfactory M-mode echocardiograms can be obtained for the majority of cats by placing the transducer over the ventral right thorax between the fourth and sixth intercostal spaces, with the cat restrained in left lateral recumbency. If the heart is not enlarged, this standard position may be awkward and uncomfortable for the technician because of the need to maintain the transducer in a ventral position along the sternum. In this situation the cat may be rotated into a more dorsal position or placed on a folded towel to lift the thorax off the table. These manipulations provide easier access to the right ventral thorax, and also enable placement of the transducer over the ventral left thorax in order to improve the quality of the study. A 5-megahertz (MHz), 6-mm, unfocused transducer is routinely used. Recordings should be made at the three standard echocardiographic positions; otherwise the study is incomplete and unsatisfactory (Fig. 18–58).

Lack of cooperation by the cat is the greatest obstacle to the recording of satisfactory echocardiograms. Struggling, growling, and purring all increase chest movements and lung excursions that detract from the quality of the recording and markedly prolong the time required. Ketamine hydrochloride, 1 to 2 mg/kg IV, is used when necessary to resolve these problems and usually provides 15 to 20 minutes of involuntary cooperation. Sedatives should be avoided for the cat with dilatative cardiomyopathy, in which cardiac output is severely depressed.

In feline cardiology, M-mode echocardiography has been most helpful in identifying dilatative cardiomyopathy and eliminating the need for VAC with its potential risks. It has been less reliable in diagnosing the other forms of cardiomyopathy and, particularly, in differentiating hypertrophic cardiomyopathy and hyperthyroidism. With more experience our ability to distinguish these two conditions should improve. Echocardiography has also been beneficial in the diagnosis of pericardial disease in cats, both pericardial effusion (Pipers and Hamlin, 1980) and congenital anomalies, and in the recognition of mitral valve disease. It is likely that with further experience and

**Table 18–12 Summary of M-Mode Echocardiographic Values in the Normal Domestic Cat**

| | PIPERS ET AL., 1979 | | | SODERBERG ET AL., 1983 | | |
|---|---|---|---|---|---|---|
| | Mean | SD | Range | Mean | SD | Range |
| LVPW Th (mm) | NR | NR | NR | 3.13 | 1.08 | 2.05–4.21 |
| LVEDD (cm) | 1.48 | 0.26 | 1.12–2.18 | 1.28 | 0.17 | 1.12–1.45 |
| LVESD (cm) | 0.88 | 0.24 | 0.64–1.68 | 0.83 | 0.15 | 0.68–0.99 |
| LVET (sec) | 0.15 | 0.02 | 0.11–0.19 | NR | NR | NR |
| % Δ D | 41.0 | 7.3 | 23–56 | 34.5 | 12.6 | 21.9–47.1 |
| AoED (mm) | 7.5 | 1.8 | 4–11.8 | 9.4 | 1.4 | 8.0–10.8 |
| LAES (mm) | 7.4 | 1.7 | 4.5–11.2 | 9.8 | 1.7 | 8.2–11.5 |
| LA/Ao | 0.99 | NR | NR | 1.09 | 0.27 | 0.82–1.36 |
| VCF (cir/sec) | 2.86 | 0.78 | 1.27–4.55 | NR | NR | NR |

Abbreviations: AoED = aortic root dimension at end-diastole; LA/Ao = left atrial to aortic root ratio; LAES = left atrium at end-systole; LVEDD = left ventricular end-diastolic dimension; LVESD = left ventricular end-systolic dimension; LVET = left ventricular ejection time; LVPW Th = left ventricular posterior wall thickness at end-diastole; NR = value not reported; VCF = velocity of circumferential fiber shortening; % Δ D = per cent left ventricular dimensional change.

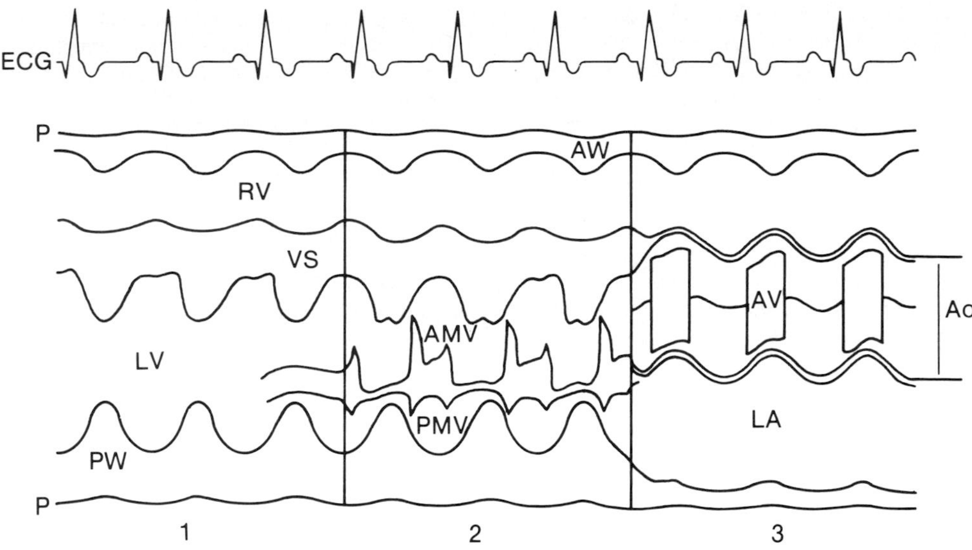


**Figure 18–58** Diagrammatic representation of the three major positions seen in an M-mode echocardiographic recording. Position 1 is recorded through the ventricles immediately below the mitral valve leaflets. Position 2 is recorded through the ventricles at the level of the mitral valve. Position 3 is centered more basally than the other positions through the aorta and left atrium. During ventricular systole, the ventricular septum moves toward the left ventricular free wall while the aorta moves toward the right ventricular free wall. Abbreviations: Ao = aorta, AV = aortic valve, AW = anterior wall or right ventricular free wall, AMV = anterior mitral valve, ECG = electrocardiogram, LA = left atrium, LV = left ventricular cavity, p = pericardium, PW = posterior wall or left ventricular free wall, PMV = posterior mitral valve, RV = right ventricular cavity, VS = ventricular septum.

the incorporation of two-dimensional echocardiographic systems into the clinical setting, the applications of echocardiography will increase. Examples of typical M-mode echocardiographic findings in the various forms of feline cardiomyopathy and other acquired cardiac disorders are presented as these subjects are discussed.

## Congenital Cardiovascular Defects*

### Occurrence

Congenital cardiovascular defects were found in 0.2 per 1000 feline admissions and 28 per 1000 feline autopsies at the Angell Memorial Animal Hospital (AMAH) during the years 1957 to 1979. The average occurrence rates for man have been reported to be 2 per 1000 among the general population and 10 per 1000 autopsy cases (Fontana and Edwards, 1962). A prospective study, however, reported 7.7 per 1000 human live births (Mitchell et al., 1971). An extensive study revealed a rate of 6.8 cardiovascular anomalies per 1000 canine hospital admissions (Patterson, 1968). Occurrence rates provided by different investigators among different species are virtually impossible to compare because of differing criteria for inclusion in study, sample population, and sampling methods. The occurrence rates of cardiovascular anomalies in dogs at AMAH (where the same criteria and methods were applied and the same geographic area studied as for rates in cats) were very similar to those in cats (0.2 per 1000 admissions and 23 per 1000 autopsies). It does not appear that cats have vastly fewer cardiovascular defects than dogs, as has often been stated.

The occurrence of specific congenital cardiovascular defects of cats at AMAH, those reported from The Animal Medical Center (AMC), and a compilation of anomalies reported by others is given in Table 18–13. It is clear that atrioventricular (AV) valve malformations, ventricular septal defects (VSD), patent ductus arteriosus (PDA), and endocardial fibroelastosis (EFE) are the most commonly diagnosed anomalies. Each species seems to have a somewhat different ranking of the various defects. The most common anomalies in humans are VSD, pulmonary stenosis, atrial septal defect (ASD), PDA, and tetralogy of Fallot (Mitchell et al., 1971). Serious human defects include complete transposition of the great vessels, valvular atresias, and coarctation of the aorta (Fontana and Edwards, 1962), all of which are quite uncommon in cats. If, however, cats received the same medical attention afforded human neonates and infants, the incidence of various anomalies, especially serious anomalies associated with early mortality, might also be quite similar. The only other species to receive detailed study in this regard is the dog. The most common cardiovascular anomalies in dogs are PDA, pulmonary stenosis, aortic stenosis, persistent right aortic arch, and VSD (Patterson, 1968). Large-scale studies have not been reported on the occurrence of various defects in other species, but commonly reported anomalies include VSD in chickens (Siller, 1958) and subaortic stenosis in swine (Emsbo, 1955).

*By Bernard C. Zook

**Table 18–13 Occurrence of Congenital Heart Defects in Cats**

| DEFECT | AMAH* | AMC† | OTHERS | TOTAL |
|---|---|---|---|---|
| Atrioventricular valve malformations | 8 | 37 | 3+ | 48 |
| Ventricular septal defects | 16 | 13 | 14 | 43 |
| Endocardial fibroelastosis | 14 | 7 | 12 | 33 |
| Patent ductus arteriosus | 7 | 7 | 18 | 32 |
| Aortic stenosis | 3 | 12 | 3 | 18 |
| Tetralogy of Fallot | 2 | 7 | 9 | 18 |
| Atrial septal defects | 7 | 2 | 4 | 13 |
| Common atrioventricular canal | 1 | 11 | 0 | 12 |
| Anomaly of vena cava or of other major veins | 0 | 1 | 11 | 12 |
| Persistent right aortic arch | 3 | 0 | 10 | 13 |
| Pulmonary stenosis | 1 | 2 | 7 | 10 |
| Pericardial sac defect | 2 | 3 | 3 | 8 |
| Double-outlet right ventricle | 1 | 1 | 5 | 7 |
| Truncus arteriosus | 0 | 2 | 1 | 3 |
| Ebstein's anomaly | 2 | 0 | 0 | 2 |
| Stenosis of common pulmonary vein | 2 | 0 | 0 | 2 |
| Taussig-Bing complex | 0 | 0 | 1 | 1 |
| Other | 5 | 1 | 6 | 12 |
| Total | 74 | 106 | 107+ | 287 |
| Percentage of admissions | 0.02 | 0.10 | — | — |
| Percentage of autopsies | 2.90 | 1.95 | — | — |

*AMAH = Angell Memorial Animal Hospital.
†AMC = The Animal Medical Center, NYC (Liu, 1977).

The causes of cardiovascular malformations are largely unknown. In humans, maternal infection with rubella virus and thalidomide taken during the first two months of pregnancy are the only certain causes. Thalidomide also induces a variety of cardiovascular defects in cats (Khera, 1975). The familial occurrence of certain defects is suggestive of hereditary transmission, but only 5 per cent of cases are clearly genetic. Both hereditary and environmental influences are suspected of contributing a share in many anomalies (Shaffer, 1975). The mechanism of genetic transmission is known for several cardiovascular defects in dogs. It seems probable, on the basis of knowledge gained in the excellent studies done of dogs (Patterson, 1968), that we will discover more genetically transmitted anomalies in the future.

Congenital cardiovascular defects are reported more commonly in Siamese cats than in other breeds (Liu, 1968; Severin, 1967; van der Linde–Sipman et al., 1973; Zook, 1974). A familial occurrence of aortic stenosis and PDA (Severin, 1967), EFE (Severin, 1967; van der Linde–Sipman et al., 1973; Zook, 1974), and atrioventricular valve malformations (Wilkinson, 1967) is reported in the Siamese breed. At the AMAH, 9 of 14 cats with EFE were Siamese (some related), 3 were Burmese, and 2 were domestics. Two of six cats with mitral valve malformation (where breed was recorded) were Siamese, and two of three cats with aortic stenosis were Siamese. No excess of breed or coat color type was noted among other anomalies; however, it was observed that no Burmese cats were found to have heart defects other than EFE. The only feline cardiovascular defect known as yet to be genetically transmitted is EFE in Burmese cats (Paasch, 1979; Paasch and Zook, 1980; Zook et al., 1978, 1981), a breed distantly related to the Siamese.

Nearly twice as many male as female cats appear in the AMAH series. Males with malformed AV valves outnumber females 5:1, those with aortic stenosis 3:0, and those with EFE 9:5. The number of males seems excessive in relation to females for almost all defects. Human males are also more often affected with congenital cardiovascular disease than females (Fontana and Edwards, 1962), but no overall sex difference is seen in dogs (Patterson, 1968). The age at which cats develop signs varies primarily with the severity of the anomaly and its effect on circulation, rather than with the specific anatomic type of defect.

## Specific Defects and Their Signs

Clinical signs in kittens with congenital cardiovascular defects include retarded growth, poor condition, and decreased activity. Owners commonly report that their cats play little and tire easily with any exertion. They often report difficulty with breathing and may believe that their cat has a "cold." Sometimes owners even notice a palpable throbbing heartbeat. However, in a number of cases the first evidence of a congenital anomaly is detected by the clinician when the cat is presented for examination, vaccination, or castration. Cyanosis present at or shortly after birth is not often reported, perhaps because kittens so affected die soon after birth or are not thought "worth" the expense of professional care. Cyanosis is not always a sign of right-to-left shunt, as it may develop rapidly with severe respiratory embarrassment. The development of cyanosis months or years after birth usually indicates deficient oxygenation of blood due to heart failure–induced lung changes. Less often, a reversal of shunt occurs owing to the development of pulmonary hypertension.

Signs of congenital heart or vascular disease in cats are principally related to heart failure. Left-sided failure is characterized by dyspnea, rales, hydrothorax fluid line, radiographically enlarged left heart and elevated trachea, and electrocardiographic evidence of left ventricular hypertrophy. Right-sided heart failure is associated with distended pulsating jugular veins, ascites, hepatomegaly, radiographically enlarged right heart, and electrocardiographic right axis deviation. Shunts and anomalous valves cause murmurs. Cardiac catheterization and measurement of blood pressures and oxygen tension in various areas or angiocardiography may be necessary to establish the specific diagnosis and determine appropriate treatment.

**PRIMARY ENDOCARDIAL FIBROELASTOSIS.** This anomaly has been observed in a number of Siamese (Harpster, 1977; Liu, 1977; Severin, 1967; van der Linde–Sipman et al., 1973; Zook, 1974) and Burmese cats but is not commonly reported in other breeds or in domestic cats. The disease occurs with some frequency in humans but is uncommon in dogs. A family of Burmese cats are known to hereditarily transmit primary EFE. All offspring of a certain pair and most offspring of another pair are affected with the disease (Paasch, 1979; Paasch and Zook, 1980; Zook et al., 1978, 1981).

The clinical signs of this disease develop usually between three weeks and four months of age. Owners report

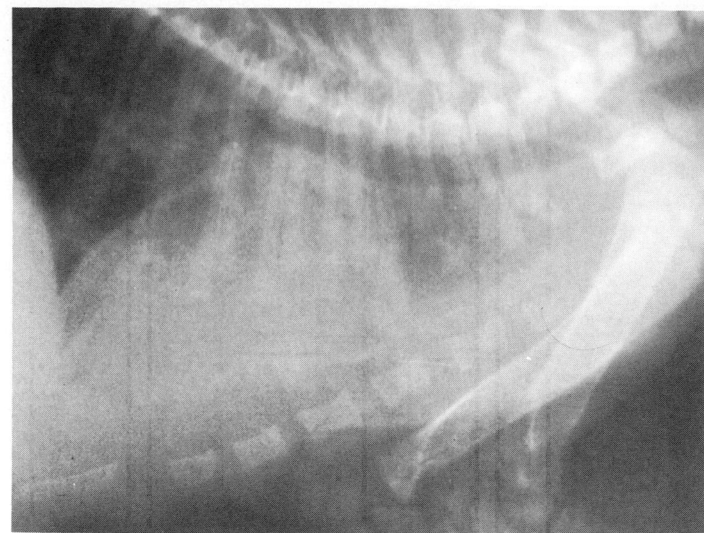

**Figure 18–59** Endocardial fibroelastosis, Burmese kitten. The heart is enlarged and the trachea elevated.

difficult respiration, sometimes open-mouth breathing, and often cyanosis apparent on exertion. Sudden death with few or no signs also occurs. Auscultation may reveal a systolic murmur due to mitral insufficiency, but gallop rhythms, tachycardia, and hydrothorax often make auscultation difficult. Phonocardiograms often reveal a diamond-shaped holosystolic murmur, especially late in the course. The heart, particularly the left atrium and left ventricle, is severely enlarged on radiography, and the trachea is usually elevated (Fig. 18–59). Electrocardiography (ECG) may reveal high R waves, altered T waves, and sometimes conduction disturbances. Angiocardiography would be expected to reveal a dilated left side of the heart with incomplete ventricular ejection and mitral regurgitation as the course advances. Systolic time intervals would probably be lengthened. The diagnosis of EFE is often made by exclusion. Once defects with shunts and aortic stenosis are excluded, the aforementioned signs in a two-week- to three-month-old with left heart failure are highly suggestive. Endocardial biopsy has been done in humans and may confirm the diagnosis. The course is generally short and the outcome fatal.

At autopsy, hydrothorax is usually present and is often of sufficient degree to cause atelectasis of the edematous lungs (Fig. 18–60). Hydropericardium is also common, but ascites is much less frequent. The heart is much enlarged, weighing 0.9 to 1.5 per cent of body weight. The left ventricle and to a lesser degree the left atrium are dilated, and the walls seem thin, although hypertrophy is evident by the heart's increased weight. Dilatation is often severe, resulting in dilatation of the mitral valve ring and mitral incompetence. The endocardium of the left side of the heart is diffusely thickened. Whereas one can clearly see the red-brown myocardium beneath normal endocardium, in EFE the endocardium becomes gray-white and opaque (Fig. 18–61). Some cases of EFE may not be recognizable grossly, and some diagnoses may even be overlooked microscopically (Williams and Emery, 1978). Less severe cases are being found in adults as well as neonates in both cats and man. It is suspected that the disease is underdiagnosed and may be much more common than generally thought (Williams and Emery, 1978; Zook et al., 1981).

Microscopically, the endocardium is thickened from 10 to 200 μm by fibrous and elastic tissue (Figs. 18–62 and 18–63). Dilated lymphatics and endocardial edema may be found in early cases, suggesting lymphatic obstruction as a possible pathogenetic mechanism (Paasch and Zook, 1980). Experimental ligation of lymphatics draining the heart has induced the disease (Miller et al., 1963; Paasch, 1979). Electron microscopic studies indicate that an ex-

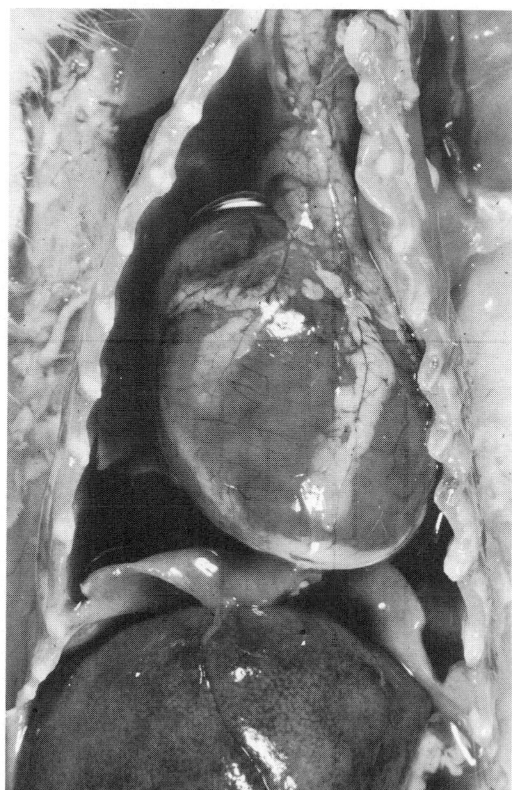

**Figure 18–60** Endocardial fibrosis, Siamese kitten. The enlarged heart nearly fills the thorax. Note the hydrothorax and atelectatic lungs.

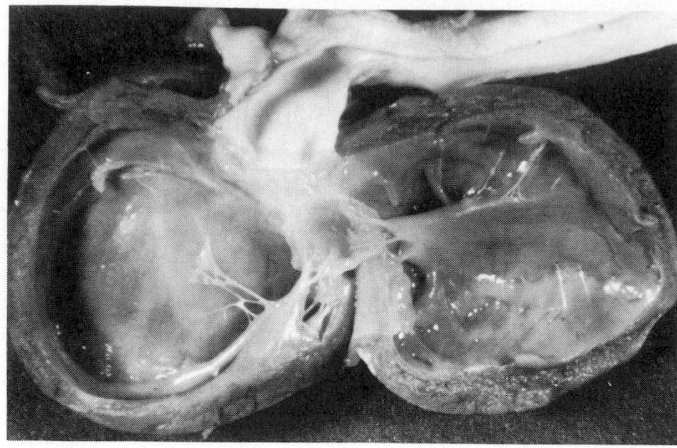

**Figure 18–61** Endocardial fibroelastosis. Marked dilatation and moderate thickening of the endocardium of the left ventricle.

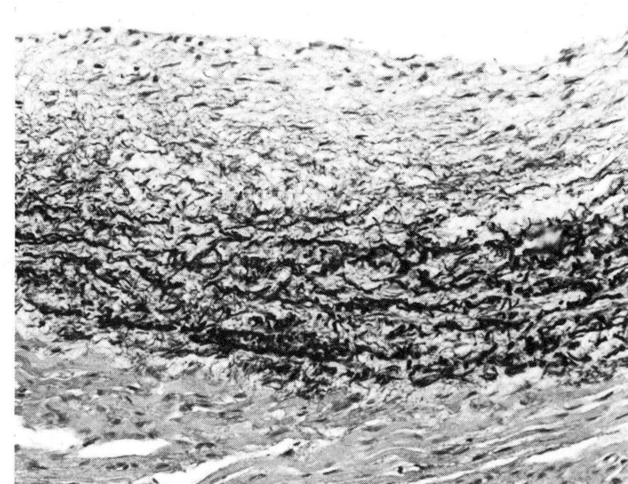

**Figure 18–62** Endocardial fibroelastosis, three-week-old Burmese. Microscopically, the endocardium is severely thickened by two layers of collagenous and elastic fibers (upper layer of thin fibers and lower layer of thick fibers).

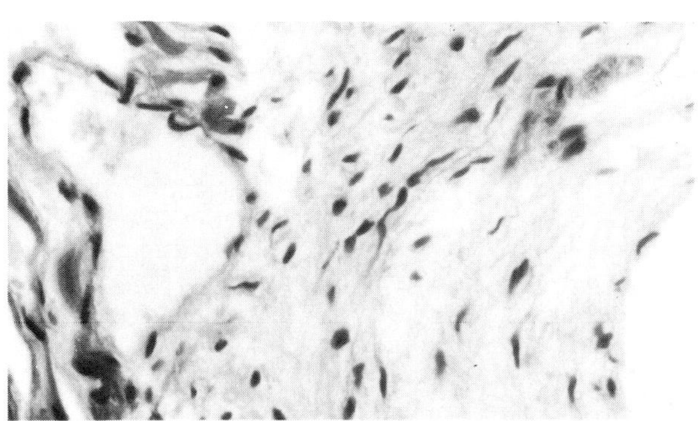

**Figure 18–63** Dilated lymphatics at the endomyocardial junction of cats with endocardial fibroelastosis support the pathogenetic role of lymphedema.

cessive number of fibroblasts in the endocardium lay down collagen fibers and later elastic fibers, which rapidly mature and organize into thicker bundles than are seen in age-matched controls. The dense connective tissue seems to limit the contractility of the left ventricle, and the endocardial connective tissue may surround Purkinje fibers, which subsequently atrophy, and may cause conduction disturbances. The myocardium is normal in primary EFE (Paasch and Zook, 1980).

Endocardial fibrosis develops as a condition secondary to certain viral myocarditides, fetal anoxia, and other cardiac defects such as anomalous origin of the left coronary artery (from the pulmonary artery) and coarctation of the aorta (Schryer and Karnauchow, 1974). In cats, secondary EFE may be associated with myocardiopathy (Liu, 1970) and has reportedly been associated with aortic stenosis (Eliot et al., 1958). It is not always possible to be certain whether some reported cases are of the primary or secondary type.

Treatment has rarely been successful in the past. More recent reports, however, indicate that the condition may not be severe in all human or feline patients (Paasch and Zook, 1980; Williams and Emery, 1978). In cats it appears that the condition actually begins morphologically soon after birth. It may be possible to arrest the development of the disease process if lymphedema is an inciting cause and the treatment is early enough. It must be kept in mind that survivors enhance the possibility of hereditary propagation of the defect unless affected cats are rendered sterile.

**PATENT DUCTUS ARTERIOSUS.** The ductus arteriosus is a vessel that connects the pulmonary trunk and aorta in the fetus and allows oxygenated blood to bypass the nonfunctional lungs. Persistence of the duct is a common anomaly in many species. A female sex predilection observed with PDA in dogs and man (Patterson, 1968; Zook, 1974) is not evident in cats. There may be a slightly higher occurrence in the Siamese breed. The onset of signs varies from one month to five years of age. Two major anatomic types occur. Most often the ductus is relatively small, and owing to the higher pressure in the aorta the vessel shunts blood during both systole and diastole into the pulmonary artery, producing a palpable thrill in the pulmonic area and a continuous, "machinery" murmur (Figs. 18–64 and 18–65).

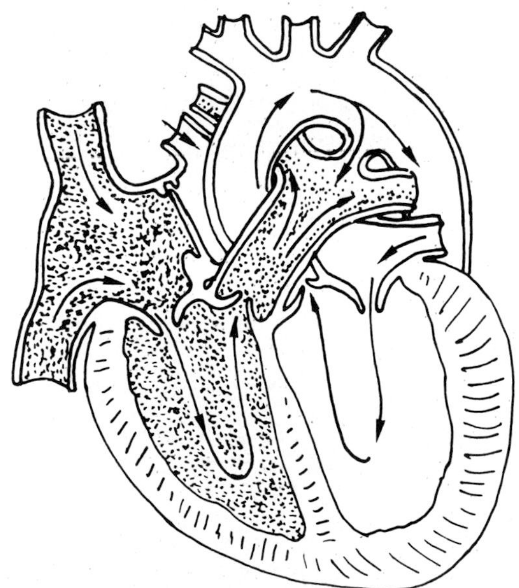

**Figure 18–64** Most cases of patent ductus arteriosus in cats are characterized by a small ductus with predominantly left-sided heart involvement.

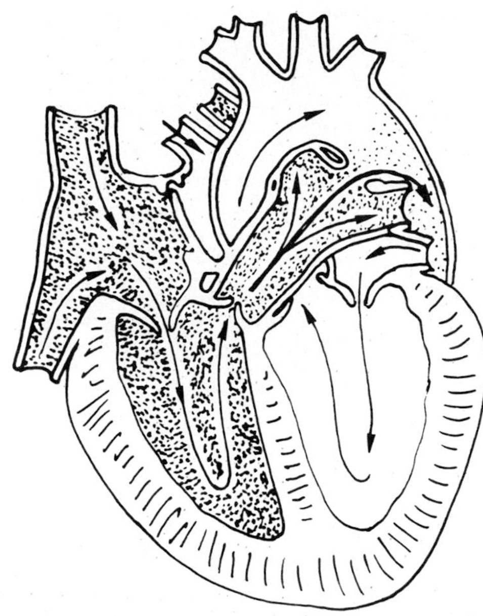

**Figure 18–65** Some cats with patent ductus arteriosus have a large ductus and pulmonary hypertension, causing a right-to-left shunt with weakness and cyanosis in the caudal parts of the body.

There is usually dilatation of the aorta and sometimes of the pulmonary artery caused by turbulence of blood flow, and jet lesions often develop in the pulmonary artery where blood strikes its wall, predisposing that vessel to infection and thrombosis. The short-circuiting of blood through the lungs causes a volume overload that results in dilatation of the left side of the heart and sometimes of the mitral valve ring, causing mitral incompetence. To maintain the systemic circulation the left ventricle must pump an increased volume of blood, causing an excess workload that induces left ventricular hypertrophy and eventually left-sided heart failure. Dyspnea and a characteristic "bounding" pulse are usually present. Radiographic features include enlarged pulmonary vascular markings, enlarged heart, and elevated trachea. The ECG is usually indicative of left ventricular enlargement. The PDA is demonstrated angiocardiographically by injection of contrast medium into the left ventricle or ascending aorta. Uncommonly, pulmonary hypertension develops with time and induces a reversal of the shunt with cyanosis in the caudal portions of the body.

In the other anatomic form of PDA, occurring in about 15 to 20 per cent of cases, the ductus is very large, about equal in size to the ascending aorta. Associated with this anomaly are right ventricular hypertrophy and signs of right-sided heart failure. The pulmonary arterioles are constricted much as they are in the normal fetus. Associated with persistence of the fetal pulmonary vasculature is pulmonary hypertension, causing the shunt to be intermittent (bidirectional) or right-to-left, usually with a systolic murmur. The flow of partially unoxygenated blood from the pulmonary artery into the aorta occurs distal to the arteries supplying the cranial part of the body, so no cyanosis occurs in the head, but weakness occurs in the hind legs with exercise and cyanosis may be evident in the claws (Fig. 18–66). Other possible features are syncope and polycythemia. The increased resistance to pulmonary blood flow causes right ventricular hypertrophy with associated radiographic and electrocardiographic findings. Similar anatomic forms of PDA occur in dogs (Zook, 1974).

Ligation of the ductus arteriosus is a common surgical procedure in man and dogs and has been carried out in cats (Cohen et al., 1975; Jeraj et al., 1978; Harpster, 1977; Jones and Buchanan, 1981). Surgical treatment should be undertaken only if angiocardiography reveals the shunt is left-to-right and no other cardiac defects for which the PDA may be life-sustaining are present. Ductal ligation should be performed early to prevent left heart failure or possible development of pulmonary hypertension.

**VENTRICULAR SEPTAL DEFECT (VSD).** This anomaly is common in many species including cats. The defect is nearly always high in the membranous portion of the interventricular septum just distal to the left aortic semilunar valve (Fig. 18–67) but may involve any part of the muscular septum. The VSD is a part of a number of complex anomalies including tetralogy of Fallot, common AV canal, double outlet right ventricle, truncus arteriosus, and Taussig-Bing complex and is often associated with other defects such as pulmonary stenosis. Occurring as an isolated defect, the size of the defect and thus the shunt of blood from left to right is directly related to clinical effects. A small VSD may induce a loud, crescendo-decrescendo systolic murmur but causes little circulatory disturbance. A large defect, on the other hand, may force the left ventricle to pump a greater volume of blood (the required aortic flow plus the "lost" volume shunted to the right ventricle). This leads to left ventricular dilatation (to hold the increased volume of blood) and hypertrophy, as increased work is required to pump this larger than usual volume (Fig. 18–68). The right ventricle and pulmonary arteries often dilate somewhat, since they receive excess blood. Thoracic radiographs and an ECG may be normal or show enlargement of both atria and ventricles. Demonstration of the defect may be possible by selective angiocardiography or echocardiography.

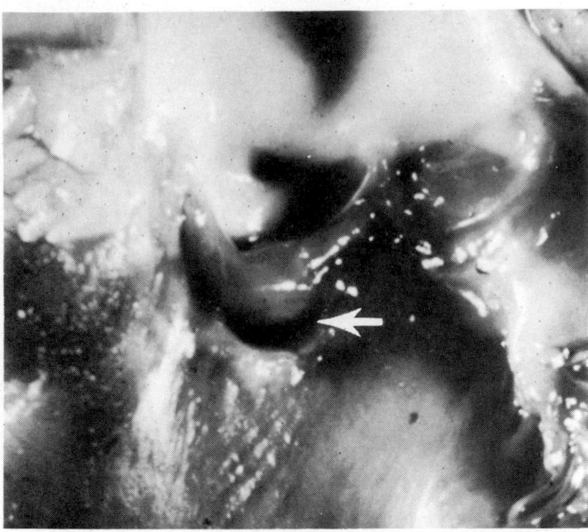

**Figure 18–67** Interventricular septal defects, such as this small one, are usually located high in the membranous part of the septum just beneath the left cusp of the aortic valve of cats.

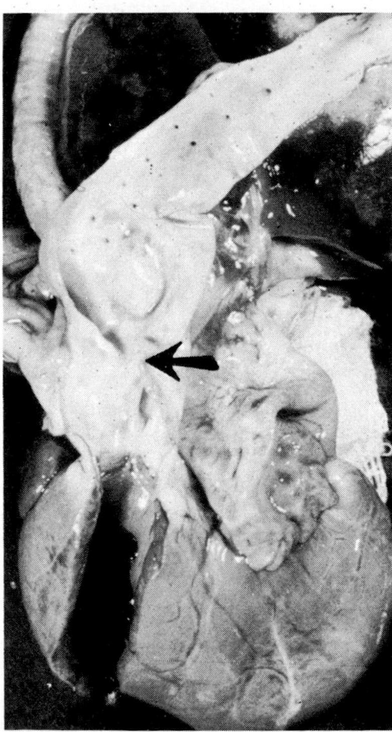

**Figure 18–66** The heart from a two and a half year old cat has a ductus (arrows) that is open and is so large that in this photograph it seems to continue the pulmonary artery into the aorta. Note the aneurysm of the aorta.

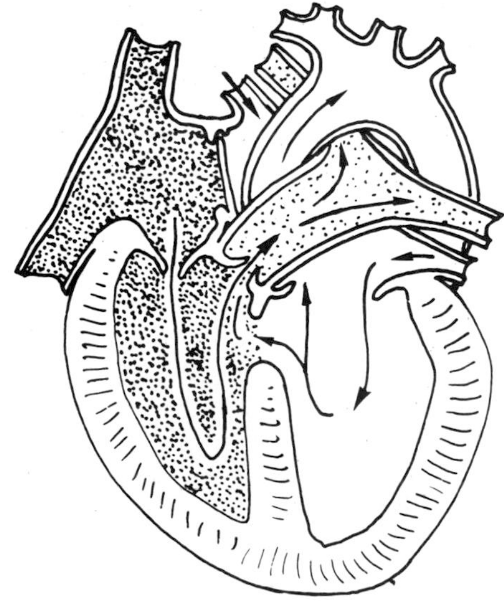

**Figure 18–68** Ventricular septal defects usually cause a left-to-right shunt.

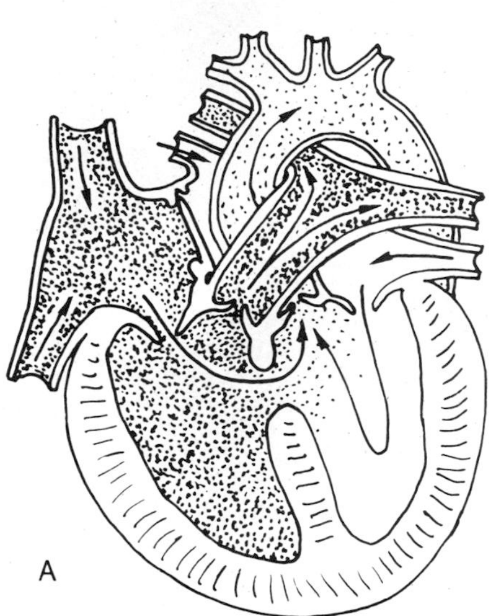


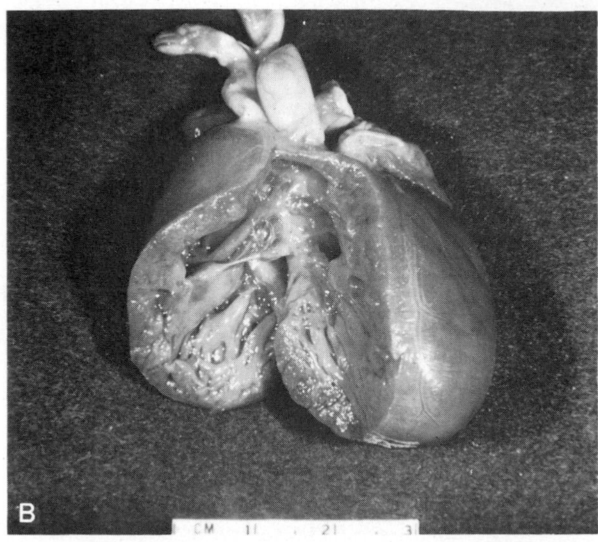


**Figure 18–69** *A*, Excess blood flow to the lungs via a ventricular septal defect may be associated with increased pulmonary vascular resistance and pulmonary hypertension causing right-to-left shunt with late-developing cyanosis. *B*, Eisenmenger's complex, eight-week-old male domestic cat. Note the septal defect and tremendous hypertrophy of the right ventricular wall.

Pulmonary vascular constriction, which may or may not develop as a result of excessive pulmonary blood flow, may induce right ventricular hypertrophy (Fig. 18–69). This complication, sometimes referred to as Eisenmenger's complex or syndrome, is a reason for early surgical repair of VSD in humans, as is also the prevention of left-sided failure. Spontaneous closure of VSD is apparently quite common in humans (Shaffer, 1975). We have observed a number of small interventricular defects occluded by a thin membrane in otherwise normal feline hearts.

Pulmonary artery banding has been used successfully in the cat to decrease pulmonary artery outflow resulting from VSD (Eyster et al., 1977b; Mann et al., 1971). Congestive heart failure may respond to medical treatment.

**AORTIC AND PULMONIC STENOSIS.** Aortic stenosis constricts the left ventricular outflow, and the severity of clinical signs is directly related to the degree of obstruction. Obstruction occurs in the ascending aorta just above the aortic valve (supravalvular) (Fig. 18–70) (Liu, 1968) or involves the valve cusps (valvular), or a constricting fibrous ring may be located just below the valve (subaortic) (Fig. 18–71) (Severin, 1967). The stenosis forces the left ventricle to perform excess work, and like any muscle that must work hard, the left ventricle hypertrophies. The left ventricular chamber does not dilate (there is no requirement to pump excess blood) until ventricular failure increases end-diastolic volume. The ascending aorta may develop a radiographically recognizable poststenotic dilatation (a fusiform aneurysm) as a result of turbulent blood flow. There may be a prominent precordial thrill, sometimes extending into the carotid arteries. Ejection murmur heard in the aortic-pulmonic area and signs of left heart failure are common.

Pulmonic stenosis causes similar effects in the right ventricle with poststenotic dilatation of the pulmonary artery and signs of right heart failure.

Surgical correction of life-threatening stenosis of either valve requires specialized resources not ordinarily available.

**TETRALOGY OF FALLOT.** The principal anomaly in this complex is pulmonary stenosis that constricts the pulmonary outflow tract. The membranous septum cannot join the aortic valve ring because the aorta is located too far to the right (dextroposition), thus overriding the septum, and right ventricular hypertrophy is secondary to pulmonary stenosis. The high right ventricular pressure also maintains patency of the VSD as it shunts unoxygenated blood into the left ventricle (Fig. 18–72). This defect is the most common cause of cyanosis from birth in cats, as well as in most other species, and is typically associated with polycythemia and stunted growth (Bolton et al., 1972; Kirby and Gillick, 1974). The retinal vessels may be distended and tortuous (see the chapter on the eye).

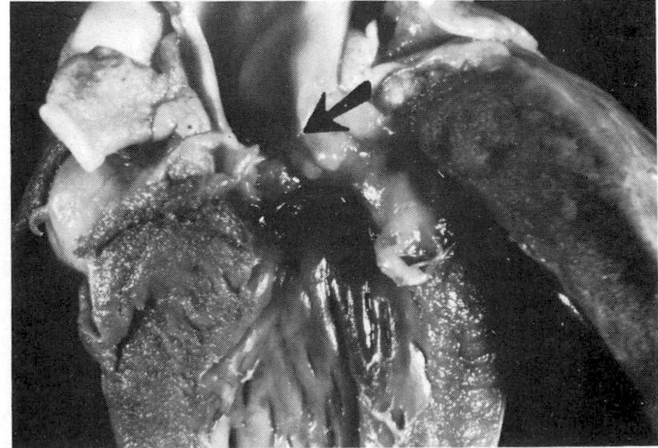

**Figure 18–70** Supravalvular aortic stenosis is seen as a constriction (arrow) just above the aortic valve.

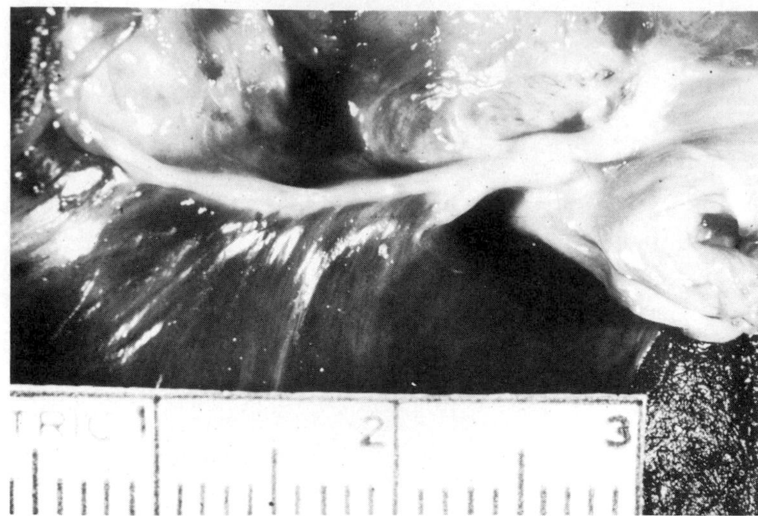

**Figure 18–71** Subaortic stenosis is caused by a fibrous band just beneath the aortic valve.

A systolic thrill and a systolic murmur are due to the pulmonic stenosis. Characteristic radiographic findings are pronounced right ventricular enlargement, pulmonary artery hypoplasia, and decreased pulmonary vascularity. The ECG reveals right axis deviation. Angiocardiography may facilitate a definitive diagnosis.

Treatment of a severely affected animal would require surgical correction of both the VSD and the pulmonic stenosis. Palliation may be attempted by creation of a shunt (Bush et al., 1972; Miller et al., 1985).

Severe pulmonary stenosis with VSD or atrial septal defect (ASD) may cause signs nearly identical to those of tetralogy of Fallot.

**ATRIOVENTRICULAR VALVE DEFECTS.** Anomalies of the mitral and tricuspid valves are not commonly reported in any species except, it seems, in cats in the northeast United States (Liu, 1977). Alterations in valves include shortened, thickened, and misshapen valve leaflets and chordae tendineae; muscular leaflets; and abnormal papillary muscles. Valves often appear "tied-down," and valve rings are dilated and usually incompetent (Fig. 18–73). Signs correspond to the severity of the valvular incompetency and to the side of the heart most affected.

**COMMON ATRIOVENTRICULAR CANAL.** In this anomaly a low ASD and a high VSD combine to form a single passageway through which all chambers communicate (Bolton and Liu, 1977; Liu, 1977; Liu and Ettinger, 1968). The mitral valve is continuous with the tricuspid valve through the large septal defect (Figs. 18–74 and 18–75). This endocardial cushion defect results from arrested development quite early in the formation of the heart. Signs of heart failure occur at an early age. Loud systolic murmur and dyspnea are common (Harpster, 1977). Conduction disturbances, especially heart block, may occur as a result of interruption of the conduction fibers by the septal defect. In radiographs the heart may appear normal or enlarged. Dye injected into the area of the defect outlines all chambers simultaneously (Fox et al., 1983).

**ATRIAL SEPTAL DEFECTS (ASD).** In the formation of the interatrial septum, a hole (the foramen primum) in the cranioventral portion of the septum primum closes as a second opening (the ostium secundum) opens in the mid-dorsal region. A second interatrial septum, the septum secundum, forms just to the right of, and fuses with, the first septum, leaving an oblique passage (the foramen ovale) through to the ostium secundum. A remnant of the septum primum forms the valve of the foramen ovale on the left side; this closes after birth as pressure on the left exceeds that on the right. Any anomaly associated with high pressure in the right atrium, e.g., tricuspid insufficiency, causing blood to flow through the foramen ovale from right to left after birth will tend to keep the valve from sealing, causing a patent foramen ovale. A defect in the fossa ovalis region where no valve remnants remain has been called a persistent ostium secundum. Less often the ostium primum does not close, leaving a persistent foramen primum. The clinical effect of any of these types of ASD is similar to that of a VSD

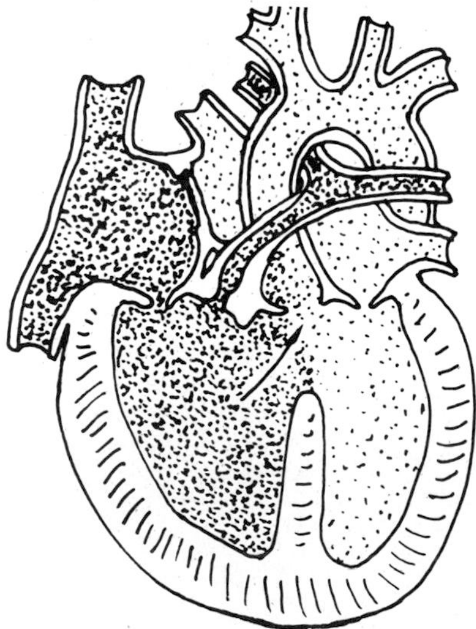

**Figure 18–72** Tetralogy of Fallot is characterized by pulmonary stenosis, right ventricular hypertrophy, ventricular septal defect, overriding aorta, and cyanosis from birth.

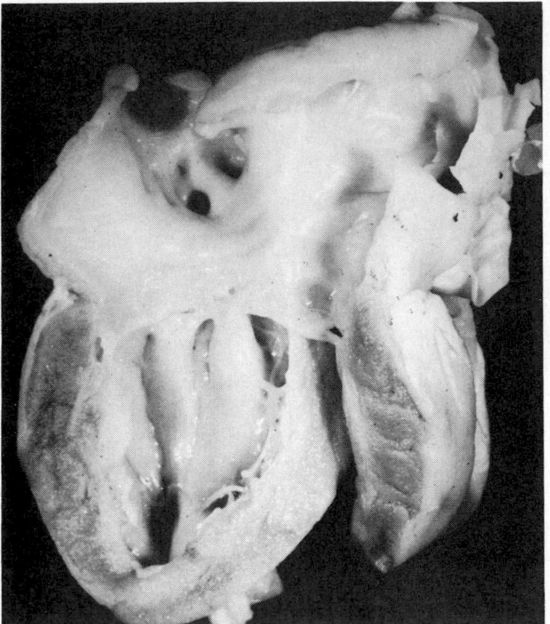

**Figure 18–73** Atrioventricular valve malformations, as in the mitral valve of this Siamese, have thickened valves improperly attached to irregular papillary muscles, rendering them incompetent. Note the dilated left atrium.

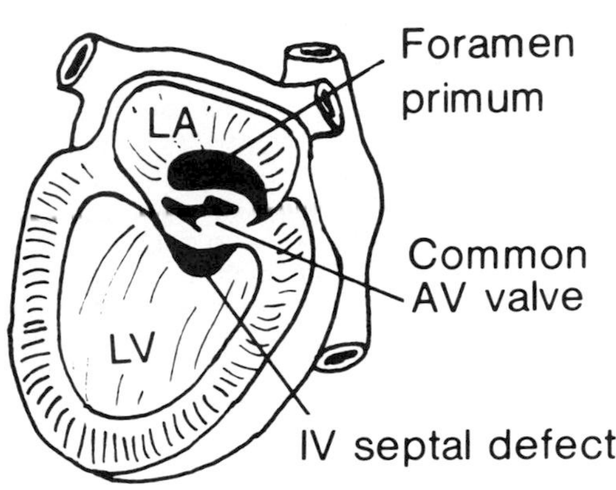


**Figure 18–74** Atrioventricular canal consists of a low atrial septal defect (foramen primum) and high ventricular septal defect with common atrioventricular valve.

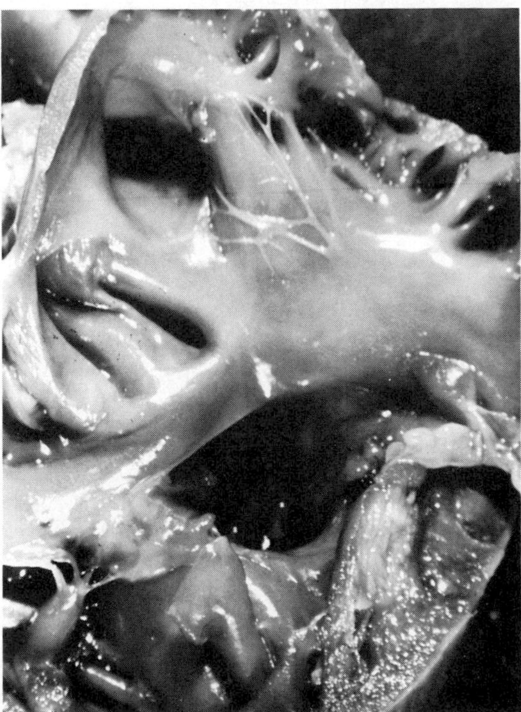

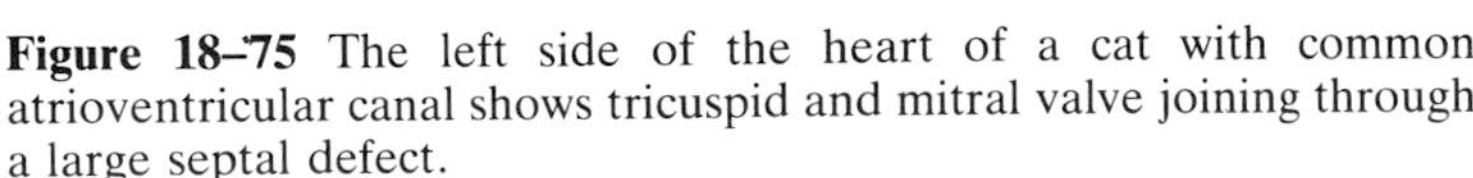

**Figure 18–75** The left side of the heart of a cat with common atrioventricular canal shows tricuspid and mitral valve joining through a large septal defect.

and depends largely on the size of the defect and shunt and on any associated anomalies. In addition, the foramen primum may by its location interrupt the conduction system or involve the mitral valve.

**COR TRIATRIATUM.** In this rare anomaly, reported in a six-month-old domestic cat with pulmonary congestion (Gordon et al., 1982), the pulmonary veins enter an accessory left atrial chamber caudal to the true left atrium. The two chambers communicate through an opening, which, if sufficiently narrow, obstructs pulmonary venous return. The result is pulmonary arterial hypertension and right ventricular hypertrophy. Radiographs and an ECG in this case gave evidence of right ventricular and left atrial enlargement.

**UHL'S ANOMALY.** Congenital hypoplasia of the myocardium of the right ventricle has been reported in the cat (Atwell, 1980). The decreased output of the right side of the heart results in severe right-sided decompensation.

**SITUS INVERSUS.** This rare anomaly was an incidental finding in a cat destroyed for urolithiasis (Vogel, 1979). The thoracic and abdominal viscera were a mirror image of the normal position.

**PERICARDIAL ANOMALIES.** Partial or complete absence of the pericardium is an occasional incidental finding (e.g., Walker and Zessman, 1952). Peritoneopericardial diaphragmatic hernia is sometimes asymptomatic, but cardiac function can be impaired if abdominal viscera are displaced within the pericardial sac. Strangulation of a liver lobe or of small intestine is a life-threatening complication. Pericardial anomalies are discussed together with acquired pericardial disorders later in this chapter.

**PERSISTENT RIGHT AORTIC ARCH.** One of the more frequent anomalies, this is the result of development and formation of the aorta by the right fourth embryonic arch instead of its left counterpart. The aorta passes to the right of the trachea and esophagus, while the pulmonary trunk and ductus arteriosus follow their normal course over the left side of the trachea and esophagus, and the ductus joins the aorta (de Lahunta and Habel, 1986). The resulting vascular ring does not impair circulation, but in time the esophagus becomes constricted and will not allow solid food to pass, and projectile vomiting results. Diagnosis is confirmed by contrast radiography (Fig. 18–76). Surgical transection of the ductus arteriosus (ligamentum arteriosum) may be curative (Lawther, 1970; Reed and Bonasch, 1962; Uhrich, 1963; Wheaton et al., 1984).

Esophageal obstruction has also been associated with a double aortic arch (van der Linde–Sipman et al., 1973) and a vascular ring formed by a left aortic arch, right ligamentum arteriosum, and part of the right dorsal aorta (van der Linde–Sipman, 1981). In a cat at AMAH, the esophagus was obstructed by a retroesophageal right subclavian artery. The obstruction was relieved surgically.

**OTHER VASCULAR ANOMALIES.** Transposition of the great arteries has been reported (e.g., Straw et al., 1985); transposition of the great vessels has also been induced by thalidomide (Khera, 1975).

Double-outlet right ventricle, described in a kitten, was successfully repaired with an aortic homograft (Northway, 1979).

Arteriovenous fistulae, shunts between an artery and a vein, cause circulatory congestion. A fistula of the aorta and caudal vena cava was described as causing congestive heart failure (Bolton et al., 1976), and an intrahepatic arteriovenous communication resulted in ascites (Legendre et al., 1976). Arteriovenous fistulae are discussed later in this chapter among causes of hyperkinetic heart disease.

Venous anomalies are often reported in the anatomic literature as incidental findings in dissections or are asymptomatic lesions found at autopsy. Rarely they may be symptomatic and even lethal. An eight-month-old Siamese that experienced sudden distress and died was found at autopsy at AMAH to have stenosis of a common pulmonary vein; associated findings were dilatation of the right ventricle and of the right atrium. Persistent left cranial vena cava has been reported (Eales, 1938; Zeiner, 1957) and in one cat was associated with tetralogy of Fallot and retinal detachment (Lombard and Twichell, 1978).

Duplication of the caudal vena cava is a common anomaly encountered in dissections and incidentally at autopsy (e.g., Tisseur and Barone, 1944). After persistent patent ductus arteriosus it is the most frequently observed vascular anomaly not directly involving the heart among cats coming to autopsy at AMAH. In a seven-year-old domestic spayed female followed at AMAH for over a year, it proved to be a life-threatening lesion. When first presented the cat wobbled on its hind legs but eventually dragged them. Three months later the muscles of the hind legs were greatly swollen and warm, and the cat could move them only slightly. Sores were present on the dorsal surface of the tail at the tip. Almost a year later the cat underwent surgery for relief of a fecal impaction. When the abdomen was clipped for surgery, distended vessels and subcutaneous edema were evident. An enlarged and tortuous double vena cava extended forward to within 2 cm of the diaphragm, where the two parts were united in a stricture so severe that the obstructed flow of blood could be heard. An attempt was made to free the vessel of constricting fibrous tissue, but the cat did not survive the surgery.

Congenital portosystemic shunts have been reported in a few cats (e.g., Gandolfi, 1984; Levesque et al., 1982; Rothuizen et al., 1982; Vulgamott et al., 1981). Signs included stunting, aggression, ataxia, and ptyalism. Blood ammonia is elevated, and there may be ammonium biurate crystals in the urine.

Instances of portal vein anomalies are on record at AMAH. A portacaval shunt in a four-month-old male domestic shorthair was associated with a small liver, ascites, and distended abdominal veins. A five-year-old neutered male Persian with bizarre behavior that included attacks on its owner proved at autopsy to have a portal shunt that emptied ultimately into the cranial thoracic vena cava. A six-month-old domestic shorthair that had portal vein hypoplasia diagnosed by liver biopsy manifested intermittent blindness, hyperesthesia, tremors, and chewing-type seizures attributed to hepatic encephalopathy. In a five-year-old neutered male Persian with a diaphragmatic peritoneopericardial hernia, the portal vein was hypoplastic in the three hypoplastic liver lobes that were incarcerated within the hernial sac.

## ACQUIRED CARDIAC DISEASE*

Less than 20 years ago many veterinary school graduates entered practice with the concept that heart disease did

*By Neil K. Harpster.

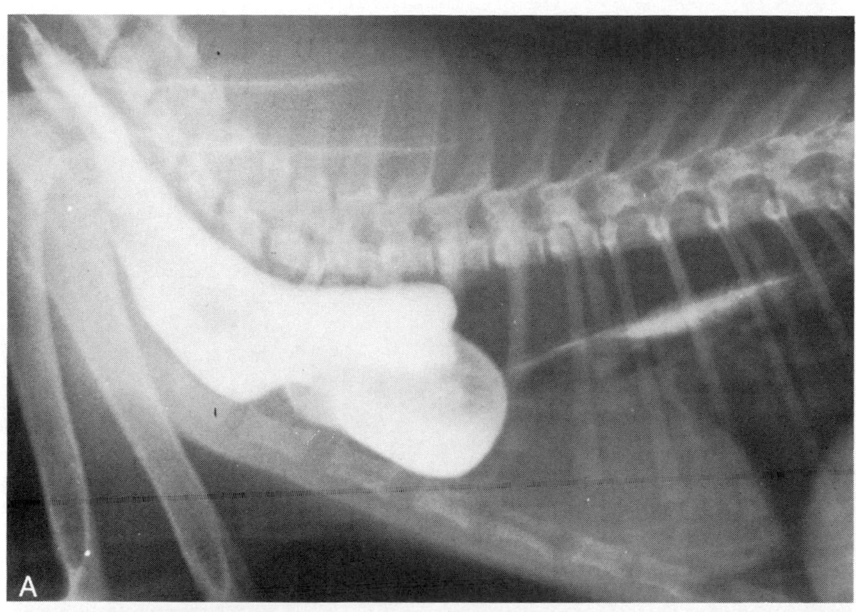


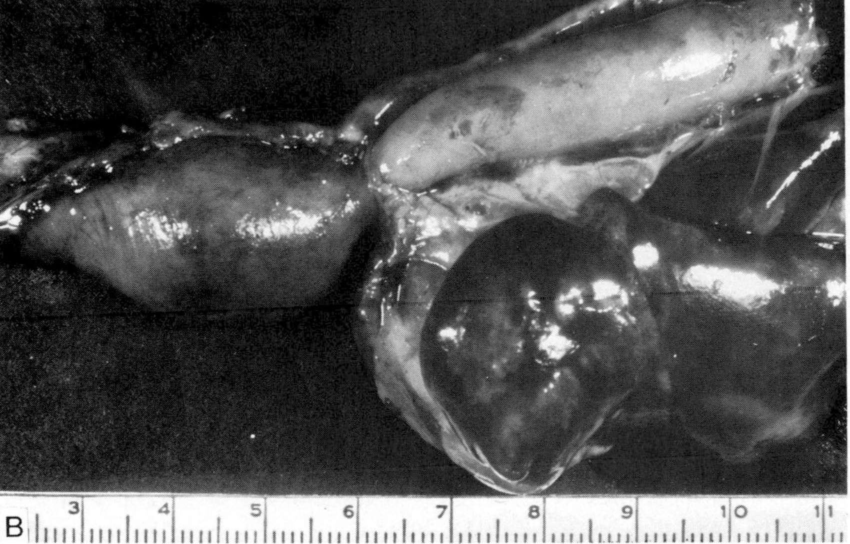


**Figure 18–76** *A*, A persistent right aortic arch constricts the esophagus at the base of the heart, permitting only a small amount of barium to pass. The esophagus cranial to the constriction is dilated. *B*, In the same three-month-old female domestic longhair, the ligamentum arteriosum was excised at surgery, but a thin band of fascia persisted, producing a moderate constriction over the dorsal aspect of the esophagus. The dilated portion of the esophagus measured about 3.0 cm in diameter. The kitten failed to recover from anesthesia.

not exist in cats, except for a low incidence of congenital cardiovascular anomalies. Now, however, this concept is no longer acceptable as the number of references at the conclusion of this chapter will attest. Whether our mentors of two decades ago were correct or whether acquired heart disease has become more common is not easily resolved. The latter explanation seems by far the stronger. At the present time the incidence of feline cardiovascular disease in a busy referral small animal practice nearly approximates that seen in dogs. If this trend continues, it is foreseeable that before the end of this decade acquired heart disease may become as commonplace as the upper respiratory diseases and urolithiasis in our feline patients.

Table 18–14 summarizes the various types of acquired heart disease currently recognized in the cat. It is acknowledged that this list is far from complete and will need revision in the future. The discussion that follows will deal with the conditions listed and our currently accepted, somewhat limited knowledge of these subjects.

## Primary Myocardial Disease

For over a decade attention has been focused on the primary myocardial diseases owing to a relative or absolute increase in the number of cats affected. Primary myocardial disease is defined as a primary disorder of the heart muscle (myocardium). However, it is not unusual for the endocardium and epicardium to be secondarily involved. It has been recommended that the term cardiomyopathy be limited to primary myocardial diseases of undetermined origin (Oakley, 1974; Schlant, 1972).

**ENDOMYOCARDITIS.** The term endomyocarditis (EM) should be reserved for heart disease in the cat characterized by diffuse mononuclear and polymorphonuclear inflammation of the endocardium and myocardium unassociated with bacteria or other identifiable infectious agents. Endomyocarditis is a histopathologic diagnosis and is not easily recognized in the living cat. On the evidence of microscopic changes it is considered to result from viral infection (Tilley, 1977), but this etiology has yet to be proved.

**Table 18–14 Types of Acquired Cardiac Disease Recognized in the Domestic Cat**

| |
|---|
| **PRIMARY MYOCARDIAL DISEASE** |
| Endomyocarditis |
| Cardiomyopathy |
| Hypertrophic |
| Intermediate (restrictive) |
| Dilatative |
| Excessive left ventricular moderator bands |
| **SECONDARY MYOCARDIAL DISEASE** |
| (See Table 18–18) |
| **VALVULAR HEART DISEASE** |
| Acquired valvular heart disease |
| Bacterial endocarditis |
| **HYPERKINETIC HEART DISEASE** |
| Anemia, chronic |
| Hyperthyroidism |
| Arteriovenous fistula |
| **PULMONARY HEART DISEASE** |
| Congenital cardiovascular shunts |
| Dirofilariasis |
| Medial hypertrophy of the pulmonary arteries |
| **OTHER HEART DISEASE** |
| Cardiac arrhythmias |
| Pericardial disorders |

In the clinical setting, endomyocarditis affects cats at a younger average age than with any of the recognized forms of cardiomyopathy. Liu (1977) reported an average age of 2.6 years (range 2.5 months to 8 years) in a group of 25 cats. The usual clinical signs result from fairly acute left-sided heart failure, which may be preceded by a brief period of lethargy and weight loss. By the time affected cats are presented for veterinary attention, difficulty in breathing is readily apparent to the owner and is often the primary reason for presentation.

In addition to polypnea, dyspnea, and fine moist inspiratory rales, systolic heart murmurs over the left or right apex, diastolic gallop rhythms, arrhythmias, or combinations of these abnormalities are frequently auscultated. Apical murmurs and arrhythmias predominate. In thoracic radiographs taken during active heart failure, the cardiac silhouette is usually partly obliterated by superimposed pulmonary edema, which may be diffuse or limited to a perihilar and dorsal caudal lobe position. Cardiac enlargement is associated with mild tracheal elevation, an increased area of cardiosternal contact, and mild left atrial enlargement. The liver often extends 2 to 4 cm behind the costal arch. Electrocardiographically, cardiac arrhythmias and conduction disturbances are frequent, with ventricular premature beats and repetitive ventricular tachyarrhythmias predominating.

A diagnosis of endomyocarditis is not easily made. In fact, there are no clearly defined diagnostic tests or procedures that permit indisputable differentiation between EM and feline hypertrophic cardiomyopathy, including venous angiocardiography.

Gross post-mortem findings in EM reveal increased thickness of the left ventricular free wall and the interventricular septum, with some reduction in the left ventricular chamber dimensions. The left atrium may be mildly dilated and thick-walled. Focal or diffuse subendocardial hemorrhages are common in the left ventricle. In some cats, a light tan fibrinous material adheres to various sites over the left ventricular endocardium. Microscopically, the earliest findings are muscle fiber degeneration and necrosis with extravasation of red blood cells and a prominent focal or diffuse cellular infiltration consisting of neutrophils, plasma cells, and macrophages. In areas of endocardial involvement, the normal surface is destroyed and replaced by necrotic tissue with cellular debris and fibrin deposition. In more advanced lesions the endocardium and myocardium are replaced by granulation tissue associated with a predominance of mononuclear cells and eventually mature fibrous tissue.

The management of cats with EM is poorly defined, mainly because of the difficulty in establishing the diagnosis in the living cat. In addition, relatively few cats with EM have been studied. My approach has been to control the heart failure initially with diuretics and once this is accomplished, to perform nonselective angiocardiography. As the majority of cats with EM have a thickened left ventricular free wall and a large ejection fraction, this study alone does not permit differentiation between EM and hypertrophic cardiomyopathy. Nonetheless, I have used propranolol (Inderal) with some success (2.5 to 5.0

mg b.i.d. or t.i.d.). Propranolol offers the potential benefits of improved left ventricular filling by slowing the heart rate (i.e., it prolongs left ventricular filling time) and of control of both supraventricular and ventricular arrhythmias. Long-term management includes propranolol, diuretics in dosages to control fluid retention, and antithrombotic agents (e.g., aspirin or aspirin-Maalox combinations at 2½ grains every three days).

The long-term prognosis for cats with EM is difficult to project because of the uncertainty of the diagnosis and our limited experience in treating cats with proven disease. Complications encountered during attempted management are sudden death due presumably to fatal tachyarrhythmias and thromboembolism.

It should be noted that the incidence of endomyocarditis has gradually diminished over recent years to a point at which it no longer appears to occur. The reason for this is no clearer than a cause for the disease itself. One possibility is that EM may represent an active, acute process that is recognized weeks, months, or even years later as restrictive cardiomyopathy.

**CARDIOMYOPATHY.** Cardiomyopathy is a primary disorder of the myocardium that alters structure or function, or both. Secondary focal involvement of the endocardium and epicardium is not unusual owing to extension of the underlying myocardial process. Since the term cardiomyopathy denotes a condition of undetermined cause, it is diagnosed on the basis of characteristic structural and functional abnormalities (Oakley, 1974). Three distinct forms are recognized: (1) hypertrophic (characterized by ventricular hypertrophy without dilatation, failure of diastolic compliance, or resistance to ventricular filling); (2) restrictive or obliterative (distinguished by ventricular dilatation without compensatory hypertrophy and typically associated with substantial deposition of endocardial and subendocardial fibrosis; primary failure of diastolic filling, although alterations in systolic performance may also be present); (3) dilatative (characterized by ventricular dilatation with some compensatory hypertrophy; failure of systolic pump function). In hypertrophic cardiomyopathy the hypertrophy is a primary abnormality and does not occur secondary to outflow obstruction or increased afterload (i.e., the pressure against which the ventricle must empty). Dilatative cardiomyopathy is the least distinct of the three forms, as ventricular dilatation with secondary hypertrophy can occur as a normal compensatory mechanism to a variety of cardiac disorders. The diagnosis must be one of exclusion.

Despite the extensive studies and literature reports that have focused on feline cardiomyopathy (FCM), little has been established regarding the cause of this disease in the majority of cats. A coronavirus has been suggested as being responsible for a dilatative-like disorder in FIP-positive cat colonies (Scott et al., 1979), although this is reported primarily in newborn and young kittens under the "kitten mortality complex" umbrella. The possibility that hypertrophic cardiomyopathy is an inherited condition in Persian cats has also been suggested (Tilley, 1977).

There is considerable overlapping of the clinical signs among the forms recognized. In brief, clinical manifestations are the result of cardiac arrhythmias, congestive heart failure (CHF), or arterial embolism. In a small group of cats, cardiomyopathy can be identified before the development of clinical signs, usually from auscultatory abnormalities (e.g., heart murmurs, arrhythmias, gallop rhythms). But a diagnosis of FCM cannot be made by the presence of auscultatory abnormalities alone. Further diagnostic procedures must be carried out in a logical sequence. Our current approach to the asymptomatic cat consists initially of a noninvasive cardiac study, including an electrocardiogram, thoracic radiographs, and laboratory tests (CBC, SMA profile, and urinalysis). If the results of these tests are normal, reevaluation in four to six months is recommended. If arrhythmias are present or if the heart (especially the left atrium) appears enlarged in thoracic radiographs, either echocardiography or nonselective angiocardiography is recommended. Treatment is determined by the form of the disease indicated by these studies. Left atrial enlargement is a particularly significant radiographic finding, for this implies chronic left ventricular filling abnormalities or chronic mitral valve insufficiency, or both.

As causes of signs in cats with symptomatic cardiomyopathy, congestive failure and embolism are of nearly equal frequency (Harpster, 1977a), although the incidence of each of these manifestations depends somewhat on the specific form of cardiomyopathy present. Congestive heart failure may occur as acute left-sided failure (with pulmonary edema) or biventricular failure (with pleural effusion and ascites). Auscultatory abnormalities frequently accompanying congestive failure include systolic or holosystolic murmurs over the left or right cardiac apex, or both (mitral area); diastolic gallop rhythms; cardiac arrhythmias; or combinations of these. Some degree of hepatomegaly is usual in both left-sided and biventricular failure.

The incidence of arterial embolism in FCM may approach 50 per cent at the time of initial presentation in some clinical surveys, although it is usually somewhat lower than this (Harpster, 1977a). Thromboembolism and its sequelae are also major concerns in the long-term management of these cats and significantly affect the long-term prognosis. The left auricular endocardium is the most frequent site of thrombus formation, most likely because of the combined effect of static blood flow due to left ventricular filling abnormalities and mitral valve incompetence and because of extension of myocardial lesions to the underlying endocardium. Far less often a thrombus develops on the left ventricular endocardium owing to stasis of blood flow or endocardial inflammation. Arterial embolism occurs when a thrombus breaks free from its site of origin in the left heart. (In rare instances, pulmonary embolism results from right-heart thrombus formation.) And while the emboli may be carried anywhere within the arterial circulation, the descending aorta, especially at its terminal bifurcation, is the most common site of occlusion. (At post-mortem, smaller emboli and subsequent infarction are frequently found in the renal and coronary circulations and less commonly in the celiac and superior mesenteric arteries. It is suspected that coronary artery embolic disease plays a significant role in the origin of cardiac arrhythmias, precipitation of heart failure, and occurrence of sudden death in some cats.) Hindlimb weakness, ataxia, paralysis, or combinations of these findings follow occlusion at the aortic bifurcation. Complete flaccid paralysis may develop within minutes accompanied by substantial pain and discomfort, coolness of the extremities, and increased firmness of the gastrocnemius muscles. When ischemia of the hindlimbs is severe, local spinal reflexes will be absent.

In affected cats, considerable discomfort may be present

on initial evaluation. Pain is particularly severe when aortic occlusion occurs at or proximal to the origin of the renal arteries, probably the result of renal or small bowel ischemia. Neurologic abnormalities of the hindlimbs are similar, notwithstanding the level of aortic occlusion. Confirmation of aortic occlusion is based on the absence of femoral pulses and cool, painless distal extremities. When the status of circulation to the hindlimbs is questionable owing to low cardiac output, evaluation of external iliac pulses by rectal examination is helpful. Lastly, nonselective angiocardiography, with the x-ray beam centered over the abdomen and radiographic exposure made at 10 to 15 seconds after injection of radiopaque dye, will confirm the presence of aortic occlusion and establish its position when the diagnosis is unclear by other methods (Fig. 18–57).

The severity of ischemia to the hindlimbs following aortic bifurcation occlusion is not due to the obstruction alone. It has been demonstrated experimentally that absence of collateral circulation via lumbar, epigastric, and urethral-umbilical arteries plays a significant role in the clinical syndrome (Butler, 1971; Schaub et al., 1976). The local release of vasoactive substances has been suggested as a cause for reduction in collateral blood flow. Five-hydroxytryptamine (serotonin) has been identified as the major vasoactive substance responsible (Butler, 1971).

For best management of cardiomyopathy it is important that the specific form of the disease be identified. The distinguishing clinical features of the three forms are outlined in Table 18–15.

**Hypertrophic Cardiomyopathy.** Hypertrophic cardiomyopathy (HCM) predominates in young to middle-aged male cats but occurs occasionally in young females and elderly males. The usual signs on initial presentation are those of acute left heart failure and arterial embolism. The incidence of embolism is greater in HCM than in the other forms, because restricted left ventricular filling predisposes to stasis of blood flow in the left atrium. Hemodynamic studies have demonstrated the elevated left ventricular end-diastolic pressures that occur in HCM (Lord et al., 1974). In addition to dyspnea and moist rales, systolic and holosystolic murmurs over the mitral valve area, diastolic gallop rhythms, and cardiac arrhythmias are common. Of these auscultatory abnormalities, heart murmurs are the most frequent. The heart rate is usually accelerated (i.e., > 200/min) even in the absence of cardiac arrhythmias.

Thoracic radiographs show mild to moderate cardio-

**Table 18–15 Distinguishing Clinical Features of the Three Forms of Cardiomyopathy Recognized in the Cat***

| CLINICAL FEATURES | HYPERTROPHIC (31)† | INTERMEDIATE (11)† | DILATATIVE (31)† |
|---|---|---|---|
| Average age (Range) | 4.86 (8 mo–14 yr) | 11.27 (7–19 yr) | 7.81 (5 mo–14 yr)‡ |
| M:F ratio (% males) | 6.75 (87.1) | 1.20 (54.5) | 0.72 (41.9) |
| Breed: No. (%) | | | |
| Domestic shorthair | 22 (71.0) | 7 (63.6) | 13 (41.9) |
| Domestic longhair | 9 (29.0) | 1 ( 9.1) | 5 (16.1) |
| Siamese | — | 1 ( 9.1) | 10 (32.3) |
| Burmese | — | — | 2 ( 6.4) |
| Persian | — | 2 (18.2) | 1 ( 3.2) |
| Clinical signs: No. (%) | | | |
| Dyspnea | 15 (48.4) | 7 (63.6) | 21 (67.7) |
| Arterial embolism | | | |
| At entry | 5 (16.1) | — | 4 (12.9) |
| Later complication | — | 1 ( 9.1) | 2 ( 6.5) |
| Syncope | — | — | 2 ( 6.5) |
| Lethargy/anorexia | 6 (19.4) | 2 (18.2) | 5 (16.1) |
| Abdominal enlargement | — | 2 (18.2) | — |
| Cough | 2 ( 6.5) | — | — |
| Asymptomatic | 3 ( 9.7) | — | — |
| Cardiovascular findings: No. (%) | | | |
| Apex murmur | | | |
| >Left apex | 13 (41.9) | 1 ( 9.1) | 7 (22.6) |
| >Right apex | 4 (12.9) | 1 ( 9.1) | 1 ( 3.2) |
| Left = Right | 4 (12.9) | — | 1 ( 3.2) |
| *Total* | 21 (67.7) | 2 (18.2) | 9 (29.0) |
| Diastolic gallop rhythm | 12 (38.7) | 3 (27.3) | 21 (67.7) |
| Arrhythmias | 8 (25.8) | 6 (54.5) | 10 (32.3) |
| Hepatomegaly | 6 (19.4) | 3 (27.3) | 9 (29.0) |
| Ascites | — | 2 (18.2) | 1 ( 3.2) |
| Heart Rate: No.(%) | | | |
| <150 | 4 (12.9) | 2 (18.2) | 4 (12.9) |
| 150–199 | 9 (29.0) | 3 (27.3) | 10 (32.3) |
| 200–250 | 15 (48.4) | 5 (45.5) | 16 (51.6) |
| >250 | 3 ( 9.7) | 1 ( 9.1) | 1 ( 3.2) |

*Values are based on the analysis of clinical data from 73 consecutive cats seen over a three and a half-year period with proven cardiomyopathy.

†Numbers in parentheses indicate the number of cats in each group.

‡Young kittens fulfilling the criteria for "kitten mortality complex" were omitted from this study.

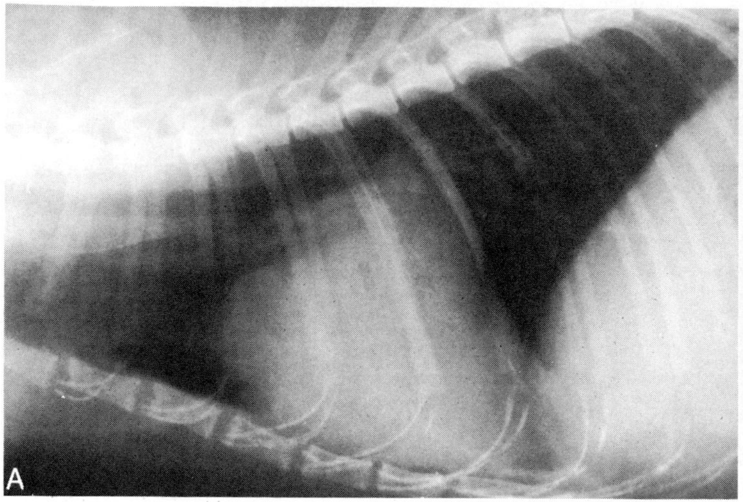


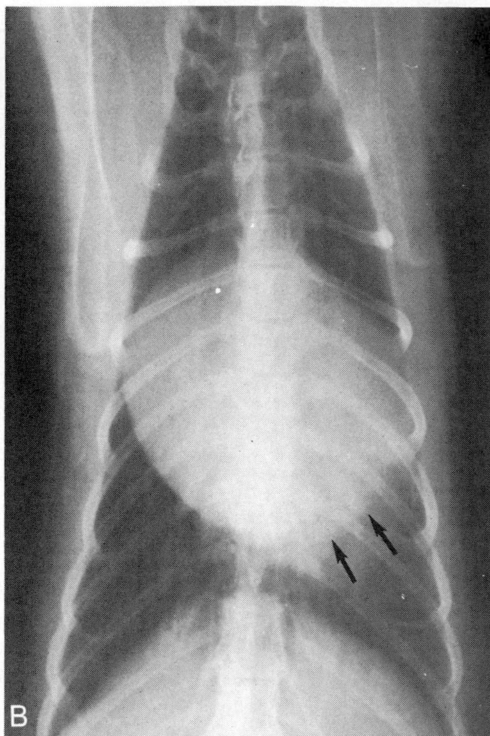


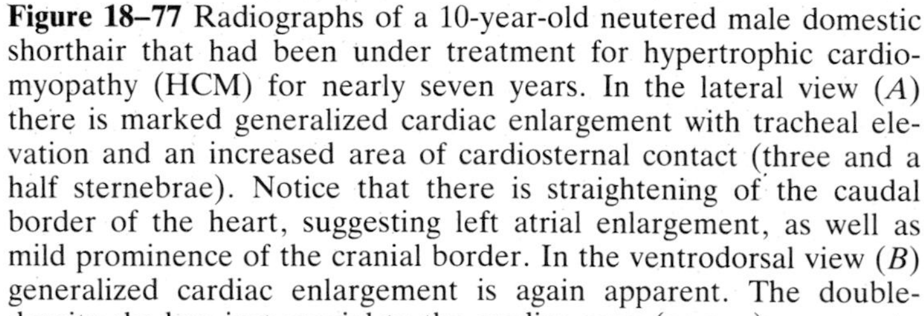
**Figure 18–77** Radiographs of a 10-year-old neutered male domestic shorthair that had been under treatment for hypertrophic cardiomyopathy (HCM) for nearly seven years. In the lateral view (*A*) there is marked generalized cardiac enlargement with tracheal elevation and an increased area of cardiosternal contact (three and a half sternebrae). Notice that there is straightening of the caudal border of the heart, suggesting left atrial enlargement, as well as mild prominence of the cranial border. In the ventrodorsal view (*B*) generalized cardiac enlargement is again apparent. The double-density shadow just cranial to the cardiac apex (arrows) represents the enlarged caudal aspect of the left atrium. A diagnosis of HCM was established by nonselective angiocardiography.

megaly, predominantly left-sided, with substantial left atrial enlargement (LAE), which appears in the lateral view as loss of caudal waist and in the ventrodorsal view as a left auricular appendage bulge over the left cardiac border at the one to three o'clock position (Fig. 18–77). The cardiac apex in the ventrodorsal view is frequently pointed. Pulmonary edema tends to be most prominent about the hilus and dorsally in the caudal lobes, and interlobar fissure lines may be present. The liver often extends 1 to 2 cm behind the costal arch.

Scalar electrocardiography may help in differentiating HCM from the other forms of cardiomyopathy. Intraventricular conduction abnormalities are characteristic of the hypertrophic form and may occur as left bundle branch block, preexcitation syndrome, and left anterior fascicular block. Of these, only the last occurs with any degree of frequency (Figs. 18–34 and 18–78). However, conduction disturbances are not limited to cats with HCM (Table 18–16). In other cats with HCM, electrocardiographic evidence of left ventricular hypertrophy is expressed as an increase in the amplitude of R waves in certain leads along with prolongation of the QRS interval. Criteria for the LVH pattern are listed in Table 18–17. Cardiac arrhythmias occur in over 50 per cent of cats with HCM, and although a variety of arrhythmias may occur, ventricular premature beats and ventricular tachyarrhythmias predominate.

Laboratory tests are of little help in diagnosis or in differentiating between the various forms of cardiomyopathy in cats. However, complete laboratory testing should be performed routinely to establish solid baselines on body organ function and to identify any other existing abnormalities that may affect a response to treatment. After major thromboembolic episodes, the majority of measurable serum muscle enzyme tests are substantially elevated (e.g., aspartate aminotransferase [SGOT], lactic dehydrogenase, creatine phosphokinase, aldolase), whatever the form of cardiomyopathy. In a small percentage of cats, hyperglycemia, glycosuria, and proteinuria are found shortly after major arterial embolism. The hyperglycemia and glycosuria are usually of short duration, are not accompanied by either ketonuria or ketonemia, and do not require treatment.

In an attempt to provide optimal management for cats with cardiomyopathy, it is important that the specific form of the disease be determined. This can be done most easily by nonselective angiocardiography (Harpster, 1977b; Owens and Twedt, 1977) or echocardiography (Pipers and Hamlin, 1980). The major disadvantage of both these procedures is equipment expense if optimal results are to be obtained. The risk of either procedure is negligible in cats with HCM, provided that heart failure is stabilized with diuretic therapy before the study.

The reader should review the section on cardiac diagnostics for standard techniques used in performing these procedures. Nonselective angiocardiography is superior to M-mode echocardiography in HCM, affording less chance for errors in interpretation. However, it may be difficult to differentiate normal cats from those with HCM by a single radiographic exposure after the injection of a radiopaque dye. Studies are improved when a rapid film or cassette changer or equipment for performing 70-mm, rapid-sequence spot films is available. M-mode echocardiographic findings in HCM have been reported (Soderberg et al., 1983).

The characteristic findings in HCM as seen with non-

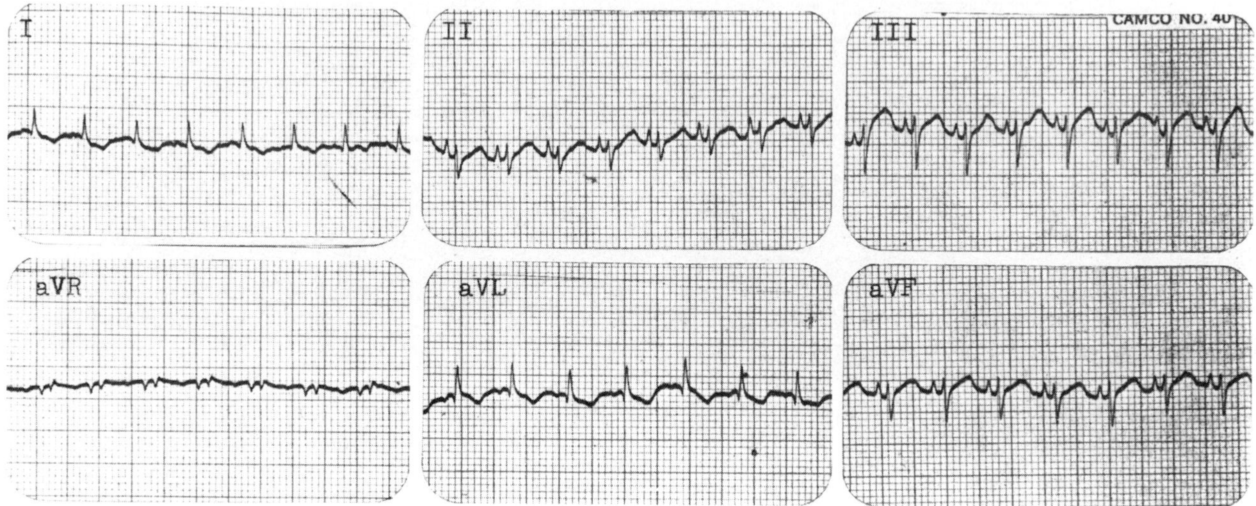


**Figure 18–78** Typical left anterior fascicular block–like conduction abnormality in a one and a half year-old neutered male domestic shorthair with hypertrophic cardiomyopathy (confirmed at autopsy). The progressive decrease in R-wave amplitude in leads I through III, accompanied by a progressive increase in S-wave depth, is the expected finding. The presence of qR complexes in aVL and deep S waves in aVF are also anticipated. The prominent amplitude of P waves in lead II (0.25 mV) suggests atrial enlargement. Compare the findings in these strips with those in Figure 18–34. 25 mm/sec; 1.0 mV = 1.0 cm.

**Table 18–16 Comparison of the Electrocardiographic Findings in 73 Cats With Three Forms of Cardiomyopathy**

| ECG FINDINGS | HYPERTROPHIC (31) No. (%) | INTERMEDIATE (11) No. (%) | DILATATIVE (31) No. (%) |
|---|---|---|---|
| P wave—Lead II | | | |
| >0.04 sec | 3 ( 9.7) | 3 (27.3) | 6 (19.4) |
| ≥0.2 mV | 6 (19.4) | 1 ( 9.1) | 2 ( 6.5) |
| QRS interval >0.04 sec | 11 (35.5) | 6 (54.5) | 22 (71.0) |
| LVH pattern | 12 (38.7) | 3 (27.3) | 12 (38.7) |
| Conduction disturbances | | | |
| Sinoatrial block | — | 1 ( 9.1) | 1 ( 3.2) |
| Left axis deviation* | 8 (25.8) | — | — |
| Left anterior hemiblock* | 4 (12.9) | 1 ( 9.1) | — |
| Left bundle branch block | — | — | 1 ( 3.2) |
| Right bundle branch block | — | — | 1 ( 3.2) |
| Other intraventricular | 2 ( 6.5) | 1 ( 9.1) | 1 ( 3.2) |
| Wolff-Parkinson-White pattern | 1 ( 3.2) | — | 1 ( 3.2) |
| Total (all types) | 15 (48.4) | 3 (27.3) | 5 (16.1) |
| Arrhythmias† | | | |
| Supraventricular: | | | |
| Premature beats | 4 (12.9) | 3 (27.3) | 3 ( 9.7) |
| Paroxysmal tachycardia | 1 ( 3.2) | — | 1 ( 3.2) |
| Atrial fibrillation | 1 ( 3.2) | 2 (18.2) | — |
| Ventricular: | | | |
| Premature beats | 11 (35.5) | 5 (45.5) | 15 (48.4) |
| Paroxysmal tachycardia‡ | 4 (12.9) | 2 (18.2) | 4 (12.9) |
| AV dissociation | 1 ( 3.2) | 1 ( 9.1) | 2 ( 6.5) |
| Total (all types) | 17 (54.8) | 7 (63.6) | 19 (61.3) |

*Electrocardiographic differentiation between left axis deviation (normal: ≤0.04 sec) and left anterior hemiblock (prolonged to >0.04 sec) was based on the duration of the QRS interval.

†More than one arrhythmia was recorded in 12 (16.4%) cats.

‡The criterion for this category was the occurrence of two or more repetitive ventricular premature beats.

**Table 18–17 Criteria for Electrocardiographic Left Ventricular Hypertrophy (LVH) Pattern in the Cat**

| LEAD | CRITERION |
|---|---|
| II | R >0.9 mV |
| $CV_6LU$ | R >1.0 mV |
| $V_6$* | R >0.5 mV |
| Base/Apex† | R >1.2 mV |
| $V_{10}$ | R/Q >1.0 |

*A precordial lead recorded with the electrode positioned in the left 6th intercostal space on a line with the point of the shoulder.

†A precordial lead recorded with the RA electrode positioned over the spine of the 7th thoracic vertebra and the LA electrode positioned over the left 6th intercostal space at the costochondral junction. The ECG is recorded with the lead selector at the Lead I position.

selective angiocardiography can be recognized in both end-systolic and end-diastolic phases of the cardiac cycle, but only when the phase of the cycle is known. (In HCM the left ventricular end-diastolic chamber size and conformation can be similar or identical to that of the normal cat in end-systole. If the phase of the cardiac cycle is unknown, as when only a single film is available for interpretation, the opportunity for error in diagnosis is obvious.) For optimal diagnosis it is also important that an unobstructed view of the left ventricle be obtained. Ideally, the right side of the heart should be empty of dye at the time of radiographic exposure, to eliminate superimposition of dye in the right and left ventricles in the lateral view. In diastole the left atrium is enlarged, with widening and apparent tortuosity of the pulmonary veins. The left ventricular free wall is thickened, and the chamber is prominently indented cranially and caudally by the respective papillary muscles (Fig. 18–79). In systole the left atrium is further enlarged and the main pulmonary veins more prominently distended. The left ventricular free wall is markedly thickened. The left ventricular chamber is diminutive, often with only a small cone-like area of dye remaining immediately below the aortic valve. Infrequently, a thin stream of dye extends from the base of the left ventricular chamber to the apex, where a small, irregular pocket of dye is present. The aorta is of normal size.

Echocardiographically, the features observed in HCM include a small left ventricular chamber with thickening of the septum and left ventricular free wall (LVFW). The amplitude of the anterior leaflet of the mitral valve is reduced, there is overlapping of the anterior leaflet and septum during diastole, and there may be systolic anterior motion of the anterior leaflet (Fig. 18–80). The left atrium (LA) is usually dilated. The aorta is of normal width with increased amplitude (i.e., exaggerated movement during ventricular systole). Systolic motion of both the septum and the LVFW remains normal so that in the presence of a small left ventricular cavity, left ventricular functional indices are increased. It is not unusual to find the percentage change in dimension (%ΔD) greater than 60 per cent and the ejection fraction exceeding 90 per cent.

At autopsy the left ventricular free wall and the interventricular septum are thickened. The left ventricular papillary muscles are enlarged and contribute further to a reduction in dimensions of the left ventricular chamber. In a few cats the basilar parts of the interventricular septum are disproportionately thickened and cause some obstruction to outflow from the left ventricle (i.e., asymmetric hypertrophic cardiomyopathy [Liu, 1977]). The left

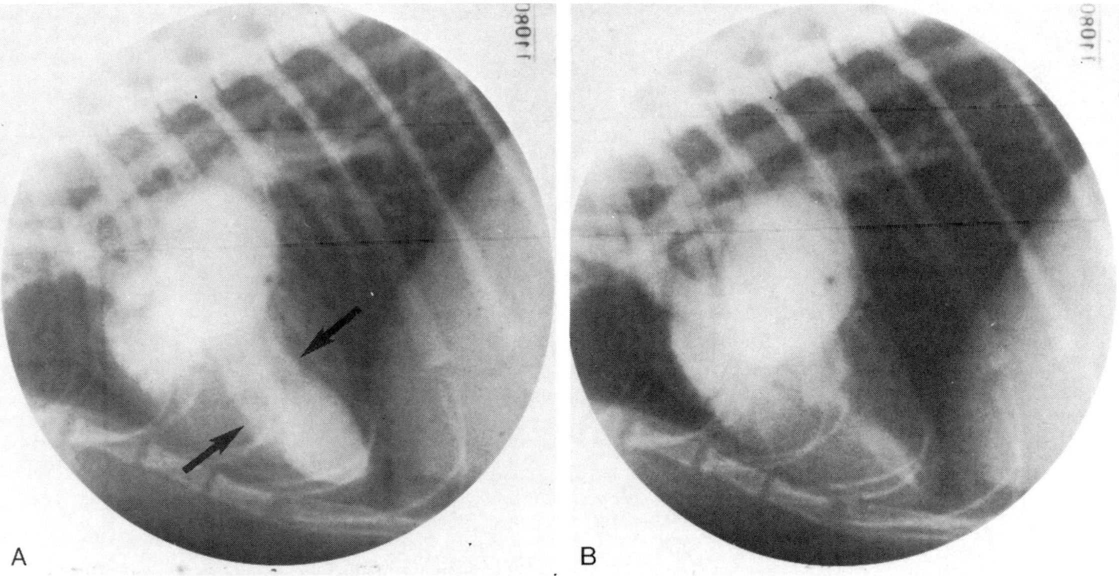


**Figure 18–79** Hypertrophic cardiomyopathy, nonselective angiocardiography, one and a half year-old neutered male domestic shorthair. In diastole (*A*) the left ventricular chamber appears elongated and reduced in size, with increased thickness of the posterior wall. The apparent filling defects seen anteriorly and posteriorly (arrows) are the result of papillary muscle prominence. During systole (*B*) only a thin stream of dye remains in the left ventricular chamber, and the posterior wall is markedly thickened. Notice the increased size and opacification of the left atrium. The radiopaque density cranial and ventral to the left atrium and ascending aorta is the right auricular appendage. 70-mm, rapid-sequence spot films.

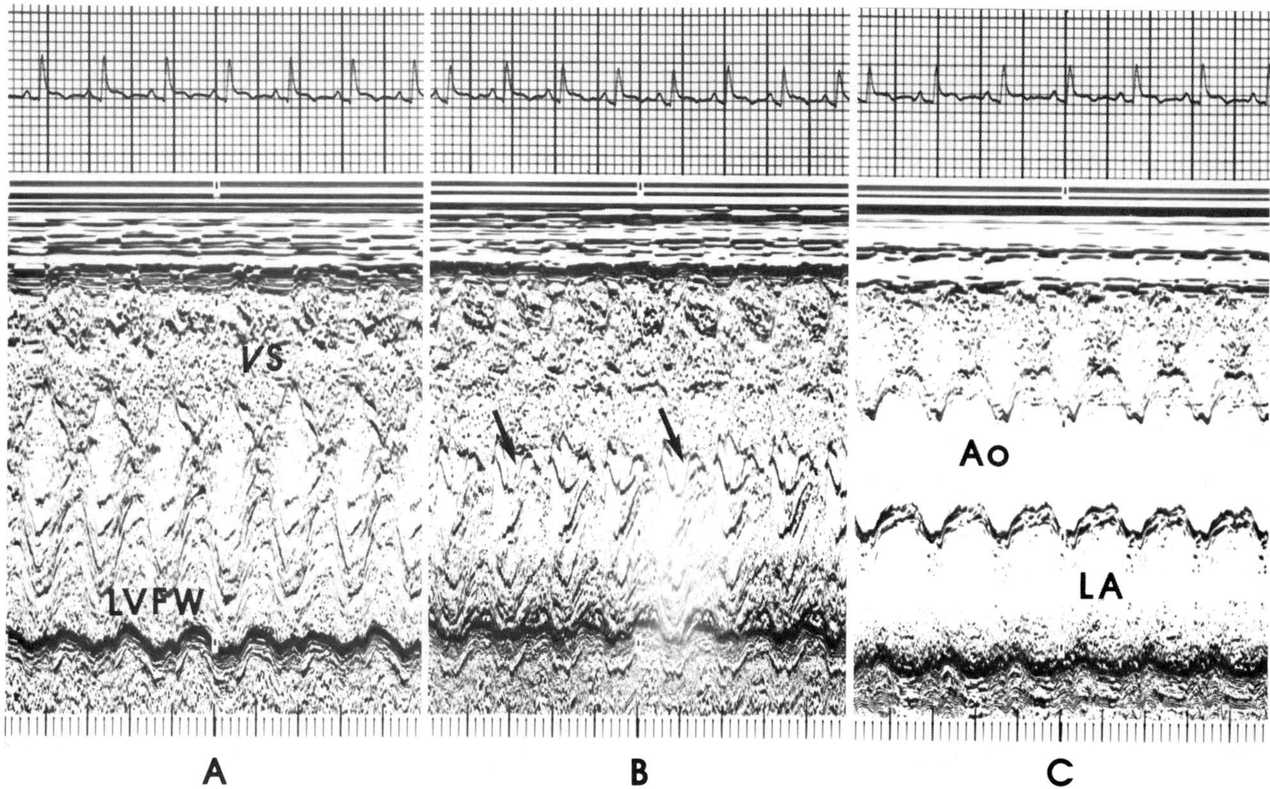


**Figure 18–80** M-mode echocardiogram of a two-year-old neutered male domestic shorthair presented because of recent development of a grade 4/6 holosystolic murmur over the mitral area. In *A*, taken through the left ventricle below the mitral valve, both the left ventricular free wall (LVFW) and the ventricular septum (VS) are slightly thickened (5.54 mm) with exaggerated systolic motion (percentage change in dimension [%ΔD] = 74.8%; ejection fraction = 99.7%). The lines between the LVFW and VS represent chordae tendineae. In *B*, taken through the mitral valve, there is systolic anterior motion of the anterior leaflet of the mitral valve (arrows), and amplitude of the anterior leaflet is diminished. Notice that there is overlapping of the VS and anterior mitral valve leaflet. In *C*, taken through the aorta (Ao) and left atrium (LA), there is normal aortic amplitude, and the LA is of normal size (LA/Ao ratio = 1.22). These echocardiographic findings are diagnostic for hypertrophic cardiomyopathy when congenital heart disease can be excluded. 50 mm/sec. ECG: 1.0 mV = 1.0 cm. The small vertical lines are 1-cm marks.

atrium is dilated, and its endocardium may be pale and thickened. Less often, thrombi of varying size are present, usually attached by a stalk arising from the endocardium of the left auricular appendage (Plate 18–1*A*). The left AV valve leaflets are frequently thickened and opaque with nodules along their free edges. The chordae tendineae may also be thickened.

Microscopically, the muscle fibers are enlarged, with prominent hyperchromatic nuclei. Foci of interstitial fibrosis are usual and may be accompanied by atrophy and lysis of muscle cells and in some instances mild mononuclear cell infiltration. In asymmetric hypertrophic cardiomyopathy, muscle fibers in the interventricular septum may be hypertrophied and irregularly arranged, and interstitial connective tissue may be increased. In the left ventricular outflow tract, just below the aortic valves, there is both endocardial and subendocardial fibrosis (Liu, 1977). Myxomatous degeneration of the left AV valve and the chordae tendineae is evident microscopically.

The prognosis for HCM is better than for other forms of cardiomyopathy but only when cardiac arrhythmias and thromboembolism can be controlled.

Routine management of HCM combines a beta-adrenergic blocking agent and diuretics. Propranolol (Inderal) is administered at 2.5 to 5.0 mg b.i.d. or t.i.d. The dosage is adjusted to maintain the heart rate under 180 per

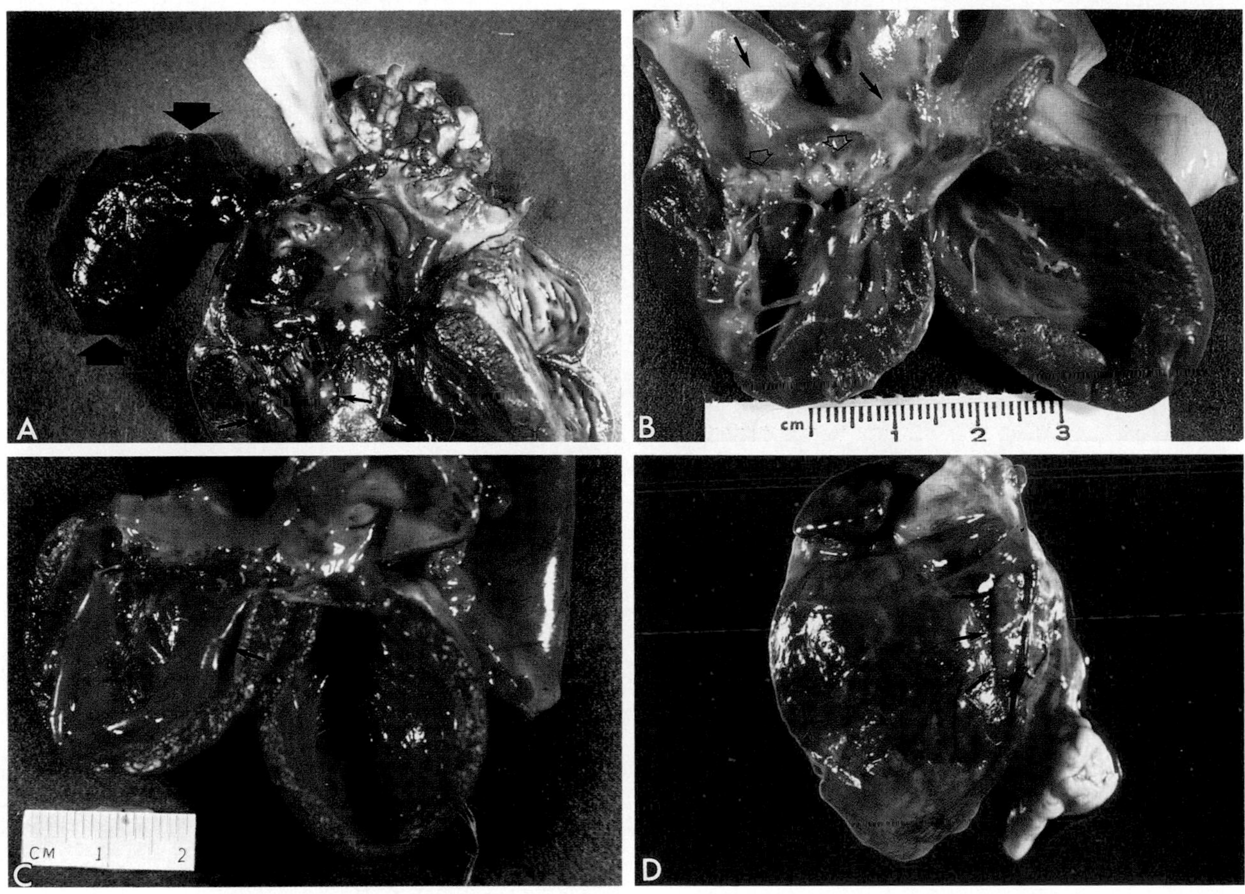


**Plate 18–1** *A*, Hypertrophic cardiomyopathy, four-year-old male domestic shorthair. A large left atrial thrombus (arrowheads) arises from the left auricular appendage. Notice the large, dilated left atrium and the small, thick-walled left ventricular cavity, which is filled with large, bulky papillary muscles (arrows). *B*, Intermediate (restrictive) cardiomyopathy, six-year-old neutered male domestic longhair. The left atrium is dilated. Its endocardial surface is generally pale and contains several large, raised plaques (arrows) representing subendocardial and endocardial fibrosis. The left ventricular wall is of normal thickness with mild chamber dilatation. Multifocal lesions of endocardial and subendocardial fibrosis are prominent over the papillary muscles and adjacent myocardium. The mitral valve leaflets (arrowheads) are thickened and nodular. Histologically, these valvular changes are characteristic of myxomatous transformation. Collectively these findings are typical of intermediate (restrictive) feline cardiomyopathy. *C*, Dilatative cardiomyopathy, seven-year-old spayed female domestic shorthair. The left ventricular chamber is dilated and its walls thin. The papillary muscles (arrows) are flattened and blend imperceptibly at their bases into the surrounding left ventricular myocardium. *D*, Pericarditis secondary to feline infectious peritonitis, five-year-old neutered male Maine coon cat. Notice the pale tan, raised fibrin deposits on the pericardium and the right atrial and ventricular epicardium. Dense adhesions can be seen on the ventricular apex and the caudal border of the left ventricle, including the left auricular appendage (arrows). An M-mode echocardiographic study disclosed small cranial and caudal echo-free spaces with preservation of normal systolic motion of both ventricular septum and left ventricular free wall.

minute. Diuretics are given in amounts to reduce fluid accumulation; in many cats an intermittent regimen (e.g., every 48 to 72 hours) is adequate. Management and prevention of thromboembolism are discussed separately.

**Intermediate Cardiomyopathy.** The intermediate form of feline cardiomyopathy (ICM), also termed restrictive (Liu, 1977), occurs mainly in middle-aged and old cats. Liu (1977) reported a male predominance at The Animal Medical Center, but the slight male predominance at AMAH is statistically insignificant. Differences in total numbers and methods of establishing the diagnosis probably account for these dissimilar findings.

As with HCM, congestive heart failure and thromboembolic episodes are the chief causes of clinical signs. In the intermediate form, however, heart failure tends to be less acute, and is often preceded by varying periods of lethargy, reduced appetite, weight loss, and, rarely, coughing. The heart failure may be manifested by pulmonary edema, pleural effusion, or, rarely, ascites alone.

The predominant findings on physical examination, in addition to abnormalities of ventilation (i.e., polypnea, dyspnea), are heart murmurs, diastolic gallop rhythms, and arrhythmias. Of these, arrhythmias are most frequent. Low cardiac output, if also present, causes weakness, lethargy, subnormal temperature, and cool extremities. The heart rate tends to be increased in the majority of cats but may be normal with hypothermia.

Generalized heart enlargement and significant prominence of the left atrium are the characteristic findings in thoracic radiographs (Fig. 18–81). Heart failure is sometimes evidenced by pulmonary edema but more often by substantial pleural effusion. These may obliterate part of the cardiac silhouette, making radiographic interpretation difficult. Varying degrees of hepatomegaly are usual.

The electrocardiographic patterns in ICM are neither specific nor distinct. Both intraventricular conduction abnormalities and the LVH pattern occasionally occur. The QRS interval tends to be mildly prolonged, sometimes with notching of major deflections, as well as multiwave forms in some leads (M and W waves). Supraventricular premature beats, supraventricular tachyarrhythmias, ventricular premature beats, and, less frequently, bradyarrhythmias (sinus arrest, atrioventricular block) occur in some cats.

The results of nonselective angiocardiography tend to be varied, probably because of (1) a marked variation in the disease itself, particularly as regards site and extent of endocardial fibroplasia, and (2) our tendency to assign to this group all cats whose VAC patterns are not typical of either the hypertrophic or the dilatative form. In the classic example of ICM, filling defects can be easily identified in the left ventricle with nonselective angiocardiography (Fig. 18–82). In diastole the left atrium is enlarged, and the main pulmonary veins widened and prominent. The left ventricular chamber is normal or reduced in size, the left ventricular free wall is of normal thickness, papillary muscles are normal or decreased in size, and filling defects over the apex are common. The aortic diameter is frequently reduced. In systole the size of the left atrium and the prominence of the main pulmonary veins are exaggerated. Systolic motion of the left ventricle appears somewhat depressed, the left ventricular free wall remains of normal thickness, and filling defects in the apex persist. The papillary muscles are usually

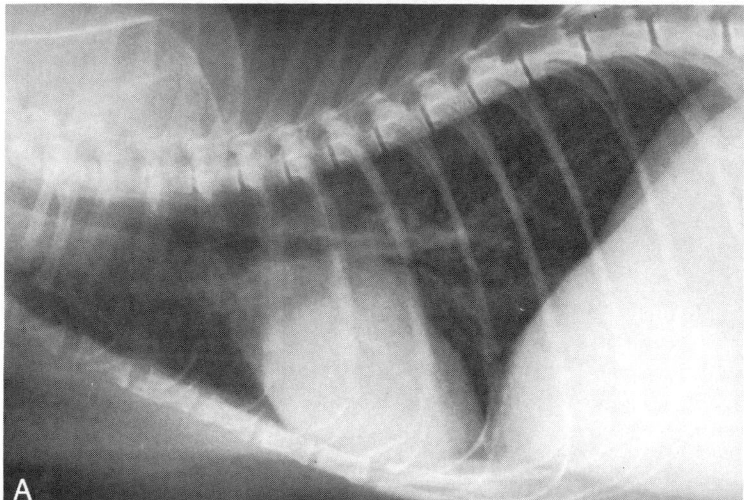


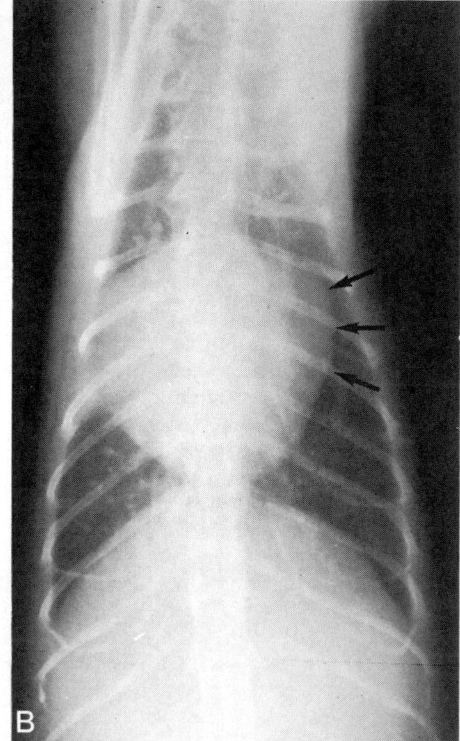


**Figure 18–81** Intermediate (restrictive) cardiomyopathy, 13-year-old neutered male domestic longhair. The lateral view (*A*) shows moderate generalized cardiomegaly with mild tracheal elevation and an increase in the area of cardiosternal contact (three and a half sternebrae). The loss of caudal waist suggests left atrial dilatation. The diffuse interstitial lung densities are characteristic of interstitial pulmonary edema. *B*, In the ventrodorsal view the cardiac silhouette assumes a broad valentine-like configuration with the left cranial prominence (arrows) resulting from enlargement of the left auricular appendage. Poor visualization of the right cranial cardiac border and mild blunting of the right costophrenic angle result from mild pleural effusion.

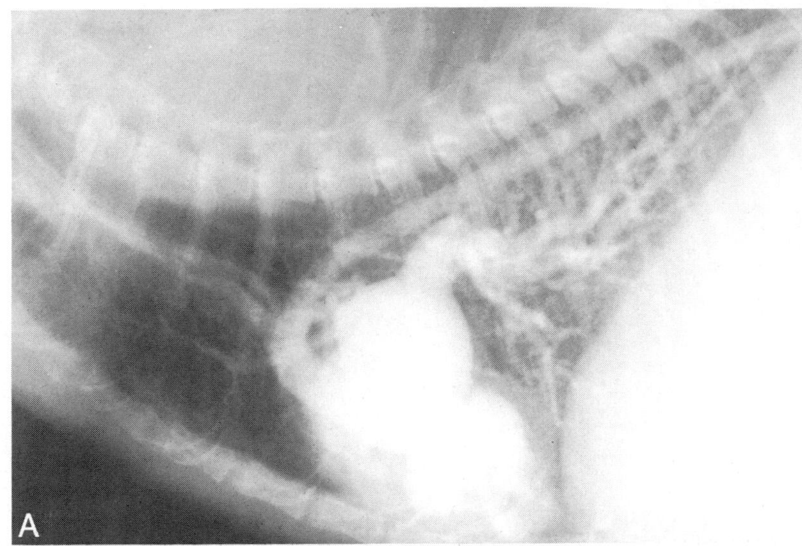


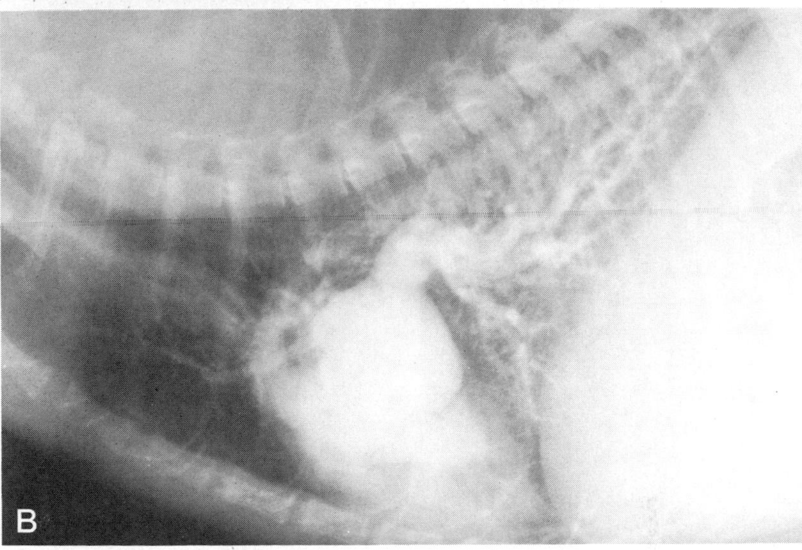


**Figure 18–82** Intermediate (restrictive) cardiomyopathy, nonselective angiocardiography, 13-year-old neutered male domestic longhair. In diastole (*A*) the left ventricular chamber appears small and assumes an irregular contour, suggesting the presence of multiple filling defects. The posterior wall is of normal thickness. At end-systole (*B*) the left ventricular chamber is diminutive, with dye remaining only in the basal half of the chamber beneath the mitral and aortic valves. In this view also, the posterior wall is of normal thickness. The papillary muscles are never clearly seen during either end-diastole or end-systole phases. The enlargement of the left atrium and the enlarged, tortuous pulmonary veins strongly suggest resistance to the left ventricular filling and should be compared with the findings in Figures 18–79 and 18–87. This study was carried out with a rapid film changer. If all phases of the cardiac cycle had not been recorded, the findings at end-systole could easily have been mistaken for those of HCM. Plain thoracic radiographs of this cat can be reviewed in Figure 18–81.

reduced in size. The aortic diameter may be less than expected.

M-mode echocardiography discloses normal left ventricular dimensions in diastole, normal septal and LVFW thickness, and mild to moderate reduction of systolic motion (Fig. 18–83). The anterior leaflet of the mitral valve approximates or is slightly separated from the septum during diastole. The left atrium is moderately dilated. The aorta tends to be of normal diameter with decreased amplitude. Because of a mild to moderate decrease of left ventricular systolic motion, left ventricular functional indices (%$\Delta$D, ejection fraction) tend to be somewhat depressed. Although these findings appear distinct, I have not studied a sufficient number of cats by both echocardiography and nonselective angiocardiography to be totally confident of the diagnosis by echocardiography alone. At this time my impression is that nonselective angiocardiography is the better method for diagnosing ICM.

Autopsy of cats with ICM discloses large, pale foci of endocardial thickening (Plate 18–1*B*). Bands of similar tissue may extend between adjacent foci or even across the left ventricular chamber. On cut section the pale endocardial foci can be seen to extend into the myocardium in some areas. The left ventricular papillary muscles are of about normal size but are frequently pale and deformed, especially where the chordae tendineae attach. The left atrium is usually dilated. The left AV valves are thickened and opaque and their edges nodular.

Microscopically, large areas of endocardium and myocardium are replaced by fibrous connective tissue. Beneath the areas of endocardial fibrosis and in some myocardial foci there may be necrosis of muscle fibers and lysis of muscle cells, accompanied by a mild infiltration of histiocytes, plasma cells, and lymphocytes. Interstitial fibrosis and atrophy of muscle fibers may be found in many sites but are almost always in the free edges of the left ventricular papillary muscles. Myxomatous change is the predominant finding in the left AV valve leaflets.

The long-term prognosis for cats with ICM is guarded. Difficulties encountered include stabilization of heart failure and control of cardiac arrhythmias, as well as the ever-present threat of thromboembolism. If these problems can be resolved, the prognosis should be improved.

When substantial pleural effusion is present, thoraco-

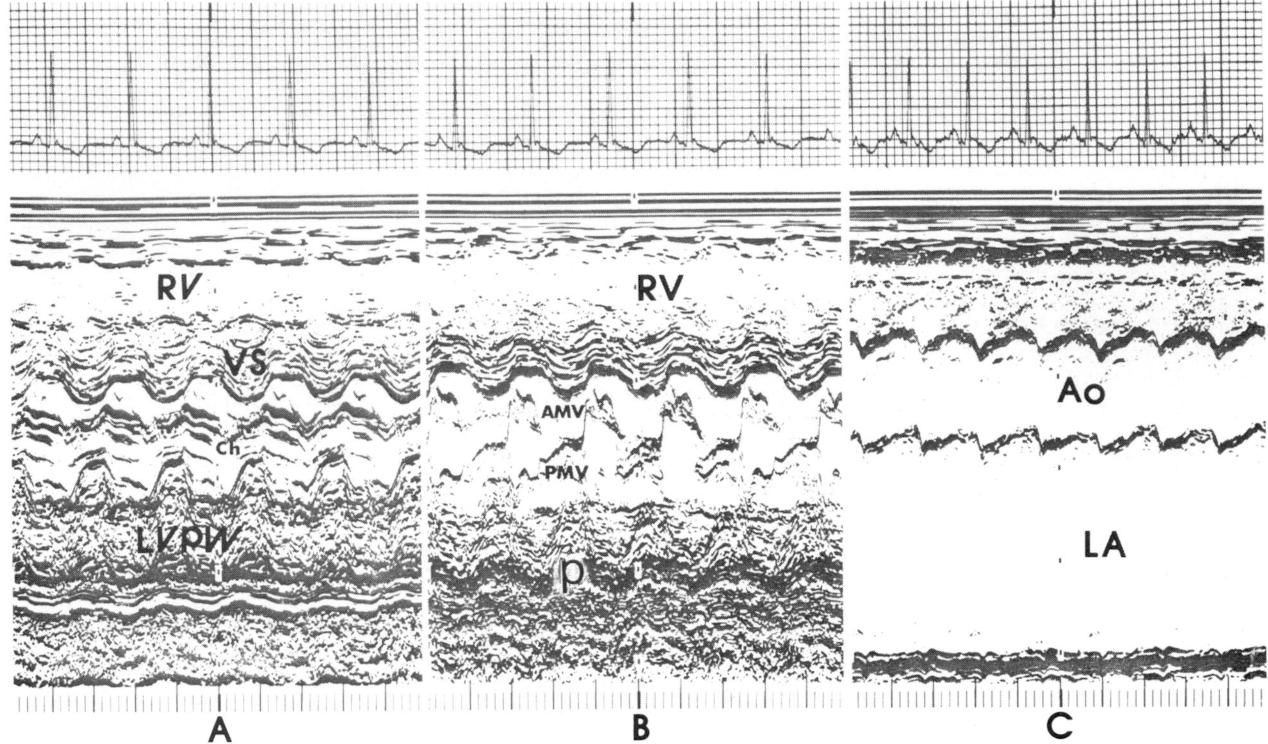


**Figure 18–83** Intermediate (restrictive) cardiomyopathy, M-mode echocardiogram, in an adult neutered male domestic shorthair. In *A*, taken through the ventricles below the mitral valve, there is thickening of the left ventricular posterior wall (LVPW), while the ventricular septum (VS) is of normal thickness. Systolic wall motion of the LVPW and VS are well preserved with normal functional indices (% Δ D = 50.1%; ejection fraction = 84.9%). However, the circumferential fiber-shortening rate (VCF) is mildly depressed (2.95), and there is right ventricular dilatation. In *B*, recorded at the level of the mitral valve, both anterior (AMV) and posterior mitral valve (PMV) leaflets are clearly visualized, suggesting mild left ventricular dilatation. The right ventricle remains dilated at this level. In *C*, at the aortic and left atrial position, aortic amplitude is depressed (2.05 mm), suggesting depressed left ventricular performance. The left atrium is markedly dilated (left atrial:aortic ratio = 2.30). AMV = anterior mitral valve, Ao = aorta, Ch = chordae tendineae, LA = left atrium, LVPW = left ventricular posterior wall, p = pericardium, PMV = posterior mitral valve, RV = right ventricle, VS = ventricular septum. 50 mm/sec; ECG: 1.0 mV = 1.0 cm.

centesis should be carried out for therapeutic and diagnostic purposes; any peritoneal effusion should also be aspirated and submitted for laboratory examination. At present, ICM is managed with digitalis glycosides and diuretics. Digoxin is given at 0.004 to 0.008 mg/kg/day divided into two doses. If arrhythmias are frequent after digitalization and resolution of active heart failure, antiarrhythmic agents can be added—either propranolol (2.5 to 5.0 mg b.i.d. or t.i.d.), quinidine sulfate (5.5 to 11.0 mg/kg t.i.d.), or procainamide hydrochloride (8 to 20 mg/kg t.i.d.). Diuretics are given in dosages to reduce excess fluid. When congestive heart failure does not respond to these measures, vasodilator agents should be tried. (See the later section on cardiac therapy.) Management and preventive measures for thromboembolism will be discussed separately.

**Dilatative Cardiomyopathy.** The dilatative form of feline cardiomyopathy (DCM) appears to have been on the increase in recent years, whereas the hypertrophic form is recognized less often. Dilatative cardiomyopathy occurs chiefly in middle-aged or old cats. While a slight predominance in females has been evident at AMAH, Liu (1977) reported a greater prevalence in males at The Animal Medical Center.

The clinical signs of symptomatic DCM are similar to those discussed for the other forms of cardiomyopathy. However, as with the intermediate form, overt signs of congestive failure may be preceded by a variable period of lethargy, depressed appetite, and weight loss. Both acute thromboembolic episodes and cardiovascular syncopal episodes may occur suddenly without premonitory signs.

Pleural effusion due to biventricular failure is the major cause of polypnea and dyspnea on presentation. Heart sounds are muffled bilaterally, as are ventral lung sounds. Despite these impediments to auscultation, cardiac abnormalities can be detected in the majority of cats. Heart murmurs over the mitral valve area, diastolic gallop rhythms, and arrhythmias are characteristic, with diastolic gallop rhythms predominating. Some degree of hepatomegaly is usual, but ascites is rare. The femoral pulses are usually weak, and the rectal temperature is frequently subnormal.

In initial thoracic radiographs, bilateral pleural effusion

may interfere significantly with interpretation. After resolution of the effusion varying degrees of generalized heart enlargement are seen, as well as mild left atrial enlargement (Fig. 18–84). Heart size varies tremendously in cats with DCM but is within the upper limits of normal in some cats. Hepatomegaly is usually evident.

Common electrocardiographic abnormalities include LVH pattern and prolongation of the QRS interval over 40 milliseconds. However, neither of these findings is limited to dilatative cardiomyopathy. Of greater significance are the cardiac arrhythmias, which may be present in over 80 per cent of cats in this group (Table 18–17).

Nonselective angiocardiography is distinctive and diagnostic (Fig. 18–85). Because of poor myocardial function, circulation of radiopaque contrast material is very slow. The left ventricular chamber is enlarged, its free wall is thin, and the left ventricular papillary muscles are difficult to distinguish even at end-systole. Left ventricular dimensions change little during systole because of severe depression of contractility. The left atrium is moderately dilated, and the aortic diameter is reduced.

Echocardiographic studies in DCM frequently demonstrate biventricular dilatation. Left ventricular dilatation is evidenced by wide separation of the anterior leaflet of the mitral valve from the septum in diastole (Fig. 18–86). Additional findings are thinning of the septum and LVFW, with depressed systolic motion of each, and moderate to marked left atrial dilatation. The aortic diameter is reduced and the amplitude decreased. Left ventricular functional indices are moderately to severely depressed (e.g., $\%\Delta D < 20\%$, ejection fraction $< 40\%$) because of the reduced left ventricular contractility.

Despite the presence of biventricular dilatation and heart failure in most cats with DCM, left-sided abnormalities predominate and are the most distinguishing features in both nonselective angiocardiography and M-mode echocardiography. Nonselective angiocardiography and M-mode echocardiography are equally useful in the diagnosis of DCM, but because of the increased risk with nonselective angiocardiography for cats with dilatative cardiopathy (profound bradycardia and cardiac arrest), M-mode echocardiography is the procedure of choice.

Autopsy discloses biatrial and left ventricular dilatation. The endocardium of the left atrium and especially of the left ventricle tends to be pale and thickened (Plate 18–1*C*). The left ventricular free wall and interventricular septum are thinned, and the left ventricular papillary muscles are small and tend to be displaced basally. The left AV valves are usually opaque and thickened along their edges.

Microscopically, the muscle fibers in some cats are thinner than normal and diffusely separated by fine interstitial connective tissue. In some areas they assume a wavy pattern. More often the myocardial fibers are of normal size, except in focal or diffuse areas of interstitial fibrosis, where myocardial atrophy is characterized by marked variation in the size of the fibers. Foci of muscle fiber degeneration and muscle cell lysis may undergo a mild mononuclear infiltration. The endocardium is thickened in some areas by deposits of dense collagenous connective tissue. The major finding in leaflets of the left AV valves is myxomatous change.

The prognosis for cats with DCM is poor, probably because of the severely depressed myocardial contractility; however, some cats do respond for a considerable time to proper management.

Treatment is similar to that for ICM. When pleural

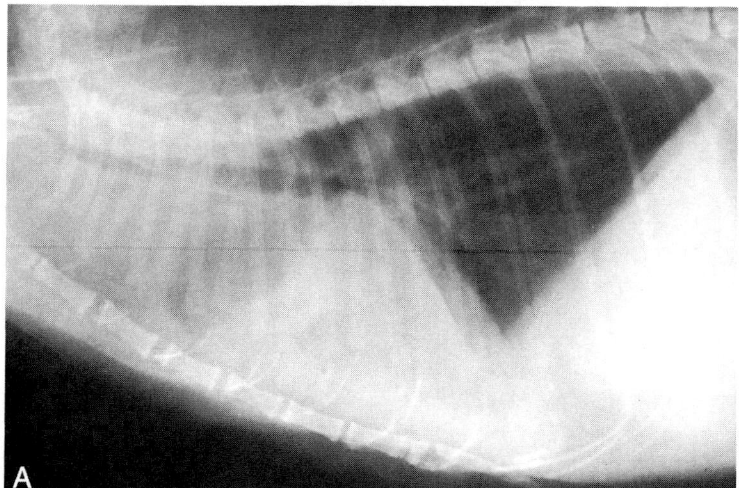


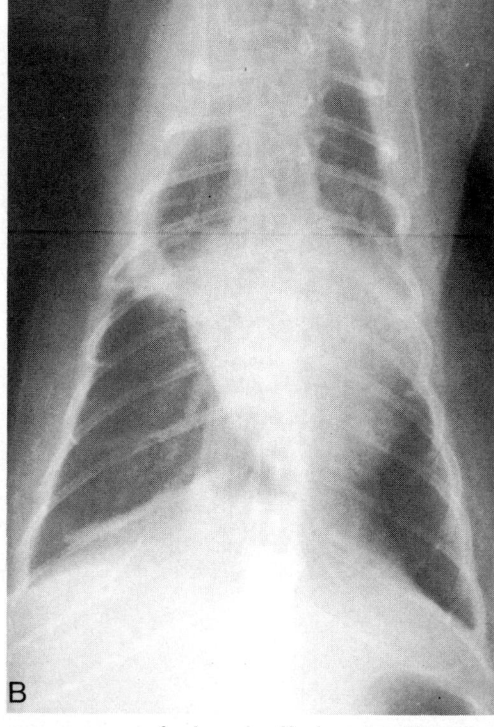


**Figure 18–84** Dilatative cardiomyopathy, 14-year-old neutered male domestic shorthair. In the lateral view (*A*) the cardiac silhouette is partly obscured owing to pleural effusion. Cardiomegaly is assumed from the tracheal elevation. In the ventrodorsal view (*B*) left ventricular enlargement predominates with shifting of the apex to the left. Bilateral pleural effusion is indicated by bilateral blunting of the costophrenic angles, incomplete visualization of the left cardiac border, and incomplete expansion of the right cranial lung lobe. A cranial mediastinal mass can be ruled out by normal width of the cranial mediastinum. These radiographs demonstrate the common occurrence of pleural effusion in dilatative cardiomyopathy. A definitive diagnosis was established by M-mode echocardiography.

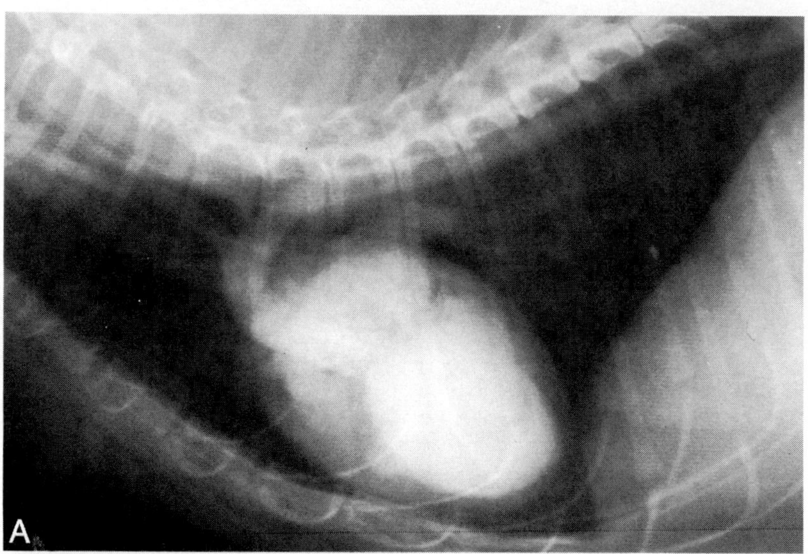


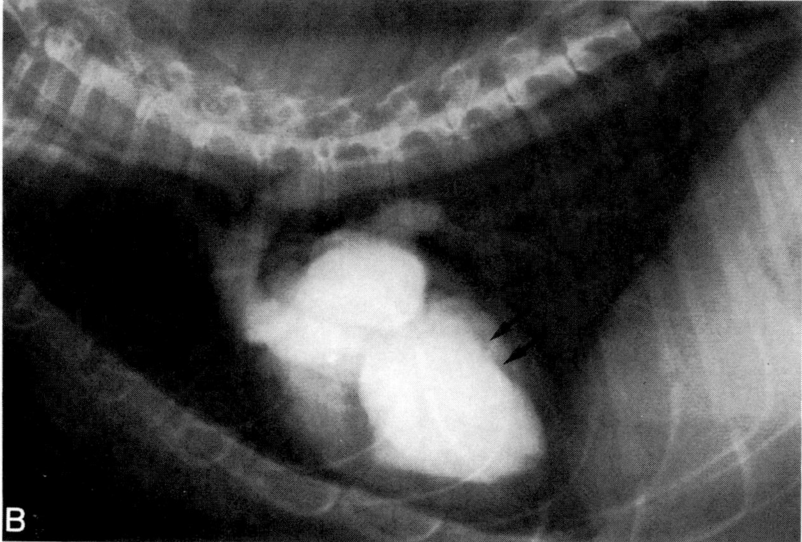


**Figure 18–85** Dilatative cardiomyopathy, nonselective angiocardiography, five-year-old neutered male domestic longhair. During diastole (*A*) there is dilatation of the left ventricular chamber and thinning of the posterior wall. The papillary muscles cannot be clearly visualized. At end-systole (*B*) the left ventricular cavity remains large and somewhat rounded and the posterior wall thin. A thin filling defect over the posterior border represents the "displaced" posterior papillary muscle (arrows). The small differences between the left ventricular end-diastolic and end-systolic chamber dimensions evident here are characteristic of dilatative cardiomyopathy. These radiographs were taken with a rapid film changer.

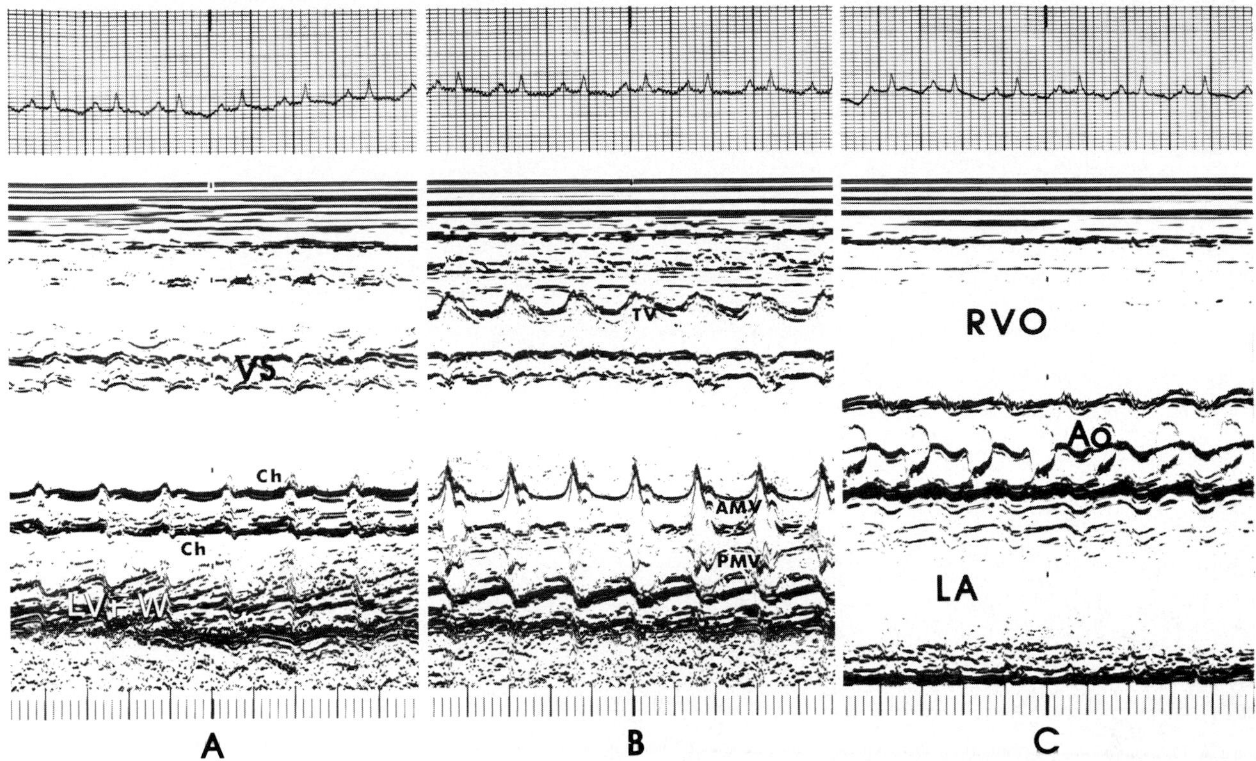


**Figure 18–86** Dilatative cardiomyopathy, M-mode echocardiogram, 11-year-old spayed female domestic shorthair. In *A*, recorded at the fringe of the mitral valve toward the apex, the left ventricle is markedly dilated, with thinning of both the left ventricular free wall (LVFW) and the ventricular septum (VS) and depressed systolic motion (%ΔD = 9.62%; ejection fraction = 22.8%). There is also right ventricular dilatation. The two parallel linear structures within the left ventricular cavity are chordae tendineae and the edges of the anterior (AMV) and posterior (PMV) leaflets of the mitral valve. These can be seen more clearly in *B*, taken through the left ventricle at the mitral valve. The wide separation between the anterior mitral valve and the ventricular septum is additional evidence of left ventricular dilatation, as these two structures should normally touch, or nearly so. The right ventricle remains dilated at this position, and the anterior leaflet of the tricuspid valve (TV) can be visualized. In *C*, recorded at the level of the aorta and left atrium, both the right ventricular outflow tract (RVO) and the left atrium (LA) are dilated (LA/Ao ratio = 1.86). The aorta is of normal dimensions with reduced amplitude, suggestive of decreased cardiac performance. Ch = chordae tendineae.

effusion is present, thoracocentesis should always be performed at the outset for therapeutic and diagnostic purposes. Digoxin is given at 0.004 to 0.008 mg/kg/day divided into two doses along with diuretics. The short-term use of other inotropic agents, such as dopamine and dobutamine, has been of some benefit in temporarily improving myocardial performance but has had little effect on the long-term prognosis. Vasodilator agents may also effect some improvement in cardiac performance and peripheral circulation and are currently being evaluated (see later section on cardiac therapeutics). Diuretic therapy must be carefully tailored to the individual's needs. Overzealous use of diuretics can cause circulatory volume depletion. The resulting reduction in cardiac output and effective peripheral circulation may lead to renal dysfunction.

**Management and Prevention of Thromboembolism.** The incidence of thromboembolism as a primary cause of clinical signs and manifestations of CM has been reported to range from 33 to 50 per cent (Harpster, 1977a; Tilley et al., 1974). After congestive heart failure, thromboembolism is the most common cause of clinical signs. In a recent review of 55 cats with cardiomyopathy thoroughly studied over a three-year period, thromboembolism was a primary clinical manifestation in only 16.4 per cent. However, this figure was falsely lowered owing to euthanasia of a significant number of cats with thromboembolism, which consequently were never seen by the cardiology service.

**Management of Acute Arterial Embolism.** My experience favors an initial 8- to 12-hour medical approach utilizing heparin and acetylpromazine maleate (acepromazine). Before this treatment is started there should be a baseline clotting time determination and neurologic evaluation of the affected limb(s). Initially, 1000 USP units of heparin are given intravenously and 0.25 to 0.5 mg/kg of acepromazine subcutaneously. After three hours 50 USP units/kg of heparin are given subcutaneously at six- to eight-hour intervals. This dosage is adjusted to prolong the clotting time two or two and a half times beyond the baseline value. The dosage of acepromazine is adjusted to maintain mild sedation.

Hydralazine (0.4 to 0.6 mg/kg orally or intramuscularly) may be substituted for the acepromazine, the purpose being to enhance circulation to affected limbs by improving blood flow through collateral vascular channels. Heparin therapy is used as described. With this approach, medical management is continued for 24 to 48 hours before surgical intervention is considered. Although the results of this regimen seem promising, too few cases have been treated in this way to justify recommending its routine use.

During initial medical treatment of thromboembolism, attention should also be focused on resolution of any cardiac problems that coexist (i.e., congestive heart failure, arrhythmias), renal function (e.g., urine production, azotemia), neurologic status of the affected, ischemic limb(s), and maintenance of body temperature. Every effort should be made to evaluate and deal with secondary complications before surgical intervention is contemplated. The cause of the embolic episode must not be disregarded in the course of its management; nonselective angiocardiography or echocardiography should be carried out in every cat before embolectomy.

Indications for embolectomy include (1) progressive worsening of limb ischemia over a 24- to 48-hour period of adequate medical management; (2) oliguria or anuria that is resistant to intravenous furosemide (Lasix) administration (4 to 8 mg/kg), or deterioration in renal function; and (3) persisting exertional ischemia of 10 to 14 days' duration that shows no evidence of improvement. The major contraindications to surgical intervention are unstable congestive heart failure and the presence of serious cardiac arrhythmias. Surgical removal of emboli within the abdominal aorta is best accomplished by laparotomy and direct aortotomy (see chapter on soft tissue surgery). I have attempted to remove emboli at the aortic bifurcation by insertion of an embolectomy catheter in the femoral artery; however, this has not proved successful owing to technical difficulties that have not so far been resolved. Surgical results have been improved by minimizing surgery time, maintaining body temperature, and preventing declamping shock during surgery by the administration of 2 mEq/kg of sodium bicarbonate by slow intravenous infusion. The greatest problem after embolectomy is the development of a low cardiac output syndrome, with death occurring 12 to 24 hours after surgery. The administration of inotropic agents is sometimes of benefit, but they are not routinely effective. This major complication has yet to be satisfactorily resolved. Identification, before surgery, of the specific form of cardiomyopathy present is desirable and should offer some options in management of complications postoperatively (e.g., propranolol for HCM vs. inotropic agents for ICM and DCM). This is my current approach to the management of cats with this complication. (See Table 18–18 for an outline of emergency and long-term management of thromboembolism associated with cardiomyopathy.)

**Prevention of Thromboembolism.** The prevalence of thromboembolism as both a cause of primary clinical signs and a common complication in cats being treated for cardiomyopathy has a major, negative effect on prognosis. Thus the need for preventive measures can be more than justified. My choice of agents depends on whether or not thromboembolism is known to have occurred in the past.

For cats receiving treatment for cardiomyopathy but with no history of thromboembolism, mild antithrombotic agents are recommended. Aspirin or an aspirin-Maalox combination is given at 2½ grains twice weekly. The antithrombotic effects of aspirin are reported to last for up to seven days. Dipyridamole (Persantine) has been suggested as an alternative to aspirin (Tilley et al., 1974).

**Table 18–18 Management of Thromboembolism Associated with Cardiomyopathy**

**ACUTE OCCLUSION OF AORTA**
Establish diagnosis
- Absence of femoral pulses, absence of external iliac pulses on rectal examination
- Aortography (nonselective angiocardiography)

Medical management
- Prevent clot extension with heparin USP 1000 units IV, then 50 units/kg SC every 6 to 8 hours
- Adjust dosage to maintain clotting time at 2 to 2½ times normal value
- Improve collateral circulation with hydralazine 0.4 to 0.6 mg/kg PO or IM every 8 hours
- Stabilize heart failure and arrhythmias with diuretics and antiarrhythmic agents. Avoid propranolol (mild vasoconstriction)

Define underlying form of cardiomyopathy
- Nonselective angiocardiography or echocardiography

Surgical intervention (embolectomy)
- Avoid barbiturate anesthesia (arrhythmogenic)
- Indications
  - Progressive hindlimb ischemia over 24 to 48 hours despite adequate medical measures
  - Anuria, oliguria: consider embolus at or proximal to origin of renal arteries. Define by aortography.
  - Long-standing exertional ischemia

**PREVENTIVE MEASURES**
Good control of heart failure
Measures to retard thrombus formation
- Antithrombotic agents. Clinical efficacy unproven; ineffective clinically in cats previously experiencing an acute thromboembolic episode
  - Aspirin—2½ grains twice weekly
  - Persantine (dipyridamole). No clinical experience
  - Warfarin-type anticoagulant agents. Inadequate studies to evaluate efficacy; appear superior to antithrombotic agents in limited clinical trials
    - Potential for adverse reactions, i.e., active, internal bleeding
    - Must avoid accidental injuries; keep cat indoors
    - Expense factor, i.e., need to evaluate prothrombin time periodically
    - Coumadin 0.1 mg/kg PO once daily. Adjust dosage to prolong the prothrombin time to twice the baseline value at 8 to 10 hours after administration. Requires 48 to 72 hours to develop an effective clinical response.

Although the efficacy of such agents is difficult to assess, the risks that attend the use of more potent drugs are hard to justify for this group of cats.

For cats that have experienced an embolic episode the mild antithrombotic agents appear to be totally inadequate. In the past I have tried short-term (i.e., one to three months) use of heparin with some apparent benefit, but long-term, frequent, subcutaneous administration is difficult for an owner to carry out. At present I am evaluating warfarin-type anticoagulants for long-term administration. The dosage is adjusted to prolong the prothrombin time to twice the normal value. The dosage for most cats ranges from 0.5 to 1.0 mg daily (0.1 mg/kg orally). Although conclusive results are not yet available, warfarin appears to be a possible alternative to heparin.

**Management of Arrhythmias.** Arrhythmias are the third most common cause of clinical signs and complications in cardiomyopathy. The prevalence of arrhythmias in the several forms of feline cardiomyopathy is shown in

Table 18–16. Frequent or persistent arrhythmias may substantially depress myocardial performance and precipitate congestive heart failure. On the other hand, intermittent or suddenly developing tachyarrhythmias or bradyarrhythmias can cause cardiovascular syncopal episodes by transient but marked reduction in cardiac output.

The tachyarrhythmias are most frequent: supraventricular premature beats, supraventricular tachyarrhythmias (e.g., paroxysmal supraventricular tachycardia, atrial fibrillation), ventricular premature beats, accelerated idioventricular rhythm, and paroxysmal ventricular tachycardia. Unless a tachyarrhythmia is contributing significantly to the development of congestive heart failure, specific treatment is usually postponed until heart failure is stabilized, the form of cardiomyopathy is defined, and the effects of treatment for it are evaluated. Digoxin and propranolol alone are often effective in controlling the heart rate in atrial fibrillation in DCM and in terminating paroxysmal supraventricular tachycardia in HCM, respectively. While the ventricular tachyarrhythmias may be reduced by similar measures, other antiarrhythmic drugs may be needed. Both quinidine sulfate (5.5 to 11 mg/kg t.i.d.) and procainamide hydrochloride (8 to 20 mg/kg t.i.d.) have been used with some success.

The bradyarrhythmias are much less frequent and are often associated with fairly severe biventricular failure. Attempts to manage these arrhythmias with combinations of sympathomimetic agents (e.g., isoproterenol, ephedrine sulfate) and diuretics have usually been disappointing. Permanent pacemaker therapy could offer some of these cats a chance for improvement, although this has not been reported.

**EXCESSIVE LEFT VENTRICULAR MODERATOR BANDS.** Moderator bands (trabeculae septomarginales) are single or branched fibromuscular strands that extend from the interventricular septum to insert on a papillary muscle or, much less often, on the right ventricular free wall adjacent to a papillary muscle (Truex and Warshaw, 1942). They are frequent in the right ventricle and rare in the left. At one time they were considered important in the prevention of excessive dilatation of the right ventricle during diastole. However, current opinion is that they play a morphologic role in conducting Purkinje fibers from the septum to the ventricular free wall, thus facilitating rapid spread of ventricular conduction and coordinated ventricular contraction (Evans and Christensen, 1979).

A specific condition in which an excessive number of left ventricular moderator bands were believed responsible for cardiac dysfunction has been reported in the cat (Liu et al., 1982). The clinical signs in a group of adult cats were indistinguishable from those of cardiomyopathy, as were many of the other findings. Congestive heart failure was the predominant reason for presentation, with nearly equal numbers of cats having left heart failure with pulmonary edema or biventricular failure with pleural effusion. Paraparesis secondary to aortic bifurcation embolization and syncopal episodes was also observed. Cardiomegaly was a consistent radiographic finding. Disturbances in impulse generation and conduction were the most frequent electrocardiographic abnormalities, and included right bundle branch block, left anterior fascicular block, atrioventricular conduction abnormalities, and sinus bradycardia. Cardiac catheterization in two cats demonstrated marked elevation of the left ventricular end-diastolic pressure (30 to 40 mm Hg). At autopsy, left ventricular dilatation was found in some cats and left ventricular hypertrophy in others; however, the ratio of heart weight to body weight (gm/kg) in both groups was less than expected in cats with comparable forms of cardiomyopathy. The microscopic myocardial changes were similar to those in the various forms of feline cardiomyopathy.

Guidelines for the management of cats with excessive left ventricular moderator bands have not been established. Because it may be difficult to differentiate this condition from cardiomyopathy by current noninvasive and invasive diagnostic procedures, until further information becomes available it would seem reasonable to follow the same course of therapy as discussed for cardiomyopathy. When the left ventricle is shown by echocardiography or nonselective angiocardiography to be dilated, the use of digitalis glycosides, diuretics, and vasodilator agents should be considered. However, when these studies show the left ventricular cavity to be small and the septum and left ventricular free wall thickened, propranolol and diuretic therapy should be instituted. Antithrombotic agents may be useful in the prevention of thromboembolism.

The question must be raised as to whether the excessive moderator bands alone are wholly responsible for the cardiac dysfunction ascribed to this condition, or whether cardiomyopathy is superimposed on cats with excessive left ventricular moderator bands. If the moderator bands alone are at fault, why should there be such a distinct difference in age between cats with left ventricular hypertrophy (mean 4.0 years) and those with left ventricular dilatation (mean 8.7 years [Liu et al., 1982])? The heart weight:body weight ratios, smaller than expected in comparable forms of feline cardiomyopathy, could represent an interference in normal cardiac compensatory changes caused by restrictions in diastolic dimensions imposed by the moderator bands.

## Secondary Myocardial Diseases

It has become common practice in human cardiology to reserve the term secondary myocardial disease for conditions of known cause or association (Oakley, 1974). The list of identified causes of myocardial disease is extensive. Included are infectious agents, metabolic disorders, neuromuscular diseases, autoimmune diseases, neoplasms, toxins, drug reactions, and hypersensitivity disorders. While no such extensive list of secondary myocardial disorders has been identified for the cat, there is no reason why the feline myocardium could not be affected by the same influences. Compared with what we know for man, our current understanding of both primary and secondary feline myocardial diseases is quite limited. Additional studies are needed to broaden our knowledge.

**INFECTION.** In man, myocardial involvement has been recognized as a rare to common complication of all known infectious agents. These include viruses, bacteria, spirochetes (syphilis, leptospirosis), rickettsiae (typhus, Rocky Mountain spotted fever, Q fever), fungi (many genera), protozoa (trypanosomiasis [Chagas' disease], toxoplasmosis, malaria, amebiasis, leishmaniasis, balantidiasis, sarcosporidiosis), and helminth parasitisms (trichinosis, echinococcosis, schistosomiasis, ascariasis, filariasis, paragonimiasis, strongyloidiasis, cysticercosis) (Wenger, 1972).

For the domestic cat ***viruses*** have often been suggested as a cause of myocardial disease, including the cardiomyopathies, but proof is lacking. A coronavirus has been proposed as a possible agent in the development of a dilatative cardiomyopathy–like disorder in kittens as part of the "kitten mortality complex" (Scott et al., 1979; Norsworthy, 1979). We have also studied several adult cats in which feline infectious peritonitis appeared to be the cause of multifocal myocardial lesions due to vasculitis, a lesion more often observed in other organs (e.g., liver, kidneys) and the pathophysiologic mechanism responsible for the development of meningoencephalitis and anterior uveitis (Plate 18–1*D*).

***Bacterial myocarditis*** is a well-recognized sequel to bacterial endocarditis in the cat (Shouse and Meier, 1956) and other mammalian species (Bornstein, 1971; Wenger, 1974). Myocardial involvement develops by extension of infection from involved valves or by hematogenous spread of bacteria and small septic emboli to the coronary circulation, and it is responsible for the cardiac arrhythmias that are commonly present. The combination of myocardial dysfunction, cardiac arrhythmias, and valvular incompetence may lead to congestive heart failure, particularly when highly virulent bacteria are responsible. Early diagnosis by appropriate laboratory tests, bactericidal antibiotic therapy based on in-vitro susceptibility tests, and control of arrhythmias by electrocardiographic monitoring and judicious use of antiarrhythmic agents are crucial in the successful management of affected cats, and in minimizing the short- and long-term deleterious effects on the heart and other organs. (The reader should refer to the section on valvular heart disease for further information regarding the diagnosis and management of primary bacterial infections involving the heart.)

***Toxoplasmosis*** is an infectious disease having well-recognized effects on the myocardium. It is caused by *Toxoplasma gondii*, a small intestinal coccidian of cats with oocysts ranging in size from 10 to 12 μ. Many species of birds and a variety of mammals, including cats, are susceptible. Infection may occur by ingestion of the oocyst, especially in herbivores and birds, by ingestion of the cyst in infected meat, and occasionally by transplacental transmission (Frenkel, 1977). Most organs can become involved by localization of tachyzoites via hematogenous and lymphogenous spread from the intestinal tract. In chronic infection, clinical signs may follow the rupture of cysts and subsequent release of bradyzoites. The incidence of myocardial lesions in a group of cats with acute and chronic toxoplasmosis was reported to be 41.7 per cent and 30.0 per cent, respectively (Petrak and Carpenter, 1965).

A review of the pathology records at AMAH for a 13-year period (1967 through 1979) identified 23 cats with toxoplasmosis. Of this group the heart was examined histologically in 20. Myocardial lesions compatible with toxoplasmosis were found in 12 cats. Characteristic microscopic lesions included focal myocardial necrosis in nine, mononuclear inflammation in two, granulomatous inflammation in one, and focal myocardial fibrosis in two. Focal interstitial hemorrhage was also common. *Toxoplasma* cysts and bradyzoites were rarely found in myocardial lesions. Thus the diagnosis of *Toxoplasma* myocarditis was usually one of inference, being strongly influenced by histopathologic lesions found in other tissues. The extent of the myocardial changes varied widely among these cats, being severe in only one. Clinical signs of heart disease were usually absent. In two cats a low-intensity heart murmur was present over the left cardiac apex, but other clinical evidence of heart disease was lacking. An electrocardiogram performed in a single cat demonstrated ST-T changes that persisted over a period of nine days without the occurrence of other abnormalities (Fig. 18–87). These observations are similar to those reported for *Toxoplasma* myocarditis in man, although congestive heart failure, pericarditis, arrhythmias, and conduction disturbances have been observed (Wenger, 1972).

If these limited observations are valid, *Toxoplasma*

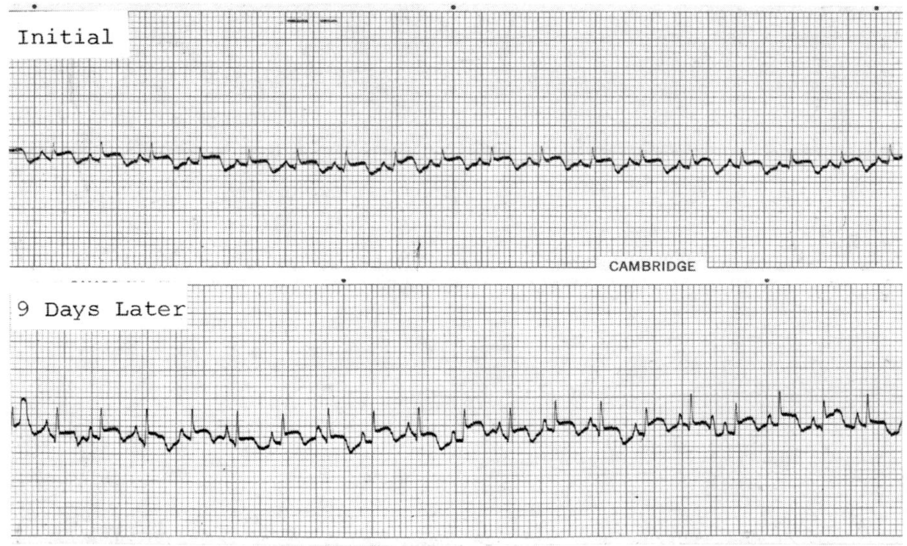


**Figure 18–87** Lead II electrocardiograms from a three-year-old male domestic shorthair presented with a history of recurrent fever (to 41.2° C) and intermittent left foreleg lameness over the preceding two and a half months. In the initial tracing the basic rhythm is normal sinus rhythm at approximately 162/minute. There is mild S-T segment elevation and prolongation of the Q-T interval (220 to 240 milliseconds). Nine days later, the heart rate had increased slightly to 167/minute and the S-T segment elevation was more impressive; however, the Q-T interval had shortened to 200 milliseconds. Myocardial ischemia and noneffusive pericarditis were considered possible causes of these abnormalities. Autopsy three days after the second tracing disclosed mild pericardial effusion and multiple tan foci in the lungs, heart, liver, and kidneys. Histologically there was necrotizing and granulomatous myocarditis. *Toxoplasma* organisms were not found in the myocardium but were present in sections of lung, liver, and periarticular tissues.

myocarditis can be considered of less significance than the other myocardial disorders discussed previously. In rapidly progressive toxoplasmosis, lung, central nervous system, and reticuloendothelial system involvement seems to dominate the clinical picture but may also obscure cardiac manifestations of the disease. Unless additional information is forthcoming, the myocardial effects of systemic toxoplasmosis would appear to be of less importance than changes in other organs.

Ante-mortem diagnosis of toxoplasmosis depends on the demonstration of a high or rising titer of *Toxoplasma* antibodies in the serum. Several serologic tests are available, including the Sabin-Feldman dye test and indirect fluorescent antibody, indirect hemagglutination, and complement fixation. While a high titer is suggestive of a recent active infection, a rising titer over a two- to three-week period provides indisputable evidence of active infection. Because of the rapid progression of toxoplasmosis in many naturally occurring cases, a diagnosis is more often made at autopsy.

Treatment combines sulfadiazine (60 mg/kg/day divided into four to six doses) and pyrimethamine (0.5 to 1.0 mg/kg/day in a single dose). These drugs are synergistic inhibitors of folate metabolism, and folinic acid, 1.0 mg/kg/day, should also be given to prevent toxic side effects. When organ involvement is severe, response to this therapeutic regimen is unlikely.

**NONINFECTIOUS CAUSES.** Secondary myocardial diseases of noninfectious origin are infrequently recognized in the cat, and, when suspected, differentiation from the primary myocardial diseases (i.e., the cardiomyopathies) may prove difficult. Of these, drug-induced cardiotoxic reactions and abnormal body-temperature states have been advanced as most common (Fox, 1983). However, metabolic abnormalities and immune-mediated diseases may also be responsible, and these could be of greater importance among elderly cats (Table 18–19).

Numerous drugs may have an adverse effect on myocardial performance. This may be a direct effect of the drug, in which case the magnitude of the toxic reaction tends to be dose-related, or it may be the result of a hypersensitivity reaction. Toxic effects may be transient or may cause permanent myocardial damage. These can range from arrhythmias without microscopic changes (e.g., digitalis glycosides, propranolol), cardiac dilatation with subendocardial hemorrhage (e.g., hyperthermia, hypothermia), interstitial deposition of acid mucopolysaccharide with myofibrillar degeneration (e.g., chronic administration of phenothiazine tranquilizers), and acute myocarditis with focal myocardial necrosis and infarction (e.g., sympathomimetic amines), to severe, diffuse myocardial degeneration (e.g., doxorubicin). Aspirin and dipyridamole offer some protection against experimental myocardial necrosis by catecholamines, suggesting that platelet aggregation plays a major role. The diffuse myocardial degeneration that can complicate chemotherapy with the anthracycline group of drugs (e.g., doxorubicin, daunorubicin) results in congestive heart failure that is refractory to therapy.

**Table 18–19 Causes of Secondary Myocardial Disease in the Cat**

**INFECTIOUS AGENTS**
- Viral
  - Feline infectious peritonitis
  - Others?
- Bacterial
- Protozoal
  - Toxoplasmosis

**NONINFECTIOUS CAUSES**
- Drug-Induced
  - Digitalis glycosides
  - Propranolol
  - Doxorubicin (Adriamycin)
  - Tranquilizers, sedatives
  - Anesthetic agents
  - Sympathomimetic amines
- Physical agents
  - Hyperthermia
  - Hypothermia
- Metabolic disorders
  - Diabetes mellitus
  - Chronic renal insufficiency
  - Hyperthyroidism
- Immune-mediated disease
  - Periarteritis nodosa

Of the metabolic disorders having proven adverse effects on myocardial performance, only hyperthyroidism occurs with any frequency in the cat. This abnormal metabolic state also affects the peripheral vascular system. It will be discussed with hyperkinetic heart disease.

Both diabetes mellitus and chronic renal failure have been thought to be responsible on rare occasions for the development of a cardiomyopathy-like syndrome in the domestic cat. In chronic renal failure, systemic hypertension and chronic anemia probably play major roles in the evolution of a cardiomyopathy characterized by heart murmurs, gallop rhythms, cardiomegaly, arrhythmias, and even overt congestive heart failure (Fox, 1983). Left ventricular hypertrophy, indistinguishable from hypertrophic cardiomyopathy, is found at autopsy. In man the cardiovascular effects of diabetes mellitus are well established (Williams and Braunwald, 1980). The vascular effects include lesions of large vessels (e.g., accelerated atherosclerosis and arteriosclerosis) and also arteriolar lesions (e.g., microangiopathic or endothelial proliferative changes). When advanced, these vascular changes can lead to the development of systemic hypertension and myocardial ischemia. More recently, myocardial disease, unassociated with significant coronary vascular lesions, has been recognized in humans with diabetes mellitus. These are characterized histologically by the interstitial deposition of glycoproteins, including collagen, triglycerides, and cholesterol; and functionally by shortening of the left ventricular ejection time, prolongation of the preejection period, and elevation of the ratio of the preejection period to the left ventricular ejection time (PEP/LVET). These changes are thought to be quite specific and have been termed diabetic cardiomyopathy (Ahmed et al., 1975; Hamby et al., 1974; Seneviratne, 1977). Although a dilatative cardiomyopathy–like disorder has been observed in diabetic cats, its histologic characteristics are not well defined, and it has not been clearly separated from idiopathic dilatative feline cardiomyopathy. The few cats we have treated have responded well to a combination of digitalis glycoside and diuretic therapy, along with insulin injections for control of the diabetic state. One cat lived for more than two years.

Lastly, the immune-mediated disorders deserve mention as potential causes of myocardial disease in the cat.

While these diseases are still infrequently diagnosed, they are being recognized more often. With the exception of feline infectious peritonitis, which histologically represents an immune-mediated arteritis, only polyarteritis nodosa has been reported as a true autoimmune disease resulting in myocardial involvement in the cat (Altera and Bonasch, 1966; Lucke, 1968). However, renal and joint involvement predominate in the clinical picture along with other systemic signs (e.g., fever, lethargy, anorexia), and myocardial involvement appears to be an incidental finding at post-mortem examination.

## Valvular Heart Disease

Acquired valvular heart disease refers to disorders in which one or more valves are affected by a primary pathologic process. Ideally this term should be reserved for those conditions in which the valve leaflets or semilunar cusps are affected primarily, rather than being involved secondarily in some myocardial, endocardial, or vascular process. However, this distinction is not easily made even with extensive physiologic and hemodynamic studies. For instance, left AV valve incompetence may result from deformity of the valve leaflets (i.e., primary disease) or may be secondary to annular ring dilatation, abnormally shortened or lengthened chordae tendineae, papillary muscle dysfunction, or even abnormal left ventricular contraction. These various components that are responsible for the proper closure of the left AV valves and the maintenance of their competence make up the mitral valve apparatus (Perloff and Roberts, 1972). In a similar fashion the aortic valves may undergo degenerative changes (e.g., mucoid degeneration, fibrosis) secondary to congenital or acquired obstructive processes proximal or distal to the cusps. Chronic turbulent blood flow is the best explanation for the valvular changes in this setting.

Primary acquired valvular heart disease in most mammals can be ascribed either to infectious agents or to degenerative processes, although connective tissue diseases and other antigen-antibody responses are additional recognized causes in man (Fowler, 1973). Bacterial and fungal endocarditis has been recognized in most species. Degenerative processes affecting the mitral valve leaflets have been reported in man and the dog (Buchanan, 1977; Mills et al., 1977).

The prevalence of degenerative changes affecting the left AV valve leaflets in the cat is significant, for myxomatous degeneration is common in all forms of cardiomyopathy. However, myxomatous degeneration can also be found in some cats not exhibiting the classic or clear-cut findings of cardiomyopathy. What role this pathologic process plays as a cause of left AV valvular incompetence and symptomatic heart disease in the cat has not been established.

Bacterial endocarditis is infrequently reported in the domestic cat (Harpster, 1977a; Joshua, 1959; Liu, 1977; Shouse and Meier, 1956). This seems somewhat incongruous in a species so often affected by bite wounds, abscesses, and a variety of other bacterial infections. The low incidence of congenital and acquired valvular heart disease may be a partial explanation, as valve abnormalities are believed to predispose to bacterial implantation following an episode of bacteremia (Beeson, 1967). As in man (Beeson, 1967) and the dog (Dear, 1977), the left AV valves are most often involved (Shouse and Meier, 1956). Clinical signs in affected cats tend to be nonspecific, with lethargy and anorexia predominating. Findings on examination suggestive of endocarditis include fever, newly found or changing heart murmurs, cardiac arrhythmias, and clinical evidence of systemic arterial occlusion. Other clinical evidence of endocarditis includes a history of recent bacterial infection or nonsterile surgery, concurrent localized bacterial infection, immunosuppression with or without the use of chemotherapeutic agents, a regenerative neutrophilia, and mild anemia. Many other conditions can be confused with bacterial endocarditis in the cat. Included in the differential diagnosis should be the myeloproliferative diseases, feline infectious peritonitis, toxoplasmosis, upper respiratory viral diseases, panleukopenia, hemobartonellosis, and localized bacterial infections. The features differentiating bacterial endocarditis and FCM are outlined in Table 18–20.

A firm diagnosis of bacterial endocarditis can be made only on the basis of positive blood cultures. Three to six cultures should be obtained over a 12- to 24-hour period before the start of antibiotic therapy. Ideally, the same bacteria should be isolated from two or more cultures to eliminate the possibility of contamination. Recent administration of antibacterial agents will markedly reduce the chance of obtaining a positive culture. Once the diagnosis is confirmed, therapeutic guidelines as outlined for the management of bacterial endocarditis in man should be followed (Bornstein, 1971; Kaye, 1973). Only bactericidal antibiotics of in-vitro demonstrated effectiveness should be used, and they should be given at full therapeutic dosages. When Gram-positive organisms of low-grade pathogenicity are isolated (e.g., alpha-hemolytic *Streptococcus* spp, beta-hemolytic *Streptococcus* spp, *Enterococcus* spp), antibiotics should be continued for four weeks. However, when highly virulent Gram-positive (e.g., *Staphylococcus* spp) or Gram-negative organisms are isolated, effective antibiotics should be administered for six

**Table 18–20 Features Differentiating Bacterial Endocarditis and Cardiomyopathy in the Cat**

| CLINICAL FINDINGS | BACTERIAL ENDOCARDITIS | CARDIO-MYOPATHY |
|---|---|---|
| Clinical onset | Usually protracted course, nonspecific | Varies with form, frequently acute |
| Fever | Present | Absent |
| Heart murmur | ± early<br>+ late | Variable<br>50–60% |
| Arrhythmias | Frequent | Frequent |
| Gallop rhythms | Unknown* | 25–30% |
| Congestive heart failure | Late, if it occurs | Early |
| Hepatosplenomegaly | + + | + |
| Icterus | ± | – |
| Arterial embolism | Common | Common |
| Cardiomegaly (x-ray) | Variable | Present |
| Hematocrit | Anemia common | Normal |
| Complete blood count | Neutrophilia with left shift | Stress neutrophilia |

*Two few cats with endocarditis to permit conclusion.

to eight weeks. After termination of antibiotic therapy the temperature should be monitored daily and blood cultures taken at weekly intervals for a month.

The major complications encountered in bacterial endocarditis include widespread sepsis with formation of microabscesses, arterial embolism and development of septic infarcts, and cardiac injury. Cardiac damage in endocarditis may result from extensive valvular destruction and deformity with subsequent incompetence and from myocardial involvement. This latter complication may occur by the extension of infection to the myocardium from affected valvular tissue or by hematogenous spread of septic emboli to the coronary circulation. The sequelae of these combined insults to the heart may be life-threatening cardiac arrhythmias or even congestive heart failure. Aortic valve involvement, in particular, results in a poor long-term prognosis.

## Hyperkinetic Heart Disease

A normal or increased cardiac output in the presence of congestive heart failure is the expected finding in hyperkinetic or high-output heart disease (Fowler, 1974). Since cardiac output is the product of heart rate and stroke volume, it may be increased by a rise in either or both of these variables. "Changes in heart rate are usually brought about by changes in the level of autonomic nervous system activity. Stroke volume is increased by an increase in myocardial contractility, a decrease in peripheral vascular resistance or intramyocardial resistance, an increased venous return of blood to the heart, or some combination of these factors" (Goodkind, 1971).

In man, hyperthyroidism (Graettinger et al., 1959), thiamine deficiency (Akbarian et al., 1966), anemia (Duke and Abelmann, 1969), and arteriovenous fistula (Muenster et al., 1959) are commonly reported and thoroughly studied causes of hyperkinetic heart disease. Less frequent causes have also been reported, including an idiopathic hyperkinetic cardiovascular syndrome that is thought to be the result of a hypersensitive response of the beta-adrenergic receptors (Frohlich et al., 1966; Gorlin et al., 1959). While similar underlying conditions have been recognized in the cat, hemodynamic studies to confirm a hyperkinetic cardiovascular state are lacking. However, common pathophysiologic mechanisms are assumed to exist on the evidence of clinical observations and noninvasive cardiovascular findings.

**ANEMIA.** The hemodynamic effects of chronic anemia include a rapid circulation time, tachycardia, decreased peripheral vascular resistance, reduced blood volume, and increased arteriovenous oxygen differences, as well as the aforementioned increase in cardiac output. A reversal of the high-output state following peripheral vasoconstriction by either physiologic or pharmacologic intervention suggests that redistribution of blood volume and vasodilatation play dominant roles in the hyperkinetic circulatory response to chronic anemia (Duke and Abelmann, 1969).

Chronic, severe anemia (i.e., hematocrit $< 20$ per cent) in the cat is frequently accompanied by systolic or holosystolic murmurs over the left cardiac apex and mild to moderate degrees of cardiomegaly. Cardiac dilatation and relative insufficiency of the left AV valves are probable causes for these findings. Less commonly, diastolic gallop rhythms, systolic ejection murmurs over the left cardiac base, and bruits over the carotid arteries may be present. These auscultatory abnormalities will disappear and cardiac size will gradually return to normal after correction of the anemia.

Severe chronic anemia is usually well tolerated in cats unless significant underlying heart disease exists. Then the added cardiac burden associated with the anemia may precipitate heart failure. Management of heart failure in these circumstances should be accomplished as rapidly as possible, as the fluid retention accompanying the heart failure effects a relative reduction in the hematocrit. The digitalis glycosides are of reported benefit in this condition (Davis et al., 1957). Blood transfusions should be avoided until the heart failure is stabilized, and then packed cells rather than whole-blood transfusions should be administered. A concerted effort should be made to identify the cause of the anemia and institute corrective measures when possible.

**HYPERTHYROIDISM.** The excessive production of physiologically active thyroid hormones is a well studied and extensively reported cause of hyperkinetic heart disease in man (de Groot, 1972; Goodkind, 1971; Graettinger et al., 1959). While causes for increased serum thyroid hormone levels are varied, the effects of increased levels on the cardiovascular system are similar in most species studied, with tachycardia and increased peripheral blood flow being the hallmarks of the hyperthyroid state. The increase in resting heart rate is the combined result of a direct effect of thyroid hormone on the myocardium and a stimulating effect on the sympathetic nervous system. An increase in myocardial contractility accompanies the tachycardia. The increase in peripheral blood flow is predominately the result of vasodilation of blood vessels to the skin and skeletal muscles, the organ systems with the largest vascular supply. Total peripheral vascular resistance is decreased. The end result of these changes is an increase in venous return and cardiac output, the latter being proportional to the degree of the hyperthyroid state (i.e., the elevation of circulating thyroid hormones above normal).

Adenomatous goiter has been reported as a cause of hyperthyroidism in cats (Holzworth et al., 1980). Weight loss despite normal or increased appetite, hyperactivity, increased frequency of defecation with soft stools, occasional vomiting, and polydipsia and polyuria are the predominant clinical signs. However, several perceptive owners noticed a rapid heart rate, and on physical examination cardiac abnormalities are frequently the most significant finding leading to diagnosis. The principal cardiovascular findings are tachycardia, systolic or holosystolic murmurs over the cardiac apex, arrhythmias, and prominent femoral pulses. In thoracic radiographs, mild degrees of cardiomegaly are usually present. The significant cardiovascular findings in 12 cats with laboratory-proven hyperthyroidism are summarized in Table 18–21. Congestive heart failure has been an infrequent complication of this condition, even when it has been thought to exist for several years. When heart failure has been present, underlying organic heart disease has been assumed to coexist, although this still needs to be clarified.

A diagnosis of adenomatous goiter is based on the presence of typical clinical signs, a palpable nodule in the area of one or both thyroid lobes, and, most importantly, an elevated serum level of triiodothyronine ($T_3$) or thyroxine ($T_4$), or both. In the majority of affected cats the $T_3$ and $T_4$ levels are both above normal. When cervical

**Table 18–21 Signalment and Significant Cardiac Findings in 12 Cats With Adenomatous Goiter**

| CARDIAC FINDINGS | RESULTS | |
|---|---|---|
| Average age (range) | 12.9 yr | (9–20) |
| Male:female ratio (% males) | 2.0 | (66.7) |
| Heart rate: Av (range) | | |
| Auscultation | 215 | (180–300) |
| Electrocardiogram | 237 | (206–286) |
| Heart murmurs: No. (%) | | |
| Left apex | 4 | (33.3) |
| Right apex | 4 | (33.3) |
| Total* | 9 | (75.0) |
| Electrocardiographic findings: No. (%) | | |
| P waves† | | |
| Duration >0.04 sec | 1 | (10.0) |
| Amplitude ≥0.2 mV | 6 | (50.0) |
| QRS interval >0.04 sec | 8 | (66.7) |
| LVH pattern‡ | 7 | (58.3) |
| Arrhythmias | | |
| Supraventricular premature beats | 4 | (33.3) |
| Supraventricular tachyarrhythmias§ | 2 | (16.7) |
| Ventricular premature beats | 3 | (25.0) |
| *Total*‖ | 7 | (58.3) |
| Conduction disturbances | | |
| Right bundle branch block | 1 | ( 8.3) |
| Intraventricular conduction abnormality | 1 | ( 8.3) |
| Congestive heart failure: No. (%) | 2 | (16.7) |

*In one cat a low-intensity murmur was heard over the cranial sternum.

†P waves could be identified in only ten cats.

‡See Table 18–17 for criteria.

§One cat was in atrial tachycardia and one in atrial fibrillation.

‖Both supraventricular and ventricular premature beats were present in two cats.

thyroid enlargement is not clinically detectable, the position of the hyperfunctioning thyroid tissue can be defined by radioisotope studies (i.e., radioscans) utilizing either $^{131}$I or technetium 99m($^{99m}$Tc) (dos Remedios et al., 1971; Turrel et al., 1984) (Fig. 18–88). In most instances the affected thyroid lobe lies at the thoracic inlet and can be felt with dorsal extension of the neck when its exact position is known from the radioisotope study. Small but discrete nodules of adenomatous goiter have been found in ectopic thyroid tissue in several cats that have gone to post-mortem examination several years after the initial diagnosis and treatment. Although the hyperthyroid state has not recurred in these cats, the potential for recurrence via ectopic thyroid tissue does exist.

Attempted medical management has produced less than optimal results. The administration of propylthiouracil at 5 to 10 mg/kg t.i.d. has been beneficial in eliminating some of the clinical signs and in preventing additional weight loss. However, significant weight gain has not been realized during short-term therapy, besides which a hemolytic anemia and thrombocytopenia have been reported in a small percentage of cats receiving this drug (Peterson et al., 1984). More recently, methimazole (Tapazole) has been recommended as an alternative to propylthiouracil for the medical management of cats with hyperthyroidism (Peterson, 1984). In our limited experience, methimazole seems to be a more effective thyroid-suppressive agent than propylthiouracil (although causing vomiting in some cats), and may be a satisfactory alternative to surgery in the long-term management of adenomatous goiter. The initial dosage is 5.0 mg t.i.d.; however, it can frequently be reduced to 5.0 mg b.i.d. after two to four weeks with good maintenance of the euthyroid state.

Propranolol is another agent that has proved useful in the short-term medical and presurgical management of hyperthyroidism in the cat. Its main indications are for the reduction of heart rate in severe sinus tachycardia (i.e., heart rate > 240/minute) and as an antiarrhythmic agent in the control of both supraventricular and ventricular arrhythmias. Effective doses range from 0.5 to 1.0 mg/kg b.i.d. or t.i.d.

The present treatment of choice for adenomatous goiter is surgical excision of all affected thyroid tissue. In most instances this means bilateral thyroidectomy, for even though only one lobe may be palpably enlarged, at surgery the opposite lobe is usually affected to a lesser degree. Grossly, affected thyroid tissue is greenish rather than the normal tan-pink, and multiple nodules of varying sizes can be seen. Both thyroid lobes should routinely be removed unless one is smaller than normal (i.e., atrophied), is of normal color, and has no grossly identifiable nodules. Subcapsular excision of the affected glands has proved most effective in preserving blood supply and normal function of the parathyroid glands. If congestive heart failure complicates the hyperthyroid state and makes

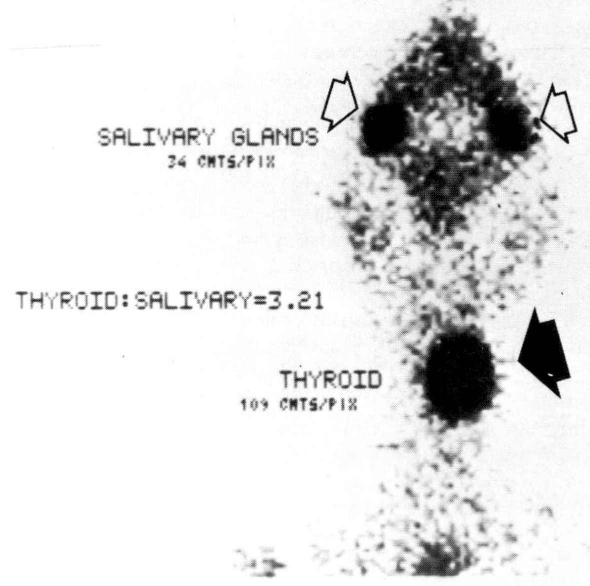


**Figure 18–88** Hyperthyroidism, sodium pertechnetate ($^{99m}$Tc $O_4$) thyroid scan of a 12-year-old neutered male domestic shorthair with a history of weight loss over a two-year period despite an excellent appetite. Although an enlarged left thyroid lobe was palpable on physical examination, serum levels of thyroid hormones were normal ($T_3$ 69 ng/dl; $T_4$ 3.3 μg/dl). The thyroid scan indicates increased size and activity of the left lobe (solid arrowhead). The two areas of increased activity in the head (open arrowheads) are the salivary glands. The right lobe was markedly atrophied at surgery and was not removed. The cat responded well to removal of the left lobe.

surgical intervention an undue risk, an acceptable alternative is a trial of methimazole or else radioisotope therapy with $^{131}I$ (Turrel et al., 1984; see also the chapter on management of tumors).

After surgical excision of hyperfunctioning thyroid tissue the euthyroid state is usually attained in 24 to 72 hours, depending on the presurgical level of $T_4$ (the half-life of thyroxine in the cat approximates 20 hours). Thyroid replacement therapy is started 48 hours after surgery with sodium levothyroxine at 0.05 to 0.1 mg daily, divided into two doses. Adjustments in replacement therapy are based on serum levels of $T_3$ and $T_4$ determined one month later and periodically thereafter.

With few exceptions, the results of surgical treatment are extremely gratifying. Immediate regression of clinical signs and substantial weight gain are usual. The heart rate returns to normal within a few days, there is disappearance or marked reduction in cardiac arrhythmias, and heart murmurs either disappear or are reduced in intensity. The only complication that has been recognized is hypoparathyroidism, due to inadvertent excision or ischemia of functional parathyroid tissue. This is most likely to happen when both thyroid lobes are considerably enlarged at surgery, making identification of parathyroid tissue more difficult. The resulting hypoparathyroidism usually develops within 24 to 48 hours after surgery and is characterized by trembling, muscle fasciculations, or even grand mal seizures. Impending hypocalcemia is detected early by measuring serum calcium levels at 24 and 48 hours after surgery. If serum calcium levels remain normal at 48 hours, the likelihood of surgically induced hypoparathyroidism is extremely remote. The hypocalcemia that develops is usually transient, provided that proper surgical protocol has been followed. It can be successfully managed by a combination of calcium lactate (2½ grains b.i.d. or t.i.d.) and vitamin $D_3$ supplement (calcitriol, cholecalciferol [Rocaltrol, Roche] 0.25 μg daily). Once serum calcium levels become normal, monitoring should be carried out weekly. This ensures maintenance of a normal serum calcium level and early detection of hypercalcemia due to excessive therapy or return of parathyroid function. In most cats, normal parathyroid function returns within two to eight weeks after surgery.

**ARTERIOVENOUS FISTULA.** An abnormal communication between an artery and a vein without an interposed capillary bed is termed an arteriovenous fistula. Congenital malformations, surgical procedures, and penetrating wounds are the reported causes for these abnormal vascular shunts (Taussig, 1960). In man, congenital arteriovenous fistulae commonly involve the pulmonary, hepatic, and coronary artery circulations (Goodkind, 1971).

The hemodynamic alterations occurring in arteriovenous fistulae are almost directly proportional to the flow through the shunt (Frank et al., 1955). In small fistulae these changes are negligible, but with moderate or large fistulae cardiac output is increased. This is thought to be the result of increased venous return with concomitant increased ventricular filling and stroke volume, as the heart rate tends to remain normal. In addition, the accompanying decrease in total peripheral vascular resistance, due to the shunting of blood through the fistula, permits greater systolic emptying of the left ventricle and further augmentation of stroke volume. In order for the peripheral vascular system to accommodate to the shunt and maintain relatively normal arterial pressure, blood flow to other parts of the body must adjust. Renal vascular resistance is increased and is accompanied by reduced excretion of salt and water (Epstein et al., 1953). However, coronary vascular resistance is decreased, attended by an increase in coronary blood flow. Myocardial oxygen consumption is increased in proportion to the increase in coronary blood flow.

The effects of a moderate- to large-sized arteriovenous fistula on the cardiovascular system are chronic volume overloading of the heart and a widened pulse pressure. Bounding or "water-hammer" pulses are expected. A palpable thrill and an auscultable continuous murmur can be detected at the site of an arteriovenous communication that is in a peripheral, accessible location. Digital occlusion of the artery proximal to the shunt results in a slowing of the heart rate, a reduction in the pulse pressure, and a transient increase in the blood pressure (Branham's sign) (Branham, 1890). Heart murmurs may be present owing to increased cardiac blood flow and cardiac dilatation. Right-sided congestive heart failure may be the end result.

The prevalence of arteriovenous fistulae in the feline population is assumed to be low on the basis of the paucity of reports in the veterinary literature. With the exception of patent ductus arteriosus, arteriovenous communications in the cat are usually peripheral, the apparent result of previous injury or surgery (Harari et al., 1984; Slocum et al., 1973). However, centrally located, congenital arteriovenous fistulae have been reported in several cats (Bolton et al., 1976; Legendre et al., 1976). When an arteriovenous fistula is present in a limb, the usual findings are subcutaneous edema and superficial venous distention distal to the shunt. Exudation of tissue fluid may occur through the intact skin owing to high local venous pressure; skin ulceration with periodic bleeding may result from ischemia distal to the fistula. In most instances the limb distal to the fistula is warmer than the opposite, unaffected limb. However, if distal blood flow is compromised, the limb may be cooler distally than the opposite one, indicating the existence of ischemia and the potential development of gangrene.

The accepted method for correction of arteriovenous fistulae is surgical extirpation of all arterial communications, as well as a portion of the affected venous system. This is not always easy, particularly with congenital malformations, in which multiple arteriovenous communications are usually present. Before surgical intervention, an arteriographic study is mandatory to define the anatomic distribution of the communications. However, small arteriovenous fistulae may not require correction. In fact, correction of larger fistulae may even be contraindicated when the surgical risk is high (usually because of the anatomic location of the fistula), and when clinical signs are absent or minimal. Indications for mandatory surgical intervention even in high-risk patients are three: heart failure caused by massive shunting of blood, pain caused by large lesions encroaching on major nerves or weight-bearing surfaces, and hemorrhage caused by a large lesion extending through the skin and becoming vulnerable to trauma (Fry, 1974). After successful surgical closure of all communications, blood flow distal to the fistula and cardiac output should return to normal. If congestive heart failure existed before surgery, this should now be more easily controlled by appropriate medical methods.

## Pulmonary Heart Disease

Cor pulmonale (pulmonary heart disease) is defined most simply as right ventricular enlargement resulting from disorders that affect the structure or function of the lungs (Robbins et al., 1984). Conditions that may lead to pulmonary heart disease are pulmonary embolization, diffuse pulmonary vascular involvement such as occurs in systemic hypersensitivity states, any chronic disease that may increase pulmonary vascular resistance or induce intrapulmonary vascular shunts, pulmonary or mediastinal tumors that compress the vessels, and skeletal or neuromuscular disorders that interfere with the bellows function of the chest.

The basic pathophysiologic process that leads to cor pulmonale is fairly straightforward. The initiating factor is either a primary pulmonary disorder that destroys many pulmonary blood vessels and thereby reduces the cross-sectional area of the pulmonary vascular bed or a primary pulmonary vascular disorder that decreases the luminal diameter of the pulmonary vessels. Both these factors can lead to increased pulmonary vascular resistance with subsequent pulmonary hypertension, which in turn increases the work of the right ventricle. If pulmonary or pulmonary vascular disease progresses, the eventual result is right ventricular hypertrophy and even right heart failure. In certain instances, acute, transient right heart failure may complicate chronic, stable pulmonary disease because of superimposed disease processes. Pneumonia, asthmatic attacks, and pulmonary embolism are common examples of these potentially reversible complications.

**CONGENITAL CARDIOVASCULAR SHUNTS.** Despite the common occurrence of diffuse pulmonary disease in the domestic cat, notably that resulting from hypersensitivity reactions (e.g., chronic allergic bronchitis, "asthma"), pulmonary heart disease has rarely been reported (Harpster, 1977a; Scratcherd and Wright, 1961). Of the possible causes, moderate-sized, chronically persisting left-to-right congenital cardiovascular shunts most often lead to pulmonary hypertension and right heart failure (e.g., Jeraj et al., 1978).

In man, pulmonary vascular disease associated with congenital cardiac shunts has been termed plexogenic pulmonary arteriopathy. The earliest recognized histologic change is muscularization of pulmonary arterioles to resemble systemic arterioles. This is characterized by a distinct tunica media of circular muscle between the inner and outer elastic laminae. The second response of the pulmonary arterioles to increased pressure is cellular proliferation. Cells responsible for this response are thought to originate from vasoformative reserve cells within the subintima. This response ultimately evolves to intimal fibrosis and intimal fibroelastosis with occlusion of small pulmonary arteries and arterioles. As the pulmonary hypertension progresses, diffuse dilatation of the pulmonary arterial tree develops. Localized dilatation of muscular pulmonary arteries results in characteristic lesions, the most distinctive of which is the plexiform lesion. The final stage in the progression of plexogenic pulmonary arteriopathy is the development of necrotizing arteritis. This is characterized by fibrinoid necrosis of the media and an acute inflammatory reaction about the damaged smooth muscle cells (Heath and Smith, 1977).

These vascular changes are the consequence of long-standing increased pulmonary blood flow. Potentially, any moderate-sized left-to-right congenital cardiac shunt may be responsible (e.g., ventricular septal defect, patent ductus arteriosus, common atrioventricular canal, and atrial septal defect with or without partial anomalous pulmonary venous drainage); however, I have observed these complications only with ventricular septal defects (Fig. 18–89) and patent ductus arteriosus.

Clinical signs may result from fixed pulmonary blood flow with reduced cardiac output (e.g., exercise intolerance, syncopal episodes), progressive pulmonary hypertension culminating in right heart failure (e.g., abdominal distention), or shunt reversal (e.g., cyanosis, tachypnea and dyspnea at rest or with minimal exertion). In advanced stages, right-sided intracardiac pressures (intravascular in the case of patent ductus arteriosus) are elevated to equal those on the left side, resulting in balancing or reversal of the shunt. At this stage, previously detected heart murmurs are usually diminished in intensity, changed in character, or absent, and both diagnosis and management of the underlying cardiac anomaly become substantially more difficult. Cardiac catheterization must now be carried out to define the exact cause of the

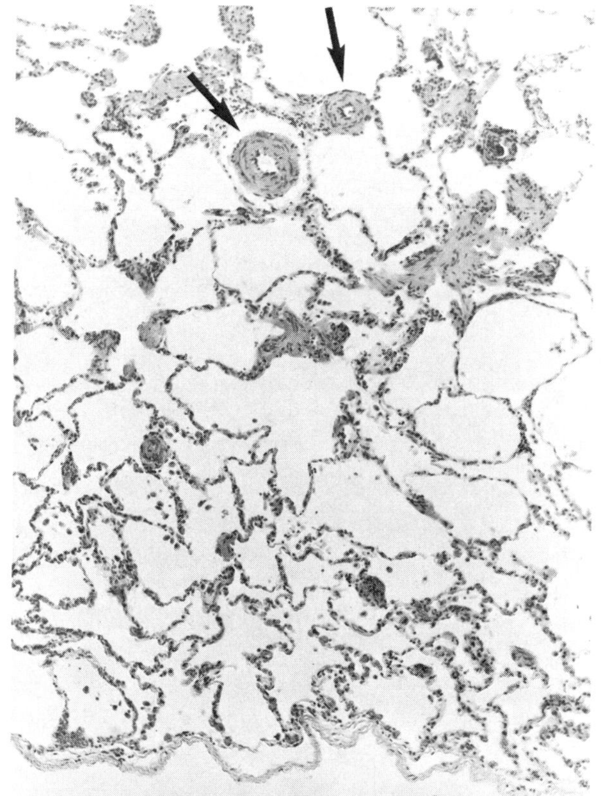

**Figure 18–89** Hypertrophy of pulmonary arteries and smooth muscle in a seven-year-old spayed female domestic shorthair presented for progressive abdominal enlargement over a two-week period. The small pulmonary arteries (arrows) are markedly thickened, resembling small systemic arteries. Alveolar septa have increased cellularity, and the alveoli contain an excessive number of macrophages. Autopsy disclosed a ventricular septal defect 5 mm in diameter in the membranous septum below the aortic valve. H & E, × 50.

cat's problem. Attempts at surgical correction are usually confounded by further elevations in pulmonary artery pressure leading to acute right heart failure and rapid deterioration in the cat's condition.

**DIROFILARIASIS.** The development of endothelial proliferation of the pulmonary arteries is a well-recognized complication of parasitism with the nematode *Dirofilaria immitis* in dogs and other members of the Canidae (Knight, 1977). These vascular changes commonly cause significant luminal narrowing of small peripheral vessels, resulting in increased pulmonary vascular resistance, pulmonary hypertension, and even right heart failure. Clinical signs are coughing, reduced exercise tolerance, classic right heart failure (e.g., hepatomegaly, ascites), and sudden death.

It has long been recognized that the cat can be parasitized by *D. immitis*. The occurrence is low, compared with that in dogs, to judge from surveys in which the incidence has ranged from 0.0 to 8.0 per cent (Ash, 1962; Holmes and Kelly, 1973; Lillis, 1964; Mann, 1955; Mann and Fratta, 1952; Rosen, 1954; Todd et al., 1976). (The incidence in dogs in these same surveys ranged from 3.2 to 37 per cent.) Unlike man, the domestic cat can serve as a definitive host, with the parasite reaching sexual maturity and propagating microfilariae.

Feline dirofilariasis experimentally induced by adult worm transplantation or subcutaneous inoculation of third-stage infective larvae (Donahoe, 1975; Donahoe et al., 1976a, b; Fowler et al., 1972; Mann and Fratta, 1953) has provided further information on the incidence of microfilaremia and on hematologic and radiographic alterations. Neither the number of infective larvae inoculated nor the number of adult worms found at autopsy correlated well with the occurrence of microfilaremia (Donahoe, 1975; Fowler et al., 1972). An explanation for these observations is not apparent. Hematologic changes included eosinophilia 90 days after inoculation and leukocytosis with neutrophilia 50 to 120 days later (Donahoe et al., 1976a). The leukocytosis, which was accompanied by a second peak of eosinophilia, was attributed to a response of the cats to maturation of the parasite. Radiographic abnormalities were evident in all cats three to seven months after inoculation: increased visibility of the main pulmonary arteries, diffuse or focal areas of density in the pulmonary parenchyma, and right-sided heart enlargement (Donahoe et al., 1976a). These changes were greatest in male cats, cats with microfilaremia, and cats inoculated with a dose of 100 or more infective larvae. When these same cats were subjected to pulmonary arteriography (Donahoe et al., 1976b), enlargement, tortuosity, and blunting of the pulmonary arteries were the most common findings. Defective filling of the right pulmonary artery was also frequent. In a few cats, adult worms could be distinguished as linear filling defects in blood vessels.

A review of the English-language veterinary literature turned up reports of 38 cats with naturally occurring dirofilariasis. The clinical and pathologic findings reported are summarized in Table 18–22. The higher incidence in males may be related to greater outside activity and therefore more exposure to infected mosquitoes. Outstanding clinical signs were sudden onset of dyspnea, sudden death, or a rapid progression of the former to the latter; in 12 cats (42.9 per cent) the presence of adult worms was considered to be directly responsible for death.

**Table 18–22 Feline Dirofilariasis: Summary of Literature Reports of 38 Naturally Occurring Cases**

| CLINICAL FINDINGS | TOTAL NO. REPORTED | NO. AFFECTED (RANGE) | PER CENT (MEAN) |
|---|---|---|---|
| Age | 20 | (<1 to 7.0) | (3.15) |
| Sex | 20 | — | — |
| Male | | 16 | 80.0 |
| Female | | 4 | 20.0 |
| Clinical signs | 28 | — | — |
| Cough | 28 | 4 | 14.3 |
| Dyspnea | 28 | 7 | 25.0 |
| Acute death | 28 | 10 | 35.7 |
| CNS signs | 28 | 4 | 14.3 |
| Other* | 28 | 6 | 21.4 |
| Microfilaria-positive† | 17 | 9 | 52.9 |
| Number of adult parasites | 29 | (1 to 12) | (3.0) |

*Unrelated to the presence of adult parasites or their effects.
†Includes cats in which peripheral blood was not examined but gravid female worms were found at autopsy.

In four of these cats a single adult worm in the brain was responsible for signs of central nervous system disturbance and progression to death or euthanasia (Cusick et al., 1976; Donahoe and Holzinger, 1974; Faries et al., 1974; Mandelker and Brutus, 1971).

The finding of either circulating microfilariae in the peripheral blood or gravid adult female worms at autopsy in as many as 52.9 per cent of the cats in which these were reported seemed surprising. However, these data are comparable to those reported for cats experimentally inoculated with third-stage larvae (Donahoe, 1975). The small numbers of adult worms found at autopsy in individual cats (mean 3.0) can be interpreted variously. Most likely the cat is a less than satisfactory host for this parasite and completion of the life cycle is difficult owing to the lack of species specificity. Possibly too the small number of adults worms together with the early age at the onset of clinical signs (mean 3.15 years) indicates that even small numbers of adult worms are lethal to the cat and that early onset of clinical signs does not permit time for more worms to develop to full maturity. The low incidence of dirofilariasis in the feline population, the presence of few mature adult worms at post-mortem examination, and the relative absence of immature parasites make the first explanation more likely.

Histologically, the pulmonary arterial changes in cats with symptomatic heartworm disease are similar to those reported for the dog (Knight, 1977). Hyperplasia of the tunica media was a consistent finding in literature reports (Abbott, 1966; Stackhouse and Clough, 1972; Todd et al., 1976). However, of greater pathophysiologic significance were papillary proliferation of the intima; intimal fibrosis; vascular and perivascular infiltration of eosinophils, neutrophils, lymphocytes, and occasional epithelioid cells; and thrombus formation (Fig. 18–90). Less frequent findings were bronchial wall thickening accompanied by inflammation, mild alveolar edema with macrophage proliferation, and pulmonary fibrosis.

It can be concluded that the domestic cat is an unnatural or atypical host for *D. immitis*. However, in certain instances the life cycle can be completed, so that the cat can serve as a reservoir for this parasite. Dirofilariasis should be considered in the differential diagnosis in any

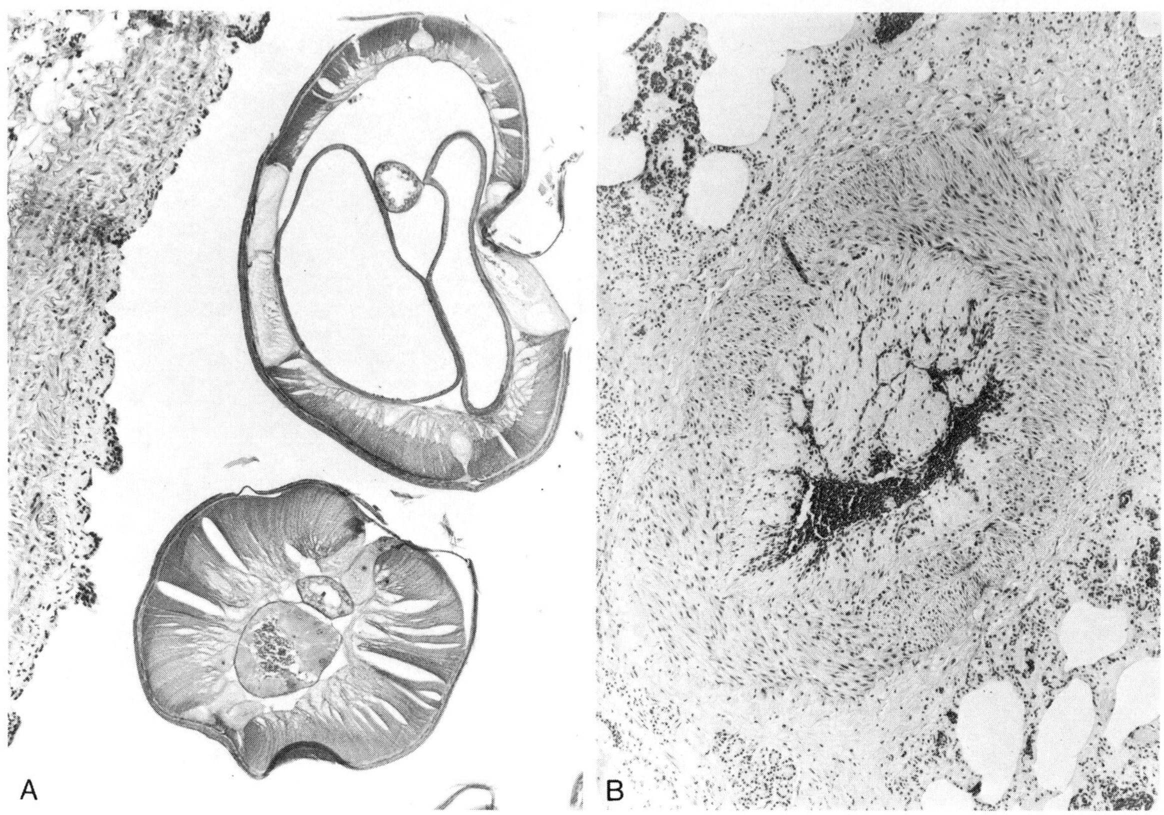


**Figure 18–90** Dirofilariasis, 16-year-old spayed female Persian presented for lethargy, anorexia, and labored breathing of two days' duration. *A*, Two transverse sections of an adult nematode can be seen in the lumen of a large pulmonary artery that exhibits mild proliferative villous endarteritis. *B*, Severe proliferative endarteritis. The lumen has been reduced to a small irregular channel. Eosinophilic and mononuclear pneumonitis (upper left and lower right corners) and hyperplasia of bronchial glands (upper left corner) were other prominent findings. Peripheral blood from this cat was positive for microfilariae. Twenty adult heartworms were found in the right ventricle and main pulmonary arteries at autopsy. H & E, × 50.

cat from an endemic area presented with acute onset of difficulty breathing in which supportive radiographic changes are found (Donahoe et al., 1976a). Owing to the much higher incidence of occult heart worm disease in the cat than reported in the dog (Wong et al., 1973), venous angiocardiography (Hawe, 1979) or pulmonary arteriography (Donahoe et al., 1976b) may be required to confirm the diagnosis. When the parasitism is diagnosed in the living cat, successful treatment has been carried out with the filaricidal agent thiacetarsamide sodium (Caparsolate) (0.22 ml/kg IV b.i.d. on two consecutive days), followed four to six weeks later by dithiazanine iodide (Dizan) (6 to 20 mg/kg orally) until the peripheral blood is negative for microfilariae (Schwartz, 1975). Levamisole has also been used successfully as a microfilaricide. Because the cat seems to be relatively resistant to infective larvae, there is no need for preventive measures at this time, except in unusual circumstances. However, preventive therapy with diethylcarbamazine should be considered for cats that have been successfully treated for dirofilariasis and perhaps even for other unaffected cats in the same household.

An excellent review of the current knowledge of feline dirofilariasis and of its manifestations in an endemic area is that of Dillon (1984). For definitive diagnosis of occult parasitism an angiogram demonstrates the distinctive sign of enlarged pulmonary arteries with ill-defined margins. Right-sided cardiac enlargement and failure are infrequent. The IFA test, when positive (in about a third of cases), is diagnostic. The ELISA test has promise, but false-positive results related to cross-reactivity are possible; also titers may vary from laboratory to laboratory depending on the method used.

**MEDIAL HYPERTROPHY OF THE PULMONARY ARTERIES.** Hypertrophic and hyperplastic alteration of the tunica media in small pulmonary arteries has long been recognized as a common histopathologic finding in cats of all ages (Dahme, 1960; Marcato, 1940, 1941; Olcott et al., 1946; Rubarth, 1940; Stünzi et al., 1966). The incidence of these changes in a number of autopsy studies has ranged from 2.0 per cent (Olcott et al., 1946) to 68.8 per cent (Tashjian et al., 1965). Frequently, associated thickening (hyperplasia) of the intima results from deposition of collagenous connective tissue between the intima and media (Fig. 18–91). Islands of hypertrophied smooth muscle, primarily distributed in terminal bronchioles and in the region of alveoli of respiratory bronchioles, have also been reported (Scratcherd and Wright, 1961). There is often an eosinophilic periarteritis (Stünzi et al., 1966).

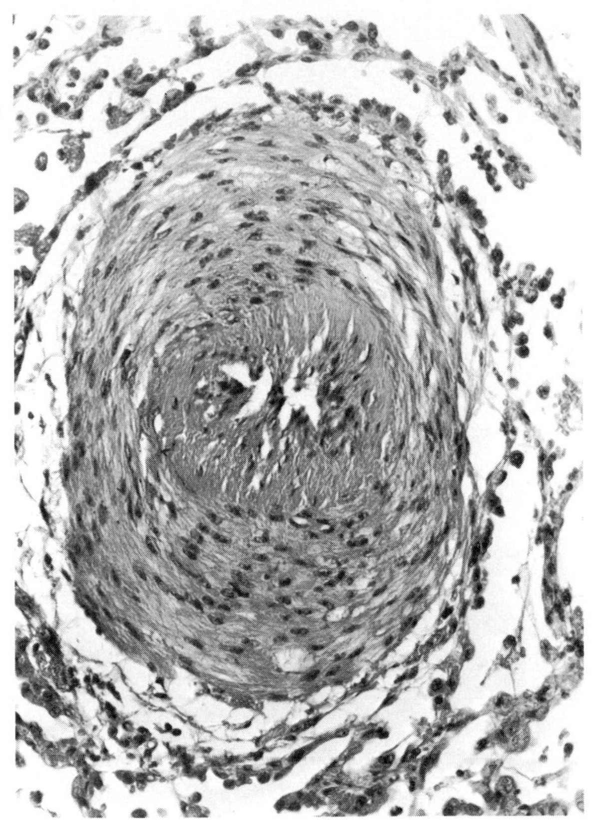

**Figure 18–91** Intimal and medial hyperplasia of a branch of a lobar pulmonary artery in a seven-year-old neutered male domestic shorthair with hypertrophic cardiomyopathy. The circularly arranged smooth muscle cells are increased in size and number. The diminutive, stellate lumen (center) is surrounded by a thickened intima composed of excess collagen. Numerous macrophages are within the adjacent alveoli. A one-year course of heart disease in this cat terminated in death from thromboembolism and pulmonary edema. H & E, × 200.

Jones and Zook (1965) reported a segmental distribution of these vascular changes and suggested undefined aging processes as a possible cause. However, Tashjian et al. (1965) considered an active process to be responsible because of the presence of identical lesions in a number of young kittens. Similar changes were also described in cats parasitized with the lungworm *Aelurostrongylus abstrusus* (Damiano and Galati, 1967; Mackenzie, 1960; Martin, 1962; Pritchett, 1938). Since these initial descriptive reports, experimental studies have attributed medial hypertrophy and hyperplasia of the feline pulmonary arteries to parasitic infestation with both *Toxocara cati* (Swerczek et al., 1970) and *Aelurostrongylus abstrusus* (Hamilton, 1970). Carpenter (1974) reported similar histologic findings in a small group of cats with bronchial asthma and Rogers et al. (1971) in specific pathogen–free cats. At present the evidence is strong that pulmonary parasitism is partly, if not totally, the cause of these pulmonary vascular lesions. What other factors or influences are capable of causing similar changes has yet to be established.

Despite the extensive distribution, and sometimes severity, of these vascular changes, related clinical signs are not recognized. Only Scratcherd and Wright (1961) reported a measurable increase in the thickness of the right ventricular free wall, which they attributed to medial hyperplasia and hypertrophy in the most severely affected cats.

Although the character of the changes in the pulmonary arteries in parasitism with *A. abstrusus* suggests that there might be right-sided heart strain, an experimental study could find no evidence of pulmonary hypertension or of an associated right ventricular response (Rawlings et al., 1980).

The role of the vascular lesion in cats with acute asthma and chronic bronchitis is unclear.

**PULMONARY ARTERIAL EMBOLISM.** This is an infrequently recognized problem in the domestic cat. Pulmonary artery embolization has been reported as a variable post-mortem finding in feline cardiomyopathy (Harpster, 1977b; Liu, 1974; Liu et al., 1970). As a rule the emboli are small, have minimal influence on pulmonary function, and probably contribute little to the morbidity and mortality associated with this disease. They tend to originate from small thrombi in the right side of the heart, particularly within the auricular appendage.

## Other Heart Disease

This category includes a group of unrelated conditions that can be considered either uncommon primary cardiovascular diseases or as representing cardiovascular effects of primary systemic diseases. Inclusion in this group should not detract from their importance; rather, a special category has been created to permit inclusion of all recognized forms of feline cardiovascular disease.

**CARDIAC ARRHYTHMIAS.** The occurrence of arrhythmias is unexpected in the normal cat. Tachyarrhythmias, when present, most often result from cardiomyopathy or hyperthyroidism. With cardiomyopathy ventricular arrhythmias predominate (e.g., ventricular premature beats, accelerated idioventricular rhythm, paroxysmal ventricular tachycardia), whereas hyperthyroidism is characterized by supraventricular arrhythmias (e.g., supraventricular premature beats, paroxysmal supraventricular tachycardia). Atrial fibrillation in the cat is usually associated with cardiomyopathy, most often the hypertrophic form (Tilley, 1985). Tachyarrhythmias may also occur in cats with bacterial endocarditis, after blunt chest trauma (Fig. 18–92), and with certain congenital cardiac defects (e.g., common atrioventricular canal, Ebstein's anomaly) (Fig. 18–93).

When tachyarrhythmias persist despite specific therapy directed at the underlying cardiac condition (e.g., control of heart failure in cardiomyopathy and congenital heart disease; establishment of euthyroid state in hyperthyroidism; administration of in-vitro effective antibiotics in bacterial endocarditis), or when aggressive, life-threatening tachyarrhythmias develop during the management of these cats, the administration of antiarrhythmic agents is indicated. Although these drugs have been used infrequently in cats and our understanding of their effects and tolerance is limited, some progress in this area has been made (Erichsen et al., 1978; Roye et al., 1973). The reader should refer to the later section on cardiovascular therapy.

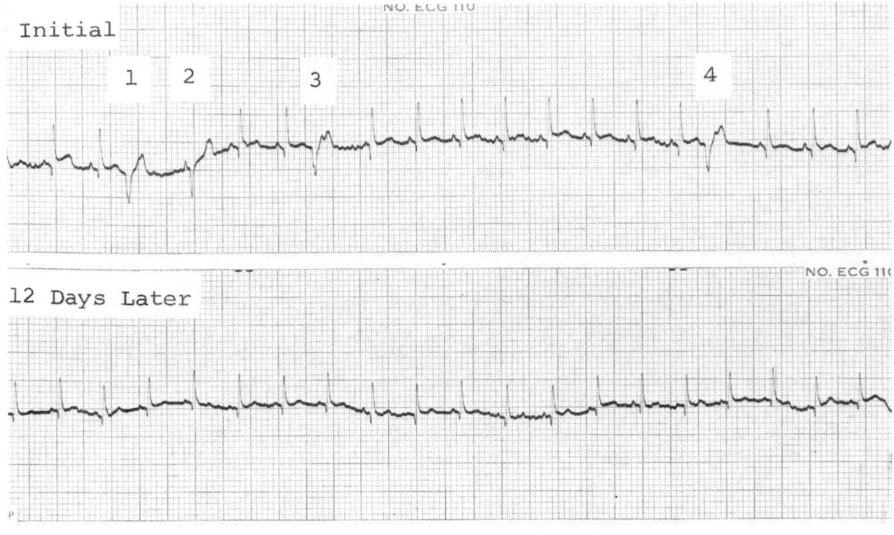


**Figure 18–92** Blunt chest trauma, lead II electrocardiograms from a six-year-old spayed female domestic shorthair. The initial tracing, taken 24 hours after an automobile injury, exhibits frequent unifocal ventricular premature beats (numbered complexes) characterized by bizarre, widened QRS complexes that differ substantially from the normal sinus QRS complexes. The second ventricular premature beat is narrower than the others and is preceded by a P wave, changes suggestive of a fusion beat. Normal sinus QRS complexes are mildly prolonged (45 to 50 milliseconds), suggesting prolonged ventricular depolarization. In a tracing taken 12 days later, no ventricular premature beats are recorded. The QRS interval is now within normal limits (40 milliseconds). No treatment was given for the arrhythmias observed initially. 25 mm/sec; 1.0 mV = 1.0 cm.

Bradyarrhythmias due to hyperkalemia are common in cats with urethral obstruction. Additional myocardial effects result from the associated hyponatremia, hypocalcemia, and metabolic acidosis. These alterations in serum electrolytes and acid-base balance are usually well developed within 24 to 48 hours of total obstruction. T-wave spiking, P-R interval prolongation, sinus arrest, widening of the QRS interval, and an idioventricular rhythm are the sequence of electrocardiographic abnormalities (Fig. 18–94). Management first requires relief of the obstruction. Then an isotonic, balanced electrolyte solution is administered intravenously to correct existing dehydration and maintain fluid balance in the face of an expected postobstructive diuresis. The first 24-hour fluid require-

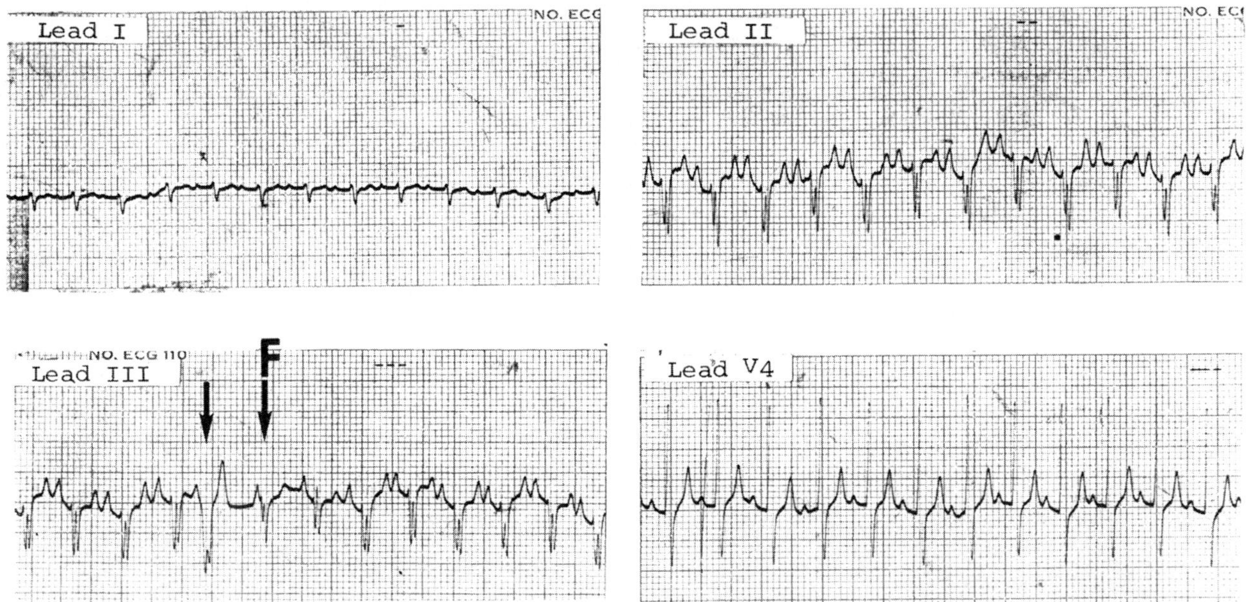


**Figure 18–93** Common atrioventricular canal, multiple-lead ECG from a 16-month-old male Himalayan. A single ventricular beat in lead III (arrow) is followed by a fusion beat (F). Notice the short P-R interval and deformity of the QRS complex associated with the fusion beat. Cardiac arrhythmias are surprisingly rare in most types of congenital heart disease until marked cardiac enlargement develops or congestive heart failure intervenes; then both supraventricular and ventricular arrhythmias are frequent. Such was the status of this young cat presented with dyspnea due to pleural effusion. The P waves are widened and of increased amplitude, suggesting biatrial enlargement. The bizarre QRS complexes are prolonged (0.99 second) owing to an intraventricular conduction abnormality. 25 mm/sec; 1.0 mV = 1.0 cm.

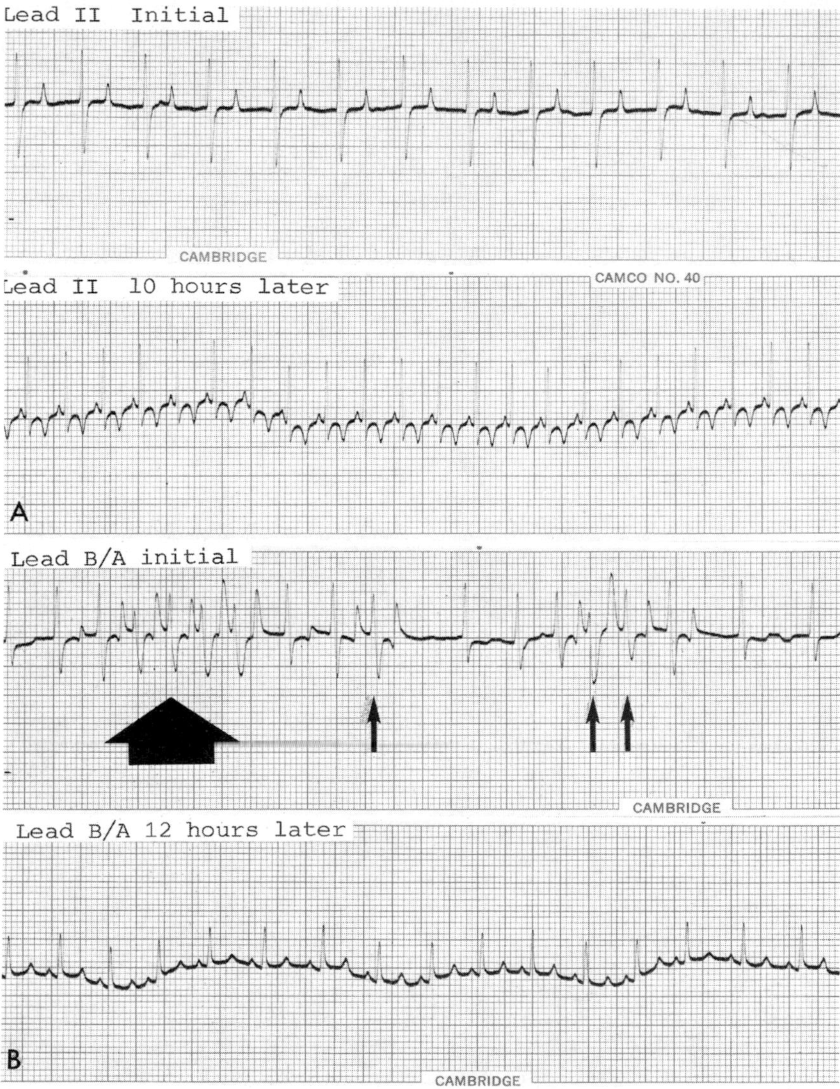


**Figure 18–94** Urethral obstruction, electrocardiographic abnormalities resulting from electrolyte and acid-base alterations. In *A*, recorded from a four-year-old neutered male Russian Blue with obstruction of three days' duration, the initial strip demonstrates a regular rhythm at 133/minute. P waves are absent and the QRS interval is prolonged (0.09 second), suggesting sinus arrest with an AV junctional rhythm and an intraventricular conduction abnormality. T waves are narrow and spiked. In a tracing taken 10 hours later, P waves are present and appear to be controlling the rhythm at 230/minute. Notice inversion of the T waves as compared with the initial tracing. The P-R interval is short, while the high-amplitude R waves and persisting S waves suggest that some intraventricular conduction abnormality is still present. After relief of the obstruction, therapy consisted of normal saline solution given IV with sodium bicarbonate (44 mEq/500 ml) and calcium gluconate 10 percent (500 mg/500 ml) added. Serum electrolytes at the time of the initial tracing were calcium 6.2 mg/dl, phosphorus 14.0 mg/dl, sodium 148 mEq/l, potassium 9.9 mEq/l. In *B*, from a one-year-old male domestic shorthair after a weekend of urethral obstruction, the underlying mechanism appears similar, with absence of P waves and widened, bizarre QRS complexes. In addition, however, there are AV junctional premature beats (arrows), as well as a short run of paroxysmal AV junctional tachycardia (arrowhead). The QRS interval widens with increased prematurity of the premature beats owing to further aberrancy of ventricular conduction. A tracing 12 hours later shows a return to normal sinus rhythm. This cat was treated similarly to the cat in *A*. Serum electrolytes at the time of the initial tracing were calcium 5.6 mg/dl, phosphorus 15.2 mg/dl, sodium 150 mEq/l, potassium 9.4 mEq/l. 25 mm/sec; 1.0 mV = 1.0 cm.

ments can be calculated by totaling the initial estimated deficit (per cent dehydration × kg body weight × 80 ml/kg), daily maintenance fluid requirement (60 ml/kg), and replacement of any contemporary losses (i.e., from vomiting or diarrhea). When postobstructive diuresis is intense, as is common in cats obstructed for 36 hours or longer, fluid therapy can be managed best by continuous monitoring of urine production and periodic measurement of serum sodium and potassium. In most instances the electrocardiographic abnormalities rapidly disappear with adequate fluid replacement and correction of the metabolic acidosis with sodium bicarbonate (1 to 2 mEq/kg over 10 to 15 minutes). If these measures prove ineffective or if life-threatening arrhythmias exist, the use of regular insulin and glucose has been recommended (Schaer, 1977). Regular insulin is added to intravenous fluid solution along with 2 gm of glucose for each unit of insulin. This solution is infused at a rate to supply the needs of the cat as discussed above.

**VENTRICULAR PREEXCITATION.** Ventricular preexcitation (Wolff-Parkinson-White [WPW] syndrome) has been reported in the cat (Flecknell et al., 1979; Harpster, 1977a; Ogburn, 1977; Tilley, 1985). It is a conduction abnormality in which impulses arising in the sinus node pass into the ventricles over an accessory atrioventricular (AV) pathway before passing through the AV node. Because decremental conduction (i.e., the normal mode of transmission in the AV node that is responsible for slowed conduction) does not exist in the accessory pathway, AV conduction is rapid, and reciprocating ventriculoatrial (VA) conduction may occur over either existing pathway, leading to supraventricular tachycardia or other supraventricular tachyarrhythmias.

In man, Wolff-Parkinson-White syndrome and other ventricular preexcitation syndromes are thought to result in the majority of patients from embryologic faults in partitioning of the atrium from the ventricle, with persisting muscular bridges passing through the faulty ring

(Gallagher et al., 1976). Wolff-Parkinson-White syndrome has been associated with other congenital cardiovascular anomalies in over 50 per cent of affected patients, as well as with hypertrophic cardiomyopathy of familial origin (Kariv et al., 1971). Supraventricular tachyarrhythmias that are fairly resistant to medical management and sudden death are well recognized complications of WPW syndrome in man.

In the cat the pathogenesis and natural causes of WPW syndrome are not well understood. Tilley (1985) has reported the association of WPW syndrome with hypertrophic cardiomyopathy and certain congenital cardiac defects (i.e., atrial septal defect, Ebstein's anomaly). The electrocardiographic features of WPW syndrome in the cat are similar to those reported for man (Estes, 1974): a short P-R interval, a widened QRS complex (> 0.06 second), and a slurred onset of the QRS complex (delta wave). The QRS complex resembles that of bundle branch block and may be accompanied by ST and T wave changes similar to those in bundle branch block (Figs. 18–36 and 18–95). Although sustained or symptomatic supraventricular tachyarrhythmias have not been reported in cats with ventricular preexcitation, one cat did have frequent atrial premature beats (Ogburn, 1977).

Treatment of WPW syndrome is not warranted unless supraventricular tachyarrhythmias are recorded or syncopal episodes have occurred. In man, initial treatment is directed at control of the recurrent tachyarrhythmias with

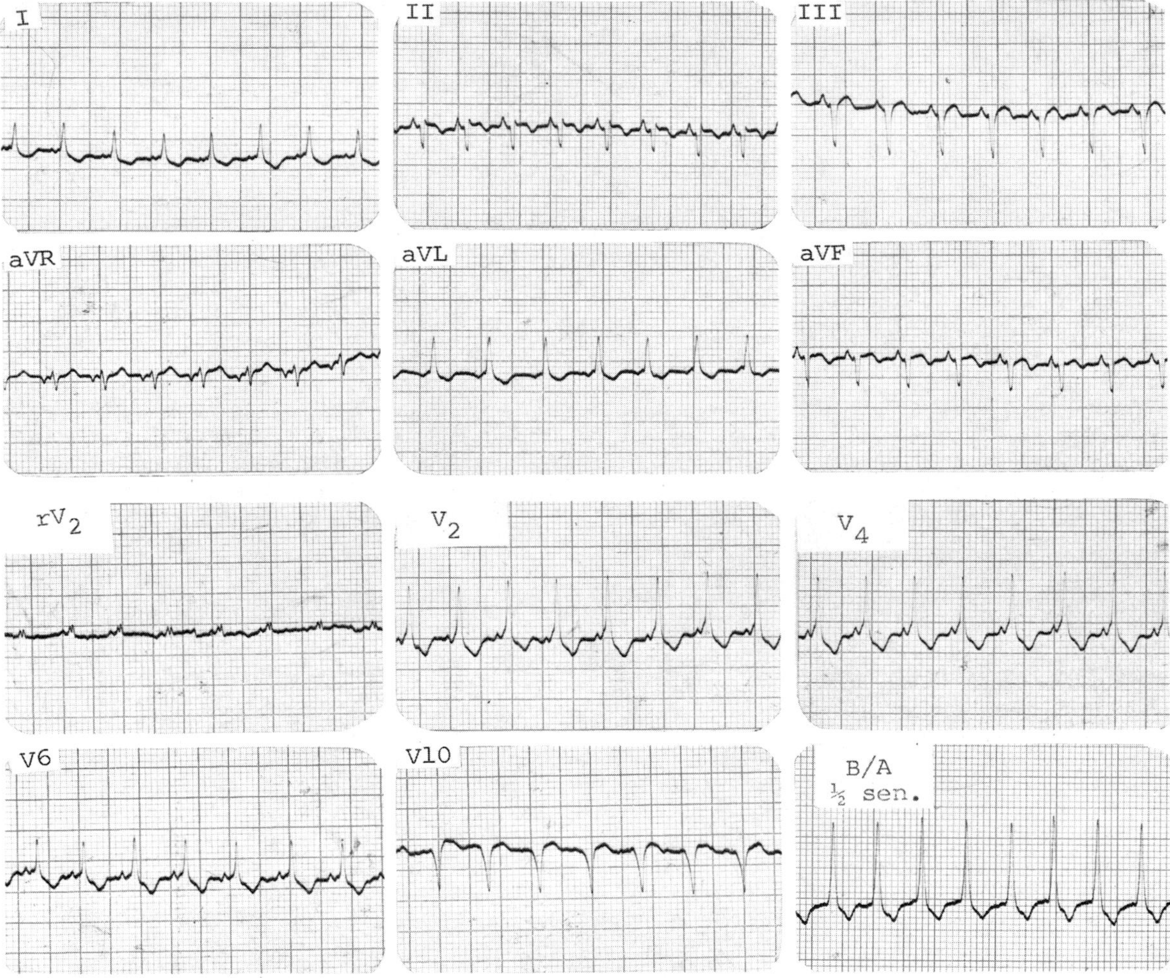


**Figure 18–95** Preexcitation syndrome in a five-year-old neutered male domestic longhair presented for chronic dysuria and hematuria, the result of a cystic calculus. An ECG was performed because of a previous report of a heart murmur and the presence of premature beats on auscultation. In the limb leads a ventricular conduction abnormality is suggested by the prolonged QRS interval (60 msec in lead II) and the abnormal configuration of the QRS complexes in leads II, III, aVL, and aVF (frontal plane mean electrical axis is − 49°). However, the short P-R interval is not readily apparent, and the diagnosis could easily be missed if only limb leads were recorded. The diagnosis becomes certain in the precordial leads, where the short P-R interval, delta waves, and prolonged QRS interval collectively fulfill the criteria for the preexcitation syndrome. The pattern seen here is the one that we have seen most often in cats and is consistent with the type A form described in man. The reader should compare this recording with that in Figure 18–36. In a seven-year period this cat never demonstrated signs referable to heart disease. A nonselective angiocardiogram suggested mild left ventricular hypertrophy but without associated left atrial enlargement. 25 mm/sec; 1.0 mV = 1.0 cm.

**Table 18–23 Peritoneopericardial Diaphragmatic Hernia in the Cat: A Summary of Literature Reports**

| REFERENCE | BREED | AGE | SEX | CLINICAL SIGNS | HERNIATED ORGANS |
|---|---|---|---|---|---|
| Reed (1951) | Domestic | NR | NR | None | Greater omentum; left lateral and medial, caudate, and right medial liver lobes |
| Barrett and Kittrell (1966) | Persian | 4 mo | F | Anorexia, vomiting | Greater omentum, spleen, liver, pyloric antrum, duodenum |
| Riffel et al (1967) | NR | 8 mo | M | Lethargy, anorexia* | Left and right medial liver lobes |
| Frye and Taylor (1968) | Siamese X | 5 mo | M | Enlarging abdomen | Right medial liver lobe |
| Jackson (1969) | DSH | 6 days | F | Acute death | Four liver lobes |
| Atkins (1974) | DSH | 7 yr | SF | Vomiting, exercise intolerance | Greater omentum, small intestine, left medial liver lobe |
| Bolland et al (1978) | Siamese | 2 yr | CM | Vomiting, weight loss | Small intestine, liver |
| Evans and Biery (1980) | DSH | 10 yr | F | None | Pylorus, spleen, right liver lobes, gallbladder |
| Evans and Biery (1980) | Persian | 10 yr | F | Vomiting | Small intestine, ? other† |
| Evans and Biery (1980) | DSH | 2 mo | F | Dyspnea | Small intestine, ? other† |
| Evans and Biery (1980) | Persian | 8 yr | SF | Seizures | NR |
| Willard and Aronson (1981) | DSH | 8 mo | CM | Lethargy, anorexia, diarrhea | Single liver lobe |
| Wilkes (1981) | Persian | 2 yr | CM | Anorexia, vomiting | Left lateral and medial liver lobes |
| Thomas (1983) | NR | 2 yr | NR | NR | Greater omentum, small intestine, portions of liver and colon |
| Mims and Mathis (1984) | DLH | 2 yr | NR | None | Right medial, quadrate, and portion of right lateral liver lobes |

*Clinical signs were probably unrelated to the congenital defect.
†Neither surgery nor autopsy performed to establish extent of herniated viscera.
NR = Not reported.

antiarrhythmic agents, either singly or in combination (Gallagher et al., 1976). If the tachyarrhythmias are refractory to medical therapy, a pacemaker is implanted or surgical interruption of the accessory pathway(s) is attempted.

**PERICARDIAL DISORDERS.** By comparison with man and the dog, the cat rarely suffers from pericardial disorders. Congenital defects, notably peritoneopericardial diaphragmatic hernia, have been most often reported (see references listed in Table 18–23), while feline infectious peritonitis is the most frequently recognized cause of acquired pericardial disease. Other reported causes have included mesothelioma (Tilley et al., 1975), lymphosarcoma (Owens, 1977), dilatative cardiomyopathy causing restrictive pericarditis (Bunch et al., 1981), and primary bacterial infection (Owens, 1977). Tashjian et al. (1965) reported five cases of pericarditis and four of pericardial effusion but provided no information on the causes of these conditions.

The pericardium (pericardial sac) is a fibroserous membrane that surrounds the heart and the most proximal parts of the great vessels. Although not required for proper functioning of the heart and the cardiovascular system, it provides a number of distinct benefits that are lacking when it is absent. It forms a smooth, frictionless compartment in which the heart functions, maintains the heart in an optimal functional position by preventing abnormal or excessive cardiac mobility, protects against acute cardiac dilatation and other sudden changes in heart size, retards the spread of infection from foci in adjacent intrathoracic structures to the heart and other intrapericardial tissues, and protects against exsanguination when acute bleeding develops from lesions within the pericardial sac.

**Congenital Anomalies.** Abnormalities arising from defective embryologic development of the pericardium include partial or complete absence, cysts, diverticula, and peritoneopericardial diaphragmatic hernia. In man the most common anomalies are complete absence or absence of the left part of the pericardium (Winters and Cortes, 1971). ***Incomplete development*** of the pericardium is believed to be related to premature atrophy of the duct of Cuvier, which results in an incomplete pleuropericardial membrane (Winters and Cortes, 1971). Nearly 75 per cent of such defects in humans occur in males, and 30 per cent are associated with other congenital anomalies (e.g., bronchogenic cysts, congenital heart disease, diaphragmatic hernia, aberrant pulmonary lobe). Partial defects are most frequent over the left atrium or pulmonary artery (Fowler, 1962). Such defects rarely cause clinical signs, although cardiac symptoms and even death have occurred after herniation of part of the heart through a pericardial defect (Chang and Leigh, 1961; Sunderland and Wright-Smith, 1944; Tucker et al., 1963). In the cat pericardial defects have rarely been reported (Harpster, 1977a; Liu, 1977; Walker and Zessman, 1952; Zook, 1974). No clinical signs have been reported as a consequence of these defects.

***Pericardial cysts*** are most often unilocular. They may be pericardial, pleuropericardial, bronchial, or cystic hygromas in origin (Winters and Cortes, 1971). Pericardial diverticula are believed to result from a congenitally weak area in the parietal pericardium. They become radiographically apparent owing to prolonged increase in intrapericardial pressure, usually secondary to pericardial effusion. Large cysts may evoke pericardial effusion by intrapericardial irritation; however, small cysts and diverticula are usually asymptomatic. They tend to mimic mediastinal tumors radiographically and echocardiographically, and surgical exploration is usually necessary to establish a definitive diagnosis. Neither pericardial cysts nor diverticula have been reported in the cat.

***Peritoneopericardial diaphragmatic hernia (PPDH)*** is a congenital anomaly that permits comunication between the pericardial and abdominal cavities. Developmentally, it probably represents a partial arrest of ventral body wall closure, as the defect in the diaphragm is usually in a ventral position (i.e., along the sternum) and is occasionally accompanied by sternal and ventral abdominal wall defects (Evans and Biery, 1980; Thomas, 1983). Clinical signs, when present, arise from the passage of abdominal viscera into the pericardial sac. Owing to the usually small size of the hernial ring, small bowel herniation often results in partial or complete (and commonly intermittent) obstruction with gastrointestional signs (anorexia, intermittent vomiting, diarrhea). Herniation of abdominal viscera may culminate in pericardial effusion or cardiac tamponade because of passive congestion or intrapericardial irritation. Hepatic cirrhosis in a dog was reported as a probable sequel to chronic ischemia of a herniated liver (Evans and Biery, 1980). Table 18–23 summarizes the clinical signs and other features of PPDH in the cat as reported in the literature.

The findings on physical examination are varied depending on the extent of abdominal organ herniation and its effect on cardiac position. A systolic or holosystolic murmur over the left cardiac apex may be the only abnormality found. More often there is unilateral muffling of heart sounds, while over the opposite chest wall the heart sounds are shifted to a more dorsal position than normal. When abdominal organ herniation is extensive, bilateral diminution of heart sounds may be evident, accompanied by a relative absence of abdominal viscera on abdominal palpation. A bilateral reduction in heart sounds may also occur when venous drainage of herniated organs is compromised, causing pericardial effusion.

A diagnosis of PPDH should be considered when an enlarged, irregular cardiac silhouette is present in both standard views in plain thoracic radiographs. A small or indistinct liver shadow is also a common radiographic finding, owing to the frequent herniation of one or more liver lobes (Fig. 18–96). When gas patterns overlie the cardiac silhouette in both projections (the result of small intestine or pyloric antrum herniation), the diagnosis is firmly established. More often, however, liver lobe herniation is alone responsible for the abnormal cardiac silhouette, and confirmation of the diagnosis is more difficult. Other useful diagnostic aids are gastrointestinal positive-contrast radiography (Evans and Biery, 1980), nonselective angiocardiography (Willard and Aronson, 1981), echocardiography (Fig. 18–97), pneumoperitoneography (Evans and Biery, 1980; Thomas, 1983), pneumopericardiography, and thoracic tomography (Evans and Biery, 1980). However, nonselective angiocardiography, echocardiography, and thoracic tomography may be insufficiently sensitive to differentiate between herniated abdominal organs and intrinsic intrapericardial masses. An upper gastrointestinal barium study will be diagnostic only when the small intestine is herniated or when herniation of other abdominal organs results in cranial displacement of the pyloric antrum.

Surgical intervention should be recommended for any cat with PPDH, provided that no other life-limiting disorder exists. (I have known an adult dog with a single herniated liver lobe to die acutely of clostridial septicemia that developed when the lobe became ischemic. Hence I advise surgery even for simple asymptomatic liver herniation.) I prefer a midline abdominal incision extending from the xiphoid process to the umbilicus. Elevation of the cat's foreparts causes the abdominal viscera to gravitate from the area of surgical concentration. In most instances the hernial ring must be enlarged to permit

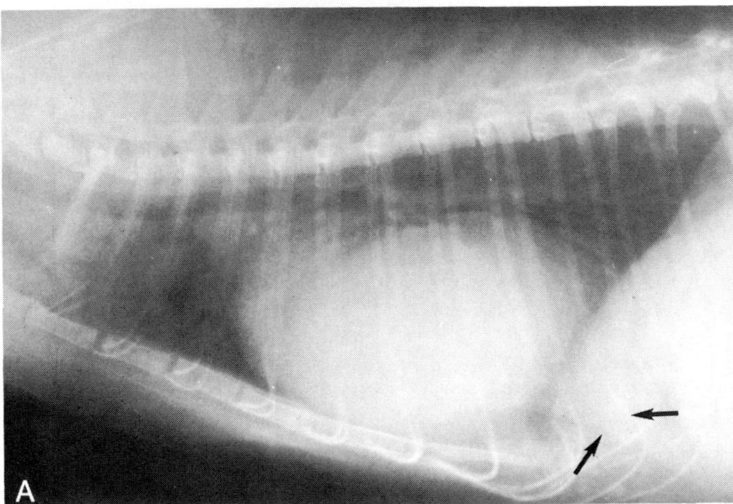


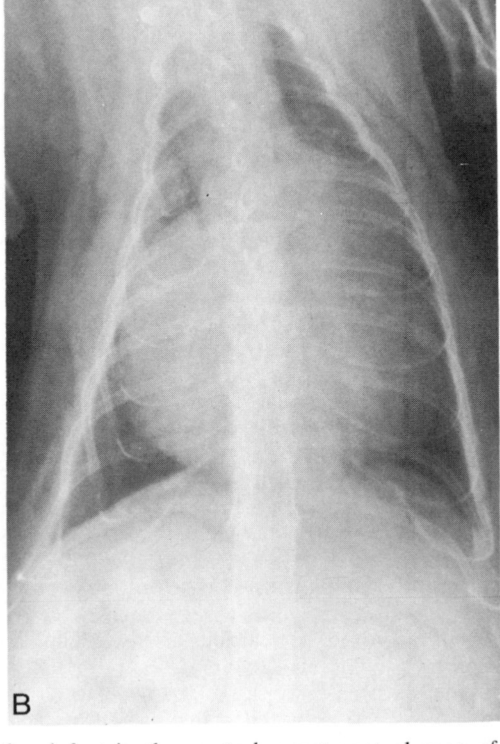


**Figure 18–96** Peritoneopericardial hernia, in an asymptomatic five-year-old female Persian with a low-intensity heart murmur auscultated in a routine physical examination. The lateral view (*A*) shows an enlarged, ovoid cardiac silhouette and tracheal elevation. Pulmonary vascularity is prominent. In the ventrodorsal view (*B*) the cardiac silhouette is somewhat irregularly rounded and entirely fills the right and left sides of the thoracic cavity. Notice the diminutive size of the liver shadow in the lateral view (arrows). At surgery all the right liver lobes were present within the pericardial sac by way of a defect in the central, most ventral area of the diaphragm.

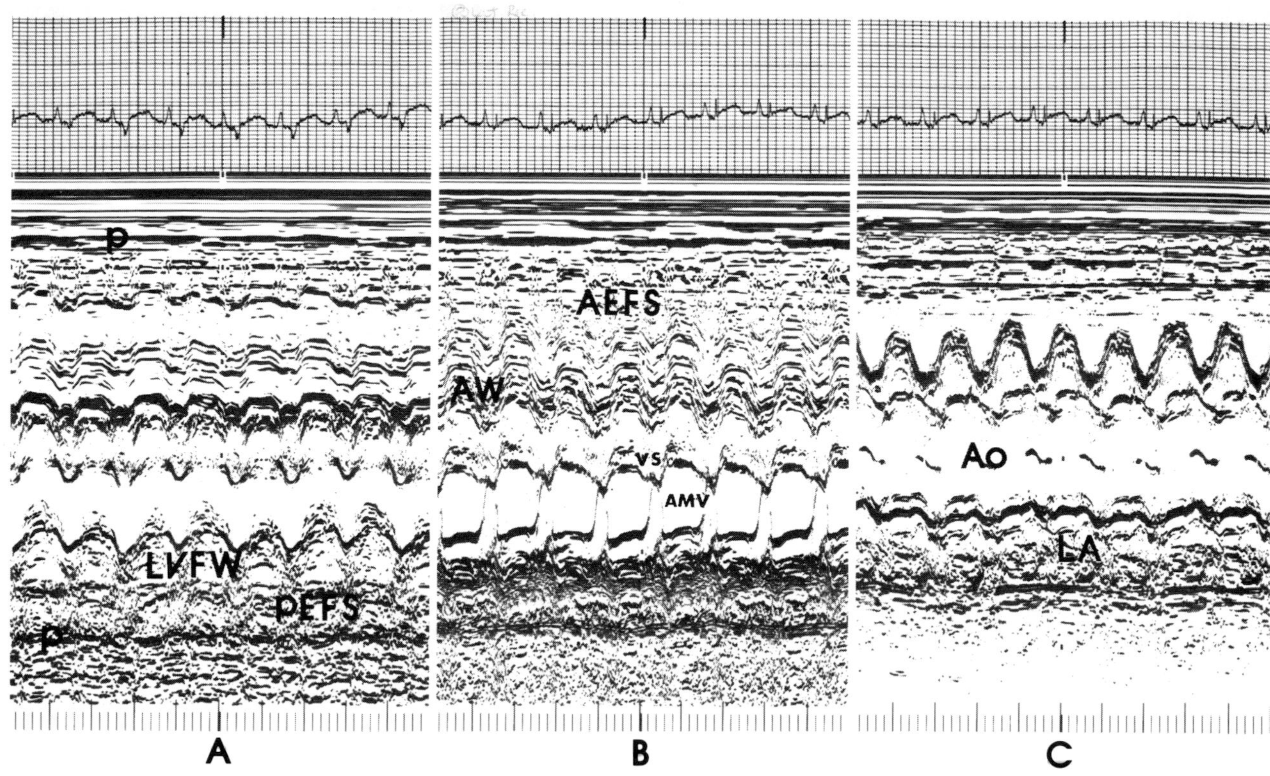


**Figure 18–97** M-mode echocardiogram of a nine-year-old spayed female Himalayan with peritoneopericardial diaphragmatic hernia confirmed at surgery. In all three positions (*A*, left ventricle below mitral valve; *B*, left ventricle at level of mitral valve; *C*, through aorta and left atrium) the most prominent abnormality is a large anterior echo-free space. However, the epicardial surfaces of the left ventricle and left atrium are never clearly seen, suggesting the presence of echo-dense tissue posteriorly as well. The left atrial (LA) dimensions are reduced (left atrial:aortic ratio = 0.63). AEFS = anterior echo-free space, AMV = anterior mitral valve, Ao = aorta, AW = anterior wall or right ventricular free wall, LA = left atrium, LVFW = left ventricular free wall or posterior wall, p = pericardium, PEFS = posterior echo-free space, VS = ventricular septum. 50 mm/sec. ECG: 1.0 mV = 2.0 cm. Small vertical marks are 1.0 cm apart.

replacement of the herniated organs in their normal positions. If replacement is still impossible owing to congestion of herniated organs or the presence of adhesions, the incision should be extended cranially by a median sternotomy. The surgeon can then see both sides of the diaphragm and can locate and break down adhesions. When all organs are restored to their normal positions, the hernial ring is closed. With small defects the free edges of the ring are abraded and then apposed with simple interrupted sutures of monofilament, nonabsorbable suture material. In the rare instance in which a large defect prevents direct apposition of free edges of the hernial ring, the pericardium has been used successfully to close the defect. As with small defects the free edges of the ring should be abraded before suturing to the pericardium with monofilament, nonabsorbable suture material.

**Acquired Pericardial Disorders.** Pericardial effusion is usually responsible for the development of clinical signs in acquired pericardial disease. This may be a response to inflammatory or noninflammatory, localized or systemic disease processes or active bleeding into the pericardial space. The clinical signs depend on the rate and volume of fluid accumulation, as well as the distensibility of the pericardial sac (Fig. 18–98). Acute bleeding usually leads to ***cardiac tamponade.*** Rapid accumulation of blood in the pericardial sac causes cardiac compression, the thin-walled right ventricle being most severely affected. This results in a decrease in the right ventricular end-diastolic dimensions and an elevation in the right ventricular end-dystolic pressure, so that venous return and cardiac output are reduced. The cardiovascular responses to these alterations are an increase in heart rate, representing an attempt to improve cardiac output, and an intense peripheral vasoconstriction to maintain central blood flow. These compensatory mechanisms, however, are often inadequate, owing to continued intrapericardial bleeding and further deterioration in cardiac performance. Shock and death follow, unless a diagnosis is made and appropriate measures are undertaken to reverse this progression.

In ***chronic pericardial effusion,*** fluid accumulates more gradually, causing less severe elevations in intrapericardial pressure and therefore less interference with venous return and cardiac output. Time is permitted for the full development of compensatory mechanisms—mild to moderate peripheral vasoconstriction, sodium and water retention by renal conservatory mechanisms, and progressive enlargement of the pericardial sac (Fig. 18–102). The resulting excessive fluid retention further increases the

ascribed to these agents are reduced myocardial oxygen demands and increased left ventricular diastolic compliance (Chatterjee, 1983). The principal action of the ***venodilators*** is a reduction in venous capacitance tone. This results in a venous pooling of blood, especially in the splanchnic bed, thus leading to a redistribution of intravascular blood volume from the central to the peripheral reservoirs and a decrease in venous return. The primary benefit of these agents lies in the reduction of cardiac filling pressures (i.e., a decrease in the left ventricular end-diastolic pressure and volume) and relief of the clinical signs associated with elevated pulmonary capillary pressures (Cohn and Franciosa, 1977). The effects of venodilators on cardiac performance depend on the initial level of left ventricular filling pressure. If the left ventricular filling pressure is normal, a further reduction of filling pressure will tend to decrease stroke volume and even cardiac output unless accompanied by an increase in heart rate. On the other hand, when the initial left ventricular filling pressure is high, a reduction in filling pressure will not significantly reduce stroke volume and may favorably influence cardiac performance by decreasing left ventricular diastolic volume. Other vasodilators affect both the peripheral arterioles and the venules. They tend to have the beneficial effects of both groups previously discussed, including a decrease in peripheral arteriolar resistance (i.e., reduced afterload), a decrease in pulmonary venous pressure (i.e., reduced preload), and an increase in cardiac output.

Many peripheral vasodilators are currently available for clinical use. The following discussion will consider only those with which the author has clinical experience with the cat. For additional information on these agents the interested reader should review articles in the veterinary (Kittleson, 1983) and human medical (Chatterjee, 1983; Frankl et al., 1984; Smith and Braunwald, 1980) literature.

**HYDRALAZINE.** This vasodilator has long been used in human medicine for the management of hypertension. Strictly an arteriolar dilator, it exerts its effect by relaxing smooth muscle in precapillary arterioles. Peripheral vascular resistance is reduced to a greater extent in arterioles of the splanchnic, coronary, cerebral, and renal circulations than elsewhere in the body. It has no direct action on the myocardium.

Hydralazine has been used in cats mainly for the long-term management of DCM. It has usually been added to the therapeutic regimen when there is recurrence of pleural effusion that was initially responsive to a combination of digoxin and a diuretic. Doses have ranged from 0.75 to 1.5 mg/kg b.i.d. The results of this approach have been gratifying in the majority of cats treated. I have observed lethargy and weakness in a significant number of cats when therapy is started, a response similar to that ascribed in man to vasodilation and a fall in blood pressure (Kelleher et al., 1984). This reaction usually lasts for only two or three days. If it persists longer or is accompanied by anorexia, the dose should be reduced. I have not observed the febrile response or the autoimmune syndromes reported in man with long-term therapy (Kelleher et al., 1984).

**NITROGLYCERIN.** Venodilation is the predominant peripheral vascular response to nitroglycerin and other chemically related nitrate vasodilators, although mild arterial dilatation also occurs. These drugs act at specific nitrate receptors in the vascular smooth muscle wall to cause vascular relaxation. Thus the major hemodynamic effect of agents in this group is redistribution of circulating blood volume, resulting in a decrease in venous return and subsequent decreases in left ventricular end-systolic and end-diastolic volume and pressure (Abrams, 1980). The accompanying arterial dilation may sufficiently lower afterload to increase stroke volume; however, this is not a constant effect, and reduction in stroke volume may occur in the presence of normal or modest increases in left ventricular filling pressure. In addition, nitroglycerin dilates the large epicardial coronary arteries. This has little effect on coronary vascular resistance, as the intramural arteries and arterioles are unaffected.

Nitroglycerin ointment has been reported to provide favorable clinical responses in DCM when used in combination with digoxin and furosemide (Fox, 1983). The recommended dose was ¼ inch applied to the skin t.i.d. or q.i.d. I have used doses of ⅛ to ¼ inch t.i.d. or q.i.d., but with inconsistent results. However, most of my experience has been in cats with severely depressed left ventricular contractility that have not responded to any therapeutic measures. Overdosage of nitroglycerin ointment can cause hypotension, as can all other peripheral vasodilators.

**CAPTOPRIL (CAPOTEN).** The primary mechanism of action of this vasodilator is inhibition of angiotensin-converting enzyme, which decreases serum concentrations of angiotensin II and aldosterone. Furthermore, captopril inhibits the degradation of bradykinin—evidence that bradykinin-induced vasodilatation may be partly responsible for the actions of this drug and possibly explaining its sustained effectiveness in patients whose plasma renin activity is not elevated (Cohn, 1980). Vasodilator actions involve both the precapillary arterioles and the postcapillary venules, evoking what is termed a balanced vasodilator response, the effects being to decrease venous return and increase cardiac output. Captopril may also have diuretic activity owing to its inhibition of aldosterone release.

I have used this agent in a small group of cats with DCM that have become resistant to therapy with digoxin and diuretics. Doses have ranged from 3.25 to 6.5 mg t.i.d. (⅛ to ¼ of a 25 mg tablet). The clinical responses have been favorable without significant side effects. However, the group of cats treated was too small to establish meaningful guidelines. The serum potassium level must be followed closely when captopril is used in conjunction with potassium-sparing diuretics.

## Antiarrhythmic Drugs

The occurrence of cardiac arrhythmias and their electrocardiographic characteristics have been well documented in the cat (Harpster, 1977a; Peterson et al., 1982; Tilley, 1985). They occur most often with cardiomyopathy and hyperthyroidism, conditions in which ventricular arrhythmias and supraventricular arrhythmias, respectively, predominate. Other causes of cardiac arrhythmias are rare and include bacterial endocarditis, other myocardial disorders, congenital cardiac defects, and chest trauma. However, despite the frequency of cardiomyopathy and hyperthyroidism, the indications for antiarrhythmic drug therapy and its efficacy have rarely been reported.

Both lidocaine and phenytoin (diphenylhydantoin) are contraindicated for the cat until safe methods for their administration can be developed. Adverse cardiovascular reactions have been reported during intravenous lidocaine infusions (< 2 mg/kg), including conduction disturbances, bradyarrhythmias, and hypotension (Tilley and Weitz, 1977). Decreased hepatic metabolism due to congestive heart failure and liver congestion may have contributed to these sometimes fatal reactions. As for phenytoin, relatively small doses administered orally or intramuscularly resulted in high plasma concentrations and clinical toxicity (Roye et al., 1973). It was suggested that this intolerance of phenytoin reflected the sensitivity of cats to phenolic compounds and an inability to hydroxylate the phenyl ring structures of the phenytoin molecule.

Only propranolol has so far been found to be an effective and safe antiarrhythmic drug in the cat (Fox, 1983; Tilley and Weitz, 1977) for countering the antiarrhythmic effects of digoxin in the management of supraventricular arrhythmias. It has been reported effective in controlling thyrotoxicosis-induced arrhythmias (Holzworth et al., 1980), in terminating ventricular arrhythmias (Tilley and Weitz, 1977), and in retarding atrioventricular conduction in atrial fibrillation and other supraventricular tachyarrhythmias (Harpster, 1977b; Tilley and Weitz, 1977). Its use together with digitalis may enhance its effect on atrioventricular conduction.

The electrophysiologic effects of beta-blocking agents, such as propranolol, on the heart are complex, as these agents both decrease adrenergic transmitter action and have a direct effect. At the doses normally used clinically, the antiarrhythmic activity of propranolol is thought to result largely from its inhibition of adrenergic stimulation of the heart. At higher serum concentrations (3 μg/ml or greater) it depresses the maximum rate of depolarization (V max), action potential amplitude, membrane responsiveness, and conduction in normal atrial, ventricular, and Purkinje fibers (quinidine-like effect). Propranolol also accelerates repolarization and shortens action potential duration of Purkinje fibers (lidocaine-like action). The resting membrane potential is unaltered (Roberts and Frankl, 1984).

The antiarrhythmic effects of propranolol in the cat at the doses normally used for the effective control of heart rate in HCM (2.5 to 5.0 mg b.i.d. or t.i.d.) have not been studied. Most likely, benefits from both its beta-blocking and its direct actions are realized at the higher doses. High doses may be necessary to maximize its antiarrhythmic actions. Intravenous administration in increments of 0.1 mg have been suggested for the termination of ventricular arrhythmias (Tilley and Weitz, 1977).

I have had some success with both quinidine sulfate (5.5 to 11.0 mg/kg t.i.d.) and procainamide hydrochloride (8 to 20 mg/kg t.i.d.) in controlling supraventricular and ventricular arrhythmias. However, the pharmacokinetics and toxicity of these agents have not been established for the cat, and their use must be considered experimental.

## Antithrombotic Agents

The efficacy of antithrombotic drugs in the prevention of thromboembolism in feline cardiomyopathy has not been established, although they are often recommended for this purpose (Fox, 1983; Harpster, 1977b; Tilley, 1976; Tilley and Weitz, 1977). Aspirin has been most commonly used, but other antithrombotic agents have been mentioned (Tilley and Weitz, 1977).

Aspirin interferes with collagen-induced platelet aggregation by inhibiting the release of endogenous ADP. It also prevents the release of ATP, serotonin, and platelet factor 4. However, aspirin may exert its greatest antithrombotic effect by the inhibition of prostaglandin synthesis (Weiss, 1976). Many other drugs have been reported to have antithrombotic properties and have been extensively evaluated in man. Combinations of these agents may be more effective than any one used alone (Weiss, 1976).

In my experience it has become painfully clear that aspirin is not an effective antithrombotic agent in cats that have experienced a thromboembolic episode. It also seems to be ineffective for prevention, as nearly 100 per cent of the cats with HCM that I have treated prophylactically with aspirin and have followed for a year or longer have eventually developed thromboembolic disease. Obviously a better preventive approach needs to be developed to reduce the prevalence of this major complication.

## Acquired Vascular Disease

The most frequent acquired vascular lesion in the cat is medial hypertrophy of the medium-sized pulmonary arteries (already discussed with pulmonary heart disease). In itself it appears to be asymptomatic but is of concern to the radiologist because, when pronounced, it could be mistaken for disseminated granuloma or tumor.

**ARTERIAL EMBOLISM.** Arterial embolism, next in frequency among vascular lesions of the cat, is most often a sequel of cardiomyopathy, less often of endomyocarditis and endocarditis, and gives rise to striking signs.

Embolism of the aorta appears to have been first described by Collet (1930), in a vivid report of a case in which it was associated with vegetative mitral endocarditis. Whether thromboembolism occurred with increasing frequency over succeeding years or simply went undiagnosed will never be known, but since the report 25 years later of 11 cases at the Angell Memorial Animal Hospital (Holzworth et al., 1955) arterial thromboembolism has come to be recognized as a common and catastrophic consequence of feline heart disease and a significant cause of mortality among domestic cats. Why the cat, so much more often than man or other animals with the same heart disorders, should suffer so disproportionately from thromboembolism is not clear.

Most studies have reported a higher incidence of thromboembolism in males than in females, but cats of both sexes from young adults to the elderly may be victims. Some have had infectious diseases, dental disease, or bite wounds, but many are well cared for indoor cats with no history of illness whatsoever. In many cats, heart disease has been previously diagnosed, as discussed earlier in this chapter, or there may be a history that a cat has had one or more episodes of weakness, when it would for a time partly or entirely lose the use of its hindlegs and drag itself about feebly. Such cats may have atrophied gastrocnemius muscles, stretched calcaneal (Achilles) tendons, and occasionally hairless calluses on the plantar surface of the metatarsals or partial hairlessness of the hindlegs (Holzworth et al., 1955).

Most embolic episodes, however, are so sudden and spectacular in onset that owners recognize the existence of an emergency and seek veterinary help within minutes or hours. Typically the veterinarian is presented with a cat in acute distress—dyspneic, cyanotic, with pupils dilated, and sometimes retching, crying out, or writhing in agony. Usually both hindlegs, occasionally a foreleg as well, are weak or paralyzed. The owner often reports that the cat was found in this condition, indoors or out, although it had shortly before appeared to be in normal health and had had no opportunity for injury. Occasionally the owner has actually seen the cat suddenly lose the use of its hindlegs and collapse in great distress. In an unusual case at AMAH, an aortic embolism occurred in a cat during hospitalization for a fever of unknown cause.

The footpads of the functionless limbs are cold, the toenails are cyanotic, and motor reflexes are suppressed. Sometimes the tail hangs limply. the heartbeat is usually weak and rapid, often with arrhythmias. The temperature is subnormal.

The higher an embolus lodges in the aorta and the more major abdominal arteries are occluded (celiac, mesenteric, renal), the greater the cat's distress, the deeper the shock, and the poorer the chance for survival. In such cases, the signs can be confused with those of spinal injury.

If the cat does not die shortly from a high embolism or from primary heart disease, a characteristic sequence of events occurs in the legs. The gastrocnemius muscles become swollen, hard, and painful. As circulation is reestablished by way of collateral vessels or recanalization of the embolus, the swelling subsides. As the cat regains the use of its legs, it is at first able to advance only the thighs, the distal parts of the legs trailing limply behind. Then it goes through a stage of hobbling on the tibiotarsal joints. An occasional cat progresses no further, and permanent contracture of the flexor tendons develops. Many, however, are eventually able to walk normally. In some the calf muscles are left atrophied and the calcaneal tendons stretched and weak, so that the cat walks "down on the hocks." Prolonged wear on the underside of the metatarsus then results in loss of fur and callus formation. In rare cases in which there is no reestablishment of circulation in the hindlegs, muscle and skin become necrotic.

As discussed earlier in this chapter, stabilization of the cat's condition by medical management should be the first consideration. Treatment must be adapted to the individual case and is influenced by clinical developments and what can be learned from diagnostic studies.

As more and more has been learned about the serious primary heart disease responsible for thromboembolism, fewer veterinarians have been tempted to perform emergency embolectomy. The indications for embolectomy would seem to be two. In the case of a high thromboembolism that occludes circulation to the digestive tract and kidneys, embolectomy would be lifesaving, but a cat so affected often dies before such surgery can be carried out or is in such unstable condition that surgery is not attempted. The other, less urgent indication for embolectomy is persistent ischemia of the hindlegs when an embolus is lodged in the terminal aorta. Fortunately circulation is reestablished in many cats and embolectomy is therefore not commonly required.

The strong possibility of recurrent embolism as a result of the primary heart disease is a further deterrent to surgery.

**"ARTERIOSCLEROSIS."** In man, "hardening of the arteries" is the major cause of illness and death worldwide. Three forms are distinguished: atherosclerosis, characterized by intimal formation of fibrofatty plaques in which cholesterol is an important component; medial calcific sclerosis, characterized by ringlike calcifications within the media of medium-sized and small muscular arteries; and hyaline or hyperplastic arteriolosclerosis involving the media and intima of small arteries and arterioles and related at least in part to elevated blood pressure.

Atherosclerosis has been produced experimentally in cats by feeding of a high-cholesterol diet (Manning and Clarkson, 1970). When cholesterol (in the form of lard) constituted 2 per cent of the diet, the serum cholesterol rose to a level of 260 mg/dl, and fatty streaks and elevated plaques developed in the aorta and, less often, in coronary arteries.

Spontaneous vascular disease is encountered occasionally in cats. Naturally occurring xanthomatosis of the arterial system was observed in an eight-year-old male (Dahme, 1965).

In a random group of 36 cats, both young and old, obtained from a shelter and from veterinary hospitals, there were 18 instances of "arteriosclerosis" in the form of intimal plaques in the aorta and coronary arteries. Aortic sclerosis ("Monckeberg type") was described in an eight-year-old neutered male (Simpson and Jackson, 1963) and intrarenal and intramural coronary arteriosclerosis in a 12-year-old neutered male with chronic pyelonephritis and uremia (Buss et al., 1972).

A fairly common lesion found at autopsy in cats with chronic renal failure is arteriosclerosis characterized by calcification of the internal elastic lamina and necrosis and calcification of the tunica media of elastic and large muscular arteries. In an extreme case observed at AMAH, all the large and medium-sized arteries were rigid, with a circumferential banding pattern of calcification. In another aged uremic cat, pulmonary hemorrhage appeared to result from fracture of calcified basement membranes and elastic fibers. The arteriosclerosis that accompanies chronic renal failure has been noted to be severe in cats with hypercholesterolemia and in cats given vitamin preparations containing vitamin D. In some uremic cats, calcification of the aorta and carotid arteries is so dense that it can be seen in radiographs.

Intimal fibrous plaques and medial necrosis and mineralization are present in the aorta of some cats with hypertrophic cardiomyopathy.

***Arteriolosclerosis*** is a rare lesion that has been observed occasionally in uremic cats at AMAH. In one ten-year-old spayed female domestic shorthair there were also signs of hypertension (nosebleed and episodes of hyphema). The heart was enlarged, and there was a murmur. Autopsy disclosed clotted blood in the nose, kidneys, and eyes. One retina was detached. Microscopically, there was arteriolosclerosis of brain, retina, tongue, heart, kidney (Fig. 18–103), spleen, pancreas, adrenals, and gastrointestinal submucosa. There was fibrinoid necrosis of some arterioles. Ruptured vessels in many organs gave further evidence of hypertension.

**ANGIOENDOTHELIOSIS.** A rare vascular disorder in man is variously described as neoplastic angioendotheliosis, angioendotheliomatosis, malignant angioendotheliomatosis, and angioendotheliomatosis proliferans–

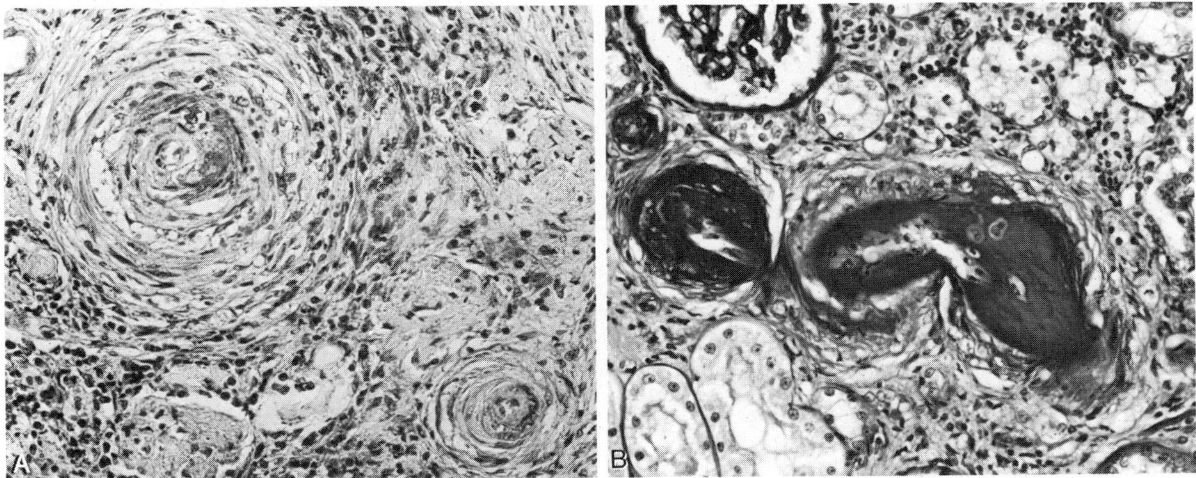


**Figure 18–103** Arteriolosclerosis of renal arteries in a 10-year-old spayed female domestic shorthair with signs of hypertension. *A*, Concentric fibrous intimal thickening, medial hypertrophy, and vacuolation of smooth muscle cells are accompanied by mononuclear and neutrophilic inflammation. H & E, × 75. *B*, The enlarged and tortuous interlobular artery (center) has undergone fibrinoid necrosis and has abundant intimal PAS–positive material. Mononuclear cell inflammation and fibrosis surround the vessel and lie next to proximal convoluted tubules (lower left) and a glomerulus (upper left). PAS, × 100. (Courtesy Dr. Charles Mohr.)

neoplastic type. It is characterized by an exuberant proliferation of endothelium that virtually fills the lumens of small arteries.

A similar lesion was found in a six-year-old male domestic shorthair with signs of central nervous disorder: absence of postural responses, reduced cranial nerve reflexes, nonresponsive pupils, and apparent blindness (Rothwell et al., 1985). At autopsy the lumens of small arteries in most organs were almost obliterated by tightly packed endothelial cells.

**PERIARTERITIS (POLYARTERITIS) NODOSA.** This disorder has been reported in a few cats (see the chapter on immunology). Several suspected cases at AMAH proved on review to be infectious feline peritonitis.

**VASCULITIS.** Fibrinoid arteritis and phlebitis are found most often in feline infectious peritonitis and are believed to represent an immune reaction (see the chapter on viral diseases).

**DISSEMINATED INTRAVASCULAR COAGULATION (DIC).** This thrombohemorrhagic disorder is a secondary complication in numerous diseases. It is precipitated by release of thromboplastic substances into the circulation and by damage to vascular endothelium. Among conditions in which it is known to occur in the cat are panleukopenia, feline infectious peritonitis, Gram-negative septicemias (notably salmonellosis), and aortic thromboembolism (Fox and Dodds, 1982). Management of DIC is discussed in the chapter on the hematopoietic system.

**VENOUS THROMBOSIS.** An unusual instance of symptomatic venous thrombosis was observed at AMAH in a seven-year-old neutered male Siamese with sudden onset of posterior paresis. On admission the cat would walk "down on the hocks" but within hours was unable to support weight on its hindlimbs. Femoral pulses were normal. The owner chose to have the cat destroyed. At autopsy a fresh thrombus measuring 1.5 × 0.5 cm and accompanied by hemorrhage was found in the left vertebral sinus at the level of L3–L4. Other lesions were focal gastric ulceration, hemorrhage, and purulent inflammation; mild multifocal lymphocytic myocarditis, and mild intestinal lymphocytic perineuritis. No underlying cause was discovered.

**VENOUS PARASITISM.** Parasitism and thrombosis of the veins of the spinal cord by a metastrongylid worm, *Gurltia paralysans,* has been described as causing posterior paralysis in cats in Chile (Wolffhügel, 1934).

**VASCULAR TRAUMA.** Aortic tears, resulting from violent injury, occur most often at the diaphragmatic-aortic hiatus. Bizarre instances of BB shot entering the aorta have been reported (Horton and Renfroe, 1978; Roumanis, 1981).

Post-traumatic fat embolism has been described (Matis, 1980). Fatal postsurgical pulmonary embolism may follow mastectomy in cats with fibroadenomatous hyperplasia (see the chapter on tumors and tumor-like lesions).

The principal damage inflicted on feline veins is by needles and the substances that they inject. When a vein must be entered repeatedly, or if clotting at venepuncture sites is impaired, a firm pressure bandage applied after each venepuncture helps to prevent hematoma formation, thrombosis, and phlebitis.

Extensive sloughs involving skin and subcutis and obliterating the vein may occur if irritant drugs are accidentally injected outside rather than into a vein. Barbiturate sloughs may often be prevented by infiltration of the injection area with a few milliliters of physiologic saline solution or 2 per cent procaine.

Calcium gluconate solution spilled outside a vein may cause a slough so extensive that a skin graft is required.

## REFERENCES

### Anatomy

Bourdelle E, Bressou C: Anatomie Régionale des Animaux Domestiques. IV Carnivores Chien et Chat. Paris, Librairie J-B Baillière et Fils, 1953.

Johnston FB: Closure of the foramen ovale in the heart of the

domestic cat, *Felis domesticus*. Anat Rec 81 (1941) Suppl 117.
Joseph DR: The ratio between the heart weight and body weight in various animals. J Exp Med 10 (1908) 521–528.
Latimer HB: The prenatal growth of the cat. XII. The weight of the heart in the fetal and in the adult cat. Growth 6 (1942) 341–349.
Liu S-K: Pathology of feline heart diseases. Vet Clin North Am 7 (1977) 323–339.
Nogalski S, Szuba Z: [The weight of the heart and its variability in the cat]. Stettin Wyzsza Szkola Roln Zeszyty 36 (1971) 213–218.
Orr TG Jr, Latimer HB: The collateral circulation in the hind limb of the cat. Trans Kans Acad Sci 42 (1939) 481–482.
Paasch LH: The comparative pathology of endocardial fibroelastosis in Burmese cats. The George Washington University, PhD dissertation, 1979.
Paasch LH, Zook BC: Estructura del endocardio en dos humanos y siete gatos en crecimiento. Veterinaria Méx 11 (1980) 133–140.
Qayyum MA: Anatomy and histology of the specialized tissues of the heart of the domestic cat (*Felis catus*). Acta Anat 82 (1972) 352–367.
Reighard J, Jennings HS: Anatomy of the Cat. New York, Henry Holt and Company, 1935.
Schummer A, Wilkens H, Vollmerhaus B, Habermehl K-H: The circulatory system, the skin, and the cutaneous organs of the domestic mammals. *In* Nickel R, Schummer A, Seiferle E (eds): The Anatomy of the Domestic Animals. New York, Springer-Verlag, 1981.
Spector WS (ed): Handbook of Biological Data. Philadelphia, WB Saunders Company, 1956.
Stünzi H, Teuscher E, Bolliger O: Systematische Untersuchungen am Herzen von Haustieren. I. Mitteilung: Untersuchung am Herzen der Katze. Zentralbl Veterinärmed 6 (1959) 101–117.
Truex RC, Warshaw LJ: The incidence and size of the moderator band in man and in mammals. Anat Rec 82 (1942) 361–372.
Welsch: Herzknorpel von Hund und Katze. Dissertation, Berlin, 1921. Cited by Ellenberger and Baum, Handbuch der Vergleichenden Anatomie der Haustiere, 18th ed. Berlin, Springer-Verlag, 1943.
Zook BC: Some spontaneous cardiovascular lesions in dogs and cats. Adv Cardiol 13 (1974) 148–168.

**Congenital Anomalies**

Atkins CE: Suspect congenital peritoneopericardial diaphragmatic hernia in an adult cat. J Am Vet Med Assoc 165 (1974) 175–176.
Atwell RB: Uhl's anomaly in a cat associated with severe right-sided cardiac decompensation. J Small Anim Pract 21 (1980) 121–127.
Barrett RB, Kittrell JE: Congenital peritoneopericardial diaphragmatic hernia in a cat. J Am Vet Radiol Soc 7 (1966) 21–26.
Bates PD: Patent ductus arteriosus with pulmonary hypertension in a cat. J Am Vet Med Assoc 173 (1978) 799–800.
Bohn FK, Buchanan JW, Kelly DF: Clinico-pathologic conference [endocardial fibroelastosis]. J Am Vet Med Assoc 157 (1970) 1360–1377.
Bolland E, Goverts JT, Osinga EC: What is your diagnosis? Tijdschr Diergeneeskd 103 (1978) 1076–1079.
Bolton GR, Liu S-K: Congenital heart diseases of the cat. Vet Clin North Am 7 (1977) 341–353.
Bolton GR, Edwards NJ, Hoffer RE: Arteriovenous fistula of the aorta and caudal vena cava causing congestive heart failure in a cat. J Am Anim Hosp Assoc 12 (1976) 463–469.
Bolton GR, Ettinger SJ, Liu S-K: Tetralogy of Fallot in three cats. J Am Vet Med Assoc 160 (1972) 1622–1631.
Buergelt CD, Suter PF, Kay WJ: Persistent truncus arteriosus in a cat. J Am Vet Med Assoc 153 (1968) 548–552.
Bush M, Pieroni DR, Goodman DG, White RI, Thomas V, James AE Jr: Tetralogy of Fallot in a cat. J Am Vet Med Assoc 161 (1972) 1679–1686.
Chang CH, Leigh TF: Congenital partial defect of the pericardium associated with herniation of the left atrial appendage [in a child]. Am J Roentgenol 86 (1961) 517–522.
Cohen JS, Tilley LP, Liu S-K, DeHoff WD: Patent ductus arteriosus in five cats. J Am Anim Hosp Assoc 11 (1975) 95–101.
Danilowicz DA, Ross J Jr: Congenital heart disease. *In* Conn HL Jr, Horwitz O (eds): Cardiac and Vascular Diseases. Philadelphia, Lea & Febiger, 1971.
Das KM, Patnaik AK, Liu S-K, Irschlinger S: Cardiovascular pathology of the dog and cat: A study of 1,000 consecutive necropsies. J Am Vet Med Assoc 147 (1965) 1648–1649.
Dear MG: An unusual combination of congenital cardiac anomalies in a cat. J Small Anim Pract 11 (1970) 37–43.
de Lahunta A, Habel RE: Applied Veterinary Anatomy. Philadelphia, WB Saunders Company, 1986.
Douglas SW, Walker RG, Littlewort MCG: Persistent right aortic arch in the cat. Vet Rec 72 (1960) 91–92.
Eales NB: Paired precaval veins in a kitten. Anat Anz 86 (1938) 68–71.
Eliot TS Jr, Eliot FP, Lushbaugh CC, Slager UT: First report of the occurrence of neonatal endocardial fibroelastosis in cats and dogs. J Am Vet Med Assoc 133 (1958) 271–274.
Emsbo P: Subaortal stenose. Komparative studier over medfodt subvalvulaer aortastenose (Venstresidig Konusstenose) hossvin og menneske. Copenhagen, Dansk Videnskabs Forlag, 1955.
Erwin WG: An unusual combination of vascular anomalies in a domestic cat. Proc Louisiana Acad Sci 11 (1948) 42–43.
Evans SM, Biery DM: Congenital peritoneopericardial diaphragmatic hernia in the dog and cat: A literature review and 17 additional case histories. Vet Radiol 21 (1980) 108–116.
Evans I, Keatts WH: Surgical correction of persistent right aortic arch in a cat. Vet Med Small Anim Clin 66 (1971) 1091–1092.
Eyster GE, Weber W, McQuillan W: Tetralogy of Fallot in a cat. J Am Vet Med Assoc 171 (1977b) 280–282.
Eyster GE, Whipple RD, Anderson LK, Evans AT, O'Handley P: Pulmonary artery banding for ventricular septal defect in dogs and cats. J Am Vet Med Assoc 170 (1977a) 434–438.
Fontana RS, Edwards JE: Congenital Cardiac Disease: A Review of 357 Cases Studied Pathologically. Philadelphia, WB Saunders Company, 1962.
Fowler NO: Congenital defect of the pericardium. Its resemblance to pulmonary artery enlargement. Circulation 16 (1962) 114–120.
Fox PR, Tilley LP, Liu S-K: The cardiovascular system. *In* Pratt PW (ed): Feline Medicine. Santa Barbara, American Veterinary Publications, Inc, 1983.
Frontera JG: Anomalous persistent left anterior cardinal system draining the coronary blood in a domestic cat. Anat Rec 106 (1950) 127–130.
Fry WJ: Surgical considerations in congenital arteriovenous fistula. Surg Clin North Am 54 (1974) 165–174.
Frye FL, Taylor DON: Pericardial and diaphragmatic defects in a cat. J Am Vet Med Assoc 152 (1968) 1507–1510.
Gandolfi RC: Hepatoencephalopathy associated with patent ductus venosus in a cat. J Am Vet Med Assoc 185 (1984) 301–302.
Godglück G: Misbildungen des Herzens bei Tieren. Dtsch Tierärztl Wochenschr 69 (1962) 98–102.
Goodman DC: A persistent left superior vena cava and anomalous anastomosing mediastinal vein in a domestic cat. Anat Rec 108 (1950) 415–420.
Gordon B, Trautvetter E, Patterson DF: Pulmonary congestion associated with cor triatriatum in a cat. J Am Vet Med Assoc 180 (1982) 75–77.
Grant SB: A persistent superior vena cava sinistra in the cat transmitting coronary blood. Anat Rec 13 (1917) 45–49.
Hamlin RL, Tashjian RJ, Smith CR: Diseases of the cardiovascular system. *In* Catcott EJ (ed): Feline Medicine and

Surgery. Santa Barbara, American Veterinary Publications, Inc, 1964, 218–236.
Hare WCD: Two cases of an atypical arrangement of the caudal vena cava in the cat. Br Vet J 107 (1951) 87–93.
Harpster NK: Cardiovascular diseases of the domestic cat. Adv Vet Sci Comp Med 21 (1977) 39–74.
Hartig F, Hebold G: Seltene Herzmisbildung bei einer männlichen Katze: Beitrag zum Taussig-Bing Komplex. Zentralbl Veterinärmed A 20 (1973) 469–475.
Hathaway JE: Persistent right aortic arch in a cat. J Am Vet Med Assoc 147 (1965) 255–259.
Hawe RC: ECG of the month [interventricular septal defect]. J Am Vet Med Assoc 182 (1983) 364–365.
Hawe RS, Witter WR, Wilson JB: Tetralogy of Fallot in a five-year-old cat. J Am Anim Hosp Assoc 15 (1979) 329–333.
Hunt CE, Formanek G, Levine MA, Castaneda A, Moller JH: Banding of the pulmonary artery, Results in 111 children. Circulation 43 (1971) 395–406.
Jackson OF: Congenital abnormalities in kittens [pericardial diaphragmatic hernia]. Vet Rec 84 (1969) 76.
Jeraj K, Ogburn PN, Jessen CA, Miller JD, Schenk MP: Double outlet right ventricle in a cat. J Am Vet Med Assoc 173 (1978) 1356–1360.
Jeraj K, Ogburn P, Lord PF, Wilson JW: Patent ductus arteriosus with pulmonary hypertension in a cat. J Am Vet Med Assoc 172 (1978) 1432–1436.
Jessop L: Persistent right aortic arch in the cat causing oesophageal stenosis. Vet Rec 72 (1960) 46–47.
Jones CL, Buchanan JW: Patent ductus arteriosus and surgery in the cat. J Am Vet Med Assoc 179 (1981) 364–369.
Khera KS: Fetal cardiovascular and other defects induced by thalidomide in cats. Teratology 11 (1975) 65–72.
Kirby D, Gillick A: Polycythemia and tetralogy of Fallot in a cat. Can Vet J 15 (1974) 114–119.
Lawther WA: Diagnosis and surgical correction of persistent right aortic arch and oesophageal achalasia in the dog and cat. Aust Vet J 46 (1970) 326–329.
Legendre AM, Krahwinkel DJ, Carrig CB, Michel RL: Ascites associated with intrahepatic arteriovenous fistula in a cat. J Am Vet Med Assoc 168 (1976) 589–591.
Levesque DC, Oliver JE, Cornelius LM, Mahaffey MB, Kolata RJ: Congenital portacaval shunts in two cats: diagnosis and surgical correction. J Am Vet Med Assoc 181 (1982) 143–145.
Lilleengen K: Hjärtmisbildningar hos djuren. Skand Vet Tidskr 24 (1934) 495–555.
Liu S-K: Supravalvular aortic stenosis with deformity of the aortic valve in a cat [also endocardial fibrosis]. J Am Vet Med Assoc 152 (1968) 55–59.
Liu S-K: Acquired cardiac lesions leading to congestive heart failure in the cat. Am J Vet Res 31 (1970) 2071–2088.
Liu S-K: Pathology of feline heart disease. *In* Kirk RW (ed): Current Veterinary Therapy V, Philadelphia, WB Saunders Company, 1974, 341–344.
Liu S-K: Pathology of feline heart disease. Vet Clin North Am 7 (1977) 323–339.
Liu S-K, Ettinger S: Persistent common atrioventricular canal in two cats. J Am Vet Med Assoc 153 (1968) 556–562.
Liu S-K, Tilley LP: Dysplasia of the tricuspid valve in the dog and cat. J Am Vet Med Assoc 169 (1976) 623–630.
Liu S-K, Tashjian RJ, Patnaik AK: Congestive heart failure in the cat. J Am Vet Med Assoc 156 (1970) 1319–1330.
Lombard CW, Twichell MJ: Tetralogy of Fallot, persistent left cranial vena cava and retinal detachment in a cat. J Am Anim Hosp Assoc 14 (1978) 624–630.
Lord PF, Zontine WJ: Radiologic examination of the feline cardiovascular system. Vet Clin North Am 7 (1977) 291–308.
Lord PF, Liu S-K, Carmichael JA: Congenital tricuspid stenosis with right ventricular hypoplasia in a cat. J Am Vet Med Assoc 153 (1968) 300–306.
Lucam F, Barone R, Flachat C, Cottereau P, Valentin F: Malformations cardiaques congénitales chez un chien et chez un chat. Rev Méd Vét 107 (1956) 674–682.
Mann PGH, Stock JE, Sheridan JP: Pulmonary artery banding in the cat: A case report [ventricular septal defect]. J Small Anim Pract 12 (1971) 45–48.
McClure CFW: On the frequency of abnormalities in connection with the postcaval vein and its tributaries in the domestic cat (*Felis domestica*). Am Naturalist 34 (1900) 185–198.
Miller AJ, Pick R, Katz LN: Ventricular endomyocardial changes after impairment of cardiac lymph flow in dogs. Br Heart J 25 (1963) 182–190.
Miller CW, Holmberg DL, Bowen V, Pharr JW, Kruth S: Microsurgical management of tetralogy of Fallot in a cat. J Am Vet Med Assoc 186 (1985) 708–709.
Mims JP, Mathis PD: Diagnosing a peritoneopericardial hernia. Vet Med Small Anim Clin 79 (1984) 911–914.
Mitchell SC, Korones SB, Berendes HW: Congenital heart disease in 56,109 births: Incidence and natural history. Circulation 43 (1971) 323–332.
Northway RB: Use of an aortic homograft for surgical correction of a double-outlet right ventricle in a kitten. Vet Med Small Anim Clin 74 (1979) 191–192.
Paasch LH: The comparative pathology of endocardial fibroelastosis in Burmese cats. The George Washington University, PhD dissertation, 1979.
Paasch LH, Zook BC: The pathogenesis of endocardial fibroelastosis in Burmese cats. Lab Invest 42 (1980) 197–204.
Palenscar JR: What is your diagnosis? [persistent right aortic arch]. J Am Vet Med Assoc 177 (1980) 366–368.
Patterson DF: Epidemiologic and genetic studies of congenital heart disease in the dog. Circ Res 23 (1968) 171–202.
Perkins RL: Multiple congenital cardiovascular anomalies in a kitten. J Am Vet Med Assoc 160 (1972) 1430–1431.
Priester WA, Glass AG, Waggoner NS: Congenital defects in domesticated animals: General considerations. Am J Vet Res 31 (1970) 1871–1879.
Reed CA: Pericardio-peritoneal herniae in mammals, with description of a case in the domestic cat. Anat Rec 110 (1951) 113–119.
Reed JH, Bonasch H: The surgical correction of a persistent right aortic arch in a cat. J Am Vet Med Assoc 140 (1962) 142–144.
Richmond BT: A case of persistent right aortic arch in the cat. Vet Rec 83 (1968) 169.
Riffel DM, Hendrickson TD, Acre KE: What is your diagnosis? [pericardial hepatocele]. J Am Vet Med Assoc 150 (1967) 1027–1028.
Rothuizen J, van den Ingh ThSGAM, Voorhout G, van der Luer RJT, Wouda W: Congenital porto-systemic shunts in sixteen dogs and three cats. J Small Anim Pract 23 (1982) 67–81.
Saperstein G, Harris S, Leipold HW: Congenital defects in domestic cats. Feline Pract 6 (4) (1976) 18–43.
Schryer MJP, Karnauchow PN: Endocardial fibroelastosis: Etiologic and pathogenetic considerations in children. Am Heart J 88 (1974) 557–565.
Severin GA: Congenital and acquired heart disease. J Am Vet Med Assoc 151 (1967) 1733–1736.
Shaffer AB: Congenital heart disease. *In* Silber EN, Katz LN (eds): Heart Disease. New York, Macmillan Publishing Company, 1975, 565–696.
Siller WG: Ventricular septal defects in the fowl. J Pathol Bacteriol 76 (1958) 431–440.
Smallwood WM: Some vertebrate abnormalities. Anat Anz 29 (1906) 460–462.
Solinger RE: Ultrasound in congenital heart disease. *In* Gramiak R, Waag RC (eds): Cardiac Ultrasound. St Louis, The CV Mosby Company, 1975, 185–209.
Spann JF, Lemole GM: Pulmonary artery constriction in the cat: A model for ventricular hypertrophy and congestive heart

failure. *In* Harmison LT (ed): Research Animals in Medicine. Washington DC, DHEW Pub NIH 72-333, 1973, PHS, NIH 141–155.

Straw RC, Aronson EF, McCaw DL: Transposition of the great arteries in a cat. J Am Vet Med Assoc 187 (1985) 634–636.

Sunderland S, Wright-Smith RJ. Congenital pericardial defects. Br Heart J 6 (1944) 167–175.

Tashjian RJ, Das KM, Palich WE, Hamlin RL, Yarns DA: Studies on cardiovascular disease in the cat. Ann NY Acad Sci 127 (1965) 581–605.

Tashjian RJ, Pensinger RR, Das KM, Reid CF, Crescenzi AA: Feline cardiovascular studies—a preliminary report. Proc Am Vet Med Assoc 100 (1963) 112–123.

Tilley LP: Erkrankungen des Kreislaufsystems. *In* Kraft W, Dürr UM (eds): Katzenkrankheiten: Klinik und Therapie. Verlag M&H Schaper, Hannover, 1979, 169–194.

Tisseur [H], Barone [L]: Duplicité de la veine cave postérieure chez une chatte. Bull Soc Sci Vét Lyon NS 3 (1944) 80–84.

Treadwell AL: An abnormal iliac vein in a cat (*Felis domestica*). Anat Anz 11 (1896) 717–718.

Tucker DH, Miller DE, Jacoby WJ Jr: Congenital partial absence of the pericardium with herniation of the left atrial appendage. Am J Med 35 (1963) 560–565.

Uhrich SJ: Report of a persistent right aortic arch and its surgical correction in a cat. J Small Anim Pract 4 (1963) 337–338.

van der Linde–Sipman JS: Vascular ring caused by a left aortic arch, right ligamentum arteriosum and part of the right dorsal aorta in a cat. Zentralbl Vet Med A 28 (1981) 569–573.

van der Linde–Sipman JS, van den Ingh TSGAM, Koeman JP: Congenital heart abnormalities in the cat: a description of sixteen cases. Zentralbl Veterinärmed A 20 (1973) 419–425.

van der Linde–Sipman JS, van der Luer RJT, Stokhof AA, Wolvekamp WThC: Congenital subvalvular pulmonic stenosis in a cat. Vet Pathol 17 (1980) 640–643.

van Heerden J, Lourens DC: Tetralogy of Fallot in a two-and-one-half-year old cat. J Am Anim Hosp Assoc 17 (1981) 129–130.

van Nie CJ, van Messel MA, Straatman TJD: Congenital bicuspid stenosis with left ventricular hypoplasia in a kitten. Vet Quart 2(1) (1980) 58–62.

Vogel O: Situs inversus bei einer Katze. Berl Münch Tierärztl Wochenschr 92 (1979) 48–49 (abstr Vet Bull 49 [1979] 4668).

Vulgamott JC, Turnwald GH, King GK, Herring DS, Hansen JF, Booth HW: Congenital portacaval anomalies in the cat: two case reports. J Am Anim Hosp Assoc 16 (1981) 915–919.

Walker WF Jr, Zessman JE: A case of an incomplete pericardial cavity in the cat. Anat Rec 113 (1952) 459–465.

Webster JA, Buckland GW, Lee SF: What is your diagnosis? [persistent right aortic arch corrected surgically]. J Am Vet Med Assoc 176 (1980) 1387–1388.

Wheaton LG, Blevins WE, Weirich WE: Persistent right aortic arch associated with other vascular anomalies in two cats. J Am Vet Med Assoc 184 (1984) 848–851.

Wilkinson GT: Dyspnoea in the cat—I Aetiology [familial defect of tricuspid valve in Siamese]. J Small Anim Pract 8 (1967) 543–549.

Will JA: Subvalvular pulmonary stenosis and aorticopulmonary septal defect in the cat. J Am Vet Med Assoc 154 (1969) 913–916.

Williams RB, Emery JL: Endocardial fibrosis in apparently normal infant hearts. Histopathology 2 (1978) 283–290.

Zeiner FN: Two cases of coronary venous drainage by a persistent left superior vena cava in cat. Anat Rec 129 (1957) 275–277.

Zook BC: Some spontaneous cardiovascular lesions in dogs and cats. Adv Cardiol 13 (1974) 148–168.

Zook BC, Kenney RA, Bailey JM, Patterson DF: Congenital endocardial fibroelastosis in Burmese cats (abstr). Publication 78–4, Am Assoc Lab Anim Sci, 29th Ann Session, Sept 1978.

Zook BC, Paasch LH, Chandra RS, Casey HW: The comparative pathology of endocardial fibroelastosis in Burmese cats. Virchows Arch [Pathol Anat] 390 (1981) 211–227.

**Acquired Cardiovascular Disorders**

Abbott PK: Feline dirofilariasis in Papua. Aust Vet J 42 (1966) 247–249.

Abrams J: Current concepts: Nitroglycerin and long-acting nitrates. N Engl J Med 302 (1980) 1234–1237.

Ahmed SS, Jaferi GA, Narang RM, Regan TJ: Preclinical abnormality of left ventricular function in diabetes mellitus. Am Heart J 89 (1975) 153–158.

Akbarian M, Yankopoulos NA, Abelmann WH: Hemodynamic studies in beriberi heart disease. Am J Med 41 (1966) 197–212.

Altera KP, Bonasch H: Periarteritis nodosa in a cat. J Am Vet Med Assoc 149 (1966) 1307–1311.

Ash LR: Helminth parasites of dogs and cats in Hawaii. J Parasitol 48 (1962) 63–65.

Beeson PB: Bacterial endocarditis. *In* Beeson PB, McDermott W (eds): Textbook of Medicine, 12th ed. Philadelphia, WB Saunders Company, 1967.

Beglinger R, Heller A, Lakotos L: Elektrokardiogramme, Herzschlagfrequenz und Blutdruck der Hauskatze (Felis catus). Zentralbl Veterinärmed A 24 (1977) 252–256.

Bigger JT Jr: Mechanisms and diagnosis of arrhythmias. *In* Braunwald E (ed): Heart Disease. A Textbook of Cardiovascular Medicine. Philadelphia, WB Saunders Company, 1980.

Bisgard GE: Pulmonary hypertension in cattle. Adv Vet Sci Comp Med 21 (1977) 151–172.

Blok J, Boeles JTF: The electrocardiogram of the normal cat. Acta Physiol Pharmacol Neerland 6 (1957) 95–102.

Bolton GR, Liu S-K: Congenital heart disease of the cat. Vet Clin North Am 7 (1977) 341–353.

Bornstein DL: Bacterial endocarditis. *In* Conn HL Jr, Horowitz O (eds): Cardiac and Vascular Diseases. Philadelphia, Lea & Febiger, 1971.

Branham HH: Aneurismal varix of the femoral artery and vein following a gunshot wound. Int J Surg 3 (1890) 250–251.

Buccino RA, Pool PE, Spann JF Jr, Sonnenblick EH, Braunwald E: Influence of the thyroid state on the intrinsic contractile properties and energy stores of the myocardium. J Clin Invest 46 (1967a) 1669–1682.

Buccino RA, Sonnenblick EH, Spann JF Jr, Friedman WF, Braunwald E: Interactions between changes in the intensity and duration of the active state in the characterization of inotropic stimuli on heart muscle. Circ Res 21 (1967b) 857–867.

Buchanan JW: Chronic valvular disease (endocarditis) in dogs. Adv Vet Sci Comp Med 21 (1977) 75–106.

Bunch SE, Bolton GR, Hornbuckle WE: Pericardial effusion with restrictive pericarditis associated with congestive cardiomyopathy in a cat. J Am Anim Hosp Assoc 17 (1981) 739–745.

Burch GE: A Primer of Cardiology, 4th ed. Philadelphia, Lea & Febiger, 1971.

Burch GE, Winsor T: A Primer of Electrocardiography, 5th ed. Philadelphia, Lea & Febiger, 1966.

Buss DD, Pyle RL, Chacko SK: Clinico-pathologic conference [chronic kidney disease with intrarenal and intramural coronary arteriosclerosis]. J Am Vet Med Assoc 161 (1972) 402–410.

Butler HC: An investigation into the relationship of an aortic embolus to posterior paralysis in the cat. J Small Anim Pract 12 (1971) 141–158.

Calvert CA, Coulter DW: Electrocardiographic values for anesthetized cats in lateral and sternal recumbencies. Am J Vet Res 42 (1981) 1453–1455.

Carpenter JL: Bronchial asthma in cats. *In* Kirk RW (ed): Current Veterinary Therapy V. Philadelphia, WB Saunders Company, 1974.

Carpenter JL, Holzworth J: Thymoma in 11 cats. J Am Vet Med Assoc 181 (1982) 248–251.

Chatterjee K: Vasodilators. *In* Sleight P, Jones JV (eds): Scientific Foundations of Cardiology. London, William Heinemann Medical Books, Ltd, 1983.

Cohn JN: Progress in vasodilator therapy for heart failure. N Engl J Med 302 (1980) 1414–1416.

Cohn JN, Franciosa JA: Drug therapy: Vasodilator therapy of cardiac failure: N Engl J Med 297 (1977) 27–31.

Colcolough HL: A comparative study of acute myocardial infarction in the rabbit, cat and man. Comp Biochem Physiol A49 (1974) 121–125.

Collet P: Thrombose de l'aorte postérieure chez un chat. Bull Soc Sci Vét Lyon 33 (1930) 136–143.

Coulter DB, Calvert CA: Orientation and configuration of vectorcardiographic QRS loops from normal cats. Am J Vet Res 42 (1981) 282–289.

Coulter DB, Duncan RJ, Sander PD: Effects of asphyxia and potassium on canine and feline electrocardiograms. Can J Comp Med 39 (1975) 442–449.

Cowgill LD, Kallet AD: Recognition and management of hypertension in the dog. *In* Kirk RW (ed): Current Veterinary Therapy VIII. Philadelphia, WB Saunders Company, 1983.

Crevasse L, Wheat MW, Wilson J, Leeds RF, Taylor WJ: The mechanism of the generation of the third and fourth heart sounds. Circulation 25 (1962) 635–642.

Cusick PK, Todd KS Jr, Blake JA, Daly WR: *Dirofilaria immitis* in the brain and heart of a cat from Massachusetts. J Am Anim Hosp Assoc 12 (1976) 490–491.

Dahme E: Der Gestaltwandel der Lunge und arteriellen Lungenstrombahn bei Störungen des kleinem Kreislaufes. Berl Münch Tierärztl Wochenschr 73 (1960) 333–336.

Dahme EG: Atherosclerosis and arteriosclerosis in domestic animals. Ann NY Acad Sci 127 (1965) 657–670.

Damiano S, Galati P: [Definition of "intimal arteriosclerosis in the lungs of the cat," with reference to other pulmonary arteriopathies described in this species.] Acta Med Vet Napoli 13 (1967) 435–445 (abstr Vet Bull 38 [1968] 3761).

Darsee JR, Braunwald E: Diseases of the pericardium. *In* Braunwald E (ed): Heart Disease. A Textbook of Cardiovascular Medicine. Philadelphia, WB Saunders Company, 1980.

Davis JO, Goodkind MJ, Ball WC Jr: Functional changes during high-output failure produced by daily hemorrhage in dogs with pulmonic stenosis. Circ Res 5 (1957) 388–394.

D'Cruz IA: Pericardial disease. *In* Talano JV, Gardin JM (eds): Textbook of Two-Dimensional Echocardiography. New York, Grune & Stratton, 1983.

Dear MG: Bacterial endocarditis. *In* Kirk RW (ed): Current Veterinary Therapy VI. Philadelphia, WB Saunders Company, 1977.

deGroot WJ: Cardiomyopathy associated with endocrine disorders. Cardiovasc Clin 4(1) (1972) 305–331.

Dillon R: Feline dirofilariasis. Vet Clin North Am 14 (1984) 1185–1199.

Donahoe JMR: Experimental infection of cats with *Dirofilaria immitis*. J Parasitol 61 (1975) 599–605.

Donahoe JMR, Holzinger EA: *Dirofilaria immitis* in the brains of a dog and a cat. J Am Vet Med Assoc 164 (1974) 518–519.

Donahoe JMR, Kneller SK, Lewis RE: Hematologic and radiographic changes in cats after inoculation with infective larvae of *Dirofilaria immitis*. J Am Vet Med Assoc 168 (1976a) 413–417.

Donahoe JMR, Kneller SK, Lewis RE: *In vivo* pulmonary arteriography in cats infected with *Dirofilaria immitis*. J Am Vet Radiol Soc 17 (1976b) 147–151.

dos Remedios LV, Weber PM, Jasko IA: Thyroid scintiphotography in 1000 patients: rational use of $^{99m}$Tc and $^{131}$I compounds. J Nucl Med 12 (1971) 673–677.

Duke M, Abelmann WH: The hemodynamic response to chronic anemia. Circulation 39 (1969) 503–515.

Edwards NJ: Canine mitral valve disease. *In* Kirk RW (ed): Current Veterinary Therapy VI. Philadelphia, WB Saunders Company, 1977.

Epstein FH, Post RS, McDowell M: The effect of an arteriovenous fistula on renal hemodynamics and electrolyte excretion. J Clin Invest 32 (1953) 233–241.

Erichsen DF, Harris SG, Upson DW: Plasma levels of digoxin in the cat: Some clinical applications. J Am Anim Hosp Assoc 14 (1978) 734–737.

Estes EH Jr: Examination by means of electrocardiography. *In* Hurst JW (ed): The Heart, Arteries and Veins, 3rd ed. New York, McGraw-Hill Book Company, 1974.

Evans HE, Christensen GC (eds): Miller's Anatomy of the Dog. Philadelphia, WB Saunders Company, 1979.

Fairley KF, Laver M: High dose furosemide in chronic renal failure. Postgrad Med J 47 (April) (1971) 40–41.

Faries FC Jr, Mainster ME, Martin PW: Incidental findings of *Dirofilaria immitis* in domestic cats. Vet Med Small Anim Clin 69 (1974) 599–600.

Feigenbaum H, Zaky A, Waldhausen JA: Use of ultrasound in the diagnosis of pericardial effusion. Ann Intern Med 65 (1966) 443–452.

Fisch C, Knoebel SB, Feigenbaum H: The effect of potassium, acetylcholine, and digitalis on atrioventricular conduction. *In* Dreifus LS, Likoff W (eds): Mechanisms and Therapy of Cardiac Arrhythmias. New York, Grune & Stratton, 1966.

Flecknell PA, Gruffydd-Jones TJ, Brown CM, Kelly DF: A case of suspected ventricular pre-excitation in the cat. J Small Anim Pract 20 (1979) 57–61.

Fowler JL, Matsuda K, Fernau RC: Experimental infection of the domestic cat with *Dirofilaria immitis*. J Am Anim Hosp Assoc 8 (1972) 79–80.

Fowler NO: The secondary cardiomyopathies. *In* Fowler NO (ed): Myocardial Diseases. New York, Grune & Stratton, 1973.

Fowler NO: High cardiac output states. *In* Hurst JW (ed): The Heart, Arteries and Veins, 3rd ed. New York, McGraw-Hill Book Company, 1974.

Fox PR: Feline myocardial diseases. *In* Kirk RW (ed): Current Veterinary Therapy VIII. Philadelphia, WB Saunders Company, 1983.

Fox PR, Dodds WJ: Coagulopathies observed with spontaneous aortic thromboembolism in cardiomyopathic cats. Sci Proc Am Coll Vet Intern Med, 1982, 83.

Frank CW, Wang HH, Lammerant J, Miller R, Wegria R: An experimental study of the immediate hemodynamic adjustments to acute arteriovenous fistulae of various sizes. J Clin Invest 34 (1955) 722–731.

Frankl WS, Roberts J, Lathers CM: Congestive heart failure. *In* Frankl WS, Roberts J, Lathers CM (eds): Cardiovascular Therapeutics in Clinical Practice. New York, John Wiley & Sons, 1984.

Frazier HS, Yager H: Drug therapy: The clinical use of diuretics. N Engl J Med 288 (1973) 246–249, 455–457.

Frenkel JK: Toxoplasmosis. *In* Kirk RW (ed): Current Veterinary Therapy VI. Philadelphia, WB Saunders Company, 1977.

Frohlich ED, Dustan HP, Page IH: Hyperdynamic beta-adrenergic circulatory state. Arch Intern Med 117 (1966) 614–619.

Fry WJ: Surgical considerations in congenital arteriovenous fistula. Surg Clin North Am 54 (1974) 165–174.

Furneaux RW, Pharr JW, McManus JL: Arteriovenous fistulation following dewclaw removal in a cat. J Am Anim Hosp Assoc 10 (1974) 569–573.

Gallagher JJ, Svenson RH, Sealy WC, Wallace AG: The Wolff-Parkinson-White syndrome and the pre-excitation dysrhythmias. Med Clin North Am 60 (1976) 101–123.

Goldberg M: The renal physiology of diuretics. *In* Orloff J, Berliner RW (eds): Handbook of Physiology, Section 8, Renal Physiology. Am Physiol Soc 1973, 1003–1031.

Goldberg M, Beck LH, Puschett JS, Schubert JJ: Sites of action of benzothiadiazines, furosemide and ethycrynic acid. *In* Lant AF, Wilson GM (eds): Modern Diuretic Therapy in the Treatment of Cardiovascular and Renal Disease. Amsterdam, Excerpta Medica, 1973.

Gompf RE, Tilley LP: Comparison of lateral and sternal recumbent positions for electrocardiography of the cat. Am J Vet Res 40 (1979) 1483–1486.

Goodkind MJ: High output heart disease. *In* Conn HL Jr,

Horwitz O (eds): Cardiac Vascular Diseases. Philadelphia, Lea & Febiger, 1971.

Gordon DB, Goldblatt H: Direct percutaneous determination of systemic blood pressure and production of renal hypertension in the cat. Proc Soc Exp Biol Med 125 (1967) 177–180.

Gorlin R, Brachfeld N, Turner JD, Messer JV, Salazar E: The idiopathic high cardiac output state. J Clin Invest 38 (1959) 2144–2153.

Graettinger JS, Muenster JJ, Silverstone LA, Campbell JA: A correlation of clinical and hemodynamic studies in patients with hyperthyroidism with and without congestive heart failure. J Clin Invest 38 (1959) 1316–1327.

Gregory LF Jr, Durrett RR, Robinson RR, Clapp JR: The short-term effect of furosemide on electrolyte and water excretion in patients with severe renal disease. Arch Intern Med 125 (1970) 69–74.

Haft JI, Horowitz MS: Clinical Echocardiography. Mount Kisco, NY, Futura Publishing Company, 1978.

Hahn AW: Digitalis glycosides in canine medicine. *In* Kirk RW (ed): Current Veterinary Therapy VI. Philadelphia, WB Saunders Company, 1977.

Hamby RI, Zoneraich S, Sherman L: Diabetic cardiomyopathy. J Am Med Assoc 229 (1974) 1749–1754.

Hamilton JM: The influence of infestation by *Aelurostrongylus abstrusus* on the pulmonary vasculature of the cat. Br Vet J 126 (1970) 202–208.

Hamlin RL, Smetzer DL, Smith CR: The electrocardiogram, phonocardiogram, and derived ventricular activation process of domestic cats. Am J Vet Res 24 (1963a) 792–802.

Hamlin RL, Smetzer DL, Smith CR: Radiographic anatomy of the normal cat heart. J Am Vet Med Assoc 143 (1963b) 957–961.

Hamlin RL, Tashjian RL, Smith CR: Diseases of the cardiovascular system. *In* Catcott EJ (ed): Feline Medicine and Surgery. Santa Barbara, American Veterinary Publications Inc, 1964.

Harari J, MacCoy DM, Johnson AL, Tranquilli WJ: Recurrent peripheral arteriovenous fistula and hyperthyroidism in a cat. J Am Anim Hosp 20 (1984) 759–764.

Harlton BW: Treatment of dirofilariasis in a domestic cat. (A clinical report.) Vet Med Small Anim Clin 69 (1974) 1440–1441.

Harpster NK: Cardiovascular diseases of the domestic cat. Adv Vet Sci Comp Med 21 (1977a) 39–74.

Harpster NK: Feline cardiomyopathy. Vet Clin North Am 7 (1977b) 355–371.

Harpster NK: Clinical evaluation of the feline cardiovascular system. Vet Clin North Am 7 (1977c) 241–256.

Harpster NK: The pericardium. *In* Gourley IM, Vasseur PB (eds): General Small Animal Surgery. Philadelphia, JB Lippincott Company, 1985.

Harris SG, Ogburn PN: The cardiovascular system. *In* Catcott EJ (ed): Feline Medicine and Surgery, 2nd ed. Santa Barbara, American Veterinary Publications Inc, 1975.

Hawe RS: The diagnosis and treatment of occult dirofilariasis in a cat. J Am Anim Hosp Assoc 15 (1979) 577–582.

Heath D, Smith P: Pulmonary vascular disease. Med Clin North Am 61 (1977) 1279–1307.

Hoffman BF: The electrophysiology of heart muscle and the genesis of arrhythmias. *In* Dreifus LS, Likoff W (eds): Mechanisms and Therapy of Cardiac Arrhythmias. New York, Grune & Stratton, 1966.

Holmes PR, Kelly JD: The incidence of *Dirofilaria immitis* and *Dipetalonema reconditum* in dogs and cats in Sydney. Aust Vet J 49 (1973) 55.

Holzworth J, Simpson R, Wind A: Aortic thrombosis with posterior paralysis in the cat. Cornell Vet 45 (1955) 468–487.

Holzworth J, Theran P, Carpenter JL, Harpster NK, Todoroff RJ: Hyperthyroidism in the cat: Ten cases. J Am Vet Med Assoc 176 (1980) 345–353.

Horan LG, Flowers NC: Electrocardiography and vectorcardiography. *In* Braunwald E (ed): Heart Disease: A Textbook of Cardiovascular Medicine. Philadelphia, WB Saunders Company, 1980.

Horton CR, Renfroe BJ: Surgical removal of a BB shot from the abdominal aorta of a cat. Vet Med Small Anim Clin 73 (1978) 321–323.

Inhoff RK: Production of aortic occlusion resembling acute aortic embolism syndrome in cats. Nature 192 (1961) 979–980.

Jeraj K, Ogburn P, Lord PF, Wilson JW: Patent ductus arteriosus with pulmonary hypertension in a cat. J Am Vet Med Assoc 172 (1978) 1432–1436.

Jones TC, Zook BC: Aging changes in the vascular system of animals. Ann NY Acad Sci 127 (1965) 671–684.

Joshua JO: Some clinical aspects of cardiovascular diseases in cats and dogs. Vet Rec 71 (1959) 941–947.

Kariv I, Kreisler B, Sherf L, Feldman S, Rosenthal T: Familial cardiomyopathy. A review of 11 families. Am J Cardiol 28 (1971) 693–706.

Kaye D: Changes in the spectrum, diagnosis and management of bacterial and fungal endocarditis. Med Clin North Am 57 (1973) 941–957.

Kelleher GJ, Frankl WS, Gerard-Ciminera J, Roberts J: Hypertension. *In* Frankl WS, Roberts J, Lathers CM (eds): Cardiovascular Therapeutics in Clinical Practice. New York, John Wiley & Sons, 1984.

Kittleson M: Drugs used in the management of heart failure. *In* Kirk RW (ed): Current Veterinary Therapy VIII. Philadelphia, WB Saunders Company, 1983.

Knight DH: Heartworm heart disease. Adv Vet Sci Comp Med 21 (1977) 107–149.

Lant AF, Wilson GM: Modern Diuretic Therapy in the Treatment of Cardiovascular and Renal Diseases. Amsterdam, Excerpta Medica, 1973.

Lillis WG: *Dirofilaria immitis* in dogs and cats from south-central New Jersey. J Parasitol 50 (1964) 802.

Lindsay S, Chaikoff IL: Arteriosclerosis in the cat. Arch Pathol 60 (1955) 29–38.

Liu S-K: Acquired cardiac lesions leading to congestive heart failure in the cat. Am J Vet Res 31 (1970) 2071–2088.

Liu S-K: Pathology of feline heart disease. *In* Kirk RW (ed): Current Veterinary Therapy V. Philadelphia, WB Saunders Company, 1974.

Liu S-K: Pathology of feline heart disease. Vet Clin North Am 7 (1977) 323–339.

Liu S-K, Fox PR, Tilley LP: Excessive moderator bands in the left ventricle of 21 cats. J Am Vet Med Assoc 180 (1982) 1215–1219.

Liu S-K, Peterson ME, Fox PR: Hypertrophic cardiomyopathy and hyperthyroidism in the cat. J Am Vet Med Assoc 185 (1984) 52–57.

Liu S-K, Tashjian RJ, Patnaik AK: Congestive heart failure in the cat. J Am Vet Med Assoc 156 (1970) 1319–1330.

Lord PF, Wood A, Tilley LR, Liu S-R: Radiographic and hemodynamic evaluation of cardiomyopathy and thromboembolism in the cat. J Am Vet Med Assoc 164 (1974) 154–165.

Lown B, Ganong WF, Levine SA: The syndrome of short P-R interval, normal QRS complex and paroxysmal rapid heart action. Circulation 5 (1952) 693–706.

Lucke FM: Renal disease in the domestic cat [polyarteritis]. J Pathol 95 (1968) 67–91.

Luisada AA, Weisz L, Hantman HW: A comparative study of electrocardiograms and heart sounds in common and domestic mammals. Cardiologia 8 (1944) 63–84.

Mackenzie A: Pathological changes in lungworm infestation in two cats with special reference to changes in pulmonary arterial branches. Res Vet Sci 1 (1960) 255–259.

Mandelker L, Brutus RL: Feline and canine dirofilarial encephalitis. J Am Vet Med Assoc 159 (1971) 776.

Mann PH: Additional information pertaining to the incidence of heartworms and intestinal helminths in stray cats and dogs in Bergen County, northern New Jersey. J Parasitol 41 (1955) 637.

Mann PH, Fratta I: The incidence of coccidia, heartworms and intestinal helminths in dogs and cats in northern New Jersey. J Parasitol 38 (1952) 496–497.

Mann PH, Fratta I: Transplantation of adult heartworms, *Dirofilaria immitis*, into dogs and cats. J Parasitol 39 (1953) 139–144.

Manning PJ, Clarkson TB: Diet-induced atherosclerosis of the cat. Arch Pathol 89 (1970) 271–278.

Marcato A: Arteriosclerosi intimale nel polmone del gatto. Nuova Vet 18 (1940) 75–83.

Marcato A: Ulteriori ricerche per l'arteriosclerosi intimale del gatto. Nuova Vet 19 (1941) 12–13.

Martin J: Systematische Reihenuntersuchungen über das Vorkommen sklerosierenden Prozesse in den Pulmonalgefässen bei Katzen. Monatsh Veterinärmed 17 (1962) 341–344.

Massmann VW, Opitz H: Das Katzen—EKG. Cardiologia 24: (1954) 54–64.

Matis U: Zur posttraumatischen Fettembolie. Kleintierpraxis 25 (1980) 155–160, 162.

Middleton DJ, Ilkiw JE, Watson ADJ: Arterial and venous blood gas tensions in clinically healthy cats. Am J Vet Res 42 (1981) 1609–1611.

Mills P, Rose J, Hollingsworth J, Amora I, Craige E: Long-term prognosis of mitral valve prolapse. N Engl J Med 297 (1977) 13–18.

Moe GK: On the multiple wavelet hypothesis of atrial fibrillation. Arch Int Pharmacodyn 140 (1962) 183–192.

Muenster JJ, Graettinger JS, Campbell JA: Correlation of clinical and hemodynamic findings in patients with systemic arteriovenous fistulas. Circulation 20 (1959) 1079–1086.

Muth RG: Diuretics in chronic renal insufficiency. *In* Lant AF, Wilson GM (eds): Modern Diuretic Therapy in the Treatment of Cardiovascular and Renal Disease. Amsterdam, Excerpta Medica, 1973.

Nadeau RA, Colebatch HJH: Normal respiratory and circulatory values in the cat. J Appl Physiol 20 (1965) 836–838.

Nanda NC, Gramiak R: Clinical Echocardiography. St. Louis, The CV Mosby Company, 1978.

Norsworthy GD: Kitten mortality complex. Feline Pract 9(2) (1979) 57–60.

Oakley CM: Clinical recognition of the cardiomyopathies. Circ Res 35 (1974) 152–167.

Ogburn PN: Ventricular pre-excitation (Wolff-Parkinson-White syndrome) in a cat. J Am Anim Hosp Assoc 13 (1977) 171–175.

Olcott CT, Saxton JA, Modell W: Medial hyperplasia in pulmonary arteries of cats. Am J Pathol 22 (1946) 847–853.

Owens JM: Pericardial effusion in the cat. Vet Clin North Am 7 (1977) 373–383.

Owens JM, Twedt DC: Nonselective angiocardiography in the cat. Vet Clin North Am 7 (1977) 309–321.

Parks J: Electrocardiographic abnormalities from serum electrolyte imbalance due to feline urethral obstruction. J Am Anim Hosp Assoc 11 (1975) 102–106.

Parmley WW, Sonnenblick EH: Cardiac muscle function studies. *In* Schwartz A (ed): Methods in Pharmacology. New York, Appleton-Century-Crofts, 1971.

Pensinger RR: Cardiovascular examination of the cat: heart sounds. J Am Anim Hosp Assoc 4 (1968) 213–223.

Perloff JK, Roberts WC: The mitral apparatus. Functional anatomy of mitral regurgitation. Circulation 46 (1972) 227–239.

Peterson ME: Canine and feline endocrinology. Proc Am Anim Hosp Assoc 51 (1984) 101–109.

Peterson ME, Hurvitz AI, Leib MS, Cavanagh PG, Dutton RE: Propylthiouracil-associated hemolytic anemia, thrombocytopenia, and antinuclear antibodies in cats with hyperthyroidism. J Am Vet Med Assoc 184 (1984) 806–808.

Peterson ME, Keene B, Ferguson DC, Pipers FS: Electrocardiographic findings in 45 cats with hyperthyroidism. J Am Vet Med Assoc 180 (1982) 934–937.

Petrak M, Carpenter JL: Feline toxoplasmosis. J Am Vet Med Assoc 146 (1965) 728–734.

Pipers FS, Hamlin RL: Clinical use of echocardiography in the domestic cat. J Am Vet Med Assoc 176 (1980) 57–61.

Pipers FS, Reef V, Hamlin RL: Echocardiography in the domestic cat. Am J Vet Res 40 (1979) 882–886.

Pritchett HD: Lungworms in a kitten. J Am Vet Med Assoc 92 (1938) 692–694.

Rawlings CA, Losonsky JM, Lewis RE, Hubble JJ, Prestwood AK: Response of the feline heart to *Aelurostrongylus abstrusus*. J Am Anim Hosp Assoc 16 (1980) 573–578.

Reeves JT, Grover EB, Grover RF: Circulatory responses to high altitude in the cat and rabbit. J Appl Physiol 18 (1963) 575–579.

Robbins SL, Cotran RS, Kumar V: Pathologic Basis of Disease. Philadelphia, WB Saunders Company, 1984.

Roberts J, Frankl WS: Cardiac arrhythmias. *In* Frankl WS, Roberts J, Lathers CM (eds): Cardiovascular Therapeutics in Clinical Practice. New York, John Wiley & Sons, 1984.

Rogers WA, Bishop SPL: Electrocardiographic parameters of the normal domestic cat: A comparison of standard limb leads and an orthogonal system. J Electrocardiol 4 (1971) 315–321.

Rogers WA, Bishop SP, Rohovsky MW: Pulmonary artery medial hypertrophy and hyperplasia in conventional and specific-pathogen–free cats. Am J Vet Res 32 (1971) 767–774.

Rosen L: Observations on *Dirofilaria immitis* in French Oceania. Ann Trop Med Parasitol 48 (1954) 318–328.

Rothwell TLW, Xu F-N, Wills EJ, Middleton DJ, Bow JL, Smith JS, Davis JS: Unusual multisystemic vascular lesions in a cat. Vet Pathol 22 (1985) 510–512.

Rotta A, Canepa A, Hurtado A, Velasquez T, Chavez R: Pulmonary circulation at sea level and at high altitudes. J Appl Physiol 9 (1956) 328–336.

Roumanis J: Pellet blockage of the aorta [letter]. J Am Vet Med Assoc 179 (1981) 206.

Roye DB, Serrano EE, Hammer RH, Wilder BJ: Plasma kinetics of diphenylhydantoin in dogs and cats. Am J Vet Res 34 (1973) 947–950.

Rubarth S: Lokale hyperplastische Prozesse in der Art. pulmonalis der Katze. Skand Vet Tidskr 30 (1940) 489–514.

Schaer M: Hyperkalemia in cats with urethral obstruction. Electrocardiographic abnormalities and treatment. Vet Clin North Am 7 (1977) 407–414.

Schaub RG, Meyers KM, Sande RD, Hamilton G: Inhibition of feline collateral vessel development following experimental thrombolic occlusion. Circ Res 39 (1976) 736–743.

Schlant RC: Physiology of idiopathic cardiomyopathies. Cardiovasc Clin 4(1) (1972) 61–76.

Schwartz A: Two cases of feline heartworm disease. Feline Pract. 5(4) (1975) 20–28.

Scott FW, Weiss RC, Post JE, Gilmartin JE, Hoshino Y: Kitten mortality complex (neonatal FIP?). Feline Pract 9(2) (1979) 44–56.

Scratcherd T, Wright DE: Medial hypertrophy and hyperplasia in cat pulmonary artery. Arch Pathol 72 (1961) 703–708.

Selzer A, Sudrann RB: Reliability of the determination of cardiac output in man by means of the Fick principle. Circ Res 6 (1958) 485–490.

Seneviratne BIB: Diabetic cardiomyopathy: The preclinical phase. Br Med J 1 (1977) 1444–1446.

Shouse CL, Meier H: Acute vegetative endocarditis in the dog and cat. J Am Vet Med Assoc 129 (1956) 278–289.

Siegenthaler W, Beckerhoff R, Vetter W, et al.: Diuretics in Research and Clinics. Stuttgart, George Thieme Publishers, 1977.

Simpson CF, Jackson RF: Aortic sclerosis in a cat. J Am Vet Med Assoc 142 (1963) 282–284.

Slocum B, Colgrove FJ, Carrig CB, Suter PF: Acquired arteriovenous fistula in two cats. J Am Vet Med Assoc (1973) 271–275.

Smith TW, Braunwald E: The management of heart failure. *In* Braunwald E (ed): Heart Disease: A Textbook of Cardiovascular Medicine. Philadelphia, WB Saunders Company, 1980.

Smith TW, Haber E: Medical progress: Digitalis. N Engl J Med 289 (1973a) 945–952.

Smith TW, Haber E: Medical progress: Digitalis. N Engl J Med 289 (1973b) 1010–1015.

Soderberg SF, Boon JA, Wingfield WE, Miller CW: M-mode echocardiography as a diagnostic aid for feline cardiomyopathy. Am Vet Radiol Soc J 24 (1983) 66–77.

Sonnenblick EH: Force velocity relations in mammalian heart muscle. Am J Physiol 202 (1962a) 931–939.

Sonnenblick EH: Implications of muscle mechanics in the heart. Fed Proc 21 (1962b) 975–990.

Sonnenblick EH: Active state in heart muscle. Its delayed onset and modification by inotropic agents. J Gen Physiol 50 (1967) 661–676.

Spann JF Jr, Buccino RA, Sonnenblick EH: Production of right ventricular hypertrophy with and without congestive heart failure in the cat. Proc Soc Exp Biol Med 125 (1967a) 522–524.

Spann JF Jr, Buccino RA, Sonnenblick EH, Braunwald E: Contractile state of cardiac muscle obtained from cats with experimentally produced ventricular hypertrophy and heart failure. Circ Res 21 (1967b) 341–354.

Stackhouse LL, Clough E: Clinical report: five cases of feline dirofilariasis. Vet Med Small Anim Clin 71 (1972) 1309–1310.

Stünzi H, Teuscher E, Pericin-Rauhut D: Die Hyperplasie der Arteria pulmonalis bei Feliden [cat and ocelot]. Pathol Vet 3 (1966) 461–473.

Swerczek TW, Nielsen SW, Helmboldt CF: Ascariasis causing pulmonary arterial hyperplasia in cats. Res Vet Sci 11 (1970) 103–104.

Tafur E, Cohen LS, Levine HD: The normal apex cardiogram. Its temporal relationship to electrical acoustic and mechanical cardiac events. Circulation 30 (1964) 381–391.

Talano JV, Gardin JM: Textbook of Two-Dimensional Echocardiography. New York, Grune & Stratton, 1983.

Tashjian RJ, Das KM, Palich WE, Hamlin RL, Yarns DA: Studies on cardiovascular disease in the cat. Ann NY Acad Sci 127 (1965) 581–605.

Taussig HB: Congenital Malformations of the Heart. Cambridge, Harvard University Press, 1960.

Thomas WP: Pericardial disease. *In* Ettinger SJ (ed): Textbook of Veterinary Internal Medicine, 2nd ed. Philadelphia, WB Saunders Company, 1983.

Tilley LP: Feline cardiology. Vet Clin North Am 6 (1976) 415–432.

Tilley LP: Feline cardiomyopathy. *In* Kirk RW (ed): Current Veterinary Therapy VI. Philadelphia, WB Saunders Company, 1977.

Tilley LP: Essentials of Canine and Feline Electrocardiography: Interpretation and Treatment, 2nd ed. Philadelphia, Lea & Febiger, 1985.

Tilley LP, Gompf RE: Feline electrocardiography. Vet Clin North Am 7 (1977) 257–272.

Tilley LP, Weitz J: Pharmacologic and other forms of medical therapy in feline cardiac disease. Vet Clin North Am 7 (1977) 415–428.

Tilley LP, Bond B, Patnaik AK, Liu S-K: Cardiovascular tumors in the cat. J Am Anim Hosp Assoc 17 (1981) 1009–1021.

Tilley LP, Lord PF, Wood A: Acquired heart disease and aortic thromboembolism in the cat. *In* Kirk RW (ed): Current Veterinary Therapy V. Philadelphia, WB Saunders Company, 1974.

Tilley LP, Owens JM, Wilkins RJ, Patnaik AK: Pericardial mesothelioma with effusion in a cat. J Am Anim Hosp Assoc 11 (1975) 60–65.

Todd KS, Byerly CS, Small E, Krone JV: Heartworm infections in Illinois cats. Feline Pract 6(2) (1976) 41–44.

Turrel JM, Feldman EC, Hays M, Hornof WJ: Radioactive iodine therapy in cats with hyperthyroidism. J Am Vet Med Assoc 184 (1984) 554–559.

Vidt DG: Diuretics: Use and misuse. Postgrad Med 59 (1976) 143–151.

Weiner DE, Verrier RL, Miller DT, Lefer AM: Effect of adrenalectomy on hemodynamics and regional blood flow in the cat. Am J Physiol 213 (1967) 473–476.

Weiss HJ: Antiplatelet drugs—A new pharmacologic approach to the prevention of thrombosis. Am Heart J 92 (1976) 86–102.

Wenger NK: Infectious myocarditis. Cardiovasc Clin 4 (1972) 167–185.

Wenger NK: Myocarditis. *In* Hurst JW (ed): The Heart, Arteries and Veins, 3rd ed. New York, McGraw-Hill Book Company, 1974.

Wilkes, RD: What is your diagnosis? [pericardial diaphragmatic hernia]. J Am Vet Med Assoc 178 (1981) 1297–1298.

Willard MD, Aronson E: Peritoneopericardial diaphragmatic hernia in a cat. J Am Vet Med Assoc 178 (1981) 481–483.

Williams GH, Braunwald E: Endocrine and nutritional disorders and heart disease. *In* Braunwald E (ed): Heart Disease. A Textbook of Cardiovascular Medicine. Philadelphia, WB Saunders Company, 1980.

Winters WL, Cortes FM: Pericardial disease. *In* Conn HL, Horwitz O (eds): Cardiac and Vascular Diseases. Philadelphia, Lea & Febiger, 1971.

Wolffhügel K: Paraplegia cruralis parasitaria durch *Gurltia paralysans* Nov. gen. Nov. sp (Nematoda). Z Infektionskr Haustiere 46 (1934) 28–47.

Wong MM, Suter PF, Rhode EA, Guest MF: Dirofilariasis without circulating microfilariae: a problem in diagnosis. J Am Vet Med Assoc 163 (1973) 133–139.

Wood GL: Canine myocardial diseases. *In* Kirk RW (ed): Current Veterinary Therapy VIII. Philadelphia, WB Saunders Company, 1983.

Zipes DP, McIntosh MD: Cardiac arrhythmias. *In* Conn HL Jr, Horwitz O (eds): Cardiac and Vascular Diseases. Philadelphia, Lea & Febiger, 1971.

Zook BC: Some spontaneous cardiovascular lesions in dogs and cats. Adv Cardiol 13 (1974) 148–168.

**Additional Reading**

Allen DG, Nymeyer D: A preliminary investigation on the use of thermodilution and echocardiography as an assessment of cardiac function in the cat. Can J Comp Med 47 (1983) 112–117.

Allen DG, Johnstone IB, Crane S: Effects of aspirin and propranolol alone and in combination on hemostatic determinants in the healthy cat. Am J Vet Res 46 (1985) 660–662.

Bolton GR, Powell W: Plasma kinetics of digoxin in the cat. Am J Vet Res 43 (1982) 1994–1999.

Bonagura JD, Pipers FS: Diagnosis of cardiac lesions by contrast echocardiography. J Am Vet Med Assoc 182 (1983) 396–402.

Bond BR, Fox PR: Advances in feline cardiomyopathy. Vet Clin North Am 14 (1984) 1021–1038.

Dyson DH, McDonell WN, Horne JA: Accuracy of thermodilution measurement of cardiac output in low flows applicable to feline and small canine patients. Can J Comp Med 48 (1984) 425–427.

Essler WO, Folk GE Jr, Adamson GE: 24-hour cardiac activity of unrestrained cats. Fed Proc 20 (1961) 129.

Fazzalari NL, Mazumdar J, Ghista DN, Allen DG, de Bruin H: A study of the first heart sound spectra in normal anesthetized cats: possible origins and chest wall influences. Can J Comp Med 48 (1984) 30–34.

Fox PR, Bond BR, Peterson ME: Echocardiographic reference values in healthy cats sedated with ketamine hydrochloride. Am J Vet Res 40 (1985) 1479–1484.

Harwood ML: Paroxysmal atrial tachycardia and left superior bundle branch blockage in a cat. Vet Med Small Anim Clin 65 (1970) 862–866.

Hill BL, Tilley LP: Ventricular preexcitation in seven dogs and nine cats. J Am Vet Med Assoc 187 (1985) 1026–1031.

Hilwig RW: ECG of the month [pacemaker abnormality]. J Am Vet Med Assoc 174 (1979) 364–365.

Jacobs G, Knight DH: M-mode echocardiographic measurements in nonanesthetized healthy cats: effects of body weight, heart rate, and other variables. Am J Vet Res 46 (1985) 1705–1711.

Jacobs G, Knight H: Change in M-mode echocardiographic values in cats given ketamine. Am J Vet Res 46 (1985) 1712–1713.

Kimman TG, van der Molen EJ: Pathaloog anatomische bevindingen bij negentien katten met idiopathische cardiomyopathie. Tijdschr Diergeneeskd 109 (1984) 132–141 (abstr Vet Bull 54 [1984] 3521).

Lacuata AQ, Yamada H, Nakamura Y: ECG of the month [tricuspid valvular endocarditis]. J Am Vet Med Assoc 177 (1980) 524–525.

McConnell MF, Huxtable CR: Pseudochylous effusion in a cat with cardiomyopathy. Aust Vet J 58 (1982) 72–74.

McLeish I: Doppler ultrasonic arterial pressure measurement in the cat. Vet Rec 100 (1977) 290–291.

Messow C: Morphologische Veränderungen am Herzen von Katzen nach Herzpunktion. Dtsch Tierärztl Wochenschr 74 (1967) 164–166.

Nobel TA, Neumann F, Klopfer U: Histopathology of the myocardium in 50 apparently healthy cats. Lab Anim 8 (1974) 119–125.

Olmstead ML, Butler HC: Five-hydroxy-tryptamine antagonists and feline aortic embolism. J Small Anim Pract 18 (1977) 247–259.

Orsini D, Buss DD: Complete atrioventricular block in a cat. J Am Vet Med Assoc 172 (1978) 158–160.

Richtig JW, Tilley LP, Liu S-K: Persistent atrial standstill [dilated cardiomyopathy]. J Am Vet Med Assoc 185 (1984) 1512–1513.

Robertson BT, Figg FA, Ewell Wm: Normal value for the electrocardiogram in the cat. Feline Pract 6(2) (1976) 20–22.

Robins GM, Wilkinson GT, Menrath VH, Atwell RB, Riesz G: Long-term survival following embolectomy in two cats with aortic embolism. J Small Anim Pract 23 (1982) 165–174.

Schaub RG, Gates KA, Roberts RE: Effects of aspirin on collateral blood flow after experimental thrombosis of the feline aorta. Am J Vet Res 43 (1982) 1647–1650.

Toal RL, Losonsky JM, Coulter DB, DeNovellis R: Influence of cardiac cycle on the radiographic appearance of the feline heart. Vet Radiol 26 (1985) 63–69.

Toman JEP, Everett GM, Oster RH, Smith DC: Origin of cardiac disorders in thiamine-deficient cats. Proc Soc Exp Biol Med 58 (1945) 65–67.

van Vleet JF, Ferrans VJ, Weirich WE: Pathologic alterations in hypertrophic and congestive cardiomyopathy of cats. Am J Vet Res 41 (1980) 2037–2048.

Yamaguchi RA, Pipers FS, Gamble DA: Echocardiographic evaluation of a cat with bacterial vegetative endocarditis. J Am Vet Med Assoc 183 (1983) 118–120.

# INDEX

Numbers in *italics* refer to illustrations; numbers followed by (t) refer to tables.